DISEASES AND ICD-9CM CODES

Acne   706.1
Adrenal Insufficiency   255.4
Alcoholism   303.9
Alopecia   704.00
Altered Mental State   780.9
Altitude Sickness   993.2
Alzheimer's Disease   331.0
Amebiasis   006.9
Amenorrhea   626.0
Anaphylaxis   995.0
Anemia, Megaloblastic   281.9
Anemia, Sickle Cell   282.60
Angina   413.9
Angioedema   995.1
Animal Bites   879.8
Ankle Fractures   824.8
Anorexia Nervosa   307.1
Anuria   788.5
Aortic Dissection   441.00
Appendicitis   541
Arrhythmias   427.9
Arthritis, Rheumatoid   714.0
Ascaris Infection   127.0
Ascites   789.5
Asthma   493.9
Atelectasis   518.0
Atrial Fibrillation   427.31
Bacteremia   790.7
Basal Cell Carcinoma   173.9
Bell's Palsy   351.0
Bladder Cancer   188.9
Blastomycosis   116.0
Bleeding Disorders   287.9
Blood Transfusion, Adverse Reaction to   999.8
Bowel Obstruction (small and large bowel)   560.9
Brain Tumor   239.6
Breast Cancer   174.9
Bronchiectasis   494
Bronchiolitis   466.1
Bronchitis   490
Bulimia Nervosa   307.51
Burns   949.0
Bursitis   727.3
Calluses   700
Cancer Screening   V76.9
Cardiac Arrest   427.5
Cardiomyopathy   425.4
Carpal Tunnel Syndrome   354.0
Cellulitis   682.9
Cellulitis, Orbital   376.01
Cervical Cancer   180.9
Cervicitis   616.0
Cheilitis   528.5
Cheilitis, Angular   528.5
Cholecystitis   575.1
Chronic Fatigue Syndrome   780.7

Chronic Obstructive Pulmonary Disease   496
Cirrhosis   571.5
Claudication   443.9
Coccidioidomycosis   114.9
Colorectal Cancer   153.9
Condyloma Acuminata   078.11
Congestive Heart Failure   428.0
Conjunctivitis   372.30
Constipation   564.0
Contraception   V25.09 Family Planning Advice
                V25.0 General Counseling
Corneal Ulceration   370.00
Corns   700
Costochondritis   733.6
Crohn's Disease   555.9
Croup   464.4
Cushing's Syndrome/Disease   255.0
Decubitus Ulcer   707.0
Deep Venous Thrombosis   453.8
Dementia   294.8
Depression   311
Dermatitis, Atopic   691.8
Dermatitis, Contact   692.9
Dermatitis, Seborrheic   690.10
Diabetes Mellitus, Type I   250.01
Diabetes Mellitus, Type II   250.02
Diarrhea, Acute   787.91
Diarrhea, Chronic   787.91
Diarrhea, Infectious   009.2
Disseminated Intravascular Coagulation   286.6
Diverticulitis   562.11
Domestic Violence   995.81
Drug Allergy   995.2
Dysfunctional Uterine Bleeding   626.8
Dyslexia   784.61
Dysmenorrhea   625.3
Dysuria   788.1
Earache   388.70
Ectopic Pregnancy   633.9
Edema, Leg   782.3
Elbow Dislocations   832.00
Endocarditis   424.90
Endometrial Cancer   182.0
Endometriosis   617.9
Endometritis   615.9
Enuresis   788.30
Epicondylitis   726.32
Epididymitis   604.90
Epistaxis   784.7
Erysipelas   035
Erythroplasia   233.5
Fecal Impaction   560.39
Fetal Alcohol Syndrome   760.71
Fetal Lung Immaturity   770.4
Fever and Chills   780.6
Fever of Unknown Origin (FUO)   780.6
Fibrocystic Disease of the Breast   610.1

Listing continues on the back end paper.

Saunders
Manual
of Medical
Practice

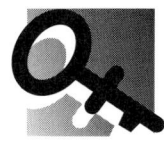

Saunders Manual of Medical Practice

ROBERT E. RAKEL, MD

Richard M. Kleberg, Sr., Professor and Chairman
Department of Family Medicine
Associate Dean for Academic and Clinical Affairs
Baylor College of Medicine
Houston, Texas

Illustrations by Jan Redden
and
Foreword by Roger C. Bone, MD

W. B. SAUNDERS COMPANY
A Division of Harcourt Brace & Company
Philadelphia, London, Toronto, Montreal, Sydney, Tokyo

W.B. SAUNDERS COMPANY
A Division of Harcourt Brace & Company

The Curtis Center
Independence Square West
Philadelphia, Pennsylvania 19106

Library of Congress Cataloging-in-Publication Data

Saunders manual of medical practice / [edited by] Robert E. Rakel; foreword by Roger C. Bone.

p.   cm.

ISBN 0–7216–5192–5

1. Internal medicine—Handbooks, manuals, etc.   I. Rakel, Robert E.   II. Title: Saunders Manual of medical practice.

[DNLM: 1. Clinical Medicine—handbooks.   2. Delivery of Health Care—handbooks.   WB 39 S257 1996]

RC55.S325   1996

616—dc20

DNLM/DLC   95-6354

Any five-digit numeric *Physicians' Current Procedural Terminology,* fourth edition (CPT) codes, service descriptions, instructions and/or guidelines are copyright 1994 (or such other date of publication of CPT as defined in the federal copyright laws) American Medical Association. All Rights Reserved.

CPT is a listing of descriptive terms and five-digit numeric identifying codes and modifiers for reporting medical services performed by physicians. This presentation includes only CPT descriptive terms, numeric identifying codes and modifiers for reporting medical services and procedures that were selected by W.B. Saunders Company for inclusion in this publication.

The most current CPT is available from the American Medical Association.

No fee schedules, basic unit values, relative value guides, conversion factors or scales or components thereof are included in CPT.

W.B. Saunders Company has selected certain CPT codes and service/procedure descriptions and assigned them to various specialty groups. The listing of a CPT service or procedure description and its code number in this publication does not restrict its use to a particular specialty group. Any procedure or service in this publication may be used to designate the services rendered by any qualified physician.

The American Medical Association assumes no responsibility for the consequences attributable to or related to any use or interpretation of any information or views contained in or not contained in this publication.

NOTICE

Medicine is an ever-changing field. Standard safety precautions must be followed, but as new research and clinical experience broaden our knowledge, changes in treatment and drug therapy become necessary or appropriate. The editor of this work has carefully checked the generic and trade drug names and verified drug dosages to ensure that the dosage information in this work is accurate and in accord with the standards accepted at the time of publication. Readers are advised, however, to check the product information currently provided by the manufacturer of each drug to be administered to be certain that changes have not been made in the recommended dose or in the contraindications for administration. This is of particular importance in regard to new or infrequently used drugs. It is the responsibility of the treating physician, relying on experience and knowledge of the patient, to determine dosages and the best treatment for the patient. The editor cannot be responsible for misuse or misapplication of the material in this work.

THE PUBLISHER

PROCEDURE NOTICE

Every effort has been made to review all procedures within this manual and present the information in an accurate and understandable manner. No students should perform any procedure for the first time, except under the direction of a qualified instructor. Some procedures are more complex than others and it is recommended that physicians seek out seminars or expert guidance with any new or unfamiliar procedures. No written procedure can ever take the place of an instructor or experience.

Contributors

NABIL ABOU-SHALA, M.D.
Consultant Intensivist, Department of Medicine, King Faisal Hospital, Riyadh, Saudi Arabia
Tuberculosis

LOUISE S. ACHESON, M.D.
Assistant Associate Professor of Family Medicine and Coordinator of the Obstetrics/Gynecology, Curriculum Case Western Reserve University School of Medicine and University Hospitals of Cleveland, Cleveland, Ohio
Endometrial Biopsy

JIMMY D. ACKLIN, M.D.
Associate Professor of Family and Community Medicine and Assistant Director of Family Practice Residency, University of Arkansas for Medical Sciences, Area Health Education Center-Fort Smith. Staff Physician, Sparks Regional Medical Center, Fort Smith, Arkansas
HIV-Associated Infections

DAVID M. ADELSON, M.D.
Clinical Instructor, University of Oklahoma College of Medicine. Chief, Section of Dermatology, St. John's Medical Center, Tulsa, Oklahoma
Fungus Infections of the Skin

DAVID C. AGERTER, M.D.
Assistant Professor of Medicine, Mayo Family Practice Program Director, Mayo Medical School, Mayo Clinic, Rochester, Minnesota
Whiplash

OSMAN AHMED, M.D., Ph.D.
Assistant Professor, Department of Community Health and Family Medicine, College of Medicine, University of Florida, Gainesville. Assistant Clinical Coordinator, Florida Medical Quality Assurance Program, Inc., Tampa, Florida
Angina

SYED M. AHMED, M.D., M.P.H., Ph.D.
Assistant Professor of Family Medicine and Director, Division of Community Oriented Studies, Center for Healthy Communities, Wright State University School of Medicine. Faculty, Family Practice Residency, Miami Valley Hospital, Dayton, Ohio
Acute Urinary Tract Infection in Children

KHALED AL-ASAD, M.D.
Chief Resident and Assistant in Clinical Medicine, Boston University School of Medicine. Pulmonary/Critical Care Fellow,

American Board in Internal Medicine, Boston University Medical Center and Affiliated Hospitals, Boston, Massachusetts
Polycythemia

MICHAEL ALLON, M.D.
Associate Professor of Medicine, University of Alabama at Birmingham School of Medicine. Staff Nephrologist, University of Alabama at Birmingham Hospital, Birmingham, Alabama
Glomerulonephritis

JATIN AMIN, M.D.
Postgraduate Research Fellow, Department of Physiology, Loyola University Stritch School of Medicine. Emergency Room Physician, Loyola University Medical Center, Maywood, Illinois
Central Venous Catheter Insertion

DAVID M. AMRON, M.D.
Division of Dermatology, Department of Medicine, University of California, San Diego, School of Medicine, San Diego, California
Kaposi's Sarcoma

MARGO K. ANDERSON, M.D.
Volunteer Faculty, University of Nebraska Medical Center. Staff, Volunteer Residency Faculty, Clarkson Hospital, Omaha, Nebraska
Fetal Alcohol Syndrome

LINDA B. ANDREWS, M.D.
Assistant Professor, Department of Psychiatry and Behavioral Sciences, Associate Residency Director in Psychiatry, and Director of Medical Student Education in Psychiatry, Baylor College of Medicine. Director, Outpatient Psychiatry Clinic, Ben Taub General Hospital, Houston, Texas
Schizophrenia

MOHAMMAD ISHAQ ARASTU, M.D.
Chief of Endocrinology, St. Luke's Hospital, Bethlehem, Pennsylvania
Hirsutism

DAVID ARAUJO, M.D.
Academic Faculty, Kaiser Fontana Family Medicine Residency Program, Southern California Permanente Medical Group, Fontana, California
Vasectomy: Traditional Method

THURAYYA ARAYSSI, M.D.
Chief Resident, University of Rochester School of Medicine, Rochester, New York
Hip Pain

JACK L. ARBISER, M.D., Ph.D.
Howard Hughes Fellow, Department of Dermatology, Harvard Medical School, Boston, Massachusetts
Acne

ROBILA ASHFAQ, M.D.
Resident, Baylor College of Medicine, Houston, Texas
Phobia

JOHN N. AUCOTT, M.D.
Assistant Professor of Medicine, Case Western Reserve University School of Medicine. Section Head, General Internal Medicine, Cleveland Veterans Affairs Medical Center, Cleveland, Ohio
Food Poisoning

CAROL A. BAASE, M.D.
Assistant Professor, Department of Family and Community Medicine, Pennsylvania State University College of Medicine, Hershey. Coordinator of Obstetrics/Gynecology Curriculum, Pennsylvania State University/The Good Samaritan Hospital, Family and Community Medicine Residency Program, Lebanon, Pennsylvania
Amenorrhea

GREGORY BAHTIARIAN, D.O.
Family Practice Residency Staff, Department of Family Practice, Womack Army Medical Center, Fort Bragg, North Carolina
Seborrheic Dermatitis

KENNETH A. BALLEW, M.D.
Assistant Professor, University of Virginia School of Medicine, Charlottesville, Virginia
Cardiac Arrest

JAMES R. BARRETT, M.D.
Assistant Professor of Family Medicine and Director, Primary Care Sports Medicine, University of Oklahoma Health Science Center, Oklahoma City, Oklahoma
Ankle and Foot Pain

KATHLEEN C. BARRY, M.D.
Private Practice Physician, St. Petersburg, Florida
Chest Tube Insertion

JEFFREY BASA, M.D.
Resident in Internal Medicine, Johns Hopkins University/Sinai Hospital of Baltimore, Baltimore, Maryland
Hiccups

ROBERT L. BASS, M.D.
Associate Professor of Family Medicine, University of Nebraska Medical Center. Active Staff, University Medical Associates, University of Nebraska Hospital, Omaha, Nebraska
Ingrown Toenail

DENNIS J. BAUMGARDNER, M.D.
Associate Professor, Department of Family Medicine, University of Wisconsin Medical School. Program Director and Research Director, St. Luke's Family Practice Residency Program, St. Luke's Medical Center, Milwaukee, Wisconsin
Blastomycosis

LEE A. BEATTY, M.D.
Clinical Assistant Professor, University of North Carolina at Chapel Hill School of Medicine, Chapel Hill. Director, Family Practice Center, Department of Family Practice, Carolinas Medical Center, Charlotte, North Carolina
Plantar Fasciitis

JOAN M. BEDINGHAUS, M.D.
Assistant Professor, Department of Family Medicine, Case Western Reserve University School of Medicine, Cleveland, Ohio
Breast-Feeding

DIANE K. BEEBE, M.D.
Associate Professor and Family Medicine Residency Director, University of Mississippi Medical Center, Jackson, Mississippi
Abnormal Vaginal Bleeding

JOSHUA BENDITT, M.D.
Assistant Professor, University of Washington Medical School. Medical Staff, University of Washington Medical Center, and Harborview Medical Center, Seattle, Washington
Pneumothorax

ROBERT L. BENZ, M.D.
Clinical Associate Professor of Medicine, Thomas Jefferson University School of Medicine, Philadelphia. Medical Director, Haverford Dialysis Unit, and Director, Lankenau Hospital Internal Medicine Residency Program, Lankenau Hospital and Research Center, Wynnewood, Pennsylvania
Chronic Renal Failure

MICHAEL DAVID BERNSTEIN, M.D.
Assistant Professor of Medicine, Health Science Center at Brooklyn. Attending Physician, Gastroenterology Division, Coney Island Hospital, Brooklyn, New York
Hyperbilirubinemia

PAUL E. BETTENCOURT, M.D., C.M.
Assistant Professor, Department of Medicine, Tufts University School of Medicine. Home Staff Manager, Faulkner Hospital; Chief, General Internal Medicine, Lemuel Shattuck Hospital, Boston, Massachusetts
Chronic Obstructive Pulmonary Disease

JAMES R. BLACKMAN, M.D.
Clinical Professor of Family Medicine, University of Washington School of Medicine, Seattle, Washington. Program Director, Family Practice Residency of Idaho, Boise, Idaho
Animal Bites

REID B. BLACKWELDER, M.D.
Assistant Professor, Department of Family Medicine, East Tennessee State University Quillen College of Medicine. Member, Medical Staff, Holston Valley Hospital and Medical Center, Kingsport, Tennessee
Wrist Fractures

GREGORY H. BLAKE, M.D., M.P.H.
Chairman, Department of Family Medicine, University of Tennessee Medical Center at Knoxville, Knoxville, Tennessee
Aphthous Stomatitis

WOLFE BLOTZER, M.D.
Clinical Assistant Professor, University of Pennsylvania College of Medicine, Philadelphia, Pennsylvania. Clinical Associate Professor, University of Maryland, School of Medicine, Baltimore, Maryland. Program Director, Internal Medicine Residency, York Hospital, York Health System, York, Pennsylvania
Osteoarthritis

LORETTA BOBO-MOSLEY, M.D.
Clinical Associate Professor of Medicine, University of Tennessee School of Medicine, Memphis. Staff Physician, Diggs-Kraus Center for Sickle Cell Disease, Regional Medical Center, Memphis, Tennessee
Sickle Cell Anemia

WILLIAM Z. BORER, M.D.
Associate Professor, Department of Pathology, Anatomy, and Cell Biology, Thomas Jefferson University. Director, Clinical Chemistry Section, Thomas Jefferson University Hospital, Philadelphia, Pennsylvania
Reference Intervals for the Interpretation of Laboratory Tests

WAYNE A. BOTTNER, M.D.
Chief, Division of Hematology, Gundersen Clinic, Ltd., La Crosse, Wisconsin
Megaloblastic Anemia

MARK D. BRACKER, M.D.
Clinical Professor, Department of Family and Preventive Medicine, University of California, San Diego, School of Medicine, La Jolla, California
Patellofemoral Pain Syndrome

RAYMOND C. BREDFELDT, M.D.
Associate Professor of Family and Community Medicine, University of Arkansas for Medical Sciences, Little Rock. Residency Director, Northwest Arkansas Family Practice Residency, Fayetteville, Arkansas
Chronic Serous Otitis Media

WALTER BRIDGES, M.D.
Clinical Faculty, Departments of Pediatrics and Internal Medicine, Texas Tech University School of Medicine and Health Sciences Center. Private Practice, University Pediatric Group Foundation, Amarillo, Texas
Earache/Ear Pain

STEPHEN A. BRIETZKE, M.D.
Clinical Assistant Professor, University of Southern Alabama School of Medicine, Mobile, Alabama. Program Director, Internal Medicine Residency, Keesler Medical Center, Keesler Air Force Base, Mississippi
Diabetes Mellitus, Type I

GARY M. BROCKINGTON, M.D.
Associate Professor, Department of Medicine, Tufts University School of Medicine. Staff Cardiologist, Faulkner Hospital, Boston, Massachusetts
Mitral Valve Disease

PETER BRODERICK, M.D.
Assistant Clinical Professor, Department of Family Practice, University of California, Davis, School of Medicine, Sacramento, California
Insomnia

MICHAEL S. BRONZE, M.D.
Associate Chairman, Department of Medicine, and Associate Professor of Medicine, University of Tennessee College of Medicine. Program Director, Internal Medicine Residency, University of Tennessee, Memphis, Tennessee.
Endocarditis

MICHAEL JON BROOKS, M.D.
Fellow in Gastroenterology, Medical College of Pennsylvania and Hahnemann University, Philadelphia, Pennsylvania
Diverticulitis

LEE K. BROWN, M.D.
Associate Professor of Clinical Medicine, University of Arizona College of Medicine, Tucson. Director, Sleep Disorders Center, and Associate Program Director, Professional Services, Department of Internal Medicine, St. Joseph's Hospital and Medical Center, Phoenix, Arizona
Sleep Apnea

WARD M. BROWN, M.D.
Assistant Clinical Professor, Department of Medicine, University of Wisconsin School of Medicine, Madison. Chief, Department of Cardiovascular Diseases and Head of Arrhythmia Services, Wisconsin Heart Institute, Gundersen Clinic/Lutheran Medical Center, La Crosse, Wisconsin
Syncope

ELIZABETH E. BROWNELL, M.D.
Assistant Professor of Family and Community Medicine, Medical College of Wisconsin, Milwaukee. Staff Physician, Waukesha Memorial Hospital, Waukesha; Private Practice, Waukesha Medical Center, Brookfield, Wisconsin
Rosacea

DOUGLAS G. BROWNING, M.D.
Assistant Professor of Family Medicine and Associate in Surgical Sciences–Orthopedics/Sports Medicine, Bowman Gray School of Medicine of Wake Forest University. Staff Physician, North Carolina Baptist Hospital, Winston-Salem, North Carolina
Wrist and Hand Pain

SUZANNE BRUCE, M.D.
Associate Professor of Dermatology, Baylor College of Medicine, Houston, Texas
Dry Skin

SUSAN C. BRUNSELL, M.D.
Clinical Assistant Professor, Uniformed Services University of Health Sciences, Bethesda. Staff Family Physician, Family Practice Residency, Malcolm Grow USAF Medical Center, Andrews Air Force Base, Maryland
Urinary Incontinence

STEPHEN A. BRUNTON, M.D.
Clinical Professor, Department of Family Medicine, University of California, Irvine, School of Medicine, Irvine. Director, Family Medicine Residency Program, Long Beach Memorial Medical Center, Long Beach, California
Gastroesophageal Reflux

JAMES K. BUCK II, M.D.
Senior Clinical Fellow, Division of Allergy and Clinical Immunology, Department of Medicine, University of Tennessee, Memphis, College of Medicine, Memphis, Tennessee
Anaphylaxis

FRANK BURWICK, M.D.
Clinical Educator, Departments of Pediatrics and Internal Medicine, Texas Tech University School of Medicine and Health Sciences Center, Amarillo, Texas
Sore Throat

MARK BYLER, M.D.
Assistant Professor, Department of Community Medicine and Family Practice, University of Missouri-Kansas City School of Medicine. Teaching Staff, Truman Medical Center-East, Kansas City, Missouri
Local and Regional Anesthesia of the Lower Extremity; Ascaris and Hookworm Infection

LISA M. CANNON, M.D.
Chief Resident, Danbury Hospital, Danbury, Connecticut. Pulmonary Fellow, Mount Sinai Hospital of the City of New York, New York, New York
Bronchiectasis

LAURA CARBONE, M.D.
Instructor, Department of Medicine, University of Tennessee College of Medicine, Memphis, Tennessee
Systemic Lupus Erythematosus

LEE M. CARTER, M.D.
Instructor in Medicine, Department of Family Medicine, University of Tennessee, Memphis, College of Medicine, Memphis, Tennessee
Dilatation and Curettage of the Uterus

FRANK S. CELESTINO, M.D.
Associate Professor and Director of Geriatrics, Department of Family and Community Medicine, Bowman Gray School of Medicine of Wake Forest University, Winston-Salem, North Carolina
Frostbite

ASHISH CHABRA, M.D.
Professor of Clinical Medicine, St. Joseph's Hospital, Family Practice Residency Program, Phoenix, Arizona
Corneal Ulceration

BENJAMIN H. CHADI, M.D.
Instructor in Medicine, Mount Sinai School of Medicine of the City of New York. Attending Physician, Division of Cardiology, Department of Medicine, Beth Israel Medical Center, New York, New York
Shock; Cardiomyopathy

S. SHEKAR CHAKRAVARTHI, M.B.
Assistant Professor, East Carolina University School of Medicine, Greenville, North Carolina
Hyperparathyroidism

JASON CHAO, M.D.
Associate Professor, Department of Family Medicine, Case Western Reserve University School of Medicine. Medical Director, Department of Family Practice, University Hospitals of Cleveland, Cleveland, Ohio
Abnormal Liver Function Tests

ANTHONY L-T. CHEN, M.D.
Clinical Assistant Professor, University of Washington School of Medicine. Medical Director, Downtown Family Medicine; Assistant Residency Director, Swedish Family Practice Residency, Seattle, Washington
Fatigue

EUGENE Y. CHENG, M.D.
Associate Professor of Anesthesiology and Medicine and Director, Critical Care Medicine, Department of Anesthesiology, Medical College of Wisconsin, Milwaukee, Wisconsin
Local and Regional Anesthesia: Head and Neck

MARC J. CHERNOFF, D.O.
Chief Medical Resident and Instructor, Milton S. Hershey Medical Center/Pennsylvania State University School of Medicine, Hershey. Chief Resident and Instructor, Harrisburg Hospital, Harrisburg, and Lebanon Veterans Administration Hospital, Lebanon, Pennsylvania
Leukemia

LORENA S. CHICOYE, M.D.
Assistant Professor and Medical Director of the Teen and Young Adult Clinic, Department of Family Medicine, Medical College of Wisconsin, Milwaukee, Wisconsin
Pelvic Inflammatory Disease

ROBERT TAO-PING CHOW, M.D.
Assistant Professor, Department of Medicine, Johns Hopkins University School of Medicine. Co-Director, Division of General Internal Medicine, Sinai Hospital of Baltimore, Baltimore, Maryland
International Travel Disease Prevention

LILI CHURCH, M.D.
Assistant Professor, Department of Family Medicine, University of Washington School of Medicine. Staff Physician, University of Washington Medical Center, Seattle, Washington
Dysfunctional Uterine Bleeding

TODD J. COHEN, M.D.
Assistant Professor of Medicine, Cornell University Medical College, Ithaca. Director of Electrophysiology, North Shore University Hospital, Manhasset, New York
Defibrillation

MARILEE C. S. COLE, M.D.
Assistant Clinical Professor, Georgetown University School of Medicine, Washington, D.C.
Acute Diarrhea; Chronic Diarrhea

JOSEPH V. CONNELLY, M.D.
Clinical Assistant Professor, New York Medical College, Valhalla, New York. Residency Director, St. Joseph's Medical Center, Stamford, Connecticut
Rubella; Measles

MICHAEL A. COOK, D.O.
Internist and Diagnostic Radiology Resident, St. Vincent's Medical Center of Richmond, Staten Island, and New York Medical College, Valhalla, New York
Appendicitis; Scrotal Pain/Mass

JOHN B. COOMBS, M.D.
Professor of Family Medicine and Pediatrics and Associate Dean, Regional Affairs and Rural Health, University of Washington, School of Medicine. Associate Vice President of Medical Affairs, University of Washington, Seattle, Washington
Loss of Appetite

DAVID J. COOPER, M.D.
Assistant Professor of Medicine, Cornell University Medical College, New York. Associate Chairman, Department of Medicine, North Shore University Hospital, Manhasset, New York
Parenteral Nutrition

JANE E. CORBOY, M.D.
Assistant Professor of Family Medicine, Baylor Colllege of Medicine. Director, Park Plaza Family Practice Center and Park Plaza Family Practice Residency Track, Park Plaza Hospital, Houston, Texas
Exercise Prescribing

SCOTT CORLISS, M.D.
Clinical Instructor of Family Medicine, University of Colorado School of Medicine, Denver. Associate Director and Director of Clinical Affairs, North Colorado Family Medicine Residency Training Program, Greeley, Colorado
Preterm Labor

JACK L. COX, M.D.
Associate Clinical Professor, Department of Family and Preventive Medicine, University of Utah School of Medicine, Salt Lake City. Director, Utah Valley Family Practice Residency, Utah Valley Regional Medical Center, Provo, Utah
Nicotine Dependence

BICKLEY CRAVEN, M.D.
Assistant Professor, Department of Family Medicine, East Tennessee State University Quillen College of Medicine, Johnson City. Attending Physician, Holston Valley Hospital and Medical Center, Kingsport, Tennessee
Pregnancy

PAUL T. CULLEN, M.D.
Clinical Assistant Professor of Family and Community Medicine, Pennsylvania State University College of Medicine, Hershey Adjunct Assistant Professor, Department of Medicine, Medical College of Pennsylvania, Pittsburgh. Program Director, Family Practice Residency Program, Washington Hospital, Washington, Pennsylvania
Tinnitus

T. K. CUMARASAMY, M.D.
Assistant Professor of Oral and Maxillofacial Surgery, University of Manitoba Faculty of Dentistry, Manitoba, Canada. Resident in Family Medicine, West Jersey Health System, Voorhees, New Jersey
Temporomandibular Joint (TMJ) Syndrome

ANNE CATHER CUTLIP, M.D.
Assistant Professor, Department of Family Medicine, West Virginia University School of Medicine, Morgantown. Staff Physician, University Health Service and Ruby Memorial Hospital, Morgantown, West Virginia
Cervical Biopsy/LEEP; Condyloma Accuminata

TIMOTHY P. DAALEMAN, D.O.
Assistant Professor, Department of Family Medicine, University of Kansas School of Medicine. Attending Physician, University of Kansas Hospital, Kansas City, Kansas
Undescended Testicle; Disseminated Intravascular Coagulation

DIANA S. DARK, M.D.
Associate Professor, University of Missouri–Kansas City School of Medicine. Associate Program Director, Internal Medicine Residency Program, Department of Medical Education, St. Luke's Hospital, Kansas City, Missouri
Coccidioidomycosis; Malnutrition

DENIS F. DARKO, M.D.
Associate Adjunct Professor, University of California, San Diego, School of Medicine. Associate Member, Department of Neuropharmacology, Scripps Research Institute; Member, Division of Psychiatry, Scripps Clinic and Research Foundation, La Jolla, California
Depression

MARC A. DARR, M.D.
Clinical Assistant Professor, Department of Family and Community Medicine, University of Arizona College of Medicine, Tucson. Assistant Director, Family Practice Residency Program, St. Joseph's Hospital and Medical Center, Phoenix, Arizona
Vitiligo

MARK D. DARROW, M.D.
Assistant Professor, Geriatric Division, Department of Family Medicine, East Carolina University School of Medicine. Staff Physician, Pitt County Memorial Hospital, Greenville, North Carolina
Impotence

DANIEL T. DAVISON, D.O.
Clinical Associate Professor of Family Medicine, Chicago College of Osteopathic Medicine, Downers Grove; Assistant Professor of Family Practice, Rush Medical College, Chicago, Illinois
Tendinitis

PETER DeMARTINO, M.D.
Director of the Emergency Department, Naval Medical Center, Oakland, California
Snakebite

MARVIN A. DEWAR, M.D., J.D.
Associate Professor of Family Medicine, University of Florida College of Medicine, Gainesville, Florida
Breast Cancer

SHIRLEY L. DICKINSON, M.D.
Faculty Physician, Family Practice Residency, Natividad Medical Center, Salinas, California
Menopause

DIANE L. DIETZEN, M.D.
Assistant Professor, Temple University School of Medicine, Philadelphia. Associate Program Director, Scranton Temple Residency Program, Scranton, Pennsylvania
Pulmonary Embolus

ROBERT A. Di TOMASSO, Ph.D.
Adjunct Associate Professor of Psychology In Education Division, University of Pennsylvania College of Medicine, Philadelphia, Pennsylvania. Associate Director of Behavioral Medicine, West Jersey Health System Family Practice Residency, Tatem-Brown Family Practice Center, Voorhees, New Jersey
Deep Muscle Relaxation Exercises

JON DIVINE, M.D.
Chief Resident, Baylor Family Practice, Baylor College of Medicine, Houston, Texas
Joint Aspiration and Injection

DAVID DOVNARSKY, M.D.
Clinical Instructor, Department of Family Medicine, Robert Wood Johnson Medical School, University of Medicine and Dentistry of New Jersey, New Brunswick. Associate Director, West Jersey Family Practice Residency, Voorhees, New Jersey
Hyperlipidemia

HOWARD G. DUBIN, M.D.
Clinical Assistant Professor, Department of Medicine, Brown University School of Medicine. Director, Division of Critical Care Medicine, Memorial Hospital of Rhode Island, Providence, Rhode Island
Cardiopulmonary Resuscitation (CPR)

MARSHA DuPREE, M.D.
Assistant Professor of Dermatology and Dermatopathology, Albany Medical College, Albany, New York
Basal and Squamous Cell Carcinoma

JERRY M. EARLL, M.D.
Professor of Medicine, Georgetown University School of Medicine. Director of Geriatrics, Georgetown University Medical Center/Hospital, Washington, D.C.
Peripheral Neuropathy

ABBAS Y. EL-KHATIB, M.D.
Senior Resident, Department of Internal Medicine, William Beaumont Hospital, Royal Oak, Michigan
Hypokalemia

CAROL L. ELLIS, M.D.
Assistant Professor and Clerkship Director, Department of Medicine, University of Tennessee Medical Center, Knoxville, Tennessee
Cellulitis

JOHN W. ELY, M.D., M.S.P.H.
Assistant Professor, University of Iowa Hospitals and Clinics, Iowa City, Iowa
Excision of a Sebaceous (Epidermal) Cyst

RANDOLPH W. EVANS, M.D.
Clinical Assistant Professor, University of Texas Medical School and Baylor College of Medicine. Chief of Neurology Section, Park Plaza Hospital, Houston, Texas
Postconcussion Syndrome; Hyperventilation Syndrome

JACQUELINE EWING, D.O.
Staff Physician, West Jersey Hospital–Voorhees Division, Voorhees, New Jersey
Lymphadenopathy

GEORGE T. FANTRY, M.D.
Assistant Professor of Medicine, University of Maryland School of Medicine. Director, Clinical Gastroenterology, Baltimore Veterans Affairs Medical Center. Baltimore, Baltimore Maryland
Peptic Ulcer Disease

RAYMOND H. FEIERABEND, Jr., M.D.
Associate Professor, Department of Family Medicine, East Tennessee State University, Quillen College of Medicine, Johnson City. Faculty, Bristol Family Practice Residency, Bristol, Tennessee
Rheumatoid Arthritis

JOEL FEIGIN, M.D.
Clinical Associate Professor of Family Medicine, Robert Wood Johnson Medical School, University of Medicine and Dentistry of New Jersey, New Brunswick. Associate Program Director, Clinical Director, and Director of Procedural Medicine, Warren Hospital Family Practice Residency Program, Phillipsburg, New Jersey
Vasectomy (No-Scalpel)

DEBRA FELDMAN, M.D.
Assistant Professor of Medicine and of Community and Preventive Medicine, Medical College of Pennsylvania and Hahnemann University, Philadelphia, Pennsylvania
Irritability

EUGENE A. FELMAR, M.D.
Clinical Professor of Family Medicine, University of California, Los Angeles, School of Medicine, Los Angeles. Director, Family Practice Residency, Santa Monica Hospital Medical Center, Santa Monica, California
Hemorrhoids; Hemorrhoid Sclerotherapy, Infrared Coagulation, and Banding

BRADLEY W. FENTON, M.D.
Clinical Associate Professor of Medicine, University of Pennsylvania School of Medicine. Staff Physician, Benjamin Franklin Clinic of Pennsylvania Hospital, Philadelphia, Pennsylvania
Infectious Diarrhea

DANIEL S. FICK, M.D.
Assistant Professor, Family Practice and Orthopaedic Surgery, University of Iowa College of Medicine, Iowa City, Iowa
Runner's Injuries

CLIFFORD FIELD, M.D.
Department of Family Medicine, Idaho State University. Medical Director, Bannock Urgent Care, Bannock Regional Medical and Geriatric Center, Pocatello, Idaho
Flexible Sigmoidoscopy/Colonoscopy

MITCHELL F. FINNIE, M.D.
Private Practice Physician; McLennan County Medical Education and Research Foundation, Waco, Texas,
Atopic Dermatitis

BRUCE FLAREAU, M.D.
Clinical Assistant Professor, University of South Florida School of Medicine, Tampa. Director, Family Practice Residency, Morton Plant Mease Healthcare Systems, Clearwater, Florida
Aquatic Injuries

A. STEVEN FLEISHER, M.B., B.Ch.
Resident, Department of Medicine, Sinai Hospital of Baltimore, Baltimore, Maryland
Hodgkin's Disease

GRANT C. FOWLER, M.D.
Associate Professor, University of Texas Medical School. Residency Director, Hermann/Lyndon Baines Johnson Hospitals Family Practice Residency, Houston, Texas
Hydrocele/Spermatocele

MICHAEL J. FREELAND, M.D.
Clinical Assistant Professor, Department of Medicine, Brown University School of Medicine, Providence. Staff Intensivist, Division of Critical Care Medicine, Memorial Hospital of Rhode Island, Pawtucket, Rhode Island
Endotracheal Intubation

KEITH A. FREY, M.D., M.B.A.
Clinical Associate Professor, Department of Family Medicine, University of Washington School of Medicine, Seattle. Director, Saint Peter's Hospital Family Practice Residency Program, Saint Peter's Hospital, Olympia, Washington
Infertility

JAN FRONEK, M.D.
Clinical Instructor, University of California, San Diego, School of Medicine. Attending Surgeon, Scripps Clinic and Research Foundation, Head Team Physician, San Diego Padres Baseball Club, San Diego, California
Patellar Dislocations

ERNEST FRUGÉ, Ph.D.
Assistant Professor, Department of Family Medicine, Baylor College of Medicine, Houston, Texas
Substance Abuse

JUAN GALARRAGA, M.D.
Instructor in Medicine, Johns Hopkins University School of Medicine. Co-Director, Division of General Internal Medicine, Department of Medicine, Sinai Hospital of Baltimore, Baltimore, Maryland
Preoperative Evaluation

NICHOLAS J. GALIOTO, M.D.
Associate Director, Family Practice Residency Program, Broadlawns Medical Center, Des Moines, Iowa
Croup

ELLEN T. GEMINIANI, M.D.
Assistant Professor of Family and Community Medicine, Pennsylvania State University College of Medicine. Assistant Professor of Family and Community Medicine, Department of Family and Community Medicine, Milton S. Hershey Medical Center, Hershey, Pennsylvania
Finger Dislocations

ROBERT M. GERBO, M.D.
Assistant Professor of Family Medicine, West Virginia University School of Medicine, Morgantown, West Virginia
Small and Large Bowel Obstruction

WILLIAM A. GHALI, M.D., M.P.H.
Fellow, Section of General Internal Medicine, Boston University Medical Center, Boston, Massachusetts
Use of Blood Products

REBECCA GLADU, M.D.
Assistant Professor, University of Texas at Houston, Medical School, Houston, Texas
Abnormal Pap Smear

BEN L. GLASPEY, D.O.
Family Practice Resident, University of Florida/Shands Hospital/Alachua General Hospital, Gainesville, Florida
Ankle Sprain

LISA A. GLEASON, M.D.
General Internal Medicine Staff and Director, Internal Medicine Clinic, Naval Medical Center, Oakland, California
Pregnancy-Induced Hypertension; Recurrent Infections

LYNNE J. GOEBEL, M.D.
Assistant Professor of Medicine, Marshall University School of Medicine, Huntington, West Virginia
Eye Pain

CHRIS GOERDT, M.D., M.P.H.
Assistant Professor, Division of General Medicine, Clinical Epidemiology, and Health Services Research, Department of Internal Medicine, University of Iowa Hospitals and Clinics, Iowa City, Iowa
Peripheral Arterial Disease

ROLAND A. GOERTZ, M.D.
Associate Professor, University of Texas–Houston Medical School. Vice President, Medical Affairs, OneCare Health Industries, Inc., Houston, Texas
Palpitations

GARY A. GOFORTH, M.D., M.T.M.H.
Associate Professor of Family Medicine, Medical University of South Carolina, Charleston. Faculty, Montgomery Center for Family Medicine, Self Memorial Hospital, Greenwood, South Carolina
Malaria

MARLENE GOLDWEIN, M.D.
Assistant Professor of Medicine, Medical College of Pennsylvania and Hahnemann University. General Internal Medicine Faculty, Medical College of Pennsylvania, Philadelphia, Pennsylvania
Gynecomastia

THOMAS B. GOLEMON, M.D.
Assistant Professor of Clinical Family Practice, University of Illinois College of Medicine at Peoria. Director, Family Practice Residency, Methodist Medical Center of Illinois, Peoria, Illinois
Osteomyelitis

RUSSELL PATRICK GOLLARD, M.D.
Clinical Fellow, Division of Hematology and Oncology, Scripps Clinic and Research Foundation, La Jolla, California
Neutropenia

HAL E. GORDON, M.D.
Medical Director, Big Muddy River Men's Correctional Center, Ina, Illinois
Heartburn and Indigestion

ALISON GRANN, M.D.
Resident in Radiation Therapy, Memorial-Sloan Kettering Cancer Center, New York, New York
Oncologic Emergencies

LELAND GRAVES, III, M.D.
Assistant Professor of Medicine, Division of Endocrinology, Diabetes, and Metabolism, University of Missouri, Kansas City, School of Medicine, Kansas City, Missouri
Hypocalcemia

BRUCE D. GREENWALD, M.D.
Assistant Professor, University of Maryland School of Medicine, Baltimore, Maryland
Ulcerative Colitis

DAWN M. GRINENKO, M.D.
Clinical Assistant Professor and Director, Adolescent/Young Adult Program, University of Florida School of Medicine, Gainesville, Florida
Anorexia and Bulimia Nervosa

EDWARD J. GURZA, M.D.
Assistant Professor, Department of Medicine, Division of General Internal Medicine, Loyola University Stritch School of Medicine, Maywood, Illinois
Thyroiditis

GEOFFREY PETER GUSTAVSEN, M.D.
Faculty, Phoenix Baptist Family Practice Residency, Phoenix Baptist Hospital, Phoenix, Arizona
Burns

DAVID E. GUTSTEIN, M.D.
Fellow in Cardiology, Mount Sinai Medical Center of the City of New York, New York, New York
Acute Heart Failure; Chronic Heart Failure

DAVID HALL, M.D.
Volunteer Clinical Supervisor, Department of Family Medicine, Baylor College of Medicine. CIGNA Healthcare Staff Physician, CIGNA Greenpark II Health Clinic, Houston, Texas
Bladder Cancer

MARY NOLAN HALL, M.D.
Clinical Assistant Professor, University of North Carolina at Chapel Hill School of Medicine. Residency Director, Department of Family Practice, Carolinas Medical Center, Charlotte, North Carolina
Pelvic Pain

NEIL K. HALL, M.D.
Clinical Associate Professor, Department of Family Practice, Health Sciences Center at Syracuse Clinical Campus at Binghamton, Binghamton. Medical Director and Director of Geriatrics Education and Research, Ideal Senior Living Center, Endicott, New York
Benign Prostatic Hyperplasia

JIMMY H. HARA, M.D.
Associate Clinical Professor, Family Medicine Division, University of California, Los Angeles, School of Medicine. Residency Program Director, Department of Family Practice, and Multi-

Disciplinary Pain Clinic Director, Kaiser Los Angeles Medical Center, Los Angeles, California
Myofascial Syndromes (Fibromyalgia and Myofascial Trigger Points)

THOMAS P. HARDER, M.D.
Program Director, Internal Medicine Education, Grant Medical Center, Columbus, Ohio
Gout

KISHORE J. HARJAI, M.D.
Fellow, Department of Cardiology, Alton Ochsner Medical Foundation, New Orleans, Louisiana
Guillain-Barré Syndrome

MICHAEL B. HARPER, M.D.
Professor of Clinical Family Medicine, and Residency Program Director, Louisiana State University Medical Center, Shreveport, Louisiana
Nasogastric Intubation

JOHN J. HART, M.D.
Clinical Associate Professor, Department of Family and Community Medicine, University of Kansas School of Medicine. Associate Director, Family Practice Residency, Wesley Medical Center, Wichita, Kansas
Myasthenia Gravis

ROBERT L. HATCH, M.D., M.P.H.
Assistant Professor, Department of Community Health and Family Medicine, University of Florida School of Medicine, Gainesville, Florida
Foot Fractures

VAN B. HAYNE, M.D.
Associate Professor of Medicine, Division of Endocrinology and Metabolism, University of Alabama School of Medicine. Clinical Faculty, The Kirklin Clinic, Birmingham, Alabama
Ketoacidosis

JAMES W. HAYNES, M.D.
Chief, Family Practice, 65th Medical Group, Lajes Field, Azores, Portugal
Alopecia

CHRISTOPHER L. HAYS, M.D.
Fellow, Primary Care Sports Medicine, Methodist Sports Medicine Center, Indianapolis, Indiana
Bursitis

ROBERT M. HEILIGMAN, M.D.
Associate Professor of Clinical Medicine, University of Arizona College of Medicine. Associate Program Director for Curricular Affairs, Internal Medicine Residency Program, St. Joseph's Hospital and Medical Center, Phoenix, Arizona
Bone Marrow Aspiration and Biopsy

SCOTT T. HENDERSON, M.D.
Assistant Professor of Family Practice and Associate Program Director, University of Wyoming Family Practice Residency Program at Cheyenne. Active Staff, United Medical Center, Cheyenne, Wyoming
First Trimester Bleeding

THOMAS HERCHLINE, M.D.
Chief, Infectious Diseases, Keesler Medical Center, Biloxi, Mississippi
Toxic Shock Syndrome

ARTHUR H. HEROLD, M.D.
Associate Professor of Family Medicine, University of South Florida College of Medicine. Chief of Family Practice, Tampa General Hospital, Tampa, Florida
Rectal Bleeding

CARLOS R. HERRERA, M.D., M.P.H.
Assistant Professor, University of Texas Medical School; Adjunct Faculty Member, University of Texas School of Public Health; and Fellow, Health Services Research, American Association of Medical Colleges. Physician, Hermann Hospital, Houston, Texas
Hypertension

HILARY I. HERTAN, M.D.
Assistant Professor of Medicine, New York Medical College, Valhalla. Attending Physician, Department of Gastroenterology and Clinical Nutrition, Our Lady of Mercy Medical Center, Bronx, New York
Nutritional Assessment in Clinical Practice

KARL R. HERWIG, M.D.
Clinical Associate Professor, Department of Surgery, University of California, San Diego, School of Medicine. Head, Division of Urology, Green Hospital of Scripps Clinic, La Jolla, California
Urinary Stones; Hypercalciuria

ROGER R. HESSELBROCK, B.S., M.D.
Clinical Assistant Professor, Department of Psychiatry and Neurology, Tulane University School of Medicine, New Orleans, Louisiana. Chief, Neurology Section, 81st Medical Group, Keesler Medical Center, Keesler Air Force Base, Mississippi
Bell's Palsy

JOE E. HIMES, M.D.
Director of Sports Medicine and Primary Care Sports Medicine Fellowship Director, Deaconess Family Medicine Residency, St. Louis, Missouri
Shoulder Dislocations

ROBERT M. A. HIRSCHFELD, M.D.
Titus H. Harris Distinguished Professor and Chairman, Department of Psychiatry and Behavioral Sciences, University of Texas Medical Branch, Galveston, Texas
Personality Disorders (Borderline, Dependent)

HOWARD A. HOLTZ, M.D.
Associate Professor of Clinical Medicine, University of Medicine and Dentistry of New Jersey Robert Wood Johnson Medical School, New Brunswick. Associate Chairman, Department of Medicine, St. Barnabas Medical Center, Livingston, New Jersey
Domestic Violence

DAVID O. HOUGH, M.D.
Professor of Family Practice and Director of Sports Medicine, Michigan State University School of Medicine, East Lansing, Michigan
Ankle Fractures

ROBERT M. HOWSE, Jr., M.D.
Adjunct Clinical Assistant Professor, Pennsylvania State University College of Medicine, Hershey. Assistant Director and Director of Geriatrics, Pennsylvania State University/The Good Samaritan Hospital, Family and Community Residency Program, Lebanon, Pennsylvania
Punch and Shave Biopsy

MARK E. HRONCICH, M.D.
Clinical Assistant Professor of Medicine, Loyola University Stritch School of Medicine, Maywood. Attending Physician, MacNeal Hospital, Berwyn, Illinois
Paget's Disease of Bone

PAUL J. HUGHES, M.D.
Clinical Assistant Professor of Family and Community Medicine, Pennsylvania State University School of Medicine, Hershey, Pennsylvania
Altitude Sickness

THOMAS K. HUNT, M.D.
Associate Clinical Professor, University of California, Davis, School of Medicine, Sacramento. Clinical Faculty, Family Practice Residency Program, Stanislaus Medical Center, Modesto, California
Stomatitis

CHARLEEN ISÉ, M.D.
Assistant Director, Bayfront Family Practice Residency Program, Bayfront Medical Center, St. Petersburg; Assistant Clinical Professor of Family Medicine, University of South Florida School of Medicine, Tampa. Attending Physician, Bayfront Medical Center, St. Petersburg, Florida
Percutaneous Incision and Drainage of Abscess

VAL GENE IVEN, M.D.
Team Physician, University of Tennessee Athletics Department, University of Tennessee, Knoxville, Tennessee
Costochondritis

NICOLA J. JACOBUCCI, M.D.
Assistant Clinical Professor of Family Medicine, Case Western Reserve University School of Medicine. Laboratory and Procedure Coordinator, Center for Family Medicine and Fairview General Hospital, Cleveland, Ohio.
Fine-Needle Aspiration of the Breast

LOUIS B. JACQUES, M.D.
Director of Predoctoral Education, Department of Family Medicine, Georgetown University School of Medicine, Washington, D.C.
Pinworms; Giardiasis

RAM JADONATH, M.D.
Staff Electrophysiologist, North Shore University Hospital and Cornell Medical College, Manhasset, New York
Arrhythmias

HARRIET A. JAKOB, M.D.
Assistant Clinical Professor of Medicine, Case Western Reserve University School of Medicine, Cleveland, Ohio.
Melanoma

STEPHEN P. JAMES, M.D.
Professor, Department of Medicine, University of Maryland School of Medicine. Head, Division of Gastroenterology, Baltimore Veterans Affairs Medical Center, Baltimore, Maryland
Crohn's Disease

ARMANDO JOSE JARQUIN, M.D.
Staff Physician, Department of Family Medicine, Kelsey Seybold Clinic, Houston, Texas
Lyme Disease

PAUL JASTER, M.D.
Assistant Professor, University of Kansas School of Medicine, Wichita. Associate Director, Smoky Hill Family Practice Residency Program; Salina, Kansas
Typhoid Fever

PHILIP C. JOHNSON, M.D.
Associate Professor and Director, Division of General Medicine, The University of Texas Medical School. Section Chief of General Medicine, Hermann Hospital, Houston, Texas
Late Symptomatic HIV Infection

ROBERT L. JOHNSON, M.D.
Member, Lubbock Diagnostic Clinic; Active Staff and Director, Diagnostic Laboratory, Methodist Hospital, Lubbock, Texas
Thoracentesis

WILLIAM M. JOHNSON, M.D.
Fellow, Pulmonary and Critical Care, University of Iowa Hospitals and Clinics, Iowa City, Iowa
Sepsis/Bacteremia

JAI H. JOSHI, M.D.
Instructor in Medicine, Department of Medicine, Johns Hopkins University School of Medicine. Division of Oncology, Department of Medicine, Sinai Hospital of Baltimore, Baltimore, Maryland
Metastatic Cancer of Unknown Origin

STEVEN J. JUBELIRER, M.D.
Clinical Professor of Medicine, West Virginia University–Charleston Division, School of Medicine. Medical Director, Cancer Center of Southern West Virginia, Charleston Area Medical Center, Charleston, West Virginia
Bleeding Disorders

GREGORY JUCKETT, M.D.
Assistant Professor of Family Medicine, Robert C. Byrd Health Sciences Center of West Virginia University. Staff Physician, Ruby Memorial Hospital, Morgantown, West Virginia
Tapeworm Infections

LEAH B. KALTMAN, M.D.
Assistant Program Director, Department of Medicine, St. Barnabas Medical Center, Livingston, New Jersey
Chronic Fatigue Syndrome

LINDA E. KANARVOGEL, M.D.
Instructor in Medicine, The Long Island Campus for Albert Einstein College of Medicine of Yeshiva University, Bronx, New York
Hematuria

IRVING KAUFMAN, M.D.
Clinical Instructor, Department of Family Medicine, Robert Wood Johnson Medical School, University of Medicine and Dentistry of New Jersey, New Brunswick. Private Practice, Somerset, New Jersey
Removal of Impacted Cerumen

MICHAEL D. KAUFMAN, M.D.
Director, Multiple Sclerosis Center, Carolinas Medical Center, Charlotte, North Carolina
Multiple Sclerosis

RICK KELLERMAN, M.D.
Associate Professor, University of Kansas School of Medicine, Wichita. Program Director, Smoky Hill Family Practice Residency, Salina, Kansas
Immunization Schedules

JOHN I. KENNEDY, Jr., M.D.
Associate Professor, Division of Pulmonary and Critical Care Medicine, University of Alabama at Birmingham School of Medicine. Director, Medical Intensive Care Unit, University of Alabama Hospital, Birmingham, Alabama
Ventilator Support

BHARAT KHANDHERIA, M.D.
Assistant Professor, Department of Internal Medicine, Texas Tech University Health Sciences Center School of Medicine. Attending Physician, Northwest Texas Hospital and Veterans Affairs Medical Center, Amarillo, Texas
Trouble Swallowing

GEORGE E. KIKANO, M.D.
Assistant Professor of Family Medicine, Case Western Reserve University School of Medicine. Director of Clinical Affairs, University Hospitals of Cleveland, Family Medicine Foundation, Cleveland, Ohio
Lead Poisoning

DAVID E. KING, M.D.
Clinical Assistant Professor, Department of Radiology, Baylor College of Medicine. Director of Magnetic Resonance Imaging, The Methodist Hospital, Houston, Texas
MRI or CT in CNS Imaging

LISA G. KING, M.D.
Physician, Internal Medicine, Crest Family Care, Tulsa, Oklahoma
Salmonellosis

JUDITH KINZY, M.D.
Assistant Professor University of Tennessee Medical Center at Knoxville, Knoxville, Tennessee
Sexually Transmitted Diseases

MICHAEL O. KIRKPATRICK, M.D.
Assistant Professor, Department of Family and Community Medicine, Texas A&M University School of Medicine. Senior Staff, Scott and White Clinic, Temple, Texas
Prostatitis

ISAAC KLEINMAN, M.D.
Clinical Associate Professor of Family Medicine, Baylor College of Medicine, Houston, Texas
Corneal Foreign Body Removal; Goiter

AUBREY L. KNIGHT, M.D.
Associate Professor of Clinical Family Medicine, University of Virginia School of Medicine, Charlottesville. Associate Director of Family Practice Education, Roanoke Memorial Hospitals, Roanoke, Virginia
Fecal Impaction

JOSEPH C. KONEN, M.D., M.S.P.H.
Vice Chair and Associate Professor, Bowman Gray School of Medicine, Wake Forest University, Winston-Salem, North Carolina
Health Maintenance Protocols

KAREN W. KRIGGER, M.D.
Assistant Professor, Department of Family and Community Medicine, University of Louisville School of Medicine, Louisville, Kentucky
Penile Discharge

ELANA NUDEL KRIPKE, M.D.
Assistant Professor of Medicine, Medical College of Pennsylvania, Philadelphia, Pennsylvania
Nipple Discharge

LINDA L. KRISHNA, M.D.
Baylor Family Practice Resident, Baylor Family Practice, Houston, Texas
Early Symptomatic HIV Infection

LINDA KURIBAYASHI, M.D.
Assistant Clinical Professor of Medicine and Program Director, Transitional Year Residency, University of California, San Francisco, Fresno Medical Education Program. Director, General Internal Medicine, Valley Medical Center, Fresno, California
Pleural Effusions

MARY ANN KUZMA, M.D.
Assistant Professor of Medicine and Director, Division of Ambulatory Care Education, Medical College of Pennsylvania/Hahnemann University, Philadelphia, Pennsylvania
Oliguria/Anuria

YONG LIE LAM, M.D.
Volunteer Faculty, University of California, San Diego, School of Medicine, San Diego. Staff Physician, San Diego Family Clinic, National City, California
Dyslexia

THOMAS L. LEAMAN, M.D.
Professor Emeritus, Department of Family and Community Medicine, Milton S. Hershey Medical Center, Hershey, Pennsylvania
Generalized Anxiety Disorder

THOMAS C. LEE, M.D.
Clinical Fellow, Scripps Clinic and Research Foundation, La Jolla, California
Iron Deficiency Anemia

MICHAEL J. LEVY, M.D.
Fellow in Gastroenterology, University of Southern Alabama College of Medicine, Mobile, Alabama
Cirrhosis

STEVEN A. LEVY, M.D.
Assistant Professor of Internal Medicine, Medical College of Pennsylvania and Hahnemann University, Philadelphia. Director of Internal Medicine Education and Associate Director, Hamot Family Practice Residency, Hamot Medical Center, Erie, Pennsylvania
Advance Directives

MICHAEL LEWKO, M.D.
Assistant Professor of Internal Medicine and Family Practice, Seton Hall University of Graduate Medical Education, South Orange. Assistant Clinical Professor of Family Practice, University of Medicine and Dentistry of New Jersey Robert Wood Johnson Medical School, New Brunswick. Chief of Geriatrics, St. Joseph's Hospital and Medical Center, Paterson, New Jersey
Temporal Arteritis

JOSEPH J. LIEBER, M.D.
Assistant Professor of Medicine, Mount Sinai School of Medicine of the City of New York, New York. Associate Attending in Medicine and Nephrology; Chief, Medical Consultation Service; and Educational Coordinator, Department of Medicine, Elmhurst Hospital Center, Elmhurst, New York
Proteinuria

JANET C. LINDEMANN, M.D.
Assistant Professor, Department of Family and Community Medicine, Medical College of Wisconsin. Associate Director of Family Health Center, John L. Doyne Hospital, Milwaukee, Wisconsin
Premenstrual Syndrome

MARTIN S. LIPSKY, M.D.
Predoctoral Director, Department of Family Medicine, Medical College of Pennsylvania and Hahnemann University, Philadelphia, Pennsylvania
Jaundice: Neonatal, Adult; Hypercalcemia; Ascites

ANNE R. LOCKETT, M.D.
Assistant Professor, Department of Family and Community Medicine, Eastern Virginia Medical School, Norfolk. Clinical Faculty, Family Practice Residency, Portsmouth Family Medicine, Portsmouth, Virginia
Contact Dermatitis

DAVID P. LOSH, M.D.
Associate Professor and Residency Program Director, Department of Family Medicine, University of Washington School of Medicine, Seattle, Washington
Decubitus Ulcer

BRIAN M. LOTT, M.D.
Clinical Assistant Professor of Family Medicine, Ohio State University College of Medicine. Faculty Instructor, Grant Family Medicine Residency, Grant Medical Center, Columbus, Ohio
Epididymitis

REGGIE LYELL, M.D.
Private Practice Physician, Corydon, Indiana
Exercise Stress Testing

VIPUL N. MANKAD, M.D.
Professor and Chairman, Department of Pediatrics, University of Kentucky College of Medicine, Lexington, Kentucky
Thalassemia Syndromes

SARAH S. MARLOWE, M.D.
Clinical Instructor of Family Medicine, University of Washington School of Medicine, Seattle. Faculty, Family Practice Residency, and Chief, Soldier Care Service, Madigan Army Medical Center, Tacoma, Washington
Back Pain

F. ALLAN MARTIN, M.D.
Assistant Professor, and Department of Family and Community Medicine, University of Arkansas for Medical Sciences. Faculty, Northwest Arkansas Family Practice Residency, and Staff Physician, Washington Regional Medical Center, Fayetteville, Arkansas
Altered Mental State/Dementia (Delirium)

JOAN B. MARTIN, M.D.
Associate Professor, Idaho State University, Pocatello, Idaho
Hair Disorders

JOSEPH R. MASCI, M.D.
Associate Professor of Medicine, Mount Sinai School of Medicine of the City of New York, New York. Associate Director, Department of Medicine, Elmhurst Hospital Center, Elmhurst, New York
Erysipelas

ANDREW D. MASSEY, M.D.
Associate Professor, Department of Neurology, University of Kentucky Medical Center, Lexington, Kentucky
Seizure Disorder

DALE A. MATTHEWS, M.D.
Associate Professor of Medicine, Georgetown University School of Medicine, Washington, D.C.
Somatoform Disorders

ROBERT MAURER, Ph.D.
Assistant Clinical Professor, University of California, Los Angeles, School of Medicine, Los Angeles. Director of Behavioral Sciences, Family Practice Residency Program, Santa Monica Hospital Medical Center, Santa Monica, California
Suicide Assessment

E. J. MAYEAUX, Jr., M.D.
Assistant Professor of Family Medicine and Clinical Assistant Professor of Obstetrics and Gynecology, Louisiana State University Medical Center, Shreveport, Louisiana
Endometrial Cancer

JOHN J. McCARTHY, M.D.
Assistant Professor of Hematology and Internal Medicine, Baylor College of Medicine. Attending Physician, Methodist Hospital, Houston, Texas
Thrombocytopenia

DOUGLAS C. McCRORY, M.D., M.Sc.
Associate Professor, Division of General Internal Medicine, Duke University Medical Center. Staff Physician, Ambulatory Care, Durham Veterans Affairs Medical Center, Durham, North Carolina
Stroke

JAMES P. McKENNA, M.D.
Adjunct Assistant Professor of Family Medicine and Clinical Epidemiology, University of Pittsburgh School of Medicine, Pittsburgh. Clinical Assistant Professor of Family and Community Medicine, Pennsylvania State University College of Medicine, Hershey. Director, Family Practice Residency Program, The Medical Center, Beaver, Pennsylvania
Parasthesias

KEVIN McKOWN, M.D.
Assistant Professor of Medicine, University of Tennessee, Memphis, College of Medicine, Memphis, Tennessee
Neck Pain

BARRY R. MEISENBERG, M.D.
Director, Bone Marrow Transplant Program, Scripps Clinic and Research Foundation, La Jolla, California
Lymphoma

DOMINICK J. MEMOLI, M.D.
Associate Physician, Greater Baltimore Medical Center, Baltimore, Maryland
Anemia Workup

LINDA N. MEURER, M.D., M.P.H.
Assistant Professor and Associate Director, Academic Fellowship, Department of Family and Community Medicine, Medical College of Wisconsin, Milwaukee, Wisconsin
Developmental Surveillance

JOHN MEYERHOFF, M.D.
Assistant Professor of Medicine, Johns Hopkins University School of Medicine. Clinical Scholar in Rheumatology, Sinai Hospital of Baltimore, Baltimore, Maryland
Polymyalgia Rheumatica

JOSEPH L. MICCA, M.D.
Active Staff, Decalb Hospital and Decatur Hospital, Atlanta, Georgia
Acute Pulmonary Edema

GIULIA MICHELINI, M.D.
Assistant Professor, Division of General Internal Medicine, Department of Medicine, University of California, Los Angeles, School of Medicine, Los Angeles. Medical Director of Urgent Care, Los Angeles County Harbor–UCLA Medical Center, Torrance, California
Allergic Rhinitis

THOMAS C. MICHELS, M.D., M.P.H.
Clinical Associate Professor of Family Medicine, Uniformed Services University of the Health Sciences, Bethesda, Maryland. Family Practice Residency Program Director, Dewitt Army Community Hospital, Fort Belvoir, Virginia
Insects and Spiders

ETAN C. MILGROM, M.D.
Associate Professor of Clinical Family Medicine and Clinical Allergy/Immunology, University of Southern California School of Medicine, Los Angeles, California
Rhinolaryngoscopy

LAWRENCE H. MILLER, M.D.
Associate Professor of Family Medicine and Program Director, Kingsport Family Practice Residency, East Tennessee State University Quillen College of Medicine, Johnson City. Active Medical Staff, Department of Family Practice, Holston Valley Hospital and Medical Center, Kingsport, Tennessee
Osteochondrosis (Osgood-Schlatter Disease); Lipoma

JEFFREY F. MINTEER, M.D.
Clinical Assistant Professor of Family and Community Medicine, Pennsylvania State University College of Medicine, Hershey. Associate Director, Family Practice Residency, Washington Hospital, Washington, Pennsylvania
Raynaud's Phenomenon

KIMBERLY L. MORRIS, M.D.
Assistant Professor, Department of Internal Medicine, University of Tennessee Medical Center at Knoxville, Knoxville, Tennessee
Orbital and Periorbital Cellulitis

EARLE E. MORTON, M.S., M.D.
Department of Family Practice, Womack Army Medical Center, Fort Bragg, North Carolina
Leprosy

ROBERT J. MOSS, M.D.
Clinical Associate Professor of Medicine, University of Chicago Pritzker School of Medicine, Chicago. Director of Geriatrics, Department of Family Practice, Lutheran General Hospital, Park Ridge, Illinois
Alzheimer's Disease

MARY KAY MROZ, M.D.
Assistant Professor of Family Medicine, University of Kansas School of Medicine, Wichita, Kansas
Vaginal Discharge

VASKAR MUKERJI, M.D.
Professor of Medicine, Division of Cardiology, University of South Alabama School of Medicine, Mobile, Alabama
Chest Pain

BRIAN S. MURPHY, M.D., M.P.H.
Clinical and Research Fellow, Department of General Internal Medicine, Harvard Medical School. Clinical Fellow, Department of General Internal Medicine, Massachusetts General Hospital, Boston, Massachusetts
Paracentesis and Abdominal Diagnostic Tap

VISHWANATHA S. NADIG, M.D.
Resident, Department of Internal Medicine, Foster McGaw Hospital, Loyola University Medical Center, Maywood, Illinois
Pericarditis

LAETH NASIR, M.D.
Assistant Professor, Department of Family Medicine, University of Nebraska Medical Center, Omaha, Nebraska
Impetigo

RICHARD NEILL, M.D.
Director of Graduate Medical Education, Department of Family Practice, University of Kentucky College of Medicine, Lexington, Kentucky
Upper Respiratory Infection

KEVIN R. NELSON, M.D.
Associate Professor of Neurology, and Director, Electromyography Laboratory, University of Kentucky College of Medicine, Lexington, Kentucky
Carpal Tunnel Syndrome and Other Nerve Entrapments

STEPHEN L. NELSON, M.D., M.P.H.
Fellow, Department of Family and Community Medicine, University of Arizona School of Medicine, Tucson, Arizona
Meniere's Disease

GARY NEWKIRK, M.D.
Clinical Professor, Department of Family Medicine, University of Washington School of Medicine, Seattle. Associate Director, Family Medicine Spokane Residency Program, Spokane, Washington
Colposcopy

J. MICHAEL NIEHOFF, M.D.
Associate Director, Department of Family Practice, Franklin Square Hospital Center, Baltimore, Maryland
Casting Techniques

W. ANDERSON NISH, M.D.
Private Allergist-Immunologist, Allergy and Asthma Clinic of Northeast Georgia, Gainesville, Georgia
Food Allergy

TOM E. NORRIS, M.D.
Assistant Dean, Regional Affairs and Rural Health, and Associate Professor of Family Medicine, University of Washington School of Medicine, Seattle, Washington
Diagnostic Upper GI Endoscopy

ANDREW J. NORTON, M.D.
Assistant Professor, Department of General Internal Medicine, Medical College of Wisconsin, Milwaukee, Wisconsin
Cushing's Syndrome/Disease

JIM NUOVO, M.D.
Residency Director, Department of Family Practice, University of California, Davis, School of Medicine, Sacramento, California
Cervical Cancer

FRANCIS G. O'CONNOR, M.D.
Director, Primary Care Sports Medicine, and Assistant Clinical Professor, Family Medicine, Uniformed Services University of the Health Sciences, Bethesda, Maryland. Director, Primary Care Sports Medicine, Fort Belvoir, Virginia
Elbow Pain

JOSEPH O'GORMAN, D.O.
Internal Medicine Resident, Department of the Air Force, Keesler Air Force Base, Mississippi
Kidney Cancer

JOHN G. O'HANDLEY, M.D.
Clinical Assistant Professor of Family Medicine, Ohio State College of Medicine, Columbus. Program Director, Mount Carmel Family Practice Residency, Columbus, Ohio
Acute Otitis Media; Excision of Thrombosed Hemorrhoid

ELLEN M. OKUN, M.D., M.P.H.
Internist, Division of General Internal Medicine, Sinai Hospital of Baltimore, Baltimore, Maryland
Psoriasis

CHERI L. OLSON, M.D.
Instructor, Mayo Graduate School of Medicine. Associate Director, St. Francis–Mayo Family Practice Residency, LaCrosse, Wisconsin
Dysuria

CHERYL A. ONCKEN, M.D., M.P.H.
Assistant Professor, University of Connecticut Health Center, Farmington, Connecticut
Osteoporosis

DONALD A. OPILA, M.D.
Assistant Professor of Clinical Medicine, University of Arizona School of Medicine, Tucson. Associate Program Director, Ambulatory Services, St. Joseph's Hospital and Medical Center, Phoenix, Arizona
Gallstones and Cholecystitis

JAMES T. PACALA, M.D., M.S.
Assistant Professor, Program in Geriatrics, Department of Family Practice and Community Health, University of Minnesota School of Medicine. Staff Physician, University of Minnesota Hospital and Clinics, Minneapolis, Minnesota
Falls in the Elderly

KRISHNAN PADMANABHAN, M.D.
Assistant Professor of Clinical Medicine, State University of New York Health Science Center at Brooklyn. Associate Director, Department of Pulmonary Medicine, Coney Island Hospital, Brooklyn, New York
Atelectasis

DAVID M. PARISER, M.D.
Professor and Chief, Division of Dermatology, Eastern Virginia Medical School. Chief, Department of Dermatology, Sentara Hospitals, Norfolk, Virginia
Hyperhidrosis

MARK A. PARKULO, M.D.
Instructor, Mayo Medical School. Senior Associate Consultant, Mayo Clinic, Rochester, Minnesota
Varicose Veins; Sclerotherapy of Varicose Veins

RAY PASTORINO, Ph.D., J.D.
Behavioral Scientist, Department of Family Medicine, Idaho State University, Pocatello, Idaho
Marital Discord

SANDESH R. PATIL, M.D.
Assistant Professor, Texas Tech University School of Medicine and Health Sciences Center, Amarillo, Texas
Bone Pain and Swelling

STEPHEN PAUL, M.D.
Clinical Instructor, Emergency Department, University Medical Center. Clinical Staff, Student Health Service, University of Arizona, Tucson, Arizona
Dysmenorrhea

DOUGLAS J. PEARCE, M.D.
Assistant Professor, Department of Medicine, University of Alabama at Birmingham School of Medicine. Director, Coronary Care Unit, and Co-Director, Chest Pain Evaluation Unit, University Hospital, Birmingham, Alabama
Acute Myocardial Infarction

CYNTHIA M. PEARMAN, M.D.
Clinical Assistant Professor, University of North Carolina at Chapel Hill. Faculty, Moses H. Cone Family Practice Residency Program, Greensboro, North Carolina
Scabies

THOMAS R. PELLEGRINO, M.D.
Professor of Neurology, Eastern Virginia Medical School. Staff Neurologist, Sentara Norfolk General Hospital, Norfolk, Virginia
Tremor

ROBERT MICHAEL PEPPER, D.O.
Assistant Professor, Department of Family and Community Medicine, University of Alabama–Birmingham School of Medicine, Birmingham, Alabama
Dizziness

JOHN L. PFENNINGER, M.D.
Director, National Procedures Institute, Midland; Clinical Professor of Family Medicine, Michigan State University School of Medicine, East Lansing, Michigan
Laceration Repair

GREGORY L. PHELPS, M.D., M.P.H.
Associate Professor, Family and Community Medicine, Mercer University School of Medicine. Medical Director, Occupational Health Center, Medical Center of Central Georgia, Macon, Georgia
Pulmonary Function Testing

LISA J. PIERCE, M.D.
Assistant Professor of Clinical Family Medicine, University of Missouri, Columbia, School of Medicine, Columbia, Missouri
Endometriosis

PIERRE PINCETL, M.D.
Assistant Professor of Medicine and Computer Medicine, George Washington University Medical School. Assistant Vice President for Information Technology and Chief Information Officer, George Washington University Medical Center, Washington, D.C.
Colorectal Cancer

ANDY PINSON, M.D.
Assistant Professor of Internal Medicine, Medical College of Virginia. Assistant Professor of Internal Medicine, Medical College of Virginia Hospital, Richmond, Virginia
Pyelonephritis

C.S. PITCHUMONI, M.D., M.P.H.
Professor of Medicine and Community and Preventive Medicine, New York Medical College, Valhalla. Director of Medicine and Chief of Gastroenterology, Our Lady of Mercy Medical Center, Bronx, New York
Pancreatitis

J. STEVEN POCETA, M.D.
Staff Physician, Divisions of Neurology and Sleep Disorders, Scripps Clinic and Research Foundation, La Jolla, California
Sleep Disorders

MARTIN H. POLESKI, M.D.
Associate Clinical Professor, University of California, San Diego, School of Medicine. Member, Scripps Clinic Medical Group, Scripps Clinic and Research Foundation, La Jolla, California
Pancreatic Carcinoma

JOHN B. POPE, M.D.
Assistant Professor of Family Medicine, Louisiana State University Medical Center, Shreveport, Louisiana
Nausea and Vomiting; Gastritis

THOMAS P. POWER, M.B.
Fellow in Cardiovascular Diseases, Allegheny General Hospital, Pittsburgh, Pennsylvania
Aortic Dissection

JANET L. PURKEY, M.D.
Assistant Professor, Department of Medicine, and Assistant Director, Ambulatory Resident Clinic, University of Tennessee School of Medicine. Section Chief, General Internal Medicine, University of Tennessee Memorial Hospital, Knoxville, Tennessee
Hoarseness; Calluses and Corns

RIFFAT QADIR, M.D.
Assistant Professor of Otolaryngology, Department of Surgery, University of Kentucky Chandler Medical Center, Lexington, Kentucky
Cheilitis and Angular Cheilitis

DAVID P. RAKEL, M.D.
Medical Staff, Teton Valley Hospital, Driggs, Idaho
Controlling Epistaxis

ROBERT E. RAKEL, M.D.
Richard M. Kleberg Senior Professor and Chairman, Department of Family Medicine, and Associate Dean for Academic and Clinical Affairs, Baylor College of Medicine. Attending Physician, St. Luke's Episcopal Hospital and The Methodist Hospital, Houston, Texas
Circumcision: Plastibell

TIMOTHY RAMER, M.D.
Associate Professor, Department of Family Practice and Community Health, University of Minnesota Medical School. Family Practice Medical Staff, Fairview Riverside Medical Center, Minneapolis, Minnesota
Circumcision: Gomco

ERIC D. RASMUSSEN, M.D.
Director, House Staff Education, Department of Medicine, Navy Medical Center, Oakland. Assistant Clinical Professor of Medicine, Department of Medicine, University of California San Francisco School of Medicine, San Francisco. Director, Inpatient Medical Services, Department of Medicine, and Director, House Staff Education, Department of Medicine, Navy Medical Center, Oakland, California
Arterial Puncture; Intracostal Anesthesia

NORMAN H. RASMUSSEN, Ed.D.
Assistant Professor, Mayo Medical School. Consultant, Division of Psychology and Department of Psychiatry and Psychology, Mayo Clinic, Rochester, Minnesota
Obsessive Compulsive Disorder

ROSE A. RECCO, M.D.
Assistant Professor of Medicine, State University of New York Health Science Center, Brooklyn. Director, Department of Infectious Diseases, Coney Island Hospital, Brooklyn, New York
Nongonococcal Urethritis

MANTHANI J. REDDY, M.D., M.P.H.
Senior Physician, Department of Family Practice, Cook County Hospital. Medical Director, Jorge Prieto Health Center, Chicago, Illinois
Headache

VINCENT A. RELLA, M.D.
Chief Resident, Ambulatory Medical Clinic and Danbury Hospital, and Hematology-Oncology Fellow, Columbia Presbyterian Hospital and State University of New York Health Sciences Center, Syracuse, New York
Hemolytic Anemia

ROXANNA RHODES, M.D.
Austin, Texas
Hepatitis

PHILLIP K. RHYNE, M.D.
Assistant Professor of Community Science, Mercer University School of Medicine, Macon, Georgia
Abdominal Pain

MARC RINGEL, M.D.
Private Practice Physician and Consultant, Telemedicine and Continuing Medical Education, Holyoke, Colorado
Enuresis

VIRGINIA E. ROBERTSON, M.D.
Clinical Assistant Professor, Department of Family Practice, State University of New York Health Science Center at Brooklyn. Predoctoral Coordinator and Assistant Attending Physician, Department of Family Practice, Long Island College Hospital, Brooklyn, New York
Varicella Infections; Warts and Nevi

AMY L. ROBINSON, M.D.
Community Preceptor for Family Practice Students, University of New Mexico Family Practice Clerkship, Albuquerque. Medical Staff, Acoma-Canoncito-Laguna Hospital, San Fidel, New Mexico
Vomiting and Diarrhea

JOHN DAVID ROGERS, M.D.
Cardiology Fellow, Scripps Clinic and Research Foundation, La Jolla, California
Swan-Ganz Monitoring

CECILIA M. ROMERO, M.D.
Associate Professor, Department of Family Medicine, and Director, Predoctoral Education, University of Texas Medical Branch. Attending Physician, John Sealy Hospital and St. Mary's Hospital, Galveston, Texas
Diaphragm Fitting

JAMES K. RONE, M.D.
Clinical Assistant Professor, University of South Alabama School of Medicine, Mobile, Alabama. Chief, Endocrinology Service, Keesler Medical Center, Keesler Air Force Base, Mississippi
Adrenal Insufficiency

J. GREGORY ROSENCRANCE, M.D.
Associate Professor of Medicine, Robert C. Byrd Health Sciences Center of West Virginia University Charleston Division. Medical Director, West Virginia Poison Center, Robert C. Byrd Health Sciences Center of West Virginia University, Charleston, West Virginia
Poisonings

JO ANN ROSENFELD, M.D.
Associate Professor of Family Medicine, Bristol Family Practice Residency Program, East Tennessee State University Quillen College of Medicine, Bristol, Tennessee
Episiotomy and Vaginal Laceration Repair

JOSEPH E. ROWANE, D.O.
Clinical Associate Staff, Cleveland Clinic Foundation, Cleveland, Ohio
Hemoptysis

MICHAEL P. ROWANE, D.O.
Assistant Professor, Department of Medicine, Case Western Reserve University School of Medicine. Residency Faculty, University Hospitals of Cleveland, Cleveland, Ohio
Bronchiolitis; Endometritis

AARON RUBIN, M.D.
Director, Kaiser Permanente/S.P.O.R.T. Sports Medicine Fellowship, and Academic Faculty, Family Medicine Residency, Kaiser Permanente Medical Center, Fontana, California
Epicondylitis; Head Injuries in Sports

TERRY S. RUHL, M.D.
Assistant Clinical Professor, Michigan State University College of Human Medicine, East Lansing. Associate Director, Mid-Michigan Regional Medical Center Family Practice Residency Program, Midland, Michigan
Itching

SHELLIE A. RUSSELL, M.D.
Assistant Professor, Department of Family Practice and Community Medicine and Assistant Professor, Department of Pediatrics, University of Texas Health Science Center. Attending Physician, Memorial Southwest Hospital, Houston, Texas
Fetal Lung Immaturity; Bladder Tap

JERRY RYAN, M.D.
Assistant Professor, Department of Family Medicine, and Medical Director, Physician Assistant Program, University of Wisconsin at Madison School of Medicine, Madison, Wisconsin
Shoulder Pain

CONSTANTINE SAADEH, M.D.
Associate Professor and Regional Chairman, Department of Internal Medicine, Texas Tech University Health Sciences Center. Chief of Rheumatology, Allergy, and Immunology and Staff Physician, Department of Veterans Affairs Medical Center and Northwest Texas Hospital, Amarillo, Texas
Urticaria and Angioedema

STEPHEN D. SAGLIO, M.D.
Assistant Clinical Professor, University of California, San Francisco, School of Medicine, San Francisco. Faculty Physician, Family Practice Residency, Natividad Medical Center, Salinas, California
Pityriasis Rosea

WILLIAM R. SCHEIBEL, M.D.
Professor of Family Medicine, University of Wisconsin School of Medicine, Madison, Wisconsin
Infectious Mononucleosis

DAWN SCHISSEL, M.D.
Associate Professor, University of Iowa School of Medicine, Iowa City. Faculty Physician, Broadlawns Medical Center, Des Moines, Iowa
Meningitis

MICHAEL SCHOOFF, M.D.
Associate Clinical Professor, Uniformed Services University of the Health Sciences, Bethesda, Maryland. Staff Family Physician, Womack Army Medical Center, Fort Bragg, North Carolina
Intussusception

E. ROBERT SCHWARTZ, M.D.
Associate Professor and Chair, Department of Family Medicine, School of Medicine, State University of New York, Stonybrook. Chief of Service, Department of Family Medicine, University Medical Center, Stony Brook, New York
Varicocele

ROBERT J. SCHWARTZMAN, M.D.
Professor and Chairman and Director, Residency Training Program, Department of Neurology, Jefferson Medical College. Active Medical Staff, Thomas Jefferson University Hospital, Philadelphia, Pennsylvania
Reflex Sympathetic Dystrophy

JOSEPH B. SELBY, M.D.
Assistant Professor and Director of Behavioral Medicine, Department of Family Medicine, West Virginia University School of Medicine. Resident, Department of Psychiatry, West Virginia University School of Medicine, Family Practice Center, Morgantown, West Virginia
Panic Disorder

ANIL SHAH, M.B.B.S.
Clinical Instructor in Medicine, Tufts University School of Medicine. Chief Medical Resident, Department of Medicine, Faulkner Hospital, Boston, Massachusetts
Aortic Valve Disease

CYNTHIA L. SHORT, M.D.
Assistant Professor of Medicine, Dartmouth Medical School. Assistant Professor of Medicine, Dartmouth-Hitchcock Medical Center, Lebanon, New Hampshire
Acute Renal Failure

GARY J. SILKO, M.D.
Adjunct Assistant Professor of Medicine, Medical College of Pennsylvania, Philadelphia. Assistant Professor, Department of Family and Community Medicine, Pennsylvania State University College of Medicine, Hershey. Assistant Director, Family Practice Residency, The Washington Hospital, Washington, Pennsylvania
Otitis Externa

DANIELLE R. SINK, M.D.
Instructor of Clinical Medicine, University of Arizona College of Medicine, Tucson. Director of Medical Student Education and Coordinator of House Staff Affairs, Internal Medicine Residency Program, St. Joseph's Hospital and Medical Center, Phoenix, Arizona
Chronic Cough

NINA SKATTUM, M.D.
Assistant Clinical Professor, Department of Family Practice, University of California Davis. Staff Physician, Truckee Tahoe Medical Group and Tahoe Forest Hospital, Truckee, California
Elbow Dislocations

W. MICHAEL SKEENS, M.D.
Associate Professor of Medicine, Marshall University School of Medicine, Huntington, West Virginia
Flashing Lights and Floaters; Optic Neuritis

ARTHUR R. SLAUGHTER, M.D.
Associate Professor of Family Medicine, University of Virginia School of Medicine, Charlottesville. Associate Director of Family Medical Education, Carilion Health System, Roanoke Memorial Hospitals, Roanoke, Virginia
Herpes Simplex Infection; Herpes Zoster Infection

JOHN T. SLEVIN, M.D.
Professor, Departments of Neurology and Pharmacology, University of Kentucky College of Medicine. Staff Neurologist, Veterans Administration Medical Center, Lexington, Kentucky
Parkinson's Disease

DAVID L. SMITH, M.D.
Assistant Professor of Medicine and Pediatrics, Division of Allergy and Immunology, University of Southern Alabama School of Medicine, Mobile, Alabama
Drug Allergy

LAWRENCE G. SMITH, M.D.
Vice Chairman of Medicine, Mount Sinai School of Medicine of the City of New York. Attending Physician, Mount Sinai Hospital, New York, New York
Weight Loss; Obesity

GREGORY T. SOLTNER, D.O.
Private Practice Physician; Staff Physician, Abington Memorial Hospital, Abington; Chestnut Hill Hospital, Philadelphia, Pennsylvania
Miliaria

JOHN G. SPANGLER, M.D., M.P.H.
Assistant Professor, Department of Family and Community Medicine, Bowman Gray School of Medicine of Wake Forest University, Winston-Salem, North Carolina
Influenza; Leukoplakia and Erythroplasia

MICHAEL L. SPARACINO, D.O.
Clinical Assistant Professor, St. Louis University School of Medicine. Director, Obstetrical Fellowship Program, Deaconess Health System, St. Louis, Missouri
Induction of Labor

JOHN P. SPECK, M.D.
Director of Acute Dialysis, William Beaumont Hospital, Royal Oak, Michigan
Hyperkalemia

ANDERSON SPICKARD, III, M.D.
Assistant Professor, Vanderbilt University School of Medicine, Nashville Division of General Internal Medicine, Vanderbilt Medical Center, Nashville, Tennessee
Pheochromocytoma

DEBORAH SPRING, M.D.
Clinical Assistant Professor of Family Medicine, Pennsylvania State University College of Medicine, Hershey. Instructor of Family Medicine, Wyoming Valley Family Practice Residency Program, Kingston, Pennsylvania
IUD Insertion and Removal

FERNANDO F. STANCAMPIANO, M.D.
Staff Physician, Department of Internal Medicine, Cleveland Clinic Florida, Fort Lauderdale, Florida
Claudication

JOHN B. STANDRIDGE, M.D.
Family Physician, Private Practice, Mountain Family Medicine, Signal Mountain, Tennessee
Growth and Development Guidelines

J. STEPHAN STAPCZYNSKI, M.D.
Associate Professor and Chair, Department of Emergency Medicine, University of Kentucky College of Medicine. Medical Director, Emergency Department, University of Kentucky Hospital, Lexington, Kentucky
Fever and Chills

EVAN STEINBERG, M.D.
Assistant Professor, Department of Medicine, Mount Sinai School of Medicine of the City of New York, New York. Assistant Attending Physician, Department of Medicine, Elmhurst Hospital Center, Elmhurst, New York
Acute Respiratory Distress Syndrome

JAMES A. STERLING, D.O.
Assistant Professor, Department of Family Medicine, Texas A&M University College of Medicine, College Station. Senior Staff Physician, Scott and White Memorial Hospital, Temple, Texas
Histoplasmosis

TIMOTHY R. STERLING, M.D.
Staff Internist, Keesler Medical Center, Keesler Air Force Base, Mississippi
Amebiasis

MICHAEL B. STEVENS, M.D.
Associate Professor, Division of Family and Community Medicine, Department of Medicine, Stanford University School of Medicine, Palo Alto. Associate Director, Family Practice Residency Program, San Jose Medical Center, San Jose, California
Migraine Headache

TOD STILLSON, M.D.
Faculty, Family Practice Residency, Carilion Health Systems–Roanoke Memorial Hospital, Roanoke, Virginia
Ectopic Pregnancy

ERIC B. STONE, M.D.
Chief of Family Practice, Lajes Field, Azores, Portugal
Starting an Intravenous Infusion: Adult and Infant

MARIAN R. STUART, Ph.D.
Clinical Professor of Family Medicine, University of Medicine and Dentistry of New Jersey, New Brunswick, New Jersey
The BATHE Technique

FRED M. SUTTON, M.D.
Associate Professor of Medicine, Baylor College of Medicine. Chief of Gastroenterology, Ben Taub General Hospital, Houston, Texas
Irritable Bowel Syndrome

JAMES E. SVENSON, M.D., M.Sc.
Assistant Professor, Department of Emergency Medicine, University of Kentucky College of Medicine, Lexington, Kentucky
Fever of Unknown Origin

GEOFFREY R. SWAIN, B.S., M.D.
Assistant Professor, Department of Family and Community Medicine, Medical College of Wisconsin. Director of Clinics, City of Milwaukee Health Department, Milwaukee, Wisconsin
Hyperprolactinemia

TONY SWALDI, M.D.
Clinical Faculty, University of Texas Southwestern Medical School, Dallas, Texas
Fungal Infections

CARLOS M. SWANGER, M.D.
General Internist, Rochester Park Medical Group and Park Ridge Hospital, Rochester, New York
Scleroderma (Systemic Sclerosis)

STEVEN K. SWEDLUND, M.D.
Associate Clinical Professor, Wright State University School of Medicine. Associate Director, Miami Valley Hospital Family Practice Residency Program, and Associate Director, Family Health Center, Miami Valley Hospital, Dayton, Ohio
Acute Urinary Tract Infection in Adults

JOHN W. SWISHER, M.D., Ph.D.
Instructor in Medicine, Pennsylvania State University College of Medicine, Hershey, Pennsylvania
Pneumonia

DAVID J. TANAKA, M.D.
Assistant Professor, Division of Internal Medicine, Department of Medicine, University of Colorado School of Medicine, University of Colorado Health Science Center, Denver, Colorado
Deep Venous Thrombosis

EROL TAŞDEMİROĞLU, M.D.
Attending Neurosurgeon, İncirli Hospital, Neurosurgery Service, İstanbul, Turkey
Subdural Hematoma

NANCY O. TATUM, M.D.
Assistant Professor and Attending Physician, Department of Family Medicine, University of Mississippi Medical Center, Jackson, Mississippi
Asymptomatic HIV Infection

NADER TAVAKOLI, M.D.
Clinical Assistant Professor of Family Practice, Georgetown University School of Medicine, Washington, D.C. Clinical Director of Family Practice Residency Program, Prince George's Hospital, Cheverly, Maryland
Pap Smear

HARRIS C. TAYLOR, M.D.
Clinical Associate Professor of Medicine (Endocrinology), Case Western Reserve University School of Medicine. Chief, Division of Endocrinology, and Director, Endocrine–Radioimmunoassay Laboratory, Health Cleveland Lutheran Medical Center, Cleveland, Ohio
Hypoglycemia

ROSLYN D. TAYLOR, M.D.
Associate Professor of Family and Community Medicine, Mercer University School of Medicine, Macon. Associate Director, Family Practice Residency, Memorial Medical Center, Savannah, Georgia
Low Back Pain Exercises

KENNETH L. TAYLOR-BUTLER, M.D.
Faculty Physician, Trinity Family Medicine Center, Trinity Family Practice Residency, Kansas City, Missouri
Finger Fractures

MICHAEL TEMPORAL, M.D.
Assistant Professor of Community and Family Medicine, University of Missouri School of Medicine. Staff Physician, Truman Medical Center East, Kansas City, Missouri
Diseases of the Nails

JONATHAN L. TEMTE, M.D., Ph.D.
Assistant Professor, Department of Family Medicine, University of Wisconsin Medical School, Madison, Wisconsin
Abdominal Pain

ANSON L. THAGGARD, M.D.
Family Physician, Methodist Medical Clinic of Central Mississippi, Kosciusko, Mississippi
Common Protozoal Disease Symptoms

JOANNA M. THOMAS, M.B., Ch.B.
Assistant Professor, Department of Family and Community Medicine, University of Arkansas for Medical Sciences. Faculty, Northwest Arkansas Family Practice Residency, Fayetteville, Arkansas
Norplant Insertion and Removal

STEVEN THOMPSON, M.D.
Assistant Clinical Professor of Medicine, University of California, San Francisco/Fresno–Central San Joaquin Valley Medical Education Program. Member, Division of General Internal Medicine, Valley Medical Center, Fresno, California
Hypernatremia; Hyponatremia

WARREN G. THOMPSON, M.D.
Associate Professor, Department of Internal Medicine, University of Tennessee, Knoxville, College of Medicine, Knoxville. Program Director, Internal Medicine Residency, University of Tennessee Medical Center, Knoxville, Tennessee
Alcoholism

G. ALLEN TINDOL, Jr. M.D.
Clinical Instructor, Department of Medicine, Section of General Internal Medicine, Medical College of Georgia, Augusta. Associate Director, Department of Internal Medicine Education, Memorial Medical Center, Savannah, Georgia
Sarcoidosis

SHIRLENE TOLBERT, M.D., M.P.H.
Clinical Professor, University of Pittsburgh School of Medicine. Director, Community Medicine/Community Oriented Primary Care, St. Margaret's Memorial Hospital, Pittsburgh, Pennsylvania
Glaucoma

DAVID E. TRACHTENBARG, M.D.
Clinical Associate Professor, University of Illinois College of Medicine at Peoria. Associate Director of Family Practice, Methodist Medical Center, Peoria, Illinois
Stasis Ulcer

LARAMIE C. TRIPLETT, M.D.
Assistant Professor, Department of Family Medicine, and Assistant Director, Residency Division, Department of Family Medicine, University of Mississippi Medical Center, Jackson, Mississippi
Heat Exhaustion and Stroke

JOSEPH A. TRONCALE, M.D.
Director, Research and Faculty Development, Lancaster General Hospital, Lancaster, Pennsylvania
Asthma

HOWARD TUNG, M.D.
Staff Neurosurgeon, Scripps Clinic and Research Foundation, La Jolla, California
Trigeminal Neuralgia

JAVIER J. URDANETA, M.D.
Third-Year Family Practice Resident, Union Hospital, Terre Haute, Indiana
Nasal Fracture Reduction

JOSEPH VALENTINO, M.D.
Assistant Professor of Otolaryngology, Department of Surgery, University of Kentucky Chandler Medical Center, Lexington, Kentucky
Epistaxis; Cricothyrotomy/Tracheostomy

CAREY VINSON, M.D., M.P.M.
Clinical Assistant Professor of Clinical Epidemiology and Family Medicine, University of Pittsburgh School of Medicine. Director for Clinical Utilization. Faculty, Family Practice Residency Program, Forbes Health System, Pittsburgh, Pennsylvania
Vaginitis; Cervicitis

ROBERT P. VOGT, M.D.
Clinical Assistant Professor, Uniformed Services University of the Health Sciences, Bethesda, Maryland. Faculty, Family Practice Residency, Eglin Air Force Base, Florida
Swimmer's Injuries

KIMBERLE J. VORE, M.D.
Adjunct Assistant Professor of Medicine, Medical College of Pennsylvania, Philadelphia. Clinical Instructor, The Washington Hospital, Washington, Pennsylvania
Gestational Hyperglycemia/Diabetes

DIANE S. VOSS, M.D.
Assistant Professor of Medicine and Clinical Director, Red Medicine Clinic, University of Missouri, Kansas City, School of Medicine, Kansas City, Missouri
Fluid Balance

BENNET M. WANG, M.D.
Senior Fellow, Pulmonary and Critical Care Medicine, University of Washington School of Medicine, Seattle, Washington
Laryngitis

LAWRENCE L. WARD, M.D.
Clinical Assistant Professor, Department of Family and Community Medicine, University of Arizona Health Sciences Center, Tucson. Assistant Medical Director, Family Practice Residency, Phoenix Baptist Hospital and Medical Center, Phoenix, Arizona
Rib Fracture

BENJAMIN C. WARF, M.D.
Assistant Professor, Department of Neurosurgery, University of Kentucky College of Medicine. Chief, Section of Pediatric Neurosurgery, University of Kentucky Chandler Medical Center, Lexington, Kentucky
Brain Tumor

PETER WARRINGTON, D.O.
Coordinator of Obstetrics/Gynecology, Wyoming Valley Family Practice Residency. Director, Osteopathic Medical Education, Pennsylvania College of Osteopathic Medicine Rotating Internship, Nesbitt Memorial Hospital, Kingston, Pennsylvania
Third Trimester Bleeding

MICHAEL L. WATERS, M.D.
Family Physician, Baptist Medical Center, Jacksonville, Florida
Red Eye

RONALD S. WATTS, M.D.
Assistant Professor, Uniformed School of University Health Sciences, Bethesda. Chief, Endocrinology Service, 89th Medical Group/Malcolm Grow USAF Medical Center, Andrews Air Force Base, Maryland
Hypothyroidism; Hyperthyroidism

RALPH WEBER, M.D.
Instructor in Cardiovascular Medicine, Johns Hopkins University School of Medicine. Attending Physician, Divisions of Cardiology and General Internal Medicine, Department of Medicine, Sinai Hospital of Baltimore, Baltimore, Maryland
Leg Edema

KENNETH A. WELLER, M.D.
Clinical Instructor of Medicine, University of Chicago Pritzker School of Medicine, Chicago. Assistant Residency Director, Family Practice Residency, Lutheran General Hospital, Park Ridge, Illinois
Impaired Hearing; Bronchitis

MARK WELLS, M.D.
Assistant Professor, Division of Plastic Surgery, University of Kentucky College of Medicine, Lexington, Kentucky
Tattoos

HAROLD V. WERNER, M.D.
Associate Professor and Chief, Division of General Internal Medicine and Section of Endocrinology, Texas Tech Health Sciences

Center School of Medicine. Staff Physician, Northwest Texas Hospital, Amarillo, Texas
Thyroid Nodule; Thyroid Carcinoma

LORI A. WHITTAKER, M.D., Ph.D.
Assistant Professor, Department of Family Medicine, Baylor College of Medicine, Houston, Texas
Cancer Screening; Ovarian Cancer

CYNTHIA M. WILLIAMS, D.O.
Commander, Medical Corps, United States Navy, Naval Hospital, Camp Pendleton, California
Fibrocystic Disease of the Breast

JOHN W. WILLIAMS, Jr., M.D.
Assistant Professor, University of Texas Health Science Center. Director, Continuity of Care Clinic, Audie Murphy Memorial Veterans Hospital, San Antonio, Texas
Sinusitis

SEYMOUR G. WILLIAMS, M.D.
Resident, Department of Family Medicine, Baylor College of Medicine, Houston, Texas
Vulvar Pruritus

SANDRA K. WILLSIE, D.O.
Associate Professor of Medicine and Deputy Assistant Dean, University of Missouri–Kansas City School of Medicine, Kansas City, Missouri
Cancers of the Larynx and Lung

BRUCE E. WILSON, M.D.
Associate Professor and Chief, Division of Endocrinology and Metabolism, University of Nevada School of Medicine, Las Vegas, Nevada
Diabetes Mellitus, Type II

TIMOTHY J. WILT, M.D., M.P.H.
Assistant Professor of Medicine, Section of General Medicine, University of Minnesota Medical School. Staff Physician, Minneapolis Veterans Affairs Medical Center, Minneapolis, Minnesota
Prostate Cancer

ROBERT J. WITYK, M.D.
Assistant Professor of Neurology and Medicine, Johns Hopkins University School of Medicine. Co-Director, Division of Neurology, Sinai Hospital of Baltimore, Baltimore, Maryland
Transient Ischemic Attack

ANDREW M.D. WOLF, M.D.
Assistant Professor, Division of General Medicine, Department of Internal Medicine, University of Virginia School of Medicine, Charlottesville, Virginia
Constipation

IRVING D. WOLFE, M.D.
Department of Dermatology, Johns Hopkins University Hospital, University of Maryland Hospital, and Sinai Hospital of Baltimore, Baltimore, Maryland
Cryosurgery and Electrocautery of Skin Lesions

MICHAEL S. WOLKOMIR, M.D.
Assistant Professor, Department of Family and Community Medicine, Medical College of Wisconsin. Assistant Director, Family Practice Residency Program, and Obstetrics/Gynecology Education Coordinator, St. Michael Hospital, Milwaukee, Wisconsin
Postpartum Hemorrhage

LAURIE J. WOODARD, M.D.
Associate Professor of Family Medicine, University of South Florida School of Medicine. Staff Physician, Tampa General Hospital, Tampa, Florida
Lumbar Puncture

ROBERT M. WOODARD, M.D.
Family Medicine Faculty Development Fellow and Attending Physician, St. Margaret's Memorial Hospital, Pittsburgh, Pennsylvania
Conjunctivitis

JACK R. WOODSIDE, Jr., M.D.
Assistant Professor of Family Medicine, East Tennessee State University Quillen College of Medicine, Johnson City, Tennessee
Local and Regional Anesthesia of the Upper Extremity

ROBERT J. WOOLLEY, M.D.
Physician, Boynton Health Service, University of Minnesota, St. Paul, Minnesota
Contraception

DAVID H. YAWN, M.D.
Professor of Clinical Pathology, Baylor College of Medicine. Director, Transfusion Service, The Methodist Hospital, Houston, Texas
Adverse Reactions to Blood Transfusions

CRAIG C. YOUNG, M.D.
Assistant Professor and Medical Director of Sports Medicine, Departments of Orthopaedic Surgery and Family and Community Medicine, Medical College of Wisconsin, Milwaukee, Wisconsin
Knee Pain

ZOBAIR M. YOUNOSSI, M.D., M.P.H.
Senior Fellow in Gastroenterology/Hepatology, Green Hospital of Scripps Clinic and Research Foundation, La Jolla, California
Acute Upper Gastrointestinal Bleeding

MUHAMMAD K. ZAMAN, M.D.
Assistant Professor of Medicine, University of Tennessee, Memphis College of Medicine. Staff Physician, Veterans Affairs Medical Center, Memphis, Tennessee
Interstitial Lung Disease; Technique of Sputum Induction

EDWARD M. ZIMMERMAN, M.D.
Clinical Assistant Professor Department of Family and Community Medicine, Pennsylvania State University College of Medicine, Hershey. Associate Faculty, Family Practice Residency, Beaver, Pennsylvania
Purpura

THOMAS J. ZUBER, M.D.
Assistant Clinical Professor, Michigan State University School of Medicine, East Lansing. Associate Physician, Midland Family Physicians, Midland, Michigan
Wound Management; Wound Revision

CHARLES I. ZUCKER, M.D.
Associate Director, North Colorado Family Medicine, North Colorado Medical Center, Greeley, Colorado
Head, Pubic, and Body Lice

Foreword

Knowledge is of two kinds. We know a subject ourselves, or we know where we can find information upon it.

Samuel Johnson, 1775

James Boswell's quote from the *Life of Johnson* is appropriate for the world's first great lexicographer. Samuel Johnson was the first person to use illustrative historical quotations and his *Dictionary,* published in 1755, is a milestone of the English language. In the creation of his *Dictionary,* Johnson knew that the educated 18th century man or woman needed a dependable reference source.

Today, the educated physician also needs a dependable reference source. *Saunders Manual of Medical Practice* offers that source with a thoroughness and clarity that is admirable.

Dr. Johnson's method of organizing his *Dictionary* was preordained—he simply depended on the English alphabet. However, the *Saunders Manual* editors were faced with a more daunting task. They had to develop a system of organizing medical knowledge so that it became readily accessible to the diligent primary care physician as well as the overwhelmed medical student. The organization had to be as easy to use—and as dependable—as looking up the word "lung" under "L."

The editors chose to organize *Saunders Manual of Medical Practice* into 20 organ system sections. The outline format within each organ system allows for instant recognition of symptoms, laboratory tests needed, treatment, and other basic relevant medical information. While allowing for a quick look-see when appropriate, each section also contains more than enough information for extensive study, including reference follow-ups for additional information.

Dr. Johnson's *Dictionary* became famous because the author took the extra step in explaining the English language. Similarly, *Saunders Manual of Medical Practice* also takes an extra step to distinguish it from other manuals. There are 58 procedures interspersed in the text. They are highly illustrated to give physicians the opportunity to quickly review procedures which they may not have the need to do every day yet are necessarily part of the lexicon of the primary care physician.

Samuel Johnson's *Dictionary of the English Language* was not the first dictionary, the only dictionary, or even the largest dictionary of his day. Yet, it survives as one of the most famous dictionaries of all time because of its energy and illustrative language and ambition to explain words in the most precise way possible.

Similarly, *Saunders Manual of Medical Practice* is not the only medical manual available to the primary care physician or medical student. However, I believe that its ambition, scope, and organization make it an outstanding volume that will soon be the standard text in every physician's office. With *Saunders Manual,* today's physician or medical student can be comfortable with Dr. Johnson's quote—"If you don't know the answer, you'll know where to find it."

ROGER C. BONE, M.D.

Preface

This book is designed to help the busy primary care physician by providing, in a concise format, information regarding diagnosis and treatment of problems most frequently encountered in practice. Also included are those problems that may not be common but, if missed or not handled properly, can lead to considerable morbidity or death. Material is presented in outline format for ease of retrieval, and key points are highlighted and boxed to aid in identifying essential information rapidly. This is becoming increasingly important as managed care programs place added emphasis on seeing a volume of patients in limited time, making it even more essential that potentially serious problems be identified in their early, undifferentiated stage when the proper selection of tests is crucial.

There are 451 topics: 318 chapters on disease, 75 symptoms (combined into 17 numbered chapters), 58 procedures, and an appendix of normal laboratory values. Most of the 414 authors are family physicians or general internists. The two-color format enhances the key material, making it more visible and easier to access rapidly.

Diseases are usually presented in the following format: etiology, symptoms, clinical findings, laboratory tests, differential diagnosis, treatment (including medications, patient education, and prevention), and follow-up.

Symptoms are presented with the emphasis on differential diagnosis followed by key questions to ask (history), clinical findings, tests, management, and follow-up. The symptoms focus on complaints in cases in which the diagnosis may not yet be evident and on the management of the problem while the diagnostic process is continuing.

The procedures are organized by indications, contraindications, preparation, equipment needed, anesthesia, precautions, technique, and follow-up. The illustrations are by Jan Redden, an artist at Baylor College of Medicine. Using a single artist for all illustrations ensured quality, consistency, and freshness, since all illustrations of procedures are original. The procedures are of greatest value to physicians in training, those recently entering practice, and experienced physicians who wish to keep abreast of recent developments such as the no-scalpel technique for vasectomy.

Each chapter includes approximately five recent or classic references for those who desire additional information. Many tables are included to provide a maximum of information in a concise and rapidly retrievable format. Dirk Lucas, Pharm.D., reviewed all drug dosages for accuracy; nevertheless, please check the drug package insert for the manufacturer's recommended dosage.

Although most chapters discuss traditional subjects, many unusual topics are included, such as metastatic cancer of unknown origin, oncologic emergencies, the technique of sputum induction, cryosurgery and electrocautery, deep muscle relaxation exercises, aquatic injuries, colposcopy, removal of impacted cerumen, sleep apnea, bulimia, costochondritis, chronic fatigue syndrome, reflex sympathetic dystrophy, and when to use CT versus MRI. Also included are useful reference chapters such as immunization schedules, health maintenance charts, growth and development guidelines, cancer screening, and the use of advance directives.

On the inside front cover of the book is an alphabetical index of the procedures presented in *Saunders Manual of Medical Practice,* with appropriate page numbers added for quick reference. Also on the inside front cover, and continuing on the inside back cover, are alphabetical lists of diseases and ICD-9CM codes and procedures and CPT-4 codes for billing purposes.

I wish to thank the staff at the W.B. Saunders Company, especially Darlene Pedersen, former Senior Vice President and Editorial Director, and Leslie E. Hoeltzel, Manager, Developmental Editorial, for their expert help in creating this book and for maintaining their usual standards of quality. Ms. Christine Cantera was responsible for the actual design of the book. My greatest appreciation goes to my editorial assistant, Jeanne Ullian, whose excellent organizational skills made it possible to produce such a complicated book on schedule.

ROBERT E. RAKEL, M.D.

Contents

Detailed table of contents begins on following right hand page

Part IV Cardiovascular Diseases

Part XV   Infectious Diseases

Saunders
Manual
of Medical
Practice

1 Immunization Schedules

Rick Kellerman

Diphtheria, Tetanus, Pertussis (DTP, DTaP, DT, dT, DTP-HbCV)

General Information

1. DTP
   a. Combination vaccine with diphtheria and tetanus toxoids and whole-cell pertussis
   b. Administered at ages 2, 4, and 6 months (Table 1–1)
   c. May administer at ages 12 to 15 months and 4 to 6 years (DTaP preferred)
   d. Dose 5 is unnecessary if dose 4 is administered after age 4 years.
   e. Antipyretics are indicated before administration.
2. DTaP
   a. Pertussis component is acellular.
   b. Lower incidence of fever, local reactions, and systemic symptoms than with DTP

   c. Administered at ages 15 months and 4 to 6 years if the child has had three DTP doses
   d. Antipyretics are indicated before administration.
   e. Future updated immunization schedules may allow DTaP for the first, second, and third doses.
3. DT
   Substitute for DTP and DTaP if the pertussis component is contraindicated in a child under age 7 years.
4. dT
   a. Adolescent booster is given at age 11 to 16 years.
   b. Adult booster is given every 10 years after the adolescent booster.
   c. Primary series in unimmunized adults and children older than age 6 years: 0, 4 to 8 weeks, 6 to 12 months
   d. All primary series doses after age 6 years should be dT.

TABLE 1–1. RECOMMENDED CHILDHOOD IMMUNIZATION SCHEDULE, UNITED STATES—JANUARY 1995

AGE ▶ VACCINE ▼	BIRTH	2 MOS	4 MOS	6 MOS	12 MOS[5]	15 MOS	18 MOS	4–6 YRS	11–12 YRS	14–16 YRS
Hepatitis B[1]	HB-1									
		HB-2		HB-3						
Diphtheria, tetanus, pertussis[2]		DTP	DTP	DTP	DTP or DTaP at 15 + m			DTP or DTaP	dT	
H. influenzae type b[3]		Hib	Hib	Hib	Hib					
Polio		OPV	OPV	OPV				OPV		
Measles, mumps, rubella[4]					MMR			MMR	or MMR	

Vaccines are listed under the routinely recommended ages. Bars indicate range of acceptable ages for vaccination.

[1]Infants born to HBsAg-negative mothers should receive the second dose of hepatitis B vaccine between 1 and 4 months of age, provided at least one month has elapsed since receipt of the first dose. The third dose is recommended between 6 and 18 months of age.

Infants born to HBsAg-positive mothers should receive immunoprophylaxis for hepatitis B with 0.5 ml hepatitis B immune globulin (HBIG) within 12 hours of birth, and 0.5 ml of either Merck Sharpe & Dohme vaccine (Recombivax HB) or of SmithKline Beecham vaccine (Engerix-B) at a separate site. In these infants, the second dose of vaccine is recommended at 1 month of age and the third dose at 6 months of age. All pregnant women should be screened for HBsAg in an early prenatal visit.

[2]The fourth dose of DTP may be administered as early as 12 months of age, provided at least 6 months have elapsed since DTP3. Combined DTP-Hib products may be used when these two vaccines are to be administered simultaneously. DTaP (diphtheria and tetanus toxoids and acellular pertussis vaccine) is licensed for use for the 4th and/or 5th dose of DTP vaccine in children 15 months of age or older and may be preferred for these doses in children in this age group. Td (diphtheria and tetanus toxoids for persons ≥7 years of age) is recommended at 11–12 years of age, provided at least 5 years have elapsed since the last dose of DTP or DT.

[3]Three H. influenzae type b conjugate vaccines are available for use in infants: HbOC [HibTITER] (Lederle Praxis); PRP-T [ActHIB; OmniHIB] (Pasteur Mérieux, distributed by SmithKline Beecham; Connaught); and PRP-OMP [PedvaxHIB] (Merck Sharpe & Dohme). Children who have received PRP-OMP at 2 and 4 months of age do not require a dose at 6 months of age. After the primary infant Hib conjugate vaccine series is completed, any licensed Hib conjugate vaccine may be used as a booster dose at age 12–15 months.

[4]The second dose of MMR vaccine should be administered EITHER at 4–6 years of age OR at 11–12 years of age, depending upon state school requirements.

[5]Vaccines recommended in the second year of life (12–15 months of age) may be given at either one or two visits.

Approved by the Advisory Committee on Immunization Practices (ACIP), the American Academy of Pediatrics (AAP), and the American Academy of Family Physicians (AAFP)

5. DTP-*Haemophilus influenzae* type b conjugate vaccines (HbCV)

   a. TETRAMUNE allows simultaneous immunization against diphtheria, tetanus, pertussis, and *Haemophilus influenzae* type b. Use same schedule as for DTP and HibTITER (ages 2, 4, 6, and 12 to 15 months).

   b. ActHIB and OmniHIB may be reconstituted with Connaught DTP for simultaneous immunization of DTP and *H. influenzae* type b.

   c. Most convenient for child under age 15 months

   d. Separate injections of DTaP and HbCV may be preferable in the up-to-date child at ages 15 months and 4 to 6 years because DTaP has fewer side effects.

Precautions

1. Diphtheria and tetanus components

   a. Rarely cause systemic reactions

   b. May cause local reactions

   c. Reactions more common with too frequent immunization

2. Pertussis component

   a. No increased risk of permanent brain damage in neurologically normal child

   b. May induce febrile seizures

   c. Not a cause of sudden infant death syndrome

   d. Consider risk/benefit ratio of administration if previous immunization was followed by the following:

      (1) Fever $\geq$ 105° F (40.5° C) within 48 hours

      (2) Hypotonic-hyporesponsive episode within 48 hours

      (3) Persistent, inconsolable crying lasting longer than or equal to 3 hours within 48 hours

      (4) Seizures with or without fever within 3 days

Contraindications

1. Immediate anaphylactic reaction

2. Acute febrile illness

3. Pertussis component–specific contraindications

   a. Encephalopathy within 7 days of administration

   b. Neurologic disorder with progressive developmental delay or changing neurologic status

   c. Over age 6 years

Special Considerations

1. Child with uncertain or uncharacterized neurologic status: Delay pertussis component until the neurologic status is clarified.

2. Child with family history or personal history of seizures without other neurologic disorder: The child may receive the pertussis component, but there is a risk for seizure.

3. Child with stable cerebral palsy or nonprogressive developmental delay without seizure disposition: The child is not at increased risk for seizures.

4. Prolonged interval between doses: Reinitiation of the primary series is not required.

5. Patient who tests positive for human immunodeficiency virus (HIV): Patient may receive the vaccine.

Polio (OPV, eIPV)

General Information

1. OPV

   a. Live virus; administered orally

   b. Risk of paralysis: 1 per 2.5 million doses distributed

   c. Excreted in stool; nonimmune contacts have low risk of vaccine-associated paralysis

   d. Administer at ages 2, 4, and 6 to 18 months and 4 to 6 years

   e. Primary series in unimmunized person under age 18 years: 0, 4 to 8 weeks, and 6 to 12 months after the second dose

2. eIPV

   a. Enhanced, inactivated virus; administered subcutaneously

   b. Schedule is identical to that for OPV.

   c. Use if polio vaccination required after age 17, HIV positive, or immunodeficient.

   d. Use if vaccinee has a household contact who is HIV positive or immunosuppressed.

Precautions

Pregnancy. (Unless contraindicated, OPV is preferred if polio vaccine is required during pregnancy.)

Contraindications

1. Anaphylaxis

2. Moderate to severe systemic illness with or without fever

3. OPV-specific contraindications

   a. HIV infection

   b. Immunodeficiency (e.g., cancer, leukemia, chemotherapy, radiation therapy, high-dose steroids)

   c. Household contacts with HIV or known immunodeficiency

4. eIPV-specific contraindication: Anaphylaxis to neomycin, polymyxin B, or streptomycin

Special Considerations

1. Child spits out dose within 10 minutes: Administer another dose.

2. Low-to-moderate-dose steroid use: Such usage is not a contraindication to OPV.

3. Incompletely immunized adults in the United States: The primary vaccination and booster doses are unnec-

essary unless there is risk because of foreign travel or occupation.

Measles, Mumps, Rubella (MMR)

General Information
1. Combination live virus vaccine administered subcutaneously; also available as individual vaccines
2. Primary dose: age 12 to 15 months
3. Booster dose: age 4 to 6 years or 11 to 12 years
4. Arthralgias may develop 1 to 3 months after immunization, especially in women.
5. May temporarily suppress tuberculin skin test reactivity; administer the tuberculin skin test on the same day or 6 weeks after the MMR vaccine.

Precautions
Immune globulin administered within previous 3 months

Contraindications
1. Anaphylaxis to egg ingestion or neomycin
2. Moderate to severe illness with or without fever
3. Pregnancy
4. Immunodeficiency (cancer, lymphoma, leukemia, chemotherapy, radiation therapy, high-dose steroids)

Special Considerations
1. Women of childbearing age: Screen for rubella immunity, and vaccinate unless the patient is pregnant or there is some other contraindication.
2. Pregnant woman with child in need of vaccination: The child may be immunized; the vaccine is not transmitted from the vaccinee to susceptible contacts.
3. Adults born before 1957 are considered immune.
4. Health care workers, college students, and international travelers born after 1956: Give special attention to vaccination and immunity status.
5. Community epidemic: The vaccine may be administered to a child under age 12 months, but it does not count as the first dose. The child must be revaccinated at age 15 months and receive a booster dose at ages 4 to 6 or 11 to 12 years.
6. Low-to-moderate-dose steroid use: This is not a contraindication.
7. HIV positive: This is not a contraindication.

Haemophilus influenzae Type b Conjugate Vaccine (HbCV)

General Information
1. Most important in children under age 15 months to prevent *H. influenzae* meningitis
2. Five vaccines are approved for children under age 15 months.

   a. HibTITER, OmniHIB, ActHIB: The primary series is administered at ages 2, 4, and 6 months; the booster, at age 12 to 15 months.

   b. PedvaxHIB: The primary series is administered at ages 2 and 4 months; the booster, at age 12 to 15 months.

   c. TETRAMUNE (DTP-HbCV): This vaccine allows simultaneous administration of DTP and HbCV. The primary series is administered at ages 2, 4, and 6 months. It may be used for the 12-to-15-month booster, although separate DTaP and HbCV vaccines may be preferable.

   d. OmniHIB and ActHIB: When reconstituted with Connaught DTP, they allow simultaneous vaccination with DTP and HbCV.

   e. Previously unvaccinated child, 15 to 59 months: Give a single dose of any HbCV vaccine.

   f. After age 5 years: HbCV vaccination is unnecessary unless a special circumstance, sickle cell disease, or asplenia is present.

3. When possible, the same HbCV should be used throughout the primary series. If different vaccines must be administered, a total of three doses of vaccine, regardless of manufacturer, should be administered for primary vaccination of a child under age 15 months. No precautions necessary.

Contraindications
1. Anaphylaxis
2. Moderate to severe systemic illness with or without fever
3. Specific for OmniHIB or ActHIB reconstituted with DTP or TETRAMUNE: See DTP Precautions and Contraindications.

Special Considerations
1. Day care centers: Special attention should be given to vaccinating all children.
2. Children under age 24 months with a history of invasive *H. influenzae* disease: do not develop immunity to natural disease; ensure vaccination.
3. Children under age 15 months, incompletely immunized: Consult package insert for dosing interval.

Hepatitis B Virus (HBV)

General Information
1. Two licensed hepatitis B vaccines: Recombivax HB and Engerix-B. Equally immunogenic
2. May be used interchangeably in their respective recommended dosages
3. Consult package insert for dosage administration because of differing formulations and schedules
4. Administered intramuscularly

5. Because of safety, it is liberally recommended, especially for sexually active teenagers and young adults.

Indications

1. All infants born to hepatitis B surface antigen (HBsAg)-negative mothers
2. All infants born to HBsAg-positive mothers in combination with hepatitis B immune globulin (HBIG)
3. Health care and public safety workers
4. Clients and staff of institutions for the developmentally disabled; inmates of correctional facilities
5. Hemodialysis patients; recipients of certain blood products
6. Injecting drug users
7. Multiple sex partners; sexually active homosexual and bisexual men; high-risk adolescents (teen pregnancy and sexually transmitted diseases are "red flags"); prostitutes
8. Household contacts, sex partners of HBV carriers
9. International travelers, especially if they are staying for more than 6 months in an area with a high rate of HBV
10. Adoptees from countries where HBV is endemic

Precautions

1. Serious active illness; severely compromised cardiopulmonary status
2. Pregnancy

Contraindications

Anaphylaxis to previous vaccination or common baker's yeast

Special Considerations

1. Periodic serologic testing—no consensus
2. Periodic revaccination—no consensus
3. Health care workers, dialysis patients, infants born to HBsAg-positive mothers, anticipated suboptimal response (HIV, immunosuppressed): Consider serologic testing.
4. Patient does not respond to the initial three-dose regimen: Revaccinate with one or more doses.
5. Elderly people, smokers, obese people: These people are less likely to develop immunity.
6. Pregnancy: Routinely screen for HBsAg.

Varicella Vaccine

General Information

1. Live, attenuated vaccine
2. Most common side effect: Injection site pain, redness, swelling
3. Fifteen per cent report fever; febrile seizures not clearly associated

4. Some vaccinees report upper respiratory illness, cough irritability, joint pain, diarrhea.
5. Five per cent or less develop generalized chickenpox rash with a median of five lesions or injection site rash within 3 weeks.
6. Cost-benefit analysis shows $5.40 of societal savings for every dollar invested in varicella vaccine, based on medical and parental work-loss costs.
7. Within 3 years, 1 per cent of children immunized will develop chickenpox, a 93 per cent decrease compared to expected attack rates; most cases are milder.
8. Pregnancy: Avoid for 3 months postvaccination.

Indications

1. Age 12 months and older if without history of natural chickenpox
   a. Age 12 months to 12 years: One dose
   b. Adults and adolescents age 13 years or older: Two doses, administered 4 to 8 weeks apart

Contraindications

1. Hypersensitivity to any component of the vaccine, including gelatin
2. Anaphylaxis to neomycin
3. History of blood dyscrasias, lymphoma, leukemia, or other malignant neoplasms of the bone marrow or lymphatic system (may not apply to children with acute lymphoblastic leukemia in remission)
4. Use of immunosuppressants
5. Primary or acquired immune deficiencies including acquired immunodeficiency syndrome (AIDS)
6. Family history of congenital or hereditary immunodeficiency unless immune competence is clear
7. Active untreated tuberculosis, febrile illness, or infection
8. Pregnancy

Pneumococcal Vaccine

General Information

1. Contains capsular polysaccharides of the 23 most prevalent pneumococcal types
2. Administered only once a lifetime, except in
   a. Adults who received 14-valent pneumococcal vaccine more than 4 years previously and are at highest risk (asplenic)
   b. Adults who received 23-valent pneumococcal vaccine more than 6 years previously with nephrotic syndrome, renal failure, or organ transplantation
   c. Children at high risk (asplenia, sickle cell disease, nephrotic syndrome), especially if under age 10 years: Revaccinate 3 to 5 years after the first dose.

Indications

1. Age over 65 years

2. Those at risk for influenza
3. Chronic disease—cardiovascular, respiratory, hepatic, and renal diseases; diabetes; immunosuppression; cancer; lymphoma; multiple myeloma; leukemia; organ transplantation
4. HIV positive
5. Native American
6. Asplenia (anatomic or sickle cell disease)
7. Chronic alcohol abuse
8. Closed groups; nursing home and institutionalized
9. Chronic cerebrospinal fluid leakage

Precautions
1. Febrile illness or active infection
2. Pregnancy

Contraindications
Anaphylaxis to vaccine or hypersensitivity to any vaccine component

Special Considerations
1. Children with chronic illness (e.g., asthma, cardiovascular disease): Vaccinate if over age 2 years.
2. Under age 2 years: Vaccination is not effective.

Influenza

General Information
1. Killed virus; cannot cause influenza
2. Needed yearly because of antigenic variation
3. Split-virus vaccine preferred over whole-virus vaccine; fewer reactions; give to children and adults

Indications
1. Over age 65
2. Chronic lung or heart disease, including children; asthma
3. Chronic illness: renal failure, diabetes, hemoglobinopathy, and immunosuppression, including AIDS
4. Residents of nursing homes and other chronic care facilities
5. Children and teenagers receiving long-term aspirin therapy; at risk for Reye's syndrome after influenza
6. Those capable of transmitting influenza to high-risk patients: health care workers, home care volunteers, household members

Precautions
1. Immunosuppression may decrease immunogenic response.
2. Pregnancy

Contraindications
1. Anaphylaxis to previous vaccination, chicken eggs, or aminoglycosides

2. Past history of Guillain-Barré syndrome
3. Acute febrile illness

Special Considerations
1. Children under age 6 months: Vaccine is not approved for use in this age group.
2. Children aged 6 months to 9 years not previously vaccinated: Give two doses of split-virus vaccine 4 weeks apart.
3. Northern hemisphere: Vaccinate in the fall.
4. Except for the 1976–1977 swine influenza vaccine, subsequent vaccines have not been clearly associated with Guillain-Barré syndrome.
5. If vaccine cannot be given to a high-risk patient, amantadine or rimantadine may be used for prophylaxis.

Rabies

General Information
1. Inactivated virus vaccine
2. Two vaccines are available: Human diploid cell vaccine (HDCV) and rabies virus absorbed (RVA)
3. Pre-exposure prophylaxis indications
   a. Veterinarians, animal handlers
   b. Cave explorers
   c. Certain rabies laboratory workers
   d. People visiting or living in countries where the rabies risk is high
4. Postexposure treatment of previously unvaccinated
   a. Thoroughly clean wound.
   b. Administer a five-dose series (1.0 ml intramuscularly) of HDCV or RVA on days 0, 3, 7, 14, and 28; the deltoid muscle is preferred.
   c. Administer human rabies immune globulin (Imogam), 20 IU/kg. Infiltrate one half around the wound; give the other one half intramuscularly, avoiding HDCV/RVA injection sites.
5. Postexposure treatment of previously vaccinated
   a. Thoroughly clean wound.
   b. Administer a two-dose series of HDCV or RVA on days 0 and 3; the deltoid muscle is preferred.
   c. Do not administer human rabies immune globulin.

Precautions
1. Immunosuppression may interfere with immunity; monitor rabies antibody response.
2. Pregnancy
3. Postexposure treatment: hypersensitivity

Contraindications
1. Pre-exposure prophylaxis: anaphylaxis
2. Pre-exposure prophylaxis: acute illness, with or without fever

Special Considerations

1. Bite by wild skunk, bat, fox, coyote, raccoon, bobcat, other carnivores: Regard the animal as rabid unless laboratory test results are negative.
2. Bite by squirrel, hamster, guinea pig, gerbil, chipmunk, rat, mouse, other rodent, livestock, rabbit, hare: Consider individually; consult public health officials; such bites seldom require rabies treatment.
3. Bite by dog or cat
   a. Rabid or suspected rabid: postexposure treatment
   b. Healthy and available for 10 days of observation: Observe the animal. No treatment is required unless the animal is rabid; destroy the animal for laboratory testing if there is any doubt.
   c. Unknown or escaped: Consult public health officials; postexposure treatment may be required.

Meningococcal Polysaccharide Vaccine

General Information

1. Contains serotypes A, C, Y, W135
2. Does not include serotype B and is not effective against serotype C in children under age 2 years. These serotypes are those most likely to cause disease in U.S. children.

Indications

1. Asplenia
2. Sickle cell anemia
3. Terminal complement component deficiencies
4. Travelers to endemic areas

Precautions

Pregnancy

Contraindications

1. Anaphylaxis
2. Moderate illness with or without fever

Special Considerations

Not routinely recommended for U.S. children

Tetanus Prophylaxis in Wound Management

General Information

1. Thoroughly clean wound; debride if necessary.
2. If the patient is over age 6 years, dT is preferred.
3. If the patient is under age 7 years, review the immunization record; use the incident as an opportunity to update immunizations.
4. For passive immunization, human tetanus immune globulin (TIG) is indicated; adult dose is 250 units intramuscularly.
5. In the U.S., tetanus is a disease of elderly people; pay attention to the immunization status of such patients; ensure completion of primary immunizations.

Indications for TIG

1. Patients who require immediate immunity against tetanus toxoid, especially those with little or no active immunity
2. Treatment for active case of tetanus

Precautions

TIG: Do not use for skin testing; reaction is easily misinterpreted.

Contraindications

TIG: anaphylaxis to previous gamma globulin or thimerosal

Special Considerations

1. Clean minor wound, more than or equal to three dT immunizations: Immunization is unnecessary if the last dT injection was given within the past 10 years; if it was not given within the past 10 years, update the immunization status with dT.
2. Clean minor wound, unknown status or fewer than three dT immunizations: Update the immunization status with dT and schedule the patient for the remaining primary series; TIG is unnecessary.
3. Contaminated, dirty wound, puncture, avulsion, crush, burn, frostbite, more than or equal to three dT immunizations: Administer dT if 5 years have passed since last dose; TIG is unnecessary.
4. Contaminated, dirty wound, puncture, avulsion, crush, burn, frostbite, unknown status or fewer than three dT immunizations: Update the immunization status with dT and schedule the patient for the remaining primary series; administer TIG.

 ## Bibliography

AAFP, AAP and ACIP collaborate in the development of a simplified childhood immunization schedule. Am Fam Physician 1994;50:1826.

Anderson DC, Stiehm ER: Immunization. JAMA 1992; 268:2959–2963.

Centers for Disease Control: General recommendations on immunization: Recommendations of the Advisory Committee on Immunization Practices. MMWR 1994;43(No.RR-1):1–38.

Thompson RF: Travel and routine immunizations: A Practical Guide for the Medical Office. Milwaukee, Shoreland Medical Marketing, 1994.

Zimmerman RK, Giebink GS: Childhood immunizations: A practical approach for clinicians. Am Fam Physician 1992;45:1759–1772.

2 Health Maintenance Protocols

Joseph C. Konen

Health Maintenance Protocol Systems

1. Health maintenance charts, protocols, and other documentation systems are essential elements in systematic approaches to the provision of clinical preventive services.
2. Both paper- and computer-based charting systems may be used by
   a. Health providers (health maintenance charts, flow sheets)
   b. Patients (hand-held medical records)
3. Health maintenance protocols prompt health care providers
   a. To perform or order clinical preventive services such as
      (1) Risk assessments
      (2) Physical examinations
      (3) Laboratory testing
      (4) Counseling/health guidance
      (5) Immunizations
   b. To document the delivery and results of these services
4. Such systems may also prompt, guide, and empower patients and their families to
   a. Request preventive services
   b. Document the delivery and results of these services

Periodic Health Examinations

1. The provision of clinical preventive services should be performed at every opportunity including
   a. During any encounter in which health care is delivered
   b. Especially during periodic health maintenance examinations
2. The periodic health examination is conducted for the purposes of reviewing an individual's health status, establishing risk factors for future illness and injury, and providing an opportunity for screening for asymptomatic disease, counseling or health guidance, and updating immunizations. The periodicity of these examinations should be determined by each individual's unique health status and risk assessment, as well as by age and gender.

Health Maintenance and Screening Recommendations

1. Current rational and systematized guidelines for providing clinical preventive services have evolved from recommendations proposed by a variety of authorities.

2. The most thoroughly reviewed evidence-based recommendations for the provision of clinical preventive services are those of the USPSTF (1989).
3. Health maintenance recommendations can often be summarized into single-page flow sheets or age-specific check lists. The most useful paper-based systems are those that
   a. Can be prominently positioned in the medical record
   b. Involve the office staff in design, planning, and maintenance

U.S. Preventive Services Task Force

1. The U.S. Preventive Services Task Force (USPSTF) was commissioned in 1984 by the U.S. Department of Health and Human Services (DHHS) and issued its *Guide to Clinical Preventive Services* in 1989 with an update in 1995.
2. The principal findings of the USPSTF are
   a. Interventions that address personal health practices of patients are among the most effective interventions available to clinicians to reduce the leading causes of disease in the United States.
   b. Greater selectivity should be used in providing preventive services. Consideration of the individual risk profile is important in determining which activities should occur during a clinical encounter.
   c. Traditional clinical activities, such as diagnostic testing, may be less valuable than activities such as counseling and patient education.
   d. The roles of health care providers and patients are changing with more patients taking an increasingly active responsibility in their own health.

Patient-Held Medical Records

1. Hand-held medical records are available for patients to review recommendations for preventive services, record their participation in specific clinical maneuvers, and track trends for such parameters as weight, blood pressure, and cholesterol. These mini-records have the potential to build collaborative preventive relationships among health providers, office staff, and patients.
2. Immunization records for children are a common example of these systems.
3. *The Personal Health Guide* (DHHS) is a more extensive example of a pocket-sized booklet that provides guidance about common preventive strategies, and allows patients to track results of screening tests and immunizations.

Integrated Systems

Offices with systems that integrate a variety of approaches to the provision of clinical preventive services are more effective than offices without such systems.

A. Computer-Based Systems

Several computer-based systems are available that incorporate prevention reminders, documentation, and tracking into office systems with or without support for patient care notes and billing systems. Such systems also allow for the generation of patient reminders and summarize the health provider's preventive activities.

B. Put Prevention Into Practice

Integrated systems, such as *Put Prevention Into Practice,* developed by the Office of Disease Prevention Health Promotion (DHHS), target health providers, patients, and office staffs through

1. Provider materials
   a. Clinician Handbook gives concise information on clinical preventive services.
   b. Examination room posters serve as references for clinicians and educational tools for patients.
2. Patient materials
   a. *Personal Health Guides* provide information and prompt patients to obtain as well as to record results of preventive services.

b. Waiting room posters promote the office's importance in dealing with preventive aspects of health care.
3. Office system materials
   a. Patient chart flow sheets assist in the tracking and prompting of preventive services.
   b. Patient chart alert stickers alert providers and staff to specific risk factors and patient needs.
   c. Prevention prescription pads help providers and staff to prescribe indicated preventive services and make referrals for further evaluations.
   d. Reminder postcards remind patients of their need for further preventive services.

Adult and Child Preventive Care Time Lines

1. Preventive care time lines have been proposed to suggest when age-specific periodic health examinations should occur as well as the content of these examinations. Recommendations by all major authorities and by some minor authorities have been collated in the DHHS *Put Prevention Into Practice* and appear in Figures 2–1 and 2–2.
2. However, the content of each specific periodic health maintenance examination must be tailored to individual needs of the patient.

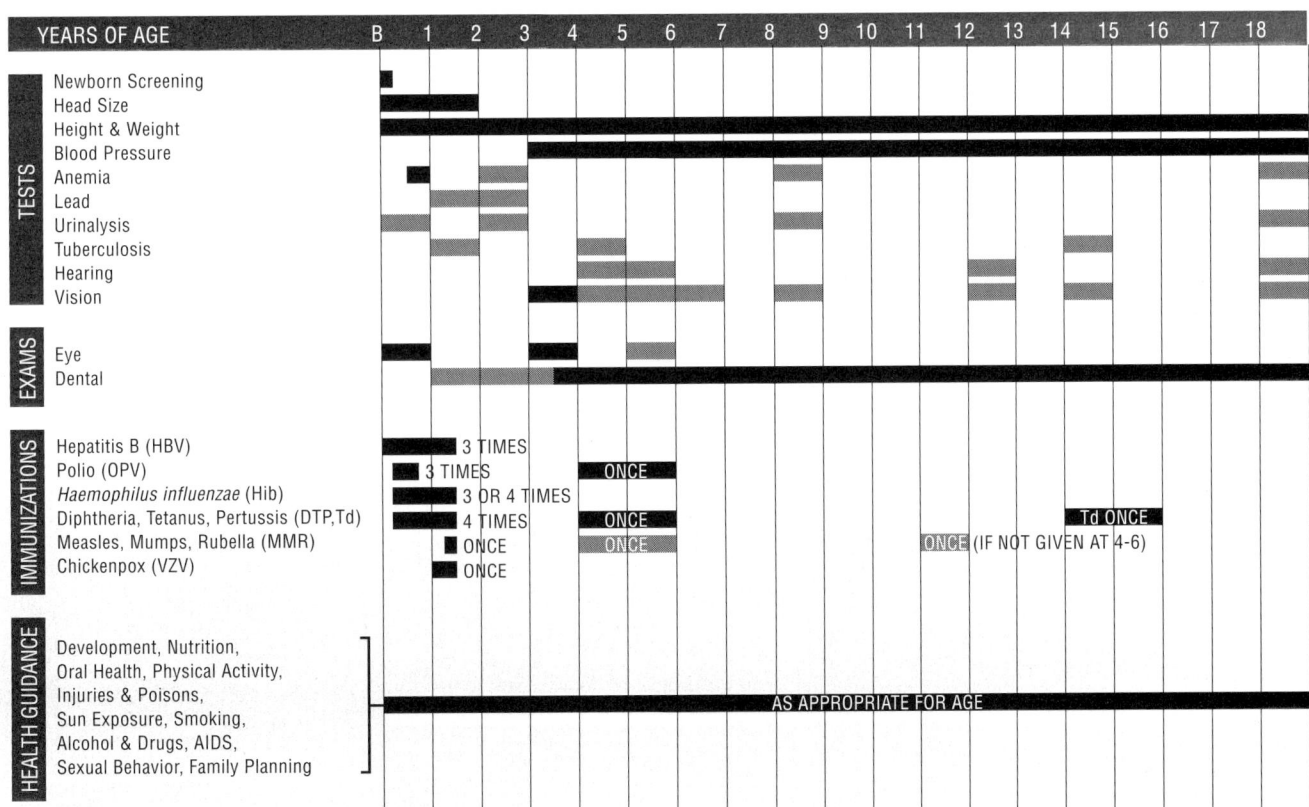

Key:
■ Recommended by all major authorities.
▨ Recommended by some major authorities.

Figure 2–1 Child preventive care time lines: Recommendations of major authorities. (From Clinician's Handbook of Preventive Services. Put Prevention Into Practice. Washington, D.C., U.S. Public Health Service, Department of Health and Human Services, 1994.)

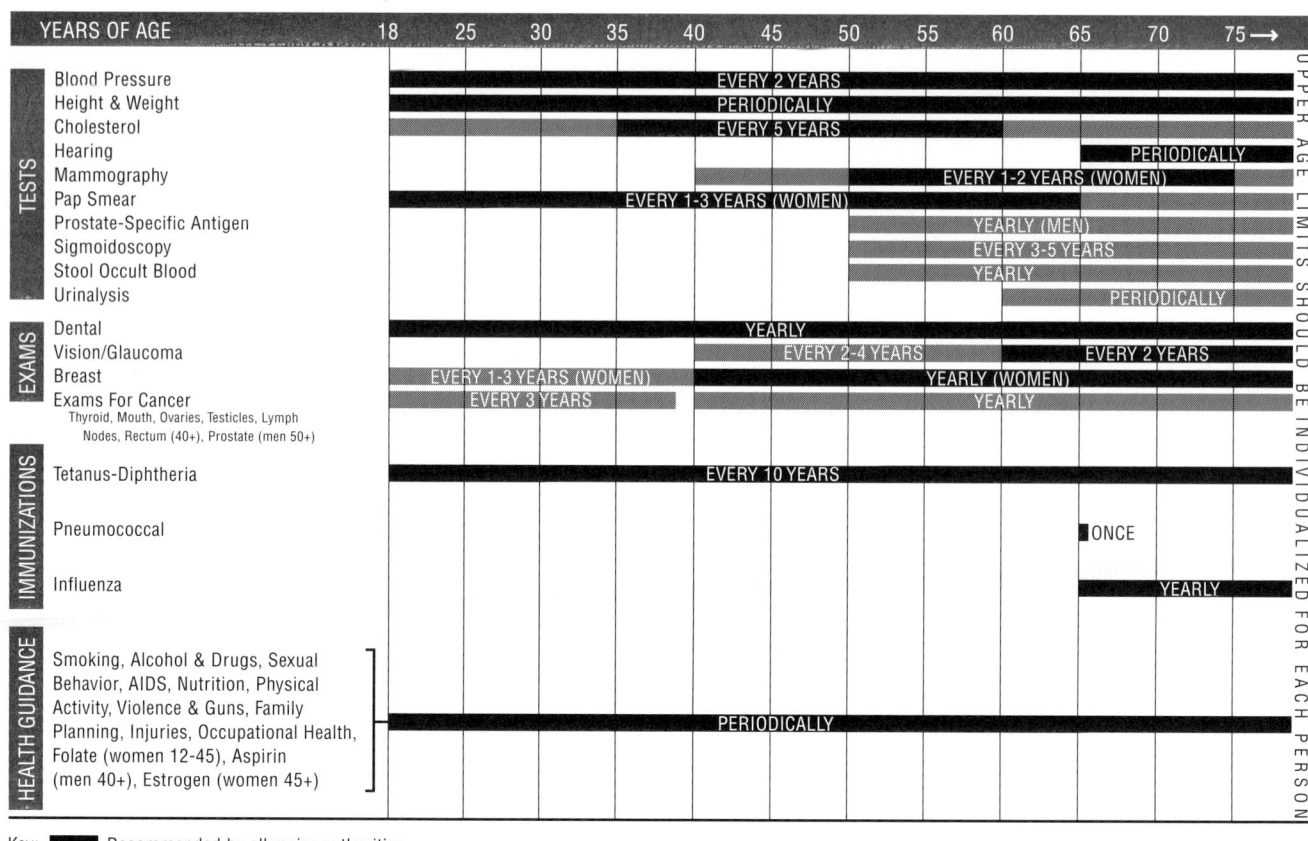

Key:
■ Recommended by all major authorities.
▓ Recommended by some major authorities.

Figure 2–2 Adult preventive care time lines: Recommendations of major authorities. (From Clinician's Handbook of Preventive Services. Put Prevention Into Practice. Washington, D.C., U.S. Public Health Service, Department of Health and Human Services, 1994.)

3. Individual patient characteristics of race and sex, and other risk factors such as lifestyle behaviors, genetic predisposition, and current health state (including ongoing medical problems and such changeable characteristics as age, height, weight, blood pressure, and cholesterol), determine the most likely leading causes of future illness and injury.

4. Screening and other health maintenance interventions should be chosen on the basis of their demonstrated effectiveness in preventing targeted conditions.

5. Although complex algorithms may be necessary to accurately account for individual risk factors in the development of specific health maintenance recommendations, these preventive care time lines summarize clinical preventive service protocols and give

reasonable first approximations to guide the clinician in the delivery of clinical preventive services.

 Bibliography

For more information on a systems approach to preventive services, see
Walsh JM, McPhee SJ: A systems model of clinical preventive care: an analysis of factors influencing patient and physician. Health Ed Quart 1992;19:157–175.
For more information on the clinical preventive service recommendations of the U.S. Preventive Services Task Force, see
U.S. Preventive Services Task Force: Guide to clinical preventive services: An assessment of the effectiveness of 169 interventions. Report of the U.S. Preventive Services Task Force. Baltimore, Williams & Wilkins, 1989.
For more information on patient-held health maintenance records, see
Dickey LL: Promoting preventive care with patient-held mini-records: A review. Patient Educ Counsel 1993;20:37–47.
For more information on computerized health maintenance systems, see
Garr DR, Ornstein SM, Jenkins RG, Zemp LD: The effect of routine use of computer-generated preventive reminders in a clinical practice. Am J Prevent Med 1993;9:55–61.
For more information on adult and child preventive care time lines, see
The Clinician's Handbook of Preventive Services. Put Prevention Into Practice. Washington, D.C., U.S. Public Health Service, U.S. Department of Health and Human Services, 1994.

WARNING

Provision of health maintenance and screening services should be based on individual risk assessments that include detailed knowledge of lifestyle behaviors, family history, genetic predisposition, and current health state.

3 Growth and Development Guidelines

John B. Standridge

Natural History

1. Normal growth is a dynamic process that requires adequate genetic, hormonal, nutritional, and psychosocial components.
2. Normal growth occurs in three distinct phases.
   a. In utero and in infancy—very fast and then decelerates
   b. Ages 2 through 10—steady but slower growth rate with linear growth gradually slowing and growth in weight gradually increasing
   c. Pubertal phase—rapid, up to 4 inches a year. Menarche, around age 13, signals the slowing of linear growth for females. Males reach peak growth velocity around age 14 and plateau around age 18.

Detection of Abnormal Growth

1. Height and weight measurements are a fundamental and necessary part of every office visit.
2. Abnormal growth patterns are recognizable only through sequential plotting of growth data (see chapter appendix for normal height and weight growth charts).
3. Regardless of cause, the best treatment occurs when early recognition leads to timely mobilization of resources.

Interpreting Abnormal Growth

1. Remeasure and reweigh the child, and rechart the data (see chapter appendix for abnormal height and weight growth charts).
2. Inquire about recent illness, caloric intake, stature and weight of siblings, and stature and weight of parents.

Key Features That Differentiate Abnormal Growth Patterns

A. Short, looks normal—low growth velocity
   1. Organic failure to thrive
      a. Neurologic—mental retardation, cerebral palsy, diencephalic syndrome
      b. Endocrine—hypothyroidism, panhypopituitarism, adrenogenital syndrome; radiography for bone age, somatomedin C (insulin-like growth factor I)
      c. Gastrointestinal—pyloric stenosis, celiac disease; growth delay may precede diarrhea and abdominal distention; jejunal biopsy
      d. Genitourinary—pyelonephritis, renal tubular acidosis; elevated creatinine and blood urea nitrogen levels; acidosis, anemia, hyperphosphatemia, hypocalcemia
      e. Cardiac—patent ductus arteriosus, coarctation of the aorta, septal defects; cyanosis, murmur; abnormal electrocardiogram and echocardiogram
      f. Pulmonary—recurrent pneumonia, tracheomalacia, cystic fibrosis; malabsorption, positive sweat chloride test
      g. Chronic infection—tuberculin test; cultures of urine, blood, and stool; erythrocyte sedimentation rate
      h. Miscellaneous—immune disorders, tumors, hematologic disease, multiple congenital abnormalities
   2. Malnutrition—listlessness, apathy, decreased lean body mass and adiposity, pallor, hair thin or sparse, hypotonia, protuberant abdomen; swallowing dysfunction (neurologic), esophageal stricture, gastroesophageal reflux, small stomach, partial obstruction, defective assimilation
   3. Nonorganic failure to thrive (psychosocial)
      a. Inadequate nutritional information (maternal)
      b. Disturbance in attachment (deficiency in care), parental inadequacy: drug and alcohol abuse, marital or family discord, neglect, mental illness, depression, or mental retardation
      c. Disturbance in separation-individualization (food refusal on the part of the child)
   4. Chromosomal—appearance, trisomy 13 and 18
B. Short, looks normal—growth velocity normal
   1. Intrauterine growth retardation—term birth weight less than 2000 gm or preterm size small for gestational age
      a. Fetal factors—chromosomal, congenital infections
      b. Placental factors—implantation or vascular abnormalities
      c. Maternal factors—malnutrition, toxemia, drugs, uterine malformations, severe diabetes mellitus
   2. Genetic short stature—family history, normal bone age. Exclude genetic growth disorder in parents
   3. Constitutional delay—family history; slowing of the growth rate between ages 1 and 3, delay in physical maturation and bone age. Growth normalizes but remains 2 to 3 years behind chronologic age.
C. Short, looks abnormal—proportionate growth
   Short stature syndromes

1. Noonan's syndrome—features similar to Turner's syndrome but more often male; normal karyotype
2. Russell-Silver syndrome—intrauterine growth retardation, craniofacial dysostosis, short limbs, triangular face, variable features

D. Short, looks abnormal—disproportionate growth
   1. Skeletal disorders
      a. Achondroplastic dwarfism—short upper arms and thighs, large head and forehead, small nose, normal intelligence
      b. Hypochondroplasia—milder form, short limbs, normal face
      c. Other skeletal dysplasias—number more than 50; bone films
   2. Chromosomal abnormalities
      a. Trisomy 21 (Down syndrome)—mental retardation, delayed bone maturation, characteristic physical features
      b. Turner's syndrome—female, variable stigmata, short limbs, no adolescent growth spurt; confirm with karyotype

E. Tall, looks normal—increased growth velocity
   1. Precocious puberty—secondary sex characteristics before age 8 in girls and before age 9 in boys
   2. Excess growth hormone—coarse facial features, organ enlargement, abnormal glucose tolerance test, abnormal hand and skull radiographs
   3. Hyperthyroidism—goiter, staring, lid lag, dermopathy; abnormal thyroid function studies

F. Tall, looks normal—normal growth velocity
   Genetic tall stature—family history, tall parents

G. Tall, looks abnormal—proportionate growth
   Cerebral giantism—birth weight and height above the 90th percentile, mental retardation, advanced bone age

H. Tall, looks abnormal—disproportionate growth
   1. Marfan syndrome—long limbs, narrow hands, arachnodactyly; arm span exceeds height; dissecting aortic aneurysm common
   2. Klinefelter's syndrome (XXY)—hypergonadotropic hypogonadism

Failure to Thrive Syndrome

1. Hallmark is failure to gain weight at an expected rate for the age of the child; may include evidence of malnutrition, delayed development, abnormal behaviors, organic disorders
2. Etiology (see previous section)
   a. Nonorganic (psychosocial)
   b. Feeding problems or malnutrition
   c. Organic
3. Evaluation
   a. History and physical-neurologic assessment

b. Developmental evaluation—Denver Developmental Screening Test
c. Calorie count, intake and output, frequent weight measurement
d. Laboratory tests—complete blood count; multichemistry profile; glucose tolerance test; urinalysis; Venereal Disease Research Laboratory (VDRL) test; thyroxine, thyroid-stimulating hormone, insulin-like growth factor I, and immunoglobulin levels; stool for pH; reducing substances and fat; sweat test; chromosomal studies
e. Radiologic—left wrist for bone age, chest, intravenous pyelography, trauma survey, upper and lower gastrointestinal series, various scans
f. Electrocardiogram and echocardiogram

4. Indications for hospitalization
   a. Strong suspicion of organic cause
   b. Signs of physical abuse
   c. Suspected neglect—poor infant hygiene (e.g., severe cradle cap, diaper rash, long dirty fingernails), parental unconcern, no previous medical attention
   d. History of frequent vomiting or diarrhea
   e. Infant over age 2 months and still near birth weight
   f. Infant between ages 3 and 6 months with minimal weight gain over previous 2 months
   g. Potentially life-threatening malnutrition
   h. Mother overtly depressed or rejecting baby
   i. History of bizarre diet
   j. Insignificant weight gain after 1 month of outpatient management

5. Management
   a. Approach the parents or caregivers with a sense of urgency to determine whether they are willing to make the required changes. If not, change the caregiving situation.
   b. Identify and then eliminate or reduce environmental stresses.
   c. Find supportive, empathetic relatives and neighbors.
   d. Find parenting classes or self-help groups.
   e. Find professional counseling or therapy, drug or alcohol treatment programs, and so on, when indicated.
   f. Find age-appropriate day care programs, respite centers, and so on, for the child.
   g. Find a social worker, psychologist, nurse, or other human services provider who can become intensely involved with the family for 1 to 2 years.

Anticipatory Guidance to Promote Normal Growth and Development

1. Diet and exercise
2. Injury prevention measures

3. Reassurance of safety and self-worth
4. Parental advice, counseling, and moral support

 Bibliography

Behrman RE, Kliegman RM (eds): Nelson Textbook of Pediatrics, 14th ed. Philadelphia, WB Saunders, 1992.

Brunader RE, Moore DC: Evaluation of the child with growth retardation. Am Fam Physician 1987;35:165–176.
Sturtz GS: Common Sense Guide to Growth and Nutrition. Watertown, NY, Hojack Publishing, 1991.
Sturtz GS: Parents' Guide to Growth and Nutrition. Utica, NY, Hojack Publishing, 1992.
Tanner JM, Whitehouse RH: Clinical longitudinal standards for height, weight, height velocity, weight velocity, and stages of puberty. Arch Dis Child 1976;51:170.

GROWTH AND DEVELOPMENT CHARTS

1 Growth at the 50th percentile. Average United States boy. (From Sturtz GS: Common Sense Guide to Growth and Nutrition, p 37. Watertown, NY, Hojack Publishing Company, 1991.)

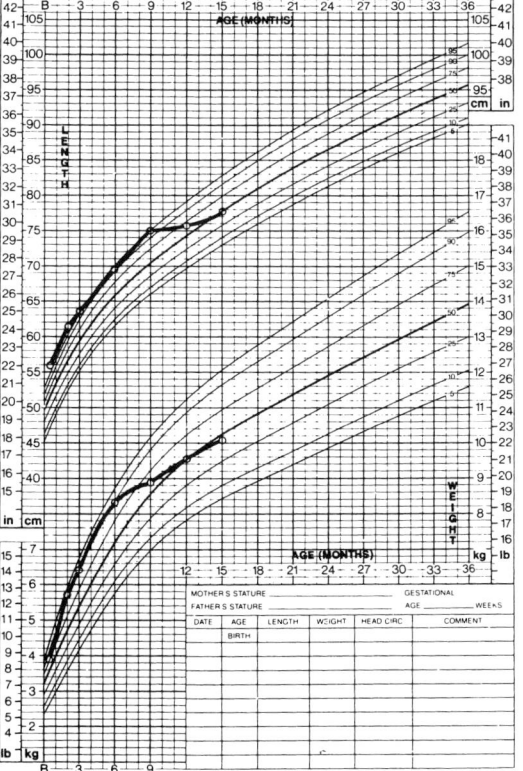

2 Neonatal growth near the 95th percentile regressing to the 50th percentile by age 15 months. (From Sturtz GS: Common Sense Guide to Growth and Nutrition, p 81. Watertown, NY, Hojack Publishing Company, 1991.)

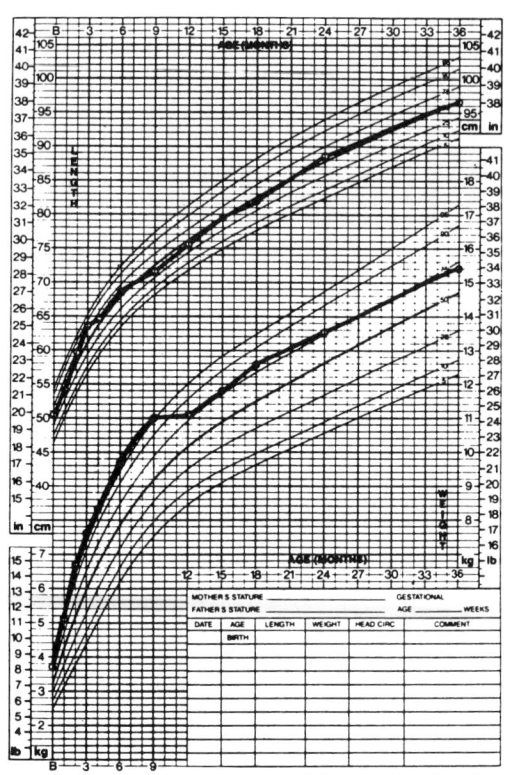

3 Breast-fed male infant with rapid weight gain that regressed toward the 50th percentile. (From Sturtz GS: Common Sense Guide to Growth and Nutrition, p 87. Watertown, NY, Hojack Publishing Company, 1991.)

4 Length is at the 25th percentile. Weight is below the 5th percentile. The small, thin son of small, thin parents. (From Sturtz GS: Common Sense Guide to Growth and Nutrition, p 52. Watertown, NY, Hojack Publishing Company, 1991.)

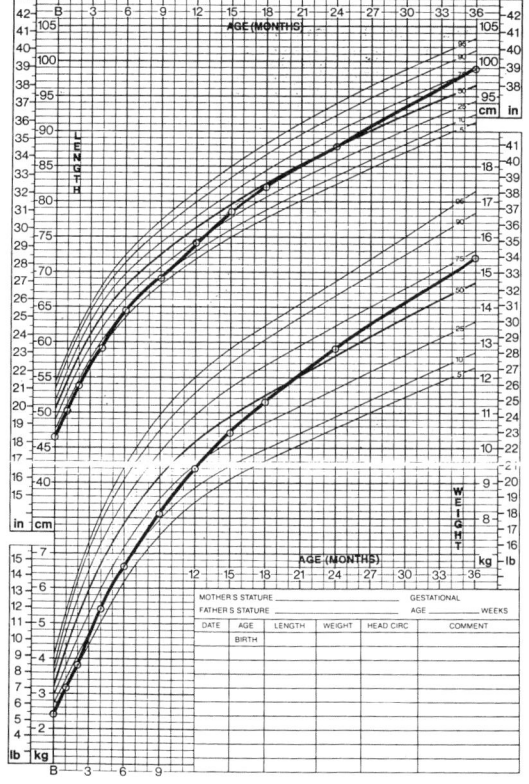

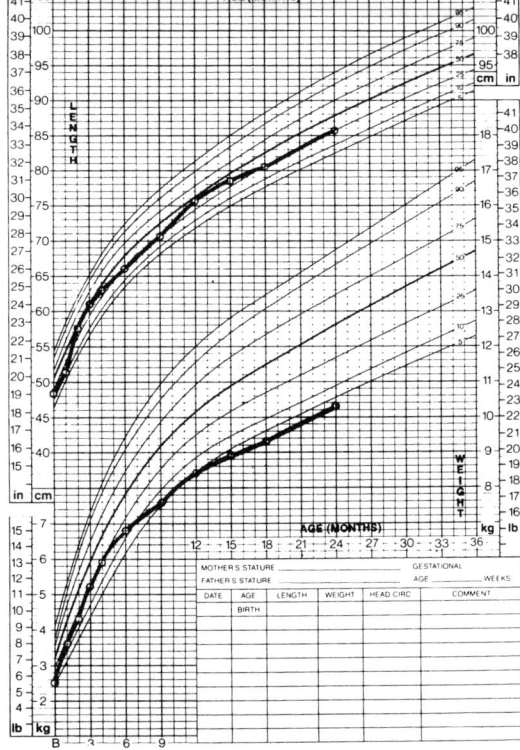

5 Catch-up growth in an infant at the 5th percentile at birth. (From Sturtz GS: Common Sense Guide to Growth and Nutrition, p 42. Watertown, NY, Hojack Publishing Company, 1991.)

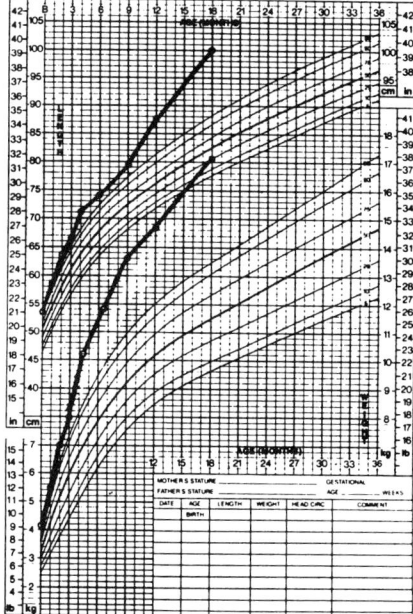

6 Enormous child who was fed enormous amounts of food despite dietary counseling. (From Sturtz GS: Common Sense Guide to Growth and Nutrition, p 54. Watertown, NY, Hojack Publishing Company, 1991.)

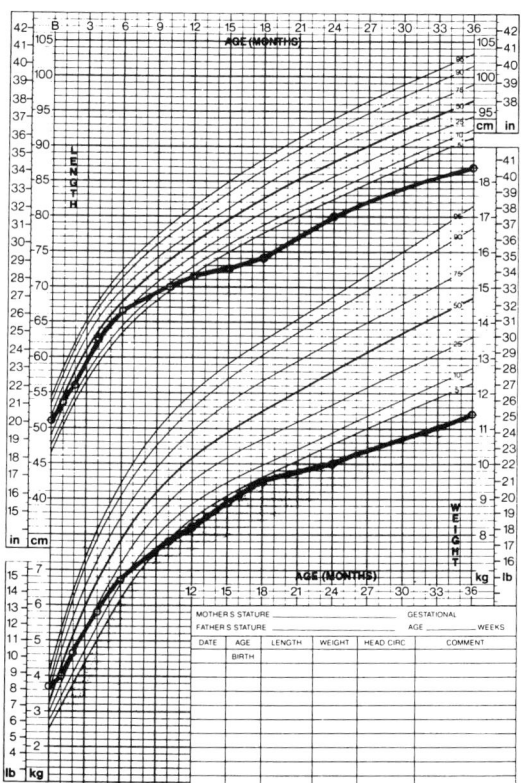

7 Length and weight fell below the 5th percentile in this boy with familial short stature. (From Sturtz GS: Common Sense Guide to Growth and Nutrition, p 91. Watertown, NY, Hojack Publishing Company, 1991.)

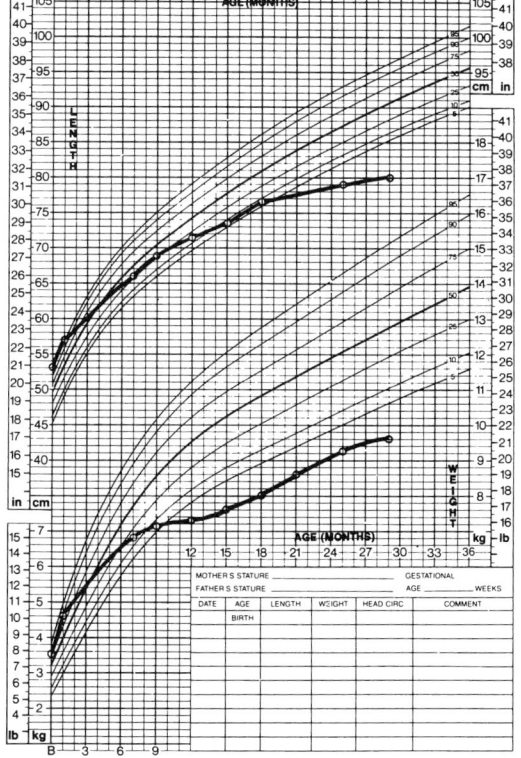

8 Classic case of failure to thrive. (From Sturtz GS: Common Sense Guide to Growth and Nutrition, p 66. Watertown, NY, Hojack Publishing Company, 1991.)

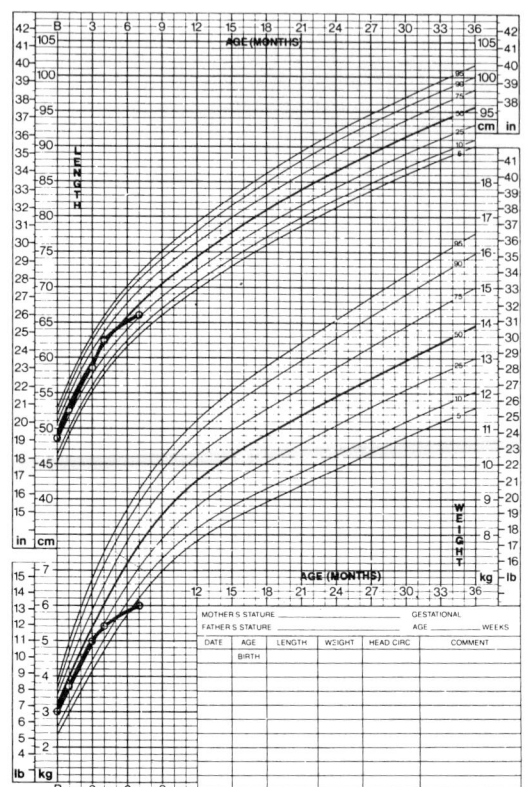
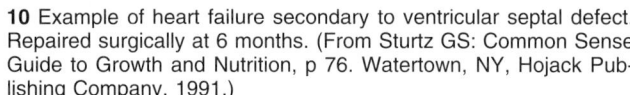

9 Example of heart failure secondary to patent ductus arteriosus. Closed surgically at age 7 months. (From Sturtz GS: Common Sense Guide to Growth and Nutrition, p 65. Watertown, NY, Hojack Publishing Company, 1991.)

10 Example of heart failure secondary to ventricular septal defect. Repaired surgically at 6 months. (From Sturtz GS: Common Sense Guide to Growth and Nutrition, p 76. Watertown, NY, Hojack Publishing Company, 1991.)

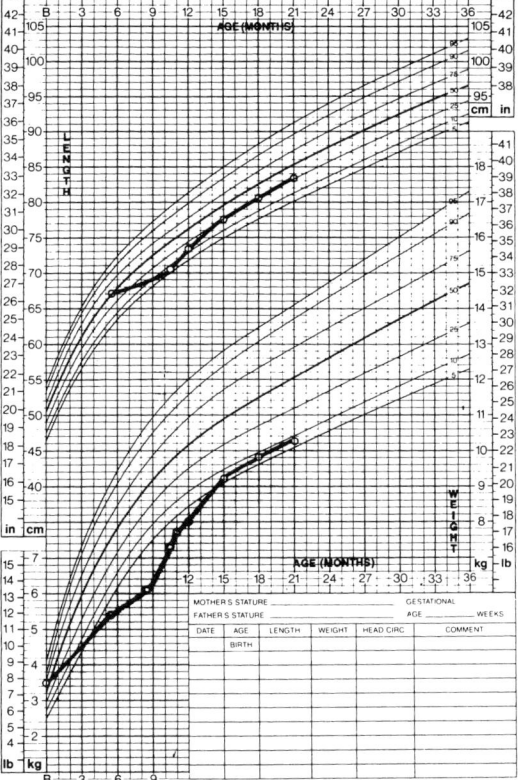

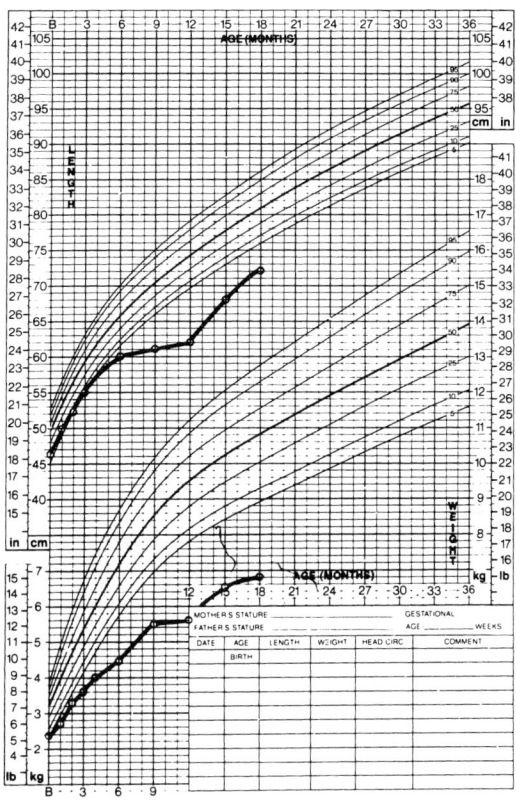

11 Example of giardiasis (contaminated family water supply) treated at age 12 months. (From Sturtz GS: Common Sense Guide to Growth and Nutrition, p 61. Watertown, NY, Hojack Publishing Company, 1991.)

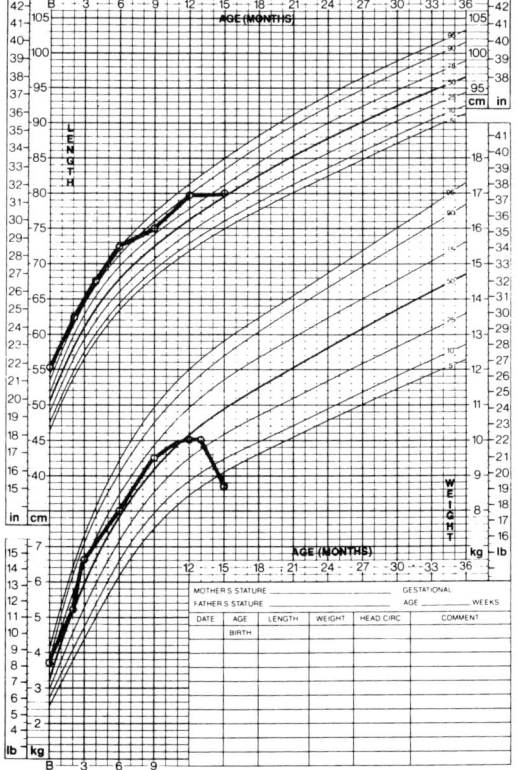

12 Example of celiac disease, beginning at 12 months and diagnosed at 15 months. Gluten-free diet led to appropriate weight gain. (From Sturtz GS: Common Sense Guide to Growth and Nutrition, p 93. Watertown, NY, Hojack Publishing Company, 1991.)

4 Developmental Surveillance

Linda N. Meurer

Etiology

1. Definitions
   a. Developmental screening—assessment of whole populations of children to identify those at high risk for developmental delay for whom more intensive investigation may be warranted; may involve the administration of brief tests
   b. Developmental surveillance—flexible, continuous process whereby knowledgeable professionals longitudinally monitor a child's development in the context of his or her environmental and medical risk factors. Providers elicit and attend to parental concerns, review relevant developmental milestones, and make clinical judgments based on careful, skilled observation of age-appropriate tasks. Formal screening tests are sometimes used as adjuncts to clinical evaluation.
   c. Developmental assessment—detailed multidisciplinary investigation of demonstrated or suspected developmental delay, designed to be diagnostic and provide prognoses
   d. Developmental delay—broad term referring to a failure to reach developmental milestones appropriately. Children develop at different rates but acquire their developmental skills in a strikingly similar and predictable sequence. Delay may occur in any or all of several domains, including fine or gross motor (e.g., cerebral palsy), language, social (e.g., infantile autism), and cognitive skills (e.g., mental retardation).

2. Epidemiology of developmental delay
   a. Two to 5 per cent of children suffer from potentially reversible visual deficits.
   b. One to 2 per cent of infants and children have hearing deficits that may interfere with the development of language, social, and cognitive skills if not identified early.
   c. Gross motor delays are the easiest to identify very early and may be associated with other developmental delays. The level of motor delay, however, does not predict future cognitive abilities.
   d. An estimated 8.5 per cent of children under age 3 years have significant language delays. Disorders of communication are the most sensitive early predictors for cognitive and school difficulties.
   e. Although advocated for all, less than 15 per cent of children under age 5 receive regular screening for vision, hearing, language, and other developmental milestones. Providers fail to identify up to 95 per cent of preschool children with speech and language disorders.

3. Risk factors
   a. Medical
      (1) Hereditary disorders—gene and chromosomal aberrations, such as fragile X and Down syndromes, inborn errors of metabolism
      (2) Perinatal morbidity—fetal alcohol syndrome, fetal malnutrition, prematurity, hypoxic encephalopathy, low birth weight, intrauterine growth retardation
      (3) Acquired childhood diseases—infection, brain trauma, lead poisoning, iron deficiency, malnutrition
   b. Environmental
      (1) Social deprivation
      (2) Parents with emotional disturbances, mental retardation, substance abuse
      (3) Low socioeconomic status—associated with many other risk factors

Presentation and History

1. Developmental delay may be suspected by health professionals because of parental concerns, a history of risk factors, medical conditions, or physical findings likely to be associated with delays or demonstrated delays at the time of observation.
2. History for every child elicits potential risk factors and includes the following:
   a. Family history
   b. Pregnancy, labor, delivery
   c. Neonatal problems
   d. Illnesses and accidents
   e. Diet and growth
   f. Developmental milestones
   g. Family and home environment
3. Parental description of a child's development may be inaccurate and must be supplemented by the direct, skilled observation of professionals.
4. Developmental history can serve as an educational intervention by introducing developmental stages and stimulatory methods to parents.

Clinical Findings

Physical examination includes the following:
1. General examination with observation for malformations or dysmorphology
2. Growth pattern
3. Neurologic examination
4. Hearing and vision tests (see below)
5. Direct observation of developmental milestones in the various domains

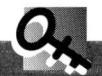

Key Components of Screening Process

- Sensitive attention to parental concerns
- Thoughtful inquiry about parental observations
- Observations of a wide variety of child's behaviors
- Examination of specific developmental attainments
- Use of all encounters for observing and recording developmental status
- Screening of vision and hearing to rule out sensory impairment as cause
- Observation of parent-child interaction

American Academy of Pediatrics Committee on Children with Disabilities

Screening Tests

1. All children should be screened for hearing deficits by age 3 and for vision, amblyopia, and strabismus by ages 3 to 4. Auditory brain stem response testing should be considered for neonates at high risk for hearing impairment. Vision and hearing deficits should be considered in any child with suspected developmental delay.

2. Developmental screening tests should be viewed as one of many sources of information obtained over multiple points in time to monitor child development.

   a. They are meant to identify children at high risk or with suspected delay who may benefit from further developmental assessment.

   b. They are not diagnostic or designed to predict function or IQ.

   c. Major pediatric organizations in the United States and Great Britain do not advocate routine administration of formal screening tests to all children but recommend their use to reinforce suspicions of delay and to monitor children at risk for developmental problems.

3. The Denver Developmental Screening Test (DDST), revised as the Denver II, is the best known instrument and is used worldwide (Fig. 4–1). Features of the DDST are as follows:

   a. Designed to be used with apparently well children between birth and age 6 years

   b. Administered by assessing a child's performance on age-appropriate tasks in four areas

      (1) Personal-social—getting along with people and caring for personal needs

      (2) Fine motor–adaptive—eye-hand coordination, manipulation of small objects, problem solving

      (3) Language—hearing, understanding, using language

      (4) Gross motor—sitting, walking, jumping, overall large muscle movement

   c. The DDST also serves as a valuable aid to provider memory and helps to communicate interest in the child's development and encourage parents to raise questions.

4. Other useful screening instruments include the following:

   a. Minnesota Child Development Inventory—for screening general development and conceptual, number, fine motor, and language skills

   b. Early Language Milestones (ELM)—for testing language skills in children under age 3

   c. Clinical Linguistic and Auditory Milestones Scale (CLAMS)—for testing language development in all children and cognitive development in children with motor delays

   d. Milani-Comparetti scale—for assessing motor skills

   e. Simultaneous Technique for Acuity and Readiness Testing (START)—for testing vision and general development

   f. Stanford-Binet—for estimating intelligence

   g. Home Screening Questionnaire (HSQ)—for identifying high-risk home environments

5. Additional tests may be necessary to determine the cause of an identified developmental delay and might include chromosomal and DNA testing, metabolic screening, thyroid studies, imaging studies such as computed tomography and magnetic resonance imaging, and others.

Interventions

1. Primary prevention

   a. Educate pregnant women as to the importance of good nutrition and avoidance of alcohol and drugs.

   b. Improve parental understanding of normal child development and developmental expectations, assist understanding of the individual developmental characteristics and temperament of their child, and encourage parental feelings of confidence and competence to affect their child's development.

2. Secondary prevention

   a. Perform developmental surveillance in all children, using all encounters as opportunities to observe developmental progress.

   b. Recognize high-risk medical and environmental situations and early delay.

   c. Obtain a complete developmental assessment of children with suspected delay.

   d. Rescreen periodically as expectations change.

3. Tertiary prevention

   a. Maintain updated information on community resources for children and families at risk for or with developmental delay.

   b. Maintain linkages with these resources and coordinate patient care with them.

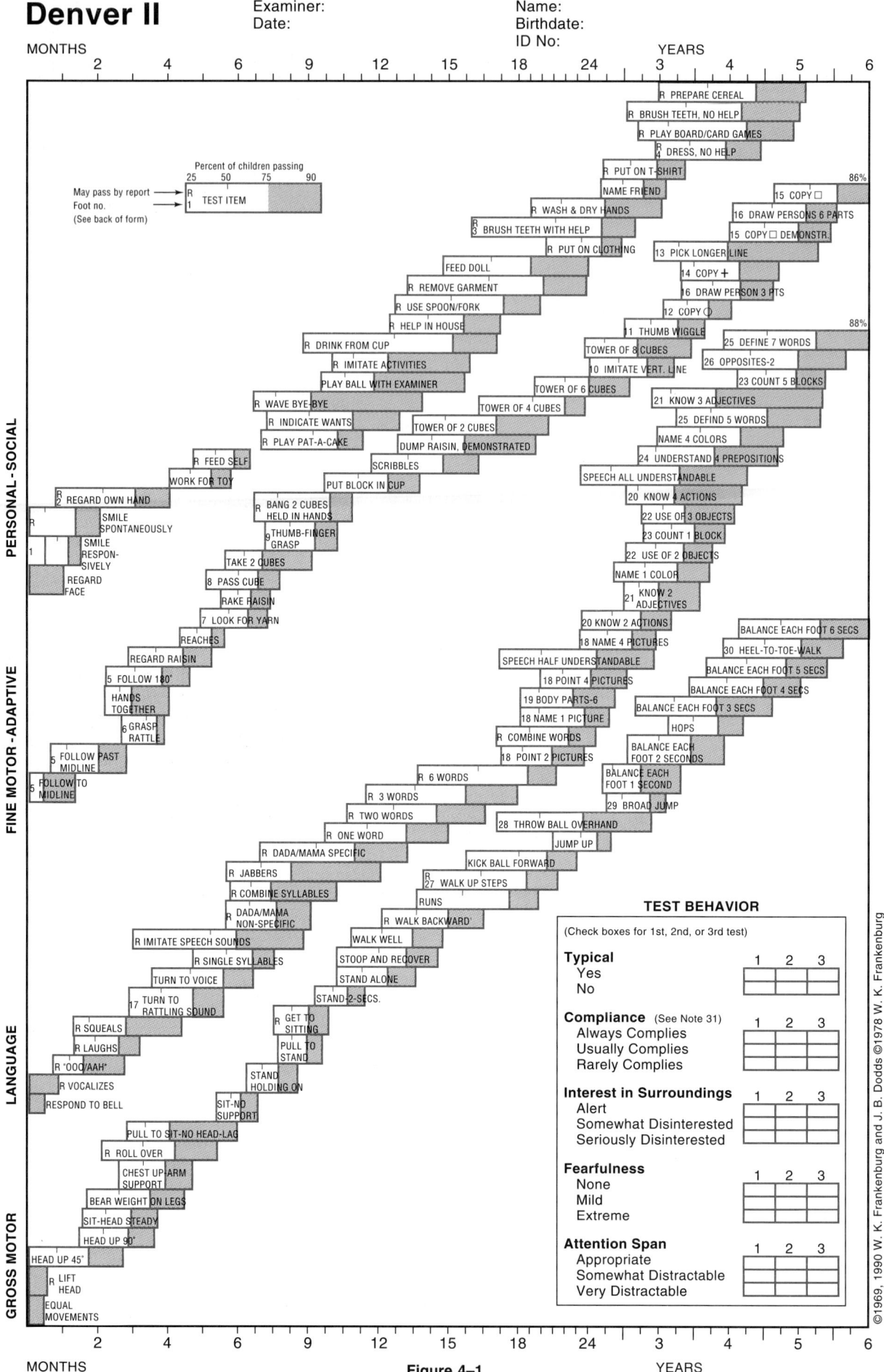

Figure 4–1

20

DIRECTIONS FOR ADMINISTRATION

1. Try to get child to smile by smiling, talking or waving. Do not touch him/her.
2. Child must stare at hand several seconds.
3. Parent may help guide toothbrush and put toothpaste on brush.
4. Child does not have to be able to tie shoes or button/zip in the back.
5. Move yarn slowly in an arc from one side to the other, about 8" above child's face.
6. Pass if child grasps rattle when it is touched to the backs or tips of fingers.
7. Pass if child tries to see where yarn went. Yarn should be dropped quickly from sight from tester's hand without arm movement.
8. Child must transfer cube from hand to hand without help of body, mouth, or table.
9. Pass if child picks up raisin with any part of thumb and finger.
10. Line can vary only 30 degrees or less from tester's line.
11. Make a fist with thumb pointing upward and wiggle only the thumb. Pass if child imitates and does move any fingers other than the thumb.

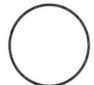 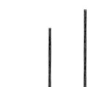 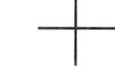 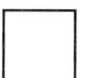

12. Pass any enclosed form. Fail continuous round motions.
13. Which line is longer? (Not bigger.) Turn paper upside down and repeat. (pass 3 of 3 or 5 of 6)
14. Pass any lines crossing near midpoint.
15. Have child copy first. If failed, demonstrate.

When giving items 12, 14, and 15, do not name the forms. Do not demonstrate 12 and 14.

16. When scoring, each pair (2 arms, 2 legs. etc.) counts as one part.
17. Place one cube in cup and shake gently near child's ear, but out of sight. Repeat for other ear.
18. Point to picture and have child name it. (No credit is given for sounds only.)
    If less than 4 pictures are named correctly, have child point to picture as each is named by tester.

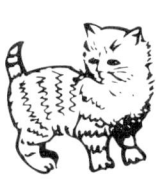 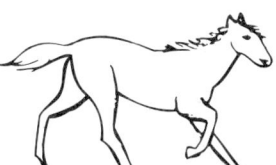 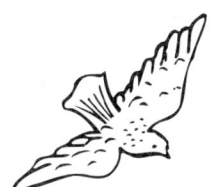 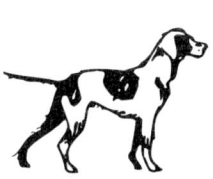 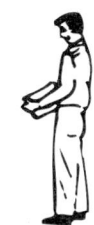

19. Using doll, tell child: Show me the nose, eyes, mouth, hands, feet, tummy, hair. Pass 6 of 8.
20. Using pictures, ask child: Which one flies?... says meow?... talks?... gallops? Pass 2 of 5, 4 of 5.
21. Ask child: What do you do when you are cold?... tired?...hungry? Pass 2 of 3, 3 of 3.
22. Ask child: What do you do with a cup? What is a chair used for? What is a pencil used for? Action words must be included in answers.
23. Pass if child correctly places <u>and</u> says how many blocks are on paper. (1, 5).
24. Tell child: Put block **on** table; **under** table; **in front of** me, **behind** me. Pass 4 of 4. (Do not help child by pointing, moving head or eyes.)
25. Ask child: What is a ball?... lake?... desk?... house?... banana?... curtain?... fence?... ceiling?... Pass if defined in terms of use, shape, what it is made of, or general category (such as banana is fruit, not just yellow). Pass 5 of 8, 7 of 8.
26. Ask child: If a horse is big, a mouse is__? If fire is hot, ice is__? If the sun shines during the day, the moon shines during the__? Pass 2 of 3.
27. Child may use wall or rail only, not person. May not crawl.
28. Child must throw ball overhand 3 feet to within arm's reach of tester.
29. Child must perform standing broad jump over width of test sheet (8 1/2 inches).
30. Tell child to walk forward, ⊂∞⊂∞⊂∞ ➔ heel within 1 inch of toe. Tester may demonstrate. Child must walk 4 consecutive steps.
31. In the second year, half of normal children are non-compliant.

OBSERVATIONS:

Figure 4–1 *Continued*

B Bibliography

American Academy of Pediatrics Committee on Children with Disabilities: Screening infants and young children for developmental disabilities. Pediatrics 1994;93(5):863–865.

Casey PH, Bradley RH, Caldwell BM, Edwards DR: Developmental intervention: A pediatric clinical review. Pediatr Clin North Am 1986;33(4):899–923.

Dworkin PH: British and American recommendations for developmental monitoring: The role of surveillance. Pediatrics 1989;84(6):1000–1010.

Frankenburg WK, Dodds J, Archer P, et al: Denver II Training Manual, 2nd ed. Denver, Denver Developmental Materials, 1992, pp 1–4.

United States Department of Health and Human Services: Healthy people 2000: National health promotion and disease prevention objectives. Washington, DC, DHHS Publication No. (PHS) 91-50212, 1990.

5 Preoperative Evaluation

Juan Galarraga

Cardiac Risks of Noncardiac Surgery

Background

The major risk factors for perioperative cardiac complications, such as acute myocardial infarction (MI) and sudden cardiac death, are the following:

1. Active congestive heart failure (CHF)
2. Unstable angina
3. MI within the previous 6 months
4. Critical aortic stenosis
5. Dysrhythmias, ventricular and supraventricular

Symptoms

1. Shortness of breath at rest or on exertion
2. Chest pain or other anginal equivalent
3. Prolonged palpitations, syncope, presyncope

Clinical Findings

1. Pulmonary crackles, increased jugular venous pressure
2. Gallop rhythm, irregular rhythm
3. Systolic murmur second right intercostal space, left sternal border, with or without carotid radiation; delayed carotid upstrokes

Tests

Dependent on history and clinical findings

1. Patients under age 40 with negative medical history and normal examination generally do not require preoperative testing.
2. Electrocardiogram should be obtained in patients with known cardiac history or symptoms suggestive of angina or dysrhythmia.
3. Echocardiogram is needed in patients with known or suspected aortic stenosis.
4. Twenty-four-hour electrocardiographic monitoring may be indicated in patients with known dysrhythmia or in those with suspected cardiogenic syncope.
5. Stress testing should be performed if there is suspicion of undiagnosed coronary disease; chronic stable angina is not an indication for preoperative stress testing.

Management

1. In general, all usual cardiac and antihypertensive medications should be taken on the morning of surgery with a sip of water. Some clinicians withhold diuretics to enhance volume status and thereby minimize anesthesia-induced hypotension.
2. Elective surgery should be postponed in patients who have had an MI within the previous 6 months; if postponement is not an option, there is evidence that an aggressive approach consisting of cardiac catheterization and angioplasty may reduce cardiac risk to an acceptable level.
3. Active CHF should be treated in the usual manner until well compensated; in the hospitalized patient, placement of a Swan-Ganz catheter may optimize this process and may help with intraoperative fluid management. Well-compensated CHF is not a contraindication to surgery.
4. Unstable angina should be treated in the usual manner; elective surgery should be postponed. Either optimized medical management or invasive testing may be pursued, depending on the patient's course. Chronic stable angina is not a contraindication to surgery.
5. In patients with critical aortic stenosis (commonly defined as peak systolic pressure gradient greater than 70 mm Hg or a valve area less than 0.6 cm/m^2 of body surface), consideration should be given to valve replacement or valvuloplasty before elective procedures.
6. Dysrhythmias
   a. Treatment of dysrhythmias known to exist preoperatively should be continued. Chronic atrial fibrillation increases perioperative morbidity and mortality, and chemical or electrical conversion should be considered before elective surgery if fibrillation is of short duration (usually less than 12 months) and left atrial size is preserved (usually less than 4.5 cm in diameter).
   b. Sustained or complex dysrhythmias that occur acutely in the intraoperative or postoperative period warrant complete evaluation of metabolic causes (arterial blood gas analysis, electrolyte panel with Ca^+ and Mg^+); acute MI, exacerbation of CHF, and pulmonary embolism should also be considered.

Special Situations

1. Patients undergoing peripheral vascular procedures or those known to have peripheral vascular disease have a high incidence (up to 60 per cent) of concurrent coronary disease; these patients should be screened

preoperatively with pharmacologic stress testing that includes an imaging modality (e.g., dipyridamole-thallium) to evaluate the extent of the myocardium at risk.

2. Similarly, carotid stenosis has been found to be a fairly good marker for coronary disease (up to 35 per cent); it is prudent to screen these patients noninvasively with stress testing as well.

The Bleeding Patient

Background

Although prolonged postoperative bleeding is clinically uncommon, all patients undergoing preoperative evaluation should be specifically asked regarding previous spontaneous or prolonged surgical bleeding, including dental procedures. When confronted with a bleeding patient, the first task is to differentiate between coagulation disorders and disorders of platelet numbers or function. The most common conditions are the following:

1. Inherited coagulation disorders
   a. Hemophilia A and B
   b. Von Willebrand's disease (VWD)
2. Acquired coagulation disorders
   a. Vitamin K deficiency
   b. Disseminated intravascular coagulation (DIC)
   c. Liver disease
   d. Drugs, especially warfarin and some second-generation cephalosporins (e.g., cefamandole [Mandol])
3. Quantitative platelet disorders—thrombocytopenia
4. Qualitative platelet disorders
   a. Aspirin and nonsteroidal anti-inflammatory drugs
   b. Renal insufficiency, uremia

Symptoms and Clinical Findings

1. Bleeding into soft tissues or retroperitoneum with hematoma formation suggests coagulation defects.
2. Mucosal bleeding suggests platelet disorders, as does the presence of petechiae or purpura.
3. The occurrence of arterial or venous thrombosis in a bleeding patient suggests DIC.

Tests

1. Prothrombin time (PT) and activated partial thromboplastin time (APTT). These tests should be done in patients with known coagulation disorders or in those undergoing major procedures (e.g., intrathoracic, intra-abdominal). Although the hemophilias cause an elevation of the APTT with a normal PT, a more common cause of this finding in otherwise healthy people is the presence of antiphospholipid antibodies ("lupus anticoagulant"). Despite an elevated APTT, these antibodies predispose to thrombosis rather than bleeding, and their presence does not contraindicate surgery. Patients with VWD may or may not have an elevated APTT; their PT is normal. Vitamin K deficiency, DIC, and liver disease may show an increase in one or both tests, depending on severity.

2. Platelet count should also be obtained in patients with a history of a bleeding disorder or those undergoing major procedures. The differential diagnosis of thrombocytopenia is extensive and will not be discussed here. It is usually part of the DIC picture and may be seen in liver disease due to splenic sequestration.

3. The bleeding time measures platelet function and is typically prolonged (greater than 10 minutes) by aspirin and nonsteroidal anti-inflammatory drugs, renal insufficiency or uremia, cirrhosis, and VWD. It should be obtained in selected patients, not routinely.

4. Other useful tests include fibrinogen, which is usually decreased in DIC and liver disease; fibrin degradation products are increased in DIC.

Management

1. Desmopressin (DDAVP) infusion at a dose of 0.3 μg/kg over 15 to 30 minutes is temporarily effective in achieving hemostasis in hemophilia A, VWD, and uremia. Its effect lasts about 6 hours, and tachyphylaxis may develop with continued use; it is most useful in emergency situations.

2. Patients with hemophilia A and VWD should receive an initial dose of cryoprecipitate of 0.1 to 0.5 bags/kg (1 bag = 15 ml, approximately) preceding surgery, followed by a maintenance dose of 0.1 to 0.3 bags/kg q 12 to 24 hr. Patients with hemophilia A may instead be given factor VIII concentrate at an initial dose of 30 units/kg followed by maintenance at 10 to 20 units/kg q 12 hr. VWD may also be treated with fresh frozen plasma (FFP) at an initial dose of 10 to 15 ml/kg followed by 10 to 15 ml/kg q 24 hr (1 unit FFP = 250 ml, approximately), although cryoprecipitate is favored. Factor VIII concentrate is not useful in the treatment of VWD.

3. Patients with hemophilia B are treated with FFP at an initial dose of 40 ml/kg followed by a maintenance dose of 10 to 15 ml/kg q 12 hr.

4. Vitamin K deficiency may be corrected by subcutaneous injection of 2.5 to 10 mg of vitamin K daily; intravenous administration may be used to achieve more rapid correction but must be given no faster than 1 mg/min because of the risk of anaphylaxis. In acute bleeding, FFP should be given at an initial dose of 10 to 20 ml/kg followed by maintenance at 10 ml/kg q 6 to 12 hr. This latter regimen also applies to coagulopathy due to liver disease, which fails to correct with vitamin K therapy.

5. Treatment of DIC is aimed at the underlying illness. Bleeding is treated with FFP in the same initial and

maintenance doses used in vitamin K deficiency. Platelet transfusions may also be required, typically when platelets fall below the 10,000 to 20,000/mm³ range; 6 to 8 units of platelets are given initially and platelet counts are followed. In rare instances, thrombosis occurs in DIC, and full heparinization is necessary. Concurrent bleeding and thrombosis present a difficult problem; therapy must be individualized in these cases.

6. Abnormal surgical bleeding is said to be unusual at platelet counts greater than 75,000/mm³. Some authorities contend that minor procedures may be performed with counts as low as 50,000/mm³; this probably represents the minimum requirement, and every effort should be made to increase platelet counts beyond the 50,000/mm³ value before emergency surgery. Platelet transfusions are usually given in 6- to 8-unit increments and counts are followed.

The Patient with Lung Disease

Background

Asthma and chronic obstructive pulmonary disease (COPD) are the most common chronic pulmonary illnesses. In COPD, some studies suggest a slightly increased mortality (up to 8 per cent versus 0 to 2 per cent in non-COPD patients); other studies do not show a significant difference. What is clear, however, is that patients with obstructive lung disease have a higher incidence of pulmonary complications (about 30 per cent in most studies). The most common complications are as follows:

1. Asthma—bronchospasm and inspissated secretions
2. COPD—atelectasis and postoperative purulent bronchitis

Symptoms

1. Dyspnea, wheezing, rhonchi
2. Productive cough—best clinical predictor of postoperative complications

Clinical Findings

1. Barrel chest, hyperresonance, intercostal retractions, cyanosis, clubbing, active wheezing, rhonchi
2. Smoking history in pack-years may be a clue to subclinical disease.

Tests

1. Except in patients undergoing lung resection, the use of preoperative pulmonary function tests (PFTs) is controversial, even in patients with known disease. Although some authorities recommend PFTs for high-risk patients (e.g., over age 60, history of asthma or COPD, smoker, anesthesia requirement longer than 2 hours, upper abdominal or thoracic surgery), others emphasize that the ability of PFTs to predict morbidity and mortality in the general surgical patient is unproven.

2. A minimum pulmonary reserve in terms of PFTs has been identified as necessary for general anesthesia: forced expiratory volume at 1 second (FEV_1) greater than 500 ml and forced vital capacity (FVC) greater than 1 L. Again, these are bare minimum values, and all but the most end-stage pulmonary patients should be able to meet these requirements.

3. As with PFTs, the use of routine preoperative arterial blood gas analyses and chest radiographs is not established and must be individualized.

4. Patients undergoing lung resection (pneumonectomy, lobectomy, segmental resection) should have preoperative PFTs. For pneumonectomy, the patient must fulfill the following criteria:
   a. FEV_1 greater than 2 L
   b. Maximum breathing capacity greater than 50 per cent of predicted
   c. FVC greater than 50 per cent of predicted

5. If all criteria are met, the patient can tolerate pneumonectomy. If any of the criteria is not met, the patient must undergo split-function pulmonary studies. Quantitative perfusion lung scanning most commonly is done to determine the relative contribution (expressed as a percentage) of each lung to the total pulmonary capacity. A prediction of the patient's postoperative FEV_1 is obtained using the following formula: measured FEV_1 × percentage of perfusion in remaining lung. An estimated postoperative FEV_1 of 800 to 1000 ml is considered necessary for any type of lung resection.

Management

1. Stop smoking 2 weeks before an elective procedure.
2. Aggressive use of postural drainage, chest physiotherapy, and incentive spirometry can reduce pulmonary complications in COPD patients.
3. Administration of β_2-agonist bronchodilators should be continued by means of a nebulizer both preoperatively and postoperatively.
4. Patients who have taken systemic steroids within the past year should receive stress doses of parenteral steroids to avoid adrenal crisis. Patients taking inhaled steroids may need parenteral steroid coverage to avoid exacerbation of their pulmonary disease during the perioperative period.
5. Theophylline has become the second- or third-line

treatment in obstructive lung disease; therefore, it is unlikely to be used intraoperatively. When doing so, levels should be reduced because its toxicity may be enhanced by general anesthetics.

6. Patients with preoperative productive cough should be given a short course of broad-spectrum antibiotics. Although antibiotics do not decrease postoperative pulmonary infections, they do decrease the volume of secretions in COPD patients.

7. In the asthmatic patient, it is especially important to avoid drying of secretions by the liberal use of preoperative intravenous hydration.

Bibliography

Huber KC, Evans MA, Bresnahan JF, et al: Outcome of noncardiac operations in patients with severe coronary disease treated preoperatively with coronary angioplasty. Mayo Clin Proc 1992;67:15–21.

Maziak DE, et al: Preoperative cardiac evaluation of the patient with vascular disease. Can J Surg 1994;37:95–103.

Messmore HL Jr, et al: Medical assessment of bleeding in the surgical patient. Med Clin North Am 1994;78:625–634.

Wong T, Detsky AS: Preoperative cardiac risk assessment for patients having peripheral vascular surgery. Ann Intern Med 1992;116:743–753.

Zibrak JD, O'Donnell CR, Marton K: Indications for pulmonary function testing. Ann Intern Med 1990;112:763–770.

6 Advance Directives

Steven A. Levy

If I should become terminally ill and incompetent to make my own decisions, this declaration reflects my firm commitment to refuse life-sustaining treatment. I direct my attending physician to withhold or withdraw life-sustaining treatment that serves only to prolong the process of my dying.

How aggressive should we be in treating people with terminal conditions when they are no longer able to make their own decisions? Advance directives can help us answer this question. An advance directive is a legal document that allows competent adults to express their intentions regarding medical treatment if they should lose decision-making capacity secondary to terminal illness. Two types of advance directives exist:

1. Treatment directive (living will)
2. Proxy directive (durable power of attorney)

Living Will

In a living will, a person states his or her preference for various forms of medical treatment (Fig. 6–1). A general statement (as in the example above) is often followed by a list of procedures, including but not limited to the following:

1. Cardiopulmonary resuscitation (CPR)
2. Mechanical ventilation
3. Dialysis
4. Surgery
5. Antibiotic therapy
6. Blood administration
7. Nutrition

The person states which, if any, of these interventions is to be performed in a terminal illness.

Such conditions as severe and irreversible dementia and persistent vegetative state often are considered as terminal illness. Vague terms such as "heroic and extraordinary measures" and "artificial life support" that appeared in earlier forms of living wills have been replaced by a list of specific procedures.

Durable Power of Attorney

The most common type of proxy directive is a durable power of attorney. An individual (a principal) names a person (surrogate) to act on his or her behalf if he or she should become incompetent. A durable power of attorney differs from a power of attorney. In the former, the authorization to act includes times when the principal lacks decision-making capacity. In the latter, the surrogate is no longer empowered to act once the principal's competency is lost. Indeed, some durable power of attorney documents do not take effect until the principal becomes incompetent.

In contrast to living wills, which deal only with end-of-life decision making, a durable power of attorney for health care usually applies to a broader range of clinical decisions (i.e., admission to hospital, various medical and surgical procedures).

Patient Self-Determination Act

On December 1, 1991, Congress enacted the Patient Self-Determination Act, which sought to heighten people's awareness of advance directives. Many states have similar laws. The act mandates that health care facilities: 1. inform patients of their right to decide whether or not they want various medical and surgical therapies, and 2. provide information on advance directives. Under this law, however, people are not required to formulate or possess advance directives. The federal act applies to all health care facilities that receive Medicare and Medicaid funds. This includes hospitals, health maintenance organizations, nursing homes, hospices, and home care programs.

Good Faith

When presented with an advance directive, a physician may, as a matter of conscience, be unable to comply with its provisions. A physician also may not agree that such a document applies to the given clinical situation. Some states confer immunity on physicians in such cases, provided that they are acting in good faith. Acting in good faith includes notifying the family or surrogate of one's moral objection to withdrawing or withholding a therapy. It also includes attempting to transfer the patient to another physician who will comply with the directive. Under these circumstances, various states will confer immunity from civil and criminal liability on a noncomplying physician.

Applications of Living Wills

The important feature to remember about living wills is that they only apply when a patient lacks decision-making capacity *and* is in a terminal condition (i.e., metastatic cancer, end-stage AIDS, persistent vegetative state). For instance, if an otherwise healthy 18-year-old is unconscious after a motor vehicle accident and in shock from a ruptured spleen, a living will is not applicable. This patient has a treatable problem, despite the fact that he or she lacks decision-making capacity. Conversely, a debilitated, cachectic nursing home patient with metastatic lung cancer who is alert, oriented, and responding appropriately is able to answer for himself or herself. The family and physician need not consult a living will.

LIVING WILL

I, _____, being of sound mind, willfully and voluntarily make this declaration to be followed if I become incompetent. This declaration reflects my firm and settled commitment to refuse life-sustaining treatment under the circumstances indicated below.

I direct my attending physician to withhold or withdraw life-sustaining treatment that serves only to prolong the process of my dying, if I should be in a terminal condition or in a state of permanent unconsciousness.

I direct that treatment be limited to measures to keep me comfortable and to relieve pain, including any pain that might occur by withholding or withdrawing life-sustaining treatment.

In addition, if I am in the condition described above, I feel especially strong about the following forms of treatment:

I ( ) do ( ) do not want cardiac resuscitation.
I ( ) do ( ) do not want mechanical respiration.
I ( ) do ( ) do not want tube feeding or any other artificial or invasive form of nutrition (food) or hydration (water).
I ( ) do ( ) do not want blood or blood products.
I ( ) do ( ) do not want any form of surgery or invasive diagnostic tests.
I ( ) do ( ) do not want kidney dialysis.
I ( ) do ( ) do not want antibiotics.

I realize that if I do not specifically indicate my preference regarding any of the forms of treatment listed above, I may receive that form of treatment.

OTHER INSTRUCTIONS:

I ( ) do ( ) do not want to designate another person as my surrogate to make medical treatment decisions for me if I should be incompetent and in a terminal condition or in a state of permanent unconsciousness. Name and address of surrogate (if applicable):

Name of Surrogate: _____

Address of Surrogate: _____
_____
_____
_____

Name and address of substitute surrogate (if surrogate designated above is unable to serve):

Substitute Surrogate: _____

Address of Substitute: _____
_____
_____
_____

I made this declaration on the _____ day of _____ (mo) _____ (yr)

Declarant's signature: _____

Declarant's address: _____
_____
_____
_____

The declarant or the person on behalf of and at the direction of the declarant knowingly and voluntarily signed this writing by signature or mark in my presence.

Witness's signature: _____

Witness's address: _____
_____
_____
_____

Witness's signature: _____

Witness's address: _____
_____
_____
_____

Figure 6–1

Concept of Futility

The concept of futility inevitably enters the conversation when making end-of-life decisions. A physician is under no ethical obligation to provide a diagnostic or therapeutic intervention, even if specifically requested, if it would be futile to do so. However, the term "futility" has many interpretations. They include the following:

- No physiologic benefit results from an intervention because the patient's vital signs are deteriorating despite maximum therapy or, as in the case of resuscitation,
- No survivors after CPR have been reported under the given circumstances in well-designed studies.

The process of defining futility should respect patient autonomy whenever possible. Judgments about what is or is not futile are most appropriate when the informed patient is able to participate in the decision-making process. People vary in their beliefs about what is beneficial or a desirable goal. In the absence of a competent, informed patient, a living will or proxy directive can help a physician make end-of-life decisions. Otherwise, physicians face a most challenging decision: how to apply their own values and beliefs in the best interest of a terminally ill, incompetent patient.

 Bibliography

Annas GJ: The health care proxy and the living will. N Engl J Med 1991; 324:1210–1213.

Bennett AJ: When is medical treatment "futile"? Issues Law Med 1993; 9:35–45.

Ethical considerations in resuscitation—guidelines for CPR. JAMA 1992;268(16):2282–2288.

Guidelines for the appropriate use of do-not-resuscitate orders. Council on Ethical and Judicial Affairs, American Medical Association. JAMA 1991; 265(14):1868–1871.

Healey JM: The emerging legal consensus about end of life decisions. Conn Med 1993; 57:351–352.

7 Cancer Screening

Lori A. Whittaker

Colorectal Cancer

Risk Factors

1. Age greater than 50
2. Personal history of colorectal cancer, colorectal adenomas, inflammatory bowel disease, Peutz-Jeghers syndrome, or breast, ovarian, endometrial, or prostate cancer
3. Family history of colorectal cancer, cancer family syndrome, familial polyposis, or Gardner's syndrome
4. High-fat and/or low-fiber diet

Screening Guidelines

1. General screening

   - Digital rectal examination annually after age 40
   - Fecal occult blood testing annually after age 50
   - Flexible sigmoidoscopy every 3 to 5 years after age 50

2. High-risk patients: screening at an earlier age, more frequently, or with full colonoscopy

Future Perspectives

1. Genetic testing in families with inherited colorectal cancer syndromes (e.g., familial polyposis [gene-cloned])
2. Detection of oncogenes or other biologic markers in stool or serum of patients with early colorectal cancers

Breast Cancer

Risk Factors

1. Age over 50
2. Personal history of breast, colon, endometrial, or ovarian cancer
3. Family history of breast cancer or cancer family syndrome
4. Cellular atypia or lobular carcinoma in situ on breast biopsy
5. Nulliparity or low parity; greater than age 30 at first live birth; early menarche or late menopause

Factors not shown to increase risk include oral contraceptive use, hormone replacement therapy, and high-fat diet.

Screening Guidelines

1. General screening

   - Monthly breast self-examination beginning at age 20
   - Professional breast examination every 3 years at ages 20 through 39 and then annually after age 40
   - Annual mammogram after age 50

   Benefits of screening mammography before age 50 and after age 70 are controversial. Screening in these age groups should be individualized.

2. High-risk women: earlier or more frequent screening

Future Perspectives

Genetic testing in high-risk families (e.g., for *BRCA1*, a gene on chromosome 17q implicated in many inherited breast cancers and breast–ovarian cancer syndrome)

Cervical Cancer

Risk Factors

1. Infection with human papillomavirus types 16, 18, 31, 33, 35, 45, 51, 52, 56
2. Early age at first intercourse
3. Multiple sexual partners
4. Male partner in a high-risk group
5. Low socioeconomic status
6. Smoking

Screening Guidelines

General screening: annual Pap smear and pelvic examination at onset of sexual activity or by age 18
Some clinicians opt to perform Pap smear less frequently after three consecutive normal Pap smears.

Future Perspectives

1. Improved sensitivity with adjuncts to the Pap smear (e.g., cervicography, fluorescent spectroscopy)
2. Human papillomavirus typing to identify patients at high risk
3. Identification of biologic markers that correlate with increased risk

Endometrial Cancer

Risk Factors

1. Menopause
2. History of infertility or anovulatory cycles
3. Obesity
4. Late menopause
5. History of unopposed estrogen replacement
6. Tamoxifen therapy

Decreased risk is associated with the use of oral contraceptives.

Screening Guidelines

1. General screening: not recommended
2. High-risk or symptomatic women: endometrial biopsy at menopause or at onset of symptoms such as abnormal uterine bleeding in women over age 40

Ovarian Cancer

Risk Factors

1. Personal history of breast, endometrial, or colon cancer
2. Family history of ovarian, breast, endometrial, or colon cancer
3. History of infertility or use of infertility drugs
4. Nulliparity
5. Perineal talc exposure

Screening Guidelines

1. General screening: annual pelvic examination beginning at age 18
2. High-risk screening: no current recommendations

Screening modalities such as transvaginal pelvic ultrasound, color flow Doppler of ovarian vessels, and determination of Ca-125 levels may be appropriate in high-risk patients (studies ongoing).

Future Perspectives

Genetic testing in high-risk families (e.g., *BRCA1* gene in breast–ovarian cancer syndrome)

Prostate Cancer

Risk Factors

1. Age greater than 50
2. African-American descent
3. Family history of prostate, breast, endometrial, or colon cancer
4. Personal history of colon cancer
5. High-fat diet
6. Occupational exposure to cadmium or rubber
7. Previous vasectomy (possible)

Screening Guidelines

General screening

- Annual digital rectal examination after age 40
- Annual prostate specific antigen level after age 50

Future Perspectives

Studies ongoing to determine the value of early prostate cancer detection

Testicular Cancer

Risk Factors

1. Ages 15 through 40 and after 60
2. White race
3. Undescended testis

Screening Guidelines

General screening

- Monthly testicular self-examination beginning at ages 13 to 14
- Annual professional testicular examination beginning at age 15

Lung Cancer

Risk Factors

1. Exposure to tobacco smoke (direct or secondhand)
2. Exposure to asbestos, radon gas, polyhydrocarbons

Screening Guidelines

No current recommendations
Frequent chest radiography or sputum cytology has not been shown to reduce mortality from lung cancer.

Future Perspectives

1. Detection of oncogenes, growth factors, or biologic markers in sputum samples of high-risk individuals
2. Identification of premalignant lesions by bronchoscopy in high-risk individuals and use of chemopreventive agents to halt progression of these lesions

Skin Cancer (Melanomatous and Nonmelanomatous)

Risk Factors

1. Cumulative sun exposure
2. Fair skin that burns easily; red or blond hair; freckles
3. History of blistering sunburns in childhood
4. Congenital nevi
5. Dysplastic nevi (high risk for melanoma if dysplastic nevi are present in an individual with a family history of melanoma)
6. History of skin cancer or preneoplastic lesions (e.g., actinic keratoses)
7. Xeroderma pigmentosum, albinism, basal cell nevus syndrome
8. Exposure to hydrocarbons, arsenic, or ionizing radiation

Screening Guidelines

1. General screening

   - Monthly thorough skin self-examination
   - Annual professional skin examination

2. High-risk screening: more frequent clinical examina-

tions suggested (e.g., up to every 4 months in patients with familial malignant melanoma–dysplastic nevus syndrome)

 Bibliography

For more information on general cancer screening, see
Daly MB: Cancer screening. *In* Weiss GR (ed): Clinical Oncology. E Norwalk, CT, Appleton & Lange, 1993, pp 35–40.

Maltese-McGill L: Cancer screening. Patient Care 1993; 27(4):34–67.

Morse RM, Heffron WA: Preventive health care in family practice. *In* Rakel RE (ed): Textbook of Family Practice, 4th ed. Philadelphia, WB Saunders, 1990, pp 232–238.

For more information on breast cancer screening, see
Harris JR, Lippman ME, Veronisi LL, et al: Breast cancer. N Engl J Med 1992;327:319–328.

For more information on colon cancer screening, see
Winawar SJ: Biologic basis for early detection of colorectal cancer. Adv Oncol 1992;9:9–13.

8 International Travel Disease Prevention

Robert Tao-Ping Chow

Each year, an estimated 8 million United States citizens travel to countries where tropic diseases are endemic. Most of these diseases are preventable through limiting exposure to infectious agents, obtaining appropriate vaccinations, and anticipating possible health hazards. When asked to provide advice to international travelers, physicians should carefully consider the travel itinerary as well as the pre-existing medical history of the traveler. Chronic obstructive lung disease, for example, may exacerbate at high altitudes, and achlorhydria increases susceptibility to enteric pathogens. After assessing the traveler's medical condition and the rigors of the proposed itinerary, the physician should provide counsel regarding the following:

1. Vaccinations (required and suggested)
2. Prevention of traveler's diarrhea
3. Malaria prophylaxis, if appropriate
4. Environmental illnesses

Vaccinations

Routine Vaccinations

1. Regardless of their destinations, travelers should be current with routine immunizations. These include the influenza, pneumococcal, measles, mumps, rubella, diphtheria, tetanus, and polio vaccinations. The recommended dosages and schedules appear in Chapter 1.
2. Tetanus and polio vaccinations warrant further comment. Certain high-risk travelers may need tetanus booster immunization every 5 years rather than every 10 years because patients with possible tetanus infection require either tetanus immune globulin or booster if they were vaccinated more than 5 years previously. Travelers who anticipate being in close contact with citizens of developing countries where polio may be endemic should consider immunization against polio. For those who received the primary series during childhood, one dose of the oral (OPV) or inactivated (IPV) polio vaccine conveys immunity. In adults, IPV is recommended over OPV because of the rare but real risk of vaccine-related paralytic polio.
3. A dosage schedule of required and recommended vaccines for adult travelers is provided in Table 8–1. Patients may receive multiple immunizations on the same day without apparent loss of efficacy. However, it is recommended that patients receive at most three live vaccines at one sitting, and live vaccines should be given at least 2 weeks before or 6 weeks after hepatitis A immunoglobulin.

Required Vaccinations

Certain countries require incoming travelers to provide proof of vaccination against yellow fever or cholera, as regulated by the World Health Organization (WHO). These vaccines are provided at state-designated vaccination centers and are charted on an official yellow "International Certificate of Health."

1. Those who travel to equatorial Africa or the jungle regions of South America should receive the yellow fever vaccine, irrespective of whether it is required. The vaccine is effective and confers immunity for 10 years.
2. The cholera vaccine has an estimated efficacy of only about 30 to 50 per cent. Although the primary cholera series requires two shots given at least 1 week apart, most healthy travelers are given a single dose because this vaccination suffices for WHO regulations. Cholera can be largely prevented by following hygienic precautions regarding proper use of food and water.

Recommended Vaccinations

1. Typhoid fever vaccination should be considered for travelers who will be exposed to potentially contaminated food or drink. Two forms of the vaccine exist: a parenterally administered inactivated form that requires two injections at least 4 weeks apart and an oral live, attenuated form taken over 1 week. The latter appears to confer a longer-lasting immunity than the inactivated form and has a lower incidence of side effects.
2. Epidemics of meningococcal meningitis have occurred in sub-Saharan Africa and Nepal. Travelers to these areas who anticipate significant contact with the local populace should receive meningococcal vaccine.
3. Rabies and plague vaccinations are recommended only for travelers who may have contact with potentially rabid animals or with wild rodents or rabbits. Plague occurs during warm, humid weather and is found in rural areas throughout the world. Candidates for vaccination include such people as farm workers, veterinarians, and hunters.
4. Japanese B encephalitis is transmitted by mosquitoes and has caused epidemics in the Far East, especially during the summer months. A killed vaccine should be administered in three shots with at least 1 week between each shot. The vaccine is available at health centers in Asia but not yet in the United States.
5. Hepatitis B vaccination is recommended for travelers who may contact the blood or secretions of infected

TABLE 8–1. VACCINE SCHEDULES FOR ADULT TRAVELERS

Vaccine	Dose	Boosters	Comments
Cholera	0.2 ml ID on days 0 and 7	Every 6 months; give concurrently with yellow fever vaccine or separate by 3 weeks	Rarely indicated; efficacy <30–50%; not recommended unless required by law at destination country
Hepatitis B	1.0 ml IM on day 0, 1 month, and 6 months	Every 5–7 years as needed based on titers	High prevalence in Asia and sub-Saharan Africa
Immune globulin	0.02 ml/kg (2.0 ml) IM 0.06 ml/kg (5.0 ml) IM	Every 3 months Every 5 months; give with or 2 weeks after live vaccines	Recommended for all travelers visiting developing countries, unless they have had hepatitis A
Measles-mumps-rubella	0.5 ml IM	Once if no booster given since 1980 and birth date after 1957	Worldwide risk; live vaccine
Meningococcal	0.5 ml SC	Every 3 years; polysaccharide vaccine	Risk in sub-Saharan Africa, the Himalayas, and for travelers to Mecca
Poliovirus, inactivated	0.5 ml SC	In adults (>12 years of age), one booster lasts for life	High risk in Asia and Africa; minimal risk in Americas
Poliovirus, oral/live	Single-dose unit	One adult booster; live vaccine	See above; potential for mutation of live virus to a paralytic strain
Rabies pre-exposure	1.0 ml IM on days 0, 7, and 21 or 28 0.1 ml ID on days 0, 7, and 28	Every 2 years or based on titers; if exposure occurs, 2 additional doses are needed	For occupational risk or children, especially long-term overseas residents
Tetanus-diphtheria	0.5 ml IM	Every 10 years or at 5 years with exposure	Recommended for all travelers
Typhoid injectable	0.5 ml SC on day 0 and 1 month later	Every 3 years with 0.1 ml ID	High risk for most travelers
Typhoid live/oral Ty21a	One capsule every other day for 4 doses	Every 5 years; live bacteria vaccine	Fewer side effects and better efficacy than injectable
Yellow fever	0.5 ml SC	Every 10 years; live vaccine; give with or 3 weeks apart from cholera vaccine	Required by some countries; risk in sub-Saharan Africa and Amazon basin

ID, intradermally; IM, intramuscularly; SC, subcutaneously.
Reprinted from the American Family Physician, published by the American Academy of Family Physicians, 1991; 44:1345.

people. Southeast Asia and sub-Saharan Africa have a high prevalence of hepatitis B.

6. Hepatitis A is prevalent throughout the developing world, and passive immunization is recommended for travelers to these regions. The dose is 0.02 ml/kg intramuscularly for visits less than 3 months and 0.06 ml/kg for those more than 3 months (repeat every 4 to 6 months). However, active immunization with hepatitis A vaccine (Havrix) is preferred. It is given as 1.0 ml intramuscularly 15 days before travel and a 1.0-ml booster dose in 6 to 12 months.

Traveler's Diarrhea Prevention

About 25 to 50 per cent of travelers to developing countries contract traveler's diarrhea. Because it is transmitted by way of the fecal-oral route, most cases can be prevented through careful hygienic measures. The clinical syndrome is described in more detail in Chapter 231.

1. Travelers should be counseled to avoid tap water, ice made from tap water, unpeeled fruits, raw vegetables, unpasteurized milk, dairy products, raw meat, and raw seafood. Tap water can be purified by boiling or by using iodine or chlorine additives (available at camping supply stores and pharmacies).

2. Foods should be cooked thoroughly and served steaming hot.

3. Bottled carbonated beverages, canned fruit juices, and beer and wine are usually safe.

4. Pharmacologic prophylaxis against traveler's diarrhea is controversial. Travelers at high risk may benefit from doxycycline, 100 mg once daily; trimethoprim-sulfamethoxazole (Bactrim, Septra), one double-strength tablet twice a day; or bismuth subsalicylate (Pepto-Bismol), two tablets four times a day. It is generally recommended that antibiotics be reserved for use if diarrhea occurs.

Malaria Prevention

1. Transmitted by the bites of infected female anopheline mosquitoes, malaria is caused by four species of the genus *Plasmodium*. It is endemic to many developing tropical countries, including Central America, South America, sub-Saharan Africa, India, Southeast Asia, and Oceanic Asia. Travelers to these areas should be instructed to use mosquito repellent that contains *N,N*-diethyl-*m*-toluamide, or DEET, daily and liberally, minimize exposed skin surfaces, sleep in screened or netted areas, and be especially vigilant during the evening or nighttime hours, when anopheline mosquitoes usually feed.

2. Pharmacologic prophylaxis is recommended in addition to these preventive measures. For travelers to Central America or the Middle East and Egypt, chloroquine (for adults, 300 mg of the base or 500 mg of the phosphate salt) should be taken weekly, starting the week before entering and continuing until 6 weeks

after leaving the endemic area. *Plasmodium falciparum* in the remainder of the world has become chloroquine-resistant. Adult travelers to those areas should take mefloquine (Lariam), 250 mg, once a week for 4 weeks and every other week thereafter. Mefloquine should be started 1 week before entering and continued for 4 weeks after leaving the endemic area. Travelers who have experienced heavy mosquito exposure should be considered candidates for a 2-week course of primaquine after finishing chloroquine or mefloquine, to prevent relapse caused by the exoerythrocytic hepatic phase of *Plasmodium vivax* or *Plasmodium ovale*. The clinician should be familiar with the potentially serious side effects and drug interactions of these agents before administration.

3. Physicians with specific questions regarding malaria prophylaxis and other travel-related infections should call the Centers for Disease Control hotline at (404) 332-4555.

Other Travel-Related Conditions

Travelers should be aware of the high prevalence of *sexually transmitted diseases* in developing countries and be counseled to take appropriate preventive measures. These diseases include gonorrhea (especially penicillinase-producing *Neisseria* gonorrhea), syphilis, chancroid, granuloma inguinale, and human immunodeficiency virus infection.

Sudden disruption of the body's sleep-wake cycle may cause fatigue, insomnia, anorexia, constipation, headache, and mild incoordination. A short-acting benzodiazepine or a feast-fast–feast-fast dietary schedule may alleviate the symptoms of *jet lag*.

Rapid ascent to high altitudes (>10,000 ft) may cause a syndrome of headache, nausea, anorexia, dyspepsia, insomnia, and fatigue. *Acute mountain sickness* (AMS) is usually self-limiting, but rare patients can develop altitude-related pulmonary or cerebral edema. The immediate treatment is descent to a lower altitude, followed by symptomatic supportive care. Those who have previously experienced AMS or anticipate rapid ascents have benefited from acetazolamide (Diamox), 500 mg two times daily, to be initiated before ascent.

Despite the plethora of potential infectious agents, the most common cause of death among international travelers is *trauma,* usually sustained in motor vehicle accidents. Unfamiliar with local road conditions and traffic patterns, travelers must also cope with the unavailability of safety devices, such as seat belts, motorcycle helmets, and traffic signals. Travelers should proceed cautiously and select safe and reliable means of transportation.

Emergency Medical Care

If medical care is needed abroad, the American embassy or consulate can usually provide names of hospitals and physicians. The quality of health care varies in developing countries, and travelers should be cautioned against consenting to blood transfusion, injection with a previously used needle, and placement of an intravenous catheter. Once stabilized, the patient should consider transportation to a modern medical facility or to the United States.

Bibliography

DuPont HL, Ericsson CD: Prevention and treatment of traveler's diarrhea. N Engl J Med 1993;328:1821–1827.

Jong EC: The Travel Tropical Medicine Manual. Philadelphia, WB Saunders, 1987.

U.S. Public Health Service, Centers For Disease Control: Health Information for International Travel. HHS Publication No. (CDC) 93-8280. Published annually.

World Health Organization: International Travel and Health Vaccination Requirements and Health Advice 1993. Geneva, World Health Organization. Published annually.

Wyler DJ: Malaria chemoprophylaxis for the traveler. N Engl J Med 1993;329:31–37.

9 Common EENT Symptoms

Michael L. Waters

Symptom	Red Eye

Scleral infection, or the "red eye," can be a sign and symptom of a variety of underlying abnormalities of the eye. Infection, allergy, drugs, chemical exposure, trauma, and systemic disease may cause scleral infection as well as many other ocular manifestations.

Differential Diagnosis

1. Conjunctivitis
   a. Bacterial (most common: *Staphylococcus aureus,* pneumococcus, *Haemophilus influenzae*)—purulent conjunctival discharge with a gritty foreign body sensation and matting of the lids and lashes.
   b. Viral (most common: adenovirus)—serous conjunctival discharge with erythematous, edematous eyelids and palpable preauricular lymphadenopathy.
   c. Allergic—watery conjunctival discharge with pruritus.
2. Drug-induced (marijuana, alcohol, benzodiazepines)—decreased or absent pupillary light reaction, corneal glaze, nystagmus, nonconvergence.
3. Chemical exposure—eye pain; burning with lid edema and possible burn of periocular skin.
4. Blepharitis—erythematous, edematous lid margins with crusting.
5. Subconjunctival hemorrhage—asymptomatic blood underneath conjunctiva.
6. Ophthalmia neonatorum—mucopurulent/purulent conjunctival discharge during first month of life.
7. Corneal abrasion—eye pain, photophobia, and history of injuring eye.
8. Corneal foreign body—foreign body sensation with blurred vision.
9. Canaliculitis—tearing with tenderness over nasal aspect of lower or upper eyelid.
10. Acute angle-closure glaucoma—halos around lights with nausea, vomiting, and frontal headache. Increased intraocular pressure (IOP).
11. Scleritis/Episcleritis—bluish hue of sclera(e) with severe pain radiating to forehead and/or jaw.

> Refer to Ch. 14, Corneal Ulceration; Ch. 13, Conjunctivitis; Procedure on Corneal Foreign Body Removal (after Ch. 14); Ch. 19, Allergic Rhinitis; Ch. 12, Glaucoma; Ch. 301, Meningitis; and Ch. 321, Substance Abuse.

12. Anterior uveitis—eye pain, photophobia with diminished vision. Light to uninvolved eye is painful to involved eye.

History: Key Questions to Ask

When a patient presents complaining of a red eye, a thorough history alone can often lead to the diagnosis.

1. When did the redness appear?
2. Is there pain, burning, visual changes, foreign body sensation, photophobia, discharge, pruritus, excessive or diminished tearing?
3. Are there systemic symptoms such as fever, upper respiratory involvement, nausea, vomiting, joint pain, rash, urethral or vaginal discharge?
4. Was there precipitating injury, drug use, or chemical exposure?
5. Do any family members or contacts have similar symptoms?
6. Have you had any previous eye disease?
7. Do you have any other medical problems?

These questions pertain to the most common etiologies for scleral infection and can help the primary care physician arrive at a differential diagnosis.

Clinical Findings

For any eye complaint, a thorough examination of both eyes should be performed to evaluate:

1. Visual acuity—should be tested with glasses or contacts if possible. Also, testing should be performed prior to treatment except in chemical burns when emergent irrigation is essential.
2. Extraocular eye movements
3. Pupil size/reaction—various street drugs cause concomitant scleral infection and pupillary size/reactivity changes.

In addition to the gross eye examination outlined above, microscopic evaluation with a slit-lamp is sometimes indicated. Chemical burn, corneal abrasion, foreign body, acute angle-closure glaucoma, scleritis, episcleritis, and anterior uveitis are all causes of scleral infection requiring slit-lamp examination for accurate diagnosis and therapy. For this reason, patients in whom these possible diagnoses are considered should be referred for ophthalmologic evaluation after gross eye examination and initial treatment have been instituted.

Management

A. Conjunctivitis

1. Bacterial—Conjunctiva(e) should be swabbed for Gram's stain, culture, and sensitivity. Topical ciprofloxacin (Cipro), erythromycin, or bacitracin should be instituted for 5 to 7 days. *H. influenzae* conjunctivitis should be treated with oral amoxicillin/clavulanate (Augmentin) (20–40 mg/kg/day t.i.d.) because of occasional concomitant otitis media, pneumonia, or meningitis. In hyperacute (onset within 12 hours) bacterial conjunctivitis possibly from *Neisseria gonorrhoeae*, single-dose ceftriaxone (Rocephin), 1 gram intramuscularly; oral tetracycline, erythromycin, or doxycycline for 2 to 3 weeks (for associated chlamydia); and topical ciprofloxacin, erythromycin, or bacitracin are all indicated. If corneal involvement is present, ophthalmologic consultation is indicated for hospitalization and intravenous ceftriaxone. The patient needs to be re-evaluated every 1 to 2 days until definite improvement is seen and then every 3 to 5 days until completely resolved. Antibiotic therapy may need to be altered depending on culture results and patient response.

2. Viral—Treatment consists of artificial tears and cool compresses 4 to 8 times per day for 1 to 3 weeks. If itching is severe, use naphazoline/pheniramine (Naphcon-A), q.i.d. Patients should be advised that symptoms may worsen for the first 4 to 7 days and may not resolve for 3 weeks. Patients should be educated on contagiousness of conjunctival secretions, which may last 2 weeks after onset. Follow up if symptoms worsen.

3. Allergic—If possible, remove the precipitating allergen. Artificial tears and cool compresses 4 to 8 times per day are adequate in mild cases. More severe cases may require naphazoline/pheniramine, q.i.d., and diphenhydramine, 25 mg t.i.d. or q.i.d. If patient response is inadequate, ophthalmology referral is indicated for topical steroid therapy. Follow up if symptoms worsen.

B. Chemical exposure

With any chemical exposure, vigorous irrigation should be instituted immediately. If possible, anesthetize the eye with any topical agent (e.g., proparacaine [Ophthaine]). Evert the upper lid and pull down the lower lid to expose the fornices. Irrigate quickly with one liter of Ringer's lactate, normal saline, or even unsterile water. Check conjunctival pH by placing litmus paper in inferior cul-de-sac and irrigate until pH is 7. Make sure fornices are clean and then apply a cycloplegic (cyclopentolate 1% [Cyclogyl]), a topical antibiotic ointment (erythromycin or bacitracin), and a pressure patch for 24 hours. If IOP is elevated from a severe burn, ophthalmologic consultation should be obtained for in-hospital monitoring. If IOP and remainder of eye examination are normal, patient can be sent home, with follow-up by an ophthalmologist in 24 hours.

C. Blepharitis

Treatment consists of scrubbing the eyelid margins with mild shampoo (e.g., Johnson's Baby Shampoo) twice a day and applying warm compresses t.i.d. or q.i.d. If severe, apply antibiotic ointment (erythromycin or bacitracin) to the eyelid(s) at night. Follow up if symptoms worsen.

D. Subconjunctival hemorrhage

No treatment is required. If eye irritation is present, artificial tears 4 times a day is adequate. However, hypertension, bleeding diathesis, and eye trauma must be ruled out. The hemorrhage usually resolves spontaneously within 2 weeks. Return for follow-up if bleeding does not resolve or with recurrence.

E. Ophthalmia neonatorum

Initial therapy is based upon results of Gram's and Giemsa stains. Gram-positive bacteria without suspicion of gonorrhea and no corneal involvement require erythromycin ointment for 2 weeks. Gram-negative bacteria without suspicion of gonorrhea and no corneal involvement require gentamicin ointment for 2 weeks. If bacteria are present on Gram's stain and the cornea is involved, obtain ophthalmologic consultation for hospitalization and treatment. If no information can be obtained from Gram's or Giemsa stains, then treat with erythromycin ointment and erythromycin syrup 50 mg/kg/day in divided doses for 2 to 3 weeks and modify according to culture results. If chemical (e.g., silver nitrate) toxicity is presumed, no treatment is indicated except 24-hour follow-up. If chlamydia is suspected, treat with erythromycin ointment and erythromycin syrup 50 mg/kg/day for 2 to 3 weeks. If chlamydia is confirmed by immunofluorescent stain or culture, remember to treat mother and sexual partner(s). If *Neisseria gonorrhoeae* is suspected, then hospitalize for evaluation and possible treatment of disseminated gonococcal infection as well as ophthalmologic consultation.

Obviously, daily follow-up of the infant is indicated until clinical response is seen. If the condition worsens or corneal involvement develops, re-culture, hospitalize, and obtain ophthalmologic consultation.

All of the remaining causes of the red eye require ophthalmologic consultation for slit-lamp evaluation. The size of a corneal abrasion must be measured and its location diagrammed for a baseline necessary in evaluating a therapeutic response. In addition, an anterior-chamber reaction must be ruled out. A corneal foreign body must be removed under slit-lamp with a foreign body spud or rust-ring drill. The punctal concretions present in canaliculitis must be removed under slit-lamp and possibly via surgical canaliculotomy for complete success. Acute angle-closure glaucoma requires continuous IOP monitoring as well as gonioscopy of anterior-chamber angles. Scleritis and episcleritis require slit-lamp examination for diagnosis and may need steroid therapy and/or surgery for resolution. Finally, anterior uveitis has a multitude of causes; therefore, accurate diagnosis is essential before extensive work-up is indicated.

Bibliography

Cullom RD Jr, Chang B: The Wills Eye Manual: Office and Emergency Room Diagnosis and Treatment of Eye Disease, 2nd ed. Philadelphia, JB Lippincott, 1994.

Gutmann E: Red eye: When to treat, when to refer. Modern Medicine 1986;54:52–69.

Potts AM: Diagnostic eye instruments for the general physician. J Florida Med Assoc 1994;81:234.

Tennant F: The rapid eye test to detect drug abuse. Postgrad Med 1988;84(1):108–114.

Zimmerman TJ: Topical ophthalmic beta blockers: a comparative review. J Ocular Pharm 1993;9:373–384.

Symptom **Eye Pain** *Lynn J. Goebel*

Decide whether the pain is coming from the eye itself or is referred from surrounding structures.

Differential Diagnosis

A. Intrinsic eye pain

The lid, conjunctiva, cornea, and uveal tract are richly innervated by the ophthalmic nerve. The retina, the vitreous, and the optic nerve, in contrast, are less well innervated and thus seldom are a source of pain.

1. Pain with swelling around the eye

    a. Stye or hordeolum—on lid margin, inflammation of glands of Zeis or Moll

    b. Chalazion—points away from lid margin, usually chronically inflamed meibomian gland

    c. Dacryocystitis and dacryoadenitis—inflammation of lacrimal system

    d. Orbital and preseptal cellulitis—may need computed tomographic scan to differentiate the two; orbital cellulitis requires parenteral antibiotics

2. Pain with foreign body sensation, usually referred to outer portion of upper eyelid regardless of location of lesion

    a. Conjunctivitis—red eye, bright red vessels located peripherally

    b. Corneal abrasion—ingrown lashes, contact lens overuse, trauma

    c. Corneal ulcer—requires referral

    d. Foreign matter on lid or surface of eye

    e. Ultraviolet overexposure (sun, sun lamp, welding)

    f. Trauma

PEARL

A drop of local anesthetic in the conjunctival sac alleviates the pain from superficial abrasion and foreign body but not that from deeper structures.

3. Pain with burning or itching

    a. Conjunctivitis

    b. Allergy

    c. Dry eyes—may be secondary to collagen vascular disease (sicca syndrome)

    d. Overuse or fatigue—seen in people who work with video display terminals because of infrequent blinking

    e. Chemical injury—history of exposure

4. Deep pain

    a. Anterior uveitis—purplish red vessels around the limbus of the cornea, miotic pupils, blurred vision, cell and flare in anterior chamber with slit-lamp

    b. Glaucoma—purplish red vessels around the limbus of the cornea; midposition fixed pupils; decreased vision; steamy cornea

    c. Scleritis and episcleritis—scleritis causes

more severe pain and may perforate; episcler-itis is easily confused with conjunctivitis, but dilated vessels are more purple and do not disappear with topical decongestants

5. Pain on movement of eyes
   a. Retrobulbar optic neuritis—some loss of central vision; swollen disk; positive swinging-flashlight test (afferent pupillary defect)
   b. Orbital pseudotumor—idiopathic orbital inflammatory syndrome; pain, lid edema, chemosis, proptosis; no fever or leukocytosis
   c. Posterior scleritis—decreased vision, disk edema
   d. Myositis—diplopia
6. Pain with no or subtle signs
   a. Eye strain
   b. Astigmatism
   c. Tonic pupil

B. Referred pain
Referred pain can be either from contiguous structures or from structures innervated by the recurrent meningeal branches of the ophthalmic nerve.

1. Headaches—migraine, sinus, cluster, tension; subarachnoid hemorrhage; pseudotumor cerebri
2. Sinusitis
3. Temporal arteritis
4. Pituitary apoplexy
5. Herpes zoster ophthalmicus prodrome or post-herpetic neuralgia
6. Trigeminal neuralgia
7. Occipital neuralgia
8. Cavernous sinus thrombosis—idiopathic, inflammatory, tumor; causes cranial nerve palsies and sensory loss in V1 and V2
9. Orbital tumors—proptosis, decreased vision, diplopia; severe pain suggests cancer
   a. Lymphoid tumors
   b. Dermoid cysts—can rupture spontaneously or with trauma and cause intense pain
   c. Metastatic tumors—lung and breast in adults
   d. Locally invasive paranasal tumors—nasopharyngeal carcinoma, squamous cell carcinoma of sinuses
10. Dissecting aneurysm of extracranial internal carotid
11. Carotid cavernous fistula
12. Aneurysm of posterior communicating artery
13. Dissection of vertebral artery
14. Stroke—parieto-occipital or thalamic infarct
15. Pontine tumors and other brain stem lesions such as Wallenberg's syndrome and multiple sclerosis
16. Increased intracranial pressure—boring pain worse with Valsalva maneuver, associated vomiting, papilledema
17. Temporomandibular joint pain

Refer to Ch. 12, Glaucoma; Ch. 13, Conjunctivitis; Ch. 14, Corneal Ulceration; Ch. 15, Optic Neuritis; Ch. 19, Allergic Rhinitis; Ch. 20, Sinusitis; Ch. 21, Oribital and Periorbital Cellulitis; Ch. 209, Polymyalgia Rheumatica; Ch. 210, Temporal Arteritis; and procedure on Removal of Ocular Foreign Body following Ch. 14.

History: Key Questions to Ask

1. Quality, timing, progression, onset, and duration of pain?
2. Relieving or exacerbating factors?
3. Associated symptoms, such as nausea or vomiting?
4. Loss of vision, diplopia, photophobia, discharge, history of trauma, exposure to ultraviolet light, possible foreign bodies, use of contact lenses?
5. History of headache, sinus problems, cancer, joint problems, rash?

Clinical Findings

1. Decreased visual acuity
2. Erythema or swelling of eyelids or conjunctiva
3. Extraocular muscle palsy or pain with movement
4. Decreased pupillary response or positive swinging-flashlight test
5. Papilledema on funduscopic examination
6. Steamy cornea or defect in cornea
7. Narrow anterior chamber or cell and flare present on slit-lamp examination

---

PEARLS

Refer to ophthalmologist if any of the following is present:

- Decreased vision
- Trauma
- Corneal ulcer
- Herpes zoster ophthalmicus
- Metallic foreign body with rust ring
- Any condition that requires topical steroid treatment
- Patient not improved with conservative management

8. Visual field defect
9. Temporal artery tenderness or swelling
10. Sinus tenderness
11. Proptosis
12. Sensory deficits
13. Unequal carotid pulses

Tests

Diagnostic tests should be carried out based on clinical suspicion. Common office tests include the following:

1. Fluorescein dye—to detect for corneal defects
2. Tonometry—to measure intraocular pressure
3. Slit-lamp examination—to detect cell and flare in the anterior chamber

Computed tomographic and magnetic resonance imaging scans, if indicated

Management

Depends on specific diagnoses

Bibliography

Kohrman B, Warfield C: Eye pain: ocular and nonocular causes. Hosp Pract 1987;22(12):33–50.

Newell FM: Ophthalmology Principles and Concepts, 7th ed. St Louis, CV Mosby, 1992.

Rosenblatt M, Sakol P: Ocular and periocular pain. Otolaryngol Clin North Am 1989;22(6):1173–1203.

Vaughan D, Asbury T, Riordan-Eva P: General Ophthalmology. E Norwalk, CT, Appleton & Lange, 1992.

Symptom | **Flashing Lights and Floaters** | *W. Michael Skeens*

The subjective complaints of flashes of light and floaters are usually of different origins. Light perception by the occipital cortex is commonly due to stimulation of the retina and less frequently due to cerebral causes. Photopsia is the subjective sensation of sparks or flashes of light induced by mechanical or electrical retinal stimulation. The visualization of floaters is primarily due to changes in the vitreous and seldom due to foreign bodies in the anterior aspect of the eye.

Differential Diagnosis

A. Flashes
   1. Bilateral photopsia (unformed visual hallucinations) is of cerebral origin.
      a. Static light and stars arise from the occipital cortex and association areas.
      b. Luminous colored flashes and rings arise from the parastriate area 18.
      c. Other cerebral areas may produce formed images.
   2. Monocular
      a. Simple traction of the vitreous on the sensory retina (Moore's lighting streak)
      b. Vitreous detachment causing a fluid-filled optically empty space between the vitreous and the retina, seen especially in women aged 55 through 65
      c. Retinal hole, possibly with hemorrhage from a small vessel tear
      d. Detachment of the retina—may be due to diabetic proliferative retinopathy causing surface wrinkling of the retina
      e. Cataracts
      f. Migraine headache
      g. Epilepsy
      h. Oculodigital phenomenon
      i. Flick phosphene of quick eye motion
      j. Retinal microembolization
      k. Retinitis (e.g., cytomegalovirus infection)
      l. Vertebral basilar insufficiency
      m. Multiple medications, including clomiphene citrate (Clomid) and many antibiotics
      n. Poisonings—mushroom, cannabis, mescaline, mullet fish, gasoline, *Myristica* (nutmeg), ololiuqui (morning glory seed)

B. Floaters
   1. Tear film debris
   2. Material in the vitreous—principally remnants of the embryonic hyaloid vascular system (muscae volitantes)
   3. Degenerative vitreous changes—syneresis (fluid replacement in part or whole of the vitreous)
      a. Myopic
      b. Aging
      c. Post-traumatic
   4. Hemorrhages
      a. Peripheral—floater
      b. Central—red haze and decreased visual acuity
      c. Due to neovascularization from diabetes, tumor, or inflammation or rupture of a subhyaloid retinal hemorrhage secondary to a subarachnoid hemorrhage (Tenson's)
   5. Corneal foreign body
   6. Carbon tetrachloride poisoning

Refer to Ch. 159, Diabetes Mellitus, Type I; Ch. 160, Diabetes Mellitus, Type II; Ch. 288, Migraine Headache; and Ch. 289, Seizure Disorder.

History

A rapid onset of flashing lights (especially a shower of them) is more suspicious of retinal detachment. The rapid onset of floating opacities is more indicative of vitreous or retinal hemorrhages and, possibly, formation of a retinal hole.

Key questions to ask:

1. Unilateral versus bilateral: Do the symptoms change or go away if one or the other eye is closed?
   a. If the symptoms change with closure of one eye, this suggests that the abnormality is relative to one eye only.
   b. If the symptoms do not change with closure of one eye, the problem is central (cerebral) in origin or, less likely, due to bilateral involvement (in this case, it should generally be asymmetrical).
2. If lights are reported, are they colored rings or halos, or are they flashes or streaks?
3. Has there been any change in overall visual acuity aside from the lights or floaters?
4. For floaters, does blinking clear or change the appearance of the opacity? If so, the opacity would be in the rear film layer.
5. For floaters, do the dots dart away when the patient tries to fixate on them? If so, this probably represents hyaloid vascular system remnants (muscae volitantes).
6. If diabetes is present, there is increased risk of hemorrhage from proliferative vessels.

Clinical Findings/Tests

1. A dilated examination, including indirect ophthalmoscopy, is required for any sudden onset of flashing lights or floaters to rule out retinal detachment or hemorrhages.
2. The presence of hyaloid artery remnants on the posterior aspect of the lens capsule (Mittendorf's dot) or on the center of the optic nerve head (Bergmeister's papilla) is not symptomatic.
3. Multiple shiny calcium-lipid deposits in the vitreous on ophthalmoscopy (asteroid hyalosis), usually unilaterally, is also a normal variant that does not cause symptoms.
4. The presence of pus in the conjunctiva and tear film

or a foreign body in the cornea can be the cause of floating or fixed densities, respectively.

5. The presence of densities seen while focusing through the vitreous during ophthalmoscopy usually is indicative of benign floaters, which may shift out of the visual axis with further degenerative changes within the vitreous.
6. Myopic patients are at increased risk for spontaneous retinal detachment because of increased traction of the attachment points of the vitreous on the retina.

Management

1. For benign floaters, no treatment is necessary or effective. With further changes and shifts in the vitreous, the densities may shift out of the visual axis, although in time they frequently return.
2. Rapid diagnosis of retinal holes or detachments is necessary for stabilization of holes or reattachment of the retina because the sensory retina cannot survive long without its vascular supply. Therapies include scleral buckling, laser therapy, cryotherapy, diathermy, encircling rod, and silicon or air injection into the vitreous.
3. The responsible drug or medication should be withdrawn.
4. For hemorrhages, vitrectomy may be required to clear the visual axis.
5. For diabetic patients, routine screening ophthalmologic examinations and good glycemic control are paramount in minimizing the risk of hemorrhages and detachments.

Bibliography

Braunwald E, Isselbacher KJ, Petersdorf RG, et al (eds): Harrison's Principles of Internal Medicine, 11th ed. New York, McGraw-Hill, 1993, pp 73, 2036.

Newell FW: Ophthalmology Principles and Concepts, 7th ed. St Louis, CV Mosby, 1992.

Roy FH: Ocular Differential Diagnosis, 5th ed. Malvern, PA, Lea & Febiger, 1993.

Spalton DJ, Hitchings RA, Hunter PA, et al: Atlas of Clinical Ophthalmology, 2nd ed. St. Louis, Mosby Year–Book Europe, 1994.

Vaughan D, Asbury T, Riordan-Eva P: General Ophthalmology, 13th ed. E Norwalk, CT, Appleton & Lange, 1992.

Symptom **Earache/Ear Pain**   *Walter Bridges*

Otalgia (ear pain) is a common complaint of adults as well as children. Although infection is the most common primary cause of earache, it should not be assumed to be the sole cause. Secondary causes are myriad because of the complex sensory innervation of the ear. Branches from the trigeminal, facial, glossopharyngeal, and vagus nerves combine to provide sensory innervation of the ear. Sensory branches from the cervical plexus (C2, C3) also contribute. Evaluation of secondary or referred otalgia requires careful examination and assessment of structures of the face, the pharynx, larynx, and other anatomic sites innervated by these nerves.

Differential Diagnosis

A. Primary causes

1. External ear

    a. Infection: bacterial (*Staphylococcus, Streptococcus, Pseudomonas, Proteus*) and fungal (*Candida, Aspergillus*)

    b. Trauma—cotton-tipped swab, hairpin; may become secondarily infected

    c. Foreign body or cerumen impaction

    d. Bullous myringitis (*Mycoplasma*)

2. Middle ear, mastoid

    a. Acute otitis media—*Haemophilus influenzae, Streptococcus pneumoniae, Moraxella catarrhalis*

    b. Barotrauma—sudden change in pressure (diving, flying) causing acute closure of the eustachian tube with extravasation of blood into the middle ear

    c. Chronic otitis media with cholesteatoma (ingrowth of epithelial cells) that appears as a gray to white mass behind the tympanic membrane. Bone erosion may occur.

    d. Eustachian tube obstruction—usually caused by neoplasm in adults

B. Secondary causes

1. Orofacial

    a. Dental—infection

    b. Muscle spasm

    c. Sinus pain

2. Temporomandibular joint syndrome—either structural or pain-dysfunction syndrome; caused by bruxism, malocclusion, emotional tension, trauma, arthritis

3. Visceral—cranial nerves IX and X; pharyngitis, tonsillitis, peritonsillar abscess

4. Trigeminal neuralgia or tic douloureux—intense stabbing pain in the mandible and maxillary branches of the trigeminal nerve; tends to occur in middle-age but consider multiple sclerosis in young adults

5. Ramsay Hunt syndrome—herpetic infection of cranial nerves VII and VIII with extension of lesions to ear; associated with facial paralysis, vertigo, and hearing loss

6. Eagle syndrome—caused by compression of the carotid artery by an elongated styloid process. Symptoms include sore throat, otalgia, and pain on swallowing.

Refer to Ch. 16, Acute Otitis Media; Ch. 17, Chronic Serous Otitis Media; Ch. 18, Otitis Externa; Ch. 20, Sinusitis; and Ch. 293, Trigeminal Neuralgia.

History

1. Predisposing factors—swimming, trauma, upper respiratory tract infections

2. Associated symptoms—discharge, hearing loss, vertigo, sore throat, toothache

3. Pain on chewing and swallowing

Clinical Findings

1. Erythema of auricle—cellulitis, furuncle, external otitis

2. Altered shape of auricle—suggestive of mastoiditis

3. Pain on movement of auricle, indicating external otitis or otitis media

4. Ear discharge, usually purulent green or yellow—external otitis, perforated tympanic membrane

5. Tympanic membrane appearance—light reflex is diffuse to dull in otitis media. Membrane may be thickened with yellow fluid behind it. Bluish discoloration of the tympanic membrane suggests blood in the middle ear.

6. Tenderness over temporomandibular joint on palpation, also eliciting otalgia

7. Swelling of parotid or thyroid gland with tenderness

8. Tooth pain on palpation

9. Tenderness of temporomandibular joint on biting of tongue blade on contralateral side

Tests

1. Myringotomy with evaluation and culture of middle ear effusion is helpful in evaluation of chronic otitis media.

2. Audiometry is useful in differentiating conductive versus sensory hearing loss.

3. Computed tomographic scan of the head may be necessary to evaluate for mastoiditis, brain abscess, and other complications of otitis media.

Diagnosis of otalgia can be accomplished most often by otoscopic examination. Examination of the oropharynx and neck (especially the thyroid) is essential in the initial evaluation of secondary otalgia. Indirect examination of the larynx and piriform sinus should be performed in any patient with normal ear examination and otalgia on swallowing because a neoplasm is likely to be present.

Management

1. Cerumen impaction

    a. Wax softeners—carbamide peroxide (Debrox), two to three drops twice a day; Colace drops (10 mg/ml), one to two drops twice a day

    b. May be removed with pulsating irrigation device or ear loop

2. Topical analgesics or antibiotic

    a. Auralgan (combination of benzocaine and antipyrine), 10 ml; fill ear canal as needed for pain

b. Cortisporin Otic or Pedi-Otic drops (combination of polymyxin B sulfate, neomycin sulfate, hydrocortisone), 10 ml, four drops three or four times a day. Use the suspension if perforation is suspected.

c. VōSol Otic drops (acetic acid), 15 ml, 30 ml; acidifies ear canal; three to five drops twice a day

3. Commonly used systemic antibiotics

a. Amoxicillin (Amoxil)—child: 125 or 250 mg/5 ml, 30 to 50 mg/kg/day orally three times a day; adult: 250 or 500 mg three times a day

b. Pediazole pediatric suspension (erythromycin ethylsuccinate 200 mg and acetyl sulfisoxazole 600 mg) per 5 ml, 8 to 12 mg/kg/day four times a day

c. Erythromycin—adult: 333 mg three times a day or 500 mg twice a day; child: 30 to 50 mg/kg/day in three to four equal doses

d. Bactrim suspension (trimethoprim 40 mg and sulfamethoxazole 200 mg per 5 ml), 8 to 12 mg/kg/day of trimethoprim in two equal doses; adult: Bactrim DS (trimethoprim 160 mg and sulfamethoxazole 800 mg), 1 tablet twice a day

e. Augmentin—child (amoxicillin 125 or 250 mg and clavulanic acid 31.25 or 62.5 mg per 5 ml): 30 mg/kg/day three times a day; adults (amoxicillin 250 or 500 mg and clavulanic acid 125 mg per tablet): one tablet three times a day

f. Cephalosporins—several preparations available; more expensive

4. Temporomandibular joint syndrome

a. Soft diet and heat are helpful.

b. Most pain can be controlled with nonsteroidal anti-inflammatory drugs.

c. Dental appliances or splints and surgery are options.

5. Tic douloureux

a. Medical management: phenytoin (Dilantin), 300 to 400 mg/day; carbamazepine (Tegretol), 600 to 1200 mg/day

b. Surgical resection of trigeminal roots may be necessary.

6. Ramsay Hunt syndrome—acyclovir (Zovirax), 200 mg orally five times a day; amitriptyline, 75 mg orally at bedtime

Patient Education

1. Ear plugs should be worn while swimming, especially if the tympanic membrane is perforated.

2. Use peroxide or alcohol drops to dry the ear canal after swimming or showering.

> **PEARL**
>
> The tympanic membrane must be seen in otalgia. If cerumen obscures visualization of the tympanic membrane, it must be removed.

 Bibliography

For more information on the sensory innervation of the ear, see
Adams RD, Victor M: Principles of Neurology, 5th ed. New York, McGraw-Hill, 1993, p 167.
For more information on otalgia and referred otalgia, see
Lucente FE, Shechtman F, Pantell J: Ear pain. In Lucente FE, Sabol SM (eds): Essentials of Otolaryngology, 3rd ed. New York, Raven Press, 1993, pp 101–112.
Paparella MM, Jung TTK: Otalgia. In Paparella M, Shumrick DA, Gluckman JL, Myerhoff W (eds): Otolaryngology, 3rd ed. Philadelphia, WB Saunders, 1991, pp 1237–1242.
Schuller DE, Schleuning AJ: DeWeese and Saunders' Otolaryngology-Head and Neck Surgery, 8th ed. St Louis, Mosby-Year Book, 1994, pp 518–519.
Wazen JJ: Referred otalgia. Otolaryngol Clin North Am 1989;22(6):1205–1215.

Symptom	**Impaired Hearing**	*Kenneth A. Weller*

Hearing loss is a common problem that affects about 10 per cent of the population and as many as 35 per cent of people over age 65. The prevalence increases significantly with age. Subtle hearing loss may be unrecognized, but with proper diagnosis, patients may benefit substantially. Impaired hearing should be classified as either a conductive hearing loss (usually implying a reversible cause) or a sensorineural hearing loss.

Differential Diagnosis

A. Conductive hearing loss

1. Otitis media with effusion—common cause of acquired hearing loss, especially in children

2. Impacted cerumen (or foreign body)—common cause in all ages

3. Chronic or serous otitis media—typically causes immobility of the tympanic membrane

4. External otitis—inflammation and exudate in the external auditory canal can lead to temporary loss of air conduction

5. Perforation of tympanic membrane—prevents normal sound translation to mechanical impulses

6. Otosclerosis—produces fixation of the stapes over the oval window, preventing transmission of sound to the inner ear. This finding is present at autopsy in 1 out of every 10 adults but clinically significant in only 1 out of 100.

7. Exostoses—bony outgrowths in the external auditory canal; may be associated with repetitive exposure to cold water, such as with ocean swim-

ming; needs correction (surgical) only if the condition produces significant narrowing of the canal

8. Developmental defects—canal atresia (such as Treacher Collins syndrome) and malformation of the ossicles. These defects may or may not be present with abnormalities of the pinna.

9. Glomus tumors—rare, benign, highly vascular tumors that produce a middle ear mass effect, leading to hearing loss

B. Sensorineural hearing loss

1. Presbycusis—most common cause of hearing loss; also called age-related hearing loss; multifactorial etiology; produces a typical high-frequency loss that is bilaterally symmetrical and irreversible

2. Noise-induced—produced by chronic exposure to high levels of sound, usually at a specific frequency (typically around 4000 Hz); irreversible cause of hearing loss but preventable with the use of earplugs or other protective devices

3. Drug-induced—most common ototoxic drugs: aminoglycosides, quinidine, furosemide, and salicylates. Salicylate toxicity is reversible.

4. Meniere's disease—causes fluctuating hearing loss (usually unilateral) associated with vertigo and tinnitus. Hearing loss begins as a low-frequency loss and commonly develops after the vertigo and tinnitus.

5. Acoustic neuroma—rare but important tumor of cranial nerve VIII that causes unilateral constant or progressive hearing loss, possibly associated with headache; requires surgical removal

6. Congenital sensorineural loss—may occur from hereditary defects (e.g., Waardenburg's syndrome), prenatal maternal infections (e.g., rubella, syphilis), or perinatal causes (e.g., erythroblastosis fetalis, anoxia)

7. Acquired infections—syphilis or viral illnesses

History

1. Hearing loss. Some patients present with a complaint of impaired hearing. Others are unaware of a problem, although those close to the patient (family members or coworkers) may have noticed it and raise their concern with the physician or to the patient.

2. Associated symptoms

a. Tinnitus, earache, or vertigo may be present.

b. Impaired ability to hear normal conversation

(1) Sensorineural loss. Patients may say that they think they hear fine, but they have difficulty understanding speech (or state that other people do not speak clearly). Noisy environments make hearing more difficult.

(2) Conductive loss. Patients complain of muffled

hearing and may actually hear better than expected in a noisy room.

3. Developmental history—especially important for children. Speech development, perinatal infections or problems, and school difficulties are important.

Clinical Findings

1. Ear

a. External auditory canal—look for obstruction, deformities, trauma

b. Tympanic membrane—intact, retracted, middle ear fluid?

2. Cranial nerves

3. Office testing

a. Weber test—vibrating 512-Hz (or higher) tuning fork placed in midline of the skull. Normally, the sound should be equal in both ears.

(1) Sensorineural loss—louder in the *unaffected* (or less affected) ear

(2) Conductive loss—louder in the *affected* ear

b. Rinne test—vibrating tuning fork placed on the mastoid process. When the sound dies away, the fork is promptly placed (without restriking it) over the external auditory meatus. Normally, by way of air conduction, the sound can be heard for twice as long as in bone conduction.

(1) Sensorineural loss—ratio of air conduction to bone conduction remains normal (2 to 1)

(2) Conductive loss—ratio becomes closer to 1 to 1, or even reversed

c. Schwabach test—bone conduction of the patient (using a vibrating tuning fork over the mastoid process) is compared with that of the examiner

(1) Sensorineural loss—patient's bone conduction is present for a *shorter* time than the examiner's

(2) Conductive loss—patient's bone conduction is present for a *longer* time than the examiner's

d. Whispering—qualitative attempt to test impaired hearing. A whisper heard from about 2 ft away is a good screen for intact hearing. Patients with a sensorineural loss have great difficulty hearing a whisper because of the high-frequency loss.

Tests

1. Office screening audiometry. Sound-generating otoscopes are available and produce sounds at 20, 25, and/or 40 decibels at frequencies of 500, 1000, 2000, and 4000 Hz. This test helps to screen for hearing loss or determine if impaired hearing is present. A loss greater than 20 decibels is considered significant.

2. Audiometry. This is the best test for determining the extent and nature of a hearing loss. It is available for

all ages, but is most useful when used with older children and adults. It can be performed in hospital speech and hearing departments as well as in physicians' offices.

3. Brain stem auditory evoked response. This study is used to detect sensorineural loss caused by retrocochlear pathology (e.g., acoustic neuroma). It is also used for neonatal screening.

4. Computed tomographic and magnetic resonance imaging scans. These tests help to detect tumors, such as acoustic neuroma and glomus tumor, and traumatic injuries.

Management

1. Sensorineural loss. Most types of sensorineural loss are not correctable, but some steps can be taken to improve hearing and avoid further damage.
   a. Noise-induced—avoid occupational exposure and wear earplugs or other protective equipment around noisy machinery.
   b. Loss secondary to medication—stop all ototoxic drugs.
   c. Acoustic neuroma—surgical removal of the tumor
2. Conductive loss. Treatment of the underlying disorder (e.g., removal of cerumen or foreign bodies, treatment of otitis media or externa, surgery for otosclerosis or tympanic membrane perforation) usually results in resolution of the hearing loss.
3. Hearing aids. These devices are useful for patients with irreversible sensorineural loss or with conductive loss when surgical correction is not chosen. Patients with a flat threshold and good speech discrimination usually respond most favorably to hearing amplification, although almost all patients benefit to some degree.

PEARLS

- Determine whether loss is conductive or sensorineural.

- Use audiometry to test hearing.

- Treat if cause is reversible.

- Prescribe a hearing aid if indicated (and loss is irreversible).

 Bibliography

For overview of impaired hearing, see
Brechtelsbauer DA: Adult hearing loss. Prim Care 1990; 17(2):249–265.
For more information on impaired hearing (otolaryngologist's viewpoint), see
Hearing loss, tinnitus, and dizziness. *In* Dayal VS (ed): Clinical Otolaryngology. Philadelphia, JB Lippincott, 1981, pp 71–106.
For more information on impaired hearing, see
Hughes GB, Nodar RH, Kay PP: Clinical evaluation of hearing loss. *In* Hughes GB (ed): Textbook of Clinical Otology. New York, Thieme-Stratton, 1985, pp 91–96.
For more information on detailed differential diagnosis, see
Nadol JB Jr: Hearing loss. N Engl J Med 1993;329(15):1092–1102.
For more information on pediatric hearing problems, see
Rapin I: Hearing disorders. Pediatr Rev 1993;14(2):43–49.

Symptom	**Tinnitus**		*Paul T. Cullen*

Tinnitus is an abnormal sound that is perceived in the ear or the head area and is unrelated to an external source. Almost 40 million Americans suffer from sustained tinnitus, and 20 per cent of this group report a significant decrease in their quality of life as a result of the symptom. The sound is usually described as a hissing, ringing, or buzzing. It is most commonly a benign disorder associated with high-frequency sensorineural hearing loss. It can be seen in more serious disorders, including acoustic neuroma. Sound transmitted from turbulent blood flow in nearby abnormal or narrowed blood vessels may cause "pulsatile" tinnitus. Neuromuscular spasms of the palate, nasopharynx, and middle ear result in vibratory tinnitus. Anxiety and depressive disorders are frequently found in patients with intractable tinnitus.

Differential Diagnosis

1. Sensorineural hearing loss of aging (presbycusis)
2. Noise-induced hearing loss
3. Meniere's disease (low-pitched, associated with vertigo)
4. Drugs: aspirin, nonsteroidal anti-inflammatory drugs, quinine, tricyclic antidepressants, aminoglycoside antibiotics
5. Muscle spasms of palate and middle ear
6. Uncontrolled hypertension
7. Carotid occlusive disease (pulsatile)
8. Traumatic head injury
9. Acoustic neuroma

About 90 per cent of tinnitus is due to otologic causes. High-frequency hearing loss with deficits at 3000 to 8000 Hz is most common. Meniere's disease is an exception with low-frequency tinnitus. Other otologic causes include otosclerosis and chronic suppurative otitis. Medical problems, including uncontrolled hypertension, have been associated with tinnitus that resolves when the blood pressure is lowered. Less frequent medical causes include hypothyroidism and hyperlipidemia.

> Refer to Ch. 53, Hypertension, and Ch. 303, Meniere's Disease.

History

1. Define the duration of symptoms; *acute-onset, short-duration* tinnitus is probably due to an acute process, such as otitis media, traumatic head injury, labyrinthitis, and noise exposure.
2. Define the nature of the sound. A pulsatile noise synchronous with the pulse results from turbulent flow in abnormal blood vessels (e.g., arteriovenous malformation, internal carotid stenosis). A vibratory intermittent noise with a beating or clicking quality is often due to spasm of the tensor tympani, stapedius, or palatine musculature.
3. Determine whether the tinnitus is unilateral. Although 50 per cent of patients with high-frequency sensorineural loss report symptoms in one ear, it should raise concern about a retrocochlear lesion—typically, acoustic neuroma.
4. Determine whether the tinnitus is continuous or fluctuating. Fluctuating tinnitus with fluctuating hearing loss and vertigo is typical of Meniere's disease.
5. Inquire about symptoms of depression. Sleep disorder, loss of interest, feelings of hopelessness and sadness, and trouble concentrating are often found in patients with intractable tinnitus.
6. Determine the medications, both prescription and over-the-counter, that the patient is taking. The most common drug that provokes tinnitus is aspirin.
7. Screen for associated neurologic symptoms that might suggest a more serious cause. Vertigo, abnormalities of facial nerve function, and symptoms of a transient ischemic attack should prompt a more detailed evaluation.

Clinical Findings

1. In the majority of cases due to cochlear disease, there are no specific abnormal findings.
2. If symptoms of pulsatile tinnitus are elicited, careful auscultation of the neck, mastoid, and skull for bruits is indicated.
3. In all cases, perform a careful examination of the tympanic membrane.
4. A directed examination of the cranial nerves and cerebellum is indicated, especially if symptoms suggest a neurologic cause.

Tests

1. Complete audiometric testing, including air and bone conduction, is mandatory in the evaluation of all patients with tinnitus. The most common abnormality is bilateral high-frequency (3000 to 8000 Hz) sensorineural loss. Some patients have significant loss into the range of normal speech (500 to 2000 Hz). A unilateral significant abnormality on audiography should be investigated for the possibility of a retrocochlear lesion (i.e., acoustic neuroma).
2. Blood pressure should be measured and treated if elevated.
3. Consider measurement of hemoglobin, blood glucose, and serum lipid levels as well as a serologic test for syphilis and thyroid function tests in selected circumstances. Only a small number of patients with tinnitus have one of these disorders as the primary cause of tinnitus.
4. In pulsatile tinnitus, computed tomography of the brain and temporal bone, duplex ultrasound examination of the carotid bifurcation, and, possibly, cerebral angiography should be performed.

Management

1. Eliminate all medications that may be contributing to the tinnitus.
2. Avoid the use of stimulants—especially nicotine and caffeine—which may worsen the symptom.
3. If a bilateral high-frequency loss is detected and the patient's primary complaints occur at bedtime, suggest a radio at a low volume to mask the tinnitus.
4. If significant hearing loss and tinnitus coexist, referral to an audiologist and evaluation for a hearing aid and masking device are indicated.
5. If depression or an anxiety disorder exists, vigorously treat with appropriate antidepressants, antianxiety drugs, and psychotherapy.
6. In patients without confirmed anxiety or depression, alprazolam, nortriptyline, biofeedback, and relaxation therapy have been used with varying degrees of success.

Patient Education

1. Although the symptom can be quite disturbing, in most cases, tinnitus is a symptom of a benign disorder. The patient should be reassured after evaluation that the symptom is not caused by a life-threatening problem.
2. Tinnitus often decreases with time.
3. Avoid noise exposure.
4. In addition to the therapies above, some patients find relief in support groups. Information can be obtained from the American Tinnitus Association, P.O. Box 5, Portland OR, 97207.

Follow-Up

Depends on the degree of the patient's dysfunction and the results of initial diagnostic tests

---

PEARLS

- Complete audiometric testing should be performed on all patients.

- Pulsatile tinnitus requires a complete evaluation for intracranial and extracranial vascular disease.

- Depression and anxiety commonly coexist in patients with intractable tinnitus.

Bibliography

Alleva M, Loch E, Paparella M: Tinnitus. Prim Care 1990; 17(2):289–297.

Marion M, Cevette M: Tinnitus. Mayo Clin Proc 1991;66:614–620.

Meyerhoff W, Ridenour B: Tinnitus. *In* Meyerhoff W, Rice D (eds): Otolaryngology Head and Neck Surgery. Philadelphia, WB Saunders, 1992, pp 435–446.

Schleuning A: Management of the patient with tinnitus. Med Clin North Am 1991;75(6):1225–1237.

Sismanis A, Smoker W: Pulsatile tinnitus: recent advances in diagnosis. Laryngoscope 1994;104:681–687.

Sullivan M, Katon W, Dobie R, et al: A randomized trial of nortriptyline for severe chronic tinnitus. Arch Intern Med 1993;153:2251–2259.

Symptom   Epistaxis

Joseph Valentino

Most people have at least one bout of epistaxis. The vast majority of nosebleeds never come to medical attention. The cause is usually local trauma to the anterior portions of the nose; however, epistaxis may be an early sign of a more significant systemic illness. Epistaxis often is intermittent, making it frustrating for both the patient and the physician. Significant bleeding, although unusual, is possible and can be life-threatening. All primary care physicians should be familiar with and be able to institute basic treatment as well as temporize severe bleeding until the otolaryngologist arrives.

Differential Diagnosis

A. Trauma

1. Self-inflicted trauma to Kiesselbach's area, such as digital manipulation, blowing, and wiping of the nose, can mechanically traumatize this area.

2. Decreased environmental humidity is associated with mucosal drying and cracking, which occur predominantly during the winter months.

3. External nasal trauma can cause tearing of intra-nasal mucous membranes. Fractures of the facial skeleton can disrupt major facial vessels.

4. Septal deformity or septal perforation can cause turbulent airflow, leading to excessive drying and disruption of the nasal mucosa.

5. Chemical irritation can result from caustic agents or drugs.

B. Inflammation

1. Rhinosinusitis—induces vascular engorgement of the nose, producing an increased friability of the mucosa. These patients are then subject to traumatization of Kiesselbach's area.

2. Allergic and vasomotor rhinitis—the mechanisms are identical to those for rhinosinusitis.

3. Bacterial and parasitic infection (e.g., typhoid, nasal diphtheria, pertussis, malaria).

C. Vascular disorders

1. Atherosclerotic peripheral vascular disease—causes elderly patients and those with hyperten-

sion to lose the adventitial and muscular integrity of the larger posterior nasal vessels. Uncontrolled hypertension exacerbates a bleed, making control difficult, but it is seldom the cause.

2. Vasculopathy (e.g., hereditary hemorrhagic telangiectasia [Osler-Weber-Rendu syndrome], Wegener's granulomatosis)

D. Clotting disorders and blood dyscrasias

1. Iatrogenic (e.g., coumadin, aspirin, heparin, nonsteroidal anti-inflammatory drugs)

2. Factor deficiencies (e.g., hemophilia, hepatic failure, vitamin K deficiency)

3. Blood dyscrasias (idiopathic thrombocytopenic purpura, leukemia, polycythemia vera)

4. Others (disseminated intravascular coagulation)

E. Tumors

1. Benign tumors (e.g., hemangioma, juvenile nasopharyngeal angiofibroma, meningioma)

2. Cancer (e.g., squamous cell carcinoma, adenocarcinoma, lymphoma, olfactory neuroblastoma)

F. Others (e.g., atrophic rhinitis, ozena, vicarious menstruation)

Refer to procedure on Nose Bleed; Ch. 19, Allergic Rhinitis; Ch. 20, Sinusitis; and Ch. 154, Bleeding Disorders.

History: Key Questions to Ask

1. Can you estimate the volume of blood lost?

2. Which side is bleeding? If both sides, which side began bleeding first?

3. Are you swallowing blood?

4. Seek signs of hypotension and hypovolemia (i.e., dizziness, level of consciousness, last void).

5. What drugs, including over-the-counter medications, are you taking?

6. History of nasal or facial trauma? Surgery?

7. Past medical history—previous epistaxis, coagulopathy, easy bruising, bleeding, complications of trauma or surgery, hypertension, liver disease?

8. History of rhinosinusitis or allergic rhinitis?

Clinical Findings

1. Vital signs
2. Examine face for fractures of the craniofacial skeleton, ecchymosis, cutaneous petechiae.
3. Intranasal examination
   a. Localize the origin of bleeding. If the patient's bleeding has stopped, the site is often a prominent erythematous vessel.
   b. Identify predisposing conditions (septal deformity, tumor, or draining mucopurulence).
4. Oral cavity—examine for bleeding from the nasopharynx.
5. General physical examination—signs of hypovolemia, cutaneous hemangioma, petechiae, neck mass.

Tests

If the bleeding is minor and not a recurring problem, no testing is indicated. For more substantial bleeding or recurrent bleeding, the following may be useful:

1. Complete blood count, including platelet count
2. Bleeding time
3. Prothrombin time and partial thromboplastin time

The hematocrit does not truly reflect the degree of acute blood loss until the patient has had sufficient volume replacement. It can show anemia from chronic blood loss and serve as a baseline to compare future laboratory values. The complete blood count reveals blood dyscrasias. Aspirin use, von Willebrand's disease, and many platelet-based bleeding disorders elevate the bleeding time. Coagulation times are elevated in hemophilia, but more often they reveal liver disease and vitamin K deficiency.

Management

Most episodes of epistaxis are mild, self-limited, and resolve spontaneously. Excessive blood loss and recurrent bleeding mandate additional intervention. Before treatment, the physician should attempt to examine the nose to determine the cause of the bleeding. First, clear the nose of blood and clot with suctioning. Then apply a topical vasoconstricting and anesthetic agent for 5 to 10 minutes. This greatly facilitates examination.

A. Anterior epistaxis
  1. Firmly grasp the nose between the thumb and forefinger and compress for 10 to 20 minutes. *If unsuccessful, then:*
  2. Chemically cauterize the site of bleeding. *If unsuccessful, then:*
  3. Cauterize the bleeding site with diathermy. *If unsuccessful, then:*
  4. Pack the nose unilaterally. *If unsuccessful, then:*
  5. Pack the nose bilaterally with gauze packing. *If unsuccessful, then:*
  6. Intervene surgically (vessel ligation, septoplasty, and/or embolization).

B. Posterior epistaxis
  1. Pack the nose unilaterally. *If unsuccessful, then:*
  2. Consider diathermy with endoscopic guidance. *If unsuccessful, then:*
  3. Pack the nose unilaterally, both anteriorly and posteriorly, using one of the following:
     a. Indwelling (Foley) catheter in the nasopharynx with an anterior gauze pack (see p. 56)
     b. Anterior/posterior balloon catheter (follow manufacturer's instructions)
     c. Formal posterior gauze or lamb's wool pack with an anterior gauze pack. *If unsuccessful, then:*
  4. Intervene surgically (vessel ligation and/or embolization).

PEARLS

- Before examining the patient, gather the following equipment: head light or head mirror, nasal speculum, Frazier tipped suction canula, bayonet forceps, cotton strips or $\frac{1}{2} \times 3$-inch cottonoids, 4% cocaine solution or a combination solution to provide anesthesia and vasoconstriction of the nose.

- Provide the usual discharge instructions:
  –Vasoconstricting sprays (oxymetazoline or phenylephrine for 2 to 3 days)
  –*Thou shall not* blow, wipe, or pick the nose.
  –No heavy lifting, straining, or exertion
  –Recommend using saline nasal spray, humidifying the environment, and applying a water-in-oil cream (e.g., Vaseline).

- Patients with coagulopathy need to have it corrected to control the bleeding. Diffuse oozing from multiple areas is common, and the manipulation during packing may exacerbate the bleeding. Expandable foam nasal tampons are useful in these patients.

- Do not cauterize both sides of the nasal septum because this may lead to septal perforation.

- Significant oxygen desaturation may accompany posterior packing. Admit and monitor these patients.

Bibliography

Ableson TI: Epistaxis. *In* Paparella MM, Shumrick DA, Gluckman JL, Meyerhoff WL (eds): Otolaryngology, vol 3. Philadelphia, WB Saunders, 1991, pp 1831–1841.

LePore ML: Epistaxis. *In* Bailey BJ (ed): Head and Neck Surgery—Otolaryngology. Philadelphia, JB Lippincott, 1993, pp 428–460.

McGarry G, Moulton C: The first aid management of epistaxis by accident and emergency department staff. Arch Emerg Med 1993;4:298–300.

Rubin J, Rood SR, Myers EN, Johnson JT: The management of epistaxis. A self-instructional package. Alexandria, VA, American Academy of Otolaryngology—Head and Neck Surgery Foundation, 1990.

Symptom Hoarseness *Janet L. Purkey*

Hoarseness results from an abnormality that involves the larynx. The structures of the larynx include the glottis, or the true vocal cords. The supraglottic area incorporates the ventricular folds (false cords), arytenoids, aryepiglottic folds, and the laryngeal surface of the epiglottis. The subglottic area begins at the lower border of the true cords and extends 1 cm distally. Many benign causes of hoarseness respond readily to conservative treatment. The patient with persistent or recurrent hoarseness must receive a thorough evaluation to rule out neoplasm.

Differential Diagnosis

1. Acute laryngitis
   a. Viral etiology, self-limiting
   b. Environmental irritants
2. Excessive voice use
   a. Screamers and singers
   b. Persistent coughing
3. Neoplasms
   a. Malignant tumors
      (1) Squamous cell carcinoma is most common.
      (2) Despite low incidence, 5-year survival rate is poor because of advanced stage at the time of diagnosis.
      (3) Must be ruled out in a patient with hoarseness that persists longer than 2 to 3 weeks
      (4) Referral to specialist without hesitation
   b. Benign tumors
      (1) Papilloma
      (2) Hemangioma
4. Chronic laryngitis
   a. Smokers
      (1) Irritation from smoke
      (2) Hyperkeratosis as a protective function of the true cords
      (3) Leukoplakia recognized as precancerous
   b. Abuse of vocal cords, as noted above
5. Nodules and polyps
   a. Usually seen in singers
   b. Can develop from area of prior traumatic injury or infection
6. Gastroesophageal reflux disease (GERD)
7. Neurologic disorders
   a. Myasthenia gravis
   b. Peripheral neuropathy after cerebrovascular accident
   c. Unilateral recurrent laryngeal nerve paralysis
      (1) After a surgical procedure in the neck or chest
      (2) Local tumor invasion
   d. Spastic dysphonia
8. Hormonal derangement
   a. Hypothyroidism
   b. Addison's disease
   c. Testosterone excess
9. Tuberculous laryngitis
10. Fungal laryngitis
11. Post intubation and other direct trauma
12. Functional or psychogenic (e.g., conversion disorder)

> Refer to Ch. 75, Gastroesophageal Reflux; Ch. 259, Basal and Squamous Cell Carcinoma; Ch. 269, Leukoplakia and Erythroplasia; and Ch. 298, Myasthenia Gravis.

History: Key Questions to Ask

1. Smoker?
2. Ethyl alcohol use or abuse?
3. Voice habits, such as loudness, singing, quantity of use?
4. Constitutional symptoms of upper respiratory tract infection or cold?
5. Timing of onset and progression of hoarseness?
6. Does hoarseness progress during the day?
7. Painful or painless?
   a. Pain is usually associated with an inflammatory process, such as viral or GERD-related.
   b. Pain occurs late in laryngeal carcinoma.
   c. Neurologic and hormonal causes do not produce pain.
8. Have other people noticed a change in voice quality?

The history of cigarette use or abuse places the patient at high risk for acute or chronic laryngitis. Such a patient is also at high risk for laryngeal neoplasm. Alcohol is a cocarcinogen in head and neck cancers. A history compatible with voice abuse or viral laryngitis directs the therapy toward a conservative approach. If the duration of hoarseness is longer than 2 to 3 weeks, prompt referral to an otolaryngologist is warranted. Patients with myasthenia gravis often have a normal voice in the morning with progression of hoarseness during the day.

Clinical Findings

A complete head and neck examination is warranted on all patients who complain of hoarseness. Primary care physicians should master the technique for direct or indirect examination of the larynx. It is imperative that a patient with chronic hoarseness be examined by an experienced physician. The physician must know when to refer to an otolaryngologist.

1. Acute laryngitis
   a. Edematous vocal cords with hyperemia
   b. Obvious irritation of the glottis and, possibly, the supraglottic area
2. No pathology may be noted in benign cases.
3. Whitish plaques are suggestive of leukoplakia.
4. Smooth nodules on the cords are suggestive of polyps or nodes.
5. Ulcerations may arise from GERD, traumatic injury, or contact of the cords from overuse.
6. Mass lesions with irregular borders are highly suspicious for cancer.
7. Lymph nodes in the neck raise the index of suspicion.
   a. Painful nodes are associated with an inflammatory process.
   b. Painless nodes are suspicious for malignant tumors.
8. The thyroid as well as the posterior pharynx must be thoroughly examined for adjacent tumors.

Tests

1. Indirect laryngoscopy
2. Direct laryngoscopy is an excellent tool for assessing the upper airway, pharynx, and larynx.
3. Other pertinent testing is based on the history and laryngeal examination.

Management

1. For acute onset, therapy is conservative.
   a. Voice rest
   b. Humidification
   c. Except in unique cases, no analgesics should be used because they allow the patient to use his or her voice and delay healing.
   d. Antihistamines dry the mucosa and should not be used.
   e. Antibiotics when appropriate (not indicated for viral infection)
   f. Cough suppression (e.g., guaifenesin and dextromethorphan or codeine)—avoid syrups that contain atropine or an antihistamine
   g. No smoking
2. If a malignant tumor is ruled out in chronic hoarseness, therapy is directed toward the cause.
   a. Smoking cessation
   b. Removal of chemical irritants
   c. Humidification and voice rest
   d. Histamine$_2$ blockers and, possibly, cisapride therapy, as appropriate, for GERD
   e. Appropriate therapy for endocrine and neurologic disorders
3. Malignant causes
   a. Surgical resection with improved outcomes if diagnosed early
   b. Radiation therapy
   c. Combination therapy of the above

PEARLS

- Voice rest and humidification are essential in acute hoarseness.

- Persistent hoarseness must be evaluated to rule out cancer.

- The physician must listen for voice quality and question the patient closely because slowly progressive hoarseness may go unnoticed by the patient.

Bibliography

Dettelbach M, et al: Hoarseness from viral laryngitis to glottic cancer. Postgrad Med 1994;95:143–162.

LaBlance GR, Maves MD, Scialfa TM, et al: Comparison of electroglottographic and acoustic analysis of pitch perturbation. Otolaryngol Head Neck Surg 1992;107:617–621.

MacKenzie K: Diagnosis and treatment of hoarseness. Practitioner 1994;238:475–478.

Sanderson RJ, Maran AGD: The quantitative analysis of dysphonia. Clin Otolaryngol 1992;17:440–443.

Simpson DM, Sternman D, Graves-Wright J, Sanders I: Vocal cord paralysis. Muscle Nerve 1993;16:952–957.

Hiccups, or singultus, is a phenomenon characterized by repetitive, sharp inspiratory sounds associated with spasm of the glottis and diaphragm. Unlike cough or sneezing, hiccups serves no identifiable purpose. It is usually transient, lasting seconds to minutes. Although it typically is benign, prolonged bouts may be the harbinger of a more serious condition. Hiccups can also be intractable and debilitating, requiring emergency treatment or hospitalization. Treatment approaches range from unorthodox to scientific. Patients commonly attempt unconventional therapies before they seek traditional medical attention. Prognosis for eradication of hiccups depends on the underlying cause, but it is generally very good.

Differential Diagnosis

1. There are more than 100 known causes of hiccups, divided into the following categories:

   a. Disorders that affect the central nervous system

   b. Disorders that affect peripheral nerves

   c. Metabolic or drug-related causes

   d. Infectious causes

   e. Psychogenic causes

   f. Idiopathic causes (Table 9–1)

2. The most common cause of hiccups is irritation of the vagus or phrenic nerve, the latter serving as the main innervation of the diaphragm. Hiccups caused by such irritation is usually benign and self-limiting.

3. Other common causes of benign hiccups include gastric distention, sudden changes in temperature, and alcohol ingestion.

4. Less common causes include pneumonia, myocardial infarction, thoracic tumors, pleurisy, and pericarditis.

5. Causes of hiccups related to the central nervous system include neoplasms, structural abnormalities, intracranial traumatic injuries, infections, and surgical manipulations. Although the exact mechanism is not fully understood, it is related to the release of normal inhibitory tone on the central reflex arc. This arc comprises the afferent and efferent limbs of the vagus and phrenic nerves, the sympathetic chain from the 6th to the 12th thoracic segments, and the ''hiccup center,'' located between the 3rd and 5th cervical segments.

6. Both the peripheral and the central nervous system pathways can be affected by metabolic disorders or

Refer to Ch. 29, Bronchitis; Ch. 34, Pneumonia; Ch. 57, Acute Myocardial Infarction; Ch. 66, Pericarditis; and Ch. 76, Gastritis.

TABLE 9–1. CAUSES OF HICCUPS

Irritation of vagus nerve
  Pharyngeal branches
    Pharyngitis
  Auricular branches
    Hair or foreign body
  Thoracic branches
    Pneumonia
    Pleuritis
    Aortic aneurysm
    Pericarditis
    Chest tumors
    Myocardial infarction
  Abdominal branches
    Distention
    Gastritis
    Ulcer disease
    Abdominal abscess
    Gallbladder disease
    Tumors
Diaphragmatic irritation
  Gastric distention
  Hiatal hernia
  Splenomegaly
  Hepatomegaly
  Subphrenic abscess
Central nervous system
  Structural lesions
  Neoplasms
  Multiple sclerosis
  Brain stem tumors
  Syringomyelia
  Trauma
  Infection (meningitis, encephalitis)
  Vascular disease
Postoperative causes
  General anesthesia
  Suppression of normal inhibition
  Stimulation of oropharynx or glottis
  Traction on viscera
  Gastric distention
  Neck extension
Toxic-metabolic
  Alcohol
  Drugs
  Uremia
  Diabetes mellitus
  Electrolyte imbalance (sodium, potassium, carbon dioxide)
Psychogenic
  Stress
  Excitement
  Conversion reaction
  Hysterical neurosis
  Malingering
Infectious causes
  Meningitis
  Encephalitis

Loft LM, Ward RF: Hiccups: A case presentation and etiologic review. Arch Otolaryngol Head Neck Surg 1992;118:1115–1119. Modified from Lewis JH: Hiccups: Causes and cures. J Clin Gastroenterol 1985;7(6):539–552.

toxic reactions to drugs. They commonly cause intractable hiccups that mandates hospitalization and an aggressive therapeutic approach. Examples include uremia, alcohol intoxication, and electrolyte abnormalities.

7. Although unusual, some reports have implicated meningitis, encephalitis, and neurosyphilis as causes of hiccups. In these cases, the hiccups usually abates once the infection is controlled.

Clinical Evaluation

1. An extensive history should be taken. It should include the onset, duration, and severity of the attack; previous episodes with aggravating and relieving factors; associated medical or surgical illnesses; and a careful history of medications or toxin exposure. Because the condition is commonplace, its occurrence can be overlooked by clinicians. A complete history usually reveals potential causes and leads to appropriate diagnosis and therapy.

2. In addition to a complete history, a thorough and systematic physical examination should be performed, with emphasis on the ears, nose, throat, chest, and abdomen. A complete neurologic examination should also be done, with special attention paid to the head and neck region. Psychogenic causes of hiccups should be ruled out.

Tests

Laboratory tests or ancillary procedures are done only to confirm the suspected cause or differential diagnosis. The practice of ordering extensive laboratory and ancillary studies is strongly discouraged, except in extreme cases when no cause can be found.

Management

1. The list of treatments for hiccups, both conventional and otherwise, is as long and diversified as the list of potential causes, ranging from folklore to scientifically proven. Most attacks are benign and self-abating, raising skepticism as to whether measures such as breathing into a paper bag or breath holding are truly efficacious. Nevertheless, treatments can be grouped into four major headings:

   a. Physical maneuvers

   b. Pharmacologic therapy

   c. Surgical therapy

   d. Miscellaneous (Table 9–2)

2. Although many of the physical maneuvers may seem unusual or frivolous, some have a physiologic basis through interruption of the central reflex arc, achieved by local stimulation of afferent nerve endings or counterirritation of end organs. However, most of the physical maneuvers reported anecdotally as being successful have no scientific basis.

3. When physical maneuvers fail to stop hiccups, a trial of drug therapy may be considered. As with physical maneuvers, the rationale for pharmacotherapy is not a result of clinical trials but rather anecdotal clinical observations. Therapeutic agents include antipsychotic medications, local anesthetics, muscle relaxants, and calcium channel blockers.

TABLE 9–2. TREATMENT OF HICCUPS

Physical maneuvers
  Swallowing granulated sugar
  Breathing into bag
  Catheter stimulation of oropharynx, nasopharynx
  Carotid sinus massage
  Gastric lavage, aspiration, induced emesis
  Traction on tongue
  Ice water gargles
  Drinking from opposite side of glass
  Valsalva maneuver
  Noxious odors or tastes
  Fright
  Ocular compression
  Breath holding
Drug therapy
  Antipsychotics
    Chlorpromazine
    Haloperidol
  Local anesthetics—nerve blocks
    Lidocaine
    Bupivacaine
  Muscle relaxants
    Cyclobenzaprine
    Baclofen
  Gastric motility agents
    Metoclopramide
  Inhalation agents
    5% Carbon dioxide
  Tricyclic antidepressants
    Amitriptyline
  Anticonvulsants
    Diphenylhydantoin
    Carbamazepine
    Valproic acid
  Antiarrhythmic
    Quinidine sulfate
  Central nervous system stimulant
    Methylphenidate
Miscellaneous
  Hypnosis
  Psychotherapy
  Acupuncture
  Phrenic nerve disruption

Loft LM, Ward RF: Hiccups: A case presentation and etiologic review. Arch Otolaryngol Head Neck Surg 1992;118:1115–1119.

4. Chlorpromazine (Thorazine) is probably the most common first-line agent used in intractable hiccups. It works as a centrally acting major tranquilizer and dopaminergic blocker, but its precise mechanism of action in hiccups remains unclear. The intravenous route is most effective, although it may be administered orally or intramuscularly. The usual adult dose is 25 to 50 mg diluted in 500 to 1000 ml of saline and infused slowly, while monitoring the patient for side effects such as hypotension and sedation. If this is effective, a maintenance dose of 25 to 50 mg orally three to four times daily should be given for 7 to 10 days.

5. Haloperidol (Haldol), another antipsychotic agent, has been reported to be effective. Its advantages lie in its efficacy when administered intramuscularly and in its lower potential for hypotension, especially

in the elderly. The recommended initial adult dose is 2 to 5 mg, and the maintenance dose is 1 to 4 mg orally three times daily. Side effects include sedation and extrapyramidal symptoms.

6. Metoclopramide (Reglan), a gastric motility agent and dopamine antagonist, is considered as the second drug of choice after chlorpromazine. The dose is 10 mg given intravenously over 1 to 2 minutes. Maintenance dose is 10 mg orally three to four times daily.

7. Studies have shown that baclofen (Lioresal), a gamma-aminobutyric acid analogue, is effective in controlling or stopping hiccups. It acts by decreasing the transmission of monosynaptic extensor and polysynaptic flexor reflexes at the spinal cord level. Optimal dosage is reached gradually, starting at 5 mg orally every 8 to 12 hrs, increasing by 15-mg increments every 3 days to a maximum of 75 mg daily. Treatment should be gradually tapered and should not be suddenly discontinued.

8. Other drugs that have been used include nifedipine, amantadine, amitriptyline, and methylprednisolone.

9. Surgical treatment can be tried as a last resort to stop clinically debilitating or intractable hiccups. This can be done by phrenic nerve crushing, ligation, or blocking with a local anesthetic. Care should be taken in performing these procedures because bilateral disruption may lead to significant pulmonary embarrassment and respiratory failure.

10. As an alternative, unorthodox measures may also be considered. They include acupuncture, hypnosis, and psychotherapy, with anecdotal cases supporting such interventions.

Bibliography

Askenasy JJM: About the mechanism of hiccup. Eur Neurol 1992; 32:159–163.

Kolodzik PW, Eilers MA: Hiccups (singultus): Review and approach to management. Ann Emerg Med 1991;20:565–573.

Launois S, Bizec JL, Whitelaw WA, et al: Hiccup in adults: An overview. Eur Respir J 1993;6:563–575.

Lewis JH: Hiccups: Causes and cures. J Clin Gastroenterol 1985;7(6):539–552.

Loft LM, Ward RF: Hiccups: A case presentation and etiologic review. Arch Otolaryngol Head Neck Surg 1992;118:1115–1119.

Procedure | REMOVAL OF IMPACTED CERUMEN

Irving Kaufman

Indications
1. Decreased hearing
2. Discomfort
3. Foreign body sensation

Contraindications
1. Perforated tympanic membrane
2. Otitis externa
3. Myringotomy tubes

Preparation
1. Soften cerumen plug
   a. Carbamide peroxide (Debrox), two drops three times per day for 3 to 5 days
   b. Mineral oil or olive oil, two drops three times per day for 3 to 5 days
2. Patient's hearing may decrease after instillation of drops in the ears. Some patients prefer that only one ear be irrigated at a time.

Equipment
1. Modified oral jet irrigator device
   a. Model 47 WaterPic
   b. Northern Electric
   c. Sears, and similar brands.

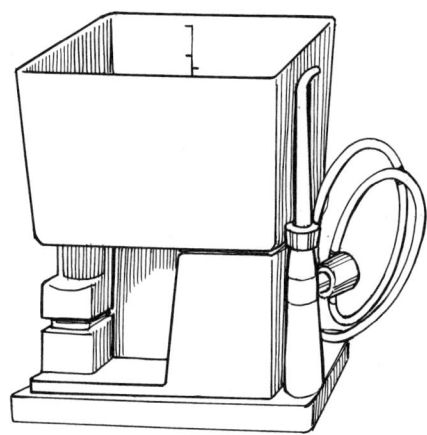

> **WARNING**
>
> **Only machines with variable settings from 1 to 10 should be used.**

2. Irrigator tip
   a. Direct-spraying oral irrigator tips work very well but they are not approved by the Food and Drug Administration (FDA)
   b. Indirect-spraying irrigator tips (e.g., Grossan Ear Irrigator) are FDA approved but do not work as well

> **WARNING**
>
> **Direct-spraying oral irrigator tips must be used with caution because of the risk of perforating the tympanic membrane.**

3. Emesis basin
4. Ear curette
5. Curved forceps
6. Gown or drape

Anesthesia
Not necessary

> **WARNING**
>
> **Severe pain is a cause to stop the procedure.**

Precautions
1. Tell the patient that the procedure will be loud but should not be painful.
2. Ask the patient to remove large, dangling earrings.
3. Warn the patient that he or she may experience transient dizziness or vertigo.
   a. May last for a few minutes
   b. Be able to lay the patient down if dizziness occurs
4. Cerumen plug should be tan to brown.
   a. White or creamy plugs may indicate perforation.
   b. Curettage only or referral to an otolaryngologist if necessary.
5. The procedure is simple and fast.
   a. Unsuccessful irrigation after 30 to 45 seconds at one-third maximal power level requires re-evaluation.
   b. In most cases, the cerumen plug was inadequately softened.

> **WARNING**
>
> **Prolonged or excessive irrigation at maximal power settings can cause severe otologic damage.**
> **a. Permanent hearing loss**
> **b. Severe vertigo**

Technique

1. Ask the patient to sit on the examination table.
2. Examine the ear with an otoscope.
3. Place an absorbent drape or gown between the patient's neck and the collar of clothing.
4. Prepare the modified oral jet irrigator.
   a. Fill the basin with warm (37° C) water.
   b. Set the power level at one-third maximum.
   c. Check that the length of tubing easily reaches the level of the patient's ear.
      (1) Tall patients may have to assume a slouched posture.
      (2) Place the irrigator on the examination table.
   d. Test the irrigator by directing the water jet into the water reservoir.

WARNING

Use only FDA-approved irrigator heads e.g., Grossan Ear Irrigator, HydroMed, Inc.; P.O. Box 91273, Los Angeles CA 90009. Tel (310) 372-8001; Fax (310) 322-3243.

---

5. Place the emesis basin under the ear being irrigated.
   a. Make a gentle seal between the smaller curve of the basin and the patient's neck.
   b. The patient may hold the basin with whichever hand is more comfortable.
6. Straighten ear canal.
   a. Pull pinna up and out.
   b. Grasp pinna of the patient's right ear with the left hand and vice versa.
7. Irrigate ear canal
   a. Place irrigator tip about 5 mm from the external auditory meatus.

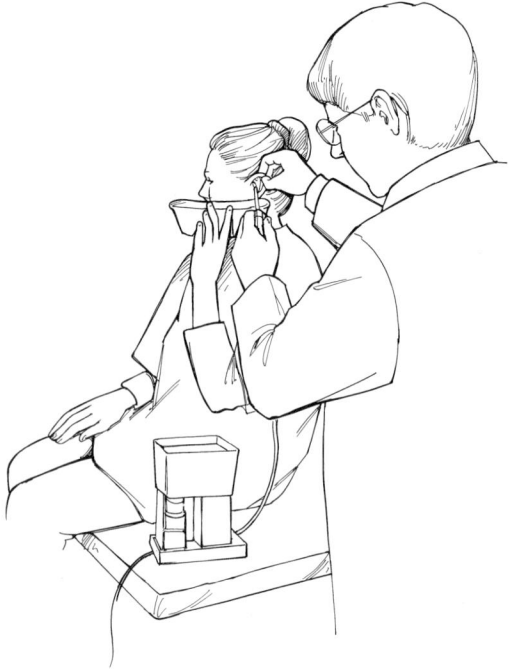

WARNING

Never place the irrigator tip in the ear canal.

---

8. Remove large chunks of partially extruded wax.
   a. By gentle traction of the plug with a curved forceps
   b. By gentle curettage
9. The procedure is finished when the water returning from the ear is clear.
10. Gently dry the ear with a tissue or cotton ball.

Follow-Up

1. Postprocedure otoscope evaluation should demonstrate a clear ear canal with an intact tympanic membrane.
2. Perforation of the tympanic membrane requires systemic antibiotics and referral to an otolaryngologist.
3. Irritation or bleeding of the ear canal with an intact tympanic membrane can be treated with polymyxin B sulfate, neomycin, and hydrocortisone (Cortisporin Otic Suspension), two drops three times per day for 5 days, and recheck the ear in 1 week.
4. Malignant otitis externa caused by *Pseudomonas* is a rare complication in diabetic or immunocompromised patients.

B Bibliography

For a review of other cerumen plug treatments, including a useful "Ear Irrigation Plan Sheet," see
Zivic R, King S: Cerumen-impaction management for clients of all ages. Nurse Pract 1993; 18(3):29–37.
For case reports of rare, severe complications, see
Dinsdale R, Roland P, Manning S, et al: Catastrophic otologic injury from oral jet irrigation of the external auditory canal. Laryngoscope 1991;101:75–78.
Lewis-Cullinan C, Janken J: Effect of cerumen removal on the hearing ability of geriatric patients. J Adv Nurs 1990;15:594–600

The most important aspect of managing epistaxis is localizing the site of bleeding. Ninety per cent of bleeds are anterior and arise from Kiesselbach's plexus (or Little's area) on the nasal septum. Anterior bleeding usually responds to local therapy, but sometimes an anterior pack is required. If the bleeding is posterior, both an anterior and a posterior pack are often needed. Posterior bleeding is usually arterial, is more severe, and arises from the spheno-palatine and the ethmoid arteries. Posterior bleeding can be associated with hypertension, atherosclerosis, and conditions that decrease platelet and clotting functions. Such bleeding is much more common in elderly people. One would suspect that the site is posterior if there is extensive bleeding into the oropharynx while pinching the anterior nose or when bleeding is from both nostrils.

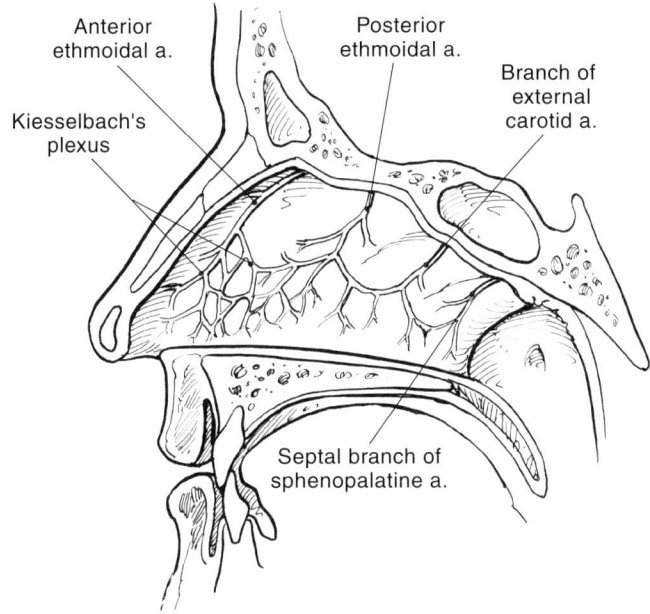

Indications
1. Local therapy—anterior bleeding
2. Anterior packing
   a. Anterior bleeding unresponsive to local therapy
   b. Posterior bleeding
3. Posterior packing—posterior bleeding
   Note: The posterior packing acts as a buttress against which the anterior packing is placed to tamponade the bleeding site.

Contraindications
1. A history of a coagulopathy is a contraindication to cautery; thus, an anterior pack should be used.
2. Obstruction of the oral airway and a history of tumor in the nasopharynx are contraindications for posterior packing.

Preparation
1. Reassure the patient.
2. Wear a protective gown. The patient should also wear a gown.
3. Position the patient upright with the head forward in a sniffing position.
4. Have the patient blow his or her nose to clear it of all clots so that it is easier to localize the bleeding site.

Equipment
A. Local therapy
   1. Headlight
   2. Suction with a No. 8 to No. 10 French tip
   3. Nasal speculum
   4. Cotton balls soaked in topical anesthetic and vaso-constrictor (see Anesthesia)
   5. Cautery tools
      a. Silver nitrate sticks
      b. Electrocautery
   6. Lidocaine 1% (Xylocaine) with 1:100,000 epi-nephrine if local injection will be attempted
B. Anterior pack
   1. Bayonet forceps
   2. Petrolatum (Vaseline) gauze or Nu-Gauze packing (½ × 72 inch)
   3. Antibiotic ointment (bacitracin or neomycin)
C. Posterior pack
   1. Foley catheter No. 12 or No. 13 French with 30-ml balloon
   2. 20-ml syringe
   3. Umbilical clamp
   4. Padding (4 × 4) to place between umbilical clamp and nose
   5. Tape to secure catheter
   6. Tongue blade

Anesthesia
A. Local therapy and anterior packing
   Cotton balls soaked in phenylephrine 1% (Neo-Syn-ephrine) and lidocaine 4% or tetracaine 2% (Ceta-caine). When placed in the nasal cavity for about 5 minutes, good anesthesia and vasoconstriction are produced.
B. Posterior packing
   If sedation is required, use morphine sulfate, 5 to 12 mg intramuscularly or intravenously, with or without midazolam (Versed), 1 to 2 mg intravenously. Watch for respiratory depression.

Precautions
1. Patients with nasal packing are at increased risk for infection, such as otitis media, sinusitis, and toxic shock syndrome. They should be placed on prophy-

lactic antibiotics (e.g., amoxicillin/clavulanate potassium [Augmentin]). The packing materials should also be covered with an antibiotic ointment.

2. Patients who require posterior packing should be admitted to the hospital and watched closely for evidence of cardiac arrhythmia and for respiratory failure.

3. Hypoxia is common in patients with posterior packs. Low-flow humidified oxygen should be given by face mask.

Technique

A. Local therapy

1. Ask the patient to blow his or her nose free of clots.

2. Determine the site of the bleeding.

3. Place medicated cotton pledgets in the bleeding nostril, and ask the patient to sit forward, pinching the nostril for about 5 minutes.

4. Remove the cotton pledgets and see if site is still bleeding.

5. If the bleeding continues, apply cautery either with silver nitrate sticks or electrocautery.
Note: Excessive electrocautery can lead to nasal septal perforation.

6. If the nose is still bleeding, inject lidocaine 1% with epinephrine using a 27-gauge needle around the bleeding site.

7. If the bleeding persists, insert an anterior pack.

B. Anterior packing

1. Open the nose with a nasal speculum.

2. With the bayonet forceps, grasp the packing 2 to 3 cm from its end, placing it in the nose in an "accordion" manner so that part of each layer is near the front of the nose.

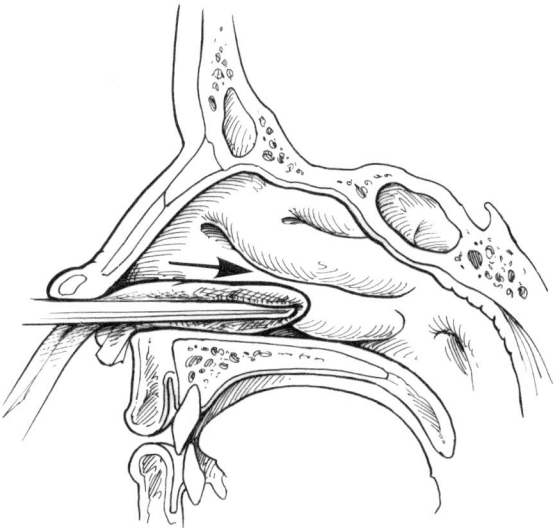

Note: The free ends of packing near the back of the nose can fall into the posterior nasopharynx, which can cause gagging.

3. After several layers have been placed, push the packing down with the bayonet forceps, making it tighter and more secure. Six feet of packing may be required for an adequate pack on the side that is bleeding.

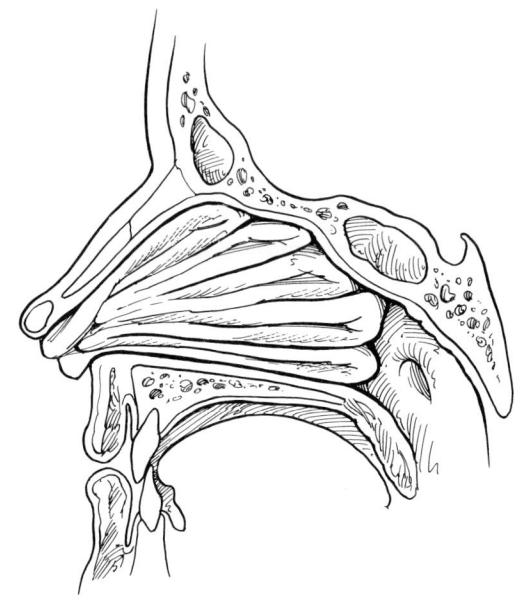

C. Posterior packing

1. Sedate the patient if necessary.

2. Take a No. 12 or No. 13 French Foley catheter, and cut off the tip distal to the balloon.

3. Advance the catheter along the floor of the nostril with the heaviest bleeding until you see the tip in the pharynx.

4. Inflate the balloon with 5 to 10 ml of water. Then apply gentle traction until the balloon lodges in the choana.

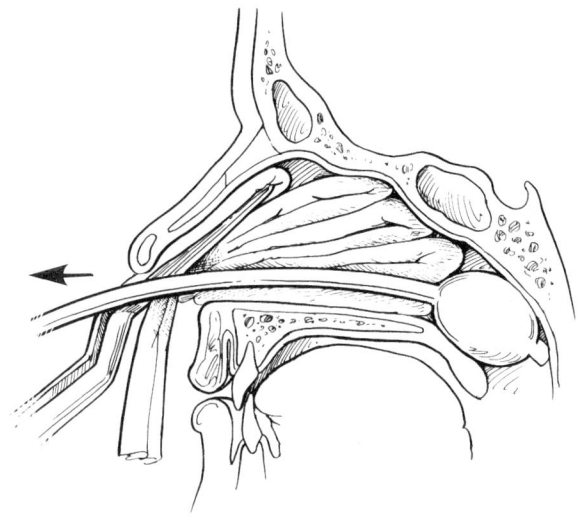

5. Add an additional 10 to 15 ml of water to the balloon. If the soft palate is grossly displaced inferiorly or there is significant pain, the balloon should be slightly deflated.

6. Have an assistant apply gentle traction on the catheter while you insert an anterior pack.

7. Fix the catheter in place using the umbilical clamp. Apply adequate padding (4 × 4) between the clamp and the nose to prevent pressure necrosis.

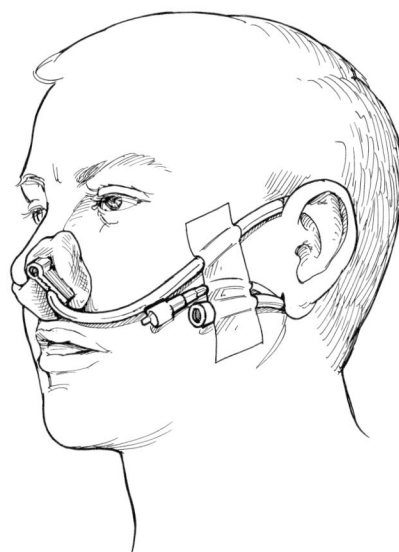

8. Secure the catheter around the ear, as shown.

Note: If bleeding continues, refer the patient to an otolaryngologist for possible arterial ligation.

Follow-Up

1. Instruct the patient to apply Vaseline to the nasal mucosa three times per day to prevent drying and cracking.

2. Recommend air humidification.

3. Tell the patient not to take aspirin.

4. Remove anterior packing in 1 to 3 days, depending on the severity of the bleeding.

5. For posterior packing, once the bleeding has stopped, deflate the balloon and leave the catheter in place for 2 to 3 hours. Reinflate the balloon if the bleeding starts again.

 Bibliography

Parretta LJ, Denslow BL, Brown CG: Emergency evaluation and treatment of epistaxis. Emerg Med Clin North Am 1987;5:265–277.

Randall DA, Freeman SB: Management of anterior and posterior epistaxis. Am Fam Physician 1991;43:2007–2014.

Rosen P, Barkin RM: Emergency Medicine; Concepts and Clinical Practice, 3rd ed. St Louis, Mosby-Year Book, 1992, pp 2465–2468.

Schlesselman LR, Iriarte RI: Controlling posterior epistaxis. *In* Driscoll CE, Rakel RE (eds): Procedures for Your Practice, 2nd ed. Los Angeles, Practice Management Information Co, 1991, pp 373–377.

Weymuller EA, Mulvaney TJ, Partlow RC: Epistaxis. *In* Wilkins EW Jr, Dineen JJ, Gross PL, et al: Emergency Medicine; Scientific Foundations and Current Practice, 3rd ed. Baltimore, Williams & Wilkins, 1989, pp 854–860.

Procedure RHINOLARYNGOSCOPY

Etan C. Milgrom

Flexible fiberoptic rhinolaryngoscopy is a safe, convenient, and effective procedure for examining the upper airway. By using rhinolaryngoscopy, physicians can easily examine areas in the nose and pharynx that were previously inaccessible. The vocal cords, larynx, pharynx, and surrounding structures can be more readily and comfortably visualized than with indirect mirrors or rigid telescopes.

Indications
1. Chronic sinusitis, sinus discomfort
2. Chronic postnasal drip
3. Chronic rhinitis
4. Nasal obstruction
5. Suspected nasopharyngeal or laryngeal tumor (neck masses)
6. Recurrent epistaxis (not active)
7. Foreign body (nasal or laryngeal)
8. Nasal polyps
9. Chronic cough
10. Chronic or recurrent hoarseness
11. Recurrent serous otitis media
12. Unexplained nasopharyngeal pain
13. Halitosis
14. Snoring
15. Dysphagia
16. Stridor
17. Phonation disturbances
18. Post-traumatic evaluation
19. Postsurgery evaluation
20. Caustic ingestion
21. History of regional radiation therapy
22. Psychogenic disorders (globus hystericus)

Contraindications
1. Acute epiglottitis
2. Impending airway obstruction
3. Blood dyscrasias
4. Hypersensitivity to topical anesthetics
5. Severe hypertension

Equipment
1. Nasal speculum
2. Ephedrine 1%, oxymetazoline (Afrin), phenylephrine 0.05% (Neo-Synephrine), or cocaine 0.5% in spray dispenser
3. Lidocaine 4% (mixed in cromolyn sodium [Nasalcrom] or flunisolide [Nasalide] sprayer, 1:1 dilution; end up with a 2% mixture); benzodiazepines and narcotics not necessary
4. Viscous lidocaine to apply to scope for lubrication (optional)
5. Fiberoptic rhinolaryngoscope with appropriate light source

Technique

1. Carefully explain indications and technical procedure to the patient.
2. Discuss patient consent form, and then witness it being signed.
3. Address drug hypersensitivity.
4. Perform routine speculum examination to identify most accessible and patent nasal passage.

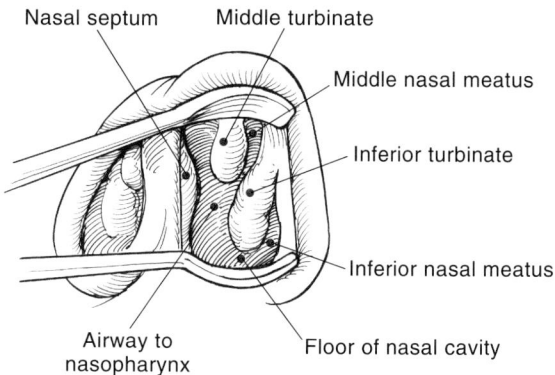

5. Apply two sprays of ephedrine 1% to each nostril to induce vasoconstriction. This should be followed by lidocaine 2% to 4% spray to each nostril (mix in Nasalcrom or Nasalide sprayer [see Equipment section]).
6. Apply viscous lidocaine 2% to scope for lubrication.
7. Place the patient in a sitting position with the head leaning against the head rest or wall (to avoid sudden jolting away from rhinolaryngoscope). The scope should rest in the clinician's hand on the angle between the first finger and thumb, so that the first finger is free to manipulate the angulation tip on the scope. The other hand should gently rest against the patient's face and help guide the scope through the nasal passage. The latter hand actually controls the movement of the scope through the nasal passage. Therefore, contact between the patient's face, the clinician's hand, and the scope should be maintained throughout the procedure.

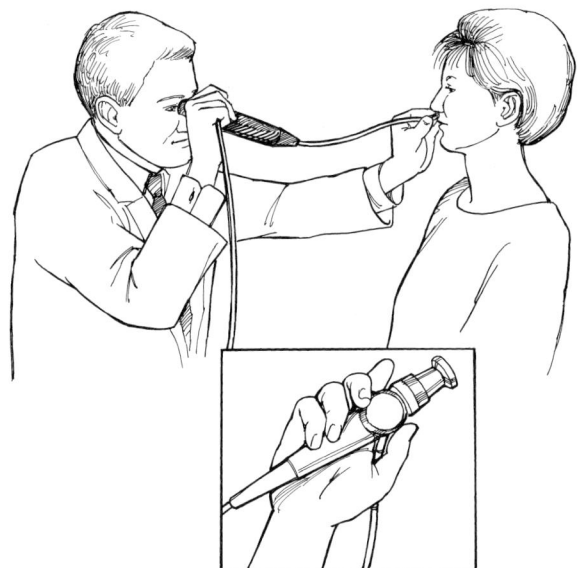

9. Suggested examination sequence
   a. Withdraw the scope once the end point has been reached.
   b. Observe the structures in the larynx.
      (1) Piriform sinuses
      (2) Arytenoids
      (3) False vocal cords
      (4) True vocal cords—ask the patient to say "Eeee" to observe vocal cord movement.

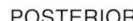
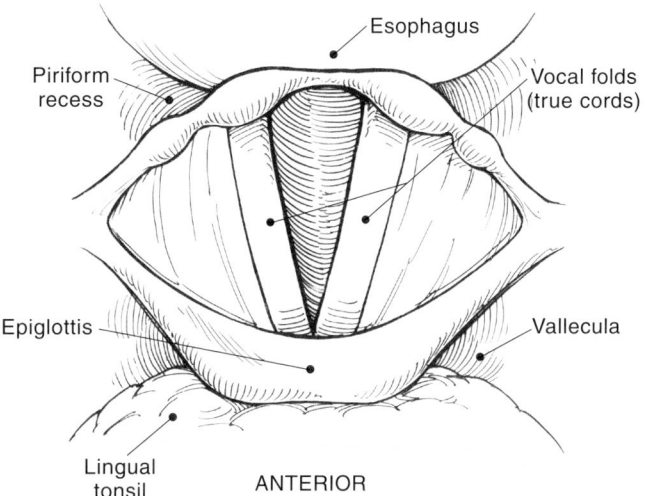

c. Pharynx. The patient should be asked to try not to swallow during the procedure. However, the patient should be reassured that if he or she swallows, it will not interfere with the procedure and will not cause harm. It is better to have the patient breathe through the mouth during the procedure because nasal breathing is more likely to fog the scope.

8. It is recommended to advance the scope to the end point and to observe the anatomy and structures in a methodical manner as the scope is withdrawn. Be sure to advance the scope along the floor of the cavity below the turbinates. Avoid making contact with the scope against the nasal septum because this causes discomfort to the patient. Also try to avoid touching the scope against the pharynx because this induces the gag reflex, making the examination more difficult for both the patient and the physician. Advance the scope along the posterior pharyngeal wall (without touching it) and over the uvula until the larynx is in full view. The angulation tip should be pushed forward to move the scope tip inferiorly. This is the end point of the scope insertion and where careful examination should begin.

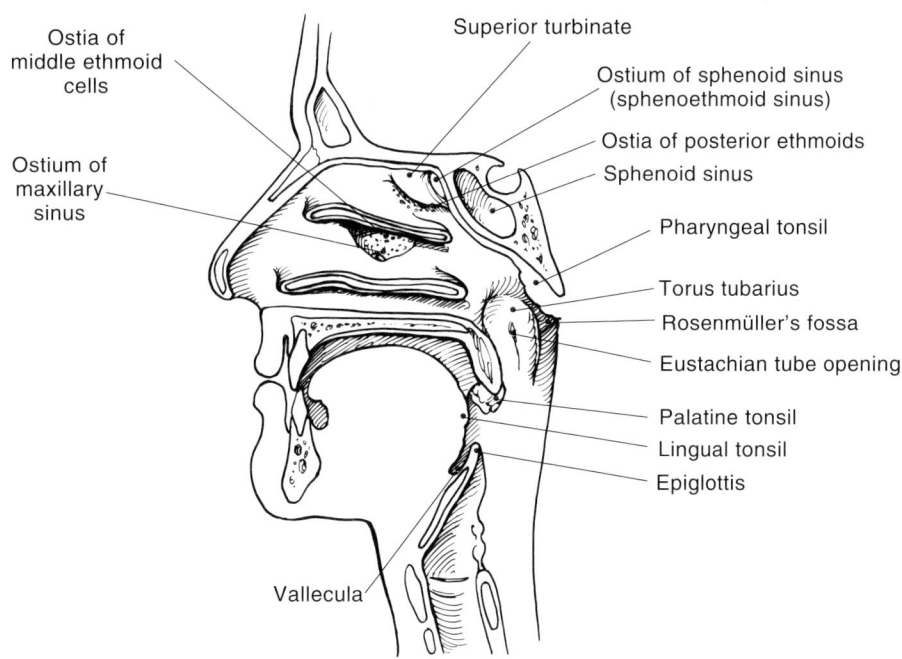

(1) Oropharynx
  (a) Glossal, epiglottic, lateral glottic folds
  (b) Epiglottis
  (c) Vallecula
  (d) Posterior tongue, lingual tonsils
  (e) Posterior pharyngeal wall
  (f) Soft palate
  (g) Lateral pharyngeal walls
(2) Nasopharynx
  (a) Rosenmüller's fossa (most common area for pharyngeal cancer)
  (b) Torus tubarius—both sides ("eeee" for function of veli palatini). The scope tip should be maintained in the flexed position, and the hand holding the eyepiece portion of the scope should should be turned to force the flexed scope tip to view the contralateral torus tubarius.
  (c) Adenoidal pad (palatine tonsil)
d. Choana (opening to pharynx); flex tip upward, view:
  (1) Introitus, ostea of sphenoid sinus, ostea of posterior ethmoids
  (2) Superior (supreme) turbinate
  (3) Sphenoethmoidal recess
e. Nasal floor, move anteriorly, view choana
f. Nasal roof (go over middle turbinate, flex tip upward)—cribriform plate
g. Middle turbinate (flex tip upward underneath turbinate, if possible; usually this is not possible)
  (1) Maxillary sinus ostium
  (2) Polyps

h. Superior portion of anterior nose
i. Nasal vestibule, septum, nasal floor, inferior turbinate (viewed from vestibule)
10. The procedure itself is not hard to perform. The difficult part is developing the skill and experience to differentiate normal anatomy from abnormal pathology. Aside from identifying abnormal structures, pay special attention to color, appearance, mobility, and function of each pertinent structure (i.e., vocal cords). Also take note of abnormal exudates that may help identify pathology (i.e., sinusitis, gastroesophageal reflux).

Complications
1. Gagging
2. Bleeding
3. Sneezing
4. Coughing
5. Laryngospasm
6. Anesthesia reaction

 Bibliography

Corey GA, Hocutt JE, Rodney WM: Preliminary study of rhinolaryngoscopy by family physicians. Fam Med 1988; 20(4):262–265.

Curry RW Jr: Flexible fiberoptic nasolaryngoscopy. Fam Pract Recertification 1990;12(6):21–36.

DeWitt DE: Fiberoptic rhinolaryngoscopy in primary care. Postgrad Med 1988;84:85.

Netter FH: Atlas of Human Anatomy, plates 32, 75. W Caldwell, NJ, Ciba-Geigy, 1989.

Selner JC: Concepts and clinical application of fiberoptic examination of the upper airway. Clin Rev Allergy 1988;6:303–320.

10 Aphthous Stomatitis

Gregory H. Blake

Etiology

1. Prevalence
   a. Affects 20 per cent of the general population; particularly common in North America
   b. Highest rates in upper socioeconomic classes with a slight predilection for females
2. Causative factors
   a. Family history
      (1) Prevalence increased by 20 per cent if both parents are affected
      (2) If positive, occurs more often and at an earlier age
      (3) Some reports of associations with human leukocyte antigens
   b. Infective agents
      (1) Possible link with L-forms of streptococci
      (2) Fourfold rise in antibody titers to varicella
      (3) Adenovirus association noted but no antibody response present
   c. Immunologic aspects
      (1) Ulcer stages
         (a) Preulcerative—predominantly mononuclear infiltrate of large granular lymphocytes and CD4 + T lymphocytes (helper-inducer cells)
         (b) Ulcerative—predominantly CD8 + T lymphocytes (cytotoxic-suppressor cells)
         (c) Healing—return to local CD4 + predominance
      (2) Circulating immune complexes with immune deposits in the stratum spinosum plus leukocytoclastic or immune complex–mediated vasculitis have been found, suggesting antibody-dependent cellular cytotoxicity.
      (3) Increases in serum IgA, IgG, IgD, and IgE levels
      (4) Altered peripheral blood CD8 + T-lymphocyte counts imply defective immunosurveillance.
   d. Local factors
      (1) Minor mucosal trauma may be causal in susceptible people.
   e. Systemic factors
      (1) Twenty per cent of patients appear to have iron deficiency, but not all respond to iron replacement.
      (2) Stress
      (3) Related to luteal phase of menstrual cycle; possibly modulated by changes in progesterone levels present in a minority of females
      (4) Found in Behçet's syndrome, Sweet's syndrome, periodic neutropenia, human immunodeficiency virus (HIV) infection, gluten-sensitive enteropathy

Symptoms

1. Prodrome of burning and tingling at ulcer site
2. Oral lesion producing pain

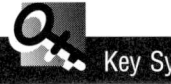

Key Symptom

Oral pain

Clinical Findings

1. Minor aphthous ulcers—80 per cent of patients
   a. Begin during childhood or adolescence
   b. Occasional 0.5-cm round or ovoid ulcer with a yellow to gray pseudomembrane; frequently surrounded by a distinct erythematous halo
   c. Located on tongue or unattached mucosa
   d. Heal without scarring in 10 to 14 days
   e. Most patients have fewer than six recurrences per year
2. Major aphthous ulcers—10 per cent of patients (Sutton's disease or periadenitis mucosa necrotica recurrens)
   a. Generally larger than 1 cm and often lasting up to 6 weeks
   b. Lesions are often continuous, involve various stages of healing, and may heal by scar formation.
   c. Accompanying facial edema and submandibular lymphadenopathy may interfere with eating, sleeping, speaking, and oral hygiene.
3. Herpetiform aphthous ulcers—10 per cent of patients
   a. Begin with up to 100 pinhead-sized lesions on unattached mucosa; coalesce to form an irregularly shaped ulcerative area
   b. Healing time of individual lesions is usually 7 to 10 days.

Key Sign

Oral ulcers on unattached mucosa

Differential Diagnosis

1. Herpes simplex virus
2. Behçet's syndrome
3. Crohn's disease
4. Mucocutaneous disease with ulcerative manifestations
   a. Erythema multiforme c. Cicatricial pemphigoid
   b. Erosive lichen planus d. Pemphigus vulgaris

Treatment

Medication

1. General
   a. If sufficiently concentrated, local treatments may decrease pain by cauterizing superficial tissues.
   b. Local treatment does not promote healing or prevent recurrences.
2. Mouth rinses and topical preparations
   a. Chlorhexidine gluconate (Peridex) can reduce number of ulcer days, increase ulcer-free days, and increase intervals between bouts of ulceration.
   b. Camphor and phenol in alcohol or oil (Cold Sore Lotion or Campho-Phenique)
   c. Carbamide peroxide 10% in anhydrous glycerol (Cankaid)
   d. Copper sulfate, iodine, potassium iodide, and alcohol 1.5% (ORA5)
3. Topical corticosteroids
   a. All can reduce symptoms.
   b. Fluocinonide (Lidex) reduces duration of ulcers and increases time between recurrences.
   c. Available in adhesive topical preparation (Kenalog in Orabase)
   d. Apply during formative stages for maximum benefit.
   e. Use as a 5-ml oral rinse after meals and at bedtime.
4. Topical tetracycline
   a. Decreases pain and duration of ulcers
   b. Empty 250-mg capsule in 50 ml of water; rinse mouth and then swallow three or four times a day for 5 to 7 days.
5. Immunomodulators
   a. Levamisole (Ergamisol)
      (1) Subjective improvement; clinical improvement seldom noted
      (2) Side effects discourage use.
   b. Systemic steroids
      (1) Promote healing of long-standing lesions
      (2) Useful in HIV-positive patients
      (3) 15-mg prednisone equivalent heals ulcers within 7 to 10 days
      (4) Do not alter recurrence rates
      (5) Administer 40 mg of prednisone daily for 5 days and then 20 mg every other day for 7 days.

6. Other
   a. Thalidomide (investigational drug in the US)
      (1) 50 to 400 mg/day may cause remission in 7 to 10 days; more rapid remission at higher dosages
      (2) Effective in severe oropharyngeal ulceration in HIV disease
   b. Prostaglandin E_2 gel (Prepidil) (not FDA approved for this application)
      (1) Reduction in number of new lesions implies a prophylactic effect.
      (2) Apply 0.5 gm of gel twice daily for 10 days.
   c. Pulsed neodymium:yttrium-aluminum-garnet (Nd: YAG) laser
      (1) Ablates lesion in 30 to 45 seconds
      (2) Provides immediate pain relief
   d. Tannic acid 7% in denatured alcohol (Zilactin Medicated)
      (1) Hydroxypropyl cellulose forms adherent, durable film on oral mucosa; protects ulcer.
      (2) Single application is beneficial up to 6 hours.
      (3) Benzocaine can be added as topical anesthetic ZilaDent.
   e. Cyanoacrylate
      (1) Glue hardens on ulcer within seconds, resulting in pain relief within 5 minutes.
      (2) Healing occurs in 5 to 7 days.

 Key Treatment

None is consistently effective; multiple choices

Diet

1. Avoid chemical irritants in toothpastes and mouthwashes.
2. Citrus fruits, strawberries, and tomatoes may exacerbate.

Follow-Up

1. As necessary to screen for other diseases
2. Symptomatic

 ## Bibliography

Jasmin JR, Muller-Giamarchi M, Jonesco-Benaiche N: Local treatment of minor aphthous ulceration in children. J Dent Child 1993; Jan–Feb 72:26–28.

MacPhail LA, Greenspan D, Greenspan JS: Recurrent aphthous ulcers in association with HIV infection: Diagnosis and treatment. Oral Surg Oral Med Oral Pathol 1992;73:283–288.

Porter SR, Scully C: Aphthous stomatitis—an overview of aetiopathogenesis and management. Clin Exp Dermatol 1991;16:235–243.

Rodu B, Mattingly G: Oral mucosal ulcers: Diagnosis and management. J Am Dent Assoc 1992;123:83–86.

Vincent SD, Lilly GE: Clinical, historic, and therapeutic features of aphthous stomatitis: Literature review and open clinical trial employing steroids. Oral Surg Oral Med Oral Pathol 1992;74:79–86.

11 Cheilitis and Angular Cheilitis

Riffat Qadir

Etiology

Cheilitis

1. Contact dermatitis
   a. Irritant
      (1) Chemicals, tomatoes, or citrus fruits
      (2) Hot beverages or foods; cold, dry weather
   b. Allergic: lip salves, lipsticks, toothpastes, foods
   c. Atopic
      (1) Commonly present in atopic individuals
      (2) Most commonly involves upper lip
2. Actinic or sun exposure
   a. This is a precancerous condition if this is the cause.
   b. Most patients are fair-complexioned with a long history of exposure.
   c. Smoke exposure, especially pipe, may be an exacerbating factor.
3. Xerostomia and Sjögren's syndrome—may be accompanied by candidal superinfection
4. Factitial and exfoliative
   a. Characterized by persistent and recurrent scaling
   b. Contact dermatitis, exposure, and xerostomia are negative, and there are emotional disturbances.
   c. Usually secondary to habitual lip-licking and/or manipulation
   d. Can be accompanied by secondary fungal infection
5. Infectious
   a. Causative agents similar to those of angular cheilitis
   b. Uncommon, except candidal secondary infection
6. Granulomatous cheilitis
   a. Lips infiltrated with noncaseating epithelioid granulomas
   b. Lymphedema produces fluid retention, susceptibility to infection.
   c. May become secondarily infected with *Candida* or *Staphylococcus*
7. Cheilitis glandularis
   a. Lip and salivary gland hyperplasia with superinfection, crusting, and ulceration
   b. Lip becomes enlarged, firm, and everted.
   c. Variable association with squamous cell carcinoma
8. Plasma cell cheilitis
   a. Plasma cell infiltration of lips that may be secondary to irritative stimulus
   b. Appears as glistening, red, edematous mass
   c. This is a rare entity; myeloma needs to be considered.

Angular Cheilitis

1. Synonyms include rhagades, perlèche, angular cheilosis
2. Infectious
   a. Fungal
      (1) Usually *Candida albicans*
      (2) Often associated with oral candidiasis
      (3) Patients with diabetes mellitus and immunosuppression have an increased incidence of candidal infections.
   b. Bacterial: impetigo; staphylococcal and/or streptococcal
   c. Viral: usually herpes simplex type I
3. Anatomic characteristics
   a. Flaccid, sagging cheeks with deepened labial angles
   b. Decreased vertical dimension of occlusion in edentulous patients due to lack of or ill-fitting dentures, leading to constant retention of moisture in the angles and predisposing to secondary infection
4. Nutritional deficiencies
   a. Vitamin B, especially riboflavin; *associated findings:* glossitis, keratitis, dermatitis
   b. Iron deficiency anemia; *associated findings:* glossitis, splenomegaly, spooning of the nails
5. Xerostomia and Sjögren's syndrome
6. Sun exposure
   a. Actinic changes can cause precancerous lesions in the angles.
   b. Chronic irritation (e.g., smoking) may exacerbate.

Symptoms

1. Sensation of dryness
2. Irritation, burning, or discomfort of the lips or corners of the mouth
3. Intermittent bleeding

Key Symptoms	
• Burning	• Discomfort
• Irritation	• Bleeding

Clinical Findings

1. Contact dermatitis: erythema, scaling, vesiculation
2. Actinic cheilitis
   a. Dry lips with scaling and crusting
   b. Gray-white discoloration with an atrophic appearance
   c. Vermilion may become indistinct.
   d. Later lesions can become elevated and ulcerated.
   e. Induration and ulceration suggest possible malignant transformation.
3. Exfoliative and factitious cheilitis: persistent or intermittent scaling that can be severe
4. Granulomatous cheilitis
   a. Lips generally enlarged; severity of edema can vary.
   b. May be somewhat nodular
   c. Associated findings of sarcoidosis (lymphadenopathy, nodular nasal mucosa), Crohn's disease, or Melkersson-Rosenthal syndrome (facial nerve paralysis, fissured tongue)
5. Infectious cheilitis and angular cheilitis
   a. Presence of pustules suggests *Staphylococcus aureus*.
   b. Vesicles suggest viral etiology.
   c. *Candida* may present with erythema and scaling.
6. Angular cheilitis
   Corners of the mouth reveal:
   a. Erythema
   b. Wrinkled, macerated skin
   c. Superficial exudative crusts
   d. Deep fissures: these do not involve mucosal surface of commissures

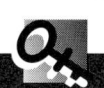

Key Signs

- Erythema
- Scaling
- Fissures

Laboratory Tests

1. Complete blood count to rule out or determine type of anemia
2. Serum glucose to rule out diabetes mellitus
3. Consider serum tests to evaluate nutritional parameters, including serum albumin and vitamin B levels.
4. Consider smear or swab for culture to determine causative agent.
5. Consider human immunodeficiency virus (HIV) testing or tests for other forms of immunosuppression.
6. Consider biopsy to help establish diagnosis and rule out cancer or precancerous condition.

Key Tests

- Complete blood count
- Culture
- Serum glucose
- Biopsy

Differential Diagnosis

1. Dysplasia and carcinoma in situ
   a. This may appear clinically as leukoplakia; this is a white patch that cannot be scraped.
   b. Alternatively, erythroplakia may be noted; this is a reddish patch with poorly defined borders and has a higher incidence of severe dysplasia or carcinoma in situ.
   c. These are precancerous conditions that result from sun exposure, tobacco, chronic infection, or chronic irritation.
   d. Causative factors must be eliminated and severe dysplasia and carcinoma in situ treated; lesser lesions may be observed.
2. Squamous cell carcinoma
   a. Lower lip is the most common site for oral cavity squamous cell carcinoma.
   b. Early biopsy leads to earlier detection and superior outcome.
3. Basal cell carcinoma
   a. Most common cancer in humans
   b. Sun exposure is the primary causative factor.
   c. Typically appears as raised, nodular lesion with pearly, smooth border and telangiectasia
   d. More commonly occurs on the upper lip
4. Lichen planus
   a. Inflammatory dermatosis in which about 50 per cent of patients have mucosal lesions
   b. Lesions can occur on the lips, although buccal mucosa is the most frequent site.
   c. Lesions most commonly reveal a reticular pattern with interlacing whitish streaks; however, papules, plaques, or ulcerations can be present.
   d. Diagnosis is established with biopsy and direct immunofluorescence.
   e. Lesions can be asymptomatic but at times may require topical or intralesional steroids, topical retinoic acid, or cyclosporine.
5. Lichenoid drug eruptions: associated with nonsteroidal anti-inflammatory drugs, thiazide diuretics, methyldopa, phenothiazines, gold
6. Pemphigus and pemphigoid
   a. Blisters and erosions are characteristic.
   b. Generally, there is diffuse involvement of the oral cavity.

c. Therapy generally consists of systemic corticosteroids.

7. Orofacial granulomatosis: associated with the following underlying conditions:
   - Crohn's disease
   - Sarcoidosis
   - Melkersson-Rosenthal syndrome

8. Immunosuppression
   a. Generally, this leads to increased incidence of opportunistic infections; candidal infection is common.
   b. Patients with HIV infection can present with only oral manifestations.

9. Chronic mouth breathing: this can lead to drying and fissuring of the mouth, resulting in a "furrowed mouth."

Treatment

1. Treatment varies, depending on the specific cause.

2. Cryosurgery, carbon dioxide laser vaporization, or surgical excision (vermilionectomy) may be indicated in cases of severe dysplasia or carcinoma in situ.

3. Refractory granulomatous cheilitis or glandular cheilitis also may benefit from surgical reduction.

Medication

1. Antimicrobial agents
   a. Viral: topical acyclovir (Zovirax) can abort progression
   b. Bacterial
      (1) Topical and, possibly, oral antistaphylococcal antibiotic (e.g., mupirocin)
      (2) Continue treatment 1 week after clinical resolution.
   c. Fungal
      (1) Topical imidazole antifungal agent (e.g., clotrimazole [Mycelex])
      (2) Consider adding topical steroid or oral nystatin suspension (Nilstat)

2. Emollients: useful for dryness, crusting

3. Vitamin B and iron supplementation: usefulness only documented in cases of deficiency

4. Corticosteroids: useful in contact cheilitis, granulomatous cheilitis, and plasma cell cheilitis

Key Treatment

Must be directed at specific cause

Diet
Unless a deficiency exists, modification is not indicated.

Activity
1. Good oral hygiene is important in controlling infection.
2. If dentures are worn, they should be cleaned well and left out at night.

Patient Education
Patient understanding of disease and contributing factors is essential in controlling disease.

Follow-Up

1. If the disease is acute and severe, the patient may need to be seen every 1 to 2 weeks to assess response to treatment.

2. Once the disease is stabilized, the patient may be evaluated less frequently.

3. If the lesion is suspected to be precancerous, a biopsy is indicated and then follow-up every month initially and then less frequently if lesion improves or stabilizes.

Bibliography

Heagerty A, Gilkes J: Lip dermatoses. Practitioner 1991;235:49–54.

Rogers RS III, Mehregan DA: Disorders of the oral cavity. In Moschella SL, Hurley HJ (eds): Dermatology, 3rd ed. Philadelphia, WB Saunders, 1992, pp 2087–2121.

12 Glaucoma

Shirlene Tolbert

Etiology

The glaucomas are a group of ocular disorders that are among the most common causes of blindness in the United States and the most common cause of blindness among African Americans. Its prevalence is 2 to 5 per cent, increasing with age to affect as much as 10 per cent of the population by age 80. It is thought that glaucomatous changes result from a pressure that is too high for normal functioning of the eye. Normal intraocular pressure (IOP) is 10 to 21 mm Hg. This number results from the difference between the production of aqueous humor and the normal resistance to drainage of aqueous humor. Aqueous humor, which nourishes the eyes, normally is produced by the ciliary body and moves out peripherally from the posterior chamber to the anterior chamber through the trabecular meshwork, canal of Schlemm, and scleral veins and out to the venous circulation. Increase in IOP results from either an overproduction or an altered drainage of aqueous humor. This causes peripheral visual field loss as the optic nerve degenerates. With progression of this optic nerve damage, blindness ultimately results as central vision is destroyed.

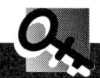
Key Symptom

Blurred vision
(Be aware that symptoms usually are not present until significant visual loss has occurred.)

Glaucoma is classified as either primary or secondary. Primary glaucoma exists when the cause of glaucomatous changes in the eye is unknown. Secondary glaucoma results from a known factor, such as trauma or a systemic illness.

1. Primary: open-angle glaucoma, closed-angle glaucoma, and infantile glaucoma
2. Secondary: glaucoma associated with pigment disorders, systemic illnesses, trauma, or acute angle-closure glaucoma

Key Signs

- Visual field loss
- Increased cup/disk ratio
- Decreased visual acuity

Risk Factors

A. Major
   1. Elevated IOP—most important risk factor
   2. Age—incidence is severalfold higher in people over age 60
   3. Race—blindness from glaucoma is six to eight times more common in blacks than in whites, especially those over age 35
   4. Family history—prevalence may be as high as 40 per cent among first-degree relatives
   5. Diabetes mellitus
   6. Myopia
B. Other important risk factors (especially for the secondary glaucomas)
   1. Previous eye surgeries or trauma
   2. History of cataracts
   3. Alcohol consumption
   4. Prolonged mechanical ventilation (rare)
   5. Medications (e.g., topical or oral corticosteroids)

Open-angle glaucoma is the most common form in adults.

Open-Angle Glaucoma

Etiology

Unknown but associated with the following:
1. Abnormal IOP
2. Optic nerve degeneration
3. Visual field loss

Although, as previously stated, glaucomatous changes are usually the result of increase in IOP, speculation continues as to the cause of optic nerve degeneration and visual field loss in normal-tension glaucoma (glaucomatous damage despite normal IOP) and low-tension glaucoma. This speculation varies from greater sensitivity of these people to even normal or low eye pressures to a variation in blood flow to the retinal nerve cells of the eye.

Symptoms

High index of suspicion is necessary because of glaucoma's insidious nature.
1. Usually not identified until significant visual loss has occurred
2. Patient complaint of blurred vision attributed to needing new glasses.

Tests

The aim is to diagnose glaucoma in its earliest stages. The diagnosis is based on evaluation of the IOP, appearance of the optic nerve, and function of the visual system. Diagnostic tools include the following.
1. Ophthalmoscopy—used to determine cup/disk ratio (cup usually about one third the size of the disk). Asymmetry in the size or contour of the cup is a highly suspicious sign. Increases in cup/disk ratio greater than 0.6 are consistent with glaucoma.

2. Gonioscopy
   a. Performed using a hand-held lens to visualize the iridocorneal angle (outflow area of the aqueous humor)
   b. Differentiates open- from closed-angle glaucoma
3. Tonometry—measures IOP of the eye by assessing amount of pressure necessary to depress the cornea
   a. Contact tonometry
      (1) Schiøtz tonometer
         (a) Hand-held device that is easy to use in the portable or supine positions
         (b) Accuracy is affected by lid squeezing (reduced by using a topical anesthetic) or improper placement on the cornea.
         (c) Sterilization between patients is important to decrease the risk of transmitting human immunodeficiency virus or other infections.
      (2) Goldmann's applanation tonometer
         (a) Major type used by ophthalmologists
         (b) Attached to a slit lamp and requires the use of a topical anesthetic
   b. Noncontact tonometry with pneumotonometer (an air-puff tonometer)
      (1) Measures pressure using a jet of air to depress the globe
      (2) Good for screening large groups of patients
      (3) May require several readings for accuracy
4. Perimetry (visual field testing)
   a. Measures integrity of the visual system and is used for definitive diagnosis of glaucoma
   b. White target lights are presented, with abnormality assessed by areas where targets were not detected
   c. Sometimes limited by time, patient cooperation, and existing eye diseases
5. Image analysis
   a. Helps to quantify the optic disk to neuroretinal rim area (changes seen before visual loss occurs)
   b. May be good for diagnosis of low- versus normal-tension glaucoma or as a follow-up tool
   c. Limited by expense of the equipment

Controversy exists concerning the most effective tool for diagnosing glaucoma. Consequently, family physicians may need to be aware of these tests but concentrate instead on becoming more skilled at identifying individual patients who require referral based on history of risk factors, ophthalmoscopic examination, and/or Schiøtz tonometry testing.

Treatment

Goal—prevent progression of disease

1. *Medication*—primary modality for treatment of glaucoma. All drugs act by decreasing IOP (see Table 12–1). Surgery is indicated for some forms of glaucoma and failed medical therapy.
2. Laser trabeculoplasty
   a. Good for elderly patients who are unfit for surgery or in whom surgical complications (anesthesia) must be avoided.
   b. Long-term results may be disappointing.
3. Surgery
   Filtering surgery may soon be the treatment of choice in glaucoma, especially in patients for whom compliance is a problem. This results from the following:

TABLE 12–1. DRUGS USED TO TREAT OPEN-ANGLE GLAUCOMA

BETA ANTAGONISTS (e.g., timolol maleate [Timoptic])*	MIOTICS (e.g., pilocarpine HCl [Pilocar])	SYMPATHOMIMETICS (e.g., epinephrine HCl [Epifrin])	CARBONIC ANHYDRASE INHIBITORS (e.g., acetazolamide [Diamox])	HYPEROSMOTICS (e.g., mannitol)
Uses: POAG, chronic open-angle glaucoma; adjunctive therapy in AACG, some secondary glaucomas	*Uses:* POAG, acute narrow-angle glaucoma, some secondary glaucomas	*Uses:* POAG—adjunctive therapy	*Uses:* adjunctive therapy	*Uses:* adjunctive therapy; AACG (may be important for use while patient awaits preparation for surgery)
Comments: caution should be used in chronic obstructive pulmonary disease, asthma, heart failure, heartblock, insulin-dependent diabetes mellitus	*Comments:* watch for cholinergic effects in elderly patients (dry mouth, blurred vision)	*Comments:* gonioscopy required before initiation of treatment; may not use in closed-angle glaucoma	*Comments:* many adverse effects, including kidney stones or acidosis, depression, seizures, and fatal aplastic anemia	*Comments:* may cause renal insufficiency, cardiac failure, and intracranial hemorrhage
Dose: 1 drop twice daily	*Dose:* 1 drop 1–6 times a day	*Dose:* 1–2 drops once or twice daily	*Dose:* 250-mg capsule once to four times daily	*Dose:* 1 to 2 gm/kg as a 20% solution over 30–60 min (1gm/kg usually effective)
Route: topical	*Route:* topical	*Route:* topical	*Route:* PO	*Route:* IV

*Drug of choice.
AACG, acute angle-closure glaucoma; POAG, primary open-angle glaucoma.

a. Medications not readily available

b. Time-consuming schedules

c. Visual problems, especially in elderly patients; good long-term results when compared with laser therapy

Closed-Angle Glaucoma

Less common than open-angle glaucoma and results from a narrowed or occluded anterior chamber angle. Etiology, symptoms, diagnosis, and management are similar to those for open-angle glaucoma.

Infantile Glaucoma

Glaucoma that occurs within the first 3 years of life (considered congenital if the disease is present at birth). This type represents one half of all glaucomas in children under age 3.

Etiology
Unknown but has a multifactorial inheritance pattern and results from a developmental anomaly of the iridocorneal angle.

Symptoms
1. Mother may give history of noticing corneal clouding and enlargement.
2. Excess tearing, photophobia (light sensitivity), and blepharospasm (voluntary eyelid closure)

Clinical Findings
1. Corneal horizontal diameter greater than 13 mm
2. Cup/disk ratio greater than 0.3 or asymmetry of the cup/disk ratio between the two eyes
3. Irregular corneal reflex

Treatment
Usually surgery to control the IOP. Goniotomy and/or trabeculotomy has an 80 per cent success rate.

Secondary Glaucomas

Etiology
More common in older children and have numerous causes, including traumatic injury, previous surgeries, Sturge-Weber syndrome, Marfan syndrome, congenital rubella syndrome, Lowe syndrome, plus many more structural, metabolic, and inflammatory diseases

Symptoms
Depend on the cause

Tests
Similar to those for open-angle glaucoma

Treatment
Treat underlying cause. May decrease IOP using methods similar to those used to treat open-angle glaucoma.

Acute Angle-Closure Glaucoma

This form is uncommon, but when it does occur, it is considered an ocular emergency.

Etiology
1. Angle crowding
2. Pupillary block
3. Neovascularization
4. Inflammatory membrane pulling the angle closed
5. Mechanical closure of the angle due to anterior displacement of the lens-iris diaphragm
6. Can be precipitated by labor (rare), sneezing, laser therapy or surgery, traumatic injury, and some medications

Symptoms
1. Severe eye pain
2. Blurred vision
3. Conjunctival injection
4. Complaints of colored halos around lights
5. Nausea and vomiting
6. Blindness in a few hours to a few days if not diagnosed and treated immediately

Clinical Findings
1. Based on history and test results to detect visual acuity, which is markedly decreased
2. Shallow anterior chamber
3. Closed angle in the involved eye
4. Increased IOP
5. Semidilated pupils that are nonreactive

Treatment
1. Laser therapy or surgery to relieve IOP caused by narrow angle
2. Medications (miotics, osmotics [e.g., mannitol])

 Bibliography

Dayluk AW, Paton D: Diagnosis and management of glaucoma. *In* Clin Symp 1991;43:4.

Jay JL: Rational choice of therapy in primary care open angle glaucoma. Eye 1992;6:243–247.

Rakel RE: Glaucoma. *In* Conn's Current Therapy. Philadelphia, WB Saunders, 1994, pp 915–916.

Tucker JB: Screening for open-angle glaucoma. Am Fam Physician 1993;48:75–80.

Wagner R: Infantile glaucomas. Pediatr Clin North Am 1993;40(40):855–867.

13 Conjunctivitis

Robert M. Woodard

Definitions

1. Conjunctivitis is defined as inflammation of the conjunctiva. When there is associated inflammation of the cornea, it is keratoconjunctivitis.

2. The conjunctiva is a thin, transparent mucous membrane that covers the posterior aspect of the tarsus (the eyelid) and the anterior surface of the sclera. The tarsal covering is the palpebral conjunctiva and the covering over the sclera is the bulbar conjunctiva. The conjunctiva protects the eye against foreign materials and microorganisms.

Etiology

1. Bacterial. Most common—*Staphylococcus aureus, Streptococcus pneumoniae, Haemophilus influenzae, Neisseria gonorrhoeae, Proteus, Klebsiella pneumoniae*

2. Viral
   a. Herpes simplex virus, usually type I
   b. Adenovirus—sporadic and epidemic
   c. Enterovirus 70—acute hemorrhagic conjunctivitis
   d. Varicella zoster—spreads down the ophthalmic nerve

3. Chlamydial—causes adult inclusion conjunctivitis, ophthalmia neonatorum, and trachoma; sexually transmitted or from passage down birth canal; usually develops 7 to 10 days after exposure

4. Allergic (atopic)
   a. Seasonal allergic conjunctivitis or hay fever conjunctivitis; usually caused by grass pollens in May and June and by ragweed pollens in August and September
   b. Vernal keratoconjunctivitis—usually occurs in childhood and youth in people with a family history of atopy
   c. Atopic keratoconjunctivitis—usually occurs in the late teen years

5. Ophthalmia neonatorum—all can lead to systemic illness if not treated
   a. Bacterial—usually *N. gonorrhoeae*
   b. Chlamydial infection
   c. Herpes simplex virus

Symptoms

1. Symptoms are somewhat variable, depending on cause, but generally are itching, watering, and redness of the eyes; foreign body sensation; and a sense of fullness around the eyes.

2. Adenovirus causes a foreign body sensation, red and watery eyes that may lead to pain, and photophobia in 5 to 7 days, when the cornea becomes involved. Also, family members may be affected.

3. Associated upper respiratory tract infection symptoms may point to a viral cause.

4. Bacterial infections, such as *S. aureus,* may produce significant stickiness of the eyelids, especially in the morning.

5. Visual loss, photophobia, and severe eye pain may suggest corneal involvement.

 Key Symptoms

• Itching	• Redness
• Foreign body sensation	• Watery eyes

Clinical Findings

1. General findings (Table 13–1)
   a. Tearing—derives from the sensation of a foreign body
   b. Hyperemia—redness that is usually greatest in the fornix and decreases toward the limbus
   c. Exudation—may have gumming of the lids on awakening. If the discharge is thick and copious, the cause is probably bacterial or chlamydial.
   d. Lid skin swelling—may cause pseudoptosis

2. More specific findings (Table 13–1)
   a. Follicles—represent areas of lymphoid tissue hyperplasia that appear as dome-shaped elevations with blood vessels on their surface. Follicles are present in many types of conjunctivitis. If they are prominent in the upper tarsus, they usually indicate a viral etiology, such as adenovirus, or *Chlamydia.*
   b. Papillae—minute elevations with vascular cores that may coalesce to form large papillae. Papillae form in response to inflammation and may be seen on the superior tarsal plate, where they usually represent vernal keratoconjunctivitis, adenovirus, or herpes simplex virus conjunctivitis.
   c. Preauricular nodes—usually noted in viral etiologies, such as herpes simplex virus and adenovirus, in chlamydial infections, and in *N. gonorrhoeae.* These nodes are less prominent in bacterial etiologies and may be tender to palpation.
   d. Subconjunctival hemorrhage—may be seen in bacterial conjunctivitis or in enterovirus 70 conjunctivitis
   e. Corneal involvement—increased in *N. gonorrhoeae,* adenovirus, and vernal keratoconjunctivitis; may appear as punctate epithelial lesions

TABLE 13–1. DIFFERENTIATION OF THE COMMON TYPES OF CONJUNCTIVITIS

CLINICAL FINDINGS AND CYTOLOGY	VIRAL	BACTERIAL	CHLAMYDIAL	ALLERGIC
Itching	Minimal	Minimal	Minimal	Severe
Hyperemia	Generalized	Generalized	Generalized	Generalized
Tearing	Profuse	Moderate	Moderate	Moderate
Exudation	Minimal	Profuse	Profuse	Minimal
Preauricular adenopathy	Common	Uncommon	Common only in inclusion conjunctivitis	None
In stained scrapings and exudates	Monocytes	Bacteria, PMNs	PMNs, plasma cell inclusion bodies	Eosinophils
Associated sore throat and fever	Occasionally	Occasionally	Never	Never

PMNs, polymorphonuclear cells.
From Vaughan D, Asbury T, Riordan-Eva P: General Ophthalmology, 13th ed. E Norwalk, CT, Appleton & Lange, 1992, p 99.

f. Membrane formation—a film that covers and adheres to the entire surface of the conjunctival epithelium. If the membrane is removed, a bleeding surface is left behind. This sign is usually associated with epidemic keratoconjunctivitis, herpes simplex virus, and *S. pneumoniae,* and *N. gonorrhoeae* conjunctivitis.

3. Ophthalmia neonatorum

   a. *Chlamydia*—usually presents 3 to 10 days after birth as a bilateral conjunctivitis with a mucopurulent discharge, moderate to severe infiltration of the palpebral conjunctiva, and marked swelling and erythema of the eyelids. The cornea is usually unaffected. It is occasionally associated with otitis media and pneumonitis.

   b. *N. gonorrhoeae*—usually presents 2 to 4 days after birth as a hyperacute conjunctivitis with significant purulent exudate and injection. The conjunctivitis may lead to corneal ulceration and visual problems.

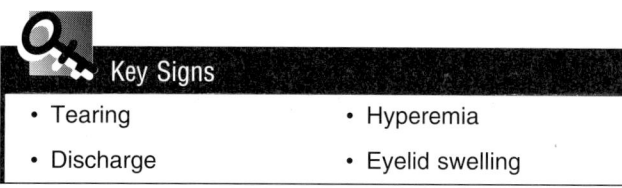

Key Signs

- Tearing
- Discharge
- Hyperemia
- Eyelid swelling

Tests

1. Record visual acuity on all patients.
2. If there is any concern for corneal involvement or suspicion of traumatic injury, stain conjunctiva with fluorescein and use blue penlight illumination to observe for corneal scratches, corneal dendrites (which represent herpes simplex virus), or corneal ulceration. Use anesthetic drops before staining the eye.
3. Gram's stain and culture of the conjunctival discharge should be done if one suspects *N. gonorrhoeae* conjunctivitis, such as in hyperacute purulent conjunctivitis. Other indications for Gram's stain and culture are for conjunctivitis that fails to respond to antibiotic therapy, ophthalmia neonatorum, membranous conjunctivitis, and severe and prolonged conjunctivitis.

4. If chlamydial infection is suspected, one can obtain *Chlamydia* cultures and/or perform fluorescent antibody tests.
5. Giemsa stain may help to differentiate causes in persistent cases of conjunctivitis. The tarsal plate is scraped and the tissue that is removed is smeared on a slide and stained with Giemsa. Microscopic evaluation may reveal neutrophils, which may represent bacterial infection; mononuclear cells, which may suggest viral infection; and eosinophils, which may represent allergic conjunctivitis.

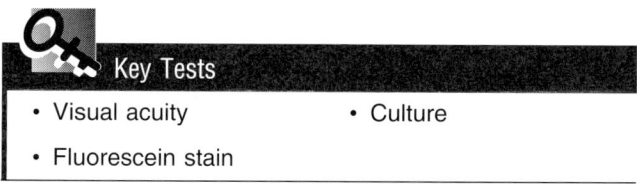

Key Tests

- Visual acuity
- Fluorescein stain
- Culture

Differential Diagnosis

Other common causes of "red eye." The following represent ophthalmic emergencies.

1. Anterior uveitis—usually presents with ocular pain, photophobia, blurred vision, injection in the limbus area, and deposits in the cornea
2. Acute glaucoma—occurs mainly in elderly people and may present with eye pain, headache, nausea, abdominal pain, blurred vision, and decreased visual acuity

Treatment

General considerations

1. Suggest warm compresses, lubrication of the eyes with artificial tears, and cleaning of the lid margins.
2. Avoid wearing contact lenses during the time of infection.
3. Avoid using topical anesthetics except before fluorescein staining and ocular pressure measurements.
4. Most cases of infectious conjunctivitis are treated initially as bacterial infection without obtaining cultures, even though many are viral or allergic in origin. The key to successful treatment is close follow-up.

Medication

1. Bacterial—unless this is a hyperacute, purulent conjunctivitis in patient at risk for *N. gonorrhoeae,* these infections are treated with topical antibiotics without sending a culture or Gram's stain.

   a. Gentamicin ophthalmic ointment or solution (Garamycin Ophthalmic)—ointment every 4 h or 1 drop every 2 h first day then every 4 h

   b. Sulfacetamide sodium 10% (Sodium Sulamyd) ophthalmic ointment or solution—ointment every 4 h; 1 drop every 2 h first day then every 4 h. Contraindicated in patients allergic to sulfa.

   c. Newer topical agents with increased spectrum —ciprofloxacin and norfloxacin

2. *N. gonorrhoeae* conjunctivitis in adults—requires systemic antibiotics as well as topical antibiotics. Also, treat *Chlamydia* presumptively.

   a. Ceftriaxone sodium (Rocephin)—1 gm intramuscularly once

   b. Penicillin G—10 million U intramuscularly once daily for 5 days

3. *Chlamydia* conjunctivitis in adults—requires systemic treatment

   a. Tetracycline—500 mg three times per day for 3 weeks

   b. Doxycycline—100 mg twice daily for 3 weeks

   c. Erythromycin—250 mg four times per day for 3 weeks

   d. Some clinicians add erythromycin ointment as well.

4. Viral—most cases are treated as bacterial conjunctivitis. If dendritic ulcers are obvious on the cornea (which is visible with fluorescein staining), this indicates herpes simplex keratoconjunctivitis, which requires initiation of topical antiviral agents, such as idoxuridine, vidarabine, or trifluridine, as well as immediate referral to an ophthalmologist. For other forms of viral conjunctivitis, treatment is mostly supportive. Topical vasoconstrictors and steroids must be avoided.

5. Allergic conjunctivitis

   a. Avoidance of offending agent

   b. Prophylactic drugs such as cromolyn sodium

   c. Topical vasoconstrictors, such as naphazoline 0.1% solution—1 to 2 drops every 3 to 4 h

   d. Topical vasoconstrictor with a topical histamine, antihistamine, such as Naphcon-A solution—1 to 2 drops q 3 to 4 h

   e. Topical nonsteroidal anti-inflammatory drugs that have good anti-inflammatory action with minimal side effects, such as ketorolac tromethamine (Acular) solution (1 drop q.i.d.) and diclofenac sodium (Voltaren) ophthalmic solution (1 to 2 drops q.i.d.). Use for up to 1 week

   f. Topical steroids—use only in the most severe and recalcitrant cases and where the diagnosis is confirmed

6. Ophthalmia neonatorum—treatment is based on culture diagnosis and consists of systemic treatment for *Chlamydia* or *N. gonorrhoeae* and eye irrigation. The drug of choice for infants is oral erythromycin estolate (Ilosone), 10 mg/kg t.i.d., or erythromycin ethylsuccinate (EES), 50 mg/kg/day in four divided doses combined with topical erythromycin ointment q.i.d. or topical tetracycline drops q.i.d. or sulfacetamide sodium drops q.i.d. for 2 to 3 weeks.

Activity

1. Patient should not go to work or attend school during acute infectious conjunctivitis.

2. Do not patch the affected eye.

Patient Education

1. Emphasize importance of good personal hygiene during acute infection.

2. Viral conjunctivitis may persist for 3 to 4 weeks and may worsen before improving.

Key Treatment

- Warm compresses

- Gentamicin (Garamycin), sulfacetamide sodium or agent-specific medication

Follow-Up

1. All patients with conjunctivitis should be followed for 24 to 72 hours to ensure proper treatment and resolution of the infection. If the condition worsens, re-evaluate the problem, obtain cultures of the discharge, and seek consultation if necessary. Potential complications include corneal abscess and keratitis.

2. Consult or refer the patient with conjunctivitis if any of the following is present:

   a. Hyperacute, purulent infection

   b. Corneal involvement with ulceration

   c. Orbital cellulitis

   d. Persistent symptoms despite adequate treatment

   e. Increasing ocular pain

   f. Decreasing visual acuity

   g. Membrane development across the upper tarsal plate

   h. Increasing corneal opacities

 ## Bibliography

Hirst LW: Conjunctivitis. Aust Fam Physician 1991;20:797–804.

O'Hara MA: Ophthalmia neonatorum. Ped Clin North Am 1993; 40:715–725.

Ragge NK, Easty DL: Immediate Eye Care. St Louis, Mosby Year Book, 1990, pp 53–67.

Syed NA, Hyndiuk RA: Infectious conjunctivitis. Infect Dis Clin North Am 1992;6:789–805.

Vaughan D, Asbury T, Riordan-Eva P (eds): General Ophthalmology, 13th ed. E Norwalk, CT, Appleton & Lange, 1992, pp 58–76.

14 Corneal Ulceration

Ashish Chabra

Etiology

1. Infection of the cornea by bacteria, virus, or fungi as a result of breakdown in the protective epithelial barrier
2. Dry eyes, contact lenses, burns, abrasions, or foreign body entry to the eye (i.e., trauma)
3. Inappropriate use of topical anesthetics or antiviral or antibiotic medications
4. Diabetes, thyroid disease (fifth-nerve palsy)
5. Chronic blepharitis, conjunctivitis, or herpes simplex keratitis
6. Immunosuppression or immunosuppressive drugs
7. Vitamin A or protein malnutrition
8. Defective closure of the eyelids (lagophthalmos)
9. Infectious agents include the following:
   a. Gram-positive organisms (e.g., staphylococci, streptococci, bacilli)
   b. Gram-negative organisms (e.g., rods, diplococci)
   c. Anaerobes
   d. Viruses (e.g., herpes)
   e. *Pseudomonas*
   f. Sexually transmitted diseases (trachoma, gonorrhea)

Symptoms

1. Red eyes
2. Sensation of foreign body in affected eye
3. Blurred vision
4. Discharge from affected eye (i.e., mucopurulent or serous if viral)
5. Pain in the eye, especially with movement
6. Photophobia
7. Blepharospasm

Key Symptoms

- Foreign-body sensation
- Eye discharge
- Blurred vision
- Pain

Clinical Findings

1. Inflammation and edema of eyelid
2. Conjunctival injection or inflammation
3. Discharge from affected eye (i.e., mucopurulent versus serous)
4. Dull, grayish, circumscribed superficial infiltration that may progress to necrosis and ulcer formation

Key Signs

- Edema and inflammation
- Mucopurulent discharge
- Ciliary injection
- Blepharospasm

Tests

1. Fluorescein stain to confirm ulcer
2. Culture
3. Scrapings for Gram's and Giemsa stains to identify bacteria, yeast, or intranuclear inclusions

Key Tests

- Fluorescein stain
- Culture

Differential Diagnosis

1. Identify infecting organism to determine if viral, bacterial, or fungal
2. Corneal abrasion
3. Corneal foreign body
4. Conjunctivitis
5. Keratitis
6. Blepharitis
7. Dacrocystitis

Treatment

1. Immediate institution of aggressive topical antibiotic treatment
2. Prompt referral to an ophthalmologist
3. Topical cycloplegics to help reduce inflammation and pain
4. Daily evaluation

WARNING

- **Topical steroids should never be used.**
- **Do not bandage the eye.**

Medication

1. Topical gentamicin (Garamycin) and tobramycin (Tobrex) for aerobic gram-negative organisms, *Enterobacter, Klebsiella,* and *Pseudomonas*
2. Topical cephalosporins (Cefazolin [Kefzol]) for gram-positive organisms
3. Sulfacetamide 10% (Cetamide Ophthalmic) only for low-grade infections
4. Ciprofloxacin (Cipro) for *Pseudomonas* infections
5. Fungal infections need to be treated with parenteral amphotericin B (Fungizone); may also require ketoconazole (Nizoral), clotrimazole (Lotrimin), or miconazole (Monistat).
6. Vidarabine (Vira-A Ophthalmic) or trifluridine (Viroptic Ophthalmic Solution 1%) for herpes simplex infection

Diet

If the patient is vitamin A–deficient or protein-malnourished, increase supplements of these in the diet; otherwise, no special dietary requirements.

Activity

Limit sports or heavy physical activities until healing is complete and vision returns to normal.

Patient Education

1. Proper handling of contact lenses
2. Prevention of abrasions or injury

Key Treatment

- Ophthalmologic referral
- Aggressive use of topical antibiotics
- Combination aminoglycosides and cephalosporins as initial therapy

Follow-Up

Daily follow-up with physician

Bibliography

Newell FW: Ophthalmic Pathology: Principles and Concepts, 7th ed. St Louis, CV Mosby, 1991.

Tahija SG, Chandler JW: Corneal ulceration: Have we advanced in the last 20 years? (review). Int Ophthalmol Clin 1990;30(1):33–35.

Whitcher JP: Corneal ulceration (review). Int Ophthalmol Clin 1990;30(1):30–32.

Procedure CORNEAL FOREIGN BODY REMOVAL   *Isaac Kleinman*

Epidemiology

1. Foreign bodies were involved in 57 per cent of all eye injuries and accounted for 3.6 per cent of all emergency department visits to one hospital; 31 per cent were due to wind and dust, 30 per cent due to grinding, 8.5 per cent due to drilling, 6.4 per cent to wood cutting, and 4.3 per cent to welding.

2. Occupational exposure is the major risk factor, along with contact lenses and failure to wear protective goggles.

Symptoms

The principal symptoms of corneal foreign body or abrasion are pain, scratchy sensation, and burning. Any time the patient presents with such symptoms, foreign body should be suspected and searched for regardless of whether the patient complains of a foreign body.

Evaluation

1. Examine both eyes with magnification (binocular loupe, ophthalmoscope, slit-lamp). This is essential to determine whether a foreign body is superficial or deep. The use of a slit-lamp is highly desirable.

2. Evert the tarsal plate of the affected eye to look for foreign material.

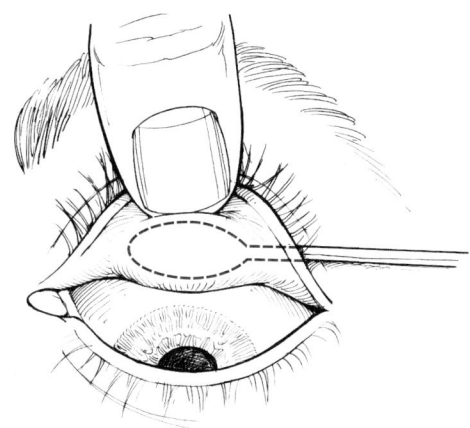

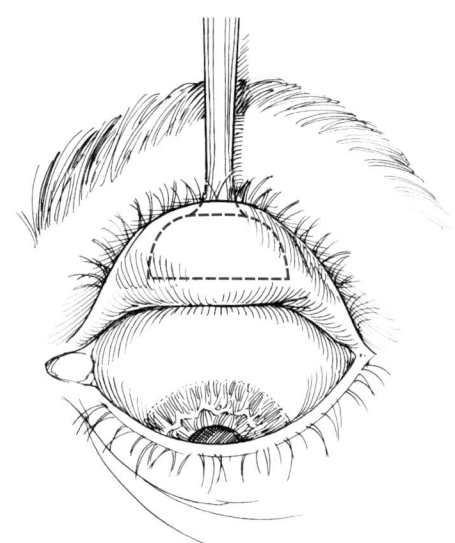

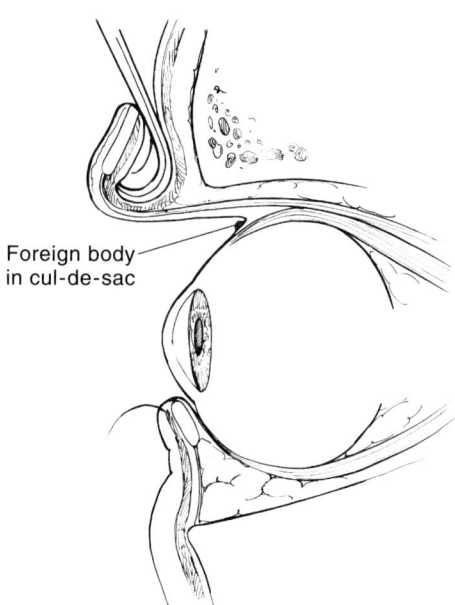

Foreign body in cul-de-sac

Double eversion of the tarsal plate may be necessary to look high into the cul-de-sac. If a Desmarres retractor is not available, a bent large paper clip will suffice. Pull down on the upper lid, "hook" the superior edge of the tarsal plate, and evert upward and outward. Vertical scratches on the cornea suggest a foreign body in the superior palpebral conjunctiva. Keep in mind that injury from wind and blast (explosion) may result in the presence of more than one foreign body in the eye.

3. Most foreign bodies are superficial and lie on or within the epithelium. If they are beneath the epithelium and if Bowman's membrane has been injured, foreign body removal is usually best done under an operating microscope by an ophthalmologist.

4. Signs of globe perforation include decreased tone on tactile examination, shallowing of the anterior chamber, altered pupil size, and a positive percolation test (i.e., continuous washing of fluorescein from the site of injury by a stream of aqueous humor leaking through the cornea [Seidel's sign]). If perforation is found, avoid manipulation, protect the eye with a shield, and refer to an ophthalmic surgeon.

5. Note any signs of anterior uveitis (cells or clouding within the anterior chamber).

6. Always test and record visual acuity before performing any procedure or manipulation.

7. If no foreign body is found, search for an inturned eyelash or eyelid (entropion). Be sure to evert the tarsal plate and look under it. If nothing is seen, anesthetize the eye surface with a drop of fluorescein from an impregnated fluorescein strip that has been moistened with a few drops of a topical anesthetic, such as proparacaine 0.5%. Wait a few minutes, and then irrigate the eye obliquely with saline solution.

8. Examine again under magnification. If no ulceration, abrasion, or foreign body can be found, examine the

eye by means of a slit-lamp or refer for slit-lamp examination. If a lesion is not acute, there may be signs of infection, such as hypopion, edema and corneal clouding, purulent discharge, or ulceration exceeding the size of the foreign body. Such signs indicate the need for urgent hospitalization.

> **WARNING**
>
> • **When a foreign object, especially a metallic foreign body, is found on the cornea, always obtain orbit radiographs to rule out an unsuspected foreign body within the orbit. This is especially true if the particle has come from a high-velocity source, such as a grinding wheel or a hammer strike.**
>
> • **Wood, plastic, and pencil lead produce intraocular foreign bodies that may not show up on radiography of the orbit; use magnetic resonance imaging or ultrasound.**

> • *Avoid magnetic resonance imaging if there is any possibility of a metallic foreign body within the eye.*
>
> • **Document all findings (e.g., visual acuity in both eyes, location of the foreign body [peripheral or central] or abrasion, signs of infection, presence of rust rings).**
>
> • **Avoid use of steroids because they retard healing and can be disastrous in the circumstance of infection.**
>
> • **Never dispense take-home topical anesthesia for pain relief because it delays corneal healing and masks symptoms.**
>
> • **Use sterile single-dose anesthesia and fluorescein.**

Technique

1. If a foreign body is seen on the cornea, it is best removed with the patient lying supine with eyes fixed on the ceiling at a point that makes the foreign body become the uppermost point of the globe.

2. Caution the patient about the need to remain still. Children may require restraint.

3. First try to blot the foreign body from the cornea with a sterile cotton-tipped applicator moistened with normal saline solution. Be careful not to use force or abrasion. Most foreign bodies come away in this manner.

4. If this fails, gently scrape the foreign body from the cornea with an eye spud or a hypodermic needle using a *tangential* approach. Select a needle size appropriate for the size of the foreign body. Having the needle attached to the barrel of a plastic syringe may help achieve hand stability. Resting the hand on the patient's cheek keeps any movements of face and hand in tandem and reduces the risk of injury. Use magnification (binocular loupe).

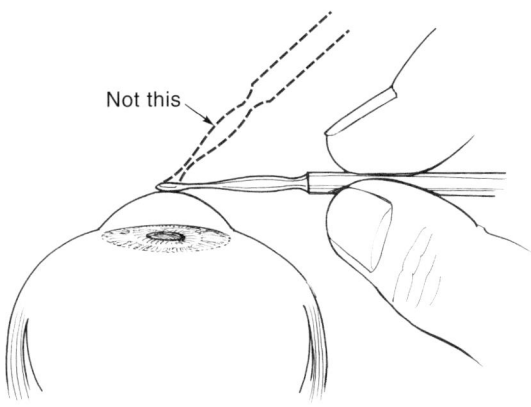

Not this

5. If the foreign body is ferrous, check carefully for a rust ring. If found, it must be removed. This can be done by gently scraping with the spud or by gentle rotation of a dental burr of appropriate size. (This method is not suitable for rust that is in the center of the cornea or for deep rust.) If an ophthalmic magnet is available, it may be used to lift off ferrous foreign bodies.

6. Instill an ophthalmic antibiotic ointment (tobramycin or gentamicin). Patch an anesthetized eye for 2 hours post examination or have the patient wear protective lenses. This provides protection against unrecognized foreign body entry while the eye is insensitive. Schedule follow-up in 24 hours and restain the cornea. Do not omit the 24-hour follow-up examination. Failure to show prompt healing requires referral. Give special attention to cases of vegetable foreign body or contaminated substances because they are prone to infection.

7. Cases in which multiple foreign bodies are driven into the cornea, such as blasts or explosions, are best referred. Tropicamide (Mydriacyl) or cyclopentolate hydrochloride (Cyclogyl), one drop in the affected eye, reduces the effects of secondary iridocyclitis and makes the eye more comfortable.

 Bibliography

Ban DH, Hedge JR: Corneal foreign body removal and treatment. Optom Clin 1991;1:59–70.

Fogle JA, Spyker DA: Chemical and drug injury to the eye. *In* Haddad LM, Winchester J (eds): Clinical Management of Poisoning and Drug Overdose. Philadelphia, WB Saunders, 1983.

Kruger RA, et al: Emergency eye injuries. Austral Fam Physician 1990;19:934–936.

Reich JA: Removal of corneal foreign bodies. Austral Fam Physician. 1990;19:719–721.

Roberts JR, Hedges JR: Clinical Procedures in Emergency Medicine. Philadelphia, WB Saunders, 1985, pp 893–900.

15 Optic Neuritis

W. Michael Skeens

Optic neuritis is due to inflammation, demyelination, or infection that affects the optic nerve at or anterior to the optic chiasm. This disorder is subdivided into papillitis and retrobulbar neuritis. The division is made based on whether the intraocular portion of the optic nerve is involved, causing the papillitis. If the adjacent retina is also involved, it is referred to as optic neuroretinitis. The primary group of entities that optic neuritis must be differentiated from are the disorders that cause optic neuropathy. As well, the papillitis may be confused with papilledema. Optic neuropathy may result from ischemia, compression, or toxic effects. These problems include arteritis, systemic lupus erythematosus, syphilis, accelerated hypertension, diabetes, collagen vascular diseases, sickle cell disease, migraine headaches, carotid artery disease, acute hypotension (as in sudden gastrointestinal hemorrhage), polycythemia vera, radiation, compression, and atherosclerosis. This also includes entities such as tobacco-alcohol amblyopia.

Etiology

1. Demyelination
   a. Multiple sclerosis
      (1) Fifteen per cent of patients with multiple sclerosis present with optic neuritis
      (2) Among all patients with multiple sclerosis, 33 per cent develop optic neuritis during some stage of their disease process
   b. Felty's syndrome (rheumatoid arthritis and hypersplenism)
   c. Behr's disease (hereditary optic atrophy)
   d. Schilder's disease (diffuse periaxial encephalitis)
   e. Diffuse cerebral sclerosis (e.g., metachromatic leukodystrophy)
   f. Brown-Marie syndrome (hereditary ataxia)
   g. Acute disseminated encephalomyelitis
   h. Neuromyelitis (Devic) bilateral with transverse spinal cord myelitis optica
2. Inflammation (including secondary due to infection)
   a. Systemic lupus erythematosus
   b. Autoimmune encephalitis
   c. Meningitis
   d. Syphilis
   e. Tuberculosis
   f. Mumps
   g. Chickenpox
   h. Infectious mononucleosis
   i. Herpes zoster
   j. Vasculitis, including Stevens-Johnson syndrome,

Henoch-Schönlein purpura, multiple myeloma (Kahler disease), temporal arteritis, Raynaud's disease, and periarteritis nodosa
   k. Lyme disease (may also present as papilledema with increased cerebrospinal fluid pressure appearing similar to pseudotumor cerebri)
3. Infection
   a. Intraocular keratitis, endophthalmitis, and chronic uveitis
   b. Orbital region infections
      (1) Orbital cellulitis
      (2) Orbital abscess (Rollet's syndrome)
      (3) Spread from spheroid and ethmoid sinuses
      (4) Wegener's granulomatosis
      (5) Tolosa-Hunt syndrome (painful ophthalmoplegia)
   c. Systemic infections, including bacterial, fungal, protozoal, helminthic, rickettsial, and viral (e.g., Guillain-Barré syndrome, hepatitis, influenza, polio)
4. Systemic diseases
   a. Diabetes (Willis' disease)
   b. Acquired immunodeficiency syndrome
   c. Alcohol ingestion
   d. Amyloidosis
   e. Sarcoidosis
   f. Behçet's disease
   g. Pregnancy
   h. Chronic glomerulonephritis
   i. Multiple medications
   j. Multiple other disease processes and tobacco use
5. Etiology unknown—frequent

Symptoms

1. Acute monocular vision loss ranging from mild decreased visual acuity to monocular blindness; abrupt onset, usually over hours, seldom over weeks
2. Color vision is affected more severely than the overall visual acuity, which is not true in optic neuropathies.
3. Primary vision loss is central in nature. It occurs primarily in the 20-to-50 age group and equally in both sexes.
4. Pain on motion of the affected eye (especially in the lateral direction) is found with retrobulbar optic neuritis.
5. Elderly patients may present with acute papilledema and monocular vision loss. Anterior ischemic optic neuropathy secondary to arteritis is more common.

Key Symptoms

- Acute monocular vision loss
- Loss of some color vision
- Primary vision loss
- Pain on motion of affected eye

Clinical Findings

1. Retrobulbar optic neuritis
   a. Pain on eye movement
   b. Tenderness on palpation of the globe with the eyelid closed
   c. Diffuse swelling and enhancement of the optic nerve on computed tomographic (CT) scan
   d. Normal ophthalmoscopy
2. Papillitis (anterior optic neuropathy)
   a. Swollen optic disk with blurred margins giving the appearance of a smaller disk, dilated retinal veins, and, possibly, flame hemorrhages
   b. If severe, an oval pattern of yellow exudates may be seen around the fovea centralis and inflammatory cells may be present in the adjacent vitreous.
   c. May advance to optic atrophy with gliosis over the disk, causing a pale nerve head, permanent visual dysfunction, and distortion of vessels
3. Papillitis and retrobulbar optic neuritis
   a. Causes are the same.
   b. Color vision is more severely affected than overall visual acuity.
   c. Afferent pupillary defect (APD; Marcus Gunn pupil)
   d. Central or paracentral scotoma
   e. Acute-onset monocular vision loss

Key Signs

Retrobulbar Optic Neuritis

- Pain on eye movement
- Tenderness on palpation of globe with eyelid closed
- Diffuse swelling of optic nerve

Papillitis

- Swollen optic disk
- Oval pattern of yellow exudate seen around fovea centralis
- Inflammatory cells present in adjacent vitreous

Tests

1. Color testing
2. Visual acuity (including pinhole to rule out refractive component) before and after shining a penlight in the affected eye. This further decreases visual acuity in patients with retinal diseases but does not affect the vision of a patient with optic neuritis.
3. CT scan of the orbit when retrobulbar optic neuritis is suspected
4. Visual fields to demonstrate the central or paracentral scotoma
5. Swinging light test to detect APD
6. Visual evoked potentials are abnormal.

Key Tests

- Color testing
- Visual acuity
- CT scan of orbit when retrobulbar optic neuritis suspected

Differential Diagnosis

1. Optic neuropathy—does not have the early loss of visual acuity seen in optic neuropathy
2. Amaurosis fugax—should resolve quickly over a short period.
3. Cystoid macular edema—central serous choroidopathy also present with painless loss of vision with central scotoma, but there is no APD and color vision is not as severely affected.
4. Papilledema must be differentiated from papillitis. Papilledema does not have the early loss of visual acuity and tends to be bilateral.

Treatment

1. Remove or treat the inciting cause, if known.
2. If optic neuritis is retrobulbar and caused by demyelinating disease, recovery usually is spontaneous within 2 to 6 weeks. Some residual optic atrophy that affects the papillomacular bundle may occur.
3. Extremely high-dose steroids may benefit some patients.

Key Treatment

- Remove or treat inciting cause.
- High-dose steroids may benefit some patients.

Bibliography

Braunwald E, et al (eds): Harrison's Principles of Internal Medicine, 11th ed, New York, McGraw-Hill, pp 73, 2036.

Gorbach SL, Bartlett JG, Blacklow NR: Infectious Diseases. Philadelphia, WB Saunders, 1992.

Roy FH: Ocular Differential Diagnosis, 5th ed. Malvern, PA, Lea & Febiger, 1993.

Spalton DJ, et al: Atlas of Clinical Ophthalmology. London, Gower Medical Publishing, 1984.

Vaughan D, Asbury T, Riordan-Eva P: General Ophthalmology, 13th ed. E Norwalk, CT, Appleton & Lange, 1992.

16 Acute Otitis Media

John G. O'Handley

Etiology

1. Eustachian tube dysfunction

   a. The peak incidence of acute otitis media is between ages 6 months and 24 months because of developmental changes that surround the eustachian tube. They include persistent collapse due to abnormal tubal compliance, as well as delayed innervation of the tensor veli palatini muscle, which opens and closes the eustachian tube.

   b. Infection ascends through the eustachian tube.

   c. Normal eustachian tube

      (1) Maintains atmospheric pressure in the middle ear

      (2) Protects the middle ear from reflux of secretions from the nasopharynx

      (3) Clears the middle ear secretions into the nasopharynx by ciliary activity

   When these functions are altered, middle ear infection can result.

2. Infective organisms

   a. The typical occurrence of acute otitis media comes 5 to 7 days after an upper respiratory tract infection. Although adequate studies that indicate a viral origin are lacking, viruses are believed to play a role in the pathogenesis of this common condition. However, bacterial cultures are positive in 75 per cent of middle ear aspirates from children with acute otitis media.

   b. Bacterial pathogens

      (1) *Streptococcus pneumoniae* and *Haemophilus influenzae* make up about 60 per cent of isolates from the middle ear.

      (2) *Moraxella catarrhalis, Streptococcus pyogenes, Staphylococcus aureus,* and anaerobic organisms, either alone or in combination, make up the rest of the 90 per cent of organisms recovered from middle ear fluid in acute otitis media.

      (3) In adults, similar organisms are found, although the incidence of *H. influenzae* in some studies is higher than that of *S. pneumoniae.*

3. Risk factors

   a. Male sex

   b. Bottle feeding, especially in the supine position

   c. Exposure to upper respiratory tract infections (e.g., day care setting, winter season)

   d. Genetic factors

   e. Ethnic factors (e.g., Inuit and Native Americans)

   f. Parental smoking

   g. Allergy

   h. Craniofacial abnormalities (e.g., cleft palate)

   i. Previous episode of acute otitis media, particularly during the preceding 3 months

Signs and Symptoms

These are due to inflammation and fluid in the middle ear.

   a. Otalgia

   b. Ear-pulling

   c. Diminished hearing

   d. Fever

   e. Loss of appetite

   f. Irritability

   g. Vomiting

   h. Vertigo

   i. Tinnitus

   j. Otorrhea

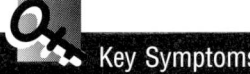 Key Symptoms

- Otalgia
- Hearing loss
- Fever

Clinical Findings

Appearance of tympanic membrane

   a. Lack of landmarks

   b. Limited mobility or complete immobility

   c. Erythema

   d. Bulging

> **Note**
> Bullae on the tympanic membrane are a nonspecific reaction to middle ear infection and are not pathognomonic for *Mycoplasma pneumoniae* infection, which seldom causes acute otitis media.

Tests

Complete blood count and blood culture only when patient is considered toxic

Differential Diagnosis

1. Myringitis—red tympanic membrane without exudate

2. Pharyngitis or tonsillitis—can cause referred pain to the ear

3. Teething

4. Referred pain from temporomandibular joint syndrome

Treatment

Medication

1. Drug of choice: amoxicillin—40 mg/kg/d in three divided doses for 10 days (adult dose is 250 mg q 8 h)

2. Alternative drugs

   a. Amoxicillin/clavulanate (Augmentin)—40 mg/kg/d in three divided doses for 10 days (adult dose is 250 mg q 8 h)

   b. Cefaclor (Ceclor)—40 mg/kg/d in three divided doses for 10 days (adult dose 250 mg q 8 h)

   c. Cefuroxime axetil (Ceftin)—children under 2 years, 125 mg twice daily; children 2 years or over, 250 mg twice daily for 10 days

   d. Trimethoprim-sulfamethoxazole (Bactrim, Septra) —8 mg/kg trimethoprim and 40 mg/kg sulfamethoxazole per 24 hrs given in divided doses every 12 hrs for 10 days

   e. Erythromycin and sulfisoxazole (Pediazole)—50 mg/kg/d erythromycin and 150 mg/kg/d sulfisoxazole in four divided doses for 10 days

   f. Cefixime (Suprax)—8 mg/kg/d as a single daily dose for 10 days

   g. Cefprozil (Cefzil)—30 mg/kg/d in two divided doses for 10 days

3. Anhydrous glycerol eardrops or similar eardrops provide symptomatic relief. Acetaminophen may also be used for pain.

4. Systemic decongestants and expectorants

Alternative drugs should be used:
- When resistant organisms have been identified on culture of middle ear fluid
- In previous treatment failure with amoxicillin
- If patient is hypersensitive to penicillin

Note
Antihistamines are not recommended for the resolution of acute otitis media because they lead to decreased ciliary motility.

Surgical Treatment

1. Tympanocentesis can be used if antibiotics are not effective.

WARNING

Determine compliance with medication before performing tympanocentesis.

---

2. Myringotomy with polyethylene tube placement if antibiotics and tympanocentesis fail to resolve an effusion lasting 3 months and there is concern over hearing or speech delay.

Diet

As tolerated

Activity

1. Pain and fever preclude going to school or work.

2. There are no restrictions after pain and fever are gone.

3. Avoid barotrauma (e.g., flying, scuba diving).

Patient Education

1. Parents should avoid bottle feeding of infants in the supine position. This practice can cause reflux of oral contents into the eustachian tube.

2. Parents should be informed that tobacco smoke increases the risk of middle ear infections in children.

3. Allergens in the home, such as pets, house dust, and mold, should be eliminated as much as possible for people who have an allergic diathesis.

Follow-Up

1. Patients require follow-up in 4 to 6 weeks. Ninety per cent of middle ear effusions have resolved by that time, and pneumatic otoscopy can determine if fluid is still present.

2. Tympanometry is another method of follow-up but increases cost. It is useful in those patients who are unable to cooperate for pneumatic otoscopy and provides an objective measurement of the status of the middle ear.

3. For patients who have had three episodes of acute otitis media in the past 6 months or four episodes in the past 12 months, prophylaxis with amoxicillin (20 mg/kg in a single dose or two divided doses) or sulfisoxazole (50 mg/kg/d at bedtime) is recommended during the winter season.

B Bibliography

Bluestone CD: Current therapy for otitis media and criteria for evaluation of new antimicrobial agents. Clin Infect Dis 1992;14:(S2)S197–203.

Bluestone CD, Klein JO: Diagnosis. *In* Bluestone CD, Klein JO (eds): Otitis Media in Infants and Children. Philadelphia, WB Saunders, 1988, pp 69–119.

Kligman EW: Treatment of otitis media. Am Fam Physician 1992;45:242–250.

Legler JD: An approach to difficult management problems in otitis media in children. J Am Board Fam Pract 1991;4:331–339.

Thoene DE, Johnson LE: Pharmacotherapy of otitis media. Pharmacotherapy 1991;11(3):212–221.

17 Chronic Serous Otitis Media

Raymond C. Bredfeldt

Etiology

1. Definition—persistence of secretions within the middle ear due to failure of the eustachian tube to effectively drain this space
2. Epidemiology
   a. Middle ear effusions are common after episodes of allergic rhinitis, upper respiratory tract infection, and acute otitis media. Although these effusions often resolve within 1 week in the setting of otitis media, effusions can persist for up to 12 weeks.
   b. Persistent serous effusions often are associated with low-grade bacterial infections with the same organisms that caused acute otitis media.

Symptoms

1. Fullness in the ear
2. Painless, low-grade hearing loss in the 15- to 20-dB range
3. Hearing loss may present with delayed language development in young children and decreased school performance in older children.
4. Middle ear effusions can result in repeated episodes of acute otitis media.

Key Symptoms

- Ear fullness
- Mild hearing loss

Clinical Findings

1. The tympanic membrane may appear dull, opaque, or normal.
2. Mobility of the tympanic membrane is decreased or absent as determined by pneumatic otoscopy and/or tympanography.
3. The tympanic membrane may appear retracted. Air/fluid levels or bubbles may be visualized behind the membrane.

Key Signs

- Dull and poorly mobile tympanic membrane
- Abnormal tympanogram

Tests

1. Pneumatic otoscopy carries high false-negative and false-positive rates with regard to the diagnosis of middle ear effusions. Tympanography is, therefore, an essential adjunct in the diagnosis of chronic serous otitis media.
2. Tympanography measures the relative compliance of the middle ear as air pressure is altered in the external ear canal.
3. The key to accurate interpretation of a tympanogram is based on the presence and shape of the compliance peak and the pressure at which this peak occurs.
4. Normal ears (type A) have a tall compliance peak (0.2 to 2.0 ml of displaced air) located between +100 and −150 mm H_2O (Fig. 17–1, curve A).
5. Type B tympanograms have no compliance peak indicating a lack of tympanic membrane mobility usually secondary to middle ear effusions (Fig. 17–1, curve B).
6. Type C tympanograms have a peak that occurs below the normal limit of −150 mm H_2O (Fig. 17–1 curve C). These tympanograms indicate that some degree of eustachian tube dysfunction is present and are considered to be intermediate between type A and type B. During the recovery from acute otitis media, the tympanogram may progress from type B to type C to type A.
7. Often a compliance curve may not fit the classic A,

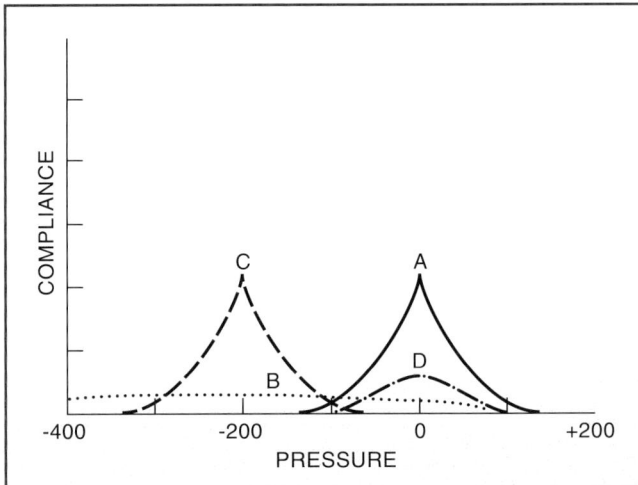

Figure 17–1 System of tympanogram classification. Type A (normal) tympanograms (curve A) are characterized by a tall compliance peak at a pressure of greater than −150 mm H_2O. Type B tympanograms are flat, indicating the presence of a middle ear effusion (curve B). Type C tympanograms (negative pressure-recovery phase) have near-normal compliance, while the peak occurs below −150 mm H_2O (curve C). Frequently the peak does not fit the classic A, B, or C patterns. Curve D shows a flattened curve often occurring during the recovery phase. (Redrawn from Adams GL, Boies LR Jr, Hilger PA [eds]: Boies Fundamentals of Otolaryngology, 6th ed. Philadelphia, WB Saunders, 1989, p 58.)

B, or C pattern type. Such curves may be somewhat flattened and occur at normal or negative pressure. These curves also represent various stages in recovery from acute otitis media with middle ear effusion (Fig. 17–1, curve D).

Key Tests

- Pneumatic otoscopy
- Tympanography

Differential Diagnosis

1. The major differential lies in distinguishing whether or not fluid is present in the middle ear.
2. Other causes of flat tympanograms in the setting of painless hearing loss include cerumen impaction and a previously perforated tympanic membrane. These conditions should be obvious on otoscopic examination.

WARNING

Treatment with prednisone discussed below should only be used along with coexisting antibiotic coverage because prednisone may increase the likelihood of infection. Its use should be avoided if varicella is prevalent in the community.

Treatment

1. Because middle ear effusions may persist for several weeks after acute otitis media, expectant management is generally indicated. Exposure to passive tobacco smoke should be strongly discouraged. Serial (monthly) examinations to monitor for the resolution of the effusion are a reasonable approach.
2. If the effusion persists for 12 weeks, a 14- to 28-day course of an antibiotic such as amoxicillin/clavulanate potassium (Augmentin), cefaclor (Ceclor), erythromycin plus sulfisoxazole (Pediazole), or co-trimoxazole (Bactrim, Septra) should be given at therapeutic doses rather than at the lower doses used in prophylaxis of recurrent otitis media. Although not universally accepted, studies indicate that the addition of prednisone, 1 mg/kg/day for 7 days, during this time increases the likelihood of resolution.

3. For effusions that persist beyond 16 weeks, consider referral to an otolaryngologist for hearing evaluation and, possibly, tympanostomy tube placement.
4. Most reports fail to show the effectiveness of oral decongestants or antihistamines.
5. For children who have recurrent otitis media (three episodes within a 6-month period), consider antibiotic prophylaxis, which should be maintained until the effusion resolves. Potential antibiotics include either amoxicillin, 20 mg/kg/day, or sulfisoxazole, 70 mg/kg/day, both in two divided doses.

Key Treatment

- Watchful waiting for 12 weeks
- If the effusion persists longer than 12 weeks, give an antibiotic that covers β-lactamase–producing organisms for 14 to 28 days. During the antibiotic therapy, the addition of prednisone for 7 days may increase the likelihood of resolution.
- Otolaryngologic referral should be considered for effusions that last longer than 16 weeks.

Follow-Up

1. Middle ear effusion after acute otitis media should be re-evaluated at 4-week intervals. The patient should return sooner if fever or earache develops.
2. Serial tympanography and pneumatic otoscopy should be considered at follow-up visits until the effusion recovers or an otolaryngologic referral is made.
3. Final follow-up should be considered 1 month after resolution of a prolonged effusion.

Bibliography

Berman S, Grose K, Nuss R, et al: Management of chronic middle ear effusion with prednisone combined with trimethoprim-sulfamethoxazole. Pediatr Infect Dis J 1990; 9:533–538.

Bredfeldt RC: An introduction to tympanometry. Am Fam Physician 1991;44:2113–2118.

Howard AJ, Dunkin KT: Bacteriology of otitis media with effusion. J Laryngol Otol 1989;103:253–256.

Legler JD: An approach to difficult management problems in otitis media in children. J Am Board Fam Pract 1991;4:331–339.

U.S. Department of Health and Human Services: Clinical Practice Guideline No. 12. Otitis media with effusion in young children. AHCPR Publication No. 94-0623, July 1994.

18 Otitis Externa

Gary J. Silko

Etiology

1. Seborrheic external otitis
2. Eczematoid external otitis caused by:
   a. Allergic hypersensitivity
   b. Contact dermatitis
   c. Atopic dermatitis
   d. Psoriasis
3. Infectious external otitis
   a. Acute localized external otitis—furuncle caused by staphylococci
   b. Acute diffuse external otitis
      (1) *Pseudomonas aeruginosa*
      (2) *Staphylococcus aureus*
      (3) *Streptococcus pneumoniae*
      (4) Gram-negative species
   c. Chronic diffuse external otitis
      (1) *Aspergillus*
      (2) *Actinomyces*
      (3) *Mucor*
      (4) *Candida*
   d. Necrotizing external otitis—severe osteomyelitis caused by *P. aeruginosa*

Symptoms

A. Seborrheic or eczematoid
   1. Itching in canal and outer ear
   2. Flaking, crusting, or weeping of skin
B. Infectious
   1. Itching in canal
   2. Ear pain
   3. Muffled hearing if the swelling is enough to occlude the canal
   4. Watery or thick discharge from the ear

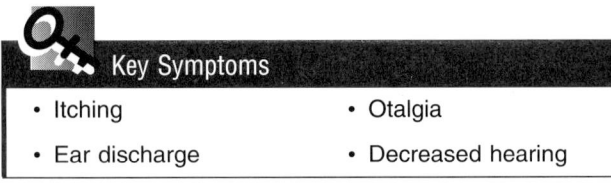

Key Symptoms

- Itching
- Ear discharge
- Otalgia
- Decreased hearing

Clinical Findings

A. Seborrheic or eczematoid
   1. Crusting or scaling of outer ear
   2. Weeping of skin
   3. Hyperemia and edema of outer ear

B. Infectious
   1. Pain accentuated by tragus pressure
   2. Erythema and swelling of canal (localized in case of furuncle, otherwise diffuse)
   3. Debris in canal
   4. Discharge—scanty to purulent; black or dark if fungal
   5. Red, "granular" tympanic membrane
   6. Lymphadenopathy—periauricular and cervical

Key Signs

- Tragal tenderness
- Debris and drainage in canal
- Narrowing of canal
- Local lymphadenopathy

Tests

1. Potassium hydroxide preparation of discharge if fungal infection is suspected
2. Cultures only if the patient is immunosuppressed or does not respond to standard therapy
3. If necrotizing otitis externa is suspected
   a. Erythrocyte sedimentation rate
   b. Complete blood count
   c. Computed tomographic scan

Differential Diagnosis

1. Seborrheic dermatitis—look for other signs, including scalp and facial involvement
2. Contact dermatitis—history may reveal offending agent
3. Infection
   a. Furuncle—focal swelling or tenderness
   b. Bacterial—pain and inflammation in canal
   c. Fungal—black or dark discharge, white if yeast
   d. Cellulitis—fever, erythema usually well delineated
   e. Necrotizing—usually in elderly, diabetic, or immunocompromised patients; can present with facial paralysis (cranial nerve VII palsy)
   f. Ramsay Hunt syndrome—herpes zoster involving the tongue and palate; can also present with facial paralysis
4. Relapsing polychondritis—systemic signs involving other cartilaginous structures

Treatment

In all cases of otitis externa—whatever the cause—management should include cleaning and drying of the canal and pain relief.

1. Cleaning may be accomplished by gentle suction or the use of cotton-tipped applicators.
2. If much debris is present (especially if moist or soggy), gentle irrigation with 3% saline solution, hydrogen peroxide 3%, or dilute alcohol solution can be performed. Gentle suction drying should follow.
3. If a simple furuncle with an obvious point is present, needle drainage should be attempted.
4. When substantial narrowing of the canal is present or response to treatment is slow, introducing a cotton wick deep in the canal by means of forceps facilitates delivery of antibiotic drops.
5. Necrotizing external otitis requires hospitalization and surgical consultation.

Medication

A. Seborrheic external otitis
   1. Treat underlying seborrhea (e.g., of the scalp) with selenium sulfide shampoo weekly.
   2. Apply midpotency topical steroid lotion or ointment to the outer ear.
B. Eczematoid external otitis
   1. Apply topical steroid lotion or ointment to the outer ear.
   2. Add steroid or antibiotic solution if secondary infection is suspected.
C. Infectious external otitis
   1. Acute localized external otitis (furuncle)—oral antistaphylococcal antibiotic for 7 to 10 days
   2. Acute diffuse external otitis (bacterial)—acetic acid 2% (VōSol Otic, Domeboro Otic); hydrocortisone, neomycin, and polymyxin B (Cortisporin Otic); neomycin, colistin sulfate, hydrocortisone, and thonzonium bromide (Coly-Mycin S). Apply any of the above four times per day for 10 days. Consider adding oral antibiotics if cellulitis is also present.
   3. Chronic diffuse external otitis (fungal or yeast)—acetic acid 2% (VōSol Otic, Domeboro Otic)
   4. Necrotizing external otitis—intravenous anti-*Pseudomonas* antibiotic and an aminoglycoside for 6 weeks

> **Note**
> Neomycin sensitivity has been reported in as much as 10 per cent of the general population. Drops that contain neomycin can occasionally increase symptoms.
> Steroid-containing solutions are not always necessary and may be reserved for those patients with substantial inflammation or itching.

Activity

Restrict swimming until symptoms begin to subside. When swimming is resumed, keep out water with earplugs—preferably the wax-moldable type.

Patient Education

Recurrent infections are common, so patients should be informed of the following preventive measures.

1. Avoid scratching the ear or other trauma such as might be induced by cotton-tipped applicators.
2. Avoid prolonged exposure to moisture.
3. Dry the ear with an alcohol solution or a hand-held hair dryer after contact with water.
4. If the infection recurs several times, diluted alcohol can be used three times per week.

Follow-Up

1. For acute external otitis in which response is rapid, follow-up appointments usually are not necessary.
2. Patients who fail to improve should be re-examined in 3 to 5 days for possible further cleaning of the canal.
3. Patients who require oral antibiotics should be re-examined in 3 to 5 days.
4. Necrotizing external otitis requires prolonged and careful follow-up.

Bibliography

Amundson LH: Disorders of the external ear. Prim Care 1990;17(2):223–227.

Austin DF: Diseases of the external ear. *In* Ballenger JJ (ed): Diseases of the Nose, Throat, Ear, Head, and Neck, 14th ed. Philadelphia, Lea & Febiger, 1991, pp 1073–1078.

Boies LR: Diseases of the external ear. *In* Adams GL, Boies LR, Hilger PA (eds): Fundamentals of Otolaryngology, 6th ed. Philadelphia, WB Saunders, 1989, pp 80–86.

Evans P, Hofmann L: Malignant external otitis. Am Fam Physician 1994;49:427–431.

Lucente FE: Fungal infections of the external ear. Otolaryngol Clin North Am 1993;26:995–1006.

19 Allergic Rhinitis

Giulia Michelini

Etiology

1. In genetically susceptible individuals, nasally inhaled allergens cause an IgE-mediated hypersensitivity response.
2. Symptoms may be seasonal, depending on the allergen and the geographical area.
   a. Ragweed—mid-August to the first frost
   b. Tree pollen—March to May
   c. Grass pollen—May to early July
3. In perennial allergic rhinitis, allergens are present year round.
   a. Dust mites
   b. Molds
   c. Animal dander or saliva
   d. Cockroach antigen
4. Irritants and other stimuli may also trigger symptoms.
   a. Smoke, air pollutants
   b. Perfumes, detergents, or soaps
   c. Solvents or fumes
   d. Changes in air temperature, light, or atmospheric pressure
   e. Emotion

Symptoms

1. Paroxysmal sneezing often occurs in the morning.
2. Nasal itching may result in frequent nose rubbing (allergic salute).
3. Nasal congestion may lead to loss of taste or smell.
4. Acute or chronic sinusitis may complicate nasal obstruction.
5. Rhinorrhea is usually watery (may be profuse and continuous).
6. Chronic postnasal drip may cause cough and/or sore throat.
7. Palatal itching, dry mouth, and halitosis also occur.
8. Conjunctivitis causes ocular itching, redness, and tearing.
9. General symptoms include fatigue and disrupted sleep.

Key Symptoms	
• Sneezing	• Nasal congestion
• Nasal discharge	• Conjunctivitis
• Postnasal drip	• Cough

Clinical Findings

Clinical signs cannot be relied on for diagnosis.

1. Pale or bluish, swollen nasal mucosa (in 50 to 60 per cent)
2. Clear, thin nasal discharge
3. Edematous turbinates
4. Allergic salute
5. Lymphoid hyperplasia in posterior oropharynx (cobblestoning)
6. Erythematous throat
7. Conjunctival and scleral injection
8. Chemosis of conjunctivae
9. Dark circles under the eyes (allergic shiners)

Key Signs	
• Pale, swollen nasal mucosa	• Turbinate edema
	• Conjunctival injection
• Allergic shiners	• Allergic salute
• Nasal discharge	

Tests

A. Nasal smears

   Cytology is examined using a Wright or Hansel stain.

   1. The presence of nasal eosinophils suggests allergy.
   2. Predominance of neutrophils suggests an infectious cause.

B. Allergy testing

   1. Skin testing is useful if the diagnosis is uncertain.
      a. An allergen is applied with a prick or intradermal injection.
      b. A wheal and flare reaction can confirm the allergen that is triggering the symptoms.
   2. Radioallergosorbent testing (RAST) is an in vitro test to measure a person's level of IgE to an allergen. It is more expensive and less sensitive than skin testing.

Key Tests	
• Nasal smears	• Skin testing
• Radioallergosorbent testing	

Differential Diagnosis

A. Infectious causes
   1. Rhinitis
      a. Viral
      b. Bacterial
      c. Fungal
   2. Sinusitis
B. Noninfectious, nonallergic causes
   1. Vasomotor rhinitis is a perennial rhinitis in response to nonspecific irritants and other stimuli (e.g., smoke, air pollutants).
   2. Rhinitis medicamentosa is caused by the local or systemic effect of drugs on the nasal mucosa.
      a. Sympathomimetic nasal drops or sprays
      b. Cocaine
      c. Antihypertensives (reserpine, guanethidine, hydralazine)
   3. Mechanical nasal obstruction can cause a secondary rhinitis.
      a. Nasal polyps
      b. Deviated septum
      c. Nasal neoplasms
   4. Systemic conditions can result in nasal symptoms.
      a. Rhinitis of pregnancy
      b. Hypothyroidism
      c. Granulomatous disease (Wegener's, sarcoid)
      d. Ciliary dysfunction (cystic fibrosis, Kartagener's)

Treatment

Medication

1. Antihistamines relieve sneezing, rhinorrhea, and pruritus.
   a. The five classes of the first-generation antihistamines differ in sedative and anticholinergic side effects.
   b. For better effect, use before allergen exposure: alkylamine class—chlorpheniramine, 4 mg orally three or four times per day
   c. Newer agents have longer action and reduced side effects.

WARNING

Rare QT prolongation and arrhythmias have occurred with the use of terfenadine or astemizole with erythromycin, clarithromycin, ketoconazole, and itraconazole and in patients with significant hepatic dysfunction.

---

   (1) Loratadine (Claritin), 10 mg orally daily
   (2) Terfenadine (Seldane), 60 mg orally twice per day
   (3) Astemizole (Hismanal), 10 mg orally daily
2. Decongestants are useful for obstructive symptoms (congestion)—pseudoephedrine hydrochloride (Sudafed), 30 to 60 mg orally q.i.d.
3. Topical nasal steroids are the most effective drugs available.
   a. Beclomethasone (Beconase, Vancenase), one spray (42 μg) per nostril b.i.d. to q.i.d.
   b. Flunisolide (Nasalide), two sprays (50 μg) per nostril b.i.d.
   c. Triamcinolone (Nasacort), two sprays (110 μg) per nostril daily

Note: Side effects (of all) include irritation and, rarely, nasal ulceration.

4. Cromolyn sodium (Nasalcrom) (a mast cell stabilizer), one spray (5.2 mg) per nostril three or four times per day. This drug has a less predictable response and should be used with regular (prophylactic) dosing.

Immunotherapy

1. Specific allergens (identified by skin tests or RAST) are injected weekly or monthly.
2. Reserved for patients with severe rhinitis who do not respond to or who cannot or will not take medications.
3. The best response is seen with seasonal allergies to pollens.

Patient Education

Avoidance of precipitating allergens is vital.

1. Dust mites
   a. Keep humidity below 50 per cent.
   b. Wash sheets in hot water at least once a week.
   c. Encase mattress, boxspring, and pillows in plastic.
   d. Dust floors (remove carpets) and surfaces frequently.
2. Mold
   a. Lower the humidity (as above).
   b. Vent and clean bathrooms with fungicides.
   c. Remove books and plants from the bedroom.
   d. Install air filter units.
3. Animal allergens
   Remove pets from the house or at least from the bedroom.
4. Pollen
   a. Avoid outdoor exposure.
   b. Keep the bedroom windows closed (use air conditioning).
   c. Install air filter units.

Key Treatment

Drugs of Choice	Alternative Drugs
• Chlorpheniramine	• Loratadine
• Topical nasal steroids	• Nasal cromolyn
	• Pseudoephedrine

Follow-Up

1. If response to treatment is poor and an anatomic or a secondary disorder is a consideration, refer to a head and neck specialist.

2. If the diagnosis seems correct but the response to treatment is poor, refer to an allergist.

Bibliography

Naclerio RM: Allergic rhinitis. N Engl J Med 1991;325:860–869.

Nalebuff DJ: Allergic rhinitis. *In* Cummings CW (ed): Otolaryngology-Head and Neck Surgery, 2nd ed. St Louis, CV Mosby, 1993, pp 765–774.

Ricketti AJ: Allergic rhinitis. *In* Patterson R, Grammer LC, Greenbeyer PA, et al (eds): Allergic Diseases: Diagnosis and Management, 4th ed. Philadelphia, JB Lippincott, 1993, pp 225–253.

| Procedure | NASAL FRACTURE REDUCTION | *Javier J. Urdaneta* |

Indications

1. History of recent nasal trauma, within 5 days
2. Clinical and/or radiologic confirmation

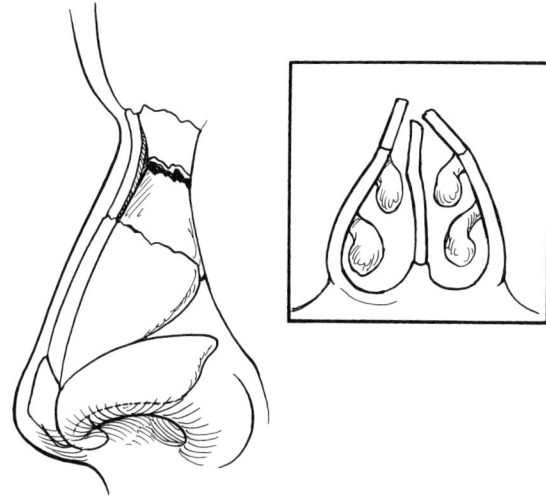

3. Unilateral compromise of the bony pyramid
4. Bilateral fractures with demonstrable integrity of the septum

Contraindications

1. Suspected or confirmed ethmoidal involvement with or without cerebrospinal fluid (CSF) leakage
2. Bilateral or complex fractures of the nasal pyramid involving the septum with or without hematoma
3. Nasal fractures with suspected or confirmed facial bone compromise

Diagnosis

1. Clinical examination
   a. External examination of the nasal pyramid and face
      (1) Inspect for deformities, asymmetry, hematomas, anterior nasal discharge versus bleeding, hypertelorism, and diplopia. Check ocular movements.
      (2) Palpate the nose and face to detect deformities and instability as well as bony crepitus and subcutaneous emphysema.
   b. Internal examination of the nose and pharynx
      (1) Perform anterior rhinoscopy with the help of a nasal speculum. Suction all the blood, apply a local vasoconstrictor, and observe carefully for CSF leakage, septal deviation or hematoma, and septal dislocation or fracture. Refer the patient if any of these are present.
      (2) Examine the oropharynx, and look for posterior nasal bleeding. If present, consider referral.
2. Radiographic examination
   a. Order standard radiographs of the nasal pyramid, and search for fractures. If more extensive lesions are suspected, radiographs of the facial bones and sinuses should be obtained and referral considered.
   b. Obtain computed tomographic scan only for complicated and extensive injuries or suspected CSF fistula.

Equipment

1. Headlamp or other good light source
2. Suction equipment with nasal cannulas
3. Nasal speculum
4. Walsham or Asch forceps or any other surgical blunted heavy instrument, such as a scalpel handle or a large hemostat wrapped with gauze at the tip to protect the nasal mucosa
5. Bayonet forceps

Anesthesia

1. Topical
   a. Intranasal
      (1) Cocaine 4% or 10% solution
      (2) Tetracaine 2% with 1:100,000 epinephrine spray
      (3) Benzocaine 20% spray with a topical vasoconstrictor, such as naphazoline hydrochloride 0.05%
   b. Extranasal: EMLA (eutectic mixture of local anesthetics) cream, optional (lidocaine 2.5% and prilocaine 2.5%)
2. Sedation with short-acting benzodiazepines (lorazepam or diazepam) when necessary

Precautions

1. Certainty of the diagnosis
2. Absence of contraindications
3. Awareness and understanding of the procedure for compliance and cooperation
4. Consent form must be signed before the procedure.

Technique

1. Have the patient sit on a chair with a posterior head support.
2. Perform an external and internal examination as described above.
3. Soak 46 cm (18 in) of ½-inch plain cotton gauze packing in any of the topical intranasal agents described, and layer it in the nasal cavity using the bayonet forceps. Remove this packing in 5 minutes.
4. Apply EMLA cream on the nasal pyramid skin 30 minutes before the procedure (optional), and cover it with an occlusive plastic dressing.
5. Give diazepam (Valium), 5 mg, or lorazepam (Ativan), 1 mg, orally 30 minutes before the procedure.
6. Insert the instrument chosen in the nostril of the affected side under the nasal bone with the dominant hand.

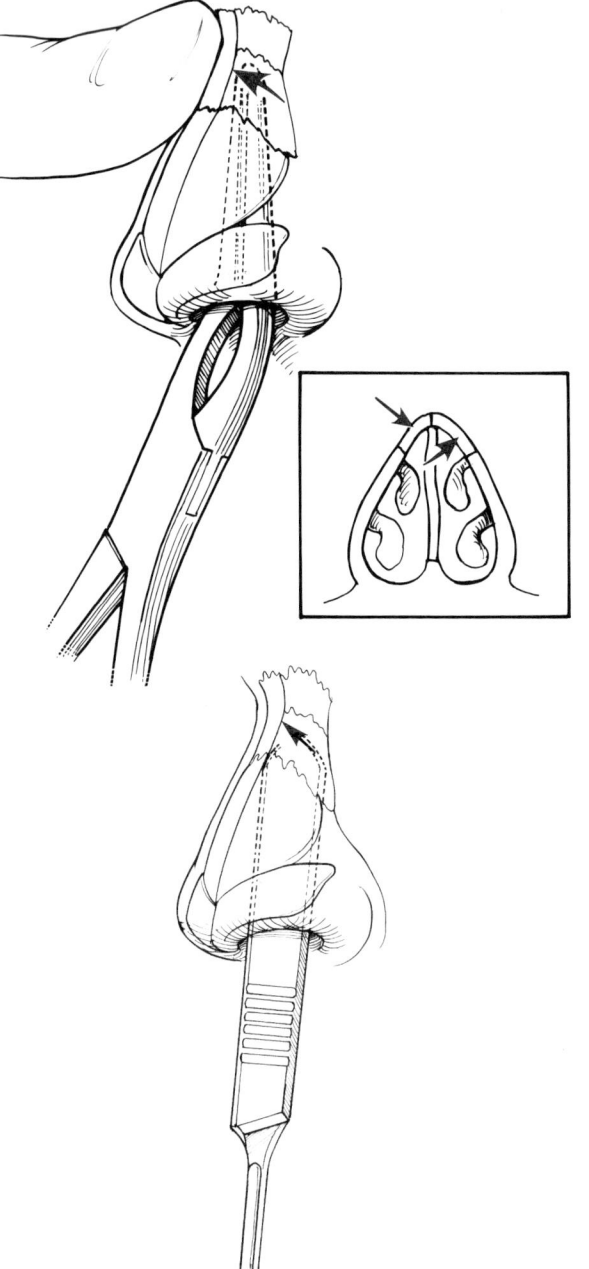

7. Reduce the fracture by pushing anteriorly and superiorly with the instrument while the nondominant hand verifies the proper position of the nasal bone.
8. In bilateral fractures, insert both blades in the side of the greatest deformity and use the nondominant hand to apply pressure on the contralateral nasal bone.
9. Inspect and palpate the nasal pyramid. It should appear aesthetically adequate for both the physician and the patient. Then perform anterior rhinoscopy, and be sure that both nasal passages look symmetric, allowing good air flow, and that the septum is midline without hematoma.
10. Proceed with layered anterior nasal packing for support and hemostasis with as little petrolatum (Vaseline) gauze as possible to avoid displacement of the fracture.
11. Place an external thermoplastic nasal splint or use cast materials. To prepare a splint, proceed as follows:
    a. Apply benzoin to the dorsum of the nose followed by layered paper tape and cotton adhesive tape.
    b. Cut four or five layers of cast material to the shape of the nose and moisten them. Apply and mold the material to the proper position.

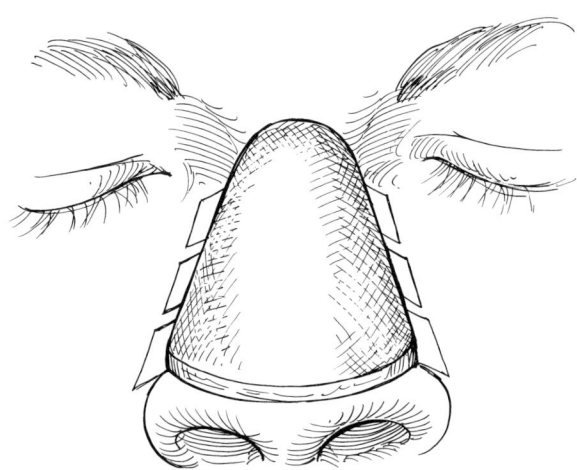

12. Observe for 15 minutes, and verify the absence of anterior or posterior nasal bleeding.
13. Prescribe a broad-spectrum oral antibiotic, such as amoxicillin or cephalexin (Keflex).

Follow-Up

1. Instruct the patient to watch for posterior nasal bleeding, hematemesis, fever, persistent headache, visual disturbances, dizziness, or any other late neurologic sign suggestive of a more complicated lesion.
2. Re-evaluate in 48 to 72 hours, and remove the nasal pack.

3. Remove the external nasal splint in 7 days.

4. Recheck the patient in 1 month, and consider possible referral if results are unsatisfactory.

 Bibliography

Drezner DA: Thermoplastic splint for use after nasal fracture. Otolaryngol Head Neck Surg 1994;111(1):146–147.

El-Kholy A: Manipulation of the fractured nose using topical local anesthesia. Laryngol Otol 1989;103:580–581.

Haug HR, Prather JL: The closed reduction of nasal fractures, an evaluation of two techniques. J Oral Maxillofac Surg 1991;49:1288–1292.

Nigam A, Goni A, Benjamin A, Dasgupta AR: The value of radiographs in the management of the fractured nose. Arch Emerg Med 1993;10(4):293–297.

Paparella MM, Shumrick DA, Gluckman JL, Meyerhoff WL: Otolaryngology, Vol 3. Philadelphia, WB Saunders, 1991, pp 1823–1830.

Weisman RA, Stanley RB: Current issues in head and neck trauma. Otolaryngol Clin North Am 1991;24(1):195–201.

20 Sinusitis

John W. Williams, Jr.

Etiology

1. Sinusitis is defined as inflammation of one or more paranasal sinuses but usually refers to infection of the sinuses. The maxillary sinuses are the most frequently infected, either alone or in combination with the ethmoid or frontal sinuses. Isolated sphenoid sinusitis is rare and constitutes a medical emergency. The maxillary sinus drains through a narrow channel, the ostiomeatal complex, that is easily obstructed by inflammation or edema. Obstruction is followed by decreased ciliary action, increased mucus production, and bacterial proliferation. In 5 to 10 per cent of cases, maxillary sinusitis is associated with dental abscess and is thought to result from contiguous spread of bacteria.

2. Factors that predispose to ostial obstruction include viral upper respiratory tract infection, allergic rhinitis, overuse of topical decongestants, deviated nasal septum, nasopharyngeal intubation, nasal polyps, and tumors. Immunodeficiency and bronchiectasis may also predispose to sinusitis.

3. The microbiology of sinusitis is best considered in relation to the duration of symptoms. In adults with acute sinusitis, the most common organisms are *Streptococcus pneumoniae* (35 per cent), *Haemophilus influenzae* (35 per cent), *Streptococcus pyogenes* and α-hemolytic streptococcus (10 per cent), viruses (9 per cent), *Staphylococcus aureus* (6 per cent), and *Moraxella catarrhalis* (5 per cent). β-lactamase–producing strains of *H. influenzae* and *M. catarrhalis* are amoxicillin-resistant but are not prevalent in acute sinusitis. In chronic sinusitis, anaerobic organisms are much more common (more than 50 per cent), and infections are more likely to be polymicrobic.

Symptoms

1. There may be a high degree of overlap between symptoms of acute or chronic sinusitis and other causes of nasal congestion, such as allergic or viral rhinitis. No single symptom or sign is pathognomonic. Despite diagnostic difficulties, the overall accuracy of the clinical evaluation is about 78 per cent and is based on the recognition of a pattern of symptoms and signs.

2. Acute sinusitis should be high on the differential when a patient has a prolonged "cold" (> 7 to 10 days) or an unusually severe "cold." Colored rhinorrhea, cough, and pain in the upper teeth are characteristic symptoms. Unilateral facial pain and failure to improve with over-the-counter decongestants or antihistamines increase the likelihood of sinusitis.

3. Chronic sinusitis presents as a protracted course of respiratory symptoms, including nasal congestion and cough. Facial fullness, headache, and nasal drainage may be prominent, but fever is uncommon.

Key Symptoms

- Maxillary toothache

- Colored rhinorrhea

- Poor response to over-the-counter nasal decongestants and antihistamines

Clinical Findings

1. A focused examination is useful diagnostically and to evaluate for predisposing causes. Most commonly the patient is afebrile or has a low-grade fever and does not appear very ill.

2. The focused examination consists of the following:

    a. Examine the nasal mucosa for color, edema, and character of nasal secretions; polyps; and structure of the nasal septum. Purulent secretion, particularly when seen coming from the middle meatus, is predictive of sinusitis.

    b. In a completely darkened room, transilluminate the maxillary sinuses by placing a Welch-Allyn Finnoff transilluminator or Mini Mag-Lite over the infraorbital rim, and judge light transmission through the hard palate. Normal and equal light transmission from side to side makes sinusitis much less likely. Decreased light transmission on either side makes sinusitis more likely but also may be due to polyps or a hypoplastic sinus.

    c. Percuss the maxillary teeth with a tongue blade to check for a dental source of sinusitis.

    d. Facial tenderness elicited by palpation is an unreliable sign for maxillary sinusitis but may be useful for frontal sinus infection.

Key Signs

- Mucopurulent or purulent nasal secretion
- Abnormal transillumination

When none of the key symptoms or signs is present, the probability of sinusitis is less than 10 per cent; when all are present, the probability of sinusitis exceeds 90 per cent.

Tests

1. Sinusitis is usually diagnosed clinically, but when considerable uncertainty persists after the clinical

evaluation or the patient fails an initial course of therapy, diagnostic testing may be useful.

2. Radiographic evaluation is the most useful diagnostic test for nonspecialists.

   a. Compared with sinus aspiration and culture, conventional radiographs are about 90 per cent sensitive and 75 per cent specific for maxillary sinusitis. A single Waters view is less expensive and correlates highly with the standard four-view sinus series. However, conventional radiographs visualize the ethmoid sinuses poorly.

   b. Sinus computed tomography is more sensitive (90 to 100 per cent) and images the ethmoid sinuses well but may have poor specificity (60 per cent; therefore, many false positives). It is best used for evaluating chronic sinusitis as well as complications of sinusitis, such as orbital cellulitis and cerebral abscess.

3. Nasal cytology may be useful for evaluating chronic nasal symptoms. A sample can be obtained by having the patient blow his nose into wax paper or by using a cotton-tipped applicator to swab the nasal mucosa. The specimen should be stained with a modified Wright-Giemsa or Hansel stain and examined at high power. Five or more neutrophils per high-power field (HPF) has 86 per cent sensitivity and 40 per cent specificity for radiographic evidence of sinusitis. Five or more eosinophils per HPF makes allergic rhinitis or nasal polyposis more likely than sinusitis.

4. Cultures of nasal secretions do not correlate with cultures from sinus antral aspirates and should not be done. Sinus aspiration and culture is the "gold standard" for establishing sinusitis but is most useful for draining the sinus and guiding antibiotic coverage in patients with complicated or refractory sinusitis.

5. Flexible rhinopharyngoscopy is most commonly used by otolaryngologists or allergists and allows a detailed inspection of the nasal cavity and posterior nasopharynx. It is most useful for establishing the diagnosis of chronic sinusitis and for identifying anatomic abnormalities that may predispose to recurrent sinusitis.

Key Tests

- Conventional radiographs are useful for confirming acute maxillary sinusitis.

- Rhinoscopy and computed tomography are most useful for evaluating chronic symptoms.

Differential Diagnosis

1. The differential diagnosis for nasal symptoms is long but can be grouped into three broad categories: inflammatory, noninflammatory, and mechanical causes.

   a. Inflammatory: allergic rhinitis (seasonal or perennial), acute viral infection, acute or chronic bacterial sinusitis, nasal polyps, Wegener's granulomatosis, sarcoidosis

   b. Noninflammatory: idiopathic vasomotor rhinitis, drug-induced vasomotor rhinitis (reserpine, guanethidine, prazosin, angiotensin-converting enzyme inhibitors, cocaine abuse), rhinitis medicamentosa, hormonal (pregnancy, hypothyroidism)

   c. Mechanical: deviated septum, nasal polyps, tumor, foreign body

2. In the primary care setting, the most common causes of nasal symptoms are allergic rhinitis, acute viral infection, acute or chronic sinusitis, idiopathic vasomotor rhinitis, rhinitis medicamentosa, and deviated nasal septum.

Treatment

The management of acute sinusitis is aimed at improving drainage of the sinuses and eradicating bacterial infection.

Medication

1. Antibiotic choice is based on the duration of symptoms, costs, and evidence of efficacy from randomized controlled trials. For acute sinusitis (symptoms present less than 30 days), 7 to 10 days of trimethoprim-sulfamethoxazole (Bactrim, Septra), 160/800 mg b.i.d., or amoxicillin, 500 mg t.i.d., leads to 80 to 90 per cent clinical response rates and these are the drugs of choice. In geographic areas with a high prevalence of β-lactamase–producing *H. influenzae* or *M. catarrhalis,* an agent with a broader spectrum, such as amoxicillin/clavulanate (Augmentin), cefaclor (Ceclor), cefuroxime axetil (Ceftin), or azithromycin (Zithromax), is appropriate. For patients with protracted symptoms, a longer course (2 to 3 weeks) of antibiotics is probably indicated.

2. Topical and systemic decongestants promote sinus drainage and ventilation and may be used safely in patients with mild to moderate hypertension. Prolonged use of topical decongestants may lead to rebound vasodilation and rhinitis medicamentosa. For adults, prescribe oxymetazoline (Afrin) nasal spray 0.05%, two sprays b.i.d. for 3 to 5 days; pseudoephedrine (Sudafed) extended release, 120 mg b.i.d.; or phenylpropanolamine extended release, 75 mg b.i.d.

3. Mucolytics and ciliator activators may thin secretions and promote sinus drainage. Evidence from one clinical trial suggests that guaifenesin, 30 ml q.i.d., speeds recovery.

4. Nasal corticosteroids have a limited role in acute sinusitis but may be useful for selected patients with underlying allergic rhinitis. Nasal steroids inhibit inflammatory responses without inducing adrenal suppression and act to decrease edema of the ostiomeatal complex.

5. Nasal saline or steam may decrease nasal crusting and liquefy secretions, thus facilitating sinus drainage.

6. Antihistamines may thicken nasal secretions, and therefore, they are not routinely indicated in the initial treatment of acute sinusitis. For patients with underlying allergic rhinitis, the nonsedating antihistamines are less likely to thicken secretions and may be useful ancillary treatment when topical corticosteroids have failed.

Patient Education

1. Most patients feel substantially improved or cured after 5 to 6 days of effective therapy.

2. Emphasize that prolonged use of topical decongestants may cause rebound vasodilation and worsening symptoms.

3. For patients with underlying allergic conditions, avoidance of environmental allergens may be helpful.

4. When prescribing nasal steroids, instruct the patient that it may take 1 to 2 weeks to achieve maximal effect.

Key Treatment

- Drugs of choice: trimethoprim-sulfamethoxazole or amoxicillin; oxymetazoline nasal spray

- Alternative drugs: amoxicillin/clavulanate, cefaclor, cefuroxime axetil, azithromycin

Follow-Up

1. For most patients, the initial course of therapy leads to clinical cure, and no specific follow-up is needed.

For patients who do not improve with initial treatment or have recurrent disease, further evaluation and therapy are indicated.

2. Patients who do not respond to an initial course of treatment should be re-evaluated. If not previously done, sinus radiographs should be taken to confirm the diagnosis. Once confirmed, a longer course of a broad-spectrum antibiotic that is effective against β-lactamase–producing organisms should be prescribed.

3. In patients with sinusitis that recurs three or more times a year, further evaluation by an otolaryngologist is indicated. This evaluation should include a search for anatomic factors that may predispose to sinusitis.

Bibliography

For more information on the bacteriology of acute sinusitis, see

Ylikoski J, Savolainen S, Jousimies-Somer H: The bacteriology of acute maxillary sinusitis. ORL J Otorhinolaryngol Relat Spec 1989;51:175–181.

For more information on the diagnosis of sinusitis, see

Williams JW Jr, Simel DL: Does this patient have sinusitis? Diagnosing acute sinusitis by history and physical examination. JAMA 1992;270:1242–1246, and Gwaltney JM, Phillips CD, Miller RD, et al: Computed tomographic study of the common cold. N Engl J Med 1994;330:25–30.

For more information on the treatment of sinusitis, see

Coates ML, Rembold CM, Farr BM: Does pseudoephedrine increase blood pressure in patients with controlled hypertension? J Fam Pract 1995;40:22–26, and Willet LR, Carson JL, Williams JW Jr: Current diagnosis and treatment of sinusitis. J Gen Intern Med 1994;9:38–45.

21 Orbital and Periorbital Cellulitis
Kimberly L. Morris

Etiology

1. Sinusitis is the most common predisposing condition in patients with orbital cellulitis. The ethmoid sinuses are most frequently involved, followed by the maxillary sinuses.

   a. Children under age 4 years

      (1) *Haemophilus influenzae,* type B—most common pathogen; consider concomitant, life-threatening infections such as meningitis, epiglottitis, and pneumonia

      (2) *Streptococcus pneumoniae*

   b. Older children and adults

      (1) Acute sinusitis—*H. influenzae, S. pneumoniae, Branhamella catarrhalis, Staphylococcus aureus, Streptococcus pyogenes,* and viridans streptococci.

      (2) Chronic sinusitis is often caused by polymicrobial infection with both aerobic and anaerobic bacteria, including *Bacteroides* sp., *Peptostreptococcus,* and *Fusobacterium* sp.

2. Orbital cellulitis may also occur as a result of contiguous spread from adjacent structures by way of the valveless facial veins.

   a. Dental infection—anaerobes

   b. Facial infection

   c. Infection of the globe or eyelids

   d. Lacrimal system

3. Less common causes of orbital cellulitis include direct trauma to the eye, often with implantation of a foreign body, and, rarely, postsurgical infection. *S. aureus* is the most common pathogen in both situations.

4. Hematogenous spread from distal infection may occur and should be considered in patients with serious underlying diseases, such as diabetes, cirrhosis, and immunosuppression.

5. Tumor resulting in sinus obstruction must also be considered in the older patient, particularly in smokers.

Symptoms

1. Pain, erythema, eyelid edema

2. Symptoms of sinusitis, such as facial tenderness, purulent nasal secretions, fever, headache, halitosis

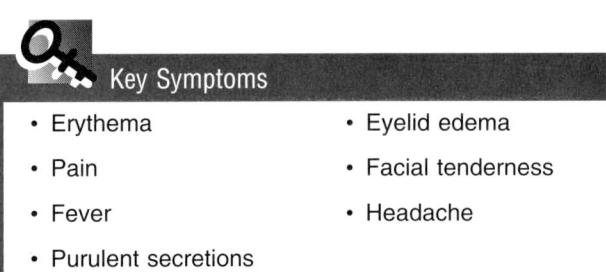

Key Symptoms

• Erythema	• Eyelid edema
• Pain	• Facial tenderness
• Fever	• Headache
• Purulent secretions	

Clinical Findings

1. Specific signs of orbital involvement include proptosis, limited extraocular movement, and vision loss.

2. Conjunctival edema (chemosis) and injection are seen frequently. Eyelid edema is a nonspecific finding.

3. A bluish skin discoloration is often seen in children with *H. influenzae* infection.

4. Ominous signs of cavernous sinus and meningeal involvement include sensory loss in the ophthalmic branch of the trigeminal nerve, cranial neuropathy, afferent pupillary defect, and mental status changes.

Key Signs

• Proptosis	• Ophthalmoplegia
• Vision loss	• Chemosis
• Pupil abnormality	• Cranial neuropathy

Tests

A. Laboratory tests

   1. White blood cell count with differential

      a. In adults, a range of 10,000 to 15,000/mm³ is common.

      b. In children, the white blood cell count may exceed 20,000/mm³.

   2. Blood cultures

   3. Drainage from all wounds should be cultured.

   4. In general, cultures from the conjunctivae, eyelids, and nasal passages are not helpful.

   5. Aspiration of orbital contents is not recommended because of the low yield of cultures and the risk of the procedure.

B. Other tests

   1. Computed tomography with axial and coronal cuts through the orbit is indicated and may provide additional information that can aid in selecting treatment.

2. Plain radiographs may assist in ruling out dental abscess in patients with maxillary sinus opacification by computed tomography.

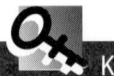

Key Tests

- Computed tomography must be performed if signs of orbital infection are present.
- Blood cultures must be obtained.

Differential Diagnosis

1. Preseptal cellulitis may cause pain, redness, eyelid edema, chemosis, and conjunctival injection. Structures anterior to the orbit are involved. A patient with these findings in the absence of orbital signs can be managed more conservatively. However, complications such as meningitis may occur in young children, and therefore hospitalization is warranted.

2. Subperiosteal abscess may involve the medial wall of the orbit. Displacement of the medial rectus muscle by the periosteum may be seen by computed tomography.

3. Blunt trauma to the eyelid with orbital foreign body or local infection

4. Orbital pseudotumor may present with eyelid edema, proptosis, and ophthalmoplegia, but the characteristic signs of infection are absent.

5. Dacryocystitis can be seen with acute mumps infection or chronic sarcoidosis.

6. Allergic reactions are usually accompanied by pruritus and are nontender and recurrent.

7. Orbital tumors such as rhabdomyosarcoma may be seen in children.

WARNING

Mycotic orbital infection must be suspected in diabetic patients or in those with metabolic acidosis. Necrosis of the palate or nasal mucosa is presumptive evidence.

Treatment

1. The patient should be hospitalized with empiric intravenous antibiotic treatment. Antibiotic selection should be made on the basis of the most likely cause.

   a. In children, a second-generation cephalosporin with gram-positive coverage and *H. influenzae* coverage would be reasonable.

   b. In adults, ceftriaxone (Rocephin), cefuroxime (Kefurox, Zinacef), or ampicillin/sulbactam (Unasyn) is suggested. In patients with immediate-type hypersensitivity reactions to β-lactam antibiotics, clindamycin (Cleocin) combined with ciprofloxacin (Cipro) or aztreonam (Azactam) would be reasonable.

   c. Amphotericin B is the drug of choice if *Mucor* sp. or *Rhizopus* sp. is suspected.

2. A multispecialty approach is optimal and should include a physician who is knowledgeable in antibiotic use, an otolaryngologist, and an ophthalmologist. Surgical intervention may be necessary if clinical response is inadequate or abscess is present.

Key Treatment

- Antibiotic selection must be based on the likely cause in view of specific patient characteristics.

Follow-Up

1. Close clinical follow-up is mandatory. Signs of orbital involvement should be assessed twice daily. Repeat computed tomographic scanning may be indicated if the clinical course is suboptimal.

2. Surgical drainage of the sinuses and orbital exploration may be necessary.

Bibliography

Davis JP, Stearns MP: Orbital complications of sinusitis. Postgrad Med J 1994;70(820):108–110.

Harley RD: Disorders of the orbit. *In* Harley RD (ed): Pediatric Ophthalmology, 2nd ed, vol 1. Philadelphia, WB Saunders Company, 1983, pp 349–388.

Lessner A, Stern GA: Preseptal and orbital cellulitis. Infect Dis Clin North Am 1992;6:933–952.

Martin-Hirsch DP, Habashi S, Hampton AH, Kotecha B: Orbital cellulitis. Arch Emerg Med 1992;9(2):143–148.

Steinkuller PG, Jones DB: Preseptal and orbital cellulitis and orbital abscess. *In* Linberg JV (ed): Oculoplastic and Orbital Emergencies. E Norwalk, CT, Appleton & Lange, 1992, pp 51–66.

Procedure | **LOCAL AND REGIONAL ANESTHESIA: HEAD AND NECK** | *Eugene Y. Cheng*

Indications

1. Surgical or dental procedures
2. Pain control: postoperative; terminal cancer
3. Facilitation of orotracheal or nasotracheal intubation
4. Diagnosis and treatment of tic douloureux and trigeminal neuralgia

Contraindications

1. Practitioner's lack of knowledge of anatomic landmarks and local anesthetic characteristics
2. Allergies to all local anesthetics
3. Poor patient cooperation
4. Infection of injection site, severe coagulopathy, lack of clearly identifiable landmarks

Preparation

1. Educate patient about pain on injection and limits of pain control.
2. Premedicate using parenteral sedatives, hypnotics, and/or opioids.
3. Have airway management and cardiopulmonary resuscitative equipment and resuscitation drugs available.

Equipment

1. Syringes (5 to 10 ml) and needles (22 to 27 gauge)
2. Skin preparation materials (sponges, iodine solution, alcohol)
3. Field sterility materials (mask, cap, drapes, gloves)

Anesthesia

1. Lidocaine (Xylocaine)
   a. Standard local anesthetic used for skin infiltration and most peripheral nerve blocks
   b. Lidocaine 1% to 2% solutions are usually used; solutions stronger than 1% may cause motor block. Upper dose limit is about 6 mg/kg.
   c. Epinephrine (1:200,000 to 1:250,000 concentration) slows the rate of systemic absorption.
2. Bupivacaine (Marcaine)
   a. Duration of action is two to three times longer than that of lidocaine.

b. More toxic (dose limit 2 to 3 mg/kg) than lidocaine
c. For peripheral nerve blocks, 0.25% to 0.50% solutions are typically used.

3. Cocaine
   a. Topical anesthetic primarily for the nose and throat; vasoconstrictive effect decreases swelling and bleeding.
   b. Total dose should not exceed 200 mg (e.g., 5 ml of 4% solution), regardless of application method.

Precautions

1. Central nervous system toxicity of local anesthetics
   a. Manifested by dysequilibrium, obtundation, confusion, seizures, or respiratory arrest
   b. Symptoms can occur with rapid absorption of perineural-injected local anesthetic or direct injection into the cerebrovascular circulation.
   c. Diazepam (Valium), 5 to 10 mg; midazolam (Versed), 2 to 6 mg; or thiopental (Pentothal Sodium), 2 to 4 mg/kg, is effective in treating local anesthetic-induced seizures.
2. Cardiotoxicity
   a. Cocaine can cause intense vasospasm leading to cardiac ischemia and infarction.
   b. Bupivacaine can cause cardiac arrest if upper dosage limits are exceeded.
3. Vasovagal response can occur with the pain of local anesthetic injection or the anticipation of injection.

WARNING

- **Severe pain with needle advancement or injection of local anesthetic could mean intraneural needle placement. Withdraw the needle and reinsert.**
- **Aspirate before local anesthetic injection. Withdraw the needle and reinsert if blood or cerebrospinal fluid is aspirated.**

Techniques

1. Brow and forehead block
   a. Blocking the supraorbital and supratrochlear nerves (terminal branches of the first division [ophthalmic nerve] of the trigeminal nerve) anesthetizes the ipsilateral forehead from eyebrow to vertex and from the midline to the temporal region.
   b. Procedure

   (1) Prepare the block site in a sterile manner.
   (2) Above the eyebrow over the medial aspect, raise a skin wheal with a local anesthetic.
   (3) Insert a small-gauge needle through the skin wheal, and infiltrate 2 to 3 ml of local anesthetic over the medial half of the eyebrow.
2. Upper lip block
   a. Blocking the infraorbital nerve (peripheral nerve of the second [maxillary] division of the trigeminal

nerve) anesthetizes the lower eyelid, cheek, lateral aspect of the nose, upper lip, and part of the temple.

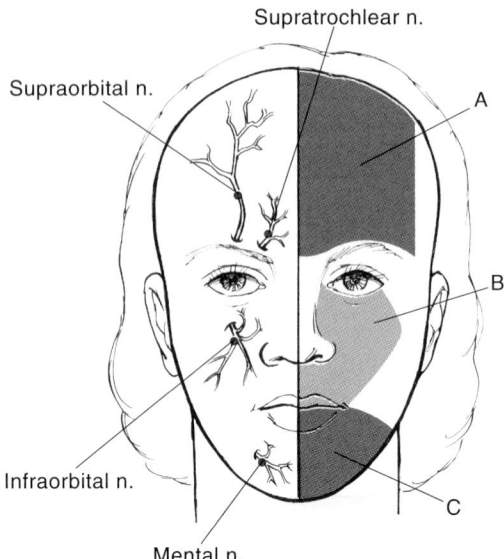

Supratrochlear n.

Supraorbital n.

A

B

Infraorbital n.

Mental n.

C

b. Procedure
   (1) Prepare the block site in a sterile manner.
   (2) The infraorbital nerve is located 1 finger-breadth below the orbital rim in the same vertical plane as the pupil with the eye looking forward. Raise a skin wheal over this site.
   (3) Insert the needle through the wheal slightly cephalad and lateral toward the infraorbital foramen. Infiltrate 2 to 3 ml of local anesthetic in the general area.

3. Lower lip block
   a. Blocking the mental nerve (peripheral branch of the mandibular nerve [third division of the trigeminal nerve]) anesthetizes the ipsilateral lower lip and chin.
   b. Procedure
      (1) Prepare the injection site in a sterile manner.
      (2) The foramen through which the mental nerve emerges is found in the same vertical plane as the pupil and slightly above or on the superior aspect of the mandibular ramus. Raise a skin wheal over the mental foramen.
      (3) Insert the needle medially through the wheal, and inject 2 to 3 ml of local anesthetic.

4. External nose block
   a. The external nose is primarily innervated by the infratrochlear and external nasal nerves (terminal branches of the ophthalmic nerve; the lateral portion of the nose is innervated by the infraorbital nerve).
   b. Procedure
      (1) Prepare the injection site in a sterile manner.
      (2) The infratrochlear and external nasal nerves are found about 1 cm above the inner canthus and just lateral to the medial wall of the orbit. Place a skin wheal over this site.

   (3) Direct the needle posteriorly and slightly medially to a depth of about 2.5 cm. Inject 2 to 3 ml of local anesthetic.
   (4) If anesthesia is also required over the lateral part of the nose, the infraorbital nerve should be blocked, as in upper lip block.

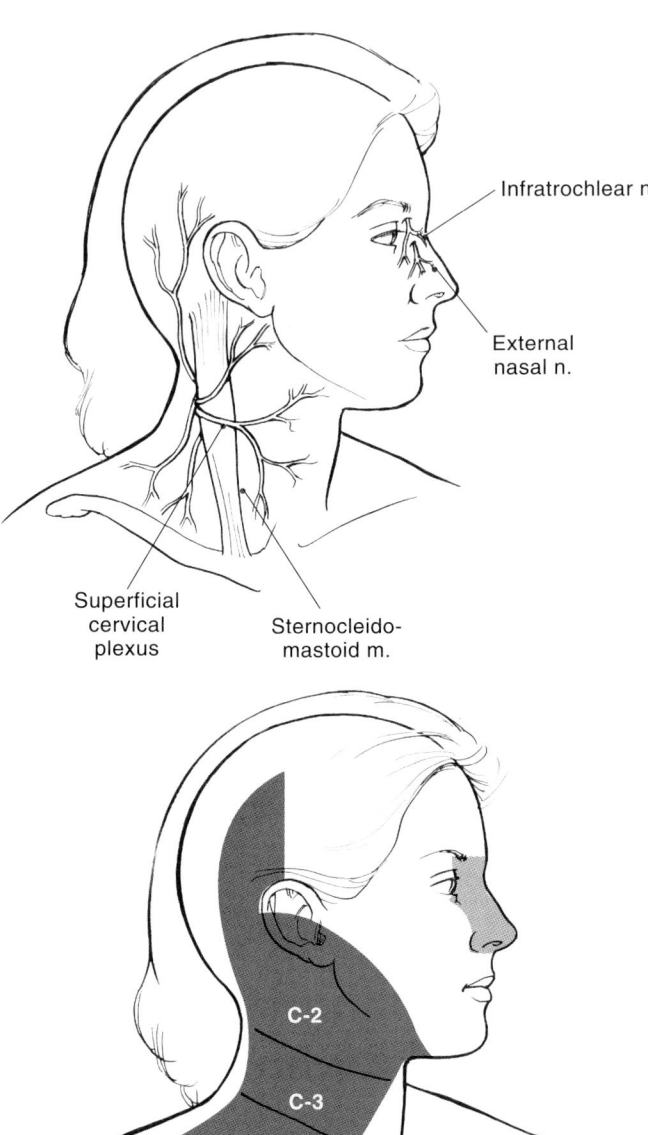

Infratrochlear n.

External nasal n.

Superficial cervical plexus

Sternocleido-mastoid m.

C-2

C-3

C-4

5. Neck block
   a. The superficial cervical plexus (see above) is derived from the anterior rami of cervical nerves 2–4 (C_{2-4}). Blocking the superficial cervical plexus anesthetizes the skin of the neck from midline to posterior.
   b. Procedure
      (1) Prepare the block site in a sterile manner.
      (2) The superficial cervical plexus (see above) is found in the posterior triangle of the neck emerging at the midpoint of the posterior border of the sternocleidomastoid muscle.

(3) Locate the posterior aspect of the sternocleido-mastoid muscle and superficially infiltrate 3 to 4 ml of local anesthetic over the middle third.

Follow-Up

1. Obtain a neurology consult if sensation or motor function does not return within the expected time period (2 to 4 hours with lidocaine; 6 to 10 hours with bupivacaine).

2. Instruct the patient to return immediately for evaluation if redness or exudation occurs at the injection site.

3. Hospitalize patients for adverse systemic reactions, such as seizures; respiratory arrest; or severe allergic reactions.

4. If peripheral nerve blocks are only partially effective, nerve root or first division nerve blocks will provide better analgesia.

Bibliography

Carron H, Korbon GA: Common nerve blocks in anesthetic practice. Semin Anesth 1983;2:30–49.

de Jong RH: Local anesthetics. *In* Raj PP: Practical Management of Pain with Special Emphasis on Physiology of Pain Syndromes and Techniques of Pain Management. Chicago, Year Book Medical Publishers, 1986, pp 539–556.

Ehlert TK, Arnold DE: Local anesthesia for soft-tissue surgery. Otolaryngol Clin North Am 1990;23:831–844.

Murphy TM: Somatic blockade of head and neck. *In* Cousins MJ, Bridenbaugh PO (eds): Neural Blockade in Clinical Anesthesia and Management of Pain, 2nd ed. Philadelphia, JB Lippincott, 1988, pp 533–560.

Quail G: Nerve blocks for the face. Aust Fam Physician 1991;20:830.

22 Common Respiratory Symptoms

Chronic cough is the fifth most common reason for office visits, leading to 30 million outpatient evaluations every year. The 20 per cent prevalence of chronic cough in nonsmoking adults increases markedly in patients who smoke or who have occupational exposure to fumes and dust. Chronic cough is traditionally defined as a cough present for greater than 3 weeks. Most researchers, however, require 8 weeks of cough for inclusion in studies.

Differential Diagnosis

1. Postnasal drip
2. Asthma
3. Chronic bronchitis
4. Gastroesophageal reflux

Other less common causes include congestive heart failure, occupational or environmental exposure, chronic lung infection, tumor, bronchiectasis, interstitial lung disease, recurrent aspiration, use of angiotensin-converting enzyme (ACE) inhibitors, cerumen impaction, psychogenic conditions, and foreign body. The most common cause of cough in smokers is chronic bronchitis. Allergic rhinitis, nonallergic rhinitis, and sinusitis all cause postnasal drip, which is the most common cause of persistent cough in nonsmokers. Reactive airways disease may present with cough as the only symptom. Likewise, patients with reflux may not have any complaint except cough.

> Refer to Ch. 19, Allergic Rhinitis; Ch. 20, Sinusitis; Ch. 28, Asthma; Ch. 29, Bronchitis; Ch. 31, Chronic Obstructive Pulmonary Disease; Ch. 60, Chronic Heart Failure; and Ch. 75, Gastroesophageal Reflux.

History

1. Duration, frequency, and severity of cough
2. Smoking history
3. Sensation of ''something dripping down the throat'' or frequent throat clearing consistent with postnasal drip
4. History of seasonal allergies, purulent nasal discharge, or facial pain
5. Presence of wheezing, shortness of breath, or worsening of cough with exercise or exposure to cold air suggestive of asthma
6. History of heartburn, sour taste in back of throat, or previous diagnosis of reflux
7. Sputum production and color and presence of hemoptysis
8. Exacerbation of cough at night. Postnasal drip, gastroesophageal reflux, and congestive heart failure all worsen while supine. Psychogenic cough does not disturb sleep.
9. Medication history, including previous treatment for cough and the use of ACE inhibitors for blood pressure control or congestive heart failure.
10. Weight loss or night sweats, which may occur with cancer or chronic infection

A carefully acquired history focuses on differentiating among the likely causes of chronic cough and can determine the cause of cough in most patients. Eighty per cent of people with postnasal drip report frequent throat clearing or a dripping sensation. Patients should be questioned regarding a history of recent respiratory tract infection, occupational or environmental exposure, tuberculosis exposure, and symptoms of congestive heart failure. Smokers should be asked if there has been a change in their cough pattern.

Clinical Findings

1. Findings consistent with postnasal drip include the following:
   a. Mucoid or mucopurulent secretions in the oropharynx or nasopharynx
   b. Cobblestoning of the posterior pharynx
   c. Edematous, hyperemic nasal mucosa
   d. Tenderness or diminished transillumination of the sinuses
2. Expiratory wheezing is suggestive of asthma.
3. A local wheeze may be present in bronchogenic cancer.
4. Cerumen or a hair on the tympanic membrane may irritate cough receptors.
5. Crackles, elevated jugular venous pulse, or an S_3 gallop indicates congestive heart failure.

Tests

1. Pulmonary function testing before and after the administration of bronchodilators
2. Methacholine inhalation challenge if pulmonary function tests are normal
3. Sinus radiography if sinusitis is suspected or if a patient with postnasal drip continues to cough on treatment

4. Barium swallow or esophagogastroduodenoscopy

5. 24-hour pH monitoring if barium swallow is normal and reflux is suspected

6. Chest radiography if the patient has fever, weight loss, hemoptysis, or a significant smoking history

7. Sputum cytology in a smoker with a normal chest radiograph if cancer is suspected

The history and physical examination should direct the patient evaluation. Because postnasal drip is by far the most common cause of cough in the otherwise healthy nonsmoker, an empiric trial of an antihistamine-decongestant combination may be the most cost-effective approach. In other settings or if the patient fails to respond to initial therapy, pulmonary function testing before and after the administration of bronchodilators is recommended as the next diagnostic test, followed by methacholine inhalation challenge if initial testing is normal.

Bronchoscopy has a low yield even in smokers unless they have an abnormality on chest radiography, hemoptysis, or a history suggestive of cancer. Some of the rare causes of cough may be diagnosed by bronchoscopy if the history, physical examination, and less invasive work-up do not point to a diagnosis and empiric treatment does not relieve symptoms. Psychogenic cough is a diagnosis of exclusion and, thus, may require bronchoscopy.

Management

A. Chronic bronchitis

1. Stop smoking

2. Inhaled ipatropium bromide (Atrovent)

B. Postnasal drip

1. Oral antihistamine/decongestant twice daily

2. Nasal corticosteroids twice daily if coughing persists despite oral medication or if allergic rhinitis is suspected

3. Oxymetazoline (Afrin) nasal spray for 3 days and antibiotics up to 6 weeks in addition to the above medications for chronic sinusitis

C. Asthma

1. Inhaled β_2 agonists, two puffs four times per day. Adjust dose according to response.

2. Consider 1-week course of oral steroids (i.e., prednisone, 60 mg daily) if β_2 agonists are inadequate.

3. Consider inhaled corticosteroids or oral bronchodilators.

D. Gastroesophageal reflux

1. Conservative measures, including elevating head of bed and not ingesting food for 2 hours before bedtime

2. Antacids

3. Oral histamine$_2$ antagonists

As defined above, treatment should be tailored to the specific cause of cough. Conservative measures are tried initially and then further treatment is added as needed.

Cough caused by reflux may require 1 to 6 months of therapy before full relief is attained. All patients should be counseled that each of these conditions is a long-term problem, and thus, therapy may need to be continued indefinitely.

Specific treatment leads to complete or marked resolution in more than 90 per cent of compliant patients, so nonspecific measures are usually unnecessary. Codeine and dextromethorphan are effective and may be used for symptomatic relief, particularly at night, if needed. Many other antitussives have not shown efficacy in trials.

Follow-Up

1. The treatment success rate in correctly diagnosed patients is high. The most common cause for treatment failure in the compliant patient is the presence of two causes for the cough.

2. If cough persists after treatment, the same diagnostic protocol should be used, looking for a second factor contributing to cough.

3. Asthma commonly coexists with postnasal drip or reflux.

4. The addition of therapy for the second diagnosis may lead to complete resolution of cough.

PEARLS

- Smoking cessation has been 100 per cent successful in resolution or marked improvement in cough within 1 month.

- Antihistamine/decongestant combination treatment alone is successful in more than 50 per cent of nonsmokers.

- Airway hyperactivity may persist in normals for 8 weeks after an upper respiratory tract infection. Consider bronchodilators or a brief course of steroids, but do not misdiagnose "asthma" in this setting.

 Bibliography

Corrao WM: Chronic cough: when to take the less traveled path. J Respir Dis 1993;14:273–280.

Irwin RS, Corrao WM, Pratter MR: Chronic persistent cough in the adult: the spectrum and frequency of causes and successful outcome of specific therapy. Am Rev Respir Dis 1989;123:413–417.

Irwin RS, Rosen MJ, Braman SS: Cough: a comprehensive review. Arch Intern Med 1977;137:1186–1191.

Pratter MR, Bartter T, Akers S: An algorithmic approach to chronic cough. Ann Intern Med 1993;119:977–983.

Zervanos NJ, Shute KU: Acute, disruptive cough: symptomatic therapy for a nagging problem. Postgrad Med 1994;95:153–164.

| Symptom | **Sore Throat** | *Frank Burwick* |

Sore throat is, in its most common form, more or less a nuisance that afflicts humans throughout life. More common in childhood, adolescence, and young adulthood, sore throat can occur at any age. Although it most commonly is a benign disease that need not—and cannot—be treated except with some soothing over-the-counter medications or home remedies of questionable value, sore throat can be a prelude to severe debilitating disease and, on rare occasions, can be a fatal disease if not recognized and treated correctly. The throat, with its lymphoglandular tissue (Waldeyer's tonsillar ring), is the first line of defense against an onslaught of external factors, be they of physical, chemical, or microbial origin.

Differential Diagnosis

1. Infectious
   a. Viral—most common; all ages, all seasons, but more prevalent during winter
   b. Bacterial—most important group A β-hemolytic streptococci; most common from ages 5 to 15 years
   c. Fungal—*Candida*
2. Environmental—tobacco smoke, smog, dust, allergens
3. Drainage from "above" or "below"
   a. Postnasal drip
   b. Gastroesophageal reflux
4. Rare causes
   a. Hypothyroidism or hyperthyroidism
   b. Thyroiditis
   c. Foreign body
   d. Leukemia, agranulocytosis
   e. Diphtheria
   f. Gonorrhea in 10 per cent of patients with anogenital gonorrhea
5. Sore throat with pharyngeal ulcers
   a. Canker sores (aphthous stomatitis)
   b. Herpangina
   c. Herpes simplex
   d. Fusospirochetal infection
   e. Candidiasis
   f. Herpes zoster
   g. Chickenpox
   h. Primary or secondary syphilitic ulcerations (usually not painful)

One can argue whether environmental factors or infections are the most common causes of sore throat. For the physician, the infectious reasons and their correct recognition are of greater importance. However, to stress the importance of environmental factors is an important part of patient awareness and education. Among infectious agents that cause sore throat, viruses far outnumber bacteria. Fungal causes are rare but on the rise as the acquired immunodeficiency syndrome epidemic continues unchecked.

Bacterial pharyngitis is often caused by group A β-hemolytic streptococci. Sudden onset of sore throat, general malaise, a temperature that is usually high (104° F [40° C] in adults and even higher in children), and suppurative and nonsuppurative sequelae make recognition of this pathogen extremely important, especially since acute rheumatic fever has become more common.

PEARLS

- Exudate is not specific for streptococcal tonsillitis; viral tonsillitis can look the same.

- Strep throat is extremely rare in children under age 3 years, and if it occurs, it is associated with purulent rhinitis.

- *Arcanobacterium haemolyticus* (formerly *Corynebacterium haemolyticum*) causes pharyngitis and tonsillitis quite similar to group A β-hemolytic streptococci infection with anterior neck lymphadenitis as well as scarlatiniform rash that often, as in strep throat, proceeds to desquamate.

- Sore throat becomes worse on swallowing, but throat examination is normal. Palpate the thyroid: thyroiditis?

Infectious mononucleosis causes about 5 per cent of sore throats. Most often it is caused by Epstein-Barr virus and rarely by cytomegalovirus. Usually a disease of adolescents and young adults, it can, on inspection, mimic strep throat, but the history is different: gradual onset, low-grade temperature, mild pharyngeal symptoms, more pronounced systemic symptoms. Enanthema and petechiae on the palate are almost diagnostic for infectious mononucleosis. Posterior cervical lymphadenitis points strongly toward infectious mononucleosis or other viral cause.

PEARLS

- For the Monospot test, there are essentially no false-negative results except in children under age 6 years. However, false-positive results are found in 10 per cent of children in this age group. Complete blood count with at least 50 per cent lymphocytes and at least 10 per cent atypical lymphocytes also confirms the diagnosis.

- Throat culture, the *gold* standard for the diagnosis of strep pharyngitis, should be performed in patients at high risk for complications even when the probability of strep throat is low (i.e., patients with diabetes mellitus or a history of rheumatic fever and during outbreak of a nephrogenic strain).

- Pharyngeal exudate is not diagnostic for strep tonsillitis; only 50 per cent of patients with strep throat have exudate, and of all patients with exudate, only 50 per cent have strep throat.

Refer to Ch. 10, Aphthous Stomatitis; Ch. 19, Allergic Rhinitis; Ch. 165, Thyroiditis; and Ch. 236, Infectious Mononucleosis.

History

In addition to inquiry about onset of symptoms, exposure to other cases with similar symptoms, and so on, it is important to take note of the time of year and age of the patient. Certain diagnoses are common in certain seasons and age-groups. The questions to ask are a logical consequence of the patient's signs and symptoms, which might include the following:

- Fever—high and sudden onset, low-grade and insidious onset
- Pain—where? Referred pain?
- ? Dysphagia
- ? Drooling
- ? Preferred position
- ? Pain on extension of the neck

Clinical Findings

1. Inspection
   a. Pharyngeal erythema
   b. Enlargement of tonsils
   c. Asymmetry, position of uvula
   d. Exudate—does it wipe off?
   e. Pseudomembrane
   f. Enanthema
   g. Postnasal drip
   h. Posterior or lateral swelling
   i. Ulcers
2. Palpation
   a. Enlarged and tender anterior cervical nodes suggest a bacterial infection.
   b. Enlarged and tender posterior cervical nodes suggest a viral infection.
   c. Check the thyroid gland if throat inspection is normal.

Tests

1. In patients whose clinical picture is consistent with influenza, common cold, or irritants, no further laboratory tests are needed.
2. A rapid strep test should be done in patients with an intermediate likelihood of strep throat and in patients at high risk for complications, even when the likelihood is small.
3. Obtain a Monospot test or complete blood count if infectious mononucleosis is suspected. If mononucleosis is confirmed, perform liver function tests and antiglobulin (Coombs') test.
4. Obtain a lateral neck radiograph if drooling is present. Look for epiglottitis?
5. Order a computed tomographic scan of the neck or a magnetic resonance imaging scan if there is retropharyngeal or peritonsillar abscess.

Management

1. Viral—symptomatic only with aspirin (acetaminophen in children), lozenges, saltwater gargling, and plenty of fluids. Avoid giving antibiotics; they are ineffective for viral sore throat and expensive, and they carry the risks of adverse effects and induction of allergy.
2. Bacterial (e.g., strep throat)—if typical presentation (rapid onset, high fever, exudate on tonsils, tender swollen anterior cervical lymph nodes), treat with penicillin (or erythromycin in penicillin allergy). The presence of cough and coryza makes viral infection much more likely.
3. Candidiasis (oral thrush)—nystatin solution or ketoconazole
4. Diphtheria—rare but possible even in societies with high immunization rates. Give diphtheria antitoxin within 48 hours of disease onset.
5. Retropharyngeal or peritonsillar abscess—requires surgery and intravenous clindamycin (Cleocin) or nafcillin (Unipen).

Follow-Up

Usually not necessary. Recurrences are common. Penicillin for strep throat prevents nonsuppurative sequelae if treatment is started within 48 hours.

 Bibliography

Del Mar C: Managing sore throat: A literature review. Making the diagnosis [review]. Med J Aust 1992;156(8):5672–5675.

Dippel DW, Touw-Otten F, Habbema JD: Management of children with acute pharyngitis. J Fam Pract 1992;32(2):149–159.

Goldstein MN: Office evaluation and management of the sore throat [review]. Otolaryngol Clin North Am 1992;25(4):837–842.

Lang SD: The sore throat. When to investigate and when to prescribe [review]. Drugs 1990;40(6):854–862.

Vukmir RB: Adult and pediatric pharyngitis: A review [review]. J Emerg Med 1992;10(5):607–616.

Hemoptysis, the expectoration of blood, ranges from blood-tinged sputum or scant hemoptysis to large amounts of blood and clots. Epidemiologic studies demonstrate that hemoptysis is responsible for 6.8 per cent of all patient visits, 11 per cent of hospital admissions, 15 per cent of pulmonary consults, and 38 per cent of thoracic surgical referrals. Making the distinction between true hemoptysis, which usually originates from the rupture of the bronchial arteries, and bleeding from other anatomic sites, such as oropharyngeal and gastrointestinal sources, requires complete history, physical examination, and appropriate studies.

Hemoptysis is broken down into scant hemoptysis (blood-tinged sputum), or frank hemoptysis, which is less than 600 ml of blood in 24 hours, and massive hemoptysis, measuring greater than 600 ml of blood in 24 hours. Because measurement of the volume can be unreliable, a clinical definition demonstrating the magnitude of effect, including the risk of aspiration, airway obstruction, or hypotension, is considered massive.

Differential Diagnosis

A. Scant or frank hemoptysis
1. Bronchitis (vigorous coughing)
2. Bronchiectasis
3. Carcinoma of the lung
4. Active tuberculosis
5. Chronic necrotizing pneumonia
6. Pulmonary emboli with pulmonary infarction
7. Congestive heart failure

B. Massive hemoptysis
1. Tuberculosis
2. Bronchiectasis
3. Necrotizing pneumonia
4. Lung abscess
5. Fungal lung infection
6. Bronchogenic carcinoma

Diagnostic advances and changes in the occurrence of disease have led to an inconsistent spectrum for causes associated with hemoptysis. The differential diagnosis for hemoptysis varies with the amount of blood expectorated. Massive hemoptysis is rare, occurring in less than 5 per cent of all cases. Overall causes associated with hemoptysis are due to tracheobronchial disorders, local or diffuse parenchymal disease, cardiovascular disease, hematologic disorders, and iatrogenic sources.

Tracheobronchial disorders include disorders that affect the bronchial lining, such as bronchitis, bronchiectasis, bronchial adenoma, bronchogenic carcinoma, and endobronchial tuberculosis. Pneumonia, abscess, tuberculosis, and fungal diseases are associated with local parenchymal disease; Goodpasture's syndrome, legionnaires' disease,

Wegener's disease, and other connective tissue diseases are associated with diffuse parenchymal disease. Cardiovascular causes include pulmonary emboli with infarction, mitral stenosis, and congestive heart failure. Hematologic causes include coagulopathy, thrombocytopenia, and other blood dyscrasias. Iatrogenic causes include trauma from intubation, tracheoinnominate fistula with long-standing tracheostomy tube, and pulmonary artery rupture from pulmonary artery catheter infarct.

> Refer to Ch. 29, Bronchitis; Ch. 30, Bronchiectasis; Ch. 34, Pneumonia; Ch. 36, Pulmonary Embolus; Ch. 38, Acute Pulmonary Edema; Ch. 43, Cancers of the Lung and Larynx; Ch. 46, Tuberculosis; and Ch. 60, Chronic Heart Failure.

History

1. Cough—severity
2. Sputum production—color, frothy
3. Occurrence of bloody sputum, character, amount, timing
4. Fever, chills, night sweats, weight loss
5. Chest pain
6. Gurgling in chest, wheezing
7. Upper respiratory tract symptoms, nasal congestion, rhinorrhea, recurrent sinusitis
8. History of smoking tobacco
9. History of rheumatic fever
10. Recent travel history to Africa, Asia, or South America

The history needs to focus initially on the cause, site, and quantity of hemoptysis. Questions detailing the amount of hemoptysis are cumbersome and must distinguish between cough and vomiting. Ask questions regarding a long history of sputum production as in chronic bronchitis, acute onset of sputum production as in acute bronchitis, or no sputum production as with bronchogenic carcinoma. Fever, mucopurulent cough, and pleuritic chest pain preceding hemoptysis suggest pneumonia; pleuritic chest pain, dyspnea, and hemoptysis suggest pulmonary emboli. The scenario of fever, night sweats, and weight loss suggests tuberculosis. A history of tobacco smoking in a patient over age 40 with recurrent hemoptysis suggests cancer, whereas recurrent hemoptysis in a young nonsmoking woman suggests bronchial adenoma. A history of hematuria associated with hemoptysis must suggest Goodpasture's syndrome, legionnaires' disease, and other connective tissue diseases, such as lupus, or recurrent sinusitis, as seen in Wegener's disease. Travel history to underdeveloped regions suggests parasitic infections, such as *Paragonimus westermani.*

Clinical Findings

1. Vital signs—normal or elevated temperature, increased heart rate, low blood pressure or hypotension, tachypnea
2. General—anxiety, pallor, possibly increased respiratory effort
3. HEENT—nasal ulcerations, purulent nasal drainage, poor dentition, lip and oral telangiectases
4. Neck—supraclavicular adenopathy
5. Chest—localized wheezing and crackles, diastolic murmur of mitral stenosis
6. Extremities—cyanosis, clubbing, edema

Clinical findings vary with each presentation of hemoptysis.

Tests

1. Chest radiography (compare with old films)
2. Complete blood count with differential (hematocrit, hemoglobin, white blood cell count with differential, platelets)
3. Type and crossmatch, screening
4. Coagulation profile (prothrombin time; partial thromboplastin time; fibrinogen level)
5. Chemistry profile (blood urea nitrogen and creatinine levels and electrolytes)
6. Arterial blood gas analysis (hypoxia, hypercapnia, acidosis)
7. Urinalysis (red blood cells, casts, protein)
8. Sputum analysis (pH, Gram's stain, acid-fast stain, cultures, cytology)
9. Echocardiography (if a diastolic murmur is present)
10. Fiberoptic bronchoscopy versus rigid bronchoscopy
11. Purified protein derivative (tuberculin; PPD) and controls
12. Ventilation scan
13. Contrast computed tomography and technetium scan (debatable)

Management

A. Scant or frank hemoptysis
    1. Order antibiotic trial if the focus of infection is present.
    2. Antitussive (nonsedating doses) may be beneficial.
    3. Treat underlying condition.
    4. Use supplemental oxygen with a compromised patient.
B. Massive hemoptysis
    1. Assess ABCs.
        a. Airway
        b. Breathing
        c. Circulation
    2. Oxygen therapy
        a. 100% with mask
        b. Orotracheal intubation if there is a threat of asphyxia (large endotracheal tube greater than 8 mm, if possible)
        c. The use of double-lumen Carlen-type endotracheal tube or selective intubation is controversial.
    3. Volume resuscitation to stabilize altered hemodynamics
        a. Intravenous fluids—normal saline (use at least 16-gauge needle; 14-gauge preferred)
        b. Transfuse packed red blood cells, 2 to 6 units, over 2 to 6 hours.
    4. Foley catheter
    5. Patient position
        a. Known site or localized bleeding—position patient with bleeding site dependent
        b. Unknown site or diffuse bleeding—place patient in Trendelenburg position
    6. Rigid bronchoscopy
        a. Packing material to tamponade bleeding
        b. Iced saline lavage
        c. Placement of Fogarty catheter with inflatable balloon
        d. Suction and removal of blood, clots, and foreign bodies
    7. Mild sedation to suppress cough and avoid continued bleeding and rebleeding
    8. Correct coagulopathy
    9. Begin appropriate anti-infectious agents if there is evidence of infection—antibiotics, antifungals, antituberculin agents
    10. Angiographic occlusion of source vessels
    11. Surgical evaluation and management

Medication

A. Scant or frank hemoptysis
    1. Antibiotics (e.g., tetracycline, ampicillin, or amoxicillin)—1 to 2 gm/day for 10 days
    2. Antitussives—codeine, 15 to 30 mg q 4 to 6 h; hydrocodone (Hycodan), 5 mg q 4 to 6 h
B. Massive hemoptysis
    1. Intravenous vasopressin (0.2 to 0.4 units/min continuous)
    2. Desmopressin (DDAVP), 0.3 μg/kg in 50 ml of normal saline solution intravenously over 30 minutes
    3. Antitussives
    4. Antibiotics

Diet

A. Scant or frank hemoptysis
    1. As tolerated

2. Maintain good hydration.

B. Massive hemoptysis

1. Nothing by mouth

2. Intravenous fluids to ensure appropriate volume status

Activity

A. Scant or frank hemoptysis

1. Rest

2. Limit activity, depending on severity of hemoptysis

B. Massive hemoptysis

1. Bed rest

2. Position—lateral decubitus Trendelenburg with bleeding side down

Patient Education

A. Scant or frank hemoptysis

1. Monitor amount of hemoptysis.

2. Advise gentle, not forceful, coughing.

3. Report PPD results.

4. No smoking

B. Massive hemoptysis. All patients in a hospitalized or an intensive care situation should be informed and reassured of status.

Follow-Up

A. Scant or frank hemoptysis

1. Depending on the severity, the patient may be seen the next day, in a few weeks after appropriate work-up and completion of treatment, or earlier with worsening condition.

2. Repeat chest radiography.

3. Consider elective bronchoscopy for failed resolution after initial treatment.

B. Massive hemoptysis—hospitalization or intensive care

PEARLS

- Hemoptysis resulting from bronchogenic cancer occurs as blood-smeared sputum caused by small, irritative mucosal lesions or massive hemoptysis caused by a large endobronchial tumor that is friable, necrotic, or eroding a central vessel.

- Metastatic tumor tends to enlarge within the lung parenchyma and seldom causes massive hemoptysis.

- Death results from asphyxiation, not exsanguination.

- Pseudohemoptysis or blood originating from another source besides the lower respiratory tract can be differentiated by inspection of the nasopharynx or analysis of bloody secretions (i.e., blood from the tracheobronchial tree is usually bright red and alkaline, demonstrates alveolar macrophages, and is mixed with frothy or purulent sputum; blood from a gastrointestinal source is dark red with acidic pH and mixed with food particles).

- Tuberculosis in patients infected with the human immunodeficiency virus is usually present with extrapulmonary disease or disseminated miliary tuberculosis. When present in the lungs of patients with acquired immunodeficiency syndrome, it is probably secondary to reactivation.

- Old cavitary lesions of tuberculosis may become colonized with an intracavitary aspergilloma, thus amounting to a rare cause of hemoptysis.

- Hemoptysis caused by pulmonary emboli is uncommon because of the rich blood supply to the lungs, but it can occur in settings of underlying cardiovascular disease that minimizes the blood supply, influencing infarction.

- Hemoptysis is a late symptom of cancer.

- Chest examination is usually normal initially.

Bibliography

Albert RK: Lung hemorrhage and hemoptysis. *In* Hall JB, Schmidt GA, Wood LDH (eds): Principles of Critical Care. New York, McGraw-Hill, 1992, pp 1736–1739.

Jones D: Massive hemoptysis. Br Med J 1990;300:889–890.

Karlinsky JB, Lau J, Goldstein RN: Decision Making in Pulmonary Medicine. Philadelphia, BC Decker, 1991, pp 10–11.

Morrisey JD, Winter SM: The causes and management of hemoptysis. Contemp Intern Med 1994;6:10–26.

Stoller JK: Diagnosis and management of massive hemoptysis: A review. Respir Care 1992;37(6):564–578.

23 Upper Respiratory Infection

Richard Neill

Etiology

1. The common cold is the single most common upper respiratory tract infection, accounting for more restricted activity days than any other illness.
2. Rhinoviruses (more than 100 serotypes) and coronaviruses (more than 3 types) account for 40 to 45 per cent of colds annually, with parainfluenza virus, respiratory syncytial virus, influenza virus, and adenovirus accounting for 10 to 15 per cent as a group.
3. Mild group A streptococcal pharyngitis is difficult to distinguish from viral infection and may account for 10 to 15 per cent of colds.
4. Up to 35 per cent of colds have no identified viral or bacterial cause.
5. Incidence of the common cold is highest from late August, when school begins, to late spring.
6. Transmission occurs by way of droplet and surface-to-surface (e.g., hand to hand, hand to nose) contact.
7. The primary reservoir is young children, who contract viral infections in school or day care and pass them on to family members.
8. Adults average two to four colds per year. Children average eight to ten colds per year from birth to age ten.

Symptoms

1. Common symptoms include the following:
   a. Nasal congestion and drainage
   b. Sore throat
   c. Cough
   d. Sneezing
2. Less common complaints include the following:
   a. Eye burning, conjunctivitis—more common in adenovirus or enterovirus infections
   b. Ear pressure or popping—often a result of eustachian tube obstruction
   c. Headache—often caused by sinus obstruction
   d. Malaise or fatigue—variable
3. Fever and adenopathy are more common in children.
4. Incubation period is 2 to 5 days, with symptoms lasting 6 to 10 days.

Key Symptoms

• Rhinorrhea	• Nasal congestion
• Sneezing	• Sore or scratchy throat
• Cough	

Clinical Findings

1. Minimal in adults, more prominent in children
2. Rhinorrhea, nasal crusting, pharyngeal erythema, and postnasal drip are all common.
3. Cervical adenopathy, pharyngeal exudate, and fever increase the likelihood of streptococcal pharyngitis.
4. Clear nasal drainage may be blood-streaked or turn yellow later in the course of illness.

Key Signs

- Often absent!
- Clear, watery nasal discharge
- Crusting of nostrils in children

Tests

1. Viral cultures for identification typically are reserved for research purposes.
2. Blood counts and chemistry profiles are normal.
3. Imaging studies (plain film radiography and computed tomography) of sinuses may show mucosal hypertrophy that reverses without intervention.

Differential Diagnosis

1. Allergic rhinitis—differentiate by seasonal nature, prominence of sneezing and rhinorrhea, and lack of fever or adenopathy; unusual in children under age 2 years. Nasal smear may show numerous eosinophils. Nasal polyps suggest allergy.
2. Sinusitis, acute or chronic—differentiate by duration of symptoms, more rapid onset of symptoms, fever in the presence of unilateral intense facial pressure or pain, malodorous nasal discharge, and upper teeth pain (which implies maxillary sinus involvement). Sinus congestion is common in colds and typically resolves spontaneously.
3. Influenza—myalgias, headache, and malaise are more prominent, accompanied by rhinitis, cough, sneezing, and fever. Gastrointestinal symptoms are uncommon with true influenza. Predominance is late fall to early spring with uncomplicated infections lasting for less than 1 week.
4. Group A streptococcal pharyngitis—combination of fever, pharyngeal exudate, and cervical adenopathy increases suspicion; often accompanied by headache or abdominal pain in children; peak ages 5 through 15. Patients with a history of recent contact with other strep cases, a history of strep or rheumatic

105

fever, or current scarlet fever are good candidates for antibiotic treatment.

5. Bronchiolitis—differentiate by the presence of increased respiratory rate, wheezing, crackles, and intercostal and subcostal retractions. These findings typically develop after a 2- to 3-day prodrome of upper respiratory tract symptoms; typically caused by respiratory syncytial virus, which affects the upper airways first and then the bronchi and bronchioles. The peak age range is 2 to 8 months. Other viruses and *Mycoplasma* are less common causes.

6. Bronchitis—differentiate by the prominence of cough, increased sputum production, less prominent nasal symptoms, and the presence of rhonchi or wheezes on lung examination. Chronic bronchitis is empirically defined by the presence of cough or sputum production on most days for at least 3 months of the year for a minimum of 2 years. Smokers are particularly susceptible.

7. Croup (laryngotracheobronchitis)—gradual onset of distinctive barking cough in nontoxic-appearing toddler (under age 3 years) that resolves in a cooler, humid environment. Low to moderate fever commonly accompanies the cough in the absence of nasal symptoms. Stridorous breathing with retractions and intercostal muscle use is common. Predilection for winter.

8. Epiglottitis—rapid onset of high fever in toxic-appearing older child (over age 3 years) accompanied by drooling, occasionally stridor, and rarely coughing. Lung findings are minimal. Patients characteristically prefer forward-leaning position while sitting. Lateral neck radiograph may show ''thumbprint'' sign.

9. Otitis media—dull, red, bulging tympanic membrane and purulent drainage in the ear canal are the best predictors. Fever, ear pulling, and irritability are less predictive. Children with upper respiratory tract symptoms are prone to middle ear infection because of the anatomy of the eustachian tube in childhood.

10. Mononucleosis—early Epstein-Barr viral infection can present with exudative pharyngitis, adenopathy, and low-grade fever with less prominent nasal symptoms. Palatal petechiae and posterior cervical adenopathy are suggestive. The duration of illness and later development of moderate to low-grade fever with abdominal symptoms differentiate from common cold.

11. Foreign body—profuse malodorous rhinorrhea in the absence of other findings is suggestive. More common in young children. Examination of nostrils confirms diagnosis.

12. Atypical pneumonia

    a. *Mycoplasma* pneumonia—persistent, minimally productive cough in adolescents or young adults in the absence of other symptoms suggests *Mycoplasma*. The duration of illness is typically 7 to 21 days. Patchy infiltrates on chest radiographs in the absence of physical examination findings are suggestive. Cold agglutinins performed in the office is suggestive, although test results are often negative.

    b. *Chlamydia* pneumonia (TWAR strain)—often asymptomatic; gradual onset of sore throat, nonproductive cough, and, occasionally, hoarseness. Nasal symptoms are more common than in other atypical pneumonias, with sinus tenderness to percussion in up to 25 per cent.

    c. *Legionella* pneumonia—one-day prodrome of myalgias and headache followed by acute onset of high fever, nonproductive cough, and occasionally pleuritic chest pain in the absence of typical upper respiratory tract symptoms makes this type of pneumonia easy to differentiate. Gastrointestinal symptoms are common with *Legionella*.

Treatment
Medication

1. Most colds require only general measures with no medication.

2. Little evidence exists to support medication use in younger children. Certain single agents have been effective in older children as well as adults.

3. If medication is used, follow these general guidelines:

    a. Treat symptoms with medication specific to the symptoms. Relief of symptoms is the goal.

    b. Choose products with fewer (one or two at most) active ingredients to minimize adverse effects.

    c. Be aware of coexisting conditions (e.g., hypertension, diabetes, arrhythmias, alcoholism, prostate hypertrophy, pregnancy, thyroid disease) and other medications being taken.

4. Drugs of choice for rhinorrhea and nasal congestion

    a. Oral decongestants

    (1) Pseudoephedrine (Sudafed), 60 mg every 6 hours; children: 4 mg/kg for 24 hours q 6

    (2) Phenylpropanolamine, 25 mg every 4 hours. Cardiovascular adverse effects are greater than with pseudoephedrine.

    (3) Restrict use in patients with uncontrolled hypertension. Short-term use of pseudoephedrine in patients with controlled hypertension is safe.

    b. Topical decongestants

    (1) Oxymetazoline (Afrin, Dristan), 0.025% or 0.05% solution, two to three drops or sprays twice daily

    (2) Phenylephrine (Neo-Synephrine) 0.125% to

0.5% solution, one to two drops or sprays one to two times every 4 hours

(3) Ephedrine, naphazoline, and xylometazoline are also available as drops or spray.

(4) Restrict use to 3 to 4 days at a time to avoid rebound phenomenon.

(5) Dosage in children under age 6 years has not been established.

c. Antihistamines

(1) Effectiveness in colds not proven

(2) Helpful in allergic rhinitis or when sedative effect is desired

(3) Common over-the-counter antihistamine ingredients include diphenhydramine (Benadryl), chlorpheniramine (Chlor-Trimeton), and brompheniramine (Dimetane). See Chapter 19 for more information.

5. Drugs of choice for cough

a. Antitussives

(1) Codeine, 10 to 20 mg every 4 to 6 hours. Gastrointestinal upset limits its effectiveness in a minority of patients; potential for abuse.

(2) Dextromethorphan (Delsym), 10 to 30 mg every 4 hours; available as lozenges, syrup, and chewy squares. Delsym liquid is alcohol-free.

(3) Benzonatate (Tessalon Perles), one or two capsules three times daily; can cause local numbness in mouth if chewed

b. Expectorants

(1) Guaifenesin (Robitussin, Humibid L.A.), 100 to 400 mg every 3 to 6 hours. Reduce dose by one half for children aged 6 to 12 years.

(2) Iodides: potassium iodide, 300 to 600 mg after meals two or three times daily or iodinated glycerol, 60 mg four times a day (give children up to half the adult dose, based on weight). Rashes, nodular enlargement of the thyroid, and parotid swelling occur in up to 50 per cent of patients.

6. Drugs of choice for pain (sore throat, myalgias, headache) and fever

a. Acetaminophen (Tylenol), 325 to 500 mg every 4 to 6 hours

b. Ibuprofen (Motrin), 200 to 600 mg every 4 to 6 hours

c. Avoid aspirin use in younger patients with upper respiratory tract infection because of its association with Reye's syndrome.

7. Alternative drugs—alpha interferon and vitamin C have been investigated in the prophylaxis and treatment of colds with varying results.

Diet

Increased fluid intake to compensate for increased insensible losses with fever; otherwise, no dietary modification necessary

Activity

1. Limited only by symptoms

2. Deferral from work may be necessary for patients taking codeine or antihistamines if concentration is necessary for the performance of job duties.

3. Deferral from school or day care typically is limited to purulent conjunctivitis, fever, or persistent severe cough.

Patient Education

1. Hand washing is the single most effective means to reduce transmission.

2. Notify health care provider in event of the following:

a. Symptoms that persist longer than 10 days

b. Temperature above 101° F (38° C)

c. Persistent vomiting, especially in infants

d. Wheezing, shortness of breath, or chest pain

Key Treatment

- For rhinorrhea and nasal congestion—oral decongestants, topical decongestants, antihistamines

- For cough—antitussives, expectorants

- For pain and fever—acetaminophen, ibuprofen

Follow-Up

Typically unnecessary

Bibliography

Bryant BG, Lombardi TP: Selecting OTC products for coughs and colds. Am Pharm 1993;33:19–24.

Gwaltney J: The common cold. *In* Mandell G, Douglas R, Bennett J (eds): Principles and Practice of Infectious Disease, New York, Churchill Livingstone, 1990, pp 489–493.

Hemila H: Does vitamin C alleviate the symptoms of the common cold? A review of the current evidence. Scand J Infect Dis 1994;26:1–6.

Hilding DA: Literature review—the common cold. Ear Nose Throat J 1994;73:639–647.

Smith MB, Feldman W: Over-the-counter cold medications. A critical review of clinical trials between 1950 and 1991 [see comments]. JAMA 1993;269:2258–2263.

24 Laryngitis

Bennet M. Wang

Etiology

The history is key to determining the cause of laryngitis and should include any specific inciting events (e.g., vocal abuse, upper respiratory tract infection, intubation), any infectious or toxic exposure (see below), and any associated gastrointestinal or pulmonary complaints. A wide variety of infectious and inflammatory (noninfectious) processes can cause laryngitis.

A. Infectious
  1. Acute infection (symptoms less than 2 to 3 weeks)
    a. Viral
      (1) Influenza A and B, parainfluenza
      (2) Adenovirus, rhinovirus, coronavirus
      (3) Epstein-Barr virus (usually in association with pharyngitis)
    b. Bacterial
      (1) *Mycoplasma pneumoniae* and *Chlamydia* species
      (2) *Haemophilus influenzae* (as in children, can cause epiglottitis in adults)
      (3) *Streptococcus pneumoniae, Staphylococcus aureus,* group A streptococcus (usually secondary to primary pharyngitis, sinusitis, or tonsillitis)
      (4) *Moraxella catarrhalis*
      (5) *Corynebacterium diphtheriae* (usually in association with pharyngitis)
  2. Chronic infection (symptoms extending over weeks to months)
    a. Bacterial
      (1) Tuberculosis (see Bibliography)
      (2) Leprosy (rare)
      (3) Syphilis (particularly secondary and tertiary stages)
      (4) Rhinoscleroma (gram-negative rod infection of the nose extending to the larynx; endemic in Central and South America, south and central Europe, Egypt, and southwest Asia)
      (5) Actinomycosis
    b. Fungal
      (1) Histoplasmosis
      (2) Blastomycosis
      (3) Candidiasis (usually in association with esophageal or disseminated candidiasis)
B. Inflammatory (noninfectious)
  1. Excessive use of the voice (can lead to vocal cord nodules or "singer's nodules")

  2. Gastroesophageal reflux (see Bibliography)
  3. Exposure to irritating agent
    a. Tobacco smoke
    b. Alcohol
    c. Chemicals (e.g., acid or petroleum fumes)
    d. Acute thermal injury (e.g., smoke inhalation, steam injury)
    e. Radiation injury
  4. Intubation granuloma (after endotracheal intubation)

Symptoms

1. Hoarseness or a change in the voice is usually the primary symptom.
2. Dysphonia or an aberration in vocal quality can be mild and intermittent initially and later more noticeable and prolonged.
3. Cough can result from laryngeal irritation. (*Note:* hemoptysis is rare.)
4. Pain may be localized to the larynx and throat but can be referred to the ear.
5. Dyspnea, stridor, dysphagia, and odynophagia are late symptoms and suggest more serious disease.

Key Symptoms	
• Hoarseness	• Cough
• Dysphonia	• Throat or ear pain

Clinical Findings

1. Fever is sometimes present in laryngitis, particularly when caused by infection.
2. A thorough head and neck examination, including gag and swallowing reflexes, is essential and may reveal lymphadenopathy; signs of inflammation on the pharynx, sinuses, and lungs; and focal neurologic abnormalities.
3. Indirect (mirror) or fiberoptic laryngoscopy is the key to visualization of the larynx to assess for:
  a. Laryngeal mucosa ulcers, edema, and/or erythema
  b. Mass lesions
  c. Vocal cord dysfunction
  d. Structural abnormalities

Key Signs
• Laryngeal ulcers, edema, and/or erythema
• Mass lesions of the larynx
• Vocal cord dysfunction

Tests

1. A white blood cell count with differential may be useful if infection is suspected.
2. Cultures from the throat, larynx, or blood and other specific tests, such as rheumatoid factor or C1 esterase levels, may be indicated in selected cases.
3. Laryngeal tissue biopsy by means of direct laryngoscopy also may be useful when noninvasive studies are not diagnostic.

Key Tests

- White blood cell count (if infection suspected)
- Cultures
- Laryngeal tissue biopsy (when noninvasive studies are not diagnostic)

Differential Diagnosis

1. Vocal cord dysfunction, in particular secondary to recurrent and/or superior laryngeal nerve dysfunction, can also present as hoarseness.
2. Neoplasms of the larynx
   a. Papilloma (benign; juvenile and adult forms)
   b. Squamous cell carcinoma (typically presents between ages 50 and 70; increased risk associated with tobacco and alcohol use)
3. Systemic disorders that affect the larynx
   a. Sarcoidosis
   b. Amyloidosis
   c. Systemic lupus erythematosus
   d. Rheumatoid arthritis of cricoarytenoid joint
   e. Allergic angioedema
   f. Acromegaly
   g. Myxedema
   h. Pemphigus vulgaris
4. Functional disorders
   a. Psychogenic aphonia (history of emotional disturbance often present)
   b. Vocal weakness (typically seen in older patients; complaint of lack of usual vigor or tone to voice; usually results from vocal cord bowing and muscle atrophy, part of the normal aging process)

Treatment

1. The goals of treatment are to treat the underlying cause if identified and to eliminate or diminish any factors that may have contributed to the laryngitis.
2. For most cases of acute laryngitis, the voice eventually returns to baseline spontaneously. Careful management can speed recovery and lessen the risk for permanent damage.
   a. Voice rest. Shouting, long telephone conversations, and prolonged whispering are prohibited. The goal should be to use as few words as possible.
   b. Elimination of throat clearing. Laryngeal edema leads to the misconception of "something in the throat," which leads to repetitive throat clearing, which can perpetuate the laryngeal damage.
   c. Humidification and hydration. The goal is to increase the lubrication of the laryngeal mucosa. One suggestion for adequate fluid intake is at least eight glasses of water a day.
   d. Cough suppression. For irritative coughs, an over-the-counter preparation of dextromethorphan can be useful.
   e. Relief of nasal obstruction. Because the nose functions to help humidify the inhaled air, nasal decongestants such as topical or oral sympathomimetics can be beneficial.
   f. Treatment of gastroesophageal reflux laryngitis if present. Use high-dose histamine$_2$ blockers or omeprazole.
   g. Antibiotics in selected patients. Use when fever, pain, productive cough, or purulent sputum suggests primary or superimposed bacterial infection.

Key Treatment

- Voice rest
- Elimination of throat clearing
- Humidification and hydration
- Cough suppression
- Relief of nasal obstruction
- Treatment of gastroesophageal reflux if present
- Antibiotics in selected patients

Follow-Up

With appropriate conservative management, most patients with acute laryngitis recover their voice within 2 to 3 weeks. (*Note:* It may take up to 8 weeks for gastroesophageal reflux laryngitis to resolve completely.) For those patients with acute laryngitis who do not improve with therapy or for those with chronic laryngitis of unknown cause, referral to an otolaryngologist is indicated.

 Bibliography

For more information on laryngitis, see
Fried M, Shapiro J: Acute and chronic laryngeal infections. *In* Paperella MM, Shumrick DA (eds): Otolaryngology, vol 3, 3rd ed. Philadelphia, WB Saunders, 1991, pp 2245–2256.

For more information on laryngeal disorders, see
Banovetz JD: Benign laryngeal disorders. *In* Adams GL, Boies LR, Hilger PA (eds): Boies Fundamentals of Otolaryngology, 6th ed. Philadelphia, WB Saunders, 1989, pp 392–411.

For more information on laryngeal tuberculosis, see
Riley EC, Amundson DE: Laryngeal tuberculosis revisited. Am Fam Physician 1992;46(3):759–762.

For more information on reflux laryngitis, see
Sataloff RT, Speigel JR, Hawkshaw M, et al: Gastroesophageal reflux laryngitis. Ear Nose Throat J 1993;72(2):113–114.

For more information on the treatment of laryngitis, see
Woodson GE: Hoarseness and laryngitis. *In* Rakel RE (ed): Conn's Current Therapy 1994. Philadelphia, WB Saunders, 1994, pp 21–26.

25 Croup

Nicholas J. Galioto

Etiology

1. Predominantly disease of viral etiology
   a. Parainfluenza 1 virus is the most common type and accounts for about 75 per cent of cases.
   b. Parainfluenza 2 and 3 virus
   c. Influenza serotype A virus
   d. Respiratory syncytial virus
   e. Rhinovirus
2. Mycoplasmal pneumonia is implicated in 3 to 4 per cent of cases.
3. Most commonly occurs in the fall and early winter

Symptoms

1. Occurs primarily in children aged 6 months to 3 years but may be seen in children up to age 6 years
2. Several-day history of progressive upper respiratory tract infection
3. "Barking" or "seal-like" cough developing on the 2nd to 3rd day of illness, especially at night
4. Hoarseness
5. Low-grade fever; generally less than 102.2° F (39° C)

Key Symptoms

- Age: 6 months to 3 years
- Upper respiratory tract infection prodrome
- Barking cough
- Hoarseness
- Low-grade fever

Clinical Findings

1. Inspiratory and expiratory stridor
2. Barking cough
3. Mild wheezing may be present on auscultation in 5 per cent of cases.
4. Position has no effect on airway obstruction.
5. Evaluate for respiratory distress
   a. Color—normal, dusky, or cyanotic
   b. Increased respiratory rate
   c. Stridor—mild or severe
   d. Retractions—supracostal, substernal, or intercostal
   e. Nasal flaring
   f. Air entry on auscultation—normal or decreased
   g. Decreased level of consciousness

If two or more signs of respiratory distress are present, the patient may require further observation and/or hospitalization.

110

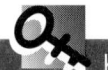

Key Signs

- Stridor
- Barking cough
- Presence or absence of respiratory distress
- Position has no effect on obstruction

Tests

1. Diagnosis is generally made on the basis of clinical findings.
2. White blood cell count is usually normal or only mildly elevated. It is greater than 15,000/mm^3 in about 20 per cent of patients.
3. Lateral and anteroposterior radiographs of the neck
   a. An anteroposterior view may demonstrate a narrowed subglottic region or the "steeple" sign in 40 to 50 per cent of cases.
   b. A lateral view may show widening of the hypopharynx and may be helpful in making the diagnosis of epiglottitis, bacterial tracheitis, or retropharyngeal abscess.
4. Arterial blood gases will help assess the adequacy of ventilation and oxygenation, especially in the setting of severe respiratory compromise.
5. Pulse oximetry may be helpful in determining oxygen saturation but needs to be interpreted in conjunction with clinical presentation. Oxygen saturations greater than 90% may be noted even in the presence of marked hypercapnia.

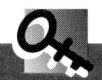

Key Test

- Diagnosis usually is made on the basis of clinical findings.

Differential Diagnosis

1. Epiglottitis—must always be considered because it can rapidly lead to complete airway obstruction
2. Spasmodic croup
3. Bacterial tracheitis
4. Peritonsillar abscess
5. Retropharyngeal abscess
6. Foreign-body aspiration
7. Diphtheria
8. Caustic ingestion
9. Laryngeal web
10. Laryngomalacia

> **WARNING**
>
> **The child who presents with rapid onset of disease, absence of cough, and drooling and is leaning forward should alert the physician to the possibility of epiglottitis.**

Treatment

1. Hospitalization is based on the degree of stridor, severity of retractions, pulse rate, respiratory rate, and evidence of cyanosis.
2. Frequent reassessments
3. Oxygen if necessary
4. Humidified air
   a. Mist tent in hospital
   b. Cool-mist vaporizer, humidifier, or bathroom steam at home
5. Hydration
   a. Intravenous fluids in hospitalized patient (intravenous flow should be based on maintenance plus ongoing losses secondary to decreased oral intake, increased respiratory rate, and fever)
   b. Encourage increased oral fluid intake at home.

Medication

1. Racemic epinephrine, 0.25 to 0.50 ml in 2 to 3 ml normal saline solution given by aerosol
   a. Onset of action is rapid and clinically detectable within 10 minutes of treatment.
   b. Mechanism of action is through its α-adrenergic effects, causing mucosal vasoconstriction and decreased tracheal edema.
   c. Medication may be repeated as necessary and is limited by the development of tachycardia (greater than 180 beats/min).
   d. Overuse may result in rebound swelling and increased stridor.
   e. Patients who receive racemic epinephrine should be considered for hospitalization. If outpatient management is still contemplated, then patients need to be observed for at least 2 hours for signs of rebound and/or worsening symptoms.
2. Corticosteroids—single dose of dexamethasone, 0.6 mg/kg, given intramuscularly or intravenously
3. Antibiotics—generally not indicated in the treatment of viral croup except for superimposed bacterial infections, such as otitis media

Diet

1. If hospitalized with respiratory distress, patients should receive nothing by mouth and intravenous fluids should be provided.
2. For outpatient treatment or once respiratory distress has resolved, start clear liquids and advance diet as tolerated.

Activity—level of activity limited by patient's clinical condition

Patient Education

1. Review signs and symptoms of worsening distress.
2. Provide humidified air either through cool-mist vaporizer or bathroom steam.
3. Walking outside in the cool air may also decrease acute stridor.
4. Giving extra oral fluids is important.
5. Order acetaminophen for fever at a dose of 10 to 15 mg/kg every 4 hours as needed.
6. Avoid preparations that increase tenacity of tracheal secretions or have a drying effect (i.e., antihistamines, cold and cough preparations).

Key Treatment

- Humidified air
- Oxygen if necessary
- Racemic epinephrine
- Corticosteroids
- Hydration

Follow-Up

1. Close follow-up is often indicated by telephone or office visit within 24 hours.
2. Parents should be encouraged to report any change in the child's condition.

 Bibliography

Cressman WR, Myer CM III: Diagnosis and management of croup and epiglottitis. Pediatr Clin North Am 1994;41(2):265–276.

Custer JR: Croup and related disorders. Pediatr Rev 1993;14(1):19–29.

Quan L: Diagnosis and treatment of croup. Am Fam Physician 1992;46(3):747–755.

Skolnik N: Croup. J Fam Pract 1993;37(2):165–170.

Stern RC: The respiratory system. *In* Behrman RE, Vaughan VC, Nelson WE (eds): Nelson Textbook of Pediatrics, 13th ed. Philadelphia, WB Saunders, 1987, pp 888–890.

26 Bronchiolitis

Michael P. Rowane

Etiology

1. Acute respiratory illness precipitated by a viral infection that results in obstruction of small airways
   Most common in children aged 2 to 12 months; unusual after age 2 years
2. Respiratory syncytial virus (RSV)
   a. Most common infectious agent (more than 50 per cent of cases)
   b. Seasonal occurrence in winter and spring
3. Parainfluenza 1 and 3 viruses
   a. Second most common agent
   b. Autumn and spring epidemics occur before and after RSV outbreaks
4. Other viruses—influenza serotype A, adenoviruses, rhinovirus
5. Rarely other organisms: *Mycoplasma pneumoniae, Chlamydia, Ureaplasma, Haemophilus influenzae, Bordetella pertussis,* and *Pneumocystis*
6. Contagious period is 24 to 48 hours before the onset of symptoms and several days after exposure.

Symptoms

1. Initial symptoms, days 1 and 2
   a. Fever—usually low grade unless concurrent otitis is present
   b. Rhinorrhea, nasal congestion
   c. Cough
2. Subsequent symptoms
   a. Wheezing
   b. Rapid breathing
   c. Poor feeding
   d. Cough deeper and more frequent
3. Risk factors for developing bronchiolitis
   a. Sick contact (e.g., older sibling with a viral respiratory illness)
   b. Low socioeconomic status (more common)
   c. Living in crowded conditions (most common variable)
   d. Passive exposure to cigarette smoke at home
   e. Infants who have not been breast-fed

Clinical Findings

1. Mild
   a. General appearance—playful and alert
   b. Well hydrated (good fluid intake)
   c. Wheezing
   d. Respiratory rate less than 50 breaths/min
   e. Mild retractions
   f. Good air exchange characterized by a normal inspiratory/expiratory ratio (2:1)
2. Moderate
   a. General appearance—active and slightly irritable
   b. Wheezing
   c. Tachypnea (respiratory rate 50 to 70 breaths/min)
   d. Mild to moderate retractions
   e. Decreased air exchange with prolonged expiratory phase
3. Severe
   a. General appearance
      (1) Lethargic with difficulty arousing
      (2) Cyanosis and pallor
      (3) Dehydrated—poor peripheral perfusion with mottling and delayed capillary refill (more than 2 seconds)
      (4) Low blood pressure
   b. Pulmonary findings
      (1) Crackles, rhonchi, expiratory wheezing
      (2) Tachypnea (respiratory rate greater than 70 breaths/min)
      (3) Severe retractions with nasal flaring, grunting, hoarseness, stridor
      (4) Shallow breathing pattern with prolonged expiratory phase, suggesting poor air exchange
   c. Cardiac—tachycardia
   d. Very severe respiratory distress—respiratory failure, prolonged or recurrent apnea, respiratory arrest
   e. Apnea is seen in 20 to 25 per cent of RSV bronchiolitis cases.
4. Acute otitis media is often seen with bronchiolitis.

Key Symptoms	
• Wheezing	• Cough
• Rapid breathing	

Key Signs	
• Tachypnea	• Prolonged expiratory phase
• Tachycardia	

Tests

1. Chest radiography
   a. Peribronchial thickening and patchy atelectasis with or without streaky infiltrates
   b. Hyperinflation with flattened diaphragms
   c. Segmental or lobar atelectasis can develop later.
2. Complete blood count—normal or elevated white blood cell count (complete blood count recommended in patient under age 3 months and/or with fever present)
3. Pulse oximetry
   a. Oxygen saturation below 90 requires supplemental oxygen.
   b. Pulse oximetry can assist in classifying severity of bronchiolitis.
      (1) Mild—more than 90 per cent oxygen saturation
      (2) Moderate—88 to 90 per cent oxygen saturation
      (3) Severe—below 88 to 90 per cent oxygen saturation
4. Viral rapid diagnosis and culture (immunofluorescent staining and enzyme-linked immunosorbent assay) on nasopharyngeal secretions
5. Arterial blood gas analysis for signs of respiratory failure
   a. Inability to maintain PaO_2 greater than 50 mm Hg with FiO_2 greater than 80 per cent
   b. Inability to keep carbon dioxide less than 55 mm Hg
   c. Inability to maintain oxygen saturation greater than 88 per cent
   d. Persistent cyanosis

Key Tests

- Chest radiography
- White blood cell count
- Viral rapid diagnosis and culture
- Pulse oximetry

Differential Diagnosis

1. Bronchial asthma
2. Congestive heart failure
3. Foreign body in the trachea
4. Pertussis
5. Organic phosphate poisoning
6. Cystic fibrosis
7. Bacterial bronchopneumonia associated with generalized obstructive emphysema

WARNING

- **Bronchial asthma is the condition most commonly confused with bronchiolitis.**
- **Fewer than 5 per cent of recurrent attacks have a viral cause. Consider another diagnosis with repeated episodes of apparent bronchiolitis.**
- **Identify any focus of infection (i.e., acute otitis media, sinusitis, pneumonia).**

Treatment

A. Mild—home care
   1. Encourage fluids with normal diet.
   2. Use cool-mist vaporizer or humidifier.
B. Moderate—home care versus hospitalization
   1. Therapeutic trial—two doses at 20-minute intervals of the following:
      a. Nebulized bronchodilator (e.g., albuterol [Proventil, Ventolin]) *or*
      b. Epinephrine or terbutaline (Brethine, Bricanyl) subcutaneously
   2. Home care with oral β-adrenergic agents if the patient responds to the therapeutic trial
C. Severe—hospitalization
   1. Closely monitor.
   2. Initial supportive care
      a. Nebulized bronchodilator (e.g., albuterol)
      b. Epinephrine or terbutaline subcutaneously
   3. Intravenous fluid repletion with poor fluid intake—maintenance, dextrose 5 per cent and ¼ normal saline solution with potassium chloride
   4. Humidified oxygen in tent
   5. Corticosteroid use is controversial; most infants respond satisfactorily without it.
   6. Theophylline in cases of respiratory failure
   7. Intubation in very severe cases
   8. Reserve ribavirin (Virazole) for high-risk cases.

All patients at high risk (i.e., underlying cardiopulmonary disorders, neuromuscular conditions, immunodeficiency disorders, or premature infants under age 12 weeks) should be considered to have severe bronchiolitis and treated as such.

Medication

1. Nebulized bronchodilator (e.g., albuterol)
2. Oral albuterol (2 mg/ 5ml), 0.1 mg/kg every 8 hours
3. Epinephrine, 0.01 ml/kg of 1:1000 dilution subcutaneously. Response favors a diagnosis of asthma.
4. Corticosteroids
   a. Not adequately studied

b. If used, doses less than that for asthma are probably adequate (asthma dose—prednisone, 0.5 to 2 mg/kg/day up to 20 to 40 mg/day for 3 to 5 days).

c. Infants with mild bronchiolitis do well without steroids.

d. Reserve for more severe forms of bronchiolitis.

5. Antibiotics

a. Beneficial only if a source for a secondary bacterial infection is evident (i.e., pneumonia, otitis media)

b. May not affect the clinical course because bacterial infections are seldom concurrently present

6. Ribavirin

a. Decreases the severity of an RSV infection if used early in the course of bronchiolitis

b. Reserve for high-risk patients because this therapy is expensive.

c. Dose—6 gm in 300 ml of water aerosolized in a croup tent for 16 to 20 hours per day for 3 to 6 days

d. May be teratogenic; thus, avoid exposure with pregnant health care workers

7. Theophylline

a. No benefit

b. Reserve for infants in respiratory failure.

8. Do not use antihistamine-decongestant mixtures.

Diet

1. Encourage fluids.

2. Regular diet if tolerated

Activity

1. Avoid excess activity.

2. Rest

Patient Education

1. Return if condition worsens (i.e., tachypnea, retractions, cyanosis, persistent fever, fever if patient is under age 3 months, poor oral intake).

2. Potential for developing asthma later in life

3. Minimize risk factors.

a. Tobacco smoke

b. Close contact with sick siblings—crowding effect

4. Hand washing is key to prevention.

5. One-half of hospitalized infants have recurrent episodes of wheezing.

Key Treatment

Mild	**Severe**
• Home care	• Hospitalize and closely monitor
• Encourage fluids	• Humidified oxygen
• Normal diet	• Nebulized bronchodilator
Moderate	• Epinephrine or terbutaline
• Nebulized bronchodilator	• Intubation if indicated
• Epinephrine or terbutaline	• Ribavirin

Follow-Up

1. Mild or moderate

a. Recheck (phone versus visit) in 24 to 48 hours.

b. Office follow-up in 7 to 14 days

2. Severe

a. Hospitalize and monitor closely.

b. Office follow-up 24 to 48 hours after discharge

Bibliography

For more information on bronchiolitis in an excellent reference text of pediatrics, see

Stern RC: Acute bronchiolitis. *In* Behrman RE, Kliegman RM, Nelson WE, Vaughan VC (eds): Nelson Textbook of Pediatrics, 14th ed. Philadelphia, WB Saunders, 1992, pp 1075–1076.

For more information on the general approach to bronchiolitis, see

Welliver JR, Welliver RC: Bronchiolitis. Pediatr Rev 1993;14(4):134–139.

For more information on the use of albuterol in bronchiolitis, see

Gadomski AM, Lichenstein R, Horton L, et al.: Efficacy of albuterol in the management of bronchiolitis. Pediatrics 1994;93(6):907–912.

For more information on bronchiolitis using an algorithmic method, see

Berman S: Pediatric Decision Making. Philadelphia, BC Decker, 1991, pp 104–107.

For more information on bronchiolitis with emphasis on practical therapeutics, see

Horst PS: Bronchiolitis. Am Fam Physician 1994;49:1449–1456.

27 Fetal Lung Immaturity

Shellie A. Russell

Etiology

1. Surfactant deficiency—primary cause of death in premature infants
2. The surfactant deficiency is compounded by immature lung structure, which leads to poor lung compliance. Poor lung compliance causes hypoxemia and hypercapnia.
3. The deficiency is usually compounded by capillary leaks, which cause worsening lung perfusion and gas exchange.

Risk Factors

1. Identifying babies at risk can change management both antenatally and postnatally.
2. Factors that correlate with increased likelihood of fetal lung immaturity include the following:
   a. Preterm delivery
   b. Male sex
   c. Maternal diabetes
   d. Cesarean delivery
   e. Caucasian heritage
   f. Perinatal asphyxia
   g. Lecithin/sphingomyelin ratio less than 2:1
3. The more preterm an infant is, the greater the chance of lung immaturity.

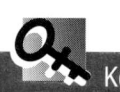

Key Risk Factors	
• Preterm infant	• White race
• Maternal diabetes	• Lecithin/sphingomyelin ratio less than 2:1
• Perinatal asphyxia	
• Male sex	

Clinical Findings

Respiratory distress syndrome is a clinical diagnosis. Clinical findings include the following:

1. Respiratory—grunting, nasal flaring, retractions, apnea, tachypnea, cyanosis, poor air flow
2. Circulatory—hypotension, tachycardia
3. Poor tone and activity
4. Low Apgar scores

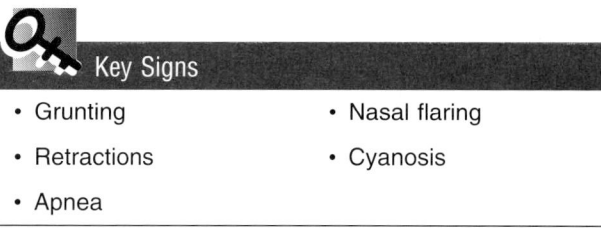

Key Signs	
• Grunting	• Nasal flaring
• Retractions	• Cyanosis
• Apnea	

Tests

1. Analysis of cord blood gases or arterial blood gases shows low pH, hypoxemia, and hypercapnia.
2. Chest radiography
   a. "Ground-glass" or "reticulogranular" appearance
   b. Diffuse atelectasis
   c. Loss of lung volume
   d. Air bronchography

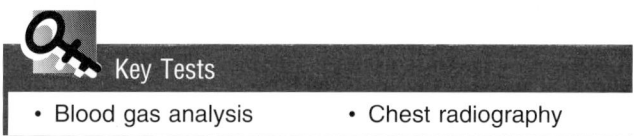

Key Tests	
• Blood gas analysis	• Chest radiography

Differential Diagnosis

1. Pulmonary considerations
   a. Pneumonia
   b. Transient tachypnea of the newborn
   c. Pulmonary hemorrhage
   d. Meconium aspiration
   e. Pneumothorax
   f. Persistent fetal circulation
2. Extrapulmonary considerations
   a. Congenital heart disease
   b. Diaphragmatic hernia
   c. Tracheoesophageal fistula

Treatment

1. Oxygen—desired PaO_2 60 to 70 mm Hg
2. Surfactant administration
   a. Colfosceril palmitate (Exosurf Neonatal), 5 ml/kg intratracheally over 20 minutes; dose should be repeated in 12 hours
   b. Numerous types of synthetic and natural surfactant are available commercially.
   c. Although well recognized to be effective in most neonates with lung immaturity, there still is debate about the most appropriate dosage and frequency as well as prophylactic or rescue therapy strategies.

3. Mechanical ventilation
   a. Used to correct hypercapnia
   b. There is a variety of ventilation now available, including pressure ventilators, high-frequency ventilators, and extracorporeal membrane oxygenation.
4. If the mother is followed closely for preterm labor, the administration of a glucocorticoid 24 to 48 hours before delivery can enhance lung maturity.
5. Health care maintenance includes warming, fluid and electrolyte balance, and nutritional enhancement.

Key Treatment

- Oxygen
- Surfactant administration
- Mechanical ventilation

Follow-Up

Complications of treatment for respiratory distress syndrome include the following:

1. Lung barotrauma—air leak (e.g., pneumothorax, bronchopulmonary dysplasia)
2. Patent ductus arteriosus
3. Intraventricular hemorrhage, especially in neonates who are less than 32 weeks' estimated gestational age
4. Pulmonary hemorrhage, especially in neonates receiving surfactant therapy
5. Infection secondary to invasive monitoring
6. Retinopathy of prematurity secondary to oxygen toxicity in neonates who weigh less than 1500 gm
7. Neurologic impairment, including cerebral palsy

 Bibliography

Berry D, Pramanik A, Philips J III, et al: Comparison of the effect of three doses of a synthetic surfactant on the alveolar-arterial oxygen gradient in infants weighing ≥ 1250 grams with respiratory distress syndrome. J Pediatr 1994;124:294–301.

Hyaline membrane disease. *In* Behrman R, Kliegman R, Nelson W, et al (eds): Nelson Textbook of Pediatrics, 14th ed. Philadelphia, WB Saunders, 1992, pp 463–469.

Mercier C, Soll R: Clinical trials of natural surfactant extract in respiratory distress syndrome. Clin Perinatol 1993;20(4):711–734.

Pramanik A, Holtzman R, Merritt TA: Surfactant replacement therapy for pulmonary diseases. Pediatr Clin N Am 1993;40:913–936.

Wiswell T, Mendiola J: Respiratory distress syndrome in the newborn: Innovative therapies. Am Fam Physician 1993;47(2):407–414.

28 Asthma

Joseph A. Troncale

Etiology

1. Asthma is a disease of increased irritability of the tracheobronchial tree. It is, by definition, a reversible obstructive airway disease with the following components:

    a. Airway obstruction

    b. Airway hyperresponsiveness

    c. Airway inflammation

    Asthma affects about 10 per cent of children and 5 per cent of adults. Data suggest that the prevalence and severity of asthma are increasing. Theories for increased severity include increased air pollutants and overuse of β-adrenergic agonists.

2. The classic definition of asthma includes two types, intrinsic and extrinsic. These distinctions are not easily made in practice, and there may be considerable overlap in most patients.

    a. Intrinsic asthma is seen in patients who have no history of allergies or hyperresponsiveness to allergens of various types. Provocation tests may be unrewarding, and there may be no family history of asthma. This type of asthma may be triggered by sinusitis, upper respiratory tract infections, or psychological stress.

    b. Extrinsic asthma, also called allergic asthma, is characterized by symptoms that occur with exposure to an allergen. Patients with extrinsic asthma may have positive skin testing, elevated serum IgE levels, a family history of allergic conditions, and attacks based on allergen exposure.

3. Other subtypes include exercise-induced and drug-induced asthma. Exercise-induced asthma is a phenomenon seen mostly in adolescents as well as in some adults who experience bronchospasm a few minutes after starting exercise. It usually goes away about 30 minutes after exercise ends. Drug-induced asthma is seen in patients with sensitivity to certain substances, both medicinal and nonmedicinal. Common offenders include β-blockers, aspirin, cyclo-oxygenase–inhibiting nonsteroidal anti-inflammatory drugs, radiocontrast material, and sulfites found in certain foods and beverages.

4. Severity ranges from mild to severe. Experienced asthma patients may be able to manage milder attacks on their own with the help of home devices such as peak flowmeters and aerosol machines. Asthma attacks may occur suddenly and be severe, however. Such attacks are best treated in a monitored environment. Asthma that lasts for days to weeks without improvement is known as status asthmaticus. This condition requires aggressive treatment and, frequently, hospitalization.

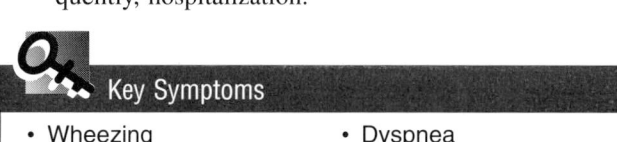

Key Symptoms

- Wheezing
- Dyspnea
- Cough

Clinical Findings

1. In most patients, the key symptoms are found either alone or in combination. Physical findings include increased inspiratory and expiratory phases of respiration. In severe cases, wheezing may be absent because air is not moving in sufficient quantity or with sufficient velocity to create sound. The chest may be hyperresonant on percussion. Accessory respiratory muscles may be used.

2. Fatigue and pulsus paradoxus (an inspiratory decline in systolic blood pressure of at least 10 mm Hg) are important late signs. These signs may signal the need for critical types of intervention, including intubation and ventilatory support.

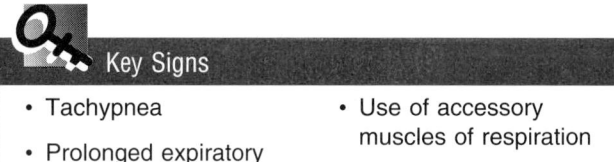

Key Signs

- Tachypnea
- Use of accessory muscles of respiration
- Prolonged expiratory phase of respiration

Tests

1. Laboratory testing in asthma may be undertaken for both diagnostic and prognostic purposes. A number of tests are helpful in the diagnosis and management of acute and chronic asthma.

2. Patients may present with a history compatible with asthma, or they may present with some of the aforementioned signs and symptoms. The following tests may be helpful in determining whether there is obstructive disease as well as whether the problem is reversible.

    a. Pulmonary function studies—demonstration of an increased forced expiratory volume at 1 second (FEV_1) of at least 15 per cent

    b. Methacholine (Provocholine) challenge test—specialized version of pulmonary function testing in which the patient is allowed to inhale a bronchoconstricting agent. The PD20, the dose at which the FEV_1 falls by 20 per cent, is measured.

Less specific tests include the following:

   a. IgE determination—may indicate extrinsic asthma

   b. Complete blood count—eosinophilia may be seen in atopic patients

   c. Examination of the sputum may show casts (Curschmann's spirals), Charcot-Leyden crystals, and eosinophils

3. The following tests may be helpful in acute situations in a symptomatic patient who presents in the office or emergency department with acute symptoms.

   a. Arterial blood gas analysis should be obtained only in reasonably severe cases. Hypoxemia is expected, but normal or increased $PaCO_2$ may indicate severe obstruction. Acidosis may also indicate impending respiratory compromise.

   b. Chest radiography—not necessary in all cases; may be helpful if the patient is febrile and suspected of having pneumonia, pneumothorax, or atelectasis

   c. Sinus radiography—sinusitis may precipitate asthma in some patients

   d. Pulse oximetry—useful in monitoring oxygen saturation intermittently or continuously when blood gas analysis is not obtained

   e. Peak flowmeter determination—used when spirometry is not available or when a quick determination of air movement is desired; also useful for measuring response to treatment; inexpensive and fast

   f. Theophylline blood level (if patient is taking medication)

Key Tests

- Pulmonary function studies and peak flowmeter determination
- Blood gas analysis and oximetry
- Chest and/or sinus radiography

Differential Diagnosis

1. Asthma must be differentiated from other diseases that may present with wheezing, cough, or dyspnea. There is an old adage: "All that wheezes is not asthma." In practical terms, a limited number of common diseases mimic asthma to a significant degree.

2. The most common diseases that must be considered include the following:

   a. Congestive heart failure

   b. Chronic obstructive pulmonary disease

   c. Pulmonary embolism

3. Other entities to be differentiated from asthma include the following:

   a. Upper or lower airway obstruction caused by foreign body or tumor

   b. Pneumonia

   c. Vocal cord dysfunction

   d. Wegener's granulomatosis (rare)

Treatment

1. As more is understood about asthma, the treatment has evolved into one that attempts to reduce the underlying airway inflammation and break the cycle of chemical mediators that contribute to bronchospasm. Specifically, the trend has been to use glucocorticoid preparations sooner and more frequently and to use methylxanthines somewhat less than in the past.

2. Treatment of acute attacks in the office or emergency department usually begin with a determination of severity by the history, physical examination, and the tests mentioned above. If the patient is determined to be in a status asthmaticus, aerosolized albuterol may be given and flow determinations obtained before and after treatment. If after three aerosol treatments the patient fails to respond significantly, admission to hospital may be required. At this time, intravenous fluids, intravenous methylprednisolone bolus, and oxygen may be given, if not already started earlier. If the patient is receiving a theophylline preparation and the blood level is found to be subtherapeutic, the patient may be given additional medication.

3. Patients who respond to aerosol therapy in the acute setting should be considered for outpatient treatment with tapering steroids and/or additional modes of therapy, including additional drugs or home aerosol treatment.

Medication

There are essentially five classes of medications (not including oxygen) that are used for asthma. Newer drugs are appearing that have longer half-lives, but the following classes are the most commonly used:

   a. β-adrenergic agonists

      (1) Metaproterenol (Alupent, Metaprel)

         (a) Adults: 20 mg orally q.i.d.; inhalation, two or three puffs q 3 to 4 hr

         (b) Children: 2 mg/kg/day of syrup divided into three doses

      (2) Terbutaline (Brethine, Bricanyl)—adults: 5 mg orally q.i.d.; inhalation, two metered-dose sprays q.i.d.

      (3) Albuterol (Proventil, Ventolin)

         (a) Adults: 4- or 8-mg extended-release tablets orally q 12 hr; inhalation, 2.5 mg by nebulization t.i.d. or q.i.d.; metered-dose inhalation: two puffs q 6 hr

         (b) Inhalation in children: safety and effectiveness of nebulized albuterol have not been established but used commonly in children effectively in proportionately smaller doses; 2 mg/5 ml of syrup may be given as 0.1 mg/kg orally t.i.d.

    (4) Salmeterol (Serevent)—adults: two inhalations twice daily

b. Glucocorticoids

    (1) Methylprednisolone—60 to 80 mg intravenous bolus q 6 to 8 hr

    (2) Hydrocortisone—2 mg/kg bolus q 4 hr

    (3) For ambulatory patients, a prednisone taper may be given. Various regimens may be used at the physician's discretion. A typical schedule might be 50 to 60 mg of prednisone per day tapered by 10 mg q 2 or 3 days.

    (4) Inhaled steroids as metered-dose inhalation—two to four puffs b.i.d. or t.i.d.

c. Methylxanthines

    (1) Theophylline—intravenously or orally in doses to achieve a serum level between 10 and 20 μg/ml

    (2) The following drugs increase theophylline levels: allopurinol, cimetidine, ciprofloxacin, erythromycin, oral contraceptives, and propranolol.

    (3) The following drugs decrease theophylline levels; phenytoin and rifampin.

    (4) Theophylline increases the renal excretion of lithium.

d. Anticholinergics

    (1) Ipratropium (Atrovent) is not officially indicated in asthma, but in smokers with a history of chronic bronchitis or chronic obstructive pulmonary disease, ipratropium may be useful.

    (2) Metered-dose inhalation—two puffs q.i.d.

e. Cromolyn sodium (Intal)

    (1) May be given by metered-dose inhalation, inhaled powder, or nebulizer solution

    (2) Metered-dose inhalation (1 mg/puff)—two puffs b.i.d. or q.i.d.

    (3) Powder inhaler (20 mg/capsule)—one capsule b.i.d. or q.i.d.

    (4) Nedocromil (Tilade)—two inhalations q.i.d.

Diet

Except for patients with food allergies that affect their asthma, no specific dietary recommendations are indicated.

Activity

It is recommended that patients with asthma maintain normal activities as much as possible. The only exception to this is in exercise-induced asthma, in which pretreatment with medications or moderation of activity may be required.

Patient Education

As with any chronic illness, education is extremely important in proper management of asthma. Important areas of education include teaching the patient about the nature of asthma and goals of therapy, warning signs of attacks, medication use, correct use of inhalers, correct use of peak flowmeters, and communication with family and significant institutions, such as school or work.

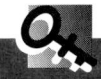

Key Treatment

- β-Agonists
- Theophylline
- Glucocorticoids

Follow-Up

1. The patient with asthma is best served by flexible health care providers who are able to work closely with the patient to manage the unpredictability of the illness. In practice, this is accomplished by the following:

    a. Monitoring peak flow determinations on a regular basis

    b. Judiciously adjusting medications and ensuring that the patient has prescriptions

    c. Monitoring theophylline blood levels when indicated

    d. Seeing patients on an as-needed basis to aggressively treat exacerbations

2. In children, follow-up requires close communication with parents or caregivers—much the same as with other chronic conditions. Significant family system issues exist with asthma, and a wise clinician will work to decrease the anxiety of the family system. This control of anxiety may be accomplished with clinical control of the illness balanced with a sensitivity to what may be fragile emotional boundaries in families with high anxiety levels. Meeting with parents and caregivers to answer questions and to allay fears may be the most important management tool in certain situations.

Bibliography

Bochner BS, Togias A, Lichtenstein LM: The outpatient management of asthma. *In* Wilson JD, Eisselbacher KJ, Braunwald E, et al (eds): Harrison's Principles of Internal Medicine, 13th ed. New York, McGraw-Hill, 1993, pp 1167–1172.

Crapo RO: Pulmonary-function testing. N Engl J Med 1994;331:25–30.

Expert Panel Report: Executive summary: Guidelines for the diagnosis and management of asthma. Bethesda, MD, National Institutes of Health, 1991.

Khan DA, Li JTC: Asthma in adolescents and adults. *In* Rakel RE (ed): Conn's Current Therapy. Philadelphia, WB Saunders, 1994, pp 707–716.

Kolski GB, Orfan NA: Asthma in children. *In* Rakel RE (ed): Conn's Current Therapy. Philadelphia, WB Saunders, 1994, pp 716–726.

29 Bronchitis

Kenneth A. Weller

Etiology

1. Acute bronchitis is a commonly seen problem, resulting from an infectious process that causes inflammation of the tracheobronchial tree.
2. A variety of organisms have been implicated.
   a. Viruses—rhinovirus most common. Cause the vast majority of cases.
   b. Atypical organisms—*Mycoplasma* and *Chlamydia* strains have been identified as causes in young adults.
   c. Bacteria—unclear what role they play. Most of the bacteria implicated (*Haemophilus influenzae, Streptococcus pneumoniae, Moraxella catarrhalis*) are also normal oral flora.
3. Higher incidence is seen in the following:
   a. Smokers—both passive and active
   b. Seasonal—more common in winter
   c. Age—more common in young children and older adults

Symptoms

1. Cough is the most common symptom, usually productive and worse in the morning.
2. Sputum production may be purulent. Purulence does not indicate a bacterial infection.
3. Mild to moderate fever may be present, usually without chills.
4. Mild dyspnea may be present at times.
5. Rhinitis, postnasal drip, and other symptoms of upper respiratory tract infections may precede or accompany the lower respiratory symptoms.

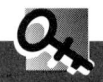
Key Symptom

- Cough

Clinical Findings

1. Auscultation of the lungs may be normal. Wheezing may be present, especially with forced expiration. Signs of consolidation should be absent.
2. Temperature may be elevated.
3. Other signs of upper respiratory tract infection may be present, such as rhinorrhea, erythema of the pharynx, and cervical lymphadenopathy.

Tests

Seldom necessary.
1. Radiography is not routinely performed, but it may be indicated to differentiate bronchitis from pneumonia in some patients.
2. Sputum Gram's stain and culture are not helpful.
3. Blood tests (culture, complete blood counts) are not indicated.

Differential Diagnosis

1. Lower respiratory tract infections
   a. Pneumonia
   b. Bronchiolitis (young children)
2. Cough with upper respiratory tract infections
   a. Sinusitis, acute or chronic
   b. Nasopharyngitis
3. Cough from noninfectious causes
   a. Asthma
   b. Medications
   c. Neoplasm
   d. Other

Treatment
Medication

1. β-agonists such as albuterol (Ventolin, Proventil) inhaler, one or two puffs every 4 to 6 hours, provide symptomatic improvement in patients with bronchitis
2. Cough suppressants (narcotic) such as guaifenesin and codeine (Robitussin A-C), 2 tsp every 4 hours as needed, especially to improve sleep with nocturnal cough
3. Antibiotics—not recommended. Although studies have not consistently demonstrated their effectiveness in either smokers or nonsmokers, physicians still commonly prescribe them.

Patient Education

1. Symptomatic treatment
   a. Over-the-counter medications

Key Treatment

Drug of Choice

- None

Alternative Drugs (symptomatic treatment)

- β-Agonists
- Cough suppressants
- Over-the-counter medications

(1) Cough suppressants (non-narcotic)—as needed

(2) Expectorants—not shown to be useful

(3) Antihistamines—avoid; dry secretions, harder to clear infection

b. Fluids—increase intake and room humidity

2. Smoking cessation—encourage in all patients

3. If not improved as expected (7 to 10 days, longer in smokers), return for re-evaluation.

Follow-Up

Needed only if symptoms significantly worsen or do not improve as expected.

 Bibliography

Hueston W: A comparison of albuterol and erythromycin for the treatment of acute bronchitis. J Fam Pract 1991;33(5):476–480.

Orr PH, Scherer K, Macdonald A, Moffatt MEK: Randomized placebo-controlled trials of antibiotics for acute bronchitis: A critical review of the literature. J Fam Pract 1993;36(5):507–512.

Prichard JG, Tierney LM Jr: Acute bronchitis. *In* Rakel RE (ed): Textbook of Family Practice, 4th ed. Philadelphia, WB Saunders, 1990, pp 506–507.

Acute bronchitis, tracheitis, and tracheobronchitis. *In* Seaton A, Seaton D, Leitch AG: Crofton and Douglas's Respiratory Diseases, 4th ed. Oxford, Blackwell Scientific, 1989, pp 276–277.

Verheij TJM, Kaptein AA, Mulder JD: Acute bronchitis: Aetiology, symptoms and treatment. Fam Pract 1989;6:66–69.

30 Bronchiectasis

Lisa M. Cannon

Bronchiectasis is defined as irreversible dilation of airways caused by inflammatory destruction.

Etiology
1. Postinfectious insults
   a. Mycobacterial tuberculosis
   b. Allergic bronchopulmonary aspergillosis
   c. Virulent bacterial and viral infections (e.g., severe pertussis, measles)
2. Bronchial obstruction
   a. Intraluminal obstruction secondary to an aspirated foreign body, neoplasm, or broncholiths
   b. Compressive obstruction secondary to adenopathy or neoplastic disease
3. Abnormal host defense
   a. Panhypogammaglobulinemia
   b. Defective mucociliary clearance
      (1) Kartagener's syndrome
      (2) Young's syndrome
      (3) Rheumatoid arthritis
   c. Chronic granulomatous disease
4. Genetic defects: cystic fibrosis
5. Congenital structural defects
   a. Bronchomalacia
   b. Mounier Kuhn syndrome
   c. Williams-Campbell syndrome

Pathology
1. Cylindrical bronchiectasis
2. Varicose bronchiectasis
3. Saccular bronchiectasis

Symptoms
1. Purulent sputum and cough
2. Hemoptysis
3. Dyspnea in severe disease
4. Fetid breath
5. Emaciation
6. Fatigue
7. Recurrent infections

Key Symptoms
- Purulent cough
- Hemoptysis
- Recurrent infections

Clinical Signs
1. Chest auscultation
   a. Moist crackles
   b. Rhonchi
   c. Wheezing
2. Extrathoracic signs
   a. Clubbing
   b. Metastatic abscesses
   c. Nasal polyps
   d. Amyloidosis
3. Radiographic findings
   a. Bronchial thickening (i.e., "tram tracks" or "ring shadows")
   b. Segmental atelectasis
   c. Cystic spaces
   d. Honeycomb pattern in severe disease

Key Sign
- Moist crackles

Laboratory Tests
1. Initial testing
   a. Complete blood count
   b. Serum protein electrophoresis
   c. Sputum for Gram's stain and AFB
2. Advanced testing
   a. Immunoglobulin quantitation
   b. Sinus radiography
   c. Spirometry
   d. Antibody tests for aspergillosis
   e. High-resolution computed tomography scan
   f. Bronchoscopy to rule out obstruction if indicated by spirometry
   g. Bronchography if surgery is contemplated

Key Tests
- High-resolution computed tomography scan
- Bronchography

Differential Diagnosis
1. Foreign body aspiration
2. Chronic bronchitis

3. Tuberculosis

4. Chronic lung abscess

Treatment

1. Basic supportive measures

   a. Postural drainage

   b. Adequate hydration

   c. Bronchodilators

   d. Oxygen therapy for hypoxemia

2. Antimicrobial therapy

   a. Culture-guided therapy

   b. If sputum culture is not diagnostic, consider empiric therapy with ampicillin or trimethoprim-sulfamethoxazole.

3. Annual influenza vaccination

4. Resectional surgery for:

   a. Disease unresponsive to medical therapy

   b. Massive hemoptysis

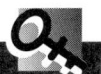

Key Treatment

• Supportive Measures

• Antimicrobial Therapy

Follow-Up

Follow-up as needed during disease exacerbations.

Bibliography

Barker AF, Bardara EJ Jr: Bronchiectasis: Update of an orphan disease. Am Rev Respir Dis 1988;137:969–978.

Baum GL, Hershko EP: Bronchiectasis. *In* Baum GL, Wolinsky E (eds): Textbook of Pulmonary Diseases. 5th ed, vol I. Boston, Little, Brown, 1994, pp 623–646.

Fraser RG, Paré PD, Fraser RS, Generaux GP (eds): Diagnosis of Diseases of the Chest. 3rd ed, vol III. Philadelphia, WB Saunders, 1990, pp 2186–2203.

McGuinnes G, Naidich DP, Lehman BS, et al: Bronchiectasis: CT evaluation. Am J Roentgenol 1993;160:253–259.

Murray JF, Nadel JA: Textbook of Respiratory Medicine, 2nd ed. Philadelphia, WB Saunders, 1994, pp 1398–1417.

31 Chronic Obstructive Pulmonary Disease

Paul E. Bettencourt

Etiology

A. Chronic bronchitis
1. Cigarette smoking
2. Occupational exposure

B. Emphysema
1. Cigarette smoking
2. α_1-Antiprotease deficiency

Symptoms

A. Chronic bronchitis
1. Cough and sputum production 3 months of the year for 2 years
2. Dyspnea on exertion
3. Wheeze
4. Leg edema

B. Emphysema
1. Dyspnea on exertion
2. Minimally productive cough
3. Leg edema

Key Symptoms

Chronic bronchitis
- Cough and sputum production
- Leg edema

Emphysema
- Dyspnea on exertion

Clinical Findings

A. Chronic bronchitis
1. Cyanosis
2. May be obese
3. Barrel chest
4. Rhonchi, wheeze
5. Prolonged expiration
6. Cor pulmonale—leg edema, elevated jugular vein pressure, right ventricular heave, tricuspid insufficiency

B. Emphysema
1. Pursed-lip breathing
2. May be thin
3. Depressed diaphragm
4. Hyperresonant to percussion
5. Prolonged expiration

6. Diminished breath sounds
7. Wheeze may be present
8. Signs of cor pulmonale—late

Key Signs

Chronic bronchitis
- Wheeze, rhonchi
- Signs of cor pulmonale

Emphysema
- Depressed diaphragm
- Diminished breath sounds

Tests

A. Chronic bronchitis
1. Chest radiography
   a. Increased anteroposterior dimension
   b. Thickened bronchial markings
   c. Enlarged right side of heart
2. Pulmonary function tests
   a. Reduced forced expiratory volume at 1 second and/or forced vital capacity; may be some reversibility after bronchodilator therapy
   b. Normal to elevated total lung capacity and residual volume
   c. Normal diffusing capacity
3. Arterial blood gas analysis—hypoxemia, hypercapnia

B. Emphysema
1. Chest radiography
   a. Depressed diaphragm
   b. Hyperlucent lung fields
   c. "Pruning" of vascular markings
   d. Vertical heart
2. Pulmonary function tests
   a. Fixed reduction in forced expiratory volume at 1 second and/or forced vital capacity
   b. Increased total lung capacity and/or residual volume
   c. Reduced diffusing capacity
3. Arterial blood gas analysis—normocapnia, mild to moderate hypoxemia
4. α_1-Antiprotease—blood level may be low

Key Tests

Chronic bronchitis

- Pulmonary function tests, chest radiography, arterial blood gas analysis

Emphysema

- Pulmonary function tests—abnormal diffusing capacity helps distinguish from other obstructive lung diseases
- Arterial blood gas analysis, chest radiography
- α_1-Antiprotease

Differential Diagnosis

A. Chronic bronchitis—asthma, bronchiectasis, cystic fibrosis, emphysema

B. Emphysema—chronic bronchitis

Treatment

A. Chronic bronchitis
1. Drugs of choice
   a. β-Agonist (e.g., albuterol [Proventil, Ventolin], metaproterenol [Alupent, Metaprel]) 2 puffs q.i.d. as needed generally given by inhalation; may also be given orally or parentally
   b. Anticholinergic aerosol (ipratroprium [Atrovent]), 2 puffs q.i.d., may be preferred
   c. Corticosteroids—inhaled, oral, or parenteral
   d. Antibiotics—for exacerbations
   e. Theophylline to maintain a serum level of 10 to 15 μg/ml, aminophylline
   f. Oxygen—if P_{O_2} is less than 55 mm Hg at rest, exercise, nocturnally, or if cor pulmonale is present
2. Alternative drugs
   a. Expectorants—controversial
   b. Digoxin (Lanoxin)—controversial because of risk of toxicity
   c. Diuretics—if cor pulmonale is present
3. Activity
   a. Pulmonary rehabilitation—exercise training
   b. Pulmonary toilet—chest physiotherapy, postural drainage
4. Patient education
   a. Stress importance of using oxygen.
   b. Advise the patient to inform the physician of exacerbation early.

B. Emphysema
1. Drugs of choice
   a. β-Agonist (e.g., albuterol, metaproterenol) 2 puffs q.i.d. as needed generally given by inhalation; may also be given orally or parenterally
   b. Anticholinergic aerosol (ipratroprium) 2 puffs q.i.d. as needed
2. Alternative drugs
   a. Corticosteroids—inhaled, oral, or parenteral (minimally effective)
   b. Antibiotics—for exacerbations
   c. Theophylline
   d. Oxygen—if P_{O_2} less than 55 mm Hg at rest, exercise, nocturnally, or if cor pulmonale is present
   e. Digoxin (Lanoxin)—controversial because of risk of toxicity
   f. Diuretics—if cor pulmonale is present
   g. α_1-Antiprotease replacement—if deficient
3. Activity—pulmonary rehabilitation; exercise training
4. Patient education
   a. Stress importance of using oxygen.
   b. Advise the patient to inform the physician of exacerbation early.

Follow-Up

A. Chronic bronchitis
1. Periodic pulmonary function tests, arterial blood gas analysis, and chest radiography (annually)
2. Reduce oral steroids to the lowest possible dose.
3. Observe for the development of cor pulmonale and bronchogenic carcinoma.
4. Give pneumococcal and influenza vaccine.

B. Emphysema
1. Periodic pulmonary function tests, arterial blood gas analysis, and chest radiography (annually)
2. Reduce oral steroids to the lowest possible dose.
3. Observe for the development of cor pulmonale and bronchogenic carcinoma.
4. Give pneumococcal and influenza vaccine.

Bibliography

Canadian thoracic society workshop group: Guidelines for the assessment and management of chronic obstructive pulmonary disease. Can Med Assoc J 1992;147:420–428.

Dantzker DR, Pingleton SK, Pierce JA, et al: Standards for the diagnosis and care of patients with chronic obstructive pulmonary disease (COPD) and asthma. Am Rev Respir Dis 1987;136:225–243.

Dubois P, Jamart S, Machiels J, et al: Prognosis of severely hypoxemic patients receiving long-term oxygen therapy. Chest 1994;105:469–474.

Snider GL: Emphysema: The first two centuries—and beyond. Am Rev Respir Dis 1992;146:1334–1344, 1615–1622.

Vaz Fragoso CA, Miller MA: Review of the clinical efficacy of theophylline in the treatment of chronic obstructive pulmonary disease. Am Rev Respir Dis 1993;147:540–547.

32 Pulmonary Function Testing

Gregory L. Phelps

Indications

Pulmonary function testing is indicated in the basic evaluation of the following:

1. Lung function
2. Smoking cessation motivation
3. Evaluation of therapeutic interventions
4. Disability determinations
5. Occupational screening, including mandated exposure screening
6. Respirator fitness

Pulmonary testing can get extremely sophisticated with various measurements, flow loops, methacholine challenges, carbon dioxide diffusion, and so on.

Contraindications

Absolute contraindications to pulmonary function testing are almost nonexistent. Relative contraindications might include the following:

1. Large pulmonary blebs or bullae
2. Severe, effort-related bronchoconstriction
3. History of marked vasovagal responsiveness
4. History of spontaneous pneumothorax
5. Uncontrolled hypertension
6. Recent myocardial infarction

Equipment

1. The basic machine measures expired air against time. To most experts, the equipment falls into two basic types:

   a. a volume-dependent spirometer

   b. a flow-measuring instrument technically called a pneumotachograph

   Both serve essentially the same functions. Each must extrapolate complementary information. Information obtained from the machine readings is compared with normative values that include age, sex, height, and race. Most equipment now sold is computer-controlled. It automatically compares the crude reading with the normative values and then reads the results in percentage of predicted equivalents. The normative standard is slightly less than the usual two standard deviation, bell-shaped curve, encompassing 95 per cent of values. Instead, normal is defined as 80 to 120 per cent of the predicted values. (This standard has come under fire from the American Thoracic Society [ATS].) Probably more important than the predicted value is the patient's previous test results.

2. Because of the legal mandates related to asbestos, cotton dust, and other material, there are National Institute of Occupational Safety and Health (NIOSH) requirements for spirometers. They include manual start pins and size and storage of tracings. The ATS has promulgated updated standards in 1987 and commentary on reference values in 1991. In a recent testing series, only 27 of 53 (51 per cent) computer-controlled systems met the ATS standards. Calibration is another essential aspect of pulmonary function testing. Ideally, there are 24 different computer-generated waveform settings that may be run. At the minimum, the equipment should be tested each day of use with a standardized 3-L syringe. Results should remain within ± 3 per cent. The timing of the writer should also be checked with a stopwatch. The system should be routinely checked for leaks. (For a further discussion of standards, the reader is strongly encouraged to review the ATS standards listed in the bibliography.)

Testing

1. Pulmonary function testing is an effort-dependent assessment. Well-trained staff are essential. Three-day pulmonary function testing seminars are available to meet Occupational Safety and Health Administration (OSHA) requirements for technician training.

2. In general, a patient forcefully exhales a minimum of three times into the machine. The two best tracings should not vary by more than 100 ml, or 5 per cent, thus indicating a consistent best effort. Coughing, intratest breathing, or tongue blocks may invalidate some tests and must be individually evaluated.

3. To avoid patient fatigue, most experts recommend limiting the number of repetitions to eight forced breaths. The best tracing for each individual value is then assessed. For valid testing, the tracing needs to last at least 6 seconds with at least 2 seconds of plateau. Spirometers need to have at least a 7-L and 15-second strip capacity.

4. Principal values assessed (Fig. 32–1)

   a. Forced vital capacity (FVC). This is the maximal volume that can be expelled after deep inspiration. This value is represented by the top point or plateau of the tracing. When the FVC is diminished, the patient often suffers from a restrictive lung disease that inhibits maximal expansion of the lung, such as sarcoidosis, or a fibrotic process like asbestosis (Fig. 32–2).

   b. Forced expiratory volume at 1 second (FEV_1). This value, when compared with the total volume (FEV_1/FVC), is usually 75 per cent of the total volume. Obstruction is indicated by an inability to expel this large percentage of total volume in the 1st second. It is represented by a longer, gentler slope often coupled with a slightly lower FVC

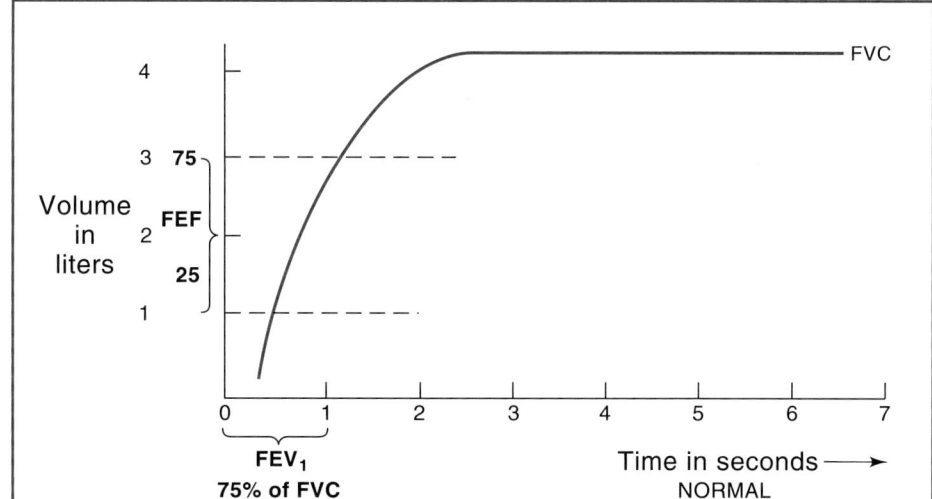

Figure 32–1 Normal values in pulmonary function tests.

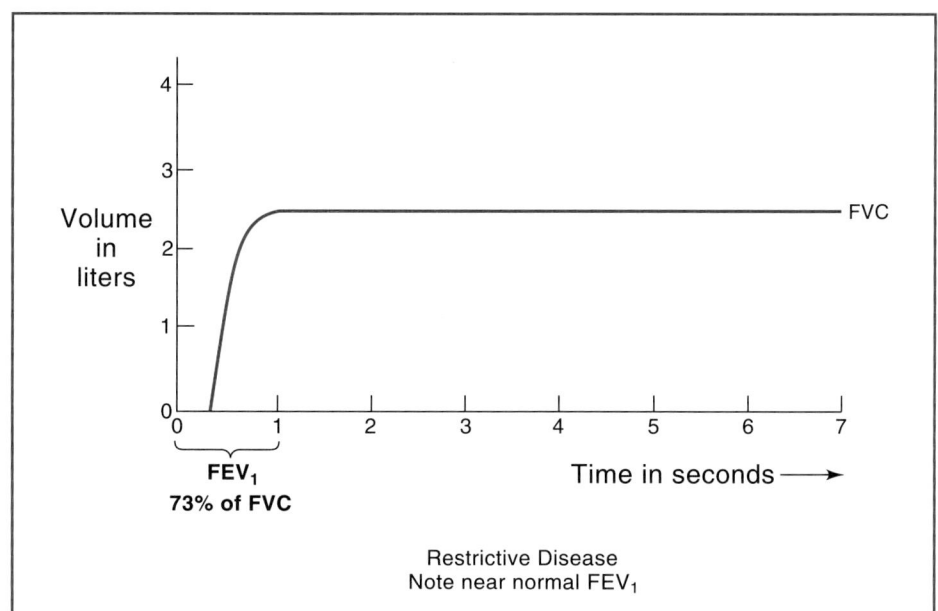

Figure 32–2 Pulmonary function test values in restrictive disease.

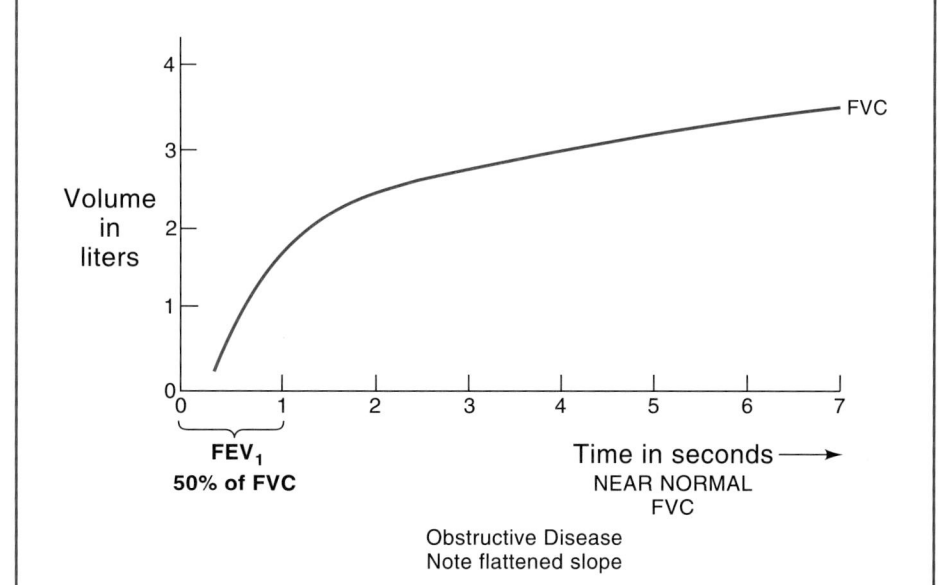

Figure 32–3 Pulmonary function test values in obstructive disease.

TABLE 32–1. CLASSES OF RESPIRATORY IMPAIRMENT

	CLASS 1: 0%, NO IMPAIRMENT OF THE WHOLE PERSON	CLASS 2: 10–25%, MILD IMPAIRMENT OF THE WHOLE PERSON	CLASS 3: 26–50%, MODERATE IMPAIRMENT OF THE WHOLE PERSON	CLASS 4: 51–100%, SEVERE IMPAIRMENT OF THE WHOLE PERSON
FVC FEV$_1$ FEV$_1$/FVC (%) D$_{CO}$	FVC $\geq$ 80% of predicted; and FEV$_1$ $\geq$ 80% of predicted; and FEV$_1$/FVC $\geq$ 70%; *and/or* D$_{CO}$ $\geq$ 70% of predicted.	FVC between 60 and 79% of predicted; or FEV$_1$ between 60 and 79% of predicted; or D$_{CO}$ between 60 and 69% of predicted.	FVC between 51 and 59% of predicted; or FEV$_1$ between 41 and 59% of predicted; or D$_{CO}$ between 41 and 59% of predicted.	FVC $\leq$ 50% of predicted; or FEV$_1$ $\leq$ 40% of predicted; or D$_{CO}$ $\leq$ 40% of predicted.
	or	or	or	or
$\dot{V}$O$_2$ Max	> 25 ml/(kg · min); *and/or* > 7.1 METS	Between 20 and 25 ml/(kg · min); or 5.7–7.1 METS	Between 15 and 20 ml/(kg · min); or 4.3–5.7 METS	< 15 ml/(kg · min); or < 1.05 L/min; or < 4.3 METS

(Guides to the Evaluation of Permanent Injury. American Medical Association, copyright June 1993.)

FVC, forced vital capacity; FEV$_1$, forced expiratory volume in the 1st second; D$_{CO}$, diffusing capacity of carbon monoxide. The D$_{CO}$ is primarily of value for patients with restrictive lung disease. In classes 2 and 3, if the FVC, FEV$_1$, and FEV$_1$/FVC ratio are normal and the D$_{CO}$ is between 41 and 79 per cent, then an exercise test is required.

$\dot{V}$O$_2$ Max, or measured exercise capacity, is useful in assessing whether a person's complaint of dyspnea is a result of respiratory or other conditions. A person's cardiac and conditioning status must be considered in performing the test and in interpreting the results.

(Fig. 32–3). This result is typical of an obstructive disease such as asthma, byssinosis, or chronic obstructive pulmonary disease. Although the ATS is now advocating relative rather than absolute standards, most experts agree that an FEV$_1$/FVC ratio of less than 70 per cent is abnormal.

c. Forced expiratory flow 25 to 75 per cent. Formerly called the midexpiratory flow, this value is often an early indicator of small airway obstructive disease. It is a little less reliable and has a wider accepted range of variation.

Interpretation

A systematic approach to interpretation is best.

1. Review the test information. It indicates patient information, test variation, duration of effort, position during testing (sitting or standing), and whether nose clips (recommended but not required) were used.

2. Evaluate the strips themselves to determine whether there is adequate duration, plateau, and best effort. Pay particular attention to the initial slope of the FEV$_1$ and then look at the FEV$_1$/FVC ratio. If available, review old strips.

3. Review the printouts that compare the patient's results with standardized norms. Remember that because the results are done in percentages of predicted, an exceptionally fit set of lungs might have to deteriorate 40 per cent of their capacity to fall out of normal range.

Variations

1. Generally, FEV$_1$ declines 20 to 30 ml per year. Some authors allow 40 to 50 ml for smokers. A change of more than 15 per cent per year is abnormal. For work-relatedness, most experts argue that a decline of 5 or more per cent in tests from before-shift to after work warrants close supervision and investigation. When testing for the therapeutic effect of bronchodilators, the patient should experience a before-to-after improvement of at least 12 to 15 per cent and 200 ml. The patient should abstain from bronchodilator inhalation for a period of time before the test.

2. For respirator evaluation, the overall cardiorespiratory condition of the patient, the patient's mental state (claustrophobia), the type of respirator and conditions for respirator use, and a pulmonary function test result must be considered. There are no specific pulmonary function values promulgated by OSHA for respirator clearance. Most experts use 50 to 70 per cent of predicted for both values as a cut-off to mandate a more intensive evaluation of respirator fitness.

3. Pulmonary function testing is one of the key measurements in evaluating lung-based disability. The American Medical Association has promulgated a series of pulmonary function test–based results to assist with interpretation (Table 32–1). The FVC is considered to hold the stronger prognostic implication. The use of pulmonary testing in patients with asthma can be frustrating when attempting to determine disability because of the day-to-day variation in results. Generally, the patient's care should be optimized before testing. Up to 50 per cent of patients with occupational asthma may have symptoms that persist longer than 2 years. Periodic pulmonary function testing is helpful in determining recovery. Determination of permanent disability should be deferred until 2 years after the onset of disease.

Bibliography

American Thoracic Society: Lung function testing: Selection of reference values and interpretive strategies. Am Rev Respir Dis 1991;144:1202–1218.

American Thoracic Society: Standardization of spirometry—1987 update. Am Rev Respir Dis 1987;136:1286–1298.

Committee of Occupational Lung Disorders of the American College of Occupational and Environmental Medicine: Spirometry in the occupational setting: Notes for guidance. J Occup Med 1992;34:559–561.

Guides to the Evaluation of Permanent Impairment, 4th ed. Chicago: American Medical Association, 1993, pp 159–167.

Scheid JA, Onion DK: Use of respirators in the workplace. J Fam Pract 1989;29(1):21–28.

State of the Art Reviews: Occupational medicine. Spirometry 1993;8:2.

Indications
1. Sampling for blood gas determination
2. After failure of venous access for phlebotomy

Contraindications (relative)
1. Coagulopathy, including therapeutic anticoagulation and thrombolysis
2. Cutaneous injury at the available sites (e.g., infection, burn)
3. Previous surgery in the puncture area
4. Severe atherosclerosis
5. Decreased collateral flow (positive Allen's test)

There are *no* absolute contraindications.

Preparation
1. Arterial site
   a. Radial (usual for single sampling, but painful)
   b. Ulnar
   c. Brachial
   d. Axillary

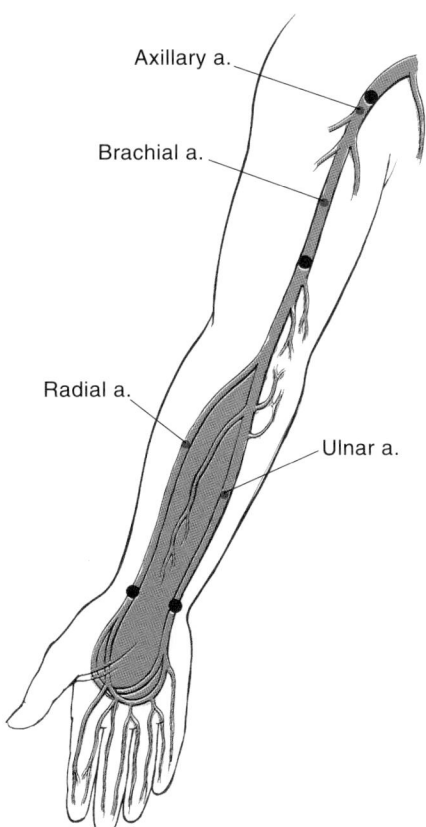

   e. Dorsalis pedis

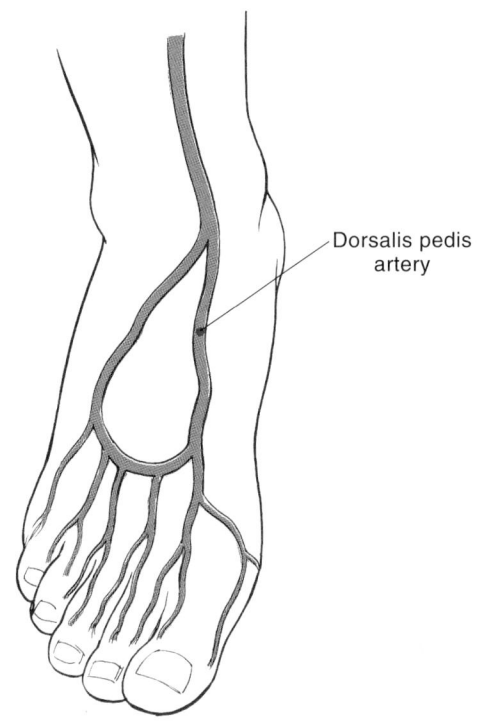

   f. Femoral (excellent for otherwise difficult access, and relatively less painful)

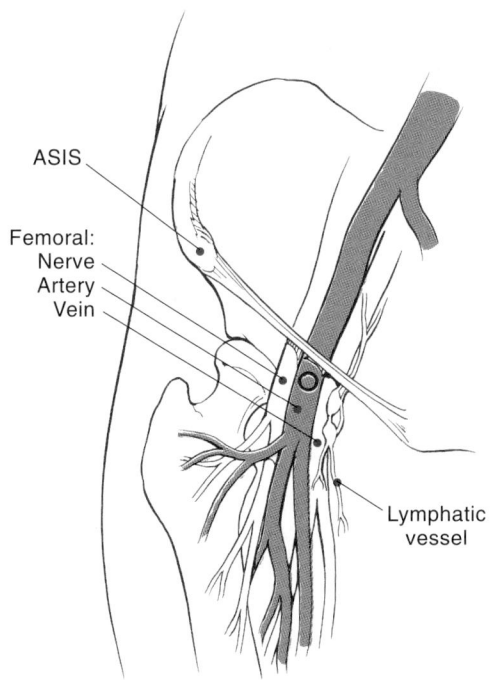

2. Detailed explanation to the patient and signing of a consent form (institution option)

Equipment

An arterial blood gas kit is often available and contains these items:

1. Alcohol pads
2. Iodophor solution and ointment
3. Adhesive tape
4. Heparinized syringe for blood gas sampling
5. 5-cc or 10-cc syringe for large-volume chemistries or hematology
6. 22-gauge needle for blood sampling (a 25-gauge or 27-gauge needle is adequate and more humane for radial ABGs, and should be substituted)
7. 2×2 dry sterile gauze
8. A small adhesive dressing
9. A cup of ice-water slush for transport
10. An adhesive label with the patient's ID

Anesthesia

Lidocaine 1% or similar, without epinephrine: Use a 1-cc syringe with a 27-gauge needle.

Precautions

1. **Don gloves before any invasive procedure.**
2. Ensure ulnar arterial flow for radial access (Allen's test).

Technique

1. Palpate the arterial pulse to locate the vessel.
2. Prepare the site with an iodophor solution.
3. Anesthetize the site with a wheal of lidocaine without epinephrine through a 27-gauge needle, then infuse a small amount *slightly* deeper than the wheal, avoiding vascular structures. To be honest, there are no reliable data that show pH, Pco_2, or Po_2 is altered by pain or anxiety, but simple compassion dictates that anesthesia be used.
4. Massage the site to re-establish landmarks and regain a clear pulse.
5. If a preheparinized syringe is used, discard all liquid heparin through the arterial puncture needle (excess heparin in the syringe may cause a falsely low Pco_2).
6. Isolate the pulse with the *nondominant* hand by straddling the wheal, using near-occluding pressure distally to distend the vessel, and merely localizing the pulse proximally. The finger separation should be about 1 cm, with pulses present under each finger.
7. Puncture the skin through the anesthetic wheal, holding the needle at about a 45-degree angle to the skin, aiming for the pulse under the proximal finger and holding the syringe with the dominant hand.

8. Once the needle has entered the arterial lumen and advanced 1 or 2 mm, the syringe plunger may be designed to rise simply under arterial pressure, without operator assistance. If not, rest the syringe-holding dominant hand on the patient's limb and, with the nondominant hand, assist the filling by gentle aspiration.
   a. If there is no flow of bright red blood into the syringe, the needle may have gone through both vessel walls. Withdraw the needle slowly while aspirating gently. If you must redirect the needle, do so only when the needle is just barely under the skin.
   b. If liquid heparin was used, at least 3 cc should be obtained for a blood gas sampling to minimize the effect of excess liquid heparin in the needle. If the syringe was preloaded with powdered heparin, only 1 cc of blood is required.

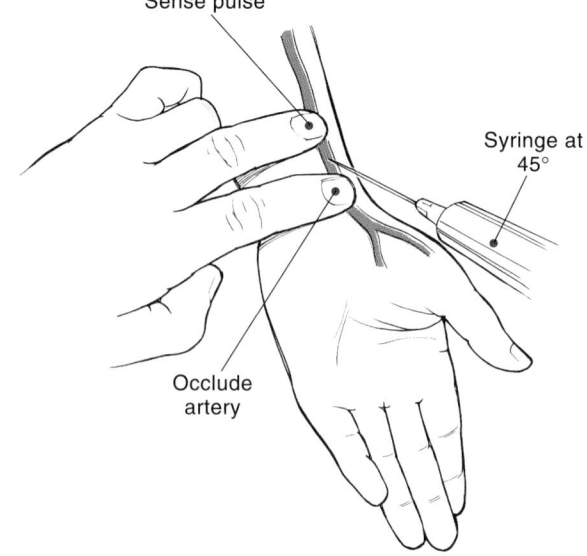

Sense pulse

Syringe at 45°

Occlude artery

Follow-Up

1. *Hold occlusive direct pressure* at the site for at least five solid minutes.
   a. Fifteen minutes or more may be necessary for those with a coagulopathy.
   b. Use a folded 2×2 sterile gauze and an adhesive strip as a dressing during direct pressure.
2. Blood gas samples must be handled carefully.
   a. All air bubbles must be *completely* expelled immediately to avoid a falsely high Po_2 after the air is evacuated (Po_2 can rise as much as 11 mm Hg in 20 minutes if air is available). One technique for expelling air is as follows.
      (1) Remove the needle.
      (2) Point the syringe at the ceiling.
      (3) Pull back on the plunger to fill the remainder of the syringe with air.

(4) Flick the syringe with your finger to break up the air bubbles.

(5) Cover the hub opening with a 2×2 gauze, and push down on the plunger to empty the air from the syringe, until a meniscus of blood is seen at the hub.

(6) Cap the syringe with an airtight seal.

b. Once capped, the sample-filled syringe should be stored in an ice-slush, where the P_{O_2}, P_{CO_2}, and pH will remain reliable for up to about an hour. They will then deteriorate fairly rapidly.

c. Label the syringe and take it to the analyzer as quickly as possible.

d. Check the patient's hand in 10 minutes for perfusion and hematoma formation.

 Bibliography

For more details on the techniques used in arterial puncture, see

Arterial puncture and cannulation. *In* Roberts JR, Hedges JR (eds): Clinical Procedures in Emergency Medicine. Philadelphia, WB Saunders, 1991, pp 255–268. Emergency procedures. *In* Knighton D, Locksley RM, Mills J (eds): Current Emergency Diagnosis and Treatment. E Norwalk, CT, Appleton & Lange, 1990, pp 801–802. Vascular cannulation. *In* Civetta JM, Taylor RW, Kirby RR: Critical Care. Philadelphia, JB Lippincott, 1992, pp 165–167.

For more information on the effects of external influences on blood-gas results, see

Madiedo G, Sciacca R, Hause L: Air bubbles and temperature effect on blood-gas analysis. J Clin Pathol 1980; 33(9):864–867. Ordog GJ, Wasserberger J, Balasubramaniam S: Effect of heparin on arterial blood gases. Ann Emerg Med 1985;14(3):233–238.

33 Interstitial Lung Disease

Muhammad K. Zaman

Etiology

1. Diverse, with nearly 200 disease entities sharing common clinical, physiologic, imaging, and pathologic features. Idiopathic pulmonary fibrosis, sarcoidosis, collagen vascular disease–associated interstitial lung disease, cryptogenic organizing pneumonia, and hypersensitivity pneumonitis constitute more than two-thirds of all cases, whereas other entities, such as pulmonary alveolar proteinosis, are distinctly rare.

2. Classification (partial list)
   a. Unknown etiology
      (1) Sarcoidosis
      (2) Idiopathic pulmonary fibrosis
      (3) Cryptogenic organizing pneumonia
      (4) Eosinophilic granuloma
      (5) Wegener's granulomatosis
      (6) Pulmonary hemorrhage syndromes
      (7) Eosinophilic pneumonia
      (8) Pulmonary alveolar proteinosis
   b. Occupational and environmental exposure
      (1) Chemical fumes and gases
      (2) Organic dusts (pneumoconioses)
      (3) Inorganic dusts (hypersensitivity pneumonitis)
   c. Collagen vascular disease
      (1) Rheumatoid arthritis
      (2) Scleroderma
      (3) Systemic lupus erythematosus
      (4) Polymyositis and dermatomyositis
      (5) Mixed connective tissue disease
      (6) Sjögren's syndrome
   d. Drug- or treatment-induced
      (1) Cytotoxic drugs
      (2) Noncytotoxic drugs
      (3) Radiation
      (4) Oxygen toxicity
   e. Infectious (clinically resemble true interstitial lung disease)
      (1) *Pneumocystis* pneumonia
      (2) Viral and atypical pneumonias
      (3) Mycobacterial and fungal pneumonias
   f. Neoplastic (clinically resemble true interstitial lung disease)
      (1) Lymphangitic carcinomatosis
      (2) Bronchoalveolar cell carcinoma
      (3) Pulmonary lymphoma

Symptoms

1. Progressively worsening dyspnea on exertion is the most common symptom.
2. Cough, usually nonproductive, may be prominent in diseases that are more bronchocentric.
3. Chest pain is uncommon but may be of pleuritic nature.
   a. Pleural involvement (e.g., collagen diseases)
   b. Pneumothorax (e.g., eosinophilic granuloma)
4. Hemoptysis is uncommon and suggests alveolar hemorrhage syndromes, underlying carcinoma, pulmonary embolism, bronchiectasis, mycetoma, and lymphangiomyomatosis.
5. Fever with acute presentation, consider infection, acute idiopathic pulmonary fibrosis, acute eosinophilic pneumonia, hypersensitivity pneumonitis, and cryptogenic organizing pneumonia.

Key Symptoms
- Chronic progressive dyspnea
- Nonproductive cough

Clinical Findings

1. Look for history of the following:
   a. Detailed occupational and environmental exposure
   b. Exposure to drugs or radiation
   d. Presence of multisystem disease
   e. Mineral oil–based nosedrops
   f. Gastroesophageal reflux
   g. Tobacco exposure
      (1) Inductive in eosinophilic granuloma and respiratory bronchiolitis
      (2) Protective in hypersensitivity pneumonitis and sarcoidosis
   h. Family history (e.g., familial pulmonary fibrosis)
2. Physical examination
   a. Bibasilar end-inspiratory dry ''Velcro'' crackles
      (1) Most characteristic finding; correlates with fibrosis; common in idiopathic pulmonary fibrosis
      (2) Often absent in sarcoidosis and other granulomatous diseases

b. Clubbing
   (1) Indicates advanced fibrosis
   (2) Particularly common in idiopathic pulmonary fibrosis
   (3) May indicate complicating carcinoma
c. Cutaneous and joint involvement—collagen disease, sarcoidosis
d. Cyanosis, late sign of advanced disease

Key Signs

- Bibasilar inspiratory crackles
- Clubbing
- Associated cutaneous or joint involvement

Tests

1. Chest radiographs—and comparison with previous films
   a. Vast majority (90 per cent) have abnormal chest radiographs
      (1) Reticulonodular bilateral interstitial pattern is most common.
      (2) Air bronchograms and air alveolograms suggest active disease.
      (3) Honeycombing suggests extensive fibrosis.
   b. Adenopathy—sarcoidosis, lymphoma
   c. Nodules—granulomatous disease, silicosis, neoplasm
   d. "Radiographic negative of pulmonary edema"—eosinophilic pneumonia
   e. Kerley B lines—pulmonary edema, lymphangitic carcinomatosis
   f. Pleural disease—collagen vascular disease, asbestosis
   g. Pneumothorax—eosinophilic granuloma, advanced fibrosis
   h. Upper lobe predominance—sarcoidosis, silicosis, eosinophilic pneumonia
2. High-resolution computed tomographic scan is an evolving technique and is not recommended for routine use. It is useful for the following purposes:
   a. Detects early interstitial lung disease with normal chest radiograph
   b. Assesses the extent, distribution, and severity of disease
   c. Offers clues to differentiate various interstitial lung disease by morphologic criteria
   d. Guides site of lung biopsy
3. Gallium-67 scanning is not recommended for routine evaluations.
4. Serology

a. Routine battery of serologic tests is not recommended.
b. Serology for collagen vascular disease, pulmonary-renal syndromes, and muscle function studies as clinically indicated.
c. Studies of hepatic, hematologic, and renal function are useful in some diseases.
d. Always consider human immunodeficiency virus (HIV) serology.
5. Pulmonary function testing (spirometry, lung volumes, and diffusing capacity for carbon monoxide)
   a. Routinely performed as baseline and followed at intervals
   b. May be abnormal with normal chest radiograph
   c. Classically reveals restrictive disease with decreased forced vital capacity, diffusing capacity for carbon monoxide, total lung capacity, and compliance with normal flow
   d. Obstructive disease with decreased forced expiratory volume in 1 second and forced vital capacity in some diseases
   e. Valuable in determining the presence and severity of disease and monitoring the progression of disease and response to therapy
6. Arterial blood gas analysis
   a. Most commonly reveals mild hypoxemia and respiratory alkalosis
   b. Carbon dioxide retention is rare even in late stages.
   c. Exercise desaturation may occur in the absence of resting hypoxemia and may be the most sensitive marker of disease severity and progression.
7. Bronchoscopic studies—should be the initial diagnostic procedure for most patients except those in whom the cause is known
   a. Bronchoalveolar lavage
      (1) Procedure of choice for assessment of infectious entities
      (2) Based on the number and percentage of neutrophils, lymphocytes, or eosinophils, the interstitial lung disease may be subcategorized and the differential diagnosis narrowed.
      (3) Increased lymphocytes suggest response to corticosteroid therapy; increased eosinophils coupled with increased neutrophils suggest a lack of such response in idiopathic pulmonary fibrosis.
   b. Transbronchial biopsy
      (1) Small sample size limits diagnostic utility, except in granulomatous diseases
      (2) Combined with bronchoalveolar lavage (BAL), can diagnose most infectious and neoplastic diseases
8. Open lung biopsy or open thorascopic lung biopsy

a. Allows large tissue sample for adequate evaluation of airways, alveoli, and vessels

b. Should be performed if expected result will alter patient therapy or outcome

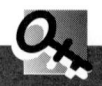

Key Tests

- Chest radiographs and comparison with previous films
- Pulmonary function tests
- Bronchoscopy with BAL and biopsy
- Open lung biopsy

Differential Diagnosis

Infectious and neoplastic diseases that resemble true interstitial lung diseases (see classification) must be excluded by appropriate tests.

Treatment

1. Depends on the ultimate diagnosis and the activity of disease—inflammatory versus end-stage fibrosis versus mixed histology

2. Avoid known exposures in all cases.

3. Always stop smoking.

4. Corticosteroids: Initial drug of choice for most noninfectious, non-neoplastic interstitial lung diseases when treatment is indicated. The usual starting dose is 1 mg/kg/d of prednisone except in sarcoidosis (0.5 mg/kg/d). Response is good in granulomatous, vasculitic, and inflammatory processes.

5. Cytotoxic medications—when steroids fail or as initial therapy with steroids when BAL cytology suggests unresponsiveness to steroids (see above). Azathioprine (Imuran) and cyclophosphamide (Cytoxan) are commonly used, but controlled trials are lacking.

6. Lung transplantation for selected end-stage patients

Key Treatment

Drug of Choice	Alternative Therapy
• Corticosteroids	• Cytotoxic agents

Follow-Up

1. Frequency depends on diagnosis and treatment.

2. Subjective and serial radiographic scoring

3. Serial pulmonary function testing, arterial blood gas analysis, or exercise saturation

4. Cardiopulmonary exercise testing in selected cases

5. Deterioration is usually due to disease progression, but one should think of congestive heart failure, bronchoalveolar cell carcinoma, pulmonary embolus, and infectious pneumonia.

 ## Bibliography

For more in-depth information on all clinical aspects of interstitial lung disease, see

Raghu G (ed): Interstitial lung diseases. Semin Respir Crit Care Med 1993;14(5):323–416 and 1994;15(1):1–96.

For more information on the immunopathogenetic approach to interstitial lung disease, see

Crystal RG, Bitterman PR, Rennard SI, et al: Interstitial lung diseases of unknown cause: Disorders characterized by chronic inflammation of the lower respiratory tract. N Engl J Med 1984;310:154–166, 235–244.

For more information on the clinicopathologic correlation of interstitial lung disease, see

Fulmer JD, Katzenstein AA: The interstitial lung diseases. Pulmonary Crit Care Med 1993;2(M-1):1–15.

For more information on an overview of sarcoidosis, see

Izumi T: Sarcoidosis. Pulmonary Crit Care Med 1993;2(M-5):1–9.

For more information on follow-up, see

Watters LC, King TE, Schwarz MI, et al: A clinical radiographic and physiologic scoring system for the longitudinal assessment of patients with idiopathic pulmonary fibrosis. Am Rev Respir Dis 1986;133:97–103.

34 Pneumonia

John W. Swisher

Etiology

Pneumonia may be caused by infection with a wide array of microbial pathogens (Table 34–1). Some pathogens are more likely to be associated with pneumonia in the setting of certain comorbid conditions (Table 34–2). Occupational, travel, and animal or bird exposure histories are important in identifying unusual causative pathogens.

TABLE 34–1. COMMON PATHOGENS THAT CAUSE PNEUMONIA

Bacteria

Community-acquired
Streptococcus pneumoniae
Haemophilus influenzae
Moraxella catarrhalis
Staphylococcus aureus
Klebsiella pneumoniae
Legionella spp.
Anaerobic bacteria
Bacteroides spp.
Fusobacterium spp.
Peptostreptococcus spp.
Peptococcus spp.

Nosocomial
Enterobacteriaceae
Escherichia coli
Klebsiella pneumoniae
Enterobacter spp.
Serratia spp.
Pseudomonas aeruginosa
Staphylococcus aureus

Bacteria-like organisms
Mycoplasma pneumoniae
Chlamydia pneumoniae (TWAR)

Virus
Influenza A and B
Adenovirus
Respiratory syncytial viruses
Parainfluenza viruses

Fungus

Community-acquired
Histoplasma capsulatum
Blastomyces dermatitidis
Coccidioides immitis
Cryptococcus neoformans

Nosocomial
Aspergillus spp.
Candida spp.

Mycobacteria
Mycobacterium tuberculosis

Parasites
Pneumocystis carinii

TABLE 34–2. PATHOGENS ASSOCIATED WITH COMORBID CONDITIONS

CONDITION	PATHOGEN
Altered consciousness or suspected aspiration	Anaerobic organisms
Chronic obstructive lung disease	*Streptococcus pneumoniae* *Haemophilus influenzae* *Moraxella catarrhalis*
Nursing home residents	Enterobacteriaceae Methicillin-resistant *Staphylococcus aureus* *Mycobacterium tuberculosis* Respiratory viruses
Immunodeficiency	*Pneumocystis carinii* Cytomegalovirus *Mycobacterium tuberculosis* *Cryptococcus neoformans* *Nocardia* spp.
Cystic fibrosis	*Pseudomonas aeruginosa* *S. aureus*
Influenza epidemic	*S. aureus*

Symptoms

A. Bacterial pneumonia (bacteria, *Legionella*)
   1. Rigors and fever
   2. Dyspnea
   3. Cough productive of purulent sputum
   4. Pleuritic chest pain
B. Atypical pneumonia (e.g., virus, fungus, *Mycoplasma, Legionella*)
   1. Often preceded by upper respiratory tract infection
   2. Fever without rigors
   3. Dyspnea
   4. Nonproductive cough
   5. Headache
   6. Myalgia and arthralgia
C. In elderly patients
   1. Nonspecific deterioration in general behavior
   2. Altered mental status, confusion, delirium
   3. Decompensation of stable pre-existing medical condition
   4. May present with fever, dyspnea, cough, or pleuritic chest pain as in younger patients

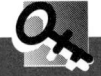

Key Symptoms	
• Fever and chills	• Dyspnea
• Cough	• Pleuritic chest pain

Clinical Findings

1. Fever in sustained or intermittent pattern
2. Tachypnea and labored respiration
3. Cyanosis
4. Focal crackles or consolidation on chest examination

Key Signs
• Fever
• Tachypnea
• Cyanosis
• Crackles or consolidation on chest examination
• Diminished breath sounds and percussion dullness if pleural effusion is present

5. Diminished breath sounds or dullness on chest percussion if pleural effusion is present

6. Chest examination findings may be minimal or diffuse in atypical lung infections.

7. Elderly patients may present with any of the typical findings or only altered level of consciousness.

Tests

1. Total and differential leukocyte counts

2. Blood cultures. Bacteremia may allow the identification of causative pathogen and aid antibiotic selection if sputum culture is nondiagnostic.

3. Sputum Gram's stain and culture

   a. Gram's stain showing greater than or equal to 25 neutrophils and less than or equal to 10 epithelial cells per low-power (100×) field is considered relatively free of oropharyngeal contamination.

   b. Observation of predominant organisms on Gram's stain can aid selection of appropriate empiric antibiotics until culture and sensitivity data become available.

4. Special sputum stains (Table 34–3)

5. Chest radiography

   a. Segmental or lobar infiltrate suggests bacterial pneumonia.

   b. Atypical pneumonia may result in diffuse or patchy infiltrate.

   c. Pleural effusion may be associated with infectious parenchymal process.

6. Bronchoscopy (may be useful if less invasive studies are inconclusive)

   a. Bronchoalveolar lavage—may be contaminated by upper airway flora

   b. Transbronchial protected brush specimen with quantitative culture—minimizes contamination by upper airway flora

   c. Transbronchial biopsy—required for confirmation of infection by organisms such as virus and fungus that have high incidence of airway colonization or contamination, especially in immunosuppressed patients

TABLE 34–3. SPECIAL STAINS FOR UNUSUAL LUNG PATHOGENS

STAIN	PATHOGEN
Acid-fast stain	Mycobacteria
Modified acid-fast stain	*Nocardia* spp.
Direct fluorescent antibody	*Legionella* spp.
	Pneumocystis carinii
	Influenza
	Respiratory syncytial virus
Silver stain	*Pneumocystis carinii*
	Fungus
Potassium hydroxide	Fungal hyphae or pseudohyphae

7. Transtracheal aspiration—bypasses oropharyngeal flora but is associated with substantial risks such as hemoptysis, soft tissue infection, and pneumothorax in unskilled hands

8. Transthoracic needle aspiration or biopsy

9. Open lung biopsy

10. Pleural fluid analysis

    a. Gram's stain and culture of pleural fluid associated with an infectious parenchymal process may be diagnostic.

    b. Evidence of pleural fluid infection is an indication for tube thoracostomy drainage.

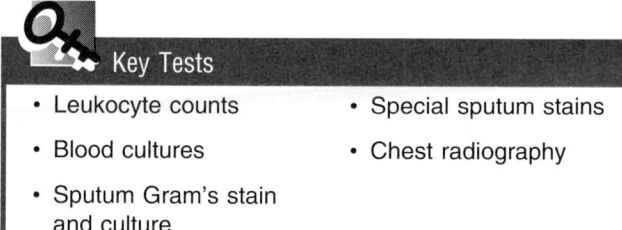

Key Tests

- Leukocyte counts
- Blood cultures
- Sputum Gram's stain and culture
- Special sputum stains
- Chest radiography

Differential Diagnosis

1. Pulmonary embolism or infarction
2. Neoplasm
3. Pulmonary hemorrhage
4. Leukoagglutinin reaction
5. Hypersensitivity pneumonitis
6. Drug-induced lung injury
7. Toxic inhalation
8. Alveolar proteinosis
9. Vasculitis
10. Sarcoidosis
11. Goodpasture's syndrome
12. Wegener's granulomatosis

Treatment

1. Hospitalization may be required based on social circumstances, comorbid conditions, and severity of illness factors, such as those listed as follows:

   a. Poor functional status and absence of a responsible caregiver

   b. Age greater than 65 with multiple medical problems

   c. Altered mental status or decreased level of consciousness

   d. Supplemental oxygen requirement (PO_2 less than 60 mm Hg while breathing room air)

   e. Mechanical ventilation

   f. Hypotension or septic shock

   g. Existence of multiorgan dysfunction

2. Supportive measures may include the following:

   a. Correct hypoxemia

TABLE 34–4. ANTIBIOTIC THERAPY FOR PNEUMONIA

SUSPECTED OR PROVEN ORGANISM	ANTIBIOTIC OF CHOICE	ALTERNATIVE ANTIBIOTICS	DURATION OF TREATMENT
Streptococcus pneumoniae	Penicillin G	Second-generation cephalosporin; macrolide	7–10 days
Haemophilus influenzae	Cefuroxime or other second-generation cephalosporin	Co-trimoxazole, amoxicillin/clavulanate	7–10 days
Staphylococcus aureus	Synthetic penicillin	First-generation cephalosporin; vancomycin	14 days
Anaerobes	Clindamycin, cefoxitin	Penicillin G or synthetic penicillin	10–14 days
Enterobacteriaceae	β-Lactam plus aminoglycoside or aztreonam	Fluoroquinolone; imipenem	10–14 days
Pseudomonas aeruginosa	β-Lactam plus aminoglycoside or aztreonam	Ciprofloxacin	10–14 days
Legionella pneumophila	Erythromycin	Tetracycline; co-trimoxazole; rifampin	14 days
Mycoplasma pneumoniae	Macrolide	Tetracycline	10–14 days
Chlamydia pneumoniae	Tetracycline	Macrolide	10–14 days

b. Control pain

c. Relieve cough

d. Control fever

e. Maintain intravascular volume

f. Chest percussion and drainage to aid secretion clearance

3. Antibiotic therapy (Table 34–4)

4. Investigate pleural effusions. Tube thoracostomy drainage if pleural fluid has quality of frank pus, microorganisms are identified on Gram's stain, or pH is less than 7.2.

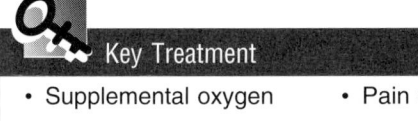

Key Treatment

- Supplemental oxygen
- Adequate hydration
- Pain control
- Antibiotic therapy

Follow-Up

1. With appropriate antibiotic therapy, improvement in clinical condition is noted in 48 to 72 hours; hence therapy should not be changed in the first 72 hours.

2. Fever and leukocytosis may persist for 4 days or longer with more severe infection.

3. Chest radiographic abnormalities may persist for 4 weeks or longer, depending on the pathogens involved.

4. When clinical and radiographic findings persist or the clinical condition worsens in the setting of antibiotic therapy, alternative pathogens or diagnoses should be considered.

Bibliography

For more information on the cause of acute pneumonia, see

Donowitz GR, Mandell GL: Acute pneumonia. *In* Mandell GL, Douglas RG Jr, Bennett JE (eds): Principles and Practice of Infectious Diseases, 3rd ed. New York, Churchill Livingstone, 1990, pp 540–555.

For more information on management of community-acquired pneumonia, see

Guidelines for the initial management of adults with community-acquired pneumonia: Diagnosis, assessment of severity, and initial antimicrobial therapy. Am Rev Respir Dis 1993;148:1418–1426.

For more information on lung infection in immunocompromised patients, see

Respiratory disease in the immunosuppressed patient. Ann Intern Med 1992;117(5):415–431.

For more information on atypical pneumonia syndromes, see

Winterbauer RH: Atypical pneumonia syndromes. Clin Chest Med 1991;12(2):203–213.

For general review of respiratory infections and their management, see

Niederman MS: Pneumonia: pathogenesis, diagnosis, and management. Med Clin N Am 1994;78.

35 Atelectasis

Krishnan Padmanabhan

Atelectasis means imperfect expansion and denotes a state of airlessness of the lung. Atelectasis is best defined as collapse or loss of volume of a lung, lobe, or segment.

Classification

1. Obstructive (resorption) atelectasis (most common)
2. Relaxation (passive) atelectasis
3. Contraction (cicatrization) atelectasis
4. Adhesive (nonobstructive—micro) atelectasis

Obstructive atelectasis occurs on occlusion of the main stem, lobar, or segmental bronchus by intraluminal obstruction or extrinsic bronchial compression. The involved portion diminishes in volume and becomes radiopaque as air distal to the obstruction is absorbed into the capillary blood, usually within 18 to 24 hours. Resorption rate is accelerated when a gas mixture containing a high concentration of oxygen is inspired. If concurrent transudation of capillary blood and fluid occurs, the volume loss is minimal or nil. The fluid-filled, airless lung appears intensely radiopaque, the "drowned lung." Adequate collateral alveolar ventilation and collateral air drift distal to the site of total bronchial occlusion can prevent atelectasis.

Relaxation atelectasis is the result of unopposed elastic recoil of the lung that occurs in the presence of an intrathoracic space-occupying lesion, such as pneumothorax or pleural effusion. The collapsed lung is not airless.

Contraction atelectasis occurs when pulmonary fibrosis leads to a diminution of lung volume and to radiopacification. In contrast to the uniform opacification of obstructive atelectasis, pockets of air trapped within fibrotic areas are often visible.

Adhesive atelectasis, or diffuse microatelectasis, is alveolar collapse due to intra-alveolar changes; occurs despite a patent bronchus. Although the mechanism is unclear, surfactant loss or dysfunction occurring after diffuse alveolar injury probably plays a dominant role. The resulting impairment of alveolar surface tension–lowering ability facilitates alveolar collapse. Continuous small tidal-volume breathing, low end-expiratory volume, and removal of alveolar nitrogen are other factors responsible for microatelectasis seen in low lung compliance states, postoperatively with diaphragmatic dysfunction, and during mechanical ventilation. Although peripheral, linear plate-like densities due to subsegmental atelectasis may be seen on the chest radiograph, volume loss without radiopacification is the hallmark. When diffuse radiopacification occurs, it is due to concomitant alveolar edema or the formation of hyaline membranes seen in diffuse alveolar injury states.

138

Etiology

A. Obstructive atelectasis
    1. Endobronchial obstruction
        a. Mucous plugs
            (1) Bronchial asthma
            (2) Allergic bronchopulmonary aspergillosis
            (3) Cystic fibrosis
            (4) Chronic bronchitis
            (5) Postoperative state
            (6) Postintubated state
        b. Endobronchial neoplasm
            (1) Bronchogenic carcinoma
                (a) Squamous cell
                (b) Small cell
            (2) Bronchial adenoma—carcinoid tumor
            (3) Endobronchial metastasis, primary
                (a) Kidney
                (b) Breast
                (c) Colon
            (4) Endobronchial lymphoma
        c. Foreign body
        d. Infection
            (1) Endobronchial tuberculosis
            (2) Broncholithiasis
                (a) Tuberculosis
                (b) Histoplasmosis
    2. Extrinsic bronchial compression
        a. Neoplasm
            (1) Lung carcinoma
                (a) Large cell
                (b) Adenocarcinoma
            (2) Mediastinal tumors
                (a) Thymoma
                (b) Teratoma
                (c) Germ cell tumors
        b. Cardiovascular—compression of left lower lobe bronchus by aneurysm of ascending aorta, by enlarged left atrium in mitral stenosis
    3. Trauma—tracheobronchial rupture secondary to blunt anterior chest wall injury
    4. Congenital—bronchial atresia: left upper lobe bronchus
    5. Tracheobronchial cartilage disorders
        Dynamic airway occlusion

a. From relapsing polychondritis

b. From tracheobronchomegaly

c. From tracheomalacia

B. Relaxation atelectasis

   1. Large pleural effusion

   2. Pneumothorax

   3. Expanding bullae

C. Contraction atelectasis
Pulmonary fibrosis caused by

   1. Tuberculosis

   2. Silicosis

   3. Sarcoidosis

D. Adhesive atelectasis

   1. Diffuse alveolar injury caused by

      a. Toxic fume inhalation

      b. Gastric acid aspiration

      c. Endotoxin injury

   2. Prolonged ventilatory support

Atelectasis from mucous plugging as in asthma and the postoperative state, airway occlusion from bronchogenic carcinoma, compression as a result of a large pleural effusion, and diffuse microatelectasis due to surfactant dysfunction constitute the more common causes of atelectasis. Extrinsic mass compression, endobronchial tuberculosis, and pulmonary fibrosis are less common causes, and congenital bronchial atresia, tracheobronchial rupture, and tracheobronchial cartilage disorders are rare causes.

Symptoms

1. Primarily those of the responsible underlying disease rather than atelectasis itself

2. Cough and exertional dyspnea from altered lung compliance and hypoxia

3. Dyspnea at rest when a whole lung collapses acutely

Key Symptoms

- Cough

- Exertional dyspnea

- Acute dyspnea at rest

Clinical Findings

Signs of atelectasis reflect the decreased ventilation in the involved area and the ipsilateral mediastinal shift as a result of the reduced lung volume. Hypoxia results from increased venous admixture because of perfusion of nonventilated alveoli. Reduced lung compliance leads to hyperventilation and respiratory alkalosis. Extensive atelectasis, however, can cause hypoventilation and respiratory acidosis.

Key Signs

- Decreased chest wall movement

- Impaired chest percussion note

- Decreased vocal fremitus

- Decreased vocal resonance

- Decreased or absent breath sounds

- Ipsilateral tracheal shift

- Tachypnea, tachycardia, hypoxia

- Hyperventilation and respiratory alkalosis

- Hypoventilation and respiratory acidosis

Tests

1. In most instances, diagnosis can be made by chest radiography. The lateral view is essential to recognize middle lobe and lingular atelectasis, whereas the apical lordotic view visualizes well the collapsed right middle lobe.

2. Not only can computed tomographic (CT) scanning establish the diagnosis of atelectasis, but it can also show the endobronchial tree, lung parenchyma, and the mediastinum and thereby help determine the cause.

3. Fiberoptic bronchoscopy under local anesthesia provides excellent visualization of the endobronchial tree, allowing for biopsy and aspiration of endobronchial and parabronchial lesions.

Diagnostic Chest Radiographic Signs

1. Major signs

   a. Displacement of the respective interlobar septum or fissure

   b. Radiopacity of the atelectatic segment, lobe, or entire lung

2. Minor signs

   a. Displacement of the hilum in the direction of the atelectatic lobe

   b. Ipsilateral shift of mediastinal structures (e.g., trachea and heart)

   c. Elevation of the ipsilateral hemidiaphragm

   d. Compensatory hyperaeration of the adjacent lung parenchyma

   e. Crowding of ribs due to a decrease in size of the thoracic cage

Demonstration of volume loss by adjoining interlobar septum or fissure displacement is essential to the diagnosis. Displacement of the hilum is also a useful sign of volume loss. The hilum is displaced upward in upper lobe atelectasis and downward in lower lobe atelectasis.

Right upper lobe atelectasis is best visualized on a posteroanterior (PA) chest radiograph as an inverted triangular opacity in the right upper zone. The minor fissure is displaced superiorly and medially.

Left upper lobe atelectasis is also best visualized on a PA chest radiograph. The opacity seen is less intense and less well demarcated and appears as a hazy density over the left upper and midzone that obliterates the left mediastinal and cardiac border. When the lingular bronchus is patent, the left cardiac border remains well defined.

Right middle lobe atelectasis is best seen on the lateral chest radiograph as a band density, formed by the displaced minor and major fissures, extending from the hilum to the base of the sternum. The collapsed right middle lobe appears as a paracardiac spiculated opacity on an apical lordotic chest radiograph.

Lower lobe atelectasis is best identified on a PA chest radiograph as a retrocardiac triangular opacity that obliterates the margin of the diaphragm. In the case of the left lower lobe, the outer margin of the descending thoracic aorta is also obscured. On the lateral view, the collapsed lower lobe is seen as a faint opacity in the paravertebral region and obscures the involved hemidiaphragm.

Right middle and *lower lobe atelectasis* is seen on the PA film as an opacity in the right midzone and base silhouetting the cardiac border and hemidiaphragm. On lateral view, the opacified atelectatic lung and adjoining cardiac shadow form a band density that extends across the chest, covering the midzones and base of the lung.

Total lung atelectasis is characterized by opacification of the entire hemithorax and marked ipsilateral shift of mediastinal structures.

Special Radiographic Signs

1. S sign of Golden—refers to the convex appearance of the outer margin of the atelectatic right upper lobe when the proximal portion of the displaced minor fissure is pushed outward by a tumor

2. Double lesion sign of Felson—refers to atelectasis of more than one lobe that cannot be explained by a single endobronchial occlusive lesion, as in right upper and right middle lobe atelectasis. This radiographic finding is suggestive of a non-neoplastic cause for the atelectasis.

3. Open bronchus sign of Felson—refers to atelectasis in the presence of a patent proximal airway and confirms a non-neoplastic cause

4. Comet tail sign is seen in round atelectasis—a lesion that presents as a round or helical pleural-based density, densest at its periphery, with contiguous pleural thickening. The regional bronchovascular structures can be seen bundled together and curving into the mass resembling a comet tail. This "comet tail" sign is best visualized on CT scanning, which often also demonstrates an air bronchogram in the central part of the mass and oligemic hyperinflated parenchyma adjacent to the mass. Pleural thickening and fibrosis, as seen in asbestosis, causing contraction of adjacent lung parenchyma, and lung tissue initially compressed

by pleural effusion and later becoming adherent to the parietal pleura, are possible mechanisms for the development of round atelectasis.

Key Tests

- Chest radiography—posteroanterior, lateral, and apical lordotic views

- Computed tomographic scan of the chest

- Fiberoptic bronchoscopy

Differential Diagnosis

1. Encapsulated pleural effusion
2. Displaced or dilated right brachiocephalic vein
3. Left pulmonary ligament abnormalities
4. Bronchogenic carcinoma in patients with round atelectasis

Interlobular effusion in the right major fissure can resemble right middle lobe atelectasis on a lateral chest radiograph. A loculated pleural effusion can mimic right middle and lower lobe atelectasis on a PA chest radiograph. A displaced or dilated right brachiocephalic vein can appear on the PA film as atelectasis of the right upper lobe, especially when the minor fissure is not seen. Thickening of or fluid accumulation in the left pulmonary ligament can be misdiagnosed as left lower lobe atelectasis on a PA radiograph. Bronchogenic carcinoma and round atelectasis resemble each other on the conventional chest radiograph. In most instances, additional chest radiographic views and CT scanning of the chest will establish the diagnosis.

Treatment

Lung expansion is best achieved by treating the underlying disease and correcting the mechanisms responsible for volume loss. Modalities include the following:

1. Chest physiotherapy—to facilitate high-volume breaths and the expectoration of airway secretions. It is both preventive and therapeutic, especially in critically ill patients and postoperative state, and includes the following:

   a. Effective pain relief and deep-breathing exercises

   b. Use of the incentive spirometer

   c. Bronchodilator therapy

   d. Postural drainage and chest percussion

   e. Nasotracheal suctioning

   f. Humidification of inspired air

   g. Use of mucolytic agents, such as iodinated glycerol, by mouth or nebulized acetylcysteine (Mucomyst) or recombinant human DNase (Dornase Alfa)

   h. Possible use of nebulized or intratracheally instilled artificial surfactant in diffuse microatelectasis

i. Endotracheal intubation to facilitate vigorous airway suctioning with isotonic saline solution instilled into airways

The role of mucolytic agents is not clear. Acetylcysteine (Mucomyst) can cause bronchospasm. The use of Dornase Alfa to cleave extracellular DNA from degenerating polymorphonuclear cells and to convert the gelatinous sputum to a more liquid form has shown promise in patients with cystic fibrosis.

2. Positive pressure breathing

   a. Continuous positive airway pressure by face mask

   b. Positive end-expiratory pressure in patients on mechanical ventilation

These techniques enable the recruitment of alveoli in states of diffuse microatelectasis and thereby increase functional residual capacity, help prevent atelectasis, and improve gas exchange. Positive pressure of 5 to 10 cm H_2O is usually adequate. The risks of positive-pressure breathing, such as barotrauma, hypotension, gastric distention, and aspiration, are the drawbacks.

3. Bronchoscopy

   a. Fiberoptic—indication is re-expansion of lung in recurrent atelectasis, especially in postintubated states; also used for foreign-body removal

   b. Rigid—method of choice for endobronchial foreign-body removal

4. Surgery—removal of the resectable neoplasm by thoracotomy

5. Endoscopic laser therapy

   a. Curative for benign endobronchial neoplasm

   b. Palliative for nonresectable malignant tumors

6. Radiotherapy—may restore airway patency in radiosensitive tumors. In most patients, the intent of radiation is palliation.

7. Chemotherapy—most effective in re-establishing airway patency in lymphoma and small-cell carcinoma

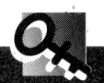

Key Treatment

- Chest physiotherapy
- Positive-pressure breathing

Bibliography

Celli BR: Physiologic and mechanical aids to lung expansion. Clin Chest Med 1993;14(2):257–260.

Gamsu G: Atelectasis and bronchial obstruction. In Moss A, Gamsu G, Genant HC (eds): Computed Tomography of the Body, 2nd ed, vol 1. Philadelphia, WB Saunders, 1992, pp 27–32.

Goldin JA, Wang KP, Keith FM: Intensive care and fiberoptic bronchoscopy, foreign body removal and laser therapy. In Murray JM, Nadel JA (eds): Textbook of Respiratory Medicine, 2nd ed, vol 1. Philadelphia, WB Saunders, 1994, pp 737–769.

Parenchymal atelectasis. In Fraser RG, Pare JAP, Pare PD, et al (eds): Diagnosis of Diseases of the Chest, 3rd ed, vol 1. Philadelphia, WB Saunders, 1988, pp 472–537.

Webb WR: Atelectasis. In Rakel RE (ed): Conn's Current Therapy. Philadelphia, WB Saunders, 1994, pp 157–159.

36 Pulmonary Embolus

Diane L. Dietzen

Etiology

1. Pulmonary embolus indicates lodging of embolic material in the pulmonary circulation. The most common material is thrombus from a distant site, although fat and foreign material can also be embolized. Pulmonary infarction is more rare and a result of complete occlusion of the circulation to an area without usual pulmonary collateral circulation.

2. Risk factors for pulmonary embolus are risk factors for the creation of thrombi in the circulation: stasis, hypercoagulability, and vascular damage. Prevention of these risks can prevent deep venous thrombosis and pulmonary embolus. Of the 650,000 cases that occur each year, about 50,000 result in death.

Risk Factors

- Surgery, especially orthopedic surgery; other major surgery
- Immobilization
- Cancer
- Prior deep venous thrombosis
- Congestive heart failure
- Pregnancy
- Hypercoagulable states, including lupus anticoagulant, nephrotic syndrome, polycythemia, and inherited antithrombin 3, protein C, and protein S deficiencies

3. Most emboli arise from the deep veins of the thigh. Other rare sources include the arms, pelvis, renal veins, and right side of the heart. The veins of the calves form thrombi that seldom cause emboli.

Symptoms

1. Chest pain occurs in 80 to 90 per cent of cases. The pain is most classically described as pleuritic, but it can be of any character and in any location in the chest.

2. Dyspnea is another common symptom. It is classically described as acute in onset.

3. Other symptoms include hemoptysis, palpitations, and a feeling of apprehension.

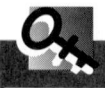

Key Symptoms

• Chest pain	• Dyspnea

Clinical Findings

1. Tachypnea (rapid respiratory rate) is the most common finding in a patient with pulmonary embolus and is found in most cases.

2. Lung examination findings of pulmonary embolus vary. The patient can have a normal lung examination, some localized wheezing or consolidation, or evidence of a pleural rub.

3. Atrial arrhythmias can be found as well as signs of congestive heart failure.

4. Signs of distal deep venous thrombosis. Looking for evidence of distal thrombosis that may have been the origin of pulmonary embolus is important in all patients with pulmonary embolus. Examination of the legs for edema, erythema, pain, or palpable vein cords is important, as is evaluation of the arms, abdomen, and pelvis.

5. Although these symptoms and clinical findings are found in patients with pulmonary embolus, no one symptom or clinical finding is diagnostic of this problem, and a high index of suspicion must be maintained to correctly pursue the diagnosis.

Key Signs

- Tachypnea
- Deep venous thrombosis

Tests

1. Arterial blood gas analysis should be done when pulmonary embolus is suspected. Hypoxia should be looked for as well as an elevated A-a gradient. These values are often normal, and if abnormal, they are not diagnostic of a pulmonary embolus. The most common finding on arterial blood gas analysis is decreased PCO_2 due to tachypnea.

2. Electrocardiography is done predominantly to look for cardiac causes of chest pain. Pulmonary embolus can produce nonspecific ST- or T-wave changes or, occasionally, evidence of strain of the right side of the heart with an incomplete right bundle branch block or an $S_1/Q_3/T_3$ pattern.

3. Chest radiography is obtained to rule out other causes of chest pain and dyspnea. The findings with pulmonary embolus are usually not a normal chest radiography; however, abnormalities are nonspecific. Occasionally, a small, wedge-shaped density indicative of a pulmonary infarct or a cutoff sign in a major vessel is seen, which increases the suspicion of pulmonary embolus.

4. Other laboratory testing commonly done on admission to the hospital is often not helpful in the diagnosis of pulmonary embolus. A baseline prothrombin time and activated partial thromboplastin time can be ordered.

5. Ventilation-perfusion (V/Q) scan. If after the initial assessment and the laboratory values discussed above, suspicion for a pulmonary embolus remains high, V/Q scanning should be pursued. V/Q scanning is done by having the patient inhale radiolabeled xenon gas and injecting radiolabeled technetium into the blood. This allows concomitant viewing of the pulmonary circulation and pulmonary ventilation, looking for areas of ventilation and perfusion mismatch. Diagnostic criteria for pulmonary embolus and V/Q scanning are best outlined by the Prospective Investigation of Pulmonary Embolism Diagnosis (PIOPED) study, although all interpretations are somewhat subjective and must be compared with clinical data. See Table 36–1 for common readings of V/Q scans and the subsequent likelihood of pulmonary embolus. Patients with low- or intermediate-probability V/Q scans still have a significant likelihood of developing pulmonary embolus. Few complications are associated with V/Q scanning.

6. Lower-extremity studies
   a. Doppler studies are the most reliable of a number of tests done noninvasively on the lower extremities to evaluate for thrombosis. As noted previously, the proximal leg is one of the most common sources of pulmonary emboli, and if thrombus is present in these veins, management is the same as if a pulmonary embolus were discovered. For this reason, if V/Q scanning is indeterminate and the results of Doppler studies are positive, anticoagulation can be done without further evaluation. Serial impedance plethysmography has also been used to detect deep venous thrombosis.
   b. Venography. In circumstances where Doppler studies or impedance plethysmography is unavailable or unreliable, consideration may need to be given to venography for detection of deep venous thrombosis. Lower-extremity Doppler

studies have few complications, but venography has a small incidence of dye reaction and venous thrombosis.

7. Pulmonary arteriography is the gold standard in the diagnosis of pulmonary emboli. The procedure is done by placing a catheter from the femoral vein into the pulmonary circulation and injecting small amounts of dye, looking for a filling defect or occlusion of a vessel by thrombus. Pulmonary arteriography should be done on those patients whose V/Q scans are not normal but of low, intermediate, or high probability when there is a need to make the definitive diagnosis. Complications of pulmonary arteriography include arrhythmia, dye reactions, and renal failure. Major complications occur in about 1 per cent of cases.

8. Echocardiography has been suggested as another method of assessing the presence of thrombus traveling to the pulmonary circulation or resulting in pulmonary hypertension. It may be of use in determining the subsequent therapy.

9. D-Dimer, a crosslink fibrin degradation product, has been studied as a possible indicator of pulmonary embolus. It may be useful in cases where it is low because it is sensitive for ongoing thrombosis and thrombolysis. It is not commonly used clinically.

10. In the appropriate clinical setting, evaluations for hypercoagulable states could be considered, including measurement of protein C, protein S, and antithrombin III levels and anticardiolipin antibody.

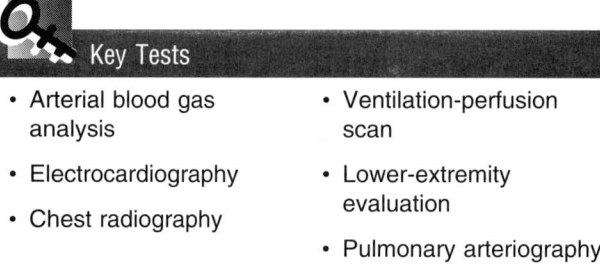

Key Tests

- Arterial blood gas analysis
- Electrocardiography
- Chest radiography
- Ventilation-perfusion scan
- Lower-extremity evaluation
- Pulmonary arteriography

Differential Diagnosis

1. Cardiac and vascular disease. Ischemic cardiac chest pain as well as chest pain of pericarditis can be mistaken for pulmonary embolus pain. Also, dissecting aortic aneurysm should remain in a differential of chest pain and shortness of breath.

2. Other pulmonary pathology. Pneumonia, pneumothorax, pleuritis, and pleural effusions can all produce similar pain and dyspnea.

3. Chest wall pain may be described as pleuritic and may produce a sensation of shortness of breath. A careful physical examination helps to evaluate this cause.

4. Gastrointestinal disorders. Esophageal rupture, gastritis, gastric ulcer, and duodenal ulcer can all produce atypical chest pain and should be considered.

TABLE 36–1. PIOPED DATA

V/Q READING	PERCENTAGE WITH POSITIVE ANGIOGRAPHY RESULTS
High probability	88
Intermediate probability	33
Low probability	12–16
Normal/near normal	4–9

Data from The PIOPED Investigators. Value of the ventilation/perfusion scan in acute pulmonary embolism. JAMA 1990;263:2753–2759.

Treatment

Medication

1. Thrombolytic therapy has been used in some patients with pulmonary embolus, but there is no evidence that it decreases morbidity or mortality. It is used in patients who are hemodynamically unstable secondary to pulmonary embolus. Patients with thrombus in the right ventricle on echocardiography or evidence of severe strain of the right side of the heart may also be candidates. Various lytic therapies have been used, including urokinase, streptokinase, and tissue plasminogen activator.

2. Heparin should be considered the drug of choice in the initial therapy of pulmonary embolus. Although it does not resolve the existing clot, it does allow the body to resolve that clot and prevents further emboli. Heparin therapy should be started at the time of suspicion of a pulmonary embolus if there are no contraindications to anticoagulation. It is empiric, and doses are adjusted to maintain activated partial thromboplastin time between 1.5 and 2.5 times control. Heparinoids, including hirudin, and dextran have been studied but are not drugs of choice. Heparin therapy should be continued for 5 to 7 days.

3. Coumadin is considered the drug of choice for the long-term therapy of pulmonary embolus. Therapy should be started 1 to 2 days after the initiation of heparin therapy. Coumadin dosing is also empiric, doses being given to maintain the prothrombin time with an international normalized ratio (INR) of two to three.

4. For patients who have contraindications to anticoagulation, various mechanical filtering devices have been developed that can be placed in the abdominal vena cava to prevent the transmission of clots from the distal extremities to the pulmonary circulation. A minor procedure is required for insertion, and they have a low complication rate. Collateral circulation eventually allows new pathways for pulmonary emboli.

The choices between the therapies above are made based on the presentation of the patient, hemodynamic stability, indications and contraindications to anticoagulation, and the patient's ability to comply with anticoagulation therapy as an outpatient. Pregnant women have a separate set of therapeutic considerations because they are normally given heparin rather than coumadin. The mortality rate decreases 75 per cent with therapy.

5. Length of therapy. Therapy for a documented pulmonary embolus is continued for at least 3 months after the event. Length of therapy after that time is based on the patient's risk factors and the likelihood of recurrent emboli as well as the risks for anticoagulation.

Activity

Patients are generally restricted to bed rest during the first 2 to 3 days of therapy for pulmonary embolus. After that time, they are ambulated gradually.

Patient Education

Patients need to be educated about the risk factors for pulmonary embolus, the underlying pathophysiology, the need for monitoring for recurrence, and the need for compliance with long-term anticoagulation therapy.

Key Treatment

- Heparin IV (drug of choice)
- Long-term coumadin therapy

Follow-Up

Follow-up is done over the long term to monitor for recurrence. With continued occurrences, evaluations for an underlying hypercoagulable state or cancer can be considered.

Bibliography

For more information about symptoms of pulmonary embolus, see

Bell WR, Simon TL, DeMets DL: The clinical features of submassive and massive pulmonary embolus. Am J Med 1977;62:355–360.

For more information about V/Q scans, see

PIOPED Investigators: Value of the ventilation/perfusion scan in acute pulmonary embolism. JAMA 1990;263:2753–2758.

For more information on all aspects of pulmonary embolus, see

Carson JL, Kelley MA, Duff A: The clinical course of pulmonary embolism. N Engl J Med 1992;326:1240–1245.

Goldhaber S, Morpuge M for the WHO/ISFC Task Force on Pulmonary Embolism: Diagnosis, treatment and prevention of pulmonary embolism. JAMA 1992;268:1727–1733.

Kelley MA, Abbuhl S: Massive pulmonary embolism. Clin Chest Med 1994;3:547–557.

37 Acute Respiratory Distress Syndrome

Evan Steinberg

Acute respiratory distress syndrome (ARDS) is difficult to define. It has many causes and varied complexities. It usually develops suddenly and is characterized by severe dyspnea, hypoxemia, diffuse pulmonary infiltrates, and stiff lungs, which follow massive acute lung injury. This often occurs in the absence of prior lung disease. ARDS is characterized by proteinaceous pulmonary edema.

Murray proposed a scoring system assessing the cause and aspects of lung injury as a definition of ARDS. Determinants of the lung injury score include the chest radiograph, the PaO_2/FiO_2 ratio, lung compliance, and the level of positive end-expiratory pressure (PEEP) used.

Etiology

Direct pulmonary trauma and/or indirect injury by way of shock of any cause can be the precipitating event.

1. Drug-related—chlordiazepoxide (Librium), colchicine (Colsalide), dextran 40 (Gentran 40), ethchlorvynol (Placidyl), fluorescein, heroin, leukagglutinin reaction, methadone, propoxyphene, salicylates, thiazides
2. Infectious
   a. Mycobacterial
   b. Pneumonia, including bacterial, fungal, viral, and *Pneumocystis carinii*
   c. Gram-negative sepsis
3. Physiochemical
   a. Diabetic ketoacidosis
   b. Inhaled toxin (nitrogen dioxide, ammonia, chlorine, cadmium, phosgene, smoke, oxygen)
   c. Near drowning
   d. Pancreatitis
   e. Uremia
4. Trauma
   a. Burns
   b. Fractures (fat embolism)
   c. Head trauma (neurogenic)
   d. Lung contusion
   e. Shock of any cause
5. Miscellaneous
   a. Amniotic fluid embolus
   b. Bowel infarction
   c. Eclampsia
   d. High altitude
6. Chronic infiltrative pulmonary diseases, such as interstitial pneumonitis and fibrosis, and left ventricular failure should be excluded.

Symptoms and Signs

1. Clinically, ARDS is manifested by tachypnea (respiratory rates typically greater than 20 per minute) and evidence of labored breathing, such as the use of accessory muscles and intercostal retractions. Radiographic abnormalities are nonspecific and include a normal examination that rapidly progresses to interstitial and later diffuse alveolar infiltration.

Key Symptom

- Tachypnea

2. Physiologic abnormalities focus on deranged oxygen transport. Overall compliance is reduced. Shunt fraction (often greater than 30 per cent) and dead-space ventilation (frequently greater than 60 per cent) are markedly increased.

Key Signs

- Interstitial infiltration
- Diffuse alveolar infiltration
- Deranged oxygen transport

Pathophysiology

The mechanisms of lung injury are difficult to define because ARDS is probably an end-stage manifestation of the pathogenetic process. The initial injury precedes the development of edema and hypoxemia, and later it is difficult to distinguish cause from effect.

1. Pulmonary edema in the presence of low left-sided heart pressures characterizes ARDS, which has been termed noncardiogenic pulmonary edema. Here, it is inferred that exchange vessels in the lung are leaking excessively and the lung vascular permeability is increased.
2. Gram-negative endotoxin or bacterial infusion, pulmonary oxygen toxicity, and ARDS increase lung vascular permeability.
3. Most acute lung injury models have demonstrated increased pulmonary neutrophil retention coincident with increased permeability. The neutrophil is equipped with substances that are directly toxic to tissue and amplify any existing inflammatory response.
4. Pulmonary hypertension is a characteristic of most acute lung injury models. Pulmonary hypertension in ARDS occurs as a spectrum, mild to severe, with

variable hemodynamic consequences that are influenced by the presence of pre-existing ischemic heart disease and/or pulmonary disease. Most diseases with which ARDS is associated are characterized by increased peripheral oxygen requirements. Inadequate oxygen availability results in anaerobic metabolism, which inefficiently satisfies adenosine triphosphate requirements; therefore, increased quantities of lactate are generated. A protracted imbalance between peripheral oxygen requirement and availability may be a contributing factor leading to multiorgan dysfunction syndrome. With an abrupt increase in pulmonary artery pressure, cardiac output may fall as right ventricular failure supervenes. The level at which increased pulmonary artery pressure significantly affects oxygen delivery in ARDS has not been determined. It is likely that hemodynamic compensation in ARDS is inadequate beyond a mean pulmonary artery pressure of 35 to 40 mm Hg.

5. The sequelae of peripheral interstitial edema in ARDS are many. Of particular importance is the possibility that interstitial edema may reduce cellular oxygen availability. ARDS is associated with an oxygen extraction defect whereby there is an apparent increase in the critical oxygen delivery threshold. Normally, oxygen consumption remains constant at a level determined by the tissue metabolic activity. If oxygen delivery decreases below the critical threshold, oxygen consumption becomes linearly dependent on oxygen delivery. In ARDS, both the critical threshold and the efficiency of oxygen extraction at any oxygen delivery may become abnormal. The reason for this includes hypoperfusion of capillaries in areas of high oxygen consumption and a limitation to the molecular diffusion of oxygen.

6. Changes in lung mechanics, specifically decreased lung compliance, and a decreased functional residual capacity are typical of ARDS. The increased resistance to airflow and decreased lung compliance may result in abnormal distribution of ventilation, disturbing the matching of ventilation to perfusion and contributing to hypoxemia.

7. Acute functional abnormalities result from the progressive accumulation of extravascular fluid in the lung. This fluid results from damage to the endothelial and epithelial membranes. The sequence of extravascular fluid accumulation in the lung is well described. The progression is similar independent of the cause of the edema. Earliest is the appearance of fluid in the loose connective tissue that surrounds the airways and pulmonary arteries. This area is most vulnerable because pressures in this region are negative relative to the alveolar wall interstitium. Initially, excess fluid is removed by lymphatic drainage, but with continued accumulation, this mechanism is overwhelmed and, eventually, there is flooding of the alveolar wall interstitium, followed by fluid spilling into the alveoli. This results in alveolar instability with increased surface forces and the alveolus fills completely, collapsing to a new volume. The consequence of these events on gas exchange depends on the stage of accumulation. Interstitial edema itself is unlikely to significantly interfere with gas transfer. Changes in the distribution of ventilation and blood flow occur with the onset of alveolar flooding. The hypoxemia of ARDS is primarily a sequela of the final stage of alveolar flooding, or pulmonary edema.

Treatment

There is no curative treatment.

1. Treat the initiating process.

2. It is imperative to maintain tissue oxygenation by improving gas exchange and blood flow. Therapeutic measures include the use of supplemental oxygen and mechanical ventilation and improvement of cardiac output.

3. The mechanism of improved gas exchange with mechanical ventilation is the increased lung volume achieved with increases in alveolar size. This spreads the liquid in the alveolus over a greater surface area and allows gas to enter the alveolus. PEEP maintains positive pressure throughout the respiratory cycle; it does not decrease extravascular water.

4. PEEP produces the following effects:
   a. Decreases the percentage of cardiac output distributed to the shunt compartment
   b. Creates units with high ventilation/perfusion ratios (because of overventilation or the diversion of blood flow from relatively normal lung units) in some patients
   c. Increases dead space caused by increased lung volume, creating zone 1 conditions (where alveolar pressure is greater than arterial pressure)
   d. Reduces shunt fraction by increasing functional residual capacity

5. Increase functional residual capacity which improves compliance

6. The major beneficial effect of PEEP on the arterial Po_2 clearly results from shunt reduction. The primary source of shunt reduction is increased alveolar volume. As PEEP increases, cardiac output decreases.

7. PEEP should not be used in patients whose acute respiratory failure is due to emphysema, chronic bronchitis, or asthma except when it is complicated by ARDS because these patients already have increased functional residual capacity, high lung compliance, and little intrapulmonary shunting. PEEP may precipitate barotrauma and depression of cardiac output, particularly in patients with bullous emphysema.

8. Reduction of PEEP should be attempted in a stable

patient with an FiO_2 less than 40 per cent, an adequate PaO_2, and an effective compliance greater than 25.

9. Fluid balance is important in patients with ARDS, and they should be kept as dry as possible without sacrificing oxygen delivery.

Key Treatment

- Treat initiating process
- Maintain tissue oxygenation through supplemental oxygen and mechanical ventilation

Prognosis

1. Overall mortality approaches 60 per cent.
2. Most survivors have few sequelae.

Bibliography

Bone RC: ARDS. *In* Bone RC, et al: Pulmonary and Critical Care Medicine, vol 2, pt R. St Louis, Mosby—Year Book, 1993, pp 1–9.

Bone RC: The pathogenesis of sepsis. Ann Intern Med 1991;115:457–469.

Lechin AE, Varon J: Adult respiratory distress syndrome (ARDS): the basics. J Emerg Med 1994;12:63–68.

Lewis JF, Jobe AH: Surfactant and the adult respiratory distress syndrome. Am Rev Respir Dis 1993;147:218–233.

Murray JF, Matthay MA, Luce J, et al: An expanded definition of ARDS. Am Rev Respir Dis 1988;138:720–723.

Procedure **ENDOTRACHEAL INTUBATION**   *Michael J. Freeland*

Indications

1. To facilitate mechanical ventilatory support in patients with respiratory failure
2. To ensure a patent airway in patients with or at risk of airway obstruction
3. To protect the bronchial tree from aspiration when airway reflexes are inadequate
4. To facilitate pulmonary toilet by providing a route for tracheal suctioning

Contraindications

1. Inadequate skill or training of the operator
2. Ability to manage the airway adequately without resort to intubation
3. Extensive facial, oropharyngeal, or laryngeal injury or instability of the cervical spine

Preparation

1. Anticipate a difficult intubation in a patient with a history of prior difficult intubation, an anatomic anomaly of the head or neck, or limited cervical mobility. A patient with a full stomach also requires special consideration to reduce the risk of aspiration.
2. Clear the airway of any foreign material (including dentures, bridges), and preoxygenate the patient with 100 per cent oxygen by mask for 5 to 6 minutes, as time permits. If spontaneous ventilation is absent and intubation cannot be performed immediately, place the patient supine, properly position the head (head-tilt/chin-lift), insert an oropharyngeal or a nasopharyngeal airway if necessary, and ventilate manually with a bag-valve mask. An assistant should apply cricoid pressure (Sellick maneuver) to prevent gastric insufflation and reduce the possibility of regurgitation and aspiration of gastric contents.
3. Confirm that all basic airway management equipment and a suction apparatus are available (see Equipment). Select an appropriately sized laryngoscope blade and endotracheal tube. A size 3 MacIntosh blade (curved) is used most often for the average-sized adult, but a size 4 may be required for adults with a long tongue. A size 2 or 3 Miller blade (straight) is usually appropriate for the average adult. Although most adults can easily accommodate a tube with an inside diameter of 8 mm (men, 8 to 9 mm; women, 7 to 8 mm), smaller-diameter tubes (6 to 7 mm) should be available in the event that the larger tube cannot be passed. The tube cuff should be tested for integrity and the laryngoscope checked to make sure the light source is working.
4. Establish intravenous access with an 18-gauge catheter and a line for infusion of normal saline or lactated Ringer's solution. A separate line should be available for administration of medications.
5. Draw up all potentially necessary drugs into syringes and clearly label (see Anesthesia).
6. Place the patient on a cardiac monitor, if possible, and closely monitor the blood pressure with a cuff or an intra-arterial catheter. Pulse oximetry should be used if available.
7. Have available a properly equipped crash cart and personnel who can perform cardiopulmonary resuscitation and/or advanced cardiac life support and can assist in manipulating the airway, suctioning, and observing monitors.

Equipment

1. Bag-valve mask ventilation device with oxygen source attachment and assorted mask sizes
2. Suction apparatus, rigid pharyngeal suction tip (Yankauer), and soft tracheal suction catheter
3. Oropharyngeal (Guedel or Berman) and nasopharyngeal airways, assorted sizes, two each
4. Endotracheal tubes, assorted sizes, two each; soft metal endotracheal tube stylets
5. Laryngoscope handles, two; Miller and MacIntosh laryngoscope blades, assorted sizes
6. Syringes, 10-ml, two, for cuff inflation
7. Magill forceps for removal of foreign material or to direct the tip of the endotracheal tube
8. Water-soluble lidocaine (2%) jelly for lubrication of the endotracheal tube and stylet
9. Tape and skin preparation solution to secure the endotracheal tube

Anesthesia

1. For unconscious orotracheal intubation, no drugs are required. Laryngoscopy with cricoid pressure, intubation, and ventilation should be performed as quickly as possible.
2. Rapid-sequence induction (crash intubation) is used in the conscious patient to decrease the risk of active regurgitation and aspiration during orotracheal intubation. This is accomplished by the simultaneous (rapid-sequence) intravenous administration of a rapid-onset, short-acting muscle relaxant and sedative hypnotic with or without a narcotic analgesic.
   a. Thiopental, 2 to 5 mg/kg intravenously. A lower initial dose (25 to 50 mg intravenously, repeated at 1- to 2-minute intervals) is recommended for patients with limited cardiovascular reserve.
   b. Succinylcholine, 1.0 to 1.5 mg/kg intravenously
   c. Optional agents (administered before the above)
      (1) Vecuronium or pancuronium, 1 mg intravenously, to prevent succinylcholine-induced fasciculations
      (2) Fentanyl, 25 to 50 μg intravenously (repeated in 1 minute if necessary), or morphine for analgesia
      (3) Lidocaine, 1 mg/kg intravenously, if intracranial pressure is increased or severe reactive airway disease is present
3. Intubation of the awake patient, using the combina-

tion of a topical anesthetic, mild sedation, and an analgesic, is advantageous because it allows the patient to remain awake and breathe spontaneously and leaves airway reflexes intact.

   a. Benzocaine (20%) aerosol can be used to anesthetize the tongue and posterior pharynx.

   b. Thiopental or a benzodiazepine (midazolam [Versed]) can be used to achieve sedation.

   c. Fentanyl and morphine are commonly used analgesics.

Precautions

1. Laryngoscopy and intubation are powerful stimuli to the autonomic nervous system and can result in hemodynamic instability, which may be detrimental to a patient with cardiovascular or cerebrovascular disease or raised intracranial pressure.

2. Drugs used to facilitate intubation may have adverse hemodynamic, neurologic, and metabolic effects that require continuous observation of any patient to whom they are administered.

3. Positive-pressure ventilation can precipitate hypotension by reducing venous return to the heart.

> **WARNING**
>
> **Endotracheal intubation should be performed only by properly trained personnel. Muscle relaxants should be used only by those experienced in their use and highly skilled in airway management.**

Technique

1. Align the oral, pharyngeal, and laryngeal axes by extending the head at the atlanto-occipital joint and flexing the neck (''sniffing'' position). A folded towel under the occiput elevates it a few inches above the level of the bed and provides proper flexion of the neck. Extension of the head is effected later when upward traction is exerted on the handle of the laryngoscope.

to bring the larynx into view. This maneuver is maintained until proper placement of the endotracheal tube is clinically ascertained.

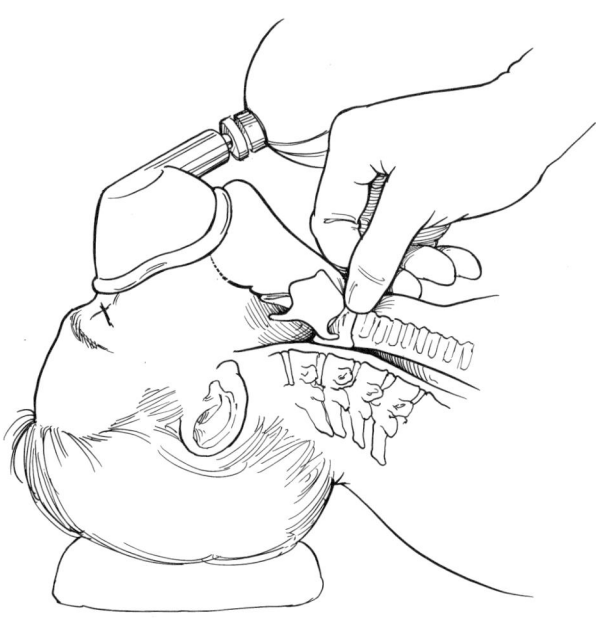

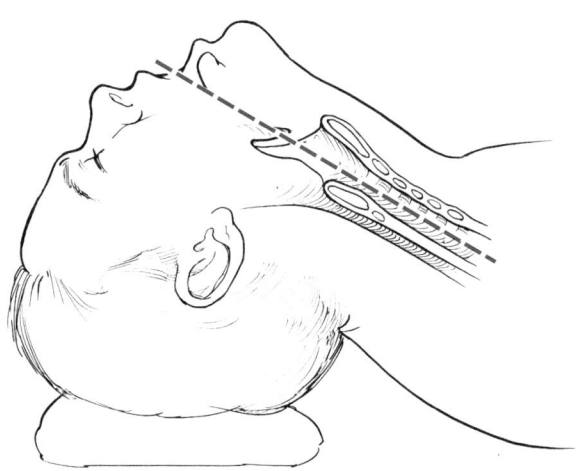

2. Sellick maneuver. Have an assistant apply backward pressure to the anterolateral rim of the cricoid cartilage with the thumb and index finger. In addition to occluding the esophagus, this maneuver often helps

3. With the laryngoscope in the left hand, open the mouth with the fingers of the right hand and insert the blade into the right side of the mouth. Advance the blade midline to the base of the tongue, sweeping the tongue leftward. If a curved blade is used, its tip should be inserted into the vallecula.

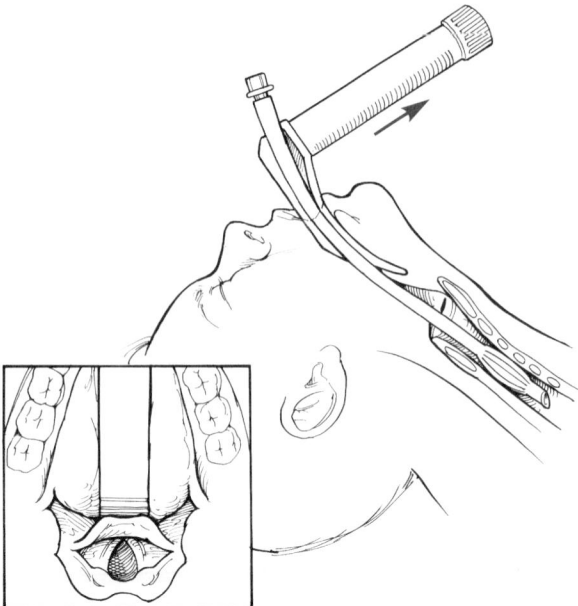

If a straight blade is used, its tip should be positioned below the epiglottis.

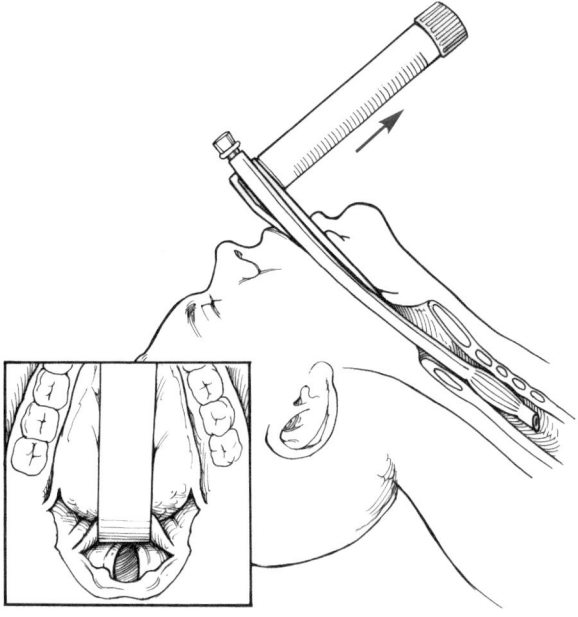

4. Lift the handle of the laryngoscope upward and forward to expose the vocal cords, avoiding pressure on the lips and teeth or entrapment of the tongue between the blade and teeth.

5. With the right hand, pass the lubricated endotracheal tube through the right corner of the mouth and advance the tip through the vocal cords under direct visualization. If the larynx is located very anterior, a curved stylet (lubricated before insertion into the tube) can aid in directing the tip to the glottic opening. When the proximal end of the cuff is at the level of the cords, the stylet should be removed and the tube advanced an additional 1 to 3 cm into the trachea before the cuff is inflated with just enough air to prevent a leak during positive-pressure ventilation. As a rule, the tube should be near the 23-cm mark at the front incisors in men and near the 21-cm mark in women for proper positioning of the tip 3 to 4 cm above the carina.

6. Assess the patient for proper tube placement. This is ascertained clinically by observation of symmetric chest expansion and auscultation of equal breath sounds during ventilation. Diminished breath sounds on the left may indicate intubation of the right mainstem bronchus (left mainstem bronchus intubation is uncommon). The epigastrium should also be auscultated. Loud, gurgling sounds with ventilation indicate esophageal intubation and require immediate removal of the tube. A rising arterial oxygen saturation by pulse oximetry and/or demonstration of a significant quantity of carbon dioxide return on exhalation by capnography is useful in confirming tracheal intubation.

7. Secure the tube with tape to the skin over the maxilla, a nonmovable body part. If the patient has a beard or facial dressings, the tube may be tied in position with cloth twill tape or intravenous tubing, making sure that the tie loops over the ears after it is brought around the neck.

Follow-Up
1. Obtain a chest radiograph to confirm the proper depth of tube placement.
2. Check the intracuff pressure with a manometer, and adjust the volume to maintain pressure below 15 to 20 mm Hg. A pressure above 25 to 30 mm Hg should be avoided to prevent mucosal ischemia and pressure necrosis.

 ## Bibliography

Benumof JL: Management of the difficult adult airway with special emphasis on awake tracheal intubation. Anesthesiology 1991;75:1087–1110.

Hee MKJ, Plevak DJ, Peters SG: Intubation of critically ill patients. Mayo Clin Proc 1992;67:569–576.

Kaplan JD, Schuster DP: Physiologic consequences of tracheal intubation. Clin Chest Med 1991;12:425–432.

Sharar SR, Bishop MJ: Complications of tracheal intubation. J Intensive Care Med 1992;7:12–23.

Stauffer JL: Medical management of the airway. Clin Chest Med 1991;12:449–482.

38 Acute Pulmonary Edema

Joseph L. Micca

Etiology

1. Imbalance of Starling forces
   a. Increased pulmonary capillary pressure ("cardiogenic" pulmonary edema)
   b. Decreased intravascular oncotic pressure
   c. Increased interstitial oncotic pressure (unknown clinical or experimental example)
2. Altered alveolocapillary membrane permeability
   a. Infection
   b. Toxins
      (1) Inhaled (e.g., phosgene, ozone, chlorine, Teflon fumes, nitrogen dioxide, smoke)
      (2) Circulating exogenous substances (e.g., snake venom, bacterial endotoxin)
      (3) Endogenous vasoactive substances (e.g., histamine, hypersensitivity pneumonitis)
   c. Aspiration of acidic gastric contents
   d. Acute radiation pneumonitis
   e. Disseminated intravascular coagulation
   f. Shock lung in association with nonthoracic trauma
   g. Acute hemorrhagic pancreatitis
3. Lymphatic insufficiency
   a. Post lung transplantation
   b. Lymphangitic carcinomatosis
   c. Fibrosing lymphangitis (e.g., silicosis)
4. Unknown or incompletely understood
   a. High-altitude pulmonary edema
   b. Neurogenic pulmonary edema
   c. Narcotic overdose
   d. Pulmonary embolism
   e. Eclampsia
   f. Post cardioversion
   g. Post anesthesia
   h. Post cardiopulmonary bypass

Symptoms

1. General
   a. Dyspnea
   b. Feeling of impending doom—anxiety
   c. Diaphoresis
   d. Tachycardia
   e. Cool and clammy extremities with high, low, or normal blood pressure
   f. Pink, frothy sputum production
2. Other symptoms, depending on cause (e.g., chest pain, palpitations)

Key Symptoms

- Severe dyspnea
- Tachycardia
- Pink, frothy sputum
- Anxiety
- Diaphoresis

Clinical Findings

1. General
   a. Tachypnea
   b. Utilization of accessory muscles of breathing
   c. Crackles, rhonchi, and/or wheezes
2. Other findings dependent on cause
   a. S_3, S_4 heart sounds
   b. Jugular venous distention
   c. Positive abdominojugular reflex
   d. Murmur
   e. Irregular or tachycardic pulse
   f. Fever
   g. Pulsus alternans

The presence of the abdominojugular reflex suggests elevated pulmonary capillary wedge pressure and thus may help to distinguish cardiogenic from noncardiogenic pulmonary edema.

Key Signs

- Pulmonary crackles, rhonchi, and wheezing
- Tachypnea

Tests

Diagnosis is made on clinical grounds, although the following are useful in the initial assessment and management of acute pulmonary edema.

1. Arterial blood gas analysis
2. Serum electrolytes, blood urea nitrogen, creatinine, and albumin; liver function tests; complete blood count
3. Electrocardiography
4. Chest radiography
5. Other tests as indicated by suspicion of cause

Echocardiography can noninvasively aid in determining cardiogenic versus noncardiogenic causes by means of an estimation of pulmonary capillary wedge pressure, quantification of valvular abnormalities, diastolic versus systolic dysfunction, atrial thrombosis or myxoma, and regional wall motion defects.

Key Tests

- Chest radiography
- Arterial blood gas analysis

Differential Diagnosis

1. Pulmonary edema
   a. Cardiogenic
   b. Noncardiogenic
2. Parenchymal pulmonary disorder
   a. Pulmonary fibrosis
   b. Sarcoidosis
3. Pulmonary embolus
4. Pulmonary infection
5. Acute asthma attack
6. Chronic obstructive pulmonary disease exacerbation
7. Hyperventilation syndrome

Treatment

Acute pulmonary edema is a medical emergency. Although identifying and treating reversible causes are essential, nonspecific therapy should be instituted to stabilize the patient while a work-up is being completed.

Physical Maneuvers

Sitting upright with the legs off the side of the bed
1. Reduces venous return, therefore decreasing preload
2. Improves breathing mechanics

Medication

1. Supplemental oxygen. Administer humidified oxygen by way of face mask, continuous positive airway pressure, or endotracheal intubation with positive airway pressure ventilatory support.
   a. Target PO_2 greater than 90 mm Hg
   b. Improved oxygenation decreases pulmonary vascular resistance.
   c. Hypoxia is arrhythmogenic.
   d. Hypoxia on arterial blood gas analysis may be minimized by compensatory tachypnea, giving a false sense of security.
   e. Hypoxia is due to a low diffusion coefficient of oxygen through the alveolar fluid.

In refractory cases, positive-pressure ventilation may be beneficial by reducing the transudation of fluid into the alveolar space and impeding venous return to the thorax.

2. Nitroglycerine, 10 μg/min—titrate to effect
   a. Reduces preload
   b. May be given sublingually until intravenous access is obtained
3. Morphine sulfate, 1 to 4 mg intravenously q 15 min
   a. Reduces preload
   b. Reduces anxiety
   c. Must monitor for respiratory depression

4. Diuretics
   a. Loop diuretic (i.e., furosemide [Lasix], 40 to 60 mg intravenously)
      (1) Initial effect is direct venodilation, which reduces preload.
      (2) Some evidence suggests afterload-reducing capabilities as well.
      (3) Diuresis begins in 5 minutes with peak effect in about 30 minutes.
      (4) Initial dose may be doubled if it is not effective.
   b. Chlorothiazide (Diuril), 250 to 500 mg intravenously, may be synergistic in producing diuresis in patients with inadequate response to loop diuretics.
5. Supplemental medications
   a. Nitroprusside sodium (Nipride), 5 μg/min intravenously—titrate to effect
      (1) Effective as both arterial and venous vasodilator; therefore, exerts both afterload and preload reduction
      (2) Consider invasive monitoring of pulmonary capillary wedge pressure, systemic vascular resistance, and systemic arterial pressures.
      (3) Use with caution in ischemia-mediated acute pulmonary edema to prevent worsening coronary ischemia by way of coronary steal syndrome.
   b. Aminophylline, bolus 5 mg/kg followed by 40 to 60 mg/h (no bolus if the patient is receiving chronic aminophylline)
      (1) May be useful when acute pulmonary edema is complicated by bronchospasm
      (2) May be useful in relieving bronchospasm and effecting diuresis but can exacerbate sinus or ectopic tachycardia
   c. Rotating tourniquets
      (1) Reduces venous return
      (2) Inflate sphygmomanometer cuffs to 10 mm Hg below the diastolic pressure on three extremities and then rotate them among the extremities every 20 minutes.
   d. Phlebotomy
      (1) Reduces preload through the removal of about 500 ml of blood
      (2) Because of the effectiveness of measures above, this measure is largely of historical interest.
   e. Digitalis
      (1) If the patient is not taking this drug, it may be of benefit in controlling ventricular response in systemic vascular resistance and in chronic management.
      (2) If the patient is taking this drug, consider

digitalis intoxication as a cause of pulmonary edema (appraise serum level, electrocardiogram, symptoms, or history of digitalis intoxication).

Special Measures: Acute Pulmonary Edema with Hypotension or Shock

1. Doses must be tailored to maintain perfusion of the brain, heart, and kidneys.
2. Consider the use of vasopressors (i.e., amrinone, dobutamine, dopamine).
3. Invasive monitoring to ascertain response of cardiac output, cardiac index (CI), pulmonary capillary wedge pressure, and systemic vascular resistance to therapeutic interventions is useful in these patients.
4. Consider the use of an intra-aortic balloon pump if ischemic heart failure is predominant.

The measures above are only temporizing in the face of repairable lesions. Therefore, immediate diagnosis of repairable lesions with surgical intervention or efforts to effect early reprofusion should not be delayed.

If acute pulmonary edema is precipitated by supraventricular tachycardia (new-onset atrial fibrillation or flutter) or ventricular tachycardia, immediate cardioversion should be considered.

Diet

Nothing by mouth until the acute phase is controlled; then diet is the same as for heart failure (see Ch. 60).

Activity

Bed rest, preferably in the sitting position

Patient Education

Depends on the precipitating cause (see Ch. 60)

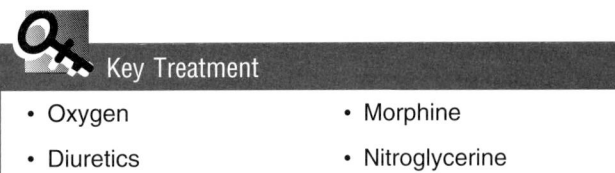

Key Treatment	
• Oxygen	• Morphine
• Diuretics	• Nitroglycerine

Follow-Up

1. Close monitoring of vital signs
2. Serial arterial blood gas analysis and/or pulse oximetry
3. Monitoring of fluid input and output
4. Further follow-up depends on cause

B Bibliography

Berger M, Bach M, Hecht SR, et al: Estimation of pulmonary arterial wedge pressure by pulsed Doppler echocardiography and phonocardiography. Am J Cardiol 1992;69(5):562–564.

Cercek B, Shah PK: Complicated acute myocardial infarction. Heart failure, shock, mechanical complications. Cardiol Clin 1991;9(4):582–583.

Ewy GA: The abdominojugular test; technique and hemodynamic correlates. Ann Intern Med 1988;109(6):456–460 [erratum, Ann Intern Med 1988;109(12):997].

Hall JB, Schmidt GA, Wood LDH (eds): Vasoactive drugs. In Principles of Critical Care. New York, McGraw-Hill, 1992, pp 1585–1597.

Rubenstine E, Federman D: Congestive heart failure. Sci Am Med 1993;8.

39 Ventilator Support

John I. Kennedy, Jr.

Mechanical ventilation is a powerful tool that can provide support for respiratory function, allowing time for other therapy to yield its effect. The decision to use this tool must be made with careful reflection on the prognosis of the underlying disease and consideration of advance directives.

Indications and Goals

1. Respiratory failure—primary indication for ventilator support. Respiratory failure may take two forms that sometimes can coexist.
   a. Hypoxemic respiratory failure results when oxygenation is impaired by ventilation-perfusion imbalance, shunt, or diffusing impairment.
   b. Hypercapnic respiratory failure results from alveolar hypoventilation. A number of mechanisms may lead to this result.
      (1) Decreased central nervous system drive may result in hypoventilation. A common example of this mechanism is sedative drug overdose.
      (2) Neuromuscular weakness (pump failure) can also result in hypoventilation. This may be due to primary neuromuscular diseases (e.g., myasthenia gravis, Guillain-Barré syndrome) or fatigue from increased workload (e.g., asthma, chronic obstructive pulmonary disease).
2. Relief of severe respiratory distress
3. Prevention or treatment of atelectasis
4. To permit the use of heavy sedation or neuromuscular blockade
5. To decrease intracranial pressure by therapeutic hyperventilation
6. To decrease oxygen consumption (e.g., in severe acute respiratory distress syndrome [ARDS], cardiogenic shock)
7. To stabilize the chest wall (e.g., severe flail chest)

Modes

1. Standard modes
   a. Assist/control (A/C). In this mode, a predetermined volume is delivered when an inspiratory effort is sensed by the ventilator or whenever the respiratory rate falls below the backup rate. If large tidal volumes are used and/or tachypnea is present, respiratory alkalosis may develop, requiring the use of sedation or rebreathing dead space.
   b. Intermittent mandatory ventilation (IMV). Breaths of preset volume are delivered to the patient at the set rate. In contrast to A/C, the patient may also inspire spontaneously without assistance from the ventilator, with the rate and tidal volume being determined by the patient's effort. Some ventilators supply gas for the spontaneous breaths by way of a demand valve that can result in increased work of breathing.
   c. Pressure support ventilation. This mode may be used alone or, more commonly, in conjunction with IMV. In contrast to A/C and IMV, no volume is set. When an inspiratory effort is sensed, airway pressure is brought to the preset level and maintained until the patient's inspiratory flow rate falls. The delivered volume is, therefore, determined by the combination of the pressure setting, patient effort, and respiratory system compliance.
2. Additional (nonstandard) modes
   a. Pressure control ventilation (PCV). PCV differs from A/C and IMV by virtue of being pressure-limited rather than volume-limited. When an inspiratory effort is sensed (or rate falls below the preset value), flow is supplied until the preset pressure is reached. PCV limits peak airway pressure and may produce salutary effects on gas exchange, but the subset of patients most likely to benefit has not been clearly identified. PCV has also been used in conjunction with inverse ratio ventilation (PC-IRV), primarily in the support of severe ARDS. Mean airway pressure is increased in PC-IRV, and significant levels of intrinsic positive end-expiratory pressure (auto-PEEP) are typically produced. Thus, the risk for barotrauma appears to be increased.
   b. High-frequency ventilation (HFV). Delivering low tidal volumes at very high rates (60 to 3000/min), HFV may be useful in selected cases of refractory hypoxemia or with bronchopleural fistulae. Results have been more promising in pediatric patients than in adults.
   c. Noninvasive ventilation using occlusive masks can be effective in respiratory failure from neuromuscular disease or kyphoscoliosis and in some patients with chronic obstructive pulmonary disease. Many patients tolerate the masks poorly, and aspiration may be a risk.
   d. Alternative modes of ventilator operation include airway pressure release ventilation, proportional assist ventilation, and mandatory minute ventilation. The advantages and roles of these modes remain to be defined.

Ventilator Settings

1. FiO_2 (fraction of inspired oxygen). In almost all situations, the initial FiO_2 should be 1.00. Subsequent downward adjustments in FiO_2 may then be made, guided by arterial blood gas analysis or pulse oximetry. The usual goal is to maintain PaO_2 equal to or greater than 60 mm Hg and oxygen saturation equal to or greater than 90 per cent with FiO_2 equal to or less than 0.50.

2. Tidal volume and rate. These parameters determine the minimum minute ventilation received. It has been customary to use tidal volumes of 10 to 15 ml/kg, but many experts now recommend more physiologic tidal volumes (5 to 8 ml/kg) to minimize overdistention of alveoli and reduce the risk of barotrauma. The rate usually should be set in a physiologic range (8 to 16). In patients with tachypnea, the work of breathing may be reduced by setting the rate at 2 to 4 breaths/min below the spontaneous rate.

3. Flow rates; inspiratory/expiratory (I:E) ratio. Some ventilators allow flow rate to be set as an independent parameter. On other machines, the I:E ratio can be set, and the flow rate depends on the ventilatory rate, tidal volume, and I:E ratio. An inspiratory flow rate of 60 L/min is adequate in most patients. Higher flow rates (80 to 100 L/min) are often helpful in patients with severe airflow obstruction, allowing more time for expiration. When the I:E ratio must be set, typical settings are 1:3 or 1:2 (inspiratory per cent = 25 to 33).

4. Sensitivity of the ventilator should be adjusted to allow the patient to trigger the ventilator with the lowest pressure that avoids autotriggering of the machine. This can usually be accomplished at about -2 cm H_2O.

5. PEEP may improve PaO_2 in some situations, particularly when terminal respiratory units are prone to collapse (e.g., ARDS), allowing FiO_2 to be reduced to nontoxic levels. Alternatively, PEEP may be adjusted in an effort to maximize systemic oxygen transport. The definition of optimal PEEP remains controversial. PEEP should be applied in increments of 2 to 5 cm H_2O and the response assessed promptly after each increase. When severe airflow obstruction exists or when IRV is used, auto-PEEP may develop. Auto-PEEP may go unrecognized and can contribute to hemodynamic compromise and respiratory distress.

Complications

1. Artificial airway complications. Endotracheal tubes may become kinked or occluded by secretions. These devices may also produce injury to the upper airway. Securing the tube so that movement is limited and using the lowest cuff pressure that achieves adequate seal help to minimize injury.

2. Ventilator malfunction. Modern ventilators are re-markably efficient and trouble-free, but problems do occur. Whenever a patient develops distress on the ventilator, it is prudent to assume that there is a malfunction and remove the patient from the machine and manually ventilate. The ease with which the patient is ventilated and the initial response to manual ventilation can provide important information in a matter of seconds.

3. Barotrauma. Disruption of alveoli from overdistention can lead to pneumomediastinum, subcutaneous emphysema, pneumoperitoneum, and pneumothorax. Of these, only pneumothorax is typically associated with important hemodynamic effects. Pneumoperitoneum may raise concern about a possible ruptured intra-abdominal viscus but is otherwise benign. Careful attention should be paid to limiting pressure and volume delivered in an effort to minimize the risk of barotrauma.

4. Cardiovascular effects. Intrathoracic pressure becomes elevated with positive-pressure ventilation, impeding venous return to the heart. This can result in significant decreases in cardiac output, which may be manifested as hypotension. Renal hypoperfusion and hepatic congestion may also result.

5. Infection. Nosocomial pneumonia is an important and serious complication of ventilator support. Elevating the patient's head and avoiding elevation of gastric pH may reduce the risk of ventilator-associated pneumonia. Prompt weaning and extubation are the most important preventive maneuvers.

Weaning

1. Timing. Selecting the appropriate time involves the assessment of multiple factors, including the following:

   a. Underlying disease. The initial problem should be improved or stabilized.

   b. Level of consciousness. The patient should be awake, alert, and cooperative. Sedative medications should be withheld before planned weaning.

   c. Gas exchange. PaO_2 should be greater than or equal to 60 mm Hg with FiO_2 less than or equal to 0.40.

   d. Ventilatory mechanics. The usual guidelines for predicting successful weaning are as follows:

      (1) Vital capacity greater than 10 ml/kg

      (2) Resting minute ventilation less than 10 L/min

      (3) Maximal minute ventilation greater than twice the resting minute ventilation

      (4) Respiratory rate divided by tidal volume (L) less than 100

      (5) Maximal negative inspiratory force less than or equal to -30 cm H_2O (i.e., more negative)

2. Techniques. A variety of approaches have been used for discontinuing ventilator support. Traditional weaning involves allowing the patient to breath spon-

taneously by way of a T tube gas supply for a period of time while observing for distress or desaturation. Alternatively, progressive reduction in IMV and/or pressure support may be used. The relative advantages of different approaches are unproven. The most important factor is that the process be carried out thoughtfully and with careful observation. The physician should be prepared to reinstitute support if needed.

B | Bibliography

For a more detailed general overview of ventilator support, see

Tobin MJ: Mechanical ventilation. N Engl J Med 1994;330:1056–1061.

For detailed, specific recommendations and guidelines on ventilator support, see

Slutsky AS: Mechanical ventilation. Chest 1993;104:1833–1859.

For more information about newer modes of ventilation, see

Sassoon CSH: Positive pressure ventilation: Alternative modes. Chest 1991;100:1421–1429.

For more information about techniques of noninvasive ventilation, see

Meyer TJ, Hill NS: Noninvasive positive pressure ventilation to treat respiratory failure. Ann Intern Med 1994;120:760–770.

For more information about discontinuation of ventilator support, see

Tobin MJ, Yang K: Weaning from mechanical ventilation. Crit Care Clin 1990;6:725–745.

Procedure | **CRICOTHYROTOMY/TRACHEOSTOMY**
Joseph Valentino

Indications

1. Prolonged need for ventilatory support by way of an endotracheal tube
2. Need for ventilatory support in a patient who cannot be safely intubated nasally or orally or who poorly tolerates an orotracheal or a nasotracheal tube
3. Obstruction of the airway in which oral or nasal intubation of the trachea cannot be performed. Examples include tumor, bilateral vocal cord paralysis, laryngeal fracture, subglottic, glottic, or supraglottic stenosis, and laryngeal edema or hematoma.
4. Prolonged need for tracheobronchial toilet

Contraindications

1. Cricothyrotomy for a laryngeal fracture
2. Cricothyrotomy in subglottic airway obstruction
3. Acute inflammation of the trachea and coagulopathy are relative contraindications to elective tracheostomy.
4. In an emergency, cricothyrotomy, a quicker and easier procedure, is strongly encouraged rather than tracheostomy.

Preparation

1. Ensure all necessary equipment is available to perform the procedure.
2. Suction, electrocautery, and adequate lighting, if available
3. A shoulder roll 3 to 7 inches in diameter is placed beneath the patient's shoulders, hyperextending the neck. This greatly facilitates tracheostomy, cricothyrotomy, or tracheostomy tube changing.
4. The skin is then prepped with antiseptic solution.

Equipment

1. Tracheostomy tube
   a. A tube with a cuff that can be inflated after insertion prevents the flow of blood from the fresh tracheostomy/cricothyrotomy wound into the airway as well as allowing for positive-pressure ventilation.
   b. If no tracheostomy tube is available, a standard endotracheal tube is an emergency substitute.
2. An emergency tracheostomy tray should include an appropriate assortment of retractors, clamps, scalpel blades, suction catheters, tracheal hooks, tracheal dilators, sponges, towels, suture material, needles, syringes, and local anesthetic.

Anesthesia

The skin and subcutaneous tissues are infiltrated with lidocaine 1% with epinephrine for local anesthesia and vasoconstriction to decrease bleeding.

Precautions

Surgical airway performed in a prepared environment with experienced personnel is always preferred.

Palpate the neck carefully for landmarks and pathology that may impede surgical procedure (i.e., a high-riding innominate artery crossing the desired tracheostomy site, a thyroid isthmus mass, or deviation of the trachea caused by previous surgery).

Technique: Cricothyrotomy

1. A 4-cm vertical incision is made through the skin into the subcutaneous fat in the midline of the neck over the thyroid and cricoid cartilages.

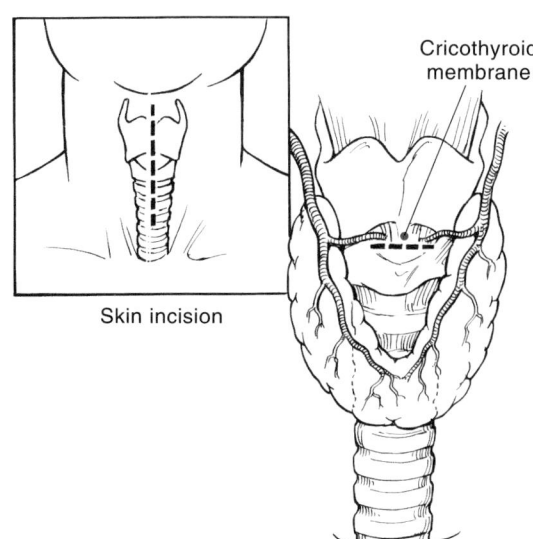

Skin incision

Cricothyroid membrane

2. Using blunt and sharp dissection, the investing cervical fascia and strap muscles are separated in the midline, vertically exposing the cricoid cartilage and thyroid lamina.

3. The cricothyroid membrane is incised with a horizontal incision, and a curved Kelly clamp is inserted into the airway and spread to open the airway widely.

4. A tracheal hook retracts the cricoid cartilage anteriorly, holding the lumen open, and the appropriate tube is inserted.

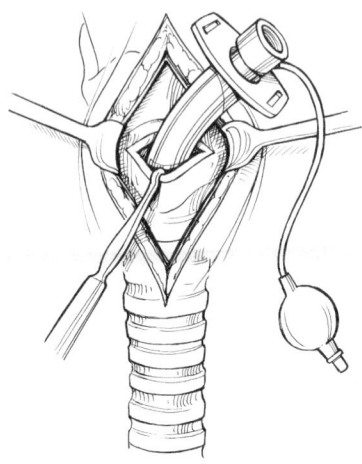

WARNING

- **A cricothyrotomy is an emergency procedure performed only when the airway has been lost and cannot be established with an orotracheal or a nasotracheal tube. Bleeding can be fully controlled after establishment of the airway. The cricothyroid cartilages, if not clearly visualized, can readily be palpated in the midline through the soft tissues or pooling blood.**

- **Hyperextension of the neck is contraindicated in patients with unstable cervical spines and severe cervical osteoarthritis.**

- **Patients with severe respiratory distress may not tolerate neck extension.**

Technique: Tracheostomy

1. A transverse incision 4 cm in length is planned midway between the cricoid cartilage and the sternal notch and is carried through the skin and subcutaneous fat to the deep cervical fascia.

2. One dissects through the investing fascia, then between the sternohyoid muscles and sternothyroid muscles in the midline to expose the thyroid isthmus.

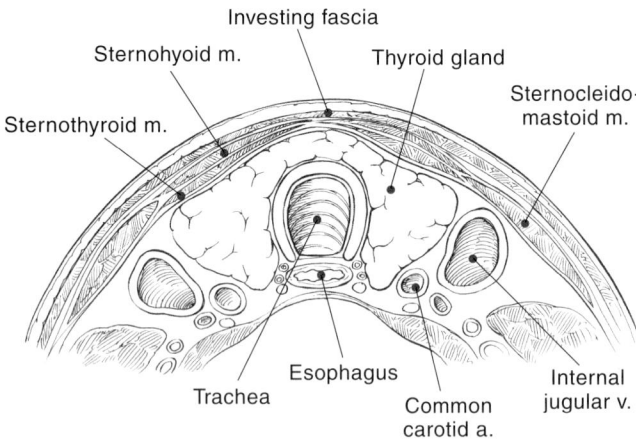

3. The thyroid isthmus usually overlies the optimal tracheostomy site. It can be retracted superiorly after ligating the inferior thyroid plexus of veins. Alternatively, the thyroid isthmus is clamped and divided and a suture ligature is applied.

4. The tracheal hook is inserted between the first tracheal ring and the cricoid cartilage to retract the cricoid cartilage superiorly and anteriorly.

5. The second or third tracheal ring is identified, and 7- to 10-mm horizontal cuts are made above and below it. The segment of tracheal ring is clamped, and a 7- to 10-mm portion of this anterior ring is removed.

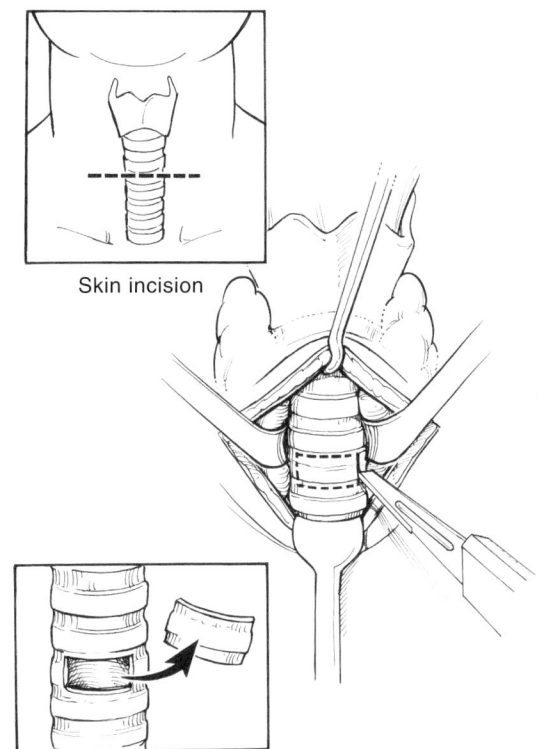

Skin incision

6. If the tracheostomy is too small, the horizontal incisions of the trachea can be extended.

7. If present, the endotracheal tube is withdrawn until only the tip can be seen at the superior aspect of the tracheostomy site.

8. The tracheostomy tube with obturator in place is inserted into the airway, and the cuff is inflated. The obturator is removed, the inner cannula of the tracheostomy tube is inserted, the ventilating tubing is connected, and the cuff is inflated.

9. Auscultate the chest bilaterally for air movement.

10. Tracheostomy ties are placed around the patient's neck and secured tight enough so that only two fingers can be inserted between the tracheostomy ties and the patient's neck in the adult.

PEARLS

- The retraction can alter the location of the trachea. Palpate the trachea! If the location of the trachea remains uncertain, aspirate for air with a needle and syringe.

- Patients often have pain despite infiltration. Use additional local anesthetic intraoperatively.

- Adequate hemostasis should be attained at each step in tracheostomy.

- Decannulation in the perioperative period can be life-threatening. Use permanent 3-0 or larger

---

sutures to secure the face plate of the tracheostomy tube to the skin of the anterior neck in addition to applying tracheostomy ties.

Follow-Up

1. Postoperative chest radiography

2. Postoperative hemorrhage is usually controlled with oxidizing packing agents or packing gauze.

3. Massive bleeding from the tracheostomy site requires surgical intervention.

4. Standard nursing care of tracheostomy tubes includes cleaning of the inner cannula, cleaning of the tracheostomy site, irrigation and suctioning of the trachea, changing of the tracheostomy sponge dressing, and changing of the tracheostomy ties.

5. A cricothyrotomy that has been performed should be converted as soon as possible to a standard tracheostomy if the patient requires more than a 1-week duration of endotracheal tube support.

6. Permanent decannulation should not be performed until the patient's airway has been fully assessed.

Bibliography

Myers EN, Stool SE, Johnson JT (eds): Tracheotomy. New York, Churchill Livingstone, 1985.

Seid AB, Gluckman JL: Tracheostomy. *In* Paparella MM, Schumrick DA, Gluckman JL, Meyerhoff WL (eds): Otolaryngology. Philadelphia, WB Saunders, 1991, pp 2429–2437.

Tracheostomy. *In* Lore JM Jr (ed): Atlas of Head and Neck Surgery. Philadelphia, WB Saunders, 1988, pp 811–818.

40 Pneumothorax

Joshua Benditt

Etiology

1. Pneumothorax (air within the pleural space) is classified etiologically as either spontaneous (occurring without immediate antecedent trauma) or traumatic. Spontaneous pneumothorax is further divided into either primary (occurring in a previously healthy person) or secondary (occurring in a person with an underlying and predisposing condition).

2. Spontaneous pneumothorax
   a. Primary
   b. Secondary
      (1) Pulmonary diseases
         (a) Airway diseases
            (I) Chronic obstructive pulmonary disease
            (II) Bronchiectasis
            (III) Asthma
            (IV) Cystic fibrosis
         (b) Interstitial diseases
            (I) Interstitial pulmonary fibrosis
            (II) Sarcoidosis
            (III) Collagen vascular diseases
            (IV) Pneumoconioses
         (c) Infections
            (I) Pneumonia (bacterial, fungal, and parasitic)
            (II) Lung abscess
            (III) Tuberculosis
         (d) Neoplastic
            (I) Lung cancer
            (II) Metastatic cancer
      (2) Extrapulmonary causes
         (a) Catamenial pneumothorax (related to menses)
         (b) Esophageal rupture
         (c) Drug abuse (e.g., inhaled use of marijuana and cocaine)
         (d) Neonatal pneumothorax

3. Traumatic
   a. Iatrogenic (e.g., central line placement)
   b. Noniatrogenic (e.g., stab wound to chest)

Symptoms

1. Predominant symptoms are chest pain that is localized to the side of the pneumothorax (usually pleuritic in nature) and dyspnea.

2. The severity of symptoms is related to the size of the pneumothorax, being more severe in larger pneumothoraces.

3. Rarely the patient may be asymptomatic.

Key Symptoms

- Chest pain
- Dyspnea

Clinical Findings

1. The physical findings are related to the size of the pneumothorax. The larger the pneumothorax, the more likely physical indications are to be found.

2. Physical findings
   a. Respiratory system
      (1) Decreased or absent breath sounds
      (2) Normal or hyperresonant chest percussion note
      (3) Unilateral enlargement of the chest
      (4) Absent tactile fremitus
      (5) Tracheal deviation (away from the side of the pneumothorax) in tension pneumothorax
   b. Cardiac system
      (1) Tachycardia
      (2) Hypotension (in tension pneumothorax)

Key Signs

- Hyperresonant chest percussion note
- Decreased or absent breath sounds
- Tachycardia

Tests

1. Chest radiography is the most important test in evaluating pneumothorax. The radiographic appearance is a sharp line representing the lung edge that usually runs parallel to the chest wall and is separated from it by a radiolucent area without lung markings, which represents air in the pleural space.
   a. Small pneumothoraces may be difficult to diagnose.
   b. In a complete pneumothorax the radiographic appearance is a grapefruit-sized opacity at the hilum.

2. An arterial blood gas analysis should be obtained in more severe pneumothoraces (greater than 20 per cent of the volume of the hemithorax) or in patients with

underlying lung disease. In these situations, significant hypoxemia may be present secondary to intrapulmonary shunting.

3. Electrocardiographic abnormalities

a. Left-sided pneumothoraces can present with findings that mimic an acute anterior non–Q-wave myocardial infarction.

(1) Right axis deviation

(2) Decreased R-wave amplitude in the precordial leads

(3) Decreased QRS amplitude

(4) Precordial T-wave inversion

b. These changes should normalize if the electrocardiogram is taken in the upright position.

Key Test

• Chest radiography

Differential Diagnosis

1. Lung-related disorders

a. Pleuritis

b. Pneumonia

c. Pulmonary embolus

d. Exacerbation of chronic obstructive pulmonary disease or asthma

e. Pulmonary infarct

2. Chest wall–related

a. Rib fracture

b. Herpes zoster that affects a thoracic dermatome

c. Bursitis of the shoulder

3. Cardiovascular system–related

a. Pericarditis or pericardial effusion

b. Myocardial infarction

c. Dissecting aortic aneurysm

d. Myocarditis

4. Intra-abdominal processes

a. Cholecystitis

b. Pancreatitis

c. Perforated peptic ulcer

d. Subphrenic abscess

Treatment

1. All patients should initially receive high-flow oxygen to increase the rate of resorption of air from the pleural space.

2. Observation alone

a. Mild symptoms or asymptomatic

b. No significant underlying lung pathology

c. Pneumothorax less than 15 per cent of the volume of the hemithorax

3. Needle aspiration of pneumothorax

a. Moderate symptoms

b. Pneumothorax greater than 15 per cent of the volume of the hemithorax

4. Tube thoracostomy

a. Significant respiratory distress

b. Significant underlying lung pathology

c. Bilateral pneumothoraces

d. Traumatic pneumothorax (especially with hemothorax)

5. Tension pneumothorax (pleural air under positive pressure with potential for hemodynamic compromise) requires the following:

a. Emergent placement of a large-bore (14-gauge) catheter in the second intercostal space on the affected side for decompression of the thorax

b. Tube thoracostomy after the thorax is decompressed with the 14-gauge catheter

Key Treatment

• Emergent decompression of the tension pneumothorax with a large-bore catheter

Follow-Up

1. The patient is treated with observation or needle aspiration.

a. Follow-up chest radiography in 6 hours. If the pneumothorax has not enlarged, the patient can go home.

b. Follow-up chest radiography in 24 hours

2. The patient is treated with tube thoracostomy.

a. Admit to hospital

b. Follow-up chest radiography immediately after a chest tube is placed

c. Follow-up chest radiography in 24 hours

3. Recurrent pneumothoraces may require definitive surgical therapy (e.g., bullectomy, pleurodesis).

Bibliography

DeMeester TR, Lafontaine E: The pleura. In Sabiston DC, Spencer FC (eds): Surgery of the Chest, 5th ed, vol 1. Philadelphia, WB Saunders, 1990, pp 444–497.

Jantz MA, Pierson DJ: Pneumothorax and barotrauma. Clin Chest Med 1994;15:75–92.

Light R: Pneumothorax. In Murray JF, Nadel JA (eds): Textbook of Respiratory Medicine, 2nd ed, vol 2. Philadelphia, WB Saunders, 1994, pp 2193–2208.

McEwen JI: Pleural disease. In Rosen P, Barkin RM (eds): Emergency Medicine—Concepts and Clinical Practice, 3rd ed, vol 2. St Louis, Mosby-Yearbook, 1992, pp 1121–1139.

Wait MA, Estera A: Changing clinical spectrum of spontaneous pneumothorax. Am J Surg 1992;164:528–531.

Procedure **CHEST TUBE INSERTION** *Kathleen C. Barry*

Indications

1. Pneumothorax—either secondary to trauma or spontaneous—causing respiratory distress
2. Hemothorax
3. Large pleural effusion causing respiratory distress

Contraindications

1. Small pneumothorax that is not causing respiratory distress and is followed with serial chest radiographs
2. Pleura adherent to the chest wall
3. Coagulopathy (relative contraindication)

Preparation

1. Explain the procedure to the patient and obtain informed consent.
2. Place the patient in the lateral decubitus position with the involved side up.
3. Prepare and drape the area of the fifth or sixth intercostal space in the midaxillary line. The midaxillary line is used because it is the least muscular part of the thorax.

Equipment

1. Skin preparation (e.g., povidone-iodine [Betadine])
2. Sterile gloves, mask, and fenestrated drape
3. 22-gauge 1½-inch needle with 10-ml syringe
4. Lidocaine 1%, 20 ml
5. No. 10 scalpel blade and handle
6. Curved clamp
7. Chest tube—type and size depend on the purpose and preference
   a. Pneumothorax—No. 22 to No. 24 French straight
   b. Hemothorax or pleural effusion—No. 32 to No. 36 French straight or right-angle
8. Multichamber water-seal suction
9. Needle holder
10. Skin suture
11. Suture scissors
12. Petroleum gauze
13. Sterile sponges
14. Elastic adhesive bandage

Anesthesia

1. Use a 22-gauge 1½-inch needle to infiltrate the subcutaneous tissue in a wheal with lidocaine 1%. This should be done along the top edge of the involved rib to avoid the neurovascular bundle that lies inferiorly.
2. Slowly advance the needle, infiltrating along the costal periosteum and down to the parietal pleura with 5 to 10 ml of lidocaine.
3. The pleural space is reached when air or fluid can be aspirated.

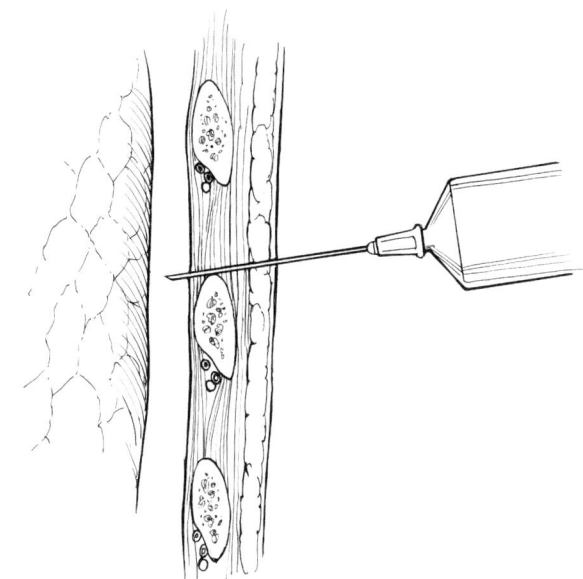

Precautions

1. Do not go lower than the fifth intercostal space to avoid perforation of the diaphragm or splenic or hepatic injury.
2. Avoid using trocars for this procedure because their use can increase the risk of injury to the pulmonary parenchyma.

Technique

1. Make a small incision through skin, fat, and muscle just superior to the lower rib of the interspace.
2. Use a curved clamp to enlarge the incision and perforate into the pleural space. Avoid lung injury by gripping the clamp so that the distance from hand to tip is just greater than the chest wall thickness. A gush of blood and/or air is to be expected on perforating the pleura.
3. Insert a finger to enlarge the tract and to confirm entry into the pleural space. Palpate the pleural surface to clean away adhesions and clots.

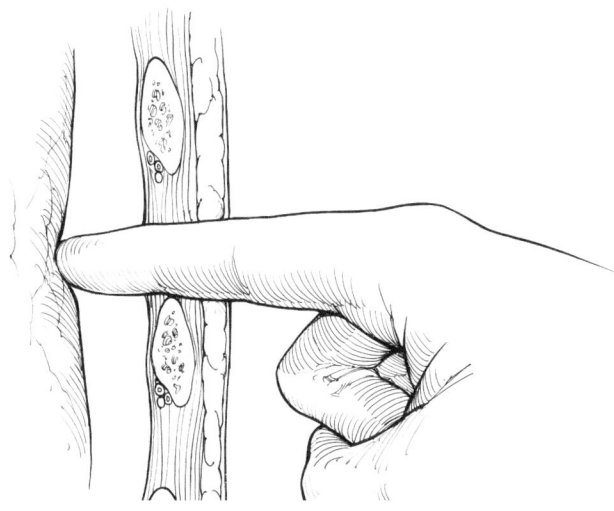

4. Grasp the chest tube with the clamp and guide it into the pleural space. Direct the tube posteriorly and toward the apex for a pneumothorax. For fluid drainage, the tube is directed posteriorly to reside in the most dependent position possible. Ensure that all drainage holes are inside the pleural space.

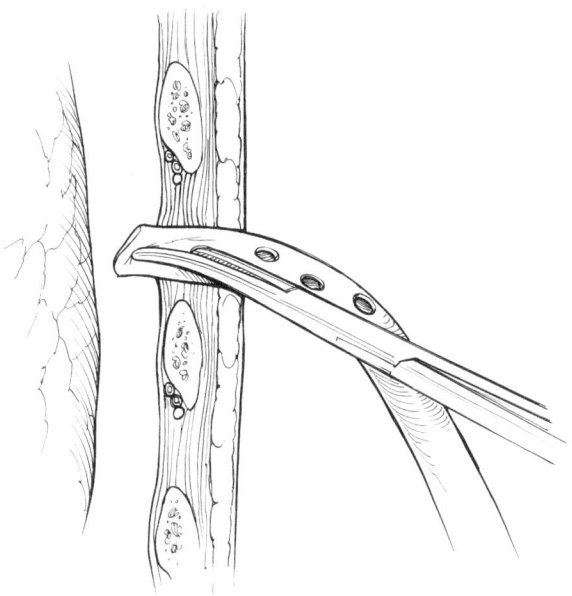

5. Attach the tube to a multichamber water-seal suction with 20 cm H_2O suction and tape the connections.

6. Place a suture through the skin and knot, leaving long ends to wrap and tie securely around the tube.

7. Place petroleum gauze around the tube exit site to make an airtight seal. Apply a split 2 × 2 sponge around the tube and apply benzoin to the surrounding skin. Place two strips of 1-inch tape over the sponge, allowing the tape to self-adhere for about 1 inch at the level of the tube. Secure the tube to these pieces of tape with additional tape. Assure that the tube stays in place by adding tape strips perpendicular to the initial strips.

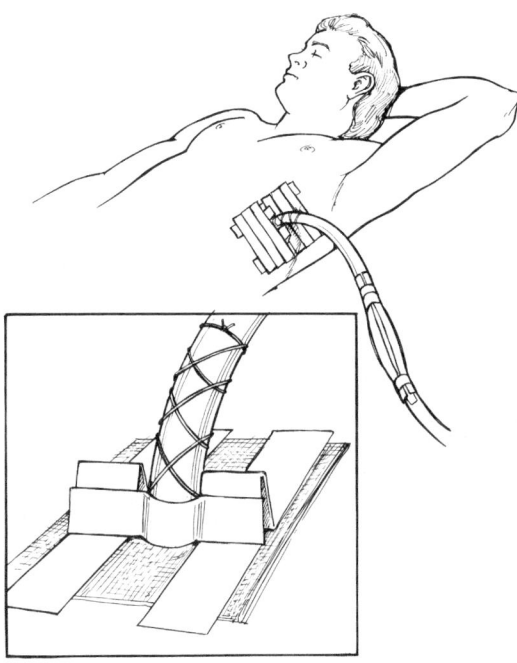

Follow-Up

Obtain a chest radiograph to confirm the position of the tube and to assess resolution of the pneumothorax or hemothorax.

 Bibliography

Arsenio JA, Barton JM, Worsetler LA, et al: Trauma: A systemic approach to management. Am Fam Physician 1988;38:96–104.

Miller AC, Harvey JE: Guidelines for the management of a spontaneous pneumothorax. Br Med J 1993;307:114–116.

Moore EE, Mattox KL, Feliciano DV (eds): Trauma, 2nd ed. E Norwalk, CT, Appleton & Lange, 1991, pp 361–362.

Spillane RM, Shepard JD, DeLuca SA: Radiographic aspects of pneumothorax. Am Fam Physician 1995;51:459–464.

Thal AP, Quick KL: A guided chest tube for safe thoracostomy. Surg Gynecol Obstet 1988;167:517–521.

41 Pleural Effusions

Linda Kuribayashi

Etiology

The accumulation of fluid in the pleural space can result from a number of mechanisms.

1. Increased hydrostatic pressure (e.g., congestive heart failure)
2. Decreased oncotic pressure (e.g., nephrotic syndrome with hypoalbuminemia)
3. Increased capillary permeability (e.g., pneumonia)
4. Decreased lymphatic drainage (e.g., carcinoma, tuberculosis)
5. Entry of fluid from a source outside the pleura (e.g., blood from trauma, chyle from rupture of the thoracic duct, crystalloid from a misplaced central line)

Symptoms

1. May be asymptomatic
2. Dyspnea
3. Pleuritic chest pain
4. Cough (often nonproductive)
5. Symptoms secondary to associated illnesses

Key Symptoms

- Often asymptomatic
- Dyspnea
- Pleuritic chest pain
- Cough

Clinical Findings

1. Physical examination reveals dullness to percussion, decreased fremitus, and decreased breath sounds at the location of the effusion.
2. Radiographic examination reveals a homogeneous density
   a. Chest radiographs: Free-flowing pleural fluid responds to gravity and causes blunting of the costophrenic angle. A meniscus sign is frequently present.
   b. Lateral decubitus radiographs: Small amounts of free-flowing pleural fluid can be seen layered along the dependent portion of the chest wall. Loculated pleural effusions do not change position.
   c. Computed tomography: Small pleural effusions can be visualized and aspirated under computed tomographic guidance.
   d. Ultrasonography: Loculated effusions can be located and aspirated using ultrasound guidance.

Key Signs

- Dullness to percussion
- Decreased breath sounds

Tests

1. Pleural fluid analysis
   a. General appearance (e.g., pus would indicate empyema, a milky appearance may indicate a chylothorax, clear yellow fluid is consistent with transudates and some exudates)
   b. Protein: Leakage of protein into the pleural space occurs with inflammation. A pleural fluid protein/serum protein ratio greater than 0.5 is characteristic of an exudate (see Table 41–1).
   c. Lactic dehydrogenase (LDH): A pleural fluid LDH/serum LDH ratio greater than 0.6 is consistent with an exudate. An absolute pleural fluid LDH greater than 200 IU is another criterion for an exudate.
   d. Cell count and differential
      (1) Leukocytosis: Elevated white blood cell count (greater than $1000/\mu l$) indicates inflammation and can be associated with infection, connective tissue disease, and pulmonary infarction. The presence of pus indicates empyema.
      (2) Red blood cell count: Grossly hemorrhagic effusions are associated with trauma, carcinoma, pulmonary infarction, and tuberculosis.
   e. Culture and smear (bacterial, acid-fast bacillus, and fungal)
   f. pH: Low pH (less than 7.30) is associated with empyema, carcinoma, connective tissue disease, tuberculosis, and esophageal rupture.
   g. Glucose: Low glucose level (pleural fluid glucose/serum glucose ratio less than 0.5) is seen more frequently in rheumatoid pleuritis and empyema.
   h. Amylase: Elevated amylase level (pleural fluid amylase/serum amylase ratio greater than 2) is associated with pancreatitis and esophageal rupture.

TABLE 41–1. CRITERIA FOR DIAGNOSING AN EXUDATE

One of the following:
1. Pleural fluid protein/serum protein > 0.5
2. Pleural fluid LDH/serum LDH > 0.6
3. Pleural fluid LDH > 200 IU

i. Cytology: Can be diagnostic for carcinoma, systemic lupus erythematosus (LE cells)

j. Lipids: Elevated lipid levels are seen with chylothorax.

2. Pleural biopsy (closed or open) can be diagnostic for carcinoma and granulomatous infections.

3. Bronchoscopy can help diagnose carcinoma and infectious causes in pleural effusions in which the diagnosis is still unclear after thoracentesis.

4. Thoracoscopy can help localize pleural disease and improve biopsy yield.

Key Test

• Thoracentesis is the definitive test.

Differential Diagnosis

1. Transudates
   a. Congestive heart failure
   b. Cirrhosis with ascites
   c. Nephrotic syndrome
   d. Hypoalbuminemia
   e. Peritoneal dialysis
   f. Superior vena cava obstruction
   g. Subclavian catheter misplacement
   h. Early mediastinal carcinoma (rare)
   i. Pulmonary embolism (rare)
   j. Constrictive pericarditis
   k. Atelectasis

2. Exudates
   a. Parapneumonic effusion
      (1) Bacterial (including tuberculosis)
      (2) Viral
      (3) Fungal
      (4) Parasitic
   b. Empyema
      (1) Bacterial (including tuberculosis)
      (2) Fungal
   c. Pulmonary embolism and infarction
   d. Carcinoma
   e. Uremia
   f. Post myocardial infarction
   g. Trauma (hemothorax)
   h. Connective tissue disease
      (1) Rheumatoid arthritis
      (2) Systemic lupus erythematosus
   i. Gastrointestinal
      (1) Pancreatitis
      (2) Esophageal rupture
      (3) Liver abscess
   j. Drug reactions (e.g., nitrofurantoin, dantrolene [Dantrium])
   k. Meigs' syndrome
   l. Chylothorax
   m. Sarcoidosis

Treatment

1. The primary treatment is therapy for the underlying disease process.

2. Unstable patients with severe dyspnea may require therapeutic thoracentesis in addition to treating the underlying cause. Removal of more than 1.5 liters of pleural fluid during a single thoracentesis is associated with the risk of re-expansion pulmonary edema.

3. Occasionally drainage by way of chest tubes or other surgical drainage procedures is required (e.g., empyema).

4. Recurrent, symptomatic pleural effusions in which the underlying disease process cannot be adequately treated (e.g., cancer) may benefit from pleurodesis.

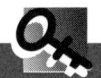

Key Treatment

• Treatment of the underlying disease process

Follow-Up

1. Appropriate follow-up is determined by the underlying cause.

2. Serial chest radiographs are often helpful in evaluating treatment response.

Bibliography

Berkman N, Kramer MR: Diagnostic tests in pleural effusion—an update. Postgrad Med J 1993;69:12–18.

Light RW: Disorders of the pleura: General principles and diagnostic approach. *In* Murray JM, Nadel JA (eds): Textbook of Respiratory Medicine, vol 2. Philadelphia, WB Saunders, 1988, pp 1703–1718.

Muller NL: Imaging the pleura. Radiology 1993;186:297–309.

Sahn SA: The differential diagnosis of pleural effusions. West J Med 1982;137:99–108.

Sahn SA: The pleura. Am Rev Respir Dis 1988;138:184–234.

Procedure THORACENTESIS

Robert L. Johnson

Indications

1. Effusion of unclear origin
2. Compromise of pulmonary status (therapeutic)
3. Contralateral mediastinal shift (therapeutic)
4. Small pneumothoraces

Contraindications

1. Hemorrhagic diathesis
2. Active local infection over area of access

Preparation

1. Obtain posteroanterior, lateral, and decubitus radiographs.
2. Position the patient on the edge of the bed.
3. Percuss the effusion to the highest and lowest levels.
4. Determine the point of access.

Equipment

1. Sterile drapes and povidone-iodine (Betadine) preparation

2. Intracath needle (14-gauge) and plasma vacuum bottles
3. Curved clamp, 50-ml syringe, three-way stopcock

Anesthesia

1. Needles—25-gauge, ⅝-inch and 22-gauge, 2-inch
2. Lidocaine 1% 10 ml

Precautions

1. Always approach from the *top* of the rib.
2. Caution and a clamp prevent overpenetration.
3. Always be prepared for a pneumothorax.

WARNING

Extreme caution must be taken to avoid puncture of the visceral pleura.

Technique

1. Position the patient on the edge of the bed with the arms supported by a table. Percuss the bottom of the effusion between the posterior axillary line and paraspinous muscles

2. Choose an access *above* the eighth rib, as low in the effusion as possible. Mark the spot with the end of a pen to indent the skin (because ink washes off) at the superior margin of the rib.

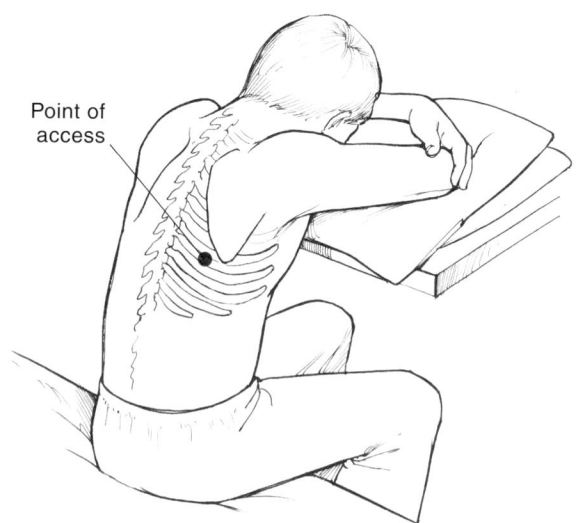

3. Prepare the skin with iodinated scrub, drape in a sterile manner, and make a "wheel" in the skin with the 25-gauge needle. Place the 22-gauge needle to

the rib, and anesthetize the periosteum as you "walk" the needle superiorly.

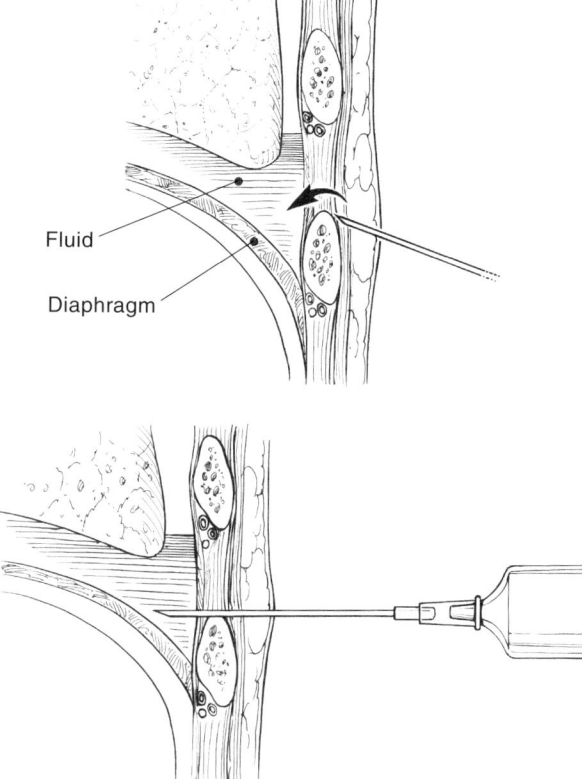

4. Advance the needle and aspirate once over the top of the rib, and carefully enter the pleural cavity. Aspirate fluid or air to confirm. Measure this depth on the needle.

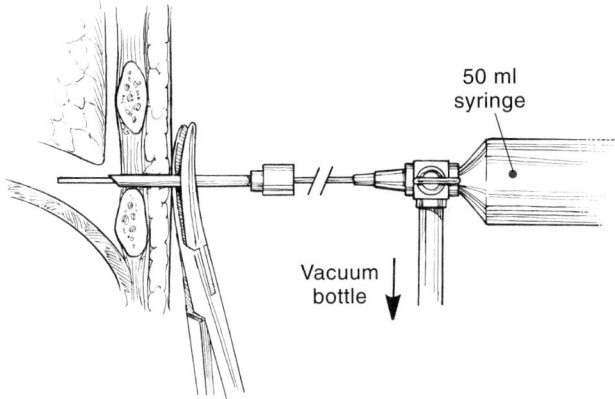

50 ml syringe

Vacuum bottle

5. Place the clamp on the intracath needle at the depth noted above. Advance the needle to the rib and again "walk" it superiorly. Aspirate as you advance past the rib to find fluid or air in the pleural space.

6. Move the clamp on the needle toward the skin, if necessary, to prevent further advancement of the needle. Remove the syringe, and advance the catheter through the needle superiorly for pneumothorax and inferiorly for effusion.

7. Attach the stopcock, tubing, and vacuum bottle and then the 50-ml syringe. Close the stopcock to the bottle and aspirate with the syringe. Close the stopcock to the catheter and empty the syringe into the bottle. Repeat above. Never remove more than 1.5 liters.

8. Remove the entire apparatus as a unit. *Never* pull the catheter back through the needle. Cover the insertion site with an elastic bandage.

Follow-Up

1. Chest radiograph
2. Pain relief as needed
3. Send fluid for studies (e.g., Gram's stain, culture and sensitivity).
4. Warning signs of the development of pneumothorax should be given to the patient.
5. Watch for bleeding and hemothorax.
6. Beware of re-expansion pulmonary edema.
7. Supportive care, rest
8. Slow, deep respirations
9. Oxygen for post-thoracentesis hypoxia, a normal and expected problem from induced ventilation-perfusion abnormalities

Bibliography

Light RW: Pleural Diseases, 2nd ed. Malvern, PA, Lea & Febiger, 1990, pp 295–304.

Pickard LR: Decision Making in Cardiothoracic Surgery. Philadelphia, WB Saunders, 1989.

Sahn SA: The pleura: State of the art. Am Rev Resp Dis 1988;138:184.

Stark P: Radiology of Thoracic Trauma. New York, Butterworth-Heinemann, 1992.

Urshel HC Jr, Cooper JD: Atlas of Thoracic Surgery. New York, Churchill Livingstone, 1994.

42 Rib Fractures

Lawrence L. Ward

Etiology

1. Direct trauma (blunt or penetrating)
   a. The rib fracture is at the site of trauma.
   b. Underlying organ injury must be considered.
   c. There is greater likelihood of a single rib fracture or at most two to three contiguous ribs being fractured.
2. Transmitted forces (rib cage compression)
   a. The rib fracture occurs at a location removed from the applied force, usually the posterior angles of ribs five through nine.
   b. Underlying organ injury is more likely to occur at the site of applied force than at the fracture site.
   c. Multiple contiguous ribs may be fractured.
3. Violent muscle contractions
   a. Fractures of the first rib at the scalene insertions and of the last three "floating" ribs are most likely of this cause.
   b. This type of fracture may be more commonly seen in athletes and in severe coughing.
4. Pathologic
   a. Osteoporosis or a bone-destroying or -replacing disease is present at the fracture site.
   b. Trauma history is minimal compared with other fracture types.

Symptoms

1. Localized pain is increased by inspiration.
   a. Pain is of abrupt onset in conjunction with the trauma involved.
   b. Pain might worsen after the first few days as the bone resorption phase of healing "loosens" the fracture fragments.
   c. Pain is aggravated by nonrespiratory thoracic muscular effort in the region of the fracture.
2. Shortness of breath
   a. Delayed onset of shortness of breath (e.g., 12 to 24 hours after injury) should suggest an underlying lung injury.
   b. The patient usually reports discomfort on deep breathing (rather than air hunger) as the reason for shortness of breath.
3. Warning signs
   Fever, cough, or hemoptysis should suggest an underlying lung injury.

Key Symptoms

- Localized pain at fracture site
- Pain aggravated by respiration
- Shortness of breath

Symptoms that suggest lung injury
- Fever, cough, hemoptysis
- Delayed-onset shortness of breath

Clinical Findings

1. Tachypnea with shallow respirations: The patient may present with hyperventilation syndrome with low P_{CO_2}.
2. Posturing so as to splint the injured side
   a. The thorax is arched toward the fractured side.
   b. The patient may be holding an arm or a pillow against the injured side.
3. Findings on palpation
   a. Careful palpation displays a discrete area of tenderness at the fracture site.
   b. There may be a cortical irregularity at the fracture site if there is any displacement.
   c. Gentle anteroposterior compression of the involved rib usually elicits pain at the fracture site.
4. Findings on auscultation
   a. Auscultation may be normal.
   b. Diminished breath sounds that are symmetric are probably due to shallow respirations.

Key Signs

- Tenderness at fracture site
- Shallow respirations, splinting
- Pain at fracture site with rib compression

WARNING

- **Below normal oxygen saturation should suggest an underlying lung injury.**
- **Asymmetric breath sounds or fremitus changes should suggest an underlying lung injury.**

Imaging Studies

1. Chest radiographs
    a. The principal importance of the plain chest film is in the diagnosis or exclusion of a suspected underlying lung or vascular injury.
    b. The posteroanterior chest view shows 90 per cent of rib fractures.
    c. Posteroanterior, lateral, and both oblique views provide optimal visualization of the cortical margins of most ribs.
    d. Cartilaginous injuries show no diagnostic findings on chest radiographs.
2. Computed tomographic (CT) scanning
    a. CT scans are not indicated for suspected *uncomplicated* rib fractures.
    b. The principal value of the CT scan is in the evaluation of suspected underlying organ injury, including the spleen, liver, kidneys, and, in some cases, great vessels.
3. Nuclear imaging (bone scan)
    a. Bone scan has no role in acute injury phase.
    b. Bone scanning may identify nondisplaced fractures not visualized on plain films by 48 to 72 hours post injury. Whether such visualization is of sufficient prognostic or therapeutic value to warrant the added expense is up to the judgment of the treating physician.

Key Test

- Chest and rib radiographs

Differential Diagnosis

1. Rib contusion
    a. Occurs only at the site of a direct blow
    b. Should have associated soft tissue swelling
    c. Pain *lessens* over days, whereas rib fracture pain usually *increases* over several days.
2. Costochondritis
    a. May have viral illness as prodrome
    b. Always painful at costochondral or costosternal articulations
    c. May result from overuse activities, seldom from trauma
3. Intercostal neuritis or neuralgia
    a. Usually gradual onset
    b. Lacks local point tenderness on rib
    c. Pain quality is often "electric-shock" or burning.
    d. May have dermatomal rash (zoster)
4. Pleurisy or pulmonary embolism
    a. Should have friction rub (contused lung may also demonstrate this)
    b. Occurs without trauma

5. Pneumothorax
    a. Spontaneous pneumothorax occurs without trauma.
    b. The affected lung displays increased tympany to percussion and decreased tactile fremitus compared with the unaffected side.

Treatment

1. Treat underlying or associated injuries such as the following:
    a. Cardiac contusion, traumatic pericarditis, laceration of great vessels or thoracic duct, rupture of esophagus. These are especially worth consideration in fractures of the sternum, clavicles, and upper two ribs.
    b. Ruptured spleen. Especially of concern in direct force fractures of the left lower posterolateral ribs.
    c. Hepatic contusion, rupture, laceration. Consider especially in direct force fractures of the right lower ribs.
    d. Pneumothorax or hemothorax. Although these may be seen with any rib fractures, the more violent the trauma or the more displaced the rib fractures, the more likely one is to find them.
    e. Pulmonary contusion. Especially likely with flail segments or multiple rib fractures. A gradual drop in Po_2 can be observed as the contusion condenses.
2. Analgesia
    a. Nonsteroidal anti-inflammatory drugs. Consider an initial regular dosage as needed because other musculoskeletal inflammation and pain may accompany the fracture site pain.
    b. Narcotics
        (1) Narcotics allow increased respiratory excursion through their analgesic effect, and their judicious use may benefit the patient's oxygenation far in excess of the risk of respiratory depression.
        (2) Beware of the presence or use of other depressants by the patient.
    c. Ice. Ice applied over the fracture site for 20- to 30-minute periods provides a topical anesthetic effect.

Key Treatment

- Pain relief

- Nonsteroidal anti-inflammatory drugs, narcotics as needed

- Ice

Overall management
- Watch for signs of lung injury.

- Order follow-up chest radiographs and arterial blood gas analysis.

d. Rib taping or belting. Some patients derive comfort from an expandable belt worn across the site of the fracture. The efficacy in pain relief is at the expense of respiratory excursion of the chest wall in all patients.

WARNING

Do not use rib belts or taping in the presence of respiratory complications such as an underlying lung injury!

---

3. Flail chest
   a. Consider the greater likelihood of injury to deeper structures.
   b. Positive-pressure ventilation by endotracheal tube may be needed if the patient's active respirations cannot maintain an acceptable oxygen saturation.
   c. Surgical stabilization of the fracture site or expectant therapy may deserve consideration, depending on the overall clinical picture.

Follow-Up

1. Patient instructions
   a. Activity
      (1) Heavy lifting and contact sports should ideally not be resumed until the patient is pain-free (3 to 6 weeks).
      (2) Most patients become reasonably comfortable and able to resume usual activities within 3 weeks.
   b. Sleeping position
      (1) Most patients feel most comfortable on their back.
      (2) Rolling over in bed is a significant source of discomfort in the first 3 weeks post fracture.
   c. Notify the physician if any of the following occur:
      (1) Fever
      (2) Increasing pain or shortness of breath
      (3) Development of productive cough
2. Revisit or re-radiograph plan
   a. If there is concern about the development of pulmonary contusion or great vessel bleeding, serial plain radiographs every 12 to 24 hours for the first few days post injury would be wise. Use serial arterial blood gas analyses or pulse oximetry to guide supplemental oxygen use.
   b. Otherwise, job restrictions and activity prescription are best guided by the clinical evaluation.
   c. Repeat plain radiographs are not indicated for the management of uncomplicated rib fractures.

Bibliography

For more information on rib fracture etiology, see

Betz P, Liebhardt E: Rib fractures in children— resuscitation or child abuse? Int J Legal Med 1994;106(4):215–218.

Mayo NE, Korner-Bitensky N, Levy AR: Risk factors for fractures due to falls. Arch Phys Med Rehabil 1993;74(9):917–921.

Szymanski S, Lieberman JA, Safferman A, Galkowski B: Rib fractures as an unusual complication of severe tardive dystonia (letter). J Clin Psychiatry 1993;54(4):160.

For more information on great vessel injuries with fractures of the upper ribs, see

Campbell DB: Trauma to the chest wall, lung, and major airways [review article: 45 refs]. Semin Thorac Cardiovasc Surg 1992;4(3):234–240.

For more information on radionuclide imaging of rib fractures, see

LaBan MM, Siegel CB, Schutz LK, Taylor RS: Occult radiographic fractures of the chest wall identified by nuclear scan imaging: report of seven cases. Arch Phys Med Rehabil 1994;75(3):353–354.

Procedure **INTRACOSTAL ANESTHESIA** *Eric D. Rasmussen*

Indications

1. Significant rib fractures
   a. Reducing splinted respirations
   b. Reducing hypoventilation
   c. Reducing atelectasis and consequent pneumonia
   d. Reducing respiratory compromise in patients with chronic obstructive pulmonary disease with little reserve
2. Post-traumatic neuralgia (including postoperative)
3. Metastatic neoplasms to vertebral bodies
4. Acute herpes zoster (not effective for postherpetic neuralgia)

Contraindications

1. Routine rib fractures in young patients are well tolerated with oral analgesics.
2. Blocks do not usually provide relief beyond 12 hours.
3. If the risks of a minor error (e.g., small pneumothorax) outweigh the benefits derived

Preparation

1. Lay the patient onto the side opposite the one to be injected.
2. Locate the 12th rib by palpation, and mark the 12th, 7th, and 3rd spinous processes.

3. T-3 is at the horizontal line linking the scapular spines; T-7 is roughly the inferior angle of the scapulae.
4. Informed consent from the patient, including that you will be anesthetizing one rib above and one below the area of pain

Equipment

1. Lidocaine 0.5% without epinephrine, 6 ml per rib, plus wheal
2. Syringe, 10 ml
3. Syringe, 3 ml
4. Needle: 8 cm spinal, 22-gauge for the block
5. Needle: 1.5-inch, 25-gauge for wheal and subdermal structure anesthesia
6. Iodophor solution
7. Alcohol swabs
8. Small adhesive bandage

Precautions

1. Risk of pneumothorax (less than 1 per 1000)
2. Risk of subarachnoid puncture (cerebrospinal fluid from the needle; rare)
3. Risk of bleeding from an intercostal vascular puncture

Technique

1. The goal is to anesthetize the lateral cutaneous branch of the thoracic nerve.
2. The thoracic nerves can be blocked from a spot 5 cm from the spinous processes, along the rib.

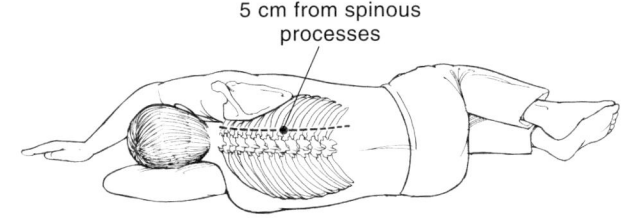

5 cm from spinous processes

3. In the subcostal groove, the nerve is lowest, the vein highest, and the artery between them.

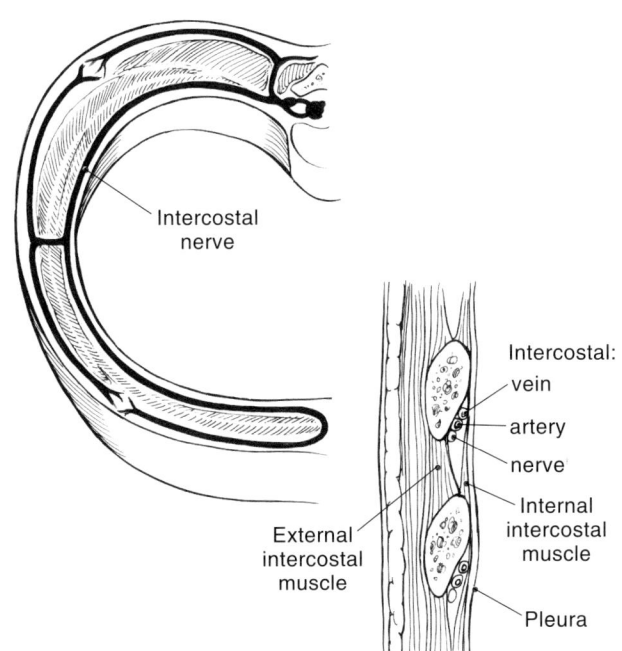

Intercostal nerve

Intercostal: vein — artery — nerve

Internal intercostal muscle

Pleura

External intercostal muscle

4. While the patient is lying on the appropriate side, curl the patient into a fetal position.

5. Place a cushion such that the spine is in optimal (straightest) alignment.

6. Clean the area appropriately.

7. With the 25-gauge needle and the lidocaine 0.5%, raise a 1-ml wheal 5 cm from the spinous process, along the affected ribs, and infuse the area with lidocaine down to the periosteum.

8. Insert the spinal needle through the wheal immediately over the rib until bone is felt. It may be helpful to use the other thumb to localize the rib and exert slight cephalad traction.

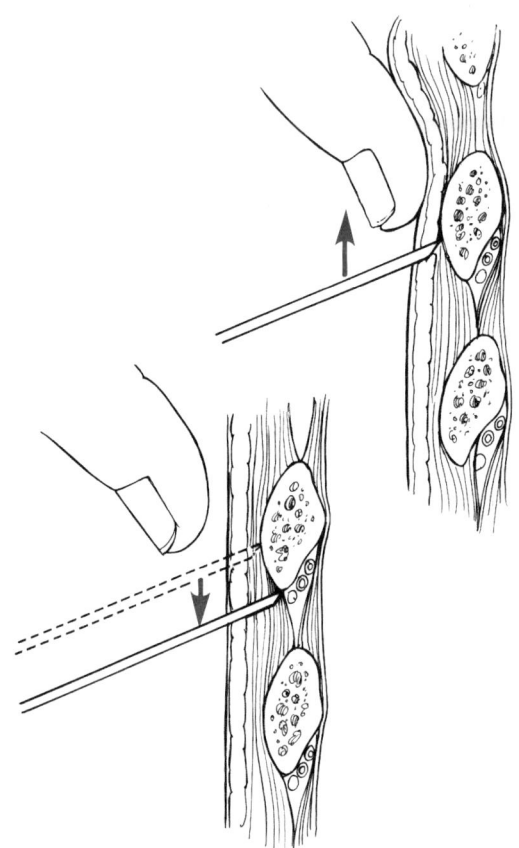

9. On finding bone, withdraw slightly, then redirect the needle so that it is pointing 45 degrees cephalad, 45 degrees medial, and 45 degrees inward toward the umbilicus. Releasing traction at this point can help position the needle appropriately and can help form a Z-track, minimizing continuity risks.

10. Advance the needle to no more than 1 cm beyond the lower border of the rib. The point should be in the intercostal space, between the external intercostal muscle and the internal intercostal fascia.

11. Inject 6 ml of lidocaine 0.5% without epinephrine, half without moving the needle, half in the area while withdrawing.

12. Inject ribs similarly, one above and one below the affected ribs, because neural overlap is extensive.

13. Cough often denotes needle penetration into the pleural space. Withdraw a few millimeters and wait until the coughing subsides.

14. Check the cutaneous hypesthesia 10 minutes after the injections, and reinject areas as needed.

Follow-Up

A chest radiograph should be done post procedure to evaluate hemopneumothorax.

Bibliography

For more information about multiple techniques for paravertebral thoracic blocks, see
Labat's Regional Anesthesia, Adriani J, Warren Green Inc., 1985, pp 300–317, 638–640.
Rivellini D: Local and regional anesthesia. Nursing implications. Nurs Clin North Am 1993;28(3):547–572.

For information regarding clinical indications, see
Jackson RP: Facet syndrome. Myth or reality. Clin Orthop 1992;279:110–121.
Skues MA, Welchew EA: Anesthesia and rheumatoid arthritis. Anesthesia 1993;48(11):989–997.
Woolf CJ, Chong MS: Pre-emptive analgesia—treating postoperative pain by preventing the establishment of central sensitization. Anesth Analg 1993;77(2):362–379.

43 Cancers of the Larynx and Lung

Sandra K. Willsie

Cancer of the Larynx

Etiology
1. Tobacco smoking and consumption of alcohol (synergistic risks)
2. Toxic or industrial exposures (prolonged)
   a. Metal or wood dusts
   b. Asbestos
   c. Hair dyes; paint, diesel, or gasoline fumes
3. Squamous cell carcinoma of the larynx accounts for about 95 per cent of all cases. Less than 5 per cent of cases are sarcomas, lymphomas, cylindromas, melanomas, or metastatic adenocarcinomas.

Symptoms
1. The most frequent presenting symptom is hoarseness or muffled voice.
2. Cough—typically nonproductive, with or without dyspnea
3. Dysphagia or odynophagia, with or without neck swelling or pain
4. Otalgia (referred pain to the ear) may occur late in the course

Key Symptoms

• Hoarseness	• Otalgia
• Odynophagia	• Cough

Clinical Findings
1. Cervical adenopathy, particularly the jugular chain
2. Fixation of the cricoid, hyoid, or thyroid cartilages
3. Stridor signifying laryngeal obstruction
4. Indirect laryngoscopy (lighted mirror) examination may reveal laryngeal irregularity, mass, edema (99 per cent of lesions are in the glottic or supraglottic location).

Key Signs

• Cervical adenopathy	• Hemoptysis
• Stridor or respiratory distress	• Fixation of hyoid, cricoid, or thyroid cartilages

Tests
1. Direct laryngoscopy with biopsy is the examination of choice.
2. Because 15 per cent of patients may have a second primary, direct laryngoscopy should be combined with bronchoscopy and esophagoscopy.

Key Test

• Inspection with biopsy is the only definitive test.

Differential Diagnosis
1. Hoarseness from other causes, including laryngeal edema, lymphatic obstruction from abscess or neoplasia, and chronic laryngitis from overuse, tobacco abuse, or syphilis
2. Upper airway obstruction from infection, cord paralysis, or thyroid enlargement

Treatment
1. Treatment of laryngeal carcinoma varies, depending on the stage of disease. Staging is by TNM (tumor, node, metastases) classification.
2. Treatment of limited disease (squamous cell carcinoma)
   a. Carcinoma in situ—vocal cord stripping or laser ablation
   b. Localized—surgical removal or radiation (90 per cent 5-year cure rate for T1 lesions)
   c. Subglottic or transglottic lesions—total laryngectomy with lymph node dissection. Consider adjunctive preoperative or postoperative radiation therapy.
3. For locally advanced lesions, experimental chemotherapy protocols should be considered versus radiation therapy with surgical extirpation following.
4. Speech rehabilitation. Many patients need subsequent speech therapy.

Key Treatment

Laryngeal Carcinoma: Treatment of Limited Disease (Squamous Cell Carcinoma)

• Carcinoma in situ—vocal cord stripping or laser ablation

• Localized—surgical removal or radiation

• Subglottic or transglottic lesions—total laryngectomy with lymph node dissection

Follow-Up

Patients should be advised to abstain from alcohol and tobacco use. Regular follow-up to look for recurrence and new lesions is necessary.

Cancer of the Lung

Etiology

1. Tobacco smoking (85 per cent of cases); secondhand smoke (implicated in 15 to 20 per cent)
2. Ionizing radiation—radon daughters
3. Occupational exposures—may be additive or synergistic with tobacco: asbestos, chromium, nickel, hydrocarbons, chloromethyl ether
4. Less well established risks—air pollution, vitamin A and E deficiencies, cigar or pipe use

Symptoms

1. Symptoms associated with bronchogenic carcinoma are often related to the cell type, location of the tumor, or rapidity of metastases—local and systemic.
2. Symptoms confined to the lung—cough, hemoptysis, hoarseness, wheezing, dyspnea, sputum production with or without fever related to postobstructive pneumonitis, chest pain

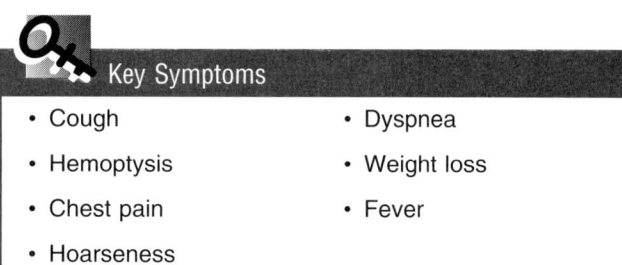

Key Symptoms

- Cough
- Hemoptysis
- Chest pain
- Hoarseness
- Dyspnea
- Weight loss
- Fever

Clinical Findings

1. Disease confined to the chest includes stridor, hoarseness, changes on examination related to atelectasis, consolidation, diaphragm paralysis or effusion, superior vena caval obstruction (cyanosis, engorgement of neck veins and lack of pulsations, enlarged neck circumference), and pericardial disease or tamponade.
2. Findings related to regional or distant metastases include adenopathy (particularly supraclavicular or scalene nodes), Horner's syndrome (supracervical ganglia involvement with miosis, ptosis, anhidrosis), and organ-specific findings.
3. Evidence of paraneoplastic syndromes or ectopic hormone production

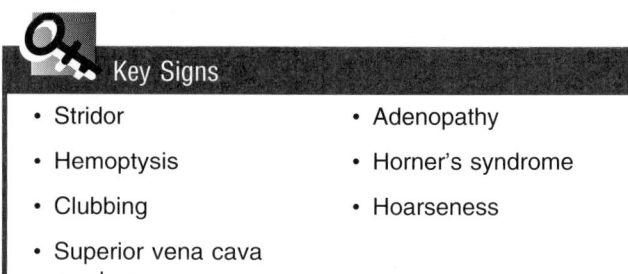

Key Signs

- Stridor
- Hemoptysis
- Clubbing
- Superior vena cava syndrome
- Adenopathy
- Horner's syndrome
- Hoarseness

Tests

1. Chest radiograph presentation classically varies according to cell type. (*Note*: This does not hold true in all cases.)
   a. Central lesions—squamous cell or small cell carcinoma
   b. Peripheral lesions—adenocarcinoma, large cell carcinoma, bronchoalveolar cell carcinoma
   c. Cavitation—squamous cell, large cell
   d. Early mediastinal, hilar involvement—small cell carcinoma
2. Sputum cytology: Negative results do not rule out carcinoma; more likely to be positive with central, endobronchial tumors.
3. Bronchoscopy—considered when sputum cytology is nondiagnostic (biopsies, needle aspiration, or lavage can be performed) and in cases of occult carcinoma (sputum cytology is positive with normal chest radiograph) preoperatively to rule out silent synchronous lesions
4. Percutaneous needle aspiration—helpful, particularly in patients with large or peripheral lesions and with negative cytology who are inoperative or bronchoscopy candidates because of the extent of disease
5. Pleural fluid should be sampled when present and sent for cytology, pH, cell counts, lactic dehydrogenase, and protein.
6. Rarely mediastinal exploration or open biopsy is needed for diagnosis.

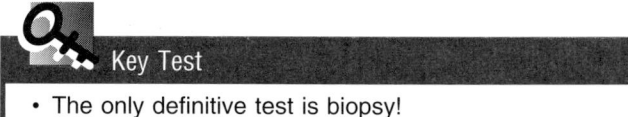

Key Test

- The only definitive test is biopsy!

Differential Diagnosis

1. Includes other diseases with similar symptomatology or chest radiograph appearance—granulomatous disease, including mycobacterial and fungal diseases and sarcoidosis; hamartomas; carcinoid tumors
2. Metastatic disease to the lung from other sites—breast, gastrointestinal tract, genitourinary tract, germ cell carcinomas, sarcomas, head and neck cancers, melanoma

Treatment

1. Treatment of bronchogenic carcinoma varies according to cell type, stage of disease (TNM classification), premorbid condition, and underlying lung function.

   a. Cell types—small cell carcinoma (SCC) and non–small cell carcinoma (NSCC). NSCC includes squamous cell, adenocarcinoma (including bronchoalveolar cell), large cell, and adenosquamous.

   b. SCC, regardless of stage, is almost always treated with chemotherapy. In the event of SCC with a solitary pulmonary nodule, excision may be performed first followed by chemotherapy.

   c. NSCC treatment is highly dependent on stage of disease.

      (1) Surgical resection is the treatment of choice for a solitary nodule or localized disease in the patient who has adequate pulmonary reserve with stage I to IIIa disease. In patients who are not surgical candidates, radiation therapy may be considered (15 to 20 per cent curative stage I disease).

      (2) Stage IIIb or IV may be considered for palliative radiation therapy or experimental chemotherapy protocols. (Chemotherapy is of uncertain benefit in NSCC; it is generally limited to young patients with good performance status.) Neoadjunctive therapy with chemotherapy with or without radiation therapy before attempted resection in stage IIIb or IV may be considered.

2. Malignant pleural effusions associated with bronchogenic carcinoma should be initially treated with therapeutic thoracentesis (if symptomatic). If there is symptomatic improvement but effusion recurs (particularly if rapid reaccumulation), pleurodesis should be considered. Pleurodesis is most likely to be effective if the pH of the fluid is greater than 7.3.

 Key Treatment

Bronchogenic Carcinoma

- Small cell carcinoma is almost always treated with chemotherapy. Small cell carcinoma with a solitary pulmonary nodule should be excised and then treated with chemotherapy.

- Non–small cell carcinoma treatment depends on the stage of disease. Surgical resection is the treatment of choice for a solitary nodule or localized disease in a patient who has adequate pulmonary reserve with stage I to IIIa disease. In patients who are not surgical candidates, radiation therapy may be considered. Stage IIIb or IV may be considered for palliative radiation therapy or experimental chemotherapy protocols.

- Malignant pleural effusions associated with bronchogenic carcinoma should be initially treated with therapeutic thoracentesis (if symptomatic). If there is symptomatic improvement but effusion recurs, pleurodesis should be considered.

Follow-Up

Close follow-up with periodic clinical examination and chest radiography should be performed to evaluate for recurrence or progression of disease.

 Bibliography

For more information on laryngeal carcinoma, see

McKenna JP, Fornataro-Clerici LM, McMenamin PG, Leonard RJ: Laryngeal carcinoma: Diagnosis, treatment and speech rehabilitation. Am Fam Physician 1991;44(1):123–129.

For more information on bronchogenic carcinoma, see

McCaughan BC: Primary lung cancer invading the chest wall. Chest Surg Clin N Am 1994;4:17–28.

For more information on staging of bronchogenic carcinoma, see

Herman SJ: Staging of bronchogenic carcinoma. World J Surg 1993;17:694–699.

44 Metastatic Cancer of Unknown Origin

Jai H. Joshi

Overview

1. Cancers of unknown origin are biopsy-proven metastatic neoplasms with histology that is inconsistent with a primary at the biopsy site. They account for about 5 per cent of cancers. Patients with this diagnosis have generally fared poorly in the past (median survival less than 6 months). Recently, however, prolonged survival has been documented in certain subgroups treated with specific therapies. Identification of these treatable subgroups using recently available diagnostic techniques such as immunoperoxidase staining, electron microscopy, and cytogenetics is crucial. It is equally important to refrain from using costly, unrewarding, and futile diagnostic and/or therapeutic interventions in subgroups for which no therapy is available.

2. Patients with cancers of unknown origin usually present with symptoms and signs referable to the multiple sites of metastatic disease—the liver, lungs, lymph nodes, and bone. Most patients also have constitutional symptoms, such as anorexia, weight loss, and fatigue. The need for obtaining adequate tissue whenever this diagnosis is considered is paramount. Open biopsy is preferable to fine-needle aspiration, and re-biopsy is mandatory whenever there is any question about the adequacy of biopsy material.

3. Findings on routine light microscopic examination of biopsy material provide a practical classification of these cancers into four groups: adenocarcinoma, squamous carcinoma, poorly differentiated carcinomas, and undifferentiated neoplasms. Most (60 per cent) are adenocarcinomas, a third (30 per cent) are carcinomas that are poorly differentiated, 5 per cent are squamous carcinomas, and 5 per cent are undifferentiated neoplasms. For undifferentiated neoplasms and poorly differentiated carcinomas, additional pathologic study is required. Rendering a specific diagnosis is important because lymphomas and germ cell tumors are highly curable when identified and specifically treated. In contrast, patients with well-differentiated adenocarcinoma and squamous carcinoma do not require additional pathologic study, except as a means of identifying treatable adenocarcinomas of the ovary, breast, and prostate. For these and squamous carcinomas of the head and neck, major palliation can be achieved, even in metastatic disease. For most other patients with adenocarcinoma, there is no effective therapy.

Undifferentiated Neoplasms

Light microscopy histology displays no lineage characteristics in this group, so that differentiation into even general neoplastic categories like carcinoma, lymphoma, melanoma, and sarcoma is impossible. Based on the extent of differentiation, these "anaplastic" neoplasms (i.e., that lack differentiation) may be further divided into undifferentiated and poorly differentiated categories. Additional pathologic study (Table 44–1) with immunoperoxidase staining, electron microscopy, and cytogenetics is mandatory because it results in specific diagnosis of treatable cancers in most patients. Two thirds have a diagnosis of non-Hodgkin's lymphoma established when leukocyte common antigen can be demonstrated in tissue by immunoperoxidase staining using monoclonal antibodies. The presence of this antigen distinguishes lymphoma from essentially all other undifferentiated tumors. Cytogenetic analyses demonstrating chromosomal translocations or immunoglobulin gene rearrangements are additionally helpful. With the implementation of chemotherapy regimens such as CHOP (cyclophosphamide, doxorubicin, vincristine, and prednisone), many patients with lymphoma diagnosed in this manner enjoy prolonged disease-free survival.

Poorly Differentiated Carcinomas

1. This heterogeneous group is distinctive in that it possesses well-defined clinical characteristics and is treatment-responsive. Epithelial features on light microscopy define the histologic criterion for inclusion in this group. In poorly differentiated, or *anaplastic, carcinoma,* the presence of epithelial features is the only lineage determinant. In poorly differentiated *adenocarcinoma,* minimal adenomatous differentiation is additionally present. This implies rudimentary gland formation or strong positivity with the histochemical stain for mucin in what otherwise is poorly differentiated carcinoma. Clearly definable glandular formation, however, must be absent because cases involving lesions with well-formed glandular structures, ducts with lumina, and mucin evident from hematoxylin-eosin staining are classified as adenocarcinomas. In poorly differentiated *small cell carcinoma (questionable neuroendocrine),* there is a cellular monotony of small cells with high nuclear/cytoplasmic ratios and displaced nuclear chromatin.

TABLE 44-1. ADDITIONAL PATHOLOGIC STUDIES

TUMOR	FINDING
Immunoperoxidase Staining	
Lymphoma	LCA(CD45) +; B, T cell markers/antigens +; (EMA ±; all other stains −)
Carcinoma	Epithelial stains (i.e., keratin and EMA) +; (LCA, S-100, vimentin −)
Sarcoma	Mesenchymal stain (i.e., vimentin) +; (epithelial stains −)
	Rhabdomyosarcoma: desmin +; myosin +
	Angiosarcoma: factor VIII antigen +
	Leiomyosarcoma: myosin +
Melanoma	S-100, HMB-45 (human melanoma black) antigen +; (epithelial stains −; mesenchymal vimentin +; NSE often +)
Neuroendocrine tumors	NSE, chromogranin +; (epithelial stains +)
Germ cell tumor	HCG, AFP +; (epithelial stains +)
Prostate cancer	PSA +; (epithelial stains +)
Breast cancer	ER, PR +; (epithelial stains +)
Thyroid cancer	Thyroglobulin +
	Medullary carcinoma of the thyroid: calcitonin +
Electron Microscopy	
Adenocarcinoma	Intercellular and intracellular lumina and surface microvilli
Squamous carcinoma	Desmosomes and prekeratin filament bundles in cytoplasm
Carcinoma	Desmosomes
Lymphoma	
Melanoma	Premelanosomes
Neuroendocrine tumors	Secretory granules
Sarcoma	Actin-myosin filaments (rhabdomyosarcoma)
Cytogenetics	
Germ cell tumors	Isochromosome 12p; 12q(−)
Lymphoma	Chromosomal translocations t(14:18); t(8:14)
Ewing's sarcoma	t(11:22)
Molecular Biology	
Lymphoma	Immunoglobulin (B-cell lymphomas), T-cell receptor gene (T-cell lymphomas) rearrangements
Neuroblastoma	*myc* oncogene
Breast carcinoma	HER-2/*neu*

+, positive result; −, negative result; LCA, leukocyte common antigen; EMA, epithelial membrane antigen; NSE, neuron-specific enolase; HCG, human chorionic gonadotropin; AFP, α-fetoprotein; PSA, prostate-specific antigen; ER, estrogen receptor, PR, progesterone receptor.

2. The clinical features that define this group include a younger age of patients, a short (less than 30-day) onset period, rapid progression, and tumor located predominantly in mediastinal, retroperitoneal, or peripheral (neck, axillary, or inguinal) lymph node groups. These findings are present in 50 per cent of patients. In others, the tumor may be located predominantly in the lung (with multiple lung masses on chest radiography and nonrevealing fiberoptic bronchoscopy results) or patients may have multiple sites of disease involvement without predominance at any one site.

3. *All* patients in this group should be treated with a chemotherapy regimen that combines cisplatin and etoposide, with or without adding bleomycin to the combination. More than 60 per cent respond, at least 25 per cent have complete responses, and most of the complete responders remain disease-free for periods in excess of 5 years, almost tantamount to "cure." Furthermore, specific subgroups identified with additional pathologic study are even more likely to respond. Patients with undiagnosed *germ cell tumors* constitute one such subgroup. This diagnosis generally remains elusive until cytogenetic studies identify the highly specific isochromosome abnormality that involves the short arm of chromosome 12 (i12p). Nonetheless, germ cell tumors should be suspected in young men who present with metastatic poorly differentiated carcinoma of unknown origin, regardless of the level of serum chorionic gonadotropin β-subunit and α-fetoprotein and even in the absence of the abnormal karyotype. With empirical treatment with cisplatin-based chemotherapy, excellent treatment responses and survival have been observed (50 per cent complete responses with 30 per cent having prolonged disease-free survival). Another subgroup with excellent prognosis is *neuroendocrine carcinoma*. This diagnosis is best established by electron microscopy (demonstrating neurosecretory granules). Positive immunoperoxidase staining for neuron-specific enolase and chromogranin is additionally helpful. Although tumors with varying clinical manifestations (from the indolent carcinoid to anaplastic small cell carcinoma) are included in the category, when neuroendocrine carcinoma masquerades as poorly differentiated carcinoma, it behaves aggressively and demonstrates a responsiveness to cisplatin-based chemotherapy.

4. Other diagnoses in cisplatin responders include malignant thymoma, melanoma, and lymphoma. *Malig-*

nant thymoma should be considered in patients with predominant mediastinal disease. *Melanoma* has been diagnosed retrospectively in cisplatin responders based on immunoperoxidase staining and electron microscopy findings. Accordingly, when melanoma is suggested in patients with poorly differentiated carcinoma, they should not be excluded from cisplatin-based chemotherapy trials because they may have uniquely sensitive tumors. *Lymphomas* can resemble anaplastic carcinoma when examined by light microscopy. Lymphomas even stain positively with epithelial markers on immunoperoxidase staining. Because the distinction between carcinoma and lymphoma can consequently affect treatment and survival, immunoperoxidase staining for leukocyte common antigen should be routinely used in all patients with poorly differentiated carcinoma.

Adenocarcinoma

1. Metastatic adenocarcinoma of unknown origin is the largest (60 per cent) group. Compared with patients having poorly differentiated carcinomas, these patients have different clinical characteristics, no extant effective therapy, and a dismal prognosis. At presentation, they have widespread metastatic disease (to the liver, lungs, and bone) and a poor performance status and are generally much older; accordingly, they should receive supportive care alone.

2. The histologic qualification for inclusion in this group is the demonstration of clearly definable glandular formation on light microscopy. This group does not include patients with poorly or moderately differentiated adenocarcinoma. This distinction is crucial. The hopeless prognosis of this group applies only to those with clearly definable glandular formation, not to those with rudimentary glandular formation or mucin positivity alone.

3. At autopsy, the most common primary sites of origin are the pancreas and lung. Because neither is treatable, attempts to find the primary are not worthwhile, and previously published large series have amply documented the futility of aggressive diagnostic testing in the pursuit of that goal. Therefore, attempts at identifying only treatable adenocarcinomas of the breast, ovary, prostate, and thyroid are appropriate. Unlike their frequency in the general population, these treatable adenocarcinomas are rare in this group. Nonetheless, given the potential therapeutic implications of such a discovery, women should be evaluated for a possible breast or ovarian primary and men for an occult prostate primary. A thyroid primary should be excluded in either sex. Additional pathologic study with immunoperoxidase staining should be pursued. Adenocarcinoma of the breast is suggested with the presence of gross cystic fluid protein or estrogen and progesterone receptors. Prostate-spe-

cific antigen (PSA) and prostate acid phosphatase staining of tissue identify prostatic adenocarcinoma. Thyroglobulin positivity identifies the thyroid as the site of origin. Radiologic evaluations should include mammography for breast cancer and either an abdominopelvic computed tomographic (CT) scan or a pelvic ultrasound for ovarian cancer. The evaluation for a prostatic primary should include an abdominal CT scan, a bone scan, and serum PSA determinations.

4. Treatable adenocarcinomas of the breast, ovary, and prostate can also be diagnosed with the recognition of specific clinical syndromes. Women with enlarged axillary nodes and adenocarcinoma on biopsy represent one such syndrome. These women should be treated as are patients with stage II breast cancer, regardless of the presence of a lesion on examination or mammography and irrespective of estrogen and progesterone receptor status in the biopsied axillary node. They should undergo modified radical mastectomy or receive breast irradiation to reduce the risk of local recurrence. In addition, they should receive adjuvant systemic hormonal (tamoxifen) chemotherapy to reduce their risk of metastatic disease. Women with malignant ascites represent the second treatable syndrome. After surgical debulking, these patients should receive cisplatin-based chemotherapy as would those with metastatic ovarian adenocarcinoma, regardless of the presence of a pelvic mass and even if normal ovaries were found at laparotomy. The third syndrome involves men with osteoblastic bone metastasis. Regardless of serum PSA levels and tissue immunoperoxidase staining, these patients should be treated with hormonal therapy as are men with metastatic (stage D) prostate cancer.

Squamous Carcinoma

1. Squamous carcinomas of unknown origin present with neck, axillary, or inguinal adenopathy. Each presentation has specific recommendations in regard to the extent of diagnostic evaluations and therapies that may be required. In patients with squamous carcinoma who present with *cervical adenopathy,* the head and neck are the most likely primary sites (especially if the patient is a heavy smoker or alcohol consumer) followed by the lungs. Diagnostic evaluation should include a complete otolaryngologic examination and chest radiography, followed by panendoscopy (laryngoscopy, nasopharyngoscopy, and esophagoscopy) and a CT scan of the head and neck to identify submucosal lesions not visualized by endoscopy. If no primary is found, blind biopsies of the nasopharynx, piriform sinuses, base of the tongue, and tonsils should be obtained. If CT scanning of the chest uncovers a lung primary, bronchoscopy should be performed. It is not necessary to search below the diaphragm for a primary. When no primary is found,

treatment should generally involve radiation therapy to the involved cervical chain combined with prophylactic irradiation of the nasopharynx, oropharynx, and larynx (the likely occult primary sites). In addition, the contralateral uninvolved neck should also be irradiated. Radiation should be administered in the same dose and fields as in patients with known primary head and neck cancers. Five-year survival rates of 30 to 50 per cent have been documented with this approach. The preference for irradiation over surgery is based on a higher relapse rate with surgery alone. Patients who present with *supraclavicular adenopathy* generally fare poorly because most have squamous carcinoma of the lung. The diagnostic evaluation for this group should include CT scanning of the chest and bronchoscopy. Again, it is not necessary to search below the diaphragm for a primary. Squamous carcinoma presenting with *inguinal adenopathy* is usually the result of metastases from an occult primary in the perineal or anorectal area. Attempts to identify them are appropriate. When no primary is found, inguinal lymph node dissection with or without irradiation is the treatment of choice. Long-term survival has been documented with this treatment approach.

2. When an occult primary squamous carcinoma is found at other sites (e.g., brain, liver, or bone), the lung is the most likely site of origin, and this is usually obvious on chest radiography. When chest radiography is unrevealing, further studies should not be undertaken because no effective therapy exists for metastatic squamous carcinoma of the lung.

ACKNOWLEDGMENT: For his succinct and prompt reviews of this article and his many excellent suggestions, I recognize the contributions of my son, Amit Joshi.

 Bibliography

Hainsworth JD, Greco FA: Carcinoma of unknown primary site. *In* Stein JH (ed): Internal Medicine, 3rd ed. Boston, Little, Brown, 1990, pp 1180–1184.
Hainsworth JD, Greco FA: Treatment of patients with cancer of an unknown primary site [review]. N Engl J Med 1993;329:257–263.
Hainsworth JD, Greco FA, Johnson DH, et al: Cisplatin-based combination chemotherapy in the treatment of poorly differentiated carcinoma and poorly differentiated adenocarcinoma of unknown primary site. Results of a 12-year experience. J Clin Oncol 1992;10:912.
Raber MN, Abbruzzese JL, Frost P, et al: Unknown primary tumors. Curr Opin Oncol 1992;4:3.
Rosen PJ: Approach to the patient with an unknown primary. *In* Kelley WN (ed): Textbook of Internal Medicine. Philadelphia, JB Lippincott, 1989, pp 1334–1336.

45 Oncologic Emergencies

Alison Grann

Although many consequences are associated with cancer, there are five oncologic emergencies that the primary care physician and house officer should look for when evaluating the patient with cancer.

Hypercalcemia

Etiology

Different tumors produce hypercalcemia by way of different mechanisms.

1. Parathyroid hormone–related peptide
   a. Commonly found in squamous cell cancers of the lung, head, and neck and in breast cancer
   b. Increased renal absorption of calcium; increased bone absorption of calcium secondary to osteoclast activation
2. Bone metastasis
   a. Many tumors; common in breast cancer
   b. Increased bone destruction leads to increased calcium levels.
3. Increased production of 1,25-dihydroxycholecalciferol
   a. Seen in lymphomas
   b. Increased gut absorption of calcium leads to hypercalcemia.
4. Cytokines—formerly known collectively as osteoclast activating factor; now known to be multiple and to include interleukin-1, tumor necrosis factor, and others
   a. Seen in myeloma and other tumors
   b. Increased bone resorption due to cytokines and impaired renal function secondary to increased calcium levels

Symptoms

Dependent on how quickly hypercalcemia develops
1. General—weakness, lethargy
2. Gastrointestinal—anorexia, nausea, vomiting, constipation, acute pancreatitis
3. Renal—polydipsia and polyuria, dehydration, nephrocalcinosis
4. Cardiovascular—ventricular arrhythmias, heart block, asystole
5. Neurologic—altered mood, depression, disturbed sleep, confusion, stupor, coma, muscle weakness

Clinical Findings

1. Renal failure
2. Hyporeflexia
3. Hypotonia
4. Stupor
5. Coma
6. Ventricular arrhythmias

Tests

1. Serum calcium: must check albumin because 50 per cent of serum calcium is bound to protein and only free ionized calcium is active
2. Serum phosphate—low in patients with parathyroid hormone–related peptide
3. Alkaline phosphate—elevated with bone metastasis
4. Electrolytes, blood urea nitrogen, creatinine
5. Electrocardiography—shortening of Q-T interval, broadening of T waves, heart block, asystole, ventricular arrhythmias

Treatment

1. Vigorous hydration with normal saline
2. Intermittent use of furosemide (Lasix) once one is well hydrated
3. Monitor for volume overload or worsening dehydration
4. Monitor cardiovascular status
5. Calcitonin—4 to 6 IU subcutaneously in 0.5 liter of normal saline over 4 to 6 hours q 12 hours
   a. Increases urinary excretion of calcium and decreases bone resorption
   b. Second-line therapy after intravenous hydration with furosemide if the patient is extremely symptomatic and calcium must be lowered quickly
   c. Limited use secondary to tachyphylaxis; can cause hypophosphatemia
6. Glucocorticoids—200 to 300 mg of hydrocortisone or its equivalent
   a. Decreases intestinal calcium absorption and inhibits bone resorption
   b. Response may be delayed up to 1 week
   c. Many adverse effects
   d. Not optimal therapy
   e. Patients with nonhematologic cancer do not respond
7. Plicamycin (mithramycin)—25 μg/kg of body weight infused over 8 to 12 hours

180

a. Inhibits ribonucleic acid synthesis of osteoclasts

b. Many toxic adverse effects, including hepatic and renal toxicity and bleeding disorders

c. Not first-, second-, or third-line therapy

8. Biphosphonates—many types, each administered differently

a. Pamidronate (Aredia)—newest compound; 90 mg given intravenously over 24 hours acts quickly and lasts for 2 to 3 weeks

b. Binds to hydroxyapatite in bone and prevents bone from being broken down

c. No significant toxicity

d. Second-line therapy after intravenous hydration and furosemide unless the patient is extremely symptomatic and calcitonin is indicated

9. Gallium nitrate (Ganite)—200 mg/m^2 body surface in dextrose 5% in water over 24 hours

a. Decreases bone resorption

b. Chief toxicity is hypophosphatemia

c. Not first-, second-, or third-line therapy

10. Phosphate causes many complications and should never be used

11. Dialysis—if therapies above do not work

Superior Vena Cava Syndrome

Etiology

Caused by partial or complete obstruction of blood flow through the superior vena cava to the right atrium

1. Mechanism of obstruction

a. Compression

b. Thrombosis

c. Fibrosis

d. Invasion

2. Most (80 to 95 per cent) of superior vena cava syndrome is caused by a mediastinal cancer, leading to compression of the superior vena cava.

Symptoms

Typically develop over 3 to 4 weeks

1. Swelling of face, trunk, and upper extremities

2. Cough

3. Hoarseness

4. Dysphagia

5. Nausea

6. Headache

7. Visual changes

Clinical Findings

1. Neck vein distention

2. Facial edema plethora

3. Tachypnea

Tests

1. Chest radiography

2. Computed tomographic scan with contrast

3. Unless impeding airway obstruction or intracerebral hemorrhage, obtain tissue

Treatment

1. Position patient upright, and maintain adequate oxygenation.

2. Diuretics

3. Steroids

4. Radiation therapy

5. Chemotherapy if tissue diagnosis

Spinal Cord Compression

Etiology

1. Occurs when metastasis to vertebral body or pedicle enlarges and compresses underlying dura

2. Most common in thoracic spine; if not in thoracic then lumbar>cervical>sacral spine

Symptoms

Depend on level of spinal cord involved

1. Back pain in 95 per cent of patients

2. Motor and sensory symptoms

3. Autonomic dysfunction with incontinence

Clinical Findings

Dependent on level of cord involved; localized back pain

Tests

1. Plain radiography

2. Magnetic resonance imaging scan of spine

3. Myelography if magnetic resonance imaging is not available

Treatment

Key to effective management is to initiate treatment before neurologic deficits develop.

1. High-dose steroids—dexamethasone (Decadron), 10 mg, intravenously followed by 4 mg q.i.d.

2. Radiation therapy

3. Surgical decompression—for patients without known cancer, those who have received maximal radiation, and those whose condition deteriorates during radiation

4. Rarely chemotherapy

Tumor Lysis Syndrome

Etiology

1. Occurs in patients who have a tumor that is extremely sensitive to chemotherapy

2. Classically seen in patients with Burkitt's lymphoma, non-Hodgkin's lymphoma, acute lymphoblastic leukemia, and acute myelogenous leukemia

3. Characterized by syndrome of hyperuricemia, hyperkalemia, hyperphosphatemia, and hypocalcemia

Symptoms and Clinical Findings

Secondary to electrolyte abnormalities and renal failure
1. Tetany
2. Ventricular arrhythmias
3. Renal failure
4. Nephrocalcinosis
5. Lethargy
6. Nausea
7. Vomiting

Tests

1. Uric acid
2. Calcium
3. Albumin
4. Potassium
5. Creatinine
6. Blood urea nitrogen
7. Phosphate

Treatment

1. Vigorous intravenous hydration before and during chemotherapy
2. Alkalinize urine with $NaHCO_3-$ for first few days of therapy.
3. Oliguric patients with bulky tumors may require dialysis during induction of chemotherapy.
4. Allopurinol before chemotherapy
   a. Decreases incidence of uric acid nephropathy
   b. Causes xanthine nephropathy
5. Monitor electrolytes every 12 to 24 hours.

Fever and Neutropenia

Etiology

Acute leukemia, intensive chemotherapy, or radiation therapy may cause neutropenia in an already immunocompromised host.
1. Worry when absolute neutrophil count is less than 500.
2. Typically, no organism is identified, but the organisms most commonly isolated are *Pseudomonas* sp., *Staphylococcus* sp., *Enterobacter* sp., *Candida* sp., *Clostridium difficile,* and *Aspergillus.*

Symptoms

1. Fever (may be only symptom)
2. Cough
3. Dysuria

4. Urinary frequency or urgency
5. Tenderness over indwelling catheter
6. Perianal pain
7. Nausea
8. Vomiting
9. Diarrhea
10. Abdominal pain

Clinical Findings

1. May find only fever
2. Pay special attention to lung examination, indwelling catheter site, perirectal area, skin, and perianal examination.

Tests

1. Blood culture
2. Urine analysis and culture
3. Chest radiography
4. Sputum culture

Treatment

1. Without immediate antibiotics, at least 50 per cent of febrile neutropenic patients die as a result of infection.
2. Empiric antibiotics with an aminoglycoside in combination with an extended-spectrum penicillin or third-generation cephalosporin
3. If there is clinical suspicion of line infection, begin vancomycin (Vancocin) immediately. If the patient remains febrile after 48 hours on only gram-negative coverage, then add vancomycin.
4. If there is suspected anaerobic infection or persistent fever after 3 to 5 days, add metronidazole (Flagyl).
5. After 7 days of persistent fever, add amphotericin B (Fungizone).
6. Consider granulocyte colony-stimulating factor. Question if some risk in leukemic patients.
7. Once the absolute neutrophil count is higher than 500, the patient is afebrile for 48 hours, and all cultures are negative, discontinue antibiotics.

Bibliography

American Society of Clinical Oncology. Recommendations for the use of hematopoietic colony-stimulating factors: evidence-based, clinical practice guidelines. J Clin Oncol 1994;12:2471–2508.

Helms SR, Carlson MD: Cardiovascular emergencies. Semin Oncol 1989;16:463–470.

Hughes WT, Armstrong D, Bodey GP, et al.: Guidelines for the use of antimicrobial agents in neutropenic patients with unexplained fever. J Infect Dis 1990;161:381–396.

Sepkowitz KA, Brown AE, Armstrong D: Empirical therapy for febrile, neutropenic patients: Persistence of susceptibility of gram-negative bacilli to aminoglycoside antibiotics. Clin Infect Dis 1994;19:810–811.

Thomas MR, Robinson WA: Oncologic emergencies in primary care. Postgrad Med 1985;78:41–49.

46 Tuberculosis

Nabil Abou-Shala

Epidemiology

1. An estimated 10 million people in the United States are infected with tuberculosis (TB). More than 20,000 new cases of TB are reported annually; 90 per cent of those arise from the previously infected pool and only 10 per cent are newly infected.
2. Since 1984, the expected decline in TB morbidity has leveled off, with more than 51,700 excess cases in 1992. This can be ascribed to the following:
   a. Human immunodeficiency virus (HIV) epidemic
   b. Deteriorating social infrastructure (homelessness, substance abuse, prisons)
   c. Poor TB control measures in hospitals, clinics, and institutions
3. More than two thirds of reported cases in the United States occur among nonwhite racial and ethnic groups. Nearly one fourth of all cases occur in foreign-born people and one third occur in the middle- and upper-income groups.

Natural History of Tuberculous Infection

1. TB is strictly a human disease.
2. Transmission of tubercle bacilli from a source case (Fig. 46–1) depends on positive sputum smear, cough frequency, ventilation, and duration of exposure.
3. Infection rate from a smear-positive case is 30 per cent of the close contacts and 15 per cent of the others.
4. An average of 1 in 10 infected persons develops the disease sometime in his or her life unless given preventive therapy.
5. Before the emergence of cellular immunity (first 2 to 4 weeks), lymphohematogenous dissemination may give rise to miliary, meningeal, or TB adenitis.
6. Once tuberculin reactivity has developed, cell-mediated immunity usually arrests the growth of tuberculin bacilli and leads to healing with granuloma formation.
7. Particularly in children and immunodeficient adults, the initial site of infection may not be contained, leading to *progressive primary TB*. Clinically, this presents with advancing pneumonitis, cavitation, pleural effusion, adenopathy, and pericarditis.
8. *Postprimary TB* develops by the following two mechanisms:
   a. Endogenous reactivation of an earlier (latent) infection
   b. Exogenous reinfection with repeated exposure to

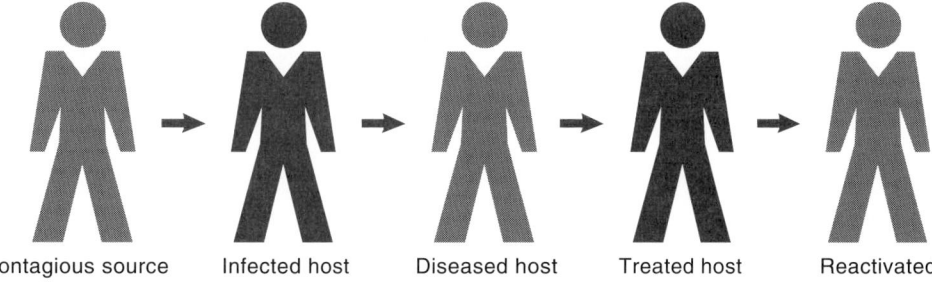

Contagious source → Infected host → Diseased host → Treated host → Reactivated

Risk of infection	Risk of progression to disease	Risk of reactivation
• Degree of contact • Age (infancy to early adult) • Sex & race:> males and nonwhites	• Time (first 2 yrs after infection) • Age (< 5 and > 60) • Dosage of infection • Size of PPD reaction • Alcoholics and IV drug users • Coexisting medical conditions: HIV, silicosis, abnormal CXR, diabetes, prolonged corticosteroid/immunosuppressive therapy, hematologic malignancies, chronic hemodialysis, intestinal bypass, postgastrectomy, malnutrition, carcinoma of the oropharynx and esophagus	• Inadequate chemotherapy • Time: shortly after treatment stopped • Extent of previous disease • Immune status

Figure 46–1. Etiologic epidemiology of tuberculosis.

highly contagious cases (such as in shelters, nursing homes) and with HIV coinfection

9. *Extrapulmonary TB* may involve nearly any organ in the body and produce signs and symptoms related to the specific site as well as systemic illness.

Key Point

- The *lifetime* risk of disease in a person infected only with TB is 5 to 10 per cent. In contrast, the risk that active TB will develop in a person coinfected with TB and HIV is about 8 per cent *per year*.

Symptoms
1. Fatigue
2. Anorexia
3. Weight loss
4. Fever with night sweats
5. Productive cough (over weeks or months)
6. Hemoptysis
7. Chest pain
8. Dyspnea (with extensive disease or massive pleural effusion)

Clinical Findings
1. The genitourinary tract may be involved (recurrent urinary tract infections, pyuria without bacteriuria, hematuria), as may the lymph nodes (intrathoracic, cervical, and supraclavicular adenopathy), bones and joints (lower spine "Pott's disease"), and meninges (insidious onset meningitis, the cerebrospinal fluid has low glucose, and increased lymphocytes). In addition, the peritoneum, pericardium, and larynx may be involved.
2. TB is a common cause of fever of unknown origin (FUO), particularly in elderly people.
3. Patients coinfected with HIV: TB usually occurs early in the course of HIV. It is difficult to separate from other HIV-related pulmonary processes. TB is characterized by rapid progression from exposure to infection to active disease, more disseminated and extrapulmonary involvement, and high fatality rate if treatment is delayed.

Key Points

- TB may simulate many other diseases.
- After TB exposure, 40 per cent of HIV-infected close contacts develop *active disease* within 4 to 8 weeks.

Radiologic Features of Pulmonary TB
1. Postprimary disease—parenchymal apical or posterior segment of upper lobes, cavitation, fibrosis

2. Primary disease—consolidation, adenopathy, pleural effusion, and normal chest radiograph

Key Point

- The chest radiograph in TB does not establish activity of disease.

Bacteriologic Evaluation
1. Sputum smears by an acid-fast procedure should be collected in early morning. The diagnostic yield is 40 per cent with one specimen and up to 80 per cent with three specimens (greater than 90 per cent if there is an open cavity).
2. Sputum induction and/or bronchoscopy may be indicated in difficult cases.
3. Regular mycobacterial cultures require 6 weeks for growth. The BACTEC procedure shortens the time to 3 weeks.

Key Points

- Bacteriology remains the "gold standard" for diagnosis of *active* disease.
- Centers for Disease Control and Prevention recommendation: All patients with TB from whom *Mycobacterium tuberculosis* is isolated should have drug susceptibility testing performed on the first isolate.

Treatment of Active Disease
1. Major antitubercular drugs
   a. Isoniazid (INH)
      (1) Ideal agent—bactericidal, relatively nontoxic, inexpensive, penetrates well
      (2) Hepatitis is the major toxic effect; more likely after age 35, alcohol use, chronic liver disease.
      (3) Peripheral neuropathy (mainly seen with diabetes, uremia, alcoholism, malnutrition, pregnancy) can be prevented with pyridoxine.
   b. Rifampin (RIF; Rimactane)
      (1) Essential drug for less than or equal to a 12-month course
      (2) Most common adverse reactions are orange discoloration of secretions and gastrointestinal upset.
      (3) Accelerates clearance of drugs metabolized by the liver (e.g., anticonvulsants, coumadin, estrogens, oral hypoglycemics, digitalis)
      (4) Intermittent administration may be associated with thrombocytopenia, an influenza-like syn-

TABLE 46–1. DOSAGES OF ANTITUBERCULAR MEDICATIONS

DRUGS	ROUTE	DAILY (MAX)	INTERMITTENT: 2 TO 3 TIMES/WEEK (MAX.)
First-Line Drugs			
Isoniazid	P.O.	5 mg/kg (300 mg)	15 mg/kg (900 mg)
Rifampin	P.O.	10 mg/kg (600 mg)	10 mg/kg (600 mg)
Pyrazinamide	P.O.	15–30 mg/kg (2 gm)	50–70 mg/kg (3 gm)
Ethambutol	P.O.	15–25 mg/kg (2.5 gm)	50 mg (2.5 gm)*
Streptomycin	I.M.	15 mg/kg (1 gm)†	25–30 mg/kg (1.5 gm)‡
Second-Line Drugs			TOXICITY
Ethionamide	P.O.	15 mg/kg (1 gm)	Gastrointestinal upset, dysgeusia, hepatitis, arthralgia
Cycloserine	P.O.	15 mg/kg (1 gm)	Mood/behavioral changes, seizures, peripheral neuropathy
Capreomycin	I.M.	15–20 mg/kg (1 gm)	Hearing loss, ataxia, nystagmus, azotemia, proteinuria
Kanamycin	I.M.	15–30 mg/kg (1 gm)	Hearing loss, ataxia, nystagmus, azotemia, proteinuria
Aminosalicylic acid	P.O.	150 mg/kg (12 gm)	Gastrointestinal upset
Ofloxacin	P.O.	400 mg b.i.d.	Abdominal distress, headache, anxiety, tremor, thrush
Ciprofloxacin	P.O.	750 mg b.i.d.	Abdominal distress, headache, anxiety, tremor, thrush

*Dosage should be 25 to 30 mg/kg (max. 2.5 gm) if given three times per week.
†In elderly patients (>60 years), dosage should be limited to 10 mg/kg/day (max. 750 mg).
‡Maximal dose is 1 gm if given three times per week.

drome, hemolytic anemia, and acute renal failure (uncommon at less than or equal to 10 mg/kg dose).

  c. Pyrazinamide (PZA)
    (1) Essential drug for a 6-month course
    (2) Adverse effects include liver injury, hyperuricemia, and arthralgias.
  d. Ethambutol (EMB; Myambutol)
    (1) Accumulates in renal insufficiency
    (2) Adverse effect—retrobulbar neuritis (dose-related in less than 1 per cent at less than or equal to 15 mg/kg/day)
  e. Streptomycin (SM)
    (1) Parenteral dosage reduction is necessary in patients over age 60 and in those with renal insufficiency.
    (2) Renal and VIIIth cranial nerve toxicities are related to total dose.
    (3) Ototoxicity is mainly vestibular (vertigo), but hearing loss may occur.
2. Dosage and adverse effects (Table 46–1)
3. Treatment regimens (Table 46–2)

TABLE 46–2. INITIAL THERAPY FOR TUBERCULOSIS*

OPTION 1
INH/RIF/PZA ± EMB or SM daily for 8 weeks, then INH/RIF ± EMB or SM daily or two or three times per week for 16 weeks
OPTION 2
INH/RIF/PZA ± EMB or SM daily for 2 weeks, then same drugs twice a week by DOT for 6 weeks, then INH/RIF twice a week by DOT for 16 weeks
OPTION 3
INH/RIF/PZA ± EMB or SM three times per week by DOT for 6 months

DOT, direct observed therapy.
*Recommendations of the Advisory Council for the Elimination of Tuberculosis.

> **Note**
> A four-drug regimen with INH, RIF, PZA, and SM or EMB is *preferred* for the initial empiric treatment in areas where the INH resistance rate is not documented to be less than 4 per cent.

Follow-Up

1. Obtain sputum for acid-fast smear and culture monthly until conversion is documented. Obtain a consult if the patient is symptomatic or the smear or culture is positive after 3 months.
2. For options 1, 2, and 3, continue treatment for at least 6 months and 3 months beyond sputum culture conversion.
3. For patients coinfected with TB and HIV, options 1, 2, and 3 can be used, but treatment regimens should continue for a total of 9 months *and* at least 6 months beyond culture conversion.
4. All regimens administered intermittently (two or three times per week) should be monitored by directly observed therapy for the duration of the regimen.
5. Obtain baseline values of liver enzymes, bilirubin, creatinine, or blood urea nitrogen and complete blood count. In addition, a uric acid level should be obtained if PZA is used and visual acuity should be assessed if EMB is used.
6. If drug susceptibility results are not available, EMB or SM should be continued for the entire course of therapy.
7. A single drug must never be added to a failing regimen.

Drug-Resistant Tuberculosis

Epidemiology

Multiple-fold increase in multidrug-resistant TB (MDRTB) in the United States from 1982 to 1991

TABLE 46-3. PEOPLE AT RISK FOR DRUG-RESISTANT TB

a. Foreign-born people from Asia, Africa, and Latin America
b. Residents in the United States from
  (1) high-prevalence areas of drug resistance or
  (2) history of hospitalization, institutionalization, or incarceration at a facility with a known multidrug-resistant TB outbreak
c. History of prior treatment for TB
d. Patients with positive bacteriology after 3 months of therapy
e. Contacts of known or suspected drug-resistant cases
f. Human immunodeficiency virus infection

1. Primary MDRTB (previously untreated) rose from 0.5 to 3.1 per cent.
2. Secondary (acquired) MDRTB increased from 3 to 7 per cent mainly in large urban areas and coastal or border communities

Risk factors for MDRTB (Table 46-3)

Etiology

1. Poor compliance with TB control guidelines
2. Increased exposure of HIV-infected patients to TB in institutional settings
3. Delayed consideration for diagnosis (leading to poor isolation measures and delayed therapy)
4. Delayed recognition of drug resistance and implementation of an appropriate drug regimen. Despite appropriate therapy, MDRTB is associated with high rates of treatment failure and mortality from the disease.

Drug regimens should include more than or equivalent to three agents (preferably a total of five) to which the organism is sensitive in vitro and/or that have not been used previously in the patient.

Preventive Therapy (Treatment of TB Infection)

1. INH decreases the likelihood of active TB developing in an infected person by 90 per cent.
  a. INH indications and duration are listed in Table 46-4
  b. Dosage
    (1) Daily: 10 mg/kg (max. 300 mg)
    (2) Intermittently: 15 mg/kg (max. 900 mg) twice weekly by direct observed therapy
  c. Duration
    (1) HIV negative
      (a) Adults—6 months

TABLE 46-4. PREVENTIVE THERAPY BASED ON PPD SKIN TEST RESULTS

HIV (−)	HIV (+)
Irrespective of Induration	
Children (<5 years) who are in close contact	Close contact with an infectious case
People with inadequately treated TB infection	Previously untreated + PPD
	Chest radiograph suggestive of untreated TB
≥5-mm Induration	
Close contacts	Any HIV-infected person not mentioned above
Chest radiograph suggestive of untreated TB	
≥10-mm Induration	
TB infection within the previous 2 years (↑ PPD by >10 mm if <35 years or by ≥15 mm if >35 years)	
Medical conditions that predispose to development of TB	
Foreign born from high-prevalence countries, medically unserved, and residents of long-term facilities (<35 years)	
≥15-mm Induration	
Low-risk population (<35 years)	

HIV, human immunodeficiency virus; PPD, purified protein derivative.

      (b) Children—9 months
      (c) Abnormal chest film—12 months
    (2) HIV positive—12 months
2. Alternative therapy (for close contacts to resistant organisms) includes the following:
  a. For INH-resistant organisms
    (1) RIF, 600 mg daily for 1 year or
    (2) RIF plus PZA for 2 months, followed by RIF alone for 4 months
  b. For multidrug-resistant organisms (with consultation of a TB medical expert)
    (1) EMB plus PZA for 6 to 12 months or
    (2) Ofloxacin (Floxin) or ciprofloxacin (Cipro) plus PZA for 6 to 12 months

B Bibliography

Abou-Shala N, Mauldin G: Tuberculosis: An old nemesis returns. J Am Acad Phys Assist 1993;6:639–648.
American Thoracic Society Statement: Treatment of tuberculosis and tuberculosis infection in adults and children. Am J Respir Crit Care Med 1994;149:1359–1374.
Barnes PF, Barrows SA: Tuberculosis in the 1990s. Ann Intern Med 1993;119:400–410.
Barnes PF, Bloch AB, Davidson PT, Snider DE: Tuberculosis in patients with human immunodeficiency virus infection. N Engl J Med 1991;324:1644–1650.
Iseman MD: Treatment of multidrug-resistant tuberculosis. N Engl J Med 1993;329:784–791.
Statement of the tuberculosis committee of the Infectious Diseases Society of America. Clin Infect Dis 1993;16:627–628.

| Procedure | **TECHNIQUE OF SPUTUM INDUCTION** | *Muhammad K. Zaman* |

Indications

When spontaneous sputum is unavailable and one of the following is suspected

A. Infectious
1. Mycobacterial disease
2. *Pneumocystis* pneumonia
3. Bacterial infection
4. Fungal infection

B. Neoplastic
1. Bronchogenic carcinoma
2. Metastasis to lungs

Contraindications

1. No absolute contraindication
2. Altered mental status and extreme dyspnea are relative contraindications.
3. Defer sputum induction in patients with untreated pneumothorax.

Preparation

1. Patient instruction: The patient must understand the technique, particularly the need for deep coughing to produce sputum. Written instructions are particularly helpful.

Patient Instructions for Sputum Induction

You are requested to provide a sputum sample that contains secretions that collect in your lungs. This sample must not contain saliva or material from your mouth or throat. It is important that the sputum is produced by several very deep coughs.

This sputum will be analyzed to find out the cause of your respiratory symptoms. It is important to follow these steps so that the sputum you produce is useful.

Clean your mouth thoroughly. Vigorously brush your teeth, gums, and tongue and the back of your mouth. Then rinse your mouth repeatedly; next, make a grunting sound to clear your throat of any material.

Deeply inhale the aerosol spray. After you clean your mouth, you will be asked to breathe in a mist of salt water through a mask for 15 minutes. Breathe slowly and deeply, and inhale as much mist as possible. Try to avoid coughing during this period.

Cough forcefully. After you have inhaled mist for 15 minutes, you will be asked to cough repeatedly as hard as you can. After several deep coughs, spit out the sputum into the cup provided. Try not to swallow before you spit! Also, please try to avoid retching or vomiting during these cough efforts.

The key thing to remember is to cough as hard and as deeply as you can. Shallow coughs produce saliva and secretions from the mouth and throat that cannot be used to make a diagnosis.

---

2. Sputum induction suite: A single-patient room, a designated sputum induction room, or a sputum induction cubicle is recommended to avoid transmission of airborne pathogens. Personnel involved in sputum induction should use respiratory precautions.

Equipment

1. Standard jet nebulizer
2. Compressed gas source (oxygen or air)
3. Corrugated wide-bore plastic tube
4. Face mask or face tent
5. Hypertonic saline solution (3% or 5%): 2 to 4 oz
6. Sputum collection cups

Precautions

1. Maintain oxygenation if the patient is hypoxemic.
2. Use respiratory precautions for contagious infections (e.g., mycobacteria).

WARNING

Use respiratory precautions to prevent transmission of airborne pathogens such as *Mycobacterium tuberculosis*.

Technique

1. Tell the patient what is involved in obtaining a good sputum sample. Explain the difference between spitting and grunting (which often yield throat contents) and deep coughing.

2. The patient should be allowed to read and understand the written instructions provided (see Patient Instructions for Sputum Induction).

3. Additional verbal reinforcement by a health care worker is usually necessary during the induction. It must be made clear that unless the patient cooperates fully and coughs forcefully, this procedure is unlikely to be successful, and in some cases, fiberoptic bronchoscopy will be necessary to make the diagnosis.

Cleaning of Oropharynx

1. The patient should brush the teeth, gum surfaces, roof of the mouth, and surface of the tongue as far back as possible.
2. This should be followed by repeated rinsing of the mouth with water and expectoration of material from the throat.

Inhalation of Hypertonic Saline

1. Prolonged inhalation of an aerosol of hypertonic saline is usually necessary to induce sputum. Patient should be sitting upright and asked to inhale an aerosol generated by a standard jet nebulizer. A saline solution (2 to 3 oz of 3% to 5%) is used in the nebulizer and aerosolized by connecting the nebulizer to a gas source. Compressed air can be used, but if the patient is hypoxic, oxygen can be used as the gas source to maintain an oxygen saturation level of greater than 90 per cent.
2. The nebulizer bottle is connected to a wide-bore tube, which in turn is connected to a face mask. The flow rate is set at 8 to 10 L/min. This high-output nebulization of saline is continued for 10 to 15 minutes while the patient breathes slowly and deeply through the mouth and nose. Coughing should be discouraged at this point.

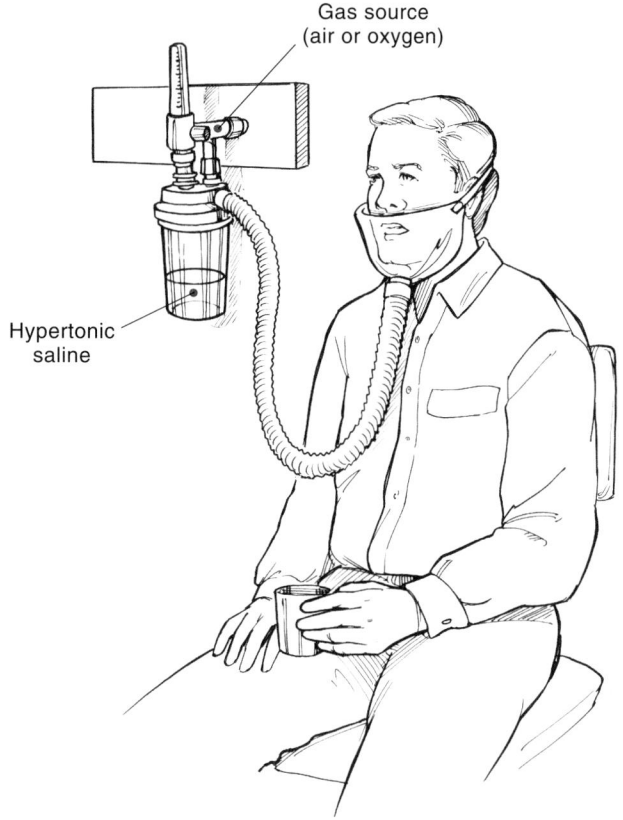

Gas source
(air or oxygen)

Hypertonic
saline

Sputum Collection and Processing

Obtaining the Specimen

1. After the patient has inhaled the aerosolized saline for at least 10 minutes, the mask is removed and the patient is instructed to expel saliva from the mouth and throat, which is discarded. A voluntary cough should then be initiated by the patient under the active supervision and encouragement of a health care worker. This person may be a physician, pulmonary function technologist, respiratory therapist, or any other person trained in the technique of sputum induction.
2. Several successive cough efforts in a stepladder manner (rapid, sequential coughs with brief pauses) are usually followed by forceful expectoration of the sputum, which is then collected in a specimen cup.
3. The patient should be encouraged to maintain forceful sequential cough efforts and not to swallow the sputum as it is raised in the throat. Several separate cough efforts should be attempted by the patient, and all sputum thus produced should be collected in one or more sputum cups.
4. If no sputum is obtained, inhalation of nebulized saline is resumed for 10 to 15 more minutes, after which coughing efforts should again be attempted. This process can be repeated once again, but if sputum cannot be obtained after two or three attempts, the induction should be terminated.

Processing the Specimen

The specimen should be stained and cultured as indicated, using standard techniques.

Follow-Up

At the end of the induction procedure, the patient is given a container and instructed to collect any subsequent sputum resulting from a deep cough. This sputum may be analyzed for appropriate pathogens or cells if initial samples are nondiagnostic.

B | Bibliography

For more information on the technique of sputum processing, see
Zaman MK, Wooten OF, Subrahmanya B, et al: Rapid noninvasive diagnosis of *Pneumocystis carinii* from induced liquefied sputum. Ann Intern Med 1988;109:7–10.

For more information on the use of sputum for the diagnosis of tuberculosis, see
Kim TC, Blackman RS, Heatwole KM, et al: Acid-fast bacilli in sputum smears of patients with pulmonary tuberculosis. Am Rev Respir Dis 1984;129:264–268.

For more information on the use of sputum for bacterial infection, see
Lipinski EM, Flakas ED, Taylor BC: An evaluation of some methods of collecting sputum from patients with bronchitis and emphysema. Am Rev Respir Dis 1964;89:760–764.

For more information on prevention of nosocomial tuberculosis during sputum induction, see
Guidelines for the Prevention of *Mycobacterium tuberculosis* in health care facilities. MMWR 1995;43:RR–13:33–36.

47 Coccidioidomycosis

Diana S. Dark

Etiology and Epidemiology

1. Coccidioidomycosis is caused by a tissue dimorphic fungus, *Coccidioides immitis*. It grows in the soil as a mold. Infection is caused by inhalation of airborne, infective arthroconidia and grows in tissues as an endosporulating spherule. When the spherule ruptures, it releases endospores that migrate through lymphatics to form additional spherules in tissue at local and distant extrapulmonary sites.

2. *C. immitis* is endemic in specific geographic areas that have short, intense rainy seasons followed by hot and dry conditions.

3. Coccidioidomycosis is found only in the Western Hemisphere. Areas of highest endemicity are the southern San Joaquin River valley in California and southern Arizona, hence the popular term for the primary pulmonary manifestation of coccidioidomycosis, valley fever. Increasingly, cases are being recognized outside the endemic areas. They occur in travelers who have visited an endemic area, or as reactivations of infections acquired earlier in former residents of endemic areas, or as infections acquired from fomites from endemic areas (fruit, cotton, and landfills are documented sources of infection).

4. Disease can occur at any age; however, most cases occur in late childhood through early middle age and show a slight male preponderance.

5. In the United States alone, about 100,000 persons are infected annually.

Symptoms

A. Primary infection

1. Most (60 per cent) of those infected have asymptomatic infections or illness indistinguishable from ordinary upper respiratory tract infections.

2. Forty per cent develop symptoms of a primary infection 1 to 3 weeks after exposure. These infections resemble a lower respiratory tract infection and/or systemic illness with some or all of the following symptoms: cough, sputum production, chest pain, malaise, headache, fever, chills, night sweats, anorexia, weakness, and arthralgias.

   a. These infections are usually mild and passed off by the patient as an influenza-like illness.

   b. In about one fourth of the symptomatic cases, the manifestations are more severe and include pleuritic chest pain. Most resolve uneventfully.

3. About 5 per cent of those infected have pulmo-nary residua, most commonly a pulmonary nodule or cavity.

4. A small number of patients develop acute progressive pneumonia, which often is fatal, or progress to chronic pulmonary disease.

5. About 0.5 per cent of patients develop disseminated (extrapulmonary) disease, which may involve almost any organ. This development is more common in an immunocompromised host.

B. Chronic pulmonary coccidioidomycosis

1. Acute pneumonia may progress to chronic pulmonary disease, usually of a cavitary nature. Patients with diabetes or with compromised immunity are more likely to develop this condition. The disease may wax and wane over many years.

2. Bronchiectasis may result from acute severe disease or chronic disease.

C. Disseminated disease

1. Disseminated coccidioidomycosis occurs in patients who are at high risk.

   a. Patients immunosuppressed as a result of steroid or cytotoxic therapy for cancer

   b. Patients who have had organ transplantation

   c. Patients with human immunodeficiency virus infection

   d. Patients with other risk factors, including dark-skinned races, extremes of age, male sex, and diabetes mellitus

2. Muscles, tendons, bones, and joints may be involved in disseminated disease.

3. Meningitis may develop and usually occurs within 6 months after the primary infection. It may also appear acutely with the primary infection. Space-occupying central nervous system lesions are rare.

4. The skin is a common target for dissemination. Skin lesions can also result from direct inoculation with contaminated materials.

Key Symptoms

- Fever
- Nonproductive cough
- Pleuritic chest pain
- Arthralgias
- Atypical skin rash (20 per cent of patients)

Clinical Findings

A. Acute coccidioidomycosis

1. Chest radiograph shows single or multiple areas of patchy pneumonitis. Hilar adenopathy is found in 20 per cent of cases. Necrosis of parenchymal lesions is common and eventually may form a characteristic thin-walled cavity.

2. Skin manifestations of primary illness are predominantly erythema nodosum and erythema multiforme.

3. Arthritis is seen in association with primary coccidioidomycosis. The ankle is the most commonly and most severely involved joint. The arthritis is usually symmetrical and self-limited; it is known as "desert rheumatism" and represents an immune complex reaction, not disease dissemination.

B. Chronic pulmonary coccidioidomycosis

1. Cavitary lesions are usually seen on chest radiographs.

2. Pulmonary fibrosis can occur.

3. Cavities can become superinfected with bacteria or aspergillus or, occasionally, rupture, causing empyema or pneumothorax.

C. Disseminated coccidioidomycosis

1. Dissemination may involve the skin, soft tissues, bones and joints, the genitourinary system, and the central nervous system.

2. Signs depend on the organ system involved.

3. Cutaneous coccidioidomycosis can present variably as papules, pustules, plaques, nodules, ulcers, abscesses, or large proliferative lesions.

Key Signs

- Single or multiple areas of patchy pneumonitis on chest radiograph

- Hilar adenopathy (20 per cent of cases)

- Paratracheal and superior mediastinal adenopathy may signal dissemination.

Laboratory Tests

A. Acute coccidioidomycosis

1. Knowledge of a patient's history of exposure through travel or residence in the endemic area is helpful.

2. Diagnosis can be confirmed by culture of the fungus on appropriate laboratory media. DNA probe identification of a suspected isolate may be helpful.

3. If a satisfactory sputum sample cannot be obtained, bronchoscopy or lung biopsy may be indicated.

4. Cultures of *C. immitis* represent a severe biologic hazard, and suspect isolates should be handled only by experienced laboratories that are prepared to deal with them.

5. The complement fixation test with *C. immitis* reacting with IgG antibody is the benchmark diagnostic test and becomes positive 2 to 6 weeks after infection.

6. There is growing experience with serum IgM precipitins, which can be demonstrated by tube precipitin, latex agglutination, or immunodiffusion method. These antibodies occur 1 to 3 weeks after onset of the symptoms of primary infection in 75 per cent of cases and disappear within 4 months. Few laboratories use this method.

7. Coccidioidin skin testing has been widely used. However, a positive skin test does not necessarily connote acute disease.

B. Chronic pulmonary coccidioidomycosis

Serum titers are often high in patients with extensive chronic pulmonary disease but typically are low or absent in the presence of a solitary lung nodule or a single, thin-walled cavity.

C. Disseminated coccidioidomycosis

1. The height of the IgG titer tends to parallel the extent of hematogenous dissemination.

2. A titer exceeding 1:16 is usually indicative of disseminated disease. However, there can be variation among laboratories. Regardless of the laboratory, failure of the titer to fall during therapy of disseminated disease has an ominous prognosis.

3. Detection of complement-fixing antibody in cerebrospinal fluid is usually indicative of coccidioidal meningitis and remains the single most useful diagnostic test for that condition.

4. Biopsy material that shows a granulomatous histopathologic response to infection and contains characteristic spherules with evidence of endosporulation may also confirm the diagnosis.

5. It is more difficult to obtain positive cultures from urine, blood, gastric aspirates, pleural effusions, and peritoneal fluid.

Key Tests

- Culture of sputum or biopsy material

- Demonstration of positive complement fixation test in serum or cerebrospinal fluid

Differential Diagnosis

Coccidioidomycosis should be differentiated from other granulomatous diseases, such as tuberculosis and histoplasmosis.

Treatment

1. Acute pulmonary coccidioidomycosis: low risk for dissemination. Patients at low risk for dissemination need no therapy other than observation.
2. Acute pulmonary coccidioidomycosis: high risk for dissemination or disseminated disease
   a. Patients with pulmonary disease at high risk for dissemination
      (1) Ketoconazole (Nizoral), 400 mg/day, or fluconazole (Diflucan), 400 mg/day, or itraconazole (Sporanox), 400 mg/day
      (2) Alternative therapy—amphotericin B (Fungizone), 0.6 mg/kg/day intravenously for 7 days then 0.8 mg/kg every other day; total dose 2.5 gm or more
      (3) Duration of therapy is unclear—usually 9 to 12 months
   b. Relapse rate after therapy for disseminated disease is 15 to 25 per cent.
3. Meningitis in adults
   Amphotericin B intravenously as for pulmonary infections above plus 0.1 to 0.3 mg/day intrathecally by way of a reservoir device. Alternative therapy is fluconazole, 400 mg/day orally for 9 to 12 months plus amphotericin B intrathecally.

 Key Treatment

Pulmonary and Extrapulmonary Disease

- **Drug of Choice**—Ketoconazole, 400 mg/day
- **Alternative Drugs**—Fluconazole, itraconazole, amphotericin B

Meningitis in Adults

- **Drug of Choice**—Amphotericin B intravenously and intrathecally
- **Alternative Drugs**—Fluconazole orally plus amphotericin B intrathecally

Follow-Up

Because the relapse rate is fairly high, patients must be followed closely long term. Immunocompromised patients may need extended duration of therapy.

 Bibliography

Coccidioidomycosis—United States, 1991–1992. MMWR 1993;42:21–24.

Einstein HE, Johnson RH: Coccidioidomycosis: New aspects of epidemiology and therapy. Clin Infect Dis 1993;16:349–356.

Stevens DA: Coccidioides immitis. In Mandell GL, Douglas RG Jr, Bennett JE (eds): Principles and Practice of Infectious Diseases, 3rd ed. New York: Churchill Livingstone, 1990, pp 2008–2017.

48 Histoplasmosis

James A. Sterling

Etiology

1. Epidemiology: Histoplasmosis is a common fungal pathogen found predominantly in the Mississippi and Ohio Valley regions of the United States.

2. Spores are found in environments inhabited by birds or bats and in recently cultivated soil contaminated by bird droppings or bat guano. With the relatively high incidence of acute symptomatic infection associated with cave exploration, the term cave fever has been applied.

3. Infection occurs when small spores (microconidia) of *Histoplasma capsulatum* are inspired into the respiratory tract and spread hematogenously throughout the reticuloendothelial system.

4. In the presence of a competent immune system, macrophages contain the infection and there are no systemic manifestations.

5. Most infections remain asymptomatic in the immunocompetent host.

6. Severe or fatal disease is rare and much more likely to occur in the immunocompromised host.

Symptoms

1. When inhaled, the fungal spores of *H. capsulatum* easily reach the terminal airways and, if the inoculum is sufficiently high, can cause disseminated disease and even death. This does not occur in most cases, however. In fact, inspiration of *H. capsulatum* spores typically produces no symptoms, with about one half of patients remaining asymptomatic.

2. If clinical disease does occur, symptoms are usually those of any nonspecific flu-like respiratory illness and include fever, chills, cough, lymphadenopathy, myalgias, and headache.

3. Symptoms typically persist for about 1 week, and the course of infection is almost always self-limited without pharmacologic intervention.

4. Chronic disease is occasionally seen and easily mistaken for tuberculosis until definitive diagnosis can be made.

5. In the chronic form, the disease is characterized by fever, malaise, night sweats, and productive cough. Cavitary pulmonary disease is seen on chest radiographs.

Clinical Findings

1. *H. capsulatum* infects certain tissues more than others. The most common presentation of infection is the asymptomatic patient who is noted to have calcified nodules on routine chest radiograph.

2. In acute infection with a large inoculum of *H. capsulatum,* infiltrates or consolidation may be seen. Because of the variability of radiographic findings, bronchoscopy is often necessary to determine the cause of the pulmonary lesion.

3. Organs most likely to show involvement are those of the reticuloendothelial system, with the most common probably being calcified granulomas within the spleen.

4. Other reported manifestations include cutaneous histoplasmosis, oropharyngeal histoplasmosis, and central nervous system involvement.

Key Signs

• Typically none	• Cutaneous granulomas
• Central nervous system involvement	• Calcified pulmonary granulomas

Laboratory Tests

1. *H. capsulatum* can be cultured from blood and tissue, and in acute disseminated histoplasmosis, blood cultures often are positive.

2. The most common diagnostic procedure is sputum culture, although it is seldom positive.

3. Specific tissue sites may be stained with Grocott methenamine–silver nitrate stain (GMS) or periodic acid–Schiff stain to directly observe *H. capsulatum* in the yeast forms; GMS staining is most diagnostic.

4. Alternatively, antigen detection (by radioimmunoassay) of blood or urine can be performed.

5. Positive tissue cultures should always be considered infectious. Positive complement fixation antibody titers in areas not highly endemic to histoplasmosis should suggest acute disease.

6. Chest radiography should always be performed, and films often reveal focal lesions. Typically, chest radiographs show single or multiple small calcified nodules.

Key Symptoms

• Asymptomatic	• Headache
• Myalgias	• Cough
• Fever, chills	• Malaise

Key Tests

- Chest radiography
- Radioimmunoassay of blood or urine
- Tissue culture
- Blood culture

Differential Diagnosis

1. Includes all granulomatous disease processes, specifically tuberculosis and coccidioidomycosis
2. Other pathogenic fungal infections, such as blastomycosis and cryptococcosis, must be considered, especially in immunocompromised hosts.

Treatment

1. Because most cases of histoplasmosis are self-limited, if not completely asymptomatic, no chemotherapy is indicated.
2. Antifungal therapy is indicated in patients with disseminated or chronic pulmonary histoplasmosis as well as those with acute pulmonary histoplasmosis and acute respiratory distress syndrome.

Medication

1. The drug of choice for nonthreatening pulmonary or localized histoplasmosis in the immunocompetent host is itraconazole (Sporanox), 200 mg/day for 9 months.
2. Until recently, the drug of choice has been amphotericin B (Fungizone) given in doses of 0.4 to 0.5 mg/kg.
3. Newer antifungal agents are now available and include ketoconazole, fluconazole, and itraconazole.
4. Amphotericin B is the alternative drug of choice in the immunocompetent host at the recommended dosage of 0.6 mg/kg/day intravenously for 7 days followed by 0.8 mg/kg intravenously every other day (or three times per week).

Diet

No specific diet is recommended.

Activity

Activity should be allowed as tolerated.

Patient Education

1. Patients at risk (spelunkers, farmers, and immunocompromised people) should be counseled to guard against exposure.

2. Patients in an immunodeficient state should be educated as to the usual signs and symptoms of the disease.

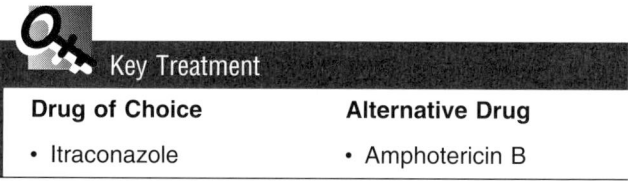

Key Treatment

Drug of Choice	Alternative Drug
• Itraconazole	• Amphotericin B

Follow-Up

1. Follow-up chest radiographs should be taken every 3 to 4 months until no further changes are noted.
2. Patients at risk (i.e., with chronic obstructive pulmonary disease or compromised immune system) who have been exposed to *H. capsulatum* should be followed up on a regular basis for their primary underlying disease process and should be educated regarding the manifestations of histoplasmosis.

ACKNOWLEDGMENT: The author thanks Jay Sanford et al for permission to use the treatment regimen for histoplasmosis as described in Sanford J, Gilbert D, Gerberding J, Sande M: The Sanford guide to antimicrobial therapy. Dallas, Antimicrobial Therapy, 1994, p 65.

 Bibliography

For more information on cutaneous histoplasmosis, see
Eidbo J, Sanchez RL, Tschen JA, Ellner KM: Cutaneous manifestations of histoplasmosis in the acquired immune deficiency syndrome. Am J Surg Pathol 1993;17(2):110–116.

For more information on oropharyngeal histoplasmosis, see
Hiltbrand JB, McGuirt WF: Oropharyngeal histoplasmosis. South Med J 1990;83(2):227–231.

For more information on central nervous system involvement of histoplasmosis, see
Wheat LJ, Batteiger BE, Sathapatayavongs B: *Histoplasma capsulatum* infection of the central nervous system, a clinical review. Medicine 1990;69(4):244–260.

For more information on pharmacologic treatment of histoplasmosis, see
Sanford J, Gilbert D, Gerberding J, Sande M: The Sanford guide to antimicrobial therapy—1994. Dallas, Antimicrobial Therapy, 1994, p 65.

For more information on imaging of thoracic histoplasmosis, see
Rubin S, Winer-Muram H: Thoracic histoplasmosis. J Thorac Imaging 1992;7(4):39–50.

49 Blastomycosis

Dennis J. Baumgardner

Etiology

1. Causative agent: *Blastomyces dermatitidis,* a dimorphic fungus that infects humans and animals
2. Endemic areas: North America (southeastern United States, Ohio and Mississippi River basins, and Canada around Great Lakes), Africa, India
3. Risk factors: Residence or visitation in a highly endemic area, especially along waterways; excavation
4. Acquisition: Except for rare inoculation disease, spores are inhaled from environment; transition to yeast form occurs in the lungs; no person-to-person or zoonotic spread (sexual and vertical transmission has been reported)

Symptoms

1. Age: All ages are affected; peak in fourth and fifth decades
2. Sex: Moderate male predominance may reflect differential exposure.
3. Pulmonary forms
   a. Acute pneumonia
      (1) Asymptomatic disease (like histoplasmosis) is common.
      (2) Mild or self-limited
      (3) Moderate to severe
   b. Chronic pneumonia
   c. Overwhelming disseminated pulmonary infection, often including adult respiratory distress syndrome

Key Symptoms

- Cough (85 per cent)
- Fever (65 per cent)
- Night sweats (61 per cent)
- Pleuritic chest pain (58 per cent)
- Weight loss (58 per cent)
- Myalgias (34 per cent)
- Hemoptysis (17 per cent)

Adapted from Baumgardner DJ, Buggy BP, Mattson BJ, et al: Epidemiology of blastomycosis in a region of high endemicity in North Central Wisconsin. Clin Infect Dis 1992;15:631. ©1992 by The University of Chicago. All rights reserved.

Clinical Findings

1. Physical pulmonary findings are nonspecific.
2. May have erythema nodosum
3. By extension or spread may involve respiratory tree, pericardium or myocardium, mediastinum
4. Disseminated disease
   a. Often not temporally related to lung disease
   b. Skin—most commonly involved
      (1) Verrucous form—sharp, raised, serpiginous border above subcutaneous abscess. Center often crusted with black dots. Tends to be on exposed peripheral areas.
      (2) Ulcerative form—often heaped borders, exudate
   c. Bone and joint—nonspecific presentation; vertebrae, ribs, skull, long bones, pelvis most commonly affected
   d. Genitourinary—prostatitis and epididymo-orchitis most common; female genital tract less common
   e. Central nervous system—epidural, cranial abscess; meningitis. Lumbar puncture not sensitive for diagnosis.
   f. Virtually every organ system and tissue has been reported. Subcutaneous abscesses and other cold abscesses may be involved.
5. Does not appear to be overrepresented in patients who are immunocompromised or who have acquired immunodeficiency syndrome, but is severe in this population

Key Signs

- No diagnostic patterns
- Air space findings most common; also mass, interstitial, miliary
- Chronic disease more apt to present as lung mass
- May have nodules, satellite lesions, cavitation, effusions, adenopathy
- Upper lobes or multiple lobes most common
- Radiographic and clinical pictures often do not correlate.

Tests

Key Tests

Prompt, reasonably sensitive diagnosis afforded by microscopic examination of sputum, exudate, or other clinical material for yeast forms (generally 8 to 15 μm) with single, broad-based (4- to 5-μm) buds.

1. Potassium hydroxide 10% and/or Calcofluor White wet preparations are useful for sputum and exudates; fungal stains are useful for most specimens.

2. Culture is definitive—takes days to weeks.

3. Older serology (CF, ID) often is unreliable, but newer antigen tests continue to be improved and may become routinely useful.

Differential Diagnosis

1. Prompt diagnosis depends on a high index of suspicion (and travel history, if nonendemic area).

2. Pulmonary disease—other fungal and pathogenic actinomycetes, especially histoplasmosis (overlapping endemic areas); tuberculosis; lung cancer; community-acquired pneumonia; sarcoidosis; silicosis; other

3. Skin disease—skin cancer, keratoacanthoma, other infections and conditions

4. Other sites—various infectious, neoplastic, and granulomatous disease

Treatment

Medication

1. Ketoconazole (Nizoral), 400 mg/day orally (at bedtime on empty stomach is best). Increase to 600 or 800 mg/day in 2 to 4 weeks if no response. Avoid any medication that reduces gastric acid. Nausea, vomiting, and headaches may occur (also hormonal abnormalities at higher doses); hepatocellular damage occurs in 1:10,000 courses (obtain baseline liver function tests and monitor while on therapy). Avoid terfenadine (Seldane) and astemizole (Hismanal). Take for minimum of 6 months. Ketoconazole has been largely replaced by the newer itraconazole as the drug of choice for oral treatment but the former is less expensive.

2. Itraconazole (Sporanox), 200 mg/day orally with breakfast; may increase to 300 or 400 mg/day if needed. Efficacy is comparable to or better than that of ketoconazole with apparently less toxicity. Obtain baseline liver function tests and follow clinically for signs of hepatic dysfunction. Avoid terfenadine (Seldane) and astemizole (Hismanal). Use for 6 months.

3. Efficacy of fluconazole (Diflucan) and other new azoles not fully tested.

4. Amphotericin B (Fungizone), total dose of 2000 mg. Use 1-mg test dose and then rapidly increase to 35 to 50 mg/day. Avoid dehydration. Premedicate with acetaminophen with or without antihistamines and/or meperidine. Monitor blood pressure during infusion, anemia, kidney and liver function, electrolytes and magnesium, gastrointestinal, thrombophlebitic, and other adverse effects.

5. Pediatrics, pregnancy—usually supportive care and amphotericin B. Consult current literature.

Diet

As tolerated. Support respiratory muscles.

Activity

As tolerated.

Patient Education

1. Advise the patient who has a history of blastomycosis to always inform the physician when ill because reactivation may occur.

2. Patients who reside or visit in a highly endemic area should know the signs and symptoms to report to the physician.

3. The use of a respirator mask when excavating in a highly endemic area is recommended but of unproven benefit.

Key Treatment

- Asymptomatic or mild acute, nonpleural pulmonary disease, stable or improving: no treatment, careful observation

- Mild to moderate acute pulmonary; chronic progressive pulmonary; extrapulmonary (non–central nervous system) disease: itraconazole

- Life-threatening or central nervous system infection; noncompliance or failure of oral therapy: amphotericin B

Follow-Up

1. Fatalities still occur, but they should be minimized by prompt diagnosis in severe cases.

2. The prognosis, after recovery, is generally good.

3. Observe for noncompliance with oral medication.

4. Be aware that reactivation may occur regardless of the severity of the initial infection or completion of a full course of therapy.

Bibliography

Al-Doory Y, DiSalvo AF (eds): Blastomycosis. New York, Plenum Medical Book Co., 1992.

Baumgardner DJ, Buggy BP, Mattson BJ, et al: Epidemiology of blastomycosis in a region of high endemicity in North Central Wisconsin. Clin Infect Dis 1992;15:629–635.

Bradsher RW: Blastomycosis. Clin Infect Dis 1992;14(Suppl 1):S82–S90.

Kauffman CA: Blastomycosis. In Rakel RE (ed): Conn's Current Therapy 1994. Philadelphia, WB Saunders, 1994, pp 176–178.

Rippon JW: Blastomycosis. In Rippon JW (ed): Medical Mycology, 3rd ed. Philadelphia, WB Saunders, 1988, pp 474–505.

50 Sarcoidosis

G. Allen Tindol, Jr.

Etiology

1. Sarcoidosis, a multisystemic disease of unknown cause, most commonly affects the lungs, lymph nodes, eyes, and skin.

2. Lesions are characterized histologically as noncaseating granulomas.

3. The disease typically affects young adults in the third and fourth decades of life and occurs more frequently in certain geographic and/or ethnic groups (e.g., Swedes, Puerto Ricans in New York City, and African-Americans in the Southeast).

Symptoms and Signs

1. Although the lungs are involved in at least 90 per cent of patients, only one half of patients with pulmonary disease are symptomatic. Pulmonary symptoms include dyspnea, dry cough, pleuritic chest pain, and, rarely, hemoptysis.

2. Skin lesions occur in at least 25 per cent of patients and include lupus pernio (frostbite-appearing lesions of the ears and hands), skin plaques, maculopapular eruptions, subcutaneous nodules, erythema nodosum, alopecia, and erythema multiforme.

   a. Granuloma formation in an old scar or tattoo is characteristic.

   b. When accompanied by fever, malaise, and polyarthralgias (as it is in about 50 per cent of cases), erythema nodosum is a good prognostic marker of mild sarcoidosis that usually resolves spontaneously in several months without corticosteroid treatment.

3. Ocular lesions occur in 15 to 25 per cent of patients. The most common eye finding is a granulomatous uveitis that may manifest as "floaters" and decreased visual acuity. Papilledema may be noted. Lacrimal gland swelling may occur.

4. Nontender, freely movable cervical lymphadenopathy is common. Splenomegaly occurs in about one fourth of patients.

5. Of neurologic manifestations, which occur in about 5 to 15 per cent of patients with sarcoidosis, cranial neuropathies are most common. A peripheral seventh-nerve palsy (Bell's palsy) is the most common single lesion and may be bilateral. Aseptic meningitis may be a manifestation of neurosarcoidosis. Seizures have been reported and generally indicate a poor prognosis.

6. Head and neck manifestations (about 10 per cent of patients) include painless parotid swelling and involvement of the upper respiratory tract, particularly the nasal mucosa.

7. Polyuria and polydipsia may stem from sarcoid involvement of the pituitary and hypothalamus or from hypercalcemia, hypercalciuria, and nephrogenic diabetes insipidus. Somnolence, insomnia, extreme variations in body temperature, progressive obesity, and marked changes in personality may also be seen with hypothalamic involvement.

8. Heart block is the most common presentation, followed by ventricular tachycardia and extrasystoles; symptomatic myocardial involvement, including myocarditis, occurs in about 5 per cent of patients.

9. Hypercalcemia is present in 10 per cent of patients with sarcoidosis, whereas hypercalciuria is three times more frequent. The abnormalities of calcium metabolism are the result of increased synthesis of dihydroxyvitamin D by the epithelioid sarcoid granulomas and enhanced absorption of calcium from the gastrointestinal tract. Hypercalcemia and hypercalciuria in patients with sarcoidosis can lead to impaired renal function, nephrolithiasis, nephrocalcinosis, chronic renal failure, and death.

10. Acute sarcoid arthritis is a commonly described syndrome characterized by symmetrical polyarthritis, with spontaneous resolution within 6 months in most patients. Chronic sarcoid arthritis is a destructive polyarthritis with waxing and waning episodes of joint inflammation.

11. Although symptomatic muscle involvement in sarcoidosis is rare, asymptomatic granulomas in skeletal muscle biopsies are frequent.

Key Symptoms

- Dyspnea
- Cough (nonproductive)
- Arthralgia/myalgia
- Blurred vision

Key Signs

- Lymphadenopathy
- Skin lesions
- Uveitis
- Splenomegaly

Tests and Findings

1. Chest radiography findings are listed in Table 50–1.

TABLE 50–1. FINDINGS ON CHEST RADIOGRAPHY AT DIFFERENT STAGES

STAGE	CHEST RADIOGRAPH
0	Clear
1	Bilateral hilar lymphadenopathy
2	Hilar lymphadenopathy plus parenchymal infiltrates
3	Parenchymal infiltrates only
4	Pulmonary fibrosis

Reprinted from Journal of Emergency Medicine, vol. 11. Pollack CV, Jorden RC: Recognition and management of sarcoidosis in the emergency department, pp 297–308, 1993. With kind permission from Elsevier Science Ltd., The Boulevard, Langford Lane, Kidlington OX5 1GB, UK.

2. The serum level of angiotensin converting enzyme is elevated in 60 per cent of patients but is nonspecific and has no prognostic value. Although serial values may grossly reflect activity of disease in some patients, they are an inaccurate reflection in many others.

3. Increased levels of a new marker, serum procollagen type III–derived peptide, have been found in bronchoalveolar lavage fluid and sera of patients with interstitial lung disease. Levels have been reported to correlate with disease activity.

4. Increased serum prolactin levels may occur in as many as one third of patients with sarcoidosis, reflecting hypothalamic involvement, although galactorrhea is much less common.

5. Typical cerebrospinal fluid findings in sarcoidosis are as follows: an elevated protein concentration in the range of 100 to 400 mg/dl, lymphocytosis with a total cell count of 10 to 60 cells/mm^3, and low cerebrospinal fluid glucose in the range of 10 to 40 mg/dl.

6. Cutaneous anergy, as demonstrated by a negative tuberculin skin test and control, is a common finding.

7. Hypercalciuria may be present with or without hypercalcemia.

8. Nephrocalcinosis may be evident on renal ultrasound.

9. Gallium scan correlates with active inflammatory processes and may indicate systemic involvement outside the lungs but has no prognostic value.

10. A computed tomographic scan of the chest may reveal mediastinal adenopathy and parenchymal fibrosis and infiltrates not visualized on chest radiograph, but it is nonspecific.

11. Pulmonary function studies reveal a restrictive pattern with reduced carbon monoxide diffusion capacity.

12. If disease has progressed to extensive lung fibrosis and pulmonary hypertension, electrocardiogram may show signs of cor pulmonale.

13. Bronchoalveolar lavage aspirate typically reveals a lymphocytic alveolar infiltrate.

14. Involved tissue is necessary for diagnosis, either from surgical removal of an accessible lymph node or from transbronchial biopsy. Open-lung biopsy is the procedure of last resort. The absence of an infectious process, such as tuberculosis and fungal, bacterial, and protozoal infections, must be demonstrated by appropriate stains and cultures.

15. In the Kveim-Siltzbach test, an antigenic extract prepared from the spleens of patients with known sarcoidosis is injected intradermally. A positive test is defined by the presence of typical sarcoid granulomata on biopsy 4 to 6 weeks later. In the era of concern for transmitting blood-borne infections, the feasibility of this test has been questioned, and it is now primarily of historical interest.

16. If muscle involvement is suspected, diagnosis is usually based on elevated serum creatine kinase levels, an electromyogram showing myopathic changes, and a muscle biopsy. Magnetic resonance imaging has been effectively used to identify nonpalpable sarcoid nodules in muscle.

Key Tests

- Chest radiography
- Pulmonary function testing
- Tissue biopsy
- Acid-fast bacillus and fungus cultures (negative)

Differential Diagnosis

1. Syphilis (especially if epitrochlear lymphadenopathy exists)
2. Acute rheumatic fever
3. Fungal infections, such as histoplasmosis, and berylliosis
4. Sarcoidosis has been described concurrently with systemic lupus erythematosus, rheumatoid arthritis, Sjögren's syndrome, spondyloarthritis, and human immunodeficiency virus.
5. Mycobacterial infection has been linked with sarcoidosis but never conclusively proved as the causative agent.

Treatment

Spontaneous remission of disease often occurs within 2 years of onset, regardless of the radiologic stage of the disease, except for fibrosis (stage 4), which is permanent.

Medication

1. Corticosteroids are the drugs of choice. Initially, 40 to 60 mg of prednisone daily, slowly tapered as tolerated over several months, usually relieves symptoms,

suppresses inflammation, slows formation of new granuloma, and resolves existing granuloma. Normalization of hypercalcemia and improvement in pulmonary function tests have been demonstrated. Alternate-day therapy is usually effective and may decrease the adverse effects of treatment; however, daily treatment may improve compliance.

2. If long-term maintenance therapy is necessary, the clinical benefits of 10 to 15 mg of prednisone daily usually far outweigh the risks associated with corticosteroids.

3. Indications for systemic treatment of sarcoidosis are listed in Table 50–2.

Key Treatment

Drugs of Choice—Corticosteroids

Alternative Drugs	*Indication*
• Chloroquine (Aralen)	• Lupus pernio, pulmonary fibrosis, hypercalcemia
• Methotrexate	• Severe skin involvement

Follow-Up

1. Asymptomatic patients with bilateral hilar lymphadenopathy (stage 1) but without extrapulmonary involvement should be left untreated. A chest radiograph should be repeated initially every 3 months and then every 6 months until the outcome of the disease is established.

2. When patients are being treated for pulmonary involvement, their course should be monitored by

TABLE 50–2. INDICATIONS FOR SYSTEMIC CORTICOSTEROIDS IN SARCOIDOSIS

Symptomatic pulmonary disease and/or significant derangement of
   pulmonary function
Neurologic lesions
Posterior ocular involvement
Uveitis or iridocyclitis not responding to local steroids
Hypercalcemia or hypercalciuria
Myocardial or endocardial disease
Symptomatic myopathy
Hypersplenism or symptomatic splenomegaly
Disfiguring or obstructive lymphadenopathy
Dry mouth or dry eye from lacrimal or salivary gland disease
Disfiguring skin lesions
Persistent constitutional symptoms
Severe acute arthralgia or arthritis or bony pain
Other significant or functional organ involvement

Reprinted from Journal of Emergency Medicine, vol. 11. Pollack CV, Jorden RC: Recognition and management of sarcoidosis in the emergency department, pp 297–308, 1993. With kind permission from Elsevier Science Ltd., The Boulevard, Langford Lane, Kidlington OX5 1GB, UK.

spirometry, diffusing capacity, chest radiograph, and serum angiotensin-converting enzyme level.

3. After initial electrocardiogram, Holter monitoring, exercise testing, and, when indicated, thallium scanning, patients with sarcoid cardiac involvement should receive yearly cardiologic evaluation.

 Bibliography

Bell NH: Endocrine complications of sarcoidosis. Endocrinol Metab Clin North Am 1991;20(3):645–654.
Mathur A, Kremer JM: Immunopathology, musculoskeletal features, and treatment of sarcoidosis. Curr Opin Rheumatol 1993;5:90–94.
Pollack CV, Jorden RC: Recognition and management of sarcoidosis in the emergency department. J Emerg Med 1993;11:297–308.
Sharma OP: Pulmonary sarcoidosis and corticosteroids. Am Rev Respir Dis 1993;147:1598–1600.
Tozman ECS: Sarcoidosis: Clinical manifestations, epidemiology, therapy, and pathophysiology. Curr Opin Rheumatol 1991;3:155–159.

51 Sleep Apnea

Lee K. Brown

Etiology

1. The respiratory disturbances associated with sleep vary by *degree.*

   a. Apnea, the cessation of airflow at the nose and mouth for 10 seconds or longer

   b. Hypopnea, a reduction in airflow at the nose and mouth

2. In addition, apneas or hypopneas may vary by *mechanism.*

   a. Obstructive: the resistance of the upper airway increases

   b. Central: respiratory effort is reduced or ceases

   c. Mixed: a period of central apnea followed by several obstructed breaths. These have the same clinical implications as purely obstructive events.

3. Following generally accepted usage, the asymptomatic disorder is defined as *sleep apnea* (central or obstructive); *sleep apnea syndrome* (central or obstructive) is diagnosed when symptoms occur. When many of the events are hypopneas rather than apneas, some clinicians classify the disorder separately as sleep apnea/hypopnea syndrome.

4. Central sleep apnea syndrome is a relatively rare entity, and the following discussion concentrates on obstructive sleep apnea syndrome. With rare exceptions, the obstruction occurs at the oropharyngeal and/or hypopharyngeal level. Several mechanisms may contribute.

   a. Reduced upper airway caliber, caused by the following:

      (1) Obesity (collections of adipose tissue have been demonstrated adjacent to the airway)

      (2) Adenotonsillar hypertrophy (usually in children)

      (3) Mandibular deficiency (e.g., micrognathia or retrognathia)

      (4) Macroglossia (usually associated with hypothyroidism)

      (5) Upper airway tumors (rare)

   b. Excessive pressure across the collapsible segment, most frequently attributed to nasal obstruction

   c. Activity of the muscles of the upper airway insufficient to maintain patency. Electromyographic studies have demonstrated reduced electrical activity of these muscles during apneas, consistent with a defect in respiratory control. The exact nature of this respiratory control instability is not known.

Symptoms

Symptoms may be either nocturnal (during sleep) or diurnal (during wakefulness).

1. Nocturnal

   a. Snoring, usually described as intermittent or *resuscitative.* Noise is produced between apneas, when large breaths are drawn through an airway that is still somewhat narrowed (almost universal).

   b. Abnormal motor activity, reflecting episodes of asphyxiation. The patients flail out and throw the bedcovers off and may sit up or get out of bed (common).

   c. Nocturia, a manifestation of diuresis and natriuresis possibly caused by increased elaboration of atrial natriuretic factor (common).

   d. Symptoms of gastroesophageal reflux, presumably from the negative intrapleural pressures developed during obstructed breaths (relatively rare).

   e. Self-reported nocturnal awakenings are rare, despite the fact that each respiratory event is generally terminated by an arousal. Occasionally, insomnia may be a presenting complaint.

2. Diurnal

   a. Excessive daytime sleepiness. Causation may be the nocturnal sleep disruption or hypoxemia (common)

   b. Cognitive impairment, including poor memory, and personality changes; correlates best with nocturnal hypoxemia (common)

   c. Morning headache, possibly of vascular origin resulting from nocturnal hypercapnia (relatively rare)

> **Key Symptoms**
> - Snoring
> - Excessive daytime sleepiness

Clinical Findings

Although a variety of physical findings may be associated with obstructive sleep apnea syndrome, none of them are specific to the disorder. They include the following:

1. Obesity

2. Macroglossia, usually associated with hypothyroidism

3. Enlarged, low-lying, edematous, or erythematous uvula

199

4. "Long" or narrow oropharynx, or oropharyngeal edema or erythema

5. Adenotonsillar enlargement (more common in children)

6. Retrognathia or micrognathia

7. Upper airway tumors

8. Systemic hypertension

9. Signs of pulmonary hypertension or cor pulmonale

10. Plethora

Tests

1. Polysomnography is the test of choice and is diagnostic if more than five obstructive apneas or hypopneas occur per hour of sleep (respiratory disturbance index >5) during at least 6 hours of nocturnal sleep. Daytime nap studies are discouraged because rapid-eye-movement sleep (which is associated with the most severe and at times the only respiratory events) seldom occurs during these studies. Unattended polysomnography in the home may be performed using portable equipment. Some systems are well validated, but all suffer from the unattended nature of the recording and some offer only a limited subset of the signals collected during a laboratory study. The following signals are recorded during the standard laboratory polysomnogram:

   a. Electrophysiologic indices of sleep stage (electroencephalogram, electro-oculogram, electromyogram)

   b. Electromechanical indices contrasting respiratory effort with actual ventilation (chest and/or abdominal movement; airflow at the nose and mouth)

   c. Consequences of apneic events, including electrocardiogram and pulse oximetry

2. Multiple sleep latency test (MSLT), a test of daytime somnolence performed by recording sleep staging parameters during four or five nap opportunities during the daytime. A reduction in mean sleep latency (average time to fall asleep for all nap opportunities) indicates pathologic sleepiness and is used to assess the efficacy of treatment. The MSLT may be diagnostic of another disorder that causes hypersomnolence, the narcolepsy/cataplexy syndrome.

3. A variety of more standard laboratory tests are useful in the overall management of these patients.

   a. Arterial blood gas analysis may reveal daytime hypercapnia, indicating coexisting pickwickian (obesity-hypoventilation) syndrome.

   b. Chest radiography and electrocardiography may reveal signs of pulmonary hypertension or cor pulmonale.

   c. Serum thyroid-stimulating hormone assay may detect unsuspected hypothyroidism.

4. Other specialized tests of use in selected patients include the following:

   a. Fiberoptic examination of the upper airway to rule out obstructing tumors

   b. Cephalometric radiography, useful in defining the anatomy of the upper airway when surgical treatment is contemplated

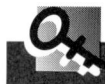

Key Test

• Polysomnography

Treatment

Treatment is generally recommended for any patient with an apnea index (number of apneas per hour of sleep) greater than 20 because this has been associated with increased mortality. Symptomatic patients with fewer respiratory events may also be treated.

1. Nasal continuous positive airway pressure (nasal C-PAP), which holds the upper airway open by a pneumatic splint effect. A tight-fitting nasal mask is attached to a flow generator, incorporating a positive end-expiratory pressure valve or other means to maintain positive airway pressure. Nasal "pillows," which fit into the nares, may be more comfortable than the mask in some patients. Nasal C-PAP is the most satisfactory treatment available. Problems with this therapy include the following:

   a. Patient compliance. Patients use the device about 4 to 5 hours per night on average; some patients may not use the device at all or use it only on alternate nights.

   b. Nasal irritation or rhinitis. This problem can be minimized by

      (1) humidification,

      (2) intranasal steroids (e.g., beclomethasone), or

      (3) intranasal disodium cromoglycate.

   c. Barotrauma, of theoretic concern whenever positive-pressure therapy is used, has been exceedingly rare.

2. Oral appliances, including a mandibular advancement orthotic (Snore Guard and others) and tongue-retaining devices, have been of limited benefit in selected patients.

3. A variety of surgical procedures have been advocated.

   a. Uvulopalatopharyngoplasty (either conventional or laser-assisted) improves oropharyngeal patency and almost always eliminates snoring. However, obstructive sleep apnea syndrome is cured (defined as respiratory disturbance index <20) in only about one half of patients, probably because of persistent hypopharyngeal obstruction. No preoperative indicators of response are known.

   b. Tonsillectomy and adenoidectomy may be of benefit in children.

   c. Midline glossectomy may be performed by conventional technique or by using the surgical laser, but only limited reports of efficacy are available.

d. Maxillofacial reconstruction, an aggressive therapy, is usually reserved for patients who fail nasal C-PAP and uvulopalatopharyngoplasty. These procedures are designed to achieve the following:

(1) Increase the size of the bony skeleton enclosing the tongue, using techniques such as inferior sagittal osteotomy of the mandible or maxillomandibular osteotomy

(2) Put traction on the base of the tongue, usually by hyoid myotomy and suspension

4. Medications with some benefit include protriptyline (Vivactil) and fluoxetine (Prozac). These nonsedating antidepressant agents suppress rapid-eye-movement (REM) sleep, when the most severe apneas characteristically occur, and may increase the tone of upper airway muscles.

5. Weight reduction may be of significant benefit in the obese patient.

6. Sleep position training. Some patients exhibit apneas predominantly in the supine position and can be induced to avoid this position by sewing a tennis ball into the back of the pajama top or through the use of electronic sensors that alarm when the patient is supine.

Key Treatment

- Nasal C-PAP

Bibliography

American Thoracic Society: Indications and standards for cardiopulmonary sleep studies. Am Rev Respir Dis 1989;139:559–568.

Brown LK: Sleep apnea syndromes: overview and diagnostic approach. Mt Sinai J Med 1994;61:99–112.

Kaplan J, Staats BA: Obstructive sleep apnea syndrome. Mayo Clin Proc 1990;65:1087–1094.

Kryger MH: Management of obstructive sleep apnea. Clin Chest Med 1992;13:481–492.

Rapoport DM: Treatment of sleep apnea syndromes. Mt Sinai J Med 1994;61:123–130.

52 Common Cardiovascular Symptoms

| Symptom | **Chest Pain** | *Vaskar Mukerji* |

Chest pain is a common symptom encountered by physicians. The causes of chest pain range from serious, potentially life-threatening diseases to relatively minor disorders that pose no threat to life but produce recurrent aggravating symptoms. Every patient complaining of chest pain should be carefully investigated. In particular, it is important not to miss the presence of serious heart disease, because the consequences of such a mistake could be disastrous. Nevertheless, the vast majority of patients coming to a physician's office with chest pain are not having an acute myocardial infarction. A working knowledge of the various conditions that may cause chest pain are crucial for the appropriate management of these patients.

Differential Diagnosis

Cardiovascular

1. Coronary artery disease
   a. Acute myocardial infarction
   b. Unstable angina pectoris
   c. Stable angina pectoris
   d. Prinzmetal's angina
2. Valvular heart disease
   a. Mitral valve prolapse
   b. Aortic stenosis
3. Hypertrophic cardiomyopathy
4. Pericarditis
5. Aortic dissection

Noncardiac

1. Pulmonary: tracheobronchitis, pneumonia, pleurisy, pulmonary embolism, lung cancer
2. Esophageal: reflux, spasm
3. Rheumatologic: fibromyalgia, costochondritis, Tietze's syndrome, arthritis (rheumatoid or osteoarthritis), injury to chest wall, spinal disease
4. Neurologic: cervical or thoracic radiculopathy, herpes zoster
5. Psychiatric conditions: panic disorder, generalized anxiety, agoraphobia and other phobias, depression, somatization, conversion, malingering, and Munchausen's syndrome
6. Breast conditions
7. Referred pain from abdominal viscera

Refer to Ch. 56, Angina; Ch. 57, Acute Myocardial Infarction; Ch. 61, Cardiomyopathy; Ch. 64, Aortic Dissection; and Ch. 66, Pericarditis.

History: Key Questions to Ask

1. What precipitates and what relieves the chest pain?
2. What is the character of the pain (location, radiation, quality, intensity, duration, frequency)?
3. Are there any associated symptoms?

Coronary artery disease primarily affects elderly and middle-aged individuals with a predilection for males. Typically the chest pain of angina pectoris occurs with exertion, anxiety, or exposure to cold and is relieved with rest or sublingual nitroglycerin. Frequently, it is accompanied by dyspnea, diaphoresis, or fatigue. Patients commonly describe the pain as a dull substernal or precordial pressure sensation radiating down the left arm or to the neck. Others describe a burning, squeezing, or tight sensation. Some patients refer to their symptom as discomfort rather than pain. Usually, an anginal episode lasts less than 15 minutes. If the pain is severe, is not relieved by sublingual nitroglycerin, and lasts more than 15 minutes, myocardial infarction should be suspected. In general, when coronary artery disease is being considered, the patient should also be questioned to determine the presence of cardiac risk factors such as smoking history, hypertension, hyperlipidemia, and diabetes.

Chest pain from other causes may be recognized by its "atypical" presentation, which may vary considerably from the preceding description. In pericarditis, the pain may be relieved with a change in position. Chest pain occurring after meals or on reclining may be indicative of gastroesophageal reflux. The presence of cough or other upper respiratory symptoms is suggestive of pulmonary disease. In rheumatologic conditions the pain may be exacerbated by upper body movements.

Clinical Findings

1. Fourth heart sound
2. Systolic click
3. Murmur—systolic or diastolic
4. Friction rub
5. Findings suggestive of noncardiac disease

Many patients with chest pain have a normal physical examination. These include patients with coronary artery disease, esophageal disorders, or psychiatric disorders. The characteristic systolic murmur can be heard in hypertrophic cardiomyopathy and in aortic stenosis. A diastolic murmur in a patient with severe chest pain may signal involvement of the aortic valve in a patient with aortic dissection. A friction rub may be heard with pericarditis. A systolic click with or without a systolic murmur may accompany mitral valve prolapse. A fourth heart sound is commonly heard in patients with coronary artery disease but may also be heard in some healthy individuals and with conditions that cause ventricular hypertrophy. The presence of abnormal breath sounds or rales or rhonchi on auscultation of the lungs suggests pulmonary disease. Musculoskeletal tenderness and pain with movement of the shoulders or spine suggest rheumatologic chest pain.

Tests

1. Chest radiograph
2. Electrocardiogram
3. Echocardiogram
4. Stress test: graded exercise test with or without thallium (or sestamibi) scintigraphy, dipyridamole thallium test, exercise echocardiography
5. Cardiac catheterization
6. Psychometric testing
7. Blood tests: complete blood count, sedimentation rate, rheumatoid factor

The chest film is useful in the diagnosis of pulmonary conditions as well as musculoskeletal disorders affecting the vertebral spine and rib cage. The cardiac shadow can be assessed for size and presence of calcification. On the electrocardiogram, ST segment depression suggests myocardial ischemia, whereas acute ST segment elevation may be diagnostic of myocardial infarction. Transient ST segment elevation during episodes of chest pain occurs with Prinzmetal angina. Exercise testing is indicated for stable patients with occasional chest pain. The use of thallium (or sestamibi) scintigraphy or echocardiography with exercise testing improves the reliability of the study. For patients who cannot exercise, the dipyridamole thallium test is a useful alternative. Coronary angiography provides the most accurate definition of the coronary anatomy and remains the gold standard for the diagnosis of coronary artery disease. Cardiac catheterization also provides important diagnostic information in valvular disorders and in hypertrophic cardiomyopathy.

Management

The management of chest pain should be directed toward the primary disorder causing the symptom.

Medication

1. Coronary artery disease: nitrates, beta-blockers, calcium channel blockers, aspirin. Percutaneous translu-minal coronary angioplasty (PTCA) or coronary artery bypass grafting may be necessary. For patients having an acute myocardial infarction, thrombolytic agents should be considered.
2. Esophageal causes: Reflux may be treated with antacids, H_2 blockers, omeprazole, or even promotility drugs. Spasm may be treated with calcium channel blockers, nitrates, or anticholinergic agents.
3. Musculoskeletal causes: nonsteriodal anti-inflamatory agents, local anesthetic injection, physical therapy. Rarely, with intractable pain, surgery may be useful.
4. Panic disorder: antidepressants (imipramine), benzodiazepines (alprazolam), serotonin uptake inhibitors.

Follow-Up

1. All patients with coronary artery disease should be followed clinically, as well as with some of the tests listed, for an indefinite period, to detect recurrence or progression of disease. Periodic adjustment of their medical regimen is necessary.
2. Most patients with chest pain and angiographically normal coronary arteries continue to complain of chest pain and physical disability, even with extended follow-up. Every effort should be made to identify and treat the cause of their chest pain.

PEARLS

- Exertional chest pain strongly suggests the presence of coronary artery disease.

- A normal physical examination, a normal electrocardiogram, or normal laboratory test results on the initial examination of a patient with chest pain does not rule out coronary artery disease.

- Noncardiac chest pain may coexist in a patient with coronary artery disease.

- When the diagnosis is unclear, it is always prudent to err on the side of caution.

Bibliography

Klinkman MS, Stevens D, Gorenflo DW: Episodes of care for chest pain: A preliminary report from MIRNET. Michigan Research Network. Fam Pract J 1994;38(4):345–352.

Mukerji B, Alpert MA, Mukerji V: Musculoskeletal causes of chest pain. Hosp Med 1994;30(11):26–39.

Mukerji V, Beitman BD, Alpert MA: Chest pain and angiographically normal coronary arteries. Tex Heart Inst J 1993;20:170–179.

Proudfit WL: Chest pain: Angina pectoris and related states. Heart Dis Stroke 1992;1(1):5–10.

Richter JE: Gastroesophageal reflux disease as a cause of chest pain. Med Clin North Am 1991;75(5):1065–1080.

Syncope is commonly defined as the transient loss of consciousness, often with the loss of postural tone, followed by spontaneous recovery without the need for resuscitative interventions. Syncope may be experienced by 30 to 50 per cent of all people at some point in their lives and accounts for approximately 3 per cent of all emergency department visits as well as at least 1 per cent of all hospital admissions. Syncope is generally of cardiovascular origin.

Differential Diagnosis

1. Neurocardiogenic vasodepressor dysfunction (NVD) —also called vasovagal reaction, vasodepressor syncope, and neurally mediated syncope—includes postmicturition syncope, carotid sinus syncope, cough syncope, heat syncope, and postprandial syncope.
2. Orthostatic hypotension
3. Tachydysrhythmias
   a. Ventricular dysrhythmias
      (1) Ventricular tachycardia (VT)
      (2) Ventricular fibrillation (VF)
   b. Supraventricular dysrhythmias
      (1) Atrial fibrillation with a rapid ventricular response
      (2) AV nodal re-entrant tachycardia (AVNRT)
      (3) Pre-excitation processes (with atrial fibrillation/flutter)
4. Bradydysrhythmias/conductive disorders
   a. AV block
      (1) Complete heart block
      (2) Mobitz II
   b. Sinus bradycardia—profound (heart rates <40 beats/min)
5. Other cardiac/vascular processes
   a. Aortic stenosis
   b. Hypertrophic cardiomyopathy (hypertrophic obstructive cardiomyopathy, idiopathic hypertrophic subaortic stenosis)
   c. Pulmonary embolus
   d. Pulmonary hypertension

Neurocardiogenic vasodepressor dysfunction (NVD) accounts for the majority of syncopal episodes experienced in the general population. If one includes light-headedness, wooziness, and near-syncope, NVD is the cause of some of the most common complaints that bring patients to medical attention. NVD is most often seen in patients with normal left ventricular (LV) function and no structural heart disease; these latter characteristics make NVD primarily a problem of younger people. The ventricular dysrhythmias are seen most often in patients with abnormal LV function (ejection fractions <40 per cent) and/or patients with structural heart disease and metabolic abnormalities. Ventricular dysrhythmias can have devastating consequences and require a thorough investigation. The high prevalence of LV dysfunction and/or structural heart disease and ischemic heart disease among older patients accounts for the high prevalence of ventricular dysrhythmias in this age group.

The other processes mentioned warrant consideration if the physical examination is abnormal (i.e., findings of aortic stenosis), the electrocardiogram (ECG) is abnormal (i.e., pre-excitation or conductive abnormality), or NVD and ventricular dysrhythmias are ruled out.

> Refer to Ch. 36, Pulmonary Embolus; Ch. 56, Angina; Ch. 61, Cardiomyopathy; and Ch. 67, Arrythmias.

History: Key Questions to Ask

1. What were you doing when the event occurred?
2. Did you actually lose consciousness (black out)?
3. Did you fall and hurt yourself?
4. How long were you out?
5. Did you lose control of your bladder or bowel?
6. Was there any seizure-like activity noted?
7. Was there any chest pain, palpitation, change in vision, or nausea before or immediately after the event?
8. Has this ever happened before?

Knowing the events surrounding the syncopal episode can help to direct the subsequent evaluation and possible treatment. For example, if the syncope occurred during micturition in a male, even though this may be a variant of NVD, addressing a potential prostate problem may be curative. Other questions that help to determine the possible severity of the syncopal problem and thus the urgency of evaluation are: Was the person able to anticipate the event and thereby prevent injury? Or was there little or no warning of the event with resultant injury? Syncope that has occurred many times before and happens with warning probably requires less urgent assessment than that which has happened without warning and has resulted in injury.

Clinical Findings

1. General appearance
2. Presence or absence of orthostatic changes
3. Evidence of aortic stenosis or hypertrophic cardiomyopathy
4. Evidence of LV dysfunction

The general appearance of the patient will help in narrowing the differential diagnosis of syncope. For example, a well-nourished young person is much more likely to have NVD than an elderly individual with a sternotomy scar. The other findings, such as those listed above, render evidence of specific diagnoses. Evidence of LV dysfunction suggests a propensity to malignant ventricular dysrhythmias (VT/VF), although it is not diagnostic for them.

Tests

1. Electrocardiogram: helps to identify or rule out conductive abnormalities/pre-excitation
2. Echocardiogram: a good method of assessing LV function and valvular state
3. Signal average ECG: in the absence of conductive abnormality on the ECG, the signal-averaged ECG (SAECG) can help predict the tendency toward VT. The SAECG is most predictive in patients with ejection fractions less than 40 per cent.
4. Head-up tilt table test: very useful test in patients with EFs greater than 40 per cent in whom NVD is suspected
5. Electrophysiologic testing: test of choice in patients suspected of having a tachydysrhythmia as the cause of syncope, especially for AVNRT and VT/VF
6. Holter monitoring and electroencephalograms are generally of very low yield and are not indicated in the initial evaluation of syncope.

Management

Of NVD

1. Maintain hydration/advise caution when changing position
2. β-blockers (divided-dose cardioselective β-blockers appear to work best)
3. Disopyramide
4. Theophylline preparations
5. Anticholinergic agents (e.g., transdermal scopolamine)

6. Serotonin reuptake inhibitor (e.g. fluoxetine [Prozac]) for patients refractory to β-blockers and/or theophylline

Of VT/VF

1. Treat/remove underlying ischemic heart disease if possible
2. Treat metabolic abnormalities
3. Consider automatic implantable cardiodefibrillator (AICD)

PEARLS

- Syncope primarily is associated with a cardiovascular problem, *not a neurologic disease.*

- NVD is most common in patients without structural heart disease.

- VT/VF is most common in patients with structural heart disease.

 Bibliography

Day SC: Evaluation and outcome of emergency room patients with transient loss of consciousness. Am J Med 1982;73:15–23.

Eagle KA: Evaluation of prognostic classifications for patients with syncope. Am J Med 1985;79:455–460.

Kapoor WN: Diagnostic evaluation of syncope. Am J Med 1991; 90:91–106.

Kosinski DJ: Neurocardiogenic syncope: A review of pathophysiology, diagnosis, and treatment. Cardiovascular Reviews and Reports. 1993; June:22–29.

Sra JS: Unexplained syncope evaluated by electrophysiologic study and head-up tilt test. Ann Intern Med 1991;114:1013–1019.

Vacek JL: Diagnosing syncope. Postgrad Med 1991;90:175–184.

Symptom | Palpitations   *Roland A. Goertz*

Palpitations are any uncomfortable awareness of the beating heart. The condition does not always imply a rapid heartbeat but can encompass any sensation in the chest described as pounding, flopping, skipping, jumping, fluttering, or thumping. The condition may be completely benign or it may be serious, demanding aggressive diagnosis and treatment. Proper evaluation includes clarifying symptom severity, defining the extent of any underlying cardiovascular disease, and determining whether a rhythm disturbance is present. A common complaint is pounding of the heart following exercise, a benign condition.

Differential Diagnosis

1. Sinus tachycardia states
   a. Anxiety, including panic disorder
   b. Exercise
   c. Fever
   d. Stress
   e. Menopause
2. Drugs that increase adrenergic tone or diminish vagal activity
   a. Coffee
   b. Nicotine
   c. Adrenergic or anticholinergic drugs
3. High cardiac output states
   a. Anemia
   b. Thyrotoxicosis
   c. Pregnancy
4. Arrhythmias
   a. Premature atrial or ventricular contractions (PACs and PVCs)
   b. Atrioventricular heart block

　　c. Bradycardias

　　d. Sick sinus syndrome

　　e. Wolff-Parkinson-White syndrome

　　f. Atrial fibrillation/flutter

　　g. Paroxysmal supraventricular tachycardia

　　h. Ventricular tachycardia

　　i. Other arrhythmias

5. Other serious conditions to be considered:

　　a. Myocardial infarction

　　b. Myocardial ischemia, unstable angina

　　c. Hypokalemia

　　d. Hypomagnesemia

　　e. Valvular heart disease

　　f. Hypoxia

　　g. Pheochromocytoma

Palpitations fall under a differential diagnosis list that encompasses normal and abnormal circumstances. Examples of normal palpitations include those related to exercise, emotion, stress, or ingestion of substances that result in any form of sinus tachycardia or increased adrenergic tone or decreased vagal activity. Caffeine, nicotine, and other related drugs must be considered. Normal palpitations by definition are those that occur in individuals who are evaluated by a physician and told they have had something happen to accelerate the normal rhythm of the heart. Many patients find a "racing" heart uncomfortable and seek medical care. Generally, palpitations not related to emotion, fever, or exercise suggest an underlying arrhythmia. Palpitations caused by clearly abnormal conditions must be discovered and appropriately treated. It is important to note that most people with arrhythmias do not present with palpitations but present with other manifestations such as syncope, angina, and shock. It is sometimes easy to overlook palpitation causes such as pregnancy, menopausal states, mitral valve disease, aortic incompetence, hypoxia, or the rare pheochromocytoma.

Refer to Ch. 57, Acute Myocardial Infarction; Ch. 67, Arrhythmias; Ch. 163, Hyperthyroidism; Ch. 315, Panic Disorder; and Ch. 316, Generalized Anxiety Disorder.

History: Key Questions to Ask

1. Under what circumstances do the palpitations start and how long do they last?

2. Is there anything you can identify that initiates them?

3. Are they related to high emotional stress or worry?

4. What do you sense or feel during the palpitations?

5. Is there chest pain or shortness of breath during the attack?

6. Do you feel dizzy or faint during the palpitations?

7. Do you drink any liquids that contain caffeine, and if so, how much?

8. Do you use nasal decongestants or have the attacks following ingestion of Chinese food?

9. Do you use any social drugs?

10. Have you had a history of heart problems?

11. What characteristics do the palpitations have when you have an episode?

The preceding questions attempt to discriminate between benign and serious palpitations. If a patient admits to having chest pain, myocardial ischemia and aortic stenosis must be considered. Shortness of breath can be an indication of anxiety with hyperventilation or a more serious condition such as mitral stenosis or cardiac failure. Dizziness and fainting are serious findings for which a more thorough investigation for serious cardiac arrhythmias is imperative.

Clinical Findings

1. Normal physical examination: a most frequent finding since palpitations frequently are not present when a patient is examined

2. Rapid heartbeat

3. Blood pressure abnormalities

4. Abnormal heart sounds

5. Irregular arterial or jugular pulsations

6. Variable findings associated with underlying etiologies

The best time to examine the patient with palpitations is during an episode. This is not usually possible, and the physical examination is generally normal. When the patient is examined during an episode, underlying cardiac etiologies may be discernible by virtue of the characteristics of the cardiac examination. Generally a pulse rate greater than 150 beats/min suggests a more serious condition. Rates that are rapid and regular but less than 150 are more likely to be sinus tachycardia and associated with exercise, fever, drugs, or thyrotoxicosis. Evidence suggestive of fever, infection, anxiety state, or depressive illnesses should be sought in addition to any findings that would reveal underlying anemia, thyroid disease, alcohol abuse, or cardiac disease.

Tests

1. Blood tests: hemoglobin, hematocrit, blood smear, thyroid function tests, serum potassium, and magnesium

2. Chest radiograph

3. Electrocardiogram (ECG)

4. Ambulatory 24-hour heart monitoring (Holter or transtelephonic)

5. Echocardiography, electrophysiology studies

6. Exercise stress test if palpitations are associated with exercise

The test most helpful in evaluating palpitations is the ECG during an episode of palpitations. Any number of specific findings from atrial fibrillation to ventricular tachycardia may be discovered with the ECG. If the cause of palpitations remains unclear after ECG, one may consider other forms of ambulatory cardiac monitoring. Transtelephonic monitoring, during which an ECG recording made by a patient during symptoms is transmitted by telephone, is often more useful and more cost-effective than Holter monitoring. A recording of normal sinus rhythm during a typical palpitation episode strongly excludes an arrhythmia. Electrophysiologic testing should be reserved for a minority of patients with palpitations and is limited to patients with sustained ventricular tachyarrhythmia, frequent symptomatic paroxysmal supraventricular tachycardia, unexplained major symptoms such as dizziness or syncope, or occupations in which a sudden loss of consciousness may be fatal to the patient or others.

Management

1. Any definable underlying cause
2. Appropriate reassurance
3. Patient education concerning possible causal activities
4. Behavior modification to include
   a. Smoking cessation
   b. Limitation of caffeine and alcohol
   c. Discontinuation of causative drugs
   d. Stress reduction

Treatment of specific underlying cardiac illnesses often requires complicated drug therapies. Situations warranting a cardiology referral include

1. Suspicion of sustained supraventricular tachycardia or ventricular tachycardia
2. An electrocardiogram indicative of Wolff-Parkinson-White syndrome (WPW)
3. Syncope or dizziness suggesting serious cardiovascular disease
4. Any unexplained arrhythmia that correlates with significant findings or symptoms

Follow-Up

Follow-up for palpitations is variable and predicated on the underlying cause. Some follow-up of patients with normal palpitations is reasonable to appropriately reassure and counsel the individual.

PEARLS

- Palpitations unrelated to anxiety, exercise, or drugs suggest an arrhythmia.

- Palpitations are a nonspecific symptom and do not necessarily imply serious illness.

- Most palpitations are benign.

- Evaluation should focus on detecting any serious arrhythmia, clarifying symptom severity, and assessing the extent of any underlying heart disease.

- The briefness and infrequency of palpitation episodes may require an ambulatory form of heart monitoring such as transtelephonic monitoring to yield useful information. Transtelephonic monitoring is often more cost-effective than Holter monitoring.

- Any patient with serious physical findings or disturbing ECG results deserves aggressive cardiac evaluation.

Bibliography

For more information on palpitations, see
Brugada P, Gursoy S, Brugada J, Andries E: Investigation of palpitations. Lancet 1993;341:1254–1258.
Kopp DE, Wilber DJ: Palpitations and arrhythmia. Postgrad Med 1992;91(1);241–251.
Smith TW: Approach to the patient with cardiovascular disease. *In* Wyngaarden JB, Smith LH, Bennett JC (eds): Cecil Textbook of Medicine. 19th ed. Philadelphia, WB Saunders, 1992, pp 147–150.
For more information on transtelephonic monitoring, and electrophysiologic studies, see
Podrid PJ, Bumio F, Fogel RI: Evaluating patients with ventricular arrhythmia. Cardiol Clin 1992;10(3):371–395.

Symptom Leg Edema

Ralph Weber

Edema is an increase in the amount of interstitial fluid (IF). Its basic determinants are *filtration* (arterial end) and *reabsorption* (venous end) at the capillary bed.

1. Four factors influence development of edema
   a. Hydrostatic pressure in capillaries and interstitial tissue
   b. Colloid osmotic pressure in plasma and interstitial tissue
   c. Permeability of capillary walls
   d. Alterations (obstruction) of lymphatic flow

The above processes are often modified by renal sodium retention.

2. Three types of leg swelling occur according to content, i.e., water, lymph, or fat (Table 52–1).
   a. Systemic edema (main component(s) similar to normal interstitial fluid)

TABLE 52–1. GENERAL FEATURES OF EDEMA

	SYSTEMIC EDEMA	LYMPHEDEMA	LIPEDEMA
Water and sodium retention	Increased	Normal	Normal
Distribution			
Bilateral	+	±	+
Foot and/or leg	Both	Both	Legs only
Toes involved before foot	−	+	−
Skin appearance			
Pitting, soft	+	*	−
General thickening	−	+	−
Toe fold thickening (Stemmer's sign)	−	+	−
Decreased with elevation of part	+	−	−

Symbols: + = present; − = absent; * = soft only if very recent onset.
Data from Spittel JA Jr, Schirger A: Edema, peripheral. *In* Taylor RB: Difficult Diagnosis. Philadelphia, WB Saunders, 1985.

    b. Lymphedema (chief component is protein)

    c. Lipedema (principal component being fat)

The distribution of edema (unilateral vs bilateral) is useful in diagnosis.

Differential Diagnosis

Bilateral (systemic) edema may be secondary to

1. Cardiac dysfunction (e.g., congestive heart failure)
2. Renal dysfunction (e.g., nephritic or nephrotic)
3. Hepatic dysfunction (e.g., cirrhosis) or, more rarely, hepatic vein thrombosis (Budd-Chiari syndrome) and portal vein thrombosis
4. Metabolic dysfunction (e.g., protein deficiency)
5. Endocrine dysfunction (e.g., Cushing's disease, thyroid disease)
6. Physiologic (e.g., pregnancy, salt overload)
7. Idiopathic cyclic edema (after other edema causes excluded): usually only in women aged 20 to 40 years, tends to involve upper extremities as well as lower, tends to have self-limited course of a few months to several years
8. Lipedema: symmetric nonpitting fat deposition in buttocks and legs but sparing feet in women
9. Microvascular capillary "leak" syndromes (e.g., exposure to temperature extremes, angioneurotic edema)

Unilateral (regional) edema may be secondary to

1. Venous disease: intrinsic (e.g., acute deep venous thrombosis, chronic venous insufficiency [CVI]); extrinsic (e.g., tumor, pressure of overlying iliac artery); traumatic interruption (e.g., surgical ligation, plication, insertion of filter)
2. Lymphedema: congenital (primary) or acquired (secondary). Most common causes are postphlebitic syndrome, tissue injury after surgery/radiation, or underlying tumor. Less frequent causes are parasitic inflammations (e.g., filariasis, lymphogranuloma venereum), syphilis, and granulomatous disease, especially tuberculosis.
3. Miscellaneous: most often the result of bacterial inflammation (e.g., cellulitis, deep tissue abscess, osteomyelitis) especially with SS disease or neuropathies, as in diabetics. Occasional causes include muscle (e.g., gastrocnemius) rupture, congenital and acquired vascular disorders, compartment syndromes.

> Refer to Ch. 60, Chronic Heart Failure; Ch. 68, Varicose Veins; Ch. 69, Deep Venous Thrombosis; Ch. 90, Cirrhosis; Chs. 129 and 130, Renal Failure; Ch. 131, Glomerulonephritis; Ch. 162, Hypothyroidism; and Ch. 166, Cushing's Syndrome/Disease.

History: Key Questions to Ask

1. Onset? Measured in hours to days: acute (e.g., cellulitis, deep venous thrombosis [DVT], compartment syndrome, gastrocnemius rupture) versus chronic (e.g., systemic process, medication, chronic venous insufficiency, lymphedema)
2. Clinical course and localization? This is usually characterized as intermittent (recurrent) versus constant.
3. Quality of pain? Painless (systemic causes or lymphedema) versus painful (cellulitis, ruptured gastrocnemius, ruptured Baker's cyst, compartment syndrome, DVT)
4. Associated systemic symptoms? Fever and chills suggest cellulitis, lymphangitis, or venous thrombosis. Symptoms associated with CHF (e.g., dyspnea, orthopnea, PND) suggest cardiac origin. Glomerulosclerosis and/or nephritis (e.g., history of recent streptococcal sore throat, recurrent cystitis, hypertension, changes in ocular fundi, urinalysis, BUN/creatinine, and serum albumin) offer a renal pathogenesis, whereas signs of acute or chronic liver disease (e.g., hepatitis, alcoholism, axillary hair loss, palmar erythema, icterus, spider telangiectasias, gynecomastia, hepatomegaly, splenomegaly, abdominal wall collateral veins, ascites, or abnormal liver function tests) are all suggestive of hepatic etiology of edema formation.
5. Medications? These include diazoxide, minoxidil, hydralazine, calcium channel blockers, α- and β-receptor blockers, reserpine, guanethidine, NSAIDs, car-

benicillin, amantadine, lithium, phenothiazines, thioridazine, monamine oxidase inhibitors, corticosteroids, testosterone, estrogen, and progesterone. Alcohol and other substance abuse? Diet faddism?

6. Endocrine diseases? These include Cushing's syndrome, thyroid dysfunction (pretibial "myxedema"), and thickened pretibial and/or foot skin during treatment of Graves' disease.

7. Miscellaneous factors? Pregnancy, salt overload, sudden cessation of laxative or diuretic abuse, carbohydrate-loading–induced antinatriuresis (diet enthusiasts after weekend binge), prolonged dependent positioning, impaired ambulation due to severe joint or neurologic disease (paraplegia)

Clinical Findings

1. Distribution: bilateral—smaller number of diseases, usually systemic; unilateral—larger number of diseases, usually regional

2. Location of swelling: calf or thigh only without feet or ankles—local cause within involved muscle groups (ruptured muscle, trauma, aneurysm, hematoma, sarcoma), or sparing of feet (lipedema)

3. Appearance of overlying skin: red (with or without tender streaks suggestive of cellulitis, phlebitis, lymphangitis): reddish-blue (DVT); slightly cyanotic and bilateral (suggestive of CHF); venous "stars" (denoting local stasis with elevated venous pressure): ecchymosis (suggestive of trauma, ruptured muscle)

4. Pitting: suggestive of systemic cause; mobility of nonchronic (i.e., <3 months in duration) pitting edema a function of tissue viscosity related to fluid protein content. When edema "pits" with little resistance and recovery is seen in <30 to 40 seconds, hypoproteinemia generally is present. *However,* if edema is chronic (>3 months), interstitial tissue fibrosis and scarring may produce prolonged pitting even if hypoproteinemia is present.

Tests

1. Serum electrolytes and biochemistry profile (including liver function tests, serum albumin, total protein, blood urea nitrogen, and creatinine)

2. Urinalysis (routine and microscopic)

3. Chest radiograph

4. Echocardiogram to assess cardiac dysfunction (prn)

5. Thyroid function tests to rule out thyroid dysfunction (prn)

6. Duplex Doppler or venography to rule out DVT (prn)

Management

1. General: Diuretics, dietary manipulation of salt and water, vasodilators, and digoxin are prescribed (see Chs. 60 and 130). Angiotensin-converting enzyme (ACE) inhibitors sometimes are helpful in the treatment of idiopathic cyclic edema, in addition to reassurance. Elastic compression with stockings, physical therapy, and intermittent pneumatic compression may be useful.

2. Specific: Treatment depends on the cause of the edema. DVT—anticoagulation with heparin followed by warfarin; CVI—sclerotherapy used in selected patients. Surgical management (ligation/stripping of incompetent perforator veins, venous reconstruction to bypass isolated obstruction or to interpose a functioning valve segment in a patent deep venous system) is applicable to <25 per cent of patients *only* after studies determine site and degree of valve dysfunction or obstruction. Surgical therapy usually is limited to patients with severe (grade III) CVI. Treatment of edema due to lymphatics is usually medical to remove as much fluid as possible (compression with stockings, physical therapy, and intermittent pneumatic compression). If medical therapy fails, palliative surgery is considered. Two types are available: excisional (debulking) and microvascular reconstruction (lymphovenous anastomosis or lymph vessel transplant). For miscellaneous inflammatory causes, antibiotics are prescribed. Abscess and osteomyelitis may warrant surgery in selected patients.

Bibliography

Abraham WT, Schrier RW: Body fluid volume regulation in health and disease. Adv Inter Med 1994;39:23–47.

Ciocon JO, Fernandez BB, Ciocon DG: Leg edema. Geriatrics 1993;48:34–45.

Ruschaupt III WF: The swollen limb. *In* Young JR, Graor RA, Olin JW, Bartholomew JR (eds): Peripheral Vascular Diseases. St. Louis, Mosby, 1991, pp 639–650.

Seller RH: Swelling of legs. *In* Seller RH: Differential Diagnosis of Common Complaints, 2nd ed. Philadelphia, WB Saunders, 1993, pp 343–350.

| Symptom | **Claudication** | *Fernando F. Stancampiano* |

The term claudication derives from the Latin word *claudicare,* to limp. In addition to its negative impact on ambulation, this condition is frequently associated with occlusive disease in other vascular areas, such as the coronary or extracranial arteries. As revealed by the Framingham study, men with intermittent claudication (IC) have a higher annual mortality rate than their normal counterparts (39/1000 versus 10/1000), mostly due to a high incidence of myocardial infarction and stroke. Although IC is usually the consequence of insufficient arterial blood supply to the lower extremities caused by arteriosclerosis obliterans (ASO), patients with lumbar canal stenosis often present with similar complaints; the latter is referred to as *pseudoclaudication.*

Differential Diagnosis

1. ASO
2. Lumbar canal stenosis and disk disease (pseudoclaudication)
3. Embolic disease
4. Buerger's disease
5. Vasculitis (Takayasu's disease, giant cell arteritis)
6. Drugs (ergot derivatives)
7. Phlegmasia (ileofemoral vein thrombosis with secondary arterial insufficiency)
8. Metabolic disease (homocystinuria)
9. Miscellanea (adventitial cyst, entrapment syndromes, fibromuscular dysplasia, reflex sympathetic dystrophy, persistent sciatic artery)

Although numerous medical and surgical conditions mimic the clinical presentation of IC, ASO of the lower extremities and aortoiliac territories is the most common etiology. Typically, patients with pseudoclaudication have pain while standing and need to change position in order to get relief, whereas in those with IC, the simple interruption of exercise is sufficient to abort the symptoms within minutes. Obvious findings consistent with ASO do not rule out pseudoclaudication, since both frequently coexist. Patients with vasculitis often have "ischemic-looking" ulcers in atypical locations.

Refer to Ch. 68, Varicose Veins; Ch. 69, Deep Venous Thrombosis; Ch. 70, Peripheral Arterial Disease; and Ch. 295, Reflex Sympathetic Dystrophy.

History

1. Pain in the lower extremities (buttocks, calves)
2. Symptoms may be unilateral or bilateral.
3. Claudication occurs with exercise and is relieved by resting within a few minutes.
4. A decrease in the claudication threshold correlates with progression of the disease.
5. Evidence of ischemia at rest is a reflection of increased severity.

At the time the diagnosis of IC is made, a significant proportion of patients are known to already have coronary and/or cerebrovascular disease. These patients commonly have a history of diabetes mellitus, tobacco abuse, and other risk factors for heart disease.

Clinical Findings

1. Diminished/absent pulses
2. Arterial bruits (femoral, Hunter's canal)
3. Diminished temperature in the affected limb(s)
4. Ischemic ulcers
5. Dependent rubor/edema
6. Muscle weakness/atrophy

Most patients with IC have absent or markedly diminished palpable pulses; however, a normal examination does not rule out the disease. Blood flow studies usually reveal one or more localized abnormalities. The typical ischemic ulcer is painful, well circumscribed, and usually located in the distal portion of the toes, interdigital areas (kissing ulcers), or pressure sites (ASO and trauma). In severe cases, atrophy and ischemic neuropathy may develop. Dependent edema and rubor tend to occur late in the course of the disease and seem to be markers of a threatened limb.

Tests

1. Arteriogram (aortogram with "runoffs")
2. Ankle/brachial systolic blood pressure index (ABI)
3. Pulse volume recordings (PVRs)
4. Other tests: plethysmography, positron emission tomography (PET), magnetic resonance imaging, digital subtraction angiography, duplex scanning
5. Risk stratification (coronary angiogram, myocardial perfusion studies)

Most cases can be diagnosed accurately on the basis of a detailed history and physical examination, combined with noninvasive methods. The simple application of basic Doppler techniques (ABI) provides valuable information regarding the severity of the disease. An ABI of <0.3 is usually associated with ischemic rest pain and impending necrosis. In PVRs, partially inflated blood pressure cuffs sense volume changes in limb segments, which are subsequently transduced and displayed as waveforms. The same techniques can be applied to document the outcome of a revascularization procedure. The angiographic evaluation of the lower extremities is not indicated in every patient but becomes mandatory when a surgical intervention is considered. Myocardial infarction significantly contributes to the postoperative mortality among patients who undergo aortofemoral or femoropopliteal reconstruction. Therefore, the status of the coronary circulation should be evaluated in all patients by means of a coronary angiogram or noninvasive nuclear techniques (Dipyridamole 201-Tl, 82-Rb PET scanning). Findings consistent with high ischemic risk warrant myocardial revascularization before surgery in the lower extremities.

Management

1. Conditioning exercises
2. Smoking cessation
3. Pharmacologic treatment
4. Revascularization procedures (angioplasty, stent placement, surgery)

It is well documented that a training program of walking exercises improves resting blood flow, reduces the onset of claudication symptoms, and increases maximal walking time. Unfortunately, the use of vasodilating drugs has yielded disappointing results. Most vasodilators reduce systemic blood pressure and increase collateral vessel resistance. The current literature does not support their widespread use. One randomized study in the United States recommends the use of pentoxifylline (Trental); however, several others did not find it to be of benefit. A long list of drugs have been tried—mostly without success—including ketanserin, heparan sulfate, prostaglandin I₂, ticlopidine, calcium channel blockers, EDTA, isradipine, fish oil, dipyridamole, and ridogel. The most important operative indications for lower extremity ischemia include ischemic rest pain or tissue loss (ulceration and/or gangrene), disabling claudication, and lack of response to an adequate trial of medical therapy. Ongoing trials are aimed at defining the role of fibrinolytic therapy in patients with peripheral arterial disease.

Patient Education

1. Lifestyle modification (smoking cessation, exercise)
2. Foot care (daily inspection, skin care)
3. Use of professionally customized shoes/orthotics

PEARLS

- Consider non-ASO causes of IC in patients with atypical features.

- Objectively assess the patient's functional capacity and status of the circulation in the lower extremities (exercise PVRs).
- Provide positive feedback to reinforce lifestyle changes.
- Try to establish the proper timing for a surgical intervention.

Bibliography

Bergqvist D, Karacagil S: Femoral artery disease. Lancet 1994; 343:773–778.

Brand F, Abbott R, Kannel W: Diabetes, intermittent claudication, and risk of cardiovascular events. The Framingham Study. Diabetes 1989;38:504–509.

Porter J: Chronic lower extremity ischemia. Curr Probl Surg 1991;28:3–179.

Strandness DE, Carter S: Outcome criteria in patients with peripheral arterial disease. Ann Vasc Surg 1993;7:491–496.

Yeager R: Nonatherosclerotic claudication. Semin Vasc Surg 1993;6:24–35.

Symptom **Shock** *Benjamin H. Chadi*

Shock is defined as the *state of hypoperfusion of vital organs associated with hypotension and a critical prognosis.* Ohm's law:

Flow = (Pressure gradient afferent-efferent)/
(Resistance in vascular bed)

is valid for individual organs and for the circulatory system as a whole. Areas of higher resistance, such as the kidneys and stenosed coronary arteries, require a higher perfusion pressure (blood pressure) for flow to occur. Above this minimal pressure, many organs such as the brain can autoregulate blood flow to maintain a relatively constant perfusion at varying blood pressures.

Reduced organ perfusion can occur because of a loss of vascular resistance (distributive), inability to generate a pressure (cardiogenic), inadequate blood volume (hypovolemic), or block to flow in the circuit (obstructive).

Differential Diagnosis

Distributive (generalized systemic vasodilatation)

1. Sepsis: bacterial (gram-positive, gram-negative), fungal, rickettsial (Rocky Mountain spotted fever), and toxins (toxic shock)
2. Anaphylaxis: drug reaction—penicillins; stings of bees, wasps, scorpions; snakebites
3. Neurogenic: spinal shock—trauma, anesthesia; vagotonic—related to procedures, sight of blood

4. Drugs: α blockers, β agonists, and vasodilators including nitroprusside, captopril, nifedipine

Cardiogenic (low cardiac output due to right or left ventricular pump failure)

1. Myocardial infarction with large areas of myocyte necrosis
2. Acute myocardial ischemia in a large area, a sign of left main or severe three-vessel coronary artery disease
3. Cardiomyopathy with progressive pump failure
4. Ischemia associated with hypotension of another cause
5. Acute coronary spasm (Prinzmetal's angina or related to drugs, cocaine)
6. Tachyarrhythmias (ventricular or supraventricular tachycardia [VT or SVT]) with inadequate time for chamber filling or loss of vasoconstrictor reflexes
7. Bradyarrhythmias including heart block
8. Ventricular free wall rupture
9. Ventricular septal defect (postinfarction)
10. Papillary muscle necrosis with acute mitral regurgitation
11. Congenital heart disease with associated sepsis
12. Severe valvular heart disease (aortic or mitral stenosis) or subaortic stenosis (IHSS) or supravalvular

stenosis with inability to increase cardiac output in response to stress (e.g., infection, vasodilator)

Hypovolemic (loss of preload)

1. Acute hemorrhage or blood loss (gastrointestinal, trauma, surgery, anticoagulants)
2. Dehydration due to fever, vomiting, diarrhea, nasogastric suction, diabetic ketoacidosis, peritonitis
3. Intravascular depletion due to third spacing including postsurgical states and hypoalbuminemia
4. Adrenal insufficiency, pheochromocytoma

Obstructive (massive increase in afterload)

1. Aortic dissection with obliteration of true lumen
2. Pericardial tamponade
3. Pulmonary embolism
4. Tension pneumothorax
5. Valvular obstruction: prosthesis malfunction, prolapse of atrial myxoma, or valve obstruction by ball valve thrombus

---

Refer to Ch. 57, Acute Myocardial Infarction; Ch. 58, Cardiac Arrest; Ch. 59, Acute Heart Failure; Ch. 60, Chronic Heart Failure; Ch. 61, Cardiomyopathy; Ch. 65, Endocarditis; Ch. 67, Arrhythmias; Ch. 195, Anaphylaxis; and Ch. 229, Sepsis/Bacteremia.

History

1. Hypotension: fatigue, dizziness, syncope
2. Poor perfusion: slow mentation, decreased urination, decreased appetite
3. Etiology: infection, fever, new drug, hypersensitivity, sting, heart attack, chest pain, shortness of breath, trauma, bleeding, melena, diarrhea, fluid losses

Clinical Findings

1. Hypotension: systolic blood pressure less than 90 mm Hg except when there is severe vasoconstriction and low output with cardiogenic shock, or a unilateral pulse deficit in aortic dissection
2. Pulse: tachycardia occurs with fever, pain, hypoxia, hyperthyroidism, or stress (adrenaline). Tachycardia increases cardiac output (C.O. = stroke volume × heart rate), increases myocardial oxygen demand (and ischemia in coronary stenosis), and shortens diastole (and ventricular filling time). Very rapid heart rates can significantly reduce stroke volume, cardiac output, and blood pressure. Bradycardia may symptomatically drop cardiac output, as in the sick sinus syndrome. In high-grade and complete heart blocks, atrioventricular dissociation further impairs ventricular filling. In hypervagotonia such as with vasovagal syncope, carotid sinus hypersensitivity, or the Bezold-Jarisch reflex noted in inferior myocardial infarction, a vasodepressor component (vasodilation) frequently accompanies the cardioinhibitory component (bradycardia), resulting in hypotension. Peripheral vasodila-

tion alone (without bradycardia) causes orthostatic hypotension in the Shy-Drager syndrome.

3. Fever: in sepsis, anaphylaxis, and adrenal insufficiency
4. Organ hypoperfusion: cold, clammy skin (except for distributive shock, in which skin is warm), pallor or cyanosis, poor mentation, decreased bowel sounds, oliguria
5. Jugular veins: flat in hypovolemic and distributive shock (<6 cm); distended in cardiogenic and obstructive shock (>8 cm water)
6. Pulmonary rales, edema, effusion: in cardiogenic or obstructive shock; in acute respiratory distress syndrome or pneumonia in any type of shock
7. Heart sounds:
   a. Distant in tamponade
   b. Loud P_2 in pulmonary hypertension
   c. Delayed A_2 in aortic stenosis
   d. S_3 and diffuse impulse in cardiogenic
   e. S_4 and prominent impulse in obstructive
   f. Murmurs of mitral regurgitation, IHSS, aortic stenosis, aortic insufficiency, ventricular septal defect
   g. Rub (two- or three-component) of pericarditis
   h. Pericardial knock of constriction
   i. Diastolic tumor plop of myxoma
   j. Muffling of metallic prosthetic valve clicks

Tests

Shock must be diagnosed immediately and its cause determined accurately, so that lifesaving therapy can be initiated immediately to correct the reversible causes of this otherwise rapidly fatal state. Monitoring, diagnosis, and therapy often have to occur simultaneously, with frequent updates and rapid response and action necessary by health care personnel. The duration of hypotension measured in minutes and hours often determines the degree and reversibility of organ system damage and sequelae. Tests include

1. Electrocardiography: Evaluate for VT, SVT, heart blocks, ST elevations of acute infarction, spasm, pericarditis, ST depressions of ischemia, Q waves of old infarctions, new right axis in pulmonary embolism, right-sided chest leads for RV infarction.
2. Chest roentgenogram: Evaluate for cardiomegaly, progressive enlargement in tamponade, evidence of pulmonary congestion, dilated aortic arch in dissecting aneurysm, pulmonary vascular plethora in septal defects, effusions in heart failure, pulmonary embolism, and other states.
3. Complete blood count: Hematocrit drops after hydration in acute blood loss; hemoconcentration in dehydration; leukocytosis, left shift, and toxic granulations in sepsis; thrombocytopenia or coagulopathies in bleeding diatheses; and schistocytes in disseminated intravascular coagulation.

4. Arterial blood gases and electrolytes: Rule out and correct hypoxia, respiratory and metabolic acidosis, hyper- and hypokalemia, natremia, calcemia, magnesemia, and glycemia, whether primary or secondary to the shock. Consider naloxone (Narcan) and flumazenil (Mazicon).

5. Blood cultures for aerobic, anaerobic, acid-fast, and fungal organisms

6. Urinalysis and culture: pyuria, casts in urosepsis, acute tubular necrosis

7. Assays: creatine kinase and MB elevation in myocardial infarction; elevated lactate dehydrogenase levels in myocardial infarction, and hemolysis (prosthetic valve dysfunction); documentation of serum amylase and lipase, renal and hepatic function including albumin, and phosphorus; serum cortisol and drug levels

8. Echocardiography with Doppler: evaluate pericardial effusion and diastolic RA, RV collapse in tamponade with respiratory variation in the mitral and aortic flow Doppler tests; evaluate for a cardiomyopathy with generalized hypokinesis or for infarctions with focal wall motion abnormalities; calculate pulmonary artery pressures and cardiac output, valve function, chamber sizes, and septal defects.

9. Transesophageal echocardiography can diagnose pulmonary artery thromboembolus, aortic dissection, septal defects, and congenital heart diseases.

10. Ventilation perfusion scanning for pulmonary embolism

11. Cardiac catheterization
   a. Arterial line to monitor blood pressure
   b. Central venous line to monitor right heart pressure (CVP)
   c. Swan-Ganz catheterization to evaluate pulmonary artery pressures and pulmonary capillary wedge pressure (PCWP, left heart preload) with measurements of cardiac output by thermodilution or Fick (oxygen uptake) methods and calculation of systemic vascular resistance
   d. Oximetry with oxygen saturations from the central vein compared to the pulmonary artery oxygen saturations with a significant step-up indicating a left-to-right shunt
   e. Coronary angiography to evaluate location and severity of coronary stenoses and occlusion of vessels in acute infarctions with evidence of reperfusion or ongoing necessity for revascularization
   f. Left ventriculography to evaluate function, regurgitation
   g. Aortography to evaluate for dissection, regurgitation
   h. Pulmonary angiography to evaluate for thromboembolism
   i. Fluoroscopic evaluation of prosthetic valve function

12. Continuous monitoring of vital signs, blood pressure, oxygen saturations, and electrocardiography (ECG) for arrhythmias

Management
Medical Therapy
Treatment depends on cause. Control of the airway and oxygen may be necessary.

1. Hypovolemic: Large-bore intravenous lines are used for fluid support (saline, packed red blood cells, albumin). Monitor hematocrit, central venous pressure, rales, PCWP (in cardiomyopathy). Find source of blood loss and stop bleeding (vascular compression, endoscopy, surgery if necessary, consider platelets or fresh frozen plasma).

2. Distributive: Intravenous saline and fluids are given to replete intravascular volume; then consider vasopressors (norepinephrine, phenylephrine, metaraminol, methoxamine) via central line if ventricular function is normal. Antibiotics for sepsis (consider antifungal drug if patient is already on several broad-spectrum antibiotics, especially for more than one to two weeks and especially if immunocompromised). Give antihistamines (H_1 and H_2) and steroids for anaphylaxis. Consider atropine for vagotonia.

3. Cardiogenic: Relieve ischemia (oxygen, nitrates, heparin). Perform thrombolysis of acute infarction (less successful in shock). Intra-aortic balloon counterpulsation (IABP) with emergency angioplasty or bypass surgery is recommended in the setting of an acute myocardial infarction and ongoing chest pain or hemodynamic instability. Perform valve repair or replacement in acute papillary muscle rupture with mitral regurgitation, and surgical repair of ventricular free wall rupture or septal defects. Inotropes including dopamine, dobutamine, amrinone, and milrinone may be given; avoid digoxin or isoproterenol in the acute infarct setting (increases myocardial oxygen demand). In end stage, consider stronger β agonists (epinephrine) via central venous line. Optimize preload. Antiarrhythmic therapy and rapid cardioversion are used to treat unstable ventricular tachycardia and primary SVT (treat underlying cause; look for hypovolemia; avoid calcium blockers in hypotension or treat overdose with intravenous calcium). For long-term treatment, consider need for diuretics, nitrates, angiotensin-converting enzyme inhibitors, and digoxin.

4. Obstructive: Immediate removal of the cause of obstruction is imperative.
   a. Pulmonary embolectomy or prolonged thrombolytic infusion for pulmonary embolism
   b. Aortic root and arch repair for type I aortic dissection
   c. Pericardiocentesis at bedside using ECG with a

grounded V lead attached under asepsis to the needle (and ideally echo or fluoroscopic guidance) for tamponade

Supportive Therapy

1. Diet: NPO; low-cholesterol/low-salt diet when tolerated
2. Activity: Bed rest immediately; gradual ambulation after treatment
3. Patient education: Condition is critical unless rapidly reversed

Follow-Up

1. Intensive care unit care with (invasive) hemodynamic monitoring until blood pressure, systemic vascular resistance, and cardiac output have normalized off drips
2. Meticulous attention to line sterility with frequent replacement (every three to four days) to avoid super-infection
3. Observe for recovery of function of brain, kidneys, and intestine as shock resolves.

Bibliography

Effron MB, Chernow B: Shock. *In* Rubenstein E, Federman D (eds): Scientific American Medicine. New York, Scientific American, 1992, 1:III:1–12.

Weil MH, von Planta M, Rackow EC: Acute circulatory failure (shock). *In* Braunwald E (ed): Heart Disease: A Textbook of Cardiovascular Medicine, 4th ed. Philadelphia, WB Saunders, 1992, pp 569–587.

Califf RM, Bengston JR: Cardiogenic shock. N Engl J Med 1994;330:1724–1730.

Nawas YN, Balk RA: General approach to shock. Clin Geriatr Med 1994;10:185–196.

Erstad BL: Oxygen transport goals in the resuscitation of critically ill patients. Ann Pharmacother 1994;28:1273–1284.

Procedure | **CARDIOPULMONARY RESUSCITATION (CPR)** | *Howard G. Dubin*

1. The chain of survival (early access, early CPR, early defibrillation, early care) should be initiated immediately for all patients in cardiopulmonary arrest.

2. The first step for the single rescuer coming upon an adult who is collapsed and/or unresponsive is to activate the emergency medical system (EMS). For pedi-atric emergencies, the first step is to access the patient and provide approximately 1 minute of rescue support before activating EMS.

3. The recommended sequence for adult CPR is *Airway*, *Breathing*, and *Circulation*.

Technique

1. The airway should be opened by head-tilt or jaw thrust maneuver.

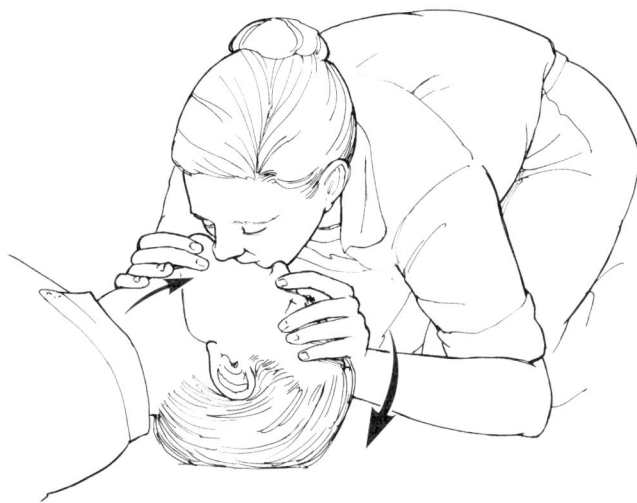

2. Ventilation time should be 1 to 2 seconds per breath. Most of the time should be spent in patient inspiration.

3. Proper hand placement is on the lower half of the sternum 2 finger breadths above the tip of the sternum. Recommended chest compression technique in an average-sized adult is to depress the chest 1½ to 2 inches, so that a carotid or femoral pulse can be palpated.

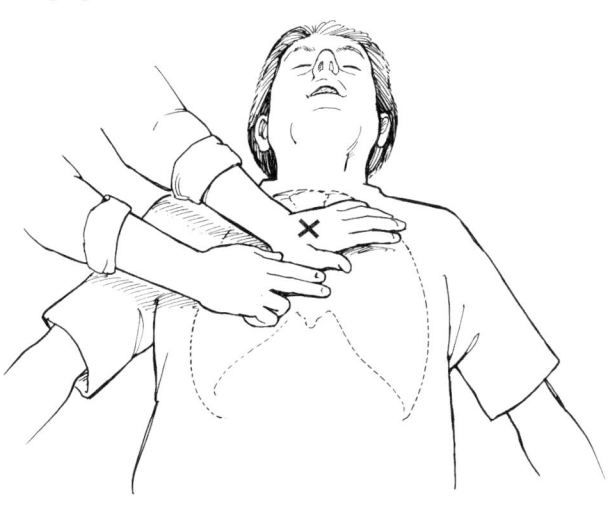

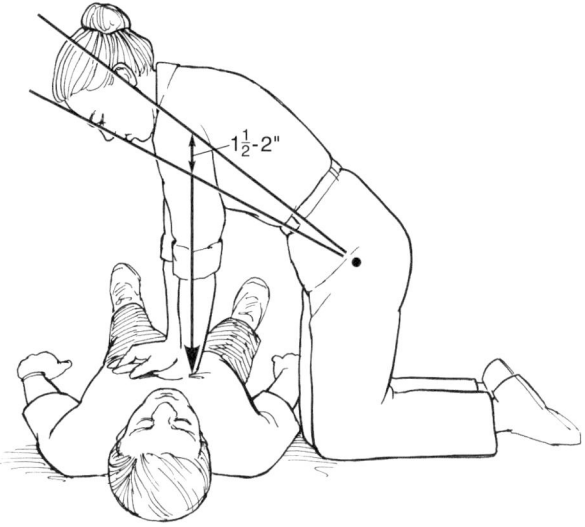

Single-Rescuer Technique
The recommended rate of chest compressions is 80 to 100 per minute, and the recommended ratio is 15 chest compressions: two breaths.

Two-Rescuer Technique
1. A second rescuer should activate the EMS system if this was not already done and perform one-rescuer CPR when the first rescuer becomes fatigued.

2. The chest compression rate for two-rescuer CPR is 80 to 100 per minute and the compression ratio for two-rescuer CPR is five chest compressions: one breath.

Alternative CPR Techniques
1. Interposed abdominal compression (IAC-CPR), active compression/decompression (ACD-CPR), and vest CPR are not recommended for routine clinical use at this time.

2. IAC-CPR remains controversial, and multiple studies show no significant outcome improvement over standard CPR technique.

3. ACD-CPR utilizes a suction cup technique to perform active compression and active decompressions according to American Heart Association standards. Early studies suggest improved cerebral, myocardial, and renal blood flow as compared with standard CPR techniques. Outcome data also suggest improvement in 24-hour survival in patients so treated. This technique may hold promise for improved perfusion during CPR as well as improved ventilation in nonintubated patients; further studies are in progress.

Foreign Body Airway Management

1. A Heimlich maneuver (abdominal thrust) should be used only if the rescuer suspects that foreign matter is obstructing the airway or if the victim does not respond appropriately to mouth-to-mouth ventilation.
2. A chest thrust is recommended for victims in advanced pregnancy or for those who are markedly obese.

Management of the Near-Drowning Victim

AHA recommendation is that an abdominal thrust should not be used routinely in victims of submersion. The standards and guidelines advise that the Heimlich maneuver be "performed on the near-drowning victim as described in the treatment of foreign body airway obstruction (unconscious, supine), except that in a near-drowning victim, the victim's head should be turned sideways." The victim's head is turned sideways to allow water forced from the lungs to flow out of the mouth. In contrast, when the Heimlich maneuver is used to treat a supine, choking person, the head must not be turned because twisting the throat may prevent expulsion of a solid foreign body.

Technique for the Heimlich Maneuver

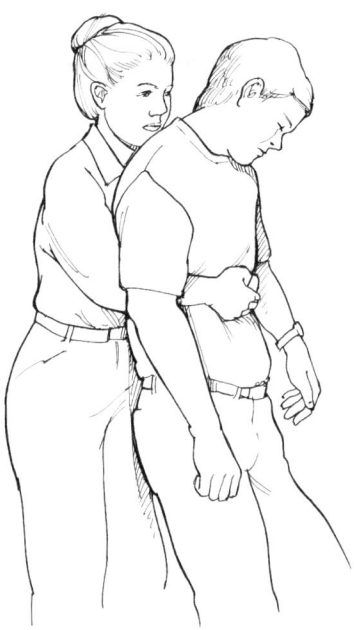

Situation 1: The victim is standing or sitting. Stand behind the victim and encircle his or her waist with your arms, place the thumb side of your fist above the navel but below the rib cage, and with the other hand over it, give a sharp upward thrust. If the obstructing object is not expelled, repeat the maneuver.

Situation 2: The victim is on the floor, unconscious. Roll the person on his or her back, face up, kneel astride the hips, place the heel of one hand between the navel and rib cage and with the other hand over it depress quickly with an upward thrust. Repeat the maneuver until the obstruction is expelled.

Situation 3: If the victim is an infant under 1 year of age, place the child face up on a firm surface, or sit the infant on your lap facing away from you. Position the index and middle fingers of both your hands just under the rib cage. Then with a quick but gentle motion apply an inward/upward thrust.

Situation 4: If the unconscious person is a near-drowning victim and the Heimlich maneuver is desired: Place the victim on his or her back, face to the side. While kneeling astride the hips place one hand atop the other over the victim's diaphragm. Push the heel of the bottom hand upward under the rib cage until all the water is expelled.

Risks

There is extremely low likelihood of disease transmission during CPR training and actual performance of mouth-to-mouth resuscitation. No cases of confirmed HIV transmission have been reported. Rare incidence of herpes transmission in the field has been reported. The emergence of multi-drug–resistant tuberculosis in some areas does raise concern.

It may be advantageous for rescuers involved in unsuccessful rescue attempts to participate in an incident stress debriefing, to discuss their thoughts and feelings about the team's performance.

After successful restoration of spontaneous circulation, the patient should be placed in the recovery position (if there is no suspected trauma) to minimize unrecognized airway obstruction. This consists of rolling the victim onto his or her side as a unit (without twisting).

 ## Bibliography

Babbs CF, Sack JB, Kern KB: Interposed abdominal compression as an adjunct to cardiopulmonary resuscitation. Am Heart J 1994;127:412–421.

Cohen TJ, Goldner BG, Maccaro PC, et al: A comparison of active compression-decompression cardiopulmonary resuscitation with standard cardiopulmonary resuscitation for cardiac arrests occurring in the hospital. N Engl J Med 1993;329:1918–1921.

Guidelines for cardiopulmonary resuscitation and emergency care. Emergency Cardiac Care Committee and Sub-Committee, American Heart Association, JAMA 1992;268:2171–2195.

Halperin HR, Tsitlik JE, Gelfand M, et al: A preliminary study of cardiopulmonary resuscitation by circumferential compression of the chest with use of a pneumatic vest. N Engl J Med 1993;329:762–768.

Tucker KJ, Savitt M, Idris A, Reldberg RF: Cardiopulmonary resuscitation. Arch Intern Med 1994;154:2141–2150.

Indications

To gain peripheral intravenous access for the infusion of fluids, blood, or medicine

Contraindications

Peripheral intravenous infusion cannot be used when hypertonic solutions such as total peripheral nutrition (TPN) are needed. This requires central venous access.

Preparation

1. All materials should be gathered and set up before beginning the procedure.
2. Gloves should always be worn when starting an intravenous infusion.

Equipment

1. Intravenous cannula (catheter over-the-needle type or a butterfly needle)
   a. 14 to 21 gauge common for adults
   b. 21 to 27 gauge common for infants and small children
2. Intravenous fluid
3. Intravenous tubing
4. Tape (pre-torn in the sizes needed)
5. Alcohol or povidone-iodine swab
6. Tourniquet (surgical Penrose tubing works well)
7. Latex gloves (nonsterile)

Extra Equipment for Infants and Children

8. Arm board (Tongue blades padded and taped together work well for infants.)
9. Clear intravenous site protector (*Tip:* The catheter package may be cut in half and placed over a successful intravenous site.)
10. Rubber band (cut) works as a tourniquet on infants.
11. Neonatal transilluminator (a high-intensity light that shines through the hands of infants) (optional)

Anesthesia (optional)

1% Lidocaine without epinephrine

Precautions

1. Intravenous cannulation should be avoided on an extremity with compromised circulation or lymph drainage such as an arm on the side on which a mastectomy has been performed.
2. An intravenous catheter should not be placed through an active infection in the skin or distal to a thrombosed vein.
3. Avoid using vessels over a joint.
4. Minimize the time the tourniquet is applied.
5. Take care not to cannulate arteries for intravenous infusions.
6. Take care not to secure intravenous tubing or arm board too tightly.

Technique

1. Locate a site:
   a. Usually the upper extremity is the site of choice. The forearm

or the dorsum of the hand

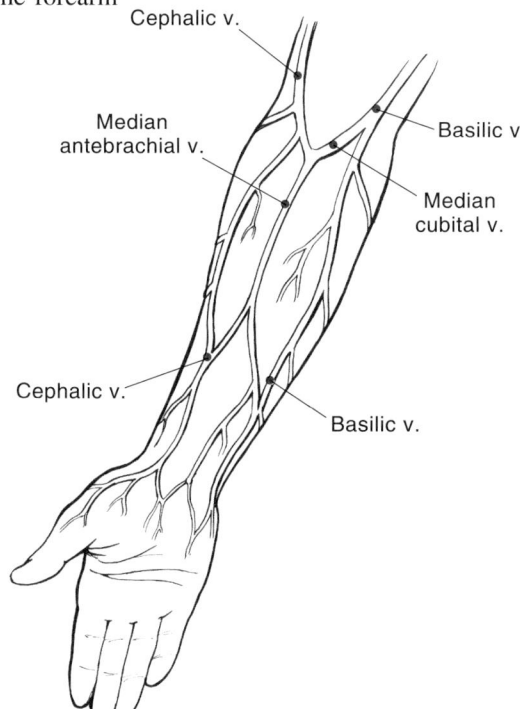

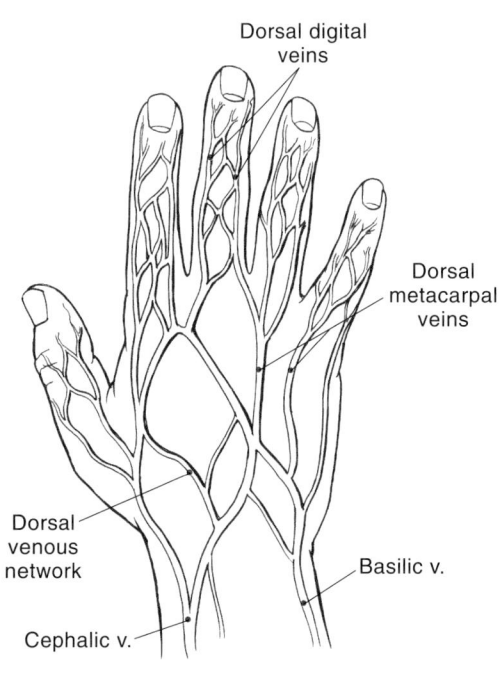

217

is commonly used. It is best to choose a distal site so that if the intravenous line infiltrates, it can be restarted more proximally.

b. In infants it is sometimes necessary to use scalp veins because they are large and easily accessible.

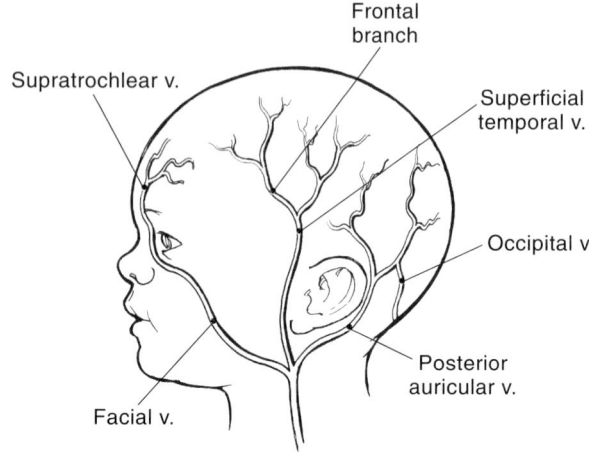

A patch of hair may need to be shaved to readily expose the veins.

WARNING

Avoid using the lower extremity in adults because there is an increased risk of thrombophlebitis.

---

2. Apply tourniquet: Firmly apply the tourniquet proximal to the chosen site of insertion. Be careful to not apply so tightly as to cut off arterial blood flow.

3. Clean site: Clean the insertion site with alcohol or povidone-iodine.

4. Anesthesia (optional): For large-bore intravenous catheters 14 to 18 gauge, you may wish to infuse a small amount of 1% lidocaine subdermally. Be careful not to infuse into a vein or infuse so much that it distorts the anatomy.

5. Insert:

   a. Stabilize the distal portion of the chosen vein with the thumb of your free hand while grasping the extremity.

   b. Insert the chosen over-the-needle catheter into the skin directly over the vein or just parallel to it with the bevel up at approximately a 30-degree angle to the skin for adults (approximately 20 degrees for infants).

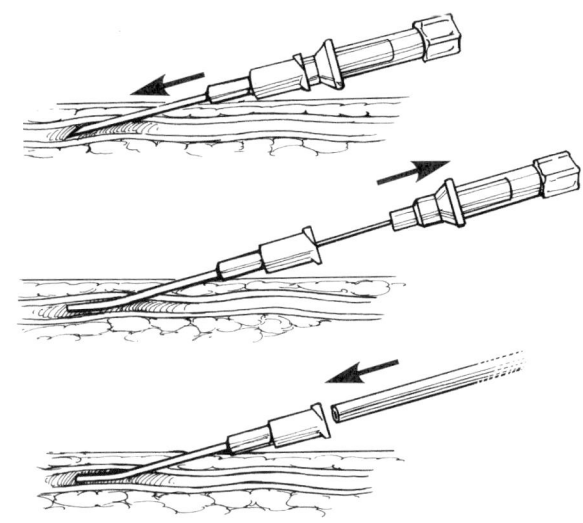

Then direct the tip of the needle into the vein until blood is seen in the flash chamber. Advance a few more millimeters to ensure that the catheter tip is completely in the lumen of the vein. *(Note: Penetration of the skin and vein is often carried out in two steps. Penetration of both in one motion seldom works except in large, stable veins.)*

   c. While stabilizing the needle, gently push the catheter over the needle into the vein.

   d. Remove the tourniquet and then remove the needle from the catheter.

WARNING

Never push the needle back into the catheter or pull the catheter back over the needle as this may shear off the catheter tip, causing a catheter embolism.

---

6. Connect tubing: After ensuring there is no air in the tubing, connect the intravenous tubing to the catheter hub. Allow the intravenous fluid to gently flow into the vein while observing the site for any induration that may indicate improper catheter placement.

7. Secure the site:

   a. Secure the catheter and intravenous tubing to the patient with the pre-torn tape. (Note: Never let go of a successful intravenous until it is secured in place.)

   b. With infants and children, consider utilizing a clear plastic site protector and an arm board.

Follow-Up

1. Check the site at least daily if not more often for induration, swelling, or signs of infection and to ensure that the line is functioning properly.

2. The intravenous site should be changed every 72 hours to lessen the risk of infection and formation of a thrombus. This can be extended to 96 hours with

close observation in those patients with difficult intravenous access.

Tips to Increase Your Success

1. Make yourself comfortable (sit if possible). This tip alone brings the most success.
2. Place the extremity in a dependent position below the level of the heart to increase vasodilation.
3. Warm the extremity with a heating pad or a warm moist towel.
4. Firmly stroke the vein. This causes vasodilation and is more comforting to the patient than slapping the vein.
5. Raise the patient's legs above the level of the heart to make more blood available to fill the veins in the arm.
6. Use the help of an assistant and/or the aid of a restraining device such as a papoose board for the child too young to cooperate.

Bibliography

Gomella LG, et al (eds): Procedures: Clinicians Pocket Reference, 5th ed. E Norwalk, CT, Appleton-Century-Crofts, 1986, pp 53–55.

MacDonald MG, Eichelberger MR: Peripheral Intravenous (PI) Line Placement. *In* Fletcher MA, MacDonald MG (eds): Atlas of Procedures in Neonatology. Philadelphia, JB Lippincott, 1983, pp 115–124.

Short BL, Avery GB: Venipuncture. *In* Fletcher MA, MacDonald MG (eds): Atlas of Procedures in Neonatology. Philadelphia, JB Lippincott, 1983, pp 58–62.

Simon RR, Brenner BE: Vascular procedures. *In* Simon RR, Brenner BE: Emergency Procedures and Techniques, 3rd ed. Baltimore, Williams & Wilkins, 1994, pp 380–384, 412–418.

Van Way CW, Buerk CA: Surgical Skills in Patient Care. St. Louis, CV Mosby, 1978, pp 85–91.

53 Hypertension

Carlos R. Herrera

Etiology

1. Hypertension occurs in 10 to 20 per cent of persons aged 25 to 45 years and 30 to 40 per cent of persons aged 55 to 74 years.
2. Risk factors include excessive dietary salt and calories consumed, and stress. It is more prevalent in African Americans, in those who are overweight, and in those who have a family history of hypertension.
3. The major system affecting blood pressure is the renin-angiotensin pathway. Renin, from the juxtaglomerular apparatus, leads to the formation of angiotensin I, which is converted in the lungs to a powerful vasoconstrictor, angiotensin II.
4. The leading pathophysiologic hypotheses are
   a. Stress and high sodium intake lead to high sympathetic activity and high renin/angiotensin, which lead to sodium reabsorption and elevated blood pressure.
   b. A primary membrane defect leads to raised intracellular calcium resulting in increased vascular tone and reactivity, then increased vascular resistance and elevated blood pressure; also, an inherited defect in sodium transport along with high sodium intake may trigger this pathway.

Symptoms

1. Patients are typically asymptomatic. They may have headaches, dizziness, vertigo, visual problems, malaise, chest pain, dyspnea, claudication, sweating, tremors.
2. Occasionally neurologic symptoms are seen: numbness or weakness of extremities, diplopia, eyelid weakness, decreased visual acuity, slurred speech, altered mental status.

Clinical Findings

1. *Retinal:* thickened arterial walls, compression of a vein where an artery crosses it, blurred disk margins, focal areas of white exudate
2. *Cardiac:* lateral displacement of point of maximal impulse, S_3, S_4
3. *Neurologic:* cranial nerve palsies, focal weakness or numbness, altered mental status
4. *Vascular:* decreased peripheral pulses; femoral, abdominal, or carotid bruits
5. *Secondary hypertension:* edema, striae, truncal obesity, hyperpigmentation, numbness of extremities, foot ulcers, muscle weakness, tachycardia

Laboratory Tests

1. *Blood pressure measurement:* The patient should be asked to return three to 5 times to verify measurements. For proper measurement, the patient should sit at rest for 5 minutes in a quiet room. The clothing should be removed from the arm and not bunched up along the deltoid. Use the proper-sized blood pressure cuff and bell of the stethoscope.
2. The basic workup is: electrolytes, blood urea nitrogen, creatinine, calcium, albumin, liver profile, cholesterol, urine analysis for leukocytes and protein, and electrocardiogram for left ventricular hypertrophy.
3. Patients with renal insufficiency, creatinine greater than 1.2 mg/dl, may warrant 24-hour urine collection for protein and creatinine, renal ultrasonography, renal nuclear scan, or captopril renin stimulation test (measure peripheral renin after oral captopril). In patients with progressively worsening renal function, renal arteriograms and renal vein renin determination may be necessary to document the need for renal artery angioplasty or surgery.
4. Other atypical presentations may be widely fluctuating blood pressure or electrolyte abnormalities, indications for a computerized tomography scan of the adrenal glands in search of pheochromocytoma or adrenal tumors respectively. Several 24-hour urine collections for catecholamine and metanephrines occasionally are helpful in detecting a pheochromocytoma. A dexamethasone suppression test may be indicated in a person with hypokalemia and striae to rule out Cushing's syndrome.
5. Ambulatory blood pressure monitoring is indicated when the patient has episodic, fluctuating blood pressures, difficult to control blood pressure, hypotensive symptoms with medications, or autonomic dysfunction.

 Key Test

- Blood pressure greater than 140/90 on three successive visits

Differential Diagnosis

1. *Temporary condition:* pain, anxiety, alcohol use, improper blood pressure measurement
2. *Renal hypertension:* nephrosclerosis, interstitial nephritis which can be caused by prolonged hypertension, medications, diabetes, collagen vascular disease, infection, or ischemia (Chapters 129 and 130)
3. *Renovascular disease* such as fibromuscular dysplasia and atherosclerotic plaque obstruction
4. *Endocrine hypertension* includes many conditions, but the most common are aldosteronism, Cushing's

disease, pheochromocytoma, and oral contraceptive use (see Part 10, Metabolic and Endocrine Diseases).

Treatment

Medication

1. Consider history of medication intolerance and cost of medications. Least costly medications: diuretics, verapamil. Short-acting verapamil can be given twice daily in the elderly.

2. *First-line agent:* diuretic, angiotensin-converting enzyme inhibitor, or calcium channel blocker. If hypertension not controlled on a first-line medication, then maximize dose; if still not controlled, then switch to another agent. If continued poor control, then add another first-line agent. In asymptomatic patients allow 2 to 4 weeks between dose changes or switches for complete efficacy.

   a. *Diuretics:* hydrochlorothiazide, 12.5 to 50 mg by mouth daily; chlorthalidone, 12.5 to 50 mg by mouth daily; chlorothiazide, 125 to 500 mg by mouth daily (higher doses of these three diuretics may frequently cause hypokalemia and hyponatremia); or indapamide, 2.5 to 5 mg by mouth daily. (These are frequently combined with potassium-sparing diuretics such as spironolactone.) Diuretics are preferred in the elderly. *Adverse effects:* hypokalemia, dehydration, hyperlipidemia.

   b. *ACE inhibitors:* enalapril, 2.5 to 20 mg by mouth twice a day; lisinopril, 5 to 40 mg by mouth daily; fosinopril, 10 to 40 mg by mouth daily. ACE inhibitors are preferred in diabetic patients. *Adverse effects:* hyperkalemia, facial swelling, cough, reversible renal failure.

   c. *Calcium channel blockers:* nifedipine XL, 30 to 120 mg/day by mouth; diltiazem CD, 180 to 360 mg/day by mouth; verapamil SR, 120 to 480 mg/day by mouth; amlodipine, 2.5 to 10 mg/day by mouth; felodipine, 5 to 20 mg/day by mouth. *Adverse effects:* bradycardia, pedal edema, cardiac failure with verapamil, tachycardia, orthostatic hypotension, constipation.

3. *Second line:* β-blockers, clonidine, doxazosin, terazosin, and methyldopa.

4. *Acute treatment:* nifedipine, 10 mg short-acting, swallowed whole every hour; captopril, 10 mg by mouth every hour; or clonidine, 0.1 mg by mouth every hour. Intravenous therapy is rarely needed.

WARNING

Be careful! Do not lower blood pressure rapidly below 140/80!

Diet

Patients should eat less salt, cholesterol, and calories. The amount of meat on the plate should be about the size of a deck of cards and the rest of the plate vegetables and starch. Insist on multiple visits with nutritionist.

Activity

Daily exercise helps with weight loss, reduces stress, and improves cardiovascular performance. Walking, stretching while sitting, and water aerobics are good ways to start sedentary patients on an exercise program.

Patient Education

Hypertension can be prevented. Once present it is a lifelong battle with diet, exercise, and medications. Small, long-term dietary changes are preferable. Crash or fad diets are dangerous. Blood pressure should be monitored at home or by visits to the local pharmacy.

Avoid wide fluctuation of blood pressure. This may cause an acute stroke or medication intolerance owing to dizziness, palpitations, and pain.

 Key Treatment

- First-line agent: diuretic, angiotensin-converting enzyme (ACE) inhibitor, or calcium channel blocker

Follow-Up

1. The goal of therapy is to reduce pressure below 140/90 without adverse effects.

2. If blood pressure above 140/90 and below 160/100, institute behavioral therapy (low salt diet, exercise, weight reduction) and check blood pressure every two months.

3. If blood pressure is above 160/100 and below 180/110, follow every 2 weeks until controlled; more frequent follow-up if renal damage is progressing. If cardiac ischemia or neurologic phenomena occur, then hospitalize.

4. If blood pressure is above 180/110, follow weekly; if above 210/120, hospitalize.

Bibliography

Black HR: Treatment of mild hypertension. The more things change . . . JAMA 1993;270:6:757–759.

Joint National Committee on Detection, Evaluation, and Treatment of High Blood Pressure: The fifth report of the Joint National Committee on detection, evaluation, and treatment of high blood pressure (JNC V). Arch Intern Med 1993;153:154–183.

Kaplan NM: Clinical Hypertension. 5th ed. Baltimore, Williams & Wilkins, 1990.

Mulrow CD, Cornell JA, Herrera CR, Kadri A, Farnett L, Aguilar C: Hypertension in the elderly: Implications and generalizability of randomized trials. JAMA 1994;272:1932–1938.

Rimmer JM, Gennari FJ: Atherosclerotic renovascular disease and progressive renal failure. Ann Intern Med 1993;118:712–719.

54 Hyperlipidemia

David Dovnarsky

Etiology

1. Primary hyperlipidemia
   a. Genetic disorders of lipoprotein metabolism
2. Secondary hyperlipidemia
   a. Excess dietary intake of fat, calories, or alcohol
   b. Concurrent illnesses
   c. Medications

Symptoms

1. No symptoms until significant atherosclerosis has developed late in course of disease, and then may include
   a. Angina
   b. Claudication
   c. Amaurosis fugax, weakness, or numbness (symptoms of transient ischemic attack or stroke)
2. Extreme elevations of triglycerides (>1000 mg per dl) may cause abdominal pain due to pancreatitis.

Clinical Findings

Xanthomas may be present on extensor tendons and xanthelasmas present periorbitally in familial cases.

Laboratory Tests

1. Lipid profile (total cholesterol [T-chol], high-density lipoprotein [HDL], estimated low-density lipoprotein [LDL], and triglycerides [TG]) or random cholesterol may be used for screening.
   a. Screening is recommended every five years in all adults.
   b. Screening is controversial in children.
2. If initial test abnormal, lipid profile recommended and at least two readings averaged to make treatment decision.

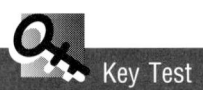

Key Test

Lipid profile

Differential Diagnosis

Secondary causes of hyperlipidemia should be screened for and treated. These include

1. Obesity
2. Hypothyroidism
3. Diabetes mellitus
4. Nephrotic syndrome or uremia
5. Drugs
   a. Corticosteroids
   b. Diuretics
   c. β blockers
   d. Oral contraceptives
   e. Alcohol

Treatment

1. Goals for cholesterol levels are noted in Table 54–1. Goals for LDL cholesterol (Table 54–2) are set on the basis of the presence of other risk factors for coronary heart disease (CHD) (Table 54–3) in combination with the LDL.
2. Classification of triglyceride levels is: <250 mg/dl, normal; 250 to 500 mg/dl, borderline; >500 mg/dl, high.

Treatment of hypertriglyceridemia is more controversial. Medication may be considered if diet and exercise fail and levels remain greater than 500 mg/dl. Medication is strongly recommended for levels over 1000 mg/dl to prevent pancreatitis.

Diet

Diet is the mainstay of therapy and should be used initially in all cases.

1. A step 1 diet (total fat ≤30 per cent of total calories, <300 mg cholesterol, 8 to 10 per cent saturated fat) should be tried for three to six months.
2. If target not reached, consider step II diet (consult dietitian) or medication.

Activity

Exercise program should be recommended routinely unless contraindicated, minimum recommendations of 20 to 30 minutes of aerobic exercise three times a week. Exercise has been shown to reduce triglycerides and increase HDL cholesterol.

Key Treatment

- Diet
- Exercise

TABLE 54–1. INITIAL CLASSIFICATION BASED ON TOTAL CHOLESTEROL AND HDL CHOLESTEROL LEVELS

Cholesterol Level	Initial Classification
Total Cholesterol	
<200 mg/dl (5.2 mmol/L)	Desirable blood cholesterol
200–239 mg/dl (5.2–6.2 mmol/L)	Borderline–high blood cholesterol
≥240 mg/dl (6.2 mmol/L)	High blood cholesterol
HDL Cholesterol	
<35 mg/dl (0.9 mmol/L)	Low HDL cholesterol

TABLE 54–2. TREATMENT DECISIONS BASED ON LDL CHOLESTEROL LEVEL

PATIENT CATEGORY	INITIATION LEVEL	LDL GOAL
Dietary Therapy		
Without CHD and with fewer than two risk factors (see Table 54–3)	≤160 mg/dl (4.1 mmol/L)	<160 mg/dl (4.1 mmol/L)
Without CHD and with two or more risk factors	≥130 mg/dl (3.4 mmol/L)	<130 mg/dl (3.4 mmol/L)
With CHD	>100 mg/dl (2.6 mmol/L)	≤100 mg/dl (2.6 mmol/L)
Drug Treatment		
Without CHD and with fewer than two risk factors	≥190 mg/dl (4.9 mmol/L)	<160 mg/dl (4.1 mmol/L)
Without CHD and with two or more risk factors	≥160 mg/dl (4.1 mmol/L)	<130 mg/dl (3.4 mmol/L)
With CHD	≥130 mg/dl (3.4 mmol/L)	≤100 mg/dl (2.6 mmol/L)

TABLE 54–3. RISK STATUS BASED ON PRESENCE OF CHD RISK FACTORS OTHER THAN LOW-DENSITY LIPOPROTEIN CHOLESTEROL

Positive Risk Factors

Age, years
  Male ≥45
  Female ≥55 or premature menopause without estrogen replacement therapy
Family history of premature CHD (definite myocardial infarction or sudden death before 55 years of age in father or other male first-degree relative, or before 65 years of age in mother or other female first-degree relative)
Current cigarette smoking
Hypertension (blood pressure ≥140/90 mm Hg confirmed by measurements on several occasions or taking antihypertensive medication)
Low HDL cholesterol (<35 mg/dl confirmed by measurements on several occasions [0.9 mmol/L])
Diabetes mellitus

Negative Risk Factors

High HDL cholesterol (≥60 mg/dl [1.6 mmol/L])

Medication

A. Drugs of choice
  1. Bile acid sequestrants e.g., cholestyramine (Questran), 4 g 1–3 doses twice daily (decreases LDL cholesterol). Gastrointestinal (GI) side effects may limit use; may increase triglycerides.
  2. Niacin e.g., nicotinic acid 1–3 g t.i.d.—start with 100 mg t.i.d. (decreases total cholesterol, decreases LDL, decreases TG, increases HDL). Side effects include flushing and GI distress. Dose should be increased gradually. Aspirin taken before dose may reduce side effects. Follow liver function tests.

B. Alternative drugs
  1. HMG Co-A reductase inhibitors e.g., lovastatin (Mevacor) 20–80 mg/day (decreases total cholesterol, decreases LDL). Are generally well tolerated. Follow liver function tests, and if greater than three times normal, discontinue drug (1 to 2 per cent).
  2. Fibric acid derivatives e.g., gemfibrozil (Lopid) 600 mg b.i.d. (decreases TG, increases HDL, decreases LDL)

  3. Probucol (Lorelco) 500 mg b.i.d. (decreases T-chol, decreases LDL, decreases HDL). May prolong QT interval.
  4. Estrogen replacement therapy e.g., conjugated estrogen (Premarin) 0.625 mg daily (decreases LDL, increases HDL, increases TG) should be considered in postmenopausal women.
  5. Combinations of medications may be used for resistant cases.

Patient Education

1. Explain link between hyperlipidemia and atherosclerosis.
2. Make patient aware of asymptomatic nature of condition until disease has progressed.
3. Stress compliance with diet, exercise, and medication (if used).
4. Discuss concomitant CHD risk factor reduction (smoking cessation, control of diabetes and hypertension).

Follow-Up

1. If screening test is normal, rescreen in five years.
2. If treatment initiated, follow cholesterol or lipid profile every three to six months based on results and particular regimen used.
3. Monitor compliance with diet and medication because this is often key to successful treatment.

 ## Bibliography

Choice of Cholesterol-Lowering Drugs. The Medical Letter 1993;35(891):19–22.

The Expert Panel: Report of the National Cholesterol Education Program expert panel on detection, evaluation and treatment of high blood cholesterol in adults. Arch Intern Med 1988; 148:36–69.

Expert Panel on Detection, Evaluation and Treatment of High Blood Cholesterol in Adults: Summary of the second report of the National Cholesterol Education Program (NCEP) expert panel on detection, evaluation and treatment of high blood cholesterol in adults (Adult Treatment Panel II). JAMA 1993; 269:3015–3023.

McBride PE, Underbakke G: Dyslipidemias. In Taylor RB (ed): Family Medicine; Principles and Practice, 4th ed. New York, Springer-Verlag, 1994, pp 956–963.

NIH Consensus Development Panel on Triglyceride, High-Density Lipoprotein, and Coronary Heart Disease: Triglyceride, high-density lipoprotein, and coronary heart disease. JAMA 1993;269:505–510.

55 Exercise Prescribing

Jane E. Corboy

Definitions

1. Fitness: a general term describing a level of cardio-vascular function that results in increased energy reserves for optimum performance and well-being
2. Endurance: the ability to work for long periods of time and resist fatigue
   a. Muscular endurance—endurance of specific muscle group
   b. Cardiovascular endurance—total body endurance
3. VO_2 max (maximum aerobic power): the capacity of the oxygen transport system
   a. Other terms include maximum oxygen uptake, cardiovascular endurance capacity, aerobic capacity
   b. Mathematical definition of VO_2 maximum is

   Cardiac output $\times$ A-VO_2 difference
   or
   (HR $\times$ SV) $\times$ A-VO_2 difference
4. Conditioning: an increase in energy capacity through exercise which produces adaptation of the cardiovascular system and muscle

Benefits of Exercise (Indications)

1. Cardiovascular effects
   a. Myocardial
      (1) Increased stroke volume and cardiac output
      (2) Decreased myocardial oxygen demand at rest
      (3) Increased tolerance for given workload
   b. Peripheral vascular
      (1) Increased capillary flow
      (2) Decreased peripheral vascular resistance
      (3) Decreased resting blood pressure
   c. Oxygen-carrying capacity
      (1) Increased blood volume and hemoglobin
      (2) Enhanced muscle extraction of oxygen
2. Musculoskeletal effects
   a. Muscle-tendon unit
      (1) Increased blood flow to muscle
      (2) Increased muscle strength
      (3) Increased tolerance for a given workload
   b. Bones and joints
      (1) Increased bone mass with weight-bearing exercise
      (2) Increased blood flow to synovium
3. Metabolic/endocrine effects
   a. Glucose metabolism
      (1) Increased muscle utilization of glucose (non–insulin-dependent transport)
      (2) Decreased blood glucose levels
   b. Lipid metabolism
      (1) Increased utilization of triglycerides
      (2) Increased levels of HDL cholesterol
      (3) Lowered levels of total cholesterol
      (4) Improved overall lipid profile
4. Obstetric-gynecologic effects
   a. Labor and delivery
      (1) Improved tolerance of labor
      (2) Shortened first and second stages of labor
   b. Gynecologic effects–lessened dysmenorrhea
5. Psychological effects
   a. Improved sense of well-being
   b. Stress reduction

Risks of Exercise

1. Cardiovascular risks
   a. Patients with ischemic heart disease
      (1) Precipitation of angina or prolonged ischemia
      (2) Precipitation of arrhythmia
   b. Patients with structural heart disease
      (1) IHSS—sudden death due to arrhythmia
      (2) Marfan's syndrome—aortic dissection
2. Musculoskeletal risks
   a. Acute effects
      (1) Muscle soreness
      (2) Traumatic injury—sprains, contusions
   b. Chronic effects—overuse injuries
3. Endocrine and metabolic risks
   Patients with *uncontrolled* conditions such as diabetes and thyroid disease may have worsened control due to increased autonomic activity with exercise.
4. Obstetric-gynecologic risks
   a. Obstetric
      (1) Decreased exercise tolerance with advanced pregnancy
      (2) Decreased uterine blood flow during exercise
      (3) Thermal stress on fetal development
      (4) Uterine contractions after exercise—may increase risk of premature labor
      (5) Risks to fetus with high-intensity exercises
   b. Gynecologic: amenorrhea
      (1) Occurs only with combination of intense exercise and weight loss (to below 10 per cent body fat)
      (2) May *increase* risk of osteoporosis/stress fractures

5. Psychologic risks
   a. Obsessive-compulsive disorder
   b. Anorexia equivalent

The Exercise Prescription (Technique)

1. Assess current fitness level
   a. History
   b. Physical examination
   c. Exercise testing: patients with more than two coronary risk factors or symptoms suggestive of cardiovascular disease, if planning vigorous exercise
2. Assess motivation for exercise
   a. Medical
   b. Social
   c. Psychological
3. Assess barriers to exercise
   a. Medical
      (1) Health conditions
      (2) Medications
   b. Social/work-related
   c. Concerns
4. Give prescription: be specific
   a. Mnemonic:
      (1) *Frequency*
      (2) *Intensity*
      (3) *Timing* (duration)
      (4) *Type* of exercise
      (5) *Energizing* (warm-up)
      (6) *Relaxing* (cool-down)
   b. Frequency: three to five days per week
   c. Intensity
      (1) 50 to 85 per cent of maximum heart rate reserve
      (2) Calculation of target heart rate range
         (a) Method 1:
(220 − age) × 50%
(220 − age) × 85% = target HR Range
         (b) Method 2:
(220 − age − resting HR) × 50% + resting HR
(220 − age − resting HR) × 85% + resting HR
Method 2 gives a narrower range and is better for patients with higher fitness levels. For methods 1 and 2, count pulse for six seconds and multiply by 10.
         (c) Method 3: rating of perceived exertion (Table 55–1) (Best for patients who are familiar with the feeling of appropriate intensity of exercise.)
   d. Duration: 15 to 60 minutes
      (1) The aerobic portion should be at least 15 minutes.
      (2) The lower the intensity, the longer the duration needed.
   e. Type of exercise

TABLE 55–1. RATING OF PERCEIVED EXERTION SCALE

3.	Extremely light	
5.	Very light	
7.	Light	
9.	Rather light	
11.	Neither light nor hard	
13.	Rather hard	"Conversational pace"
15.	Hard	
17.	Very hard	Target heart rate zone
19.	Extremely hard	

Use of the scale: The exercise level associated with the "rather hard" to "very hard" rating of exertion generally correlates with the target heart rate zone. This range is also the pace at which most people can carry on a conversation with moderate breathlessness.

      (1) Goal—increased cardiovascular endurance: *aerobic exercise*
         (a) Uses large muscle groups in continuous rhythmic manner
         (b) Examples: walking, jogging, bicycling (stationary or regular), swimming, aerobic dance, cross-country skiing, rowing, rope-jumping
      (2) Goal—increased flexibility: *stretching*
         (a) Sustained static stretches, no bouncing
         (b) Major target areas are hamstrings, quadriceps, calves, and low back
      (3) Goal—increased muscle strength: *resistance training*
         (a) High tension, low repetition
         (b) May create anaerobic environment; avoid Valsalva maneuver
      (4) Goal—increased muscle endurance: *light weights or gravity*
         (a) Low tension, high repetition
         (b) "Sport-specific"
         (c) "Cross-training"—using different aerobic activities will increase endurance in different muscle groups
   f. Warm-up
      (1) 5 minutes of light exercise
      (2) 5 minutes of gentle stretching
   g. Cool-down
      Similar to warm-up activities, but increased stretching to decrease soreness later

Modifications for Particular Illnesses or Health Conditions (Precautions)

1. Cardiovascular disease
   a. Angina—stable: exercise at 5 to 10 beats under heart rate
      (1) "Ischemic threshold"
      (2) Use nitroglycerin
      (3) Supervised programs
   b. Hypertension: avoid isometric exercise; aerobic and low resistance exercise beneficial

c. Valvular disease: mild to moderate is permissible after valve repair or replacement; anticoagulants; no contact sports

d. Cardiac medications:

(1) β blockers—blunt HR response

(2) Diuretics may increase risk of dehydration, hypokalemia, and muscle cramps

e. Peripheral vascular disease: claudication limits exercise

(1) Exercise increases functional capacity

(2) Walk to onset of pain, rest, then resume

2. Pulmonary disease

a. COPD: Exercise improves functional capacity, mainly walking.

b. Exercise-induced asthma: worse with cold weather, dry air; may need to pretreat with cromolyn or β-adrenergic inhalers

3. Musculoskeletal disability

a. Arthritis—severe

(1) May prefer swimming, non–weight-bearing exercises

(2) Importance of stretching and range of motion exercises

b. Spinal cord injury: wheelchair sports, arm exercises have different cardiovascular response (lower muscular efficiency so higher oxygen consumption than with leg exercises)

4. Metabolic/endocrine

a. Diabetes

(1) Type 1: adjust insulin dose/exercise/medications to avoid hypoglycemia

(2) Type 2: chronic; be sure to emphasize foot care, no ballistic exercises with retinopathy

b. Obesity: Start with lower intensity to minimize musculoskeletal injuries

5. Pregnancy

a. Avoid exercise in patients with vaginal bleeding, history of premature delivery, incompetent cervix

b. Avoid supine position after 20th week of pregnancy

c. Avoid core temperature over 102° F (39° C) throughout pregnancy

 Bibliography

For more information on psychological effects of exercise, see

Anthony J: Psychological aspects of exercise. Clin Sports Med 1991;10(1):171–180.

For more information on exercise in pregnancy, see

Artal R: Exercise and pregnancy. Clin Sports Med 1992; 11(2):363–377.

For more information on exercise in hypertension, see

Gordon NF, Scott CB, et al: Exercise and mild essential hypertension: Recommendations for adults. Sports Med 1990; 10(6):390–404.

For more information on exercise prescription, see

Blair SN, Kohl HW, Gordon NF, Paffenbarger RS Jr: How much physical activity is good for health? Ann Rev Pub Health 1992;13:99–126.

Levine GN, Balady GJ: The benefits and risks of exercise training: The exercise prescription. Adv Intern Med 1993;38:57–79.

56 Angina

Osman Ahmed

Etiology

1. Definition: Angina is one of several clinical presentations of coronary artery disease. The hallmark of "typical" angina is exertional chest pain. Angina is often suspected in those with underlying risk factors for coronary artery disease (CAD) including: middle or old age, male, suggestive family history, smoking, diabetes, dyslipidemia, hypertension, sedentary lifestyle, and obesity. Controversy still persists whether personality type is an independent risk factor for CAD. There are four distinct types of angina: stable, unstable, Prinzmetal's, and angina equivalents. This chapter will address only medical management of angina pectoris in an ambulatory care setting.

2. Epidemiology: Coronary artery disease claims the lives of 500,000 Americans annually. The estimated prevalence of angina pectoris ranges between 5 and 7 per cent in individuals aged 44 to 75 years and increases with age. Menopausal women not receiving hormonal replacement therapy are also at increased risk of angina.

Symptoms

Chest pain is the cardinal symptom of angina. Anginal pain is retrosternal or substernal, dull, heavy, or crushing in nature, radiating to the jaw or left arm, associated with diaphoresis, nausea, or vomiting, and often relieved by rest or nitroglycerin. Note that many patients may have less typical symptoms and many others may be asymptomatic.

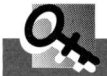

Key Symptom

- Chest pain

Clinical Findings

1. Physical examination findings are usually normal. The purpose of physical examination is to exclude other causes of chest pain.
2. S_4 gallop may be audible on auscultation.
3. Signs of congestive heart failure as S_3 gallop, jugular venous distention, and edema of the lower extremities may be present.

Diagnostic Tests

1. Electrocardiography (ECG): ECG may show changes (mainly nonspecific ST segment flattening or depression, or T wave inversion). However, normal ECG does not exclude angina.
2. Exercise tolerance testing (ETT): ETT is indicated to estimate severity of the disease and for risk stratification before referral to a specialist or for invasive testing. A positive test is characterized by a downsloping or horizontal ST segment depression of at least 1 mm for a duration of 80 msec (see the Procedure on Exercise Stress Testing). Useful diagnostic information can be obtained if chest pain occurs during ETT. Hypotension is a poor diagnostic sign indicative of ventricular failure. ETT has a sensitivity of 70 per cent and specificity of 85 per cent.

3. Dipyridamole stress test: The indications are the same as for ETT plus the presence of limiting factor to perform treadmill exercise (i.e., severe arthritis, morbid obesity, stroke, and peripheral arterial disease). The sensitivity and specificity are 80 to 90 per cent. Stress echocardiogram may demonstrate wall motion abnormalities.

4. Radionuclide scans: Thallium imaging is used instead of a standard 12-lead ECG to diagnose myocardial ischemia. The sensitivity and specificity may reach as high as 90 per cent. Multiple-gated acquisition scans are particularly useful in evaluating wall motion abnormalities and ejection fraction. Regional wall motion abnormalities and diminished ejection fraction are indicative of advanced CAD. Radionuclide scans are particularly valuable in women.

5. Coronary angiography: Cardiac catheterization is indicated in angina when there is high risk of noninvasive testing (ETT, or thallium stress test), unstable angina, or angina unresponsive to medical management. Angiography visualizes the extent, severity, and location of the disease. Prinzmetal's angina may be diagnosed if a spasm of coronary arteries is documented during the procedure.

Key Tests

- ETT
- Radionuclide scan
- Coronary angiography

Differential Diagnosis

1. Cardiac: Myocardial infarction, dissecting aortic aneurysm, pericarditis, and valvular diseases (particularly aortic stenosis and mitral valve prolapse)
2. Pulmonary: Pulmonary embolism, pleurisy, tracheobronchitis, and pneumonia
3. Gastrointestinal: cholecystitis, peptic ulcer disease, and hiatal hernia
4. Musculoskeletal: costochondritis, myalgia, and rib fracture
5. Neurologic: neuropathy and cervical disk disease

6. Psychogenic: anxiety, hyperventilation, and panic disorder

Treatment

Risk Factor Modification

1. Tobacco use: Smoking cessation reduces the risk of CAD by at least 50 per cent within 5 years of quitting.

2. Physical inactivity: Regular physical exercise significantly reduces the risk of CAD. Exercise increases high-density lipoprotein, lowers blood pressure, and improves glucose tolerance and myocardial efficiency.

3. Obesity: Maintenance of ideal body weight reduces the risk of CAD by 45 per cent. A low-calorie diet rich in fiber and low in fat combined with exercise should be recommended by primary care physicians.

4. Hypertension and diabetes: Control of hypertension and diabetes by weight management, daily exercise, and drug therapy may retard the progression of CAD.

5. Dietary interventions: Sodium restriction and, to a lesser extent, potassium supplementation may have a blood pressure–lowering effect. Antioxidants may be protective in angina and CAD and have been recommended in the following daily doses for patients with risk factors: vitamin E 100, 400 units; beta carotenes, 25 to 50 mg; and ascorbic acid, 500 to 1000 mg.

Medication

1. Aspirin: ASA in daily doses ranging from 75 to 325 mg is effective in secondary prevention of CAD in patients with angina. The use of aspirin in primary prevention of CAD is still debated. ASA inhibits platelet aggregation and lowers the risk of coronary events.

2. Nitrates: Nitrates reduce preload and afterload. They may also act by dilating the coronary arteries. Many preparations are commercially available. Sublingual nitrates are short acting with immediate effects (30 seconds) and peak action (2 minutes); dose is 0.15 to 0.6 mg on PRN basis. Lingual aerosol (Nitrolingual) may be used as 1 or 2 doses (0.4 mg/metered dose) sprayed on tongue on PRN basis. Transdermal preparations, 2.5 to 15 mg q 24 hr with variable release rates, are effective. Patients should observe a daily nitrate-free interval of 8 to 10 hours. Many oral sustained-release preparations (e.g., isosorbide mononitrate [ISMO]) are effective in preventing the acute episodes of angina.

Nitrates may cause headache, which often can be reduced by reducing the dose. Tolerance to these drugs may develop after repeated doses, particularly when no nitrate-free intervals are observed.

3. β-Adrenergic blockers: These are effective antianginal agents for decreasing heart rate, contractility, and overall myocardial work. β-blockers are likely to be useful in exercise-induced angina. Cardioselectives are preferable to nonselective blockers. Atenolol (Tenormin), 50 to 200 mg/day, or metoprolol (Lopressor), 50 to 100 mg/day, is more commonly used today than propranolol. Contraindications include asthma, symptomatic bradycardia, heart failure, and severe peripheral arterial disease.

4. Calcium channel blockers (CCBs): CCBs increase coronary perfusion and diminish afterload. Recommended daily doses are nifedipine (Procardia), 30 to 90 mg, diltiazem (Cardizem), 120 to 360 mg, and verapamil (Calan, Isoptin), 240 to 360 mg. Preference is based on side effects, drug interactions, and effects on coexisting disease. Dihydropyridines (nifedipine, felodipine [Plendil], nicardipine [Cardene], and isradipine [DynaCirc]) may cause headache, flushing, dependent peripheral edema, orthostasis, and tachycardia. Side effects of nondihydropyridines vary. Verapamil may produce AV conduction defects and constipation. Diltiazem may be associated with headache, dizziness, fatigue, and AV conduction defects.

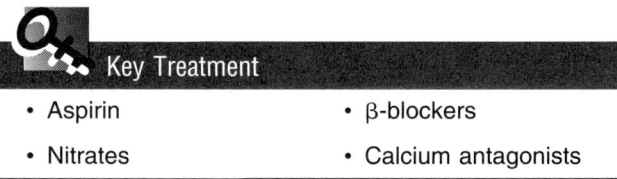

Key Treatment

- Aspirin
- Nitrates
- β-blockers
- Calcium antagonists

Bibliography

Fraser GE (ed): Preventive Cardiology. New York, Oxford University Press, 1986, pp 3–168.

Hurst JW: Recognition and treatment of four types of angina pectoris and angina equivalents. *In* Hurst JW, et al (eds): The Heart. 7th ed. vol 1. New York, McGraw-Hill, 1990, pp 1046–1052.

Manson JE, Tosteson H, Ridker PM, et al: The primary prevention of myocardial infarction. N Engl J Med 1992;326:1406–1416.

Simon BH: Patient-directed, nonprescription approaches to cardiovascular disease. Arch Intern Med 1994;154:2283–2296.

Procedure **EXERCISE STRESS TESTING**   *Reggie Lyell*

Indications

1. Assisting in the evaluation and diagnosis of chest pain
2. Screening for ischemic heart disease in asymptomatic men at risk
3. Evaluating dysrhythmias which may be exacerbated with stress
4. Determining exercise capacity and generating exercise programs
5. Establishing prognosis of patients with ischemic heart disease*
6. Evaluating antianginal or antihypertensive therapy*
7. Evaluating patients after myocardial infarction*

Contraindications

1. Evolving myocardial infarction, unstable angina, or uncontrolled heart failure
2. Uncontrolled hypertension
3. Cardiomyopathy, myocarditis, pericarditis, or suspected aortic aneurysm
4. Recent embolic phenomena (cerebral, pulmonary, or systemic)
5. Severe aortic stenosis or idiopathic hypertrophic subaortic stenosis

---

*These indications carry a higher risk, and consultation with a cardiologist should be considered.

6. Rapid dysrhythmias or conduction defects greater than first-degree heart block
7. Patient unwilling or unable to give informed consent

Preparation

1. Choose patients carefully. Thoroughly explain procedure, risks, and benefits.
2. Have informed consent document signed by patient.
3. Evaluate for signs of heart failure or pericarditis.
4. Determine predicted end point. This could be limited by symptoms or heart rate. Maximal (220 minus age) or submaximal (maximal × 85 per cent) heart rates can be used.

Equipment

1. Treadmill: Those with varying speeds and grade are preferred.
2. Monitor: Three-lead continuous monitoring preferred.
3. ECG machine: Twelve leads preferred.
4. Emergency resuscitation kit: Rapid access to advanced cardiac life support (including medications and defibrillation) is necessary.

Technique

1. Obtain pretest resting 12-lead ECG in both supine and standing positions, along with a baseline heart rate and blood pressure.
2. Demonstrate to the patient the method for starting the exercise test.
3. Have the patient begin exercising, increasing speed or grade of exercise (depending on protocol) at three-minute intervals.

4. During the last minute of each three-minute stage, record a 12-lead ECG, heart rate, and blood pressure. Likewise, ask the patient to rate his or her exertion on a scale of 0 to 10 (0 being no exertion and 10 being maximal exertion).
5. Stop the test for any of the following reasons
   a. Patient is unwilling or unable to continue (exhaustion, severe dyspnea, chest pain).
   b. Significant ST segment deviation (2 mm or more horizontal, downsloping, or delayed upsloping ST segment depression or ST segment elevation).

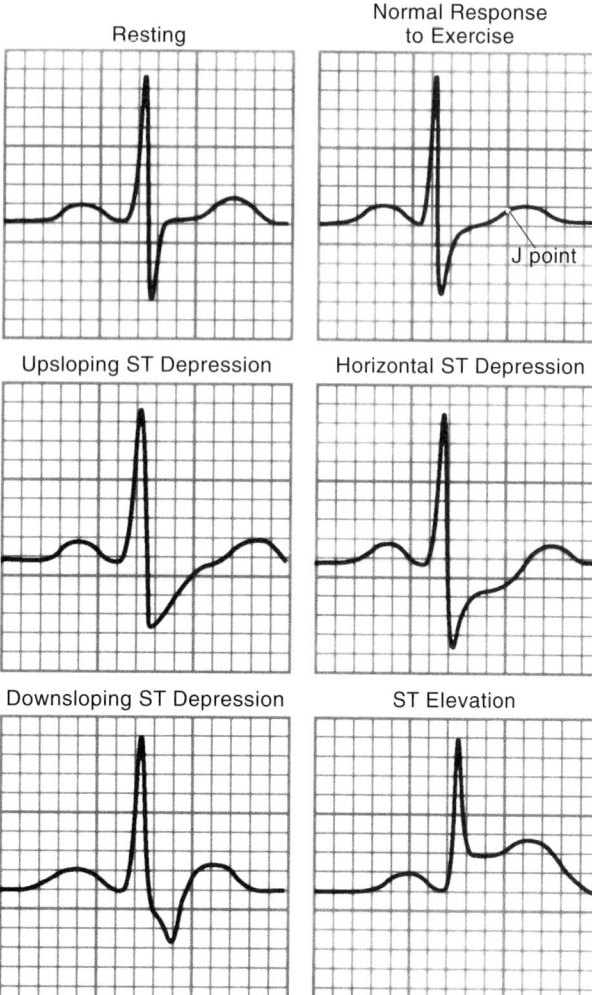

Resting

Normal Response to Exercise

J point

Upsloping ST Depression

Horizontal ST Depression

Downsloping ST Depression

ST Elevation

f. Development of acute chest pain

g. Significant hypertension (>240/110)

6. Record ECG, heart rate, and blood pressure immediately upon termination of test while standing or walking (slowing down).

7. Obtain ECG, heart rate, and blood pressure readings at 2, 5, and 10 minutes after termination of test.

8. Monitor patient until full recovery from any precipitated ischemia.

Follow-Up/Interpretation

1. Evaluate the entire test when reporting the results. Note the blood pressure and heart rate response, the amount of work performed in metabolic equivalents (METs), any dysrhythmias, any symptoms, and lastly the presence or absence of ECG changes.

2. ECG criteria suggestive of a positive test include

   a. Horizontal or downsloping ST depression >1 mm.

   b. J-point depression and upsloping ST depression that does not return to baseline within 80 msec

   c. Any J-point or ST elevation >1 mm

3. Note that the normal ECG response to exercise is a depressed J point with the ST segment returning to baseline within 80 msec. The baseline is considered to be the PQ junction, and the J point is considered the junction of the QRS complex and the ST segment.

4. Other criteria suggestive of ischemia include hypotension, frequent exercise-induced ectopy, or exercise-induced angina.

Bibliography

Chaitman B: Exercise stress testing. *In* Braunwald E (ed): Heart Disease: A Textbook of Cardiovascular Medicine. 4th ed. Philadelphia, WB Saunders, 1992, pp 161–179.

Evans CH, Karunaratne HB: Exercise stress testing for the family physician: Part I. Performing the test. Am Fam Phys 1992;45:121–132.

Evans CH, Karunaratne HB: Exercise stress testing for the family physician: Part II. Interpretation of results. Am Fam Phys 1992;45:679–688.

Marriott HJL: Coronary insufficiency. *In* Practical Electrocardiography. 8th ed. Baltimore, Williams & Wilkins, 1988, pp 455–464.

c. Appearance of bundle branch block or any exercise-induced heart block or dysrhythmia (including atrial fibrillation or flutter, ventricular tachycardia or fibrillation, second- or third-degree heart block)

d. VPCs induced or exacerbated by exercise (>25 per cent of beats)

e. Decreasing systolic blood pressure with increasing workload

57 Acute Myocardial Infarction

Douglas J. Pearce

Etiology

Myocardial oxygen supply is inadequate to meet demand.

1. Ninety-five per cent of myocardial infarctions (MI) result from coronary atherosclerosis with superimposed thrombosis and total, or near total, occlusion of an epicardial coronary artery.
2. Five per cent are the result of multiple less common causes including coronary artery spasm, nonatherosclerotic coronary artery disease (e.g., Kawasaki's disease, Takayasu's disease, polyarteritis nodosa), coronary artery emboli, congenital coronary artery anomalies, carbon monoxide poisoning, thyrotoxicosis, and severe aortic stenosis.

Symptoms

1. Pain
   a. Crushing substernal chest pain frequently radiates to the anterior chest, neck, and arms
   b. Less commonly, the pain may originate in or be confined to the epigastrium, neck, jaw, arm, wrist, or interscapular region
   c. Typically severe, lasts 30 minutes or longer, and is not relieved by rest or sublingual nitroglycerin.
   d. Frequently accompanied by diaphoresis and dyspnea.
2. Nausea and vomiting in 50 per cent of patients; occasionally diarrhea.
3. Less commonly, presenting symptoms may be limited to weakness, dizziness, or lethargy.
4. Twenty per cent of MI patients may have no identifiable symptoms at all (particularly in diabetics).

Key Symptoms

- Crushing substernal chest pain or pressure
- Diaphoresis
- Nausea and vomiting
- Dyspnea

Clinical Findings

1. General appearance
   a. Anxious, restless, diaphoretic
   b. Patient may clutch the chest over the sternum or describe pain using a clenched fist (Levine's sign) held against sternum.
   c. If cardiac output is compromised
      (1) Pallor
      (2) Acral cyanosis
      (3) Impaired mentation
   d. If pulmonary edema present
      (1) Dyspnea
      (2) Gasping respirations
      (3) Pink frothy sputum
2. Vital signs
   a. Heart rate may vary from profound bradycardia to tachycardia.
   b. Blood pressure is generally normotensive but may be hypotensive or hypertensive.
   c. Ventricular ectopy is common.
   d. Tachypnea is generally present.
3. Cardiovascular examination
   a. Jugular venous distention is unusual in the absence of right ventricular involvement.
   b. Palpation of the precordium
      (1) May be normal or silent
      (2) If a large area of dyskinetic myocardium is present, there may be a systolic bulge along the left sternal border.
      (3) Palpable S_4 is common.
   c. Auscultation
      (1) S_1 and S_2, usually soft
      (2) Loud S_4 frequently present
      (3) S_3 occasionally heard
      (4) A blowing murmur of mitral regurgitation, presumably secondary to papillary muscle dysfunction, may be heard.
      (5) Occasionally, a harsh holosystolic murmur heard throughout the precordium indicates papillary muscle rupture.
      (6) Less commonly, a similar harsh holosystolic murmur is secondary to septal perforation.
      (7) Pericardial friction rubs
         (a) May be heard as early as 24 hours, but most frequently at 48 to 72 hours
         (b) Generally thought to represent transmural infarction

Key Signs

• Diaphoresis	• Dyspnea
• Pallor	• Presence of an S_4
• Bradycardia or tachycardia	

231

(c) Frequently transient and intermittent

(d) May occasionally be heard for days

Laboratory Tests

1. Electrocardiogram (ECG)

   a. Myocardial infarctions are usually categorized as Q-wave (transmural) or non–Q wave (nontransmural) based on ECG.

   b. Patients ultimately developing Q waves usually have ST segment elevation during the initial hours of their infarction.

2. Enzymes

   a. Serial measurement of the MB isoenzyme of creatinine kinase (CK-MB) is the standard measured every eight hours for the first 24 hours. It will rise and fall over a 24- to 48-hour period. CK-MB subform ratios ($CK-MB_1$:$CK-MB_2$) are positive earlier than total CK-MB and may provide an earlier diagnosis.

   b. Lactic dehydrogenase (LDH)

      (1) The LDH generally peaks in 3 to 5 days and the LDH_1/LDH_2 ratio is greater than 1.0.

      (2) Routine measurement not needed but may be of value when CK-MB may have returned to normal due to late presentation.

   c. Troponin-T, an intracellular protein, equals CK-MB in sensitivity, is more specific for cardiac damage, and elevated levels may persist for 6 days postinfarction.

   d. Aspartate aminotransferase (AST) (SGOT): Although once used for diagnosis of acute MI, this enzyme is too nonspecific to be of value.

3. Radionuclide imaging studies

   a. Technetium-pyrophosphate scan

      (1) Occasionally, diagnosis of acute MI is difficult based on ECG and cardiac enzymes, as in a patient with a left bundle branch block on ECG who presents several days after onset of symptoms, at which time the enzymes may have returned to normal.

      (2) The technetium-pyrophosphate scan is most sensitive during the first 24 to 72 hours and is generally negative by 5 to 6 days after.

   b. Indium-labeled antimyosin FAB fragments

      (1) Imaging is performed about 24 hours after injection.

      (2) Increased sensitivity and specificity compared with technetium-pyrophosphate scanning

   c. Myocardial perfusion imaging: With thallium 201 or with the technetium-99m labeled agents sestamibi and teboroxime

4. Echocardiography: A two-dimensional echocardiogram obtained emergently at the bedside is useful for assessing regional and global ventricular function and can be particularly helpful in detecting wall motion abnormalities when ECG is nondiagnostic.

Key Tests

- Electrocardiogram
- Cardiac enzymes (CK-MB, LDH)
- Troponin-T
- Echocardiogram

Differential Diagnosis

1. Aortic dissection: Pain is severe, frequently described as tearing, is continuous, and often radiates to the back. Physical examination may reveal neurologic changes, absence of pulses in one or more extremities, and aortic insufficiency.

2. Acute pericarditis: Pain is generally sharp and associated with pleuritic features; may be preceded by a viral syndrome. Fever may be present. ECG typically shows diffuse ST elevation not corresponding to any particular vascular distribution.

3. Pleuritis: Pain is frequently sharp, exacerbated by inspiration, and positional in nature.

4. Pulmonary embolism: Pain is typically pleuritic; dyspnea is prominent.

5. Musculoskeletal pain: Pain is generally localized, stabbing, and reproduced by palpation or body motion.

6. Gastroesophageal disorders: Pain is typically exacerbated by lying supine and may be relieved by antacids. ECG should be normal.

7. If there is any doubt about the cause of the symptoms, the patient should be admitted for further observation.

WARNING

Acute MI can accompany aortic dissection secondary to the dissection extending into a coronary artery. Treatment is generally surgical, and great harm could be done by administering anticoagulant or thrombolytic agents.

Treatment

Medication

1. Aspirin (160 mg minimum) chewed and swallowed

2. Intravenous heparin

3. Nitrates

4. β blocker

5. Thrombolysis: Key in treating patients with acute cardiac ischemia is the presence or absence of ST elevation (or new left bundle branch block) on ECG. In the absence of ST elevation, or new left bundle

TABLE 57-1. SUGGESTED THROMBOLYTIC REGIMENS

Alteplase (tPA, Activase)
  Aspirin, 325 mg, chewed and swallowed
  Heparin, 5000 U IV, followed by constant infusion at 1000 U/hr*
  Alteplase 100 mg total
    15 mg IV bolus over 1–2 minutes
    0.75 mg/kg (maximum amount 50 mg) infused over first 30
    minutes
    0.50 mg/kg (maximum amount 35 mg) infused over subsequent 60
    minutes
Anistreplase (APSAC, Eminase)
  Aspirin, 325 mg, chewed and swallowed
  Anistreplase 30 U IV bolus over 2 to 5 minutes
Streptokinase (SK, Streptase)
  Aspirin, 325 mg, chewed and swallowed
  Streptokinase, 1,500,000 U IV, infused over 60 minutes
  Heparin, 5000 U IV, followed by constant infusion at 1000 U/hr
    —begin at completion of SK infusion*

*The activated partial thromboplastin time (APTT) should be checked every 6 hours and be maintained between 60 and 90 seconds.

branch block on ECG, management is the same as for unstable angina—aspirin, heparin, nitrates, and β blockers. Patients who present within 12 hours of the onset of symptoms consistent with MI and who have ST elevation or new left bundle branch block on ECG should generally receive reperfusion therapy: either thrombolytic therapy or angioplasty of the infarct-related artery. For maximal effect, reperfusion therapy must be initiated immediately. Therapy should *not* be delayed until transfer to another facility or the coronary care unit. Thrombolytic therapy may be administered as a tissue plasminogen activator (alteplase), streptokinase (SK), or anistreplase (APSAC) (Table 57–1). Absolute contraindications to thrombolytic therapy are

a. Active internal bleeding

b. Suspected aortic dissection

c. Prolonged or traumatic cardiopulmonary resuscitation

d. Recent head trauma or known intracranial neoplasm

e. Diabetic hemorrhagic retinopathy or other hemorrhagic ophthalmic conditions

f. Pregnancy

g. Previous allergic reaction to the thrombolytic agent

h. Blood pressure greater than 200/120 mm Hg

i. History of cerebral vascular accident known to be hemorrhagic

6. Angiotensin-converting enzyme (ACE) inhibitors, begun after the first 24 hours and in the absence of hypotension, decrease recurrent ischemic events and attenuate ventricular expansion.

7. Oxygen

8. Analgesia (morphine)

9. Sedation (benzodiazepines)

10. Bowel management to prevent constipation

11. Calcium channel blockers

    a. Diltiazem, Verapamil: In patients without heart failure, diltiazem and verapamil may reduce the incidence of reinfarction. Their use should be limited to patients intolerant of β blockers.

    b. Nifedipine

12. In patients with suspected right ventricular infarction, nitrates must be used with caution. Volume expansion, dobutamine, and atrioventricular sequential pacing may improve hemodynamics.

Diet

1. A light or liquid diet is given for the first 24 hours.

2. A low-cholesterol diet is generally indicated and a low-sodium diet if there is a history of hypertension or heart failure.

Activity

1. Without complications, patients require bed rest only for the first 24 to 36 hours, ambulating in the room by the third or fourth day. Activity can then slowly be increased, as appropriate for the specific patient, with resumption of normal activity at 6 weeks.

2. Isometric exercise should be avoided during initial convalescence.

Key Treatment	
• Aspirin	• Thrombolytic agent
• Intravenous heparin	• Primary angioplasty
• Nitrates	• Morphine
• β blockers	

Predischarge assessment

1. Coronary angiography—indications are

    a. Recurrent ischemic chest pain

    b. Heart failure

    c. Acute mitral regurgitation

    d. Ruptured intraventricular septum

    e. Shock

    f. Positive-graded exercise test

2. If coronary angiography is not done, there are several accepted strategies for noninvasive risk stratification. For example, in patients with an uncomplicated course, a *submaximal* graded exercise test may be done six to ten days following the MI. If positive, proceed to cardiac catheterization. If negative, the patient is discharged on medical therapy, and a *symptom-limited* exercise test, with thallium, is done at four to eight weeks. If negative, the patient remains on medical therapy. If positive, proceed to cardiac catheterization.

3. Ventricular function should be assessed by radionuclide ventriculography or echocardiography, unless previously assessed by another method.

Complications

1. Arrhythmias
2. Heart failure
3. Cardiogenic shock: mortality over 70 per cent. Current evidence suggests that *primary angioplasty* is the best method of reperfusion in cardiogenic shock. Digitalis in *not* generally beneficial acutely and may be harmful. Intra-aortic balloon pumping is frequently necessary and may be lifesaving.
4. Acute mitral regurgitation: Mitral regurgitation occurs in approximately 25 per cent of patients following acute myocardial infarction but is *rarely hemodynamically significant.*
5. Septal rupture
6. Cardiac rupture: Most commonly occurs one to four days postinfarction and is usually fatal.
7. Ventricular aneurysm: Following MI the ventricle may dilate with expansion of infarcted wall.
8. Postinfarction ischemia and infarct extension: Postinfarction ischemia occurs in 5 to 20 per cent of patients and results in a fourfold increase in mortality; it is an indication for early cardiac catheterization.
9. Thromboembolism: A frequent complication after large anterior MI. Prophylaxis is IV heparin followed by oral warfarin for 3 months.
10. Pericarditis: Common in patients with transmural infarctions and is generally seen *between days 2 and 4*; often confused with recurrent ischemia. Aspirin is the treatment of choice.
11. Dressler's syndrome: Thought to be an autoimmune phenomenon resulting in pleuropericarditis; usually seen *2 to 10 weeks* following infarction. The treatment is aspirin, and occasionally steroids.

Patient Education

1. Encourage patients to take an active role with respect to *lifestyle modification,* including a low-cholesterol prudent diet, smoking cessation, and weight loss.

2. Diabetes, hypertension, and dyslipidemia should be vigorously controlled.
3. Although the effect on mortality is debatable, cardiac *rehabilitation programs* may be beneficial in patient education and behavior modification.

Follow-Up

1. In the absence of contraindications, all patients should receive
   a. Daily aspirin (80 to 325 mg)
   b. β blocker for at least 2 years
2. There is increasing evidence that even in the absence of hypertension, treatment with an ACE inhibitor results in less ventricular enlargement and fewer recurrent ischemic events.
3. Patients with evidence of a left ventricular mural thrombus, severe heart failure, or history of thromboembolic phenomena should be discharged on Coumadin for at least 3 months. An international normalized ratio (INR) of 2.0 to 3.0 should be maintained.

Bibliography

For more information on acute myocardial infarction, see
ACC/AHA Task Force Report: Guidelines For The Early Management of Patients With Acute Myocardial Infarction. J Am Coll Cardiol 1990;16:249–292.
Harger JM, Kloner RA: Acute myocardial infarction. *In* Kloner RA (ed): The Guide to Cardiology. 2nd ed. New York, Le JACQ Communications, 1990, pp 207–239.
Pasternak RC, Braunwald E, Sobel BE: Acute myocardial infarction. *In* Braunwald E (ed): Heart Disease. 4th ed. Philadelphia, WB Saunders, 1992, pp 1200–1291.
For more information on the management of dyslipidemia, see
Summary of the Second Report of the National Cholesterol Education Program (NCEP) Expert Panel on Detection, Evaluation, and Treatment of High Blood Cholesterol in Adults (Adult Treatment Panel II). JAMA 1993;269:3015–3023.
For information on cardiac arrhythmias during acute myocardial infarction, see
Roelke M, Harthorne JW: Pacing for bradyarrhythmias: implantation, indications, and selection of pacing mode. *In* Podrid PJ, Kowey PR (eds): Cardiac Arrhythmia. Baltimore, Williams & Wilkins, 1995, pp 545–546.

58 Cardiac Arrest

Kenneth A. Ballew

Etiology

1. The incidence of sudden cardiac death in the United States is approximately 300,000 per year.
2. Coronary artery disease is the most common cause of sudden cardiac death. Cardiac arrest is the initial manifestation of coronary disease in 20 to 25 per cent of patients with coronary artery disease.
   a. Chronic ischemia with or without underlying myocardial scarring
   b. Acute myocardial infarction (MI): Only 20 per cent of out-of-hospital cardiac arrests are associated with acute MI.
   c. Congenital coronary artery anomalies
3. Left ventricular hypertrophy
4. Obstructive hypertrophic cardiomyopathy
5. Chronic congestive heart failure
6. Prolonged Q-T interval syndrome
   a. Congenital
   b. Drug-induced (antiarrhythmics, psychotropics)
7. Wolff-Parkinson-White syndrome
8. Toxic/metabolic/electrolyte disturbances
9. Proarrhythmic medications (encainide, flecainide)
10. Pulmonary embolism

Symptoms

Some patients may have prodromal symptoms such as chest pain, palpitations, dyspnea, fatigue, and lightheadedness up to several months prior to the onset of cardiac arrest.

Key Symptoms

- Chest pain
- Palpitations
- Dyspnea
- Fatigue
- Lightheadedness

Clinical Findings

1. Unresponsiveness
2. Pulselessness
3. Apnea or agonal respirations
4. Pallor or cyanosis

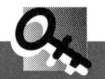

Key Signs

- Unresponsiveness
- No pulse
- Apnea or agonal respirations
- Pallor or cyanosis

Laboratory Tests

1. Electrocardiography. Findings include
   a. Ventricular fibrillation or ventricular tachycardia (VF/VT)
   b. Pulseless electrical activity (electromechanical dissociation)
   c. Asystole
2. Consider the following toxic, electrolyte, or metabolic disturbances as the cause of arrest
   a. Hypoxia
   b. Hypokalemia or hyperkalemia
   c. Hypomagnesemia
   c. Acidosis
   d. Drug overdose
   e. Proarrhythmic medications

Key Test

- Electrocardiography

Differential Diagnosis

1. Foreign body aspiration, "cafe coronary"
2. Vasovagal syncope
3. Seizure

Treatment

Basic Life Support

1. Assess responsiveness.
2. Activate emergency medical system.
3. Assess airway, breathing, and circulation. If airway obstruction is present, dislodge the object using the Heimlich maneuver (see Ch. 52).
4. If the patient is apneic and pulseless and does not have airway obstruction, initiate cardiopulmonary resuscitation.
5. Consider precordial thump if the arrest is witnessed, the patient is pulseless, and a defibrillator is not immediately available.
6. Begin advanced cardiac life support when the necessary equipment becomes available. Cardiac rhythm determines the treatment system that should be used.

Advanced Cardiac Life Support

1. Ventricular fibrillation and pulseless ventricular tachycardia (VF/VT)
   a. Immediate defibrillation prior to intubation or establishment of intravenous access is crucial to success. Defibrillation should begin using 200 joules and, if needed, repeated in rapid succession at 300 and 360 joules.

b. If the patient remains in VF/VT after three defibrillations, then intubate and place intravenous access.

c. Epinephrine 1:10,000, 1.0 mg intravenous push, repeat defibrillation at 360 joules. Repeat epinephrine followed by defibrillation every 3 to 5 minutes for continued VF/VT. If the initial dose of epinephrine does not convert VF/VT, give:

d. Lidocaine, 1.5 mg/kg intravenous push. After 30 to 60 seconds defibrillate at 360 joules. Repeat lidocaine and defibrillation after 3 to 5 minutes if unsuccessful. Once spontaneous circulation is restored, start a continuous infusion of lidocaine at 2 to 4 mg/min. If the patient remains in VF/VT, give:

e. Bretylium, 5 mg/kg intravenous push. After 1 to 2 minutes defibrillate at 360 joules. If the patient remains in VF/VT after 5 minutes, give bretylium, 10 mg/kg, and repeat defibrillation. Once spontaneous circulation is restored, bretylium can be given as a continuous infusion at 1 to 2 mg/min.

2. Pulseless electrical activity (electromechanical dissociation)

a. Intubate and obtain intravenous access.

b. Identify and treat underlying cause of arrest

(1) Hypovolemia

(2) Hypoxia

(3) Cardiac tamponade

(4) Tension pneumothorax

(5) Hypothermia

(6) Pulmonary embolism

(7) Drug overdose

(8) Hyperkalemia

(9) Acidosis

(10) Massive myocardial infarction

c. Epinephrine, 1.0 mg intravenous push

d. For bradycardia give atropine, 1.0 mg intravenous push.

3. Asystole

a. Intubate and obtain intravenous access.

b. Confirm asystole in more than one lead.

c. Consider possible causes

(1) Hypoxia

(2) Hyperkalemia or hypokalemia

(3) Acidosis

(4) Drug overdose

(5) Hypothermia

d. Epinephrine, 1.0 mg intravenous push, repeat every 3 to 5 minutes.

e. Atropine, 1.0 mg intravenous push, repeat after 5 minutes.

Key Treatment

- Basic life support
- Assess responsiveness
- Assess airway, breathing, circulation (A, B, C)
- Initiate CPR if patient is apneic, pulseless, and does not have airway obstruction
- Consider precordial thump if arrest is witnessed and patient is pulseless

Follow-Up

1. Initial management of cardiac arrest survivors includes stabilization of cardiac rhythm and hemodynamics. Provide supportive treatment of organ damage caused by cardiac arrest.

2. Further management is designed to prevent recurrence and depends on the underlying cause of the arrest.

3. For cardiac arrest unassociated with acute MI or other reversible causes

a. Evaluate coronary artery anatomy with cardiac catheterization.

b. Assess cardiac function with echocardiography.

c. Treat coronary artery disease.

(1) Aspirin

(2) β blocker and other antianginal therapy

(3) Percutaneous transluminal coronary angioplasty

(4) Coronary artery bypass graft surgery

d. Treat congestive heart failure with angiotensin-activating enzyme inhibitors.

e. Perform electrophysiologic testing.

(1) If the patient is found to have inducible VF/VT

(a) VF/VT suppressed with antiarrhythmic drugs. Treat with appropriate antiarrhythmic medications. Consider automatic implantable cardioverter defibrillator (AICD) placement, particularly if left ventricular function is reduced.

(b) VF/VT not suppressed with antiarrhythmic drugs. Place AICD, consider adding empiric amiodarone.

(2) If the patient has noninducible VF/VT

(a) If left ventricular function is abnormal, place AICD.

(b) If left ventricular function is normal, a subset of patients may merely require treatment of reversible causes of arrest, such as ischemia.

4. For cardiac arrest due to reversible causes
Generally, electrophysiologic testing and chronic an-

tiarrhythmic therapy are not required. Treat underlying cause of arrest.

a. Acute MI

b. Toxic/metabolic/electrolyte disturbances

c. Pulmonary embolism

Bibliography

For more information on the management of sudden cardiac death survivors, see

Akhtar M, Garan H, Lehmann MH, Troup PJ: Sudden cardiac death: Management of high-risk patients. Ann Intern Med 1991;114:499–512.

Pinski SL, Trohman RG: Implantable cardioverter-defibrillators: implications for the nonelectrophysiologist. Ann Intern Med 1995;122:770–777.

For more information on in-hospital cardiac arrest, see

Bedell SE, Delbanco TL, Cook EF, Epstein FH: Survival after cardiopulmonary resuscitation in the hospital. N Engl J Med 1983;309:569–576.

For more information on CPR and ACLS, see

Emergency Cardiac Care Committee and Subcommittees, American Heart Association: Essentials of ACLS. In Cummins R (ed): Textbook of Advanced Cardiac Life Support. Dallas, American Heart Association, 1994.

For more information on cardiac arrest, see

Myerburg RG, Castellanos A: Cardiac arrest and sudden cardiac death. In Braunwald E (ed): Heart Disease. A Textbook of Cardiovascular Diseases. 4th ed, vol 1. Philadelphia, WB Saunders, 1992; pp 756–789.

Indications

1. Termination of life-threatening ventricular arrhythmias
   a. Ventricular tachycardia
   b. Ventricular fibrillation
   c. Ventricular flutter
2. Termination of supraventricular tachyarrhythmias (with hemodynamic compromise)
3. Termination of refractory supraventricular tachycardia (such as atrial fibrillation)

Contraindication

The contraindication is termination of atrial fibrillation with severe digitalis toxicity. The toxicity should be alleviated before cardioversion/defibrillation.

Preparation

1. The defibrillator should be inspected regularly.
2. The defibrillator should be plugged into a standard electrical outlet that is appropriately grounded.
3. The electrocardiogram (ECG) should be monitored to determine the arrhythmia and to rule out artifact. Presence or absence of a palpable pulse and blood pressure should be confirmed.
4. For elective cardioversions, the electrolytes and hematologic laboratory values should be checked and should preferably be within normal limits.
5. Patients with an organized arrhythmia (such as ventricular tachycardia or ventricular flutter) or a more benign arrhythmia such as supraventricular tachycardia (atrial fibrillation) should receive defibrillation synchronized to the R wave of the QRS complex, which is known as cardioversion. These more organized arrhythmias require lower energies to convert as compared with the more disorganized arrhythmias such as ventricular fibrillation.
6. Defibrillation conducting gel should be available for use with paddles; skin patches suitable for defibrillation can be used as an alternative.

Equipment

1. Standard external defibrillator
2. Skin patches or defibrillator paddles
3. Conducting gel
4. ECG leads
5. Advanced cardiac life support equipment

Anesthesia

1. During hemodynamically significant arrhythmia (cardiac arrest), anesthesia is not necessary because the patient is unconscious.
2. During more stable arrhythmias, patients should be appropriately sedated with close monitoring of their oxygen saturation, respiratory rate, heart rate, and blood pressure. Anesthesia should be administered according to the recommendations of an anesthesiologist.

Precautions

1. Conducting gel and/or skin patches should be placed in discrete areas over the chest (not in continuity with one another). This is to prevent sparking between the cathode and anode.
2. The operator should avoid contact with the patient as well as touching a metal surface during defibrillation. The operator may shout "All clear" before defibrillation.
3. The defibrillator must be inspected regularly to make sure that it will function appropriately. The hospital's biomedical engineering service should be able to provide this function as a standard of care.

> **WARNING**
>
> **To perform defibrillation or cardioversion requires the delivery of high direct-current energy to the patient. It is essential that the operator or medical personnel not be in physical contact (other than through defibrillation paddles) with the patient or the electrical equipment during delivery of high voltage energy. The person performing defibrillation should make sure the paddles are well separated.**

Technique

1. The technique of external transthoracic cardioversion-defibrillation requires placement of either skin patches or defibrillation paddles in an anterior or posterior location. We routinely place the posterior skin patch between the two scapulae and the anterior patch over the left ventricular apex.

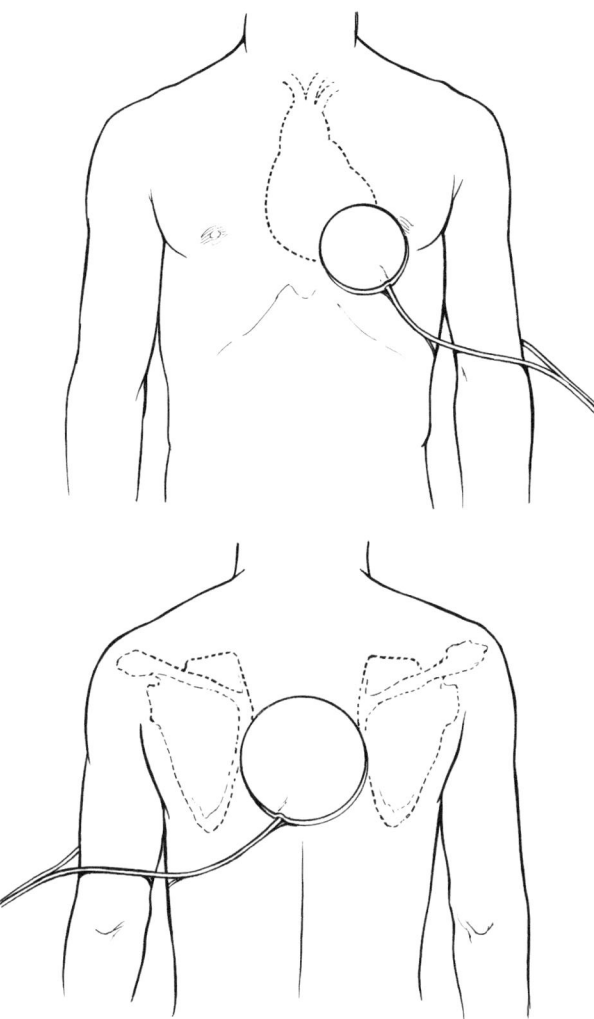

For cardioversion of atrial arrhythmias (including atrial fibrillation and atrial flutter) a more midline anterior and posterior patch placement is preferable. If one configuration fails multiple times, an alternative configuration can be utilized.

2. The defibrillator is turned on and the ECG is monitored.

3. The arrhythmia is verified perhaps by a true 12-lead ECG as well as hemodynamic data (i.e., pulse and blood pressure).

4. Before defibrillation or cardioversion, the defibrillator ECG strip should be pressed to record data, and the defibrillator should be charged to the appropriate energies.

5. Hemodynamically significant ventricular tachyarrhythmias require shocks of the order of 200, 300, and 360 joules as per advanced cardiac life support protocols. Termination of atrial fibrillation requires lower energy levels of the order of 100 joules initially. Atrial flutter may be terminated by as low as 25 joules. If unsuccessful, higher energies can be utilized.

6. The defibrillator capacitors are charged before delivery of direct current energy. This can be performed either via the paddles or via the defibrillator box itself. Once fully charged, the operator makes sure that all personnel move away from the patient and that all metal is removed from the area around the patient's bed. Defibrillation is then performed by pressing the button to discharge the capacitor.

This is to encompass as much of the myocardium as possible in order to perform a successful defibrillation. Alternatively, skin paddles can be placed over the anterior chest as well as lateral precordium.

7. After defibrillation, the ECG is then checked to determine whether there is termination of the arrhythmia as well as return of the vital signs (i.e., heart rate and blood pressure towards normal).

8. If unsuccessful, further delivery of direct energy can be performed according to advanced cardiac life support protocols.

9. If it is an elective and not an emergency case and there is hemodynamic stability, anesthesia should be used. This helps minimize the discomfort to the patient of the direct current shocks.

10. If the arrhythmia fails to be terminated by maximal energies (for treatment of refractory ventricular tachyarrhythmias), emergency rescue techniques should be considered. These techniques include emergency intracardiac defibrillation and transesophageal defibrillation. Both methods facilitate the delivery of high direct current energy in proximity to the myocardium using a standard defibrillator.

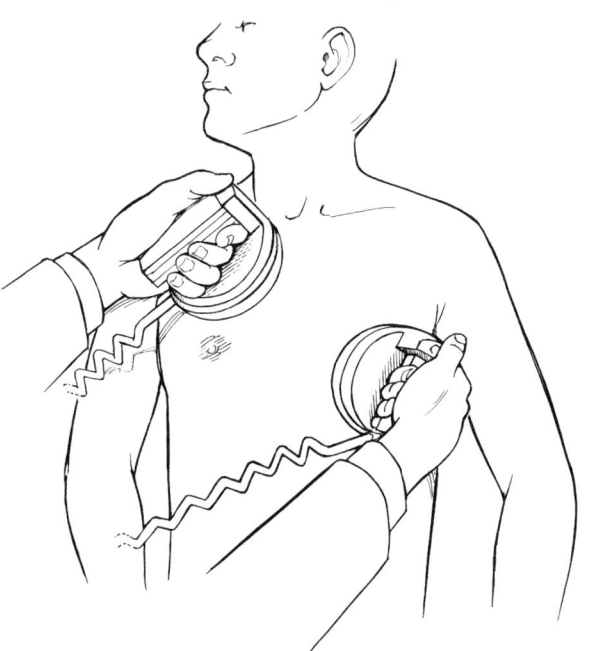

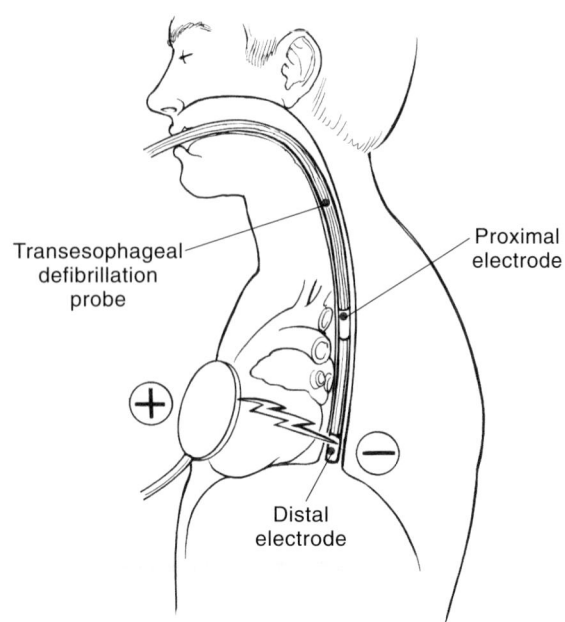

Transesophageal
defibrillation
probe

Proximal
electrode

Distal
electrode

Follow-Up

1. For all patients in the setting of significant ventricular tachyarrhythmias, critical care monitoring in an appropriate hospital facility is required. For more benign arrhythmia termination such as atrial fibrillation, atrial flutter, monitoring for at least a three-hour period by trained advanced cardiac life support nursing personnel is also prudent.

2. An appropriate 12-lead ECG should be obtained as well as follow-up by the patient's physician.

B | Bibliography

Cohen TJ: Cardiopulmonary Resuscitation. *In* American College of Chest Physicians Pulmonary and Critical Care Update Series. (Lesson 25). 1994;9:1–7.

Cohen TJ, Scheinman MM, Pullen BT, et al: Emergency intracardiac defibrillation for refractory ventricular fibrillation during routine electrophysiology study. J Am Coll Cardiol 1991; 18:1280–1284.

Cummins R (ed): Defibrillation. Advanced Cardiac Life Support. Dallas, American Heart Association, 1994, pp 4-1 to 4-22.

Eisenberg MS, Copass MD, Hallstrom AP, et al: Treatment of out-of-hospital cardiac arrests with rapid defibrillation by emergency medical technicians. N Engl J Med 1980; 302:1379–1383.

Weaver WD, Copass MK, Bufi D, et al: Improved neurologic recovery and survival after early defibrillation. Circulation 1984;69:943–948.

59 Acute Heart Failure

David E. Gutstein

Etiology

1. Definition: A sudden cardiac event with overwhelming effects on the heart's function. This results in an acute decline in cardiac output, insufficient perfusion, and acute pulmonary and systemic venous congestion.
2. Precipitating factors
   a. May arise from acute myocardial infarction, ischemia, acute mitral regurgitation or ventricular septal defect, aortic dissection causing acute aortic insufficiency, cardiac rupture, tamponade, arrhythmia, or pulmonary embolus
   b. Ischemia and infarction decrease cardiac output and compliance, resulting in increased left ventricular filling pressures and pulmonary edema, without changing total blood volume.

Symptoms

1. May develop over the course of several minutes or less, reflecting a sudden decompensation of pump function
2. The most profound symptom of acute heart failure is acute dyspnea, or sudden onset of respiratory distress.
3. May be accompanied by chest pain, palpitations, diaphoresis, and cough productive of frothy sputum

Key Symptoms

- Sudden, extreme dyspnea
- Pink, frothy sputum
- Diaphoresis

Clinical Findings

1. Patient appears grossly cyanotic, with cold and clammy skin.
2. Acute onset of hypertension and tachycardia
3. Jugular venous distention
4. New heart sounds, such as a third heart sound (S_3) or a new murmur
5. Pulmonary crackles or rhonchi. Presence of pulmonary wheezes is referred to as "cardiac asthma."
6. May rapidly progress to signs of respiratory failure and shock

Key Signs

- Tachycardia
- Cyanosis
- Jugular venous distention
- Third heart sound (S_3)
- Pulmonary rales

Diagnostic Tests

1. Hematocrit, blood urea nitrogen, and creatinine: to rule out anemia and renal failure as precipitating causes
2. Arterial blood gas and oxygen saturation: to quantitate extent of respiratory failure, assess oxygenation
3. Electrocardiogram: to evaluate for arrhythmia, ischemia, or infarction
4. Chest radiograph: Signs of heart failure include increased cardiothoracic ratio, vascular redistribution, interstitial pulmonary edema, and alveolar edema. Film may also reveal other sources of dyspnea (e.g., pneumonia, pneumothorax).
5. Echocardiogram: may reveal mitral regurgitation or ventricular septal defect in the patient with a new systolic murmur; shows focal wall motion abnormalities, significant pericardial effusion
6. Right-heart (Swan-Ganz) catheterization: to assess pulmonary artery pressures, rule out left-to-right shunt, quantitate response to therapy
7. Cardiac catheterization: evaluate coronary arteries

Key Tests

- Arterial blood gas
- Chest film
- Electrocardiography

Differential Diagnosis

Conditions that may imitate aspects of acute heart failure include reactive airway diseases (e.g., asthma, chronic obstructive pulmonary disease [COPD]), pneumonia, pneumothorax, re-expansion pulmonary edema, adult respiratory distress syndrome, high-altitude pulmonary edema, neurogenic pulmonary edema, pulmonary embolus, eclampsia, and heroin overdose.

Treatment

Medication

Treatment of "flash pulmonary edema" revolves around improving hemodynamics by reversing ischemia and reducing preload.

1. Supplemental oxygen: may require intubation for respiratory failure
2. Nitrates: nitroglycerin sublingual every five minutes × 3 initially; nitroglycerin ointment (Nitro-Bid or Nitrol ointment) 1 to 2 inches topically; or intravenous nitroglycerin drip starting at 20 μg/min. Hold for hypotension.

3. Morphine: reduces preload. Start with 2 mg IV; may repeat once or twice every few minutes. Hold for hypotension.

4. Diuretics: limited role in true ischemic flash pulmonary edema, but useful in acute-on-chronic exacerbations of heart failure. Furosemide (Lasix) may be used, starting at 20 mg intravenously. "Renal dose" dopamine (2 to 3 μg/kg/min) may improve diuresis in oliguric patients unresponsive to diuretics by dilating renal vascular beds. Hemodialysis or ultrafiltration may be needed to treat heart failure complicated by anuria.

5. Digoxin (Lanoxin): useful for slowing rapid atrial fibrillation in the setting of heart failure or shock

6. Pressors: for acute heart failure refractory to above measures. Adverse effects may include tachycardia, tachyarrhythmia and excessive vasoconstriction.

   a. Dopamine: indicated for acute heart failure with hypotension. "Beta-range" (5 to 10 μg/kg/min) has inotropic and chronotropic effects. "Alpha-range" (10 to 20 μg/kg/min) stimulates systemic vasoconstriction.

   b. Dobutamine (Dobutrex): used in refractory heart failure with poor cardiac output, but with systolic blood pressure exceeding 100. Increases contractility, decreases systemic vascular resistance. Start at 2 to 5 μg/kg/min.

   c. Norepinephrine: for heart failure with severe hypotension and normal or low systemic vascular resistance. Acts as a vasoconstrictor, positive inotrope and chronotrope. Start at 1 to 4 μg/min.

   d. Phosphodiesterase inhibitors (e.g., amrinone [Inocor], milrinone [Primacor]): effects similar to dobutamine. For milrinone, load 50 μg/kg, then maintain on 0.375 to 0.75 μg/kg/min.

7. Intra-aortic balloon pump and left ventricular assist device: indicated for cardiogenic shock refractory to inotropes. Useful for stabilizing patient before revascularization.

8. Revascularization: Thrombolysis is indicated for stabilizing heart failure in the setting of acute myocardial infarction. If unsuccessful, angioplasty or coronary artery bypass grafting may achieve revascularization.

Diet

Should include salt restriction initially. Maintenance diet depends on cause of initial event and presence of underlying risk factors.

Activity

Bed rest should be observed during treatment of acute event. Patients are often more comfortable in the sitting position during the event.

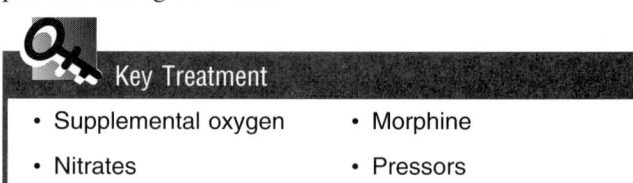

Key Treatment

- Supplemental oxygen
- Morphine
- Nitrates
- Pressors

Follow-Up

1. Prevention of recurrent events: must emphasize medical compliance, avoidance of smoking, and attention to other correctable cardiac risk factors

2. Monitoring: close observation after stabilization. If the nature of the underlying heart disease is unknown, careful work-up may reveal a correctable lesion.

3. Complications: Watch for signs of recurrent acute heart failure, development of chronic heart failure, dehydration secondary to diuresis, electrolyte abnormalities, and drug toxicity.

4. Prognosis: Acute heart failure continues to carry a high mortality, especially in the elderly. Studies have shown a 33 per cent mortality in the first three months after admission in elderly patients hospitalized for acute heart failure.

Bibliography

Braunwald E, Grossman W: Clinical aspects of heart failure. *In* Braunwald E (ed): Heart Disease: A Textbook of Cardiovascular Medicine, 4th ed. Philadelphia, WB Saunders, 1992, pp 444–463.

Fein SA, et al: Approach to ischemic heart disease, coronary care, and severe heart failure (including cardiogenic shock). Clin Geriatr Med 1994;10:145–160.

Ingram RH Jr, Braunwald E: Pulmonary edema: Cardiogenic and noncardiogenic causes. *In* Braunwald E (ed): Heart Disease: A Textbook of Cardiovascular Medicine, 4th ed. Philadelphia, WB Saunders, 1992, pp 551–568.

McGhie AI, Goldstein RA: Pathogenesis and management of acute heart failure and cardiogenic shock: Role of inotropic therapy. Chest 1992;102(supp 2):626S–632S.

Rogers WB, Frank MJ: Congestive heart failure. *In* Rakel RE (ed): Conn's Current Therapy. Philadelphia, WB Saunders, 1994, pp 276–279.

60 Chronic Heart Failure

David E. Gutstein

Etiology

1. Definition: Long-term failure of the heart to pump blood sufficiently to meet the metabolic demands of the tissues. Injury to the heart may cause loss of functioning myocardium. Compensatory mechanisms, including cardiac hypertrophy and neurohumoral processes, exert adverse long-term effects.
2. Epidemiology: Over 3 million United States citizens have chronic heart failure. Incidence increases with age and is higher in men than in women; 30 to 40 per cent of patients are hospitalized yearly.
3. Precipitating factors
   a. Injuries to the myocardium that may lead to chronic heart failure include myocardial infarction, toxins (e.g., alcohol, cytotoxic drugs), viral myocarditis, hypertensive or valvular heart disease, hypertrophy, congenital lesions, amyloidosis, hemochromatosis, pregnancy-related disorders, lipid storage disorders, and idiopathic dilated cardiomyopathy.
   b. Factors that may suddenly exacerbate chronic heart failure include medical or dietary noncompliance, uncontrolled hypertension, myocardial infarction, ischemia, valvular disorders, infection, arrhythmia, renal failure, anemia, pulmonary embolus, and thyrotoxicosis.

Symptoms

1. Chronic heart failure develops over a protracted period of time, with symptoms reflecting long-standing whole-body fluid overload.
2. Dyspnea on exertion is the most common initial symptom.
3. Orthopnea is the most sensitive clinical indicator of high filling pressures.
4. Other symptoms include fatigue, paroxysmal nocturnal dyspnea, nocturia, confusion, ankle edema, nausea, and right upper quadrant abdominal pain.

Key Symptoms
- Dyspnea on exertion
- Orthopnea
- Fatigue
- Edema
- Paroxysmal nocturnal dyspnea

Clinical Findings

1. Tachycardia and hypotension are common chronically; pulse pressure decreases as cardiac index declines.
2. Jugular venous distention with hepatojugular reflux
3. Signs of cardiomegaly; third heart sound (S_3); regurgitant systolic murmurs
4. Pulmonary rales with dullness at the bases
5. Hepatomegaly and ascites
6. Edema, cyanosis, and cachexia

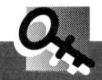

Key Signs
- Jugular venous distention
- Third heart sound (S_3)
- Pulmonary rales
- Edema

Diagnostic Tests

1. Blood tests: to rule out anemia, renal failure, hepatic and thyroid abnormalities
2. Electrocardiogram: abnormal in most advanced chronic heart failure patients, showing conduction abnormalities, infarct patterns, atrial arrhythmias, or ventricular ectopy
3. Chest film: Signs of chronic heart failure include cardiomegaly, vascular redistribution, and occasionally frank pulmonary edema.
4. Pulmonary function testing: may reveal pulmonary source of dyspnea
5. Exercise testing: evaluates for the presence of underlying ischemia; analysis of expired gas sometimes useful
6. Echocardiography, radionuclide angiography: Both estimate ejection fraction and evaluate wall motion; echo also evaluates chamber sizes and valves and estimates pulmonary pressures.
7. Electrophysiologic studies: used to evaluate recurrent serious ventricular arrhythmias
8. Cardiac catheterization (with hemodynamics, coronary angiography, and occasionally endomyocardial biopsy): used to evaluate refractory advanced chronic heart failure, unstable patients, nonischemic dilated cardiomyopathy, and heart transplant candidates

Key Tests
- Electrocardiogram
- Chest film
- Echocardiogram

Treatment

Medication

The following discussion refers to treatment of heart failure resulting predominantly from systolic dysfunction.

1. Diuretics: provide symptomatic relief. Loop diuretics include furosemide (Lasix), which is commonly started at 20 mg/day orally. Furosemide may be combined with another class of diuretic in refractory cases (e.g., metolazone [Zaroxolyn], 2.5 to 5 mg orally one half hour before furosemide).

2. Digoxin (Lanoxin): improves symptoms and hemodynamics. Digoxin is loaded with 0.75 to 1 mg in split doses over the first day, followed by maintenance at 0.125 to 0.25 mg/day orally (reduce dose in renal failure).

3. Angiotensin-converting enzyme (ACE) inhibitors: Long-term treatment improves symptoms, hemodynamics, and survival; act as peripheral vasodilators. Example: enalapril (Vasotec), 5 to 20 mg/day orally.

4. Isosorbide dinitrate (Isordil) and hydralazine (Apresoline): Combination vasodilator treatment confers greater survival benefit than placebo but less than enalapril. Isosorbide: 10 to 40 mg orally three to four times daily. Hydralazine: 10 to 60 mg orally four times daily.

5. β blockers: prolong survival in ischemic disease but may worsen heart failure. Studies in heart failure are ongoing.

6. Anticoagulation: reduces thromboembolic events in patients with severe left ventricular dysfunction, especially in the presence of atrial fibrillation

7. Short-term intravenous therapy for refractory heart failure

   a. Nitroprusside (Nipride): combined with intravenous diuretics, hemodynamic monitoring for 24 to 48 hours; oral vasodilator is added as nitroprusside is tapered. Start at 10 μg/min, increase by 5 to 10 μg/min every five minutes to a maximum of 300 μg/min. Adverse effects include hypotension and thiocyanate toxicity (especially in renal failure).

   b. "Dobutamine holiday": short-term (48 to 72 hours) infusion of dobutamine (Dobutrex) or phosphodiesterase inhibitor (e.g., amrinone [Inocor], milrinone [Primacor]) to improve cardiac function while oral medications are adjusted. Also used to maintain patients with end-stage heart failure awaiting cardiac transplantation.

8. Left ventricular assist device: increasingly used as a temporizing measure for terminally ill patients awaiting cardiac transplantation

9. Revascularization: Coronary artery bypass grafting provides survival benefit when compared with medical therapy in selected patients with poor systolic function and underlying three-vessel disease.

10. Cardiac transplantation: This may be a consideration in advanced heart failure that is not amenable to other surgical or medical therapy. Improves one-year survival to 90 per cent. Selection criteria tend to be fairly strict.

11. Diastolic dysfunction: Treatment of heart failure resulting from diastolic dysfunction, in patients with normal systolic function, differs substantially from the treatment for systolic dysfunction. Goals of treating isolated diastolic dysfunction include improving left ventricular filling and relaxation. As a result, several of the interventions discussed above (e.g., diuretics, digoxin, inotropes) may be inappropriate for treatment of the patient with diastolic dysfunction.

Diet

Weight loss, salt restriction, and abstention from alcohol are the rule. Limit fluid intake to two liters per day.

Activity

Bed rest is required during treatment of decompensated chronic heart failure.

Patient Education

1. Moderate regular exercise, being careful not to provoke dyspnea

2. Avoid smoking.

3. Regular influenza and pneumococcal vaccines

4. Explaining rationale of medical therapy may help to improve patient compliance.

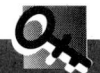
Key Treatment

- Diuretics
- Digoxin
- Angiotensin-converting enzyme inhibitors

Follow-Up

1. Prevention: ACE inhibitors have been shown to reduce the risk of developing heart failure in patients with asymptomatic left ventricular dysfunction.

2. Monitoring: Close follow-up is required if the patient is to be maintained as an outpatient.

3. Complications: These include atrial and ventricular arrhythmias, thromboembolic events, pulmonary infections, acute decompensation, electrolyte abnormalities, dehydration from overzealous diuresis, and drug toxicity.

4. Prognosis: The 5-year survival rate is 25 per cent for men, 38 per cent for women. Predictors of poor outcome include an ejection fraction <20 per cent, ischemic etiology, ventricular arrhythmias, serum sodium less than 130 mEq/L, poor functional class, low cardiac index, and high filling pressures.

Bibliography

Braunwald E, Grossman W: Clinical aspects of heart failure. *In* Braunwald E (ed): Heart Disease: A Textbook of Cardiovascular Medicine, 4th ed. Philadelphia, WB Saunders, 1992, pp 444–463.

Cody RJ: Management of refractory congestive heart failure. Am J Cardiol 1992;69:141G–149G.

Dargie HJ, McMurray JJ: Diagnosis and management of heart failure. Br Med J 1994;308:321–328.

Edwards BS, Rodeheffer RJ: Prognostic features in patients with congestive heart failure and selection criteria for cardiac transplantation. Mayo Clin Proc 1992;67:485–492.

Ho KK, et al: The epidemiology of heart failure: The Framingham study. J Am Coll Cardiol 1993;22(supp 4A):6A–13A.

Smith TW, et al: The management of heart failure. *In* Braunwald E (ed): Heart Disease: A Textbook of Cardiovascular Medicine, 4th ed. Philadelphia, WB Saunders, 1992, pp 464–519.

Ventura HO, et al: Current issues in advanced heart failure. Med Clin North Am 1992;76:1057–1082.

Procedure | **CENTRAL VENOUS CATHETER INSERTION**   *Jatin Amin*

Indications

1. Hypotension: requiring large fluid volume and rapid infusion
2. Dehydration: no peripheral intravenous access
3. Chemical: administration of special agents and nutrition not possible peripherally
4. Cardiac arrest: for intravenous antiarrhythmics and other pressor medications
5. Transducers: for measurement of central venous pressures

Contraindications

1. Thrombocytopenia
2. Increased prothrombin time or partial thromboplastin time

Preparation

1. Obtain consent from patient if patient is in stable condition; explain risks and possible complications
2. For thoracic insertions (internal jugular or subclavian), the patient should be supine or in slight Trendelenburg position. The semirecumbent position is acceptable if patient is on ventilator or in congestive heart failure.
3. Insertion site should be prepped as usual with Betadine in a circular outgoing manner.

Equipment

Central Line Kit. Most kits today contain all equipment needed for the complete insertion. Key items to include and verify are as follows:

1. Sterile gloves, drapes
2. Scalpel
3. Suture, hemostat, or driver
4. Facemask
5. Lidocaine 1% or 2% (non-epinephrine)
6. Saline flush
7. Syringes
8. Needles

Anesthesia

Procedures are generally performed with local anesthesia (e.g. lidocaine without epinephrine)

Precautions

1. Bleeding
2. Infection
3. Thrombosis
4. Pneumothorax
5. Maintenance of aspiration to avoid air embolization.
6. Arrhythmias while inserting and manipulation with guidewire.

Technique

Seldinger Technique: This method is a percutaneous approach in which a narrow gauge needle is used to locate and subsequently cannulate a guidewire into the vessel. Afterward the needle is removed and the catheter is slid over the wire into the vein. An alternative method (rarely used, mostly in trauma patients) is venous cutdown and cannulation of the cephalic vein in the upper arm.

1. Location and preparation of site (Table 60–1)

2. Preparation of the catheter: Flush all lumens and ports, uncap the distal lumen port if multi-lumen catheter (usually brown by convention).
3. Measure approximate distance that the catheter is to be advanced once in place.
4. Infiltrate intended puncture site with lidocaine without epinephrine.
5. Using continuous aspiration, the seeking needle (20-gauge) is used to locate and enter the vein.

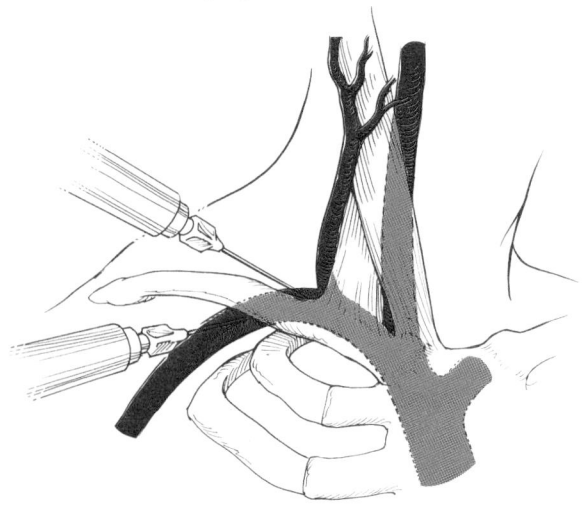
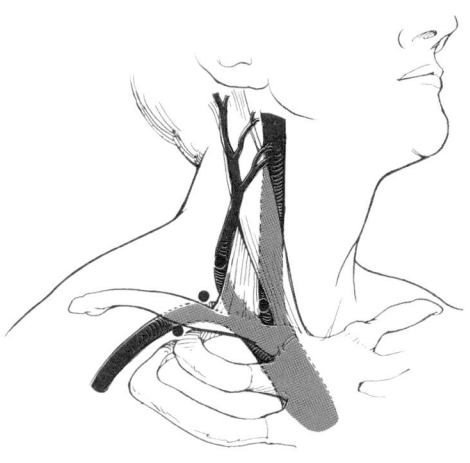

TABLE 60-1. ACCESS SITES

Site/Vein	Approach	Landmark	Benefits	Contraindications	Best Reserved for/Comments
1. Subclavian	Above or below clavicle with equal success; supraclavicular better as vein is more superficial	Insertion point is located just lateral to clavicular head of SCM, direction is to suprasternal notch	Ease of insertion and patient comfort make this the method most commonly used	Pneumothorax (1 to 2% of attempted insertions) and subclavian artery puncture (1% of attempts) are serious complications. *Rule out pneumothorax—check expiratory chest film before using opposite side approach*	Subclavian central access is ideal for long-term cannulation, TPN, and in general for stable IV cannulation; minimal overall risks
2. Int. jugular	Anterior or posterior to SCM* at base of neck; direction of needle is to ipsilateral nipple	Vein is just under SCM; seeking needle should be approx. 1 cm inferior to bifurcation	Minimal risk for pneumothorax, allows direct access for threading catheters and pacemakers	Major risk is carotid artery puncture (2–10%). Approach not suitable for platelets less than 50K, or if PT is 3 sec. greater than control. *Rule out pneumothorax, check expiratory chest film before using opposite side approach*	Disadvantage far outweighs the single advantage of lower incidence of pneumothorax; however, in patients with positive pressure ventilation, approach is suitable
3. Femoral	Medial to femoral artery below the inguinal ligament; for blind insertion, use 2/3–1/3 rule	Inguinal ligament serves the superior border; vein is 1–2 cm medial to the artery	Risk of pneumothorax eliminated, has ease of insertion; allows for blind insertion	Higher risk of infection if in place longer than 3 days; thrombosis (10%) and femoral artery punctures (5%); limits flexion at the hips, leading to discomfort if patient is conscious	Method and approach best reserved for emergency situations—cardiac arrests, short-term access in patients who are comatose or paralyzed
4. Ext. jugular	Easily identified by inspection of surface of the SCM with patient in Trendelenburg position	EJ vein passes over SCM and joins subclavian at an acute angle	Risk of pneumothorax eliminated; bleeding easily controlled	Major problem with this approach is difficulty in advancing catheter; unnecessary force should not be used as this will cause perforation of subclavian vein	In patients with severe coagulopathy, this method leads to impairment of neck mobility and is not well tolerated by conscious patients
5. Basilic/Brachial	Best if placed on top of the bicepital aponeurosis and aimed medially to basalic vein	With straight arm and tourniquet, the vein is entered by direct vision	No risk of pneumothorax and minimal risk of bleeding	High risk of infection, high rate of thrombosis, difficulty in threading catheter (<60% success); cutdowns should be avoided due to the high infection rate	Short-term IV access

*Sternocleidomastoid.

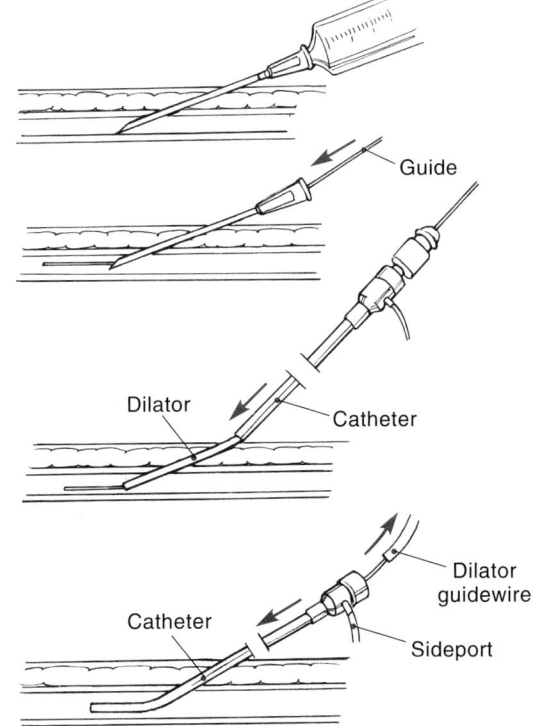

> **WARNING**
>
> **Never lose sight of the guidewire. Watch for arrhythmias if close to right atrium or right ventricle. If an attempt made on one side is not successful, an approach by way of the opposite side of chest should never be attempted without chest films to verify the absence of pneumothorax.**

6. The guidewire needle (18-gauge) is then used to cannulate the vein. The guidewire (J wire) is inserted through the needle; then the needle is removed.

7. The skin/subcutaneous tissue is cut with a scalpel to allow room for the catheter.

8. For large catheters, the tract should be widened with a dilator.

9. The catheter is placed with the distance equal to that previously measured.

10. Once flow and flush have been established, the catheter is sutured and secured.

11. Finally, an expiratory chest film should be checked to ensure correct placement and to rule out pneumothorax.

 Bibliography

Agee KR, Balk RA: Central venous catheterization in the critically ill patient. Crit Care Clin 1992;8:677–686.

Denny DF Jr: Placement and management of long-term central venous access catheters and ports. Am J Roentgenol 1993;161:385–393.

Johnson JC: Complications of vascular access devices. Emergency Med Clin N Am 1994;12:691–705.

Olson IE, Lam K, Bodey GP, et al: Evaluation of strategies for central venous catheter replacement. Crit Care Med 1992; 20:797–804.

Shimada M, Matsuma T, Wakiyama S, et al: A safe and simple technique for exchanging central venous catheters. Postgrad Med J 1993;69:139–140.

Procedure **SWAN-GANZ MONITORING** *John David Rogers*

Indications
1. Congestive heart failure
2. Respiratory failure (cardiogenic versus noncardiogenic [ARDS])
3. Shock states
   a. Cardiogenic
   b. Hypovolemic
   c. Septic
4. Complicated myocardial infarction
5. Intraoperative and postoperative fluid management
6. Fluid management in trauma, burn patients
7. Cardiac tamponade/constriction
8. Fluid management in acute renal failure and advanced cirrhosis

Contraindications
None are absolute.
1. Bleeding disorders
   a. Thrombocytopenia
   b. Profound anticoagulation
2. Infection at proposed venous access site
3. Lack of knowledgeable personnel
4. Lack of appropriate/functional equipment
5. When hemodynamic data obtained from the catheter will not make a difference in patient management

Preparation
1. Discuss procedure with the patient or family if possible to obtain informed consent.
2. Patient should be continuously monitored by electrocardiography (ECG).
3. Select and prepare a venous access site using sterile technique (see preceding procedure on Central Venous Catheter Insertion). Preferably right internal jugular or left subclavian
4. Select appropriate Swan-Ganz catheter.
5. Make certain pressure transducers are properly connected to the pressure monitors.
6. All intravenous lines, including pressure tubing, must be flushed completely to remove all the air in these lines.
7. Position the pressure transducer so that the air reference point is at the midchest (phlebostatic axis).
8. Flush all lumens of the catheter with heparinized saline. All intravenous ports should then be connected to the appropriate pressure transducer or continuous intravenous flush line. The sterile sleeve should be placed over the catheter.

Equipment
1. Percutaneous (or cutdown) introducer sheath insertion tray. This usually comes as a kit. (See preceding procedure on Central Venous Catheter Insertion for full list of supplies.)
2. Intravenous fluids (usually heparinized saline)
3. Pressure tubing and pressure transducer set-up

4. Pressurized intravenous cuff or pump
5. Swan-Ganz catheter: most commonly used has four lumens and a thermistor device

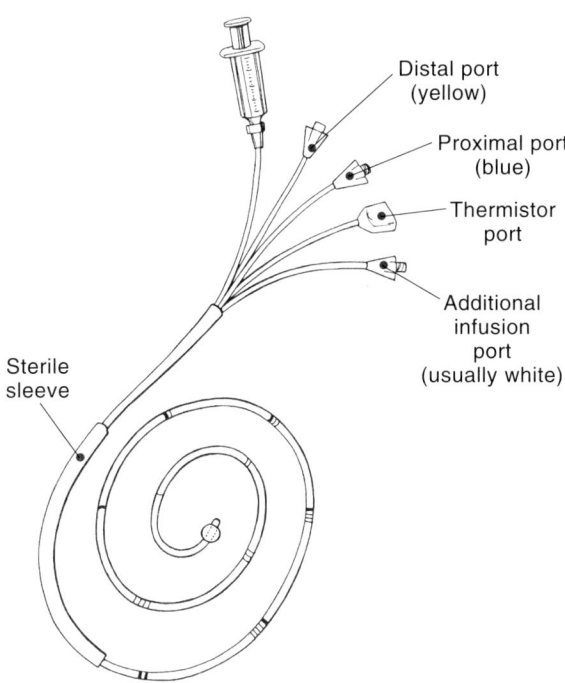

Distal port (yellow)
Proximal port (blue)
Thermistor port
Additional infusion port (usually white)
Sterile sleeve

6. Catheter sleeve (allows for sterile manipulation of catheter once it is placed)
7. Continuous ECG and pressure waveform monitor
8. Access to fluoroscopy if needed
9. ACLS equipment standing by (e.g., defibrillator, drugs)

Anesthesia
1. 1% lidocaine without epinephrine (for local infiltration)
2. Occasionally the very anxious or agitated patient may require short-acting sedation.

Precautions
1. This procedure must be performed using aseptic technique.
2. The physician performing this procedure should be familiar with the local anesthetics, including maximum dose, duration of action, and signs/symptoms of allergic reactions.
3. Only physicians experienced in obtaining central venous access, placement of Swan-Ganz catheters, and interpretation of the hemodynamic data should perform this procedure. Physicians who have such experience may supervise those who wish to learn the procedure.
4. Swan-Ganz catheter placement and hemodynamic monitoring can be performed only in certain areas such as cardiac catheterization laboratory, ICU/SICU, CCU, operating rooms, and some emergency rooms.

Technique

1. Place an introducer sheath using aseptic central venous insertion techniques (see procedure on central venous catheterization).

2. Insert the catheter into the introducer sheath and advance it into the vein. When the pressure monitor begins to show some respiratory variation, the tip of the catheter is usually in the superior vena cava. At this point the balloon can be partially inflated to assist with further advancement.

3. Once the right atrium (RA) is reached, the balloon can be fully inflated. Characteristic RA pressure waves should be seen on the monitor.

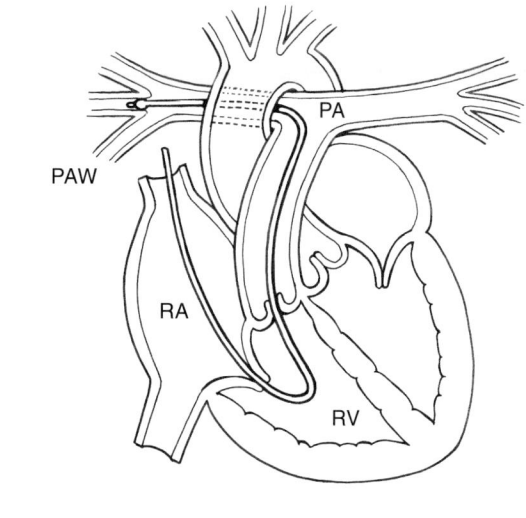

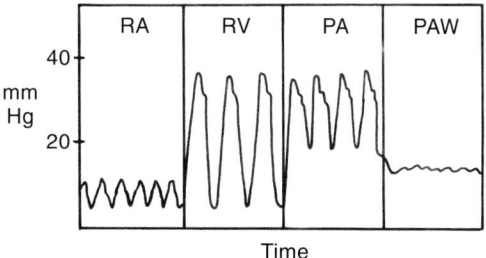

These pressures should then be recorded.

4. With the balloon fully inflated, advance the catheter into the right ventricle (RV). The ECG monitor should be watched for ventricular ectopy and arrhythmias. Once the characteristic RV pressure waves are seen, they should be recorded.

5. While the balloon is still inflated, the catheter is gently advanced until a pulmonary artery pressure (PAP) waveform is seen. This pressure should then be recorded. If a PAP waveform is not obtainable, if ventricular ectopy increases, or if the RA waveform reappears, the catheter is most likely coiling in the RV. If this occurs, deflate the balloon, slowly pulling the catheter back to the original RA position. Inflate the balloon again and gently but rapidly advance the catheter through the RV and into the PA. Once a PAP waveform is seen, stop advancing the catheter.

6. With the balloon still inflated, advance the catheter from the PA position until the waveform changes to a pulmonary artery wedge pressure (PAWP). Once this waveform is seen, stop advancing the catheter and record the pressures.

7. Allow the balloon to deflate by removing the syringe. This causes the balloon to deflate passively rather than by active suction, which may damage the delicate balloon. When the balloon is deflated, the PAP waveform should be seen. If the PAWP waveform persists after the balloon is deflated, the catheter tip is in too far and is measuring a continuous PAWP. If this occurs, keep the balloon deflated and slowly withdraw the catheter until the PAP waveform appears. The balloon can then be slowly inflated to allow the catheter to float into the PAWP position.

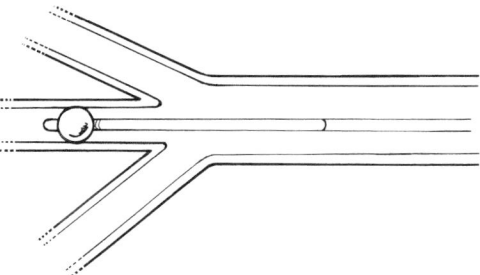

The PAWP should be measured intermittently; the catheter tip should never be kept in the PAWP position for very long.

8. Once the catheter is properly positioned, the catheter sleeve is then attached proximally to the introducer sheath, stretched out, and fastened distally to the catheter. It is important to remember that the sleeve is placed on the catheter before it is inserted into the introducer sheath.

9. Proper catheter placement is then verified by portable chest film. A properly placed catheter tip will be seen in the beginning of the PA (just beyond the edge of the vertebral bodies).

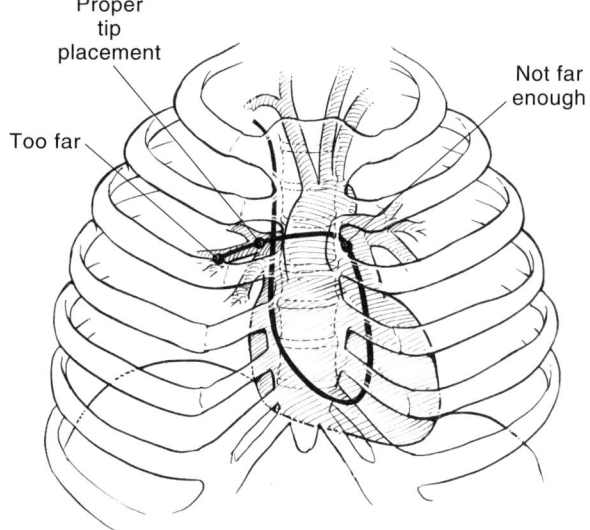

10. Each lumen of the catheter should then be flushed and the balloon locked in the deflated position.

11. If the introducer sheath has not been sutured to the skin, this should be done now.

12. Iodinated ointment should be applied to the puncture sites and a sterile dressing used.

13. After the patient is made more comfortable, the transducer should be recalibrated (see preparation) and then the pressures and cardiac outputs re-measured. Patient anxiety and agitation manifested as interrupted breathing or even breath holding (simulating a Valsalva maneuver) may give erroneous pressure readings initially. If the luxury of a few minutes' time is available, the results are generally more accurate.

Follow-Up

1. Interpretation of hemodynamic data—Normal hemodynamics
   a. RA 2–6 mm Hg
   b. RV 20–30/0–5 mm Hg
   c. PAP 20–30/8–12 mm Hg
   d. PAWP 4–12 mm Hg
   e. C.O. 3.5–5.5 L/min; C.I. 2.7–3.3 L/min/m^2
   f. SVR 900–1200 dynes/sec/cm^{-5}
2. Complications
   a. Those seen with central venous access (see procedure on Central Venous Catheter Insertion)
   b. Additional complications seen with Swan-Ganz catheterization
      (1) Cardiac arrhythmias
      (2) Thrombosis of cannulated vein and thromboembolism from catheter-associated thrombus
      (3) Pulmonary infarction and pulmonary artery rupture
      (4) Balloon rupture
      (5) Damage to the tricuspid and pulmonic valve
      (6) Knotting of the catheter

Bibliography

Devendra KA, Prediman KS, Swan HJC: The technique of inserting a Swan-Ganz catheter. J Crit Ill 1993;8:1147–1156.

Matthay MA, Chatterjee K: Bedside catheterization of the pulmonary artery: risks compared with benefits. Ann Intern Med 1988;109:826–834.

Shoemaker WC: Use and abuse of the balloon tip pulmonary artery (Swan-Ganz) catheter: are patients getting their money's worth? Crit Care Med 1990;18:1294–1295.

Spodick DH: Flow-directed pulmonary artery catheterization. Chest 1989;95:489–490.

Steingrub JS, Celoria G, Vickers-Lahti M, et al: Therapeutic impact of pulmonary artery catheterization in a medical/surgical ICU. Chest 1991;99:1451–1455.

61 Cardiomyopathy

Benjamin H. Chadi

Etiology

1. Definition: Cardiomyopathy (CMP) is heart muscle disease of unknown cause (idiopathic), although often used loosely to refer to specific heart muscle diseases (mentioned under differential diagnosis)

2. Classification

   a. Dilated (DCMP): up to 20 per cent familial; some sporadic

   b. Hypertrophic (HCMP): 50 per cent may be familial with point mutations in the β myosin heavy-chain gene on chromosome 14; others heritable or sporadic

   c. Restrictive (RCMP): primary; endocardial fibroelastosis; endomyocardial fibrosis without and with eosinophilia (as in eosinophilic leukemia, hypersensitivity states, or parasitic infestations); infiltrative disorders (as in amyloidosis, hemochromatosis, sarcoidosis)

   d. Obliterative

Symptoms

1. Heart failure: dyspnea on exertion and later at rest; subsequently paroxysmal nocturnal dyspnea, orthopnea, pedal edema, and RUQ abdominal tenderness in acute hepatic congestion

2. Arrhythmias: palpitation, tachycardia, syncope

3. Chest discomfort, cough, hemoptysis

4. Low output state with fatigue, decreased mentation, skin and gut hypoperfusion, and decreased urination

5. Embolisms: pulmonary, peripheral vasculature (stroke, renal and splenic infarcts)

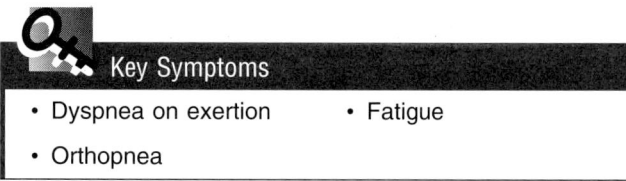

Key Symptoms

- Dyspnea on exertion
- Fatigue
- Orthopnea

Clinical Findings

1. History: family, alcohol, toxins, viral syndrome, residence in tropics

2. Examination

   a. Tachycardia with narrow pulse pressure due to low output with pulsus alternans in end-stage

   b. Jugular venous distention more than the normal 6- to 8-cm vertical height above the RA level (manubriosternal junction at the midaxillary line)

   c. Crackles, pedal edema, hepatomegaly, and ascites (quantify)

   d. Cardiomegaly with point of maximal impulse (PMI) laterally displaced and diffusely enlarged (in DCMP) or more forceful (in HCMP)

   e. Parasternal lift and heave with mitral regurgitation or with pulmonary hypertension

   f. Loud P_2 and reversed split S_2 in pulmonary hypertension

   g. Diastolic gallops: S_3 early filling and S_4 atrial kick

   h. Holosystolic murmurs of mitral regurgitation (apical to axillary or left sternal) and tricuspid regurgitation (parasternal, louder with inspiration)

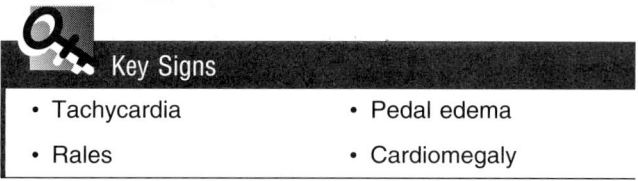

Key Signs

- Tachycardia
- Pedal edema
- Rales
- Cardiomegaly

Laboratory Tests

1. Electrocardiogram: normal or abnormal

   a. Arrhythmias: atrial and ventricular ectopies, sinus tachycardia, atrial fibrillation

   b. Increased voltage and left axis deviation in left ventricular hypertrophy; RVH and right axis deviation in pulmonary hypertension and right heart failure; low voltage in infiltrative CMP (vs. COPD, obesity, hypothyroidism); electrical alternans in pericardial tamponade

   c. Conduction abnormalities and bundle branch blocks (BBB), generally LBBB in DCMP, RBBB in Chagas' disease, and complete heart block in heredofamilial disorders

   d. Left atrial abnormality due to left atrial hypertrophy or dilatation, commonly with mitral valve or left ventricular disorders; right atrial abnormality in right arterial (RA) enlargement or hypertrophy as with severe tricuspid regurgitation or pulmonary hypertension and right ventricular (RV) failure

   e. Q waves of infarction or mimic

   f. ST/T changes of infarction, ischemia, pericarditis, myocarditis, electrolyte imbalance

   g. Prolonged QT interval

2. Chest roentgenogram

   a. Cardiomegaly with an enlarged cardiac silhouette due to dilatation, hypertrophy, or effusion; enlargement of LA, RA, and RV chambers

   b. Increased pulmonary vascular redistribution, interstitial and alveolar edema, Kerley B lines, and perihilar infiltrates

3. Doppler and echocardiography
   a. Wall thickness: markedly increased septal thickness often with evidence of dynamic outflow tract obstruction in HCMP. A ground-glass texture often accompanies the wall thickening in infiltrative disorders such as amyloidosis. Ventricular hypertrophy commonly accompanies hypertensive disorders and aortic stenosis. Apical thrombus and cavity obliteration occur in endomyocardial disease. Right ventricular hypertrophy commonly accompanies pulmonary hypertension.
   b. Wall motion abnormalities: usually hypercontractile in HCMP; global hypokinesis in DCMP or end-stage HCMP.
   c. Chamber size: left atrial enlargement is the rule in all forms of cardiomyopathy. The left ventricular cavity size is small in HCMP and RCMP, but dilated in DCMP. The right ventricle may dilate in right heart failure.
   d. Pericardial disease: the presence of an effusion and, if large, evidence for tamponade and chamber collapse; Doppler evidence for inspiratory decline in left ventricular in- and outflow suggests tamponade, pericardial restriction, or restrictive cardiomyopathy (differentiated by pulmonary venous Doppler).
   e. Valvular pathology: systolic anterior motion (SAM) of the anterior mitral leaflet in HCMP with systolic closure of the aortic valve evidence of dynamic outflow obstruction. Mitral regurgitation may be due to SAM in HCMP or to a dilated mitral annulus in DCMP. Pulmonary artery systolic pressure (P, mm Hg) can be reliably calculated from the peak tricuspid regurgitation velocity (v, m/s) by the modified Bernoulli equation

$$(P \text{ in } RV - P \text{ in } RA = 4 \, v^{**}2)$$

   The severity of accompanying valvular stenoses or regurgitation can be quantitated.
   f. The presence of congenital heart disease and shunts or abnormal flows (such as atrial septal defect, patent ductus arteriosus) can be evaluated.
   g. Specific evaluations include contrast injection and transesophageal echocardiography for better resolution of pathologic features as in HCMP or to evaluate LA thrombus, anomalous pulmonary venous return, patent foramen ovale; provocative maneuvers such as use of nitroglycerin or amyl nitrite to provoke the outflow gradient in HCMP; stress echo/Doppler to evaluate for ischemia or changes in a valvular or subvalvular gradient with exercise.
4. Radionuclide studies
   a. MUGA (radionuclide ventriculography): ejection fraction

   b. Stress thallium: rule out ischemic etiology, infarction
5. Cardiac catheterization
   a. Right heart to evaluate right atrial, pulmonary, and wedge pressures (LV preload), cardiac output by thermodilution or Fick, oximetry to evaluate for right to left shunt, and calculations of systemic and pulmonary vascular resistance
   b. Left heart catheterization to evaluate intracavitary pressures and evaluate gradients (HCMP or valve stenosis) by simultaneous measurements and by pullback
   c. Coronary angiography to evaluate coronary disease including intravascular ultrasound of suspicious lesions
   d. Ventriculography and aortography to evaluate ejection fraction and valvular regurgitation
   e. Provocation of gradient in HCMP by vasodilators, inotropes, or post-premature ventricular complexes
   f. Myocardial biopsy to rule out infiltrative disorders, myocarditis, transplant rejection, and drug toxicity
6. Blood tests
   a. ASO titer (rheumatic heart disease), Chagas' titers
   b. WESR (myocarditis)
   c. CK/MB (acute myocardial infarction, myocarditis, neuromyopathies)
   d. Screen for toxins including cocaine, alcohol
   e. Thyroid function tests, screen for pheochromocytoma

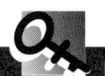

Key Tests

- Electrocardiogram
- Echocardiogram
- Chest radiograph

Differential Diagnosis

1. Specific heart muscle diseases
   a. Ischemic with myocardial infarction and hibernation (focal)
   b. Hypertensive with left ventricular hypertrophy
   c. Alcoholic with dilatation: direct toxicity or via acetaldehyde
   d. Toxicity of cocaine, catecholamines, anthracyclines (doxorubicin, daunorubicin)
   e. Nutritional deficiencies: beriberi (thiamine), Keshan's disease (selenium)
   f. Myocarditis: viral, bacterial, parasitic (Chagas' disease due to *Trypanosoma cruzi*), HIV-associated
   g. Heredofamilial: Duchenne's and Becker's muscu-

lar dystrophies, Kearns-Sayre syndrome (ophthalmoplegia, pigmentary retinopathy, cerebellar ataxia, mitochondrial gene inheritance)

   h. Metabolic errors: glycogen storage diseases

   i. Drug hypersensitivity

   j. Hormonal: pheochromocytoma, thyrotoxicosis (high output)

   k. Infiltrative disorders: amyloidosis, sarcoidosis, hemochromatosis

   l. cor pulmonale due to pulmonary hypertension associated with any etiology including idiopathic, collagen vascular disease, recurrent pulmonary embolism, COPD, methotrexate

   m. Idiopathic postpartum dilated cardiomyopathy

   n. Transplant rejection

2. Cardiac disorders mimicking heart muscle disease

   a. Valvular regurgitation, stenosis

   b. Pericardial constriction, tamponade, pericarditis

   c. Congenital heart diseases: atrial septal defect, anomalous pulmonary venous return, cor triatriatum, ventricular septal defect, tetralogy of Fallot

3. Noncardiac disorders: acute pulmonary embolism, acute respiratory distress syndrome, COPD, pneumonias

Treatment

Medication

1. Diuretics to decrease preload in DCMP with evidence of congestion. Loop diuretics such as furosemide or bumetanide can be used alone or in combination with thiazides or metolazone. Closely monitor and supplement potassium. Restrict free water intake in hyponatremia.

2. Vasodilators can increase cardiac output and survival in DCMP. The angiotensin-converting enzyme inhibitors such as captopril and enalapril can be titrated to blood pressure and help conserve potassium. Isordil and hydralazine have documented efficacy. Vasodilators can potentially worsen the dynamic obstruction in hypertrophic cardiomyopathy.

3. Digitalis increases inotropic state, improves ejection fraction, and improves symptoms in DCMP, without causing hypotension. It can control the ventricular response to atrial fibrillation. It should be avoided in infiltrative CMP of amyloid and in HCMP. Due to a narrow therapeutic index and risk for potentially life-threatening arrhythmias and toxicity, it should be monitored. Digibind Fab anti-digitalis antibodies can be used acutely in the management of intoxication.

4. β-blockers have potential for use in DCMP but may exacerbate heart failure. They are useful in HCMP to improve diastolic filling parameters.

5. Calcium blockers have negative inotropic effects and should generally be avoided in DCMP. The negative chronotropic effects improve diastolic filling in HCMP.

6. Pacemaker insertion may be necessary preventively in cardiomyopathies that progress to heart block (Kearns-Sayre syndrome and some muscular dystrophies). Dual chamber pacing has shown promise in reducing the outflow tract gradient in HCMP.

7. Surgical considerations include coronary revascularization, mitral valve replacement, myomectomy for HCMP with obstruction, thrombectomy with endocardial stripping for eosinophilic endomyocardial disease, and transplant in end-stage DCMP.

8. Anticoagulation therapy may be given in atrial fibrillation, in DCMP, and in RCMP to prevent thromboembolism.

9. Anti-inflammatory agents may be given in eosinophilic endocardial disease, but their efficacy has not been documented in myocarditis, in which 50 per cent may improve spontaneously.

10. The role of the implantable defibrillator is being defined.

Diet

1. Low sodium (2 gm/day or 500 mg in severe cases), optimize nutrition, avoid alcohol and cardiotoxins

2. Thiamine and selenium for specific states

Activity

1. Avoid heavy lifting, vigorous exertion, and hot weather.

2. Maintain a mild daily aerobic exercise regimen to improve muscle conditioning, peripheral blood flow, exercise tolerance.

Education

1. Symptoms and signs of heart failure (edema, dyspnea, loss of appetite, rapid weight gain, or stable weight with anorexia)

2. Measure body weight daily and record

3. Salt content of foods (fresh or frozen vs. processed, pickled, canned)

4. Importance of fluid balance: Water intake is generally controlled by thirst related to dietary salt intake. An adequate urinary output and brisk response to diuretic are critical to maintain homeostasis. A lack of urine output may relate to renal disease, urinary obstruction, or to worsening heart failure, with gut edema and poor diuretic absorption along with poor renal perfusion and resultant potential for serious hyperkalemia and digitalis toxicity. Anuria needs emergent evaluation.

5. Role of diarrhea in causing potassium loss or as a manifestation of hyperkalemia

6. Signs of hypokalemia including leg cramps, arrhythmias

7. Need to monitor regularly prothrombin time on war-farin, electrolytes, and periodically digoxin level

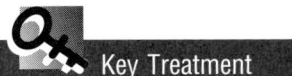

Key Treatment

- Diuretics
- Vasodilators
- Digitalis

Follow-Up

Depends on the specific etiology, preventive therapy, and severity of heart failure.

Bibliography

Brandenburg RC, et al: Myocardial disease. *In* Giuliani ER, et al (eds): Cardiology Fundamentals and Practice. St. Louis, Mosby–Year Book, 1991, pp 1773–1880.

Giles TD, Sande GE: Cardiomyopathy. Littleton, MA, PSG Publishing, 1988.

Katz AM: The cardiomyopathy of overload: An unnatural growth response in the hypertrophied heart. Ann Intern Med 1994;121:363–371.

Louie EK, Edwards LC III: Hypertrophic cardiomyopathy. Progr Cardiovasc Dis 1994;36:275–308.

Wynne J, Braunwald E: The cardiomyopathies and myocardi-tides: Toxic, chemical, and physical damage to the heart. *In* Braunwald E (ed): Heart Disease: A Textbook of Cardiovascu-lar Medicine. Philadelphia, WB Saunders, 1992, pp 1394–1450.

62 Mitral Valve Disease

Gary M. Brockington

Mitral Stenosis

Etiology

1. Rheumatic fever
2. Cardiac tumors
3. Rheumatologic disorders (e.g., lupus, rheumatoid arthritis)
4. Mucopolysaccharidoses
5. Congenital defects
6. Endomyocardial fibroelastosis
7. Malignant carcinoid

Symptoms

Orifice size of 1 cm^2 results in symptoms due to gradient across valve; rheumatic stenosis is often asymptomatic until fourth or fifth decade of life.

1. Exertional dyspnea, paroxysmal nocturnal dyspnea, orthopnea
2. Hemoptysis (secondary to severe pulmonary hypertension)
3. Systemic emboli with atrial fibrillation
4. Pulmonary edema with exertion

Key Symptoms

- Exertional dyspnea
- Hemoptysis
- Systemic emboli

Clinical Findings

1. Female predominance
2. Malar flush ("mitral facies")
3. Prominent jugular vein *a* waves (when in sinus rhythm)
4. Palpable P$_2$
5. Right ventricular lift (when significant pulmonary hypertension present)
6. Accentuated S$_1$
8. Low-pitched diastolic rumble with presystolic accentuation (heard best at the apex)
9. Edema and liver engorgement (if right ventricular failure present)

Key Findings

- Opening snap
- Diastolic rumble
- Loud S$_1$

Laboratory Tests

1. Electrocardiogram (ECG): left atrial enlargement (*p-mitrale*) if sinus rhythm present, atrial fibrillation (very common), and right ventricular hypertrophy
2. Chest radiograph: left atrial predominance, prominent pulmonary arteries, calcified mitral annulus (in some cases), interstitial edema, and elevation of left main-stem bronchus (with severe left atrial enlargement)
3. Echocardiography: left atrial enlargement, decreased excursion of mitral valve leaflets with fusion of fissures, valvular calcification, and estimation of valve area
4. Nuclear scanning: estimation of left ventricular function
5. Cardiac catheterization: accurate assessment of transvalvular gradient and degree of pulmonary hypertension; coronary angiography

Key Tests

- Electrocardiogram
- Chest radiograph
- Echocardiography
- Cardiac catheterization

Differential Diagnosis

1. Tricuspid stenosis (rarely an isolated lesion)
2. Mitral regurgitation (not associated with opening snap or accentuated S$_1$; diastolic murmur in severe states)
3. Cor triatriatum (echocardiography delineates between the two)
4. Atrial septal defect (diastolic rumble with large defect due to excessive flow across tricuspid valve)

Treatment

1. Medical

   a. Drugs: endocarditis prophylaxis, rate control if in atrial fibrillation (digitalis, β blockers), anticoagulation (warfarin [Coumadin]), diuretics

b. Activity: limitation

c. Diet: salt restriction

2. Valvuloplasty

   a. May be an open (surgical) or closed (balloon) procedure.

   b. Significant mitral regurgitation is a contraindication.

   c. Poor result anticipated if heavy valvular calcification present.

   d. Anticoagulation and/or exclusion of left atrial thrombi is necessary prior to performing balloon angioplasty.

   e. Results may be long-lasting (greater than 5 years without restenois).

3. Surgical: May be treated with either mechanical or bioprosthetic valve.

Patient Education

1. Strict adherence to prothrombin time check schedule

2. Endocarditis prophylaxis

Key Treatment

- Diuretics
- Valvuloplasty
- Control of atrial fibrillation
- Surgery

Follow-Up

1. Serial echocardiography

2. Frequent prothrombin time (PT) checks (keep international normalized ratio [INR] 3 to 4 with mechanical valve)

Mitral Regurgitation

Etiology

1. Rheumatic fever

2. Endocarditis

3. Papillary muscle dysfunction

4. Ruptured chordae tendineae

5. Myxomatous degeneration of mitral valve (i.e., mitral valve prolapse, idiopathic)

6. Mitral annular calcification

7. Collagen-vascular disease (i.e., lupus)

8. Atrial myxoma

Symptoms

1. Fatigue

2. Orthopnea, nocturnal paroxysmal dyspnea, edema

3. Frank pulmonary edema

4. Systemic emboli

Key Symptoms

- Congestive heart failure
- Fatigue
- Thromboemboli

Clinical Findings

1. Hyperdynamic apical impulse

2. Ejection or holosystolic murmur loudest at apex with radiation to axilla

3. Severe cases associated with diastolic rumble and/ or S_3

4. Crackles, liver congestion, and edema (decompensated states)

Key Signs

- Holosystolic murmur
- Congestive heart failure

Laboratory Studies

1. ECG: left atrial enlargement if in sinus rhythm, atrial fibrillation (very common), left ventricular hypertrophy, and left axis deviation

2. Chest radiograph: left ventricular predominance, left atrial enlargement, mitral annular calcification, dilated pulmonary arteries, and interstitial edema (when left ventricular decompensation has occurred)

3. Echocardiography: left atrial enlargement (common), left ventricular function (poor to hyperdynamic), and degree of regurgitation (mild, moderate, severe)

4. Radionuclide scanning: assessment of left ventricular function and degree of regurgitation (stroke volume index)

5. Cardiac catheterization: elevated left atrial and pulmonary artery pressures and large *v* wave in pulmonary capillary wedge pressure tracings; left ventriculogram quantifies degree of regurgitation and left ventricular function

Key Tests

- Electrocardiogram
- Echocardiogram
- Chest radiograph
- Catheterization

Differential Diagnosis

1. Tricuspid regurgitation (murmurs loudest at left fourth intercostal space)

2. Ventricular septal defect (murmur loudest at lower left sternal border; may vary in intensity with respiration)

3. Pulmonary regurgitation (loudest at pulmonic area; isolated pulmonic regurgitation not associated with signs of left ventricular failure)

4. Hypertrophic obstructive cardiomyopathy (ejection murmur loudest at lower left sternal border; increases with Valsalva)

Treatment

1. Medical (drugs)

   a. Diuretics, digitalis, and afterload reduction if congestive failure present

   b. Endocarditis prophylaxis

   c. Anticoagulation (Coumadin) if atrial fibrillation present

2. Surgical

   a. Mitral valve repair (may be superior to replacement)

   b. Valve replacement (either mechanical or bioprosthetic)

WARNING

Surgery is reserved for severely symptomatic patients in whom optimal medical therapy has failed or who demonstrate rapidly increasing left ventricular diastolic dimensions.

Diet
Salt restriction
Activity
Limitation if congestive heart failure
Patient Education
Education regarding risks and benefits of Coumadin; importance of endocarditis prophylaxis

Key Treatment

- Control of congestive heart failure
- Surgery

Follow-Up

Serial echocardiography; PT (aiming for INR of 3 to 4) in patients with mechanical valves

Bibliography

Braunwald E: Mitral regurgitation: Physiologic, clinical and surgical considerations. N Engl J Med 1969;281:425.

Braunwald E: Valvular heart disease. *In* Braunwald E (ed): Heart Disease. A Textbook of Cardiovascular Medicine. 4th ed, vol 2. Philadelphia, WB Saunders, 1992, pp 1007–1078.

Dajani AS, Bisno AL, Chung KJ, et al: Prevention of bacterial endocarditis: Recommendations by the American Heart Association. JAMA 1990;264:2919–2922.

Morton MJ, Rahimtoola SH: How to follow patients with prosthetic heart valves. J Cardiovasc Med 1980;5:475.

Reyes VP, Raju BS, Wynne J, et al: Percutaneous balloon valvuloplasty compared with open surgical commissurotomy for mitral stenosis. N Engl J Med 1994;331:961–967.

63 Aortic Valve Disease

Anil Shah

Aortic Stenosis

Etiology

1. Congenital aortic stenosis (major cause in patients under age 30)
2. Congenital bicuspid valve (progressive sclerosis occurs with age)
3. Rheumatic aortic stenosis (usually accompanied by disease of the mitral valve)
4. Calcific aortic stenosis (most common cause in patients older than age 60)

Symptoms

Paucity of symptoms occur until valve area of less than 1 cm^2.

1. Angina: Left ventricular hypertrophy causes increase in oxygen demand.
2. Syncope: Commonly associated with exercise.
3. Congestive heart failure (CHF): Initially diastolic failure; may progress to systolic dysfunction.

> **WARNING**
>
> **Once symptoms begin, life expectancy is significantly decreased.**

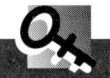

Key Symptoms

- Angina
- Syncope
- Congestive heart failure

Clinical Findings

1. Harsh crescendo-decrescendo murmur heard best at base with radiation to carotids.
2. Absent aortic component of second heart sound with severe stenosis.
3. Carotid impulses are diminished and delayed: pulsus parvus et tardus.
4. Sustained forceful apical impulse.

Key Signs

- Systolic murmur
- Pulsus parvus et tardus

Laboratory Tests

1. Electrocardiogram (ECG): left ventricular hypertrophy (most common finding), left atrial enlargement, intraventricular conduction delay, left axis deviation
2. Chest radiograph: left ventricular predominance (without gross cardiomegaly), calcification of aortic cusps and/or annulus, poststenotic dilatation of the ascending aorta, and pulmonary vascular congestion (in the presence of heart failure).
3. Echocardiography: Concentric left ventricular hypertrophy and thickening with or without calcification of the aortic cusps with decreased separation. Doppler gradient across the aortic valve (greater than 50 mm in severe cases). Valve area calculation of less than 0.8 cm^2 consistent with critical stenosis.
4. Radionuclide scanning: Gated blood pool scanning gives an accurate assessment of left ventricular function. Time to peak filling is often delayed.
5. Cardiac catheterization: direct measurement of valvular gradient; angiography to exclude concomitant coronary artery disease

Key Tests

- Electrocardiogram
- Chest radiograph
- Echocardiogram
- Cardiac catheterization

Differential Diagnosis

1. Aortic sclerosis (not associated with absent A$_2$ or diminished carotid pulses)
2. Mitral regurgitation (holosystolic murmur at apex)
3. Pulmonic stenosis (ejection murmur loudest at left sternal border)
4. Hypertrophic obstructive cardiomyopathy (ejection murmur at left sternal border, prominent pulses with bifid quality)

Treatment

1. Medical (drugs)
   a. Diuretics if CHF present
   b. Antibiotic prophylaxis for dental and surgical procedures

> **WARNING**
>
> **Avoid vasodilators; may result in profound and irreversible hypotension.**

2. Valvuloplasty: Small improvements in valve area result in significant symptom improvement. High restenosis rate within a year of procedure. Bridge procedure in patients needing noncardiac surgery with critical stenosis; palliative procedure in symptomatic patients who are poor surgical candidates.

3. Surgery: Definitive therapy in symptomatic patients. Reduced systolic function not a contraindication to surgery. Bioprosthetic or metal valves; latter requires lifetime anticoagulation.

Diet

Sodium restriction if CHF present

Activity

Moderate limitation (no competitive exercise in significant cases)

Patient Education

1. Strict compliance with diet and medication

2. Adherence to prothrombin time (PT) evaluation (warfarin [Coumadin] needed with mechanical valve).

Key Treatment

- Diuretics
- Valvuloplasty
- Salt restriction
- Surgery

Follow-Up

1. Serial echocardiography

2. PT checks with mechanical valve (aim for an international normalized ratio [INR] of 3 to 4)

Aortic Regurgitation

Etiology

1. Rheumatic fever

2. Endocarditis

3. Congenital valvular deformities (e.g., bicuspid valve)

4. Collagen-vascular disorders (e.g., ankylosing spondylitis, systemic lupus erythematosus)

5. Myxomatous degeneration (e.g., Marfan syndrome)

6. Aortic dissection

7. Trauma

Symptoms

1. Dyspnea

2. Paroxysmal nocturnal dyspnea and orthopnea

3. Edema (if biventricular failure present)

4. Chest pain and rarely syncope

Key Symptoms

- Dyspnea
- Edema

Clinical Findings

Acutely may result in pulmonary edema; chronic state may be tolerated for decades.

1. High-pitched decrescendo diastolic murmur at aortic area; radiates along left sternal border

2. Rapid and forceful carotid upstrokes with dramatic collapse (Corrigan's pulse)

3. Wide pulse pressure

4. Head bobbing with each systole (de Musset's sign)

5. Prominent pulsations of skin capillaries (Quincke's pulse)

6. Hill's sign (significantly higher popliteal artery pressure than brachial pressure)

7. Duroziez murmur (to and fro murmur heard over the femoral artery)

8. Displaced and hyperdynamic PMI

9. S_3 or S_4

Key Signs

- Diastolic murmur
- Wide pulse pressure

Laboratory Tests

1. ECG: left ventricular hypertrophy and ST-T wave changes

2. Chest radiograph: cardiomegaly (in chronic cases), pulmonary vascular congestion, aortic root dilatation, and "double-lumen" sign when aortic dissection present

---

IMPORTANT

CT or nuclear magnetic resonance scanning can be invaluable in diagnosing dissection.

---

3. Echocardiography: left ventricular chamber dilatation (chronic cases), systolic function abnormal (may be hyperdynamic in acute cases, poor in decompensated chronic cases), diastolic fluttering of anterior leaflet of the mitral valve, and Doppler estimation of degree of regurgitation (range: mild to severe).

4. Radionuclide studies: ejection fraction, stroke volume index (degree of regurgitation). Serial studies and exercise studies may help decide timing of elective valve replacement.

5. Cardiac catheterization: elevated left ventricular diastolic pressure; root flush for quantification of degree of regurgitation (1 + to 4 +); coronary angiography

Key Tests

- Electrocardiogram
- Chest radiograph
- Echocardiogram
- Radionuclide scan
- Cardiac catheterization

Differential Diagnosis

1. Pulmonic regurgitation (left ventricular prominence not seen)
2. Patent ductus arteriosus (continuous murmur heard in diastole and systole)

Treatment

1. Medical (drugs)
   a. Afterload-reducing agents
   b. Digitalis
   c. Diuretics
   d. Endocarditis prophylaxis
2. Surgical: Valve replacement is only surgical option. Indications are symptomatic patients with chronic regurgitation, severe acute regurgitation, progressive reduction in systolic function, end-systolic dimensions of left ventricle greater than 55 mm via echocardiogram, failure to increase ejection fraction with exercise

Diet
Salt restriction
Activity
Moderate restriction
Patient Education
1. Explain risks of Coumadin (needed with mechanical valve).
2. Stress prothrombin (PT) checks.

Key Treatment

- Afterload reduction
- Diuretics
- Digoxin
- Surgery

Follow-Up

1. Serial echocardiography
2. PT checks (aiming for INR of 3 to 4)

Bibliography

Braunwald E: Valvular heart disease. *In* Braunwald E (ed): Heart Disease: A Textbook of Cardiovascular Medicine, 4th ed, vol 2. Philadelphia, WB Saunders, 1992, pp 1007–1078.

Dajani AS, Bisno AL, Chung KJ, et al: Prevention of bacterial endocarditis: Recommendations by the American Heart Association. JAMA 1990;264:2919–2922.

Frank S, Johnson A, Ross J: Natural history of valvular aortic stenosis. Br Heart J 1973;35:41.

Morton MJ, Rahimtoola SH: How to follow patients with prosthetic heart valves. J Cardiovasc Med 1980;5:475.

Scognamiglio R, Rahimtoola SH, Fasoli G, et al: Nifedipine in asymptomatic patients with severe aortic regurgitation and normal left ventricular function. N Engl J Med 1994;331:689–694.

64 Aortic Dissection

Thomas P. Power

Aortic dissection occurs when blood accumulates within the media of the aorta, causing separation of the intima from the adventita. The usual initiating event is tearing of the intima and migration of the blood into the media. Rarely, rupture of the vasa vasorum within the media may lead to dissection without intimal tearing. In either case, blood tracks within and dissects the media, creating a false lumen. Aortic dissection may occur at any age (mean age is 59 years), and the ratio of males to females is 3:1. Aortic dissections are classified as follows

1. Based on the anatomic location

   a. Proximal (type A) are those dissections that involve, but are not necessarily limited to, the ascending aorta.

   b. Distal (type B) are those dissections whose involvement is limited to the distal aorta.

2. Based on the age of the dissection

   a. Acute dissections are those that have occurred within the preceding two weeks.

   b. Chronic dissections are more than two weeks old.

Etiology

While the exact cause of aortic dissection is not known, it is usually associated with an abnormality of the media. The following conditions predispose to aortic dissection

1. Hypertension

2. Congenital disorders (Marfan's syndrome, Ehlers-Danlos syndrome, Turner's syndrome, aortic coarctation).

3. Trauma (including iatrogenic trauma)

4. Inflammatory conditions (relapsing polychondritis, giant cell arthritis)

5. Pregnancy (third trimester)

Symptoms

1. Chest pain is the cardinal symptom of aortic dissection. It occurs in 89 per cent of proximal dissections and 97 per cent of distal dissections. The pain is severe, described as tearing or ripping, and is usually of sudden onset. It may migrate to the neck, jaw, arms, or back, and migration of the pain is usually associated with progression of the dissection.

2. Syncope occurs considerably less frequently than chest pain. It may be due to severe pain or hypotension, as would occur with aortic rupture or pericardial tamponade. Occasionally syncope occurs before any pain is perceived and is therefore the presenting symptom.

3. Dyspnea as a presenting symptom is unusual; how-ever, if specifically sought on history it is usually present. It may be related to cardiac tamponade, cardiac failure, or the presence of a large pleural effusion.

4. Alteration of mental status is not uncommon but is often subtle and overshadowed by chest pain. It may be due to impaired cerebral perfusion (hypotension or cerebral vessel involvement) or to the effects of previously administered narcotics.

Key Symptoms

- Chest pain; sudden, severe, tearing or ripping
- Syncope

Clinical Findings

1. Blood pressure changes. If all patients with aortic dissection are considered, hypertension is more common than hypotension at the time of presentation. However, patients with proximal dissection more commonly present with hypotension than with hypertension, and in these cases pericardial tamponade and aortic rupture must be considered. Occasionally, due to branch vessel involvement in the dissection, the cuff blood pressure may not reflect the true intra-arterial blood pressure (pseudohypotension).

2. Pulse deficits occur in about 50 per cent of patients with proximal aortic dissection and are considerably less common in distal dissection. Their presence is highly suggestive of this diagnosis. Pulse deficits are the result of either an intimal flap, which overlies and occludes the origin of a branch vessel, or propagation of the dissection into the lumen of the branch vessel.

3. Aortic valvular regurgitation, with its associated physical signs, occurs in approximately two thirds of patients with proximal aortic dissection. The presence of new aortic regurgitation in a patient with chest pain should lead one to strongly suspect aortic dissection. It should be remembered, however, that the clinical picture of acute aortic regurgitation, such as occurs with dissection, is often much less dramatic than that of chronic regurgitation. The first heart sound is often diminished due to premature closure of the mitral valve (related to the rapid rise in left ventricular diastolic pressure). The diastolic murmur may be heard best at the right sternal border in contradistinction to that of pure valvular regurgitation, in which it is heard best to the left of the sternum. Aortic regurgitation is the usual cause of

cardiac failure in both acute and chronic aortic dissection.

4. Neurologic deficits are found in 36 per cent of proximal and 6 per cent of distal dissections. Global changes result from hypotension, whereas focal signs are due to aortic branch vessel involvement (cerebral vessels, spinal arteries) or peripheral ischemic neuropathy.

5. Pericardial rub is a rare finding in aortic dissection, but when present, is an ominous sign because it is often followed by pericardial tamponade.

6. Tracheal tug due to traction on the left main bronchus during systolic expansion of the dissected aorta is also a rare but interesting sign.

Key Signs

- Hypertension
- Pulse deficit
- Aortic insufficiency

Laboratory Tests

Whenever aortic dissection is suspected, no time should be wasted in confirming the diagnosis because the mortality increases with time to treatment. Chest radiograph (showing widening of the mediastinum, left pleural effusion) and electrocardiogram (showing sinus tachycardia, low voltage) will often show abnormalities consistent with aortic dissection, but they are never diagnostic. Therefore the most easily available, most accurate, and safest test should be chosen. This choice will differ from patient to patient and from institution to institution.

1. Echocardiography. Transthoracic (TTE) and transesophageal (TEE) echocardiography are now available in most hospitals. Neither requires the use of intravenous contrast agents and both can be performed at bedside. TEE is particularly helpful in visualization of the true and false lumens, the intimal flap, and the presence of associated aortic regurgitation. It can often identify the site and extent of dissection and determine the degree of involvement of the proximal coronary arteries.

2. Computed tomographic (CT) scanning has been used since 1979 in diagnosis of aortic dissection and is now widely available. Sensitivity and specificity are high, and alternative diagnoses are often evident in those who do not have aortic dissection. However, CT scanning necessitates transportation of the patient and the use of intravenous contrast agents. It is not particularly useful in identification of associated aortic regurgitation or coronary artery involvement.

3. Aortography was considered the gold standard for diagnosis of aortic dissection, and it is still commonly used. It is particularly useful in the determination of the extent of dissection and the degree of branch vessel involvement (including the coronary arteries). Aortic regurgitation can also be identified. However, aortography is invasive, and large volumes of contrast agent are sometimes required. It necessitates transportation of the patient and assembly of a team to perform the procedure.

4. Magnetic resonance imaging (MRI) has the highest sensitivity and specificity for diagnosis of aortic dissection. However, monitoring of patients during imaging is difficult, and imaging times may be prohibitively long for unstable patients. MRI may be most useful in the diagnosis of chronic aortic dissection in stable patients or in long-term follow-up of treated patients. However, this technology is not available in many hospitals.

Key Tests

- Transesophageal echocardiography
- CT scan

Differential Diagnosis

1. Myocardial infarction (MI) is important in the differential diagnosis of aortic dissection for two reasons
   a. Administration of thrombolytic therapy to a patient with aortic dissection may have disastrous consequences.
   b. 1 to 2 per cent of proximal aortic dissections extend into the proximal coronary arteries and cause MI. Therefore, an electrocardiogram consistent with acute MI does not exclude the diagnosis of aortic dissection.

2. Aortic valvular regurgitation without dissection

3. Nondissected aortic aneurysm

4. Pericarditis

5. Musculoskeletal chest pain

6. Mediastinal tumors

Treatment

Mortality from untreated aortic dissection is high and increases incrementally with time. Prompt diagnosis and treatment are therefore of utmost importance. Treatment should begin as soon as the diagnosis is suspected. The aim of initial pharmacologic therapy is to prevent extension of the dissection by reducing shear force on the aorta during systole.

1. β blockers should be administered until the pulse rate is 60 to 70/min (e.g., propranolol, 1 mg intravenously q 5 min).

2. This should be followed by nitroprusside (25 μg/min intravenously) until the systolic blood pressure is reduced to 100 to 120 mm Hg.

3. Analgesia (morphine sulfate, 3 to 5 mg intravenously

q 10 min prn) will also help to reduce systolic shear forces.

Definitive therapy depends on the site and age of the aortic dissection. All patients with acute proximal dissection should be referred for immediate surgical correction. Chronic proximal dissection, if complicated (e.g., extension, aneurysm formation, aortic regurgitation) should also be treated surgically. Distal dissections, both acute and chronic, should be treated medically if uncomplicated and referred to surgery if complications arise. Patients with Marfan's syndrome should be treated surgically regardless of the site or age of their dissection. Medical treatment consists of rigorous blood pressure control. It must continue indefinitely for all patients, including those who have undergone surgical correction, as there is a continued risk of re-dissection.

Key Treatment

- β blockers
- Surgery

Follow-Up

All patients who survive to be discharged from the hospital require careful lifelong follow-up. Physical examination, chest film, and noninvasive imaging should be performed at three-month intervals for the first year and twice yearly thereafter. The choice of imaging modality is dependent on availability of technology and expertise.

Bibliography

Cigarroa JE, Isselbacher EM, DeSanctis RW, Eagle KA: Diagnostic imaging in the evaluation of suspected aortic dissection. N Engl J Med 1993;328:35–43.

Crawford ES: The diagnosis and management of aortic dissection. JAMA 1990;264:2537–2541.

Nienaber CA, von Kodolitsch Y, Nicolas V, et al: The diagnosis of thoracic aortic dissection by noninvasive imaging procedures. N Engl J Med 1993;328:1–9.

Slater EE, DeSanctis RW: The clinical recognition of dissecting aortic aneurysm. Am J Med 1976;60:625–633.

Treasure T: Imaging the dissected aorta. Br Heart J 1993; 70:497–498.

65 Endocarditis

Michael S. Bronze

Infective endocarditis (IE) denotes infection of the endocardial surface of the heart including the valves, septal defects, and the mural endothelium. The designations of acute and subacute endocarditis are often used, but a classification based on the microbiologic etiology is preferable as it has implications on course, complications, and appropriate therapy.

Etiology/Epidemiology

1. Microbiology
   a. Causes of IE (Table 65–1)
   b. Less common causes of IE include the following
      (1) HACEK bacterial group (*Haemophilus* sp., *Actinobacillus* sp., *Cardiobacterium* sp., *Eikenella* sp., and *Kingella* sp.)
      (2) Anaerobes, *Chlamydia*, *Rickettsia*, *Brucella*, *Legionella*
      (3) Viruses (echovirus, coxsackie, adenovirus)
   c. Culture-negative IE occurs in 3 to 5 per cent of patients and may be related to
      (1) Prior exposure to antibiotics
      (2) Fastidious organisms or nonbacterial cause (viral or fungal)
      (3) Indolent tricuspid valve disease
2. Frequency of cardiac valve involvement in IE
   a. % isolated mitral valve >aortic >tricuspid >pulmonic valve
   b. 3 to 5 per cent have simultaneous left and right heart valves involved
   c. 30 to 35 per cent have concomitant mitral and aortic valve involvement
3. Estimated risk for IE due to underlying cardiac lesion
   a. Increased risk
      (1) Prosthetic heart valve
      (2) Congenital heart disease
         (a) Patent ductus
         (b) Ventricular septal defect
         (c) Bicuspid aortic valve
         (d) Coarctation of aorta
      (3) Rheumatic valvular disease
      (4) Mitral valve prolapse with regurgitation
      (5) Prior endocarditis
      (6) Marfan's syndrome
      (7) Isolated valve dysfunction
      (8) Acquired valvular stenosis
      (9) Acquired valvular insufficiency
   b. Low to negligible risk
      (1) Coronary artery disease
      (2) Syphilitic aortitis
      (3) Permanent cardiac pacemaker
      (4) Atrial septal defect
      (5) Mitral valve prolapse without regurgitation

Symptoms

The symptoms of IE are the manifestations of the following

1. The infectious process on the valve leading to valve disruption
2. Bland or septic emboli
3. Bacteremia and metastatic infections
4. Circulating immune complexes

They are protean and include fever, chills, sweats, weight loss, malaise, fatigue, and dyspnea.

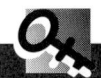

Key Symptoms

- Fever
- Chills
- Malaise

Clinical Findings

1. Similar to the symptomatology, clinical signs of IE demonstrate varying levels of sensitivity and specificity. Major physical findings include fever (90 to 95 per cent), heart murmur (>80 per cent), embolic phenomena, and signs of congestive heart failure.
2. Less common findings may include splenomegaly, retinal lesions (Roth's spots), signs of metastatic infection (pneumonia, meningitis), and cutaneous signs including splinter hemorrhages, Osler's nodes, Janeway lesions, and petechiae.

Key Signs

- Fever
- Heart murmur

TABLE 65–1. COMMON CAUSES OF INFECTIVE ENDOCARDITIS

NATIVE VALVE	PROSTHETIC VALVE	IV DRUG ABUSE
Streptococci	Staphylococci	Staphylococci
Staphylococci	Streptococci	Streptococci
Gram-negative rods	Gram-negative rods	Gram-negative rods
	Fungi	Fungi

Pathologic Findings

1. Cardiovascular finding may include intracardiac suppuration (valve ring abscess, valvular perforation and rupture, myocardial abscess), valvular stenosis due to large vegetations, systemic embolization, and mycotic aneurysms.

2. Kidney involvement is common and may consist of renal abscess, renal embolization with infarction, or glomerulonephritis.

3. The central nervous system involvement includes cerebral infarction due to embolization, cerebral vasculitis, cerebritis or abscess, meningitis, or intracranial/subarachnoid hemorrhage due to ruptured mycotic aneurysms.

Laboratory Tests

1. Routine laboratory findings may include
   a. Normocytic anemia, >70 per cent
   b. Elevated ESR, >90 per cent
   c. Leukocytosis, monocytosis, <25 per cent
   d. Proteinuria, pyuria, hematuria, <65 per cent
   e. Positive blood cultures, >93 per cent

2. Echocardiography may be useful both as a diagnostic tool and for prognosis. For the diagnosis of IE, the current debate is whether to use transthoracic (TTE) or transesophageal (TEE) echocardiography.
   a. Studies suggest that
      (1) TTE has a lower sensitivity but a highly acceptable specificity. A negative TTE does not exclude the diagnosis of IE.
      (2) TEE has improved sensitivity but may have a higher false-positive rate. Uses of TEE may include prosthetic valve endocarditis, confirming the diagnosis of IE in a patient with a negative TTE and detecting intracardiac suppurative complications such as perivalvular ring abscesses.
   b. The role of echocardiography in assessing prognosis has been the focus of several studies, especially those involving patients with right-sided IE. Echocardiographic evidence of large vegetations may indicate an increased risk of embolization, valve disruption with congestive heart failure, and a more prolonged febrile course. However, the presence of visible vegetations by echocardiography does not imply the need for surgery in all cases, treatment failure if the vegetations persist, or the specific organism involved (i.e., fungal).

3. Ancillary imaging tests with anecdotal support, but undefined clinical utility, include gallium-67, gallium-SPECT, or indium radionuclide scans.

Key Tests

- Echocardiogram
- Sedimentation rate

Treatment

Antibiotic Therapy

Antibiotic therapy for IE should include the following

- Use of parenteral antibiotics that ensure sustained drug levels
- Long-term administration usually for 4 to 6 weeks to reduce the risk of relapse
- Use of synergistic combinations to achieve a bactericidal effect
- Selection of antibiotics dictated by the isolated organism and the determined minimum inhibitory concentration (MIC) and the minimum bactericidal concentration (MBC) for the antibiotics used

1. Streptococcal infective endocarditis. Treatment of IE due to streptococci should take into consideration whether the organism is penicillin-sensitive (MIC <0.2 μg/ml) or penicillin-resistant (MIC >0.5 μg/ml). Streptococci considered to be penicillin-sensitive include most viridans streptococci, S. bovis, and group A streptococci, and exclude the group D enterococci.
   a. "Penicillin-sensitive"

---

10 to 20 million units of penicillin G IV daily for 4 weeks (may also include 2 weeks of gentamicin, 1 mg/kg q 8 hr)

or

10 to 20 million units penicillin G IV daily plus gentamicin 1 mg/kg (not to exceed 80 mg IV q 8 hr) for 2 weeks*

or if penicillin-allergic

vancomycin, 15 mg/kg IV q 12 hr for 4 weeks

---

*Two-week course is designed for patients with streptococci with MIC to penicillin, ≤0.1 μg/ml in the absence of impaired renal function, complicated course, prosthetic valve IE, or a tolerant strain.

   b. "Penicillin-resistant" (includes enterococci)

---

20 million units penicillin G IV daily plus gentamicin, 1 mg/kg, q 8 hr for 6 weeks

or

ampicillin, 2 gm IV q 6 hr plus gentamicin for 6 weeks

or

vancomycin, 15 mg/kg IV q 12 hr plus gentamicin for 6 weeks

---

2. Staphylococcal infective endocarditis
   a. Recommended regimens should take into consideration that most strains are resistant to penicillin G and may be resistant to methicillin or oxacillin.

Antibiotic regimens may include those presented in the following box.

nafcillin, 1.5 to 2.0 gm IV q 4 hr for 4 to 6 weeks, plus gentamicin, 1 mg/kg IV q 8 hr for 5 to 7 days

or

vancomycin, 15 mg/kg IV q 12 hr, plus rifampin, 300 mg PO q 12 hr for 4 to 6 weeks, plus gentamicin, 1 mg/kg IV q 8 hr for 5 to 7 days

or

cephalothin, 2 gm IV q 6 hr for 4 to 6 weeks, plus gentamicin for 5 to 7 days

   b. Recently a 2-week regimen consisting of nafcillin and tobramycin has been shown to be effective in uncomplicated right-sided endocarditis due to methicillin-sensitive *S. aureus* in intravenous drug abuse–associated IE.

3. Enteric gram-negative bacillus–associated infective endocarditis. Treatment of IE due to gram-negative aerobic bacilli (e.g., *E. coli, Klebsiella* sp., *Proteus* sp., *Pseudomonas, Serratia* sp.) should be dictated by antimicrobial sensitivities. Regimens typically include a cephalosporin or expanded-spectrum penicillin combined with an aminoglycoside continued for six weeks. Left-sided endocarditis due to *Pseudomonas* or *Serratia* sp. may require a combined medical-surgical approach for cure.

4. Prosthetic valve endocarditis. Prosthetic valve endocarditis (PVE) is often divided into "early" PVE (within 60 days of surgery) or "late" (after 60 days).

   a. Early PVE is most commonly due to *Staphylococcus epidermidis, Staphylococcus aureus, Streptococcus* sp., and gram-negative bacilli.

   b. Late PVE is most often associated with viridans streptococci, but can also be due to *Staphylococcus* sp., enterococci, and gram-negative bacilli.

   c. Antimicrobial therapy should be based on antimicrobial sensitivities of the isolated organism, but initial therapy should include vancomycin and gentamicin plus rifampin pending results of cultures.

5. Endocarditis in IV drug users. The most commonly isolated organisms include *Staphylococcus aureus,* streptococci including the enterococcus, gram-negative bacilli, and fungi. Empiric coverage pending results of cultures should include nafcillin (or vancomycin) plus gentamicin. Some would advocate adding penicillin or ampicillin for added coverage of enterococci.

Indications for Surgical Intervention in Infective Endocarditis

Generally accepted indications for surgical therapy in IE include

1. Progressive congestive heart failure

2. Recurrent major embolization

3. Uncontrolled infection or resistant infection (e.g., fungal)

4. Extravalvular intracardiac suppuration (e.g., ring abscess)

5. Selected patients with prosthetic valve endocarditis

Endocarditis Prophylaxis

1. Patients with known cardiac conditions predisposed to the development of IE or patients with previous episodes of IE who undergo certain invasive procedures should be given antibiotic prophylaxis to prevent endocarditis.

2. The decision to recommend prophylaxis is based on the risk of bacteremia from the procedure and the type of underlying cardiac condition. These conditions and procedures and the recommended antibiotic regimens have been clearly delineated by the American Heart Association (JAMA, 264:2919, 1990).

 Bibliography

Birmingham GD, Rahko PS, Ballantyne F: Improved detection of infective endocarditis with transesophageal echocardiography. Am Heart J 1992;123:774–781.

Durack DT, Lukes AS, Bright DK, and the Duke Endocarditis service: New criteria for diagnosis of infective endocarditis: utilization of specific echocardiographic findings. Am J Med 1994;96:200–209.

Durack DT: Prevention of infective endocarditis. N Engl J Med 1995;332:38–44

McKinsey DS, Ratts TE, Bisno AL: Underlying cardiac lesions in adults with infective endocarditis. The changing spectrum. Am J Med 1987;82:681–688.

Scheld WM, Sande MA: Endocarditis and intravascular infections. *In* Mandel GL, Douglas RG, Bennett KE (eds.): Principles and Practices of Infectious Diseases. 3rd ed. New York, Churchill Livingstone, 1990, pp 670–706.

66 Pericarditis

Vishwanatha Nadig

Pericarditis is the inflammatory response of the pericardium due to diverse causes. These inflammatory responses could result in acute pericarditis, pericardial effusion, or constrictive pericarditis. The incidence of acute pericarditis is 2 to 6 per cent. Men are affected more often than women and adults more often than children. Constrictive pericarditis is usually a sequela of acute pericarditis.

Etiology

A. Acute pericarditis: Most common causes of acute pericarditis are infections, myocardial infarction, cardiac surgery, malignancy, uremia, autoimmune disorders, and radiation (Table 66–1).

B. Constrictive pericarditis: Most common causes of constrictive pericarditis are idiopathic (42 per cent), cardiac surgery (29 per cent), radiotherapy (13 per cent), tuberculosis, uremia, and rheumatoid arthritis.

Symptoms

A. Acute pericarditis: Chest pain is the characteristic feature of acute pericarditis.

   1. The pain is retrosternal, sharp, intermittent, reduced by sitting up and leaning forward and increased in a supine position.

   2. With radiation to the neck or arms, the pain may simulate angina. Radiation to the superior border of the scapula is considered highly specific for pain due to pericarditis.

   3. Hemodynamically significant pericardial effusion (tamponade) with symptoms of dyspnea, oliguria, and dizziness results in cardiogenic shock.

   4. Large pericardial effusion causes hoarseness, cough, and dysphagia due to its pressure effects on the adjacent structures.

B. Constrictive pericarditis: The fibrocalcified scar in constrictive pericarditis limits the cardiac output, resulting in symptoms of right-sided heart failure with ascites and peripheral edema. The majority (90 per cent) of patients also experience dyspnea, orthopnea, and cough due to left ventricular failure.

Key Symptoms

Acute pericarditis	Constrictive pericarditis
• Sharp central chest pain may have pleuritic quality	• Exertional dyspnea, orthopnea
• Radiation to one of the trapezius ridges	• Ascites, jugular venous distention, and peripheral edema

Clinical Findings

A. Acute pericarditis: Pericardial friction rub is the characteristic sign of acute pericarditis.

   1. Classically this is a high-pitched, superficial scratching/grating sound with three components (presystolic, systolic, and diastolic). The rub is best heard adjacent to the lower left sternal border.

   2. Nonspecific findings of fever, tachycardia, and tachypnea are often present.

   3. Signs of a large pericardial effusion include absent apical impulse, distant heart sounds, dullness to percussion over inferior angle of the left scapula (Ewart's sign), and crackles over the lung bases.

   4. Presence of prominent neck veins, cold clammy skin, hypotension, and pulsus paradoxus of more than 10 mm Hg with absent heart sounds in the right setting should be further evaluated for cardiac tamponade.

B. Constrictive pericarditis: Jugular venous distention, ascites, peripheral edema, and hepatomegaly with cardiac cirrhosis are the predominant signs seen in constrictive pericarditis.

TABLE 66–1. ETIOLOGY OF PERICARDITIS

1. Idiopathic
2. Infectious agents
   a. Viral: coxsackie, varicella, influenza, HIV, hepatitis B viruses
   b. Bacterial: Staphylococcus, Streptococcus, *Mycobacterium, Pneumococcus, Gonococcus*
   c. Fungal: *Histoplasma, Candida, Blastomyces*
   d. Parasitic: *Echinococcus, Cysticercus,* ameba
3. Autoimmune disorders: Systemic lupus erythematosus, rheumatic fever, rheumatoid arthritis, and polyarteritis nodosa
4. Neoplasms: Lung cancer, breast cancer, lymphoma-leukemia
5. Radiation
6. Uremic pericarditis
7. Hypersensitivity: Postmyocardial infarction, postsurgical
8. Drugs: Procainamide, hydralazine, methysergide, penicillins, and so on
9. Miscellaneous: Myxedema, chylopericardium, sarcoidosis, amyloidosis, regional enteritis

Key Signs

Acute pericarditis	Constrictive pericarditis
• Pericardial friction rub	• Jugular venous distention, positive Kussmaul's sign
• Tachypnea	• Early diastolic pericardial knock, right ventricular failure

1. With inspiration the neck veins become more prominent (Kussmaul's sign).

2. The heart sounds are distant. An early diastolic pericardial knock is heard best along the left sternal border.

Laboratory Tests

1. Electrocardiography (ECG): Four stages of ECG changes are classically described in acute pericarditis.

   a. Stage I: Epicardial leads show ST segment elevation in 90 per cent of cases while cavitary leads aVR, V1, and occasionally V2 show ST segment depression.

   b. Stage II and III: PR segment depression and T wave inversion follow subsequently.

   c. Stage IV: Normalization of ST, PR, and T wave changes are the late findings.

   d. ECG shows low voltage with nonspecific T wave changes, electrical alternans in pericardial effusion, and constrictive pericarditis. Left atrial abnormality (P mitrale) is seen in constrictive pericarditis.

2. Routine laboratory test: Leukocytosis and an elevated erythrocyte sedimentation rate (ESR) are seen in acute pericarditis.

3. Radiography:

   a. Chest film is usually normal.

   b. Large pericardial effusion shows cardiomegaly (water bottle appearance) on the chest film.

   c. Pulmonary edema (85 per cent), pleural effusion (85 per cent), left atrial enlargement (85 per cent), cardiomegaly (65 per cent), and calcification (43 per cent) are common chest film abnormalities seen in patients with constrictive pericarditis.

   d. Computed tomographic (CT) and magnetic resonance imaging have emerged as important tools in evaluating constrictive pericarditis.

4. Cardiac catheterization: Cardiac catheterization is useful in differentiating cardiac tamponade, restrictive cardiomyopathy, and constrictive pericarditis.

   a. Preservation of x descent with absence of y descent is seen in cardiac tamponade. The pulmonary wedge pressure and left ventricular pressure are usually elevated.

   b. In constrictive pericarditis, a dip and plateau configuration ("square root sign") is seen on the ventricular tracings. The diastolic pressures in all four cardiac chambers will be equal.

5. Echocardiography: Echocardiography will detect as little as 20 ml of pericardial effusion.

   a. Moderate effusion (>300 ml) demonstrates an echo-free space both posterior and anterior to left ventricular wall, "swinging" of the heart, and mitral valve pseudoprolapse.

   b. When cardiac tamponade is clinically suspected, echocardiography is mandatory. Echocardiography easily differentiates tamponade from other causes of hypotension with jugular venous distention.

   c. In constrictive pericarditis, M-mode echocardiography demonstrates multiple dense echoes and two parallel lines (representing two pericardial layers) separated by clear space. However, CT scan may be more informative.

6. Pericardiocentesis with pericardial biopsy: Diagnostic pericardiocentesis is rarely required. Fluid should be examined for microbial agents including tuberculosis; if the fluid is serosanguinous it should be studied for neoplasia and autoimmune diseases (e.g., lupus, rheumatoid arthritis).

Key Tests	
Acute pericarditis	**Constrictive pericarditis**
• ECG: Diffuse ST segment elevation, PR segment depression, T wave inversion	• ECG: Low voltage in all the leads, P mitrale
• Echocardiogram	• Chest film: ring calcification, cardiomegaly
	• Cardiac catheterization: square root sign, equalization of diastolic pressures in all four chambers

Differential Diagnosis

A. Acute pericarditis

1. Unstable angina: Patients with postmyocardial infarction pericarditis may appear clinically to have unstable angina. However, a brief course of aspirin or indomethacin will relieve the discomfort.

2. Dissecting aneurysm: Severe sudden onset of chest pain radiating to the back along with widened mediastinum should distinguish acute pericarditis from dissection.

3. Pneumothorax: Sharp chest pain with dyspnea and scratching sound due to mediastinal air can simulate acute pericarditis. However, ECG and chest film should differentiate the two conditions.

4. Pulmonary infarction: Evidence of predisposing deep venous thrombosis, abnormal lung scans, and pulmonary arteriography should distinguish pulmonary infarction from acute pericarditis.

5. Esophageal diseases: Esophageal rupture or symptomatic hiatal hernia may occasionally simulate acute pericarditis without clinical signs of pericarditis.

B. Constrictive pericarditis: On clinical grounds, constrictive pericarditis and restrictive cardiomyopathy resemble each other, making the diagnosis difficult. Echocardiography and angiography help in distinguishing these two conditions (see above). Occasionally myocardial biopsy is required.

Treatment

A. Acute pericarditis: All patients should be hospitalized to rule out a purulent process or an evolving myocardial infarction. Analgesics such as indomethacin, 50 mg orally, t.i.d.; ibuprofen, 400 mg orally, q.i.d.; aspirin, 650 mg orally, q.i.d.; or codeine, 15 to 30 mg orally, q 4 hr are quite effective in relieving the pain. Analgesic dosage may be increased or a different analgesic chosen if the pain persists beyond 24 to 48 hours. Steroids should be used with caution since steroid withdrawal results in recurrence of the pain. Specific treatment should be directed toward the underlying cause of acute pericarditis.

B. Constrictive pericarditis: Definitive treatment of constrictive pericarditis is total pericardiectomy. Cardiac functions may not return to normal, though most patients (90 per cent) experience significant relief of symptoms after surgery. Failure to respond to surgery results from incomplete removal, extension to epicardium, or myocardial involvement. Very elderly patients with limited life expectancy should be managed conservatively since they carry significant mortality (5 to 14 per cent).

C. Diet: There are no dietary restrictions either for acute or constrictive pericarditis.

D. Activity: Patients with acute pericarditis need bed rest until their pain abates. Associated illness may prolong activity limitations as in myocardial infarction or severe rheumatoid arthritis. Constrictive pericarditis usually limits physical activity because of exertional dyspnea and orthopnea. They should not exert themselves until after the surgery.

E. Patient education: Patients should be warned against potential complications of acute pericarditis. These include recurrent pericarditis, cardiac tamponade, and constrictive pericarditis.

Key Treatment

Acute pericarditis

- Analgesics: Indomethacin, aspirin, or ibuprofen

Constrictive pericarditis

- Surgery: Pericardiectomy

Follow-Up

A. Acute pericarditis: Most episodes of acute pericarditis are self-limiting, with laboratory signs resolving in four to six weeks. Recurrent pericarditis is the most common complication (28 per cent) followed by cardiac tamponade and chronic pericarditis. Initial clinical follow-up may be as frequent as every two weeks. Prompt evaluation with echocardiography is warranted if the patient shows any clinical signs of tamponade.

B. Constrictive pericarditis: In the majority of patients (90 per cent), the hemodynamic and symptomatic relief is achieved in 2 to 6 months. Postsurgical follow-up is required to identify the 10 per cent who do not improve because of the causes mentioned above. Elderly patients, who are managed conservatively, also need frequent monitoring of their hemodynamic status.

Bibliography

For more information on constrictive pericarditis, see
Fowler NO: Constrictive pericarditis: New aspects. Am J Cardiol 1982;50:1014–1017.

For more information on hemodynamic alterations in cardiac tamponade, see
Shebetai R, Fowler NO, Guntheroth WG: The hemodynamics of cardiac tamponade and constrictive pericarditis. Am J Cardiol 1970;26:480–489.

For more information on acute pericarditis, pericardial effusion, and cardiac tamponade, see
Lorrell BH, Braunwald E: Pericardial disease. In Braunwald E (ed): Heart Disease, 4th ed. Philadelphia, WB Saunders Co., 1992, pp 1465–1516.
Shabetai R: Disease of the pericardium. In Schlant RC, Alexander RW (eds): The Heart. New York, McGraw-Hill, 1994, pp 1647–1674.
Spodick DH: Pericarditis, pericardial effusion, cardiac tamponade, and constriction. Crit Care Clin 1989;5:455–476.

67 Arrhythmias

Ram Jadonath

Arrhythmias Due to Conduction Disorders

1. First-degree atrioventricular (AV) block: Usually asymptomatic and no treatment required
2. Second-degree AV block
   a. Type I Wenckebach
      (1) Conduction defect usually supra-Hisian (AV node).
      · (2) May be transient.
      (3) Usually asymptomatic.
      (4) Can lead to dizziness, presyncope, syncope.
      (5) Treatment: None indicated if asymptomatic; prognosis good.
   b. Type II
      (1) Conduction defect usually infra-Hisian.
      (2) May be transient.
      (3) Symptoms include dizziness, lightheadedness, syncope.
      (4) More ominous prognosis.
      (5) Treatment: Permanent pacing may be required if no reversible etiology is found.
3. Complete heart block
   a. Atrial depolarizations not transmitted to ventricles.
   b. Ventricles depolarized by subsidiary pacemaker (nodal or infranodal)
   c. Etiology: degenerative diseases of conduction system, digitalis toxicity, congenital, myocardial ischemia/infarction, drugs, electrolyte imbalances, Lyme disease, infiltrative diseases, Chagas' disease
   d. Symptoms: May be asymptomatic or present with weakness, dizziness, syncope, hemodynamic instability.
   e. Treatment
      (1) If unstable: atropine, temporary pacing
      (2) If chronic or high likelihood of recurrence: permanent pacing
4. AV dissociation
   a. Atrial and ventricle beating independently.
   b. May be seen in supraventricular tachycardia (SVT), ventricular tachycardia (VT), atrioventricular (AV) block.
   c. Usually asymptomatic.
   d. Treatment: Correction of underlying cause.

Arrhythmias Involving the Sinus Node–Atrium

1. Sinus tachycardia
   a. Diagnosis
      (1) Rate is greater than 100 beats/min (bpm) and generally less than 170 bpm.
      (2) P wave precedes each QRS complex.
   b. Clinical features
      (1) Can be physiologic, pathologic, or pharmacologic.
      (2) Can lead to decreased cardiac output.
   c. Treatment
      (1) Correction of underlying etiology.
      (2) Fluid replacement in hypovolemic patient.
      (3) Low-dose β blocker in symptomatic volume-repleted patients.
2. Sinus bradycardia
   a. Diagnosis
      (1) Rate less than 60 bpm
      (2) Normal P-wave contour
   b. Clinical features
      (1) Physiologic: well-trained athletes, during sleep
      (2) Pathologic: increased vagal stimulation, increased intracranial pressure, hypothermia, myxedema, acute inferior myocardial infarction, convalescence from infection (typhoid, influenza)
      (3) Pharmacologic: usually asymptomatic for rates greater than 40 bpm
      (4) Symptoms include dizziness, weakness, fatigue, presyncope, and syncope.
   c. Treatment
      (1) If asymptomatic, no treatment necessary.
      (2) For symptomatic patients, permanent pacing may be indicated if no reversible cause found. Atropine 0.5 mg intravenously can be used acutely.
3. Sinus arrhythmia
   a. Diagnosis
      (1) Variation between longest and shortest sinus cycle length greater than 0.12 second
      (2) Phasic or nonphasic variation
   b. Clinical features
      (1) In phasic variation, cycle length accelerates with inspiration and slows with expiration.
      (2) Nonphasic variation may be related to alteration in vagal tone.
      (3) Normal findings
      (4) Symptoms unusual unless accompanied by long pauses.
   c. Treatment: usually unnecessary

271

4. Sinus pause/arrest
   a. Diagnosis: PP interval delimiting the pause is not a multiple of the basic PP interval.
   b. Clinical features
      (1) Excessive vagal tone, digitalis toxicity, degenerative fibrotic changes, acute myocardial infarction, drugs, electrolyte imbalances
      (2) Symptoms: If prolonged, can be associated with lightheadedness, dizziness, presyncope, or syncope.
   c. Treatment: Correct underlying cause. Permanent pacing may be necessary for pauses greater than 3 seconds.

5. Sinoatrial exit block
   a. Diagnosis: Duration of pause is a multiple of the basic PP interval.
   b. Clinical features
      (1) Failure of impulse propagation
      (2) Excessive vagal stimulation, acute myocarditis, myocardial ischemia/infarction, drugs, electrolyte imbalances, hyperkalemia
      (3) Symptoms: same as sinus pause.
   c. Treatment: for symptomatic patients, same as sinus pause

6. Wandering atrial pacemaker
   a. Diagnosis: variations of the RR interval, PR interval, and P-wave contour
   b. Clinical features
      (1) Excessive vagal tone
      (2) Symptoms: usually asymptomatic
   c. Treatment: None indicated, except in very symptomatic patients

7. Sick sinus syndrome
   a. Diagnosis: paroxysms of regular or irregular bradycardia and tachycardia (tachy-brady), sinus pause, sinoatrial exit block, and associated AV conduction disturbances
   b. Clinical features
      (1) Fibrotic, inflammatory, or degenerative changes involving sinus node/atria
      (2) Symptoms: dizziness, weakness, palpitations, near-syncope, or syncope
   c. Treatment: drugs to control the tachycardia and usually permanent pacing for symptomatic bradycardia or pause

8. Atrial fibrillation
   a. Diagnosis: small irregular baseline undulations at rates 350 to 600 bpm with irregular ventricular response
   b. Clinical features
      (1) Etiology depends on the type (chronic, paroxysmal, or lone). Common causes include hypertensive heart disease, valvular heart disease, cardiomyopathy, ischemic heart disease, congestive heart failure, pericarditis, pulmonary disease, pulmonary emboli, status post open heart surgery, alcoholism, infections and thyroid disease
      (2) Symptoms: palpitations, dizziness, dyspnea, other symptoms relating to decrease in cardiac output from loss of atrial contraction
   c. Treatment
      (1) Chronic anticoagulant therapy to reduce the risk of embolization. Aspirin 325 mg may be beneficial in patients younger than 75 years old with nonvalvular atrial fibrillation.
      (2) Correction of precipitating causes
      (3) Electrical cardioversion
      (4) AV node blocking drugs to slow ventricular response (digitalis, β blockers, calcium antagonists)
      (5) Class IA, IC, or III antiarrhythmic drugs for conversion and maintenance of sinus rhythm
      (6) In drug-refractory atrial fibrillation, AV node ablation with permanent pacing

9. Atrial flutter
   a. Diagnosis
      (1) Common type I: atrial rate 250 to 350 bpm. Sawtooth pattern (especially in leads II, III, aV_F). Ventricular response regular or irregular (variable block).
      (2) Uncommon type II: atrial rate 350 to 450 bpm.
   b. Clinical features: same as atrial fibrillation
   c. Treatment
      (1) Anticoagulation usually not necessary
      (2) Synchronous DC cardioversion
      (3) Rapid atrial pacing
      (4) AV node blocking drugs (digitalis, β blockers, calcium antagonists, Esmolol, intravenous diltiazem)
      (5) Class IA, IC, and III antiarrhythmics
      (6) Catheter ablation

10. Atrial tachycardia
    a. Diagnosis
       (1) Atrial rate 140 to 200 bpm. P-wave contour different from sinus rhythm, and there is an isoelectric interval between P waves.
       (2) May be secondary to increased automaticity or re-entry
    b. Clinical features
       (1) Sometimes difficult to differentiate from atrial flutter
       (2) Symptoms similar to atrial flutter
    c. Treatment

(1) Correct underlying cause (e.g., electrolytes, drug toxicity, hypoxia).

(2) Digitalis, β blockers, calcium antagonists

(3) Synchronized low-energy cardioversion in acutely symptomatic patients

(4) Class IA, IC, or III antiarrhythmic drugs for symptomatic chronic form

(5) Radiofrequency catheter ablation highly successful but the condition can recur.

11. Atrial tachycardia with block

a. Diagnosis: commonly 2:1 block but can be higher grade (4:1).

b. Clinical features: usually occur in setting of digitalis excess or toxicity, hypokalemia, lung disease

c. Treatment

(1) Potassium supplementation and hold digitalis

(2) Synchronize DC cardioversion in acutely symptomatic patients

(3) Digitalis (if not previously treated with this drug) or calcium antagonists

(4) Class IA, IC, or III antiarrhythmic drugs for chronic symptomatic form

(5) Radiofrequency catheter ablation

12. Multifocal (chaotic) atrial tachycardia

a. Diagnosis: rate 100 to 130 bpm with irregular variations in PP intervals and three or more P-wave morphologies

b. Clinical features: usually occur in setting of chronic obstructive lung disease or congestive heart failure

c. Treatment

(1) Correction of underlying cause

(2) Avoid β blockers if lung disease is present.

(3) Verapamil is effective.

(4) Digitalis tends to be ineffective.

13. Sinus node re-entrant tachycardia

a. Diagnosis

(1) Similar to sinus P wave

(2) Long RP interval, short PR interval

(3) Rates 80 to 200 bpm (generally 120 to 140 bpm).

(4) Tachycardia can persist despite AV block.

b. Clinical features

(1) Can be confused with sinus tachycardia

(2) Accounts for 5 to 10 per cent of supraventricular tachycardia

(3) Usually asymptomatic because of slower rate

c. Treatment

(1) β blockers, calcium antagonists, and digitalis are effective.

(2) Catheter ablation

Arrhythmias Involving the AV Node

1. AV junctional rhythm

a. Diagnosis

(1) Narrow complex regular or irregular escape rhythm at 30 to 60 bpm.

(2) P waves may be present (PR interval <0.12 second), absent, or retrograde.

b. Clinical features

(1) Can be stable rhythm

(2) Symptoms depend on rate and underlying heart disease.

(3) Common causes include myocardial ischemia/infarction, hypokalemia, digitalis excess/toxicity, and AV node blocking drugs.

c. Treatment

(1) Correction of underlying cause

(2) Temporary pacing if unstable

(3) Permanent pacing may be necessary.

2. AV junctional tachycardia

a. Diagnosis: nonparoxysmal, regular, narrow complex with rates 70 to 130 bpm

b. Clinical features: Common causes include digitalis toxicity, inferior myocardial infarction, myocarditis, acute rheumatic fever, and status post open heart surgery.

c. Treatment

(1) K^+ and Mg^{2+} supplementation

(2) If secondary to digitalis toxicity, withhold digoxin and administer K^+, lidocaine, or phenytoin.

(3) Class IA, IC, or III antiarrhythmic drugs or catheter ablation for chronic symptomatic type

3. Atrioventricular node re-entrant tachycardia

a. Diagnosis: narrow complex or wide complex (secondary to pre-existing or functional bundle branch block) tachycardia, 150 to 250 bpm. Two types:

(1) Typical (slow-fast) with short RP, long PR

(2) Atypical (fast-slow) with long RP, short PR

b. Clinical features

(1) Typical variety occurs in 95 per cent of cases.

(2) The P wave usually is within the QRS complex or at the end of the QRS.

(3) Frequently occurs in absence of structural heart disease.

(4) Typical symptoms include palpitations, anxiety, and presyncope.

c. Treatment

(1) Acute episode

(a) Sedation, rest, vagal maneuvers

(b) Intravenous verapamil, diltiazem, adenosine, edrophonium, or β blockers

(c) Class IA for refractory recurrent episode

(d) Rapid atrial or ventricular pacing

(e) Synchronized low-energy DC cardioversion for symptomatic drug-refractory type

(2) Prophylactic therapy

(a) Not necessary for minimally symptomatic and infrequent recurrences

(b) Catheter ablation highly successful

(c) Class IA, IC, or III antiarrhythmic drugs

(d) Antitachycardia pacing

(e) Surgical resection (now rare because of success of catheter ablation).

Arrhythmias Involving the Atrium and Ventricle

1. Atrioventricular re-entrant tachycardia

   a. Concealed (retrograde) atrioventricular bypass tract

   (1) Antegrade occurs via the AV node and retrograde conduction via the retrograde bypass tract. Narrow complex tachycardia (150 to 300 bpm) or wide complex due to pre-existing or functional bundle branch block; short RP.

   (2) Clinical features

   (a) Symptoms depend on rate

   (b) Usually no underlying heart disease

   (c) Can produce syncope

   (3) Treatment

   (a) Acute episode

   (i) Termination with vagal maneuvers, adenosine, verapamil, digitalis, β blockers, or calcium antagonists

   (ii) Low-energy synchronized DC cardioversion if unstable and unable to terminate with medications

   (iii) Rapid atrial or ventricular pacing also may terminate.

   (iv) Class IA, IC, or III antiarrhythmic drugs

   (b) Prophylactic

   (i) Class IA, IC, or III drugs

   (ii) Verapamil or digoxin not contraindicated if the bypass tract conducts retrograde only

   (iii) Catheter ablation curative

   b. Wolff-Parkinson-White (pre-excitation) syndrome

   (1) Short PR (<0.12 second). Slurring of initial portion of QRS complex (delta waves). Two types of tachycardia:

   (a) Antidromic tachycardia (wide complex) resulting from antegrade conduction via bypass tract and retrograde via AV node

   (b) Orthodromic, similar to concealed bypass tract

   (2) Clinical features

   (a) Similar to concealed bypass tract

   (b) Usually no underlying heart disease, but there is an association with Ebstein's anomaly, mitral valve prolapse, and cardiomyopathies.

   (c) Because of potential for antegrade conduction via bypass tract, patients who develop atrial tachyarrhythmias are at risk for ventricular fibrillation because of rapid antegrade conduction.

   (3) Treatment

   (a) Same as concealed bypass tract

   (b) Digitalis and verapamil contraindicated

   (c) In asymptomatic patients, no treatment may be necessary.

Ventricular Arrhythmias

1. Ventricular ectopic beats

   a. Single premature ventricular contractions (PVCs), multifocal PVCs, couplets, bigeminy, trigeminy, quadrigeminy. May or may not be associated with heart disease.

   b. Treatment

   (1) Generally not indicated unless symptomatic

   (2) Correct underlying cause (hypokalemia, hypomagnesemia, hypoxia, acidosis, fluid overload, ischemia, drug toxicity).

   (3) Lidocaine if the presentation is acute ischemia/infarction

   (4) Symptomatic patients: β blockers

   (5) Significantly symptomatic patients unresponsive to β blockers: electrophysiologic guided drug therapy.

2. Ventricular tachycardia

   a. Three or more beats in a row with QRS complex more than 0.11 second and rate 70 to 250 bpm. Usually regular but can be irregular. QRS complex may be monomorphic, multimorphic, or polymorphic. Nonsustained form lasts less than 30 seconds and sustained lasts greater than 30 seconds or associated with hemodynamic instability.

   b. Differential diagnosis: SVT with aberrancy

   c. Clinical features

   (1) Symptoms depend on rate, duration, and underlying heart disease.

   (2) Underlying causes include myocardial ischemia, infarction, congestive heart failure, cardiomyopathy, drugs, hypokalemia, and hypomagnesemia.

(3) Rarely occurs in normal heart.

d. Treatment

(1) Stable VT

(a) Precordial thump, intravenous lidocaine or procainamide

(b) If persists or unstable, synchronized DC cardioversion

(c) Correct underlying cause.

(d) Overdrive pacing

(2) Prevention of recurrences

(a) Electrophysiologic guided drug therapy (class IA, IB, IC, or III alone or in combination)

(b) Implantable cardioverter defibrillator

(c) Surgical resection, revascularization, catheter ablation

3. Other types of ventricular tachycardia

a. Torsades de pointes

(1) Changing QRS amplitude and twisting around isoelectric line. Prolong Q-T interval (>0.5 second).

(2) Etiology: congenital or acquired long Q-T; may be due to early afterdepolarization.

(3) Treatment

(a) Withhold responsible drugs (class IA, IC)

(b) Correct hypokalemia, hypomagnesemia, hypocalcemia.

(c) Temporary pacing and isoproterenol may be needed.

(d) Class IB drug may be efficacious.

(e) Other treatment as described for VT

b. Right ventricular outflow tract tachycardia

c. Bidirectional tachycardia: usually a result of digoxin toxicity

d. Bundle branch re-entrant tachycardia

e. Idiopathic left ventricular tachycardia

f. VT from arrhythmic right ventricular dysplasia

g. Accelerated idioventricular rhythm

(1) Rate 60 to 120 bpm, regular or irregular

(2) Causes: myocardial infarction, digitalis toxicity, reperfusion

(3) Clinical features: usually stable

(4) Treatment

(a) If stable and less than 100 bpm none required

(b) If unstable, same as for VT

4. Ventricular flutter and fibrillation

a. Diagnosis

(1) Rate 200 to 350 bpm

(2) Low and varying QRS amplitude and morphology

(3) Flutter has a sine wave appearance.

b. Clinical features

(1) Usually underlying heart disease present

(2) Less commonly, it can occur in normal hearts.

(3) Hemodynamic collapse invariably occurs.

c. Treatment

(1) Cardiopulmonary resuscitation and immediate nonsynchronized DC defibrillation (200 to 400 J)

(2) Correct the underlying cause.

(3) Preventing recurrences: electrophysiologic guided therapy, implantable cardioverter defibrillator

Bibliography

Josephson ME, Buxton AE, Marchlinski FE: The tachyarrhythmias. In Isselbacher KJ, Braunwald E, Wilson JD, et al (eds): Harrison's Principles of Internal Medicine, 13th ed. New York, McGraw-Hill, 1994, pp 1011–1019.

Josephson ME, Marchlinski FE, Buxton AE: The bradyarrhythmias: Disorders of sinus node function and AV conduction disturbances. In Isselbacher KJ, Braunwald E, Wilson JD, et al (eds): Harrison's Principles of Internal Medicine, 13th ed. New York, McGraw-Hill, 1994, pp 1019–1036.

Pritchett ELC: Management of atrial fibrillation. N Engl J Med 1992;326:1264–1271.

Prystowsky EN, Klein GJ: Supraventricular tachycardia. In Prystowsky EN, Klein GJ (eds): Cardiac Arrhythmias: An Integrated Approach for the Clinician. New York, McGraw-Hill, 1994, pp 99–130.

Zipes DP: Specific arrhythmias: Diagnosis and treatment. In Braunwald E (ed): Heart Disease. 4th ed. Philadelphia, WB Saunders, 1992, pp 667–725.

68 Varicose Veins

Mark A. Parkulo

Etiology

1. Definition: abnormally dilated, lengthened, or twisted superficial vessels usually caused by inefficient or defective venous valves. These vessels are most commonly found in the lower extremities.
2. Epidemiology: present in 30 to 60 per cent of adults
   a. The prevalence of the disease is higher in women. This is probably due to estrogen/progesterone influences on veins as well as changes that occur during pregnancy.
   b. There is an increasing incidence of development of varicose veins with age.
3. Risk factors
   a. Female gender
   b. History of deep venous thrombosis or insufficiency
   c. Pregnancy
   d. Local trauma
   e. Family history of varicose veins

Symptoms

1. Unsightly veins: Although this is the most common reason for patient presentation, a careful history often reveals some of the other symptoms recorded below.
2. Achy, burning legs: The pain may be disproportionate to the degree of visible pathologic change. Patients with small early varicosities may complain more than patients with large chronic ones. These symptoms are usually worse in warm weather, with prolonged standing, during menstruation, during pregnancy, with exogenous hormones, and following intercourse.
3. Night cramps
4. Restless legs
5. Leg swelling
6. Venous ulceration

Clinical Findings

1. Dilated superficial veins
2. Edema
3. Cutaneous pigmentation, stasis dermatitis
4. Cutaneous ulceration

Laboratory Tests

1. The diagnosis can usually be made by careful history and physical examination. Important historical findings not related to varicosities include history of arterial disease, diabetes, and deep venous thrombosis. Inquiries concerning the progression of the patient's disease and previous treatment are also helpful. Physical findings of concomitant arterial disease or neuropathy are important. Patients who have a history or physical findings suggestive of deep venous thrombosis (DVT), arterial occlusive disease, or diabetes require further evaluation to determine whether their symptoms are related to these processes and not due to varices.
2. Noninvasive vascular testing
   a. Continuous wave Doppler: This hand-held device is extremely helpful in the evaluation of varicose veins by an experienced operator. Evaluation of several specific sites (e.g., saphenofemoral junction, saphenopopliteal junction) in the lower extremity for patency, flow, valve competency, phasicity, pulsatility, and augmentation is helpful in determining the underlying cause of varicose veins and in the assessment for possible obstruction.
   b. If obstruction is suspected other tests such as impedance plethysmography and venous duplex scanning should be performed.
   c. Further assessment of venous insufficiency can be performed with exercise plethysmography, photoplethysmography, or venous duplex scanning.

Differential Diagnosis

1. Deep venous thrombosis
2. Arterial occlusive disease
3. Diabetes

Treatment

Treatment depends on the extent of the varicose veins, the underlying pathologic mechanisms, and the overall medical status of the patient. Pregnancy is a contraindication to treatment of varicose veins since many will resolve without treatment following the resolution of pregnancy.

1. Conservative management
   a. Hosiery: Elastic compression stockings relieve symptoms, conceal veins, and prevent deterioration but do not cure the disease. These should be graduated stockings with the greatest compression at the ankle and less compression higher. Ideally, these stockings should be individually fitted to the patient. A foam pad for increased compression, especially around the ankle, is sometimes helpful. These stockings should be worn continuously while the patient is upright. Compression bandaging is also an option, but it is often difficult to get adequate graduated compression with this method. Patient compliance with hosiery wearing is often problematic due to difficulty with placement and discomfort while wearing.
   b. Elevation of extremities
   c. Good local skin care

2. Sclerotherapy (see following procedure on Sclerotherapy of Varicose Veins): This technique of injecting varicose veins with a sclerosing substance is probably most beneficial in patients with smaller varicosities without junctional incompetence, patients with telangiectasias only, and patients with persistent or recurrent varicosities following surgery. Contraindications to sclerotherapy include pregnancy, hypersensitivity to sclerosant, moderate-to-severe arterial occlusive disease, diabetes, hypercoagulable states, and severe obesity. Complications can include hyperpigmentation, cutaneous necrosis, DVT, pulmonary embolism, and allergic reaction to sclerosant.

3. Surgical treatment: Several surgical options are available depending on the location and underlying mechanism of the varicosity. Many of these surgical procedures can have excellent cosmetic results due to the very small "stab" incisions used to perform the surgery. Indications for surgery are large varicosities, junctional reflux, and varicosities in the medial or anterior thigh. Contraindications include high-risk medical patients, moderate-to-severe arterial occlusive disease, lymphedema, skin infection, coagulopathy, and pregnancy. Complications include excessive scarring, wound infection, cutaneous pigmentation, superficial thrombophlebitis, deep venous thrombosis, pulmonary embolus, and recurrence of varicosities.

Follow-Up

1. Regular follow-up for patients who are conservatively treated is a must to assess for progression of disease and attempt to prevent cutaneous ulceration. This is especially important due to patient compliance issues.

2. Regular follow-up in the postsclerotherapy and postsurgical period is also important to assess for effectiveness of therapy and possible need for further treatment. Further sclerotherapy may be needed to obliterate remaining varicosities.

Bibliography

Gloviczki P, Merrell SW: Surgical treatment of venous diseases. Cardiovasc Clin 1992;22(3):82–98.

Goldman MP, Weiss RA, Bergan MM: Diagnosis and treatment of varicose veins: A review. J Am Acad Dermatol 1994; 31(3):393–413.

Hobbs JT: Varicose veins. ABC of vascular diseases. Br Med J 1991;303(6804):707–710.

Ramelet AA: Primer of phlebology. Int J Dermatol 1992; 31(12):833–839.

Rooke TW: The noninvasive vascular laboratory. Cardiovasc Clin 1992;22(3):27–41.

Procedure **SCLEROTHERAPY OF VARICOSE VEINS**   *Mark Parkulo*

Indications

1. Cosmesis: Although this is a common reason for patient presentation, reimbursement for this indication from insurance companies is often problematic.

2. Symptomatic varicose veins: Symptoms include aching, lower extremity pain, burning, restless legs, heavy legs. Many patients will notice improvement in these symptoms even if they are not the principal reason for their visit.

3. Signs of venous insufficiency: Signs include edema, stasis dermatitis, hyperpigmentation, and ulceration.

Contraindications

1. Pregnancy
2. Breast-feeding
3. History of deep venous thrombosis (DVT) or pulmonary embolism
4. Inability to ambulate immediately after procedure
5. Hypersensitivity to sclerosing agents
6. For patients taking Antabuse, the sclerosing agent used should not contain ethyl alcohol.

Preparation

1. Initial evaluation: History with emphasis on vascular system

   a. Previous venous surgery or sclerotherapy
   b. Lower extremity trauma or DVT
   c. Temporal progression of venous disease
   d. Symptoms and severity of symptoms
   e. Family history of venous, arterial, or lymphatic disease
   f. Allergies

2. Physical examination: Identify major reflux points.

   a. Saphenofemoral junction: usually best treated with surgical intervention
   b. Saphenopopliteal junction
   c. Incompetent perforators

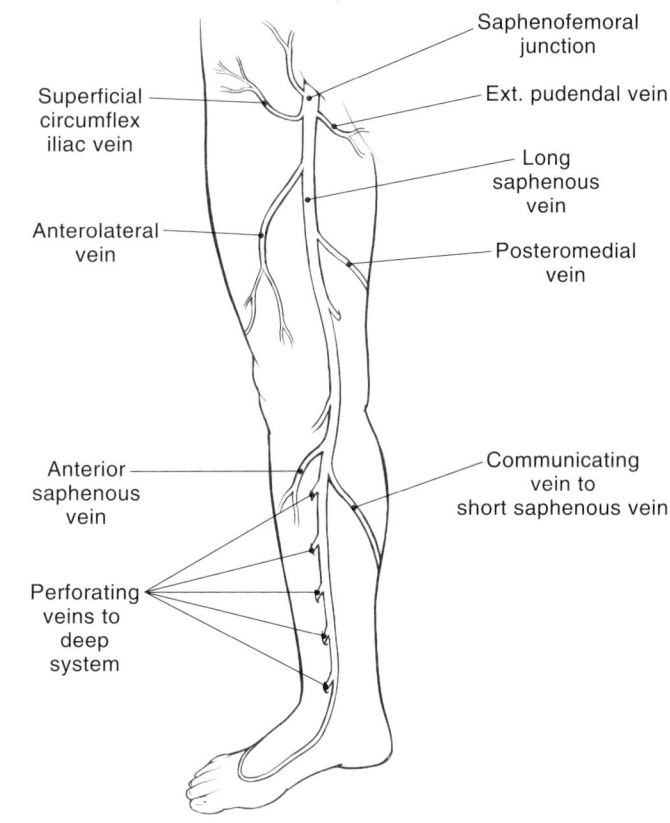

MAJOR SUPERICIAL VEINS OF LOWER
EXTREMITY–ANTERIOR

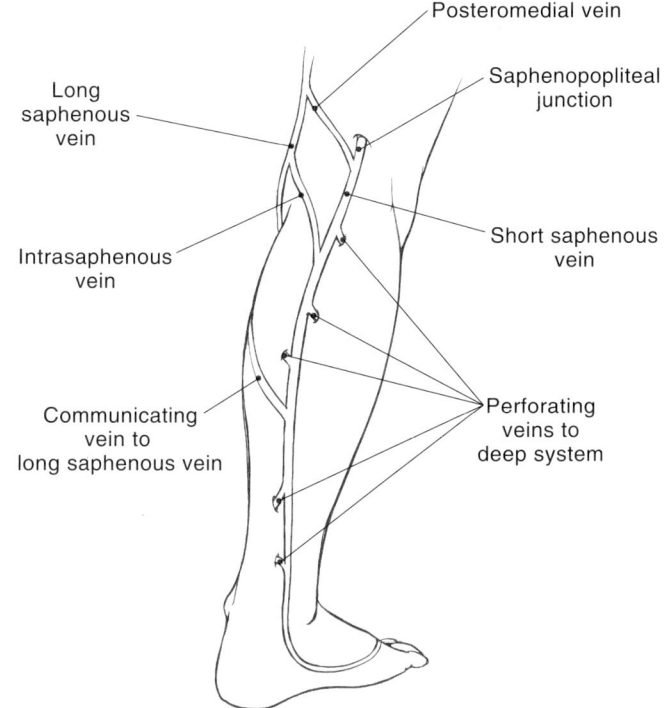

MAJOR SUPERFICIAL VEINS OF LOWER
EXTREMITY–POSTERIOR

3. Noninvasive testing: Due to the considerable anatomic variability of the venous system, noninvasive testing is extremely important in the evaluation

   a. Bidirectional Doppler evaluation

      (1) Identifies superficial junctional reflux

      (2) Can differentiate between superficial and deep venous incompetence

   b. If bidirectional Doppler is abnormal, consider duplex scanning, varicography, or photoplethysmography.

Equipment

1. Syringe

   a. Any commercially available plastic syringe can be used, preferably 3 to 5 cc in volume.

   b. Some physicians prefer an eccentric hub to facilitate easier entry into superficial veins.

   c. To facilitate needle changing, a nonlocking hub is preferable.

2. Needle or butterfly cannula

   a. Usually a small-gauge needle such as 26- to 33-gauge

   b. Almost any commercially available type can be used.

3. Alcohol swabs

4. Compression stocking: 30 to 40 mm Hg compression

5. Sclerosing solution: There are only three FDA-approved solutions in the United States. I will discuss these three and several other solutions commonly used in Europe and Canada. I will give some common dilutions of several sclerosants as a guideline. I recommend that you consult the package insert and distributor for further information. I will also give recommendations for sclerosants, although it is probably most prudent to use the sclerosant with which you are most familiar.

   a. Sodium tetradecyl sulfate (Na 1-isobutyl-4-ethyl-octyl sulfate)

      (1) *Advantages*

         (a) FDA approved

         (b) Low incidence of systemic reactions

      (2) *Disadvantages*

         (a) Epidermal necrosis if injected extravascularly, especially at higher concentrations. Correct dilution is important in limiting cutaneous reactions.

         (b) Allergic reactions have been reported occasionally.

      (3) *Concentrations commonly used*

         (a) 0.1 to 0.3% for telangiectasias up to 1 mm in diameter

         (b) 0.5 to 1.0% for veins 2 to 4 mm in diameter

         (c) 1.5 to 3.0% for larger veins, including the saphenofemoral junction and incompetent perforating veins

      (4) *Maximum recommended dose* per session is 5 cc of 3% solution.

   b. Ethanolamine oleate (synthetic mixture of ethanolamine and oleic acid)

      (1) *Advantages*

         (a) FDA approved

         (b) Low incidence of allergic reactions

      (2) *Disadvantages*

         (a) Nonspecific reactions including red blood cell hemolysis

         (b) One case of acute renal failure was reported when a large volume of solution was injected.

      (3) *Maximum recommended dosage* per session is 10 cc of 0.5% solution.

   c. Sodium morrhuate (mixture of sodium salts of fatty acids)

      (1) *Advantages*

         (a) FDA approved

         (b) Useful for large varicosities due to strong sclerosing ability

      (2) *Disadvantages*

         (a) Cutaneous necrosis if injected extravascularly

         (b) Anaphylactic reactions are reported more commonly than with other solutions. Deaths rarely have been reported.

   d. Polidocanol (hydroxypolyethoxydodecane in distilled water with ethyl alcohol 5% added to solution)

      (1) *Advantages*

         (a) Good safety profile due to quick distribution and elimination

         (b) Painless injection

         (c) Low risk of cutaneous ulceration

         (d) Lower incidence of hyperpigmentation

      (2) *Disadvantages*

         (a) Not FDA approved

         (b) Not as strong a sclerosant as some other agents used in varicosities

         (c) Rare allergic reaction

      (3) *Recommended concentration* of solution

         (a) 0.25 to 0.75% for telangiectasias

         (b) 1% for veins 1 to 2 mm in diameter

         (c) 2% for veins 2 to 4 mm in diameter

         (d) 3% for veins 4 to 8 mm in diameter

         (e) 4% for saphenofemoral junction and saphenopopliteal junction

      (4) *Maximum recommended dose* per session is 5 cc of 3.0% solution.

   e. Chromated glycerine

      (1) *Advantages*

         (a) Weak sclerosing agent, most useful for telangiectasias

         (b) Less incidence of hyperpigmentation

         (c) Less incidence of skin necrosis if injected extravascularly

(2) *Disadvantages*

(a) Not FDA approved

(b) Local pain on injection; can be overcome by adding lidocaine to solution.

(c) Hematuria or ureteral colic have been reported theoretically due to hemolysis of red blood cells. This has occurred only after injection of large volumes of solution.

(d) Transient ocular manifestations of blurred vision have also been reported.

(3) *Maximum recommended dose* is 0.1 cc of pure solution per session.

f. Hypertonic saline (18 to 30%)

(1) *Advantage:* Nonallergenic

(2) *Disadvantages*

(a) Skin necrosis if injected extravascularly

(b) Local pain. Addition of lidocaine has been reported to reduce incidence.

(c) Transient muscle cramping

(d) Increased incidence of post-treatment hyperpigmentation

(e) Ineffective in treating large varicosities

(f) Case reports of hypertension or congestive heart failure if excessive volume is used due to sodium bolus

(3) *Solution concentration* used

(a) 18 to 25% for small telangiectasias

(b) 25 to 30% for telangiectasias 4 to 5 mm in diameter

(c) Rarely effective for vessels larger than 5 mm in diameter

(4) *Maximum recommended dose* per session is 5 cc of 20% solution.

g. Hypertonic dextrose and sodium (250 mg/ml dextrose, NaCl 100 mg/ml, propylene glycol 100 mg/ml, and phenethyl alcohol 8 mg/ml)

(1) *Advantage:* Addition of dextrose and decreased concentration of sodium chloride help

to decrease pain and discomfort as compared to hypertonic saline.

(2) *Disadvantages*

(a) Similar to hypertonic saline with above noted advantages

(b) Allergic reactions to alcohol can occur.

(3) *Maximum recommended dosage per site* is 1 cc

(4) *Maximum recommended dosage per session* is 10 cc

h. **Recommendations**

(1) Of the three FDA sclerosants approved, sodium tetradecyl sulfate is the most versatile and useful with the best side effect profile when used in appropriate concentrations.

(2) Polidocanol, a widely used sclerosant in Europe, has the best side effect profile (especially for inexperienced practitioners due to a very low incidence of cutaneous necrosis when extravasated) and is especially useful for telangiectasias. It is not FDA approved, however.

6. Magnifying loops

7. Crash cart: Resuscitation equipment is essential due to the possibility of severe reactions.

8. Camera

9. Consent forms

Precautions

1. Complications of the procedure can include allergic reactions, DVT, thrombophlebitis, and cutaneous necrosis.

2. Side effects include edema, pain, cutaneous hyperpigmentation, capillary telangiectasia, localized urticaria, blisters, and folliculitis. These are usually self-limited, but hyperpigmentation can persist.

3. Inadvertent arterial injection can cause acute arterial thrombosis either at injection site or further downstream. Areas of concern include

a. Posterior tibial artery in medial malleolar region due to proximity to vein

b. Saphenofemoral junction

Technique

Telangiectasias

1. Preparation prior to injection

a. Inform patient of risks and benefits of procedure. Have patient sign consent form. (Some publications listed in the Bibliography contain examples of consent forms.)

b. Photograph areas to be treated. This is important for comparison after treatment both for medicolegal reasons and for the patient's satisfaction be-

cause patients may not remember exactly how areas appeared prior to the procedure.

2. Patient is placed in prone, supine, or lateral decubitus position, depending on the site of the vein being treated.

3. Leg may be elevated to reduce venous distention.

4. Area is cleansed with alcohol swabs.

5. Enter vein quickly. The needle may be bent at an angle to facilitate entry into cutaneous veins. The free hand is used to stabilize the vein to reduce local trauma.

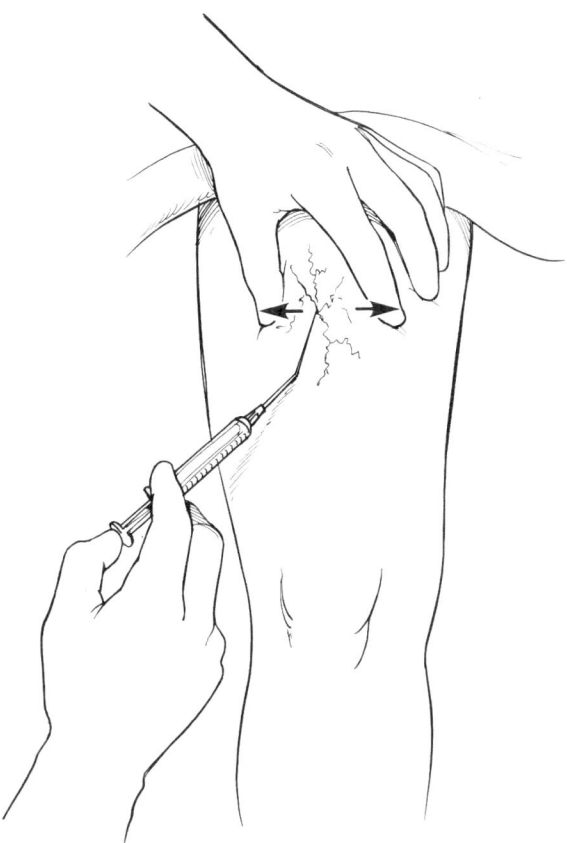

6. Withdraw on syringe plunger to assess for blood return and ensure proper placement in the vein.

7. Inject sclerosing solution. This can proceed slowly. The quantity of sclerosing solution depends on the size of the vein being treated. The typical quantity injected at one site is 0.5 to 1 cc. Often, experience is helpful in guiding the amount of sclerosant to be injected.

8. Remove needle quickly.

9. Exert pressure over area to prevent reflux into vein and enhance the chances of vein resorption. A small bandage may be placed over the injection site.

10. Postsclerotherapy compression: Although controversial, compression therapy following a session of sclerosing is theoretically effective, with few drawbacks except for cost.

    a. Compression stocking 30 to 40 mm Hg: This is probably the greatest amount of compression that patients will tolerate.

    b. Some have advocated compression bandages, but it is difficult to obtain consistent compression with a bandage alone.

    c. A small bandage and foam padding at the site of injection can also be used to increase compression, especially for telangiectasias of the thigh.

    d. The stockings are believed to be beneficial even if only telangiectasias are injected, but no controlled studies have been performed on this matter.

    e. The stocking should be worn every day, except

for bathing, for 2 to 3 days. There is disagreement as to whether the stocking should be worn at night, although some patients may not tolerate constant compression.

    f. Caution should be used in treating patients with arterial disease with compression stockings.

11. Patient should ambulate after procedure is completed.

Varicose Veins

1. Preparation of the patient should proceed as outlined for telangiectasias.

2. Several strategies are available for sclerotherapy of large varicosities. Two strategies (Tournay's and Fegan's) rely upon treatment of high-pressure inflow areas prior to treating the varicosity, whereas the Sigg technique relies upon random injection along the entire varicosity.

    a. *Tournay's technique*

       (1) Identify major reflux points through physical examination and noninvasive testing.

           (a) Saphenofemoral junction incompetence

           (b) Saphenopopliteal junction incompetence

           (c) Incompetent perforating veins

           (d) Incompetent communicating veins

       (2) Treat incompetent vessels starting with proximal vessels and continuing distally.

           (a) Most experts recommend surgical treatment for the saphenofemoral junction incompetence. Four weeks following surgical treatment, sclerotherapy can be used for remaining varicosities.

           (b) Saphenopopliteal and incompetent perforators can be effectively treated with sclerotherapy alone.

       (3) Reanalyze after several weeks and treat other smaller varicose vessels as needed.

    b. *Fegan's technique*

       (1) Identify incompetent perforating veins first and treat these areas.

       (2) Reanalyze after several weeks and treat other smaller varicosities as required.

    c. *Sigg's technique:* Treat entire varicosity with injections at several sites along vein without regard for underlying pathophysiology. This is usually performed with an injection every 4 to 6 cm along the entire varicosity.

3. Injection technique: Injection technique is variable from one phlebologist to another. Some overall guidelines are presented below. Numerous variations of these techniques also are effective.

    a. Standing/reclining technique

       (1) With patient standing and vein distended, needle is inserted quickly into the vein.

       (2) Needle is secured with tape or by hand.

(3) Patient reclines and leg is elevated to decrease venous distention.

(4) Withdraw plunger to ensure blood return and correct needle placement after movement of limb.

(5) Inject sclerosant slowly.

(6) Remove needle quickly.

(7) Apply immediate compression of area.

(8) Apply postsclerotherapy compression as outlined in section on telangiectasias.

b. Fegan's technique

(1) Similar to standing/reclining

(2) Patient sits on examination table with legs dangling. Theoretically, having the patient sit reduces the risk of a fall if vasovagal syncope occurs during needle insertion.

(3) Physician sits on low stool in front of the patient.

(4) Needle is inserted.

(5) Patient reclines, and leg is elevated and supported on physician's shoulder.

(6) The rest of the technique is the same as the standing/reclining technique.

(7) One can either insert all needles while veins are distended or insert the needles separately repeating the technique many times. If the needles are inserted separately, the veins of the previously treated areas need to be compressed distally to prevent their refilling with blood.

(8) Some physicians prefer to only mark the veins while they are distended and then to insert the needle when the patient has reclined. Others believe that it is more difficult to cannulate the vein with this technique.

Follow-Up

1. Re-evaluation in two weeks to be certain thrombosis is not present. If present the thrombus should be removed. A post-procedure photograph should be taken at this time and at the 6-week follow-up.

2. No further therapy at same site until 6 weeks following prior treatment to allow adequate healing time. It is possible to treat different sites prior to this 6-week interval, however.

3. If the vein is not completely sclerosed at 6 weeks, a second attempt can be performed with adjustment of sclerosant concentration as needed.

Bibliography

deGroot WP: Practical phlebology. Sclerotherapy of large veins. J Dermatol Surg Oncol 1991;17(7):589–595.

Duffy DM: Setting up a vein treatment center—incorporating sclerotherapy into the dermatologic practice. Semin Dermatol 1993;12(2):150–158.

Goldman MP: Sclerotherapy: Treatment of Varicose Veins and Telangiectatic Leg Veins. St. Louis, Mosby–Year Book, 1991.

Green D: Sclerotherapy for varicose and telangiectatic veins. Amer Fam Phys 1992;46(3):827–837.

Marley WM, Marley NF: Sclerotherapy treatment of varicose veins. Semin Dermatol 1993;12(2):98–101.

69 Deep Venous Thrombosis

David J. Tanaka

Etiology

1. Virchow, in 1856, cited three factors that lead to thrombosis.
   a. Stasis: Common causes of stasis are
      (1) Bed rest secondary to illness or surgery
      (2) Prolonged sitting on a plane or automobile
      (3) Paralysis or paresis
   b. Vessel wall injury or abnormality
      (1) The most common cause is hip or knee surgery. Hip or knee replacement without deep venous thrombosis (DVT) prophylaxis is associated with approximately 50 per cent incidence of postoperative DVT.
      (2) Chemical (chemotherapeutic, radiocontrast, or blood pressor agents) or infectious agents
   c. Hypercoagulability
      (1) Antithrombin III, protein C, and protein S deficiencies
      (2) Dysfibrinogenemia
      (3) Antiphospholipid antibodies (lupus anticoagulant) sometimes indicated by an increased activated partial thromboplastin time (aPTT)
      (4) Trauma and surgery
2. Other risk factors
   a. Advancing age
   b. Pregnancy and pharmacologic doses of estrogen
   c. Malignancy, especially adenocarcinoma of lung, breast, and viscera
   d. Polycythemia

Symptoms

Symptoms of DVT are often nonspecific. Many DVTs are asymptomatic.
1. Pain in a limb made worse by standing or walking and better with rest and elevation
2. Swelling of the lower extremity sometimes associated with varicosities, edema, and/or cyanosis

Key Symptoms

- Pain
- Swelling

Clinical Findings

Physical examination for DVT is insensitive and nonspecific. Proximal DVT is associated with an approximately 50 per cent incidence of pulmonary embolism, which is often asymptomatic.

1. Swelling of the affected lower extremity above or below the knee. This can be verified by measuring and comparing extremity circumferences.
2. Unilateral edema
3. Homans' sign (calf pain on dorsiflexion of the foot with the knee slightly flexed): present in only 10 to 20 per cent of the cases of DVT and also seen with any cause of calf inflammation.
4. Fever has been found in patients with proximal DVT, possibly secondary to undiagnosed pulmonary embolism.

Key Signs

- Swelling documented by measurement
- Unilateral edema
- Fever

Laboratory Tests

1. There are no blood tests for DVT.
2. Noninvasive tests: Either of these should be the initial diagnostic test for proximal DVT in a symptomatic patient.
   a. Impedance plethysmography (IPG): This test measures the rate of venous drainage from the lower extremity. If there is an acute proximal thrombosis, the drainage will be impaired and the test will be abnormal.
      (1) IPG has a sensitivity and specificity of approximately 90 per cent in diagnosing proximal DVT in symptomatic patients.
      (2) Causes of false-positive results are conditions that inhibit venous drainage, such as pregnancy, congestive heart failure, and obesity.
      (3) IPG is not useful in evaluating calf DVT.
      (4) IPG may be the noninvasive test of choice for evaluating for recurrent DVT because the majority of patients (90 per cent) normalize their IPG within 6 to 12 months after an acute DVT.
   b. Ultrasonography: The tests utilizing ultrasonography are real-time ultrasonography, duplex scanning and color-flow Doppler ultrasonography. The criteria used to diagnose DVT by these methods is the failure of the venous lumen, as identified by real-time ultrasonography to fully collapse under gentle pressure from the transducer probe.
      (1) Duplex scanning and color-flow Doppler add Doppler information to assist in identifying the venous system.

(2) Ultrasonography by real-time, duplex, or color-flow Doppler have sensitivities and specificities of 90+ per cent in diagnosing proximal DVT in symptomatic patients.

(3) They are all more operator dependent than IPG.

(4) Ultrasonography may not be as useful as IPG in evaluation of recurrent DVT because the affected veins remain incompressible in many cases.

3. Ascending contrast venography: This is the gold standard for the diagnosis of proximal and distal DVT. Venography does have many disadvantages.

a. Approximately 10 per cent of studies will be inadequate for interpretation or unable to be performed for technical reasons.

b. The test causes a DVT after approximately 2 to 3 per cent of studies.

c. There is the risk of a hypersensitivity reaction.

d. The test is uncomfortable for the patient.

e. The test may cause renal insufficiency or congestive heart failure in susceptible patients.

f. The test is the most costly of the diagnostic tests for DVT.

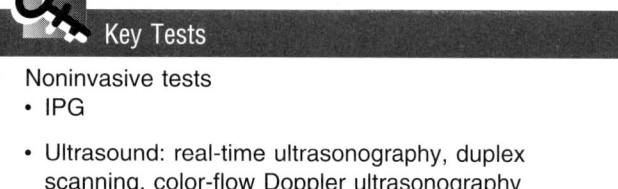

Key Tests

Noninvasive tests
• IPG

• Ultrasound: real-time ultrasonography, duplex scanning, color-flow Doppler ultrasonography

• Ascending contrast venography: Gold standard for diagnosis of DVT

Differential Diagnosis

1. Cellulitis

2. Superficial thrombophlebitis and lymphangitis

3. Ruptured popliteal synovial membrane or cyst (Baker's): The main difference between this and a DVT is that a ruptured cyst usually occurs in the setting of an arthritic knee.

4. Muscle strain or rupture (plantaris or gastrocnemius muscles): The mechanism of injury is the main differentiating clue between these disorders and DVT.

5. Postphlebitic syndrome: This is usually a chronic disorder, but can present with symptoms similar to those of an acute DVT.

Treatment

A. Treatment of choice

1. Heparin: Heparin is the treatment of choice for acute DVT. Heparin binds to antithrombin III and increases its antithrombotic activity, which prevents further thrombosis and extension of the clot.

a. Initiate heparin therapy with a 5,000 to 10,000 unit intravenous bolus and start maintenance infusion at 1300 units/hour. Check aPTT at 6 hours to keep aPTT between 1.5–2.5 times control. See Table 69–1, Guidelines for Anticoagulation, and Table 69–2, Intravenous Heparin: Monitoring and Adjusting Dosage.

TABLE 69–1. GUIDELINES FOR ANTICOAGULATION

DISEASE	GUIDELINE
Suspected	Give heparin 500 U IV and order imaging study
Confirmed	Rebolus with heparin 5–10,000 U IV and start maintenance infusion at 1300 U/hr (heparin 20,000 U in 500-ml D₅W, infused at 33 ml/hr)
	Check aPTT at 6 hr to keep aPTT between 1.5–2.5 times control
	Check platelet count daily
	Start warfarin therapy on day 1 at 10 mg daily for first 2 day, then administer warfarin daily at estimated daily maintenance dose
	Stop heparin therapy after 5 to 7 day of joint therapy when INR is 2.0–3.0 off heparin
	Anticoagulate with warfarin for 3 mo at an INR of 2.0–3.0

From Hyers TM, Hull RD, Weg JG: Antithrombotic therapy for venous thromboembolic disease. Chest 1992;102(suppl):408S–425S.

TABLE 69–2. INTRAVENOUS HEPARIN: MONITORING AND ADJUSTING DOSAGE*

APTT, s†	RATE CHANGE, ml/hr	DOSE CHANGE, U/24 hr	ADDITIONAL ACTION	NEXT APTT
≤45	+6	+5,760	Rebolus with 5,000 U	4–6 hr
46–54	+3	+2,880	None	4–6 hr
55–85‡	0	0	None	Next morning§
86–110	−3	−2,880	Stop infusion 1 hr	4–6 hr after restart
>110	−6	−5,760	Stop infusion 1 hr	4–6 hr after restart

*A starting bolus of 5000–10,000 U is given IV followed by IV infusion of 1,300 U/hr (heparin 20,000 U in 500 ml D₅W at approximately 33 ml/hr). The concentration of heparin is 40 U/ml. When aPTT is checked at 6 h or longer, steady-state kinetics can be assumed. Dosage adjustments are made according to the protocol.
†Normal aPTT range with Dade-Actin FS reagent of 27 to 35 sec.
‡The therapeutic range of 55–85 sec is roughly equivalent to a plasma heparin concentration range of 0.2–0.4 U/ml by protamine titration or to 0.35–0.7 U/ml by inhibition of factor Xa. The therapeutic range will vary with different aPTT reagents and coagulation machines.
§During the first 24 hr, repeat aPTT in 4–6 hr. Thereafter, monitor aPTT daily unless it is subtherapeutic.
From Hyers TM, Hull RD, Weg JG: Antithrombotic therapy for venous thromboembolic disease. Chest 1992;102(suppl):408S–425S.

b. Failure to achieve an adequate anticoagulant response (aPTT >1.5 times control) is associated with a 20 to 25 per cent recurrence of venous thromboembolism.

c. The main risk of heparin therapy is bleeding and thrombocytopenia. Thrombocytopenia associated with thrombosis, often arterial, is seen less commonly.

d. Osteoporosis is a risk for more prolonged heparin therapy.

2. Coumarin compounds: Warfarin or dicumarol, an oral anticoagulant, may be started once the heparin is therapeutic (usually day 1). The anticoagulant effect of coumarin compounds is measured by the prothrombin time (PT) and the international normalized ratio (INR). The therapeutic range for the INR is 2.0–3.0.

   a. Start warfarin at 10 mg for 1 or 2 days, then administer at estimated daily maintenance dose. See Table 69–1, Guidelines for Anticoagulation.

   b. Anticoagulate with warfarin for 3 months at an INR of 2.0–3.0.

Alternative Treatments

1. Inferior vena caval interruption

   a. The major indication is the presence of a proximal DVT in a patient in whom anticoagulation is contraindicated.

   b. Less common indications are

     (1) Recurrent thromboembolism despite adequate anticoagulation

     (2) Presence of a large free-floating caval thrombus

     (3) Chronic recurrent embolism with pulmonary hypertension

2. Thrombolytic agents: The use of thrombolytic agents have the theoretic advantage of lysing the thrombus and hopefully preserving the venous valves. There is conflicting evidence that thrombolytics may decrease the incidence of postphlebitic syndrome. Because of the increased risk of bleeding and inadequate evidence of benefit, thrombolytics cannot be routinely recommended at this time.

Special Cases

1. Isolated calf venous thrombosis should be treated with anticoagulation for 3 months. If anticoagulation is not given, serial noninvasive studies of the lower extremity should be performed for 10 to 14 days to assess for proximal extension of the thrombus.

2. Patients with recurrent thromboembolism or continuing risk factor (hypercoagulable state) should be treated indefinitely.

Medication

1. Patients should check their warfarin tablets to verify size and consistent manufacturer and take exactly as prescribed.

2. Warfarin should be taken at the same time every day.

3. All new medicines or changes in medicines should be reported to their doctor immediately.

Diet

The diet should contain a consistent amount of vitamin K (70 to 140 micrograms) during warfarin therapy.

1. Avoid substantial changes in diet.

2. Avoid food high in vitamin K.

   a. Liver

   b. Tea (green)

   c. Green leafy vegetables: broccoli, brussel sprouts, cauliflower, chickpeas, kale, spinach, turnip greens

   d. Permissible vegetables: lettuce, cabbage, asparagus, green beans

Activity

1. During hospitalization, the affected extremity should be elevated as much as possible and the patient may ambulate as tolerated. After discharge, the patient should gradually resume normal activities but avoid prolonged sitting or standing.

2. Avoid any contact sport that exposes the patient to risk of serious injury during warfarin therapy.

Patient Education

1. Patient compliance is crucial for effective and safe anticoagulation.

2. Patients should alert the physician if they have any unusual bleeding (e.g., excessive bleeding from gums, nose, or vagina, hematuria, melena, or excessive bruising).

3. Patients need to inform their physicians if they are planning on becoming or have become pregnant.

4. Any travel should be discussed with the physician in advance.

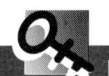

Key Treatment

Treatment of choice	Alternative treatment
• Heparin	• Inferior vena caval interruption
• Coumarin compounds	• Thrombolytic agents

Follow-Up

1. Patients need to have regular prothrombin/INR testing to monitor warfarin therapy.

2. Noninvasive venous testing is not routinely done after an acute DVT. If postphlebitic syndrome is suspected, noninvasive venous studies can document the degree and location of venous insufficiency.

Bibliography

For more information on the treatment of DVT, see
Hyers TM, Hull RD, Weg JG: Antithrombotic therapy for venous thromboembolic disease. Chest 1992;102(suppl):408S–425S.

For more information on the diagnosis of DVT, see
Richlie DG: Noninvasive imaging of the lower extremity for deep venous thrombosis. J Gen Intern Med 1993;8:271–277.

For more information on distal or calf DVT, see
Powers LR: Distal deep vein thrombosis: What's the best treatment? J Gen Intern Med 1988;3:288–293.

For more information on heparin therapy, see
Hirsh J, Dalen JE, Deykin D, Poller L: Heparin: Mechanism of action, pharmacokinetics, dosing considerations, monitoring, efficacy, and safety. Chest 1992;102(suppl):337S–351S.

For more information on warfarin therapy, see
Hirsh J, Dalen JE, Deykin D, Pollar L: Oral anticoagulants: Mechanism of action, clinical effectiveness, and optimal therapeutic range. Chest 1992;102(suppl):312S–326S.

70 Peripheral Arterial Disease

Chris Goerdt

Etiology and Epidemiology

1. Atherosclerosis causes the majority of peripheral arterial disease (PAD).

2. PAD most commonly involves the lower extremities and presents after the fifth decade of life.

3. Approximately 1 to 2 per cent of the adult population and 10 per cent of those over age 70 have symptomatic disease.

4. Risk factors: smoking (most important), diabetes, hyperlipidemia, and hypertension.

5. Ten per cent of patients with lower extremity PAD also have high-grade carotid artery stenoses and 50 per cent have high-grade coronary artery stenoses.

6. Progressive deterioration occurs in 15 to 20 per cent of patients, but less than 5 per cent require an amputation. Smoking and diabetes markedly increase the risk of deterioration and the need for surgery.

7. The presence of lower extremity PAD determined by an ankle/brachial systolic blood pressure ratio <0.9 more than triples the risk of mortality for both symptomatic and asymptomatic patients. Cardiovascular diseases cause 80 per cent of the deaths.

8. Other causes include
   a. Arteritis (connective tissue diseases, giant cell arteritis, Takayasu's disease)
   b. Thromboangiitis obliterans (Buerger's disease)
   c. Raynaud's disease
   d. Artery entrapment

9. Symptoms of abrupt onset, digit or upper extremity involvement, or in a person less than 40 years of age suggest an uncommon etiology.

Symptoms

1. Intermittent claudication is the hallmark symptom
   a. Produces cramping, pain, weakness, or numbness in affected muscles (calf discomfort is most common but may also occur in buttock, thigh, or foot)
   b. Predictably produced by walking a specific speed and distance; relieved by resting within about 5 minutes

2. Rest pain occurs in advanced disease
   a. Involves the foot, usually distal to the metatarsals (nocturnal metatarsalgia)
   b. Aggravated by leg elevation or cool temperature

3. Approximately 50 per cent of patients with clinically evident lower extremity PAD are asymptomatic.

4. Nocturnal leg cramps and "cold feet" usually do not indicate PAD

Key Symptoms

- Intermittent claudication
- Rest pain

Clinical Findings

1. Diminished or absent pulses. Dorsalis pedis pulse is congenitally absent in approximately 8 per cent of normal individuals. The posterior tibial pulse should be palpable.

2. Arterial bruits

3. Arterial insufficiency: dry, scaly, atrophic skin; extremity hair loss, brittle nails, and dependent rubor

4. Ischemic ulcers that are painful, dry, and pale, and often have a black necrotic crust. Ulcers usually occur on the heels or toes.

5. Gangrene

6. Lower extremity pallor within one minute after leg elevation to 60 degrees and return of color delayed more than 15 seconds after lowering.

7. Rest pain, ischemic ulcers, or gangrene, especially with a resting ankle systolic pressure ≤50 mm Hg, indicate limb-threatening ischemia.

Key Signs

• Diminished pulse	• Ischemic ulcer
• Arterial bruit	• Pallor with elevation

Laboratory Tests

1. Ankle/brachial index (ABI):
   a. Noninvasively assesses lower extremity arterial insufficiency by determining ratio of ankle to brachial systolic blood pressures measured by a Doppler device; can be performed at the bedside
   b. Abnormal ratio <0.9, moderate disease <0.8, severe disease <0.6, and <0.4 associated with ulcers and gangrene
   c. A 20 per cent decrease in ABI postexercise indicates disease and is useful if resting ABI is normal and yet patient has symptoms suggesting PAD.
   d. Ankle pressures in diabetics may be falsely elevated secondary to medial calcinosis of arteries.

2. Special procedures
  a. Plethysmography (PPG)
    (1) Measures pulse-volume waveforms and toe pressures
    (2) Useful in patients with diabetes who may have falsely elevated ankle pressures or disease confined to distal arterial beds
  b. Transcutaneous oxygen tension (tcPo$_2$) measurements
    (1) Assess tissue perfusion and viability
    (2) Also useful in patients with diabetes (see above)
  c. Angiography is the "gold standard" for the diagnosis of anatomic disease; used when considering an interventional procedure

> **Key Test**
>
> • Ankle/brachial index

Differential Diagnosis

1. Arthritis
2. Lumbar spinal stenosis (pseudoclaudication)
  a. Symptoms produced by walking or prolonged standing
  b. Relieved by flexing spine (sitting)
3. Herniated lumbar disk
4. Peripheral neuropathy
5. Muscle cramps
6. Restless legs syndrome
7. Shin splints
8. Venous claudication .
  a. Edema and venous stasis are present
  b. Typically produces rest pain as well
9. Other arterial diseases: arteritis, thromboangiitis obliterans, Raynaud's disease, artery entrapment.

Treatment

1. Management of PAD without limb-threatening ischemia
  a. Smoking cessation
  b. Control of diabetes, hyperlipidemia, and hypertension
  c. Regular walking for 30 minutes a day and resting when symptoms occur has improved walking distance more than any drug treatment.
  d. Special attention to foot care (see below)
  e. Optimize treatment of concurrent medical conditions (e.g., congestive heart failure, chronic obstructive pulmonary disease).
  f. Weight loss

2. Prompt surgical referral for consideration of arterial bypass or percutaneous transluminal angioplasty if clinical evidence of critical leg ischemia exists such as rest pain, ischemic ulcers, or gangrene. A concomitant resting ankle systolic pressure ≤50 mm Hg or a toe systolic pressure ≤30 mm Hg worsens the prognosis.
3. Medication
  a. Aspirin for stroke and myocardial infarction prevention
  b. Pentoxifylline (Trental), 400 mg t.i.d., has shown only modest clinical efficacy
4. Diet: As determined by risk factor status
5. Activity: Regular walking
6. Patient education
  a. Inspect and wash feet daily
  b. Check water temperature before washing feet (avoid hot water)
  c. Dry between toes to prevent maceration
  d. Apply moisturizing lotion to feet
  e. Keep nails trimmed
  f. Wear comfortable shoes
  g. Regularly inspect shoes for foreign bodies
  h. Do not smoke
  i. Do not walk barefoot
  j. Do not treat corns or calluses yourself
  k. Do not use heating pads on feet

> **Key Treatment**
>
> • Smoking cessation
> • Walking program
>
> | **Drug of Choice** | **Additional Drug** |
> | --- | --- |
> | • Aspirin | • Pentoxifylline |

Follow-Up

As needed for control of risk factors

 Bibliography

Clement DL, Shepherd JT (eds): Vascular Diseases in the Limbs: Mechanisms and Principles of Treatment. St. Louis, Mosby-Year Book, 1993.

Newman AB, et al: Morbidity and mortality in hypertensive adults with a low ankle/arm blood pressure index. JAMA 1993;270:487–489.

Porter JM: Chronic lower extremity ischemia. Part 1. Curr Probl Surg 1991;28:11–92.

Spittell JA: Diagnosis and management of occlusive peripheral arterial disease. Curr Probl Cardiol 1990;15:7–35.

Wilt TJ: Current strategies in the diagnosis and management of lower extremity peripheral vascular disease. J Gen Intern Med 1992;7:87–102.

71 Raynaud's Phenomenon

Jeffrey F. Minteer

Epidemiology and Etiology

1. Affects 3 to 5 per cent of male and 4 to 9 per cent of female population
2. It is estimated that fewer than 50 per cent ever seek medical attention.

Primary Raynaud's Phenomenon (PRP)

1. Affects younger age group (15 to 20 years old); only 24 per cent present after age 20.
2. Predominance of women (60 to 90 per cent)
3. Origin of vasospasm unknown but probably multifactorial; associated with increased sympathetic tone and/or increased sensitivity or density of α_2 receptors under central sympathetic influence; if severe, may have characteristics of endothelial damage. Endothelium-dependent venodilatation is impaired due to diminished release of nitric oxide.

Secondary Raynaud's Phenomenon (SRP)

1. Affects older age group (over 35); less sex difference
2. Associated with endothelial damage, intimal proliferation, fixed vascular obstruction, or inflammation resulting in release of vasospastic substances such as thromboxane and endothelin-1
3. Also associated: hard red cells, activated platelets, increased plasma viscosity, decreased fibrinolysis
4. Seen in 90 per cent of patients with systemic sclerosis (SS) (80 per cent present with Raynaud's), 85 per cent of those with mixed connective tissue disease, 10 to 44 per cent with systemic lupus erythematosus (SLE), 20 per cent with Sjögren's syndrome, 5 per cent with rheumatoid arthritis (RA)
5. Can be caused by drugs such as bleomycin and vincristine (see Differential Diagnosis); usually resolves after drug is discontinued

Symptoms

Primary Raynaud's Phenomenon: 70 per cent of all cases

1. Classic triphasic color changes: pallor → cyanosis → rubor; usually two are required, pallor and cyanosis being the most common (best to use the Maricq's standard color chart to get accurate history)
2. Bilateral, episodic attacks of well-demarcated pallor followed by cyanosis and rubor brought on by cold exposure or emotional stress; affects fingers (one or more but may spare the thumb) more often than toes; lasts 15 to 30 minutes after rewarming
3. May also affect toes, earlobes, lips, or tip of nose
4. May also give rise to complaints of tingling and burning sensations during reperfusion

Secondary Raynaud's Phenomenon

1. Similar color changes (cyanosis more prominent)

2. May be unilateral
3. Symptoms of precipitating disease such as sicca symptoms, dysphagia, photosensitivity, skin lesions, joint pain, telangiectasias; history of more than 5 years in high-risk occupations such as use of vibratory tools
4. Symptoms tend to be more severe with rapid progression.

Key Symptoms

- Episodic triphasic color changes
- Precipitated by cold, emotional stress

Clinical Findings

Primary Raynaud's Phenomenon

1. Pallor: vasospasm in response to cold or emotional stress
2. Cyanosis: stagnated blood flow in dilated capillaries
3. Rubor: accumulation of vasodilating agents in ischemic tissue
4. Normal examination when patient is not having symptoms; normal pulses

Secondary Raynaud's Phenomenon

1. May see digital pitting scars or gangrene
2. May see signs of primary disease such as periungual telangiectases, sclerodactyly, arthritis, signs of carpal tunnel syndrome, decreased peripheral pulses, or signs of thoracic outlet syndrome

Key Signs

- Color changes in response to cold
- Digital pitting scars

Laboratory Tests

1. Basic tests to exclude precipitating cause (all normal in primary RP)
   a. Antinuclear antibodies (ANA), sedimentation rate (SR) complete blood count
   b. Wide-field capillary microscopy of the nail folds (apply immersion oil to nail base and observe with $10\times$ magnification and inverted microscope eyepiece): capillary loss and enlarged, tortuous capillary loops
   c. Abnormal ANA and microscopy identify 95 per cent of those who will develop SS but not inevitable; 28 per cent with abnormal capillaries develop SS in six years.

2. Expanded work-up—if there are suggestive symptoms/signs or abnormal screening tests (i.e., sedimentation rate >20, ANA >1:100, or abnormal nail fold capillaries)

   a. Anti-double-stranded DNA, anti-centromere antibody (ACA), anti-topoisomerase I (Anti-Sc1-70)

   b. For signs of increased viscosity (cyanosis predominates clinical picture) add serum protein electrophoresis, cold agglutinins, cryoglobulins

   c. Add vascular studies if obstruction indicated

   d. Add nerve conduction studies if nerve entrapment suggested

   e. Pulmonary diffusion or esophageal motility studies if subclinical SS suspected

Key Tests

- Antinuclear antibodies, erythrocyte sedimentation rate
- Nail fold microscopy

Proposed Criteria for Diagnosis of PRP

- Attacks episodic with acral pallor or cyanosis
- Strong and symmetric pulses
- No evidence of peripheral pitting, gangrene, or ulcerations
- Normal nail fold capillaries
- Antinuclear antibodies (ANA) under 100
- Westergren erthyrocyte sedimentation rate under 20 mm/hr

Differential Diagnosis: Secondary Causes

1. Systemic rheumatic disorders

   a. Systemic sclerosis: suggested by signs/symptoms, abnormal nail fold capillaries, and high ANA (speckled) with positive Sc1-70 or ACA; most common connective tissue disease causing Raynaud's phenomenon; 80 per cent present with Raynaud's as the first symptom; 90 per cent have Raynaud's

   b. SLE (+ anti-double-stranded DNA), RA (? association): dermatomyositis, mixed connective tissue disease, Sjögren's—29 per cent, and possible association with SS-like syndrome associated with silicone breast implants

2. Occupational

   a. Vibration white finger—90 per cent of loggers; carpal tunnel syndrome

   b. Polyvinyl chloride

3. Drugs or chemicals

   a. β blockers (? evidence acutely), ergotamine, narcotics, birth control pills, sympathomimetics, imipramine, bromocriptine, α-interferon

   b. Heavy metals, caffeine

   c. Chemotherapy: bleomycin, vincristine, vinblastine—20 to 40 per cent

4. Occlusive arterial disease: thromboangiitis obliterans, peripheral vascular disease, thoracic outlet syndrome

5. Hyperviscosity diseases: polycythemia, cryoglobulinemias, paraproteinemias, thrombocytosis

6. Other causes: reflex sympathetic dystrophy, infections, malignant disease, cerebrovascular accident, polio, syringomyelia, pulmonary hypertension, hypothyroidism—48 per cent; Lyme disease

7. Nonspecific syndromes

   a. Blue toe syndrome: cyanotic lesions with dependent mottling from emboli, thrombosis, or vasculitis

   b. Erythromelalgia: red, warm, and painful feet made worse by warm temperatures and improved on aspirin; occurs in idiopathic myeloproliferative disorder, autoimmune disease, pregnancy, and use of vasodilator drugs

8. Associated conditions: possibly indicates systemic vasospasm

   a. 61 per cent of PRP patients have migraine syndromes.

   b. 47 per cent of PRP patients have atypical chest pain, especially those with aura-associated migraines (67 per cent).

   c. 41 per cent of females with fibromyalgia have PRP.

Treatment

Medication

1. Drug therapy for patients unresponsive to patient education measures or signs of severe disease (e.g., ulcers/gangrene)

2. Calcium channel blockers: nifedipine (Procardia), 30 to 60 mg per day or prior to precipitating events (e.g., 10 mg orally before cold exposure); others may be useful; two thirds of patients so treated have decrease in symptoms; work better for primary disease in sustained-release form

3. ACE inhibitors, peripheral vasodilators, antiplatelet drugs, pentoxifylline (controversial)

4. Serotonin receptor antagonist: ketanserin (not available in the United States) affects vasoconstriction and platelet aggregation

5. Prostacyclin analog: iloprost (not available in the United States) improved signs and symptoms in 47 per cent of patients who failed nifedipine; drug-induced hypercoagulable state a concern

Surgery

1. Cervical sympathectomy does not affect long-term course of disease and is a last resort in SRP unresponsive to medications.

2. Digital sympathectomy has shown some success in healing digital ulcers.

Diet

1. Fish oil supplements: substrate for cyclooxygenase, antiaggregative effects on platelets, no clinical support as yet

Patient Education

1. Dress appropriately in the cold

2. Stop smoking

3. Avoid over-the-counter sympathomimetics

4. Biofeedback for stress-induced symptoms (one third are stress related with 92 per cent response rate)

Key Treatment

- Patient education
- Nifedipine

Follow-Up

1. Prognosis in PRP: 38 per cent stable, 36 per cent improved, 16 per cent worse, 10 per cent disappear over a 6- to 10-year follow-up.

2. Ten to 30 per cent of those with PRP are diagnosed with a connective tissue disease within six to eight years.

3. The risk of progression of PRP to SRP is high when

    a. Onset occurs after 20 years of age.

    b. Patient has intense, painful attacks and/or digital ulcers.

    c. Attacks are asymmetric.

    d. The ANA is positive and/or nail fold capillaries are abnormal.

Bibliography

Adee AC: Managing Raynaud's phenomenon: A practical approach. Am Fam Phys 1993;47:823–829.

Klippel JH: Raynaud's phenomenon. Arch Intern Med 1991;151:2389–2393.

Ohtsuka T, Ishikawa H: Statistical definition of nail fold capillary pattern in patients with systemic sclerosis. Dermatology 1994;188(4):286–289.

Waller PA, Leroy EC: Raynaud's phenomenon and connective tissue disease. J South Carolina Med Assoc 1993;89(11):536–542.

Wigley FM: Raynaud's phenomenon. Curr Opinion Rheumatol 1993;5(6):773–784.

72 Common Gastrointestinal Symptoms

| Symptom | Abdominal Pain | *Phillip K. Rhyne* |

Abdominal pain is a common problem that may pose diagnostic challenges for the clinician. In a series of 8758 emergency department visits made by patients of a family medicine residency, approximately 13 per cent of the patients had abdominal pain. This does not accurately represent the incidence of abdominal pain because many patients do not see a physician (i.e., pain either resolves untreated or by means of over-the-counter remedies or other alternative therapies). However, this selection process does not ensure that only patients with the most pathologically significant problems will seek medical help. An understanding of the physiology of pain and basic anatomy is essential in the evaluation of abdominal pain, but determination of an etiology can be difficult owing to overlapping symptoms in pathologic processes and to the variable response of individuals to pain. The most powerful diagnostic tools are the history and physical examination and the realization that both are evolving, not static, entities. Chronicity is a key determinant of the pace of assessment. Prompt evaluation and appropriate treatment of acute abdominal pain are crucial. Chronic abdominal pain usually may be evaluated in a more unhurried manner.

Differential Diagnosis

1. Intra-abdominal disorders
   a. Inflammatory (e.g., appendicitis, pyelonephritis, abscesses)
   b. Mechanical (e.g., visceral obstructions, aneurysm, trauma)
2. Extra-abdominal (e.g., pneumonia, myocardial infarction, shingles, sickle cell anemia, diabetic ketoacidosis, depression, anxiety)

Refer to Ch. 34, Pneumonia; Ch. 57, Acute Myocardial Infarction; Ch. 77, Appendicitis; Ch. 132, Pyelonephritis; Ch. 145, Sickle Cell Anemia; and Ch. 161, Ketoacidosis.

History

1. Onset (chronic or acute)
2. Progression (improving, worsening, or stable)
3. Migration (has it moved?)
4. Localization (generalized, periumbilical, pelvic, or quadrantal)
5. Character (e.g., colicky or continuous, cramping, or stabbing)
6. Associated symptoms (e.g., nausea, vomiting, anorexia, change in bowel habits)
7. Medical history and review of systems
   a. To appreciate historical data the clinician must have a basic understanding of abdominal nociception, which consists of a localization and discrimination step and an alerting and affective step. It is not synonymous with pain. The abdominal viscera have splanchnic innervation, which recognizes only distention or stretch and is bilateral (i.e., visceral pain is felt in the midline). Somatic innervation of the parietal peritoneum is accomplished along cerebrospinal pathways at the T6–T12 dermatome levels. The visceral peritoneum is believed to have no sensory innervation. If there is a visceral insult that activates pain receptors and is of slow onset, the progression of symptoms might be an anterior, symmetric, midline pain that may advance to a combined visceral and localized somatic pain as the process involves somatic receptors of the peritoneum. Somatic pain may be so great that the original visceral pain is no longer a distinct entity. If the visceral insult is of rapid onset or sufficient magnitude, there may be a cross-over at the spinal cord level of visceral sensation to cerebrospinal tracts, producing localized symptoms without actual involvement of somatic receptors.
   b. Associated symptoms may be generalized (e.g., vasomotor symptoms, such as vomiting and diaphoresis) or specific (e.g., hematuria or hematochezia) in nature. Specific symptoms or localization of pain should prompt detailed questions about a suspect system or disease process. A history of abdominal surgery, chronic disease, or prior pelvic inflammatory disease should raise the index of suspicion for associated sequelae (e.g., small bowel obstruction due to postoperative intra-abdominal adhesions).

Clinical Findings

1. Vital signs and general appearance (e.g., fever, shock, body position, jaundice)
2. Inspection (e.g., contour, scars, pulsations, skin or vascular lesions, visible masses, or peristalsis)
3. Auscultation (e.g., murmurs or bruits, peristaltic sounds, succussion splash)
4. Palpation and percussion (e.g., light and deep, guard-

ing and tenderness, organomegaly, masses, hernias, ascites)

5. Rectal and/or pelvic examination (e.g., urethral or cervical discharge or bleeding, prostate or adnexal tenderness or masses, stool impaction, rectal bleeding)

Tests

1. Complete blood count with differential
2. Urinalysis
3. Serum electrolytes, blood urea nitrogen, creatinine, glucose if vomiting or other symptoms are present
4. Serum lipase and amylase if pancreatic process is suspected
5. Serum bilirubin (conjugated and unconjugated), transaminase levels, and albumin if hepatic process is suspected. If jaundice is present, prothrombin time and partial thromboplastin time may also be indicated.
6. Urine pregnancy test
7. Diagnostic imaging (e.g., flat and upright abdominal films, chest radiograph, abdominal/pelvic ultrasonography or CT, upper and lower bowel contrast studies)
8. Abdominal paracentesis
9. Direct visualization by endoscopy, laparoscopy, or surgery

In the evaluation of abdominal pain, there is no test that is superior to a good history and physical examination. Though this maxim is usually true, well-chosen diagnostic studies can be helpful in confirming or excluding certain processes. No test should be universally ordered in patients with abdominal pain nor should multiple tests be ordered in hopes of a serendipitous diagnosis. As the delivery of health care is scrutinized and accurate cost-benefit and risk-benefit information becomes available, protocols and other algorithmic methods to "guide" clinicians in test selection seem inevitable. These devices may or may not yield greater efficiency in ordering tests.

Management

Although the management of abdominal pain is specific to the causative pathology, the following general measures may be useful in the management of acute abdominal pain.

Medication

1. Narcotic and non-narcotic parenteral analgesics
2. Antiemetics, such as prochlorperazine (Compazine), and other symptomatic medications
3. Specific pharmacotherapy as indicated (e.g., H_2 blockers in ulcer disease)

Diet

Nothing by mouth until a diagnosis is made; thereafter, the diet is determined by the disease.

Activity

Usually bed rest (especially if there is risk of medication-related falls or aortic aneurysm)

Patient Education

1. The patient should promptly report changes in symptoms.
2. The clinician must keep the patient advised of the situation and obtain necessary informed consent before administration of narcotics or other medications that may affect decision making.

Orthodoxy holds that, for fear of masking abdominal symptoms, analgesics should not be given until a probable diagnosis is made and a course of treatment is determined. Recent information suggests that some analgesics (especially parenteral nonsteroidal anti-inflammatory drugs) may not significantly interfere with the evaluation of acute abdominal pain.

Follow-Up

1. In acute abdominal pain, even if the cause is known, follow-up may be as frequent as every few minutes.
2. In chronic abdominal pain, re-evaluation may be as infrequent as every several months depending on the patient, the suspected or confirmed cause, and the physician's degree of comfort.

PEARLS

- Determine whether pain is acute or chronic. If acute, work-up should proceed rapidly.

- History and physical examination should guide focused selection of diagnostic studies.

- Keep patients with acute abdominal pain NPO initially.

- For chronic pain, recording of symptoms on a calendar along with menses, diet, and other features may be helpful.

Bibliography

DeGowin RL: Diagnostic Examination. 6th ed. New York, McGraw-Hill, 1994, pp 463–566.

Seller RH: Differential Diagnosis of Common Complaints, 2nd ed. Philadelphia, WB Saunders, 1993, pp 1–7, 19–28.

Silen W: Cope's Early Diagnosis of the Acute Abdomen, 18th ed. London, Oxford University Press, 1991.

Swartz MH: Textbook of Physical Diagnosis: History and Examination, 2nd ed. Philadelphia, WB Saunders, 1994, pp 302–336.

Wiener SL: Differential Diagnosis of Acute Pain: By Body Region. New York, McGraw-Hill 1993, pp 215–359.

Symptom   Nausea and Vomiting
John B. Pope

Nausea is an ill-defined and unpleasant, although not painful, sensation generally perceived in the pharynx and upper abdomen. It is usually accompanied by hypersalivation and the desire to vomit, or the feeling that vomiting is imminent. It may be brief or quite prolonged and sometimes occurs in waves. Retching refers to forceful rhythmic contractions of the respiratory and abdominal musculature that sometimes precedes vomiting. Vomiting is the forceful expulsion of gastric contents through the mouth. Although generally regarded clinically as undesirable side effects, nausea and vomiting may have evolved as a survival function for eliminating potentially toxic substances from the gastrointestinal tract. This function may be triggered by various toxins recognized by sensors in the upper gut and central nervous system. The initiation and coordination of these events involves complex neurochemical interactions involving specific areas of the brain, including the vomiting center of the lateral reticular formation and the chemoreceptor trigger zone (CTZ) in the area postema in the floor of the fourth ventricle. Although generally self-limited, nausea and vomiting may be severe or protracted, leading to serious complications such as dehydration, hypokalemia, metabolic alkalosis, aspiration pneumonitis, malnutrition, dental caries, ruptured esophagus (Boerhaave's syndrome), or mucosal tears with hemorrhage (Mallory-Weiss syndrome).

Differential Diagnosis

Nausea and vomiting are manifestations of a large number of disorders not limited to the digestive system or abdomen.

1. Acute infectious diseases: virtually any infection (bacterial, viral, parasitic) can stimulate nausea and vomiting. These symptoms are common in children with systemic infections not directly involving the gastrointestinal (GI) tract.
2. Acute abdominal emergencies (appendicitis, cholecystitis, pancreatitis, peritonitis, intestinal obstruction, visceral inflammation, perforation, ischemia)
3. Drugs and toxins: many different classes of drugs and various toxins may stimulate the CTZ or directly irritate the stomach mucosa, triggering nausea (NSAIDS, digitalis, morphine, erythromycin, azathioprine, enterotoxins).
4. Intracranial disease: increased CNS pressure may cause vomiting, sometimes projectile.
5. Pregnancy usually confined to the first trimester but may be prolonged or severe.
6. Psychogenic (anorexia nervosa, bulimia, emotional upset)
7. Gastric retention (gastroparesis, dysmotility, pyloric obstruction)
8. Metabolic and endocrine disorders (diabetic ketoacidosis, adrenal insufficiency, thyrotoxicosis, uremia)
9. Chronic indigestion (peptic ulcer disease, aerophagia)
10. Labyrinthine disorders (acute labyrinthitis, Meniere's disease)
11. GI bleeding: blood in the stomach may stimulate vomiting
12. Cardiac disease (congestive heart failure, myocardial infarction)
13. Pain: more often associated with nausea than with frank vomiting

History

1. Timing and character of vomitus: helpful in delineating cause
   a. Early morning vomiting: pregnancy, alcoholic gastritis, uremia
   b. Feculent vomitus: gastrocolic fistula, distal intestinal obstruction
   c. Projectile vomiting: increased intracranial pressure, pyloric stenosis
   d. Bilious vomitus: increased bile may indicate obstruction below ampulla of Vater.
   e. Bloody vomitus: GI bleeding
2. Associated symptoms
   a. Vertigo and tinnitus: Meniere's disease, labyrinthitis
   b. Relief of abdominal pain with vomiting: peptic ulcer disease
   c. Early satiety: gastroparesis
   d. Weight loss: malignancy
3. Food ingestion
   a. Potential toxin ingestion
   b. Vomiting during or soon after eating: psychogenic cause
   c. Delayed vomiting after eating: obstruction or dysmotility
   d. Vomiting old food: impaired gastric emptying
   e. Vomiting undigested food: esophageal or Zenker's diverticulum
4. Recent use of medications
5. Other close contacts similarly affected
6. Unusual stressors, emotional upset, depression

Clinical Findings

1. Abdominal tenderness, rebound, guarding, distention, abnormal bowel sounds (hyperactive, diminished, or absent)
2. Intravascular volume depletion (bradycardia, hypotension, skin pallor)

3. Anorexia, weight loss, wasting

4. Altered autonomic activity (diarrhea, increased perspiration, hypersalivation)

5. Hematemesis, coffee-ground emesis, feculent emesis

6. Dental caries

7. Projectile vomiting

Tests

1. Plain radiographs: may suggest intestinal obstruction

2. Upper GI series: can assess motility and mucosa of proximal GI tract

3. Esophagogastroduodenoscopy: obstruction, mucosal aberrations

4. Gastric emptying scans: gastric paresis

5. Computed tomography of the brain: intracranial disorders

6. Pregnancy test

7. Electrolytes: useful for assessing volume and electrolyte status

Management

1. Correction of the underlying cause

2. Antiemetics for symptom alleviation—effectiveness variable

3. Prevention and treatment of complication development

Medication

Because of complexity of the neurophysiologic process in vomiting, it may not be possible to find a single agent that is effective for all emetic stimuli.

1. Antihistamines (dimenhydrinate, promethazine): useful in inner ear dysfunction

2. Anticholinergics (scopolamine): useful for motion sickness

3. Phenothiazines (prochlorperazine [Compazine], chlorpromazine [Thorazine]): useful for mild symptom relief but fraught with side effects (sedation, hypotension, Parkinson-like symptoms)

4. Butyrophenones (haloperidol [Haldol], droperidol [Inapsine]): useful in cytotoxic drug-induced vomiting

5. Dopamine antagonists (metaclopromide [Reglan]): useful in gastric and small bowel stasis and prophylaxis for chemotherapy-induced nausea and vomiting

6. 5HT$_3$ antagonists (ondansetron [Zofran]): excellent in cytotoxic drug-induced and radiation-induced vomiting

Diet

1. Avoid all foods for several hours; irritable stomachs respond to food with vomiting.

2. Nausea may be reduced by sucking on hard candy or popsicle, particularly in children.

3. Begin frequent, small quantities of clear liquids and slowly advance diet as tolerated.

Activity

Avoid excessive activity and overheating.

Patient Education

1. Hematemesis or other evidence of GI bleeding needs prompt medical attention.

2. Frequent or prolonged vomiting (particularly in children) may result in dehydration.

3. Persistent vomiting during pregnancy should be investigated.

4. Numerous drugs have nausea as a common side effect.

Follow-Up

1. Most cases of nausea and vomiting are mild and self-limited and require no specific follow-up once the underlying etiology is identified and corrected.

2. Follow-up, when required, should be tailored to the individual case on the basis of cause, severity, and risk of complication development.

PEARLS

• A careful history is the most important factor in determining etiology.

• Assess volume status with history of frequent or prolonged vomiting.

• Check stool for occult blood with history of hematemesis (unwitnessed).

• Obtain pregnancy test with history of vomiting and amenorrhea.

Bibliography

For more information on nausea and vomiting, see
Cooke CE: Oral ondansetron for preventing nausea and vomiting. Am J Hosp Pharm 1994;51:763–771.
Friedman LS, Isselbacher KJ: Anorexia, nausea, vomiting, and indigestion. In Wilson JD, Braunwald E, et al (eds): Harrison's Principles of Internal Medicine, 12th ed. New York, McGraw-Hill, 1991, pp 251–253.
Kousen M: Treatment of nausea and vomiting in pregnancy. Am Fam Physician 1993;48(7):1279–1284.

For more information on antiemetics, see
Allan SG: Antiemetics. Gastroenterol Clin North Am 1992; 21:597–611.

For more information on the physiology of nausea and vomiting, see
Andrews PLR: Physiology of nausea and vomiting. Br J Anaesth 1992;69(suppl 1):2S–19S.

Symptom **Trouble Swallowing**   *Bharat Khandheria*

1. The term for trouble or difficulty in swallowing, *dysphagia,* is derived from the Greek: "phagia," to eat, and "dys," difficulty or disordered.

2. Odynophagia is painful swallowing.

3. Dysphagia is relatively common, affecting up to 35 per cent of patients in the chronic care setting.

4. A patient may describe dysphagia by saying that food "sticks" or "stops" or "hangs up."

5. Dysphagia should be differentiated from "globus sensation," in which the patient feels something in the back of the throat all the time, but the sensation disappears on swallowing. Globus invariably occurs in young women who have suffered from other functional nervous afflictions such as hysterical aphonia.

Swallowing is a complex sequence of integral motor events programmed entirely within a "pattern" generator—the medullary swallow center. The swallow is not a reflex but rather a programmed response, which is initiated only when the right combination of cortical and peripheral sensory cues is given to the medulla. Successful swallowing transfers the food from mouth to stomach without regurgitation or aspiration into the respiratory tract. It is possible only with fine coordination between the different muscle groups of pharynx, larynx, and esophagus.

Differential Diagnosis

See Table 72–1.

History

1. Detailed history-taking can suggest the cause of dysphagia in almost 80 per cent of cases.

2. Patient should be asked whether dysphagia
   a. Occurs every day or intermittently
   b. Occurs with solid food or liquids or both
   c. Is associated with such symptoms as choking, coughing, regurgitation, changes in speech, heartburn, and chest pain.

Oral causes are easily recognized on simple physical examination. Historical clues readily differentiate oropharyngeal and esophageal causes.

In the oropharyngeal type, the patient is often unable to initiate swallowing and can pinpoint the site of symptoms to the cervical esophagus. Symptoms occur within one second of swallowing. In many cases saliva cannot be swallowed and the patient drools. Liquid bolus may enter the larynx or nose and cause coughing, choking, or nasal regurgitation.

The esophageal stage lasts 8 to 20 seconds. It is perceived by the patient to be in the suprasternal, retrosternal, or epigastric region. Patient may also experience heartburn and regurgitation. There may also be odynophagia. Usually, symptoms appear with the ingestion of solids, progressing later to follow ingestion of liquids as well.

Clinical Findings

1. Complete head and neck examination

2. Sensory and motor function of the cranial nerves involved in swallowing

3. Examination for systemic disorders of the nervous system, including Parkinson's disease, multiple sclerosis, myasthenia gravis, poliomyelitis, and diabetes mellitus.

Presence of masses, adenopathy, and spinal deformity should be paid particular attention. Pulmonary examination may reveal evidence of acute or chronic aspiration. Observing the patient swallowing water is mandatory and informative.

Tests

1. Modified barium swallow

2. Endoscopy

3. Manometric and motility studies

Modified barium swallow is a dynamic technique designed to evaluate swallowing function and dysfunction as it relates to the oral and pharyngeal phase of swallowing. It should be videotaped, allowing careful slow-motion replay for qualitative and quantitative assessment of different phases of the oropharyngeal swallowing processes. Endoscopy and manometric and motility studies are necessary to delineate esophageal causes of dysphagia.

Management

1. Depends on underlying cause

2. Multidisciplinary team approach

3. Gastrostomy, jejunostomy, or parenteral feeding

PEARLS

- Sometimes unexplained weight loss may be the only clue to a swallowing disorder; patients may avoid eating because of the difficulty encountered.

- Individuals with no gag reflex may be able to swallow normally, and the presence or absence of a gag reflex may not indicate anything about swallowing function.

- Thorough psychosocial questioning should be a component of every dysphagia patient's history.

- Videoradiography is the single most valuable technique in the evaluation of oropharyngeal dysphagia.

- The speech pathologist is the most important member of the multidisciplinary team in the evaluation and treatment of dysphagia.

TABLE 72-1. CAUSES OF DYSPHAGIA

	OROPHARYNGEAL CAUSES					ESOPHAGEAL CAUSES		
Oral Causes	**Nervous System Disorders**	**Muscle Abnormality**	**Inflammatory/ Infectious**	**Structural**	**Other Causes**	**Muscular Disorder**	**Structural**	**Motility Disorders**
Stomatitis	Cerebrovascular accident, especially of brain stem, or pseudobulbar palsy	Myasthenia gravis	Pharyngitis/retropharyngeal abscess	Local neoplasm in the oropharynx	Upper esophageal sphincter dysfunction (e.g., UES achalasia)	Same as oropharyngeal causes	Benign strictures (e.g., peptic, corrosive, inflammatory, radiation)	*Primary* 1. Achalasia 2. Diffuse esophageal spasm 3. Hypertonic lower esophageal sphincter
Ulcer of the tongue	Parkinson's disease	Muscular dystrophy	Botulism	Webs	Sodium fluoride poisoning		Neoplasm (e.g., esophageal carcinoma)	
Cleft palate	Multiple sclerosis	Polymyositis	Acute anterior poliomyelitis	Extrinsic compression (e.g., vertebral osteophyte)	Plummer-Vinson: occurs exclusively in females, is precancerous and disappears with treatment of anemia with iron		Webs and rings (e.g., Schatzki's ring)	*Secondary* 1. Gastroesophageal reflux disease 2. Scleroderma 3. Chagas' disease
Vitamin deficiency	Amyotrophic lateral sclerosis	Metabolic myopathy as in myxedema	Hydrophobia (e.g., rabies and tetanus)	Diverticula (e.g., Zenker's)	Radiation therapy: causes dysphagia by xerostomia and causing swelling and mucosal injury		External compression (e.g., vascular thyroid, mediastinal mass, left atrial enlargement, aortic aneurysm) Diverticula	
Sjögren's syndrome with poor salivation	Huntington's disease							
	Tumors especially of the brain stem							
	Peripheral neuropathy (diabetes mellitus, lead poisoning, diphtheria polyneuritis, alcoholism & hypercalcemia)							
	Recurrent laryngeal nerve damage							

Many swallowing problems are not easily curable or reversible, but most patients experience some improvement through the intensive efforts of a multidisciplinary team. The team should consist of a speech pathologist, primary care physician, dietitian, ENT specialist, and gastroenterologist. Speech pathologists are trained to use the functional and behavioral techniques in patients with oropharyngeal dysphagia. These techniques include changes in food consistency, sensory stimulation, motor retraining, controlled breathing, coughing, and head positioning. If all these efforts fail to provide a safe oral route of feeding, alternative routes, as mentioned above, should be considered to maintain adequate nutritional status.

Bibliography

Diamont NE: Approach to patient with dysphagia. *In* Kelley WN: Kelley's Textbook of Medicine, 2nd ed. Philadelphia, JB Lippincott, 1992, pp 597–599.
Ellis H: French's Index of Differential Diagnosis, 12th ed. Bristol, England, John Wright & Sons Ltd, 1985, pp 212–216.
Goyal R, et al: Dysphagia. *In* Harrison's Principles of Internal Medicine, 13th ed. New York, McGraw-Hill, 1994, pp 206–208.
Koch WM: Swallowing disorders. Med Clin North Am 1993; 77:571–582.
Sleisenger MH, Fordtran JS: Gastrointestinal Disease, 5th ed. Philadelphia, WB Saunders, 1993, pp 333–335.

| Symptom | **Heartburn and Indigestion** | *Hal E. Gordon* |

A Gallup survey done in 1988 found that almost 40 per cent of the United States population experience *heartburn* at least once a month and as many as 13 per cent have daily symptoms. Heartburn is a sensation of warmth, burning, or searing occurring underneath the sternum; this sensation may occur in waves with a tendency to ascend from the subxiphoid area toward the neck. Heartburn, the classic embodiment of gastroesophageal reflux disease, occurs when the sensitive chemoreceptors in the esophageal mucosa are stimulated by reflux of acidic or alkaline material originating from the gastric or gastroduodenal areas. This results from a decrease in lower esophageal sphincter tone, sometimes in combination with a large hiatal hernia. When the reflux becomes chronic, esophagitis can occur. The severity and extent of the esophagitis depend on the amount of exposure time the esophageal mucosa has to the offending agent and the resistance of the epithelium to the offending agent. Heartburn can be exacerbated by any agent that is directly irritating to the sensitive mucosa or that lowers esophageal sphincter tone so that gastric pool material is allowed to reflux into the esophagus. Some notable offending agents are tomato and citrus juices, alcohol, chocolate, coffee, onions, cigarettes, fats, sugars, spicy foods, carminatives, and medications. Increasing abdominal pressure, which occurs with bending over, lifting, tight-fitting clothes, straining upon defecation, and exercise may also cause exacerbations of heartburn.

Indigestion or *dyspepsia,* on the other hand, involves the following set of symptoms, some alone or in various combinations: abdominal pain or discomfort, postprandial fullness, abdominal bloating, belching, early satiety, anorexia, nausea with or without vomiting, any of which may be accompanied by heartburn and regurgitation. Indigestion or dyspepsia commonly results when there is a prolongation of gastric emptying time. This may result from mechanical obstruction via acute inflammation, edema, and later scarring secondary to peptic ulcer disease, tumors in the pyloric region, gastroduodenal Crohn's disease, and idiopathic hypertrophic pyloric stenosis. Nonobstructive causes, which may be intrinsic or extrinsic, include inflammatory processes such as cholecystitis, pancreatitis, hepatitis, appendicitis, peritonitis, gastroenteritis, peptic ulcer disease, and sepsis. Patients can have systemic lupus erythematosus, scleroderma, hyperplastic gastritis, sarcoidosis, neoplastic disease outside the gastrointestinal tract, congestive heart failure, pulmonary tuberculosis, or uremia. Additional causes include electrolyte abnormalities, metabolic disorders, ketoacidosis, diabetic neuropathy, paraplegia, postsurgical immobilization, vagotomy, and various drugs, most notably aspirin and NSAIDs, which directly irritate the gastric mucosa.

Differential Diagnosis (Table 72–2)

Heartburn (pyrosis)
1. Gastroesophageal reflux disease (GERD)
2. Inflammation or infection of the esophagus, stomach, or duodenum
3. Abnormal esophageal motor activity
4. Reflux secondary to pregnancy

Indigestion (dyspepsia)
1. Functional dyspepsia and irritable bowel syndrome
2. Esophagitis, gastritis, or duodenitis
3. Peptic ulcer disease
4. Gastroesophageal reflux disease (GERD)
5. Gastric malignancy
6. Cholecystitis
7. Miscellaneous—myocardial infarction, pericarditis, pancreatitis, pleurisy

Patients may have a reflux-like dyspepsia in which the symptoms of heartburn and regurgitation predominate. They may have ulcer-like dyspepsia with epigastric pain that may wax and wane, be relieved by food or antacids, and awaken them at night. They may have a dysmotility-like dyspepsia with poorly localized abdominal discomfort, bloating, early satiety, nausea, and sometimes vomiting. Finally, patients might have a functional dyspepsia in which

TABLE 72–2. DIFFERENTIAL DIAGNOSES OF HEARTBURN AND INDIGESTION

LIKELY DIAGNOSIS	HISTORY	POSSIBLE CLINICAL FINDINGS
GERD	Burning epigastric or substernal pain ascending to the neck; increased symptoms with recumbency; symptom relief with antacids or sitting upright	Patient may be obese; examination usually normal
Esophageal malignancy	Burning substernal pain; symptoms progressive; regurgitation of liquids; dysphagia	Weight loss, cachexia, possible lymphadenopathy; chest or back pain on palpation
Ulcer-like dyspepsia	Burning or gnawing epigastric pain—localized, episodic, usually 1–3 hours after eating; relieved by antacids; worsened by aspirin or NSAIDs	Epigastric tenderness, heme positive stool
Functional dyspepsia	Abdominal discomfort; bloating; nausea; symptoms worsened with increased stress; fatigue, insomnia, and anxiety not uncommon	Minimal abdominal tenderness; physical examination may be entirely normal, heme negative stool
Irritable bowel syndrome	Symptoms of functional dyspepsia, plus alteration of bowel habits; diarrhea alternating with constipation	Minimal abdominal tenderness, usually over the colon in patients with IBS; physical examination may be entirely normal

no underlying pathologic process has been found to explain the symptoms. They complain of the typical symptomology and may additionally report increasing fatigue, trouble sleeping, and anxiety. Endoscopy is usually negative, but *Helicobacter pylori* may be found in inflamed gastric mucosa. A full year of treatment does not seem to improve the symptoms in these patients unless the bacteria is eradicated.

Patients with irritable bowel syndrome will commonly complain of dyspepsia characterized by bloating but will also report alteration of their bowel functioning. Diagnostic studies will show no organic etiology for their symptoms. However, these patients may also report more anxiety or daily stress, which gives rise to a psychophysiologic response from the gastrointestinal tract. These patients, along with those who have functional dyspepsia, may account for the largest group of individuals who present with the complaint of indigestion.

History: Key Questions to Ask

When patients complain of heartburn or indigestion, it is important for the physician to clarify exactly what the patient means. Ask the patient to describe the symptom and inquire about specific aggravating factors. For *heartburn*, ask the following.

1. Where do you have the sensation?
2. When does this occur? Does it ever occur with exercise?
3. How often does this occur?
4. Do you ever experience an acidic, bitter, or sour taste in your mouth?
5. Do stomach contents ever regurgitate into the back of your throat?
6. What do you do to make it better?
7. Do you take antacids? Medications?
8. Does bending over, lying down, lifting, or straining upon defecation affect your symptom?

9. Is your symptom affected by certain foods such as citrus or tomato juice, coffee, alcohol, chocolate, spicy foods, or carminatives? (Explain these)
10. Do you smoke tobacco products?
11. Have you noticed any weight loss, trouble swallowing, loss of appetite, or darkening of your stools?

If there is a correlation of the patient's symptom with the aforementioned questions, and if the patient does not add weight loss, dysphagia, loss of appetite, or stool darkening to the description, in all likelihood he or she is describing heartburn associated with gastroesophageal reflux disease.

Questions in addition to those above should be asked of patients who complain of *indigestion*. The following may be helpful.

1. Does your symptom begin 1 to 3 hours after eating?
2. Do you ever experience nausea, vomiting, bloating, belching, pain, flatus, vague upper abdominal discomfort, changes in your bowel habits, stool consistency, or color?
3. What is the nature of your pain? Does food relieve or exacerbate it? Does it wax and wane? Does it ever awaken you at night?
4. Does stress affect your symptom?
5. Do you ever experience insomnia? Fatigue?
6. What are your bowel habits normally like? Do you ever have constipation alternating with diarrhea?

Again, questions about weight loss, dysphagia, lack of appetite, and darkening of the stool are important. By asking the right questions, you can help patients clarify their symptoms. Clarification will allow you to narrow the focus and avoid excessive diagnostic studies. However, do not eliminate tests if you are not reasonably comfortable with the diagnosis. Physicians can be cost-effective utilizers of technology by being more diligent history takers.

Clinical Findings

Patients with heartburn or indigestion generally have unremarkable physical examinations. However, certain clinical findings are important when present.

1. Epigastric or upper abdominal tenderness
2. Murphy's sign
3. Abdominal distention, organomegaly, or abdominal masses
4. Chest or back tenderness, which can be present in patients with mediastinal pathology
5. Cervical or supraclavicular lymphadenopathy, which is occasionally found in patients with metastatic esophageal malignancy
6. Pallor
7. Icterus
8. Oral or pharyngeal ulcers or thrush, which may be present in patients with infectious esophagitis caused by herpes simplex, *Cytomegalovirus,* or *Candida*
9. Tooth or gum disease in patients who might have heartburn from induced vomiting
10. Cutaneous changes, which may occur in patients with scleroderma, for example

Clinicians should always consider whether a physical finding has any relationship to the patient's symptom.

Diagnostic Tests

1. Refractory heartburn without dysphagia
   a. Esophagogastroduodenoscopy (EGD) with biopsy
   b. Ambulatory 24-hour pH monitoring (if EGD is normal)
   c. Bernstein test is used if EGD and pH monitoring are normal. Dilute hydrochloric acid is instilled into the distal esophagus. The test is positive if symptoms are reproduced during acid infusion and not during saline infusion.
2. Refractory heartburn with dysphagia: Use double-contrast barium esophagography.
3. Refractory indigestion
   a. Esophagogastroduodenoscopy with biopsy and evaluation for the presence of *Helicobacter pylori*
   b. Ultrasonography
   c. Computed tomography and magnetic resonance imaging
   d. Laboratory testing for abnormalities in fat, sugar, protein, carbohydrate and vitamin absorption if patients report indigestion consistent with malabsorption.

Controversy is abundant about the best way to approach patients with heartburn or indigestion when speaking in terms of diagnostic studies. Most physicians seem to reserve these studies for patients who have more complicated disease, atypical symptoms, or symptoms persisting longer than 2 weeks, despite dietary modification and empiric therapy with antacids. Some may also prescribe a course of H$_2$ blockers, promotility agents, or both in combination before utilizing any diagnostic studies. Physicians should try to be cost conscious and rely on a good history and physical examination before engaging in diagnostic testing.

Management

1. Antacids: Liquids are preferable.
   a. Absorbable: contain calcium bicarbonate and/or sodium bicarbonate
      (1) Tums
      (2) Titralac
      (3) Rolaids
   b. Nonabsorbable: contain aluminum hydroxide, magnesium hydroxide, or combinations of the two (may also contain simethicone for relief of gas)
      (1) Maalox
      (2) Mylanta
      (3) Riopan
      (4) Gelusil
      (5) Amphojel
      (6) Basaljel
      (7) Camalox—also contains calcium
   c. Antacid plus alginic acid (Gaviscon tablets): forms a foam that floats on top of the gastric contents, lessening the effects of any refluxed material in contact with sensitive esophageal mucosa
   d. Nonparticulate antacids and bismuth salts
2. Lifestyle modification
   a. Quitting tobacco smoking
   b. Weight loss, avoid overeating
   c. Not eating within 2 to 3 hours of bedtime
   d. Avoiding aggravating foods and alcohol
   e. Elevating the head of the bed
3. H$_2$ blockers
   a. Cimetidine (Tagamet)
   b. Ranitidine (Zantac)
   c. Famotidine (Pepcid)
   d. Nizatidine (Axid)
   e. Roxatidine: experimental, four to six times stronger than cimetidine
4. Proton pump inhibitors
   a. Omeprazole (Prilosec)
   b. Lansoprazole: experimental
5. Promotility agents: may be used as adjunct to antacids and H$_2$ blockers
   a. Metoclopramide (Reglan)
   b. Cisapride (Propulsid)
6. Mucosal coating agents (Sucralfate [Carafate]): effective in dyspepsia in peptic ulcer disease
7. Anti-infectives
   a. Antifungals for candidiasis

b. Antivirals for herpes and *Cytomegalovirus*

c. Antibacterials for *Helicobacter pylori* in addition to H$_2$ blockers or proton pump inhibitor

Various OTC agents are used by patients when they require symptomatic relief of their heartburn and indigestion, and for mild or occasional symptoms. These compounds are effective, safe, and inexpensive. Liquid agents are preferred by health care professionals, but this form presents practical problems for patients who must carry antacids with them during the day.

Depending on the nature of the patient's symptoms, some physicians may want to utilize H$_2$ blocking agents, a proton pump inhibitor, or a promotility agent in combination with an antacid or H$_2$ blocker as their initial treatment. Others might want to assess the effectiveness of antacids alone before advancing into the use of prescription medications.

In initially choosing an antacid or prescription medication, one should remember that overall effectiveness will vary from patient to patient. Cost, the patient's personal preference, and the patient's overall medical condition should be considered in guiding the decision. One must also be aware of the side effects these agents may have, especially in patients who have renal conditions or take certain medications.

Bibliography

Richter E: Heartburn, dysphagia, odonophagia and other esophageal symptoms. *In* Sleisenger MH, Fordtran JS (eds): Gastrointestinal Disease, 5th ed, vol. 1. Philadelphia, WB Saunders, 1993, pp. 331–333.

Schachter H: Indigestion and heartburn. *In* Walker HK, Hall WD, Hurst JW (eds): Clinical Methods, 3rd ed. Boston, Butterworths, 1990, pp 434–436.

Seller RH: Differential Diagnosis of Common Complaints, 2nd ed. Philadelphia, WB Saunders, 1993, pp 185–193.

Spiro HM: Clinical Gastroenterology, 4th ed. New York, McGraw-Hill, 1993, pp 100–104.

Spiro HM: Hiatus hernia and reflux esophagitis. Hosp Pract 1994;29:51–66.

| Symptom | **Acute Upper Gastrointestinal Bleeding** | *Zobair M. Younossi* |

Acute upper gastrointestinal (GI) bleeding is estimated to result in 250,000 to 300,000 hospitalizations each year. The mortality rate from upper GI bleeding has remained stable at about 10 per cent. This stable rate has been interpreted as an improvement (considering the aging population), which in turn may be a reflection of recent advances in endoscopic, medical, or surgical therapies.

The prognosis of upper GI bleeding depends largely on the source of bleeding and the clinical status of the patient. Variceal bleeding, peptic ulceration, and stigmata of recent hemorrhage (active arterial "spurting," visible vessel, and fresh blood clot) all are associated with higher morbidity and risk for rebleeding. Patient characteristics that are important prognostic factors include: older patients (more than 60 years of age), hemodynamic instability, and presence of multisystem failure.

Differential Diagnosis

The sources of an upper GI bleeding are summarized in the order of occurrence in Table 72–3.

Refer to Ch. 74, Peptic Ulcer Disease

History

The history may suggest the time of onset of bleeding, its severity, and possible causes.

1. A history of syncope and hematochezia in the presence of coffee-ground emesis would indicate severe bleeding.

2. A medication history, especially drugs such as nonsteroidal anti-inflammatory drugs (NSAIDs), would provide clues to drug-induced gastropathy or gastric ulcers as the possible source of bleeding.

3. A history of recurrent ulcers (especially duodenal) should raise the suspicion of infection with *Helicobacter pylori* or a gastrinoma as the possible factor.

4. Heavy ethanol consumption can be associated with severe gastritis, cirrhosis, and portal hypertension resulting in esophageal or gastric variceal bleeding.

5. A Mallory-Weiss tear may result from retching and vomiting.

6. A history of aortic stenosis or chronic renal failure should raise suspicion for angiomata.

7. Abdominal aortic surgery remains important as a source of gastrointestinal bleeding due to an aortoenteric fistula.

TABLE 72–3. SOURCES OF GASTROINTESTINAL BLEEDING, IN ORDER OF OCCURRENCE

	FREQUENCY (%)
1. Peptic ulcer (duodenal and gastric)	33–51
2. Esophageal and gastric varices	23–33
3. Mallory-Weiss tear	3–10
4. Gastric or duodenal erosion	1–19
5. Angiomata	0–7
6. Neoplasm	1–5
7. Dieulafoy's lesion	1.3
8. Aortoenteric fistula	<1
9. Hematobilia	<1
10. Ménétrier's disease	<1

From Jensen DM (ed): Severe nonvariceal upper GI hemorrhage. Gastrointestinal Endoscopy Clin North Am, 1991;1:211.

Clinical Findings

1. Vital signs may provide important information about the severity of blood loss. Tachycardia, hypotension, or hypovolemic shock all indicate severe, acute blood loss. The presence of orthostatic changes suggests a 20 per cent or greater blood volume loss. In those who lose over 40 per cent of their blood volume, hypovolemic shock may result.

2. Skin examination may provide evidence of the amount of blood loss (pallor of the skin) and suggest a possible etiology. Spider angiomata, palmar erythema, and icterus suggest chronic liver disease and possible variceal bleeding. Telangiectasia of the lip and perioral area suggests Osler-Weber-Rendu syndrome.

3. Nasogastric lavage provides important information in clinical assessment. The severity of bleeding can be estimated by examining nasogastric aspirate and stool color. Aspiration of bright red blood by nasogastric tube indicates active bleeding and is associated with higher mortality than melena.

4. Clinical indices such as the Baylor bleeding score (see Saeed in bibliography) help to identify patients at high risk.

Tests

1. All patients with significant GI bleeding should have blood sent for type and crossmatch, hemoglobin/hematocrit, prothrombin time, partial thromboplastin time, platelet count, electrolytes, urea nitrogen, creatinine, and liver enzymes. Although the initial hematocrit is important in determining the baseline oxygen-carrying capacity, it poorly reflects the degree and severity of blood volume loss because it takes 24 to 48 hours to equilibrate the intravascular volume.

2. An electrocardiogram in the elderly and in those with coronary artery disease may indicate ischemia related to severe anemia. Barium studies in the setting of acute upper GI bleeding are of little value. Endoscopy (both diagnostic and therapeutic) has contributed significantly in the management of patients with upper GI bleeding.

Management

1. Patients must undergo a rapid clinical evaluation with concomitant resuscitative measures. Those with significant bleeding should have two large-bore intravenous lines or a central venous access and should be admitted to the ICU for close monitoring and administration of an appropriate amount of fluids to correct the volume loss. Blood transfusion may be required depending on the volume of blood loss, age of the patient, presence of concomitant cardiorespiratory disease, and presence of continued bleeding. A reduction in oxygen-carrying capacity in those with hemoglobin below 10 gm/dl, especially the elderly, may be crucial. If coagulopathy is present, fresh frozen plasma and vitamin K should be given. Patients receiving massive blood replacement may require platelet transfusion and, rarely, calcium supplementation.

2. In those with active bleeding, airway protection is needed to avoid aspiration of blood and gastric contents. This can usually be accomplished with continuous suction and elevation of the head of patient's bed. Endotracheal intubation to reduce the risk of aspiration must be considered in those with active massive hematemesis and in those with mental status changes or shock.

3. In the past decade the role of emergency endoscopy as a diagnostic and therapeutic tool has been well recognized. Endoscopy, when available, should be considered in all patients with upper GI bleeding. It may be reasonable to omit endoscopy in patients with terminal illness and minor bleeding *or* in whom the decision to withdraw care has been made. In those presenting with upper GI bleeding, a source can be found in 95 per cent of patients. The timing of endoscopy is important, and in this respect, patients may be divided into three groups:

   a. Those with evidence of active hemorrhage. This group should have emergent endoscopy performed as soon as the patient is hemodynamically stabilized.

   b. Those with acute, self-limited bleeding without active bleeding. This group can have endoscopy within 24 hours unless they are suspected of having portal hypertension or aortoenteric fistula or have re-bled after initial stabilization.

   c. Those with chronic blood loss. Patients with chronic blood loss can have elective endoscopy.

   Unless urgent endoscopy is indicated, there is now a growing consensus among endoscopists to avoid middle-of-the-night endoscopies because of the possibility of suboptimal support. The value of endoscopy is not only to determine the source of blood loss but also to provide therapeutic and prognostic assistance in managing these patients. The Baylor bleeding score (see Saeed reference) can help to predict those patients at high risk for rebleeding. In patients with active bleeding with a negative endoscopy or those with uncontrollable bleeding, angiography may provide diagnostic and therapeutic assistance.

4. Surgical consultation in patients with significant upper GI bleeding may be necessary to coordinate the management appropriately. Further treatment depends on the source of the bleeding, the most common being peptic ulcer (see Ch. 74) and esophageal varices. Current approaches to the latter entity will be addressed here.

Variceal Bleeding

1. Patients with portal hypertension and variceal bleed-

ing have a high mortality rate and a difficult challenge to clinicians. Endoscopic treatment of esophageal varices with sclerotherapy has been shown to reduce transfusion requirement and acute mortality. Although there are multiple different sclerosant agents, 1 to 2% sodium tetradecyl sulfate is currently used in most centers. Multiple intravariceal and sometimes paravariceal injections may be required to achieve hemostasis, with a success rate of about 80 to 90 per cent. The risks of sclerotherapy include esophageal perforation, ulceration, stenosis, stricture, and necrosis, in addition to pleural effusion and mediastinitis.

2. Band ligation of esophageal varices may also be accomplished with similar success. It is associated with a lower rate of complications. The procedure requires placement of a large overtube to avoid repeated passage of the endoscope through the esophagus. In the setting of active bleeding, poor visualization of the bleeding varix may result in a slightly lower success rate.

3. Infusion of vasopressin results in a reduction of hepatic blood flow due to a decrease in portal pressure and portosystemic pressure gradient. This may lead to a reduction in variceal bleeding. The initial dose is 0.2 units/min. It is gradually increased to 0.8 units/min if there is no evidence for ischemia (especially mesenteric or myocardial). Nitroglycerin (2% ointment, 15 to 30 mg q 4 hr) is used concomitantly to reduce the risks of ischemia. Vasopressin could be used as a temporizing measure until a more definitive treatment (e.g., sclerotherapy, shunt) can be arranged. Vasopressin should not be stopped abruptly but should be tapered. Prolonged use over 12 hours is not recommended, and the presence of coronary artery disease is a relative contraindication.

4. Use of intravenous somatostatin or octreotide (Sandostatin) has been shown to decrease the risk of rebleeding without significant side effects. They have been shown to be as efficacious as sclerotherapy and more efficacious than vasopressin. The dose of somatostatin used in different trials ranges between 50 and 250 μg bolus followed by infusion of 50 to 250 μg/hr for 2 to 5 days.

5. Surgical placement of shunts reduces mesenteric flow and lowers portal pressure, and represents a valuable treatment option in patients with repeated variceal bleeding. Placement of an emergent surgical shunt in patients with advanced liver disease is often associated with high mortality. More recently, with advances in interventional radiology, transjugular intrahepatic portosystemic shunt (TIPS) accomplishes the same goal with a lower mortality. This procedure places a stent through central venous access across the hepatic parenchyma, creating a communication between the hepatic and portal venous systems, thus reducing portal pressure. TIPS is an important alternative in patients with recurrent variceal bleeding in whom sclerotherapy has failed. It is the preferred method of shunt creation in patients who are candidates for liver transplantation.

6. Balloon tamponade, using either Sengstaken-Blakemore tube or Minnesota tube (with gastric and esophageal balloons) or Linton tube (with gastric balloon), may be a useful temporizing measure in patients with esophagastric variceal bleeding. Familiarity with the use of these devices is important to avoid complications such as esophageal perforation, necrosis, and asphyxiation. Recent advances in endoscopic, medical, and surgical treatments of variceal bleeding have resulted in reduced reliance on balloon tamponade.

Bibliography

Brown KE, Peura DA: Diagnosis of *Helicobacter pylori* infection. Gastroenterol Clin North Am 1993;22:105–115.

Gupta PK, Fleischer DE: Nonvariceal upper gastrointestinal bleeding. Med Clin North Am 1993;77:973–992.

Hentschel E, Brandstatter G, Dragosics B, et al: Effect of ranitidine and amoxicillin plus metronidazole on the eradication of *Helicobacter pylori* and the recurrence of duodenal ulcer. N Engl J Med 1993;328:308–312.

Saeed ZA, Winchester CB, Michaletz PA, et al: A scoring system to predict rebleeding after endoscopic therapy of nonvariceal upper gastrointestinal hemorrhage, with a comparison of heat probe and ethanol injection. Am J Gastroenterol 1993; 88(11):1842–1849.

Sung JJY, Chung SCS, et al: Octreotide infusion or emergency sclerotherapy for variceal haemorrhage. Lancet 1993;342:637–641.

Symptom **Acute Diarrhea**   *Marilee C. S. Cole*

Most episodes of acute diarrhea are mild and self-limited. Of the fewer than 10 per cent of cases that come to the physician's attention, most simply require symptomatic oral rehydration.

Differential Diagnosis

1. Infectious diarrhea
   a. Viral diarrhea

b. Bacterial diarrhea
   (1) *Campylobacter jejuni:* often in college students
   (2) Salmonella: from contaminated beef, poultry, milk
   (3) *Shigella:* in day care centers, Native American reservations, areas of food and water contamination, homosexual males
   (4) Enterohemorrhagic *Escherichia coli:* in nurs-

ing homes, in the severely debilitated; from undercooked beef

    (5) Staphylococcal food poisoning: from unrefrigerated meat and cream-based foods

    (6) *Clostridium difficile:* with exposure to antibiotics

    (7) *Vibrio parahaemolyticus:* from exposure to raw or partially cooked seafood

    (8) Consider *Yersinia entercolitica, Vibrio cholerae, Clostridium perfringens, Bacillus cereus,* enterotoxigenic *E. coli, Aeromonas hydrophila, Plesiomonas shigelloides, Mycobacterium avium–intracellulare* under special circumstances

  c. Protozoa

    (1) *Giardia lamblia:* in day care centers, travelers, campers, homosexual males, and the immunocompromised

    (2) *Entamoeba histolytica:* predominantly in homosexual males and travelers to the tropics

    (3) *Cryptosporidium:* in young children, in the immunocompromised such as those with AIDS, and in contaminated water

2. Drugs

  a. Laxatives: phenolphthalein, magnesium citrate, senna, bisacodyl, lactulose, castor oil, milk of magnesia, polyethylene glycol purge

  b. Antibiotics: erythromycin, clindamycin, cephalosporins

  c. Antiarrhythmics: quinidine, digitalis

  d. Diuretics: furosemide, thiazide

  e. Other drugs: over-the-counter headache remedies, nonsteroidal anti-inflammatory drugs, gold, magnesium-containing antacids, thyroid medications, theophylline, stimulants, enemas, misoprostol, colchicine, anticholinesterase inhibitors, methyldopa, chemotherapy

3. Dietary items: lactose, caffeine, sorbitol, mannitol, fructose, sucrose, diet colas

4. Inflammatory bowel disease

5. Toxins: heavy metals, insecticides, mushrooms

6. Intestinal ischemia

Refer to Ch. 246, Giardiasis; and Ch. 247, Amebiasis.

History

1. Description of diarrhea: onset, duration, frequency, character of stools (soft, watery, bloody, mucus), associated nausea, vomiting, abdominal pain, tenesmus

2. Systemic symptoms: fever, chills, rigors, dry mouth, dizziness, decreased urine output, weight loss

3. Dietary history 48 hours before symptoms: ingestion of rice, milk, meat, uncooked or poorly cooked fish/ seafood, untreated water, unrefrigerated cream-based food, caffeine

4. Sexual history: homosexuality, multiple sex partners, sex with intravenous drug users, oral/anal sex, sexually transmitted diseases

5. Social history: exposure to day care center, nursing home, mental institution, poultry processing, military, travel abroad, camping, industrial toxins, farms/insecticides, Native American reservations

6. Medications: especially antibiotics

7. Medical history: sickle cell anemia, gastrectomy, thyroid disorder, malignancy, radiation, immunosuppression, malaria

Clinical Findings

1. Vital signs: temperature, blood pressure, pulse, orthostasis

2. Skin: turgor, mucous membranes, rash, erythema nodosum

3. Abdomen: distention, tenderness, bowel sounds, splenomegaly, liver, appendicitis, rectal discharge, fissures

4. General: arthritis, lymphadenopathy

Tests

1. Stool examination for white cells or blood: on moderately symptomatic patients with fever, abdominal pain, tenesmus, dehydration, diarrhea of longer than three days' duration

2. Stool cultures: on those with white cells, blood, or mucus in stool, fever, abdominal pain (use rectal swab if no stool sample is available)

3. Stool for ova and parasites: for severe or persistent diarrhea (tetracycline, sulfonamides, castor oil, magnesium hydroxide, barium, hypertonic saline, soap, tap water, bismuth, kaolin, and antiprotozoals interfere with the examination)

4. Blood tests: electrolytes; blood cultures for high fever, rigors

5. Additional tests (as indicated by type of patient and type of exposure)

  a. Day care centers: stool enzyme-linked immunosorbent assay (ELISA) for *Giardia lamblia,* modified acid-fast, *C. difficile* toxin, *E. coli* serotype 0157

  b. Travelers: enterotoxic *E. coli* toxin, *V. cholerae* (alert the laboratory), string test/ELISA *G. lamblia,* modified acid-fast (*Cryptosporidium*)

  c. Antibiotics: *C. difficile* toxin

  d. Immunosuppressed patients: modified acid-fast, HIV, *Mycobacterium avium–intracellulare*

  e. Food poisoning: culture food, vomitus, feces

  f. Seacoast: thiosulfate citrate bile salts (*Vibrio parahaemolyticus*)

  g. Weight loss: stool ELISA *G. lamblia,* ameba titers

h. Unexplained fever: *Yersinia enterocolitica* (alert lab)

i. Nursing home or hospital: enterohemorrhagic *E. coli* serotype 0157, *C. difficile* toxin

6. Sigmoidoscopy: reculture and perform biopsy in undiagnosed diarrhea

Management

1. Fluid replacement
   a. Minimally dehydrated: "drink lots of fluids" (except with vomiting, ileus)
   b. Moderately dehydrated: oral replacement therapy with glucose and electrolytes (e.g., Pedialyte, Gatorade) to 1000 ml/hour
   c. Severely dehydrated: intravenous hydration with Ringer's lactate with potassium supplement in emergency department

2. Adsorbant: Kaopectate improves stool form.

3. Antimotility agents

After removing lactose and caffeine from the diet in an afebrile patient with nonbloody diarrhea without fecal leukocytes, the following agents are useful.

   a. Loperamide (Imodium): 4 mg orally to begin and 2 mg orally after each formed stool to five doses per day
   b. Diphenoxylate hydrochloride with atropine sulfate (Lomotil): 2.5 mg to 5.0 mg orally to five doses per day
   c. Others: codeine, paregoric, deodorized tincture of opium

4. Antisecretory agent: bismuth subsalicylate (Pepto-Bismol)

5. Antimicrobials
   a. *Campylobacter jejuni:* erythromycin, 250 mg orally q.i.d. for 7 days, or ciprofloxacin (Cipro), 500 mg orally b.i.d. for 7 to 10 days; start before fourth day of illness for severe illness
   b. *Clostridium difficile:* metronidazole (Flagyl), 250 mg orally q.i.d. for 10 days (avoid in pregnancy), vancomycin, 125 mg orally to 250 mg orally q.i.d. for 5 to 10 days for severe or persistent disease if the offending antibiotics cannot be stopped.
   c. *E. coli* (traveler's diarrhea): trimethoprim/sulfamethoxazole (TMP/SMZ) (Bactrim DS, Septra DS), 160 mg TMP/800 mg SMZ orally b.i.d. for 5 days or ciprofloxacin, 500 mg orally b.i.d. for 5 days.
   d. *Entamoeba histolytica:* metronidazole, 750 mg orally t.i.d. for 10 days, followed by iodoquinol,

650 mg orally t.i.d. for 20 days to eliminate the cyst phase (do not use if patient is allergic to iodine)

   e. *Giardia lamblia:* quinacrine HCl (Atabrine), 100 mg t.i.d. for 5 days, furazolidine (Furoxone), 100 mg orally q.i.d. for 7 days, or metrinidazole, 250 mg orally t.i.d. for 7 days (avoid in pregnancy)
   f. *Salmonella enteritidis:* treat only if immunocompromised, bacteremic, younger than 1 year with ciprofloxacin, 500 mg orally b.i.d. for 7 days, or TMP/SMZ, 160 mg TMP/800 mg SMZ orally b.i.d. for 5 days (adult dosage)
   g. *Shigella:* TMP/SMZ, 160 mg TMP/800 mg SMZ orally b.i.d. for 5 days; ciprofloxacin, 500 mg orally b.i.d. for 5 days; norfloxacin (Noroxin), 800 mg orally stat

Prevention

1. Vaccines: typhoid, cholera, shigella, rotavirus
2. Travelers: "Boil it, cook it, peel it, or forget it."
3. In day care centers: handwashing after each diaper change

PEARLS

- Be sure to ask the patient to describe the frequency, liquidity, and character of the stools, as patients often misdiagnose any change in bowel habits as diarrhea.

- Look for *Giardia lamblia* in lactose-intolerant patients.

- Patients on oral hypoglycemic agents should avoid TMP/SMZ because it may lead to hypoglycemia.

B | ## Bibliography

Cheney C: Acute infectious diarrhea. Med Clin North Am 1993;77:1169–1196.

Kelly C: *Clostridium difficile colitis.* N Engl J Med 1994;330:257–262.

Kozicki M: Boil it, cook it, peel it, or forget it. Does this rule prevent travelers' diarrhoea? Int J Epidemiol 1985;14:169–171.

Mac Kenzie W: A massive outbreak in Milwaukee of *Cryptosporidium* infection transmitted through the public water supply. N Engl J Med 1994;331:161–167.

Patterson J: The pre-travel medical evaluation: The traveler with chronic illness and the geriatric traveler. Yale J Biol Med 1992;65:317–327.

Rubinoff M: Infectious diarrhea. Ann Rev Med 1991;42:403–410.

| Symptom | **Chronic Diarrhea** | *Marilee C. S. Cole* |

Chronic diarrhea lasts longer than 3 to 4 weeks and may be continuous or episodic. With the advent of AIDS, chronic diarrhea is an increasingly common and often difficult complaint to manage.

Differential Diagnosis

1. Irritable bowel syndrome
2. Diet and medications: (see preceding symptom, Acute Diarrhea)
3. Infection: *Giardia lamblia, Entamoeba histolytica, Campylobacter, Cryptosporidium, Mycobacterium avium–intracellulare* or *tuberculosis, Isospora, Cytomegalovirus, Microsporidia*
4. Malabsorption: pancreatic insufficiency, bacterial overgrowth, gluten-sensitive enteropathy (celiac disease), ileal resection
5. Carcinoma of the bowel or pancreas
6. Inflammatory bowel disease: ulcerative proctitis, ulcerative colitis, Crohn's disease, ischemic colitis, radiation colitis
7. Metabolic: hyperthyroidism, diabetes mellitus, hypoadrenalism
8. Peptide-induced gastrinoma, vasoactive intestinal polypeptide (VIP) tumor, carcinoid, villous adenoma, thyroid medullary carcinoma
9. Laxative abuse
10. Fecal impaction: especially in nursing home patients on tricyclic and anticholinergic medications

> Refer to Ch. 78, Colorectal Cancer; Ch. 81, Crohn's Disease; Ch. 82, Ulcerative Colitis; Ch. 83, Irritable Bowel Syndrome; Ch. 86, Fecal Impaction; Ch. 93, Pancreatic Carcinoma; Ch. 246, Giardiasis; and Ch. 247, Amebiasis.

History

This is key to differentiating irritable bowel syndrome, the most common cause of chronic diarrhea, from the less common forms of chronic diarrhea. Irritable bowel syndrome is characterized by frequent, incomplete evacuations and daytime diarrhea (often alternating with constipation), typically beginning in adolescence and exacerbated by stress.

1. Abdominal symptoms: age at onset; chronicity, frequency and character of stools (color, mucus, blood); presence of abdominal pain, bloating, flatulence, incontinence; inciting and ameliorating factors (time of day, foods, medicines, stress, fasting)
2. General: fever, weight loss, flushing, joint aches
3. Travel history, work history
4. Medical history: diverticulosis, diabetes mellitus, radiation therapy, ileal resection, anorectal surgery

5. Medications: consider laxative abuse, opioid withdrawal (for complete list see preceding symptom, Acute Diarrhea)
6. Sexual history: homosexuality, HIV status
7. Endocrinologic: salt craving, heat intolerance, polyuria, polydipsia, polyphagia
8. Psychiatric: increased stress, eating disorders, history of physical or sexual abuse

Clinical Findings

1. General: racial group, flushing, lymphadenopathy
2. Vital signs: fever, tachycardia
3. HEENT (eye, ear, nose, and throat): iritis, aphthous ulcers, parotid enlargement, loss of tooth enamel
4. Neck: thyroid swelling
5. Abdomen: tenderness, presence of right lower quadrant mass, perirectal fistula
6. Skin: erythema nodosum, dermatitis herpetiformis, dorsum of hand roughened, larva currens
7. Extremity: arthritis, bone fractures
8. Neurologic: peripheral or autonomic neuropathy, tetany

Tests

Before launching into an extensive evaluation, eliminate infectious causes of diarrhea. In one study in 38 per cent of patients thought to have inflammatory bowel disease the cause was infectious.

1. Exclude acute causes: (see preceding symptom, Acute Diarrhea)
2. Exclude lactose intolerance by lactose restriction or lactose tolerance test
3. Flexible sigmoidoscopy, preferably without enema prep, for culture and biopsy (or colonoscopy)
4. Plain film of abdomen: for pancreatic calcifications, obstruction
5. Air contrast barium enema (except with severe ulcerative colitis or Crohn's disease of the colon to avoid toxic megacolon)
6. Upper gastrointestinal series with small bowel follow-through to evaluate for Crohn's, celiac, and Whipple's disease
7. Blood tests: potassium, calcium, cholesterol, albumen, fasting blood sugar, 2-hour postprandial blood sugar, T_4, 8 AM cortisol, amylase, iron, prothrombin time, immunoglobulins, sedimentation rate, eosinophil count, vitamin B_{12}, HIV
8. Malabsorption work-up (for weight loss with good appetite)
   a. 72-hour fecal fat (abnormal if greater than 6 gm/day on 80- to 100-gm fat diet)

b. D-Xylose absorption (abnormal if less than 4.5 gm/five hour urine collection after ingesting 25 gm D-xylose orally)

c. Schilling or breath test for bacterial overgrowth

d. Small bowel biopsy, aspirate, culture

e. Bentiromide test for pancreatic function

f. Gluten sensitivity screen: especially for gliadin antibody

9. Stool volume, electrolytes, osmolality (especially after fasting)

10. Therapeutic trials

a. Restricted diets (e.g., gluten)

b. Antibiotics (e.g., tetracycline, metronidazole)

11. Heavy metals: arsenic, mercury, lead, cadmium

12. Urine 5HIAA, plasma gastrin, calcitonin, VIP, glucagon, somatostatin

13. Stool alkalinization for identification of laxative phenolphthalein use/abuse

Management

1. As for acute diarrheas: hydrate, eliminate causative medicines and foods, treat underlying infections, use antimotility agents when necessary (see preceding symptom, Acute Diarrhea)

2. Irritable bowel syndrome: adequate fluids and dietary fiber, stress reduction, sympathetic physician, psyllium, antispasmodics such as dicyclomine (Bentyl), 10 mg orally t.i.d.

3. Lactose-intolerant patients: remove lactose from diet, maintain dietary calcium intake with yogurt, lactose hydrolyzed milk (Lactaid), or calcium carbonate tablets (Tums)

4. Malabsorption

a. Pancreatic insufficiency: pancreatic enzyme (Pancrease), 1 to 2 capsules with each meal and 1 with snack

b. Bacterial overgrowth: antibiotics (e.g., TMP/SMZ [Bactrim DS] 160 mg TMP/800 mg SMZ orally b.i.d.

c. Celiac disease: avoid wheat, barley, rye flours

5. Inflammatory bowel disease

a. Ulcerative proctitis: hydrocortisone, 100 mg retention enema (Cortenema) at bedtime for 21 days, or mesalamine (Rowasa), 4 gm enema

b. Ulcerative colitis: prednisone, 60 mg orally daily until remission; then maintenance, 15 to 30 mg orally daily plus sulfasalazine or mesalamine (Asacol, Pentasa), orally 2 gm to 4 gm daily plus steroid enema

c. Crohn's disease: as per ulcerative colitis, plus antibacterial, vitamin supplement with folic acid, antimotility agent, occasionally elemental diet (Ensure)

6. Diabetes mellitus: clonidine, octreotide (Sandostatin)

7. Chronic secretory diarrhea: octreotide

8. Intractable diarrhea: cholestyramine

PEARLS

- Think Crohn's disease in the elderly with nonspecific symptoms and an indolent course. Time to diagnosis in one study was three times longer in the elderly than in younger patients with Crohn's disease (6.4 versus 2.4 years).

- Prepare a homemade hydrocortisone enema (cheaper than the expensive commercial preparations) by blending 100 mg hydrocortisone hemisuccinate in 60 ml of safflower oil.

- A majority of AIDS patients have had at least one diarrheal episode. Symptomatic treatment of stool-culture–negative AIDS-related diarrhea is both efficacious and cost-effective.

B ## Bibliography

Greenberger N: Diagnostic approach to the patient with chronic diarrheal disorder. Disease-a-month 1990;36:131–179.

Grimm I: Inflammatory bowel disease in the elderly. Gastroenterol Clin North Am 1990;19:361–389.

Jernigan J: Parasitic infections of the small intestine. Gut 1994;35:289–293.

Johanson J: Efficient management of diarrhea in the acquired immunodeficiency syndrome (AIDS). Ann Intern Med 1990;112:942–948.

Levine J: Decision Making in Gastroenterology. St. Louis, Mosby-Year Book, 1992, pp 12–403.

Nolte F: Practical considerations in the laboratory diagnosis of bacterial enteric infections. Am J Clin Pathol 1994;101:S14–S17.

Symptom **Constipation** *Andrew M. D. Wolf*

1. Epidemiology: Constipation is the most common digestive complaint in the United States, affecting over 4.5 million people or 2 per cent of the population. It is two to three times more common in women, and there is a marked increase in constipation after age 65, but this is a consequence of co-morbidity, environmental influences, and over-reporting, not of the aging process itself. Between 2 and 3 million people use laxatives regularly in the United States, with potentially damaging consequences and an annual expenditure approaching $400 million for over-the-counter (OTC) laxatives alone.

TABLE 72–4. CAUSES OF CONSTIPATION

Health habits	Neurologic
Low fiber/fluid intake	Parkinson's disease
Inactivity	Multiple sclerosis
Medications	Spinal cord lesions
Anticholinergics (tricyclics,	Autonomic neuropathy
neuroleptics, anti-Parkinson)	(esp. diabetes mellitus,
Antihypertensives (verapamil,	pseudo-obstruction)
diuretics, clonidine)	Hirschsprung's disease
Narcotics	Psychiatric
Antacids (with aluminum or	Depression
calcium)	Endocrine/metabolic
Iron	Hypothyroidism
Bile resins	Pregnancy/premenstrual
Sympathomimetics	Hypercalcemia
Chronic stimulant laxative use	Hypokalemia
Irritable bowel syndrome	Uremia
Structural lesions	
Tumor	
Stricture	
Hemorrhoids	
Fissure	
Rectocele	

2. Definition: The generally accepted standard is fewer than three stools/week. Passage of hard small stools, straining, and sense of incomplete evacuation are often included in the definition.
3. Etiology: Table 72–4.

History

1. Clarify "constipation": stool frequency, consistency, straining; many patients are preoccupied with their bowels but are not constipated.
2. Onset: Recent onset raises possibility of significant pathology, especially tumor.
3. Associated symptoms: Abdominal pain can suggest irritable bowel syndrome (IBS) or tumor; hematochezia, reduced caliber, and tenesmus can suggest structural lesion (tumor, hemorrhoids, fissure, stricture); constitutional symptoms can suggest malignancy, or endocrine or metabolic causes; depressive symptoms may suggest a psychiatric etiology.
4. Sexual history: As many as 50 per cent of women with functional gastrointestinal (GI) complaints have been victims of sexual abuse.
5. Medication history (see Table 72–4): Be sure to ask about OTC laxative use, as this may well contribute to chronic constipation ("cathartic" or atonic colon).
6. Brief diet/exercise screen: adequate fiber, fluids, activity

Key Questions to Ask

1. What does the patient mean by "constipation?"
2. When did symptoms begin?
3. Any associated GI symptoms?
4. Any constitutional symptoms?
5. What medications?

Clinical Findings

1. Abdominal examination: Check for tenderness, masses.
2. Rectal examination: Examine for anal tone (rule out neurologic lesion), trauma (especially in children and adolescents), hemorrhoids, fissure, stricture/stenosis, rectocele, tumor, impaction, and occult blood.
3. General examination: Look for signs of hypothyroidism and neurologic disease.

Tests

1. Blood tests: Recent onset of severe constipation warrants checking serum potassium, calcium, and thyroid-stimulating hormone. Chronic laxative users should have a complete set of electrolytes, blood urea nitrogen, and creatinine in view of the potential metabolic sequelae.
2. Endoscopy: Most middle-aged or older patients with recent onset of significant constipation should undergo flexible sigmoidoscopy at a minimum to rule out colorectal carcinoma. This may also detect other structural lesions (see above) and melanosis coli, suggestive of chronic stimulant laxative abuse. Severe constipation, concomitant abdominal pain, occult blood in the stool, and constitutional symptoms generally dictate the need for full colonoscopy or addition of barium enema to the sigmoidoscopy.
3. Radiography: Plain abdominal films are not routinely indicated but can occasionally be useful to confirm the diagnosis by demonstrating feces throughout the colon. Barium enema may also be necessary, as discussed above.
4. Colonic transit time/motility studies: rarely indicated. Reserve for instances of severe constipation unresponsive to treatment, when the results will alter management approach.

Management

1. First treat fecal impaction if present.
2. Nonpharmacologic treatment should be mainstay of therapy.
   a. Ensure adequate fluid intake (1500 cc minimum).
   b. Ensure adequate dietary fiber intake—bran cereal, beans, vegetables, fruit (14 gm crude fiber, 30 gm dietary fiber/day).
   c. Ensure adequate physical activity.
   d. Bowel retraining: Patient should attempt to defecate at the same time daily within 10 to 15 minutes of a meal (to utilize the gastrocolic reflex); may require daily suppository or enema at first.
3. Pharmacologic treatment (Table 72–5)
   a. Bulk-forming laxatives: should be used preferentially for long-term management of ambulatory patients but may be ineffective in bed-bound patients

TABLE 72–5. COMMON LAXATIVES

CATEGORY NAME (EXAMPLES)	ADULT DOSE	POTENTIAL ADVERSE EFFECTS/COMMENTS
Bulk-forming		
Psyllium (Metamucil)	1 tsp q.d.-t.i.d.	Bloating, gas, obstipation if taken without fluids
Methylcellulose (Citrucel)	1 tbsp q.d.-t.i.d.	Bloating, gas, but less than with psyllium
Stool softeners		Mucosal irritation; no evidence for true laxative effect
Docusate sodium (Colace)	50–500 mg q.d.	
Docusate calcium (Surfak)	240 mg q.d.	
Osmotic		
Lactulose	15–60 cc/day	Bloating, cramps, flatulence
Sorbitol (70%)	30–60 cc/day	Same as lactulose, much less expensive
Glycerin	1 suppository	Occasional rectal irritation
Saline		
Magnesium hydroxide (Milk of Magnesia)	30–60 cc	Cramping, diarrhea, dehydration, ↑ Mg in elderly and renal disease
Sodium phosphate (Fleet Enema, Phospho-Soda)	PO: 20–30 cc enema: 1–2/wk	Dehydration, ↑ phosphate in renal disease
Stimulants		Electrolyte imbalance, "cathartic" (atonic) colon
Phenolphthalein (Ex-Lax, Correctol)	1–2 tabs at HS	
Bisacodyl (Dulcolax)	1–3 tabs, 1 suppository (max. 3/wk)	
Senna (Senokot)	2 tabs at HS	
Cascara	1 tab at HS	
Lubricants		
(Mineral oil)	15–45 cc PO or by enema	Fat-soluble vitamin malabsorption, lipoid pneumonia if aspirated

b. Osmotic agents: preferred second-line agents because they are less toxic than other alternatives

c. Stool softeners: useful when straining should be avoided (e.g., hemorrhoids, myocardial infarction), but have no effect on stool frequency and are greatly overprescribed

d. For refractory constipation: A regimen including bisacodyl suppositories or tapwater enemas once or twice a week, together with a daily osmotic laxative, is generally safe and effective; stimulant laxatives are a last resort because of potential long-term toxicity.

e. Cisapride, a GI prokinetic drug, can be useful for slow-transit constipation but has not yet been approved for this indication.

PEARLS

* Check the list of medications for constipating drugs.

* New-onset of significant constipation requires lower GI evaluation.

* Mainstays of treatment are adequate fluids, fiber, and exercise.

* Bulk-forming laxatives should be first-line, followed by osmotic agents.

* Stool softeners have little or no laxative effect; they simply soften stool.

 ## Bibliography

Devroede G: Constipation. *In* Sleisenger MH, Fordtran JS (eds): Gastrointestinal Disease: Pathophysiology/Diagnosis/Management. 5th ed, vol 1. Philadelphia, WB Saunders, 1993, pp 837–887.

Donatelle EP: Constipation: Pathophysiology and treatment. Am Fam Physician 1990;42:1335–1342.

Harari D, Gurwitz JH, Minaker KL: Constipation in the elderly. J Am Geriatr Soc 1993;41:1130–1140.

Marshall JB: Chronic constipation in adults: How far should evaluation and treatment go? Postgrad Med 1990;88:49–63.

Wald A: Constipation and fecal incontinence in the elderly. Gastroenterol Clin North Am 1990;19:405–418.

| Symptom | **Rectal Bleeding** | *Arthur H. Herold* |

The complaint of rectal bleeding must be taken seriously. The severity of bleeding does not relate to the significance of the underlying pathology, and the same types of lesions can produce extremes in bleeding rates. The physician must first determine whether the rectal bleeding has produced hemodynamic compromise. Such patients require resuscitation and stabilization first before searching for the cause. However, episodes of rectal bleeding are usually self-limiting, and the evaluation can be carried out in a timely methodical manner. Determining the site (upper gastrointestinal [GI], small bowel, colorectal) takes precedence over identifying the source. The frequency of causes of rectal bleeding is influenced by the patient's age, whether a particular study is conducted on inpatients or outpatients, and whether the bleeding is occult, small, or massive.

Differential Diagnosis
1. Colorectal diseases (80 to 85 per cent)
   a. Diverticulosis
   b. Angiodysplasia
   c. Neoplasms
      (1) Colon cancer
      (2) Colonic polyps
   d. Inflammatory bowel disease
      (1) Ulcerative colitis
      (2) Crohn's colitis
   e. Anorectal disorders
      (1) Hemorrhoids
         (a) External
         (b) Internal
      (2) Anal fissure (fissure in ano)
      (3) Anal fistula (fistula in ano)
      (4) Rectal prolapse
      (5) Neoplasms
         (a) Rectal carcinoma
         (b) Rectal polyps
      (6) Proctitis
         (a) Ulcerative
         (b) Infectious
      (7) Cryptitis
      (8) Draining perirectal abscess, pilonidal cyst
      (9) Dermatologic conditions
   f. Colitis
      (1) Ischemic
      (2) Infectious
      (3) Radiation
2. Upper GI tract (10 per cent)
   a. Duodenal ulcer
   b. Erosive gastritis
   c. Mallory-Weiss tear
   d. Esophagitis
   e. Gastric ulcer
   f. Esophageal varices
   g. Neoplasm
   h. Biliary or pancreatic duct bleeding
3. Small intestine diseases (5 per cent)
   a. Neoplasms
   b. Crohn's disease
   c. Aortoenteric fistula
   d. Angiodysplasia
   e. Meckel's diverticulum
   f. Intussusception
4. Systemic conditions (rare)
   a. Anticoagulation therapy
   b. Thrombocytopenia
   c. Histiocytosis
   d. Amyloidosis
   e. Vasculitis
   f. Elastic tissue diseases
5. Trauma (uncommon)
   a. External abdominal
   b. Rectal

Refer to Ch. 74, Peptic Ulcer Disease; Ch. 76, Gastritis; Ch. 78, Colorectal Cancer; Ch. 80, Intussusception; Ch. 82, Ulcerative Colitis; Ch. 84, Diverticulitis; and Ch. 85, Hemorrhoids.

History
1. Character of blood: color, consistency, amount, frequency, duration
   a. Hematochezia
      (1) Bright red: usually a distal colorectal or anorectal source. Can be a proximal GI hemorrhage if brisk and associated with increased colonic motility
         (a) On toilet paper, dripping into toilet, typically limited amounts, especially with defecation: probably a perianal source
         (b) Coating a normal stool: consider a lesion in the anal canal
         (c) Streaking or mixed with a formed stool: suggests rectosigmoid or descending colon lesion
      (2) Maroon stools: source may be proximal colon, small intestinal, or distal colon if associated with constipation.

b. Melena (sticky, jet-black, tarry, foul-smelling stools)

(1) Do not confuse with

(a) Clotted blood, which will turn water red

(b) Iron or bismuth ingestion

(c) Dark but normal stools

(2) Source

(a) Significant upper GI bleeding (oral cavity, esophagus, stomach, or duodenum)

(b) May be lower GI hemorrhage if colonic motility is slow

c. Occult blood loss: The patient may present with symptoms of anemia (orthostasis, syncope, dyspnea on exertion, angina, fatigue, or pallor) but usually is asymptomatic.

2. Pain with bleeding

a. Absent: consider diverticulosis, angiodysplasia, internal hemorrhoids

b. Abdominal

(1) Epigastric: upper GI source, such as peptic or gastric ulcer, esophageal varices, Mallory-Weiss tear. Typical symptoms include hematemesis or vomiting, history of aspirin, nonsteroidal anti-inflammatory drugs (NSAIDs), alcohol, or tobacco use; peptic ulcer disease (PUD).

(2) Periumbilical: small bowel. Think ischemic bowel if there is a history of vascular or coronary artery disease.

(3) Hypogastric: colonic lesions

(4) Suprapubic: rectosigmoid lesion

(5) Generalized (but may be upper, mid, or lower abdominal): ruptured aortic abdominal aneurysm with aortoenteric fistula. (Patient is catastrophically ill, has tearing back pain during dissection.)

(6) Left lower quadrant: descending colon or sigmoid lesions

(7) Crampy with gas and bloating: inflammatory bowel disease

(8) Colicky: intussusception

c. Sacral: rectal lesions

(1) Sharp, knife-like after bowel movement: anal fissure

(2) Constant throbbing: perirectal abscess, acute thrombosed external hemorrhoids

3. Change in bowel habits with bleeding

a. Constipation

(1) Chronic: hemorrhoids

(2) Recent progressive: distal colonic annular constricting carcinoma

(3) Voluminous hard stool with pain: anal fissure

b. Diarrhea

(1) Frequent bloody bowel movements, small amounts ± mucus, weight loss: inflammatory bowel disease

(2) With pus: infectious colitis or proctitis

c. Tenesmus: anorectal lesions such as proctitis or neoplasm

d. Discharge, mucopurulent ± blood ± stool ± foul odor: proctitis, draining perirectal abscess/cryptitis, fistula in ano, pilonidal cyst

e. Change in shape of stool, decreased caliber, or flat spot: anal or rectal carcinoma

f. Sensation of rectal fullness, incomplete evacuation, or recognition of rectal mass present: rectal carcinoma or hemorrhoids

4. History of systemic disease, anticoagulation therapy, aspirin, NSAID use or symptoms of metastasis such as weight loss, anorexia, abdominal bloating or swelling, malnutrition

5. History of trauma, abuse (child, sexual, spouse), insertion of foreign objects into the rectum, or anal intercourse

The clinician must be suspicious that an underlying lesion has been unmasked when rectal bleeding occurs in an anticoagulated patient, especially if the patient is not overly anticoagulated.

Clinical Findings

1. Degree of blood loss: Evaluate general appearance and vital signs.

a. Chronic (pallor, tachycardia, postural hypotension): carcinoma

b. Acute

(1) Massive (altered mental status, hypotension, shock, gross evidence of blood loss rectally ± abdominal distention): bleeding ulcer, varices, angiodysplasia, diverticulosis, ruptured abdominal aortic aneurysm

(2) Minimal (stable vital signs): anorectal conditions, carcinoma

2. Abdominal examination

a. Distended: ruptured aneurysm

b. Pulsating mass: aneurysm

c. Tender epigastrium: ulcers

d. Hepatomegaly: metastatic colon cancer

e. Ascites: metastatic colon cancer

f. Sausage-shaped mass right side: intussusception

g. Diffuse mild tenderness without guarding: colitis

h. Left lower quadrant tenderness: sigmoid colon lesion

i. Mass along course of colon: colon cancer

j. Hyperactive bowel sounds: colitis, obstruction

3. Rectal examination

a. Anal inspection: Spread the buttocks vigorously with patient in left lateral position.

   (1) External hemorrhoids, prolapsing internal hemorrhoids, and carcinoma should be apparent.

   (2) Draining sinus tract: superior—pilonidal cyst; perianal—fistula in ano

   (3) Tear in anal skin parallel to anal canal, superior or inferior ± sentinel tag: anal fissure

b. Digital examination

   (1) Perianal mass deep in buttocks with surrounding erythema and inflammation: perirectal abscess

   (2) Pain with insertion of digit into anal canal: anal fissure

   (3) Stenosis of anal canal: constricting anal carcinoma

   (4) Solid mass in rectum: rectal carcinoma

4. Confirmation of bleeding

a. Inspect toilet or bed pan for color and amount. If stool just eliminated, hemoccult sample if presence of blood is doubtful.

b. Rule out bleeding from the vagina or urethra in women.

c. Inspect underclothes and buttocks. The presence of blood in a continent patient suggests bleeding external to the anal sphincter.

d. Inspect sample during rectal examination for presence of melena, maroon-colored blood, or bright red blood.

e. Hemoccult stool sample from rectum regardless of appearance

Tests

1. Laboratory

a. Complete blood count

   (1) Anemia: may be present when GI blood loss has been subacute or chronic and significant

   (2) Normal blood count: present when bleeding has been acute and massive because plasma volume has not equilibrated, or chronic lesions with insignificant blood loss

b. Serum iron, total iron-binding capacity, ferritin: helpful to confirm iron deficiency when patient has anemia and GI blood loss is suspected but not confirmed

c. Chemistry studies: useful if a systemic process is suspected such as inflammatory bowel disease or metastatic carcinoma

d. Fecal occult blood test: If the patient is stable and GI blood loss is questionable, give the patient three cards to collect samples at home. Hand out instructions to minimize false-positive or false-negative test results.

2. Anoscopy

a. Should be performed during the initial physical examination

b. Rules out lesions of the anus and anal canal such as hemorrhoids or fissures

3. Proctosigmoidoscopy: The clinician must be trained before attempting this procedure.

a. Examines the rectum, sigmoid and sometimes part of the descending colon

b. Useful to rule out left-sided colorectal lesions such as polyps, proctitis, colitis, and carcinoma, when brisk bleeding is not present

4. Colonoscopy: ideally inspects the entire colon

a. Limited value if lower GI bleeding is acute and massive or patient is unprepped

b. Used to diagnose slow bleeding lesions to include polyps, diverticula, angiodysplasia, carcinoma, or colitis

5. Arteriography

a. Best initial test if bleeding is rapid (must be at least 0.5 to 1.0 ml/min)

b. Allows rapid localization and possible treatment of a briskly bleeding lesion such as diverticula, angiodysplasia, carcinoma, and lesions proximal to the colon

c. Has high complication rate

6. Technetium-99m–labeled red blood cell scintigraphy

a. Order for intermittent bleeding if the patient is stable and recurrent bleeding is anticipated within 30 hours; delayed images can be obtained.

b. Slowly bleeding lesions (as low as 0.1 ml/min) can be seen to include diverticula or angiodysplasia.

c. More useful than technetium-99 sulfur colloid scan because this radionuclide is rapidly cleared, making it a poor technique for diagnosing intermittent bleeding

7. Barium enema: Do not order when vigorous bleeding is present.

a. Diagnostic for space-occupying lesions larger than 1 cm, such as polyps and carcinoma

b. Can detect moderately advanced inflammatory bowel disease

c. Cannot detect actual sites of bleeding such as angiodysplasia or bleeding from diverticulosis

d. Order this test only after performing sigmoidoscopy or if colonoscopy does not visualize the cecum.

8. Nasal gastric tube insertion

a. Should be done first if the patient has rectal bleeding, is hemodynamically compromised, and is suspected of having an upper GI bleed

b. Positive findings are active bleeding, gross blood,

blood clots or coffee grounds. Otherwise do not Hemoccult test other materials since a traumatic insertion can produce a positive result.

9. Esphagogastroduodenoscopy: order this test if
    a. Lower GI work-up is unrevealing
    b. Nasogastric tube insertion is positive
    c. Nasogastric tube insertion is negative but clinically an upper GI bleed is suspected

10. Enteroclysis: radiography of the small intestine using controlled infusion of contrast via a nasogastric tube inserted into the duodenum
    a. Order for evaluation of chronic GI bleeding when work-up of the upper GI tract and colon has not revealed the source.
    b. Low-yield test but can diagnose Meckel's diverticulum, Crohn's ileitis, and small bowel cancers

11. Miscellaneous tests
    a. Meckel's radionuclide scan: most useful in the evaluation of lower GI bleeding in children and adolescents; positive in only 60 per cent of cases
    b. Plain films of the abdomen: usually not helpful but can show an ileus from ischemic colitis or severe inflammatory bowel disease, calcification of an abdominal aneurysm, or free air from a perforated viscus

For patients older than age 50 with non-urgent rectal bleeding, order colonoscopy, because diverticulosis and angiodysplasia are high in the differential diagnosis. Middle-aged adults may have the colon assessed with fiberoptic flexible sigmoidoscopy and air contrast barium enema (ACBE) in lieu of colonoscopy. Young adults may be evaluated with just sigmoidoscopy if a source is found, such as anorectal lesions, or if there is a reasonable explanation for the bleeding.

Management

1. General
    a. Resuscitate hemodynamically compromised patients.
    b. Looking for the source of bleeding may occur concomitantly with attempts to stabilize the patient.
    c. Even if bleeding has stopped, anticipate re-bleeding.

2. Upper GI bleeding
    a. Must treat urgently since upper GI bleeding that produces rectal bleeding will be massive
    b. See other sections of the book for treatment of specific diseases of the upper GI tract.

3. Lower GI bleeding
    a. Urgent therapy: continuous bleeding or recurrent bleeding that has required more than 3 units of blood

b. Elective therapy
    (1) In about 80 per cent of acute lower GI bleeding cases, bleeding will stop spontaneously.
    (2) Most patients with anorectal conditions

c. Colonoscopic therapies
    (1) Employs various probes, forceps, or lasers
    (2) Used initially for angiodysplasia, diverticula, polyps, or small carcinomas

d. Angiographic techniques
    (1) Intra-arterial vasopressin or embolization
    (2) Used for bleeding from angiodysplasia or diverticula, which is massive or unresponsive to treatment ''c''

e. Surgical treatment: usually a segmental or subtotal colectomy
    (1) For patients with large-volume blood loss (≥ 6 units of blood), actively or recurrently, who have failed treatments ''c'' or ''d''
    (2) Patients with multiple lesions (angiodysplasia or diverticula) not amenable to treatments ''c'' or ''d''
    (3) Patients with cancers
    (4) Obscure and uncontrolled colonic bleeding

f. Specific conditions: see appropriate section under Gastrointestinal Diseases.

PEARLS

- The volume of bleeding is not related to the significance of the underlying lesion.

- The color and consistency of the blood depend on GI motility. Do not rely solely on the blood's appearance as an indicator of the level from which it is coming.

- Be skeptical of attributing rectal bleeding to just a benign anorectal source in adults ≥ 50 years of age, even if active bleeding is seen from such lesions in this area.

Bibliography

Cello JP: Diagnosis and management of lower gastrointestinal tract hemorrhage. Medical Staff Conference, University of California, San Francisco. Western J Med 1985;143:80–87.

Edmundowicz SA, Zuckerman GR: Gastrointestinal bleeding. In Dunagan WC, Ridner ML (eds): Manual of Medical Therapeutics, 26th ed. Boston, Little, Brown, 1989, pp 280–289.

Friedman LS (ed): Lower gastrointestinal bleeding. Gastroenterol Clin North Am 1994;23:1.

Marshall JB: Acute gastrointestinal bleeding. Postgrad Med 1990;87:63–70.

Peterson WL: Obscure gastrointestinal bleeding. Med Clin North Am 1988;72:1169–1176.

Procedure **NASOGASTRIC INTUBATION**   *Michael B. Harper*

Indications

1. Diagnostic evaluation and possible treatment for upper gastrointestional bleeding
2. Obstruction of small bowel or gastric outlet obstruction
3. Lavage for poisoning or overdose and administration of oral antidote
4. Enteral feeding

Contraindications

1. Maxillofacial trauma or basilar skull fracture; tube may enter the cranium
2. Bilateral nasal obstruction; oral route may be used
3. Recent surgery to the nose, pharynx, esophagus, or stomach
4. Use caution in patients with a bleeding diathesis

Equipment

1. Use the proper tube for the situation: Salem sump tube (16 to 18 Fr) for drainage of air and liquids, large-bore tube (Ewald) by oral route for overdose, specialized small-bore tubes for enteral nutrition
2. Lubricant, topical anesthetic, and topical vasoconstrictor
3. Emesis basin, 30- to 60-cc syringe with catheter tip
4. Gloves, goggles, gown, and protective sheet
5. Suction tube, tonsilar tip, and suction device
6. Tape and benzoin

Anesthesia

1. Xylocaine jelly, solution, and spray
2. Topical vasoconstrictor such as phenylephrine or cocaine

Precautions

1. Aspiration of gastric contents may cause aspiration pneumonia. Risk of this complication is high with enteral feeding (20 to 50 per cent) and may be decreased by placement of a feeding tube into the duodenum.
2. Injury to nasal mucosa may cause epistaxis.
3. Inadvertent tracheal intubation may occur and is identified by coughing, choking, and difficulty in talking. These signs are less apparent with small-bore feeding tubes.
4. Lung injury and pneumothorax may occur if enteral feeding tubes with weighted tip and/or metal stylet are passed into the trachea.
5. Vigorous attempts at passage can cause perforation of the esophagus (rare).

WARNING

In a patient with altered mental status, tracheal intubation may occur without typical signs.

Technique

1. Measure the distance from the patient's ear to umbilicus to estimate the required length of tube to be inserted.
2. Place the patient in the sitting position or left lateral decubitus with neck flexed (if no C-spine injury) to make esophageal passage more direct and avoid tracheal intubation.

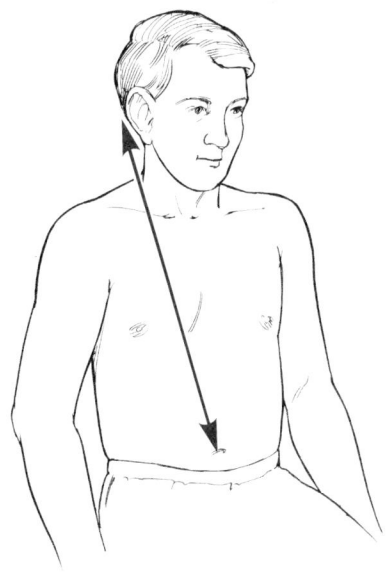

3. Select the most patent nostril and apply topical anesthetic and vasoconstrictor to nasal mucosa. Apply Xylocaine jelly to the tube.

4. Have suction ready to remove emesis or secretions, especially in obtunded patients.

5. Gently insert the tube directed toward the occiput; have the patient swallow when the tube is felt on the back of the throat (15 to 20 cm); sipping water through a straw may help.

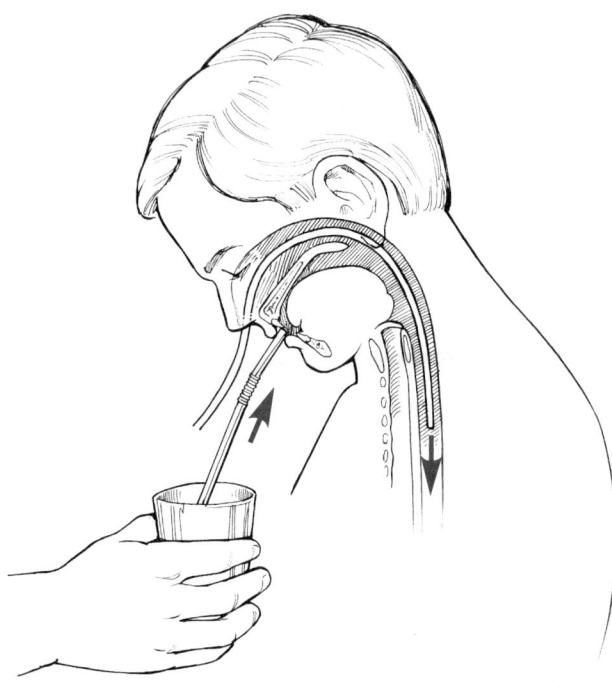

6. If passage into the mouth or coiling occurs, chill the tube with ice to increase its rigidity and help eliminate this problem.

7. If excessive gagging occurs spray the patient's throat with Xylocaine.

8. Insert the tube to the level of the stomach as previously measured (usually 40 to 50 cm).

9. Instill air with a 30- to 60-cc syringe and listen over the stomach for passage of air.

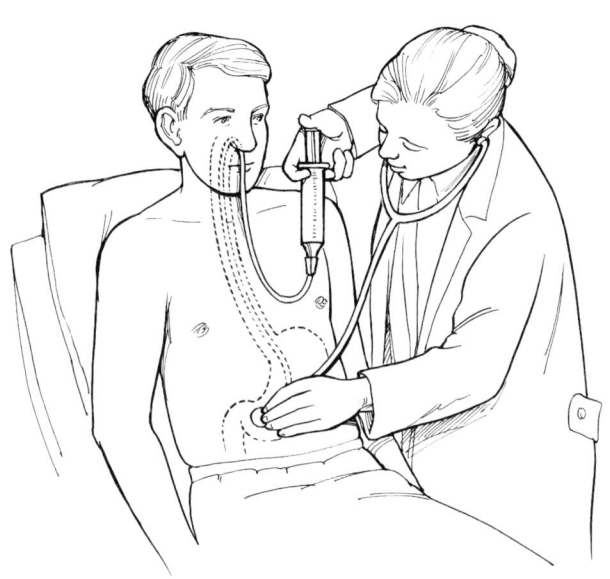

Aspiration of gastric contents and pH of aspirate (usually <5) can be used to help confirm placement.

10. Secure tube with tape and benzoin to the nose, avoiding pressure to the nostril.

11. Radiographic confirmation of placement is mandatory if any substance is to be administered through the tube or if the tube is to be left in place for any length of time.

12. Enteral feeding tubes with weighted tip may pass into the duodenum by placing the patient on the right side for 8 to 24 hours. Active passage into the pylorus using a tube with wire stylet can be performed. Duodenal location is indicated by aspiration of bile and/or aspirate with a pH over 7. Position is confirmed with radiographs.

Follow-Up

1. Check periodically to confirm proper tube functioning by observing continued accumulation of gastric fluids in the collection bottle.

2. If the tube becomes blocked, instill 20 to 30 cc of air into the sump channel to free the tube from gastric mucosa. If blockage persists, inject air or a small amount of normal saline into the main lumen. If blockage recurs, reposition the tube.

3. Periodically check for pressure necrosis of the nose and reposition the tube if necessary.

4. Remove the tube as soon as feasible to avoid complications of prolonged use. Potential problems include: gastric erosion with hemorrhage, perforation of stomach or intestine, sinusitis, otitis, pharyngitis, and laryngeal obstruction from subglottic stenosis.

Bibliography

Drickamer MA, Cooney LM: A geriatrician's guide to enteral feeding. J Am Ger Soc 1993;41:672–679.

Sagar PM, Kruegener G, MacFie J: Nasogastric intubation and elective abdominal surgery. Br J Surg 1993;79:1127–1131.

Thomas S, Raman R, Idikula J, Brahmadathan N: Alterations in oropharyngeal flora in patients with a nasogastric tube: A cohort study. Crit Care Med 1992;20:1677–1680.

Wrenn K: The lowly nasogastric tube: Still appropriate after all these years (at times). Am J Emerg Med 1993;11:84–89.

Zaloga GP: Bedside method for placing small bowel feeding tubes in critically ill patients. Chest 1991;100:1643–1646.

Procedure | **EXCISION OF THROMBOSED HEMORRHOID** | *John G. O'Handley*

Indications

1. Constant anal pain of sudden onset
2. Ulceration or rupture of the thrombosed hemorrhoid

IMPORTANT

The pain associated with a thrombosed hemorrhoid often resolves after 48 hours. The clot is gradually absorbed over seven to ten days. When this does not occur or the patient desires immediate relief, excision is an option.

Contraindications

1. Absolute
   a. If thrombosed hemorrhoid is internal (above dentate line)
2. Relative
   a. Bleeding or clotting disorder
   b. Associated infection

Preparation

1. Patient is placed either in the lateral Sims position or jackknife position.
2. Assistant to adequately expose the entire thrombosed hemorrhoid
3. The anal area is cleansed with povidone-iodine.

Equipment

1. No. 15 or No. 11 blade
2. Adson's forceps with teeth
3. Straight hemostat
4. Curved iris scissors
5. 10-cc syringe
6. 27-gauge 1¼″ needle
7. Electrocautery and/or Monsel's solution

Anesthesia

1. 0.5% bupivacaine in 1:200,000 epinephrine with 1:10 sodium bicarbonate, USP 8.4%
   a. The sodium bicarbonate is mixed with the bupivacaine just before surgery to avoid precipitation.
   b. By alkalinizing the solution, one can prevent the burning pain of the anesthetic.
2. The area surrounding the base of the thrombosed hemorrhoid is infiltrated just beneath the skin, raising a slight wheal circumferentially.
3. Adequate time is allowed (2 to 4 minutes) for the anesthetic to take effect.

Precautions

1. If the patient is hypertensive, the blood pressure should be checked following anesthesia.
2. Failure to anesthetize completely around the hemorrhoid may result in pain with the excision.
3. Failure to completely remove the clot may result in prolonged postoperative bleeding and continuing pain.

Technique

1. After exposure of the hemorrhoid, the incision is planned. The type of excision depends on the size of the hemorrhoid and the amount of skin that can be safely removed.
   a. For hemorrhoids 2 cm or larger, a radial elliptical (fusiform) incision over the top of the hemorrhoid can be made using the curved iris scissors and Adson's forceps or blade.

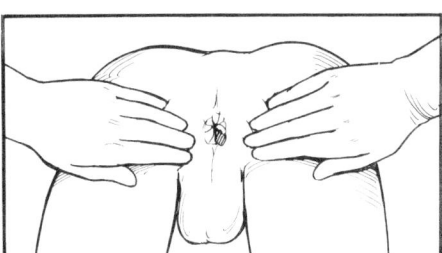

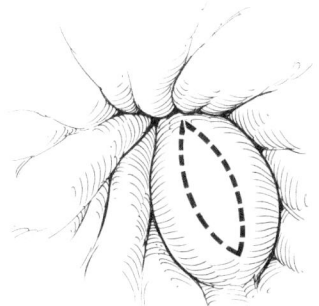

b. For hemorrhoids less than 2 cm, the entire hemorrhoid can be excised using the curved iris scissors and Adson's forceps, again utilizing a radial elliptical (fusiform) excision.

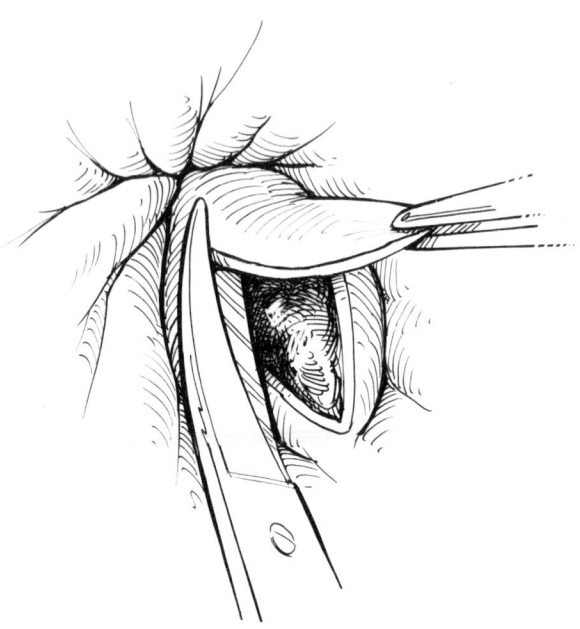

c. Express the clot by applying pressure laterally. Determine whether the entire clot has been removed by palpating over the area. If any clot remains, a straight hemostat may be used to open up any remaining clotted veins.

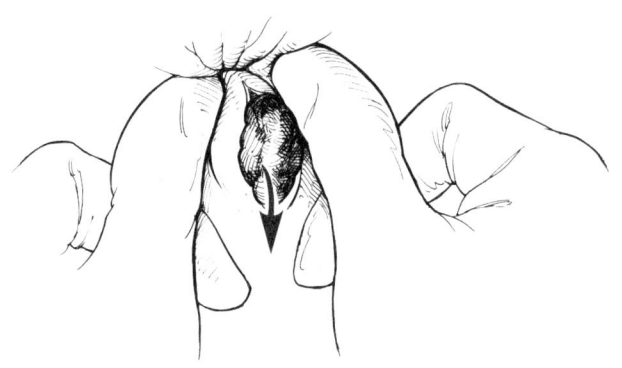

2. Hemostasis can be achieved with pressure, Monsel's solution, and/or electrocautery.
3. Packing is not required.
4. A dressing of 4 × 4s and a large pad can be applied. This should be left on for at least four hours.

Follow-Up

1. The patient is instructed to begin warm sitz baths twice a day, no sooner than 4 hours after the surgery, and continue these for 7 to 10 days.
2. Stool softeners
3. Analgesia in the form of acetaminophen plus propoxyphene hydrochloride can be given for the first few days following surgery. After that, acetaminophen should be all that is required.

IMPORTANT

If a stronger narcotic, such as hydrocodone or oxycodone, is required, the patient should be warned about its potential for causing constipation.

---

4. The patient is to report any bleeding that soaks through the dressing in the first 24 hours. Subsequently, the bleeding should gradually stop over 5 to 7 days. If it begins heavier than before, the physician must be notified.
5. Anoscopy and flexible sigmoidoscopy are recommended in 2 weeks.

Bibliography

Corman ML: Colon and Rectal Surgery, 3rd ed. Philadelphia, JB Lippincott, 1993; pp 77–78.

Goligher J: Surgery of the Anus, Rectum and Colon, 5th ed. London, Balliere Tindall, 1984, pp 143–144.

Grosy CR: A surgical treatment of thrombosed external hemorrhoids. Dis Col Rect 1990;249–250.

Salvati EP, Eisenstat TE: Hemorrhoidal disease. In Condon RE (ed): Shackelford's Surgery of the Alimentary Tract, 3rd ed, vol IV. Philadelphia, WB Saunders, 1991, p 295.

73 Stomatitis

Thomas K. Hunt

Etiology

1. Stomatitis represents a spectrum of inflammatory changes of the oropharynx, most typically ulcerative or vesicular.
2. Causes are multiple and may be *primary,* such as local infections or trauma in the oral cavity, or *secondary,* such as oral manifestations of systemic diseases. Often, no cause can be identified.
   a. The etiologic agent in the most common ulcerative oral lesion, aphthous stomatitis (''aphtha'' means ''ulcer''), is unknown and may be multiple. Proposed factors have included streptococcal and herpetic infections, minor dental trauma, stress, menstruation, and nutritional deficiencies, to name a few, but none have withstood rigorous analysis.
   b. Viral-induced oral infections are common. Herpes simplex virus type 1 causes several distinct oral diseases, among them acute herpetic gingivostomatitis and herpes simplex labialis (''cold sores''). Coxsackie A viruses cause at least two clinical entities: (1) herpangina and (2) hand-foot-and-mouth disease. Many of the childhood viral exanthems (rubella, rubeola, varicella) present with oral lesions.
   c. Other infectious causes include syphilis, tuberculosis, deep fungal infections, *Mycoplasma pneumoniae,* cytomegalovirus, and anaerobic bacteria.
   d. Stomatitis may reflect systemic disease, particularly inflammatory bowel disease, collagen vascular disease, Behçet's syndrome, Kawasaki's disease, erythema multiforme, and immunosuppressive conditions such as HIV infections.
   e. Other etiologies include trauma (from biting or ill-fitting dentures), irritants (aspirin, nicotine), chemotherapy, and carcinoma.

Symptoms

1. Aphthous ulcers or ''canker sores'' are painful and can recur four or more times a year.
2. Stomatitis caused by viral infections have classic prodromal phases of fever, chills, myalgias, arthralgias.
3. Any stomatitis can be disabling and cause anorexia.

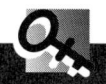
Key Symptoms

- Oral pain
- May have systemic symptoms: fever, chills, malaise, anorexia, arthralgias

Clinical Findings

1. Aphthous stomatitis (or ''canker sores'') is characterized by its painful and recurring nature. Aphthous ulcers are rarely found on oral mucosa that is bound to periosteum, such as the attached gingiva and hard palate; this provides an important distinction from herpetic ulcers. There are three variants.
   a. The *minor* form (80 per cent) is usually a solitary oval ulcer measuring less than 1 cm in diameter and lasting 7 to 10 days. Most patients are young. Disease prevalence is 20 to 50 per cent in the general population.
   b. *Major* ulcers (10 per cent) are multifocal and ragged and may be up to 2 cm in diameter; these frequently last up to 6 weeks, may scar, and are often immediately followed by a recurrent ulcer.
   c. *Herpetiform* ulcers (10 per cent) are so named because the papulovesicular lesions are grouped, simulating herpes simplex infections.
2. In *acute primary herpetic gingivostomatitis* the patient is usually young and toxic-appearing with the classic viral prodrome followed in 24 to 48 hours by mucosal vesicles, which quickly rupture and coalesce into large, painful ulcers associated with gingivitis, a white coating on the tongue, and regional lymphadenopathy. The acute phase rarely lasts more than a week. Recurrent episodes, commonly known as *herpes labialis* or ''cold sores,'' are characterized by single or multiple 2- to 4-mm vesicles around the vermilion border of the lip, frequently following prodromal ''itchiness'' or ''tingling,'' and rupturing in 36 to 48 hours to form crusts. Frequency of recurrences varies and may be influenced by sunlight, cold, and stress.

Key Signs

- Oral vesicles or ulcers
- Lymphadenopathy
- Fever
- Toxic appearance (in herpetic infections)

Laboratory Tests

1. Diagnosis of aphthous stomatitis is clinical.
2. Herpes infection can be confirmed by titers in acute and convalescent sera and by cytology showing giant cells with viral inclusion bodies.
3. Suspected syphilitic lesions can be sampled by smear for darkfield microscopy.

4. Biopsy may be required where tuberculous, fungal, or carcinomatous etiologies are considered.

Differential Diagnosis

Aphthous ulcers must be differentiated from acute herpetic gingivitis, traumatic ulcers, allergy, and ulcerations due to systemic disease:

1. Ulcerations due to herpes simplex virus infections usually follow constitutional symptoms and rupture of vesicles.
2. Traumatic and aphthous ulcers are clinically and histologically identical and are distinguished by anatomic relation to irritating structures.
3. Allergic lesions tend to be diffuse and do not ulcerate.
4. Ulcers of systemic diseases are slow to heal but rarely recur.

Treatment

1. Therapy for aphthous stomatitis is palliative and should include avoidance of hot or acidic foods, gentle rinsing with saline solution, and topical viscous lidocaine (3 ml of 2% solution held in the mouth for one to two minutes before meals). Diphenhydramine solution, sometimes mixed with Kaopectate, is also analgesic.
2. Antibacterial washes (tetracycline mouthwash or chlorhexidine gluconate oral rinse, Peridex) may diminish secondary bacterial infection.
3. Topical steroids provide relief for aphthous but not viral stomatitis. Dry the lesion first, then apply triamcinolone cream 0.1% every 4 to 6 hours mixed with, or followed by, Orabase to affix the steroid. Use systemic or locally injected steroids only in severe cases.
4. Topical acyclovir (5%) may help herpes labialis. Consider oral acyclovir during the prodrome.

5. Provide symptomatic relief for viral syndrome.
6. Treat other infections accordingly (e.g., syphilis, tuberculosis)

Diet

1. Avoid hot, acidic, irritating foods. Encourage fluid intake.
2. Role of iron, B_{12}, and folate supplementation is not clear.

Patient Education

1. Probably a role in aphthous stomatitis for stress reduction
2. Patients with herpes virus infection need to understand they are infectious.

Key Treatment

- Saline rinses
- Steroid cream applied locally

Follow-Up

Perform biopsy on any ulcer that fails to heal spontaneously in 10 to 14 days.

Bibliography

Allen CM: Diagnosing and managing oral candidiasis. J Am Dent Assoc 1992; 123(1):77–78, 81–82.

Eversole LR: Inflammatory diseases of the mucous membranes. Part 1: Viral and fungal infections; Part 2: Immunopathologic ulcerative and desquamative diseases. CDA (California Dental Association) Journal, 1994; 22(4):52–66.

Greenspan D, Greenspan JS: Oral lesions of HIV infection: Features and therapy. AIDS Clin Rev 1992;225–239.

Rogers RS III: Common lesions of the oral mucosa. A guide to diseases of the lips, cheeks, tongue, gingivae. Postgrad Med 1992; 91(1):141–148, 151–153.

Sonis ST, Fazio RC, Fang L: Principles and Practice of Oral Medicine. Philadelphia, WB Saunders, 1984.

74 Peptic Ulcer Disease

George T. Fantry

Etiology

1. *Helicobacter pylori* infection
   a. The major cause of chronic active gastritis and the primary etiologic factor in peptic ulcer disease (PUD)
   b. Associated with 95 to 99 per cent of duodenal ulcers and 70 to 90 per cent of gastric ulcers
   c. Treatment of *H. pylori* improves the healing rate and markedly decreases the recurrence rate of peptic ulcers, altering the natural history of the disease.
2. Nonsteroidal anti-inflammatory drugs (NSAIDs)
   a. May cause gastric or duodenal ulcers; addition of steroids potentiates risk
   b. Accounts for the majority of *H. pylori*-negative ulcers
3. Stress: severe physiologic stress such as burns, CNS trauma, surgery, severe medical illness
4. Hypersecretory states (uncommon): gastrinoma (Zollinger-Ellison syndrome or multiple endocrine neoplasia [MEN-1]), antral G cell hyperplasia, systemic mastocytosis, basophilic leukemias
5. Rare causes: viral (herpes, cytomegalovirus), radiation, chemotherapy-induced, vascular insufficiency (crack cocaine), duodenal obstruction
6. Diseases associated with PUD: cirrhosis, chronic pulmonary disease, renal failure, renal transplantation

Pathogenesis

1. The pathogenesis of PUD is related to an imbalance between the normal protective factors and injurious factors.
   a. Defensive factors: mucus, bicarbonate, mucosal blood flow, prostaglandins, alkaline tide, hydrophobic layer, restitution, epithelial renewal
   b. Offensive factors: *H. pylori,* acid, pepsin, bile acids, smoking, ethanol, NSAIDs, aspirin, steroids, stress
2. Risk factors: smoking
3. Genetics: familial tendency, increased frequency in persons with blood group O

Symptoms

Symptoms may vary from classic symptoms to vague symptoms to symptoms related to complications of PUD.
1. Epigastric pain
   a. Gnawing or burning
   b. Occurs one to three hours after meals
   c. Relieved by food or antacids
   d. May occur at night
   e. May radiate to back (consider penetration)
2. Nausea
3. Vomiting (may be related to partial or complete gastric outlet obstruction)
4. Dyspepsia (belching, bloating, distention, fatty food intolerance)
5. Heartburn
6. Chest discomfort
7. Anorexia, weight loss
8. Hematemesis or melena (secondary to gastrointestinal bleeding)

Key Symptoms

- Epigastric burning pain
- Dyspepsia

Clinical Findings

In uncomplicated PUD, clinical findings are few and nonspecific.
1. Epigastric tenderness
2. Guaiac-positive stool (due to occult blood loss)
3. Melena (due to acute or subacute gastrointestinal bleeding)
4. Succession splash (due to partial or complete gastric outlet obstruction)

Key Sign

- Epigastric tenderness

Laboratory Tests

1. Routine laboratory tests in most patients with uncomplicated PUD are not helpful in diagnosis but may include a complete blood count, serum creatinine, and serum calcium.
2. Diagnostic studies
   a. Upper gastrointestinal endoscopy with antral biopsy: superior sensitivity and specificity, allows for detection of *H. pylori.*
   b. Upper gastrointestinal series
3. Special studies
   a. Detection of *H. pylori* (essential in all patients with peptic ulcers): urease test (best endoscopic diagnostic test), histopathology, culture, urea breath test, serum *H. pylori* Ab

b. Serum gastrin: useful in recurrent, refractory, or complicated PUD and in patients with a family history of PUD to screen for Zollinger-Ellison syndrome (ZE syndrome)

c. Secretin stimulation test: used to distinguish ZE syndrome from other conditions with a high serum gastrin, such as achlorhydria, antisecretory therapy (see below)

d. Measurement of acid secretion: useful to distinguish ZE syndrome from other hypergastrinemic states; not useful in routine evaluation of PUD

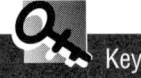 **Key Test**

• Endoscopy, diagnostic test for *H. pylori*

Differential Diagnosis

1. Gastroesophageal reflux disease
2. Nonulcer dyspepsia, gastroduodenitis
3. Drug-induced dyspepsia (theophylline, digitalis, caffeine)
4. Biliary tract disease
5. Pancreatitis
6. Musculoskeletal (back-gut syndrome)
7. Gastric cancer, duodenal cancer, pancreatic cancer
8. Crohn's disease
9. Other infectious and infiltrative lesions of the stomach and duodenum: giardiasis, sarcoidosis, tuberculosis, Menetrier's disease, lymphoma, *Mycobacterium avium–intracellulare*

> **WARNING**
>
> **Elderly patients are more likely to be asymptomatic and have an increased risk of complications such as gastrointestinal bleeding, particularly if taking NSAIDs.**

Treatment

There are multiple effective and well tolerated therapeutic regimens available to treat peptic ulcers. Considerations when choosing a regimen include compliance, drug interactions, and cost. Gastric ulcers may require a longer course of therapy than duodenal ulcers. In addition to standard ulcer therapy, all patients with peptic ulcers and *H. pylori* infection should be treated with a regimen to eradicate *H. pylori*.

Medication

A. Ulcer therapy (antisecretory, acid-dependent)
  1. H_2-receptor antagonists (H$_2$RA)
     a. Inhibit acid secretion by blocking H_2 receptors on parietal cells

b. Equal efficacy in equivalent doses (healing rate of 70 to 80 per cent at 4 weeks, 90 to 95 per cent at 8 weeks)

c. Therapeutic regimen
   (1) Cimetidine (Tagamet), 400 mg b.i.d. or 800 mg hs for 6 to 8 weeks
   (2) Famotidine (Pepcid), 20 mg b.i.d. or 40 mg hs for 6 to 8 weeks
   (3) Nizatidine (Axid), 150 mg b.i.d. or 300 mg hs for 6 to 8 weeks
   (4) Ranitidine (Zantac), 150 mg b.i.d. or 300 mg hs for 6 to 8 weeks

2. Proton pump inhibitors
   a. Inhibit the parietal cell H^+, K^+-ATPase pump, the final common pathway in acid secretion
   b. Achieve a healing rate of 80 to 100 per cent at four weeks, significantly greater than H$_2$RA
   c. Therapeutic regimen: Omeprazole (Prilosec), 20 to 40 mg daily for 4 weeks

3. Prostaglandins
   a. Inhibit acid secretion by decreasing generation of cyclic AMP in the parietal cell in response to histamine stimulation
   b. Healing rates are equal to or slightly lower than those for H$_2$RA.
   c. Primary role is as a prophylactic agent to prevent NSAID-induced ulcers, not recommended as routine therapy for PUD; use may be limited by side effects.
   d. Prophylactic regimen: Misoprostol (Cytotec), 200 μg q.i.d.

4. Antimuscarinic agents: Pirenzipine, telenzipine; not approved for use in the United States

B. Ulcer therapy (cytoprotective: enhances mucosal defense, acid-independent)
  1. Sucralfate
     a. Healing rates comparable to those of H$_2$RA
     b. Therapeutic regimen: Sucralfate (Carafate), 1 gm q.i.d. or 2 gm b.i.d. for 6 to 8 weeks
  2. Antacids (multiple aluminum, magnesium, and calcium-based antacids are available)
     a. Moderate- to high-dose antacids result in healing rates comparable to H$_2$RA
     b. Tablet and liquid forms are equally effective; four times a day dosing is adequate
     c. Therapeutic regimen: Antacid, 1 hr pc and hs for 6 to 8 weeks
  3. Bismuth

C. *Helicobacter pylori* eradication
  1. Indicated in all *H. pylori*-infected patients with PUD
  2. Therapeutic regimens

a. Triple therapy (treatment of choice, duration of 1 week is most effective; eradication rate: 85 to 90 per cent; may be limited by side effects)

   (1) Bismuth subsalicylate (Pepto-Bismol), 2 tablets q.i.d.

   (2) Metronidazole (Flagyl), 250 to 500 mg t.i.d.

   (3) Tetracycline, 500 mg q.i.d., or amoxicillin, 500 mg q.i.d.

         or

   (4) Omeprazole (Prilosec), 40 mg daily

   (5) Clarithromycin (Biaxin), 500 mg b.i.d. or t.i.d.

   (can substitute amoxicillin, 500 mg for either 2 or 3)

b. Two-drug regimen (duration 2 weeks, less effective; variable eradication rate: 50 to 84 per cent, fewer side effects)

   (1) Omeprazole, 40 mg daily

   (2) Amoxicillin, 1 gm b.i.d., or Clarithromycin, 500 mg t.i.d.

Key Treatment

Drugs of Choice	Alternative Drugs
• H$_2$-receptor antagonists	• Proton pump inhibitors
• Anti-*H. pylori* therapy	• Sucralfate, antacids

Diet

No special diet is required.

Patient Education

1. Smoking cessation

2. Avoid NSAID and aspirin use

3. Avoid heavy alcohol use

4. Stress-reduction counseling may be helpful in individual cases but not routinely needed.

Follow-Up

1. Endoscopy is required to document healing of gastric ulcers and to rule out gastric cancer.

2. Peptic ulcer disease is a chronic disease with a one-year recurrence rate of 60 to 90 per cent.

3. Maintenance therapy with half standard doses of H$_2$RA at bedtime decreases the 1-year recurrence rate of peptic ulcers to 20 to 25 per cent.

4. Eradication of *H. pylori* decreases the one-year recurrence rate to less than 10 per cent on no therapy.

5. Maintenance therapy is not required in patients who have uncomplicated ulcers and who have had *H. pylori* infection eradicated. It should be considered in patients older than 60, smokers, and patients with recurrent, refractory, or complicated ulcers, particularly those in whom *H. pylori* has not been eradicated.

 Bibliography

For more information on etiology, pathogenesis, diagnosis, and treatment of peptic ulcer disease, see

Soll AH: Gastric, duodenal, and stress ulcer. *In* Sleisenger MH, Fordran JS (eds): Gastrointestinal Disease. vol 1, 5th ed. Philadelphia, WB Saunders, 1993, pp 580–679.

For more information on *H. pylori* and its role in peptic ulcer disease, see

Dooley CP, Cohen H (eds): *Helicobacter pylori* infection. Gastroenterol Clin North Am 1993;22:1–206.

For more information on treatment of *H. pylori,* see

Chiba N, Rao BV, Rademaker JW, Hunt RH: Meta-analysis of the efficacy of antibiotic therapy in eradicating *Helicobacter pylori.* Am J Gastroenterol 1992;87:1716–1727; Graham DY, Ginger LM, Klein PD, et al: Effect of treatment of *Helicobacter pylori* infection on long-term recurrence of gastric or duodenal ulcer, a randomized, controlled study. Ann Intern Med 1992;116:705–708.

NIH Consensus Conference: *Helicobacter pylori* in peptic ulcer disease. JAMA 1994;272:65–69.

Indications

1. Upper abdominal distress (epigastric pain, heartburn, dyspepsia, or indigestion) that persists despite an appropriate trial of therapy
2. Upper abdominal distress associated with symptoms and/or signs suggesting serious organic disease (such as weight loss, anorexia, or persistent anemia)
3. Pain or difficulty in swallowing
4. Esophageal reflux symptoms that persist despite appropriate therapy
5. Persistent vomiting or nausea of unknown cause
6. Radiographic findings of a suspected neoplastic lesion, an esophageal stricture, or a gastric ulcer
7. Active upper gastrointestinal (GI) bleeding, especially when surgery is contemplated
8. When gastric or duodenal tissue or fluids must be sampled

Contraindications

1. Adult patient refuses the examination
2. Patient is moribund or has life-threatening instability of cardiopulmonary status
3. Known or suspected perforation in GI tract
4. Lack of availability of resuscitation equipment or personnel
5. Large esophageal diverticulum (relative)

Preparation

1. Patient education about the procedure (verbally and in writing) and informed consent
2. Nothing to eat or drink for 6 hours before the procedure
3. If delayed gastric emptying is suspected, use a clear liquid diet the day before the procedure.
4. Have patients arrange for transportation home (i.e., not driving themselves) with someone accompanying them after the procedure.

Equipment

1. Upper GI endoscope (fiberoptic or video)
2. Light source
3. Bite block
4. Photographic equipment (optional) (still or video)
5. IV fluids and equipment for administration
6. Medications for topical anesthesia and conscious sedation
7. Biopsy forceps and brushes
8. Suction pump or vacuum source
9. Oxygen and administration equipment
10. Pulse oximetry monitor and probes
11. Crash cart, defibrillator, and resuscitation equipment

Topical Anesthesia and Conscious Sedation

1. Topical anesthesia for oropharynx and esophagus
   a. Spray the oropharynx with benzocaine or tetracaine spray or
   b. Swab the oropharynx with viscous lidocaine and have the patient swallow and gargle with viscous lidocaine.
2. Conscious sedation
   a. Start intravenous line and use rapidly flowing fluids and a relatively large-bore catheter.
   b. Give a small test dose and then titrate to desired level of conscious sedation using diazepam or midazolam.
3. Monitor carefully during conscious sedation using vital signs and other appropriate observations. Many endoscopists use pulse oximetry for monitoring. Record all monitoring data.
4. Resuscitation equipment and appropriately trained personnel must be available. Drugs to reverse benzodiazepines (flumazenil) should be available.

Precautions

1. Know the patient's drug allergies.
2. Use caution and extra monitoring in patients with cardiopulmonary diseases.
3. Do not oversedate the patient.
4. Monitor carefully.
5. Be ready and able to provide resuscitation if needed.

Technique

1. Arrange all equipment in the room.

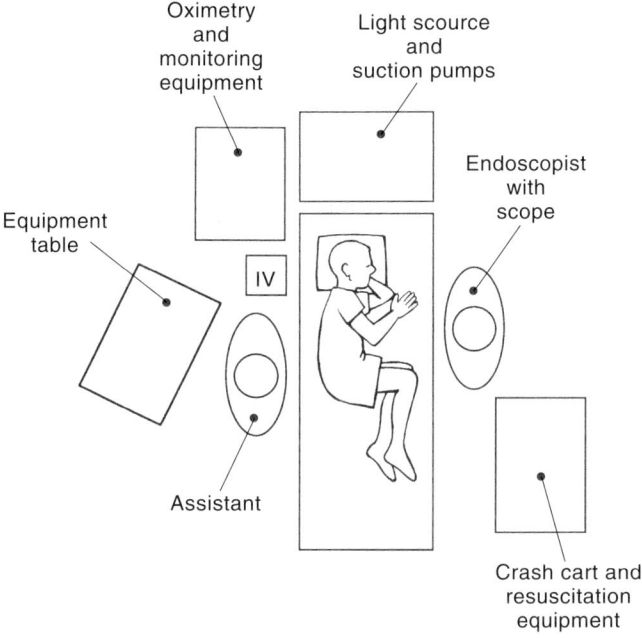

2. Thoroughly examine the oral cavity and oropharynx, recording any abnormalities noted.

3. Apply topical anesthesia and start the intravenous line.

4. Position the patient in the left lateral decubitus position.

5. Administer the drugs for conscious sedation and titrate to the desired level of sedation.

6. Insert the tip of the endoscope into the patient's mouth, either by direct observation through the endoscope or by blindly passing the tip of the scope through the operator's fingers.

7. At the level of the cricopharyngeus muscle (upper esophagus), ask the patient to swallow in order to gently pass that point of constriction. Look for tracheal intubation (indicated by cough and the visualization of the tracheal rings through the scope. If seen, remove the scope and reinsert.

8. Under direct visualization, advance the scope through the esophagus. Try to keep the lumen centered in the scope's field in order to avoid trauma to the walls. Carefully note any pathology seen (use descriptions or photographs of the abnormal areas).

9. Carefully study the distal esophagus and the esophagogastric junction. If abnormalities are noted, make a mental note to obtain biopsies as the scope is removed at the end of the procedure.

10. At this point the patient can be asked to sniff or to inhale to allow the endoscopist to see the indentation from the diaphragm on the outside of the esophagus. This procedure is useful in determining the presence of a hiatal hernia.

11. Gently inflate the lower esophagus and pass the scope into the stomach.

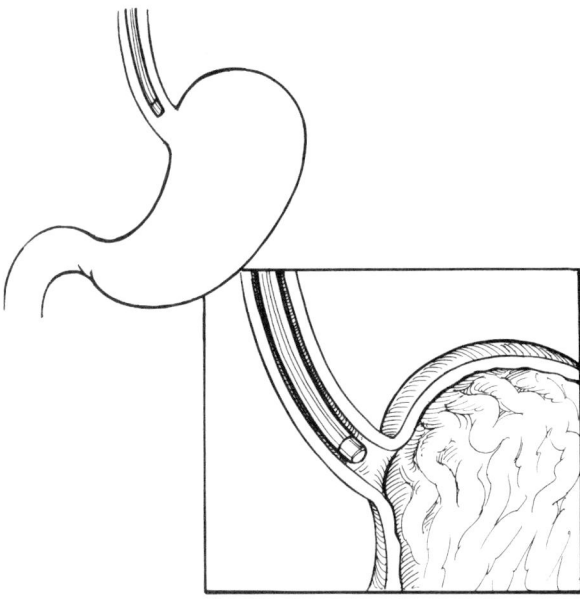

Once the stomach is entered, insufflate gently to allow visualization. Then move the tip of the scope to the greater curvature (which will be dependent) and suction the "gastric pool" of secretions.

12. Insufflate more air into the stomach, briefly view the mucosa, and move to the pylorus. Note the appearance of the mucosa and use the angularis or incisura, a fold on the lesser curvature, as a landmark.

13. Move the scope to the pylorus and, using small puffs of air and gentle pressure, pass the tip of the scope through the pylorus.

14. Carefully inspect the duodenum, noting the rings of Kerckring and the papilla of Vater. Obtain biopsies or brushings if indicated and take photographs as needed.

15. Withdraw the scope tip into the stomach and do a complete inspection of the entire gastric mucosal surface. The tip of the scope will need to be retroflexed in order to view the cardia.

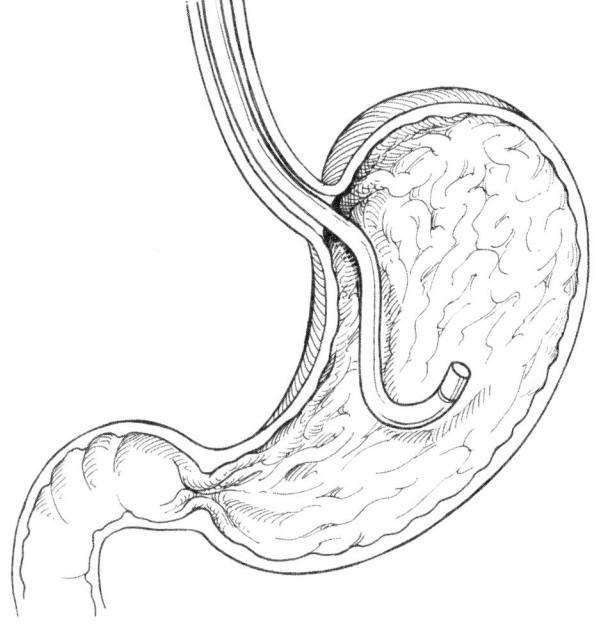

16. Take biopsies, brushings, and photographs as indicated if abnormalities are noted. This is a good time to take another look at any areas that appear abnormal.
17. Withdraw the scope and again view the esophagus. Esophageal biopsies may be obtained now.
18. Observe the patient until the sedation has diminished; remove the line and complete the monitoring record and the medical record.

Follow-Up

1. Meet with the patient (and family if appropriate) either that day after the sedation has cleared or on another day to discuss the findings and to review photographs and pathologic reports.

2. Prescribe any treatment that is indicated by the findings of the procedure and arrange follow-up.

Bibliography

Blackstone MO: Endoscopic Interpretation: Normal and Pathologic Appearances of the Gastrointestinal Tract. New York, Raven Press, 1984.

Demling L: Endoscopy and Biopsy of Esophagus and Stomach, 2nd ed. Philadelphia, WB Saunders, 1982.

Norris TE (ed): Esophagogastroduodenoscopy (EGD): A Syllabus for the Family Physician. Kansas City, American Academy of Family Physicians, 1994.

Silverstein FE, Tytgat GNJ: Atlas of Gastrointestinal Endoscopy. Philadelphia, WB Saunders, 1987.

75 Gastroesophageal Reflux

Stephen A. Brunton

Etiology

1. Predominantly a motility disorder with an incompetent lower esophageal sphincter (LES) allowing retrograde flow of stomach contents into esophagus; may also have delayed gastric emptying and impaired esophageal clearance

2. Hiatal hernia is present in approximately 80 per cent of people with reflux esophagitis, although approximately half of all people with hiatal hernia have no reflux.

Symptoms

1. The predominant symptom is heartburn (pyrosis), which may be associated with regurgitation, water brash, and odynophagia. Other symptoms that may reflect dysmotility include early satiety, abdominal fullness, bloating, and belching.

2. Atypical symptoms include chest pain or symptoms referable to the respiratory tract such as cough, laryngitis, or wheezing.

 Key Symptoms

Typical	Atypical
• Heartburn	• Chest pain
• Regurgitation	• Cough
• Water brash	• Laryngitis

Clinical Findings

The physical examination is nonspecific and usually is negative.

Laboratory Tests

1. Radiographs: Upper gastrointestinal (GI) series may be helpful to detect sequelae of gastroesophageal reflux (GER) such as ulcerations and stricture; however, it has limited usefulness in diagnosing GER without complications.

2. Upper GI endoscopy: useful for evaluation of GER sequelae such as esophagitis, ulceration, and stricture. Essential for identification of Barrett's esophagus (columnar metaplasia of esophageal squamous epithelium) or as a screen for adenocarcinoma.

3. Bernstein test—provocative test for GER: Dilute HCl alternating with normal saline dripped above LES and correlated with symptoms; highly sensitive but has low specificity

4. 24-hour esophageal pH monitor: definitive diagnostic test correlating symptoms with periods of time with pH <4 above LES.

Key Tests

- Upper GI film series
- Upper GI endoscopy
- Acid Bernstein test
- 24-hour esophageal pH monitor

Differential Diagnosis

1. Peptic ulcer disease: Pain may be epigastric and is often relieved by food.

2. Coronary ischemia: It is essential to rule out central chest pain of cardiac origin. GER and coronary ischemia may co-exist, and the pain of GER may aggravate ischemia.

Treatment

1. Phase 1
   a. Dietary modifications
      (1) Weight loss in obese
      (2) Decrease in food with high fat content
      (3) Avoidance of citrus fruits, tomato-based products, coffee (caffeinated and decaffeinated), onions, chocolate, and peppermint
   b. Smoking cessation
   c. Elevation of the head of the bed
   d. Avoiding late or large evening meals
   e. Modifying or stopping medications that decrease LES pressure, including theophylline, anticholinergics, nitrates, calcium channel blockers, progesterone-containing birth control pills
   f. Antacids

2. Phase 2
   a. H_2 antagonists
      (1) Cimetidine (Tagamet), 800 mg hs or 400 mg b.i.d.
      (2) Famotidine (Pepcid), 40 mg hs or 20 mg b.i.d.
      (3) Nizatidine (Axid), 300 mg hs or 150 mg b.i.d.
      (4) Ranitidine (Zantac), 300 mg hs or 150 mg b.i.d.
   b. Prokinetic agents
      (1) Cisapride (Propulsid), 10 to 20 mg q.i.d.
      (2) Metoclopramide (Reglan), 10 to 20 mg q.i.d.

3. Phase 3—proton pump inhibitor: omeprazole (Prilo-

sec), 20 mg q.i.d.; or Lansoprazole (Prevacid), 30 mg q.i.d.

4. Phase 4—surgery: Nissen fundoplication most frequently utilized

Patient Education

Patients should follow guidelines as listed in Phase 1 treatment.

Key Treatment

Phase 1: Lifestyle modification and antacids

Phase 2: H₂ antagonist or prokinetic agent or combination

Phase 3: Proton pump inhibitor

Phase 4: Surgery

Follow-Up

GER is a lifelong irreversible condition. The patient should be re-evaluated regularly to assess therapeutic progress. GER sequelae such as esophagitis, stricture, or Barrett's esophagus require intensive lifelong follow-up.

Bibliography

Champion GL, Richter JE: Atypical presentation of gastroesophageal reflux disease: Chest pain, pulmonary, and ear, nose, throat manifestations. The Gastroenterologist 1993;1:18–33.

Hixson LJ, Kelley CL, Jones WN, Tuohy CD: Current trends in the pharmacotherapy for gastroesophageal reflux disease. Arch Intern Med 1992;152:717–723.

Richter JE: Gastroesophageal reflux disease. *In* Winawer SJ (ed): Management of Gastrointestinal Diseases. New York, Gower, 1992, pp 2–44.

Sontag SJ: The medical management of reflux esophagitis. Gastroenterol Clin North Am 1990;19:683–712.

Traube M: The spectrum of the symptoms and presentations of gastroesophageal reflux disease. Gastroenterol Clin North Am 1990;19:609–616.

76 Gastritis

Etiology

Inflammatory changes of the gastric mucosa are classified by histology, pathogenesis, or clinical associations, and may result from various causes such as

1. *Helicobacter pylori*-associated gastritis: the major etiologic agent in chronic gastritis

   a. May result in acute inflammation with evolution into chronic superficial gastritis and ultimately chronic atrophic gastritis with intestinal metaplasia, or ulceration

   b. Over 80 per cent of chronic gastritis is associated with this organism.

   c. Pathogenesis unclear but may involve altered mucosal integrity secondary to secretion of potentially toxic enzymes or chemicals

   d. May promote development of peptic ulcer disease or gastric cancer

2. Non-*H. pylori* infectious gastritis

   a. Bacterial: any gastric bacterial infection may lead to gastritis

      (1) Syphilis—secondary and tertiary: may cause superficial gastritis to transmural infiltration

      (2) *Mycobacterium* spp: uncommon but may cause ulceration, transmural inflammation, or even fibrosis of gastric antrum

      (3) *Clostridium* and *Escherichia*: may cause emphysematous gastritis (wall gas)

      (4) *Streptococcus, Staphylococcus, E. coli,* and *Proteus*: may cause a severe purulent gastritis known as phlegmonous gastritis

   b. Viral (e.g., cytomegalovirus, herpesvirus): occurs more frequently in immunocompromised hosts

   c. Fungal (e.g., *Candida,* histoplasmosis, mucormycosis): usually seen in immunocomprised host, although rarely

   d. Parasitic: also more common in immunocompromised host

      (1) *Strongyloides stercoralis*: common worldwide; rarely affects stomach

      (2) Anisakiasis: an unusual cause of clinical acute gastritis

3. Noninfectious granulomatous gastritis

   a. Crohn's disease: clinically significant gastric disease is relatively uncommon.

   b. Sarcoidosis: although gastrointestinal involvement is rare, the stomach is most frequently affected.

   c. Eosinophilic: extensive infiltration causing wall thickening and fibrosis

4. Mucosal irritants: generally cause chronic superficial gastritis, but the gastritis may be acute with severe erosion and hemorrhage

   a. Alcohol: depletes epithelium of extracellular mucus and intracellular mucus glycoproteins, producing gastric mucosal injury

   b. NSAIDs: positively linked to chronic gastritis and gastric ulcer

5. Autoimmune disease: causes chronic atrophic gastritis

   a. Exclusive distribution in the gastric corpus and fundus; *H. pylori* rarely seen

   b. Found in 20 per cent of patients with pernicious anemia

   c. Genetic link with autosomal dominant mode of inheritance

   d. Characterized by parietal cell and intrinsic factor autoantibodies, hypergastrinemia, and eventual hypochlorhydria

6. Stress-induced gastritis: damage from gastric secretions as a result of increased mucosal susceptibility from conditions of extreme physical stress

   a. True incidence disputed, may be 80 to 100 per cent of critically ill patients evaluated endoscopically

   b. Characterized by shallow multiple erosions of proximal stomach

7. Alkaline reflux gastritis: reflux of alkaline secretions into the gastric remnant

   a. Incidence may range from 5 to 35 per cent of patients with operations obliterating sphincteric function of pylorus—most commonly Billroth II.

   b. May rarely occur in patients without gastrobiliary surgery who have reduced pyloric pressure and abnormal sphincteric response to gastrointestinal stimulation

   c. Pathogenic mechanism uncertain but may involve motility disorders and cytotoxic effects of bile and pancreatic enzymes on susceptible mucosa

8. Miscellaneous gastritis

   a. Gastric ischemia: sometimes seen with vasculitis and atheromatous embolization, but generally not recognized

   b. Ménétrier's disease: entity of unknown cause characterized by marked mucosal hypertrophy with pseudopolypoid, thickened rugal folds, protein-losing gastropathy with hypoalbuminemia, and foveolar (gastric pit region) hyperplasia

   c. Gastric antral vascular ectasia: uncommon entity characterized by dilated antral vasculature with fibrin thrombi and fibromuscular hyperplasia

d. Hypersecretory: Zollinger-Ellison syndrome with hypergastrinemia

e. Physical causes

(1) Corrosive: cardia and pylorus commonly affected with scarring and obstruction

(2) Irradiation: 1600 rads can produce marked deep gastritis.

Symptoms

1. Acute gastritis: symptoms usually mild if present and may include epigastric pain, nausea/vomiting, flatulence, excess salivation, headache, malaise

2. Chronic gastritis

   a. Frequently asymptomatic

   b. Symptoms usually nonspecific, and likelihood of symptoms may increase with depth of inflammatory involvement

      (1) Chronic abdominal pain, usually epigastric in location

      (2) Vague dyspepsia or mild ulcer-like symptoms

      (3) Nausea, anorexia

      (4) Malodorous breath

Key Symptom

- Epigastric pain (chronic gastritis is frequently asymptomatic)

Clinical Findings

Significant clinical findings are frequently absent but may include

1. Hematemesis, bloody nasogastric aspirate, or other evidence of gastrointestinal bleeding

2. Abdominal tenderness

3. Bloating, emesis, and other findings of delayed gastric emptying

4. Intravascular volume depletion and shock may be seen in stress gastritis.

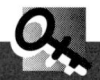
Key Sign

- Epigastric tenderness (clinical findings are frequently absent in chronic gastritis)

Laboratory Tests

1. Endoscopy with biopsy: gold standard diagnostic test providing macroscopic and histologic confirmation of inflammation, modalities for detection of etiologic agents, and evidence of complication development

2. Upper gastrointestinal radiographic study (UGI): typical radiographic features useful in diagnosis and delineation of specific etiologies

3. Nasogastric aspirate: useful in detection of bleeding, bile reflux, and infections

4. *Campylobacter*-like organism (CLO) test: useful in confirming presence of *H. pylori*

5. Vitamin B$_{12}$, gastrin, and pepsinogen levels may be affected in severe atrophic gastritis.

Key Test

- Endoscopy coupled with history is the best diagnostic test.

Differential Diagnosis

1. Peptic ulcer disease

2. Nonulcer dyspepsia

3. Gastroparesis

4. Gastric carcinoma and lymphoma

5. Gastroesophageal reflux disease

6. Pancreatitis

Treatment

1. General treatment for acute gastritis includes

   a. Removal of mucosal irritants

   b. Treatment of underlying etiologic agents

   c. Acidification prevention

2. Severe hemorrhage in acute stress gastritis is managed with a variety of surgical and nonsurgical therapies; prevention is most important.

3. Treatment of chronic gastritis is variable depending on the etiology.

   a. General treatment would include avoidance of potential etiologic agents.

      (1) Eradication of underlying infectious agents (e.g., *H. pylori* triple therapy)

      (2) Treatment of underlying chronic diseases (e.g., Crohn's, sarcoidosis)

      (3) Avoidance of potentially etiologic drugs and foods (e.g., NSAIDs, spices)

   b. Specific symptoms may be treated with antacids, acid antisecretory drugs, mucosal protective drugs, or gastric motility stimulants; response is variable.

   c. Surgical therapy may be necessary in alkaline reflux gastritis.

Medication

1. Combination of tetracycline 500 mg four times a day *or* amoxicillin 500 mg four times a day *plus* metronidazole 250 mg three times a day *plus* bismuth sulfate 525 mg four times a day for 14 days) has been over 90 per cent effective against *H. pylori* infection

2. Antacids, H$_2$-blockers, omeprazole (Prilosec), and sucralfate (Carafate) are useful with hypersecretion.

Diet

Avoidance of spicy foods

Patient Education

1. Avoidance of alcohol, tobacco, and excessive NSAID use

2. Chronic gastritis is a risk factor for the development of peptic ulcer disease.

3. Atrophic gastritis is associated with an increased risk of gastric cancer.

Follow-Up

The benefit of surveillance endoscopy for chronic gastritis has not been established.

Bibliography

For more information on *Helicobacter pylori* infection, see

Axon ATR: *Helicobacter pylori* infection. J Antimicrob Chemother 1993;32:61–68.

Fennerty MB: *Helicobacter pylori.* Arch Intern Med 1994;154(7):721–727.

For more information on stress gastritis and acute hemorrhagic gastritis, see

Chamberlain CE: Acute hemorrhagic gastritis. Gastroenterol Clin North Am 1993;22(4):843–873.

Durham RM, Shapiro MJ: Stress gastritis revisited. Surg Clin North Am 1991; 71(4):791–810.

For more information on specific types of gastritis, see

Lichtenstein JE: Inflammatory conditions of the stomach and duodenum. Radiol Clin North Am 1993;31(6):1315–1333.

77 Appendicitis

Michael A. Cook

Etiology

1. The principal cause of acute appendicitis is luminal obstruction. When the lumen becomes obstructed, the volume of fluid and pressure within the lumen increase. This causes vascular congestion and eventually edema and inflammation. Causes of luminal obstruction include

   a. Appendicolith, the most common cause, composed of fecal material

   b. Calculi

   c. Inspissated barium from a previous contrast study

   d. Pinworms, tapeworms, roundworms

   e. Carcinoid and carcinoma; rarely, metastatic disease

   f. Submucosal lymphoid hyperplasia due to viral infection

2. In immunocompromised patients, consider uncommon etiologies such as tuberculosis. In patients with AIDS, consider cytomegalovirus, *Cryptosporidium*, and Kaposi's sarcoma.

Symptoms

1. The classic symptoms are infrequently elicited and begin with epigastric or periumbilical pain that localizes to the right lower quadrant. The patient then becomes anorexic, complains of nausea, and experiences vomiting. Appendicitis should be considered in all patients who are otherwise well and present with a sudden onset of anorexia and abdominal pain. A high index of suspicion must be maintained, particularly in infants and the elderly, because they often present with vague histories and poorly localizing signs. In both groups the condition progresses rapidly, and they are more likely to develop perforation.

2. The pain localizes to the region of the appendix. If the appendix is in the pelvis, the patient may complain of pelvic or rectal pain. If the appendix is retrocecal, there is back pain or right flank pain. Malrotation can cause the appendix to be located anywhere in the abdomen, and the patient complains of pain in the respective location. The symptoms can simulate acute cholecystitis when the appendix is in the right upper quadrant.

Key Symptoms	
• Right lower quadrant pain	• Nausea
• Anorexia	• Vomiting

3. Dysuria and frequency can be present if the inflamed appendix is close to the ureter or bladder.

Clinical Findings

1. There is usually a low-grade fever. If the oral temperature is greater than 101° F, consider perforation.

2. The point of maximal tenderness depends on the location of the appendix, as previously discussed. Typically, there is right lower quadrant rebound tenderness at McBurney's point. Eventually involuntary guarding develops.

3. Hyperesthesia may be present.

4. A mass in the right lower quadrant suggests a periappendiceal abscess.

5. Classic physical signs

   a. Rovsing's sign: right lower quadrant pain on palpation on the left lower quadrant.

   b. Psoas sign: right lower quadrant pain on hyperextension of the right hip

   c. Obturator sign: right lower quadrant pain on internal rotation of the flexed right hip

6. Rectal examination reveals right-sided tenderness in the case of a pelvic appendix.

7. Pelvic examinations must be performed on all women.

Key Sign	
• Right lower quadrant rebound tenderness	

Laboratory Tests

All patients must have a complete blood count and urinalysis (UA). Women in the reproductive years should have a urine pregnancy test.

1. Complete blood count

   a. There is usually a leukocytosis between 10,000 and 20,000/mm³ with a left shift. A leukocytosis greater than 20,000/mm³ should raise the suspicion of perforation. A normal leukocyte count can be present but is misleading, particularly in immunocompromised patients. Their old records should be checked to determine their usual leukocyte count, and the blood smear should be reviewed for toxic granulations.

   b. Anemia in older patients with right lower quadrant pain should raise the suspicion of cecal carcinoma.

2. Urinalysis

   a. Dehydration will elevate the specific gravity.

   b. If the inflamed appendix abuts the ureter or blad-

der, there can be microscopic hematuria and pyuria.
3. Imaging
   a. Kidney, ureter, bladder: In the proper clinical set-
      ting, the presence of an appendicolith establishes
      the diagnosis. Radiographic signs include blurring
      of the right psoas margin, lumbar scoliosis with
      the convexity to the right, and a distended air-
      filled loop of small bowel (sentinel loop) in the
      right lower quadrant. A gas-containing abscess or
      pneumoperitoneum can occur with perforation.
   b. Graded compression ultrasonography: The appen-
      dix appears fluid-filled, is noncompressible, and is
      greater than 6 mm in diameter. Method is good in
      pregnant women, in women in the reproductive
      years, and in children.
   c. Barium enema: Complete opacification of the ap-
      pendix excludes the diagnosis. If the tip is not
      opacified, the diagnosis cannot be excluded.
   d. Computed tomography: Primary signs include the
      presence of an inflammatory mass, abscess, or
      appendicolith and a thickened appendiceal wall,
      which can enhance with intravenous contrast.

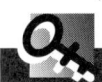

Key Tests

- CBC
- UA
- Urine pregnancy test

Differential Diagnosis

1. The list is extensive but can be narrowed considerably
   with a good history, meticulous physical examination,
   and the proper tests (e.g., intravenous pyelogram,
   barium enema, Meckel's scan, ultrasonography, computed tomography, stool guaiac).
2. Consider the following: cholecystitis, diverticulitis,
   gastroenteritis, ectopic pregnancy, acute salpingitis,
   tubo-ovarian abscess, mittelschmerz, ovarian torsion,
   ruptured or torsed ovarian cyst, ureteral calculus,
   acute pyelonephritis, perinephritic abscess, Crohn's
   disease, *Yersinia* enterocolitis, Meckel's diverticulitis,
   acute mesenteric adenitis, psoas abscess, torsion of
   an undescended testicle, perforated duodenal ulcer,
   omental torsion, perforated cecal carcinoma, muco-
   cele, strangulated inguinal hernia.
3. In patients with AIDS, consider *Mycobacterium
   avium–intracellulare* adenitis.

Treatment

1. All patients suspected of having appendicitis must be
   hospitalized and an early surgical opinion obtained.
   Patients with concurrent medical illness, electrolyte
   disturbances, and dehydration must be stabilized.
   Medical consultation must be obtained when appropriate.

2. Antibiotics (intravenous, to cover aerobic gram-negative bacilli and anaerobes including *Bacteroides frag-
   ilis*)
   a. Prophylaxis before surgery
      (1) 1 gm cefoxitin (Mefoxin), or cefotetan (Cefo-
          tan) or
      (2) Clindamycin (Cleocin) or metronidazole (Fla-
          gyl) with gentamicin (Garamycin)
   b. Treatment of established infection
      (1) Ampicillin, gentamicin, clindamycin, or met-
          ronidazole
      (2) Ampicillin/sublactam (Unasyn) or ticarcillin/
          clavulanate (Timentin)
      (3) Second-generation cephalosporin
3. Immediate appendectomy, for virtually all patients
4. If the patient is a poor surgical risk, treat with intravenous antibiotics, and as long as the symptoms are
   subsiding, elective surgery is scheduled for 4 to 6
   weeks later. In cases of perforation with periappendiceal abscess, a percutaneous drain can be placed.
   Again, if there is no improvement, the patient is
   taken to the operating room. If the patient improves,
   elective surgery can be scheduled for 4 to 6 weeks
   later.
5. Surgery should not be delayed in pregnancy.
6. Appendectomies can be performed laparoscopically.

Key Treatment

- Surgery (possibly laparoscopically) for virtually all
  patients

Prognosis

1. Prompt diagnosis, preoperative medical stabilization,
   and properly timed surgery optimize the outcome.
2. Mortality is lowest in healthy young adults without
   complications (0.7 per cent) and highest in the elderly
   with perforation or abscess who undergo emergency
   surgery (30.8 per cent).
3. The most common cause of morbidity is wound infection.
4. The length of stay is between four and six days.

Bibliography

Balthazar EJ, Birnbaum BA, Yee J, et al: Acute appendicitis:
   CT and US correlation in 100 patients. Radiology
   1994;190:31–35.
Blair NP, Bugis SP, Turner LJ, MacLeod MM: Review of the
   pathologic diagnosis of 2,216 appendectomy specimens. Am
   J Surg 1993;165:618–620.
Hubert J, Neff U, Kelemen M: Appendicitis diagnosis today.
   Clinical and ultrasonic deductions. World J Surg
   1993;17:243–249.
Schirmer BD, Schmieg RE, Dix J, et al: Laparoscopic versus
   traditional appendectomy for suspected appendicitis. Am J
   Surg 1993;165:670–675.

78 Colorectal Cancer

Pierre S. Pincetl

Colorectal cancer is the second leading cause of cancer death in the United States (approximately 61,000 in 1989) following lung cancer. In spite of increased awareness of the need to screen patients for colon cancer regularly, there has been no decline in mortality from this disease in the past 40 years among males in the United States and only a slight unexplained decline among females.

Etiology

Epidemiologic studies point to several environmental factors that appear to be components in the etiology of the majority of colorectal cancer cases.

1. Diet: Although a specific agent has not been identified, rates of colorectal neoplasms have been correlated with levels of consumption of animal fats and protein. Studies have shown a higher incidence of colorectal cancer in Western countries, which typically have higher levels of fat intake, than in countries with demonstrably lower dietary fat. Migrant populations have been observed to develop the cancer rate of the countries to which they migrate. Populations with high fiber content in their diets tend to have lower rates of colorectal cancer. Calcium is currently being evaluated as a protective agent in patients who are predisposed to colorectal cancer.

2. Genetics: There is a family history of colorectal neoplasm in 25 per cent of patients.

   a. Polyposis syndromes: The familial polyposis syndromes have been separated into two categories.

      (1) Familial adenomatous polyposis is a rare autosomal dominant disorder in which colorectal neoplasia is virtually assured to develop by the age of 40. The colon is involved with thousands of adenomatous polyps.

      (2) Familial hamartomatous polyposis syndromes have also been associated with an increased risk of neoplasia (e.g., Peutz-Jeghers syndrome, juvenile polyposis).

   b. Inflammatory bowel disease: Both ulcerative colitis and Crohn's disease have been associated with an increased risk of colorectal neoplasia.

   c. First-degree relatives: An increased risk of two- to threefold for colorectal cancer has been observed in first-degree relatives even in the absence of other associated syndromes.

3. Polyps: The majority of colorectal cancers are believed to begin as adenomatous polyps. The prevalence of adenomatous polyps increases with age to a rate of more than 25 per cent in patients over the age of 50.

4. Other etiologic factors: Uterosigmoidostomy, *Streptoccocus bovis* bacteremia, and possibly cholecystectomy have all been associated with an increased incidence of colon cancer.

5. Daily aspirin intake in one study has been associated with a diminished risk of colorectal cancer.

Symptoms

1. Bowel-specific symptoms: Owing to the elasticity of the bowel, colorectal neoplasia can often reach advanced stages without symptoms; hence the need for adequate screening and a high index of suspicion. Elderly patients presenting with a change in bowel habits, bloody rectal discharges, or abdominal discomfort should be evaluated for colon cancer. The symptoms often suggest the location of disease. Right-sided lesions may not create obstructive symptoms until late due to the liquid nature of the stool when entering the cecum. They can cause severe, symptomatic anemias through chronic blood loss. Transverse and descending colon lesions can cause abdominal pain and cramping secondary to obstruction. Rectosigmoid lesions may cause a change in the caliber of the stool, hematochezia, and tenesmus.

2. Systemic symptoms: Because of the insidious nature of colorectal neoplasms, the presenting symptoms may be systemic. Fatigue and weight loss, as well as anemias, may be the only indicators of disease. Fever may be noted in the presence of hepatic metastases.

Clinical Findings

1. Examination of the abdomen: Most often an external examination of the abdomen will be unrevealing. Abdominal tenderness or a discrete mass may be elicited, depending on tumor size and location. Rarely, a fistula may be present. If the bowel wall is penetrated, the findings could include an acute, hard abdomen.

2. Digital rectal examination: The rectal examination, combined with stool guaiac testing, is the most important component of the physical examination. Annual examinations should be performed starting at age 40. A rectal mass may be felt on examination since about 30 per cent of colorectal neoplasms arise in the rectosigmoid area.

Laboratory Tests

1. Screening tests: The American Cancer Society (ACS) and the National Cancer Institute recommend that annual stool guaiac testing be commenced at age 50. A study by Mandel et al. showed a 33 per cent reduction in mortality from colorectal cancer when participants submitted six guaiac cards annually in comparison with controls who did not have guaiac testing. His 13-year study was based on rehydrating

332

the guaiac cards and performing colonoscopy to evaluate guaiac-positive patients. Rehydrating guaiac cards has been shown to increase their sensitivity. To reduce the false-positive rate, dietary iron, animal proteins, and gastric mucosa irritants (nonsteroidal anti-inflammatory agents) should be discontinued for several days before guaiac testing. The appropriate role of flexible sigmoidoscopy in annual screening is less well defined. The ACS recommends an initial flexible sigmoidoscopy at age 50 with follow-ups every three to five years.

2. Diagnostic tests: Two modalities are available to evaluate patients with suspected colorectal cancer. The double-contrast barium enema has been the traditional method of evaluation, since a single-contrast barium enema (barium only) was shown to be inadequate. Colonoscopy has recently gained favor as it provides direct visualization and the ability to obtain a biopsy of a suspected lesion or to remove detected polyps immediately.

3. CEA: The carcinoembryonic antigen (CEA) is not recommended as a screening test for colon cancer. Many conditions can cause elevated CEAs including carcinomas at other sites, smoking, gastritis, and renal disease. In addition, not all colorectal neoplasms secrete CEA. It is useful for monitoring therapy as levels should drop after surgery, and re-elevation during follow-up suggests the possibility of a recurrence. There is a direct correlation between the level of elevation of the CEA and the Dukes' stage of the cancer. A CEA level greater than 5/ng/ml has been associated with a poor prognosis. The presence of an elevated CEA has also been correlated with a greater likelihood of recurrence.

Differential Diagnosis

1. Hematochezia: Colorectal polyps, hemorrhoids, angiodysplasia, diverticulosis, rectal fissures, and inflammatory bowel disease can all cause hematochezia. Patients presenting with hematochezia should undergo anoscopy at a minimum and probably flexible sigmoidoscopy as well.

2. Change in bowel habits: Many disorders (both functional and organic) can cause a change in bowel habits. A change in stool caliber may occur with diverticulosis but in patients over 40 years old should trigger a consideration of colorectal cancer.

3. Abdominal pain: While nonspecific, the presence of abdominal pain in high-risk patients (positive family history of colon cancer, age over 40) should generate a suspicion of colorectal cancer.

Staging

In 1929, Dukes, a pathologist at St. Mark's hospital in London, developed a classification scheme for rectal cancers based on pathologic depth of involvement. His scheme has undergone many modifications; one of the more useful was devised by Astler and Coller (Table 78–1).

After involving regional lymph nodes, colorectal cancer metastasizes primarily to the liver via the portal venous circulation. Neoplasms arising in the distal rectum can

TABLE 78–1. CLASSIFICATION OF RECTAL CANCERS

DUKES' STAGE	PATHOLOGIC INVOLVEMENT	FIVE-YEAR SURVIVAL (%)
A	Mucosal and submucosal	88
B	Extending into the muscularis	90
B2	Extending through the muscularis; no lymph node involvement	67
C1	Not penetrating the bowel wall; with lymph node involvement	65
C2	Penetrating the bowel wall; with lymph node involvement	50
D	Distant metastasis	<5

metastasize through the paravertebral venous plexus to the lungs and supraclavicular nodes.

Treatment

1. Surgery is generally the treatment of choice. Metastatic disease precludes resection for cure, but palliative surgery may still be indicated to relieve obstruction or to control hemorrhaging. A metastatic workup prior to surgery should include liver function tests, a CEA level, colonoscopy, and a chest film.

2. Chemotherapy: Chemotherapy alone has not proved to be curative. Its role is primarily palliative, but it may also increase survival. The drug-of-choice for treatment of metastatic colorectal cancer is 5-fluorouracil. The addition of levamisole HCl (Ergamisol) reduces the rate of tumor recurrence.

3. Radiation therapy: While radiation therapy is not a primary treatment, it is useful in conjunction with surgical excision of stages B2 and C rectal tumors. Rectal tumors tend to metastasize to regional lymph nodes early due to the extensive lymphatic drainage, and radiation therapy can inhibit the metastases.

Follow-Up

1. Colorectal cancer: After resection, close follow-up is indicated. Semiannual examinations, with history and physical examination, stool guaiac testing, chest radiography, liver function tests, and CEA should be performed. Annual colonoscopy, or semiannual sigmoidoscopy for rectal cancers, is also recommended.

2. Colorectal adenomatous polyps: A repeat colonoscopy should be performed one year after the excision of an adenomatous polyp. If no other polyps are noted, the examination should be repeated every three to five years.

 Bibliography

Astler VB, Coller FA: Prognostic significance of direct extension of carcinoma of the colon and rectum. Ann Surg 1954; 139:846–852.

Fleischer DE: Detection and surveillance of colorectal cancer. JAMA 1989; 261:580–586.

Mandel JS, et al: Reducing mortality from colorectal cancer by screening for fecal occult blood. N Engl J Med 1993; 328:1365–1376.

Peleg II, Maibach HT, Brown SH, Wilcox CM: Aspirin and nonsteroidal anti-inflammatory drug use and the risk of subsequent colorectal cancer. Arch Intern Med 1994; 154:394–399.

Winawer SJ, Zauber AG, May Nah Ho MS, et al: Prevention of colorectal cancer by colonoscopic polypectomy. N Engl J Med 1993; 329(27):1977–1981.

Procedure | FLEXIBLE SIGMOIDOSCOPY/COLONOSCOPY

Clifford J. Field

The techniques used in flexible sigmoidoscopy and colonoscopy are essentially the same. The following outline, except when noted, is pertinent to both. Many of the subtle techniques would require too lengthy a discussion. Additional reading and training is encouraged.

Indications

Indications for lower endoscopy:

1. Rectal bleeding
2. Unexplained abdominal symptoms
3. Equivocal or abnormal barium enema
4. Removal or search of polyps
5. Search and biopsy of undiagnosed cancer
6. Cancer surveillance
7. Intraoperative colonoscopy
8. Unexplained weight loss
9. Metastatic carcinoma of unknown primary
10. Unexplained chronic diarrhea
11. Sigmoidoscopy is also recommended for routine screening for patients over age 40.

Contraindications

1. Absolute contraindications:
   a. Patient refusal
   b. Patient is moribund
   c. A known or suspected perforation
   d. Unavailability of resuscitation
   e. Unstable cardiac condition
2. Relative contraindications:
   a. Respiratory insufficiency
   b. Diagnosis already established

Patient Preparation

1. Informed consent is necessary with these procedures. Videotapes are available to show the patient and are very useful in answering the patient's questions.
2. Pre-procedure instructions (sigmoidoscopy)
   a. The patient should avoid eating red or orange gelatin the day before. They often will cause an appearance of blood in the lumen.
   b. The patient administers a Fleet enema every half hour beginning 2 hours before on the morning of the procedure until the return is clear.
3. Pre-procedure instructions (colonoscopy)
   a. The patient should be limited to clear liquids the day before the examination and no red or orange gelatin.
   b. Metoclopramide, 10 mg at 11 A.M. and 3 P.M. the day before, will facilitate a clean colon.
   c. Start Colyte 4 liters (2 glasses every half hour) at 1 P.M. Ideally, a colonoscopy should be done in the morning.
4. Procedure preparation (sigmoidoscopy): Left lateral positioning with the right knee flexed more than left.
5. Procedure preparation (colonoscopy)

   a. Intravenous KVO, monitor (cardiac, oxygen [O_2] saturation is ideal), administer O_2 if needed.
   b. Remove the patient's dentures, if appropriate.
   c. Place the patient in a left lateral position with the right knee flexed more than left.

Equipment

Many types of flexible endoscopy equipment are available. When deciding what equipment to purchase, consider present and future needs. Inexpensive basic flexible sigmoidoscopy equipment is available; however, if you also want the ability to perform upper endoscopies and/or colonoscopies, you may need to consider a scope that could serve dual function such as a gastroscope or a small-diameter colonoscope. Whatever your choice, keep in mind:

1. The smaller the diameter the more comfort to the patient.
2. The smaller the diameter the more difficult it is to pass the scope through colon loops.
3. A biopsy channel is important.
4. The ease in which air, water, and suction are used is an important consideration.
5. Videoscopes are more expensive, give excellent pictures, and allow easy documentation.
6. A videoscope's light is less intense—an advantage because of potential harm to mucosa, a disadvantage if you use transabdominal illumination as a clue for locating your position in the colon.
7. Clean the scope thoroughly!

For colonoscopies you should also have a cardiac and O_2 saturation monitor, O_2, IV equipment, and resuscitation equipment.

Anesthesia (Colonoscopy)

1. The degree and method of sedation varies widely with each endoscopist. Most medication can irritate the veins. Keeping the intravenous line wide open at time of administration reduces this irritation. A darkened room helps facilitate sedation. Monitor the patient closely. Talk to the patient while giving sedation; adequate sedation is achieved when the patient develops slurred speech. The sedation may be reversed at the end of the procedure using naloxone (Narcan) 0.4 mg intravenously.
2. Medication
   a. Meperidine (Demerol) 50 to 100 mg intravenously
   b. Midazolam (Versed) 0.5 mg (titrate in 0.5 mg increments)
   c. Morphine 5 to 10 mg intravenously
   d. Diazepam (Valium) 5 to 20 mg intravenously
   e. Fentanyl (Sublimaze) 0.05 mg to 0.1 mg intravenously
   f. Naloxone (Narcan) and flumazenil (Mazicon) should be available if needed.

Complications/Precautions

Complications are infrequent if the examination is gentle and not rushed. Potential complications:

1. Related to preparation, related to sedation, bacteremia, hemorrhage, perforation, diastatic serosal tears, post colonoscopy distention, vasovagal reflex, splenic avulsion, cardiac abnormalities, volvulus
2. If cautery is used, additional complications could include serosal burns and explosions.

Technique

1. Do a final check of equipment and the "reach" of the connections. Reassure the patient and begin sedation if needed. Perform a digital rectal examination before insertion. Lubricate the distal 3 to 4 cm of the scope and insert the scope 5 to 10 cm. Always keep the lumen in the center of the view and do not force the instrument while advancing the scope. Loss of visualization of the lumen and blanching of the mucosa suggest impending perforation and the scope should be partially withdrawn and the lumen visualized before proceeding. Use air sparingly to keep the lumen inflated. Water is also effective to expand the lumen. Observe for mucosal irregularities and polyps and biopsy any suspicious mucosa or lesion. Random biopsies are appropriate if you suspect colitis even if the mucosa has a normal appearance. Post-procedure management includes observing the patient until awake and coordinated. Home instructions and follow-up care are discussed when the patient is fully awake. Patients are told that they may have "gas" pains and blood with the next bowel movement. They should also notify their physician if they develop pain, chills, or an elevated temperature. If they received sedation they should not drive or do anything that could be hazardous for the rest of the day.

2. A thorough examination includes the following:

   a. Rectum: Retroverting the scope is best method to visualize the rectum.

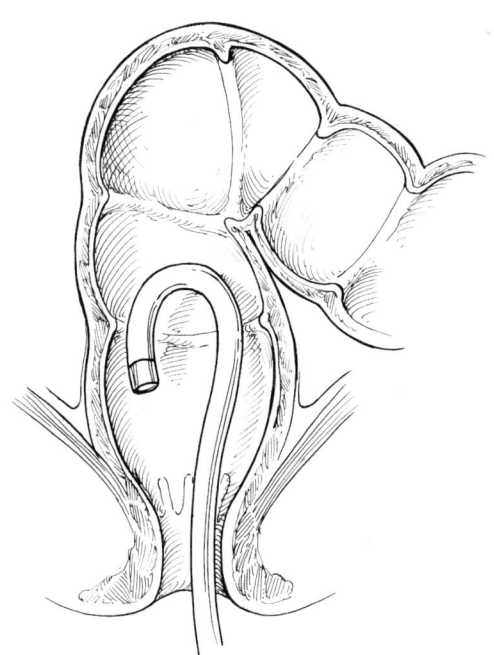

   This is accomplished by rotating the large wheel counterclockwise and the small wheel clockwise when 10 to 15 cm is reached. Gently advance the scope while torquing the scope clockwise. This should bring the scope and internal sphincter into view. Continuing the torquing motion and slight withdrawal will give an excellent view of the entire rectum. This maneuver is usually done at the end of the examination.

   b. Sigmoid: The sigmoid colon is the most likely place for "loop" formation, and diverticula. Keeping the colon inflated can be difficult. The number of diverticula and the difficulty in keeping the bowel inflated increase the risk of accidental intubation of a diverticulum.

   c. Descending colon: The descending colon is reached when the colon straightens and becomes more easily inflated. It ends at the splenic flexure and is characterized by a sharp turn.

   d. Transverse colon: The transverse colon has a triangular lumen and is usually easier to intubate with patient on the back. The hepatic flexure is often confused with the cecum. Loop formations can also occur in the transverse colon.

   e. Ascending colon: The ascending colon often has green liquid stool if there was a marginal preparation. The wall is thinner than the rest of the colon. The cecum has a bird's foot appearance and the ileocecal valve should be identified. If enteritis is suspected, intubation of the terminal ileum is important.

Scope Advancement: Loop Formations and Reduction Techniques

1. Alpha loops occur commonly in the sigmoid colon and occasionally in the transverse colon. A loop usually becomes evident when paradoxical movement is present. Paradoxical movement is occurring if the scope appears to withdraw when the scope is advanced. Loops also make passage more difficult and increase discomfort for the patient. Reduction of an alpha loop is achieved by torquing the scope clockwise while withdrawing. This often takes several attempts.

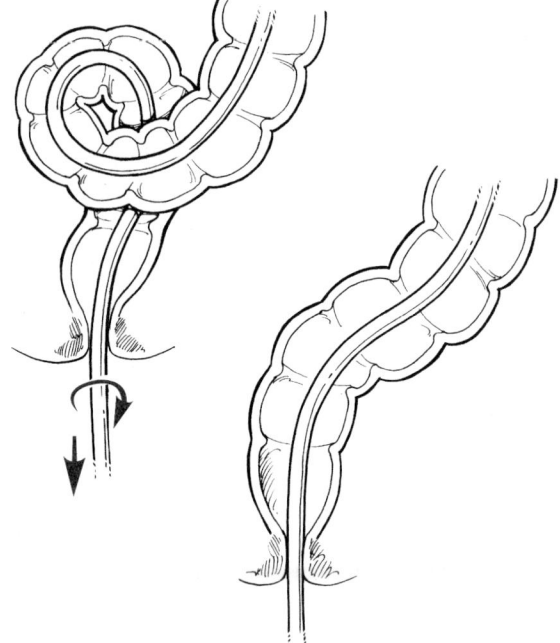

A reverse alpha loop requires counterclockwise torquing of the scope. Loops are often formed when a moderate amount of redundant bowel is present. After reduction to avoid the recurrence of the loop, the intestine should be "telescoped" on the scope. This is achieved by gently catching the side of the bowel wall with the tip of the scope and withdrawing as the scope is torqued.

2. Counter pressure: Abdominal counter pressure by an assistant is a useful technique in colonoscopy to help advance the scope. With the patient on his or her back, loops and distentions of the scope are palpated. These can be controlled by having an assistant apply abdominal pressure, pushing the scope into the quadrant in which the scope should be placed. Another counter pressure technique used to simplify advancement of the scope around the splenic flexure is to have the patient take a deep breath. The diaphragm will help "push" the scope around the corner.

3. Patient positioning: There is no rule saying that the patient must remain in the left lateral position when the scope is advanced. This is the most useful position for examination of the left colon. However, moving the patient onto the back or right side will often let gravity straighten out a sharp corner of the bowel and allow easier advancement.

Bibliography

Baillie J: Gastrointestinal Endoscopy: Basic Principles and Practice. New York, Butterworth, Heineman Ltd., 1992.

Cotton PB, Tytgat GNJ, Williams CB: Annual of Gastrointestinal Endoscopy. London, Current Science Ltd., 1991.

Keeffe EB, Schrock TR: Complications of gastrointestinal endoscopy. In Sleisenger MH, Fordtran JS: Gastrointestinal Disease. Philadelphia, WB Saunders, 1993.

Maratka Z: Illustrated Terminology, Definitions and Diagnostic Criteria in Digestive Endoscopy. Englewood Cliffs, NJ, Normed Verlag, 1992.

Silverstein FE, Tytgat NJ: Atlas of Gastrointestinal Endoscopy, 2nd ed. Philadelphia, Gower Medical Publishing, 1991.

79 Small and Large Bowel Obstruction

Robert M. Gerbo

Etiology

A. Small bowel
   1. Postoperative adhesions are the most common cause.
   2. Hernia, especially an external (abdominal wall) hernia (i.e., inguinal, femoral, umbilical, ventral or incisional hernia)
   3. Neoplasm, with the primary origin more likely to be from an intra-abdominal site such as the colon, pancreas, stomach, or a gynecologic site
   4. Other causes include intussusception, volvulus, gallstones, foreign body, bezoar, inflammatory bowel disease, intestinal worms, traumatic injury, radiation injury, meconium, and congenital intrinsic lesions
   5. There frequently may be more than one cause.

B. Large bowel
   1. Cancer is the most common cause.
   2. Volvulus
   3. Diverticulitis usually only causes partial obstruction.
   4. Other causes include inflammatory bowel disease, benign tumors, fecal or barium impaction, and congenital disorders such as Hirschsprung's disease.

Symptoms

1. Cramping abdominal pain may be localized or diffuse. Severe, constant pain suggests strangulation.
2. Nausea and vomiting are common and may even be feculent in a distal obstruction. However, vomiting may not occur at all in a large bowel obstruction.
3. Obstipation occurs with complete obstruction, although feces distal to the obstruction may still pass.
4. Bloating and distention occur late.

Key Symptoms

- Cramping abdominal pain
- Obstipation
- Vomiting

Clinical Findings

1. Tenderness is common; severe tenderness and rigidity suggest strangulation or perforation.
2. Abdominal distention may be mild or severe.
3. Bowel sounds may be high-pitched and "tinkling" or absent.

4. Fecal blood (gross or occult) may be present.
5. Fever is suggestive of strangulation or perforation.
6. Signs of dehydration may also be present.

Key Signs

- Tenderness
- Distention
- "Tinkling" or absent bowel sounds

Laboratory Tests

1. Laboratory tests are of no diagnostic value. Leukocytosis may not be present. Chemistries may indicate dehydration.
2. Plain abdominal radiographs (supine and upright) typically demonstrate dilated loops of bowel and air-fluid levels in a stepladder manner.
   a. Gas is usually absent distal to the obstruction.
   b. In large bowel obstruction, the small bowel will also be dilated if the ileocecal valve is incompetent.
   c. Free air beneath the diaphragm is an ominous sign indicating bowel perforation.

> **WARNING**
>
> **Free air beneath the diaphragm on radiograph indicates bowel perforation, and emergency surgical consultation should be obtained.**

3. In equivocal cases contrast studies (barium or water-soluble medium such as Gastrografin) confirm the diagnosis. Water-soluble contrast is safer if perforation occurs.
4. With a suspected large bowel obstruction and a "nonsurgical" abdomen, endoscopy can confirm diagnosis and aid in determining etiology.

Key Tests

- Radiography (supine and upright)
- Contrast studies

Differential Diagnosis

1. Small versus large bowel obstruction
   a. Symptoms of large bowel obstruction are slower to develop.

b. Abdominal films show dilated colon in large bowel obstruction.

2. Paralytic ileus occurs with recent abdominal surgery, peritonitis, abdominal or spinal trauma, and other associated illnesses.

   a. The pain is constant and mild, and there is abdominal distention.

   b. Radiographs show gas in both the small and large bowel.

   c. Contrast studies are useful in equivocal cases.

3. Pseudo-obstruction is a chronic, recurring syndrome of signs and symptoms of bowel obstruction due to abnormal gastrointestinal (GI) motility and not a mechanical obstructing lesion.

   a. Secondary causes are numerous and include collagen vascular disease, amyloidosis, various neurologic and endocrine disorders, various drugs, and multiple miscellaneous entities.

   b. Primary causes are characterized as familial or sporadic.

   c. Contrast studies exclude a mechanical obstructing lesion.

4. Mesenteric vascular occlusion is usually due to emboli or atherosclerosis of the mesenteric vasculature.

   a. A history of cardiac disease and/or a thromboembolic event is common with severe abdominal pain.

   b. Arteriography confirms the diagnosis.

   c. The bowel may appear dusky in color on colonoscopy.

Treatment

1. Begin with nasogastric (NG) tube decompression and intravenous fluids.

2. Prompt surgical consultation is indicated since nearly all complete obstructions require an operation.

3. Endoscopy can be an option in some nonacute settings (i.e., no peritoneal signs).

   a. In malignant large bowel obstruction, endoscopic dilatation and decompression, as well as laser fulguration, are options.

   b. Detorsion of a volvulus endoscopically is frequently successful, but the recurrence rate is high and surgical treatment is definitive.

Medication

1. Broad-spectrum antibiotic coverage against gram-positive, gram-negative, and anaerobic organisms should be considered in the perioperative period.

2. Use of cathartics or other GI stimulants proximal to a complete bowel obstruction may result in perforation and should therefore be avoided. Enemas are safer but still require caution.

> **WARNING**
>
> **Use of cathartics or other GI stimulants proximal to an obstruction may result in perforation.**

Diet
NPO status should be maintained.

Activity
Bedrest is required while the patient is acutely ill.

Patient Education

1. Although not being permitted oral intake and having an NG tube are uncomfortable, it is hoped that these measures will prevent perforation.

2. Perforation leads to spillage of bowel contents into the abdomen, resulting in life-threatening infection.

3. Refusal to have recommended surgery is life-threatening.

4. If partial bowel resection is necessary and primary reanastomosis is not possible, an ostomy will be performed with the possibility of reanastomosis at a later date.

Key Treatment

- Nothing by mouth
- Surgery
- NG suction

Follow-Up

1. Monitor for signs and symptoms of recurrence at follow-up visits.

2. If a second, elective operation is needed, begin planning and patient preparation.

3. After resection for colon cancer, colonoscopy, examination of stool for occult blood, and carcinoembryonic antigen levels should be used to monitor for recurrence.

Bibliography

Dorudi S, Berry AR, Kettlewell MGW: Acute colonic pseudo-obstruction. Br J Surg 1992;79(2):99–103.

Fabri PJ, Rosemurgy A: Reoperation for small intestinal obstruction. Surg Clin North Am 1991;71(1):131–146.

Holder WD Jr: Intestinal obstruction. Gastroenterol Clin North Am 1988;17(2):317–340.

McGregor JR, O'Dwyer PJ: The surgical management of obstruction and perforation of the left colon. Surg Gynecol Obstet 1993;177(2):203–208.

80 Intussusception

Michael Schooff

Etiology

1. Definition: intussusception (IS) occurs when one segment of bowel telescopes into the lumen of an adjacent segment. Subsequent peristalsis causes further telescoping of bowel with its accompanying mesentery and blood vessels, resulting in bowel obstruction, necrosis, and gangrene. IS may occur in any portion of the GI tract but is most common at, or proximal to, the ileocecal valve.

2. Demographics
   a. In children, IS is the most common cause of intestinal obstruction and the second most common cause of acute abdominal pain, after appendicitis.
   b. Peak incidence occurs in children 3 to 9 months old, and 80 per cent of patients are less than 2 years old. Adults account for only 5 to 10 per cent of all cases. Incidence of IS is two to four cases per 1000 live births, with a male to female ratio of 2:1.

3. Causes: IS is idiopathic in 90 per cent of cases in children. These cases may be due to a viral-induced hypertrophy of Peyer's patches. An identifiable cause is found in over 90 per cent of cases in adults. Half of these cases are due to a primary GI malignancy. Any bowel lesion that alters the normal peristaltic pattern increases the risk of IS, including
   a. Malignant tumors: colonic adenocarcinoma, small bowel leiomyosarcoma, metastatic melanoma, Kaposi's sarcoma
   b. Benign tumors: lipoma, adenomatous polyp, hemangioma, neurofibroma, hamartoma, villous adenoma
   c. Miscellaneous: AIDS, sprue, hemophilia, nephrotic syndrome, ascariasis, cystic fibrosis, Meckel's diverticulum, Henoch-Schönlein purpura, postoperative state

Symptoms

1. Classic triad of symptoms: Only 20 per cent of patients present with all three; up to 40 per cent present with only one.
   a. Intermittent crampy abdominal pain
   b. Vomiting
   c. Blood and mucus in stool ("currant jelly stool")

2. Most reliable complex: occurs in 80 to 95 per cent of cases
   a. Sudden onset of severe paroxysms of pain lasting four to five minutes and recurring at 5- to 30-minute intervals
   b. Straining, loud crying, and flexing of the hips
   c. Progressively weak and lethargic, eventually becoming febrile and shock-like

3. Other symptoms may include vomiting, irritability, poor feeding, decreased activity, altered consciousness, diarrhea, and constipation.

4. Adult IS usually presents as an insidious onset of vague colicky abdominal pains, lacking the classic symptoms, and rarely having evidence of bowel obstruction.

Key Symptoms

- Paroxysms of abdominal pain
- Loud crying
- Flexing at hips
- Becoming progressively lethargic

Clinical Findings

1. Abdominal findings: Most common findings include tenderness, distention, and abnormal bowel sounds (hyper- or hypo-active, may have "rushes" during paroxysms of pain); may have abdominal mass, which changes in size and firmness during paroxysms of pain.

2. Rectal examination: stool often is positive for occult blood. Bloody mucus in stool is a late finding.

3. Constitutional findings may include dehydration, fever, hypotonia, and weight loss.

4. Normal physical examination in up to 25 per cent of cases.

Key Signs

- Abdominal tenderness
- Abdominal mass
- Abnormal bowel sounds
- Occult or frank blood in stool
- Dehydration

Laboratory Tests

1. Abdominal radiographs
   a. Common findings include dilated loops of bowel, signs of bowel obstruction, soft tissue mass, and mass effect.
   b. Radiographs may be normal in up to 25 per cent of cases.

2. Contrast enemas may be both diagnostic and therapeutic. The classic findings in IS are a "cervix-like"

mass at the lead point and a "coiled spring" appearance of contrast material between two segments of bowel.

> **WARNING**
>
> **Contrast enemas are contraindicated in patients with signs of peritonitis, bowel perforation, or hypovolemic shock.**

3. Other radiologic studies are of limited value. Ultrasonography or computed tomography might aid in establishing the diagnosis in cases with atypical presentations and contraindications to contrast enemas.
4. Other tests: Serum electrolytes, complete blood count, and urinalysis are recommended.

Key Tests

- Abdominal radiographs

- Contrast enema (may be diagnostic and therapeutic)

Differential Diagnosis

1. The differential diagnosis of IS is essentially that of any patient with abdominal pain, and varies with the age of the patient.
   a. Neonates: congenital intestinal atresia or stenosis, motility disorders, necrotizing enterocolitis
   b. Infants and children: gastroenteritis, colic, GE reflux, sepsis, pyloric stenosis, appendicitis, malrotation, volvulus, complicated Meckel's diverticulum, adhesions, inflammatory bowel disease
   c. Adolescents and adults: as above, plus testicular or ovarian diseases, pelvic inflammatory disease, ectopic pregnancy, ruptured GI tumor
2. Initial misdiagnosis of IS has been reported in 55 to 60 per cent of cases, with the most common misdiagnosis being gastroenteritis. In adults, the correct diagnosis is made preoperatively in only 20 to 25 per cent of cases.

Treatment

> **WARNING**
>
> **Morbidity and mortality increase dramatically if intussusception is not reduced in the first 24 to 48 hours.**

A. Hydrostatic reduction under fluoroscopy
1. Initial treatment of choice in most institutions
2. Indicated in known or suspected cases of IS
3. Contraindicated in all adults, in any case with suspected pathologic lead point, and in children with signs of bowel perforation, peritonitis, or hypovolemic shock

4. Relatively contraindicated in neonates and older children
5. Successful reduction in 85 to 90 per cent of cases. Lower rate in patients with symptoms lasting over 24 hours, radiologic evidence of bowel obstruction, age over 2 years, or recurrent IS.
6. Recurrence rate is 10 per cent.
7. Less than 0.5 per cent risk of bowel perforation during reduction

B. Surgical reduction
1. Indicated in patients with contraindications to hydrostatic reduction and in cases of unsuccessful hydrostatic reduction
2. Manual reduction of IS is contraindicated if there is high possibility of malignant lead point, relatively long segment of bowel involved, or evidence of bowel ischemia.
3. Primary resection of involved segment of bowel is necessary if manual reduction is unsuccessful or contraindicated.
4. Success rate is 100 per cent.
5. Recurrence rate is 2 to 5 per cent.

C. Supportive therapy
1. Nasogastric decompression of bowel
2. Intravenous hydration and management of electrolytes
3. Broad-spectrum antibiotics if perforation or necrotic bowel is suspected

Diet
1. Feedings may begin after return of normal bowel sounds.
   a. Often same day with hydrostatic reduction
   b. Often day 2 or 3 postoperatively

Activity
1. Average length of hospital stay
   a. Hydrostatic reduction = 1.7 days
   b. Surgical reduction = 7.4 days

Patient Education
All parents need to be informed of the symptoms of IS and the importance of minimizing time from onset of symptoms to diagnosis and reduction.

Follow-Up
1. Monitor weight gain.
2. Routine wound care after surgical reduction

Bibliography

Alford BA, McIlhenny J: The child with acute abdominal pain and vomiting. Radiol Clin North Am 1992;30(2):441–453.

Bruce J, Huh YS, Cooney DR, et al: Intussusception: Evolution of current management. J Pediatr Gastroenterol Nutr 1987; 6(5):663–674.

Losek JD: Intussusception: Don't miss the diagnosis. Pediatr Emerg Care 1993;9(1):46–51.

Prater JM, Olshemski FC: Adult intussusception. Am Fam Physician 1993;47(2):447–452.

Stringer MD, Pablot SM, Brereton RJ: Paediatric intussusception. Br J Surg 1992;79:867–876.

81 Crohn's Disease

Stephen P. James

Etiology

1. Cause is unknown, but is probably multifactorial.
   a. Environmental: more common in industrial countries, with rapid increase in prevalence in 20th century (currently 20 to 40/100,000); relative risk higher in smokers
   b. Bacterial products: products of intestinal flora thought to contribute to intestinal inflammation; no unique infectious agent has been identified
   c. Genetic: There is a familial tendency and high concordance in twins; it is more common in Jews and non-Jewish Caucasians.
   d. Immunologic factors: No unique immunologic abnormality has been identified, but disease appears to be immunologically mediated.
2. Pathogenesis: Inflammatory lesions may be present anywhere in alimentary tract. There are characteristic patterns of disease.
   a. Ileocolonic Crohn's disease (40 per cent of patients): tendency to form strictures in ileum, fistula formation, abdominal abscess, perirectal disease
   b. Colonic Crohn's disease (granulomatous colitis, Crohn's colitis, 30 per cent of patients): Inflammation may occur anywhere in colon with skip areas that distinguish it from ulcerative colitis.
   c. Small bowel Crohn's disease (regional ileitis, 30 per cent of patients); tendency to form strictures, obstruction
   d. Upper gastrointestinal (GI) Crohn's disease (less than 5 per cent of patients). Inflammatory lesions of esophagus, stomach, and duodenum may resemble acid-peptic disease.

Symptoms

Symptoms are highly variable depending on site and severity of lesions.
1. Diarrhea
2. Abdominal pain
3. Fatigue
4. Weight loss
5. Rectal pain, hematochezia, purulent discharge from fistula
6. Fever
7. Growth failure (children)
8. Nausea, vomiting, dyspepsia
9. Arthralgias (joint swelling uncommon)
10. Skin ulcers (pyoderma gangrenosum), skin nodules (erythema nodosum)
11. Painful aphthous mouth ulcers

Key Symptoms

- Diarrhea
- Abdominal pain
- Fatigue
- Weight loss

Clinical Findings

Clinical findings are highly variable depending on location and severity of lesions. Some patients have no physical findings.
1. Abdominal tenderness
2. Abdominal mass
3. Abdominal distention (with partial obstruction)
4. Hyperactive bowel sounds (with partial obstruction)
5. Fever
6. Perineal fistulas with purulent drainage
7. Rectal abscess
8. Mouth ulcers
9. Extraintestinal manifestations (all relatively uncommon)
   a. Eye: episcleritis, iritis, uveitis
   b. Skin: erythema nodosum, pyoderma gangrenosum
   c. Joints: swelling, tenderness
   d. Hepatic: hepatomegaly, splenomegaly, jaundice

Key Signs

- Highly variable
- Some patients may have no physical findings
- Abdominal tenderness
- Abdominal mass

Laboratory Tests

Routine laboratory tests are helpful as a clue to underlying inflammatory disease and to assess complications of severe diarrhea, bleeding, or malabsorption.
1. Complete blood count: anemia, leukocytosis, thrombocytosis
2. Electrolytes, blood urea nitrogen, creatinine: metabolic acidosis, prerenal azotemia
3. Sedimentation rate: useful for monitoring response to therapy
4. Liver function tests: Abnormal values suggest pericholangitis or sclerosing cholangitis.
5. Nutritional status: albumin, prealbumin, B_{12}

341

6. Stool
   a. Leukocytes, occult blood often present
   b. Exclude bacterial pathogens, parasites, *Clostridium difficile* toxin
7. Blood cultures: for suspected sepsis
8. Special studies are required to make the diagnosis and for potential complications.
   a. Colonoscopy
      (1) Diagnose colonic and terminal ileal Crohn's disease; biopsies mandatory
      (2) Define extent and severity of colonic disease
      (3) Screen for colon cancer in long-standing colonic Crohn's

---

WARNING

In severely ill patients with abdominal abscess, small bowel obstruction, toxic megacolon, or suspected perforation, bowel preparations or invasive procedures may precipitate marked deterioration or complication and should be either avoided or used with extreme caution.

---

   b. Upper GI and small bowel series
      (1) For diagnosis of upper GI Crohn's disease, strictures, fistulas
      (2) Small bowel enteroclysis may provide better definition.
   c. Abdominal computed tomography with oral contrast
      (1) Define abdominal mass, abscess
      (2) Identify abdominal fistulas
   d. Abdominal ultrasound
      (1) Hydronephrosis due to oxalate stones
      (2) Gallstones associated with bile salt deficiency
   e. Upper GI endoscopy: for diagnosis, biopsy of suspected upper GI Crohn's disease

Key Tests

• Stool examination

• Colonoscopy with biopsy

• Upper GI and small bowel series

Differential Diagnosis

1. Irritable bowel syndrome
2. Other forms of colitis: ulcerative colitis, infectious colitis, pseudomembranous colitis, ischemic colitis, radiation colitis, lymphocytic colitis
3. Other causes of hematochezia: hemorrhoids, colorectal cancer, diverticular disease, ischemic colitis

4. Other causes of diarrhea
5. Other causes of small bowel narrowing, obstruction, inflammation: infectious ileitis (*Mycobacterium, Yersinia, Actinomyces*), lymphoma, carcinoma, nonsteroidal anti-inflammatory drugs, adhesions, intussusception, celiac disease
6. Other causes of right lower quadrant pain: appendicitis, pelvic inflammatory disease, ovarian mass, nephrolithiasis
7. Other causes of gastric or duodenal inflammation: peptic ulcer disease, Zollinger-Ellison syndrome, adenocarcinoma

Treatment

The disease and its complications are highly variable, and treatment must be tailored to the particular location and severity of disease. There is no universal prescription for therapy. Some symptoms may be due to obstruction, abscess, or fistulas that will not respond to anti-inflammatory therapy and require surgical intervention.

WARNING

Septic complications may be masked in patients on chronic prednisone and/or immunosuppressive drugs. Patients with prior steroid therapy with septic complications may require stress steroid doses because of adrenal insufficiency.

Medication

1. Metronidazole (Flagyl), 250 mg q.i.d.: for colonic, fistulous disease; other antibiotics have been used in uncontrolled trials (ciprofloxacin).
2. 5-ASA drugs: Sulfasalazine (Azulfidine), olsalazine (Dipentum), mesalamine (Asacol, Pentasa). Used for mild disease of colon or terminal ileum or as adjunct to prednisone. Mesalamine is useful for small bowel disease.
3. Corticosteroids
   a. 40 to 60 mg/day of prednisone orally for acute exacerbations tapered over approximately 2 months
   b. Low continuous dose may be required for maintenance.
   c. Intravenous steroids for severe exacerbations
   d. Avoid with septic complications, abscess, fistulas.
4. Immunosuppressive drugs
   a. Azathioprine (Imuran), 100 to 150 mg/day, or 6-mercaptopurine (Purinethol), 50 mg/day; indicated as steroid sparing agents; primary therapy for fistulous disease; long delay before onset of action (2 to 6 months)
   b. Methotrexate: for severe, unresponsive disease
   c. Cyclosporine: for severe, unresponsive disease

5. Adjunctive therapy
   a. Antidiarrheals: Diphenoxylate-atropine, loperamide; 1 to 2 tabs two to four times daily
   b. Vitamin B_{12}: Monthly by injection for extensive ileal disease or prior ileal resection
   c. Cholestyramine: 4 gm one to two times daily for bile salt–induced diarrhea

Surgery

Indicated for major complications: obstruction, pyogenic abscess, fistulas unresponsive to medical therapy, perforation, toxic megacolon, cancer, refractory disease, severe hemorrhage. Surgery is not curative; therefore, it should be conservative.

Diet

1. Low residue diet when obstructive symptoms present
2. Oral elemental diet or total parenteral nutrition for severe unresponsive disease or growth retardation
3. Lactose-free diet if lactase deficient

Patient Education

1. Careful education as to realistic expectations required for this chronic relapsing disease and side effects of therapy
2. Special problems: pregnancy, childhood Crohn's disease, genetic counseling
3. Patient educational materials are available through Crohn's and Colitis Foundation of America, 386 Park Ave. So., 17th Fl., New York, NY 10016

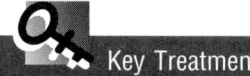

Key Treatment

- No universal prescription for therapy

Follow-Up

Prognosis is for lifelong relapsing and remitting disease that may require frequent follow-up.

1. After initial evaluation and definition of disease extent, adjustment of therapy can often be made by careful symptom assessment and examination. Reevaluation of procedures may be necessary if a major complication is suspected or if there is a lack of expected response to therapy.
2. Steroids and immunosuppressive drugs should be tapered to lowest possible dose.
3. Surgical therapy should be offered for intractable symptoms due to fixed stricture, fistulas, severe unresponsive disease. Majority of patients require surgery at some time during course.
4. Colon cancer surveillance by colonoscopy should be considered with long-standing colonic disease (more than 10 years). Screening hemoccult cards and flexible sigmoidoscopy are not useful.
5. Emotional support is required, but psychiatric evaluation is indicated only for major psychiatric diagnosis.

 ## Bibliography

For more information on etiology and pathogenesis of Crohn's disease, see
Targan SR, Shanahan F (eds): Inflammatory Bowel Disease: From Bench to Bedside. Baltimore, Williams & Wilkins, 1994.
For more information on clinical manifestations and treatment of Crohn's disease, see
Podolsky DK: Inflammatory bowel disease. N Engl J Med 1992;325:928–937.
For more information on treatment of Crohn's disease, see
Linn FV, Peppercorn MA: Drug therapy for inflammatory bowel disease. 1992; Am J Surg 164:85–89 (Part I) and 178–185 (Part II).
Singleton JW, Nanauer SB, Gitnick GL, et al: Mesalamine capsules for the treatment of active Crohn's disease: Results of a 16-week trial. Pentasa Crohn's Disease Study Group. Gastroenterology 1993;104:1293–1301.
For more information on diet and Crohn's disease see
Royall D, Jeejeebhoy KN, Baker JP, et al: Comparison of amino acid versus peptide-based enteral diets in active Crohn's disease: clinical and nutritional outcome. Gut 1994;35(6):783–787.

82 Ulcerative Colitis

Bruce D. Greenwald

Etiology

Cause is unknown, but it is probably multifactorial.

1. Environmental: more common in Scandinavian countries, Great Britain, North America
2. Genetic: familial tendency, increased concordance in twins, more common in Jews and non-Jewish Caucasians
3. Immunologic: No unique abnormality identified at this time. Anticolon antibodies are present but their significance is uncertain.

Symptoms

1. Diarrhea: usually small volume (200 ml/day or less), can be bloody
2. Hematochezia
3. Abdominal pain or cramping
4. Fever: seen in more severe cases
5. Weight loss
6. Fatigue
7. Proctitis symptoms
   a. Tenesmus (straining without passing stool)
   b. Rectal urgency
   c. Constipation
8. Extracolonic symptoms (45 per cent of cases)
   a. Joints: arthralgias and arthritis
   b. Skin
      (1) Erythema nodosum: tender red nodules, most commonly on the anterior lower legs
      (2) Pyoderma gangrenosum: painful ulcers, usually on extremities
   c. Eyes: pain or burning, blurred vision, photophobia, scleral injection

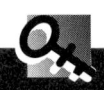

Key Symptoms

- Diarrhea
- Rectal bleeding
- Abdominal cramping

Clinical Findings

Some patients have no physical findings.
1. Abdominal tenderness
2. Hematochezia or heme-positive stools
3. Severe disease
   a. Fever
   b. Tachycardia
   c. Malnutrition and dehydration

d. Abdominal distention
4. Extracolonic manifestations
   a. Eyes: uveitis, iritis, episcleritis
   b. Skin: erythema nodosum, pyoderma gangrenosum
   c. Joints: arthritis, often migratory, affecting large joints; usually nondestructive
   d. Liver: jaundice, hepatomegaly, splenomegaly

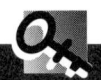

Key Signs

- Rectal bleeding
- Abdominal tenderness

Laboratory Tests

Blood tests may be normal in mild or moderate colitis.
1. Complete blood count (CBC): anemia, leukocytosis, thrombocytosis
2. Electrolytes: prerenal azotemia
3. Sedimentation rate: elevated in severe disease
4. Liver function tests: Elevated alkaline phosphatase or bilirubin suggests associated pericholangitis or sclerosing cholangitis.
5. Albumin, prealbumin, transferrin: may be low
6. Stool studies
   a. Leukocytes: frequently present
   b. Occult blood: frequently present
   c. Culture—ova and parasites, *Clostridium difficile* toxin: done to exclude other causes of colitis. Note: Culture of *Yersinia, Campylobacter,* and *Escherichia coli* O157:H7 must be specifically requested in many laboratories when sending stool cultures.
7. Abdominal radiographs: Look for colonic distention in severe disease.
8. Special studies are required to make the diagnosis and assess for complications.
   a. Colonoscopy
      (1) Define extent and severity of disease. Obtain

> **WARNING**
>
> **In severely ill patients, especially with colonic distention, bowel preparations or invasive procedures may precipitate marked deterioration or complication and should be either avoided or used with extreme caution.**

stool for culture and biopsies to exclude other causes of colitis.

    (2) Screen for colon cancer in patients with long-standing disease.

b. Barium enema: less sensitive in mild disease

c. Upper GI and small bowel series: to exclude a diagnosis of Crohn's disease

Key Tests

- Stool examination
- Colonoscopy with biopsy

Differential Diagnosis

Ulcerative colitis is a diagnosis of exclusion. Other causes of colitis must be excluded before this diagnosis is made.

1. Irritable bowel syndrome
2. Infectious colitis

    a. Bacteria: *Shigella, Salmonella, Yersinia, Campylobacter, E. coli* O157:H7

    b. Parasites: *Entamoeba histolytica, Giardia lamblia*

3. Ischemic colitis
4. Drug-induced: especially antibiotics
5. Diverticulitis
6. Colon cancer
7. Crohn's disease
8. Radiation colitis
9. HIV-associated diarrhea

Treatment

Medication

1. Mild to moderate attack

    a. Proctitis: mesalamine suppositories (Rowasa), 500 mg; hydrocortisone suppositories (Anusol-HC 25 mg); or hydrocortisone foam (Cortifoam) b.i.d. or t.i.d.

    b. Left-sided colitis: mesalamine enemas (Rowasa), 4 gm, or hydrocortisone enemas (Cortenema), 100 mg hs or b.i.d.

    c. Left-sided colitis and pancolitis:

        (1) 5-ASA preparations

            (a) Sulfasalazine, 1 gm q.i.d. (should also give folic acid, 1 mg daily)

            (b) Mesalamine (Asacol), 800 mg t.i.d.

            (c) Mesalamine (Pentasa), 1 gm q.i.d.

        (2) Prednisone, 40 to 60 mg once daily or equivalent: Use for more severe disease.

2. Severe attack

Patients with fever, tachycardia, dehydration, or severe diarrhea should be hospitalized.

    a. Methylprednisolone IV, 20 to 30 mg t.i.d. or

    b. ACTH intramuscularly, 80 units daily (Note: Efficacy is greatest with first attack or in those who have never received corticosteroids)

    c. Intravenous antibiotics to cover bowel flora (e.g., ampicillin + gentamicin + metronidazole, cefoxitin [Mefoxin], or ticarcillin/clavulanate [Timentin])

3. Maintenance therapy

The goal of maintenance therapy is to prevent relapse of disease. Most patients should receive maintenance therapy after an acute attack.

    a. Steroids are ineffective as maintenance therapy.

    b. Proctitis: Mesalamine suppositories, 500 mg; may be tapered weekly to every other night, then every third night, until the lowest dose maintaining remission is found.

    c. Left-sided colitis: Mesalamine or steroid enemas may be tapered as described above for suppositories; oral aminosalicylates as described below for pancolitis.

    d. Pancolitis

        (1) Sulfasalazine, 1 to 2 gm b.i.d. (should also give folic acid, 1 mg daily)

        (2) Mesalamine (Asacol), 800 to 1200 mg b.i.d.

        (3) Olsalazine (Dipentum), 500 mg b.i.d.

4. Immunosuppressive therapy

    a. Indicated for refractory colitis: patients unable to reduce their dose of steroids below prednisone, 5 to 10 mg daily (or equivalent), or those suffering from sequelae from chronic steroid use

    b. Drugs

        (1) Azathioprine (Imuran), 100 to 150 mg daily or

        (2) 6-mercaptopurine, 50 mg daily

    c. Both have been shown to be effective in refractory colitis.

    d. Two to six months of treatment may be needed until an effect is seen.

    e. Complications of therapy include pancreatitis (usually seen within the first month), leukopenia, allergic reactions, hepatitis.

    f. CBC with differential should be monitored monthly. Liver function tests should be monitored quarterly.

5. Antimotility agents (loperamide [Imodium], diphenoxylate [Lomotil]) should be used with caution.

Diet

1. Diet is ineffective as primary therapy. Elemental diets are ineffective as treatment of ulcerative colitis.

2. Total parenteral nutrition and bowel rest may be needed during severe attacks of acute colitis owing to incapacitating diarrhea, abdominal pain, nausea, and vomiting.

3. Nutritional supplementation may be needed for malnutrition. Oral supplements can be used.

4. Foods that induce diarrhea, such as large amounts of raw fruits and vegetables, caffeine, and spicy foods, should be avoided during acute attacks.

Surgery

1. Surgery is curative in ulcerative colitis.
2. Indications
   a. Colon perforation or obstruction
   b. Toxic megacolon
   c. Severe disease refractory to intensive inpatient medical therapy for 3 to 7 days
   d. Intractable or refractory disease
   e. Colon cancer or high-grade dysplasia

Patient Education

1. Ulcerative colitis is a chronic disease with a variable course. Surgery is curative.
2. Pregnancy planning should begin before conception.
3. Patients are at increased risk for colorectal cancer, especially those having disease beyond the rectum for longer than 10 years.
4. Patient educational materials are available through Crohn's and Colitis Foundation of America, 386 Park Ave. So., 17th Fl., New York, NY 10016.

Follow-Up

1. After initial evaluation and definition of disease extent, adjustment of therapy can often be made by careful symptom assessment and physical examination. Re-evaluation with endoscopy or barium enema may be necessary if major complication is suspected or if there is a lack of expected response to therapy noted.
2. Steroids should be tapered by 10 mg/week until 20 mg, then 5 mg/week, and halted within 3 months of initiation.
3. Colon cancer surveillance by colonoscopy is necessary in patients with disease for longer than 10 years and extending beyond the rectum.
4. Emotional support is required, but psychiatric consultation is indicated only for major psychiatric diagnosis.

Bibliography

Farmer RG, Easley KA, Rankin GB: Clinical patterns, natural history, and progression of ulcerative colitis: A long-term follow-up of 1116 patients. Dig Dis Sci 1993; 38(6):1137–1146.

Hanauer SB: Medical therapy of ulcerative colitis. Lancet 1993;342(8868):412–417.

Linn FV, Peppercorn MA: Drug therapy for inflammatory bowel disease. Am J Surg 1992;164:85–89;178–185.

Podolsky DK: Inflammatory bowel disease. N Engl J Med 1992;325:928–937; 1008–1016.

Targan SR, Shanahan F (eds): Inflammatory Bowel Disease: From Bench to Bedside. Baltimore, Williams & Wilkins, 1994.

83 Irritable Bowel Syndrome

Fred M. Sutton

Etiology

1. *Definition:* Irritable bowel syndrome (IBS) is a functional gastrointestinal disorder attributed to the intestines and associated with symptoms of pain and altered defecation and/or symptoms of bloatedness and distension.

2. *Epidemiology:* Studies from Western countries indicate that 15 to 20 per cent of patients suffer from IBS and most do not seek medical attention for their symptoms. In Western countries, 75 per cent of patients with IBS seen by a physician are female. In countries such as India and Sri Lanka, male patients predominate.

3. *Pathophysiology:* Certain motility and sensory abnormalities are found in patients with IBS as a group, and these distinguish them from healthy individuals.

   a. Various stimuli including stress, meals, and peptides alter colonic or small intestinal motor response.

   b. It is presumed that pain symptoms in patients with IBS are due to hyperactivity.

   c. These patients also have reduced sensory thresholds for stimuli such as rectal and ileal distention.

   d. Evidence that balloon distention at certain points in the small and large intestine reproduces pain confirms the gut as the site of the symptom.

Symptoms

Criteria for IBS include continuous or recurrent symptoms, for at least three months of

1. Abdominal pain or discomfort relieved by defecation or associated with a change in the frequency or consistency of stool and/or

2. An irregular pattern of defecation at least 25 per cent of the time (three or more of the following)

   a. Altered stool frequency

   b. Altered stool form (hard or loose, watery stool)

   c. Altered stool passage (straining or urgency, feeling of incomplete evacuation)

   d. Passage of mucus

   e. Bloating or feeling of abdominal distention

Key Symptoms

- Alternating diarrhea and constipation
- Abdominal pain relieved by defecation
- Abdominal bloating
- Passage of mucus

Clinical Findings

1. The physical examination in most patients with IBS is generally normal.

2. Physical examination may reveal tenderness in the area of the colon in patients with the spastic colon variety of IBS. In patients with small bowel involvement, pressure over the umbilicus or epigastrium may precipitate symptoms.

3. Most patients with IBS are between the ages of 20 and 50.

4. Patients with IBS commonly have a past history of multiple illnesses such as allergies, headache, kidney disease, joint symptoms, and in women dyspareunia.

Key Sign

- Normal physical examination findings

Laboratory Tests

1. Laboratory studies are generally normal in IBS. The diagnosis should be suspected based on the patient's symptoms and by excluding organic diseases. There are no definitive tests for a diagnosis of IBS.

2. A minimal evaluation would consist of a complete blood count and erythrocyte sedimentation rate (ESR).

3. If diarrhea is a predominant symptom, stool samples for leukocytes, culture for enteric pathogens, and examination for ova and parasites should be pursued.

4. A urinalysis should be obtained since urinary tract symptoms can mimic functional gastrointestinal disease.

5. Sigmoidoscopy offers little diagnostic information unless there is suspicion of inflammatory bowel disease. In patients with IBS, air insufflation during sigmoidoscopy often reproduces a patient's symptoms.

6. Roentgenographic studies of the small bowel or colon are generally not indicated with typical IBS symptoms. If the patient has had symptoms for more than

Key Tests

• Normal complete blood count	• Stool negative for leukocytes, blood
• Normal ESR	• Pain reproduced by sigmoidoscopy

three months or is over age 45, a barium enema or colonoscopy should be performed.

Differential Diagnosis

1. Malignancies such as colon cancer, inflammatory diseases such as Crohn's disease or ulcerative colitis, infectious diseases such as infectious colitis, diverticulitis, and parasitosis, and ischemic diseases of the gastrointestinal tract
2. Diarrhea as the predominant symptom may be due to lactase deficiency, laxative abuse, malabsorption, and hyperthyroidism.
3. Constipation as the predominant symptom may be due to hypercalcemia, hypothyroidism, and medication side effects.
4. Epigastric and periumbilical pain may be due to peptic, biliary, gastric, or pancreatic disease.

Treatment

The key to successful management of IBS is a positive diagnosis, which depends on identifying certain symptom patterns.

1. Constipation predominant
   a. Review dietary history
   b. Therapeutic trial
      (1) Increase fiber (start with one tablespoon psyllium per day or twice a day). Alternatives include polycarbophil or methylcellulose.
      (2) Osmotic laxative
      (3) Stool softener
      (4) Prokinetic agents (trial of cisapride [Propulsid], 20 mg twice daily)
2. Diarrhea predominant
   a. Review dietary history. Eliminate sorbitol products; consider lactose intolerance.
   b. Consider lactose H_2 breath test.
   c. Therapeutic trial.
      (1) Loperamide (Imodium), 2 to 4 mg every 6 to 8 hours
      (2) Diphenoxylate (Lomotil), 2.5 to 5 mg every 4 to 6 hours
   d. Fiber
3. Pain/gas/bloat predominant
   a. Review diet history
   b. Plain abdominal radiography
   c. Therapeutic trial
      (1) Anticholinergics (dicyclomine [Bentyl], 10 to 20 mg 30 to 45 minutes before meals four times a day; hyoscyamine)
      (2) Antidepressants (amitriptyline HCl [Elavil], or doxepin [Sinequan], starting with 25 to 50 mg at hour of sleep and gradually increased to 75 to 150 mg at hour of sleep as tolerated. Fluoxetine [Prozac], 20 mg, as single daytime dose is less sedating.)

      (3) Prokinetic agents, cisapride, 10 to 20 mg daily
      (4) Psychiatric intervention employing biofeedback, psychotherapy, or hypnosis is an alternative for patients with IBS refractory to standard therapeutic measures.

Diet

1. If certain products such as lactose, caffeine, fatty foods, alcohol, sorbitol, or beans are associated with symptoms, they can be eliminated to see if symptoms abate.
2. Fiber results in improvement of constipation and abdominal pain.

Activity

Low physical activity has been reported as an association with constipation.

Patient Education

1. A positive physician–patient interaction is associated with a reduced number of return visits for IBS-related symptoms.
2. Certain acute situations seem to precipitate attacks of IBS. These include acute illnesses, severe financial demand, loss of a job, a serious family crisis, or death of a close friend or relative.
3. Many patients with IBS come from families in which other members have the syndrome, suggesting that symptoms may be a learned behavior.
4. It is usually helpful to explain that IBS is a real disorder in which the intestine is overly sensitive to various stimuli such as food, hormonal changes (menses), and stress.
5. Make the patient aware that although chronic, the symptoms do not indicate serious illness, require surgery, or shorten life expectancy.
6. Setting realistic goals is extremely important.
7. The patient needs to concentrate on functioning as normally as possible and not on eliminating all symptoms.

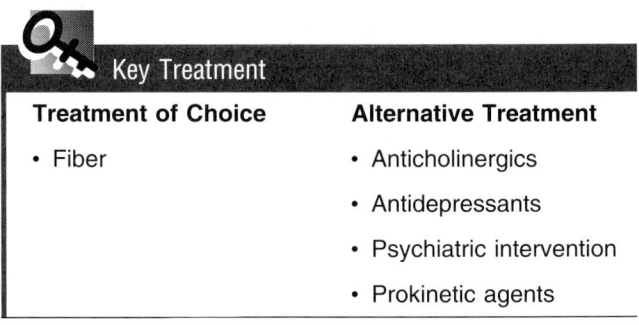

Key Treatment	
Treatment of Choice	**Alternative Treatment**
• Fiber	• Anticholinergics
	• Antidepressants
	• Psychiatric intervention
	• Prokinetic agents

Follow-Up

1. Prevention
   a. High-fiber diet and prophylactic use of medications
   b. Regular exercise
   c. Avoid products that aggravate symptoms

2. Monitoring
   a. Periodic evaluation for a change in symptoms, particularly diarrhea
   b. Regular physician visits early in treatment to reassure the patient
3. Prognosis
   a. A diagnosis of IBS persists over time, and most patients continue to have symptoms several years following the initial diagnosis.
   b. Up to 30 per cent of patients with IBS resort to alternative medicine.
   c. IBS does not predispose one to more serious diseases or shorten one's life expectancy.

Bibliography

Brannan DP, Drossman DA: Toward a newer understanding of irritable bowel syndrome. Contemp Intern Med 1991;9:73–91.

Camilleri M, Prather CM: The irritable bowel syndrome: Mechanisms and a practical approach to management. Ann Intern Med 1992;116:1001–1008.

Drossman DA, Thompson WG: The irritable bowel syndrome: review and a graduated multicomponent treatment approach. Ann Intern Med 1992;116:1009–1016.

Hasler WL, Owyang C: Irritable bowel syndrome. *In* Yamada T, Alpers D (eds): Textbook of Gastroenterology. Philadelphia, JB Lippincott, 1991, pp 1696–1714.

Owens DM, Nelson DK, Talley NJ: The irritable bowel syndrome: Long-term prognosis and the physician-patient interaction. Ann Intern Med 1995;122:107–112.

84 Diverticulitis

Michael Jon Brooks

Etiology

1. Preexisting diverticulosis
2. Microperforation and inflammation of a diverticulum
   a. Diverticulosis is a herniation of mucosa through the muscular wall of the colon, typically located where nutrient arteries penetrate the muscularis propria (Fig. 84–1).
   b. Diverticulosis develops secondary to increased intraluminal pressures that result from insufficient intake of dietary fiber.

Symptoms

1. Abdominal pain
   a. Constant in nature
   b. Typically left lower quadrant in location but may be diffuse
2. Fever
3. Altered bowel habits
   a. Constipation most often
   b. Diarrhea in some cases
4. Nausea/vomiting
   a. Mechanical causes
      (1) Localized edema/inflammation-induced obstruction
      (2) Abscess causing obstruction
      (3) Spasm
   b. Systemic causes
      (1) Sepsis
      (2) Electrolyte abnormalities
5. Malaise
6. Urinary complaints
   a. Dysuria/frequency; secondary to adjacent bladder inflammation
   b. Pneumaturia; secondary to colovesical fistula

Key Symptoms

- Constant abdominal pain; LLQ or diffuse
- Fever
- Altered bowel habits
- Nausea and vomiting
- Malaise

Clinical Findings

1. Mild/moderate abdominal tenderness (common); more often localized to lower left quadrant
2. Severe abdominal tenderness; "acute abdomen" (uncommon)
   a. Due to diffuse peritonitis
   b. Abdominal guarding and rebound often present
   c. May represent frank perforation
   d. Surgical emergency
3. Temperature over 38° C (100.4° F)
4. Abnormal bowel sounds
   a. Usually hypoactive
   b. May be high-pitched/tinkling with impending or early intestinal obstruction
   c. May be absent (ileus) with complete obstruction or frank perforation
5. Guaiac-positive stools
   a. Commonly seen
   b. Frank bleeding is rare
6. Leukocytosis (>12,000/μl) with left shift
7. Abdominal mass; may be palpated in the presence of significant abscess or inflammation

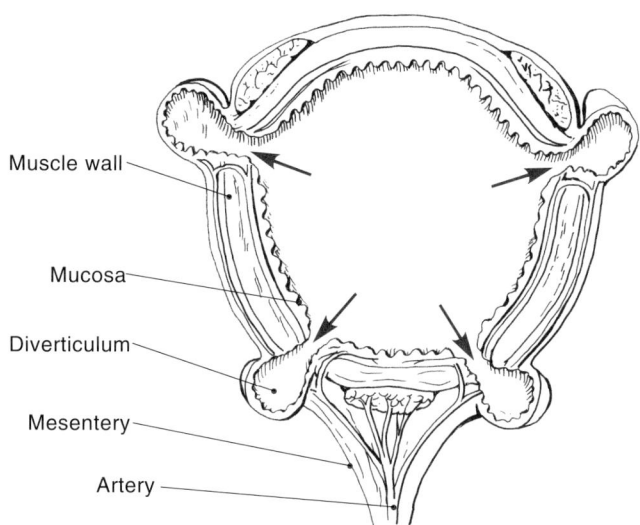

Figure 84–1 Schematic cross-section of the colonic wall showing sites of formation of diverticula at points of penetration of the vasa recta.

Muscle wall
Mucosa
Diverticulum
Mesentery
Artery

> **WARNING**
>
> **Beware of deceptively benign abdominal examinations in elderly or immunocompromised patients; further diagnostic evaluations should be pursued if clinical suspicion exists.**

Key Signs

- Abdominal tenderness (LLQ usually; ± rebound)
- Temperature >38° C (100.4° F)
- Hypoactive bowel sounds
- Guaiac-positive stools
- Abdominal mass (palpable abscess/inflammation)

Laboratory Tests

1. Complete blood count with differential; generally reveals leukocytosis with left shift
2. Plain films of abdomen
   a. Signs of obstruction
      (1) Distended bowel loops with abrupt end
      (2) Air/fluid interfaces
   b. Signs of perforated viscus (rare); free air under diaphragm
   c. Ileus (common)
   d. Extracolonic gas pattern suggestive of pericolic abscess
3. CT scan of abdomen and pelvis
   a. Diagnostic test of choice in most institutions
   b. Very sensitive for delineation of diverticular pericolic abscess versus nondiverticular causes of abdominal symptomatology
4. Barium enema with water-soluble contrast material
   a. Safe and effective to diagnose diverticulitis
   b. Yields less information concerning extracolonic pathology
5. Abdominal ultrasonography
   a. Noninvasive, safe; may be technically difficult to perform
   b. Usually provides less information than computed tomography (CT) or barium enema (BE)
6. Endoscopy: role is limited in acute diverticulitis
7. Urinalysis: presence of pyuria or hematuria may signify colovesical fistula
8. Erythrocyte sedimentation rate; almost always elevated

Key Tests

- CT scan of abdomen + pelvis or barium enema with water-soluble contrast material
- Complete blood count with differential
- Abdominal films
- Erythrocyte sedimentation rate

Differential Diagnosis

1. Intestinal ischemia
   a. Usually in patient with diffuse arteriosclerotic vascular disease
   b. Most consistent finding is pain out of proportion to examination.
2. Cancer of colon: frequently diagnosed with endoscopic biopsy after resolution of acute abdominal process
3. Intestinal obstruction
4. Appendicitis
5. Penetrating duodenal ulcer
6. Inflammatory bowel disease
7. Tubo-ovarian abscess: seen in younger, sexually active women
8. Sigmoid volvulus
9. Pancreatitis: elevated amylase and lipase should be noted

Treatment

1. Hospitalization: required in majority of patients
2. Surgical evaluation: should be obtained early in hospital course
3. Outpatient therapy is effective in selected patients
   a. Mild abdominal pain/tenderness
   b. Tolerates liquid diet/no evidence of obstruction
   c. Low-grade fever/mild leukocytosis (<12,000/μl)
   d. Failure to improve after 24 to 36 hours indicates need for inpatient treatment.
4. Nasogastric intubation for decompression if distention develops

Medication
1. Oral tetracycline or TMP/SMX (Bactrim, Septra) with metronidazole (Flagyl) in mild cases
2. Broad-spectrum parenteral antibiotics in more severe cases
   a. Ampicillin + aminoglycoside + metronidazole
   b. Ampicillin/sulbactam (Unasyn)
   c. Ticarcillin/clavulanate (Timentin)
   d. Imipenem/cilastatin (Primaxin)
3. Intravenous hydration
4. Analgesics

Diet
1. Liquid diet during treatment of mild/outpatient cases
2. NPO/bowel rest in hospitalized patients with acute disease
3. Initial low residue diet with stool softener after resolution of acute inflammation
4. Gradual increase of dietary fiber to achieve 25 to 35 gm/day

Patient Education

1. Maintenance of adequate dietary fiber intake after recovery is essential (25 to 35 gm/day)
   a. High-fiber cereals
   b. Fresh fruits/vegetables
   c. Legumes
2. Adequate fluid intake in association with dietary fiber is important to prevent constipation and bloating.
3. Low dietary fat intake is also prudent.

Key Treatment

- Hospitalization in majority of patients
- NPO/bowel rest
- IV hydration
- Parenteral broad-spectrum antibiotics
- Surgical evaluation (or intervention if indicated)
- Outpatient therapy with liquids and oral antibiotics in mild cases

Follow-Up

1. Flexible endoscopy approximately one month after recovery to evaluate extent of disease and/or associated conditions
   a. Rule out malignancy
   b. Rule out stricture
2. Alternatively, BE or CT with rectal contrast may be used in follow-up evaluation.
3. Recurrent attacks are common (up to 30 per cent).
   a. Patient awareness of presenting signs and symptoms is essential.
   b. Surgical resection of diseased segment may become necessary to prevent recurrence.

Bibliography

Cheskin LJ: Diverticular disease of the colon. *In* Barker LR, Burton JR, Zieve PD (eds): Principles of Ambulatory Medicine, 3rd ed. Baltimore, Williams & Wilkins, 1991, 465–467.

Freeman SR, McNally PR: Diverticulitis. Med Clin North Am 1993;77:1149–1167.

Jones DJ: ABC of colorectal disease and diverticular disease. Br Med J 1992;304(6839):1435–1437.

Rothenberger DA, Wiltz O: Surgery for complicated diverticulitis. Surg Clin North Am 1993;73:975–990.

Schoetz JD: Uncomplicated diverticulitis: Indications for surgery and surgical management. Surg Clin North Am 1993;73:965–974.

85 Hemorrhoids

Eugene A. Felmar

Everything that itches, bulges, bleeds, or is painful in the anal region is commonly referred to as hemorrhoids, or "piles," by the patient. Treatment on the basis of the patient's complaint alone is unacceptable. It is essential that the physician specifically identify the cause of the patient's presenting symptoms in order that an appropriate and effective intervention be planned. Nonhemorrhoidal causes of anal discomfort include pruritus ani, fissure-in-ano, abscess, fistula, and hemorrhoidal disease (both external and internal).

Etiology

1. Hemorrhoidal disease may be produced by anything that increases pressure in the hemorrhoidal veins.
2. Common etiologies are thought to include
   a. Constipation
   b. Straining at stool
   c. Valsalva maneuver during other activities such as lifting
   d. Lesions of the rectum and distal sigmoid colon that produce venous obstruction
   e. Increased venous pressure secondary to pregnancy
3. Because the internal hemorrhoidal venous plexus is one of the several areas of anastomosis of the systemic and portal circulation, internal hemorrhoids may also develop secondary to the portal hypertension produced by hepatic cirrhosis.

Symptoms

1. Internal hemorrhoids represent varicosities of the hemorrhoidal plexus of veins. The superior, middle, and inferior hemorrhoidal veins are terminal branches of the left colic vein. Anatomically, the hemorrhoidal veins lie above the pectinate line or mucocutaneous junction and above the limit of sensory pain receptors that are found primarily in the cutaneum (Fig. 85–1). For this reason, internal hemorrhoidal disease is not associated with pain unless the hemorrhoid dissects distally into tissues lying below the pectinate line. Such advancement may be produced by repeated bulging of the veins during a Valsalva maneuver or defecation, causing them to dissect and distend into the infrapectinate tissues.

Key Symptoms
- Painless rectal bleeding
- Anal pruritus
- Perianal soiling

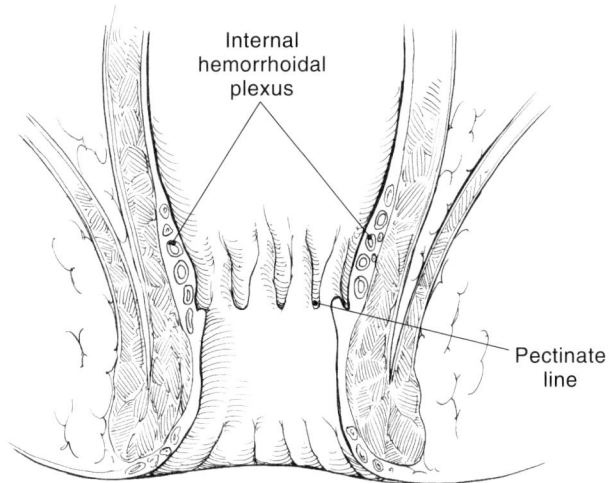
Figure 85–1 Hemorrhoidal veins above the pectinate line.

2. Internal hemorrhoids are commonly associated with complaints related to bleeding, soiling (secondary to mucosal secretions), and itching.

Clinical Findings

Internal hemorrhoids present at the right posterior-lateral, right anterior-lateral, and left lateral positions. Internal hemorrhoids are graded on the basis of their anatomic presentation (Fig. 85–2):

1. *Grade I.* The hemorrhoidal mass is swollen and projects into the anal canal.
2. *Grade II.* The hemorrhoidal mass is pendulous on defecation but reduces spontaneously.
3. *Grade III.* The hemorrhoidal mass prolapses on defecation and recedes only following manual reduction.
4. *Grade IV.* The hemorrhoidal mass is permanently prolapsed.

Key Sign
- Hemorrhoids visible in anal canal or protruding from anal orifice

Tests

Before any type of operative hemorrhoidal therapy is undertaken, a digital rectal and flexible sigmoidoscopic examination should be performed and appropriate coagulation studies (prothrombin time and partial thromboplastin time) should be obtained if clinically indicated.

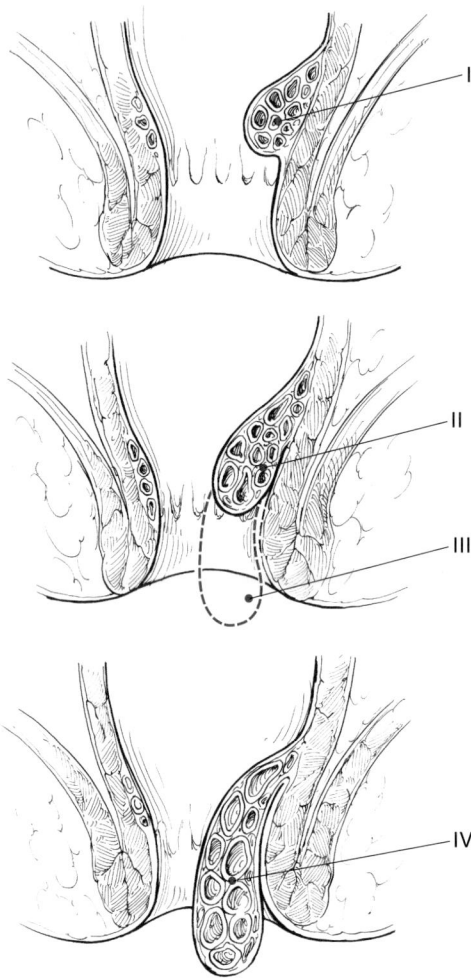

Figure 85–2 Primary hemorrhoidal groups.

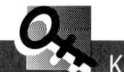
Key Tests

- Anoscopy
- Sigmoidoscopy

Treatment

1. Contrary to popular belief, there is no role for suppositories in the management of hemorrhoidal disease.
2. The treatment of grade I and grade II internal hemorrhoids consists of stool softeners and/or surface tension–decreasing agents, warm sitz baths, and improved bowel habits. This noninvasive protocol may reduce the need for more aggressive intervention in the majority of patients.

Key Treatment

- Stool softeners
- Improved bowel habits

| Procedure | **HEMORRHOID SCLEROTHERAPY, INFRARED COAGULATION, AND BANDING** | *Eugene A. Felmar* |

Sclerotherapy

Indications

Sclerotherapy has come and gone in the medical armamentarium. Because of variable outcomes and the availability of more definitive therapy, management of internal hemorrhoids by sclerotherapy should be limited to grade I and grade II (occasionally grade III) hemorrhoidal masses.

Contraindications

1. Allergy to the sclerosant solutions
2. Coagulopathy or any medical condition that would contraindicate intervention

Technique

1. The patient assumes either a jackknife or a left lateral Sims' position. The discomfort of sclerotherapy is primarily secondary to the introduction of the anoscope required for visualization and tissue manipulation. Most intraoperative discomfort can be alleviated by the topical application of lidocaine (Xylocaine) jelly to the anal tissues and the anoscope.
2. The anoscope (I prefer a Fansler or Fansler-Ives anoscope) is inserted, and the hemorrhoid to be treated is selected.
3. Sclerosis is achieved by the submucosal injection of a sclerosing solution of quinine and urea hydrochloride or 5 per cent phenol in peanut oil using a 30-gauge needle proximally at three sites. Injection of approximately 0.3 to 1.5 ml is usually sufficient for each hemorrhoid. Total sclerosant volume injected when using solutions containing quinine should not exceed 3.0 ml.

mucosally adjacent to the hemorrhoid to be treated and that they not be injected intravascularly.

Key Points

- Primarily indicated for grade I and grade II hemorrhoids
- Occasionally indicated for grade III hemorrhoids
- Inject with 30-gauge needle
- Inject sclerosant submucosally, not intravascularly
- Inject only one hemorrhoid at each visit
- Space successive treatments 3 to 4 weeks apart

Complications

1. Long-term success with sclerotherapy is variable, as recanalization may occur after a brief interval.
2. The procedure may be uncomfortable, and allergic reactions to sclerosing materials are not uncommon.
3. Sloughing, burning, and thrombosis are among the most common complications reported.

Postoperative Instructions

1. The patient is advised to use stool softeners (fiber and/or surface tension–decreasing agents) temporarily and is instructed in dietary and toilet habit modification.
2. Significant bleeding, fever, and unusual pain are to be immediately reported to the physician.

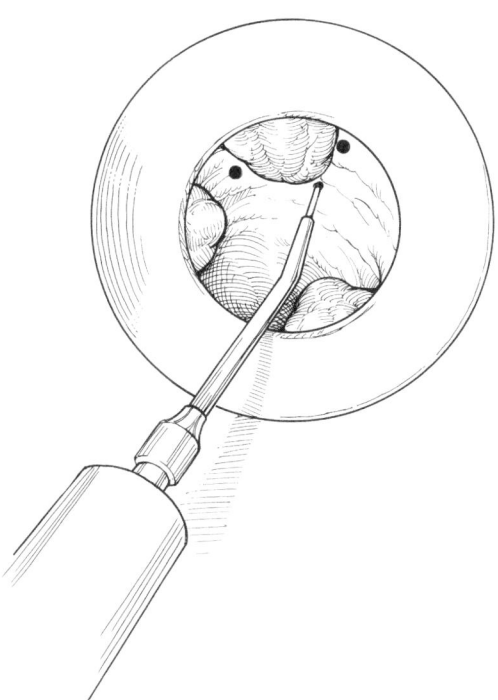

4. It is crucial that sclerosing injections be placed sub-

Infrared Coagulation

This technique, accomplished above the dentate line, requires no anesthesia. It uses an instrument that generates infrared energy with a halogen light source. The radiant energy produced is conducted to the surgical site by means of a quartz rod. The heat produced "spot welds" the mucosa to the muscularis in the tissues adjacent to the internal hemorrhoidal plexus, causing obliteration of the hemorrhoidal vein complex. Following the use of the infrared coagulator, the overlying redundant mucosal tissue shrinks as it is no longer being distracted and distended by the underlying bulging hemorrhoidal vein system. The infrared coagulation technique does not produce slough of tissue, bleeding, or stenosis.

Indications

Infrared coagulation therapy is appropriate for grades I, II, and III hemorrhoids.

Contraindications

Coagulopathy or any medical condition that would contraindicate surgical intervention.

Technique—Infrared Coagulation

1. The patient assumes the left lateral Sims' or jackknife position.
2. The anal canal is lubricated with Xylocaine jelly as is the Fansler or Fansler-Ives anoscope, which is inserted to permit visualization of the hemorrhoid to be treated.
3. The infrared coagulator is set for 1.0 to 1.5 seconds.
4. The tip of the coagulator is lightly pressed against the tissues just proximal to the hemorrhoid.

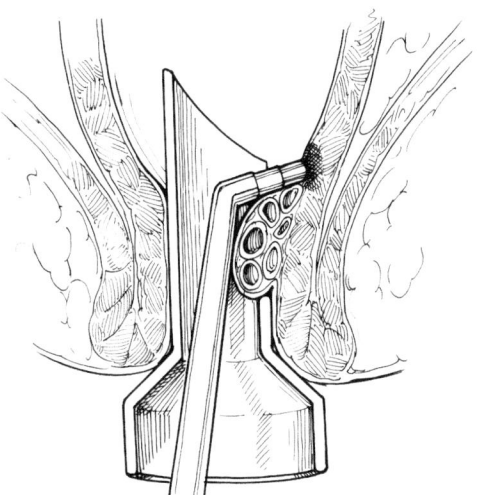

5. The coagulator is energized.
6. Repeat the process five to seven times in the area above the hemorrhoid, leaving a 2-mm untreated tissue bridge between treatment sites. Only one hemorrhoid is treated at each session.

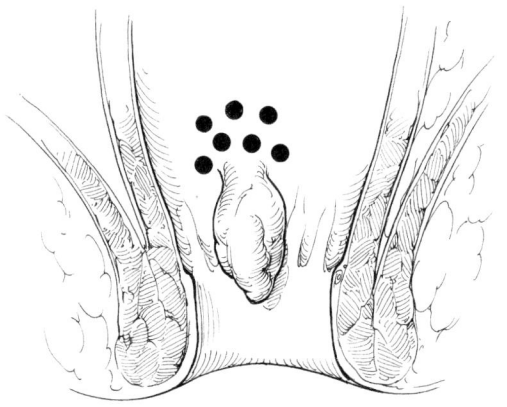

7. Successive treatment may be undertaken, one hemorrhoid at a time, every 10 to 14 days.

Key Points

- Indicated for grades I, II, and III hemorrhoids
- The most common inspiratory reserve capacity (IRC) setting is 1.5 seconds
- Place all IRC "welds" above dentate line
- Place all IRC "welds" just above the hemorrhoid in diamond or triangle pattern
- Leave 2 to 3 mm untreated tissue between "welds"
- Treat only one hemorrhoid at each visit
- Space successive treatments every 10 to 14 days

Complications

Rare postoperative pain and bleeding have been reported.

Postoperative Instructions

1. The patient is advised to use stool softeners (fiber and/or surface tension–decreasing agents) temporarily and is instructed in dietary and toilet habit modification.
2. Significant bleeding, fever, and unusual pain are to be immediately reported to the physician.

Banding Ligation

1. Rubber ring banding ligation is a procedure that ablates the internal hemorrhoidal mass through the application of a constricting rubber ring, which is intended to produce ischemia and painless sloughing of the hemorrhoid in seven to ten days. Banding should be performed on only one hemorrhoidal mass at a time. If more than one hemorrhoid is to be banded, at least 14 to 21 days should intervene between the banding procedures. Because banding is intended to be done on lesions that lie above the pectinate line, anesthesia is not required for this procedure. However, if tissues below the pectinate line are included in the rubber band ligature, severe pain will be instantly produced.

2. Banding, if properly performed, is at worst uncomfortable. Most complaints are referable to the introduction of the anoscope required for visualization and tissue manipulation. Most intraoperative discomfort is alleviated by the topical application of Xylocaine jelly to the anal tissues and the anoscope.

Indications

Banding is appropriate for grades II and III and some grade IV internal hemorrhoids.

Contraindications

Coagulopathy and certain medical conditions would contraindicate surgical intervention.

Technique—Banding Ligation

1. The patient assumes either a jackknife or left lateral Sims' position.
2. The Fansler or Fansler-Ives anoscope is inserted, and the hemorrhoid to be treated is selected. The hemorrhoidal banding instrument is "loaded" with two rubber rings.

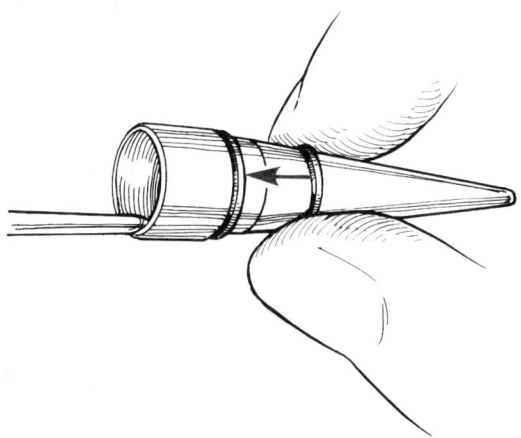

3. An alligator forceps is inserted through the banding instrument, and the hemorrhoid is grasped and placed under tension.

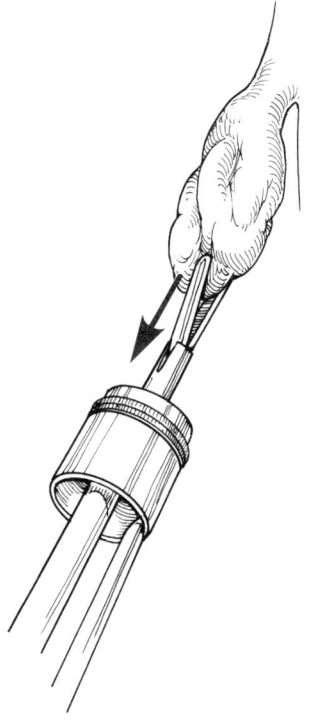

4. The banding instrument is advanced to the base of the hemorrhoid and the two rubber ring ligatures are simultaneously placed. Care must be taken to grasp and band the hemorrhoid above the dentate line or pain will be produced.

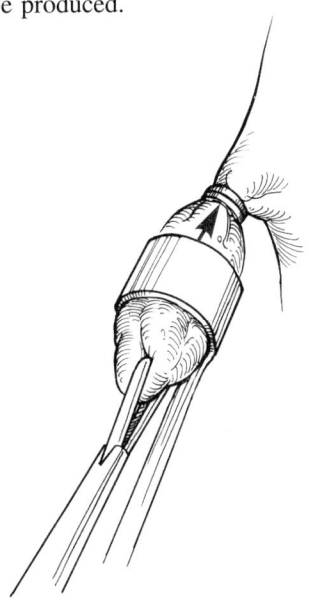

5. Only one hemorrhoid is banded at each visit. Patients who have more than one hemorrhoid will require multiple banding visits that should be spaced about 3 to 4 weeks apart.

Key Points

- Most useful for grade II and grade III hemorrhoids
- May be occasionally used for grade IV hemorrhoids
- Place all bands above the dentate line
- Place two bands on each hemorrhoid
- Treat only one hemorrhoid at each visit
- Space successive treatments at 3- to 4-week intervals

Complications

1. Common complications of the banding technique most frequently reported include ulceration, slipping or breaking of the rubber ring ligature, and pain.
2. Rarely, brisk bleeding that may require surgical intervention to establish hemostasis occurs at the time of slough.

3. Patients who have not undergone anticoagulation or have known coagulopathies may be at higher risk if they experience any postoperative bleeding.

Postoperative Instructions

1. The patient is advised to use stool softeners (fiber and/or surface tension–decreasing agents) temporarily and is instructed in dietary and toilet habit modification.

2. Significant bleeding, fever, and unusual pain are to be immediately reported to the physician.

Bibliography

Ambrose NS, Hares MM, Alexander-Williams J, Keighly MRB: Prospective randomized trial of photocoagulation and rubber band ligation of hemorrhoids. Br Med J 1983;286:1389.

American Society of Colon and Rectal Surgeons–Standards Task Force: Practice parameters for ambulatory anorectal surgery. Dis Colon Rectum 1991;34:285.

Corman M: Colon and Rectal Surgery, 3rd ed. Philadelphia, JB Lippincott, 1993.

Dennison JR, Whitston DC, Rooney S, Morris DL: The management of hemorrhoids. Am J Gastroenterol 1989;84:475.

Leicester RJ, Nichols RJ, Mann CV: Infrared coagulation: A new treatment for hemorrhoids. Dis Colon Rectum 1981;24:602.

86 Fecal Impaction

Aubrey L. Knight

Etiology

1. Definition: a large, firm, immovable mass of stool in the colon due to incomplete evacuation of feces. The impaction is usually found in the rectum but can occur in the more proximal segments of the colon.

2. Epidemiology: The elderly are at particular risk as a result of several physiologic changes that occur with aging.
   a. The total colonic transit time in elderly individuals with constipation has been shown to be prolonged.
   b. There is a decline in internal sphincter tone and external sphincter and pelvic muscle strength with aging.
   c. Subsets of elderly persons with a history of constipation or fecal impaction may have increased or decreased rectal tone. Those with increased rectal tone tend to have difficult, painful passage of hard fecal pellets. Similar rectal physiology is evident in irritable bowel syndrome. Those with decreased rectal tone require a higher volume of rectal distention to achieve sphincter relaxation and may be asymptomatic.

3. Risk factors
   a. Institutionalized elderly: This occurrence is sometimes referred to as the "terminal reservoir syndrome" and is primarily the result of immobility and a failure to respond appropriately to the urge to defecate. The gastrocolic reflex requires physical activity for its initiation.
   b. Depression
   c. Hypothyroidism
   d. Localized or generalized neurologic disorders
   e. Individuals with painful rectal conditions such as anal fissures and hemorrhoids
   f. Diet lacking in fiber or in fluids
   g. Hypokalemia and hypercalcemia
   h. Medications, such as stimulant laxatives, opiates, iron, aluminum-containing antacids, psychoactive substances, and drugs with anticholinergic potential
   i. Infants with congenital bowel obstruction caused by stenosis, atresia, or Hirschsprung's disease

Symptoms

1. The major symptoms of fecal impaction are abdominal pain and distention; the pain is frequently postprandial.

2. Paradoxically, a predominant symptom may be fecal incontinence. This is frequently misinterpreted and mistreated as diarrhea, which can worsen the problem.

3. Other symptoms include nausea, vomiting, anorexia, headache, confusion, urinary frequency and incontinence, and tenesmus.

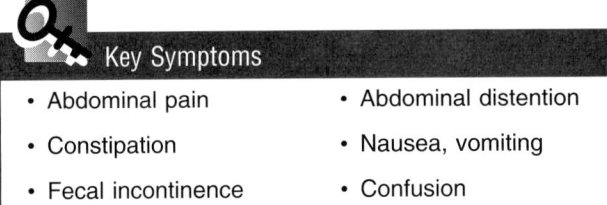

Key Symptoms

• Abdominal pain	• Abdominal distention
• Constipation	• Nausea, vomiting
• Fecal incontinence	• Confusion

Clinical Findings

1. On physical examination, one might expect to see a low-grade fever, tachycardia and tachypnea, and elevated blood pressure.

2. There may be signs of dehydration and weight loss.

3. A mass of stool may be palpable in the left lower quadrant or rectal vault.

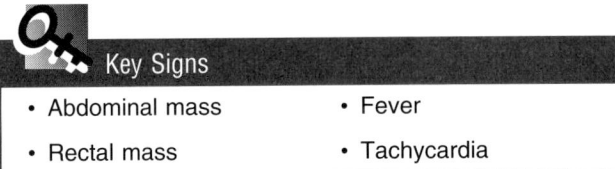

Key Signs

• Abdominal mass	• Fever
• Rectal mass	• Tachycardia

Laboratory Tests

1. The diagnosis can usually be made by careful history and physical examination. There are no specific laboratory tests, but the white blood cell count may be elevated; there may be hypokalemia and laboratory values consistent with dehydration.

2. The stool may be positive for occult blood.

3. Plain abdominal films will identify the stool or signs of obstruction when the physical examination is unrevealing. Barium enema or sigmoidoscopy may identify rectosigmoid masses that are contributory.

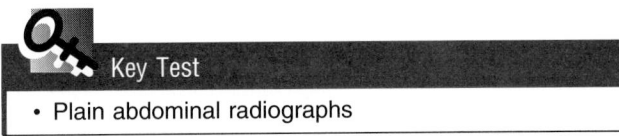

Key Test

• Plain abdominal radiographs

Differential Diagnosis

1. Irritable bowel syndrome
2. Carcinoma of the colon
3. Inflammatory colonic conditions

359

Treatment

1. Treatment of established fecal impaction involves first clearing the bowels with gentle manual fragmentation and removal of the fecal mass.
2. Enemas and suppositories may be of additional value in clearing the bowels.
3. Proximal masses may be fragmented with a water jet directed through a flexible sigmoidoscope.
4. Rarely, laparotomy is necessary.

Medications

1. There is no drug of choice for the acute treatment of fecal impaction.
2. When gentle digital evacuation is not completely successful, bisacodyl suppositories or enemas with mineral oil, tap water, or sodium phosphate may be of value. Soap suds enemas should be avoided in this situation as they may produce mucosal damage.
3. Poorly absorbed isosmotic solutions (GoLYTELY, Colyte) taken orally may be of further value.

Diet

1. Persons with fecal impaction should be maintained on a high-fiber diet.
2. A minimum intake of 1500 ml/day of fluid is recommended. This should be increased in summer.

Activity

Increased regular activity is an important aid in the initial therapy of fecal impaction and in the prevention of reimpaction.

Patient Education

1. Avoid irritant laxatives and hot water or soap enemas.
2. Establish a regular toilet time.
3. Recognize the importance of exercise, diet, and fluids.
4. Monitor bowel habits as reimpaction is likely.

Key Treatment	
Treatment of Choice	**Alternative Treatment**
• Manual disimpaction	• Isosmotic fluids orally (GoLYTELY, Colyte)
• Bisacodyl suppository	
• Enemas	

Follow-Up

1. Prevention
   a. High-fiber diet, ± fiber supplements
   b. Adequate fluid intake
   c. Regular exercise
   d. Establish a regular toilet time and evoke the gastrocolic reflex, if necessary.
   e. Stool-softening agents (e.g., Colace), if needed.
   f. Periodic suppositories or enemas
2. Monitoring
   a. Periodic rectal examination
   b. Bowel movements less often than every second to third day signify the possibility of reimpaction
3. Complications of fecal impactions include urinary tract infections, bowel obstruction, perforation, rectal bleeding, stercoral ulcers, volvulus, and weight loss. Rectovaginal fistulas have been described in elderly women and dystocia in pregnant women.
4. Prognosis
   a. Mortality is highest in the very old.
   b. Patients with a history of impaction have a higher likelihood of reimpaction. Following a bowel regimen becomes very important.

Bibliography

Barrett JA, Brockelhurst JC, Kiff ES, et al: Anal function in geriatric patients with fecal incontinence. Gut 1989;30:1244–1251.

Castle SC: Constipation: Endemic in the elderly? Med Clin North Am 1989;73:1497–1509.

Cort DHB: Miscellaneous inflammatory and structural disorders of the colon. *In* Yamada T, Alpers DH, Owyang C, et al (eds): Textbook of Gastroenterology. Philadelphia, JB Lippincott, 1991, pp 1846–1847.

Giggons JC, Levy SM: Gastrointestinal diseases in the aged. *In* Reichel W (ed): Clinical Aspects of Aging, 3rd ed. Baltimore, Williams & Wilkins, 1989, pp 195–197.

Hariri D, Gurwitz JH, Minaker KL: Constipation in the elderly. J Am Geriatr Soc 1993;41:1130–1140.

87 Common Hepatobiliary Symptoms

Jaundice is a yellowish discoloration of the skin and mucous membranes caused by excessive bilirubin. In adults, physical examination can detect jaundice at 2.5 to 3.5 mg/dl. In neonates, the threshold for visible jaundice is 5 to 6 mg/dl. Clinically, jaundice may be divided into two groups based on whether the hyperbilirubinemia is predominantly unconjugated (indirect) or conjugated (direct):

A. Unconjugated hyperbilirubinemia
1. The indirect bilirubin exceeds 80 per cent of the total bilirubin.
2. Mechanisms that cause unconjugated hyperbilirubinemia are excess bilirubin production, decreased hepatic uptake, and impaired conjugation.
3. Hemolysis or ineffective erythropoiesis causes overproduction of bilirubin.
4. An example of impaired conjugation is Gilbert's syndrome, which occurs in 3 to 7 per cent of the U.S. population and is due to decreased UDP-glucuronyl transferase activity. A mildly elevated bilirubin level in a healthy individual with a positive family history and normal liver function tests characterizes this disorder.
5. Defective uptake by immature hepatocytes leads to physiologic jaundice of the newborn.

B. Conjugated hyperbilirubinemia
1. The direct fraction of bilirubin ranges from 20 to 60 per cent.
2. Direct bilirubin elevations occur when conjugated bilirubin returns to the blood stream instead of draining into the bile ducts. Obstruction can occur at different sites, e.g., the cellular level in hepatocellular disease or at the bile duct in extrahepatic obstruction.

Differential Diagnosis

The differential diagnosis can be grouped by the age of onset.

A. Adult-onset conjugated hyperbilirubinemia
1. Hepatitis is the most common cause of jaundice in young adults, while in individuals 30 to 60 years old, cirrhosis accounts for about one third of cases. Alcoholic liver disease most commonly causes cirrhosis in the United States, while viral hepatitis, particularly type B, is the leading cause worldwide. Other types of cirrhosis include primary biliary cirrhosis, secondary biliary cirrhosis, cardiac cirrhosis, and metabolic diseases, such as α_1-antitrypsin deficiency, hemochromatosis, and Wilson's disease. Other causes of conjugated hyperbilirubinemia are
   a. Drug-induced cholestasis from medications such as estrogens or phenothiazines
   b. Primary metastatic liver cancer
   c. Congenital syndromes, such as Dubin-Johnson or Rotor syndrome
   d. Granulomatous infiltration of the liver
2. In new-onset jaundice in patients over age 60, extrahepatic obstruction from gallstones, strictures, and malignancies account for the majority of cases.
3. Hemolytic diseases, Gilbert's disease, and Crigler-Najjar syndrome cause conjugated hyperbilirubinemia. These illnesses also may also present in childhood.

B. Childhood jaundice
1. Physiologic jaundice occurs in up to 50 per cent of newborns and is the most common cause of neonatal unconjugated hyperbilirubinemia. Hemolytic disease, the most common pathologic cause of jaundice, results from ABO incompatibilities or, less likely, Rh disease, spherocytosis, or hemoglobinopathies. Other types of neonatal jaundice include breast milk jaundice, polycythemia, hematoma resorption, pyloric stenosis, and congenital hypothyroidism.
2. Neonatal conjugated hyperbilirubinemia with a direct bilirubin greater than 2.0 mg/dl may indicate more serious disorders. Causes include sepsis, neonatal hepatitis, TORCH infections, extrahepatic obstruction as seen in biliary atresia or choledocholithiasis, and metabolic diseases such as galactosemia or α_1-antitrypsin deficiency. Viral hepatitis is the most common cause of jaundice in a previously healthy child.

History

History provides clues to the cause of jaundice. Abdominal pain or a history of gallstones or biliary surgery may indicate obstructive jaundice, whereas depression and weight loss suggest an underlying malignancy. Risk factors for hepatocellular dysfunction include travel to an area endemic for hepatitis, raw shellfish consumption, excessive alcohol intake or intravenous drug use. Medications such as estrogens raise the possibility of intrahepatic cholestasis.

🔑 Key Questions

- Is there abdominal pain?
- Exposure to hepatitis?
- Previous biliary surgery?
- Travel history?
- Drug use?
- History of gallstones?

Clinical Findings

1. Palmar erythema
2. Small liver
3. Splenomegaly
4. Gynecomastia
5. Spider angiomata
6. Hepatomegaly
7. Ascites
8. Palpable gallbladder
9. Masses
10. Tenderness
11. Edema
12. Weight loss

Palmar erythema, spider angiomata, gynecomastia, testicular atrophy, ascites, and splenomegaly are findings associated with cirrhosis. A palpable gallbladder or mass may indicate an obstructive disorder. The rapid onset of mild to moderate tender hepatomegaly is most consistent with hepatocellular dysfunction. Although rare, Kayser-Fleischer corneal rings are pathognomonic of Wilson's disease.

Tests

1. A complete blood count (CBC) and liver profile are mandatory in all adult patients.

   a. The alkaline phosphatase level usually parallels the degree of cholestasis or obstruction, whereas the transaminases (ALT and AST) generally rise in proportion to the degree of hepatocellular disease. Alkaline phosphatase levels three times normal suggest obstruction, whereas AST/ALT levels five times normal generally indicate hepatocellular disease.

   b. A prothrombin time is indicated if findings are suspicious for severe liver dysfunction or obstruction.

   c. Tests for viral hepatitis, such as hepatitis A and B, are indicated in the presence of hepatocellular disease. Titers for less common infections, such as Epstein-Barr virus, hepatitis C, and cytomegalovirus, should be considered in the appropriate clinical setting.

   d. Special studies include antimitochondrial antibodies to screen for primary biliary cirrhosis, iron studies for hemochromatosis, serum ceruloplasmin for Wilson's disease, and antinuclear and anti-smooth muscle antibodies for autoimmune hepatitis.

   e. Ultrasonography is indicated in all suspected cases of extrahepatic obstruction. An ultrasound is about 90 per cent sensitive and specific for detecting mechanical obstruction. A CT scan is similarly sensitive and specific but is more expensive. CT scan is helpful if the ultrasound is unsatisfactory or to define ultrasound findings. Endoscopic retrograde cholangiopancreatography (ERCP) is an invasive procedure that images the ductal system and can provide cytologic specimens for diagnosing malignancies. ERCP also may be therapeutic by affording the removal of common bile duct stones, stent placement, or sphincterotomy.

2. Physiologic jaundice in newborns requires no testing or only a CBC and bilirubin level to confirm the clinical impression. Jaundice beginning the second to fourth day with a total bilirubin of less than 13 mg/dl, a direct bilirubin of less than 1.5 mg/dl, and a rise of less than 5 mg/dl per day characterizes physiologic jaundice. In nonphysiologic jaundice, total and direct bilirubin, CBC with differential, reticulocyte count, Coombs' test, and maternal and infant blood type are important initial tests.

   a. An elevated reticulocyte count indicates hemolysis. A positive Coombs' test indicates hemolysis caused by an ABO or Rh incompatibility. The smear may suggest a hemolytic process such as spherocytosis.

   b. If the direct bilirubin is more than 2.0 mg/dl, obtain a full liver battery and consider TORCH studies, viral studies, and if clinically indicated, a septic workup. An ultrasound is helpful to rule out biliary atresia if jaundice persists after two weeks of life.

   c. Jaundice from hypothyroidism, galactosemia, Gilbert's disease, and Crigler-Najjar syndrome usually begins on or after the fourth day of life.

Management

Treating the underlying cause is the most effective therapy for jaundice.

1. Obstructive jaundice is usually treated surgically versus medical management for nonobstructive jaundice.
2. Abstinence from alcohol and withdrawing medications are appropriate if these are contributing factors.
3. Interferon is useful in certain situations for chronic hepatitis B and C. Occasionally, hyperbilirubinemia causes pruritus.
4. Cholestyramine (one packet three times a day) or an antihistamine, such as diphenhydramine, will generally control itching.
5. Wilson's disease and hemochromatosis can be treated

effectively with penicillamine and phlebotomy, respectively.

6. In neonates, in addition to identifying the underlying cause of jaundice, the prevention of kernicterus is a consideration.

a. Although controversial, most authorities recommend phototherapy when the bilirubin reaches 5 mg/dl below the threshold for exchange transfusion. It is important to protect the infant's eyes and to promote adequate fluid intake. Exchange transfusions are rarely needed since the advent of phototherapy.

b. Physiologic jaundice requires no treatment. Breast milk jaundice requires no treatment, although some authorities recommend withholding breast-feeding if the bilirubin level approaches 20 mg/dl.

Bibliography

Kelly WN (ed): Essentials of internal medicine. *In* Approach to the Patient with Jaundice. Philadelphia, JB Lippincott, 1994, pp 189–192.

McKnight JT, Jones JE: Jaundice. Am Fam Phys 1992; 45:1139–1148

Newman TB, Maisels MJ: Evaluation and treatment of jaundice in the term newborn: A kinder, gentler approach. Pediatrics 1992;85:809–811.

Newman TB, Easterling JM, Goldman ES, Stevenson DK: Laboratory evaluation of jaundice in newborns. Am J Dis Child 1990;144:364–368.

Steiner GA, Lipsky MS: Jaundice. *In* Mengel MB, Schweibert LP (eds): Ambulatory Medicine. E Norwalk, CT, Appleton & Lange, 1993, pp 191–199.

Symptom	Ascites	*Martin S. Lipsky*

Ascites is the accumulation of excess fluid within the peritoneal cavity. Although ascites is most commonly associated with severe liver disease, there are several other possible causes. To simplify evaluation, it is useful to classify ascites based on the characteristics of the ascitic fluid:

1. *Transudates* are characterized by clear or straw-colored fluid that has a low protein content (<25 g/L), a low specific gravity (<1.016), a low cell count, and a high gradient difference in the albumin concentration between the serum and ascitic fluid (serum albumin $-$ ascites albumin >1.1). Although the precise pathophysiologic mechanisms remain uncertain, experts feel that transudates form due to a combination of increased portal pressure, increased lymph production, decreased oncotic pressure, and the impaired renal excretion of sodium and water.

2. *Exudates* are less common than transudates. Although the mechanisms of formation are uncertain, inflammatory processes that damage capillaries and disrupt the lymphatics are thought to be important factors. The inflammation causes protein to leak into the ascitic fluid, leading to an exudative or low-gradient ascites (serum albumin $-$ ascitic albumin $<$ 1.1). Sometimes a second process, such as infection, can turn a transudate into an exudate.

Differential Diagnosis

Conditions that cause abdominal swelling such as ovarian cysts, pancreatic cysts, bladder distention, or neoplasm may mimic ascites. After confirming the presence of ascites, grouping the differential diagnoses by the type of ascitic fluid is useful for determining its cause.

A. Transudative ascites

1. Cirrhosis is the most common cause of high-gradient ascites.

2. Right-sided heart failure, constrictive pericarditis, Budd-Chiari syndrome, and other disorders associated with increased portal pressure also can cause high-gradient ascites.

3. Nephrotic syndrome, hypoalbuminemia, myxedema, and Meigs' syndrome are other less common causes.

B. Exudative ascites

1. Most commonly, tumor and infection cause exudative ascites.

2. Peritonitis, pancreatitis, and a ruptured viscus are among other possible etiologies.

3. The presence of chylous ascites, or turbid milky ascitic fluid, indicates the presence of lymphatic obstruction due to trauma, neoplasm, or tuberculosis.

Refer to Ch. 60, Chronic Heart Failure; Ch. 66, Pericarditis; Ch. 90, Cirrhosis; Ch. 92, Pancreatitis; and Ch. 93, Pancreatic Carcinoma.

History

1. Whereas small amounts of ascites are frequently asymptomatic, larger accumulations increase abdominal girth and are often accompanied by anorexia, nausea, early satiety, and heartburn.

2. Extensive ascites associated with marked abdominal distention can cause shortness of breath.

3. The patient's clinical setting is often the best indicator for determining the etiology of the ascites. For example, the development of ascites in an alcoholic or a patient with chronic liver disease suggests cirrhosis.

Key Questions

- Is your waist increasing in size?
- Previous liver disease?
- Alcohol use?
- Is there a history of cancer or symptoms to suggest a malignancy?

Clinical Findings

1. The physical examination is not very sensitive for recognizing early ascites and requires at least several hundred milliliters of fluid to detect its presence.
2. Protruding flanks, shifting dullness, fluid waves, and a puddle sign are some physical findings associated with ascites.

Tests

Many cases of ascites will be part of a recognized disease such as cirrhosis, congestive heart failure, nephrosis, or malignancy. However, nearly all presenting patients require *paracentesis*. In addition, paracentesis should be considered in worsening ascites to rule out a new process such as spontaneous bacterial peritonitis or neoplasm.

1. Testing ascitic fluid for cell count and total protein and to determine the albumin gradient, culture and sensitivity, cytology, specific gravity, and amylase is helpful. An elevated amylase suggests pancreatic disease. An exudative or low-gradient ascites implies the presence of an inflammatory process such as an infection or neoplasm. An ascitic fluid total white blood cell count greater than 500 or an absolute polymorphonuclear count greater than 250 suggests infection. No further diagnostic workup may be required if the paracentesis results document a transudate in a patient with clinically evident disease (e.g., cirrhosis or congestive heart failure).
2. Occasionally, the cause may not be certain, and a patient will merit further evaluation, such as liver function tests, a liver-spleen scan, and an abdominal CT scan or other hepatic imaging procedure.
3. Patients with suspected right-sided heart failure or pericarditis need a cardiac evaluation.
4. Imaging the ovaries can rule out Meigs' syndrome or other gynecologic diseases.
5. For perplexing cases, diagnostic laparoscopy with biopsy and sampling of the peritoneal and hepatic surfaces is a more invasive option.

Management

Whenever possible, direct the treatment of ascites at the underlying cause. For example, a malignancy may require referral and surgery. More commonly, ascites develops in the presence of slowly worsening disease. Treatment goals are to prevent complications and to control the ascites. An important concept is that ascites by itself is rarely life-threatening and in the absence of complications such as respiratory embarrassment or bacterial peritonitis does not require urgent treatment. In fact, vigorous attempts to reduce ascites can do more harm than good.

1. Salt restriction and judicious use of bed rest are the cornerstones of treatment. If feasible, stop medications that can contribute to fluid retention, such as nonsteroidal anti-inflammatory drugs. If the ascites persists, start spironolactone (Aldactone), 100 mg/day. Because ascitic fluid is mobilized slowly, a reasonable goal is loss of 0.5 kg/day, or up to 1 kg/day if the patient has peripheral edema. More aggressive diuresis robs the intravascular fluid compartment and can induce renal insufficiency. Spironolactone may be increased gradually by 100 mg/day every 3 to 4 days until adequate diuresis or to a maximum dose of 600 mg/day.
2. Initiating loop diuretics, such as furosemide (Lasix), 40 mg/day, is the next step. Doses may be increased gradually to achieve appropriate weight loss. Monitor the patient carefully to avoid electrolyte imbalances and renal insufficiency.
3. Generally, only hyponatremic patients require fluid restriction.
4. Initiate treatment for patients with presumptive bacterial peritonitis with broad-spectrum antibiotics (e.g., a second- or third-generation cephalosporin) to cover gram-negative coliform bacteria and *Streptococcus.*
5. Significant ascites that fails to respond to salt restriction and diuretics may require large-volume paracentesis. Although authorities once felt that removing large amounts of ascitic fluid was dangerous, studies show that slowly removing up to 5 liters of fluid is safe. Some experts recommend administering intravenous albumin for all patients undergoing large-volume paracentesis, whereas others give albumin only if the patient becomes hypotensive.
6. In refractory cases, consider surgical consultation for placing a peritoneovenous shunt (e.g., LaVeen shunt). Unfortunately, these shunts are associated with several complications such as infection, valve failure, thrombosis, and disseminated intravascular coagulation (DIC) that limit their effectiveness. A liver transplant may be the best option in selected individuals.

 ## Bibliography

Arroyo V, Gines P, Planas R: Treatment of ascites in cirrhosis: Diuretics, peritoneovenous shunt, large-volume paracentesis. Gastroenterol Clin North Am 1992;21:237–256.

Runyon BA: Refractory ascites. Semin Liver Dis 1993;13:343–351.

Runyon BA: Care of patients with ascites. N Engl J Med 1994; 330:337–342.

Wilson JD, et al: Harrison's Principles of Internal Medicine, 12th ed. New York, McGraw-Hill, 1991.

| Symptom | **Abnormal Liver Function Tests** | *Jason Chao* |

Abnormal liver function tests are commonly discovered in asymptomatic individuals. While liver disease is often present, it is also common for patients to have results outside the "normal" range because of statistical chance. Liver disease also may be far advanced without any elevation in liver tests. Most liver or biliary tract disease generally manifests in one of two pathologic and biochemical patterns: parenchymal necrosis or cholestasis.

Differential Diagnosis

1. Patients with minor elevated liver tests (less than threefold) and no risk factors by history or physical examination are at low risk of significant liver pathology and may have follow-up liver testing in 1 to 3 months. Patients with chronic (more than 6 months) or major elevations in liver function tests should undergo further testing without delay.

2. Parenchymal liver disease typically causes elevated serum levels of alanine transaminase (ALT or SGPT) and aspartate transaminase (AST or SGOT). Lactic dehydrogenase (LDH) is a less sensitive and less specific marker of liver cell damage. Gamma glutamyl transpeptidase (GGT) is a more specific indicator of liver pathology but is also often elevated when cholestasis is present.

   a. Alcohol-induced hepatitis. Alcoholism is a lethal but treatable disease that may be first detected by abnormal liver tests.

   b. Chronic viral hepatitis B or C. Acute viral hepatitis A is self-limited. Patients with hepatitis B or C need to be followed for chronic hepatitis.

   c. Toxin-induced and drug-induced hepatitis.

   d. Obesity. Some morbidly obese patients may develop liver disease with hepatosteatonecrosis.

   e. Hemochromatosis. This treatable autosomal recessive disease may occur as a spontaneous mutation without a family history. There is an excess accumulation of iron in the liver and other organs. Transaminases are usually only moderately elevated.

   f. Autoimmune hepatitis. This disease primarily affects women between the ages of 20 and 40 years. Transaminases are quite elevated.

   g. Wilson's disease. This should be considered in patients younger than 40. There is an excess accumulation of copper that leads to liver failure and neurologic symptoms if untreated.

   h. α_1-Antitrypsin deficiency. Many patients with this autosomal recessive disease do not have chronic obstructive pulmonary disease at the time of diagnosis.

3. Alkaline phosphatase (ALP) greater than three times normal or elevated bilirubin suggests cholestatic or biliary tract disease. ALT and AST are usually less than three times normal.

   a. Biliary tract obstruction. Extrahepatic structural or mechanical obstruction of the bile ducts is most commonly due to choledocholithiasis, biliary stricture, pancreatic or periampullary carcinoma, pancreatitis, or biliary atresia.

   b. Drug-induced cholestasis.

   c. Congestive heart failure. Older patients may present with right-sided heart failure and jaundice.

   d. Intrahepatic cholestasis of pregnancy.

   e. Hemolytic anemias and ineffective erythropoiesis such as thalassemias.

   f. Gilbert's and Crigler-Najjar syndromes cause isolated hyperbilirubinemia.

   g. Hepatobiliary neoplasms. Primary benign and malignant tumors of the liver, gallbladder, and extrahepatic bile ducts and metastatic tumors to the liver may cause cholestasis.

   h. Primary biliary cirrhosis. Typical patients are middle-aged females with very high serum alkaline phosphatase levels.

   i. Primary sclerosing cholangitis. This chronic, progressive disease is more common in middle-aged males with elevated serum alkaline phosphatase levels. Most patients also have inflammatory bowel disease. It may be difficult to differentiate from a cholangiocarcinoma.

> Refer to Ch. 88, Hepatitis; Ch. 91, Gallstones and Cholecystitis; Ch. 92, Pancreatitis; Ch. 93, Pancreatic Carcinoma; and Ch. 319, Alcoholism.

History

1. Look for symptoms of liver disease, including fatigue, pruritus, jaundice, and bruising.

2. Detailed alcohol intake history. Underreporting is common among alcoholics, so a sensitive yet thorough history of alcohol consumption is necessary. Verification of the history by family or friends may be necessary.

3. Occupational or home chemical exposure to hepatotoxins. Household toxins include carbon tetrachloride, chloroform, heavy metals, and phosphorus.

4. Risk factors for viral hepatitis (blood transfusions, needle-stick injury, injected drug use, contact with patient with known hepatitis, unsafe sexual practices).

5. Family history of liver disease.

6. Past and current medications.

   a. Drug-induced hepatitis: acetaminophen, amiodarone, anesthetic agents, isoniazid, ketoconazole, nitrofurantoin, penicillins, sulfonamides, tetracyclines, methyldopa, procainamide, quinidine, propylthiouracil, niacin, vitamin A, disulfiram, dantrolene, methotrexate, carbamazepine, phenytoin, valproic acid.

  b. Drug-induced cholestasis: androgens, estrogens, carbamazepine, clavulanic acid, diazepam, disulfiram, erythromycin estolate, haloperidol, oral hypoglycemics, penicillamine, phenothiazines, propoxyphene.

Clinical Findings

1. Liver size and tenderness
2. Ascites
3. Encephalopathy

Tests

1. Further testing should be chosen based on history and pattern of abnormal test results.
2. Serologic tests for hepatitis A, B, and C, Epstein-Barr virus, and cytomegalovirus will identify viral hepatitis.
3. Elevation of serum iron, transferrin saturation, and ferritin may indicate hemochromatosis.
4. Low serum ceruloplasmin level and elevated 24-hour urinary excretion of copper may indicate Wilson's disease.
5. Low serum α_1-antitrypsin level may indicate α_1-antitrypsin deficiency. These patients often have an abnormal serum protein electrophoresis.
6. Elevated IgG and autoimmune markers such as antinuclear antibodies and anti–smooth muscle antibodies help identify autoimmune hepatitis. Other markers of collagen vascular disease may be absent.
7. Antimitochondrial antibodies are usually present in patients with primary biliary cirrhosis.
8. For parenchymal liver disease, hepatic imaging with ultrasound or computed tomography may be helpful.
9. Liver biopsy should be reserved for those with persistent elevations greater than three times normal.
10. Conjugated and unconjugated bilirubin determinations in cholestatic liver disease help differentiate causes of jaundice.
11. Prothrombin time may be prolonged in both hepatocellular and cholestatic liver disease.
12. Ultrasonographic imaging of the liver and biliary tract is recommended for initial radiologic evaluation of cholestatic liver disease.

13. Endoscopic retrograde cholangiopancreatography (ERCP) or percutaneous transhepatic cholangiography (PTC) may be necessary if extrahepatic obstruction is suspected.

Management

1. Alcohol and other hepatotoxic drugs should be avoided.
2. The underlying cause for elevated biochemical liver tests will determine further treatment.

PEARLS

- Most hepatocellular dysfunction causes the AST/ALT ratio to remain less than 1, except for alcoholic liver disease, which typically raises the ratio to greater than 2.

- Although alcoholic liver disease is very common, other treatable causes of liver disease may coexist.

- Elevated ALP may originate from bone, placenta, or bowel rather than liver.

- If the prothrombin time is prolonged, administration of a single dose of parenteral vitamin K may dramatically improve the prothrombin time in obstructive disease.

 ## Bibliography

For more information on the causes of abnormal liver tests, see
Herrera JL: Abnormal liver enzyme levels: The spectrum of causes. Postgrad Med 1993;93:113–116.
For more information on the evaluation of abnormal liver tests, see
Herrera JL: Abnormal liver enzyme levels: Clinical evaluation in asymptomatic patients. Postgrad Med 1993;93:119–130.
For more information on the usefulness of ultrasound, see
Ekberg O, Aspelin P: Ultrasonography in asymptomatic patients with abnormal biochemical liver tests. Scand J Gastroenterol 1986;21:573–576.
For more information on the usefulness of liver biopsy, see
VanNess MM, Diehl AM: Is liver biopsy useful in the evaluation of patients with chronically elevated liver enzymes? Ann Intern Med 1989;111:473–478.
For more information on screening for asymptomatic liver disease, see
Wright C, Rivera JC, Baetz JH: Liver function testing in a working population: Three strategies to reduce false positive results. J Occup Med 1988;30:693–697.

Procedure | **PARACENTESIS AND ABDOMINAL DIAGNOSTIC TAP** | *Brian S. Murphy*

1. *Ascites* is the abnormal accumulation of fluid within the abdominal cavity and *paracentesis* is an invasive procedure to remove this fluid for both therapeutic and diagnostic purposes. Epidemiologic studies have shown that formation of ascites is most commonly related to parenchymal liver disease (about 80 per cent), whereas another 5 per cent may involve a mixed pattern of liver disease and an abdominal malignancy. Less frequent causes of ascitic fluid collections are heart failure, tuberculosis, pancreatitis, myxedema, and nephrotic syndrome.

2. Patients with ascites may complain of weight gain, increasing abdominal girth, and shortness of breath, especially in the recumbent position.

3. Evidence of flank dullness on physical examination should lead to evaluation of shifting dullness in the abdomen. It has been estimated that 1500 cc of ascitic fluid need to be present in order to detect shifting dullness. The presence of a fluid wave is a less sensitive indicator of ascites. Studies have reported that abdominal ultrasonagraphy has been able to detect at least 100 cc of fluid in the abdomen.

Indications

1. Ascitic fluid analysis is valuable in helping to pinpoint the etiology of ascites.

2. Paracentesis is especially important to perform because up to 25 per cent of patients admitted with ascites have evidence of peritonitis.

Contraindications

An underlying coagulopathy is rarely a contraindication to performing paracentesis. Some patients with coagulopathies are given fresh frozen plasma and/or platelets before or during the procedure to lessen the likelihood of bleeding. There are no data to support giving blood products to prevent hematoma formation and, in fact, transfusing such products places the patient at increased risk for developing post-transfusion hepatitis.

Preparation

1. Once a site has been chosen, a sterile field should be established.

2. Although use of sterile gloves is essential, a mask, gown, and hat are not required.

3. The area should be disinfected with an iodine-based solution, and local anesthetic should be infiltrated into the skin and deeper tissues.

Equipment

1. 60-cc syringe
2. 1.5-inch 22- or 18-gauge needles
3. 1 liter evacuated collection bottle and sterile plastic tubing (if a therapeutic paracentesis is being done)
4. 3 sterile drapes
5. Iodine solution

Anesthesia

1% lidocaine solution without epinephrine

Technique

1. The site of needle insertion depends on the amount of ascites. It is often recommended that the needle be introduced approximately 2 finger breadths cephalad and 2 finger breadths medial to the anterosuperior iliac spine—whichever quadrant is most dull to percussion. Because the lower quadrants can be highly vascular, an alternative site is in the midline, caudad to the umbilicus. Because patients may have a neurogenic bladder or bladder outlet obstruction, it is recommended that the bladder be emptied before use of a midline approach to avoid bladder puncture.

2. When the area has been prepped, the needle should be introduced in a "Z" track to prevent leakage of ascitic fluid when the needle is removed. This is done by retracting the skin caudally before inserting the needle and then releasing the skin when the peritoneum is entered. The needle should be advanced in small increments (about 5 mm) and aspirated intermittently to ensure that the tip does not enter a blood vessel.

3. Needles should never be introduced into a highly vascular area, into an area midline cephalad to the umbilicus, or through or within several centimeters of scar tissue. Such placements put the patient at risk of vessel puncture and subsequent hematoma formation or a perforated viscus adherent to a surgical scar.

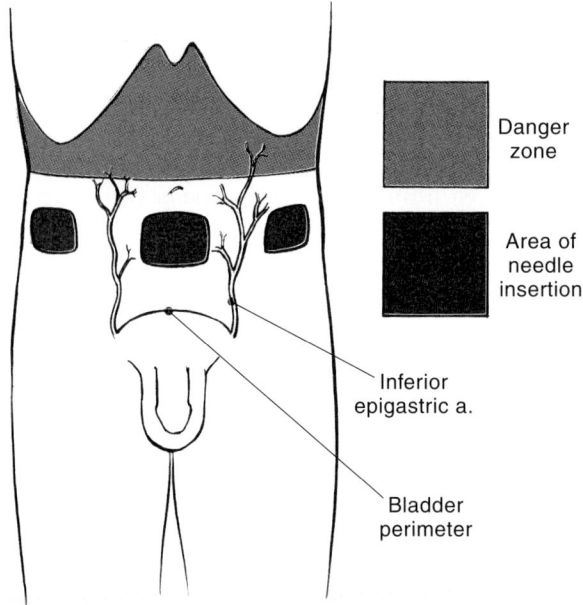

Danger zone

Area of needle insertion

Inferior epigastric a.

Bladder perimeter

Fluid Analysis

1. *Cell count:* A pre-diuresis elevation of the ascitic fluid white blood cell (WBC) count greater than 250 cells/mm^3 is seen in episodes of spontaneous bacterial peritonitis with a left shift. Lymphocytic predominance occurs in cases of tuberculous peritonitis and peritoneal carcinomatosis. In cases of a bloody fluid, 1 PMN is subtracted for every 250 red blood cells present. If the corrected WBC count is greater than 250 cells/mm^3, the fluid is presumed to be infected.

2. *Albumin:* Ascitic fluid albumin should be measured the same day as the serum albumin. When the ascitic fluid value is subtracted from the serum value, the physician obtains the serum-ascites albumin gradient (SAAG). The SAAG is determined by oncotic-hydrostatic balance. Portal hypertension produces a high hydrostatic pressure gradient between the portal bed and the ascitic fluid.

    a. An SAAG value greater than 1.1 gm/dl is consistent with portal hypertension and is associated with cirrhosis, liver metastasis, hepatic failure, alcoholic hepatitis, the Budd-Chiari syndrome, cardiac ascites, portal vein thrombosis, myxedema, fatty liver of pregnancy, or veno-occlusive disease.

    b. SAAG values less than 1.1 gm/dl are frequently associated with peritoneal carcinomatosis, biliary ascites, pancreatic ascites, tuberculous ascites, the nephrotic syndrome, bowel obstruction with in-

farct, postoperative lymphatic leakage, or serositis seen in connective tissue disease.

3. *Culture:* Studies have shown that bedside inoculation of ascitic fluid is superior to laboratory inoculation. While the majority of spontaneous bacterial peritonitis (SBP) is due to a monomicrobial infection, it is imperative to obtain both aerobic and anaerobic cultures.

Adjunctive Testing

1. *Protein:* This test has largely been replaced by the SAAG determination. It is noteworthy that patients with extremely low protein ascites have been found to be predisposed to develop SBP.

2. *Amylase:* Patients with pancreatitis or gut perforation exhibit elevated amylase levels, usually three to five times serum concentrations.

3. *Tuberculosis (TB) Testing:* TB peritonitis is often associated with negative standard cultures of ascitic fluid and a mononuclear predominance of total WBCs from the ascites. However, studies have shown that laparoscopy with histologic analysis of biopsy samples is more sensitive than culture of the ascitic fluid and smear testing for acid-fast bacilli.

4. *Cytology:* Ascitic fluid cytologic analysis has proved most sensitive in cases of peritoneal carcinomatosis. This analysis is less sensitive in conditions when tumor cells do not line the peritoneal cavity (e.g., hepatoma or lymphoma).

5. *Triglycerides:* Suspicion of chylous ascites usually arises when the ascitic fluid is milky white or cloudy. This is further supported by triglyceride levels of more than 200 mg/dl, sometimes as high as 1000 mg/dl.

6. *Bilirubin:* If the ascitic fluid bilirubin is greater than or equal to 6 mg/dl and elevated more than that found in the serum, this can indicate a biliary or upper gastrointestinal tract perforation. A dark-brown ascitic fluid is often seen in such cases.

 ## Bibliography

Mallory A, Schaeffer JW: Complications of diagnostic paracentesis in patients with liver disease. JAMA 1978;239:628.

Runyon BA: Care of patients with ascites. N Engl J Med 1994;330(5):337–341.

Runyon BA: Paracentesis of ascitic fluid: a safe procedure. Arch Intern Med 1986;146:2259–2261.

Runyon BA, et al: Comparison of the utility of the serum-ascites albumin gradient to the exudate/transudate concept in the differential diagnosis of ascites. Hepatology 1992;16:85A.

88 Hepatitis

Roxanna Rhodes

Etiology

Viral Hepatitis

1. Hepatitis A
   a. Fecal-oral transmission
   b. Endemic in underdeveloped countries
   c. Outbreaks in day care centers and residential institutions
   d. Incubation: 2 to 6 weeks
2. Hepatitis B
   a. Parenteral inoculation, sexual, or perinatal transmission
   b. 90 per cent recover
   c. Over 1 per cent develop fulminant hepatitis
   d. 10 per cent develop chronic hepatitis
   e. Incubation: 4 weeks to 6 months
3. Hepatitis C
   a. 85 per cent transfusion-associated hepatitis cases
   b. Parenteral inoculation, especially intravenous drug use
   c. >50 per cent become chronic hepatitis, which leads to cirrhosis in 20 per cent
   d. Incubation: 5 to 10 weeks
4. Hepatitis D
   a. Requires HBV for its replication; coinfects with HBV or superinfects a chronic HBV carrier
   b. Incubation: 4 weeks to 6 months
   c. Can accelerate chronic hepatitis B to cirrhosis
   d. Occasionally causes fulminant acute hepatitis
5. Hepatitis E
   a. Epidemic form of non-A, non-B hepatitis
   b. Epidemics of hepatitis in India, Southeast Asia, North Africa, Soviet Union, and Mexico
   c. Self-limited illness
   d. High mortality rate in pregnant women (20 per cent)
   e. Incubation: 2 to 9 weeks
   f. All reported cases in the United States have been imported by immigrants or visitors to endemic areas.
6. Cytomegalovirus and Epstein-Barr virus

Drugs and Toxic Hepatitis

1. Alcholic hepatitis: 10 to 15 per cent of long-term alcohol intake leads to hepatitis
2. Drugs: halothane, isoniazid, acetaminophen

Autoimmune Chronic Hepatitis

1. Most often affects young women
2. Associated with arthralgia, arthritis, skin rash, and fever

Symptoms

1. Malaise
2. Nausea
3. Anorexia
4. Fatigue
5. Vomiting
6. Diarrhea
7. Low-grade fever

Key Symptoms

- Malaise
- Nausea
- Fatigue

Clinical Findings

1. Tender hepatomegaly
2. Dark urine
3. Jaundice

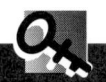

Key Sign

- Tender enlarged liver

Laboratory Tests

1. Increased ALT and AST
2. Anti-HAV
   a. IgM type: signifies current or recent infection hepatitis A
   b. IgG type: signifies current or previous infection hepatitis A and indicates immunity to hepatitis A
3. HBsAg (hepatitis B surface antigen)
   a. Positive in both acute or chronic hepatitis B infection
4. HBeAg (hepatitis B e antigen)
   a. Positive in acute hepatitis B infection and during active replication in chronic hepatitis B
   b. Reflects infectivity
5. Anti-Hbc IgM (antibody to hepatitis core antigen)
   a. Marker of HBV acute infection
6. Anti-HBc IgG
   a. Marker of chronic hepatitis and carrier state hepatitis
7. Anti-HBe (antibody to hepatitis B e antigen)
   a. Transiently positive in convalescence and in some chronic cases of hepatitis B
   b. Not protective.

8. Anti-HBs (antibody to hepatitis B surface antigen)
   a. Positive late in acute hepatitis B
   b. Protective
9. Anti-HCV (antibody to hepatitis C virus)
   a. Second-generation ELISA is 70 to 80 per cent accurate.
   b. Second-generation recombinant immunoblot assay (RIBA) is used as a confirmatory test and is 90 per cent accurate.
   c. Polymerase chain reaction (PCR) test is useful in equivocal cases and positive 2 weeks after infection.
   d. ELISA and RIBA may not be positive for 6 to 8 weeks and may take up to 12 months.
   e. Not protective.
10. Anti-HDV (antibody to hepatitis D virus)
    a. Does not become positive until 15 weeks after clinical onset
    b. Not protective
11. Inceased sedimentation rate, positive antinuclear antibody, and positive lupus cell in autoimmune hepatitis
12. Eosinophilia in drug-induced hepatitis

Differential Diagnosis

1. Acute hepatic congestion
2. Disseminated sepsis
3. Liver abscess
4. Biliary tract disease with or without cholangitis
5. Wilson's disease

Treatment

1. Hepatitis A
   a. After exposure: immune globulin, 0.02 ml/kg intramuscularly within 2 weeks plus hepatitis A vaccine (Havrix) 1 ml intramuscularly at a separate site.
   b. Travel to endemic areas
      (1) Hepatitis A vaccine (Havrix) 1 ml intramuscularly 15 days before travel (90 per cent protective)—follow with 1 ml booster dose in 6 to 12 months.
      (2) Immune globulin, 0.02 ml/kg intramuscularly for travel less than 3 months; 0.06 ml/kg intramuscularly for travel longer than 3 months (repeat every 4 to 6 months) if hepatitis A vaccine is not available
2. Hepatitis B
   a. After exposure: hepatitis B immune globulin (HBIG) plus active immunization with HBV vaccine (Recombivax HB).
      (1) After needle stick

      (2) Within 14 days after sexual exposure to a partner with acute hepatitis B infection
      (3) At birth to infants born to HBsAg-positive mothers
   b. Before exposure: recombinant hepatitis B vaccine
      (1) Health workers
      (2) Homosexual men
      (3) Household and sexual contacts of HBsAg carriers
      (4) All neonates in endemic areas
      (5) High-risk neonates in lower-risk areas
3. Hepatitis C: alpha interferon for chronic infection
   a. Three million units SC or IM three times weekly for 6 months
   b. Remission 40 to 50 per cent
4. Hepatitis D
   a. No treatment
   b. Hepatitis B vaccine is preventive
5. Hepatitis E: no treatment
6. Autoimmune chronic hepatitis
   a. Corticosteroids
   b. Azathioprine

Follow-Up

1. If tests are negative, repeat in 3 to 6 months.
2. HCV can produce fluctuations in transaminases and therefore serial testing may be required to detect a rise in ALT.
3. A liver biopsy is needed in order to treat chronic hepatitis B and C.
4. Hepatocellular carcinoma can develop with chronic hepatitis.

B | Bibliography

For more information on hepatitis, see
Agus SG: Acute liver disease and hepatitis. *In* Sachar DB, Wayne JD, Lewis BS (eds): Pocket Guide to Gastroenterology. Baltimore, Williams & Wilkins, 1991, pp 121–136.

For more information on acute hepatitis, see
Dienstag JL, Wands JR, Isselbacher KJ: Acute hepatitis. *In* Wilson JD, Braunwald E, Isselbacher KJ, et al (eds): Harrison's Principles of Internal Medicine, 12th ed. New York, McGraw-Hill, 1991, pp 1322–1337.

For more information on acute hepatitis, see
Ockner RK: Acute viral hepatitis. *In* Bennett JC, Plum F (eds): Cecil Textbook of Medicine, 20th ed. Philadelphia, WB Saunders, 1996.

For more information on chronic hepatitis, see
Ockner RK: Chronic hepatitis. *In* Bennett JC, Plum F (eds): Cecil Textbook of Medicine, 20th ed. Philadelphia, WB Saunders, 1996.

For more information on chronic hepatitis, see
Wands JR, Isselbacher KJ: Chronic hepatitis. *In* Wilson JD, Braunwald E, Isselbacher KJ, et al (eds): Harrison's Principles of Internal Medicine, 12th ed. New York, McGraw-Hill, 1991, pp 1337–1340.

89 Hyperbilirubinemia

Michael David Bernstein

Etiology

A. Unconjugated hyperbilirubinemia
1. Overproduction of bilirubin
   a. Hemolysis, intravascular: disseminated intravascular coagulation (DIC)
   b. Hemolysis, extravascular
      (1) Hemoglobinopathies
      (2) Enzyme deficiencies such as glucose-6-phosphate deficiency
      (3) Autoimmune hemolytic anemias
   c. Ineffective erythropoiesis
   d. Hematoma
   e. Blood transfusions
2. Hereditary unconjugated hyperbilirubinemia
   a. Gilbert's syndrome (autosomal dominant)
   b. Crigler-Najjar syndrome type I (autosomal recessive)
   c. Crigler-Najjar syndrome type II (autosomal dominant)
3. Drugs
   a. Chloramphenicol: neonatal hyperbilirubinemia
   b. Vitamin K: neonatal hyperbilirubinemia
   c. 5β-Pregnane-3α, 20α-diol: cause of breast milk jaundice

B. Conjugated hyperbilirubinemia
1. Inherited disorders
   a. Dubin-Johnson syndrome (autosomal recessive)
   b. Rotor syndrome (autosomal recessive)
2. Hepatocellular diseases and intrahepatic causes
   a. Viral hepatitis
   b. Alcoholic hepatitis
   c. Drug-induced hepatitis: isoniazid (INH), nonsteroidal anti-inflammatory drugs, Bactrim, zidovudine (AZT)
   d. Cirrhosis
   e. Drug-induced cholestasis: perchlorperazine, haloperidol (Haldol), estrogens
   f. Sepsis
   g. Postoperative jaundice
   h. Infiltrative liver disease: tumor, abscesses (pyogenic, amebic), tuberculosis (TB), parasites (*Toxoplasma*), *Pneumocystis carinii* pneumonia, *Echinococcus*
   i. Primary biliary cirrhosis
   j. Primary sclerosing cholangitis (PSC)
3. Extrahepatic causes
   a. Gallstone disease
   b. Pancreatitis-related stricture
   c. Pancreatic head tumor
   d. Cholangiocarcinoma
   e. PSC

Production and Elimination

Bilirubin is a waste product of heme metabolism, largely produced in the spleen, where senescent red blood cells (RBCs) are destroyed. The bilirubin is bound to albumin and transported to the liver, where it is taken up and conjugated with glucuronic acid by the enzyme UDP-glucuronyl transferase. It is then excreted into the bile. Hyperbilirubinemia can result from overproduction, failure of conjugation, or failure to excrete into bile at the level of the canaliculus or the common bile duct.

1. Indirect hyperbilirubinemia is usually the result of overproduction of bilirubin.
2. Hemolysis: Either intravascular as in DIC or extravascular as in hemolytic anemia. Transfusions of blood and resorbing hematomas also can increase bilirubin levels. The total bilirubin level rarely rises above 4 mg/dl in these states.
3. Gilbert's disease is a probable autosomal dominant disease characterized by indirect hyperbilirubinemia due to a deficiency of UDP-glucuronyl transferase. Inadequate conjugation of bilirubin leads to decreased elimination in bile and accumulation of indirect bilirubin. Levels range from 1 to 6 mg/dl. The disease is usually asymptomatic, but overt jaundice can occur at times of stress, such as starvation, intercurrent disease, or alcohol consumption. The diagnosis is made by excluding hemolysis or intrinsic liver disease. Phenobarbital will rapidly decrease serum indirect bilirubin level, but treatment is unnecessary because the disease has an excellent prognosis.
4. Crigler-Najjar syndrome type I is inherited as an autosomal recessive disease. It is manifested by the onset of severe indirect hyperbilirubinemia 3 to 4 days after birth. Levels of indirect bilirubin are in the range of 20 to 50 mg/dl.

Bilirubin encephalopathy or kernicterus usually leads to death within the first year. The disease is caused by complete or near-complete deficiency of UDP-glucuronyl transferase with failure to excrete unconjugated nonpolar bilirubin into the bile. A lack of response to phenobarbital is characteristic. Definitive treatment is liver transplantation. Phototherapy, which converts bilirubin into more polar excretable photoisomers, done over a 12-hour period may serve as temporary therapy.

5. Crigler-Najjar syndrome type II is a probable autosomal dominant inherited disease characterized by deficiency of UDP-glucuronyl transferase but associated with less severe indirect hyperbilirubinemia than in type I. Bilirubin levels range between 7 and 20 mg/dl. Type II is responsive to phenobarbital treatment (60 to 180 mg/day) with a rapid decline in plasma bilirubin level. The diagnosis rests on exclusions of intrinsic liver disease or hemolysis and a dramatic response to administration of phenobarbital. Unlike type I disease, type II disease has an excellent prognosis. It rarely requires treatment except in the newborn with seriously rising bilirubin levels.

6. Physiologic jaundice results from deficient UDP-glucuronyl transferase activity in the first week of life combined with increased destruction of red blood cells, leading to indirect hyperbilirubinemia in the newborn. This is usually benign and resolves by the first week of life.

7. Breast milk jaundice is a benign disease that results either from a β-glucuronidase that metabolizes bilirubin diglucuronide or a fatty acid in breast milk that inhibits UDP-glucuronyl transferase.

8. Post-transfusion and hematoma resorption. Indirect hyperbilirubinemia results from overproduction of unconjugated bilirubin that overwhelms the conjugating system. Intrinsic liver disease must be excluded.

9. Familial conjugated hyperbilirubinemia
   a. Dubin-Johnson syndrome, an autosomal recessive disease, is associated in Iranian Jews with factor VII deficiency. Dubin-Johnson syndrome results from defective secretion of conjugated bilirubin. Characteristically, the liver appears black due to accumulation of a black pigment contained in lysosomes. The plasma bilirubin level approaches 2.5 mg/dl but can rise as high as 20 mg/dl. Typically, total urine coproporphyrin levels are normal or slightly increased, and there is a reversal in the ratio of urinary coproporphy-

rin I to coproporphyrin III with greater coproporphyrin I levels. Additional findings include a nonvisualizing oral cholecystogram (OCG) and a second peak in sulfobromophthalein plasma levels 45 to 90 minutes after intravenous injection. Phenobarbital may lower bilirubin levels in some patients. Patients are generally asymptomatic, and prognosis is excellent.

   b. Rotor syndrome is an autosomal recessive disease that is similar to Dubin-Johnson syndrome in course and treatment. In contrast, however, black pigment does not accumulate, OCG is visualized, and the sulfobromophthalein curve, while abnormal, does not show a second plasma peak. Urinary coproporphyrin levels are increased, and the ratio is less dramatically reversed than in Dubin-Johnson syndrome.

10. Hepatocellular disease (Table 89–1)
    a. Hepatitis A, B, C, D, or E: liver cell destruction with rise in SGOT/SGPT to 10 to 50 times the upper limit of normal and possible jaundice with bilirubin ranging from 0 to 20 mg/dl, mostly direct.

    b. Drugs such as acetaminophen, INH, NSAIDs: same as above.

    c. Alcohol: with SGOT 6 to 10 times the upper limit of normal and SGPT 2 to 3 times the upper limit of normal, with increased bilirubin related to liver cell destruction.

    d. Ischemic hepatitis: very high transaminase, 100 times the upper limit of normal with increased bilirubin.

11. Cholestatic disease
    a. Drugs such as phenothiazines, sulfonylureas, allopurinol, and estrogens: alkaline phosphatase 5 to 10 times the upper limit of normal.

    b. Viral, such as cytomegalovirus, Epstein-Barr virus, hepatitis C, and cholestatic hepatitis A: alkaline phosphatase 5 to 10 times the upper limit of normal.

    c. Infiltrative disease, such as TB, lymphoma, MAI, hepatoma, metastatic carcinoma, or sarcoid, diag-

TABLE 89–1. GENERAL LABORATORY FINDINGS IN DIRECT HYPERBILIRUBINEMIA (APPROXIMATES THAT MAY BE SEEN)

DISEASE	BILIRUBIN	ALKALINE PHOSPHATASE	SGOT	SGPT	ALBUMIN
Alcoholic liver disease	0–20	5–10 × nl	5–6 × nl	2 × nl	nl or ↓
Acute viral hepatitis	0–20	2–3 × nl	10–50 × nl	10–50 × nl	nl
Drug-induced cholestasis	0–20	5–10 × nl	5–10 × nl	5–10 × nl	nl
Common bile duct obstruction	0–20	5–10 × nl	nl to 2–3 × nl	nl to 2–3 × nl	nl
Malignant bile duct obstruction	0–20	5–20 × nl	nl to 1.5–2 × nl	nl to 1.5–2 × nl	nl
Primary biliary cirrhosis	0–20	1.5–20 × nl	nl	nl	nl or ↓
PSC	0–20	1.5–20 × nl	nl	nl	nl or ↓
Ischemic hepatitis	0–20	3–5 × nl	20–50 × nl	20–50 × nl	nl

nosed by liver biopsy: alkaline phosphatase 5 to 10 times the upper limit of normal.

d. Gram-negative sepsis.

e. Primary biliary cirrhosis, diagnosed by antimitochondrial antibodies and liver biopsy.

12. Extrahepatic cholestasis

a. Gallstone disease. Ultrasound and computed tomographic (CT) findings show dilated common bile duct with possible stones. Generally, alkaline phosphatase is 5 to 10 times the upper limit of normal with smaller elevations of SGOT and SGPT and a bilirubin less than 20 mg/dl. ERCP is the "gold standard" for visualization of stones in the common bile duct.

b. Benign strictures of intra- and extrahepatic ducts. Examples include primary sclerosing cholangitis and pancreatitis-related strictures. Alkaline phosphatase is disproportionately elevated to SGOT and SGPT. ERCP is diagnostic.

c. Neoplasm: cholangiocarcinoma, Klatskin tumors, pancreatic carcinoma. Usually high alkaline phosphatase out of proportion to SGOT and SGPT. Diagnosis is made with aid of CT scan, ultrasound, and ERCP.

 Bibliography

Chopra S, Griffin PhH: Evaluation of liver disease: Laboratory tests and diagnostic procedures. Am J Med 1985;79:221.

Jansen PL, Oude Elfeink RP: Hereditary conjugated hyperbilirubinemia in Wistar rats: A model for the study of ATP-dependent hepatocanalicular organic ion transport. Adv Vet Sci Comp Med 1993;37:175–195.

Polin RA: Management of neonatal hyperbilirubinemia: Rational use of phototherapy. Biol Neonate 1990;58(suppl 1):32–43.

Schiff ER, Schiff L: Diseases of the Liver. Philadelphia, JB Lippincott, 1987.

Zakim D, Boxer TD: Hepatology: A Textbook of Liver Disease. Philadelphia, WB Saunders, 1990.

90 Cirrhosis

Etiology

1. Definition: triad of parenchymal necrosis, regenerating nodules, and fibrosis
2. Epidemiology
   a. The age of onset, incidence, and gender predominance vary among the given causes.
   b. Alcohol abuse and viral hepatitis cause most cases.

Symptoms

1. Most symptoms are nonspecific and may include easy bruising, fatigue, malaise, and weight loss.
2. Other symptoms or diseases may occur as a result of the primary disorder that caused the cirrhosis. These symptoms and diseases may be a clue to the cause and include Addison's disease, arthralgia, autoimmune disease, bone pain, diabetes mellitus, heart failure, hyperpigmentation, hypothyroidism, loss of libido, night blindness, pruritus, and steatorrhea.

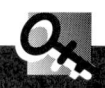

Key Symptoms

• Easy bruising	• Malaise
• Fatigue	• Weight loss

Clinical Findings

1. Physical examination abnormalities include clubbing, gynecomastia, hepatomegaly, jaundice, lacrimal and parotid gland enlargement, muscle wasting, palmar erythema, spider angioma, splenomegaly, and testicular atrophy.
2. Portal hypertension is suggested by abdominal collaterals (caput medusae), ascites, encephalopathy, esophageal varices, hemorrhoids, and splenomegaly.
3. Palpation of the liver reveals variable findings:
   a. Enlarged and easily palpable liver
   b. Regenerating macronodules along the liver border (micronodules are nonpalpable)
   c. In advanced stages the liver is often small and hard.
4. Hepatocellular carcinoma should be suspected in patients demonstrating a right upper quadrant bruit or friction rub, especially if bloody ascitic fluid is aspirated.
5. Other signs may occur as a result of the primary disorder that caused the cirrhosis. They therefore may be a clue to the cause. They include arthropathy, dermatitis, Dupuytren's contracture, dysrhythmia, ecchymosis, glossitis, hyperpigmentation, Kayser-Fleischer ring, neurologic abnormality, xanthelasma, and xanthoma.

Key Signs

• Clubbing	• Muscle wasting
• Gynecomastia	• Palmar erythema
• Hepatomegaly	• Spider angioma
• Jaundice	• Splenomegaly
• Parotid gland enlargement	• Testicular atrophy

Laboratory Tests

1. Laboratory abnormalities are often nonspecific.

Key Tests

General

• Albumin	• Bilirubin
• Alanine aminotransferase (ALT, formerly serum glutamate pyruvate transaminase [SGPT])	• Globulins
	• 5′-Nucleotidase
	• Prothrombin time
• Alkaline phosphatase (ALP)	
• Aspartate aminotransferase (AST, formerly serum glutamic-oxaloacetic transaminase [SGOT])	

α_1-Antitrypsin Deficiency

• α_1-Antitrypsin (AAT)	• Pi typing

Hemochromatosis

• Iron (hepatic, serum)	• Total iron-binding capacity
• Serum ferritin	
	• Transferrin saturation

Primary Biliary Cirrhosis

• Antimitochondrial antibodies	• Antinuclear antibody

Primary Sclerosing Cholangitis

• Cholangiography

Viral Hepatitis

• Hepatitis panel (B,C,D)

Wilson's Disease

• Ceruloplasmin	• Copper (hepatic, urine, serum)

2. Certain disease processes are associated with more specific laboratory alterations that may suggest the diagnosis.

3. Liver biopsies may identify histology unique to a given diagnosis. Unfortunately, in late-stage cirrhosis, the histology no longer differentiates the cause.

Differential Diagnosis

While most cases of cirrhosis occur secondary to alcohol abuse or viral hepatitis, the following are also implicated (Table 90–1).

Treatment

1. Therapy of cirrhosis is usually supportive and aimed at improving nutritional status, treating complications, and avoiding factors that may accelerate hepatic insufficiency.

2. When cirrhosis occurs as a result of a treatable condition, therapy should be directed at the primary disorder.

3. In a limited number of disorders, a drug or therapy of choice does exist.
   a. *Alcoholic liver disease:* Abstinence is the only established therapy.
   b. α_1-*Antitrypsin deficiency:* Liver transplantation is curative.
   c. *Hemochromatosis:* Iron removal by phlebotomy is the therapy of choice. Chelation therapy with deferoxamine (Desferal) and ascorbic acid is an alternative.
   d. *Primary biliary cirrhosis:* Liver transplantation is curative. Ursodeoxycholic acid (ursodiol [Actigall]) may offer limited benefit.
   e. *Secondary biliary cirrhosis:* Relief of biliary obstruction by endoscopy or surgery serves a preventive and therapeutic role.
   f. *Wilson's disease:* Penicillamine (Cuprimine) chelates copper and is the drug of choice. Trientine hydrochloride (Cuprid) and zinc sulfate are alternative medications. Transplantation is curative.

TABLE 90–1. DIFFERENTIAL DIAGNOSIS

ALCOHOL	**INFECTION**
BILIARY OBSTRUCTION	Hepatitis B, C, D
	Schistosomiasis
CARDIOVASCULAR	Syphilis (tertiary)
Right-sided heart failure	
Tricuspid insufficiency	**MALNUTRITION**
	Gastroplasty
DRUGS AND TOXINS	Jejunoileal bypass
Amiodarone	
Carbon tetrachloride	**METABOLIC/INHERITED**
Isoniazid	Antitrypsin deficiency
Methotrexate	Hemochromatosis
Methyldopa	Wilson's disease
Oral contraceptive	

Diet

1. Patients require a well-balanced diet high in calories.
2. Limiting protein intake is important when encephalopathy is present.
3. The use of branched-chain amino acids also may benefit patients with encephalopathy.
4. Appropriate mineral and vitamin (fat-soluble) intake is especially important when cholestasis is present.
5. Sodium restriction is indicated if sodium retention occurs.
6. Copper restriction is important in Wilson's disease and diseases that involve biliary obstruction. Patients should restrict their intake of copper-rich food such as chocolate, dried beans, organ meat, peas, shellfish, and whole wheat.

Patient Education

1. Patients should be made aware of factors (drugs, toxins, infections) that may exacerbate their liver disease.
2. Alcohol counseling benefits patients and family members.
3. Family planning and screening are important in a few diseases such as hemochromatosis and Wilson's disease.
4. The correct use, need for compliance, and possible side effects of medications should be emphasized.
5. Making patients aware of disease complications encourages them to seek prompt medical attention, allowing for early diagnosis and treatment.

Follow-Up

1. Monitor medication efficacy and side effects as well as disease progression.
2. Complications include ascites, bacterial peritonitis, bleeding varices, encephalopathy, hepatic failure, hepatoma, and hepatorenal syndrome.
3. This is a good time to re-emphasize patient education.

B Bibliography

Boyer TD: Cirrhosis of the liver and its major sequelae. *In* Wyngaarden JB, Smith LH, Bennett JC (eds): Cecil's Textbook of Medicine, vol 1, 19th ed. Philadelphia, WB Saunders, 1992, pp 786–795.

Gregory PB: Cirrhosis of the liver. *In* Rubenstein E, Federman DD (eds): Scientific American, vol 1, sec 4. New York, Scientific American, Inc, 1994, pp 1–18.

Podolsky DK, Isselbacher KJ: Alcohol-related liver disease and cirrhosis. *In* Wilson JD, Braunwald E, Isselbacher KJ (eds): Harrison's Principles of Internal Medicine, vol 2, 13th ed. New York, McGraw-Hill, 1994, pp 1483–1495.

Scharschmidt BF: Inherited, infiltrative, and metabolic disorders involving the liver. *In* Wyngaarden JB, Smith LH, Bennett JC (eds): Cecil's Textbook of Medicine, vol 1, 19th ed. Philadelphia, WB Saunders, 1992, pp 782–786.

Spiro HM, Atterbury CE, Barwick KW, et al: Cirrhosis. *In* Spiro HM, Colin EA (eds): Clinical Gastroenterology, 4th ed. New York, McGraw-Hill, 1993, pp 1153–1205.

91 Gallstones and Cholecystitis

Donald A. Opila

It is estimated that 20 million people in the United States have gallstones. The prevalence increases with age such that 10 per cent of the population over 60 years of age has gallstones. Asymptomatic patients with gallstones become symptomatic at the rate of 2 per cent per year.

Etiology

1. Bile is composed of lecithin, bile salts, and cholesterol. It is produced and excreted by the liver, concentrated and stored in the gallbladder, and released into the intestine after ingesting a meal. The majority of released bile is reabsorbed in the ileum, with a small amount passing out in the stool. This "enterohepatic" circulation constantly recycles bile and probably provides feedback to the synthesis of bile salts by the liver. Patients who have undergone cholecystectomy are thought to have nonlithogenic bile due to interruption of the enterohepatic circulation. When certain solubility characteristics of bile are exceeded in the gallbladder, stone formation occurs.

2. There are two types of gallstones: cholesterol (white, 70 per cent) and bile (pigmented, 30 per cent).

   a. Medical conditions that predispose to cholesterol gallstone formation include obesity, long-term TPN, female sex, cephalosporin or clofibrate use, and possibly diabetes mellitus.

   b. Pigmented gallstones are associated with age, hemolysis (i.e., sickle cell anemia, prosthetic heart valves), and cirrhosis.

Symptoms

The clinical dilemma of gallbladder disease is that it is a common condition that does not always present with symptoms.

1. A gallbladder attack characteristically is brought on by ingestion of a fatty meal. Obstruction of the cystic duct produces a crampy right upper quadrant/epigastric discomfort that generally lasts several hours but may continue for days. The pain may radiate around to the back or to the tip of the right scapula. There may be associated nausea and vomiting. Jaundice is not characteristic unless the stone has passed through the cystic duct and into the common bile duct, where it creates obstruction. Patients may complain of associated symptoms of belching, a sensation of bloating, flatulence, or "an acid stomach." The pain is not relieved by antacids or food. Positional changes do not affect the quality of pain. The attacks, as they increase in number and severity, often occur at night and may awaken the patient from sleep. Gallbladder stones are very common, and symptoms ascribed to

the gallbladder may not be eliminated by treatment. The main feature of gallbladder disease is pain (not belching or bloating), and hence a diagnosis of gallbladder disease without pain as a central feature is suspect.

2. Acute cholecystitis implies inflammation of the gallbladder and presents with a more toxic picture, including fever, chills, and sweats in addition to the preceding symptoms.

3. Biliary dyskinesia implies a poorly contracting gallbladder without the presence of stones.

Key Symptoms

- Right upper abdominal pain
- Nausea
- Vomiting

Clinical Findings

1. Clinical findings are present only during an acute gallbladder attack. On palpation, there is epigastric and right upper quadrant tenderness. The gallbladder is not palpable. Stool is heme-negative and should be a normal brown color.

2. With acute cholecystitis, the clinical picture is more toxic. Vital signs may reveal a fever and tachycardia. Palpation of the epigastric and right upper quadrant will demonstrate more marked tenderness, and an inspired breath will be arrested (Murphy's sign). Bowel sounds may be diminished or absent due to ileus. Guarding, both voluntary and involuntary, may be present.

3. If there is a palpable right upper quadrant mass, then it should be presumed that there is a hydrops gallbladder nearing perforation, and urgent surgery should be performed. Jaundice may be present if the pain has persisted for several days before examination or a stone has obstructed the common bile duct. Symptoms of pancreatitis may occur if the stone has passed to the sphincter of Oddi.

Key Signs

- Epigastric and right upper quadrant tenderness
- Murphy's sign present

Laboratory Tests

1. The laboratory workup (complete blood count [CBC], liver function tests, and amylase) for a gallbladder attack will usually be normal but should be done to

exclude other diseases producing similar symptoms. *Acute cholecystitis* will elevate the white blood cell count and there may be slight elevation of the liver function tests. If biliary obstruction is present, then the bilirubin, alkaline phosphatase, and amylase levels may be elevated. Marked elevation of the liver function tests, a low albumin level, or a prolonged prothrombin time would suggest another disease process.

2. A *plain film* of the abdomen is not particularly useful, since only 20 to 30 per cent of all gallstones are radiopaque. The presence of calcification in the gallstones may have therapeutic ramifications, which will be discussed later.

3. *Ultrasound* (US) of the gallbladder is technician-dependent, and body habitus (obesity) may preclude an adequate examination. The test relies on acoustic shadowing of the stones in the dependent portion of the gallbladder. In *acute cholecystitis,* there also may be a dilated gallbladder with a thickened wall and surrounding edema. The advantages of US are that it does not require any gastrointestinal preparation and is readily available.

4. *Oral cholecystogram* (OCG) requires that the patient take an oral dose of iopanoic acid and then undergo a radiograph of the abdomen 12 to 24 hours later. The dye is taken up by the liver and excreted to the gallbladder, where it is concentrated and outlines the stones. A "nonvisualization" of the gallbladder implies cystic duct obstruction. It may be necessary to take a second dose of pills (double dose) and repeat the radiograph in 48 hours to reveal the stones. A "nonvisualization" double-dose OCG is highly correlated (90 per cent) with gallbladder pathology at operation. False-positive tests may result when the patient does not take the pills as directed, if the pills are not absorbed, or if there is hepatic dysfunction (indicated by a bilirubin level greater than 3 mg/dl). Ultrasound and oral cholecystography are the diagnostic tests of choice. The sensitivity (96 versus 95 per cent) and specificity (96 versus 97 per cent) of each test are nearly equal, so the clinical situation will determine which test is done. If gallbladder disease alone is the most likely diagnosis, then US should be done first. If the differential diagnosis includes other upper GI pathology, then an OCG combined with an upper GI series may be more efficient. In the subacute/urgent situation, US should always be done first to avoid delays in diagnostic testing.

5. *Computed tomographic scanning* is less sensitive than US or OCG and therefore should not be used to diagnose gallbladder disease.

6. *Nuclear imaging* (HIDA or PAPIDA) is done to rule out acute cholecystitis. The test sensitivity is 98 per cent, and specificity is 93 per cent. A patient must fast for 2 to 4 hours before the test. The nuclear scanning agent is taken up by the liver and excreted, to be taken up into the gallbladder. If the cystic duct is obstructed, then the gallbladder will not visualize. The isotope should travel to the duodenum by 4 to 6 hours unless the common bile duct is obstructed. Nuclear scanning will *not* demonstrate gallstones but only obstruction of the cystic or common hepatic duct.

7. A CCK-stimulated HIDA with ejection fraction less than 35 per cent is helpful in diagnosing biliary dyskinesia (clinical symptoms of gallbladder disease without stones on OCG/US). Cholecystectomy will alleviate symptoms in 75 per cent of these patients.

8. *Cholangiography* (IVCA, PTCA, or ERCP) is not helpful in the diagnosis of gallstones and should be reserved for the workup of patients presenting with jaundice or other diseases of the biliary system.

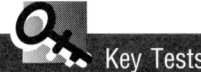

Key Tests

- Ultrasound of gallbladder
- Oral cholecystogram

Differential Diagnosis

The differential diagnosis of right upper quadrant/epigastric pain is broad. Gastric or duodenal ulcers, pancreatitis, appendicitis, hepatitis, gastroesophageal reflux, hepatic tumors, aortic aneurysm, angina, congestive heart failure, pneumonia, pleurisy, and pyelonephritis may mimic the symptoms of gallstones or cholecystitis. Nerve root irritation caused by osteoarthritis of the spine or shingles may radiate from the back to the right upper quadrant.

Treatment

1. Conservative management. Conservative management of gallstones is reasonable. Only 30 per cent of patients who present with a gallbladder attack will have a recurrent attack, so the natural history can be benign. Avoidance of a fatty diet is thought to be helpful by some patients but has yet to be proven scientifically. A low-fat diet is also generally deficient in calcium, so long-term adherence to the diet may accelerate osteoporosis in this older population.

2. Cholecystectomy
   a. Definitive treatment for a gallbladder attack is cholecystectomy—whether it be open or closed (laparoscopic). Initial experience with laparoscopic cholecystectomy is promising in selected patients, but complication rates (1 per cent bile leak and hemorrhage) may be unacceptable when compared with traditional open cholecystectomy (0.1 per cent infection). Hospital stay is generally shorter with laparoscopic cholecystectomy—4 versus 7 days.
   b. Surgical management should be individualized and

take into consideration the following: First, not all gallstones are symptomatic, and even those which are do not often progress to acute cholecystitis. Second, accelerated atherosclerotic heart disease with silent ischemia is the most frequent cause of perioperative morbidity and mortality. Elective cholecystectomy for relief of gallbladder attack symptoms without acute cholecystitis should not be taken lightly. Third, wound healing alone has not been shown to be a contributing factor to poor outcome in operating on the diabetic patient.

c. Obesity, coronary bypass surgery, long-term hyperalimentation, and heart or renal transplantation with long-term immunosuppression are situations in which some physicians recommend prophylactic cholecystectomy.

d. The initial therapy for acute cholecystitis is hospitalization for supportive therapy, including intravenous fluids, broad-spectrum antibiotics, nothing by mouth, and pain management. The average attack of acute cholecystitis lasts 7 to 10 days without surgery. Cholecystectomy should be done within 24 to 48 hours of the initial diagnostic confirmation. The tradition of a "cooling off period" for 1 to 2 months before performing an elective cholecystectomy exposes the patient unnecessarily to the risk of complications. Complications include jaundice (indicating biliary obstruction), palpable gallbladder (indicating hydrops), persistent fever (indicating abscess), or peritonitis (indicating perforation). Every patient with acute cholecystitis should have a cholecystectomy, because recurrence is inevitable. Medically high-risk patients may require an alternative procedure (i.e., cholecystotomy).

3. Dissolution

a. Two oral agents are available for gallstone dissolution. Chenodesoxycholic acid (CDCA) and ursodeoxycholic acid (UDCA) reduce the amount of cholesterol present in bile and hence allow for dissolution of the cholesterol in formed stones. CDCA blocks hepatic synthesis of cholesterol and UDCA blocks intestinal uptake, so a case can be made for concurrent use. Criteria favoring stone dissolution include radiolucency, lack of calcification, small stones (less than 2 cm), small number of stones, floating stones, and a nonobese body habitus. Diarrhea (25 to 50 per cent) is a side effect of CDCA that may affect compliance, and long-term use of CDCA elevates LDL cholesterol, which may pose an added coronary risk.

b. Unfortunately, this nonsurgical approach may take months to years and is more likely to be successful in younger patients whose stones contain cholesterol than in older patients who have pigmented and calcified stones. Most patients must remain on maintenance therapy after stone dissolution to prevent recurrence (25 per cent). The lifetime cost

of continued stone dissolution may make it a cost-ineffective option when compared with surgery.

4. Lithotripsy

a. Lithotripsy may be helpful in selected patients who are nonoperative candidates. Lithotriptors generate a large-amplitude acoustic wave within a water medium that is coupled to the skin of the patient and focused on the gallbladder. The water and body tissue do not impede the shock wave and hence are not damaged during the repetitive waves (1500 to 2000) required to fragment the stones into pieces small enough to pass through the biliary system and out into the intestine. Success is better in patients with fewer than four stones, each stone less than 3 mm, and cholesterol in content (not pigmented or calcified). The last criterion, unfortunately, eliminates many elderly patients for whom a nonsurgical approach would be desirable. The presence of a pacemaker is a contraindication for the procedure. Approximately 10 to 40 per cent of patients will require a second treatment to completely fragment remaining stones. Lithotripsy does not change the lithogenic nature of bile, however, and the stones may re-form.

b. Complications are minimal and include hematuria and biliary pain due to passage of fragments. Less than 5 per cent of patients will require cholecystectomy or ERCP with sphincterotomy. The procedure is done on an outpatient basis, and patients can resume normal activity the same day.

5. Contact dissolution. Percutaneous entry into the gallbladder and installation of methylterbutylether (MTBE) is an investigational procedure to date. Early results are promising, with 95 per cent dissolution over a 12-hour infusion.

 Key Treatment

- Conservative management is reasonable.

- Definitive treatment is cholecystectomy.

ACKNOWLEDGMENT: I gratefully acknowledge Ralph Doerr, M.D., Associate Professor of Medicine, SUNY Buffalo, for his critique of this manuscript.

 Bibliography

Greenberger NJ, Isselbacher KJ: Diseases of the gallbladder and bile ducts. *In* Isselbacher KJ, Braunwald E, Wilson JD, et al (eds): Harrison's Principles of Internal Medicine, 13th ed. New York, McGraw-Hill, 1994, pp 1504–1516.

Johnston DE, Kaplan MM: Pathogenesis and treatment of gallstones. N Engl J Med 1993;328(6):412–421.

Johnson L, Cleary PA, Lachink JM, et al: The natural history of cholelithiasis: The National Cooperative Gallstone Study. Ann Intern Med 1984;101:171–175.

Zeman RK, Garra BS: Gallbladder imaging: State of the art. Gastroenterol Clin North Am 1991;2(1):127–156.

92 Pancreatitis

C. S. Pitchumoni

Acute Pancreatitis

Etiology

1. Nearly 90 per cent of clinically acute pancreatitis is secondary to alcoholism or gallstone disease. Alcoholic pancreatitis is histologically chronic.
2. Rare causes include abdominal trauma, infections (mumps, and other viral diseases), hyperlipidemias, hypercalcemia, drugs (thiazide, furosemide, valproic acid, dideoxyinosine sulfonamides, pentamidine, and azathioprine), and ductal abnormalities (pancreas, divisum).

Symptoms

Abdominal pain in the epigastrium and left upper quadrant, radiating to the back, associated with nausea and vomiting, aggravated by eating food and partially relieved by sitting up and leaning forward, lasting for hours to days.

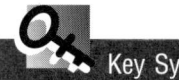

Key Symptom
• Abdominal pain

Clinical Findings

1. Physical examination findings include a low-grade fever, tachycardia, tachypnea, and basal consolidation of the lung and minimal pleural effusion on the left side.
2. Bowel sounds are often feeble or totally absent in view of paralytic ileus.
3. Low blood pressure, rapid thready pulse, diaphoresis, and tachypnea indicate shock.
4. Rare findings include jaundice (common bile duct compression), distention of the abdomen, and a bluish discoloration of flanks (Grey-Turner sign) or of the periumbilical region (Cullen's sign).

Key Signs	
• Low-grade fever	• Tachycardia
• Tachypnea	

Laboratory Tests

1. *Serum amylase elevation*
   a. Greater than four times normal is suggestive of acute pancreatitis.
   b. May be high in other conditions, such as acute cholecystitis, mesenteric thrombosis, intestinal obstruction, and perforated peptic ulcer.
   c. Does not correlate with prognosis.
   d. In hyperlipidemic pancreatitis, may not be appreciable.
2. *Urine amylase* levels are neither sensitive nor specific.
3. *Serum lipase* elevation is delayed but is more specific than amylase.
4. *Routine blood counts and biochemical tests.* Hemoglobin, hematocrit, leukocyte count, blood glucose, electrolytes, BUN, creatinine, liver function tests, and blood gas studies assist in the prognostic evaluation.

Radiologic Studies

1. *Plain film of the abdomen* in the upright position helps to exclude perforated peptic ulcer or intestinal obstruction. A dilated loop of jejunum (sentinel loop) or transverse colon (colon cutoff sign) is nonspecific.
2. *Abdominal sonogram* identifies gallbladder, stones, and the size of the common bile duct.
3. *Computed tomographic* (CT) scan of the abdomen. The size of the pancreas, extent of necrosis, and the number and size of fluid collections help in the diagnosis and assess the prognosis.

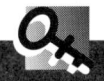

Key Tests	
• Plain film of abdomen	• CT scan of abdomen
• Abdominal sonogram	

Prognosis

An uncomplicated acute pancreatitis subsides with conservative measures in 48 to 72 hours. Mortality is nearly 10 per cent.

Treatment

1. Total elimination of oral feedings (NPO) until pain subsides
2. Nasogastric tube aspiration of the stomach in all patients except in mild pancreatitis
3. Intravenous fluids to maintain fluid and electrolyte balance. (Intravenous calcium may be needed if there is hypocalcemia.)
4. Parenteral analgesics to relieve pain. Meperidine (Demerol), 75 to 100 mg intramuscularly q 4 hr is recommended.
5. Parenteral broad-spectrum antibiotics in severe biliary pancreatitis.
6. Surgical treatment when diagnosis is not clear, abscess is suspected, or no relief with conservative

treatment. In gallstone-induced pancreatitis, cholecystectomy is to be performed during the same admission but only after pancreatitis subsides.

7. Endoscopic papillotomy with stone extraction when common bile duct is dilated and a stone is impacted in the distal duct

8. Other complications of acute pancreatitis such as noninfected pancreatic necrosis (phlegmon), pseudocyst, and pancreatic abscess need prompt diagnosis and appropriate treatment.

Key Treatment

- NPO until pain subsides
- Nasogastric tube aspiration of stomach
- Intravenous fluids
- Parenteral analgesics

Chronic Pancreatitis

Etiology

Secondary to alcoholism (80 gm of alcohol per day for more than 15 years); rarely, idiopathic, hereditary, or tropical (in Afro-Asian countries attributed to nutritional deficiency).

Symptoms

1. *Abdominal pain* is recurrent, epigastric, radiating to the back, lasting for hours to days, and often precipitated by drinking alcohol.

2. *Steatorrhea* when 90 per cent of the pancreas is destroyed.

3. *Diabetes mellitus*: a late manifestation, brittle in nature. Hypoglycemic episodes may be fatal.

4. *Other complications* include obstructive jaundice, pseudocyst, pancreatic ascites, pleural effusion, gastrointestinal bleeding (peptic ulcer, varices), and malnutrition (malabsorption, poor eating habits, and alcoholism).

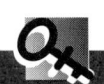

Key Symptom

- Recurrent abdominal pain

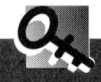

Key Sign

- Epigastric tenderness

Tests

Laboratory Tests

1. *Blood tests* are not useful. Amylase or lipase elevations occur only in acute exacerbations.

2. *Duodenal aspiration* after intravenous secretin admin-

istration to estimate the volume and bicarbonate of pancreatic secretion (secretin test) is not practical.

Radiologic Tests

1. *Flat-plate abdomen* may reveal calculi. Pathognomonic but notable only in a minority of patients.

2. *Endoscopic retrograde cholangiopancreatography* (ERCP). Dilated main pancreatic duct with strictures and intraductal filling defects and prominent side branches indicates chronic pancreatitis.

3. *CT scan of abdomen* may show calculi, ductal abnormalities, and pseudocyst.

Other Tests

Miscellaneous tests: Chymex test and stool chymotrypsin levels helpful only in the diagnosis of exocrine insufficiency.

Key Tests

- Flat-plate abdomen
- ERCP
- CT scan
- Secretin stimulation test

Treatment

Symptomatic for pain, steatorrhea, and diabetes. Complications such as pseudocyst and pancreatic ascites may need surgery.

1. *Pain*

   a. Abstinence from alcohol

   b. Nonnarcotic analgesics such as acetaminophen or aspirin

   c. Narcotic analgesics (fear of addiction)

   d. A low-fat diet

   e. Therapy with large doses of pancreatic extracts

   f. Surgical treatment when the preceding measures fail

2. *Steatorrhea*: Oral enzyme supplements with meals, low-fat diet, and medium-chain triglyceride supplementation

3. *Diabetes*: Calorie restriction is not needed, but insulin is to be administered only in small doses at frequent intervals.

Key Treatment

- Abstinence from alcohol
- Analgesics
- Pancreatic enzyme for steatorrhea
- Small doses of insulin for diabetes
- Surgery in selected cases

Bibliography

For more information on acute pancreatitis, see
Grendell JH, Cello JP: Chronic pancreatitis. *In* Sleisenger MH,

Fordtran JS (eds): Gastrointestinal Disease: Pathophysiology, Diagnosis, Management. Philadelphia, WB Saunders, 1993, pp 1654–1681.

For more information on complications of acute pancreatitis, see

Pitchumoni CS, Agarwal N, Jain NK: Systemic complications of acute pancreatitis. Am J Gastroenterol 1988;6:597–606.

For more information on chronic pancreatitis, see

Soergel KH: Acute pancreatitis. *In* Sleisenger MH, Fordtran JS (eds): Gastrointestinal Disease: Pathophysiology, Diagnosis,

Management. Philadelphia, WB Saunders, 1993, pp 1628–1653.

For more information on diagnosis of chronic pancreatitis, see

Niedron C, Grendell JH: Diagnosis of chronic pancreatitis. Gastroenterology 1985;88:1973.

For more information on chronic pancreatitis management, see

Pitchumoni CS, Badiga M: Management of pain in chronic pancreatitis. *In* Barkin JS, Rogers A (eds): Difficult Decisions in Gastroenterology. St. Louis, Mosby-Year Book, 1994.

93 Pancreatic Carcinoma

Martin H. Poleski

Etiology

1. Ductal adenocarcinomas are responsible for 90 percent of pancreatic cancers. The remaining cancers are of endocrine, connective tissue, acinar cell, epidermoid, and mixed cell origin. This chapter will consider the ductal cell cancers.

2. The incidence of pancreatic duct adenocarcinoma in the United States is approximately 10 per 100,000, with a male-to-female ratio of 1.3:1. Overall 2-year survival is 10 per cent; 5-year survival is 3 per cent. In surgical series 5 to 22 per cent of patients have resectable tumors; of these people, 15 per cent may survive 5 years.

3. Risk factors:
   a. Cigarette smoking, relative risk of 1.5
   b. Diet high in fat and/or meat, low in vegetables and fruits
   c. Chronic pancreatitis of any origin, such as alcohol, familial, standardized incidence ratio of 26.3
   d. Diabetes mellitus
   e. Exposure chronically to 2-naphthylamine, benzidine, and gasoline derivatives
   f. Age greater than 60 years

Symptoms

1. Pain is usually the earliest symptom of the disease. The pain can be vague and may be diagnosed initially as nonulcer dyspepsia. More characteristic is discomfort in the back or abdomen that is worsened by lying or relieved by sitting or crouching.

2. Weight loss and/or depression may be present with or without the pain.

3. The onset of jaundice is also characteristic, since a majority of tumors occur in the head of the pancreas.

4. New onset of glucose intolerence may begin a year before diagnosis and up to 80 per cent of patients are glucose-intolerant to some degree.

5. Other less common and nonspecific symptoms include anorexia, nausea, vomiting, and weakness.

6. Superficial thrombophlebitis (Trousseau's sign) occurs in less than 5 per cent of patients but occurs with other malignancies.

7. Obstruction of the pancreatic duct may lead to the onset of acute pancreatitis.

 Key Symptoms

- Abdominal pain
- Weight loss
- Pruritus
- Jaundice
- New-onset diabetes

8. Variceal hemorrhage is very rare and occurs with invasion or compression of the splenic or portal veins.

Clinical Findings

1. Most patients who present early in the course of the disease have no physical findings.

2. If the common bile duct is obstructed due to a mass in the head of the pancreas, jaundice and scleral icterus may be found. In this situation, a gallbladder may be palpated 30 per cent of the time (Courvoisier's sign). Those with prolonged or marked jaundice may have excoriations and lichenification of the skin due to persistent scratching.

3. Hepatomegaly may be found in association with jaundice or in advanced disease may signify the presence of metastases.

4. Ascites or peripheral edema may be a sign of portal hypertension or peritoneal metastases.

 Key Sign

- None early in the course of pancreatic carcinoma.

Laboratory Tests

1. Routine blood tests in patients with early cancer may be normal. Laboratory studies that are frequently abnormal include elevated glucose, lipase, and amylase levels, all of which can be elevated with benign diseases such as acute or chronic pancreatitis. Alkaline phosphatase and transaminases are often abnormal but are nonspecific because they are often abnormal in a variety of hepatobiliary disorders.

2. No sensitive or specific serologic marker is available to aid in screening or diagnosis of pancreatic cancer. Mucinous glycoproteins such as CA 19-9 may be elevated (>37 units/ml) in 75 per cent of pancreatic cancers but are often elevated in other gastrointestinal malignancies, acute and chronic pancreatitis, and about 6 per cent of normal individuals. CA 19-9 levels greater than 70 units/ml in people suspected of having pancreatic cancer have a positive predictive value of 59 per cent and a negative predictive value of 92 per cent. CA 50 is another muciglycoprotein with very similar sensitivity and specificity as CA 19-9.

3. Ultrasonography (US) is the best initial diagnostic imaging test in those suspected of pancreatic cancer. It is noninvasive, results in no radiation exposure, and can detect lesions as small as 2 cm, as well as pancreatic and bile duct dilations and hepatic metastases. It is also cheaper than the alternative, computed tomography (CT). CT is better at staging pancreatic cancer and providing better definition of the tumor

and its invasion of surrounding structures. CT depends less on the patient's body habitus or the operator's experience. If diagnosis is still in doubt after US and CT, endoscopic retrograde cholangiography (ERCP) and pancreatography may be performed. Magnetic resonance imaging (MRI) has no significant advantage over CT. Angiography is no longer used as a diagnostic test for pancreatic cancer, although some surgeons use it to assess resectability and vascular anatomy preoperatively.

Key Tests

- US should be initial imaging study in suspected pancreatic cancer—75 per cent sensitivity, 85 per cent specificity.

- US- or CT-guided percutaneous needle biopsy can be done to confirm diagnosis in those who are not surgical candidates.

- Preoperative pancreatic biopsy to confirm cancer is controversial.

Differential Diagnosis

1. Chronic pancreatitis
2. Cholecystitis
3. Irritable bowel syndrome
4. Other causes of jaundice, hepatitis
5. Retroperitoneal lymphoma or sarcoma
6. Carcinoma of the duodenum
7. Common bile duct stones and strictures
8. Peptic ulcer disease
9. Depression
10. Ampullary carcinoma
11. Metastatic disease to the pancreas and/or retroperitoneum

Treatment

1. Surgery is the only form of curative therapy available for pancreatic cancer. Unfortunately, only 10 to 15 per cent of tumors are surgically resectable. Recent studies suggest that of those patients who have successful resection, about 30 per cent are alive at 2 years and approximately 17 per cent at 5 years. Staging of pancreatic cancer to determine resectability requires the use of high-resolution CT scanners using a thin-section collimation (5 to 7 mm), an orally administered contrast agent to opacify the upper gastrointestinal tract, and acquisition of the scan at the dynamic phase of contrast enhancement with injection of a bolus of 150 to 180 ml of 60% iodinated contrast material. In this manner, the pancreatic tumor is best detected, as is identification of hepatic metastases and vascular involvement. CT is almost 100 per cent accurate in predicting unresectability and 70 per cent accurate in predicting resectability. Because of the latter figure, some surgeons begin pancreatectomy with laparoscopy to detect occult metastases to the liver, peritoneum, and so

on. Pancreatoduodenectomy (Whipple's operation) is still the most popular surgical technique. Total pancreatectomy is much less frequently used; occasionally, a distal pancreatectomy may be possible.

2. Some centers advocate the addition of pre- or postoperative radiotherapy with or without chemotherapy, usually 5-fluorouracil (5-FU). Intraoperative radiotherapy also has been used. Chemoradiotherapy may delay or prevent local recurrence, but it is unclear whether it improves survival.

3. Lesions of most patients are unresectable. Palliation of jaundice may be accomplished with a cholecystojejunostomy or choledochojejunostomy; duodenal obstruction can be bypassed with a gastrojejunostomy. Mean survival after palliative surgery is 5 to 6 months. Those people whose projected survival is less than 3 months due to advanced disease, or who have other factors that increase their surgical risk, can have jaundice relieved with stents. These can be placed endoscopically (ERCP). This technique is more comfortable for the patient than percutaneously placed stents. Stents may become blocked or infected and are replaced every 2 to 3 months on average.

4. *Pain management* is an important aspect of pancreatic cancer palliation. Pain often can be managed initially with acetaminophen or nonsteroidal anti-inflammatory drugs (NSAIDs). More severe pain requires the adequate use of narcotics such as morphine or codeine. Pain medications should be used on a regular basis and in combination, such as NSAIDs and codeine. In some patients, intraoperative or percutaneous neurolytic celiac plexus block can be effective in controlling pain.

5. Malabsorption may be a problem with mild to moderate steatorrhea. Pancreatic enzyme therapy with meals in an adequate dose to abolish diarrhea is usually successful.

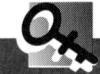

Key Treatment

- Surgery is the only curative therapy.

Bibliography

For general reference, see
Warshaw AL, Fernandez-del Castillo CF: Pancreatic carcinoma. N Engl J Med 1992;326:455–465.
For more information on the classification, see
Cubilla AL, Fitzgerald PJ: Classification of pancreatic cancer (nonendocrine). Mayo Clin Proc 1979;54:449–452.
For more information on risk factors, see
Lowenfels AB, Maisonneuve P, Cavallini G: Pancreatitis and the risk of pancreatic cancer. N Engl J Med 1993;328:1433–1437.
For more on the methods of staging with imaging techniques, see
Nghiem HV, Freeny PC: Radiologic staging of pancreatic adenocarcinoma. Radiol Clin North Am 1994;32:71–79.
For more on surgery and adjuvant therapy, see
Griffin JF, Smalley SR, Jewell W: Patterns of failure after curative resection of pancreatic carcinoma. Cancer 1990; 66:56–61.

94 Common Reproductive Symptoms

Nipple discharge is a common office complaint. It is incumbent upon the primary care physician to determine whether it requires medical or surgical intervention. Initially one must distinguish between *spontaneous* discharge and *nonspontaneous* discharge (i.e., requiring manipulation to produce). Only spontaneous discharge is clinically significant. Evaluation is based on the type of discharge: milky (galactorrhea), purulent, nonbloody, or bloody.

Galactorrhea

Differential Diagnosis

1. Normal
2. Drugs: Common culprits are oral contraceptives, tricyclic antidepressants, tranquilizers, and cannabis.
3. Hyperthyroidism or hypothyroidism
4. Pituitary adenoma: Patient will have elevated prolactin levels. Prolactin level will be normal in the first three diagnoses listed. Nonpathologic galactorrhea can occur during puberty as well as during pregnancy. It can continue after pregnancy for months or years. Pituitary adenomas can cause infertility.

> Refer to Ch. 111, Contraception; Ch. 162, Hypothyroidism; Ch. 163, Hyperthyroidism; and Ch. 169, Hyperprolactinemia.

History

1. Is the patient pubertal?
2. Careful reproductive history: pregnancy, infertility, lactation, menses
3. History of visual disturbances, headaches, and/or neurologic symptoms may suggest adenoma.
4. Medications?
5. Palpitations, weight change, changes in skin or hair may suggest thyroid disease.

Clinical Findings

1. Bilateral milky discharge
2. Visual field cut (with a pituitary adenoma)
3. Stigmata of thyroid disease

Tests

1. Prolactin level
2. Pregnancy test
3. Computed tomography scan with contrast or magnetic resonance imaging of head with attention to sella turcica *if* patient has a significantly elevated prolactin level

Management

1. Observation alone (if normal prolactin level)
2. Bromocriptine for persistent galactorrhea not secondary to an adenoma
3. Referral to an endocrinologist

Purulent Discharge

A purulent discharge is almost always noted during lactation or pregnancy and secondary to bacterial infection, usually staphylococcal. Physical examination may reveal elevated temperature, erythema, and fluctuance, as well as purulent discharge. A sample should be sent for culture, and treatment with appropriate antibiotics should be instituted. If an abscess is suspected, treatment by incision and drainage is appropriate; biopsy of the abscess wall should be obtained to rule out malignancy.

Nonbloody Discharge

This includes green, brown, and yellow heme-negative discharge. It is the most common discharge and is usually benign. Patients first notice it on their bras or nightgowns or secondary to manipulation of the breast. It often occurs in association with menses.

Differential Diagnosis

1. Duct ectasia
2. Carcinoma (rarely)

The discharge from benign ectasia is usually from multiple ducts.

History

1. Breast manipulation?
2. Relation to menses?

Clinical Findings

1. Breasts are examined to determine which duct or ducts are secreting.
2. Breasts are palpated for underlying breast mass.

Tests

1. Mammogram: should be done in women past 30 years of age or with strong family history of breast cancer
2. Cytologic examination of fluid
3. Galactogram: not very useful

Management

1. Advise patient to decrease breast manipulation.
2. If findings on palpation, mammogram, or cytologic examination are positive, prompt referral to a surgeon is appropriate.
3. Surgical transection of the mammary ducts is an option if workup is negative and the discharge interferes with the patient's life.

Bloody Discharge

Sanguineous, serosanguineous, or clear heme-positive discharge is indicative of cancer until proved otherwise.

Differential Diagnosis

1. Intraductal papilloma
2. Duct ectasia
3. Carcinoma

Refer to Ch. 97, Breast Cancer

Clinical Findings and Tests

As per nonbloody discharge.

Management

1. Excisional biopsy of any mass
2. Excision of offending duct for pathologic evaluation if no mass is found

Follow-Up

If work-up is negative
1. Monthly breast examination for one year
2. Biannual mammograms for one year

PEARLS

- Bloody discharge is cancer until proved otherwise
- Nipple discharge in *men* is cancer until proved otherwise.
- Discharge that is from multiple ducts or bilateral is rarely cancer.
- Breast cancer rarely presents as isolated nipple discharge.
- *Bilateral* discharge is usually normal or secondary to endocrine disorders or drugs.
- *Unilateral* discharge should raise suspicion of neoplasm or infection—consider surgical consultation.

Bibliography

King E, Goodson W: Discharges and secretions of the nipple. *In* Bland K, Copeland E (eds): The Breast, 1st ed. Philadelphia, WB Saunders, 1991, pp 61–67.
Leis HR Jr: Management of nipple discharge. World J Surg 1989;13:736–742.
State D: Nipple discharge in women. Postgrad Med 1991;89:65–68.

| Symptom | **Dysmenorrhea** | *Stephen Paul* |

Pain with menstruation is reported to be the most frequent reason for which young females seek medical help. Dysmenorrhea is found to be the leading cause of absenteeism for adolescent females, in addition to contributing to a significant loss of working hours. The reported prevalence is from 30 to 80 per cent, with between 10 and 18 per cent of young females experiencing pain severe enough to restrict daily activities, including missing work or school. Dysmenorrhea is divided into primary and secondary dysmenorrhea according to history, clinical findings, etiology, and treatment.

Differential Diagnosis

A. Primary dysmenorrhea
B. Secondary dysmenorrhea
  1. Endometriosis
  2. Complications of pregnancy
    a. Ectopic
    b. Spontaneous abortion
    c. Incomplete abortion
  3. Pelvic inflammatory disease (PID)
  4. Intrauterine device (IUD)
  5. Ovarian cysts
  6. Tumors
    a. Adenomyosis
    b. Fibroids (myomata uteri, leiomyoma)
    c. Malignant
  7. Adhesions
    a. Postoperative, D&C
    b. Endometriosis
    c. Infections
  8. Obstruction of the cervix
    a. Congenital
    b. Polyps

 c. Submucous fibroids

 d. Infection

 e. Postprocedural (electrocautery, cryotherapy, conization, radiation)

 9. Congenital malformations

 a. Müllerian duct

 b. Bicornate uterus

 c. Septate uterus

 d. Rudimentary uterine horn

 e. Cervical stenosis

 10. Pelvic congestion

Primary dysmenorrhea is noted for having a typical history (see below) in the absence of clinical findings or pelvic pathology. The pathophysiology of primary dysmenorrhea is related to an increase in prostaglandin ($PGF_{2\alpha}$) concentration in the endometrial lining shed during menstruation resulting in increased myometrial resting tone and pressures, frequency of contractions, uterine hypoxia, as well as smooth muscle contractions. Prostaglandin concentrations with resulting endometrial effects are greater in women with dysmenorrhea than in asymptomatic women.

Secondary dysmenorrhea is associated with pelvic pathology. Increase in prostaglandin concentration is also reported in association with IUD use and in some cases of endometriosis and uterine fibroids.

> Refer to Ch. 99, Endometrial Cancer; Ch. 101, Ovarian Cancer; Ch. 104, Pelvic Inflammatory Disease; Ch. 106, Endometriosis; Ch. 109, Ectopic Pregnancy; and Ch. 111, Procedure on IUD Insertion and Removal.

History

1. Complete menstrual history

2. Family history of dysmenorrhea

3. Sexual history, including method of contraception

4. Description of pain, including

 a. Temporal relationship of pain to age at menarche

 b. Temporal relationship (onset, duration, intensity) of pain to menses

 c. Quality, whether pain is referred to elsewhere

5. Associated symptoms such as nausea, vomiting, diarrhea, headache, dizziness, or fatigue

6. Limitation of daily activities

7. Previous treatment attempts and results

Primary dysmenorrhea becomes symptomatic after ovulation, often after the first few menstrual cycles after menarche. Eighty per cent of symptomatic females develop dysmenorrheic symptoms within the first 3 years after menarche. Incidence of primary dysmenorrhea is greatest in the teens and early twenties and declines with increasing age. The pain of primary dysmenorrhea typically begins 1 to 2 hours before menstrual flow and lasts several hours to 1 to 2 days, often decreasing with menstrual flow. The pain is usually a diffuse, dull ache centered in the midline, lower abdomen, just above the pubis, often radiating to the lower back and/or anterior thighs. Symptoms of nausea, vomiting, diarrhea, headache, dizziness, or fatigue are often associated with primary dysmenorrhea.

Secondary dysmenorrhea is typically noted either with the first menstrual cycles after menarche (congenital problems) or much later, usually after age 25. The pain of secondary dysmenorrhea often begins a few days before menstrual flow and lasts longer. Pain from secondary dysmenorrhea is atypical, sometimes chronic, and varies in description and temporal relationships depending on the etiology. With endometriosis the pain is often deep, aching, and may radiate to the rectum or the perineum, many times increasing with each successive cycle, and is often associated with dyspareunia, menorrhagia, or infertility. The pain with PID is often greatest premenstrually and decreases with menses. Pain secondary to IUD use appears after placement of the IUD. Cervical obstruction is noted for scant menstrual flow with pain throughout menses. Fibroids usually affect women in their forties and are associated with menorrhagia. Menorrhagia is also associated with endometriosis, tumors, PID, and polyps.

Clinical Findings

A. Primary dysmenorrhea

 1. Physical findings are normal.

 2. Pelvic examination may not be necessary in non–sexually active adolescents with a typical history.

B. Secondary dysmenorrhea. Pelvic examination is recommended for

 1. Non–sexually active females with an atypical history

 2. All sexually active females

 3. Rule out

 a. Endometriosis (best performed in late luteal phase), painful nodules in posterior cul de sac, restricted uterine motion

 b. Infection (bilateral adnexal and cervical motion tenderness with discharge)

 c. Placement and location of IUD

 d. Pelvic mass, uterine enlargement

 e. Adhesions (restricted uterine motion)

 f. Cervical obstruction and abnormalities (inability to pass a small probe)

 g. Pelvic congestion (engorged pelvic vasculature, uterine enlargement and tenderness)

 h. Congenital malformations

Tests

1. Pregnancy test

2. Papanicolaou smear

3. Cultures with sensitivities (include gonorrhea and chlamydia)

4. Pelvic ultrasound

5. Exploratory laparoscopy

6. Hysterosalpingogram

7. Hysteroscopy

These tests are recommended to identify specific pelvic pathology if clinically indicated by history and physical examination. A therapeutic trial of medication is often recommended first, with the following tests employed after failure of trial of treatment, unless clinically indicated. Pap smear is used to rule out cancer. Cultures are utilized to identify infection in PID. Pelvic ultrasound is used to look for pregnancy, fibroids and other tumors, ovarian cysts, and congenital malformations. Invasive tests are recommended only after noninvasive tests and trial of treatments are exhausted. Exploratory laparoscopy is the diagnostic test for endometriosis and other pelvic pathology. Hysterosalpingogram and hysteroscopy are used to identify abnormalities in the uterus such as polyps, adhesions, tumors, and congenital malformations.

Management

A. Primary dysmenorrhea

　1. Medication (see below)

　2. Transcutaneous electrical nerve stimulation (TENS) unit

　3. Investigational methods not approved or not conclusively proven by randomized, blinded clinical trials:

　　a. Calcium-channel blockers

　　b. Osteopathic manipulative treatment

　　c. Clonidine

　　d. Acupuncture

B. Secondary dysmenorrhea

　1. Trial of medication (see below)

　2. Treat cause—correct and/or treat underlying pathology

　3. Surgery is reserved for intractable, severely debilitating pain as last resort, caution to risks versus benefits of surgical procedure

　　a. Presacral neurectomy

　　b. Laser ablation of uterosacral nerves/ligaments

Medication

A. The nonsteroidal anti-inflammatory medications (NSAIDs) (prostaglandin inhibitors)

　1. Benefits

　　a. Summary of clinical trials reports successful alleviation of symptoms in 56 to 100 per cent.

　　b. Suppress $PGF_{2\alpha}$ synthesis, which decreases $PGF_{2\alpha}$ concentration in endometrium, resulting in decrease in uterine contractility and pressures, an increase in platelet aggregation, and a decrease in menstrual blood lost

　　c. May be helpful in pain associated with IUDs, endometriosis, and fibroids

　2. Instructions

　　a. Take with first symptoms or with onset of menstrual flow.

　　b. Allow 3- to 6-month trial.

　　c. If poor response, change to NSAID of different family.

　3. Medication and dosages

　　a. Naproxen (Naprosyn), 500 then 250 mg q 6–8 hr (longer duration of action)

　　b. Naproxen sodium (longer duration *and* rapid onset)

　　　(1) Anaprox, 550 then 275 mg q 6–12 hr

　　　(2) Aleve, 440 then 220 mg q 6–12 hr

　　c. Ibuprofen (Motrin), 400 mg q 6–8 hr

　　d. Fenamates (also block action of $PGF_{2\alpha}$ at target organs).

　　　(1) Mefenamic acid (Ponstel), 500 then 250 mg q 6–8 hr

　　　(2) Meclofenamate sodium (Meclomen), 100 then 50 to 100 mg q 6–8 hr

　4. Contraindications: currently pregnant or a history of hypersensitivity reaction to NSAIDs, bronchospasm, peptic ulcer disease, gastrointestinal bleeding

　5. Side effects: nausea, gastrointestinal discomfort and/or bleeding, dizziness, visual disturbances, hemolytic anemia, rash, tinnitus

B. Oral contraceptives (low-dose combination)

　1. Benefits:

　　a. Reported to be effective 80 to 90 per cent

　　b. Ideal if patient desires contraception

　　c. Inhibits ovulation

　　d. Decreases concentration of $PGF_{2\alpha}$ in menstrual fluid, decreasing uterine contractions and amount of menstrual flow.

　2. Medication and dosage—oral contraceptive of choice

　3. Contraindications and side effects as per oral contraceptive guidelines

Activity

1. No conclusive evidence with regard to exercise.

2. Aerobic exercise has been recommended, and it does not appear to worsen symptoms.

Patient Education

1. See above (medications) for instructions on treatment options. Patients should be reassured of diagnosis and response to treatment. Understanding and empathy for psychological impact of disability from symptoms should be noted along with encouraging the patient to resume normal activities.

2. Pamphlet: *Dysmenorrhea.* ACOG (1985), 600 Maryland Ave. SW, Suite 300 East, Washington, DC 20024-2588.

3. Homehealth Handbook: *Menstrual Cramps: Dysmenorrhea,* Packet 3d, Group 8, Card 45, MCMXLI, IMP BV/IMP, Inc.

4. Griffith HW: Dysmenorrhea (Menstrual Cramps). *In* Instruction for Patients, 5th ed. Philadelphia, W.B. Saunders, 1994, p 138.

PEARLS

- *Primary dysmenorrhea* is noted for onset 6 to 18 months after menarche in teens and early twenties. The pain starts 1 to 2 hours before menses, lasts 1 to 2 days, and is typically a dull ache in lower abdominal midline radiating to low back/anterior thighs and associated with nausea, vomiting, diarrhea, headache, dizziness, or fatigue.

- *Secondary dysmenorrhea* occurs with first menses or later, often in women older than age 25. The pain begins earlier and lasts longer than the pain in primary dysmenorrhea.

- Dysmenorrhea associated with menorrhagia, dyspareunia, infertility, vaginal discharge, or IUD use warrants further workup.

- Warning women to start NSAID treatment only with onset of menstrual flow will help prevent potential teratogenic effects of NSAIDs used during pregnancy.

- Counseling women using oral contraceptives of the benefit of decreased symptoms of dysmenorrhea may increase compliance.

Follow-Up

1. Assess effectiveness and/or side effects of treatment; change family of medications if necessary.
2. Investigate possible complications
   a. Decrease in daily activities secondary to symptoms may lead to depression or anxiety
   b. Sexually transmitted diseases
   c. Infertility secondary to pathology in secondary dysmenorrhea

Bibliography

For more information on epidemiology of dysmenorrhea, see
Andersch B, Milsom I: An epidemiologic study of young women with dysmenorrhea. Am J Obstet Gynecol 1982;144:655–660.
For more information on dysmenorrhea, see
Dawood MY: Dysmenorrhea. Clin Obstet Gynecol 1990;33:168–178.
For more information on dysmenorrhea, see
Menstrual problems and common gynecological concerns: Dysmenorrhea. *In* Hatcher RA et al: Contraceptive Technology, 16th ed. New York, Irvington Publishers, 1994, pp 486–490.
For more information on dysmenorrhea, see
Smith RP: Dysmenorrhea and pelvic pain. *In* Glass RH (ed): Office Gynecology, 4th ed. Baltimore, Williams & Wilkins, 1993, pp 403–414.
For more information on treatment of dysmenorrhea with nonsteroidal anti-inflammatories, see
Dawood MY: Nonsteroidal antiinflammatory drugs and reproduction. Am J Obstet Gynecol 1993;169:1255–1265.

| Symptom | **Amenorrhea** | *Carol A. Baase* |

Amenorrhea is the absence of menstruation in a woman of reproductive age. *Primary amenorrhea* occurs when there is no menses by the age of 16. In *secondary amenorrhea,* there is an absence of periods for six months in a woman in whom normal menstruation had been established.

Differential Diagnosis

1. Pregnancy: the most common explanation for amenorrhea
2. Menopause: symptoms include hot flashes, night sweats, and vaginal dryness. The follicle-stimulating hormone (FSH) and luteinizing hormone (LH) levels are elevated.
3. Hypothalamic amenorrhea including
   a. Functional amenorrhea caused by a failure of the LH surge that is required for ovulation. The FSH level and estrogen stimulation are normal. A progesterone challenge test induces withdrawal bleeding. This pattern can be caused by emotional stress, concurrent illness, sudden weight loss, or increase in exercise and will usually resolve on its own.
   b. Amenorrhea associated with anorexia causes a more severe disruption of the hypothalamic-pituitary axis. There is loss of LH release, and estrogen secretion is low. A progesterone challenge test does not induce a withdrawal bleed. Normal menstrual function is resumed with weight gain.
   c. Athlete's amenorrhea is characterized by hypothalamic suppression and a hypoestrogenic state. The progesterone challenge test fails to induce a withdrawal bleed. Energy expenditure (stress) and level of body fat both have critical roles contributing to the amenorrhea.

4. Hyperprolactinemia accounts for up to 20 per cent of the cases of secondary amenorrhea. Prolactin inhibits the release of gonadotropin-releasing hormone (GnRH) from the hypothalamus, resulting in the cessation of FSH and LH release. Only about one third of women with high prolactin levels will have galactorrhea. Causes of hyperprolactinemia include

   a. Prolactin-secreting adenomas

   b. Idiopathic hyperprolactinemia: clinically indistinguishable from adenoma except there is no tumor

   c. Hypothyroidism

   d. Drug-induced hyperprolactinemia: phenothiazines, thioxanthenes, and other dopamine antagonists

5. Other pituitary lesions are less common, but amenorrhea may be the first clue of their existence. Headache and visual defects are late signs of an expanding mass. Pituitary ischemia and infarction (Sheehan's syndrome) develop in the setting of an obstetric hemorrhage.

6. Polycystic ovarian disease (Stein-Leventhal syndrome) is characterized by amenorrhea, hirsutism, infertility, and obesity. The ovaries are enlarged, with increased stroma and a thickened capsule. Anovulation is caused by increased secretion of androgen, which is converted to estrogen in adipose tissue. This hyperestrogenic state stimulates the pituitary to secrete an elevated LH:FSH ratio, leading to further anovulation. A progesterone challenge test induces a withdrawal bleed.

7. Asherman's syndrome is generally the result of overly vigorous curettage, which results in intrauterine scarring with destruction of the endometrium.

8. Structural abnormalities typically cause primary amenorrhea and include an imperforate hymen, absence of the cervix or uterus, and absence of the vagina.

9. Chromosomal abnormalities can produce problems with gonadal development. Examples include Turner's syndrome (45 XO) and mosaicism.

10. Endocrine disorders—These include uncontrolled diabetes mellitus, severe hypo- and hyperthyroidism, and Cushing's syndrome.

Refer to Ch. 108, Menopause; Ch. 114, Disorders of Pregnancy; Ch. 162, Hypothyroidism; Ch. 169, Hyperprolactinemia; and other endocrine disorders in Part X.

History

A detailed history should include

1. Menstrual history including age of menarche, character of normal cycles, pattern and timing of periods. This is helpful in determining anovulatory periods since they tend to be irregular in interval, duration, and amount of flow.

2. Any prior pregnancies or abortions

3. History of sexual activity, contraception use, and any pregnancy symptoms

4. Changes in exercise and eating habits

5. Medications and drug use

6. Emotional stressors

7. Physical symptoms including headache, breast discharge, changes in body hair pattern, and symptoms of thyroid and adrenal disease

8. Family history of a problem similar to the patient's

Clinical Findings

1. Assessment of weight and height in search of possible anorexia, polycystic ovary disease, or genetic disorder

2. Breast development and other secondary sexual characteristics, assessing for hormonal presence

3. Body hair distribution and virilization

4. Breast examination seeking evidence of galactorrhea or darkening of the areola (occurring in pregnancy)

5. Assessment of visual fields for possible pituitary tumor

6. Pelvic examination, looking specifically for any clitorimegaly, intact patent vagina, appearance of cervix, presence and size of uterus, and size of ovaries

Tests

1. Pregnancy test: all patients should have pregnancy ruled out before proceeding further.

2. Prolactin assay should be done early in all cases of secondary amenorrhea. If elevated, a computed tomography (CT) or magnetic resonance imaging (MRI) is warranted.

3. Progestin challenge test: administer medroxyprogesterone acetate (Provera), 10 mg orally once daily for five days. After stopping the medication, the patient will either bleed or not bleed within two to seven days.

   a. Bleeding confirms that there is adequate endogenous estrogen and that the amenorrhea is caused by anovulation. If the prolactin is normal and there is no galactorrhea, further evaluation is not needed.

   b. If there was no withdrawal bleeding, further testing is needed.

4. Estrogen/progestin cycle: Administer 2.5 mg conjugated estrogen daily for 21 days. Add medroxyprogesterone acetate, 10 mg daily, for the last five days. Absence of withdrawal bleeding confirms that there is an end-organ problem (e.g., Asherman's syndrome, cervical obstruction).

   If there is withdrawal bleeding, proceed with

5. FSH: If this is elevated, the diagnosis is ovarian failure (menopause).

   If the FSH is normal or low, proceed with

6. CT scan or MRI to rule out a pituitary tumor. If normal and the prolactin is low, the diagnosis is hypothalamic amenorrhea with a hypoestrogenic state.

7. Chromosomal evaluation is reserved for those patients with ovarian failure who are under 30 years of age or for those with evidence of a genetic disorder.

Management

Anovulatory Amenorrhea

1. Medication
   a. Monthly administration of a progestational agent (10 mg medroxyprogesterone acetate daily for 10 days) every one to two months to prevent hyperplasia of the endometrium or
   b. Oral contraceptive pill for younger patients

2. Patient education
   a. Treatment for induction of ovulation is available, and fertility can be achieved.
   b. Use of the progestational agent alone does not provide contraceptive protection should ovulation occur.

Hyperprolactinemic Amenorrhea

1. Medication: Bromocriptine (Parlodel), 2.5 mg daily, to reduce the prolactin level and often control or reduce the adenoma

2. Patient education: Fertility can be achieved with the use of bromocriptine.

Hypoestrogenic Amenorrhea

1. Medication
   a. Oral contraceptives for younger patients or
   b. Conjugated estrogen, 0.625 mg daily, days 1 through 25; add medroxyprogesterone acetate, 10 mg, days 16 through 25.

2. Patient education
   a. Advise about the risk of developing osteoporosis and encourage adequate calcium intake.

b. Encourage those with amenorrhea secondary to inadequate fat stores to gain weight.

Follow-Up

1. All patients should be followed annually to review any problems or concerns.

2. Patients with hyperprolactinemia should have annual prolactin level testing and radiologic evaluation of the pituitary.

PEARLS

- Always rule out pregnancy before proceeding with an amenorrhea evaluation.

- Use the step-wise approach to evaluate all amenorrhea and a cause will be determined in the majority of patients.

- Tailor management decisions according to the cause of amenorrhea.

 Bibliography

For more information on amenorrhea, see
Galle P, McRae MA: Amenorrhea and chronic anovulation. Postgrad Med 1992; 92:255–260.
Pernoll M (ed): Current Obstetrics and Gynecologic Diagnosis and Treatment, 7th ed. E Norwalk, Connecticut/San Mateo, California, Appleton and Lange, 1991, pp 1037–1045.
Speroff L, Glass R, Kase N: Clinical Gynecological Endocrinology and Infertility, 5th ed. Baltimore, Williams & Wilkins, 1994, pp 401–456.

For more information on amenorrhea in athletes, see
Marshall L: Clinical evaluation of amenorrhea in active and athletic women. Clin Sports Med 1994;13:371–387.
Shangold M, Rebar R, Wentz A, Schiff I: Evaluation and management of menstrual dysfunction in athletes. JAMA 1990;263:1665–1669.

| Symptom | **Abnormal Vaginal Bleeding** | | *Diane K. Beebe* |

Abnormal vaginal bleeding may result from gynecologic lesions, structural abnormalities, infections, hormonal disturbances, or underlying systemic disease. Causes may differ depending on age group.

Differential Diagnosis

A. Prepubertal age group
   1. Vulvovaginitis
   2. Vaginal trauma may result from three causes:
      a. Accidents from a fall on a sharp object
      b. Foreign bodies
      c. Sexual abuse
   3. Urologic abnormalities, such as urethral prolapse

   4. Ovarian tumors. Two thirds are benign.
      a. Follicular cysts
      b. Juvenile granulosa cell tumors
      c. Carcinomas, such as embryonal cell, are rare.
   5. Vaginal
      a. Tumors, most commonly benign
      b. Polyps and hymeneal tags
   6. Hormonal stimulation
      a. Menstruation secondary to precocious puberty
      b. Exogenous estrogen exposure, most commonly oral contraceptive ingestion

B. Reproductive age group
   1. Pregnancy
      a. Early: spontaneous abortion, ectopic pregnancy, gestational trophoblastic disease (hydatidiform mole), lesions of the cervix or vagina
      b. Late: placenta previa (usually bright red, painless bleeding) and abruptio placentae (usually dark red, painful bleeding)
   2. Hormonal abnormalities
      a. Dysfunctional uterine bleeding
      b. Endocrine diseases
         (1) Ovarian dysfunction or tumor
         (2) Hyper- or hypothyroidism
         (3) Diabetes mellitus
         (4) Pituitary dysfunction
         (5) Adrenal dysfunction or tumor
   3. Infections: endometrial or cervical
   4. Uterine pathology
      a. Leiomyoma: most common benign neoplasm of the uterus. Submucosal leiomyomas are more likely to bleed than intramural ones because of disruption of endometrial vasculature.
      b. Endometrial polyps
      c. Neoplasms
      d. Use of an intrauterine device for contraception
   5. Cervical polyps, lacerations, and carcinoma
   6. Vaginal trauma, neoplasia, and atrophy
   7. Vulvar atrophy and neoplasia
   8. Underlying systemic disease
      a. Coagulopathies: thrombocytopenia, von Willebrand's disease, or vitamin K deficiency
      b. Hepatic disease
      c. Renal disease
   9. Medications: steroids, anticoagulants, oral contraceptives, anti-inflammatory agents, major tranquilizers and neuroleptics, chemotherapeutic agents, antihistamines, alcohol, local anesthetics
   10. Nutritional factors such as obesity, iron-deficiency anemia, vitamin C deficiency
C. Postmenopausal age group
   1. Hormonal disturbances
   2. Cervical lesions, including carcinoma
   3. Endometrial lesions, most benign

Refer to Ch. 98, Cervical Cancer; Ch. 99, Endometrial Cancer; Ch. 100, Dysfunctional Uterine Bleeding; Ch. 102, Vaginitis; Ch. 108, Menopause; Ch. 109, Ectopic Pregnancy, Ch. 111, Contraception; Ch. 114, Disorders of Pregnancy; Chs. 117 and 118, Bleeding Disorders; Ch. 119, Postpartum Hemorrhage; and Part X, Metabolic and Endocrine Diseases

History

1. Pattern of bleeding (onset, duration)
2. Medical illness such as thyroid, renal, liver, or blood disorders, history of bleeding or easy bruising
3. Gynecologic history such as previous or recent gynecologic disorders or infections, last menstrual period, menstrual history, associated molimenal symptoms, contraceptive use, and sexual history
4. In young children, sexual abuse questioning and access to exogenous estrogens
5. Drug use

Clinical Findings

1. Vital signs, especially blood pressure, pulse, and weight
2. Thyroid examination
3. Hirsutism or stria may suggest adrenal disease.
4. Petechia or ecchymosis for evidence of bleeding disorders
5. Cervical abnormalities such as polyps or lesions
6. Uterine size to suggest fibroids or pregnancy

Tests

1. Blood
   a. Complete blood count and platelet count
   b. Human chorionic gonadotropin
   c. Thyroid functions
   d. Prolactin, follicle-stimulating hormone, luteinizing hormone
   e. Renal/hepatic studies
2. Tissue sampling
   a. Pap smear
   b. Endometrial biopsy
   c. Dilatation and curettage
   d. Hysteroscopy
3. Imaging
   a. Pelvic sonogram
   b. Transvaginal ultrasonography
   c. Computed tomography
   d. Magnetic resonance imaging
   e. Hysterosalpingography

Management

1. Perineal hygiene, particularly in the prepubertal age group
2. Antibiotics for bacterial organisms present
3. Hormonal therapy
   a. Combination oral contraceptives. For acute bleeding, 4 pills daily for 4 days, then 3 pills daily for 3 days, followed by routine oral contraceptives for several months
   b. Oral progestins (medroxyprogesterone acetate), 10 mg daily for the first 10 days of each month on a cyclic basis

c. Gonadotropin-releasing hormone (GnRH) agonist (danazol)

d. Intravenous estrogen, 25 mg q 4–6 hr for four to six doses, usually resolves bleeding within 24 hours.

e. Transfusion for hemorrhage or a hemodynamically unstable orthostatic patient

4. Nonsteroidal anti-inflammatory drugs for pain as well as reduction of blood loss

5. GnRH agonists for pituitary-gonadal suppression in chronic anovulatory bleeding, followed by cyclic low-dose contraceptives

6. Surgery

a. Dilatation and curettage

PEARLS

- In the prepubertal age group, bleeding is most commonly associated with vulvovaginitis.

- In the nonpregnant reproductive age group, dysfunctional uterine bleeding, a diagnosis of exclusion, is most common.

- Postmenopausally, hormonal disturbances, followed by cervical and uterine abnormalities, are most common.

---

b. Endometrial ablation for refractory anovulatory bleeding. Twenty to forty per cent of women will continue to have some bleeding following the procedure.

c. Hysterectomy for uterine fibroids, endometrial hyperplasia, refractory anemia, or bleeding

---

Important Patterns of Abnormal Uterine Bleeding

- Menorrhagia—excessively heavy or prolonged menstrual bleeding

- Metrorrhagia—irregular intermenstrual bleeding

- Polymenorrhagia—menses at less than 21-day regular intervals

- Menometrorrhagia—regular but excessive uterine bleeding

 Bibliography

Fishman A, Paldi E: Vaginal bleeding in premenarchal girls: A review. Obstet Gynecol Surv 1991;46:457–460.

Galle PC, McRae MA: Abnormal uterine bleeding: Finding and treating the cause. Postgrad Med 1993;93:73–81.

Long CA, Cowan BD: Abnormal uterine bleeding. *In* Jacobs AJ, Gast MJ (eds): Practical Gynecology. Redding, MA, Appleton Lange, 1994, pp 158–164.

Mason E: Medical causes of abnormal vaginal bleeding. NAA-COGs Clin Issues 1991;2:322–327.

Weiss RM: The management of abnormal uterine bleeding. Hosp Pract 1992;Oct:55–78.

Symptom Vaginal Discharge   *Mary Kay Mroz*

Women often seek medical help with the complaint of vaginal discharge of varying color, consistency, odor, and timing. It is estimated that approximately 10 million cases of vaginitis are evaluated and treated in physicians' offices each year, with an unknown number of cases self-diagnosed and self-treated. By the time most women reach age 65, they will have experienced at least one episode of vaginitis, with many women suffering from chronic vaginitis. Vaginal discharge can be either physiologic or pathologic. A conceptual framework that uses patient age and potential etiologic agent groupings will help the clinician sort out the diagnostic possibilities. Knowing whether a female is prepubertal, menstruating, pregnant, or postmenopausal will help the clinician use the etiologic agent subgroupings of infectious, foreign body, contact/allergic, and hormonal to quickly arrive at the most likely cause so an appropriate diagnostic workup and treatment plan may begin.

Differential Diagnosis

1. Physiologic: hormonal
2. Infectious
   a. Bacterial vaginosis

b. *Candida albicans*

c. *Trichomonas vaginalis*

d. Other agents causing vaginitis/cervicitis

   (1) *Chlamydia*

   (2) *Neisseria gonorrhoeae*

   (3) *Mycoplasma*

   (4) *Ureaplasma*

   (5) Herpes simplex genitalis

   (6) Human papillomavirus

   (7) *Escherichia coli*

   (8) Group B streptococci

   (9) Pinworms

3. Retained foreign body

   a. Tampon

   b. Contraceptive sponge, diaphragm, cervical cap

   c. Other objects

4. Contact sensitivity/allergy

   a. Contraceptives: spermicides and condoms

   b. Tampons: deodorant

   c. Medications: prescription and over-the-counter

d. Douches

e. Perfumed menstrual pads, toilet paper, and feminine deodorant products

History

1. Date of last menstrual period, if postmenarchal
2. Whether patient is sexually active
3. Method of contraception
4. Onset of discharge
5. Color
6. Consistency
7. Odor
8. Pruritus
9. Medications
10. Allergies
11. Chronic diseases
12. Self-treatment attempts

Clinical Findings

1. Malodor: "Fishy" should suggest bacterial vaginosis, and "baking bread" should suggest *Candida.*
2. Erythema of the labia should suggest *Candida,* a contact/allergic reaction, or eczema.
3. Edema of the labia should suggest *Candida* or a contact/allergic reaction.
4. Vaginal discharge
   a. Grayish white, staining the undergarments: bacterial vaginosis
   b. White-curdy ("cottage cheese"): *C. albicans*
   c. Grayish yellow: *T. vaginalis*
5. Retained object visible in vagina

Tests

1. Saline wet-mount slide: Multiple white blood cells (WBCs) suggest an inflammatory process. "Clue cells" suggest bacterial vaginosis. Motile protozoans identifiable as *Trichomonas* may be seen.

2. Potassium hydroxide 10% slide: When vaginal discharge is added, a "fishy" or amine odor may occur, which should suggest bacterial vaginosis (a positive whiff test); when the slide is warmed and cell walls are allowed to disintegrate, hyphae and budding forms of *C. albicans* may be seen.

3. pH paper can be applied to the vaginal discharge. pH greater than 4.5 suggests bacterial vaginosis; if pH is between 5 and 7, consider *T. vaginalis*; and if pH is between 6.5 and 7.5 in a menopausal woman, consider atrophic vaginitis.

4. Appropriate cultures
   a. *C. albicans* on Nickerson's media
   b. *T. vaginalis* on Trichicult or Diamond's media
   c. *N. gonorrhoeae* on chocolate agar
   d. Herpes simplex genitalis on viral media
   e. Other aerobic and anaerobic bacteria as appropriate by history

5. Immunofluorescence studies can detect *Chlamydia* rapidly in the office.

6. DNA probes can detect *Chlamydia, N. gonorrhoeae,* and human papillomavirus.

7. Colposcopy can be used if condylomatous lesions are visualized on perineum or no cause is found in a recurrent or persistent vaginal discharge.

Management

1. Correctly identify the causative agent, decide if it is pathologic, and treat appropriately.
2. Stop the offending agent if one can be identified.
3. Evaluate and treat the sexual partner if appropriate.
4. Do not overlook the possibility of a systemic cause or disease process.

Medication (Table 94–1)

1. For bacterial vaginosis, consider metronidazole (Flagyl) or clindamycin (Cleocin) orally or intravaginally, ofloxacin (Floxin) orally, or, in pregnancy, ampicillin or amoxicillin.

TABLE 94–1. MEDICATIONS USED IN TREATING VAGINITIS

CAUSATIVE AGENT	MEDICATIONS	DOSAGES
Bacterial vaginosis	Metronidazole (Flagyl, Protostat, Metrogel)	250 mg t.i.d. or 500 mg b.i.d. PO or one application vaginally b.i.d. × 7 days
	Clindamycin (Cleocin)	300 mg PO b.i.d. or one application vaginally b.i.d. × 7 days
	Ofloxacin (Floxin)	300 or 400 mg PO b.i.d. × 7 days
	In pregnancy	
	Amoxicillin	250 mg PO t.i.d. × 7 days
	Ampicillin	500 mg PO q.i.d. × 7 days
Candida albicans	Imidazole derivative (Monistat, Terazol, Gyne-Lotrimin, Femstat, Mycostatin, Nizoral, Diflucan)	Suppositories: one vaginally for 1–7 days; cream: one application vaginally for 7–14 days Nizoral tablets: 200 mg PO b.i.d. for 14 days Diflucan tablet: 150 mg PO single dose
Trichomonas vaginalis	Metronidazole (Flagyl, Protostat)	250–500 mg PO t.i.d. × 7 days for patient and 2 grams PO single dose for partner
Atrophic vaginitis	Estrogen (Premarin, Ogen, Estrace)	Cream: 1–4 grams vaginally × 7 days; then 1× weekly to maintain symptom relief

2. For *C. albicans,* consider an imidazole derivative in tablet, suppository, or cream form. For recurrent or recalcitrant infections, consider ketoconazole (Nizoral) or nystatin orally.

3. For *T. vaginalis,* consider metronidazole orally for patient and partner.

4. For atrophic vaginitis, consider estrogen cream vaginally or estrogen replacement orally or topically.

5. For other identified pathogens, treat appropriately.

Activity

1. Use condoms during intercourse to avoid transmission of infectious agents.

2. For women with recurrent yeast infections, encouragement to wear loose-fitting, cotton-crotched undergarments.

Patient Education

1. Reassure the patient if the vaginal discharge is found to have a physiologic basis.

2. Instructions to avoid chemical agents such as douches, deodorants, and perfumes in the genital area.

3. Instructions to complete prescribed medications for self and partner.

4. Reinforce prompt removal of contraceptive devices from the vagina at the earliest, safest time.

5. Frequent changes of tampons during menses and removal before sleep.

Follow-Up

1. Make sure to check all cultures obtained to ensure treatment of all causative agents involved.

2. If sexually transmitted agent is identified, make sure patient's sexual partner is notified and directed to appropriate treatment.

3. For patients in whom a sexually transmitted agent has been identified, a follow-up appointment should be made to reculture as a test of cure.

4. For patients in whom no cause is found or recurrent cases of vaginitis are diagnosed despite appropriate treatment, reassurance should be given to ease the suffering these women frequently bear.

PEARLS

* The mere presence of *Gardnerella vaginalis* or *C. albicans* does not make it the responsible agent for the vaginal discharge, because both are normal flora in the female genital tract.

* Many women will not complain of vaginal discharge as the presenting indication but, when questioned, will admit to vaginal discharge, odor, or itch.

* In the reproductive age group, bacterial vaginosis, *C. albicans,* and *T. vaginalis* are the top three causative agents for vaginal discharge.

Bibliography

For more information on normal vaginal flora, see
Larsen B: Vaginal flora in health and disease. Clin Obst Gynecol 1993;36(1):107–121.

For more information on bacterial vaginosis, see
Sobel JD: Bacterial vaginosis. Br J Clin Pract Symp Suppl 1990;71:65–69.

For more information on differentiating etiologic agents, see
Sobel JD: Vulvovaginitis. Dermatol Clin 1992;10(2):339–359.

For more information on treatment options, see
Reed BD, Eyler A: Vaginal infections: Diagnosis and management. Am Fam Physician 1993;47(8):1805–1818.

For more information on unusual causes of vaginal discharge, see
Hammill HA: Unusual causes of vaginitis. Obstet Gynecol Clin North Am 1989;16(2):337–345.

| Symptom | **Pelvic Pain** | *Mary N. Hall* |

Pelvic pain is a common symptom and causes great concern and significant morbidity for many women. For a woman with pelvic pain, the clinician must determine whether the problem is acute and life-threatening or long-term and chronic, considering organic causes stemming from several organ systems as well as functional ones in the differential diagnosis.

Differential Diagnosis

Surgical emergencies must be considered first. Second, determine if the patient is pregnant. Third, assess whether pain is short term or long term.

1. Pregnancy-related pelvic pain

 a. Ectopic pregnancy must be ruled out in all patients with acute pelvic pain.

 b. Threatened or incomplete abortion

 c. Corpus luteum cyst

2. Non–pregnancy-related gynecologic pelvic pain

 a. Pelvic inflammatory disease (PID)

 b. Dysmenorrhea

 c. Pain related to ovaries

 (1) Ovarian cyst

 (2) Mittelschmerz

 (3) Adnexal torsion

 d. Pain related to uterine leiomyoma

(1) Degeneration

(2) Torsion

   e. Tumor–uncommon etiology

   f. Pain of a more chronic nature

(1) Endometriosis

(2) Adhesions

3. Nongynecologic pelvic pain

   a. Gastrointestinal

(1) Appendicitis (must be ruled out in all patients with acute pelvic pain)

(2) Irritable bowel syndrome

(3) Inflammatory bowel disease

(4) Diverticular disease

   b. Urinary tract

(1) Urinary tract infection

(2) Renal stones

   c. Musculoskeletal

(1) Abdominal wall musculature and rib–strain, contusion, or fracture

(2) Radicular pain secondary to herniated disk or a fracture or arthritis of the spine

(3) Inguinal or abdominal hernia

   d. Psychological

(1) Sexual dysfunction

(2) Sexual abuse (current or past)

(3) Somatization disorder

Refer to Ch. 77, Appendicitis; Ch. 81, Crohn's Disease; Ch. 83, Irritable Bowel Syndrome; Ch. 84, Diverticulitis; Ch. 104, Pelvic Inflammatory Disease; Ch. 106, Endometriosis; Ch. 109, Ectopic Pregnancy; Ch. 110, Premenstrual Syndrome; Ch. 128, Urinary Stones; Ch. 133, Acute Urinary Tract Infection in Adults; and Ch. 309, Marital Discord.

History

Determine if the pain is acute and life-threatening, subacute but progressive and serious, chronic, or self-limited.

1. Nature of the pelvic pain

   a. Character and intensity

   b. Location and radiation. Appendicitis moves from epigastrium to right lower quadrant, whereas PID is usually bilateral.

   c. Onset, duration, and frequency. Adnexal torsion is an intense, progressive pain, often involving a history of repetitive, transitory pain.

   d. Remissions and exacerbations

   e. Aggravating or ameliorating factors (i.e., what makes it worse or better)

   f. Associated symptoms–vaginal discharge or bleeding, urinary or gastrointestinal symptoms, fever

   g. Relationship to menstrual cycle

(1) PID typically occurs within first week of menstrual cycle.

(2) Endometriosis occurs just prior to and during menses.

(3) Ovarian cyst problems occur in midcycle.

2. Risk factors

   a. Factors associated with an increased incidence of PID include age in mid-20s, age at first intercourse 15 to 16 years, increased number of sexual partners, history of PID, use of intrauterine device (IUD), and vaginal douching.

   b. Factors associated with ectopic pregnancy include history of ectopic pregnancy, PID, IUD in place, or history of bilateral tubal ligation (BTL).

3. Gynecologic history

   a. Menstrual history

(1) Abnormal uterine bleeding absent in half the cases of ectopic pregnancy and present in a third of cases of PID and about 10 per cent of the cases of appendicitis.

(2) Missed menses suggests pregnancy-related pain.

   b. Obstetric history

   c. Birth control use

(1) IUD increases risk of PID and/or ectopic pregnancy.

(2) BTL increases the risk of ectopic pregnancy.

(3) Oral contraceptives decrease chance of ovarian cyst, ectopic pregnancy, and PID.

   d. Medical and surgical history, such as PID, any surgical procedure, infertility, appendicitis.

   e. Recent procedure, such as IUD insertion, cervical dilitation, endometrial biopsy, induced abortion

4. Sexual history. It is crucial to establish a nonjudgmental atmosphere so as to encourage the most accurate sexual history possible. Develop the habit of seeing preadolescent girls without a parent or guardian in the room. This lays the groundwork for a trusting relationship.

   a. Onset and frequency of sexual activity

   b. Number and sex of partners. Does partner have other partners? Does partner have signs of infection?

   c. Pain with intercourse

   d. History of sexual trauma

Clinical Findings

1. General appearance and vital signs. Does the patient look toxic?

   a. Fever is associated with PID and appendicitis but is not always present.

   b. Tachycardia and hypotension may be signs of sepsis or dehydration.

2. Abdominal examination

a. Ask the patient to point to the pain.
  (1) One finger is consistent with peritoneal or skin involvement.
  (2) The entire palm is consistent with a visceral etiology.
b. Focal tenderness indicates certain organs. Rebound tenderness and involuntary guarding suggest peritoneal irritation and necessitate urgent evaluation.

3. Pelvic examination is essential in any patient with pelvic symptoms.
  a. Look for vaginal and cervical erythema, discharge, and bleeding.
  b. Cervical and uterine motion tenderness (chandelier sign). Although quite sensitive for PID (97 per cent), not very specific; about 50 per cent of ectopic pregnancies and about 25 per cent of appendicitis cases involve cervical motion tenderness. Adnexal tenderness is consistent with ectopic pregnancy, PID, and appendicitis.
  c. Evaluate uterine size and consistency, thinking of pregnancy, leiomyomas, and endometriosis.
  d. Nodularity of uterosacral ligament and fixation of uterine structures are consistent with endometriosis.
  e. Adnexal masses. Absent in half the cases of ectopic pregnancy but present in 70 to 98 per cent of adnexal torsions and 25 to 50 per cent of acute PIDs.
  f. Rectal examination may pick up a retrocecal appendicitis.

Tests

1. Complete blood count, to look for signs of hemorrhage or infection; not sensitive or specific.
  a. Hematocrit is less than 30 in only 28 per cent of ectopic pregnancies.
  b. The white blood cell (WBC) count is often normal in PID and appendicitis.
  c. WBC count is elevated in 15 per cent of ectopics and 63 per cent of bleeding corpus luteum cysts. Elevation without a left shift is consistent with noninfectious physiologic stress.

2. Urinalysis, to look for signs of infection or renal stones. (WBC counts can be elevated from an inflamed appendix next to bladder or ureter or contaminated from a vaginal discharge.)

3. Pregnancy test is indicated in all women with acute pelvic pain unless the clinician has no doubt that the patient is not sexually active. Err on the side of getting this test unnecessarily rather than missing a pregnancy.
  a. Urine monoclonal antibody tests are usually sufficient and detect human chorionic gonadotropin (hCG) as low as 25 mIU/ml (96 to 100 per cent sensitive).

b. Serum quantitative radioimmunoassay for B subunit detects hCG at 5 mIU/ml (7 to 9 days after conception, 98.8 to 100 per cent sensitive). Obtain if titers need to be followed or if the urine test is negative and pregnancy is still suspected.
c. hCG is still detectable 9 to 35 days after a spontaneous abortion and 16 to 60 days after an induced abortion.
d. A positive pregnancy test still requires localization of the tissue responsible for hCG production.

4. Evaluate for chlamydia and gonorrhea
  a. Obtain chlamydia and gonorrhea cultures in all patients in whom you suspect PID. However, results are not immediately available, and these organisms are not always recovered from the cervix.
  b. Gonorrhea and chlamydia nonculture tests are widely used and are fairly sensitive and specific.
  c. Gram's stain of cervical discharge. Greater than 10 polymorphonuclear cells per oil-immersion field is consistent with mucopurulent cervicitis and supports PID.

5. Abdominal flat plate, if suspicious of renal stone or free air under the diaphragm

6. Erythrocyte sedimentation rate is not specific but is sensitive for inflammation.

7. Pelvic ultrasound (US)
  a. Essential in evaluation of pelvic pain associated with pregnancy.
    (1) Look for double decidual sign to confirm intrauterine pregnancy (IUP). Ectopic and intrauterine pregnancies rarely coexist.
    (2) Know the absolute basal hCG level at which an IUP should be seen by the ultrasonographer at your site. Studies have shown that an IUP sac is visible at as low as 3600 mIU/ml by transabdominal US and 1600 mIU/ml by transvaginal US.
    (3) A noncystic adnexal mass with fluid in the cul-de-sac is 94 per cent sensitive for ectopic pregnancy.
  b. Not as helpful in the evaluation of pelvic pain not associated with pregnancy.
    (1) There are ultrasonographic findings suggestive of PID or appendicitis but not specific.
    (2) Obtain US if a mass is palpated on pelvic examination.

8. Culdocentesis. The aspiration of fluid from cul-de-sac. Not routinely performed, but it can be helpful.
  a. Nonclotting blood—hemoperitoneum; clear flowing blood-tinged fluid—ovarian cyst; purulent fluid—PID, appendicitis, diverticular abscess
  b. Contraindicated if uterus is retroflexed or if a mass is palpated in cul-de-sac.

9. Diagnostic laparoscopy

a. The gold standard for evaluation of pelvic pain, but logistically and economically prohibitive for most patients; not without risk.

b. Indicated if

(1) The diagnosis is unclear after a comprehensive evaluation.

(2) A surgical process (ectopic, appendicitis) is suspected.

(3) In the setting of pelvic pain of 3 to 6 months' duration in one location, no etiology is determined.

Management

1. Evaluate for surgical emergency (i.e., ectopic pregnancy, incomplete abortion, appendicitis, adnexal torsion).

2. Diagnose and treat medical problems (for example):

a. An ovarian cyst may be managed expectantly, medically with oral contraceptives, or patient can be referred if cyst is not resolving.

b. PID

(1) Polymicrobial antibiotic coverage for anaerobes, gram-negative bacilli, chlamydia, and gonorrhea (per 1993 guidelines).

(2) Evaluate for other sexually transmitted diseases, including HIV.

(3) Provide safe sex counseling.

(4) Treat partners.

(5) Hospitalize patient with PID if pelvic abscess, pregnant, adolescent, severe or systemic illness, and if diagnosis is uncertain or if no response to treatment.

c. Primary dysmenorrhea. Treat with nonsteroidal medications or oral contraceptives.

d. Other nongynecologic causes should be treated accordingly.

3. If patient is not pregnant and no cause for pain is determined:

a. Watch expectantly until diagnosis declares itself or until symptoms resolve or worsen. Remember to include psychosocial factors in evaluation and treatment.

b. Treat for PID even if only minimal criteria are present (i.e., lower abdominal tenderness with cervical motion tenderness and bilateral adnexal tenderness).

c. Consider referral for diagnostic laparoscopy if there is a risk of surgical emergency, if antibiotic trial fails, or if symptoms worsen.

4. Chronic pelvic pain

a. Best managed with an integrated team approach using chronic pain specialists from onset.

b. Often associated with a history of psychosexual trauma, which must be evaluated and managed.

c. A diagnostic laparoscopy is indicated in any patient with pain in the same location for at least 3 to 6 months.

PEARLS

- All patients must be evaluated for an acute, life-threatening illness

- The history and physical examination are the most important steps in evaluation.

- No one symptom, physical finding, or laboratory test is completely sensitive or specific for one diagnosis.

- To obtain an accurate history, develop the habit of seeing preadolescent girls during routine visits, without the parent or guardian present, so as to be prepared to see them alone during an acute illness.

- Pregnancy test is essential in almost all patients with acute pelvic pain.

Bibliography

Hensel WA, Hall MN: Abdominal and pelvic pain: *In* Sloane PD, Slatt LM, Curtis P (eds): Essentials of Family Medicine, 2nd ed. Baltimore, Williams & Wilkins, 1993, pp 225–233.

McCormack WM: Pelvic inflammatory disease. N Engl J Med 1994;330(2):115–118.

Peters AAW, von Dorst E, Jellis B, et al: A randomized clinical trial to compare two different approaches in women with chronic pelvic pain. Obstet Gynecol 1991;77(5):740–744.

Quan M: Pelvic inflammatory disease: Diagnosis and management. J Am Board Fam Pract 1994;7(2):110–123.

Quan M: Diagnosis of acute pelvic pain. J Fam Pract 1992;35(4):422–432.

Roseff SJ, Murphy AA: Laparoscopy in the diagnosis and therapy of chronic pelvic pain, Clin Obstet Gynecol 1990;33 (1):137–144.

| Symptom | **Vulvar Pruritus** | *Seymour G. Williams* |

Vulvar pruritus is defined as intense itching of the female external genitalia. It is estimated that approximately 10 per cent of private-practice gynecologic patients have this as their chief complaint. More commonly it is a symptom indicating underlying local or systemic disease. Idiopathic vulvar pruritus is not uncommon; it is, however, primarily a diagnosis of exclusion. From the outset of the patient's presentation, the physician should attempt to differentiate vulvar pruritus from pain (vulvodynia) and also the role of the itch/scratch cycle (i.e., itching leading to excoriations and skin changes, which in turn cause more itching) in the cause of the patient's complaints.

Differential Diagnosis
In order of likelihood, from anecdotal evidence:
1. Vulvovaginitis
   a. Protozoal (trichomoniasis)
   b. Fungal (candidiasis)
   c. Bacterial (*Gardnerella vaginalis*) or other vaginal infections
2. Essential pruritus, localized neurodermatitis
3. Lichen simplex chronicus
4. Vulvar vestibulitis
5. Urinary tract infection
6. Atrophic vaginitis secondary to estrogen deprivation
7. Human papilloma virus (causing condylomata acuminata)
8. Lichen planus
9. Vulvar carcinoma (in situ and invasive malignancy)
10. Lichen sclerosus et atrophicus (LSA)
11. Seborrheic dermatitis
12. Fecal soilage secondary to anal incontinence
13. Contact dermatitis—irritant, allergic, and atopic
14. Parasitic infestations—crab lice, pinworms, scabies, or other insect bites
15. Neurogenic/psychiatric
16. Fox-Fordyce disease—due to apocrine sweat gland occlusion
17. Associated systemic conditions
   a. Diabetes
   b. Drug hypersensitivity
   c. Gout
   d. Pellagra
   e. Pregnancy
   f. Sjögren's syndrome
   g. Psoriasis
   h. Lymphoma
   i. Leukemia
   j. Hepatic or renal diseases
   k. Carcinomatosis or polycythemia

History: Key Questions to Ask
1. When did the symptoms begin, and is there any variation of the symptoms with sanitary or tampon use, menses, sexual activity, or vaginal cleansing routines?
2. Where else is the patient itching or has a rash?
3. What treatment has been or is presently being tried?
4. Are there psychogenic/marital stresses?

Clinical Findings
1. Visible skin changes (vulvar area especially)
2. Note color, look for warts, tumors, ulcers, and scaling
3. Do entire cutaneous examination, and check pubic hair if indicated.
4. Check for vaginal or anal discharge.
5. Colposcopic and histologic changes

Tests
1. Examination of skin and vulvar/anal region
2. Wet mount of vaginal secretions—Check for trichomoniasis and clue cells (indicative of bacterial vaginosis).
3. KOH of vaginal secretions—Rule out fungal infection.
4. Colposcopy before and after acetic acid application if indicated
5. Biopsy of all suspicious-looking lesions
6. Urine analysis with microscopy to check for bacteriuria and glycosuria; send culture if indicated.
7. Scotch tape test—Rule out pinworm, if indicated.
8. Complete blood count if indicated to check for blood dyscrasias
9. Chemistry panel—Check the glucose (do 1-hour glucose tolerance test if indicated) and for values indicating uremia and hepatobiliary problems.
10. Patch testing if indicated for contact dermatitis—for allergy testing

Management
1. Outpatient medical management and appropriate local excision is the usual. In general, patient should suspend all previous treatments and implement the indicated patient education instructions.
2. Inpatient care is reserved for intractable cases requiring ethanol injection or Mering procedure (vulvar undercutting causing denervation).
3. Some investigators have recommended laser to vaporize the vulvar epidermis or Grenz-ray therapy
Medication
1. Symptomatic
   a. Hydroxyzine (Atarax, Vistaril), 25 to 50 mg t.i.d.–q.i.d. and hs

b. Doxepin (Sinequan, Adapin), 25 to 50 mg b.i.d.–t.i.d.

c. Terfenadine (Seldane), 60 mg b.i.d.

d. Amitriptyline (Elavil), 25 mg q.h.s.

e. Topical lidocaine (Xylocaine)

f. Ice packs at night as needed.

g. Crotamiton cream (Warn patients that they will have initial burning.)

2. For chronic or idiopathic vulvar pruritus

a. Topical steroids: 1% to 2.5% hydrocortisone cream apply twice daily. Initially, it may be necessary to start therapy with a more potent steroid, for example, triamcinolone ointment (Kenalog) (0.025%) or fluocinolone ointment (Synalar) (0.025%), but therapy should be switched to hydrocortisone once improvement is noted so as to avoid anogenital atrophy.

b. Subcutaneous injection of triamcinolone acetonide (Kenalog)—for intractable cases—depends on comfort and expertise of practitioner.

3. Systemic steroids may be used in very acute self-limiting cases.

Diet

Avoidance of certain foods is advocated: those that contain caffeine; also, tomatoes and peanuts.

Activity

As tolerated

Patient Education

1. Avoid possible irritants: douches, perfumed soaps and body powders or lotions, fabric softeners and detergents, rubber condoms and diaphragms.

2. Observe regular but not overzealous perineal hygiene. Can wash anogenital area with hypoallergenic cleansing lotion.

3. Avoid tight-fitting clothes or nylon pantyhose; instead, wear loose-fitting cotton underwear.

4. Notify sexual partner to obtain treatment if experiencing similar symptoms.

5. Sitz baths (tepid water at 98° F) with a few drops of water-dispersible oil or tar emulsion as necessary.

Follow-Up

1. Need to monitor progress of therapy closely because some of the treatments can accentuate symptoms.

2. Also need to be aware of the 1 to 5 per cent malignant potential of vulvar dystrophies and that the most common presenting symptom of vulvar carcinoma is pruritus.

3. Gynecology and/or dermatology consult may be needed for specific cases.

4. The majority of patients can be managed with success on an outpatient basis with conservative medical management. With recurrent symptoms after different therapies, the possibility of a psychogenic basis should be more thoroughly investigated.

PEARL

• The primary symptom of vulvar and vaginal neoplasms is itching.

Bibliography

ACOG Technical Bulletin Number 139: Vulvar dystrophies. Int J Gynecol Obstet 1991;35(3):269–273.

Bornstein J, Pascal B, Abramovici H: The common problem of vulvar pruritus. Obstet Gynecol Surv 1993;48(2):111–118.

Kelly RA, Foster DC, Woodruff JD: Subcutaneous injection of triamcinolone acetonide in the treatment of chronic vulvar pruritus. Am J Obstet Gynecol 1993;169(3):568–570.

Pincus SH: Vulvar dermatoses and pruritus vulvae. Dermatol Clin 1992;10(2):297–308.

Stone SP: Pruritus ani and vulvae. *In* Rakel R (ed): Conn's Current Therapy. Philadelphia, WB Saunders, 1994, pp 816–818.

| Symptom | **Scrotal Pain/Mass** | *Michael A. Cook* |

Causes of scrotal pain and masses include acute and chronic factors. Diagnosis is often difficult clinically because many disorders present similarly. The most common problem is differentiating testicular torsion from acute epididymitis.

Differential Diagnosis

1. Trauma: testicular laceration, hematoma, hematohydrocele

2. Testicular torsion

3. Torsion of appendages of the testis and epididymis

4. Epididymitis

5. Viral orchitis

6. Hydrocele, hematocele, varicocele, epididymal cyst/spermatocele

7. Testicular tumor: primary and metastatic

8. Renal colic/urolithiasis

9. Inguinal hernia

10. Acute appendicitis

11. Distal abdominal aorta aneurysm, Henoch-Schönlein purpura

---

Refer to Ch. 77, Appendicitis; Ch. 123, Epididymitis; Ch. 124, Varicocele; Ch. 125, Hydrocele/Spermatocele; and Ch. 128, Urinary Stone.

History: Key Questions to Ask

1. Did the pain develop abruptly or gradually? Is the pain localized to a specific area of the testicle?

2. Is there a scrotal mass?

3. Is the patient sexually active? Is there dysuria, a urethral discharge, frequency, urgency, inguinal adenopathy, or fever?

4. Is there a history of scrotal trauma, testicular ectopia, cryptorchidism, renal lithiasis, hematuria, cancer, lymphoma, leukemia, or recent viral illness?

5. Abdominal pain, nausea, or vomiting?

Torsion of the testicle or testicular appendages presents abruptly with pain. Epididymitis, incarcerated hernia, and viral orchitis present gradually with scrotal pain. Hematuria should raise the possibility of renal lithiasis and trauma. Hydrocele, testicular tumor, varicocele, and epididymal cyst are typically painless unless there is a rapid increase in size.

Clinical Findings

1. Testicular torsion

   a. Initially, the testicle is diffusely tender with hemiscrotal edema and erythema. Eventually, the entire scrotum becomes tender, edematous, and erythematous.

   b. The testicle is elevated in the scrotum and lies in a horizontal position.

   c. Elevation of the testicle above the pubic symphysis does not relieve the pain (negative Prehn's sign).

   d. Abdominal pain, nausea, and vomiting

   e. Absent cremasteric reflex

   f. Usually in teenagers and men in their 20s

2. Torsion of testicular appendage

   a. A tender, palpable, firm nodule on the anterosuperior aspect of the testicle

   b. When the skin over the testicle is pulled tightly, a "blue dot" can appear, which represents the ischemic testicular appendage.

3. Epididymitis

   a. Epididymal tenderness; testicular tenderness if orchitis has developed

   b. A purulent discharge suggests gonococcal infection, and a clear discharge suggests nongonococcal infection.

   c. Urethritis, prostatitis, and cystitis can coexist.

   d. Usually afebrile without leukocytosis

   e. Can have pyuria and bacteria

   f. Usually in men over 25 years of age

   g. Pain relieved by elevating the testicle above the pubic symphysis (positive Prehn's sign)

4. Renal colic/urolithiasis: flank tenderness, scrotal tenderness, gross or microscopic hematuria

5. Varicocele: dilated, veins palpable above the testicle; more pronounced when the patient is standing and initiates a Valsalva maneuver, less pronounced when the patient lies down; can feel like a "bag of worms."

6. Epididymal cyst or spermatocele

   a. Usually painless mass in the head of the epididymis

   b. Clear or cloudy fluid with sperm when aspirated

7. Hydrocele

   a. Enlarged, usually painless testicle that transilluminates

   b. Aspiration produces clear fluid.

8. Hematocele

   a. Enlargement that may be painful and does not transilluminate

   b. Usually a history of trauma

9. Testicular tumor

   a. Painless enlargement that does not transilluminate

   b. Firm nontender nodule

10. Viral orchitis

    a. Diffuse testicular tenderness

    b. Parotitis antedates testicular pain by 1 to 2 weeks.

11. Inguinal hernia

    a. Bowel palpable in the scrotum or in the inguinal canal

    b. Bowel sounds may be audible in the scrotum if the hernia is incarcerated. If strangulation has occurred, bowel sounds are not audible in the scrotum, and the abdomen is likely to be tender, distended, and without bowel sounds.

Tests

1. Complete blood count (CBC)

2. Urinalysis, culture and sensitivity

3. Flat and upright abdominal radiographs

4. Testicular sonography and color Doppler examination

5. Testicular scintigraphy

6. Intravenous pyelogram (IVP)/renal sonogram

7. Abdominal sonogram and computed tomography

8. Tumor markers: human chorionic gonadotropin, α-fetoprotein

The CBC is nonspecific. If the history suggests renal colic, an IVP is indicated. An abdominal radiograph is helpful to identify bowel obstruction and to look for radiopaque renal calculi. Nuclear scrotal scintigraphy and color Doppler testicular sonography demonstrate diminished or absent flow in testicular torsion. Either test must be available within 1 hour. Tumor markers and testicular sonography must be obtained in all cases of testicular tumors prior to surgery.

Management

1. Testicular torsion is a surgical emergency.

a. Surgical detorsion must be accomplished within 4 to 6 hours. After 24 hours, the testicle has infarcted.

b. Bilateral orchiopexy is indicated to prevent recurrence.

2. Torsion of testicular appendage

a. Bed rest, analgesia, scrotal elevation

b. Surgical exploration is indicated when the diagnosis is uncertain or the pain persists.

3. Epididymitis

a. A urine and urethral specimen should be sent for bacterial and gonococcal cultures.

b. If sexually acquired, treat for *Chlamydia trachomatis* and *Neisseria gonorrhoeae*: (1) ofloxacin (Floxin), 300 mg b.i.d. for 10 days or (2) ceftriaxone (Rocephin), 250 mg intramuscularly once and doxycycline (Vibramycin), 100 mg b.i.d. for 10 days

c. If not sexually acquired, treat for *Escherichia coli, Enterococcus, Pseudomonas,* and *Proteus* species: trimethoprim–sulfamethoxazole, ciprofloxacin, amoxicillin–clavulanate, third-generation cephalosporin

4. Urolithiasis: hydration, analgesics, urologic consultation

5. Varicocele

a. No treatment in an asymptomatic young male

b. If of acute onset in an older man, consider left renal vein thrombosis from a retroperitoneal neoplasm.

c. Varicocelectomy if infertility is a problem

6. Epididymal cyst and hydrocele

a. Aspirate if painful

b. If the hydrocele develops acutely, consider testicular neoplasm, and order a testicular sonogram.

7. Testicular neoplasm: surgical exploration through an inguinal approach, radical orchiectomy, radiation and chemotherapy depending on the histology

8. Viral orchitis: bed rest, scrotal elevation, analgesics

9. Inguinal hernia and acute appendicitis: surgical consult

Follow-Up

1. Acute epididymitis. If sexually acquired, obtain serology for syphilis 3 months after last sexual contact.

2. Viral orchitis. If bilateral, infertility and gynecomastia can develop years later due to testicular atrophy. The risk of tumor in the affected testicle is slightly increased.

3. Inguinal hernia. Examine annually for recurrences.

PEARL

• Consider testicular torsion in every male who presents with either scrotal or abdominal pain.

B | **Bibliography**

Centers for Disease Control: 1993 Sexually transmitted diseases treatment guidelines. MMWR 1993;42:47–62.

Edelsberg JS, Surh YS: The acute scrotum. Emerg Med Clin North Am 1988;6:521–545.

Kim CK, Zuckier LS, Alavi A: The role of nuclear medicine in the evaluation of the male genital tract. Semin Roentgenol 1993;28(1):31–42.

Langer JE: Ultrasound of the scrotum. Semin Roentgenol 1993;28(1):5–18.

Thompson IM, Teague JL: Genitourinary tumors. In Rakel RE (ed): Conn's Current Therapy. Philadelphia, WB Saunders, 1994, pp 682–683.

95 Fibrocystic Disease of the Breast

Cynthia M. Williams

Etiology

1. Fibrocystic disease of the breast (FDB) is the most common benign breast condition in women.

2. The condition has been known by numerous names in the past, including *mammary dysplasia, chronic cystic mastitis, fibrocystic mastopathy, fibroadenosis,* and *cystic epithelial hyperplasia.*

3. A consensus conference in 1985 recommended that the term "fibrocystic disease" should be replaced by the terms "fibrocystic condition" and "fibrocystic complex," because 50 per cent of premenopausal women note breast lumps or nodularity on physical examination and about 90 per cent of postmenopausal women have pathologic evidence of benign breast disease.

4. The exact cause of FDB is unknown, but it is thought to be hormone-dependent.

   a. Estrogens and progesterones are primarily responsible for the development, growth, and function of the breast. Abnormalities in the breast may reflect abnormalities in the relative concentration of the hormones or exaggerated response to normal hormonal levels by hypersensitive tissues.

   b. Fibrocystic changes begin in a woman's mid-20s to 30s and peak before menopause. Changes are rarely seen in adolescents and postmenopausal women, unless they are using hormone replacement therapy.

   c. During the menstrual cycle, the breast undergoes cyclic changes reflecting hormonal interaction. Breasts become full and heavy and have varying degrees of pain and tenderness.

   d. Fibrocystic changes are seen most commonly in women who are nulliparous, not using oral contraceptives, have a history of early menarche and late menopause, and/or suffer from premenstrual syndrome.

Symptoms

1. FBD is usually asymptomatic. Woman may feel smooth, discrete, sometimes tender breast lumps during self-examination, as may the physician performing a breast examination. This is referred to as "physiologic nodularity."

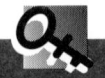

Key Symptoms

• Fullness	• Swelling
• Tenderness	• Pain

2. Over time, the breast feels more nodular and becomes more painful. Premenopausal women may have painful solitary or multiple lesions, usually in the upper-outer quadrant of the breast.

Clinical Findings

1. A woman who notes a lump or change in her breast usually seeks evaluation. The main concern of both the woman and the physician is whether the lump is cancer.

2. A thorough history is taken, including

   a. Location of lump, duration, and change in size

   b. Pain or associated tenderness

   c. Relationship to menstrual cycle, pregnancy, trauma, or medications

   d. Nipple discharge and skin changes

   e. Use of hormonal agents

   f. Previous breast disease and family history of breast cancer

   g. Previous cancer, especially of ovary, endometrium, or colon

   h. Previous breast procedures, including aspiration, biopsy, augmentation, or reduction

3. A thorough examination of the breast should be done with the patient first sitting and then supine and should include thorough inspection and palpation of each breast and axilla and an attempt to express fluid from the nipple.

4. Findings may include skin dimpling; breast asymmetry; nipple discharge; multiple bilateral, discrete, uniform, tender lumps that feel rubbery, fluctuant, or firm; thickening, especially in the upper-outer quadrant; a dominant mass that is soft, cystic, smooth, or mobile; or a dominant mass that is hard, fixed, irregular, and asymmetric.

Key Signs

- Nodularity of breast tissue
- Thickening in the upper-outer quadrant
- Lumps that feel soft, cystic or rubbery, smooth, or mobile
- Cysts, solitary or multiple

Laboratory Tests/Diagnostic Evaluation

1. Routine laboratory tests are not helpful in evaluation of FBD.

2. Diagnostic evaluation may include physical examination, large-needle breast cyst aspiration, ultrasonography, mammography, fine-needle aspiration, and excisional biopsy.

3. If examination indicates a cyst, try to aspirate it. The aspirate may be yellow to dark green or brown in color. Blood-tinged aspirate should be evaluated, and the patient should have a mammogram and tissue biopsy.

4. An ultrasound of the breast may be needed to distinguish a cyst from a solid mass, especially in a younger woman.

5. Mammography is recommended for any woman over age 35 who has a dominant breast lump that may be suspicious of cancer. The mammogram usually is obtained before tissue biopsy to characterize the mass and identify other suspicious areas.

6. First try fine-needle aspiration. If aspiration cannot be performed or is inconclusive, then perform an excisional biopsy.

Key Tests

- Large-needle aspiration
- Fine-needle aspiration
- Mammography
- Excisional biopsy
- Breast ultrasound

Differential Diagnosis

1. Fear of cancer is the primary reason women seek help for evaluation of changes in their breasts.

2. The cancer risk associated with FBD is shown in Table 95–1.

3. A family history of breast cancer in a woman with atypical hyperplasia increases her relative risk to 9.0; in women with cysts, the relative risk is 3.0.

4. Not all women whose breasts are tender and painful have FBD. Other conditions that could cause aches and pains include cervical or dorsal radiculitis, costochondritis, herpes zoster infection, trauma, other infections, and cancer.

Treatment

Symptoms usually abate with the onset of menses and need no further treatment except reassurance that changes are physiologic responses and not cancer. Some women have continued symptoms that are severe enough to warrant symptomatic treatment.

Medication

1. Low-dose oral contraceptives (low estrogen with relatively high progesterone) eliminate breast pain, usually after the first cycle of pills, and improve fibrocystic changes after 6 months of treatment.

2. Danazol (Danoctine) has been approved by the FDA for treatment of fibrocystic changes. Doses of 100 to 600 mg/day for 2 to 6 months decrease pain and nodularity in 60 to 90 per cent of patients. High doses are usually required. Side effects include amenorrhea, acne, hirsutism, deepening of the voice, atrophic vaginitis, headaches, weight gain, and edema. Symptoms usually recur when the drug is withdrawn.

3. Progestins such as medroxyprogesterone acetate (Provera), 10 mg on days 15 to 25 of the menstrual cycle, provide symptomatic relief in 80 to 85 per cent of patients.

4. Other drugs for relief of symptoms include bromocriptine (Parlodel), 5 to 7.5 mg/day, and tamoxifen (Nolvadex), 10 mg b.i.d., for perimenopausal women. Neither of these drugs has been approved specifically for FBD, but they have benefited some women.

Diet

1. Abstinence from methylxanthines, including coffee, tea, chocolate, cola, and theophylline, may be effective.

2. A low-fat, high-fiber diet is recommended as part of a healthy lifestyle.

3. A combination of vitamins E, B-complex, and C, and selenium has decreased symptoms for some women.

Activity

Aerobic activity three to four times a week for 30 minutes may be beneficial for mild breast pain. A well-fitting support bra is essential.

Patient Education

1. Patients should be taught how to do breast self-examination (BSE) and report any changes.

2. Patients also should know the warning signs of breast cancer and the recommendations for mammography to screen for breast cancer.

TABLE 95–1. RISK OF BREAST CANCER WITH FIBROCYSTIC BREAST DISEASE

% ALL BIOPSIES FOR FBD	RELATIVE RISK	PATHOLOGY
70	1.0 No increased risk	Nonproliferative (apocrine metaplasia, cysts, mild hyperplasia, fibroadenomas)
26–28	1.5 Slightly increased risk	Proliferative without atypia (papillomas, sclerosing adenosis)
2–4	4.5–5.0 Moderately increased risk	Proliferative with atypia (atypical hyperplasia)

Follow-Up

1. Women with average risk should have a clinical breast examination every 3 years until age 40 and then annually. Mammography is recommended every 2 years from ages 40 to 50 and then annually thereafter.

2. Women with painful, nodular breasts should be offered reassurance and close follow-up to help correct misinformation, interpret findings, and help eliminate the anxiety and fear of cancer produced by finding a lump in the breast.

Bibliography

Bodian C: Benign breast disease, carcinoma in situ, and breast cancer risk. Epidemiol Rev 1993;15:177–187.

Conroy C: Evaluation of a breast complaint: Is it cancer? Am Fam Physician 1994;49:445–450.

Decker P, Ricci A: Pain and lumps in the female breast. Hosp Pract 1992:Feb 28:67–94.

Dupont WD, Parl F, Brinton L, et al: Breast cancer risk associated with proliferative breast disease and atypical hyperplasia. Cancer 1993;71:1258–1265.

Gray D, Hodgkins M, Goodson W: The lumpy breast. West J Med 1988;149:226–229.

96 Abnormal Pap Smear

Rebecca Gladu

Etiology

1. Abnormal pap smears indicating precancerous cervical lesions are due to human papillomavirus (HPV) infection with subtypes 16, 18, and 31.
2. Abnormal Pap smears are reported using the Bethesda system of Pap smear reporting originated in 1988 by the National Cancer Institute:
   a. Infection: yeast (*Candida*), viral (herpes, HPV), protozoan (*Trichomonas*), or bacterial (*H. vaginalis*) can be identified.
   b. Reactive or reparative changes:
      (1) Inflammation
      (2) Changes such as those due to radiation or chemotherapy
   c. Epithelial cell abnormalities:
      (1) Atypical squamous cells of undetermined significance—epithelial cells that are seen to have an aberration of nuclear size and morphology.
      (2) Squamous intraepithelial lesions (SIL):
         (a) Low grade: cervical intraepithelial neoplasia (CIN I)—involving the lower third of the squamous mucosa
         (b) High grade:
            CIN II—the lower two thirds of the squamous mucosa
            CIN III—the entire mucosal thickness
      (3) Squamous cell carcinoma—90 per cent of all invasive cervical cancer
   d. Glandular cell abnormalities:
      (1) Endometrial cells present in an unusual circumstance (such as in a postmenopausal woman)
      (2) Atypical glandular cells
      (3) Adenocarcinoma—5 per cent of all invasive cervical cancer
   e. Other epithelial malignant neoplasm: specify
   f. Nonepithelial malignant neoplasm: specify
   g. Hormonal evaluation if these tests have been requested

Symptoms

1. Invasive carcinoma of the cervix may present with bleeding, especially after intercourse.
2. Preinvasive lesions are asymptomatic.
3. Infectious lesions causing abnormal pap smears may present with purulent vaginal discharge, pelvic pain, or dyspareunia.

Clinical Findings

1. Signs of infectious disease of the cervix, such as cervical motion tenderness, mucopurulent discharge, or condylomatous changes. Infectious etiologies such as yeast or bacterial disease can be noted on the Pap smear correlating with clinical signs.
2. There are no obvious visual signs associated with preinvasive lesions of the cervix. Occasionally, HPV infection will cause verrucous lesions (condyloma accuminata) seen on the perineum, vagina, and/or cervical mucosa. These are seen most easily using the colposcope.
3. Invasive carcinoma of the cervix is often visible to the naked eye and may bleed easily. It has a cauliflower appearance and is hard and fixed to the touch.

Laboratory Tests

1. Conventional Pap smears are prepared by sampling cells from the cervix, smearing them onto a glass slide, and then fixing them with a spray. In a new technique known as the ThinPrep method, the physician rinses the cervical sample into a small vial containing preservative. This vial is sent to the laboratory and inserted into the ThinPrep processor. Cell clusters remain intact and produce a higher-quality slide for the cytotechnologist to view. A 4 to 1 reduction in the number of false-negative readings was found in one study using the ThinPrep method over conventional slides.
2. When indicated by abnormal epithelial cell findings on Pap smear, further laboratory evaluation with colposcopically directed cervical biopsy and endocervical curettage give a specific tissue diagnosis.
3. Specific indications for colposcopy:
   a. Atypia in certain cases, as described below
   b. Persistent inflammation despite therapy
   c. Human papillomavirus (HPV) effect
   d. A visible cervical abnormality
   e. CIN I–III, carcinoma in situ, and invasive cancer
4. Always perform endocervical curettage when taking directed biopsies at the time of colposcopy to ensure complete endocervical sampling.

Key Tests (if Pap smear is abnormal)

- Colposcopy
- Cervical biopsy
- Endocervical curettage

Differential Diagnosis

Because the Pap smear report is able to give specific information about the cause of the abnormal Pap smear, a differential diagnosis is not necessary.

Treatment

1. Atypia
   a. If associated with infection, treat the infection appropriately and repeat the Pap smear every 3 months until two negative Pap tests are obtained. Three months are necessary to allow for full repair of cervical inflammatory changes.
   b. Some authors recommend colposcopy for all atypia, since an underlying CIN may be found in 19 to 56 per cent of cases. This remains controversial.
   c. Persistent atypia without response to treatment definitely should be examined by colposcopy.
2. CIN I–III, carcinoma in situ
   a. Cryotherapy—inexpensive, comparable results with those of laser therapy, available as a simple office procedure. Indications:
      (1) Satisfactory colposcopic examination
      (2) Negative endocervical curettage
      (3) No microinvasion
      (4) Pap smear and biopsy correlate within one grade
   b. Laser evaporation—expensive, precise
      (1) For large lesions that the cryoprobe will not cover
      (2) For the irregular cervix with scars and deep clefts
      (3) For lesions extending onto the vagina
      (4) For CIN with deep glandular involvement
   c. Cone biopsy—an operative procedure to excise deep cervical lesions. Indications:
      (1) Positive endocervical curettage—a deep lesion
      (2) Unsatisfactory colposcopic examination—the entire squamocolumnal junction was not seen.
      (3) Microinvasion biopsy or cytology
      (4) When there is suspicion for invasion on cytology, but directed biopsy does not show an invasive lesion
   d. Cervical loop diathermy (LEEP/LETZ)—a new simple office procedure using a heated wire to excise the cervical tissue. Indicated for the same lesions as cone biopsy but at less cost and risk.
3. Invasive cancer
   a. Staging
   b. Specific oncologic treatment—radiation, surgery as indicated
   c. Referral to a gynecologic oncologist
4. If endometrial cells are present in a postmenopausal woman or greater than 7 days after menses, perform an endometrial biopsy.
5. Indications for excisional therapy—conization or LEEP:
   a. Inadequate colposcopy
   b. Positive endocervical curettage
   c. Incompatible biopsy and cytology

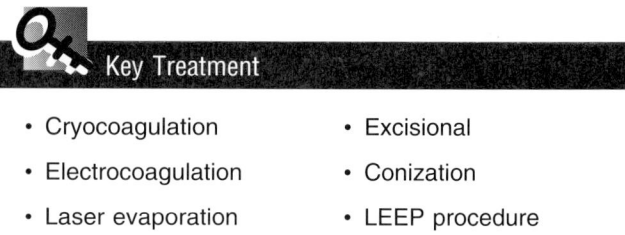

Key Treatment

- Cryocoagulation
- Electrocoagulation
- Laser evaporation
- Excisional
- Conization
- LEEP procedure

Follow-Up

1. If the Pap smear is *normal,* repeat Pap smear annually.
2. If the Pap smear is *inadequate* (usually no endocervical cells obtained), repeat Pap smear.
3. If the Pap smear shows *atypia* associated with infection or inflammation:
   a. Treat infection appropriately and then repeat Pap smear in 3 months.
   b. If negative at 3 months, repeat at 6 months.
   c. If negative a second time, repeat annually.
   d. If inflammation persists 3 months after treatment, evaluate with colposcopy.
   e. If infectious etiology is not reported on the Pap smear, repeat a physical examination and include a wet mount, KOH prep, and vaginal or cervical cultures to establish a diagnosis prior to treatment.
   f. If the causative agent cannot be established, treat with a broad-spectrum antibiotic vaginal cream and then repeat the Pap smear after 3 months to allow for repair of the inflammation.
4. If the Pap smear shows *atypia* due to HPV or does not specify the cause, perform colposcopy.
5. For CIN I–III after cryotherapy:
   a. Repeat the Pap smear at 4 months.
   b. Repeat again after 4 months.
   c. If both are normal, repeat every 6 to 12 months for life.
6. After laser therapy:
   a. Perform Pap smear at 3 months.
   b. Repeat Pap smear at 6 months.
   c. If both smears are negative, obtain a Pap smear every 6 to 12 months.
7. After cone biopsy:
   a. Perform Pap smear at 1 month.
   b. Repeat Pap smear at 4 months.
   c. Repeat annually thereafter.

Bibliography

Automated pap smear makes for easier detection of cervical cancer. Primary Care Cancer 1994;14(4):36.

Cline MK, Baxley EG, Montgomery RP: Papanicolaou smear discrepancy: Resolution by review. J Am Board Fam Pract 1994;7(1):9–13.

Gearhart JG, Davey-Sullivan BJ, Fulton LJ: Management of the abnormal pap smear. J Miss State Med Assoc 1991; 32:159–164.

Hatch KD: Handbook of Colposcopy. Boston, Little, Brown, 1989.

Himmelstein LR: Evaluation of inflammatory atypia: A literature review. J Reprod Med 1989;34(9):634–637.

Hutchinson ML, Agarwal P, Denault T, et al: A new look at cervical cytology: ThinPrep multicenter trial results. Acta Cytol 1992;36(4):499–504.

97 Breast Cancer

Marvin A. Dewar

Etiology and Clinical Epidemiology

1. Breast cancer is the most common malignant disease among women in the United States and the leading cause of cancer death in women 35 to 54 years old. The American Cancer Society estimates that 182,000 women will be newly diagnosed with breast cancer and 46,000 women will die of the disease in 1994. Overall, 12 per cent of women will develop breast cancer, and 3.5 per cent will die of the disease.

2. The *incidence* of breast cancer has been increasing at a rate of approximately 1 per cent per year since 1973, with the increase most marked in younger women. This increased incidence is related to both mammography screening with detection of early-stage disease and an underlying increase in the absolute number of breast cancer cases in women.

3. As with other cancers, the underlying *cause* of breast cancer is multifactorial, involving a complex interplay between genetic and other host factors and external cancer promoters (e.g., chemical carcinogens and lifestyle factors). Specific genetic findings associated with breast cancer have been described, including specific gene amplification and/or overexpression and point mutations. For example, the Li-Fraumeni syndrome, associated with a point mutation on the p53 tumor suppressor gene, is associated with increased risk of breast cancer, sarcoma, and other cancers.

4. Seventy-five per cent of women with breast cancer have no identifiable specific *risk factor* other than gender. Specific factors associated with an increased risk of breast cancer include
   a. Increasing age
   b. Prior personal history of breast cancer
   c. Family history of breast cancer in a first-degree relative, particularly if the family member was premenopausal and the breast cancer was bilateral
   d. Late menopause (after age 55)
   e. Early menarche
   f. Nulliparity or first pregnancy after the age of 30
   g. Benign breast disease *if* breast biopsy demonstrates proliferative epithelial changes and particularly if associated with atypia (atypical ductal hyperplasia and atypical lobular hyperplasia)

5. *Additional factors* that may be associated with an increased risk of breast cancer, but for which conflicting evidence exists, include high dietary fat, obesity, oral contraceptive use, postmenopausal estrogen replacement, and alcohol consumption. Breast-feeding, early age at first pregnancy, and early menopause (surgical) may be associated with a decreased risk of breast cancer.

Symptoms

1. A palpable, usually painless breast lump, detected by the patient, is the presenting complaint in 80 to 90 per cent of palpable breast cancers.

2. Nipple discharge (particularly if bloody and unilateral), focal breast pain, and inflammation of the skin over the breast also may be associated with breast cancer, although all these symptoms are also commonly associated with benign breast disease.

3. Symptoms such as bone pain, focal neurologic findings, abdominal pain, and jaundice are indicative of systemic breast cancer and advanced metastatic disease.

4. Increasingly, occult breast cancers are detected by screening mammography at a stage when they are not palpable and are otherwise asymptomatic.

Clinical Findings

1. Dominant breast masses should be considered highly suspicious for breast cancer.
   a. Suspicion is increased further if the dominant mass is hard or fixed to the overlying skin.
   b. Fixation of a dominant mass to skin can produce dimpling or retraction of the overlying skin when the pectoral muscles are contracted.

2. Unilateral bloody nipple discharge is particularly suspicious when found in association with a dominant mass.

3. New onset of inverted nipple should raise the possibility of breast cancer.

4. Axillary adenopathy may be indicative of node-positive breast cancer, although the clinical examination is neither sensitive nor specific for axillary metastasis.

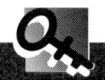 **Key Signs**

- Dominant breast mass
- Unilateral bloody nipple discharge

Screening

1. Screening strategies involving mammography, clinical breast examination, and breast self-examination are intended to detect breast cancer at an early stage when treatment options are maximized and mortality is decreased.
   a. Mammography screening of appropriately selected women has successfully decreased breast cancer mortality by almost one third and could potentially reduce breast cancer mortality by as much as 50

per cent if screening protocols were adhered to by all women.

b. Mammography is capable of detecting early-stage breast cancers less than 1 cm in size, compared with an average size of about 2.5 centimeters for breast cancers detected by women themselves.

c. Clinical breast examination and breast self-examination are also important components of breast cancer screening, since 10 to 15 per cent of palpable breast cancers are not detected on screening mammograms.

2. Quality control is critical to obtaining the promised benefit of screening mammography and should include modern equipment capable of producing high-quality mammography films with minimal radiation exposure, well-trained and experienced technicians and radiologists, and periodic audit review of mammography film interpretations. The American College of Radiology (ACR) has devised a program for evaluating and accrediting mammography screening centers in an attempt to ensure quality.

3. *Screening recommendations* vary among sponsoring organizations. Current American Cancer Society guidelines follow:

a. Breast self-examination: monthly for women 20 years and older

b. Clinical breast examination: every 3 years between the ages of 20 and 40, annually thereafter

c. Mammography: every 1 to 2 years from age 40 to 50, annually thereafter. (The data supporting the benefit of screening mammography in women between the ages of 40 and 50 are not clear, and a number of organizations do not recommend mammography screening for this age group.)

Laboratory Tests

Confirmation of a suspicion of breast cancer requires pathologic diagnosis by cytology or histology.

1. Fine-needle aspiration (FNA) of a breast mass may allow the cytologic diagnosis of breast cancer. A negative FNA (no cancer cells) is not sufficient evidence to rule out breast cancer in a suspicious lesion, however, and the technique is most useful in differentiating a solid breast mass from a breast cyst.

2. Core-needle biopsy of a solid breast mass provides material for histologic examination.

3. Open excisional biopsy of a breast mass is frequently used to diagnose breast cancer. This is usually done as a separate procedure from the definitive surgical management of a subsequently detected breast cancer.

4. Occult nonpalpable breast lesions detected by mammography may be biopsied after guidewire needle localization or stereotactically guided core-needle biopsy using mammography guidance.

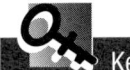

Key Tests

• FNA

• Core-needle biopsy

• Open excisional biopsy

Differential Diagnosis

1. Fibroadenomas present as hard, mobile breast nodules, usually in young women. Fibroadenomas tend to fluctuate with the menstrual cycle and pregnancy and may regress with menopause.

2. Breast cysts are most common during breast involution, which usually begins at about age 35 and continues through menopause. FNA and breast ultrasound help differentiate breast cysts from solid breast lesions.

3. Mastitis, usually due to gram-positive organisms, may produce breast changes mimicking inflammatory breast cancer. Associated signs of infection and response to antibiotics help differentiate the two diagnoses.

4. Nonpalpable suspicious mammographic findings, such as asymmetry, microcalcification, and irregular breast densities, may be seen in both neoplastic and benign breast disease. Approximately 80 per cent of nonpalpable suspicious lesions detected by mammography will be found to be benign disease on biopsy.

Treatment

1. Management of breast cancer involves the selective combined use of surgery, radiation therapy, and chemotherapy. Treatment choice for a particular patient depends on the characteristics of the breast cancer, patient preference, and local medical expertise.

a. *Breast-conserving surgery* (BCS, also called "lumpectomy") provides mortality results similar to more aggressive surgery in appropriately selected women and is cosmetically more acceptable to many women.

(1) BCS is combined with axillary dissection and examination of lymph nodes and followed by whole-breast radiation therapy.

(2) Factors weighing *against* BCS versus more aggressive surgical procedures include, but are not limited to, an unfavorable tumor/breast size ratio, multiple breast cancers, and large central versus small peripheral tumors.

b. *Modified radical mastectomy* with removal of the breast, axillary dissection, and preservation of the pectoral muscles is indicated when BCS is not used. Mastectomy may be performed with or without breast reconstruction.

2. A majority of women found to have breast cancer in

one or more *positive axillary nodes* will have disease recurrence and arc candidates for *adjuvant therapy.*

   a. Combination chemotherapy for 2 to 6 months is recommended for women younger than age 50.

   b. Tamoxifen is recommended for node-positive women older than age 50. Although the benefit of tamoxifen may be greater in estrogen and progesterone receptor–positive women, both receptor-positive and -negative women experience benefit.

3. The treatment of women with *negative axillary nodes* is an area of much current research and changing recommendations. Because 25 to 30 per cent of axillary node–negative women will experience disease recurrence, many should be considered for adjuvant therapy.

   a. Women with tumor size less than 1 cm have a recurrence risk of less than 10 per cent and may not require adjuvant therapy.

   b. The role of other prognostic factors affecting the likelihood of disease recurrence, such as receptor status, tumor grade, DNA index, and S-phase fraction, in the decision to treat node-negative women with adjuvant therapy is currently being studied.

   c. The choice of tamoxifen or chemotherapy for node-negative patients receiving adjuvant therapy depends on a number of factors, including menopausal status and tumor receptor status. When possible, women requiring adjuvant therapy should be enrolled in clinical trials.

4. *Metastatic breast cancer* and *disease relapse* are usually managed by hormonal therapy or combination chemotherapy. Some patients may be candidates for high-dose chemotherapy combined with autologous bone marrow transplantation. Where possible, women with metastatic breast cancer or treatment relapse should be enrolled in clinical trials.

Key Treatment

- Selective combination of surgery, radiation, and chemotherapy

Bibliography

American College of Obstetricians and Gynecologists: Carcinoma of the Breast. ACOG Technical Bulletin No. 158. Washington, ACOG, 1991.

Chittor SR, Swain SM: Adjuvant therapy in early breast cancer. Am Fam Physician 1991;43:453–462.

DelTurco MR, Palli D, Cariddi A, et al: Intensive diagnostic follow-up after treatment of primary breast cancer. JAMA 1994;271:1593–1597.

Harris JR, Lippman ME, Veronesi U, Willett W: Breast cancer, parts I, II, and III. N Engl J Med 1992;327:319–328, 390–398, 473–480.

Scanlon EF: Breast cancer. *In* Holleb AI, Fink DJ, Murphy GP (eds): Clinical Oncology. Atlanta, American Cancer Society, 1991, pp 177–193.

Indications

1. Palpable breast mass
2. Cystic or solid lesion of breast

Contraindications

1. Known bleeding disorder
2. Anticoagulant therapy

Preparation

1. History and physical examination
2. Informed consent

Equipment

1. Betadine or 70% alcohol solution
2. 10- or 20-milliliter syringe—standard or three-finger control
3. 1.5-inch 22-gauge needle
4. Glass slides (preferably poly-L-lysine–coated)
5. Cell filtration solution (i.e. Cytolyt), if cell filtration equipment is available. This technique allows minimal in-office handling of specimen.
6. Slide fixative or 95% ethanol, depending on preference of cytopathologist
7. Diff Quick stain—optional if planning to view air-dried slides immediately
8. 1-inch 30-gauge needle (optional for anesthetic)
9. Xylocaine without epinephrine, 0.5 to 1 ml (optional for anesthesia)
10. 3-ml syringe (optional for local anesthetic)

Precautions

1. Hematoma is the most common complication.
2. Pneumothorax—rare
3. Acute mastitis—rare
4. Tumor growth in the needle track—theoretical risk but not observed with needle sizes used in this procedure. If cancer is present, the track will likely be excised or will be included in radiation therapy field of treatment.

Technique

1. Antiseptic preparation to skin over biopsy site with alcohol or betadine
2. Optional—Xylocaine injection into dermis and subcutaneous tissue, being careful to avoid biopsy tissue. Anesthetic should be in 3-ml syringe with 30-gauge needle.
3. Use a three-finger control syringe or place a standard 10- or 20-cc syringe in pistol grip, if available.
4. Optional—withdraw plunger of syringe to 3- to 5-ml mark. This step avoids need to remove syringe after obtaining specimen for transport or slide preparation.
5. Place index and middle fingers of nonaspirating hand over mass, compressing structures over mass.
6. Spread fingers and press more firmly.

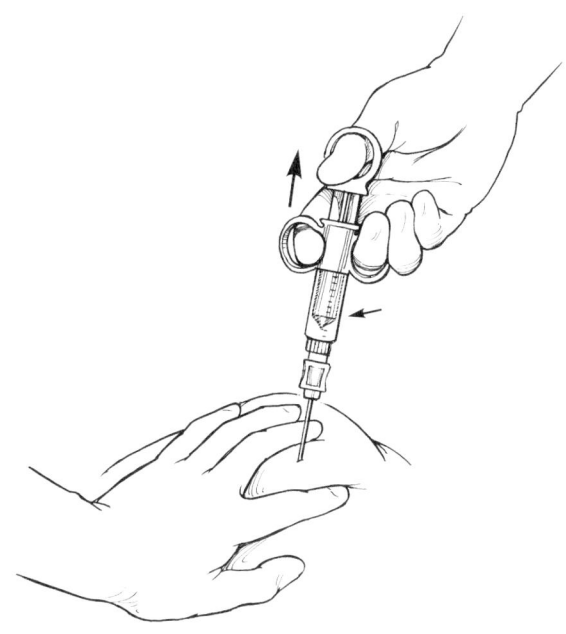

7. Introduce needle through skin and into mass. Move needle from side to side, and palpate mass. Mass should move with needle if proper placement is achieved.

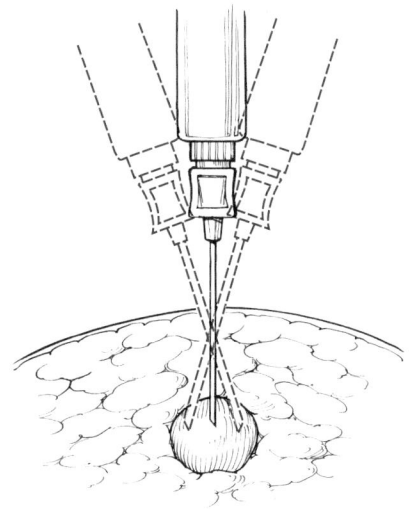

8. Apply negative pressure by withdrawing syringe plunger (see figure on p. 411).

9. Pass needle through mass 6 to 10 times, maintaining negative pressure. If fluid is obtained, remove all fluid and then re-examine for mass. If mass is present, repeat the procedure to obtain a biopsy specimen for evaluation.

10. Upon completion of multiple passes, cellular material may be noted in the hub of the needle, although this is not necessary to have an adequate specimen.

11. Release negative pressure from syringe prior to removal from mass, then remove needle from lesion.

12. Apply pressure to areas for 1 to 2 minutes to minimize occurrence of hematoma.

13. If step 4 was omitted, remove syringe from needle and withdraw plunger to fill syringe with air.

14. If using cell filtration solution (i.e., Cytolyt), contents of needle may be expressed into solution, and this can be sent for laboratory evaluation. Occasionally, solution may be drawn into syringe to ensure maximal yield of specimen when specimen is scant.

15. Slides can be prepared as with standard hematologic smear and fixed in 95% ethanol or fixative spray.

Alternatively, "book-opening technique," with one air-dried and one fixed slide, may be used. (See Wilkinson and Bland [1990] for description of "book-opening technique.")

Follow-Up

1. Positive results should be followed by open biopsy and definitive care.

2. Negative results should be evaluated. Acellular results may require rebiopsy or close clinical follow-up. Clinical suspicion of malignancy based on history and examination should be used to decide on further treatment or evaluation.

WARNING

Mammogram may be altered for up to 3 weeks after the procedure.

WARNING

All laboratory preparation and handling should be discussed with individual reference laboratory and/or pathologist to maximize information obtained from procedure.

 ## Bibliography

Erickson R, Shank JC, Gratton C: Fine-needle breast aspiration biopsy. J Fam Pract 1989;28:306.

Grundfest S: Fine-needle breast aspiration biopsy. Mod Med 1987;55:72.

Hindle WH: The use of fine-needle aspiration in the evaluation of persistent palpable dominant breast masses. Am J Obstet Gynecol 1993;168:1814.

Jackson WK, Archibald LH: Fine-needle aspiration biopsy of thyroid, neck masses and lymph nodes, and breast masses. Primary Care 1986;13:549.

Wilkinson EJ, Bland KI: Techniques and results of aspiration cytology for diagnosis of benign and malignant diseases of the breast. Surg Clin North Am 1990;70:801.

98 Cervical Cancer

Jim Nuovo

Etiology

Risk Factors

1. First sexual contact at a young age
2. Multiple sexual partners
3. A promiscuous male partner
4. History of genital warts
5. Smoking
6. Folate deficiency
7. Immunosuppression
8. Low socioeconomic status
9. A prolonged time since the last Pap smear (>5 years)

HPV Types and Extent of Cervical Disease

It has been suspected for a number of years that the agent responsible for the development of cervical cancer is contagious and sexually transmittable. The link between the human papillomavirus (HPV) and cervical cancer and its precursors (dysplasia) is strong. With the development of techniques in molecular biology allowing for the identification and classification of the HPV, it has been possible to compare specific HPV types against the extent of cervical disease. The findings from this research include the following observations:

1. Infection with HPV is extremely common, and in fact, HPV represents the most common viral sexually transmitted disease (STD). HPV infects 10 per cent of the general population and up to 30 per cent of individuals presenting to STD clinics.
2. HPV is a highly contagious disease.
3. Many patients with HPV will have "subclinical" disease, and there may be a long latency period between the time of infection and the expression of overt disease.
4. There is an association between certain HPV subtypes and the development of cervical cancer. HPV subtypes 16, 18, 31, 33, 35, and 39 are particularly associated with an increased risk. However, because patients infected with an oncogenic strain will not necessarily develop cervical cancer or dysplasia, it remains unclear whether HPV testing is worthwhile.

Symptoms

1. Cervical cancer and dysplasia usually occur without symptoms. For this reason, it is important to recommend that patients at risk for cervical cancer participate in periodic cytologic screening.
2. Among women being screened for cervical disease with a Pap smear, approximately 90 to 95 per cent will be diagnosed as normal.
3. Because of extensive screening, most women who have cervical precancers are identified by the Pap smear at a stage where the lesion is easily eradicated. The 5-year survival rate is considerably better for women with local cervical cancer (90 per cent) versus those with advanced disease (40 per cent). Therefore, the goal of screening is to detect precursors to cervical cancer and to provide an opportunity for the provider to prevent progression to invasive cancer.
4. The effectiveness of cervical cancer screening increases when Pap smear testing is performed frequently. Aggressive (dysplastic) lesions are less likely to escape detection when the interval between smears is short.
5. Pap smear screening schedule recommendations have come from many groups. The recent recommendations from the U.S. Preventive Services Task Force encompass many of the principles seen in other reports; that is, "testing should begin at the age when the woman first engages in sexual intercourse. Pap tests are appropriately performed at an interval of 1 to 3 years, to be recommended by the physician based on the presence of risk factors."
6. Another issue related to screening is that of false-negative examinations. The reported frequency has ranged from 20 to 45 per cent.
7. Two factors contributing to false-negative results include Pap smear technique and reliability of interpretation. Proper technique in the performance of a Pap smear is crucial. The proper methodology is reviewed in the first Procedure following this chapter.
8. The combined use of a cytobrush and Ayre spatula has been shown to improve the quality of the submitted smear. A cytopathologist has over 50,000 epithelial cells to review on a given Pap smear slide. Only a small percentage of the cells may be abnormal on any given slide.
9. The criteria used to define an abnormal cell include
   a. Abnormal amount for nuclear chromatin
   b. Collection of chromatin clumps in the nucleus
   c. Increased nuclear size and nuclear/cytoplasmic ratio
   d. Increased mitotic activity
   e. Increased number of nuclei
10. These criteria are subject to problems with intra- and interobserver variability. In a study of the reproducibility of cytodiagnosis of Pap smears, it was shown that agreement between two cytopathologists was achieved 75 per cent of the time and on rereview by the same pathologist 80 per cent of the time.
11. In 1988, federal Pap smear legislation was enacted

413

to improve the quality of Pap smear reporting and reduce the confusion on Pap smear terminology. Uniform standards were established in reporting cytology results. This new classification system was designated the *Bethesda system.* The new system has not been adopted by all pathologists, and therefore, it is important to be able to compare the differences between the systems. Even with the Bethesda system there remains confusion by family physicians as how to manage an abnormal result. Melnikow et al. (1993) found that family physicians were more likely to misinterpret the results of a cytology report using the Bethesda system of nomenclature and were likely to overutilize colposcopy.

Clinical Issues

1. In order to get a good cervical smear, direct visualization of the cervix during a Pap smear is an important part of the pelvic examination. However, cervical cancer and its precursors generally will not be detectable by direct inspection.

2. Colposcopy has been used to identify the specific abnormal areas, to determine the extent of a lesion, and to direct the biopsy to the areas of concern.

3. Some authors advocate acetic acid washes of the cervix as an adjunct to the Pap smear. Those patients who demonstrate areas of whitening would be advised to undergo colposcopy.

4. Cervicography, acetic acid washing followed by a standardized photograph of the cervix, also has been proposed. The ''cervigram'' is reviewed by an expert, and recommendations follow as to whether the patient needs colposcopy. It remains controversial as to whether either test offers an advantage over periodic Pap smears with colposcopy for those with dysplastic or atypical findings.

Laboratory Tests

The ''laboratory test'' in the evaluation of a patient for cervical cancer is the Pap smear report. Clarity in the reporting of Pap smear results has been an ongoing problem.

1. Systems used to report cytologic findings:

   a. Class system (classes I through V)

   b. World Health Organization system (normal; atypical; dysplasia—mild, moderate, and severe; invasive squamous cell carcinoma; and adenocarcinoma)

   c. CIN system (normal; CIN I, II, or III; invasive squamous cell carcinoma)

   d. Bethesda system (within normal limits, epithelial cell abnormalities; SIL low-grade versus high-grade, squamous cell carcinoma, and gland cell abnormalities)

2. Equivalent reports among the four systems:

   a. Normal (class I, within normal limits)

   b. Atypia (class II, atypical)

   c. Dysplasia (class III, CIN I, dysplasia—mild, SIL low-grade)

   d. Dysplasia (class IV, CIN II or III, dysplasia—moderate to severe, SIL high-grade)

   e. Carcinoma (class V, carcinoma, squamous cell carcinoma)

Key Tests

- Pap smear
- Colposcopy

Differential Diagnosis

1. Dysplasia on a Pap smear must be investigated to rule out invasive carcinoma.

2. Atypia on a Pap smear may be produced by dysplasia, infection, or repair of the cervix. Infectious processes that may produce atypia (other than HPV) include

   a. Bacterial vaginosis

   b. *Candida*

   c. *Trichomonas*

   d. *Chlamydia trachomatis*

   e. *Neisseria gonorrhoeae*

3. In the postmenopausal patient, hormone-related atrophic changes may produce atypia as well.

Treatment

1. Dysplasia. All patients with a Pap smear demonstrating dysplasia are recommended to undergo a colposcopic examination of the cervix. Management of the patient after colposcopy is dependent on the specific findings. If dysplasia is found, the patient may undergo cryotherapy, laser ablation, low-voltage loop electroexcision, or cone biopsy. The appropriate treatment and follow-up will depend on the following parameters: lesion grade, size, and whether it involves the endocervical canal.

2. Atypia. In patients who have atypia on their Pap smear, there remains a great deal of controversy as to whether a colposcopy is warranted. One may choose to re-examine a patient with atypia to assess whether there is an ongoing infection. If an infection is discovered, the patient may be treated accordingly and the Pap repeated in 3 to 4 months. There are no data to suggest that cautious follow-up with repeat Pap smears will result in a delayed diagnosis with increased morbidity.

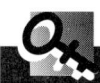

Key Treatment

- Colposcopy if dysplasia is present

Follow-Up

The appropriate follow-up for a patient with an abnormal Pap smear is dependent on the abnormality seen.

1. Dysplasia. Patients who have dysplasia should undergo a colposcopic examination. If dysplasia is detected on this examination, the patient should undergo appropriate treatment. Follow-up for these patients will be more frequent (on average every 4 to 6 months for 1 to 2 years). Repeat colposcopy is done for recurrent abnormalities. If there is a marked discrepancy between the Pap smear and the colposcopy report (e.g., high-grade dysplasia on a Pap smear and a normal or nondiagnostic colposcopy report), a repeat colposcopy should be considered.

WARNING

There is confusion among physicians as to how to interpret Pap smear reports. All women with dysplasia (or the equivalent term) should undergo colposcopy. Women with atypia may be evaluated for infection and, if present, treated and then have another Pap smear in 3 to 4 months. Persistent atypia warrants colposcopy.

---

2. Atypia. Patients with atypia may be investigated for infection. If an infection is discovered, the patient should be treated and seen again for a Pap in 3 to 4 months. Persistent atypia warrants colposcopy.

 Bibliography

For more information on cervical cancer screening, see
The U.S. Preventive Services Task Force: Screening for cervical cancer. Am Fam Physician 1990;41:853–857.

For more information on the Pap smear test, see
Koss LG: The Papanicolaou test for cervical cancer detection: A triumph and a tragedy. JAMA 1989;261:737–743.

For more information on the confusion in interpreting Pap smear reports, see
Melnikow J, Sierk A, Flocke S, Peters CA: Does the system of Papanicolaou test nomenclature affect the rate of referral for colposcopy? A survey of family physicians. Arch Fam Med 1993;2:253–258.

For more information on the human papillomavirus, see
Reid R: Biology and colposcopic features of human papillomavirus-associated cervical disease. Obstet Gynecol Clin North Am 1993;20:123–151.

For more information on the management of patients with an abnormal Pap smear, see
Nuovo GJ: Cytopathology of the Lower Female Genital Tract: An Integrated Approach. Baltimore, Williams & Wilkins, 1994.

Procedure | **PAP SMEAR**

Nader Tavakoli

Indications

The Pap smear is used primarily to screen for cervical cancer. Opinions on the frequency of Pap smears are outlined below.

1. The U.S. Preventive Services Task Force has established the following screening guidelines:

   a. Pap smear should begin at age 18 or at the age of first sexual intercourse, whichever comes first.

   b. Between the ages of 18 and 65, Pap smears should be repeated every 1 to 3 years on the basis of risk factors for cervical cancer.

   c. After the age of 65, screening tests may be discontinued if previous smears have been consistently normal.

2. The American Cancer Society and the American College of Obstetricians and Gynecologists recommend annual Pap smears beginning at age 18 or at the age of first sexual intercourse, whichever occurs first. After three or more consecutive, satisfactory annual tests with normal findings, it can be performed less frequently if recommended by the physician. I favor annual Pap smears in women with one or more risk factors for cervical cancer.

Precautions

The Pap smear should not be obtained if the patient is menstruating or has douched within 24 hours.

Equipment

1. Vaginal speculum
2. One or two glass slides
3. Wooden cervical spatula
4. Cytobrush or cotton swab moistened with normal saline solution
5. Fixative (95% ethyl alcohol or commercial spray)
6. Gloves

Technique

1. With an assistant in attendance and patient in lithotomy position, insert an unlubricated speculum (water only) to expose the cervix, and gently wipe away any excessive discharge.

2. Insert the cytobrush or cotton swab into the cervical canal, rotate 360 to 720 degrees, and roll onto the glass slide.

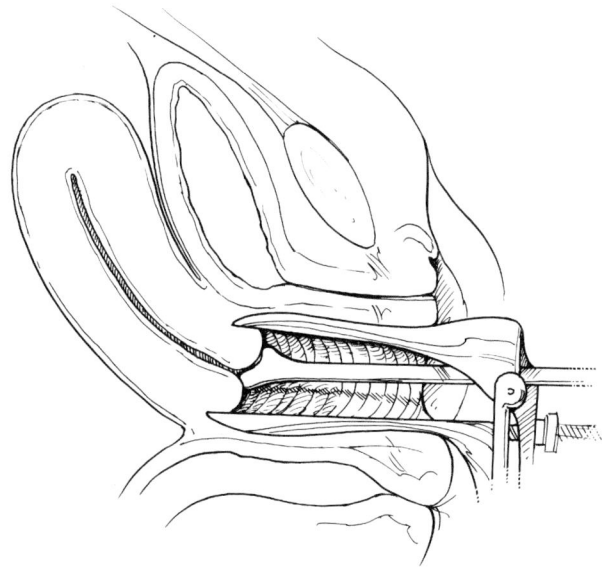

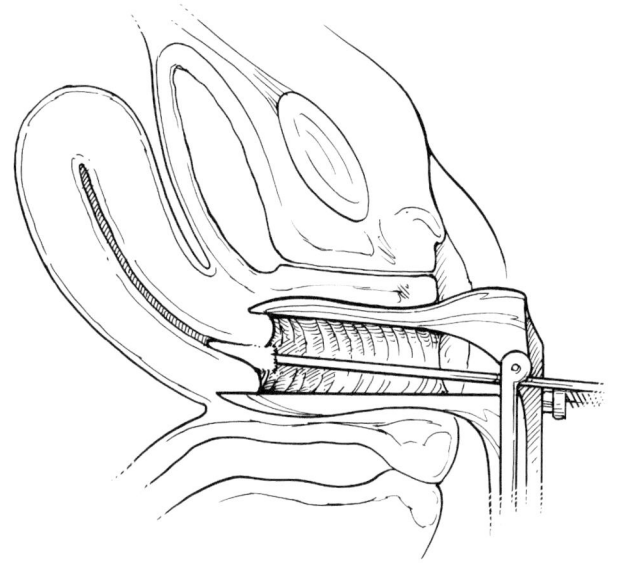

3. Rotate a wooden cervical spatula 360 degrees around the external os to obtain scraping from the squamocolumnar junction, and then roll onto the same or second slide, depending on the requirements of the cytopathologist.

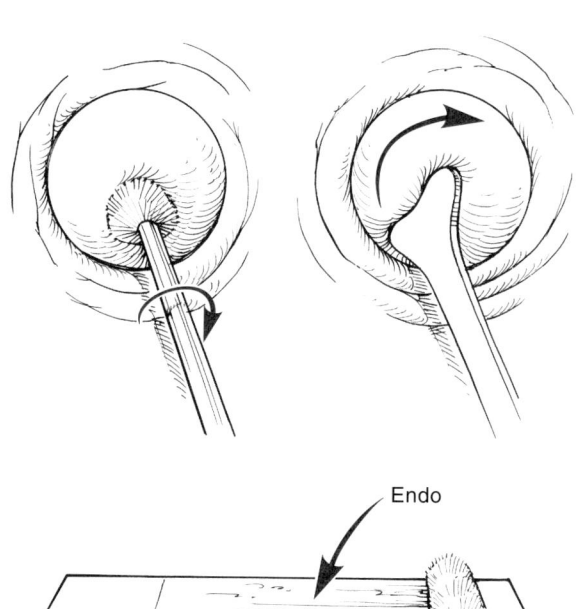

Endo

Exo

4. The slides must be fixed within 10 seconds or there will be drying artifacts.
5. Include with your slides all pertinent clinical information, such as patient age, last menstrual period, type of contraceptive, and any previous diagnosis or treatment (e.g., biopsy, laser, radiation therapy, etc.).

Follow-Up

1. Forewarn the patient that she may experience some spotty vaginal bleeding.
2. Follow-up is indicated to inform the patient of the cytologic analysis. An appropriate appointment for the patient must be made if the results are abnormal.

B | Bibliography

Committee on Gynecologic Practice: Routine cancer screening. ACOG Committee Opinion 1993;128.

Fink DJ: Change in American Cancer Society checkup guidelines for detection of cervical cancer. CA 1988;38:127–128.

Gall SA: Pap smears. Do them right and every year—forever. Postgrad Med 1989;85:235–239.

Kurman RJ: Cervical cytology: Evaluation and management of abnormalities. ACOG Tech Bull 1993;183.

U.S. Preventive Services Task Force: Screening for cervical cancer. Am Fam Physician 1990;41:853–857.

Procedure **COLPOSCOPY**   *Gary Newkirk*

Indications

1. A Papanicoloau (Pap) smear indicating dysplasia, persistent or unexplained atypia, or human papilloma virus infection
2. An observed abnormality of the cervix, vagina, or vulva
3. A history of known intrauterine diethylstilbestrol (DES) exposure

Contraindications

1. Active cervicitis
2. Heavy menses
3. Inability of patient to cooperate

Preparation

1. Signed informed consent
2. Pregnancy test as necessary
3. Midcycle time ideal (avoid menses)

Equipment

1. Colposcope

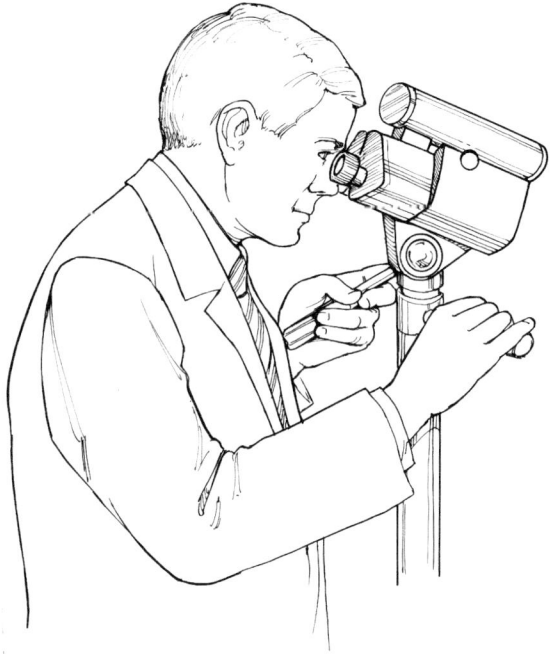

2. Vaginal and endocervical (Kogan) speculum
3. Biopsy forceps (Tischler or Kevorkian)
4. Endocervical curette (Kevorkian without basket)
5. 5% acetic acid, Lugol's solution (concentrated iodine), Monsel's paste (ferrous subsulfate), normal saline
6. Specimen bottles
7. Q-Tips, swabs
8. Pap, KOH, culture devices

Anesthesia

Optional, topical 20% benzocaine syrup (Hurricaine)

Precautions

1. Endocervical curettage is contraindicated in pregnancy.
2. Patients who require SBE prophylaxis may require antibiotics.

Technique

1. Perform careful bimanual examination.
2. Insert appropriate-sized speculum to visualize cervix.
3. Remove heavy mucus; examine the vaginal fornices and cervix for abnormal mucosa and vessel patterns.
4. Obtain KOH, cultures, Pap smear as necessary.
5. Apply normal saline to highlight vessel abnormalities.
6. Apply 5% acetic acid.

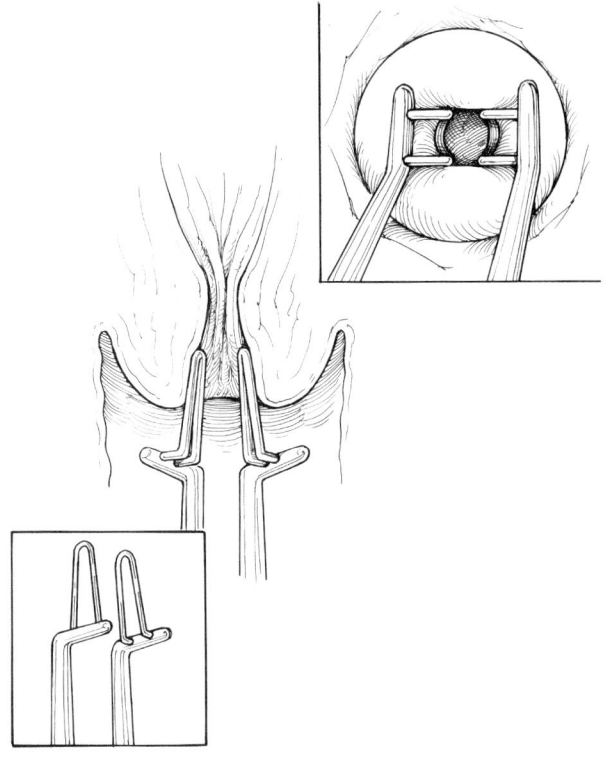

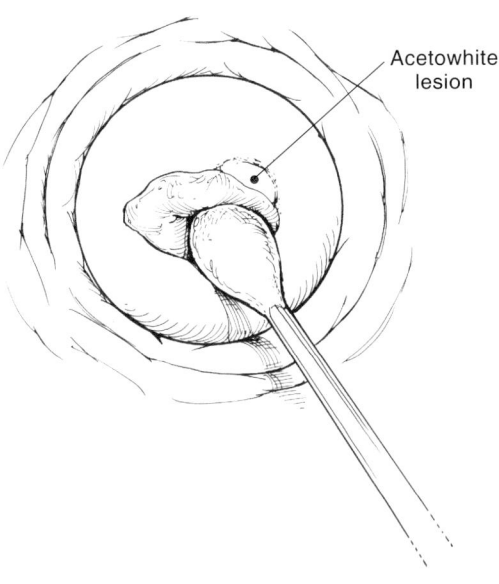

Acetowhite lesion

9. Apply Lugol's solution (optional)
10. Perform endocervical curettage (nonpregnant only).

7. Perform colposcopic examination; note abnormal areas.
   a. Normal colposcopic findings
      (1) Original squamous epithelium
      (2) Columnar epithelium
      (3) Transformation zone
      (4) Squamous metaplasia
      (5) Squamocolumnar junction
   b. Abnormal colposcopic findings
      (1) Leukoplakia (white lesion without solutions)
      (2) Acetowhite epithelium (see above)
      (3) Punctuation
      (4) Mosaic pattern
      (5) Abnormal blood vessels
   c. Other colposcopic findings
      (1) Vaginocervicitis
      (2) Epithelial erosion
      (3) Atrophic epithelium
      (4) Gross cervical condylomata
      (5) Nabothian cysts
8. Inspect endocervical canal for disease (use Kogan's speculum).

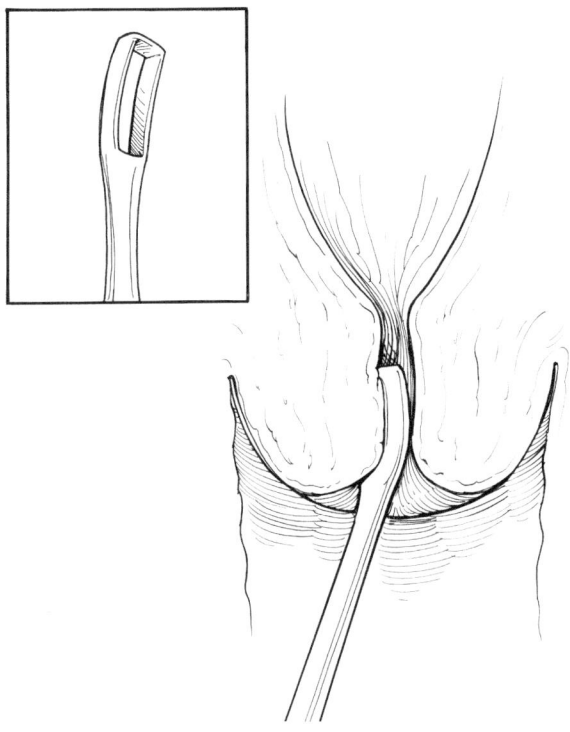

11. Perform cervical biopsies; place samples in bottles.

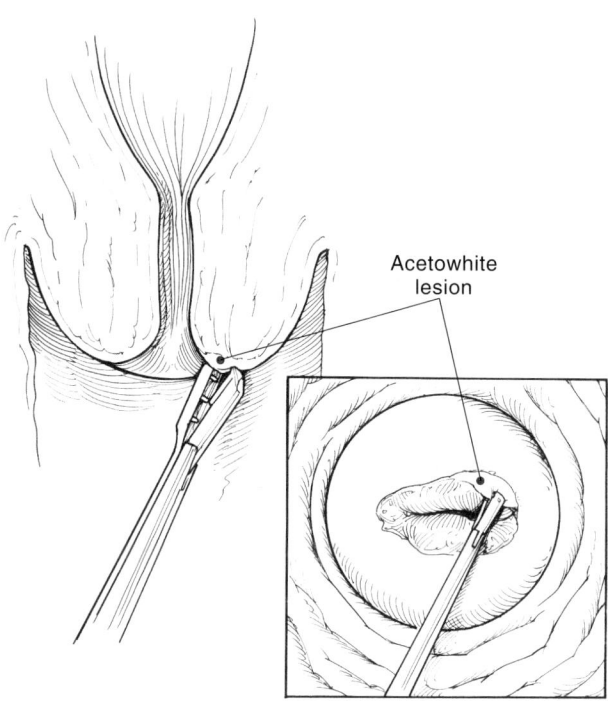

Acetowhite lesion

12. Apply Monsel's paste to control bleeding as needed.
13. Examine the vagina and vulva for abnormal areas; obtain biopsy as necessary.

14. Produce written diagram of findings and biopsy sites.
15. Complete pathology requisition forms.

Follow-Up

1. Advise patient to avoid tampons and intercourse for 5 days.
2. Patient is advised to return for excessive bleeding, odor, discharge, pain, or fever.
3. Discuss histologic pathology report when available.
4. Recommend treatment as indicated by pathology.

Bibliography

Anderson MC, et al: A Text and Atlas of Integrated Colposcopy. St. Louis, Mosby–Year Book, 1991.

Burghardt E: Colposcopy, Cervical Pathology: Textbook and Atlas. New York, Thieme Medical Publishers, 1991.

Campion MJ, Ferris DG, di Paola FM, Reid R, Miller MD: Modern Colposcopy: A Practical Approach. Augusta, Georgia, Educational Systems, 1991.

Cartier R: Practical Colposcopy. Stuttgart and New York, Fischer, 1988.

Newkirk GR: The colposcopic examination. In Pfenninger JL, Fowler GC (eds): Procedures for Primary Care Physicians. St. Louis, Mosby–Year Book, 1994, pp 616–639.

Cervical Biopsy

Indications

A biopsy should be taken from any visible, abnormal lesion on the cervix.

Contraindications

1. Acute pelvic inflammatory disease or acute cervicitis
2. Coagulopathy (biopsy should be performed in a hospital setting)

Preparation

No special preparation of the patient is typically required.

Equipment

1. Cervical biopsy punch (variety of styles and sizes; Kevorkian, Tischler-Morgan, Younge) (see previous Procedure, Colposcopy)
2. 5% acetic acid, Monsel's paste, silver nitrate sticks
3. 10% neutral buffered formalin in appropriately labeled specimen container
4. Iris hook, forceps
5. Cotton-tipped applicators, large and small

Anesthesia

1. No local anesthesia is typically used, although a paracervical block may be performed.
2. A nonsteroidal anti-inflammatory medication may be given prior to the procedure.

Precautions

Patients at risk for subacute bacterial endocarditis should receive appropriate medications beforehand.

Technique

1. Insert the speculum. Apply acetic acid to the cervix to enhance visualization of the lesion.
2. Place the biopsy punch over the lesion. A punch or bite of the lesion is taken and immediately fixed (see preceding Procedure, Colposcopy).
3. Hemostasis is obtained via pressure, application of Monsel's paste, or cautery with silver nitrate.

Follow-Up

1. Patients are instructed to place nothing in the vagina (e.g., no douching, tampons, sex) for two weeks.
2. Patients should be seen for persistent bleeding or malodorous discharge.

LEEP (*L*oop *E*lectrical *E*xcision *P*rocedure)

Indications

1. LEEP is a treatment option for cervical intraepithelial neoplasia (CIN) that entirely excises the cervical lesion and transformation zone (TZ). Current passes through a thin wire loop electrode for excision.
2. LEEP can be used as a type of cervical conization procedure.
3. LEEP may be used to treat or remove superficial benign lesions (e.g., verrucae, nevi, keratoses).
4. Advantages of LEEP include
   a. Simultaneous diagnosis and treatment of a cervical lesion during a single office visit
   b. Allowing the diagnosis of microinvasive or invasive disease missed by cytology or colposcopy
   c. Excellent patient acceptance (outpatient procedure, local anesthesia, minimal bleeding)
   d. Easily incorporated into office practice; short excision time; reasonable set-up cost
   e. Removing versus destroying tissue; the histologic specimen has minimal thermal damage

Contraindications

1. Pregnancy
2. Acute cervicitis
3. Suspected invasive or microinvasive cancer
4. Abnormal Pap test without a biopsy confirmation or a colposcopically clear-cut CIN lesion
5. Coagulopathy

Preparation

1. Various options should be discussed with the patient and informed consent obtained.
2. Good colposcopic skills are required to identify the TZ, presence of disease, and complications.
3. Experience at a "hands-on" course prior to performing LEEP is highly recommended.

Equipment

1. Electrosurgical generator (with coagulate, cut and blend modes) and a hand or foot switch
2. Loop and ball electrodes (available in a variety of sizes)
3. Patient grounding pad
4. *Nonconductive* instruments (e.g., speculum, vaginal wall retractor, forceps, hooks)
5. Smoke evacuator, tubing, and filter system
6. Colposcope
7. 5% acetic acid, Lugol's iodine solution, Monsel's paste
8. 2% Xylocaine with epinephrine (1:100,000); 27-gauge needles with extender or dental syringe
9. 10% neutral buffered formalin in container, pathology cassette for tissue specimen
10. Large GYN or rectal swabs
11. Consent form, postprocedure information sheet
12. If needed: endocervical curette (for endocervical curettage [ECC]), long needle holder, and 2-0 Vicryl (for suturing)

Anesthesia

Infiltrate the cervix superficially with a total of 3 to 5 ml Xylocaine at four to eight positions (3, 6, 9, and 12 o'clock and spaces between) at a distance of 3 mm beyond the TZ. A paracervical block is not needed.

Precautions

1. Patients can unintentionally be shocked or burned at a number of sites due to
   a. Inadvertent contact with the active electrode
   b. Inadequate patient contact with the ground pad
   c. Conduction through alternative sites (via uninsulated stirrups or instruments)

2. The smoke evacuator must be used and attached to the speculum.
   a. This helps to provide an unobstructed view.
   b. Viral particles in the plume are potentially contagious.

3. A depth of 5 mm or less at the 3 and 9 o'clock positions avoids cervical branches of the uterine arteries, which may bleed significantly. A depth of 7 to 8 mm is desirable at the center of the biopsy.

4. Cervical stenosis can occasionally occur and is more common in postmenopausal women.

5. Secondary infections are rare, occurring in one to three weeks, and respond to appropriate antibiotics.

LEEP

Technique

1. Obtain consent, place the patient in lithotomy position with the ground pad applied and insert the insulated speculum. Use the vaginal sidewall retractor as needed.

2. Stain the cervix with acetic acid to delineate the lesion, then with Lugol's solution to delineate the TZ.

3. Anesthetize the cervix with Xylocaine as described above.

4. Select the proper-sized loop based on the size of the TZ (a 20-mm wide by 8-mm deep loop is often adequate for a simple excision). Insert the loop onto the electrode handle.

6. Moisten the cervix with acetic acid before the excision.

7. Turn on the generator to the blended mode. Turn on the vacuum.

8. Begin 3 to 5 mm lateral to the TZ and apply pressure to the loop to push it perpendicularly into the tissue to a depth of 5 to 8 mm (or until the loop crossbar is reached).

9. Draw the loop across and underneath the tissue to 3 to 5 mm beyond the TZ on the opposite side. Bring the loop straight up and out of the tissue. (If the loop stalls during a pass, stop, turn off the unit, and remove and clean the loop. Reposition it and begin where you left off to complete the pass.)

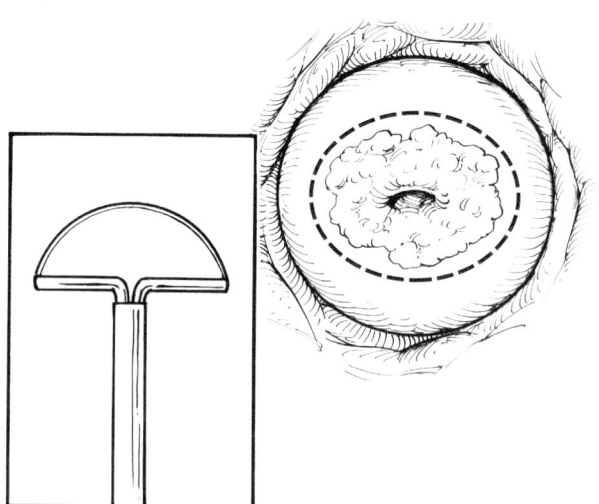

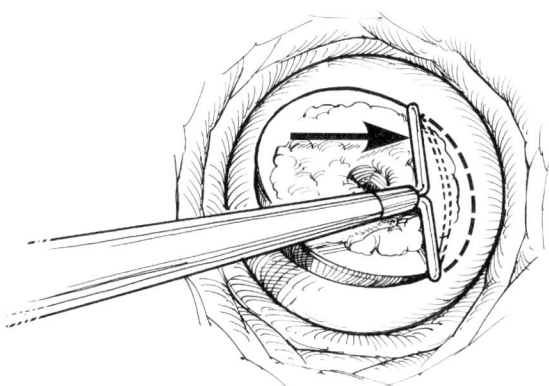

10. If a single pass does not encompass the entire TZ, it can be excised in several transverse strips.

11. Remove the tissue from the cervix, and mark it for orientation in a pathology cassette. Place in formalin. (See following page.)

12. Perform an ECC as indicated.

13. Insert the ball electrode into the handle. Set the electrosurgical generator to coagulation and lightly fulgurate the entire crater base. Treat all bleeding points. Spare the external os as much as possible.

5. Make a test pass without power to ensure that loop chosen is the correct size and the vaginal walls are clear. Move either from side to side, top to bottom, or bottom to top, but avoid a backhanded pass.

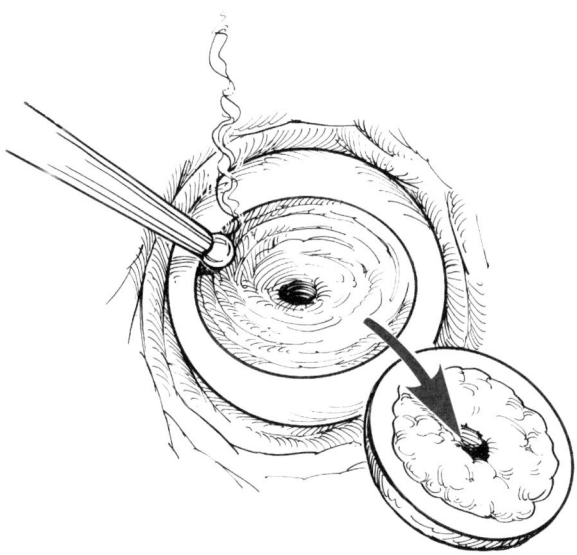

14. Apply a thick layer of Monsel's paste to the tissues. Remove the speculum after the bleeding has stopped. (Incidence of perioperative bleeding is approximately 1 per cent.)

15. A cone biopsy can be performed with a two-step LEEP approach. (See references for more detail.)

Follow-Up

1. An information sheet should make patients aware that
   a. Abdominal cramps may occur for a day or two.
   b. Brownish discharge will last for several weeks.
   c. No heavy lifting is recommended for 4 weeks.
   d. Nothing should be placed in the vagina for 4 weeks.
   e. The physician should be contacted in case of heavy bleeding or malodorous discharge.

2. Bleeding for more than a week should be evaluated. Heavy postoperative bleeding may occur several days to 3 weeks after the procedure. Treat with fulguration or Monsel's. Hospitalization is rare.

3. Patients should return for follow-up 6 months after the LEEP for colposcopy, Pap smear, and ECC.

Bibliography

Apgar BS, Wright TC, Pfenninger JL: Loop electrosurgical excision procedure for CIN. Am Fam Physician 1992;46(2):505–520.

Bloss JD: The use of electrosurgical techniques in the management of premalignant diseases of the vulva, vagina, and cervix: An excisional rather than an ablative approach. Am J Obstet Gynecol 1993;169(5):1081–1085.

Bonardi R, Cecchini S, Grazzini G, Ciatto S: Loop electrosurgical excision procedure of the transformation zone and colposcopically directed punch biopsy in the diagnosis of cervical lesions. Obstet Gynecol 1992;80(6):1020–1022.

Wright TC, Richart RM, Ferenczy A: Electrosurgery for HPV-Related Diseases of the Lower Genital Tract: A Practical Handbook for Diagnosis and Treatment by Loop Electrosurgical Excision and Fulguration Procedures. New York, Arthur Vision, 1992.

Wright TC, Gagnon S, Richart RM, Ferenczy A: Treatment of cervical intraepithelial neoplasia using the loop electrosurgical excision procedure. Obstet Gynecol 1992;79(2):173–178.

99 Endometrial Cancer

E. J. Mayeaux, Jr.

Etiology

1. Related to the amount of estrogen stimulation and endometrial hyperplasia
2. Risk factors:
   a. Age
      (1) Seventy-five per cent of cases occur after menopause, with peak incidence in the late 60s.
      (2) Relative risk at age less than 60 years = 5.2
   b. Obesity—especially upper body fat
      (1) May be secondary to increased estrogen production and bioavailability
      (2) Relative risk of obesity = 3 to 10
   c. Polycystic ovary disease relative risk = 5.2
   d. Unopposed exogenous estrogen:
      (1) Relative risk = 2 to 14
      (2) When progestins are added (oral contraceptives or with replacement therapy), relative risk is less than that for the general population. Relative risk = 0.5 to 1
   e. Diabetes (all types grouped); relative risk = 2.8
   f. Associated with a personal or family history of ovarian or breast cancer. Women who are overweight and have had breast cancer are at even greater risk.
   g. Nulliparity—higher risk than parous women. Relative risk = 1.3
   h. Late menopause—relative risk if person enters menopause after age 52 = 2.5

Symptoms

1. Postmenopausal bleeding:
   a. Prevalence of cancer may be as high as a third of cases.
   b. The presence of uterine myomas should *not* delay appropriate workup.
2. Metrorrhagia—any nonmenstrual or intermenstrual bleeding
3. Lower abdominal pain or pressure (approximately 10 per cent of cases)
4. Rare—back pain or lower extremity edema secondary to metastasis

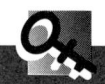

Key Symptom

• Postmenopausal bleeding is endometrial cancer until proven otherwise!

Clinical Findings

1. Most commonly, patient has normal findings on examination of vagina, uterus, and cervix.
2. Advanced disease is associated with enlarged uterus or pelvic mass.
3. Cervical and vaginal metastasis can cause cervical stenosis, pyometra, or a mucosanguineous vaginal discharge.
4. Regional metastasis may present as a bladder or rectal mass.

Key Signs

Most commonly, vaginal, uterine, and cervical examination findings are normal.

Laboratory Tests

1. Endometrial biopsy (EMB)—in-office first-line procedure
   a. Provides an adequate sample for diagnosis in 90 to 95 per cent of cases
   b. Newer methods produce equally good samples with little pain.
2. Dilatation and curettage (D&C) allow more extensive sampling.
   a. Higher sensitivity than endometrial biopsy (especially with smaller in situ lesions). Often used when EMB is inadequate or dysfunctional uterine bleeding (DUB) treatment fails
   b. When combined with endometrial biopsy, detection rate approaches 100 per cent.
   c. Fractional D&C required for staging of occult cancer.
3. Transvaginal uterine ultrasonography—still experimental
   a. New technique shows promise, especially in high-risk patients.
   b. Endometrial thickness less than 6 mm—rarely associated with cancer
4. Hysteroscopy with directed biopsy
   a. Probably more sensitive than fractional D&C
   b. May become required for staging of occult cancer
   c. May often be performed in the office setting
5. On routine Pap smear, may occasionally be detected as "endometrial cells"
   a. Unreliable for screening—less than 40 per cent of cancers will be detected on Pap smear
   b. Pap smear rarely detects endometrial hyperplasia.

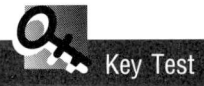

Key Test

- Endometrial biopsy

Differential Diagnosis

Other causes of postmenopausal bleeding or DUB include:

1. Endometrial hyperplasia. May be a precurser of endometrial cancer
   a. Related to estogen stimulation
   b. Risk of progression to endometrial cancer is 5 to 30 per cent depending on severity.
2. Anovulatory dysfunctional uterine bleeding may be hormonal (premenopausal) or related to menopause.
3. Endometrial or endocervical polyps
4. Cervicitis or cervical cancer
5. Atrophic vaginitis
6. Uterine fibroids

Treatment

1. Extrafascial total abdominal hysterectomy with wide vaginal cuff. Usually with salpingo-oophorectomy and retroperitoneal lymph node sampling
2. With cervical involvement, radical hysterectomy with salpingo-oophorectomy and retroperitoneal lymph node dissection
3. Radiation may be used in the uterine cavity or externally before surgery, especially in grade 3 or greater lesions. Radiation also is used for recurrences.

Medication

1. Continuous nonestrogenic progesterone derivatives usually are used with advanced or recurrent disease. Reassess response every 3 months.
2. Hydroxyprogesterone caproate 1 gm per week intramuscularly
3. Medroxyprogesterone acetate 500 mg per week intramuscularly

TABLE 99–1. SIMPLIFIED DEFINITIONS FOR FIGO STAGES AND PROGNOSIS WITH CORRECT TREATMENT

CLASSIFICATION	DESCRIPTION	5-YEAR SURVIVAL
Stage 0	Atypical endometrial hyperplasia or carcinoma-in-situ	100%
Stage 1	Carcinoma confined to the uterine corpus	73%
a	Length of uterine cavity ≤ 8 centimeters	
b	Length of uterine cavity > 8 centimeters	
Stage 2	Carcinoma involves corpus and cervix but has not extended outside the uterus	55%
Stage 3	Carcinoma extends outside the uterus but has not extended outside the true pelvis	28%
Stage 4	Carcinoma extends beyond the true pelvis or obviously involves the mucosa of the bladder or rectum	8.7%
a	Spread to adjacent organs such as bladder or rectum	
b	Spread to distant organs	

Patient Education

1. Emphasize importance of follow-up monitoring. (prognosis related to stage—5-year survival rates are shown in Table 99–1)
2. Risks and benefits of estrogen use should be explained to patients.

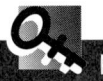

Key Treatment

- Abdominal hysterectomy
- Drugs for advanced or recurrent disease: radiation, chemotherapy, and/or continuous nonestrogenic progesterone derivatives

Follow-Up

1. Follow-up every 2 months for the first year after treatment, 3 months for the second year, 4 months for the third year, 4 months for the fourth year, 6 months for the fifth year, and then annually
   a. A careful pelvic examination should be performed with emphasis on the vaginal apex and sidewalls.
   b. Ask about any associated symptoms, especially bowel and bladder symptoms.
2. Breast examinations should be done by the physician every 6 months.
   a. The patient should perform monthly breast self-examinations.
   b. Mammograms should be performed annually.
3. Cytologic smears from the vaginal apex should be taken every 6 months for 5 years and then annually.
4. A plastic vaginal dilator may be necessary, especially when radiation has been used.
5. Sexual intercourse is permissible once healing is complete. Additional vaginal lubrication may be necessary.
6. It was once dogma that estrogen use was contraindicated after endometrial cancer.
   a. Several studies have shown no increase in recurrences with estrogen therapy.
   b. Currently, ACOG allows for its use based on prognostic indicators and the risk the patient is willing to assume.

 Bibliography

For more information on screening for endometrial and other gynecologic cancers, see

Campion MJ, Reid R: Screening for gynecologic cancer. Obstet Gynecol Clin North Am 1990;17:695–727.

For more information on endometrial cancer, see

Gilman CJ: Management of early-stage endometrial carcinoma. Am Fam Physician 1987;35:103–112.

Gronoos M, Salmi TA, Vuento MH, et al: Mass screening for endometrial cancer directed in risk groups of patients with diabetes and patients with hypertension. Cancer 1993; 71:1279–1282.

Averette HE, Steren A, Nguyen HN: Screening in gynecologic cancers. Cancer 1993;72:1043–1049.

For more information on estrogen use after treatment for endometrial cancer, see

Creaseman WT: Adenocarcinoma of the uterine corpus. Curr Opin Obstet Gynecol 1992;5:80–83.

100 Dysfunctional Uterine Bleeding
Lili Church

Etiology

1. Dysfunctional uterine bleeding (DUB) is defined as the bleeding manifestations of anovulatory cycles.
2. In a normal menstrual cycle, the endometrial lining is built up during the initial proliferatory phase due primarily to the effects of estrogen. Ovulation then occurs midcycle, followed by the secretory phase during which the endometrial lining further develops and stabilizes owing to the combined effect of both estrogen and progesterone. If ovulation does not occur, unopposed estrogen continues to stimulate the endometrial lining, causing it to thicken abnormally. In the relative absence of progesterone, however, this thickened lining is relatively unstable and results in intermittent partial sloughing of the endometrial lining.
3. Causes of DUB resulting from a thickened endometrium include:
   a. Perimenopause
   b. Puberty
   c. Polycystic ovarian disease (PCOD, or Stein-Leventhal syndrome)
   d. Obesity
   e. Unopposed estrogen replacement therapy
4. Another pattern of anovulatory cycles causing DUB occurs when estrogen is low relative to progesterone. This results in a thin and unstable endometrial lining that similarly is prone to irregular bleeding. Causes of DUB resulting from a thinned endometrium include:
   a. Progestins
      (1) Progesterone-only "minipill"
      (2) Depo-Provera
      (3) Norplant
   b. Some low-estrogen combination oral contraceptive pills (OCPs)

Symptoms

1. Dysfunctional bleeding pattern is typically amenorrhea with infrequent periods of heavy flow. In general, women whose DUB is caused by a thickened endometrium will have heavier bleeding and are at risk for acute hemorrhage. While women with a thin endometrium similarly have irregular and unpredictable bleeding, the actual blood loss is usually small, and the blood loss is usually inconvenient rather than dangerous and requires no treatment.
2. Another risk of untreated anovulation is endometrial cancer. Endometrium that is chronically stimulated with a relative excess of estrogen is prone to develop proliferative hyperplasia. This may further progress into adenomatous hyperplasia and eventually endometrial cancer.

Key Symptoms

- Irregular heavy periods
- Intermittent spotting

Clinical Findings

Clinical presentation may be acute or chronic.
1. Acutely, it may present with:
   a. Orthostatic changes in blood pressure and heart rate
   b. Pallor
   c. Vagina—large amount of blood in vault rapidly replaced with ongoing bleeding from cervical os
   d. Uterus—normal or enlarged (retained clots)
2. Chronically:
   a. Stable blood pressure and heart rate
   b. Body habitus—may reflect underlying obesity or stigmata of polycystic ovarian disease
   c. Skin—pale or normal
   d. Vagina—small amount or absence of blood
   e. Uterus—normal

Key Signs

- Pale skin
- Vaginal bleeding

Laboratory Tests

Tests obtained are individualized to each case but may include:
1. Pregnancy test
2. Hematocrit
3. Pap smear
4. Cervical cultures
5. Endometrial biopsy
6. Prothrombin time, partial thromboplastin time, platelets
7. Luteining hormone, follicle-stimulating hormone, thyroid function tests, prolactin, testosterone
8. Hysteroscopy
9. Ultrasound

Key Tests

- Hematocrit
- Pregnancy test
- Endometrial biopsy

Differential Diagnosis

There are many other causes of abnormal uterine bleeding in addition to anovulatory cycling. These must be assessed for and excluded before a patient is diagnosed to have DUB. This is accomplished by taking a careful history with particular attention to the timing and characteristics of the bleeding pattern, performing a physical examination, and utilizing individualized laboratory tests.

1. Hormonal
   a. Anovulation, that is, DUB (puberty, perimenopause, anorexia, extreme stress, obesity, hypothyroidism, prolactinoma, PCOD)
   b. Breakthrough bleeding on combination or progesterone-only OCPs (Depo-Provera, Norplant, estrogen replacement therapy or hormone replacement therapy)
2. Anatomic and physiologic
   a. Cancer (cervical, endometrial, ovarian)
   b. Polyps (cervical, endometrial)
   c. Uterine fibroids (usually submucosal)
   d. Pregnancy (miscarriage, ectopic, mole)
   e. Ovulation
   f. Postpartum (retained placental tissue, atony, subinvolution)
3. Infectious
   a. Cervicitis (e.g., chlamydia)
   b. Endometritis (e.g., postpartum)
   c. Pelvic inflammatory disease (PID) (e.g., gonococcal)
4. Hematologic—bleeding diathesis (e.g., idiopathic thrombocytopenic purpura, hemophilia)

Treatment

1. Treatment is determined by the severity and chronicity of bleeding.
   a. Acute treatment—required if the patient is hemorrhaging, with anemia present or predictable. Treatment options include:
      (1) Combination OCPs q.i.d. for 7 days
      (2) Combination OCP q.i.d. for 2 days, then t.i.d. for 2 days, then q day until 21-day pack is completed. (Then expect heavy bleeding several days after stopping pills. Warn the patient of this!)
      (3) Intravenous Premarin 25 mg q 4 hr (Note: Estrogen is indicated when the patient has had prolonged hemorrhaging resulting in a very thin and friable endometrial lining.)
      (4) Dilation and curettage (only when above fails)
   b. Subacute treatment—acute bleeding episode has already been controlled. If the endometrium is still estimated to be overall thickened, continued but controlled shedding is indicated with such treatment as combination OCP for 3 months. Many patients then resume normal ovulatory menstrual cycling on their own without further need for hormonal regulation. However, a significant number re-develop anovulation with resultant DUB and require chronic treatment.
   c. Chronic treatment—chronic treatment usually is required when the patient has an underlying predisposing cause (perimenopausal) that results in ongoing abnormal bleeding. Treatment is aimed both at preventing complications of chronic blood loss and preventing endometrial cancer. This is accomplished by regularly hormonally shedding (or surgically eliminating) the endometrial lining. Choice of treatment additionally depends on whether contraception is also desired. Options include:
      (1) Combination OCPs
      (2) Regular progestin cycling
         (a) Provera 10 mg, days 1–10 q month
         (b) Provera 10 mg, days 1–10 q 3 months
         (c) Other progestins include Norlutin 5 mg and Micronor 2 mg (same timing as Provera)
      (3) Endometrial ablation
      (4) Hysterectomy (last resort)

Key Treatment

- Combination oral contraceptive pills
- Estrogen
- Provera

Follow-Up

Close follow-up for DUB is important for both its acute and chronic presentations. DUB can be a recurrent problem for which patient education is particularly crucial. Treatment goals include:

1. Control DUB symptoms.
2. Treat anemia, if present, with dietary and/or supplementary oral iron if indicated. Monitor for initial normalization of hematocrit and whether further chronic maintenance iron is required.
3. Identify underlying cause of DUB.
4. Monitor for treatment effectiveness, compliance, and side effects.
5. Change therapy as treatment goals change, as with need for concurrent contraception.
6. Work with patients to develop mutual treatment goals.
7. Educate patients about warning symptoms and when to seek medical advice.
8. Consult gynecologist for DUB that remains unexplained or unresponsive to hormonal therapy.

Bibliography

For more information on dysfunctional uterine bleeding, see

Buletti C, Flamigni C, Prefetto RA, et al: Dysfunctional uterine bleeding. Ann NY Acad Sci 1994;734:80–90.

Fraser IS: Menorrhagia—a pragmatic approach to the understanding of causes and the need for investigations. Br J Obstet Gynaecol 1994 (Suppl) 11:3–7.

Rakel RE, (ed.): Conn's Current Therapy. Philadelphia, WB Saunders, 1995.

Shaw RW: Assessment of medical treatments for menorrhagia. Br J Obstet Gynaecol 1994 (Suppl)11:15–18.

Speroff L, Glass RH, Kase NG: Clinical Gynecologic Endocrinology and Infertility, 5th ed. Baltimore, Williams & Wilkins, 1994.

Procedure | ENDOMETRIAL BIOPSY

Louise S. Acheson

Indications

Usually performed to rule out endometrial cancer or hyperplasia.

1. Suspected anovulatory cycles and unopposed estrogen effect
2. Dysfunctional uterine bleeding in women over age 35
3. Postmenopausal bleeding
4. Abnormal bleeding in women on estrogen and progesterone or tamoxifen
5. Periodically when unopposed estrogen has been prescribed for a woman with a uterus
6. Pap smear with normal endometrial cells in a postmenopausal woman or during the latter half of the cycle in a premenopausal woman
7. After treatment for endometrial hyperplasia
8. Postmenopausal women with fluid in endometrial cavity on ultrasound
9. As part of workup for infertility or recurrent miscarriages, sample on day 25 to 26 to test for a luteal phase defect.

Contraindications

1. Acute pelvic infection
2. Pregnancy
3. Bleeding disorders
4. Circumstances when dilation and curettage (D&C) or hysteroscopy is preferable:
   a. Abnormal uterine anatomy
   b. Inability to accomplish office endometrial aspiration
   c. Endometrial hyperplasia that did not respond to treatment
   d. Pap smear with atypical or suspicious endometrial cells

Preparation

1. Timing: late luteal phase if cycling
2. Premedication may be helpful: nonsteroidal anti-inflammatory drug 1 hour beforehand

3. Obtain informed consent.

Equipment

1. Endometrial sampling devices: When successful, all have equivalent yield of endometrial neoplasms.
   a. Flexible 3-mm plastic cannula (e.g., Pipelle from Unimar, Wilton, CT, or Z-Sampler from Zinnanti, Chatsworth, CA)
   b. Rigid 3-mm cannula with syringe for suction (e.g., Explora, Tis-U-Trap from Milex)
   c. Rigid cannula with mechanical suction (e.g., Vabra aspirator from Berkeley Medevices attached to electric suction pump)
   d. Less discomfort and risk from flexible aspiration devices
   e. Use 3-mm rigid cannula if unable to pass flexible one. Have both types available.
2. Other equipment for the procedure
   a. Vaginal speculum and light
   b. Pap smear sampling devices
   c. Endocervical curette
   d. Ring forceps
   e. Large swabs or small gauze with prep solution
   f. Tenaculum
   g. Uterine sound (usually unnecessary)
   h. Scissors
   i. Specimen containers with fixative (formalin)

Anesthesia

1. Usually none
2. Paracervical anesthesia used rarely for exceptional cases (e.g., stenotic os)

Precautions

1. Consider a pregnancy test before endometrial sampling in premenopausal women.
2. Those at risk for bacterial endocarditis should have prophylactic antibiotics.

Technique

1. Bimanual examination: Ascertain axis of endometrial cavity, uterine size and contour, and adnexae.
2. Examine vulva, vagina, and cervix. Obtain Pap smear with endocervical sampling to rule out extrauterine causes of abnormal bleeding.
3. Cleanse the cervix with Betadine, Zephiran, or other antibacterial solution using large swabs or ring forceps and gauze.

4. Warn the patient of impending discomfort, usually "cramping."
5. Attempt to pass the flexible cannula through the internal cervical os. If this is unsuccessful, stabilize the cervix by grasping the anterior or posterior lip with a tenaculum and exert gentle countertraction.
6. With steady, controlled pressure, insert the flexible or rigid cannula through the internal cervical os to the depth of the endometrial cavity (typically 7 cm).

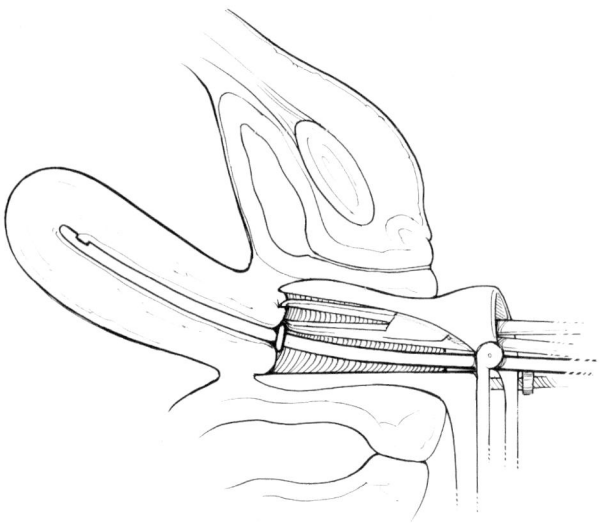

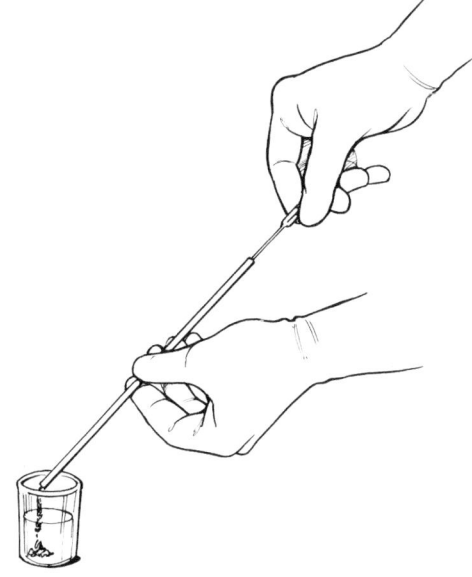

7. Flexible cannula (Pipelle or Z-Sampler):

  a. Apply suction by withdrawing the plunger most of the way. Do not allow the hole in the tip to emerge from the uterine cavity during aspiration, or all suction will be lost.

  b. Rotate the cannula at least 360 degrees while moving it from side to side and gradually withdrawing it almost to the internal os. The area sampled will be a spiral. Make more than one pass in this fashion until the cannula is full or no more tissue enters the cannula.

  c. If it is full, continue the aspiration with a new Pipelle or Z-Sampler until no more tissue is obtained.

8. Rigid cannula (e.g., Explora):

  a. Apply suction on the attached syringe; lock plunger in position.

  b. Use an in-and-out motion while rotating the cannula, never withdrawing it completely from the endometrial cavity until sampling is complete. (Sample longitudinal strips of endometrium.)

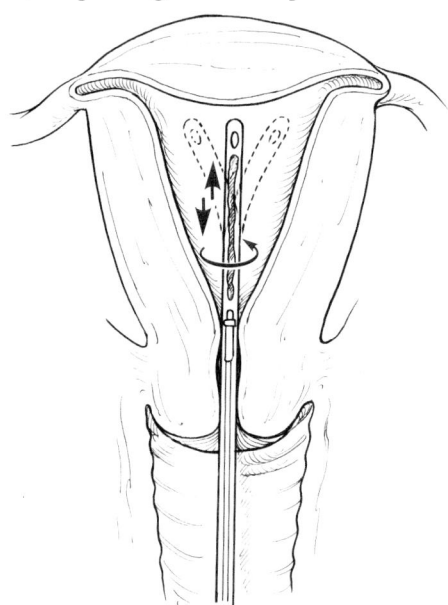

9. Using scissors, cut off the distal tip of the flexible cannula (rigid cannulas do not need to be cut). Expel the tissue sample into a container of fixative, and send it for histologic examination.

10. If a tenaculum was used, remove it and apply pressure to the site until hemostasis is achieved.

11. Remove the speculum.

12. Instruct the woman not to insert anything into her vagina for about 3 days and to contact you for hemorrhage, pain, or signs of infection.

Follow-Up

Follow-up depends on the histologic diagnosis.

1. *Insufficient tissue* may indicate *atrophic endometrium:* reassuring if technique was good and suspicion of endometrial cancer low. Transvaginal ultrasound confirming a thin (<5 mm) endometrial stripe is also reassuring. Otherwise, proceed to hysteroscopy.

2. *Proliferative endometrium* indicates unopposed estrogen effect. Cyclic progesterone may be indicated in premenopausal woman with anovulatory cycles.

3. *Endometrial hyperplasia* may be a precursor to endometrial cancer.

  a. *Adenomatous or cystic, without atypia:* usually treated with cyclic or continuous progesterone. Repeat sampling after 2 to 3 months. If hyperplasia has not resolved, a D&C and/or hysteroscopy is indicated.

  b. *Atypical hyperplasia* may be an indication for D&C and/or hysteroscopy, with or without progesterone treatment

4. *Endometrial carcinoma* requires definitive treatment.

5. *Polyp:* usually benign. If found in a *postmenopausal* woman, D&C and/or hysteroscopy indicated because of high incidence of associated endometrial neoplasia.

B Bibliography

Byyny RL, Speroff L: A Clinical Guide for the Care of Older Women. Baltimore, Williams & Wilkins, 1990, pp 87–89.

Chambers JT, Chambers SK: Endometrial sampling: When? Where? Why? With what? Clin Obstet Gynecol 1992;35(1):28–39.

Feldman S, Berkowitz RS, Tosteson ANA: Cost-effectiveness of strategies to evaluate postmenopausal bleeding. Obstet Gynecol 1993;81:968–975.

Kaunitz AM: Endometrial sampling in menopausal patients. Menopausal Med 1993;1(4):5–8.

mortality. Several large-scale prospective trials are under way to determine if screening women at high risk for ovarian cancer based on family history is more effective. Despite lack of conclusive evidence, a consensus panel of the National Institutes of Health has recommended annual pelvic examination, CA 125 levels, and transvaginal pelvic ultrasound as the preferred screening strategy for high-risk women.

   B. Preoperative staging tests in patients with suspected ovarian cancer:

      1. Chest radiograph

      2. Complete blood count and serum chemistry profile

      3. Intravenous pyelogram

      4. Cystoscopy

      5. Proctoscopy

      6. Barium enema

   C. Surgery. A definitive tissue diagnosis is made by histology on a surgical specimen. The specimen is usually obtained at laparotomy, but in selected cases, laparoscopy may be appropriate.

Key Tests

- Pelvic examination
- Serum tumor markers
- Preoperative staging tests
- Pelvic ultrasound
- Color flow Doppler of ovarian vessels
- Surgery

Differential Diagnosis

1. Benign pelvic masses

   a. Functional follicular or corpus luteum cyst

   b. Luteoma of pregnancy

   c. Benign germ cell neoplasm, such as dermoid cyst

   d. Benign mesothelial ovarian tumor, such as serous cystoma or cystadenoma

   e. Ovarian fibroma

   f. Endometriosis

   g. Tubo-ovarian abscess or cyst

2. Other pelvic or abdominal neoplasm

3. Ectopic pregnancy

Treatment

   A. Surgery. All patients with suspected ovarian cancer should undergo laparotomy to accurately diagnose and stage the lesion, debulk the tumor, and relieve any bowel obstruction

   B. Postoperative therapy

      1. Early-stage disease

         a. Stage I (tumor confined to one or both ovaries), grade I (well-differentiated), and selected cases of grade II (moderately differentiated) disease. No further treatment is required. Five-year survival is greater than 90 per cent.

         b. Stage I, grade III; stage II and stage IIIa

            (1) Melphalan (Alkeran)

            (2) Intraperitoneal ^{32}P

            (3) Whole-abdomen radiation therapy

      2. Advanced disease (stages IIIb and IIIc and IV)

         a. First-line therapy: systemic chemotherapy with cisplatin (Platinol) and cyclophosphamide (Cytoxan)

         b. Second-line therapy and alternative agents

            (1) Systemic chemotherapy

               (a) Carboplatin (Paraplatin)

               (b) Paclitaxel (Taxol) and other taxenes

               (c) Ifosfamide (Ifex)

            (2) Intraperitoneal chemotherapy

            (3) Biologic response modifiers

            (4) Autologous bone marrow transplantation

            (5) Hormonal therapy

   C. Palliative therapy

      1. Second debulking surgery

      2. Radiation therapy

      3. Nutritional support

      4. Drainage of ascites or pleural effusions

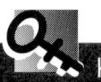

Key Treatment

Drugs of Choice	Alternative Drugs
• Melphalan or ^{32}P (early disease)	• Carboplatin
• Cisplatin and cyclophosphamide (advanced disease)	• Paclitaxel or other taxenes
	• Ifosfamide
• Surgery	• Intraperitoneal chemotherapy
• Radiation therapy	• Hormonal therapy
• Bone marrow transplantation	
• Palliative measures	

Follow-Up

1. "Second look" laparotomy to assess residual disease
2. Serial CA 125 levels

 Bibliography

For more information on epithelial ovarian cancer, see

Mann WJ: Diagnosis and management of epithelial cancer of the ovary. Am Fam Physician 1994;49:613–618.

Runowicz CD: Advances in the screening and treatment of ovarian cancer. CA 1992;42:327–349.

Cannistra SA: Cancer of the ovary. N Engl J Med 1993; 329:1550–1559.

For more information on germ cell tumors of the ovary, see

Gershenson DM: Current status of the management of malignant ovarian germ cell tumors. Cancer Bull 1990;42:93–97.

For more information on hereditary ovarian cancer, see

Lynch HT, Conway T, Lynch J: Hereditary ovarian cancer: pedigree studies, part II. Cancer Genet Cytogenet 1991;52: 161–183.

102 Vaginitis

Carey Vinson

Etiology
1. Bacterial vaginosis—*Gardnerella vaginalis, Mycoplasma hominis, Mobiluncus,* other anaerobes and gram-negative bacteria, not usually sexually transmitted
2. *Candida* vulvovaginitis. *Candida albicans* causes 85 per cent of cases.
3. *Trichomonas* vaginitis—*Trichomonas vaginalis,* flagellated anaerobic protozoan, usually sexually transmitted

Symptoms
1. Bacterial vaginosis—vaginal odor
2. *Candida* vulvovaginitis
   a. Intense itching
   b. Thick, white discharge
3. *Trichomonas* vaginitis
   a. Vaginal odor
   b. Vulvovaginal itching and irritation
   c. Urethral discharge
   d. Dyspareunia

Key Symptoms
- Vaginal itching
- Dysuria
- Vaginal odor
- Increased vaginal discharge
- Change in consistency of vaginal discharge

Clinical Findings
1. Bacterial vaginosis
   a. Positive "whiff" test—fishy odor of volatile amines when discharge mixed with potassium hydroxide
   b. Homogeneous, white, adherent discharge
   c. pH of discharge greater than 4.5
2. *Candida* vulvovaginitis—thick, white discharge
3. *Trichomonas* vaginitis
   a. Vaginal odor
   b. Gray, frothy discharge
   c. Strawberry cervix
   d. pH of discharge greater than 5.0

Key Signs
- Discharge odor: "fishy" = bacterial vaginosis
- Discharge pH: greater than 5.0 = *Trichomonas*

Laboratory Tests
1. Normal saline preparation of vaginal discharge
   a. Bacterial vaginosis—clue cells, epithelial cells studded with bacteria
   b. *Trichomonas* vaginitis—motile trichomonads, more than 10 WBCs per high-power field
2. Potassium hydroxide preparation of discharge. *Candida* vulvovaginitis—hyphae or budding spores
3. Cultures
   a. Sabouraud's or Nickerson's agar—*Candida* vulvovaginitis
   b. Modified Diamond liquid media—*Trichomonas* vaginitis

Key Tests
- Normal saline preparation: clue cells = bacterial vaginosis, motile trichomonads = *Trichomonas* vaginitis.
- Potassium hydroxide preparation: hyphae or budding spores = *Candida* vulvovaginitis.

Differential Diagnosis
1. Atrophic vaginitis
2. Allergic vaginitis
3. Cervicitis

Treatment
1. Bacterial vaginosis
   a. Metronidazole (Flagyl, Protostat), 500 mg orally twice daily for 7 days
   b. Metronidazole gel (MetroGel Vaginal), 5 gm intravaginally twice daily for 5 days
   c. Clindamycin (Cleocin) 2% cream, 5 gm intravaginally once daily for 7 days
   d. Pregnancy: clindamycin, 300 mg orally twice daily for 7 days
2. *Candida* vulvovaginitis
   a. Miconazole

(1) 200-mg suppository (Monistat 3) intravaginally at bedtime for 3 nights

(2) Vaginal cream (Monistat-Derm) 1 applicatorful intravaginally at bedtime for 7 nights or clotrimazole (Gyne-Lotrimin)

(3) 100-mg vaginal tablet intravaginally at bedtime for 7 nights

b. Butoconazole (Femstat) 2% cream, 1 applicatorful intravaginally at bedtime for 3 nights

c. For recurrent or persistent cases: fluconazole (Diflucan), 100 to 150 mg orally 1 time

d. For prophylaxis: clotrimazole (Mycelex-G) 500-mg vaginal tablet intravaginally once each month

e. For pregnancy: clotrimazole, 100-mg vaginal tablet intravaginally at bedtime for 7 nights

3. *Trichomonas* vaginitis

a. Sexual partner will need treatment.

b. Metronidazole (Flagyl, Protostat)

(1) 2 gm orally 1 time

(2) 500 mg orally twice daily for 7 days

(3) For recurrent or persistent cases: 500 mg orally twice daily for 14 days

(4) For pregnancy

(a) First trimester: clotrimazole (Gyne-Lotrimin, 100-mg vaginal tablet intravaginally at bedtime for 7 nights

(b) After first trimester: metronidazole, 2 gm orally 1 time

4. Sulfonamide creams are not reliably effective.

Key Treatment

- Bacterial vaginosis: metronidazole, 500 mg orally twice daily for 7 days
- *Candida* vulvovaginitis: miconazole, 200-mg vaginal suppository intravaginally at bedtime for 3 nights
- *Trichomonas* vaginitis: metronidazole, 2 gm orally 1 time
- Sexual partner needs treatment.

Follow-Up

For *Trichomonas* vaginitis, test for cure, test for other sexually transmitted diseases (VDRL, HIV, chlamydia and gonorrhea cultures)

Bibliography

For more information on vaginitis, see
Reed BD, Eyler A: Vaginal infections: Diagnosis and management. Am Fam Physician 1993;47:1805–1816.

For more information on bacterial vaginosis, see
Sweet RL: New approaches for the treatment of bacterial vaginosis. Am J Obstet Gynecol 1993;169:479–482.

For more information on *Candida* vulvovaginitis, see
Sobel JD: Candidal vulvoginitis. Clin Obstet Gynecol 1993;36:153–165.

For more information on *Trichomonas* vaginitis, see
Heine P, McGregor JA: *Trichomonas* vaginalis: A reemerging pathogen. Clin Obstet Gynecol 1993;36:137–144.

For more information on diagnostic methods, see
Hillier SL: Diagnostic microbiology of bacterial vaginosis. Am J Obstet Gynecol 1993;169:455–459.

103 Cervicitis

Carey Vinson

Etiology

1. *Chlamydia trachomatis* causes 30 to 60 per cent of cases.
2. *Neisseria gonorrhoeae*
3. A primary infection of herpes simplex virus may cause cervicitis along with genital herpes.
4. In up to one third of cases, an etiology cannot be determined.
5. True prevalence is usually underestimated. Cervicitis has been found in 24 to 40 per cent of female patients in sexually transmitted disease (STD) clinics and 34 per cent of patients seen routinely at a university student health clinic.

Symptoms

1. Often, cervicitis is asymptomatic or symptoms are vague, but untreated infection can lead to pelvic inflammatory disease (PID) and infertility
2. An increase in vaginal discharge
3. Vaginal bleeding or spotting, especially postcoital
4. Vague lower abdominal pain
5. Mild dyspareunia
6. Can be confused with vulvovaginitis

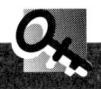
Key Symptoms

- Often asymptomatic
- Increased amount of vaginal discharge
- Postcoital bleeding

Risk Factors

1. Previous treatment for STD
2. New sexual partner
3. Male partner with urethritis

WARNING

- **Cervicitis should be considered an STD.**
- **High risk of spread of infection to sexual partners**
- **Proximal extension of infection can cause endometritis, salpingitis, infertility, chorioamnionitis, and premature rupture of membranes in pregnancy.**

Clinical Findings

1. Cervical ectopy, the appearance of endocervical epithelium on the visible exocervix, is *not* cervicitis and is *not* pathologic.
2. Yellow mucopurulent cervical discharge
3. Cervical os friable, easily produces bleeding
4. Edema of the columnar epithelium

Key Signs

- Cervical os discharge
- Friable cervix

Laboratory Tests

1. Gram's stain of cervical discharge
   a. Positive if more than 10 WBCs per high-power field
   b. Gram-negative intracellular diplococci: gonorrheal cervicitis
2. Thayer-Martin media culture: gonorrheal cervicitis
3. Enzyme-linked immunoassay (ELISA): *Chlamydia* cervicitis
4. Fluorescent monoclonal antibody test for chlamydial antigens: *Chlamydia* cervicitis
5. Nucleic acid hybridization test: *Chlamydia* cervicitis

Key Tests

- Gram's stain of cervical discharge: greater than 10 WBCs per high-power field
- Gram's stain of cervical discharge: gram-negative intracellular diplococci—gonorrhea
- Gonorrhea culture
- Immunoassay test for *Chlamydia*

Differential Diagnosis

1. Nonspecific bacterial vaginosis
2. *Trichomonas* vaginitis

Treatment

1. Sexual partner needs treatment
2. Many patients have simultaneous chlamydial and gonorrheal infections
3. *Chlamydia*
   a. Doxycycline (Vibramycin, Vibra-Tabs, Doryx), 100 mg orally twice daily for 7 days
   b. Azithromycin (Zithromax), 1 gm orally 1 time only

c. Erythromycin base (E-Mycin, Eryc, Ery-Tab), 500 mg orally 4 times daily for 7 days

d. Ofloxacin (Floxin), 300 mg orally twice daily for 7 days

e. Tetracycline (Achromycin V, Sumycin), 500 mg orally 4 times daily for 7 days

f. Pregnancy:

   (1) Erythromycin base, 500 mg orally 4 times daily for 7 days

   (2) Amoxicillin (Amoxil, Wymox), 500 mg orally 3 times daily for 10 days

   (3) Sufisoxazole (Gantrisin), 500 mg orally 4 times daily for 10 days

4. Gonorrhea. Use one of the preceding regimens plus

   a. Ceftriaxone (Rocephin), 125 mg intramuscularly 1 time

   b. Cefixime (Suprax), 400 mg orally 1 time

   c. Ciprofloxacin (Cipro), 500 mg orally 1 time

   d. Ofloxacin (Floxin), 400 mg orally 1 time

   e. Pregnancy. If allergic to β-lactamase, spectinomycin (Trobicin), 2 gm intramuscularly 1 time

Key Treatment

- *Chlamydia* cervicitis: doxycycline, 100 mg orally twice daily for 7 days; sexual partner needs treatment.

- Gonorrheal cervicitis: ceftriaxone, 125 mg intramuscularly 1 time; sexual partner needs treatment.

Follow-Up

1. Test the patient for cure after completion of therapy. Repeat the culture or test that was initially positive.

2. Test for other sexually transmitted diseases.

   a. VDRL test for syphilis

   b. ELISA anti-HIV antibody test for human immunodeficiency virus

   c. Saline wet smear test of vaginal secretions for *Trichomonas* vaginitis

Bibliography

For more information on cervicitis, see
Recommendations for the prevention and management of *Chlamydia trachomatis* infections, 1993. MMWR 1993;42(RR-11):1–36.
Rosenfeld WD, Clark J: Vulvovaginitis and cervicitis. Pediatr Clin North Am 1989;36:489–511.

For more information on chlamydial cervicitis, see
Potts JF: Chlamydial infection screening and management update, 1992. Postgrad Med 1992;91:120–126.

For more information on *Chlamydia* testing, see
Stamm WE: Toward control of sexually transmitted chlamydial infections. Ann Intern Med 1993;114:432–434.

For more information on gonorrhea cervicitis, see
Sparling PF: Gonococcal infections. *In* Wyngaarden JB, Smith LH, Bennett JC (eds): Cecil Textbook of Medicine, 19th ed. Philadelphia, WB Saunders, 1992, pp 1754–1759.

104 Pelvic Inflammatory Disease

Lorena S. Chicoye

Etiology

Pelvic inflammatory disease (PID) is an inflammatory process due to ascending microorganisms into the upper genital tract causing endometritis, oophoritis, parametritis, salpingitis, tubo-ovarian abscess, and pelvic peritonitis. The causative agents are

1. *Chlamydia trachomatis,* which may cause marked inflammation and intraluminal fibrin deposition and may account for damage within the tubes. Hormonal changes (menses, oral contraceptives, age) and mechanical manipulation of the uterus (IUD insertion, douching) may allow breach of the natural barriers and ascent of *Chlamydia.*

2. *Neisseria gonorrhoeae* exhibits the same pathogenesis except with oral contraceptives, which may have some growth-depressant effect secondary to progesterone. *N. gonorrhoeae* are believed to produce an endotoxin that may initiate tubal mucosal destruction.

3. Vaginal aerobes and anaerobes (*Escherichia coli, Haemophilus influenzae, Mycoplasma hominis, Ureaplasma urealyticum*)

Symptoms

Severity and presentation vary widely, including

1. Lower abdominal pain, usually in the week following menstruation
2. Abnormal vaginal discharge
3. Postcoital bleeding
4. Spotting between menstrual periods
5. GI symptoms (nausea, vomiting, and diarrhea)
6. Fever/chills
7. Dysuria
8. Dyspareunia

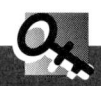

Key Symptoms

- Abdominal pain
- Vaginal discharge

Clinical Findings

1. Lower abdominal pain on palpation, often with rebound tenderness
2. Cervical motion tenderness
3. Adnexal tenderness
4. Adnexal fullness/mass
5. Fever

Key Signs

- Cervical tenderness to motion
- Lower abdominal tenderness with rebound
- Adnexal fullness and tenderness

Laboratory Tests

No laboratory tests are pathognomonic for PID.

1. Laparoscopy is the "gold standard" for diagnosis.
2. Pregnancy test
2. White blood cell (WBC) count greater than 10,500 per cubic millimeter
3. Culdocentesis with leukocytes and bacteria
4. Sedimentation rate greater than 15 mm/hr
5. C-reactive protein
5. Antigen test for *Chlamydia* (positive less than 50 per cent of the time)
6. Gram's stain for *N. gonorrhoeae* (positive less than 50 per cent of the time)
7. Endometrial biopsy to rule out endometritis
8. Pelvic ultrasound to rule out tubo-ovarian abscess

Key Tests

- Laparoscopy
- WBC count

Differential Diagnosis

1. Ectopic pregnancy
2. Appendicitis
3. Chronic pelvic pain
4. Chronic adhesive disease
5. Endometriosis
6. Ovarian torsion
7. Ovarian cysts
8. Irritable bowel syndrome
9. Somatization disorder

Treatment

The threshold for management of PID to prevent associated morbidity must be lowered. Treatment should be initiated within less than 3 days of onset of symptoms, especially when *Chlamydia* is the etiologic agent, to prevent tubal damage and infertility or ectopic pregnancies. Most treatment is performed on an outpatient basis.

Hospitalization is recommended by the Centers for Disease Control and Prevention (CDC) when

1. The diagnosis is uncertain.
2. The possibility of surgical emergencies (ectopic pregnancy or appendicitis) cannot be excluded.
3. A pelvic abscess is suspected.
4. The patient is pregnant.
5. The patient is an adolescent.
6. Severe illness precludes outpatient management.
7. The patient is unable to follow or tolerate an outpatient regimen.
8. The patient has not responded to outpatient therapy.
9. Clinical follow-up cannot be arranged within 72 hours of the initiation of antibiotic therapy.
10. Patient is known to be infected with HIV.

Medication

A. Outpatient
1. Regimen 1: either cefoxitin (Mefoxin), 2 grams intramuscularly in a single dose, plus concomitant probenecid, 1 gm orally, or ceftriaxone (Rocephin), 250 mg intramuscularly, or another third-generation cephalosporin such as ceftizoxime (Cefizox) or cefotaxime (Claforan) plus doxycycline (Vibramycin), 100 mg orally 2 times a day for 14 days.
2. Regimen 2: ofloxacin (Floxin), 400 mg orally 2 times a day for 14 days, plus either clindamycin (Cleocin), 450 mg orally 4 times a day for 14 days, or metronidazole (Flagyl), 500 mg orally 2 times a day for 14 days.

B. Inpatient
1. Regimen 1: cefoxitin, 2 gm intravenously q 6 hr, or cefotetan, 2 gm intravenously q 12 hr, plus doxycycline, 100 mg intravenously or orally q 12 hr. Continue at least 48 hours after substantial clinical improvement, after which doxycycline, 100 mg orally 2 times a day given for a total of 14 days of treatment.
2. Regimen 2: clindamycin, 900 mg intravenously q 8 hr, plus gentamicin, 2 mg/kg of body weight intravenously or intramuscularly (loading dose) followed by 1.5 mg/kg intravenously or intramuscularly q 8 hr (maintenance dose). Continue at least 48 hours after substantial clinical improvement, after which doxycycline, 100 mg orally 2 times a day, or clindamycin, 450 mg orally 4 times a day for a total of 14 days of treatment.

Patient Education

1. Medical management
   a. Take medications as directed.
   b. Follow-up within 48 hours
   c. Abstain from sex until treatment completed.
2. Prevention
   a. Limit the number of sexual partners.
   b. Question partners about high-risk behaviors, previous history of sexually transmitted diseases (STDs).
   c. Inspect genitalia of sexual partners for lesions.
   d. Use barrier methods and spermicides always.
   e. Seek medical attention immediately if suspected exposure to STD or occurrence of symptoms.
   f. Routine clinical and laboratory examination and treatment of sexual partners (even if asymptomatic) of women with acute PID

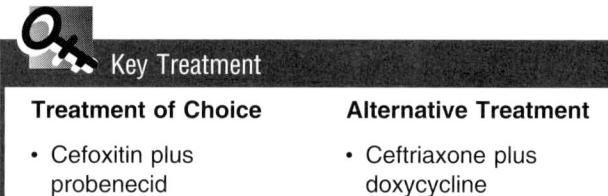

Key Treatment

Treatment of Choice	Alternative Treatment
• Cefoxitin plus probenecid	• Ceftriaxone plus doxycycline

Follow-Up

1. The patient should be reassessed 24 to 48 hours after initiation of therapy to determine clinical improvement. If no improvement, consider noncompliance or reassessment of diagnosis and hospitalization.
2. Maximize patient education and routine health maintenance checkups to prevent recurrent disease.

 ## Bibliography

For more information on the pathogenesis of PID, see
Rice PA, Schachter J: Pathogenesis of pelvic inflammatory disease. JAMA 1991;266(18):2587–2593.

For more information on the diagnosis of PID, see
Kahn JG, Walker CK, Washington AE, et al: Diagnosing pelvic inflammatory disease. JAMA 1991;266(18):2594–2604.

For more information on sequelae of delayed treatment, see
Hillis SD, Joesoef R, Marchbanks PA, et al: Delayed care of pelvic inflammatoy disease as a risk factor for impaired fertility. Am J Obstet Gynecol 1993;168(5):1503–1509.

For more information on treatment of PID, see
1993 sexually transmitted diseases guidelines. MMWR 1993;42(RR-14):75–81.

For more information on prevention of PID, see
Washington AE, Cates W, Wasserheit JN: Preventing pelvic inflammatory disease. JAMA 1991;266(18):2574–2580.

105 Sexually Transmitted Diseases

Judith Kinzy

Gonorrhea

Etiology

Neisseria gonorrhoeae: a gram-negative diplococcus

Symptoms

1. Women are usually asymptomatic. Only 10 to 20 per cent complain of vaginal discharge. Other symptoms include dyspareunia, lower abdominal discomfort, intermenstrual spotting, and menorrhagia.
2. Men may complain of urinary frequency and dysuria. Approximately 95 to 99 per cent have purulent urethral discharge, which may be eliminated or reduced with micturition.

Key Symptoms

- Vaginal or urethral discharge
- Urinary frequency
- Women usually asymptomatic
- Dysuria

Clinical Findings

1. Purulent urethral or cervical discharge
2. Red and swollen cervix or urethra
3. Tender inguinal adenopathy

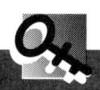
Key Signs

- Red and swollen cervix or urethra
- Tender inguinal adenopathy
- Purulent urethral or cervical discharge

Laboratory Tests

A stained smear of urethral exudate in men or endocervical smear in women may be diagnostic, particularly in patients with purulent drainage. Cultures on selective media such as Thayer-Martin, Martin-Lewis, or NYC are essential in most women.

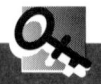
Key Tests

- Gram's stain of purulent drainage
- Culture

Differential Diagnosis

The differential diagnosis of gonorrhea includes non-gonococcal urethritis, traumatic urethritis, herpes simplex, foreign body, *Chlamydia trachomatis* infection, prostatitis, *Gardnerella* vaginitis, and *Candida albicans* infection.

Treatment
Medication

The drug of choice for gonorrhea is ceftriaxone (Rocephin), 125 mg intramuscularly once. Alternatives include cefixime (Suprax), 400 mg orally once, ciprofloxacin (Cipro), 500 mg orally once, or ofloxacin (Floxin), 400 mg orally once. Treat concurrently for *Chlamydia*. Treat sexual partner.

Patient Education

Avoid sexual intercourse for 2 days after intramuscular injection and for 5 days after oral medication.

Key Treatment

Drug of Choice

- Ceftriaxone 125 mg intramuscularly once

Alternative Drugs

- Cefixime 400 mg orally once, ciprofloxacin 500 mg orally once, or ofloxacin 400 mg orally once
- Treat for *Chlamydia*

Follow-Up

Patient should be examined 3 to 5 days after treatment. Repeat cultures particularly if the patient is thought to be noncompliant or if only one antibiotic was given.

Chlamydia
Etiology

Chlamydia trachomatis

Symptoms

1. Men complain of dysuria and/or discharge.
2. Women present with dysuria or frequency but often are asymptomatic.

Key Symptom

- Dysuria

Clinical Findings

1. Urethritis and epididymitis are the most frequent manifestations of *C. trachomatis* infection in men. Cervicitis, urethritis, endometritis, or salpingitis is

seen most commonly in women. Unexplained pyuria or culture-negative cystitis in sexually active women suggests *Chlamydia* infection.

2. Lymphogranuloma venereum caused by *C. trachomatis* serotypes L1 to L3 presents as enlarged, prominent painful lymph nodes.

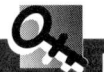

Key Signs

- Urethritis
- Culture-negative cystitis
- Epididymitis
- Cervicitis

Laboratory Tests

Culture in mammalian cell lines is the "gold standard." Use wire swabs with Dacron or cotton because wood swabs are treated with chemicals that may interfere with the culture. Swab the endocervix in women and at least 2 to 3 cm into the urethra in men and then rotate for several seconds.

Key Test

- Culture is the "gold standard."

Differential Diagnosis

Differential diagnosis of *Chlamydia* infection includes *N. gonorrhoeae, Ureaplasma urealyticum,* and herpes simplex virus.

Treatment

The drug of choice is doxycycline (Vibramycin), 100 mg orally b.i.d. for 7 days, or azithromycin (Zithromax), 1 gm orally in a single dose. Alternative drugs include erythromycin, 500 mg orally q.i.d. for 7 days, sulfasoxazole, 500 mg orally q.i.d. for 7 days, or ofloxacin (Floxin), 300 mg orally b.i.d. for 7 days. Doxycycline, other tetracyclines, and ofloxacin are contraindicated in pregnancy. Treat sexual partner.

Key Treatment

Drugs of Choice	Alternative Drugs
• Doxycycline, 100 mg b.i.d. orally for 7 days	• Erythromycin, 500 mg orally q.i.d. for 7 days
• Azithromycin, 1 gm orally once	• Sulfisoxazole, 500 mg orally t.i.d. for 7 days
	• Ofloxacin, 300 mg orally b.i.d. for 7 days

Follow-Up

Evaluate patient 1 week after treatment.

Chancroid

Etiology

Haemophilus ducreyi: a gram-negative streptobacillus

Symptoms

1. Men may complain of a painful ulcer or inguinal adenopathy.
2. Women may complain of symptoms unrelated to the ulcer, such as dysuria, dyspareunia, or hematochezia.

Clinical Findings

1. Deep necrotizing ulcerations are found on the shaft of the penis.
2. Tender unilateral lymphadenopathy is common.

Key Signs

- Deep necrotizing ulcers
- Tender inguinal lymphadenopathy

Laboratory Tests

Obtain smear and/or biopsy from undermined edges of lesion. Gram's stain reveals "schools of fish" or "railroad tracks." Culture on gonococcal agar or Mueller-Hinton agar.

Key Tests

- Gram's stain of smear
- Culture

Differential Diagnosis

Includes syphilis, herpes simplex, lymphogranuloma venereum, and granuloma inguinale.

Treatment

Drugs of choice include ceftriaxone (Rocephin), 250 mg intramuscularly once, erythromycin, 500 mg orally q.i.d. for 7 days, or azithromycin (Zithromax), 1 gm orally once. Alternatives include amoxicillin-clavulanic acid (Augmentin), 500 mg orally t.i.d. for 7 days, or ciprofloxacin (Cipro), 500 mg orally b.i.d. for 3 days.

Key Treatment

Drugs of Choice	Alternative Drugs
• Ceftriaxone, 250 mg intramuscularly one time	• Ciprofloxacin, 500 mg orally b.i.d. for 3 days
• Erythromycin, 500 mg orally q.i.d. for 7 days	• Amoxicillin-clavulanic acid, 500 mg orally t.i.d. for 7 days
• Azithromycin, 1 gram orally once	

Aspiration of fluctuant lymph nodes is necessary to prevent rupture. Avoid sexual activity for 1 week after treatment.

Follow-Up

Patients should be seen weekly until cure is achieved. They should be tested for coexisting sexually transmitted diseases, including HIV. Repeat HIV testing in 3 to 6 months.

Syphilis

Etiology

Treponema pallidum

Symptoms

1. Primary syphilis presents as a chancre, a painless ulcer at the point of inoculation.
2. Secondary syphilis presents with rash, fever, malaise, and lymphadenopathy 4 to 10 weeks after the chancre.

Key Symptoms	
Primary Syphilis	**Secondary Syphilis**
• Painless ulcer	• Rash
	• Lymphadenopathy

Clinical Findings

1. Chancre is a painless solitary lesion with raised, well-defined borders and a clean indurated base found in primary syphilis. Patients may have unilateral or bilateral regional nontender lymphadenopathy.
2. A macular, papular, annular, or follicular rash is the typical manifestation of secondary syphilis. Alopecia, condylomata lata, and shallow, painless ulcerations seen on the mucous membranes called "mucous patches" are other clinical findings.

Key Signs	
Primary Syphilis	**Secondary Syphilis**
• Chancre	• Macular, papular, or follicular rash
• Lymphadenopathy	
	• Mucous patches

Laboratory Tests

RPR and VDRL tests are recommended for screening. One can follow the response to therapy with these tests because titers diminish with treatment. Fluorescent treponemal-antibody absorption (FTA-ABS) is more sensitive but is not used for screening because it is more expensive.

Key Tests
• RPR
• VDRL

Differential Diagnosis

1. Differential diagnosis of primary syphilis includes herpes simplex, *H. ducreyi,* streptococci, staphylococci, and *Candida.*
2. Differential diagnosis in secondary syphilis includes pityriasis rosea, lichen planus, psoriasis, drug eruption, impetigo, or chickenpox.

Treatment

Medication

The drug of choice is penicillin G benzathine, 2.4 million units intramuscularly once. Alternatives for nonpregnant patients include doxycycline, 100 mg orally b.i.d. for 14 days, tetracycline, 500 mg orally q.i.d. for 14 days, or erythromycin, 500 mg orally q.i.d. for 14 days. Treat sexual contacts.

Patient Education

Avoid sexual contact for 1 week after treatment.

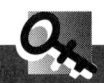

Key Treatment	
Drug of Choice	**Alternative Drugs**
• Penicillin G benzathine, 2.4 million units intramuscularly	• Doxycycline, 100 mg orally q.i.d. for 14 days
	• Tetracycline, 500 mg orally q.i.d. for 14 days
	• Erythromycin, 500 mg orally q.i.d. for 14 days

Follow-Up

Follow VDRL or RPR titers. Successful treatment should be a fourfold decrease in serum RPR at 6 months for primary syphilis and an eightfold decline within 12 months for secondary syphilis. Check HIV, since disease is linked with HIV.

Bibliography

Abramowitz M (ed): Drugs for sexually transmitted diseases. Med Lett 1994;36:1–6.

Braverman PK, Strasburger VC: Sexually transmitted diseases. Clin Pediatr 1994;33:26–37.

Centers for Disease Control and Prevention: 1993 Sexually transmitted diseases treatment guidelines. MMWR 1993;42 (RR-14):1–102.

Fiumara NJ: Pictorial Guide to Sexually Transmitted Diseases. New York, Cahners Publishing, 1989.

Hook EW, Marra CM: Acquired syphilis in adults. N Engl J Med 1992;326:1060–1069.

106 Endometriosis

Lisa J. Pierce

Etiology

1. "Endometriosis" is defined as the presence of functional endometrial tissue outside the uterine cavity.
2. Estimated to affect 5 to 20 per cent of all women of reproductive age.
3. Mean age at diagnosis is 25 to 29 years. There are no racial differences in the prevalence of the disease.
4. There is a familial tendency toward endometriosis with no specific pattern of inheritance.
5. Three main theories of pathogenesis:
   a. Retrograde transport of endometrial tissue through the fallopian tubes at menstruation leading to seeding of the peritoneal cavity.
   b. Metaplastic transformation of coelomic epithelium leading to functioning endometrial tissue at extrapelvic sites (e.g., umbilicus, appendix, diaphragm, pleural peritoneum).
   c. Spread of endometrial tissue through lymphatic and vascular channels.
6. Recent studies have investigated the possibility of an autoimmune cause and the possible role of exposure to toxic chemicals in development of endometriosis.

Symptoms

1. Pain is the most common complaint; may be manifested as secondary dysmenorrhea, worsening primary dysmenorrhea, chronic pelvic pain, backache.
2. Infertility may be due to anatomic distortion of the reproductive organs or other factors.
3. Dyspareunia is usually secondary to fixed retroversion of the uterus from scar tissue.
4. Menstrual irregularities have been attributed to anovulation caused by scarring of the ovary, although it is controversial whether this association truly exists.
5. Unusual symptoms may relate to extrapelvic sites of endometrial tissue: cyclic hemoptysis, painful defecation, cyclic headaches or seizures, sciatica, or cyclic scar pain.
6. Presence and severity of symptoms correlate poorly with degree of endometriosis seen at laparoscopy. Many women are asymptomatic despite the presence of significant pathology at the time of surgery.

Key Symptoms

- Dysmenorrhea
- Dyspareunia
- Infertility
- Menstrual irregularities
- Chronic pelvic pain

Clinical Findings

1. Bimanual examination may reveal tenderness in the vaginal cul-de-sac and fixed uterine retroversion with cervical motion tenderness.
2. Adnexal enlargement and tenderness may indicate the presence of an endometrioma (chocolate cyst) of the ovary. These cysts may grow to 15 cm in diameter and are filled with endometrial blood and debris. Rupture of these usually painless cysts can cause an acute abdomen due to spillage of the contents of the cyst. This spillage results in further scarring and progression of the disease.
3. Rectovaginal examination may demonstrate uterosacral or rectovaginal septum nodularity.
4. Pelvic examination is best done in the immediate premenstrual period.
5. Often the physical examination is normal even with moderate to severe endometriosis.

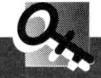

Key Signs

- Fixed uterine retroversion
- Uterosacral ligament nodularity
- Fixed ovarian mass

Laboratory Tests

1. Visualization of the disease by laparoscopy or laparotomy is considered the "gold standard" for diagnosis.
2. Because of the heterogeneic appearance of endometriotic lesions, a surgeon skilled in the diagnosis of endometriosis should perform the laparoscopy and biopsy any suspicious areas.
3. Ultrasound can be used to identify endometriomas of the ovary but is not useful in detecting focal implants.
4. Magnetic resonance imaging (MRI) has been studied, but there is no pathognomonic appearance of endometriosis, so the sensitivity and specificity of MRI in diagnosing the disease are low.
5. An elevated blood level of CA 125 has been found repeatedly in women with endometriosis, but its sensitivity and specificity are not adequate for screening. Studies looking for other serum protein markers are under way.

Key Test

Laparoscopy

445

Differential Diagnosis

1. Chronic pelvic inflammatory disease (PID) is associated with many similar symptoms.
2. Pelvic adhesions from PID or previous surgery can mimic endometriosis.
3. Ovarian cysts or tumors may simulate an endometrioma.

Treatment

1. Optimal treatment regimen depends on desired outcome: pain relief or fertility.
2. Surgery
   a. Conservative
      (1) Preserves reproductive organs.
      (2) Ablation of endometrial implants via laser or thermal cautery and/or adhesiolysis performed via laparoscopy or laparotomy
      (3) Drainage or removal of endometriomas
      (4) Used extensively in conjunction with medical therapy in an attempt to enhance fertility and reduce pain, especially in women with advanced disease.
      (5) Surgery results in significant improvement in fertility in severe endometriosis, but it is unclear whether it is beneficial in mild to moderate disease.
   b. Radical
      (1) Hysterectomy with salpingo-oophorectomy is the definitive procedure.
      (2) Eliminates pain in 90 per cent of cases.
      (3) Up to a third of women will have disease recurrence if the ovaries are not removed.
      (4) Should be considered only in women no longer desiring pregnancy.

Medication

1. Danazol (Danocrine) is a derivative of 17α-ethinyl testosterone.
   a. Prescribe 400 to 800 mg daily in 2 to 4 divided doses, adjusting based on symptoms and/or side effects.
   b. Creates a high-androgen, low-estrogen state with anovulation and amenorrhea, which inhibits the growth of endometrial tissue.
   c. May cause fetal virilization, so must have a negative pregnancy test prior to initiating therapy, and a barrier contraceptive method should be used during therapy.
   d. Length of therapy depends on response to treatment and whether surgical therapy is planned. If planning only primary medical therapy, then at least 6 months of treatment is required. If used as adjuvant therapy pre- or postoperatively, then 12 weeks is usually adequate.
   e. Improvement or resolution of dysmenorrhea, dys-

pareunia, and pelvic pain occurs in 80 to 90 per cent of cases, but there is no effect on fertility.
   f. Side effects include weight gain, hirsutism, acne, mood alterations, and adverse effects on lipid metabolism. Most of these changes are reversible within 6 months of discontinuing the drug.
2. Gonadotropin-releasing hormone (GnRH) agonists
   a. Nafarelin acetate (Synarel), 0.2 to 0.4 mg intranasally b.i.d.
   b. Leuprolide acetate (Lupron), 3.75 mg intramuscularly monthly (depot) or 0.5 to 1.0 mg subcutaneously daily.
   c. Create a hypoestrogenic, amenorrheic state.
   d. Usually well tolerated, but side effects include hot flashes, vaginal dryness, and trabecular bone loss, which is probably reversible when the drug is discontinued.
   e. Duration of treatment is usually 6 months.
   f. Addition of a progestogen may decrease the effects on bone loss and the vasomotor side effects.
   g. Between 80 and 90 per cent of women show improvement in pain symptoms, but there is no effect on fertility.
3. Progestogen
   a. Medroxyprogesterone acetate (MPA)
      (1) Depot MPA (Depo-Provera), 100 mg every 2 weeks for four doses, then 200 mg monthly for 4 months
      (2) MPA, 30 mg orally daily for 3 months
   b. Causes atrophy of endometrial tissue.
   c. Side effects include irregular bleeding, nausea, depression, and fluid retention.
   d. Depot MPA may result in prolonged anovulation and should not be used in women desiring pregnancy.
   e. Between 80 and 90 per cent of women report improvement in pain symptoms, but there is no effect on fertility.
4. Combined estrogen-progesterone
   a. Oral contraceptive pills containing 30 to 35 μg ethinyl estradiol taken continuously to produce amenorrhea. May require two or more tablets daily to prevent breakthrough bleeding.
   b. Duration of treatment is 6 to 9 months, but symptoms may worsen initially.
   c. Side effects are frequent and sometimes severe, including breast tenderness, bloating, weight gain, nausea, and edema.
   d. Less effective in relieving symptoms than other medical therapies and possibly lower pregnancy rates. Should be used only if other regimens are contraindicated.
5. Nonsteroidal anti-inflammatory drugs (NSAIDs) may be effective in pain relief.

6. Infertility has been treated with ovarian hyperstimulation and in vitro fertilization with varying success.

Key Treatment

Drugs of Choice	Alternative Drugs
• Danazol	• Estrogen-progestin oral contraceptive pills
• GnRH agonists	
• Progestogens	

Patient Education

1. Patients need to be aware of the chronic nature of endometriosis and the potential negative impact it may have on fertility. Many physicians counsel pa-tients to avoid delaying childbearing once the diagnosis is made.

2. The Endometriosis Association (800–992–3636) offers support and information to women affected by the disease.

Bibliography

Daywood MY: Considerations in selecting appropriate medical therapy for endometriosis. Int J Gynecol Obstet 1993; 40(suppl):529–542.

Kase NG, Weingold AB, Gershenson DM (eds): Principles and Practice of Clinical Gynecology, 2nd ed. New York, Churchill-Livingstone, 1990.

Kauppila A: Changing concepts of medical treatment of endometriosis. Acta Obstet Gynecol Scand 1993;72:324–336.

Olive DL, Schwarts LB: Endometriosis. N Engl J Med 1993;328(24):1759–1769.

Stenchever MA: Office Gynecology. St Louis, Mosby–Year Book, 1992.

107 Endometritis

Michael P. Rowane

Etiology

1. "Endometritis," inflammation of the endometrium, the decidual mucous membrane of the gravid uterus, is the most common postpartum infection, especially after a cesarean delivery.

2. The cellular debris and the large raw area of placental insertion are excellent media. The cervicovaginal flora, with anaerobes and gram-negative organisms, are the most common causes.

3. Microorganisms
   a. Aerobic bacteria
      (1) Gram-positives
         (a) Group A, B, and D streptococci (30 per cent of group B are completely/partially involved)
         (b) Enterococci
             Staphylococcus aureus
      (2) Gram-negatives
         (a) *Escherichia coli* (most common gram-negative)
         (b) *Gardnerella vaginitis*
         (c) *Neisseria gonorrhoeae* (2 to 8 per cent)
   b. Anaerobic bacteria (involved in 50 to 95 per cent of uterine puerperal infections)
      (1) *Bacteroides bivius* and other *Bacteroides* species
      (2) Peptostreptococci
      (3) Peptococci
      (4) *Proteus mirabilis*
   c. Other organisms
      (1) *Ureaplasma urealyticum*
      (2) *Mycoplasma hominis*
      (3) *Chlamydia trachomatis* (associated specifically with a late-onset postpartum endometritis)

Symptoms

1. *Fever*
   a. Occurs most commonly on the first or second postpartum day.
      (1) Oral temperature of greater than 38.5° C in the first 24 hours after delivery, or
      (2) Greater than 38.0° C for more than 6 consecutive days after first postpartum day.
   b. Fever can be a clue to involved organisms.
      (1) Less than 48 hours postpartum: Suspect gram-positive streptococci.
      (2) More than 48 hours postpartum: Suspect a mixed anaerobic and gram-negative infection.

2. *Chills* (Fever and chills occur more commonly in the late afternoon or evening.)
3. *Malaise*
4. *Abdominal pain*
5. Foul-smelling lochia
6. Symptoms of ileus (i.e., distention, constipation)

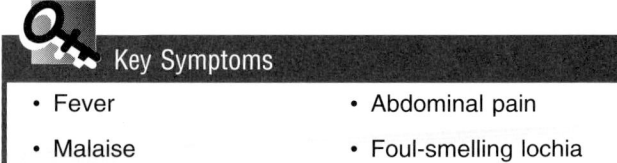

Key Symptoms	
• Fever	• Abdominal pain
• Malaise	• Foul-smelling lochia

Clinical Findings

1. Temperature above 100.4° F
2. Tachycardia
3. Abdominal:
   a. Tenderness in the lower abdomen without lateralization
   b. Infection of abdominal wound after cesarean section
   c. Fundal height same as uterus of normal puerpera
   d. Ileus with diminished/absent bowel sounds and distended
4. Pelvic:
   a. Uterus soft and tender to palpation
   b. Inspect uterus for retained material or pyometra, a collection of pus within the endometrial cavity.
   c. Adnexal mass (abscess versus infected hematoma)
   d. May or may not have a foul-smelling lochia/discharge
   e. Evaluate for infection of episiotomy
5. Severe disease: high fever, abdominal tenderness, ileus, hypotension, and generalized sepsis

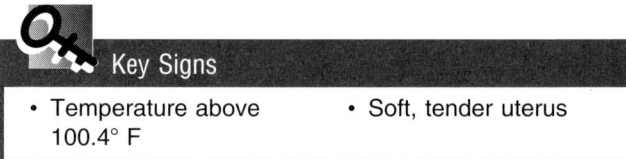

Key Signs	
• Temperature above 100.4° F	• Soft, tender uterus

Laboratory Tests

1. Cervical/endometrial cultures
   a. GC and *Chlamydia*
   b. Aerobic and anaerobic
      (1) To find resistant organisms while on broad-spectrum antibiotics
      (2) Any wound infection, abscess, or hematoma

448

2. Complete blood count (CBC) with differential (Leukocytosis may be seen.)

3. Blood cultures and sensitivities ×2

4. Electrolytes, blood urea nitrogen (BUN), and creatinine

5. Urinalysis, with urine culture and sensitivities

6. Chest radiograph (rarely of benefit unless signs and symptoms point to a possible pulmonary cause of the fever)

7. Gram's stain: genital or amniotic fluid after cesarean section

8. Ultrasound (if considering pyometra)

Key Tests

- Cervical/endometrial cultures
- CBC with differential
- Blood cultures and sensitivities ×2
- Electrolytes, BUN creatinine
- Urinalysis, with urine culture and sensitivities

Differential Diagnosis

1. Genital source:
   a. Infected mass, such as abscess and incisional hematoma
   b. Pelvic cellulitis
   c. Septic pelvic thrombophlebitis
2. Nongenital source:
   a. Urinary tract infection
   b. Pneumonia (especially smokers and after general anesthesia)
   c. Intravenous phlebitis
   d. Appendicitis
   e. Viral syndrome
   f. Drug fever
   g. Breast engorgement

Risk Factors

1. Cesarean delivery (10 to 30 per cent) versus vaginal delivery (less than 5 per cent)
2. Prolonged rupture of membranes more than 12 to 24 hours (the major risk factor after cesarean section if more than 6 hours)
3. Intrapartum and postpartum anemia
4. Multiple vaginal examinations in labor (single predictor of prophylactic antibiotic failure following cesarean section)
5. Intrauterine pressure catheters (>8 hours)
6. Fetal scalp electrode monitoring
7. Pre-existing vaginitis/cervicitis
8. Operative vaginal deliveries
9. Prolonged labor (>8 hours)
10. Coitus near term
11. Indigent patients
12. Chorioamnionitis
13. Toxemia
14. Poor nutrition
15. Obesity

Treatment

1. General principles
   a. The prognosis of postpartum endometritis is excellent with prompt therapy.
   b. Delays in diagnosis may lead to complications (e.g., pelvic abscess or septic pelvic thrombophlebitis bacterial heparinase progressing to clots in pelvic vessels, with potential septic emboli).
   c. The choice of antibiotics for treatment depends on the suspected organisms and the severity of the disease.
   d. Initial therapy requires high-dose intravenous antibiotics.
   e. For patients with known risk factors or at high risk for infection at delivery, initial therapy is with two- or three-drug regimens, preferably including clindamycin. Equal efficacy seen with a single-agent intravenous infusion of broad-spectrum agent.
   f. There are numerous acceptable antimicrobial regimes with broad-spectrum antimicrobial therapy as the mainstay.
   g. Intravenous therapy until afebrile (<38° C [99.5° F]) and pain-free for 48 hours and asymptomatic.
   h. Clindamycin is added if clinical/laboratory results suggest that *Bacteroides* species are involved.

PEARLS

- In septic abortion, *Clostridium perfringens* may cause fulminate intravascular hemolysis.

- In postpartum patients with uncertain fever and/or pulmonary emboli, consider septic pelvic vein thrombophlebitis requiring heparin and antibiotics.

- Endometritis requires the same coverage as amnionitis and septic abortion.

- Abdominal wound infections are primarily responsible for persistent fever and therefore antibiotic failure.

- With high fever and hypotension soon after delivery, think of a group B streptococcal infection.

2. Surgical

   a. Dilation and curettage (D&C) of uterus if indicated (e.g., to remove retained products of conception)

   b. Drainage of pyometra (ultrasound may assist/guide)

Medication

1. *Early postpartum,* first 48 hours: Two options to consider:

   a. Doxycycline along with one of the following agents:

     (1) Cefoxitin (Mefoxin), 2 gm intravenously q 6 hr

     (2) Ticarcillin-clavulanate (Timentin), 3.1 gm intravenously q 4–6 hr

     (3) Imipenem-cilastatin (Primaxin), 0.5 to 1 gm q 6 hr

     (4) Ampicillin-sulbactam (Unasyn), 3 gm intravenously q 6 hr

   b. Clindamycin along with one of the following agents:

     (1) Gentamicin, 120 mg (2 mg/kg) intravenous piggyback (IVPB) then 80 mg (1.5 mg/kg) IVPB q 8 hr (monitor peak and trough levels) (Note: Recent data support 1 mg/kg per dose as adequate.)

     (2) Third-generation cephalosporin

   c. After discharge, continue doxycycline or clindamycin.

2. *Late postpartum,* 48 hours to 6 weeks:

   a. Usually after vaginal delivery

   b. Doxycycline, 100 mg q 12 hr intravenously or orally for 14 days

3. *Postcesarean endometritis:* Clindamycin and gentamycin or ceftriaxone, 1 to 2 gm intravenously or intramuscularly q 12–24 hr

4. *Alternative regimen:* Add one of the following agents to gentamicin:

   a. Clindamycin, 900 mg intravenously q 8 hr

   b. Cefoxitin (Mefoxin), 2 gm intravenously q 6 hr

   c. Cefotetan (Cefotan), 2 gm intravenously q 12 hr

   d. Piperacillin-mezlocillin, 4 gm intravenously q 6 hr

   e. Ampicillin-sulbactam (Unasyn), 3 gm intravenously q 6 hr

   f. Ticarcillin-clavulanate (Timentin), 3.1 gm intravenously q 4–6 hr

5. *Single-agent therapy* also has been successful with broad-spectrum agents such as ampicillin-sulbactam, imipenem-cilastatin, ticarcillin-clavulanate, cefoxitin, cefotetan, or ceftizoxime.

6. Discontinue nursing if using tetracyclines, because they are not recommended in nursing mothers.

Diet

1. Must encourage fluids

2. Intravenous fluids if lacking adequate oral intake

3. Diet as tolerated

Activity

1. Mild to moderate endometritis: bed rest with limited activities (e.g., bathroom privileges)

2. Severe endometritis: bed rest

3. Increase activity as tolerated

Patient Education

1. Labor and delivery education/prevention:

   a. The possibility of endometritis

   b. Avoid high-risk behavior

   c. Need for last-trimester cultures

2. Stress that with antibiotic therapy and supportive management, most patients are afebrile in a few days with complete resolution

 Key Treatment

Drugs of Choice (Multiple Options)

• Gentamicin	• Ticarcillin-clavulanate
• Doxycycline	• Imipenem-cilastatin
• Clindamycin	• Ceftizoxime
• Ampicillin-sulbactam	• Cefoxitin
• Piperacillin-mezlocillin	• Cefotetan

Dilation and curettage of uterus if indicated

Follow-Up

1. Hospitalize.

2. The response to this therapy should be carefully monitored for 24 to 48 hours. Deterioration or failure to respond both clinically and on laboratory tests results requires a complete re-evaluation.

3. Office follow-up within the first week of discharge.

4. Inform patient of need to call with any complications.

 Bibliography

For more information on endometritis and other obstetrical emergencies, see

Benrubi GI: Obstetrical and Gynecological Emergencies. Philadelphia, JB Lippincott, 1994, pp 156–159.

For more information on endometritis in a good general review of obstetrics and gynecology, see

Pernoll ML, Benson RC: Current Obstetric and Gynecologic Diagnosis and Treatment. East Norwalk, CT, Appleton & Lange, 1991.

For more information on practical management guidance in obstetrics and gynecology, see

Chan PD: Current Clinical Strategies Obstetrics and Gynecology. Fountain Valley, CA, CCS Publishing, 1992, pp 55–56.

For more information on antimicrobial therapy in endometritis and other disorders, see

Sanford JP: Guide to Antimicrobial Therapy 1994. Dallas, Antimicrobial Therapy, Inc, 1994, p 13.

For more information on infections and antimicrobial therapy associated with endometritis and cesarean sections, see

Soper DE: Infections following cesarean section. Curr Opin Obstet Gynecol 1993;5(4):517–520.

108 Menopause

Shirley L. Dickinson

Definition/Epidemiology

1. Menopause is the cessation of menstruation due to the failure of ovarian follicular development in the presence of sufficient gonadotropin levels.
2. The perimenopause is characterized by a gradual decline in ovarian function and estrogen production.
   a. Declining estrogen levels result in the onset of increased rate of bone loss previously believed to start only after complete cessation of menstruation.
   b. Patients may be asymptomatic during this period or complain of symptoms typical of the menopause.
3. The average age of menopause is 51.4 years, with the age range being 40 to 60 years. Smokers may have an accelerated menopause.

Symptoms of Estrogen Deficiency

1. Prevalence
   a. Seventy-five to 80 per cent will experience some discomfort.
   b. Ten to 15 per cent have symptoms that interfere with daily functioning.
   c. Twenty-five per cent of women complain of symptoms lasting more than 5 years.
2. Menstrual cycle changes, including hypermenorrhea, oligomenorrhea, and finally amenorrhea
3. Extragenital symptoms
   a. Hot flashes
   b. Psychological manifestations may occur before and 3 to 5 years after the menopause.
      (1) Insomnia, fatigue
      (2) Irritability, anxiety
      (3) Depression, memory loss
   c. Skin thickness and collagen content are decreased, resulting in wrinkles.
   d. Osteoporosis and coronary heart disease may be silent until 10 to 15 years after the onset of the menopause. At this point significant irreversible disease may be present.

Key Symptoms

- Vasomotor flushes
- Vaginal dryness
- Urinary stress incontinence
- Cystitis-like symptoms
- Insomnia
- Irritability
- Anxiety
- Memory loss

Clinical Findings

1. Urogenital atrophy tends to occur 3 to 5 years after development of amenorrhea.
   a. *Mucosa* of the genitourinary tract is extremely sensitive to estrogen.
   b. *Vaginal atrophy:* resulting in, dyspareunia, atrophic vaginitis, an increased susceptibility to bacterial vaginitis, or vaginal bleeding
   c. *Vulvar atrophy:* resulting in pruritus vulvae, loss of pubic hair, and labial atrophy
   d. *Atrophy of urethra and bladder trigone:* resulting in symptoms of cystitis or urgency incontinence
   e. *Atrophy of the pelvic support:* resulting in uterine prolapse, cystocele, and rectocele
2. Osteoporosis
   a. Affects one third of postmenopausal women in the United States
   b. Results in a loss of bone strength resulting in an increased susceptibility to fracture primarily of the hip, vertebrae, distal forearm, humerus, and pelvis.
   c. Accounts for significant morbidity and mortality
      (1) Survivors of hip fractures are frequently severely affected and may become permanently disabled.
      (2) Mortality rate of hip fracture is 10 to 20 per cent within the first 6 months. Mortality is related either directly to the hip fracture or to surgical, embolic, or cardiopulmonary complications.
   d. Prevention in high-risk women includes early estrogen replacement, adequate calcium intake, and weight-bearing exercise.
3. Cardiovascular disease
   a. After the menopause there is a progressive increase in the incidence of coronary heart disease (CHD).
   b. Estrogen results in a 50 per cent reduction in the incidence of CHD and related mortality.
   c. Estrogen benefits the lipoprotein profile by increasing the HDL cholesterol and decreasing LDL and total cholesterol.
   d. Acts directly at the coronary arteries, resulting in vasodilatation, and inhibits the development of atheromatous plaques.
   e. Estrogen does not increase the incidence of hypertension or aggravate pre-existing hypertension.
      (1) Natural estrogens have been shown to lower diastolic blood pressure.
      (2) Conjugated equine estrogens can cause an id-

iosyncratic hypertensive response in a small percentage of patients. Changing to an alternative estrogen corrects the hypertension.

Key Sign

• Vaginal atrophy

Laboratory Tests

In general, no tests are necessary to diagnose the menopause. Symptoms and clinical evidence should suffice. When necessary to confirm, the following tests can be done.

1. FSH and estradiol
   a. During the perimenopausal period women have lower estradiol levels and rising FSH levels as the follicular phase begins to shorten.
   b. FSH levels in the postmenopausal range (>40 mIU/ml) can be seen despite continued menstrual bleeding.
   c. Decreasing estradiol levels result in early bone loss.
2. Luteinizing hormone (LH)
   a. During the perimenopausal period LH levels remain in the high normal range.
   b. Reaches a peak 1 to 3 years after the menopause, followed by a gradual decline.
3. Endometrial biopsy
   a. Baseline biopsy not necessary unless history of abnormal bleeding.
   b. Biopsy is indicated if breakthrough bleeding or heavy withdrawal bleeding occurs.

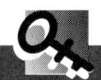

Key Tests

• FSH elevated

• LH normal to elevated

Treatment

1. Natural estrogens should be used for replacement therapy as synthetic estrogens have a profound hepatic stimulatory effect.

2. Oral estrogens undergo a first pass effect through the liver which is responsible for the beneficial effects on the lipoprotein profile. Transdermal estrogens bypass this first pass effect and are the preferred route in patients with underlying hepatic disease.

3. Generic preparations have erratic rates of absorption and poor bioavailability.

4. Estrogen can be given either unopposed or in combination with a progestin. Unopposed estrogen should be reserved for hysterectomized women due to an increased incidence of endometrial hyperplasia and cancer.

Medication (Table 108–1).

1. *Unopposed estrogen* is given on a continuous basis to hysterectomized women.

2. *Combination therapy* can be given either cyclically or continuously.
   a. *Cyclic therapy:* results in the resumption of regular menses.
      (1) Traditional method: Estrogen days 1 to 25, progesterone days 12 or 14 to 25. Results in resumption of symptoms for the 5 days off therapy.
      (2) Current method: Estrogen continuously, progesterone days 1 to 14.
   b. *Continuous therapy:* Estrogen and progesterone given daily. Often results in irregular spotting for several months before the onset of amenorrhea. If the spotting is troublesome, the progesterone dose can be temporarily increased to achieve amenorrhea sooner.

3. *Progestin only* therapy may be necessary in patients unable to take estrogens due to contraindications. Progestins can relieve vasomotor symptoms and are beneficial in maintenance of bone mass. Clonidine, 0.05 to 0.2 mg twice a day, is also beneficial.

   See Table 108–1 for recommended dosages for each regimen.

Diet

1. *Calcium:* In order to maintain zero calcium balance, women on estrogen require 1000 mg/day of calcium. The average American diet contains 500 mg/day. Untreated women require 1500 mg/day. Calcium alone or in combination with exercise will *not* prevent osteoporosis.

TABLE 108–1. ESTROGEN AND PROGESTERONE DOSAGES IN THE MENOPAUSE

Cyclic		Continuous	Progesterone Only
Estrogens	**Progesterones**		
CEE 0.625 mg, estrone sulfate 0.625 mg, estradiol 1.0 mg, or transderm estradiol 0.05 mg days 1–25 or continuously	Medroxyprogesterone acetate (MPA) 5–10 mg or norethindrone acetate (NET) 1.0 mg for 14 days each month	CEE 0.625 mg, estradiol 1.0 mg, estrone sulfate 0.625 mg, or transderm estradiol 0.05 mg and MPA 2.5 mg or NET 1.0 mg daily	MPA 10 mg daily or depo MPA 100 mg monthly

2. Dietary calcium is optimal, but when necessary supplemental calcium is appropriate.

Activity

Aerobic, weight-bearing exercise should be done three times a week.

Patient Education

1. Performance of breast self-examination every month
2. Importance of regular mammograms
3. Importance of reporting any abnormal vaginal bleeding
4. Prior to the initiation of therapy the patient should be well informed regarding the potential benefits and risks of therapy in order to make an informed choice regarding initiation of treatment.

Risks of Estrogen Replacement Therapy (ERT)

1. Endometrial cancer
   a. A four- to eightfold increase in the risk of developing endometrial cancer in users of unopposed therapy. Cancers that do develop are well differentiated and treatable.
   b. Increased risk persists for 10 years after discontinuing therapy.
   c. Adding a progestin significantly reduces risk to a level equal to that of nonusers of estrogen.
2. Breast cancer
   a. No conclusive evidence has demonstrated an *overall* increased risk; however, the risk may be increased with duration of use.
   b. Current doses of ERT known to protect against osteoporosis and cardiovascular disease are not known to be associated with an increased risk.
   c. Increased dosages of estrogen and parenteral or pellet forms may have increased risk.
   d. Estrogen users who do develop breast cancer have been shown to have decreased mortality over nonusers.
3. Thromboembolic disease: no increased risk with oral estrogens. Transdermal preparations recommended in patients with pre-existing disease as these agents bypass the first pass effect of the liver.

Contraindications to Estrogen

1. Personal history of estrogen-dependent tumors
2. Recurrent, active, or spontaneous thromboembolic disease
3. Acute severe liver disease

Key Treatment

- Natural estrogens
- Low androgenic progestins
- Calcium 1000 to 1500 mg/day
- Regular weight-bearing exercise

Follow-Up

1. Encourage patients to perform monthly breast self-examination.
2. Regular mammograms per recommended guidelines based on age and family history.
3. Regular clinical breast examinations every 6 to 12 months.
4. Endometrial biopsy if any abnormal bleeding on ERT.

 Bibliography

Harlap S: The benefits and risks of hormone replacement therapy: An epidemiologic overview. Am J Obstet Gynecol 1992;166:1986–1992.

Mishell D (ed): Menopause Physiology and Pharmacology. Chicago, Year Book, 1987.

Nabulsi AA, Folsom AR, White A, Patsch W, Heiss G, Wu KK, Szklo M: Association of hormone-replacement therapy with various cardiovascular risk factors in postmenopausal women. N Engl J Med 1993;328:1069–1075.

Notelovitz M: Estrogen replacement therapy: Indications, contraindication, and agent selection. Am J Obstet Gynecol 1989;161:1832–1841.

Williams DB, Moley KH: Progestin replacement in the menopause: Effects on the endometrium and serum lipids. Curr Opinion Obstet Gynecol 1994;6:284–292.

109 Ectopic Pregnancy

Tod Stillson

Etiology

1. Definition
   a. Blastocyst implantation anywhere except the endometrial cavity.
   b. Locations can include
      (1) Tubal—compose 99 per cent of all ectopics: 55 per cent are ampullary, 25 per cent isthmic, 17 per cent fimbrial, 2 per cent interstitial
      (2) Ovarian
      (3) Abdominal
      (4) Cervical
2. Risk Factors
   a. Pelvic inflammatory disease/salpingitis
   b. Peritubal adhesions—subsequent to postabortion, appendicitis, endometriosis, previous tubal pregnancy, tubal ligation
   c. Tubal developmental abnormalities
   d. Surgical manipulation of the tubes
   e. Tumors that distort the tube
   f. Intrauterine devices
   g. Use of ovulatory agents to induce fertility
   h. In utero exposure to diethylstilbestrol
   i. Use of Norplant or progesterone-only birth control pills

Symptoms

1. Amenorrhea, delayed menstruation
2. Vaginal bleeding—irregular, "spotting," usually scanty and dark brown
3. Severe lower abdominal pain—sharp, tearing, stabbing, may be unilateral, bilateral, lower abdominal, upper abdominal, or generalized
4. Vasomotor disturbances—range from vertigo to syncope
5. Shoulder or neck pain—secondary to diaphragmatic irritation

Key Symptoms	
• Amenorrhea	• Abdominal pain
• Irregular vaginal bleeding	• Dizziness/syncope

Clinical Findings

1. Orthostatic hypotension
2. Cervical motion tenderness
3. Adnexal tenderness

4. Abdominal tenderness—generalized or focal, peritoneal signs if ruptured
5. Palpable pelvic mass—usually posterior or lateral to uterus
6. Enlarged uterus—size increases almost appropriately for first 3 months
7. Temperature less than 38° C—in contrast to temperature in salpingitis

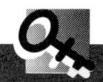

Key Signs	
• Cervical motion tenderness	• Palpable pelvic mass
	• Orthostatic hypotension
• Adnexal tenderness	

Laboratory Tests and Imaging Studies

1. Urine pregnancy test—sensitive for detecting β-human chorionic gonadotropin (β-hCG) levels greater than 50 milli-International Units (mIU)
2. Serum qualitative β-hCG—99 per cent sensitive in detecting pregnancy
3. Serum quantitative β-hCG
4. Complete blood count—Check for severe anemia; white blood cell count is nonspecific.
5. Blood type and Rh—Determine if rhogam is necessary.
6. Ultrasound—Look for absence of intrauterine pregnancy.
   a. Transabdominal—When β-hCG is greater than 6000 to 6500 mIU, 94 per cent sensitive.
   b. Transvaginal—When β-hCG is greater than 2000 mIU, is adequately sensitive.
7. Culdocentesis—withdrawal of nonclotting blood from Douglas' cul-de-sac, indicative of ectopic pregnancy. Coupled with positive pregnancy test is 95 per cent sensitive.
8. Endometrial curettage—Look for villi on histology to rule out incomplete abortion. Particularly helpful if β-hCG is less than 2000 mIU, no intrauterine pregnancy on transvaginal sonogram, and serum progesterone is less than 5.0 ng/ml.
9. Serum progesterone—Less than 15 ng/ml is suspicious for ectopic/abnormal pregnancy, and greater than 25 ng/ml is likely to be a normal intrauterine pregnancy.
10. Laparoscopy/laparotomy—diagnostic

Key Tests

- Pregnancy test— qualitative and/or quantitative
- Ultrasound
- Laparoscopy or laparotomy

Differential Diagnosis

1. Acute or chronic salpingitis/pelvic inflammatory disease—most commonly mistaken for ectopic pregnancy. Pain and tenderness usually bilateral, temperature usually greater than 38° C.
2. Threatened or incomplete abortion—Bleeding is usually heavy.
3. Ruptured corpus luteal or follicular cyst—Difficult to distinguish clinically from ectopic pregnancy.
4. Torsion of ovarian cyst
5. Appendicitis
6. Gastroenteritis
7. Discomfort from IUD—Crampy pelvic pain and bleeding are common problems.
8. Tubo-ovarian abscess
9. Ovarian tumor
10. Endometrioma

WARNING

Think ectopic!

Treatment

A. Surgical
   1. Salpingectomy
   2. Conservation of oviduct—linear salpingostomy, salpingotomy and tuboplasty, segmental resection
   3. Sterilization—Prior to surgery, check with patient about desired fertility.

B. Nonsurgical
   1. Methotrexate
      a. Qualifications
         (1) Diameter of ectopic pregnancy less than 3.5 cm
         (2) Serum β-hCG greater than 2000 mIU and

no intrauterine pregnancy on transvaginal sonogram, or

         (3) Serum β-hCG less than 2000 mIU and no villi on curettage
         (4) Without evidence of rupture or impending rupture
         (5) No evidence of hepatic dysfunction, blood dyscrasia, thrombocytopenia, or renal disease
      b. Dosage 50 mg/m² methotrexate intramuscularly once
      c. Follow-up β-hCG levels on days 4 and 7 and then weekly until less than 10 mIU
      d. About 94 per cent success rate
   2. Rhogam if patient Rh-negative
   3. Observation—in asymptomatic patients with low β-hCG (<2000) or declining β-hCG levels

Follow-Up

1. Patient monitoring
   a. Weekly serial serum quantitative β-hCG until level is less than 10 mIU
   b. Pelvic sonogram for persistent mass or increasing pain
2. Prevention
   a. Reliable contraception
   b. Risk of repeat ectopic pregnancy approximately 10 to 15 per cent
   c. Ultrasound should be used to confirm that future pregnancies are intrauterine.
3. Complications
   a. Infertility—20 to 50 per cent, or higher in nulliparous women
   b. Infection, postoperative

Bibliography

Carson SA, Buster JE: Ectopic pregnancy. N Engl J Med 1993;329:1174–1181.

Cunningham G, MacDonald P, Gant F, et al (eds): Ectopic pregnancy. *In* Williams' Obstetrics, 19th ed. Norwalk, CT, Appleton and Lange, 1993, pp 691–719.

Lawlor HK, Rubin BJ: Early diagnosis of ectopic pregnancy. West J Med 1993;159:195–199.

Rock J: Ectopic pregnancy. *In* Operative Gynecology, 7th ed. Philadelphia, JB Lippincott, 1992, pp 411–436.

Ory SJ: New options for diagnosis and treatment of ectopic pregnancy. JAMA January 1992;267(4):534–537.

110 Premenstrual Syndrome

Janet C. Lindemann

Etiology

"Premenstrual syndrome" (PMS) is the cyclic recurrence of a group of symptoms which peak premenstrually and disappear postmenstrually. While no cause has been clearly substantiated, several endocrine hypotheses exist:

1. Neurotransmitter dysfunction
2. Prostaglandin excess
3. Pyridoxine (vitamin B_6) deficiency
4. Estrogen/progesterone imbalance, especially progesterone deficiency
5. Endorphin-mediation

Symptoms

1. Multiple and diverse symptoms including but not limited to
   a. Somatic (mastalgia, bloating, headache, pelvic pain, fatigue)
   b. Mood (irritability, depression, mood swings)
   c. Cognitive (poor concentration, confusion)
   d. Behavioral (social withdrawal, impulsiveness, appetite changes)
2. At least one somatic symptom and one psychological symptom (mood, cognitive, or behavioral) is necessary for the diagnosis of PMS.
3. The cyclic premenstrual timing of the symptoms is key. The patient's pattern is repetitive and demonstrates a peak of symptom severity immediately prior to menses and a symptom-free interval following menses.

Key Symptom

Cyclic recurrence of multiple symptoms premenstrually

Clinical Findings

There are no characteristic physical signs for PMS, but a complete physical examination should be performed to rule out other illnesses.

Laboratory Tests

1. The symptom diary is the essential test for PMS and should be kept prospectively for a minimum of three months (Fig. 110–1).
2. No other laboratory tests are useful except to rule out other causes.

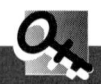

Key Test

A symptom diary is the key test for PMS.

Differential Diagnosis

1. Primary affective disorder
   a. Anxiety or depressive neuroses may have related physical symptoms and premenstrual exacerbation.
   b. Absence of symptoms will not be present postmenstrually.
2. Dysmenorrhea: Physical symptoms of pelvic cramping may begin premenstrually but peak during menses.
3. Menstrual migraine
   a. Vascular headache symptom complex with exacerbation premenstrually.
   b. Probably a separate disorder and responsive to migraine therapy.

Treatment

Medication

Unless otherwise stated, these drugs are used throughout the monthly cycle.

1. Etiology-based treatments
   a. Fluoxetine (Prozac), 20 mg daily, or sertraline (Zoloft), 50 mg daily
   b. Naproxen sodium, 550 mg b.i.d. from onset of symptoms until menses
   c. Pyridoxine (vitamin B_6), 50 to 100 mg daily
   d. Progesterone, 400-mg suppositories, up to 4 daily, or oral micronized natural progesterone, 200 mg b.i.d. from anticipated onset of symptoms until menses. While its effectiveness is not corroborated by placebo-controlled studies, progesterone is used with reported success in PMS clinics.
2. Symptomatic therapy
   a. Alprazolam (Xanax), 0.25 mg t.i.d., or buspirone (BuSpar), 5 to 10 mg t.i.d. for anxiety
   b. Spironolactone (Aldactone), 25 mg q.i.d. for fluid retention from onset of symptoms until menses
   c. Bromocriptine (Parlodel), 5 mg daily for breast pain
3. Anovulatory treatment
   a. Danazol (Danocrine), 200 mg daily
   b. Oral contraceptives

Diet

1. Patients should be encouraged to eat small meals frequently which are high in complex carbohydrates to avoid sharp fluctuations in blood glucose concentrations.
2. Limit salt and caffeine.

Month:	Jan.	Feb.	March			
1						
2						
3						
4						
5						
6		h				
7						
8						
9						
10						
11						
12						
13			H d			
14			H D			
15			H D			
16		D	H D			
17		H d	M d			
18	d	H D	M			
19	H d	H D	M			
20	D	M	M			
21	M D	M	M			
22	M D	M				
23	M h	M				
24	M					
25	M					
26	M					
27	M					
28						
29						
30						
31						

Key: M = menstruation

Use capital letters for severe symptoms and small letters for mild symptoms.

symbol	symptom
H	headache
D	depressive symptoms

Figure 110–1. Symptom diary. (From Lindemann JC: Premenstrual syndrome: A practical approach. Wis Med J 1984;83:30–32.)

Activity

Regular moderate exercise has been shown to be effective in alleviating symptoms.

Patient Education

1. Since patients may have preconceived notions about PMS from the lay media, it is essential to provide information based on medical studies.
2. The education that results from maintaining the symptom diary often reduces anxiety and other symptoms.

Follow-Up

1. Initially, the patient needs to be seen every 3 months to make the diagnosis and monitor treatment.
2. Establish realistic expectations for symptom improvement.

Bibliography

For more information on diagnosis, see
Johnson SR: Clinician's approach to the diagnosis and management of premenstrual syndrome. Clin Obstet Gynecol 1992;35(3):637–657.

For more information on endocrine theories, see
Strickler RC: Endocrine hypotheses for the etiology of premenstrual syndrome. Clin Obstet Gynecol 1987;30(2):377–385.

For more information on symptom diaries, see
Lindemann JC: Premenstrual syndrome: A practical approach. Wisc Med J 1984;83:30–32.

For more information on treatment, see
Moline ML: Pharmacologic strategies for managing premenstrual syndrome. Clin Pharmacol 1993;12:181–196.

For more information on depression and PMS, see
Bancroft J, et al: Vulnerability to premenstrual mood change: The relevance of a past history of depressive disorder. Psychosom Med 1994;56(3):225–231.

111 Contraception

Selecting a Contraceptive Method

1. The first consideration is permanent versus reversible contraception. If permanent contraception is desired, sterilization of either partner is the method of choice, if cost is not prohibitive.

2. If reversibility is desired, level of contraceptive efficacy is the next consideration. The couple must decide what degree of risk of failure their life situation can tolerate. Reversible contraception can be broadly grouped into high, medium, and low effectiveness.

   a. *High effectiveness:* Norplant, depot medroxyprogesterone acetate, intrauterine device (IUD), combined oral contraceptives, and progestin-only oral contraceptives

   b. *Medium effectiveness:* condoms, female condoms, cervical cap, diaphragm, vaginal sponge, and spermicides. (Appropriately selected combinations of these should be able to achieve effectiveness equivalent to the first category.)

   c. *Low effectiveness:* periodic abstinence, coitus interruptus. These can be recommended only in the very unusual circumstances in which all other methods are unacceptable to the couple; these will not be discussed further in this chapter.

3. Engage the patient in an honest evaluation of her ability to be consistently compliant with daily pill use or coitus-dependent actions (barrier methods). If this cannot be ensured, a long-acting method is to be strongly preferred.

4. Prepare for the patient a list of options in order of your customized recommendations for her, based on the preceding considerations. Discuss relative advantages, disadvantages, and costs, leaving the final decision to the patient. If condoms are not to be the primary contraceptive method, their use should be advised in addition to the primary method for any couple at risk of sexually transmitted disease (STD) transmission.

Male Sterilization

1. *Advantages:* Permanent, highly effective, no user action needed after azoospermia verified.

2. *Disadvantages:* Reversal expensive and inconsistently successful.

3. *Short-term complications:* Less than 2 per cent incidence of infection, hematoma, sperm granuloma, and congestive epididymitis.

4. *Long-term complications:* Possible consequences in essentially every organ system, especially cardiovascular disease, have been postulated, but none confirmed. Recent studies appear to show an increased

lifetime risk of prostate cancer, but no plausible explanatory biological mechanism is available. At present, consensus is that this possibility need not deter patients from vasectomy.

5. *Failures:* Most are due to recanalization, usually within 6 weeks. This can be detected by semen analysis 6 and 10 weeks after procedure.

Female Sterilization

1. *Advantages:* Permanent, highly effective, no user action needed after procedure.

2. *Disadvantages:* Compared with male sterilization, cost, invasiveness, complications, and failure rate are all higher. Reversal is expensive and inconsistently successful. May leave visible scars.

3. *Short-term complications:* Occasional bleeding, infection.

4. *Long-term complications:* When failure occurs, relative risk of ectopic pregnancy is increased. Hormonal and menstrual pattern changes have been reported, but a causal relationship has not been established.

Intrauterine Device (IUD)

Note: This section describes the Copper-T 380A (Paragard) IUD. A progesterone-releasing IUD (Progestasert) is also available but is generally reserved for patients experiencing menorrhagia and will not be discussed herein.

1. *Mechanism:* Exact mechanism is uncertain, but primarily prevents fertilization, probably by immobilization of sperm by copper, as well as nonspecific foreign body reaction.

2. *Effectiveness:* 0.8 per cent typical first-year failure rate; 78 per cent 1-year continuation rate.

3. *Advantages:* High effectiveness. No user action is required after insertion (though patient should check position monthly). Longest duration (10 years) and lowest annualized cost of any reversible contraception.

4. *Disadvantages:* Appropriate only for parous women in stable, monogamous relationships.

5. *Risks:* Insertion occasionally causes uterine infection or perforation. STDs more likely to result in pelvic inflammatory disease (PID) with IUD in place. In case of failure, risk of ectopic pregnancy is increased, and risk of spontaneous abortion is 25 to 50 per cent.

6. *Side effects:* Increased menstrual bleeding and cramping, usually well tolerated; cause for removal in 10 to 15 per cent of patients. Intermenstrual bleeding is common in first few months.

7. *Contraindications:* Nulliparity, risk for acquiring

STD, uterine malformations or cancer, undiagnosed unusual vaginal bleeding.

8. *Insertion and removal:* See Procedure following this chapter.

Levonorgestrel Implants (Norplant)

1. *Mechanism:* Six subdermal 34-millimeter flexible Silastic capsules release levonorgestrel over 5 years. Levonorgestrel causes genital tract changes typical of the luteal phase: increased thickness of cervical mucus, decreased uterine tube motility, disorganized endometrium. Ovulation is only inconsistently suppressed.

2. *Effectiveness:* 0.9 per cent first-year failure with both typical and perfect use. One-year continuation rate is 85 per cent (highest of any reversible method). Body weight greater than 70 kg decreases effectiveness, estimated at a cumulative pregnancy risk of 7 per cent over 5 years. This is still better use-effectiveness than oral contraceptives (OCs) or any barrier method and should not be considered a contraindication to use of Norplant.

3. *Advantages:* High effectiveness, long duration, high continuation rate, no user action needed after insertion.

4. *Disadvantages:* Frequent menstrual changes, high initial cost (though if amortized over 3 or more years, comparable to OCs), requires minor surgical procedure to insert and remove.

5. *Risks:* No tumorigenic effect known or suspected. No known adverse effect on fetus in case of failure. No known adverse effect in infant if used during breastfeeding. Relative risk of ectopic pregnancy, in case of failure, may be increased. No permanent effect on fertility; serum levels are undetectable within 48 hours of removal. Minimal or no adverse effect on blood pressure, carbohydrate metabolism, liver function tests, coagulation, or blood lipids.

6. *Side effects*

   a. Sixty per cent of women have significant changes in menstrual patterns. Bleeding may occur daily for first 6 to 9 months of use. Patient must be explicitly warned about this, since it is the leading cause of patient dissatisfaction. After this interval, irregular menses remain the rule, though total amount of bleeding per year is about the same as without hormones. Many women regain a fairly regular pattern in third or fourth year, but this cannot be ensured.

   b. Headaches; mechanism unknown. If not relieved by standard analgesics, a common cause for Norplant removal.

   c. Weight gain or loss. Neither is clearly a direct effect of the hormone.

   d. Mastalgia, galactorrhea. More common when in-

sertion occurs during lactation. Usually transitory; no treatment needed.

   e. Acne. Worst in first year. Treat in standard manner. (Antibiotics are not contraindicated.)

   f. *Other:* Ovarian cysts, hirsutism, scalp hair loss, cervicitis, vaginitis, dizziness, abdominal pain, musculoskeletal pain, insertion-site pain or pigmentation. All are usually self-limited or, if severe or prolonged, treated by removal of the Norplant.

   g. *Prediction of side effects:* A 1- to 6-month trial of norgestrel progestin-only pills (Ovrette) may predict tolerance of Norplant side effects, but this theory has not been formally tested.

7. *Contraindications:* Active thrombotic disease (though probably not worsened by Norplant), undiagnosed abnormal vaginal bleeding, active liver disease, current breast or genital tract cancer.

8. *Drug interactions:* Phenytoin and carbamazepine significantly reduce effectiveness of Norplant; their use should be considered a contraindication.

9. *Insertion and removal techniques:* See Procedure.

Depot Medroxyprogesterone Acetate (DMPA) (Depo-Provera)

1. *Mechanism:* Primary means of action is inhibition of ovulation by suppression of pituitary secretion of luteinizing hormone (LH) and follicle-stimulating hormone (FSH). DMPA also causes genital tract changes typical of the secretory phase (e.g., thickened cervical mucus, decreased uterine tube motility).

2. *Effectiveness:* 0.3 per cent first-year failure rate with both typical and perfect use; 70 per cent first-year continuation rate.

3. *Advantages:* High effectiveness. No user action is needed between injections. Use is undetectable to partner (a feature unique to this method). Can be given immediately postpartum; does not interfere with lactation. Probably protective against ovarian and endometrial cancer. Increases hemoglobin concentration. Inhibits sickling in sickle cell anemia.

4. *Disadvantages:* Return of fertility after last injection is variable: 50 per cent at 6 months, 75 per cent at 12 months, 85 per cent at 18 months, 95 per cent at 24 months. (Remainder have other causes of infertility.)

5. *Risks:* No known teratogenicity. No known carcinogenicity. Relative risk of ectopic pregnancy is increased in case of failure. Possible slight decrease in bone density with long-term use, though, if true, presumably reversible upon cessation of use. No adverse effects on glucose, lipids, or blood pressure.

6. *Side effects:* Menstrual irregularity is nearly universal; continued use usually leads to amenorrhea. About 1 in 200 women will require treatment for very heavy or prolonged bleeding; one combined oral contraceptive pill (50 or 35 μg estrogen) daily for 14 days is usually adequate. Injection soon after childbirth usu-

ally causes prolonged (weeks), but not severe, post-partum bleeding. Weight gain of 1 to 3 kg is common, but 20 to 40 per cent of patients lose weight. Premenstrual syndrome–like symptoms are common with first injection but resolve spontaneously and are less severe with subsequent shots.

7. *Contraindications:* None

8. *Drug interactions:* No known interaction with antibiotics or anticonvulsants

9. *Administration:* 150 mg injected deep intramuscularly (deltoid or gluteus). Peak serum levels occur within 24 hours. Plateau levels are maintained about 3 months, with gradual declines thereafter. First injection is ideally given in first 7 days of menstrual cycle, but it can be given any time that the absence of pregnancy can be ensured. Subsequent doses are given every 3 months. A patient presenting up to 2 weeks beyond the scheduled date can be given her shot without fear of pregnancy.

Combined Oral Contraceptives (COCs)

1. *Mechanism:* Primarily suppress ovulation by inhibition of gonadotropins. Secondarily, the progestin component produces genital tract changes of the luteal phase.

2. *Effectiveness:* 0.1 per cent first-year failure rate with perfect use; 3 per cent with typical use. One-year continuation rate is 72 per cent.

3. *Advantages:* Highly effective with proper use. Causes decreased rates of benign breast disease, endometriosis, dysmenorrhea, anemia, premenstrual syndrome, and ovarian and endometrial cancers. Can be used to treat benign menstrual irregularities, endometriosis, and polycystic ovarian disease. Mild protective effect against PID.

4. *Disadvantages:* Effectiveness is dependent on consistent daily use, which is difficult for many users, especially adolescents.

5. *Risks*
   a. Small adverse effect on lipid profile, but probably not atherogenic.
   b. Rare thrombotic effects (deep vein thrombosis, stroke, myocardial infarction). This is essentially limited to smokers and those with pre-existing (though often unknown) hypercoagulable state. In smokers over age 35, risk of death from this cause exceeds risk of death from accidental pregnancy, contraindicating COCs.
   c. Between 1 and 5 per cent of women develop hypertension, reversible with cessation of use. Previously controlled hypertension may worsen, but a trial of COCs may be attempted.
   d. *Reproductive system:* Relative risk of ectopic pregnancy is increased in case of failure. Possibly a slight (3 per cent) increase in lifetime risk of cervical cancer. Breast cancer risk probably not

increased by COCs. Conflicting evidence on whether tricyclic preparations increase risk of functional ovarian cysts.
   e. *Hepatobiliary system:* Increased incidence of gallstones. Relative risks of hepatic adenoma and hepatocellular carcinoma are increased, but absolute risk is negligible.
   f. *Teratogenicity:* Several effects postulated, none confirmed
   g. *Use during lactation:* No adverse effect on infant but may decrease quantity and quality of milk produced; progestin-only methods are preferred.

6. *Side effects*
   a. *Systemic:* Symptoms similar to early pregnancy (nausea, fluid retention, breast tenderness) may occur during first two to three cycles. Some women report libido changes, mood changes, and frank depression. Increased appetite may lead to weight gain, though weight loss is just as common.
   b. *Reproductive tract:* Breakthrough bleeding common in first three cycles. Menstrual bleeding is often scant. Amenorrhea may occur occasionally; if for two or more consecutive cycles, test for pregnancy, and then consider change of COC formulation.
   c. *Neurologic:* New onset of migraine with pill use requires discontinuation. Pre-existing common migraines are not necessarily a contraindication.
   d. *Dermatologic:* Oily skin and exacerbation of acne are fairly frequent, hair loss less so; change to a progestin of low androgenicity. Melasma occurs rarely.

7. *Contraindications*
   a. *Absolute:* Current or past thrombotic disease, cerebrovascular accident, coronary artery disease, breast, genital tract, or liver cancer, current pregnancy or impaired liver function.
   b. *Relative:* Smoker over age 35, diabetes, undiagnosed abnormal vaginal bleeding, lactation.

8. *Drug interactions*
   a. *Antibiotics:* Rifampin and griseofulvin reduce contraceptive efficacy; barrier method should be added during their use. Contrary to common belief, other commonly used antibiotics are not known to exert any clinically significant effect on COC efficacy, and additional precautions are not needed.
   b. *Anticonvulsants:* Phenytoin, carbamazepine, and barbiturates decrease COC efficacy. Alternative methods (such as DMPA) are preferred, though a 50-μg pill may be considered.
   c. *Other drugs* whose effect may be altered by COCs and must be monitored: Warfarin, thyroid hormone, corticosteroids (effect decreased); cyclosporine, tricyclic antidepressants, theophylline (effect increased).

9. *Prescribing information*

a. *Pill selection:* Clinical differences between formulations of low-dose pills (≤35 μg estrogen) are minimal. Selection can logically be made on the basis of cost (several generic formulations are available) and/or lowest total monthly hormone dose. Also, 28-day packs are to be preferred.

b. *Patient education:* Needs to emphasize consistency of use. Also include written information on when to start pills (Sunday start seems to be easiest and most common method), side effects, missed pills, warning signs of dangerous complications.

c. *Follow-up:* If possible, give three to four sample packages, and then see patient again to check blood pressure, evaluate side effects, inquire about consistency of use. Encourage phone calls for problems or questions and have well-trained nurse to handle such calls.

Progestin-Only Pills (POPs)

1. *Mechanism:* Primary mechanism is induction of genital tract changes of the luteal phase. Ovulation inconsistently suppressed.

2. *Effectiveness:* 0.5 per cent first-year failure rate with perfect use; 3 per cent with typical use. One-year continuation rate 72 per cent.

3. *Advantages:* Highly effective with consistent use. POPs eliminate estrogenic and thrombotic side effects and risks of COCs. Can be used immediately postpartum with no adverse effect on infant or lactation.

4. *Disadvantages:* Effectiveness dependent on consistent daily use, which is difficult for many users, especially adolescents. This is even more important with POPs than with COCs, a method more tolerant of occasional omissions.

5. *Risks:* Relative risk of ectopic pregnancy is increased in case of failure. No known carcinogenicity or teratogenicity. No thrombotic risks. Increased rate of functional ovarian cysts.

6. *Side effects:* Menstrual irregularity indicates consistent or intermittent anovulation (and higher efficacy); many women continue having regular ovulatory cycles. Any of the other side effects listed for COCs may occur with POPs, but with much lower incidences.

7. *Contraindications:* Undiagnosed irregular vaginal bleeding, current genital tract cancer, active liver disease.

8. *Drug interactions:* None of clinical significance.

9. *Prescribing information*

a. *Pill selection:* Only two formulations are available in the United States (norethindrone 0.35 mg, norgestrel 0.075 mg); there is no compelling reason to prefer one over the other.

b. *Patient education:* Must emphasize consistency of use. Also stress that, unlike with COCs, there are no monthly pill-free intervals and no placebo pills that can be ignored; pill ingestion is daily, without exception.

c. *Follow-up:* Same as for COCs.

Barrier Methods

1. *Condoms:* 3 per cent first-year failure rate with perfect use; 12 per cent with typical use. Provide best protection against STDs. Recommend latex, prelubricated condoms and use of additional intravaginal spermicide (any form). During patient education, include information on consistency of use, method and timing of use, and lubrication use.

2. *Female condoms* (Reality): 5 per cent first-year failure rate with perfect use; 21 per cent with typical use. Instruct patient in consistency of use, proper insertion, and use of additional spermicide.

3. *Diaphragm:* 6 per cent first-year failure rate with perfect use; 18 per cent with typical use. Increases risk of urinary tract infections (UTIs). Instruct patient in concurrent use of spermicide, timing of use, proper care of diaphragm. See Procedure following for fitting instructions.

4. *Cervical cap:* First-year failure rate 26 per cent (parous) or 9 per cent (nulliparous) with perfect use; 36 or 18 per cent, respectively, with typical use. No apparent effect on cervical dysplasia, as earlier feared. Can be left in up to 48 hours. Care is similar to that of a diaphragm. See source in Bibliography for fitting instructions.

5. *Vaginal sponge* (Today): First-year failure rate 20 per cent (parous) or 9 per cent (nulliparous) with perfect use; 36 or 18 per cent, respectively, with typical use. Can be left in through repeated acts of intercourse up to 24 hours. Relatively expensive. Distribution in the U.S. was halted in 1994 and its future is uncertain.

6. *Spermicides:* 6 per cent first-year failure rate with perfect use; 21 per cent with typical use. Can be purchased without prescription in multiple forms: creams, gels, foams, suppositories, and film. All use either nonoxynol 9 (1 to 28%) or octoxynol 9 (1 to 3%), surfactants with similar properties. Instructions for proper use are different for each product. Can be used with any other barrier method to increase efficacy. May cause local irritation and increase risk of vaginal candidiasis

Postcoital Contraception

1. *Oral contraceptives:* Two tablets of Ovral (preferred) or four tablets of Lo/Ovral, Nordette, or Levlen as one dose; repeat 12 hours later. Must be initiated within 72 hours of unprotected intercourse, preferably within 24 hours. Pregnancy risk after treatment is approximately 1.8 per cent. Nausea is frequent, 50 per cent or more. Vomiting may necessitate retreatment.

Older, high-dose estrogen regimens (including DES) are no longer recommended.

2. *Danazol:* 600 mg as a single dose, repeated 12 hours later. Must be initiated within 72 hours of intercourse. Pregnancy risk after treatment is approximately 2.0 per cent. Side effects are similar to above but less frequent.

3. *IUD insertion:* Can be performed up to 5 days after intercourse and is the most effective available method (pregnancy rate 0.1 per cent). However, it is rare to find a woman in need of emergency postcoital contraception who is both a willing and suitable candidate for an IUD.

Bibliography

Contraceptives. *In* Drug Evaluations Subscription. Chicago, American Medical Association, Fall 1993.

Choice of contraceptives. Med Lett 1995;37:9–12.

Filshie M, Guillebaud J (eds): Contraception: Science and Practice. London, Butterworths, 1989.

Hatcher RA, Trussell J, Stewart F, et al: Contraceptive Technology, 16th ed. New York, Irvington Publishers, 1994.

Shoupe D, Haseltine FP (eds): Contraception. New York, Springer-Verlag, 1993.

| Procedure | **DIAPHRAGM FITTING** | *Cecilia M. Romero* |

Advantages

1. Barrier method of contraception in which potential side effects associated with systemic medications are avoided
2. Intermittent usage, offering a woman more control over her body
3. Protection against sexually transmitted diseases (STDs), including gonorrhea, syphilis, herpes, *Trichomonas,* and *Chlamydia* when used with spermicide

Contraindications

1. Allergy to rubber, latex, or spermicides
2. Uterine prolapse, severe cystocele, rectocele, or substantial anteversion or retroversion of the uterus
3. Recurrent urinary tract infections (UTIs)
4. Inability to have diaphragm fitted correctly
5. Inability to insert or remove diaphragm
6. History of toxic shock syndrome

Preparation

1. Appropriate counseling regarding diaphragm use, advantages, and disadvantages. Strong emphasis should be placed on the fact that effectiveness depends on motivation and correct use.
2. Complete history to assess appropriateness of diaphragm as method of contraception for this patient.
3. Complete pelvic examination to rule out any pelvic abnormality that contraindicates its use
4. Clean set of diaphragm rings or full diaphragms

Equipment

1. Set of diaphragm rings or diaphragms. Set of diaphragms of the different spring types is best. Sizes range from 50 to 100 mm in diameter. Sizes increase in 5-mm increments.
2. The following diaphragms are available by spring type (see Table 111–1):
   a. Arcing spring—sizes 55 to 95
      (1) Used most often in the United States—thought to be the easiest to insert
      (2) Recommended for women with less than normal vaginal support
   b. Coil spring—sizes 50 to 95
      (1) May be used with introducer or inserter for those having trouble with insertion
      (2) Recommended for those with good vaginal support
   c. Flat spring—sizes 55 to 95
      (1) May be used with introducer or inserter for those having trouble with insertion
      (2) Suitable for smaller women, especially those with a shallow notch or pocket behind the symphysis

Precautions

1. Allergy to rubber, latex, or spermicide
2. Diaphragm users may have more frequent UTIs.
3. Toxic shock syndrome has been reported and has in most cases involved retention of the diaphragm for at least 36 hours.
4. Foul vaginal discharge and vaginal wall ulceration can be associated with prolonged retention.
5. Should not be used during the 6-week postpartum period.

TABLE 111–1. AVAILABLE DIAPHRAGMS BY SPRING TYPE AND MANUFACTURER

| SPRING TYPE (IN DESCENDING ORDER OF STRENGTH) | MANUFACTURER | | | |
	Ortho Pharmaceuticals	Holland-Rantos	Schmid Products	Milex
Arcing Spring	Allflex Sizes 55–95	Koroflex Sizes 60–95	Rames Bendex Sizes 65–95	Wide-seal Sizes 60–95
Coil Spring	Ortho Diaphragm Sizes 50–95	Koromex Sizes 50–95	Ramses Flexible Cushioned Sizes 50–95	Wide Seal Omiflex Sizes 60–95
Flat Spring	Ortho White Sizes 55–95			

From Corsaro M, Lichtman R: Barrier methods. *In* Lichtman R, Papera S (eds): Gynecology—Well-Woman Care. East Norwalk, CT, Appleton & Lange, 1990.

Technique

1. The examiner inserts gloved index and middle fingers into the patient's vagina to measure the distance from the posterior cervix to the inner aspect of the symphysis pubis. The middle finger touches the posterior vaginal wall, and the distance to the index finger at the symphysis pubis is measured using the tip of the thumb.

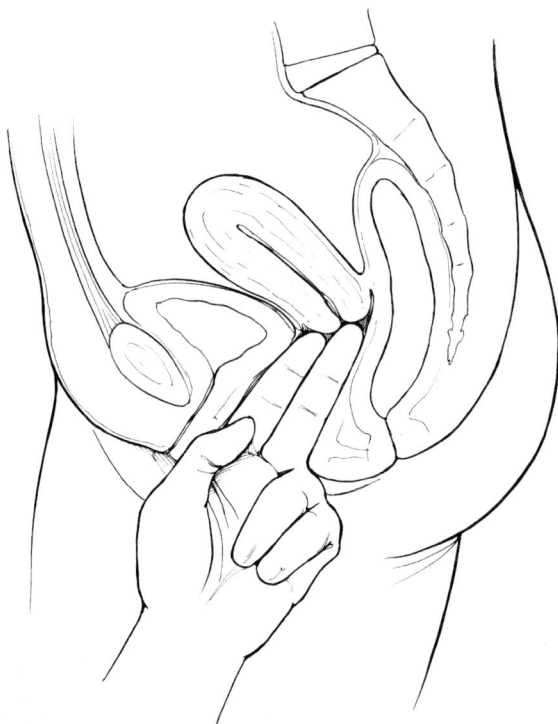

This is the approximate diameter of a diaphragm that will fit.

2. Measure the distance from the distal middle finger to the point where the inner aspect of the symphysis pubis was on the index finger. This measurement can be done directly on the diaphragm rings.

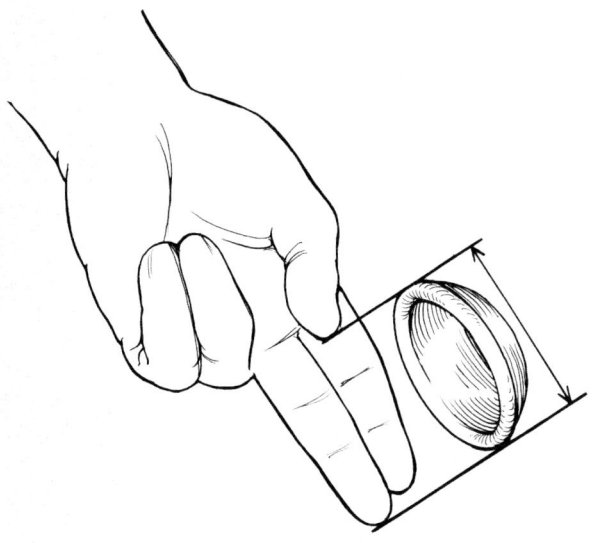

3. Match the length to the diameter of the fitting diaphragms or rings. Insert the diaphragm or ring into the vagina to check the fit. The cervix should be covered as well as the anterior rim behind the pubic bone. There should be a fingertip space between the pubic arch and the diaphragm rim or ring.

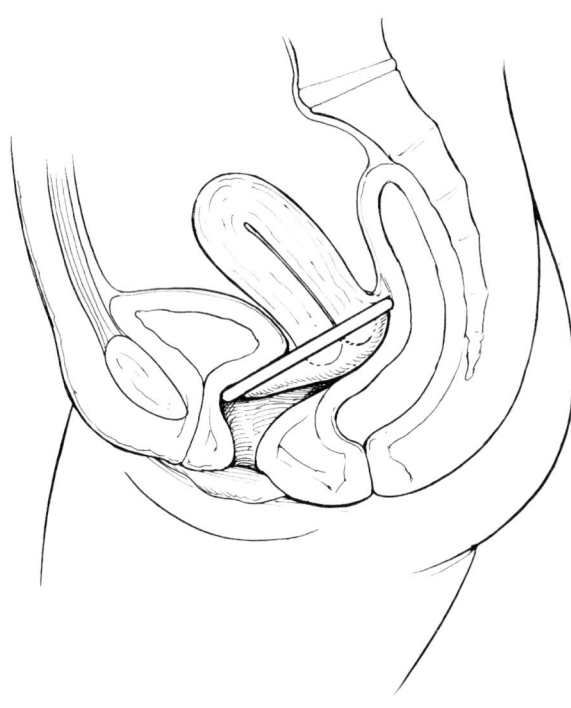

4. The initial estimate of the size of the diaphragm may change after the first attempt to fit. The correct size has been selected if the cervix is covered completely and at least but not more than one finger fits between the pubic bone and anterior rim and the sides of the diaphragm do not buckle against the vaginal side walls but are held firmly by the walls. Change size if necessary.

5. The patient should walk around for a few minutes with the diaphragm or ring in place to make sure she cannot feel it. The patient should feel inside her vagina and feel the cervix to be certain the cervix is covered.

6. The examiner should recheck to see if the diaphragm or ring is still in place.

7. The patient should be instructed on its insertion and removal. It is helpful to have the patient practice insertion and removal at this time, if possible. Reinforcement is necessary regarding the patient's need to practice insertion and removal of the diaphragm.

8. Rings or diaphragms should be washed thoroughly in mild soap and water and disinfected.

9. Write prescription for diaphragm by rim type and size.

Follow-Up

1. Patient should be instructed to practice with the diaphragm for 1 to 2 weeks and then return for a check. It may be best to recommend additional contraceptive use such as condoms, in addition to the diaphragm and spermicide during this initial period. She should use the diaphragm for at least one 8-hour period even if she does not have intercourse.

2. The practitioner should be available by phone to answer any questions the woman may have.

3. At the follow-up visit, the woman should be wearing the diaphragm or insert it during the visit. Correct placement is assessed by the examiner. The patient is encouraged to ask questions and discuss concerns at this time.

Bibliography

Brenner PF, Mishell DR Jr: Control of human reproduction: Contraception, fertilization, and pregnancy termination, *In* JR Scott, PJ DiSaia, CB Hammond, WN Spellay (eds): Danforth's Obstetrics and Gynecology, 6th ed. Philadelphia, JB Lippincott, 1990, pp 709–713.

Burkman RT: Barrier methods and spermicides. *In* Handbook of Contraception and Abortion. Boston, Little, Brown, 1989, chap 3, pp 55–59.

Corsaro M, Lichtman R: Barrier methods. *In* R Lichtman, S Papera (eds): Gynecology: Well-Woman Care. E Norwalk, Conn, Appleton & Lange, 1990, chap 6, pp 71–89.

Heaton CJ, Smith MA: The diaphragm. Am Fam Physician 1989;39(5):231–236.

Kovacs GT: Fitting a diaphragm. Aust Fam Physician 1990;19(5):713–716.

| Procedure | **IUD INSERTION AND REMOVAL** | *Deborah Spring* |

There are, currently, two products marketed in the United States: ParaGard, T380A and Progestasert.

Indications

An IUD is indicated for intrauterine contraception. It is recommended for women who

- Have at least one child
- Are in a stable, monogamous relationship
- Have no history of pelvic inflammatory disease (PID)

Contraindications

1. Pregnancy
2. Uterine abnormalities
3. Acute PID, cervicitis, or vaginitis
4. Postpartum endometritis
5. Known or suspected malignancy or abnormal Pap smear
6. Impaired resistance to infection (e.g., AIDS, diabetes, steroid use)
7. Multiple sexual partners
8. History of ectopic pregnancy
9. Known allergy to copper

Equipment

1. Sterile speculum, uterine sound, scissors, and tenaculum
2. Antiseptic solution
3. IUD insertion kit

Preparation

1. Review and sign informed consent.
2. Confirm that the patient has a normal Pap smear.
3. Evaluate for active pelvic infection; culture if indicated.
4. Instruct the patient to have insertion performed within 7 days after onset of menses. This minimizes the likelihood of pregnancy and eases insertion.
5. Antibiotics (optional)
   a. Doxycycline, 200 mg 1 hour prior to insertion, or
   b. Erythromycin, 500 mg 1 hour prior and 6 hours after insertion

Anesthesia (Optional)

Ibuprofen, 600 milligrams 2 hours prior to insertion

Precautions

1. Any intrauterine procedure can cause pain, bradycardia, and syncope.
2. Confirm that there is no evidence of acute or chronic infection.

WARNING

- **The possibility of perforation must be kept in mind during insertion. If perforation occurs, the IUD should be removed as soon as possible.**

Technique

1. Explain the procedure, risks, and complications to the patient.
2. Review informed consent with the patient, and obtain signature.
3. Perform a bimanual examination, with the patient in the lithotomy position, to determine position of the uterus and to exclude pregnancy.
4. Insert speculum and visualize the cervix.
5. Cleanse the cervix with antiseptic solution.
6. Grasp the cervix with the tenaculum. Apply traction to stabilize and straighten the uterus.
7. Sound the uterus to determine depth and direction of the canal. Depth should be equal to or greater than 6.5 centimeters.

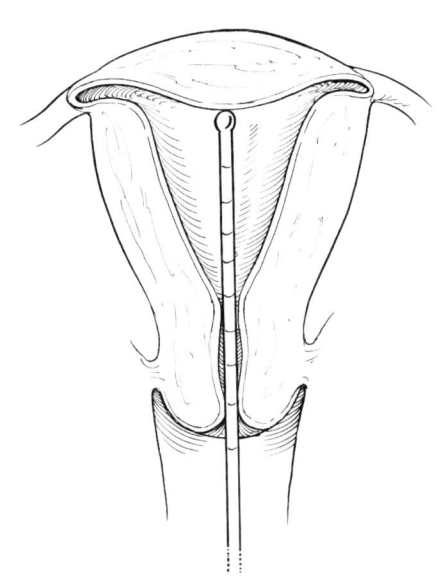

8. Follow package instruction for preparation of the IUD (ParaGard or Progestasert). Load IUD into inserter.

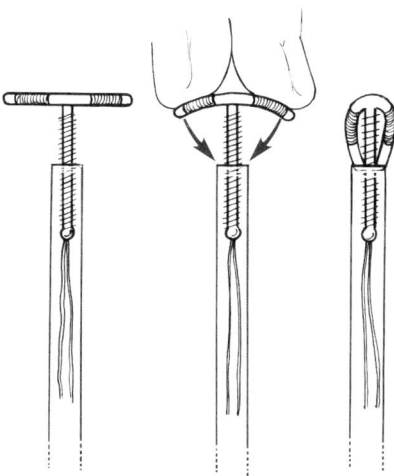

9. Advance the insertion tube to the correct depth as determined by the uterine sound.
   a. For the ParaGard T380A, refer to the plastic flange.
   b. For the Progestasert, refer to the printed gradations.
10. Introduce the loaded inserter through the cervical canal until the IUD lies in contact with the fundus.

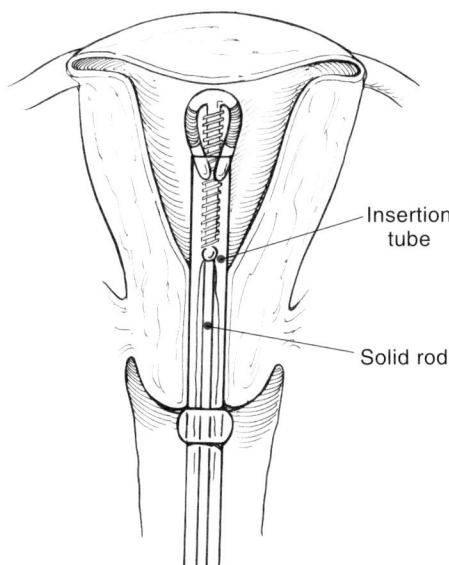

Insertion tube

Solid rod

Ensure that the horizontal arms of the IUD and the long axis of the flange lie in the same horizontal plane.
11. Release IUD.
   a. ParaGard T380A
      (1) While holding the solid rod stationary, withdraw the insertion tube approximately ½ inch to release the arms of the ParaGard.

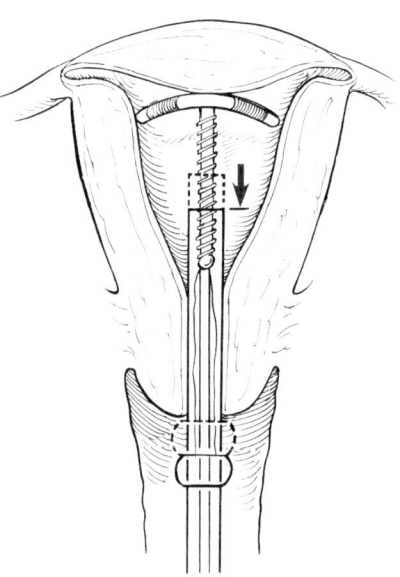

(2) Advance the insertion tube until fundal resistance is felt.
      (3) Withdraw the solid rod first and then the insertion tube.
   b. Progestasert
      (1) Squeeze the wings of the thread-retaining plug, and remove it.
      (2) Slowly withdraw the insertion tube.
12. Clip strings long (2.5 to 4 centimeters from external os).

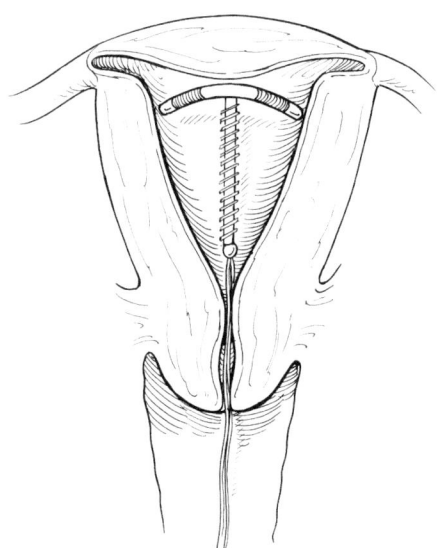

13. Observe for signs of vasovagal reactions.
14. Discharge the patient when stable.

Follow-Up

1. Re-examine the patient in 1 to 3 months to evaluate for expulsion; schedule annual examinations thereafter.

2. Educate the patient to monitor the IUD strings for evidence of expulsion.

3. Instruct the patient to have the IUD replaced at the appropriate time interval.

   a. After 8 years of use for the ParaGard T380A

   b. Not longer than 12 months of use for the Progestasert

Removal

1. Visualize the cervix and IUD strings.

2. Grasp string with forceps, and remove with steady, gentle traction.

3. If strings are not visible, gently insert a cytobrush or cotton swab into the endocervical canal and twirl while removing slowly.

> **WARNING**
>
> **Never attempt reinsertion of a partially expelled IUD; it must be removed.**

Bibliography

ParaGard T380 prescribing information, GynoPharma, Inc., Somerville, NJ, June 1993.

Progestasert prescribing information, Alza Corporation, Palo Alto, CA, May 1993.

Sivin I, Greenslade F, Schmidt F, Wadman SN: The Copper T380 Intrauterine Device: A Summary of Scientific Data. New York, The Population Council Inc., 1992.

Speroff L, Darney P: A Clinical Guide for Contraception. Baltimore, Williams & Wilkins, 1992, pp 157–182.

Norplant Insertion

Procedure time of 10 to 15 minutes.

Indications

1. A means of contraception for someone requiring reversibility but long-term effectiveness
2. Poorly compliant patient
3. Patient with contraindication to estrogen and therefore combined oral contraceptive

Contraindications

1. Pregnancy
2. Acute liver disease
3. Undiagnosed vaginal bleeding
4. Breast malignancy
5. Thromboembolic disorders

Preparation

1. Patient needs to sign informed consent form and needs full counseling on the risks of the procedure, the benefits, contraceptive efficacy, failure rate of 0.2 per cent, and alternative methods of contraception.

2. Patient also needs to be informed prior to insertion of the potential side effects of Norplant.

Equipment

1. 6-ml syringe
2. 22-gauge 1.5-inch needle, for infiltrating anesthetic agent
3. 18-gauge 1-inch needle, for drawing up anesthetic agent
4. 10-gauge 2.75-inch trocar
5. Six Silastic Norplant implants
6. Scalpel with No. 11 blade

Anesthesia

6 ml of 1% lidocaine

Precautions

1. Ensure that patient is not pregnant. A serum pregnancy test is recommended prior to insertion.
2. There may be diminished contraceptive effectiveness in patients who are taking antiseizure medications such as phenytoin or carbamazepine.

Technique—Norplant Insertion

1. Physician stencils a fanlike pattern on the medial surface of the arm 8 to 10 mm above the elbow crease.

2. The area is then cleansed with either iodine or alcohol and draped with sterile drapes.

3. Using aseptic technique, 6 ml of 1% lidocaine is drawn up into the syringe using an 18-gauge needle. Six channels of 1 ml of anesthesia are infiltrated subdermally each about 4.0 to 5.0 cm long, approximating the fan-shape configuration, using the 22-gauge needle.

4. At the base of the fan, a 3.0-ml incision is made using the blade.

5. The trocar is inserted with obturator in place through the incision (bevel up) into the subdermal plane, at a shallow angle of 30 degrees, and advanced up to the proximal notch.

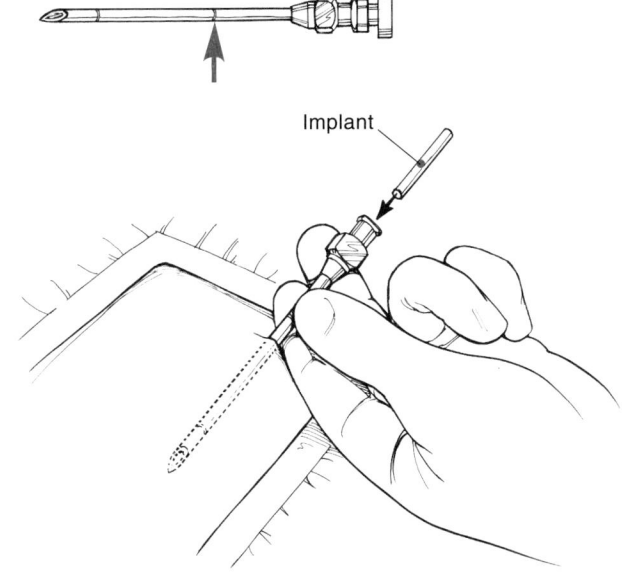

Implant

Information in Norplant system kit courtesy of Wyeth-Ayerst Laboratories, Philadelphia, Pennsylvania.

Drawings modified from Silva PD, Glasser KE: Subdermal contraceptive implants. Drug Ther 1992;22:109–115.

6. The obturator is removed and the implant placed in the trocar. The obturator is replaced and the trocar is withdrawn until the distal notch is visible. This leaves the implant in place.

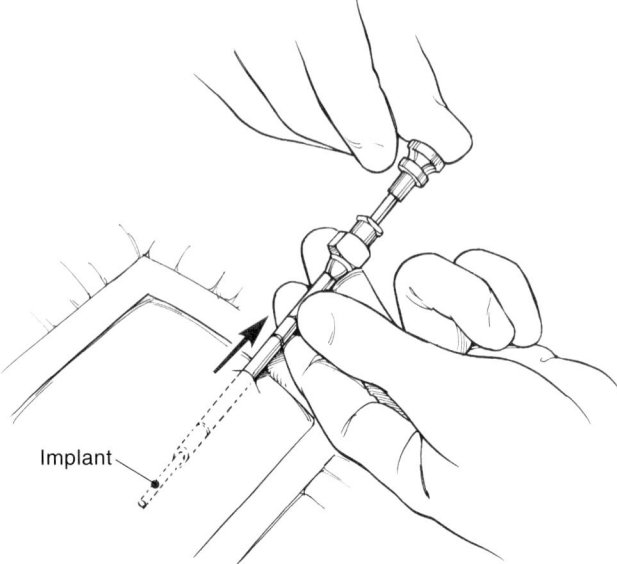

Implant

7. The procedure is then repeated for the second through the sixth implants following the fan-shape pattern traced on the skin.

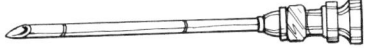

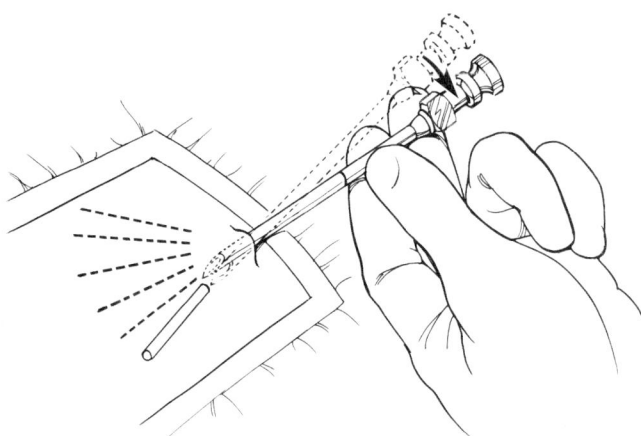

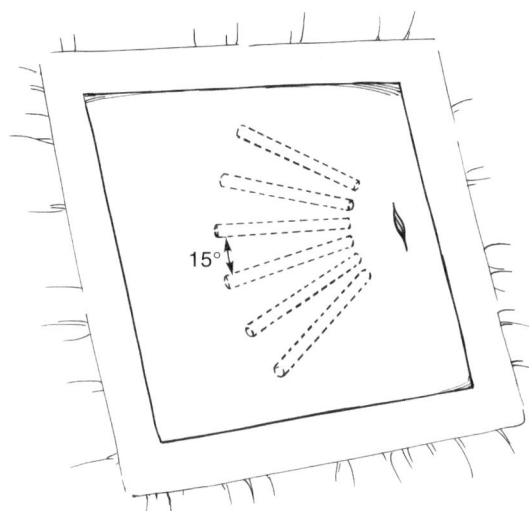

Note: Do not remove the trocar tip from the incision between insertions. Once all six capsules are in place, the trocar is removed and the incision is closed with Steri-Strips and the arm bandaged.

8. Patients are told that some bruising and mild discomfort are normal, but they should report purulent drainage and excessive pain.

9. Finally, a procedure note detailing the location should be recorded in the patient's chart.

Norplant Removal

Procedure time up to 30 minutes.

Equipment
1. Scalpel
2. Two Kelly clamps
3. Iris scissors

Precautions
1. Inform patient that removal will take longer than the insertion procedure did.
2. Obtain signed informed consent.
3. More than one incision may need to be made.

Technique—Norplant Removal

1. Prep and drape as per insertion.
2. Palpate to locate implant. Infiltrate area with 1% lidocaine.
3. A 3.0-mm incision is made where the implants converge close to the original insertion.
4. An implant is located and grasped with a Kelly clamp at the proximal tip. The fibrous capsule is dissected away using Iris scissors. The implant can then be easily grasped with the other Kelly clamp and removed.
5. If the patient wants to continue with the implant

system, the next set of six implants may be implanted through the same incision.

Alternative Removal Technique

An alternative technique has been used by some physicians and is reported to be faster and less painful than the conventional method of removal. It involves infiltrating the area through which removal is to be achieved with twice as much lidocaine, making a 1.0-cm incision, and vigorously dissecting away tissues using curved Halsted forceps, small straight mosquito Halsted forceps, and toothed tissue Adson forceps.

 Bibliography

Flattum-Riemers J: Norplant: A new contraceptive. Am Fam Physician 1991;44(1):103–108.

Mastroianni L, Robinson JC: Contraception in the 1990s. Patient Care 1994;28(1):107–119.

Norplant System Information Booklet, Wyeth-Ayerst Laboratories, December 1990.

Pierce C: New Norplant removal method: Easier, less painful. Fam Prac News 1993;Nov:22–23.

Silva PD, Glasser KE: Subdermal contraceptive implants. Drug Ther 1992;22:109–115.

Procedure | **VASECTOMY: TRADITIONAL METHOD** | *David Araujo*

Indications

1. Vasectomy is a method of permanent sterilization for the male. It is a safe and frequently performed procedure in an outpatient setting, with local anesthesia, at a considerable less expense and risk than female tubal sterilization.

2. The prevasectomy conference with the patient, and ideally his spouse, is of paramount importance. At this conference, the nature of the operation must be explained, with all the attendant implications of permanent sterilization. It must be stressed to the patient that this should be considered an irreversible and permanent procedure. While vasovasostomy is technically feasible, its success rate (10 to 40 per cent) makes it a poor option. Possible complications of vasectomy also must be discussed with the patient.

   a. The most common complications that can occur include failure with recanalization and subsequent continuation of fertility (0.5 to 5 per cent), hematoma (2 per cent), infection (1 to 3 per cent), epididymitis (2 per cent), and sperm granuloma (1 to 2 per cent). Long-term complications include the production of sperm antibodies (40 to 60 per cent), chronic orchalgia (0.01 per cent), and late failures.

   b. The reported failure rate ranges from 0.5 to 5 per cent depending on the type of occlusive technique used. Intraluminal cautery with application of a medium hemoclip, after removal of a 1- to 2-cm segment of vas, has the lowest reported recanalization rate. In my experience, I have used the technique of crushing the vas ends with a hemostat and ligature with polyglactin (Vicryl) after excision of a 1- to 2-cm segment of vas deferens, with less than a 1 per cent failure rate.

3. Informed consent must be documented in the patient's chart. Some states require separate consent forms for any sterilization procedure in addition to standard operative consent forms.

Contraindications

1. Individuals on chronic anticoagulation medications.
2. Those who express any ambivalence concerning their future desire to father children.
3. Anatomic factors that preclude performing a vasectomy under local anesthesia. These patients may require referral to a surgeon who can perform the procedure under general anesthesia.

   a. Inability to palpate bilateral vasa through the scrotal wall
   b. Individuals who have had prior scrotal content surgery or injury with resulting scarring who may require general anesthesia to allow adequate exploration of the scrotal sac to identify the vas.

Preparation

After informed consent has been obtained and the patient has been examined to determine that he is a suitable candidate for vasectomy under local anesthesia, he is given instructions on how to prepare for the procedure.

1. The patient should avoid aspirin for at least 5 days prior to the procedure.
2. On the day of the procedure, the patient should shave his scrotum of any hair.
3. He should bring an athletic supporter to his appointment to wear postoperatively.

Equipment

For vasal occlusion, the equipment used depends on the technique that is chosen (see Table 111–2).

1. Ligature occlusion with polyglactin (Vicryl) or polyglycolic acid (Chromic) after crushing the vasal ends with a mosquito clamp
2. Thermal fine-wire cautery intraluminal occlusion with or without hemoclip application
3. Hemoclip application alone
4. Any of the preceding combined with separation of the vasa into different tissue planes by fascial interposition. This involves covering either cut end of the vas with fascia and suturing the fascia closed.

Anesthesia

1. Local anesthesia is either with Xylocaine without vasoconstrictors or a combination of half and half 1% Xylocaine and 0.25% bupivacaine.
2. Preoperative medication for sedation can be given if so desired, such as a short-acting benzodiazepine. In my experience this has not been needed, and "verbal anesthesia" has been successful in calming the anxious patient.

TABLE 111–2. EQUIPMENT FOR VASECTOMY

REQUIRED	OPTIONAL (DEPENDING ON VASAL CLOSURE TECHNIQUE)
Sterile drapes and sponges	3-0 Polyglactin (Vicryl) suture
Xylocaine 1% and bupivacaine 0.5%	
10-ml 3-ring syringe and 25-gauge ⅝-inch needle	Medium hemoclips and applicator
No. 15 scalpel	Fine-wire thermal cautery
Allis clamp (2)	Electrocautery unit
Curved mosquito clamps (2)	
Toothed forceps	
Needle driver	
Suture scissors	
3-0 plain gut suture	

Technique

1. The patient is laid supine on the operating table. His groin, including the penis, is prepped with an antiseptic solution, such as povidone-iodine.
2. Sterile drapes are used to isolate the scrotum and keep the penis out of the operating field.
3. With the operator on the right side of the patient, the scrotum and its contents are briefly examined to identify the vasa bilaterally.
4. The three-finger technique is used to isolate the vas, starting with the patient's left side first.

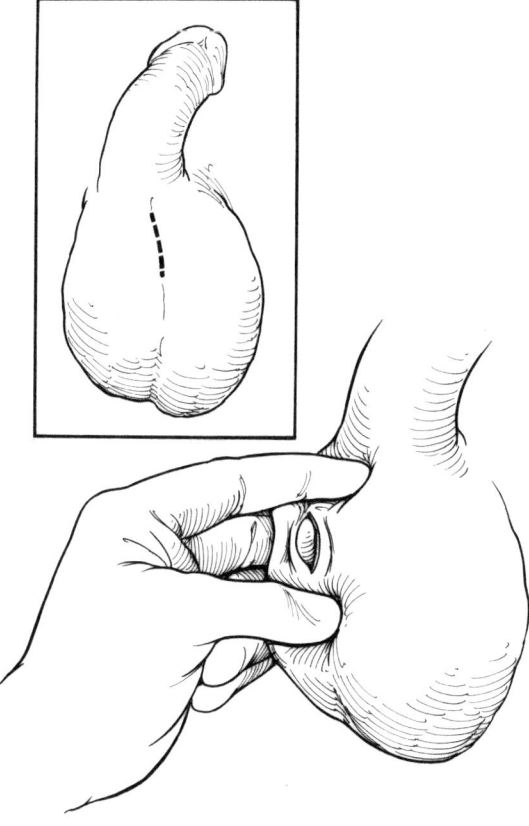

This involves draping the tube-like vas over the middle finger of the operator's left hand while stretching the scrotal skin tautly with the thumb and index finger. Since the scrotal skin is so loose, the *vas can be moved over such that the midline of the scrotum overlies the vas so that only one incision is needed.*

5. Local anesthesia is applied to the skin overlying the vas with a 25-gauge needle. While still holding the vas, the needle is then driven through the skin, and the fascia sheath surrounding the vas is pierced. Anesthetic is injected into this space. Successful vasal nerve block can be assessed by noting the patient's sensation of pain up into the ipsilateral groin.
6. While still grasping the vas, a no. 15 scalpel is used to make a 0.5-cm incision through the midline of the scrotum (see above). The vas is identified by rubbing over it with the closed end of an Allis

clamp. The vas is then grasped by opening the Allis clamp over it while pushing down on the finger over which the vas is draped. The surrounding sheath and vas are grasped securely and delivered through the skin incision.

7. The scalpel is then used to incise the vasal sheath longitudinally and expose the vas.

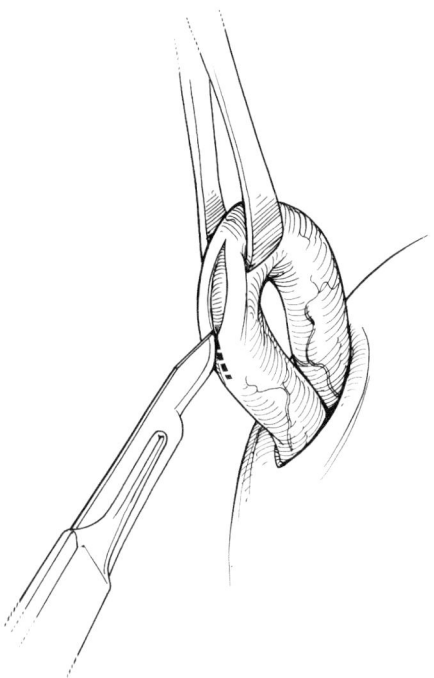

A second Allis clamp grasps the vas to bring it out of its sheath.

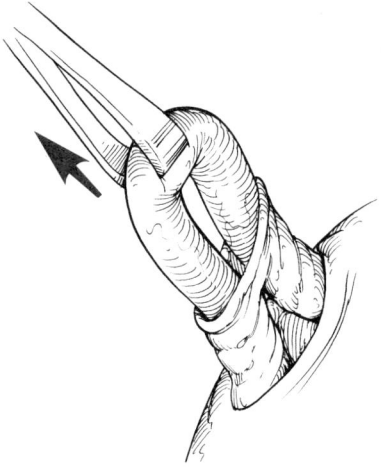

8. The next step depends on the type of occlusive technique used. My technique is to use curved mosquito clamps to tease away the connecting tissue attached to the vas, clamping the vas distally and proximally, and excising the intervening segment of 1 to 2 cm.

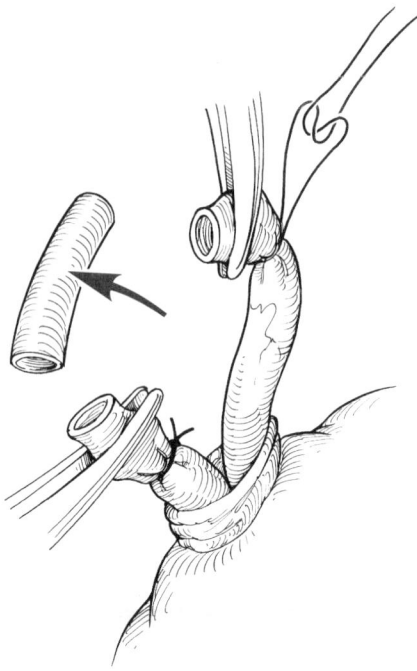

The cut ends are then tied with a ligature of 3-0 polyglactin (Vicryl). An optional step is to cover the cut end of the proximal vas with fascia, placing the two vas ends in different tissue planes.

9. The right vas is then isolated with the three-finger technique, and the scrotal skin is adjusted so that the midline incision lies over the grasped vas. The procedure is then repeated on the right vas.

10. The scrotal skin is closed with 4-0 undyed polyglactin (Vicryl) with a subcuticular stitch that closes the fascia of the scrotum.

Follow-Up

1. Postoperative instructions given to the patient include
   a. No heavy lifting greater than 25 pounds for 5 days.
   b. No sexual intercourse for 5 days.
   c. Place an ice pack on the scrotum for 20 minutes of each hour for the first 8 to 12 hours.

   d. Pain medications can be prescribed, such as acetaminophen with codeine.
2. A semen sample must be brought to the laboratory for microscopic sperm analysis 15 to 20 ejaculations after the vasectomy. Two azoospermic specimens 4 weeks apart are considered proof of sterility. Until the patient is sterile, the couple must be counseled to use an alternative form of birth control to prevent pregnancy.

WARNING: POSTOPERATIVE COMPLICATIONS

- **Hematoma—If minor, can be handled with scrotal support and bed rest; if major, may require incision and drainage, with placement of Penrose drains in the scrotum.**
- **Infection—Skin cellulitis can be treated with antibiotics (dicloxacillin or cephalexin); epididymitis, a tender erythematous warm lump usually at the site of the cut end of the testicular vas, responds well to anti-inflammatory medication and antibiotics (doxycycline or sulfamethoxazole-trimethoprim).**
- **Sperm granuloma—This occurs at the cut end of the testicular vas, often as a tender lump. It can be treated with anti-inflammatory medication. It is differentiated from epididymitis by its time of presentation, usually weeks to months after the vasectomy as opposed to days to a few weeks for epididymitis.**

 ## Bibliography

Alderman PM: Complications in a series of 1224 vasectomies. J Fam Pract 1991;33(6):579–584.

Davis JE: Male sterilization. Curr Opin Obstet Gynecol 1992;4(4):522–526.

Goldstein M: Surgery of male infertility and other scrotal disorders. In Walsh PC, Retik AB, Stamey TA, Vaughan ED (eds): Campbell's Urology, vol 3, 6th ed. Philadelphia, WB Saunders, 1992, pp 3119–3125.

Greenberg MJ: Vasectomy technique. Am Fam Physician 1989;39(1):131–138.

No-scalpel vasectomy is a refined, less invasive approach to isolation and delivery of the vas deferens.

Benefits

The benefits of no-scalpel vasectomy, compared with traditional approaches, are as follows:

1. Up to 10 times fewer complications (bleeding, hematoma, infection)
2. Less intimidating to clients
3. Less intraoperative and postoperative pain
4. Reduced operative time
5. Faster recovery

Contraindications

1. For health or personal reason(s), client is unready or inappropriate for vasectomy.
2. Inability to identify and isolate both vasa

Preparation

1. Carefully select patients during a thorough prior consultation with the prospective couple.
2. A relaxed scrotum is key to a smooth procedure. Provide a warm room (70 to 80° F).
3. Retract the penis upward onto the man's abdomen with a rubber band and clip.
4. Shave or clip the scrotal hair overlying the small operative area.
5. Wash the scrotum with a warm antiseptic solution.
6. Cover the prepared area with a sterile fenestrated drape.

Equipment

1. Extracutaneous ringed forceps ("ringed clamp") used to fix the vas deferens
2. Surgical hemostat ("dissecting forceps") used to puncture the scrotal skin, to spread underlying tissues, to dissect the sheath, and to deliver the vas deferens

Anesthesia: Vasal Nerve Block

1. Prepare a 10-ml syringe with 2% lidocaine without epinephrine attached to a 1.5-inch 27-gauge needle.
2. Using the three-finger technique, isolate the right vas from the spermatic cord vessels to a superficial position under the median raphe, fixing the vas over the middle finger of the left hand and under the index finger and thumb.
3. Inject lidocaine to raise a 1-cm superficial skin wheal.
4. Fully advance the needle within the perivasal sheath. Gently aspirate to verify that the needle is not in a blood vessel, and then slowly inject 2 to 3 ml of lidocaine around the vas. Avoid multiple injections.
5. Similarly fix and anesthetize the left vas through the initial skin puncture.
6. Pinch the original skin wheal to reduce local edema.

Technique

A. Three-finger technique to isolate and fix the vas deferens

1. Stand comfortably near the patient's scrotum on his right side, facing his head, and take one step backward toward his feet.
2. The left thumb is placed to *indicate* the juncture of the middle and upper thirds of the median raphe, in an area free of blood vessels.
3. The left middle finger *isolates* the vas from the spermatic cord and sweeps the vas from under the scrotum toward the raphe beneath the thumb.
4. The left index finger further *stabilizes* the vas when placed slightly above the thumb.

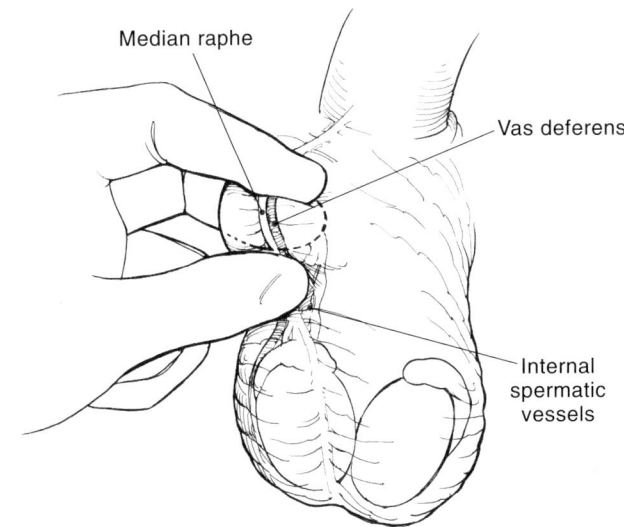

Median raphe — Vas deferens — Internal spermatic vessels

5. Upward pressure from the middle finger, combined with downward pressure from the index finger and thumb, creates a bend in the vas for better isolation and fixation.

6. To isolate the patient's left vas while standing on his right side, take one step toward the patient's head and turn the body to face his feet. Reach across the patient's abdomen with the left hand, and repeat the three-finger technique.

B. Surgical approach

1. Again, fix the right vas under the skin wheal with the left hand using the three-finger method.

2. Apply the ringed clamp perpendicularly with downward pressure, stretching the scrotal skin tightly over the vas and locking the entire vas within the clamp.

3. Place the ringed clamp in the left hand, lowering the handles to elevate the trapped vas, with the left index finger tightening the scrotal skin over the vas.

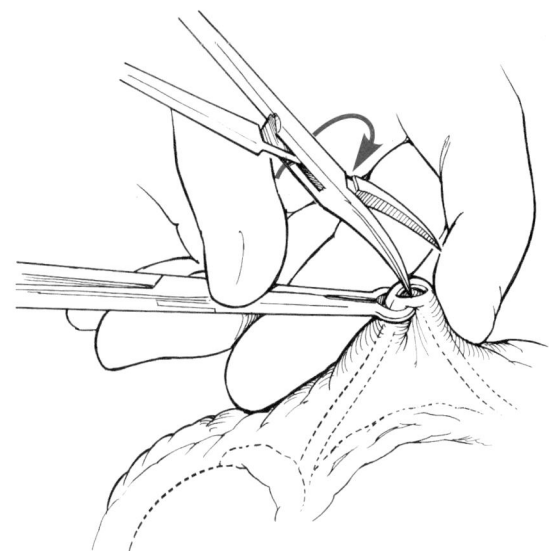

7. Grasp a partial thickness of the elevated vas at the crest of the loop with the ringed clamp.

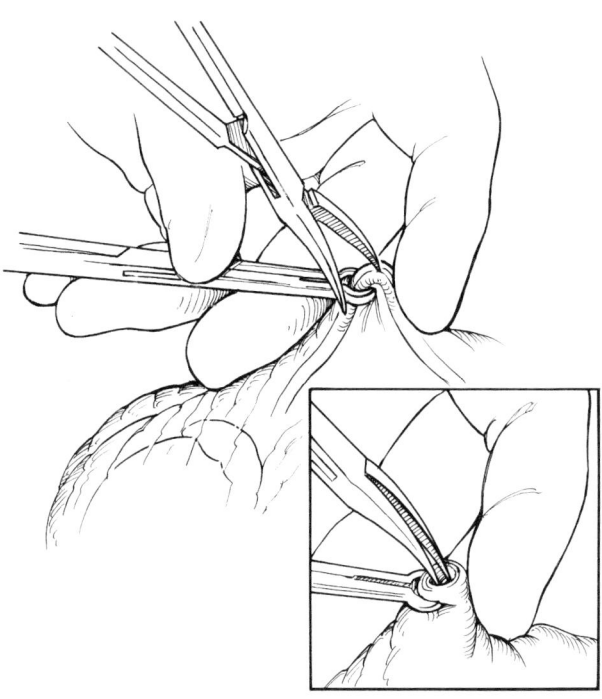

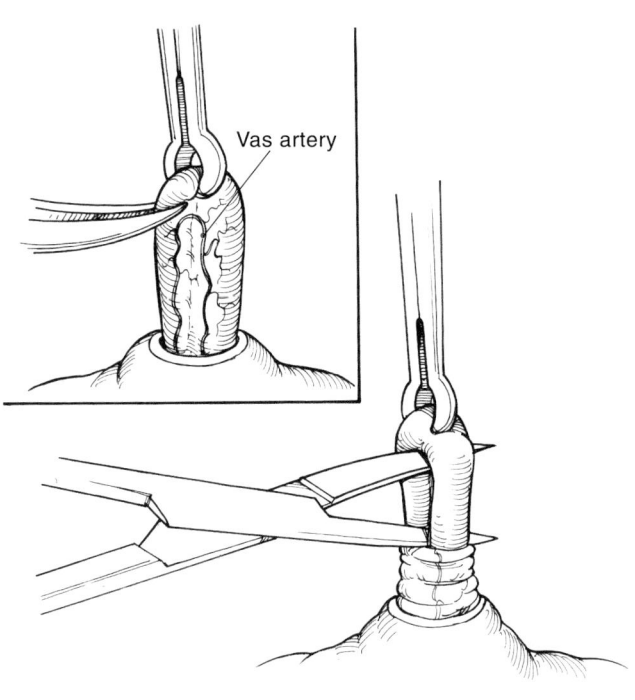

4. At the apex of the bend, pierce the scrotal skin, vas sheath, and vas wall down to the lumen at a 45-degree angle with the left blade of the dissecting forceps.

5. Using the same angle, introduce the closed tip of the dissecting forceps through the puncture to the same depth, and gently open and close the blades a few times, stretching and spreading all layers to fully expose the bare vas wall.

6. Skewer the vas wall at a 45-degree angle with the right blade of the dissecting forceps, and rotate the instrument 180 degrees, delivering the vas while the fixation clamp is simultaneously released.

8. With one tip of the dissecting forceps facing upward, puncture the vas sheath just below the vas and above the vas artery. Reintroduce the closed tip of the forceps. Spread the tips to gently strip the sheath, including the vas artery, downward to yield a clean 1-cm segment of vas.

9. Occlude and divide the right vas using a conventional method.

10. Return the fully retracted ends of the right vas to the scrotum.

11. After isolating the left vas directly under the puncture using the three-finger technique, apply the ringed clamp around the puncture or directly grasp the vas and its sheath through the puncture site.

12. The remainder of the procedure is identical to that described for the right side.

13. Pinch the puncture site, and inspect for bleeding.

14. A Band-Aid may be used to cover the small wound; a supporter is worn for comfort.

15. Observe the patient for 30 minutes following the procedure for possible bleeding or hematoma.

Hands-on training is crucial to precisely learn and ultimately master this technique.

Follow-Up

1. Patient rests for 24 to 48 hours, using a cold pack.

2. With prior permission, call the day after the procedure to check patient's progress.

3. Have patient visit 1 week following the procedure to discuss normal recovery and to emphasize instructions regarding semen analysis and postprocedure contraception.

4. Obtain two absolutely azoospermic specimens 4 to 6 weeks apart.

Bibliography

Fishman MA, Nagler HM: New options in vasectomy. Med Aspects Hum Sex 1991;25(11):33–38.

Gonzales B, Marston-Ainley S, Vansintejan G, Li PS: No-Scalpel Vasectomy: An Illustrated Guide for Surgeons. New York, Association for Voluntary Surgical Contraception, 1992.

Li S, Goldstein M, Zhu J, Huber D: The no-scalpel vasectomy. J Urol 1991;145:341–344.

Li PS, Li S, Schlegel PN, Goldstein M: External spermatic sheath injection for vasal nerve block. Urology 1992;39:173–176.

Niraputhpongporn A, Huber D, Krieger J: No-scalpel vasectomy at the king's birthday vasectomy festival. Lancet 1990; 335:894–895.

112 Infertility

Keith A. Frey

Etiology

1. There are multiple causes of infertility, and interference with the conception process may occur at various sites in the male or female reproductive system. Consider more than one cause, since 10 to 30 per cent of couples have more than one cause.
2. Common etiologies of infertility are listed in Table 112–1.

Symptoms

1. Symptoms are as varied as the etiologies.
2. It is crucial that the physician perform a detailed reproductive and sexual history and general review of systems (Table 112–2).

Clinical Findings

1. A thorough physical examination of each partner, with specific attention to the reproductive tract, is essential.
2. Observe for findings of structural abnormalities, endocrinopathy, and infection (Table 112–3).
3. Arrange a meeting with the couple early in the diagnostic workup. This provides an important opportunity to review reproductive biology and the rationale for subsequent laboratory tests.

Laboratory Tests

1. Each couple must be evaluated by a series of routine laboratory tests and appropriately timed studies to evaluate each major reproductive factor that may cause infertility.
2. Routine laboratory tests for the male and female partners are listed in Table 112–3.
3. Basal body temperature recording provides valuable information regarding both the presence and timing of ovulation and the timing of key diagnostic studies (Table 112–4).
4. The comprehensive diagnostic survey can and should be completed for most couples in 3 to 6 months.

Differential Diagnosis

1. The results of the comprehensive diagnostic survey (history, physical examination, laboratory tests, and diagnostic studies) generally identify the factor(s) contributing to the couple's infertility.
2. The more common disorders, by reproductive category, include
   a. Male factors
      (1) Varicocele
      (2) Oligospermia/azoospermia
      (3) Disorders of sperm function or motility (asthenospermia)
      (4) Abnormalities of sperm morphology (teratospermia)
   b. Ovulatory dysfunction
      (1) Hypothalamic anovulation (e.g., psychogenic trauma, anorexia nervosa, pharmacologic agents)
      (2) Pituitary anovulation (e.g., pituitary tumors, ischemia, defects)
      (3) Ovulatory anovulation (e.g., ovarian dysgenesis, premature ovarian failure, ovarian tumors)
      (4) Integrative anovulation (e.g., polycystic ovar-

TABLE 112–1. COMMON CAUSES OF INFERTILITY

ETIOLOGIC FACTOR	RANGE IN INFERTILE COUPLES (%)
Male factors	18–31
Ovulatory dysfunction	16–30
Tubal damage	12–16
Endometriosis	5–25
Cervical mucus abnormalities	3–5
Unexplained	13–28

TABLE 112–2. THE INFERTILITY WORKUP IN OUTLINE: HISTORY (MALE, FEMALE, OR BOTH)

Marriage	Occupation and Habits	Review of Systems
Duration of infertility	Exposure to radiation, chemicals,	Focus on endocrine conditions
Fertility in previous relationships	excessive heat (saunas, hot tubs, etc.)	(diabetes, thyroid disorders)
Frequency of intercourse	**Childhood Illness**	**Gynecology**
Sexual potency and techniques	Cryptorchidism	Coital frequency and techniques
Use of coital lubricants	Timing of puberty	Contraceptives use
Adult Illnesses	**Surgery**	Diethylstilbestrol use by mother
Acute viral or febrile illness in past	Herniorrhaphy	Douches and lubricants use
3 months	Retroperitoneal surgery	Exposure to radiation and chemicals
Mumps orchitis	Vasectomy	Fertility in previous relationships
Renal disease	**Drug Use**	Menarche
Radiation therapy	Alcohol, tobacco, and drugs	Menses (regularity and flow)
Sexually transmitted disease	Alkylating agents	Mittelschmerz
Radiation therapy	Hormones	
Stress and fatigue	Nitrofurantoin (Macrodantin)	
Tuberculosis		

From Frey KA: Infertility. *In* Mengel MB, Schwiebert LP (eds): Ambulatory Medicine: The Primary Care of Families. East Norwalk, CT, Appleton & Lange, 1993, p 559.

TABLE 112–3. THE INFERTILITY WORKUP (MALE AND FEMALE)

MALE		FEMALE	
Physical Examination	**Routine Laboratory Tests**	**Physical Examination**	**Routine Laboratory Tests**
Hair pattern	CBC	Breast formation	CBC
Genitalia	Semen analysis	Distribution of body fat	Pap smear
Meatus size and location	Abstinence of 2 days	Galactorrhea	Urinalysis and urine culture if
Prostate and seminal vesicles	Masturbation into sterile vessel	Hair pattern (virilization)	indicated
Scrotum	To lab (warm) within 2 hours	Height and weight	VDRL test
Testicular size (≥ 4 cm in	Results	Neurology	At-home tests
long axis)	Volume: 2–5 ml	Anosmia	Basal body temperature
Varicocele (standing and	Liquefaction: complete within 30	Visual fields	Measure temperature for 5–10
Valsalva maneuver)	min	Pelvis	min orally before arising
Neurology	Sperm count: 60–150 million/ml	External genitalia	Measure temperatures throughout
Anosmia	Sperm motility: >60%	Retrovaginal area (endometriosis)	evaluation and treatment
Visual fields	Morphology: >60% normal forms	Uterus and adnexa	Bring chart on each visit
	2–3 test as necessary	Vagina and cervix	
	Urinalysis and urine culture if indicated		
	VDRL test		

From Frey KA: Infertility. *In* Mengel MB, Schwiebert LP (eds): Ambulatory Medicine: The Primary Care of Families. East Norwalk, CT, Appleton & Lange, 1993, p 560.

ian syndrome, nonpsychogenic weight disturbances)

  c. Tubal damage

    (1) Tubal damage or obstruction (following acute salpingitis)

    (2) Adnexal adhesions

  d. Endometriosis (leading to chronic inflammation and disruption of conception)

  e. Cervical mucus abnormalities (e.g., cervical infections, previous surgery or cautery, hormonal disruptions)

TABLE 112–4. THE INFERTILITY WORKUP: FURTHER DIAGNOSTIC TESTS

Postcoital (Sims'-Huhner) Test
  Determines number and condition of sperm and their ability to penetrate cervical mucus
  Performed around time of ovulation
Hysterosalpingogram
  Preferred test of tubal patency
  Performed 2–6 days after cessation of menstrual flow
  May enhance fertility temporarily
Laparoscopy
  Performed if hysterosalpingography unproductive
  Permits examination of pelvic contents
Endometrial Biopsy
  Determines if luteal phase defect exists
  Performed 2–3 days before expected menses
  Informed consent required
  Requires histologic dating
Serum Progesterone
  May be an alternative to endometrial biopsy
  Sample drawn 5–7 days after supposed ovulation
  Serum level >3 ng/ml is compatible with ovulation

From Frey KA: Infertility. *In* Mengel MB, Schwiebert LP (eds): Ambulatory Medicine: The Primary Care of Families. East Norwalk, CT, Appleton & Lange, 1993, p 561.

Treatment

1. Generally, treatment should not be initiated until the diagnostic evaluation is completed. Therapy should proceed at a rate that the couple finds comfortable.

2. Therapy for the specific disorders identified by the comprehensive diagnostic evaluation often can be ini-

tiated by the primary care physician. For detailed descriptions of specific treatment approaches, the reader is referred to the Bibliography.

3. The workup, diagnosis, and treatment of infertility can precipitate intense emotional reactions. The physician should discuss such emotions as anger, guilt, self-doubt, depression, and grief with the couple. In addition, help the couple understand their motives for parenting. Assist the couple in the development of mutual support and an adaptive "couple-coping" style. Discuss sexual issues, and encourage the couple to nurture their intimacy. Help the couple broaden their support system, including self-help groups (e.g., Resolve, Inc.).

Follow-Up

1. The exact prognosis of infertility can be difficult to define due to the multiple potential causes.

2. Conception rates following specific therapy are favorable for most disorders.

3. "Unexplained" infertility is the persistent inability to conceive after a comprehensive diagnostic assessment fails to identify a specific diagnosis. If an etiology is not apparent or treatment is unsuccessful, referral is warranted. The primary care physician also should discuss adoption options with the couple, and the costs involved in further infertility evaluation and treatment.

 ## Bibliography

Frey KA: Infertility. *In* MB Mengel, LP Schwiebert (eds): Ambulatory Medicine: The Primary Care of Families. E Norwalk, CT, Appleton & Lange, 1993, pp 558–562.

Frey KA, Stenchever MA, Warren MP: Helping the infertile couple. Patient Care 1989;23:22.

Jones WJ, Toner JP: The infertile couple. N Engl J Med 1993;329:1710–1715.

Neumann PJ, Gharib SD, Weinstein MC: The cost of a successful delivery with in vitro fertilization. N Engl J Med 1994;331:239–243.

Speroff L, Glass RH, Kase NG: Clinical Gynecologic Endocrinology and Infertility, 4th ed. Baltimore, Williams & Wilkins, 1988.

113 Impotence

Mark D. Darrow

Etiology

1. Vascular, neurogenic, and end-organ dysfunctions become more frequent with age and in the presence of disease states.
2. Etiologies may be multifactorial:
   a. Neurogenic
   b. Medication/substance abuse
   c. Anatomic abnormalities
   d. Complex systemic disease
   e. Vasculogenic
   f. Psychogenic
   g. Endocrinologic
   h. Social/personal beliefs

Symptoms

Erectile dysfunction is significant enough to inhibit vaginal penetration and sexual satisfaction.

Key Symptoms

- Decrease in erectile frequency
- Degree of tumescence not enough for penetration
- Rapid detumescence
- Complete lack of erection
- Lack of sexual desire

Clinical Findings

1. History
   a. Medical and surgical history
   b. Family and social history
   c. Review of systems
      (1) Evidence of systemic disease
      (2) End-organ or genitourinary dysfunction
      (3) Local trauma
   d. Drug history
      (1) Prescription/oral contraceptive pills (OCP)
      (2) Alcohol
      (3) Illicit
   e. Sexual history
      (1) Baseline function
      (2) When change occurred
      (3) Regular partner/health status?
      (4) Frequency of attempts/failures

WARNING
The presence of nocturnal tumescence rules out psychogenic impotence. However, the patient may not be aware that it occurs and a negative response may not be accurate.

   (5) Quality of erection (25, 50 per cent)?
   (6) Duration of tumescence?
   (7) Nocturnal tumescence, quality?
2. General medical examination for vital signs, general appearance, and evidence of endocrine or other systemic disease
   a. Vascular—Note peripheral pulses, bruits.
   b. Genital—penis, testicular size, prostate
   c. Neurologic—general status, local reflexes
   d. Musculoskeletal—mobility, arthritis
3. If indicated or findings are unclear, consider
   a. Mini–mental state examination
   b. Depression scale
   c. CAGE test for alcoholism
   d. Other psychological screens as indicated

Laboratory Tests

1. Blood tests as indicated by history and physical examination
2. In the absence of disease, request the following:
   a. Fasting blood sugar, electrolytes, blood urea nitrogen (BUN), creatinine
   b. Complete blood count (CBC)
   c. Urinalysis
   d. Lipid profile
   e. Thyroid function tests
   f. Serum prolactin level
   g. Serum free testosterone level (if indicated)
3. Functional tests
   a. Nocturnal penile tumescence—snap gauge
   b. Psychiatric testing
   c. Intracavernosal test injection
4. Vascular tests (when indicated)
   a. Penile vessel ultrasound
   b. Penile brachial index
   c. Pelvic angiography—useful with trauma history

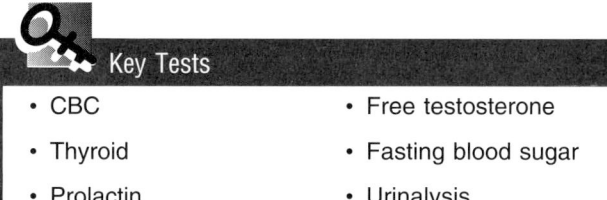

Key Tests

- CBC
- Thyroid
- Prolactin
- Free testosterone
- Fasting blood sugar
- Urinalysis

Differential Diagnosis

1. A number of medical, physiologic, social, and psychological conditions are important in considering the various causes of erectile dysfunction.

2. Differential diagnosis by etiology:

   a. Vascular causes: diabetes mellitus, atherosclerosis, vasculitides

   b. Neurologic causes: stroke, multiple sclerosis, anterior temporal lobe lesions, spinal cord syndromes and injuries, sensory nerve damage, autonomic neuropathies, diabetes mellitus

   c. Medications: anticholinergics, antiandrogens, antidepressants, antipyschotics, central-acting depressants, antihypertensives

   d. Substance abuse: alcohol, tobacco, heroin

   e. End-organ disease: Peyronie's disease, diseases of the cavernous sinuses, venous leak

   f. Endocrine disorders: testicular failure, hyperprolactinemia, thyroid disorders

   g. Psychogenic causes: depression, anxiety, psychosis

   h. Social causes: marital status, partner health and availability, personal beliefs and acceptance

Treatment

1. Counseling

   a. Normal aging, social acceptance

   b. Sex therapy, interpersonal relationships, pleasuring, awareness of physical infirmities

   c. Psychotherapy

   d. General health, smoking cessation, exercise

   e. Substance abuse counseling

2. Medical interventions

   a. Oral and other agents

      (1) Antidepressants, if patient is depressed

      (2) Yohimbine, 5.4 mg (1 tablet) 3 times daily (for psychogenic impotence)

      (3) Ointments: nitroglycerin (not effective)

      (4) Hormone replacement (Thyroid for hypothyroidism; testosterone for low free-testosterone levels only.)

      (5) Others: control diabetes, hypertension

   b. Vacuum and other support devices

      (1) External vacuum devices, in all but severe vascular compromise

      (2) Restrictive bands for venous leak

      (3) Rigid condoms (not well tolerated)

   c. Intracavernosal injection: papaverine and phentolamine and prostaglandin E_1, alone or in combination, are useful in most forms of impotence.

   d. Surgical

      (1) Implants: rigid, malleable, inflatable

      (2) Arterial reconstruction (investigational)

      (3) Venous ligation

Key Treatment

- Counseling
- Medications
- Intracavernosal injection
- Surgical
- External vacuum devices

Follow-Up

1. Long-term compliance is poor with external devices and intercavernosal injection; reasons are unclear.

2. Inflatable prostheses have a 20 per cent repair or replacement rate.

3. Follow-up is needed soon after vacuum device, injection, or medication trial to ensure proper technique, partner participation, and patient satisfaction.

   a. Encourage record keeping of attempts, failures.

   b. Assess need for additional sex therapy.

4. If current method fails, reassess, counsel, and suggest addition or substitution of another treatment method.

WARNING

The cause of impotence may be multifactorial. Treatment may unmask another cause.

Bibliography

For more information on erectile dysfunction, see
Lerner SE, Melman A, Christ GJ: A review of erectile dysfunction: New insights and more questions. J Urol 1993;149:1246–1255.

For more information on the diagnosis and treatment, see
National Institutes of Health: Impotence. NIH Consensus Statement 1992;10(4):1–33.
Johnson LE, Morley JE: Impotence in the elderly. Am Fam Physician 1988;38(5):225–240.
Kirby RS: Impotence: Diagnosis and management of male erectile dysfunction. Br J Med 1994;23;308(6936):1091.

For more information on intracavernous pharmacotherapy, see
von Heyden B, Donatucci CF, Kaula N, Lue TF: Intracavernous pharmacotherapy for impotence: Selection of appropriate agent and dose. J Urol 1993;149:1288–1290.

114 Pregnancy

Bickley Craven

Diagnosis Early in Gestation

1. Signs or symptoms: amenorrhea, nausea, fatigue, breast enlargement or tenderness
2. Human chorionic gonadotropin, β subunit (β-hCG) is detected by maternal serum and urine assays 8 to 10 days after fertilization or at 22 to 24 days' gestational age. This is before the first missed menstrual period.
3. Ultrasound
   a. Transabdominal: A normal intrauterine pregnancy may be detected at 4 to 5 weeks' gestational age.
   b. Transvaginal: Fetal cardiac activity may be detected at 40 days' gestational age

Key Signs and Symptoms

- Amenorrhea
- Nausea
- Fatigue
- Breast enlargement or tenderness

Preconception/Prenatal Care

1. Preconception and prenatal periods are an optimal time for health promotion. The process of preconception/prenatal care encompasses preventive measures in ongoing identification of risk factors, management of medical, obstetric, or psychosocial problems, and health education and promotion.
2. Information gathered during these visits must be documented completely and clearly. Many standardized "prenatal forms" are available for use. An individual patient's forms must be available to her caregivers in the office and delivery settings, especially during the second and third trimesters.

Preconception Visit

1. This visit should occur within 1 year of conception.
2. A complete history should include present and past medical history of both parents, obstetric history of the prospective mother, high-risk behaviors (smoking, drug use), infectious risks (HIV, hepatitis), and genetic and psychosocial history.
3. A complete, general physical examination should be done, including blood pressure, height and weight, pelvic examination, and pelvimetry.
4. Laboratory testing includes hemoglobin/hematocrit, Rh factor, rubella antibody titer, urinalysis, Pap smear, syphilis serology, gonorrhea culture, and hepatitis B surface antigen. For patients at risk, testing may include HIV antibody, *Chlamydia* screen, herpes simplex culture, purified protein derivative (PPD) tuberculin, and specific genetic screens.
5. The information gathered in this comprehensive examination is scrutinized to identify risks for the future mother or fetus. The medical care provider and patient develop a plan to remove or ameliorate each of the risks. Similarly, at each subsequent visit, risks to the pregnancy are sought and intervention is undertaken as necessary.
6. Health promotion and counseling include attention to risks specific to the individual, such as smoking cessation or substance abuse intervention. General counseling covers the need for early initiation of prenatal visits after conception, nutrition, avoidance of potential teratogens, safer sex, and so on.

Initial Prenatal Visit

1. The initial visit as described assumes that a comprehensive preconception visit occurred and that the information collected is available to the current prenatal care provider.
2. The initial visit is best accomplished as early as possible in the pregnancy, say, at 6 to 8 weeks' gestational age.
3. An updated medical, surgical, psychosocial history is done. The history of the current pregnancy to date is taken to include menstrual history.
4. The physical examination should include a brief general examination with attention to blood pressure, weight, and pelvic examination, including determination of uterine size and estimation of gestational age.
5. Laboratory tests include rubella antibody titer or Pap smear, if not recorded previously, hematocrit/hemoglobin, blood type, Rh screen, and urine culture. For patients with ongoing risks of sexually transmitted disease (STD), repeat syphilis serology, gonorrhea culture, or HIV antibody may be indicated. Tests for specific indications: blood glucose screen and the like.
6. Health promotion/counseling covers the frequency and content of prenatal visits, avoidance of teratogens, sexuality, safer sex, fetal growth and development, and preparation for future screening or diagnostic testing. For some patients, nutrition counseling and strategies for discomforts of pregnancy may be indicated. All patients are counseled to report "danger signs" whenever they occur (see below).
7. Organized prenatal classes or childbirth classes are helpful and, if available, should be recommended to all first-time mothers. Physical changes of pregnancy, nutrition, psychological changes, exercise, prepara-

tion for labor and delivery, and many other topics are usually covered in six to eight sessions.

Dating the Pregnancy

Determination of the most accurate estimated date of confinement (EDC) possible is an important component of prenatal care. Appropriate management in many obstetric situations depends on fetal gestational age. Documentation of the following data will allow determination of a reliable EDC in most cases:

1. The last normal menstrual period and date of the first positive pregnancy test

2. The date of the first pelvic examination and estimated gestational age

3. Fundal height in centimeters approximates the length of gestation from 20 to 30 weeks.

4. Fetal heart tones are generally audible with Doppler fetoscope at 10 to 12 weeks and with fetoscope or stethoscope examination at 18 to 20 weeks.

5. If dates are in question or the patient seeks prenatal care late, ultrasound in the first or second trimester is critical for determining the EDC.

Subsequent Prenatal Visits

1. Traditional timing of visits is as follows: every 4 weeks until 28 weeks, every 2 weeks until 36 weeks, weekly until delivery. A more flexible schedule is recommended by some authors. More frequent visits may be indicated in the first trimester if specific intervention is required such as smoking cessation. Less frequent visits may be appropriate for the low-risk, healthy woman with her second or third pregnancy.

2. Important history items will vary with the stage of gestation. In the first trimester, history of uterine cramping, vaginal bleeding, or exposure to infectious agents is important. In the second and third trimesters, fetal activity, vaginal bleeding, excessive weight gain or edema, headache, or visual changes are important history items.

3. The components of the physical examination also depend on gestational age. Weight should be determined at each visit. By convention, blood pressure and fetal heart rate are checked at each visit. Fundal height is measured and recorded from 16 weeks on. Fetal lie, presentation, and engagement and cervical examination are indicated late in the third trimester.

4. The following laboratory tests are recommended:

    a. 15 to 18 weeks: maternal serum α-fetoprotein

    b. 24 to 28 weeks: hemoglobin/hematocrit, blood glucose screen, antibody screen if Rh-negative

    c. 36 weeks: hemoglobin/hematocrit, repeat testing for STDs if indicated

    d. More frequent testing may be indicated for patients with risk factors. The tradition of testing urine for protein and glucose at each visit is not thought to be indicated.

5. Obstetric ultrasound. The issue of routine versus indicated obstetric ultrasound is under hot debate. A list of some 27 indications for ultrasound during pregnancy accepted by the American College of Obstetricians and Gynecologists (ACOG) and others results in most pregnancies being scanned at least once. Ultrasound is often indicated if the EDC is in question. Ultrasound is critical if fundal height/fetal growth is not as expected or if fetal position is in question late in pregnancy or during labor.

WARNING

Patients are counseled to report the following warning signs:
- **Any vaginal bleeding, abdominal pain, escape of fluid from the vagina**
- **Swelling of the face or fingers, severe or continuous headache, blurring of vision**
- **Persistent vomiting, chills or fever, dysuria**
- **Marked change in frequency or intensity of fetal movements**

Education/Counseling

Nutrition

1. Normal-weight women should gain approximately 20 to 30 pounds in pregnancy. More or less weight gain may be appropriate for low-weight or overweight women.

2. The pregnant woman is encouraged to eat a broad variety of foods, take in adequate liquids, and include fiber in her diet.

3. The primary care provider may explore food intake by dietary recall at intervals throughout the pregnancy.

4. Calcium supplementation may be indicated if the woman does not take three to four servings of dairy products daily. Iron supplementation at 30 to 60 mg/day and folic acid at 1 mg/day are indicated.

Exercise

1. Women may continue to exercise commensurate with their activity before pregnancy.

2. Previously sedentary women may begin a walking program.

3. Women with an active exercise routine may continue but are cautioned not to embark on a more intensive training program during pregnancy.

Work

1. In the absence of complications, pregnant women may continue to work.

2. Severe physical strain and fatigue should be avoided.

3. Women and employers should be encouraged to ensure periods of rest during working hours.

4. A history of delivering a low-birth-weight infant may

indicate a need to minimize physical work or prolonged standing.

Sexual Activity

1. In the absence of complications, common sense would suggest that sexual activity the woman finds comfortable and pleasurable is appropriate.
2. When an obstetric complication occurs, counseling regarding sexual practices must be specific.

Substance Use/Abuse

During preconception and pregnancy, many women are open to lifestyle change. During this time a woman may be particularly successful in ceasing or decreasing her use or abuse of nicotine, alcohol, caffeine, and illicit drugs, all of which affect the fetus adversely.

Bibliography

Antepartum: Management of normal pregnancy. *In* Cunningham FG, et al (eds): Williams' Obstetrics, 19th ed. East Norwalk, CT, Appleton & Lange, 1993, pp 247–271.

Jack B, Culpepper L: Preconception care. *In* Taylor RB (ed): Family Medicine Principles and Practice, 4th ed. New York, Springer-Verlag, 1993, pp 59–69.

Nagey D: The content of prenatal care. Obstet Gynecol 1989;74:516–528.

Noller K, Wertheimer R: Obstetrics. *In* Rakel RE (ed): Textbook of Family Practice, 5th ed. Philadelphia, WB Saunders, 1995, Chap 26.

Rosen M, Merkatz I, Hill J: Caring for our future: A report by the expert panel on the content of prenatal care. Obstet Gynecol 1991;77:782–787.

Procedure | EPISIOTOMY AND VAGINAL LACERATION REPAIR

Jo Ann Rosenfeld

Indications

1. Episiotomies do not decrease perineal trauma, prevent pelvic relaxation, improve postpartum perineal healing, or prevent fetal distress. Having an episiotomy increases the rate of perineal lacerations and trauma up to 50 times and predisposes women to third- or fourth-degree lacerations. Rectal injuries are 8.9 times more likely in women with episiotomies. Women without episiotomies have less postpartum pain and are more likely to resume sexual intercourse within 1 month. There has been no proven beneficial effect of episiotomies for the infant.
2. Episiotomies may help with shoulder dystocia.

Contraindications

Bleeding disorders and severe scarring on the perineum are contraindications.

Preparation

1. Sterile procedure should be maintained. The woman can be redraped after delivery.
2. The operator may wish to place a packing gauze in the vagina.
3. Inspect the cervix and vagina for lacerations after delivery, and stop bleeding, if possible.

4. The operator may need fresh sterile gloves after the delivery.

Equipment

1. Standard laceration repair equipment should be present, including pickups, long scissors, two needle holders, and 4 × 4 sponges.
2. In addition, the following specific equipment should be available: packing gauze, two Allis clamps, one Gelpi clamp, one ring forceps, a straight catheter, and lubrication.
3. Two to three packages of 3-0 or 2-0 synthetic absorbable suture material (Dexon or Vicryl). Compared with catgut, their use is associated with a 40 per cent decrease in short-term pain and need for analgesia.
4. For repair of fourth-degree lacerations, one package of absorbable 4-0 synthetic suture material is needed.

Anesthesia

1. Usually the anesthesia used for delivery is sufficient for repair of an episiotomy or lacerations.
2. Additional local anesthesia can be used. Lidocaine 1% or 2% without epinephrine infiltrated in the laceration may help immensely.

Technique

Episiotomy

1. Cut a midline episiotomy, if required, after the perineum is thinned by the pressure of the fetal head. The surgeon places index and middle fingers into the posterior vagina between the fetal head and the vagina, one finger on each side of the midline, and cuts between the fingers downward and posteriorly on the midline. One cut with scissors at this point will incise both the posterior wall of the vagina and the perineum from the posterior vaginal opening posteriorly toward but not into the rectal capsule.
2. Delivery usually occurs soon. If not, light pressure on the episiotomy incision with a 4 × 4 bandage will decrease the amount of bleeding.

Repair

1. Determine the depth and degree of episiotomy and lacerations. Lacerations are considered first-degree if only superficial skin or vaginal wall is torn and second-degree if the laceration extends into subcutaneous tissues down to fascia. A laceration is considered third-degree if it extends through the external anal sphincter (EAS) and fourth-degree if it tears through into the rectal mucosa.
2. Repair of the second-degree episiotomy requires reconstruction in layers. Start with repair of the poste-

rior vaginal wall. Place the first stitch approximately 1 cm proximal to the deepest extension of the episiotomy on the vaginal wall. Place the stitch 1 cm to each side of the midline defined by the episiotomy, and tie.

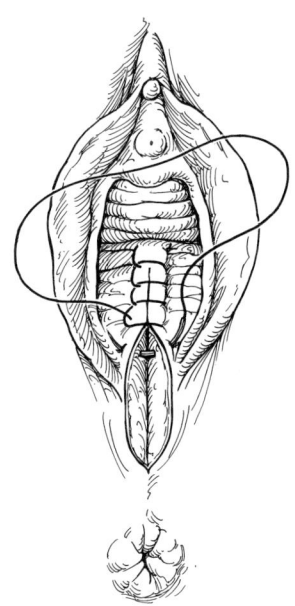

3. Using a continuous locked stitch, place sutures approximately 1 cm apart, each approximately 1 cm from the edge of the incision, working toward the introitus. Make the sutures shallow, approximately 0.5 cm below the posterior vaginal wall. Match the edges of the hymenal ring. Stop at the introitus, putting this suture down. Some experts choose to make a knot at this point.

4. Unless the episiotomy is very superficial or if there is a third- or fourth-degree laceration, the next step is to place three to four deep interrupted sutures using a new suture. These stitches should be approximately 1 cm apart; the most posterior stitch should be 1 cm above the exterior anal sphincter.

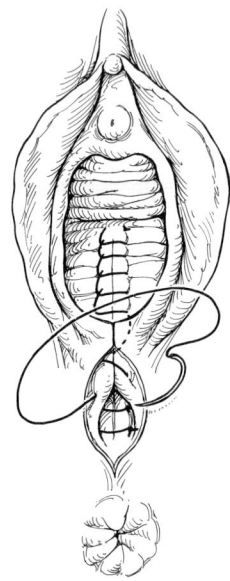

5. Then, taking up the first suture, bring the needle from the vagina under the hymen to the perineum. Sew posteriorly down the perineum with a continuous nonlocking suture, bringing the edges together; the perineum should lie closed at the end of this layer. The final layer is sewn anteriorly toward the vagina as a subcuticular continous layer. The last stitch is brought into the vagina and tied.

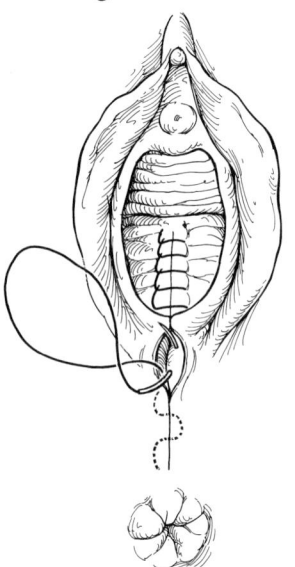

First- and Second-Degree Lacerations

1. First- and second-degree periurethral lacerations are common and usually are easily repaired. If bleeding has stopped and the edges are less than 1 cm apart, no suturing is necessary. If the lacerations are larger or hemorrhaging, one or two figure-of-eight sutures should bring the edges together and are sufficient. If the lacerations are very close to the urethra or the urethra is swollen, a red rubber intermittent catheter can be placed in the urethra while stitching is done to prevent inadvertent closure of the urethra.

2. First- and second-degree lacerations of the posterior vaginal wall should be repaired before the episiotomy is repaired. Start the repair the same way as the repair of the episiotomy. Place the first stitch 1 cm deep or proximal to the furthest extension of the tear. Tie the first stitch, and then proceed with a locking continuous repair. The suture can be tied off before episiotomy repair or continued right into the episiotomy.

Third- and Fourth-Degree Lacerations

1. Use a Gelpi clamp to hold the laceration apart, and place one Allis clamp on each edge of the torn rectal sphincter.

2. Start the repair by suturing the anterior rectal wall, if needed, with a row of interrupted sutures of 4-0 synthetic absorbable suture. Carry the stitch submucosal to the mucosa of the anterior wall of the rectum to approximate the mucosa without the suture entering the rectal lumen.

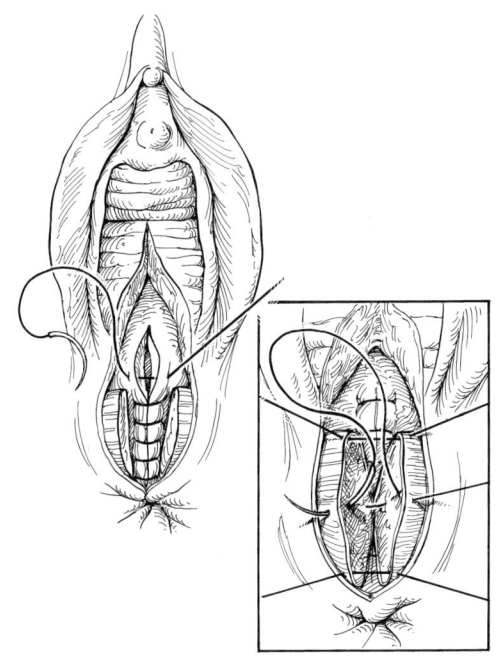

3. Then, holding the Allis clamps in one hand, place four interrupted 2-0 or 3-0 sutures into the fascial wall of the rectal sphincter. Place one below, one behind, and one above the torn muscle, and then, releasing the Allis and Gelpi clamps, place one in

front of the muscle. This will bring the donut-shaped muscle back together.

4. Repair the remaining laceration as one would a second-degree episiotomy.

Follow-Up

1. Routine follow-up includes warm sitz baths 2 to 4 times a day and local anesthetic gels if needed.

2. Infection can occur, as evidenced by foul odor and discharge. Treatment includes antibiotics, sitz baths, and possibly removal of suture material.

Bibliography

Green JR, Soohoo SL: Factors associated with rectal injury in spontaneous deliveries. Obstet Gynecol 1989;73:732–738.

Shiono P, Kleabanoff MA, Carey JC: Midline episiotomies: More harm than good? Obstet Gynecol 1990;75:765–770.

Smith MA, Acheson LS, et al: A critical review of labor and birth care. J Fam Pract 1991;33:281–292.

Sultan AH, Kamm MA, Hudson CN, et al: Anal-sphincter disruption during vaginal delivery. N Engl J Med 1993; 328:1906–1911.

Walker MPF, Farine D, Rolbin SH, Ritchie JWK: Epidural anesthesia, episiotomy and obstetrical laceration. Obstet Gynecol 1991;77:668–671.

115 Breast-Feeding

Joan M. Bedinghaus

Benefits of Breast-Feeding

1. Nutrition: Breast milk is the only food an infant needs for the first several months. It is free and convenient, requiring no mixing, warming, or sterilization.

2. Protection against infection: In developing countries, breast-feeding exerts a major protective effect against infant mortality from diarrheal and respiratory disease. In developed countries, breast-feeding has been shown to protect against diarrhea, necrotizing enterocolitis, respiratory infections, and otitis media if sustained for at least 3 months.

3. Psychosocial: Breast-fed infants have a small but measurable increase in intellectual development scores compared with those of bottle-fed infants. Breast-feeding is believed to promote close and healthy maternal-infant relationships.

4. Advantages to mothers: Breast-feeding decreases the risk of subsequent breast cancer. It also facilitates mother's return to her prepregnancy weight and can augment the effects of contraceptive methods.

Prenatal Counseling and Preparation

1. Education and support: Since the decision to breast-feed is usually made early in pregnancy, counseling and education should begin in the first trimester. Partners and key family members should be included. Childbirth education classes cannot be assumed to include breast-feeding education. Lactation consultants on hospital staffs, in WIC programs, or in private practice are useful resources. The La Leche League is a peer-support organization of breast-feeding mothers that has chapters in most communities; this organization can be easily located in a telephone directory. Peer counseling and support programs have been developed by some WIC programs. Educational videotapes effectively demonstrate breast-feeding skills.

2. Nipple preparation: Breast shells and nipple stretching exercises do not appear to be useful in preparing inverted nipples for breast-feeding. Rolling of nipples, which can be started at 35 to 36 weeks after the danger of stimulating premature labor is past, may reduce postpartum nipple soreness.

Initiation of Breast-Feeding

1. Timing: The infant should be offered the breast in the recovery room. Breast-feeding (nursing) every 2 to 3 hours in the immediate postpartum period is associated with higher continuation rates and with less neonatal jaundice. It is not necessary to limit the length of breast-feeding. Alternating infant position with each feed may help prevent nipple soreness and cracking.

2. Positioning: The infant's chest should be laid against the mother's, avoiding rotation of the infant's head. The infant may lie across the torso (cradle hold), along the flank (football hold), or alongside a supine mother (Fig. 115–1). In nursing while sitting, the mother's arms should be generously supported with cushions so that she may relax during nursing.

3. "Latching on": Proper positioning of the infant's mouth on the nipple at the start of each feed ("latching on") is essential to effective nursing. Taking advantage of the rooting reflex, the baby's mouth is stroked with the nipple or a finger. When the baby opens the mouth wide, the nipple is placed as far back in the mouth as possible. When the jaws are closed, most of the areola should be covered by the mouth. The entire mandible moves rhythmically. No lip-smacking noises will be heard; instead, swallowing noises will be apparent.

   If the infant does not latch on effectively, have the mother break suction on the nipple by sliding a finger between the infant's jaws and begin again with the rooting response. Improper latching on leads to ineffective suckling, sore and cracked nipples, and failure to stimulate the milk supply and to condition the milk ejection reflex.

4. The milk ejection reflex and milk supply: The strok-

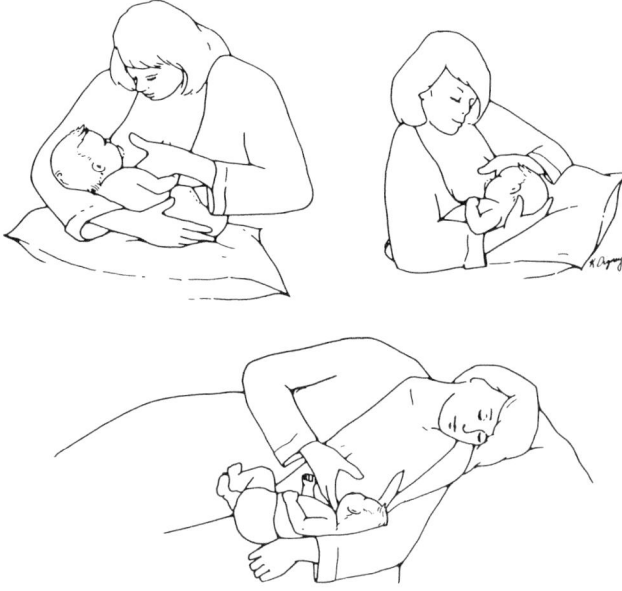

Figure 115–1 The three most common positions for breast-feeding. (From Melnikow J, Bedinhaus J: Management of common breast-feeding problems in the early postpartum weeks. J Family Pract 1994;39, Fig. 1.)

ing action of the infant's jaws and tongue on the subareolar ampullae pumps milk from the nipple; negative pressure inside the infant's mouth is not the primary stimulus to milk flow. The sensation of suckling stimulates release of oxytocin and prolactin from the maternal pituitary. Oxytocin causes contraction of the myoepithelial cells of the milk ducts, moving milk toward the ampullae, while prolactin stimulates future milk production. This neuroendocrine pathway is called the "milk ejection reflex" or "letdown."

The supply of milk made by the breast is determined primarily by the frequency of suckling (via the stimulation of prolactin release) and by the emptying of the breast. Supply is thereby regulated by demand. Frequent suckling (every 2 to 3 hours around the clock) is essential in the immediate postpartum period to stimulate early milk production. During this period, delays in offering the breast, supplementation with formula or glucose water, and feeding intervals of 4 hours or more reduce the likelihood of breast-feeding success.

5. Hospital policies that support breast-feeding include rooming-in policies that allow the mother and infant to be together around the clock, prohibition of formula supplements in the absence of a medical indication, availability of a lactation consultant or a well-trained nurse educator, and provision of an inexpensive manual breast pump instead of formula samples on discharge. Medications incompatible with breast-feeding, routine use of formula, and inappropriate feeding intervals should be eliminated from routine postpartum orders. Specific orders may be necessary to ensure that the infant is brought to the mother at 2- to 3-hour intervals and to obtain appropriate education and consultation.

6. Nipple care: To prevent cracking that can predispose to infection, nipples should be allowed to air dry after feedings. Pads worn inside the bra to absorb leaking milk should be changed when moist. No special cleansing is necessary; soap and disinfectants should be avoided. Anhydrous lanolin and vitamin E oil are commonly used as nipple emollients but may cause topical sensitivity.

Maintenance of Breast-Feeding

1. Vitamin supplements and maternal nutrition: Breast milk is somewhat low in vitamin D. Infants born in winter and dark-skinned infants may need supplementation (400 units/day) to avoid nutritional rickets, although this problem is seen mainly in older infants who have been exclusively breast-fed for more than 6 months. Where the water supply is not fluoridated, 0.25 mg/day of fluoride also may be given, though the necessity of supplementing very young infants is debated. Mothers should continue their prenatal vitamins while lactating; vitamin levels in milk reflect maternal levels. Lactating women require 250 to 750 kcal/day over baseline needs to support milk production. Rigorous weight-loss programs are not recommended during lactation.

2. Conditioning of the letdown reflex: The milk ejection reflex, or letdown, described above requires several days to weeks to become effectively conditioned. A well-conditioned letdown produces milk within a few minutes of the onset of suckling and repeats during a feed. Other stimuli such as hearing a baby's cry, thinking about the baby, sexual stimulation, manual expression, or mechanical pumping also can trigger letdown. Forceful ejection of milk sometimes causes the infant to cough or choke; manual expression of some milk before nursing can be used to avoid this problem. Troublesome leaking of milk usually subsides as breast-feeding continues for several months.

3. Inhibited letdown: Pain, embarrassment, and ineffective latching on are common causes of inhibition of the milk ejection reflex. Provide the mother with comfort, support, and privacy. Observe and correct infant body and mouth position. Pitocin nasal spray (Syntocinon, one spray in one or both nostrils 2 minutes before nursing) may be used to stimulate letdown. Its major contraindication is pregnancy, and its major side effect is headache. It should be discontinued after a few days of successful feeding.

4. Engorgement: As the breasts make the transition from colostrum to full milk production, on the second to third postpartum day, they become full, swollen, and tender. Lymphatic congestion as well as milk production contributes to initial engorgement. Emptying the breasts to relieve pressure is the most effective therapy. A breast pump or manual expression may be used after feedings to finish emptying the breasts. Emptying with a pump does not prolong the period of engorgement. Engorgement in the areolar area may make the nipple difficult for the infant to grasp; instruct the mother to manually express or pump enough to soften the breast and allow the nipple to protrude. Cool compresses, mild analgesics, and arm exercise can all be used to provide some relief of discomfort, which normally subsides within a few days.

5. Relief bottles and supplemental feeding: Bottle-feeding of expressed milk or formula should be delayed until the breast-feeding skills of mother and infant and the milk supply are well developed at about 6 weeks postpartum.

6. Returning to work: Returning to work is a common reason for discontinuation of breast-feeding. Restrictive maternity leave policies may require a mother to return to work when the infant is only 6 weeks of age. Mothers can be encouraged to continue breast-feeding by one of several methods:
   a. Locating child care near their jobs, allowing them to nurse on lunch hours and work breaks.

b. Using a mechanical pump or manual expression to collect and store milk during work breaks. Emptying the breast maintains the milk supply, and the expressed milk can be bottle-fed by other caretakers.

c. Reverse-cycle feeding: The mother nurses more frequently in the evening, night, and early morning. The infant is fed less frequently by the caretaker when the mother is working.

Common Problems

1. Sore nipples: Limiting nursing time does not prevent sore nipples. Alternating the infant's position on the breast (cradle hold, football hold, lying alongside mother) will enable the jaws to close on a different area of the nipple with each feeding.

2. Thrush nipples: Redness and burning nipple pain may accompany oral moniliasis in the infant. Treat nipples with nystatin cream while treating the infant with oral nystatin.

3. Plugged duct: a small (3- to 8-ml) tender lump in the breast that persists after nursing. Treat with local heat and massage toward the nipple.

4. Mastitis: an infection of the lactating breast, most commonly caused by *Staphylococcus aureus.* Missed feedings, cracked nipples, and excessive fatigue are predisposing factors. Symptoms may include fever and diffuse myalgias; a flulike illness in a lactating woman should prompt a breast examination. Examination reveals a tender, erythematous, wedge-shaped area. Treatment is dicloxacillin or cephalexin, 250 to 500 mg every 6 hours for 10 to 14 days, bed rest, fluids, analgesics, and frequent emptying of the breast. The bacteria that cause mastitis are usually part of the infant's oral flora, and nursing at a mastitic breast does not harm the infant. *It is extremely important to continue to empty the breast* in order to prevent the development of a breast abscess; therefore, breast-feeding should continue.

5. Breast abscess: Breast abscess complicates 5 to 10 per cent of cases of mastitis. Examination reveals a tender, hard breast mass with overlying erythema. Incision and drainage are required, followed by antibiotics, analgesics, and frequent emptying of the breast. A radial incision avoids severing the subareolar ducts. Gentle mechanical pumping of the affected breast, discarding the milk from that side, is advised for the first few days after drainage; breast-feeding from the affected breast may then resume.

6. Poor infant weight gain: Breast-fed infants should have an office or home visit for a weight check at 2 weeks of age. The infant who is obtaining adequate milk will regain birth weight by 2 weeks, will wet 6 to 12 diapers per day, and will have soft, seedy yellow stools. If the infant is not gaining weight, check for adequate latch-on and letdown. The frequency of nursing should be increased to every 2 to 3 hours around the clock. The infant should gain 2 ounces or more of weight in 2 days and show catch-up growth thereafter. If weight gain is still inadequate, or if at any time the infant appears dehydrated, breast-feeding must be supplemented with the appropriate formula. A supplemental nursing system (Lact-Aid or Medela SNS) dispenses formula during suckling through a small soft plastic tube taped near the nipple. This maintains nipple stimulation to milk production, allows the baby to control milk flow, and avoids confusing the stressed infant with switching between the breast and rubber nipples. If such a system is not available, a bottle may be offered at the end of each feed. Once the infant has regained birth weight, supplements may be decreased to every other feed and then gradually discontinued.

Sheehan's syndrome, or breast surgery that has severed the milk ducts or the innervation of the nipple, may cause lactation failure. Physiologic lactation failure is rare in a primary care population.

7. Maternal contraception and medication: Combined oral contraceptives may inhibit milk production but can be started after lactation is well established (6 to 8 weeks). Progestin implants have no adverse effects on lactation if inserted after the sixth postpartum week. All other contraceptive methods may be used in the immediate postpartum period. For most indications for maternal medication, alternatives are available that are safe during lactation. The American Academy of Pediatrics publishes a list for quick reference (see Bibliography).

8. Maternal infections: In developed countries including the United States, maternal HIV infection contraindicates breast-feeding. In developing countries, the risk of death if the infant is bottle-fed may outweigh the risk of HIV transmission. Maternal hepatitis B is a relative contraindication, though no transmission via breast milk has been documented. If the infant has received hepatitis B immune globulin (HBIG) and vaccine, breast-feeding should be safe. When the mother has active tuberculosis, separation from the infant is considered necessary until the mother's sputum is clear of acid-fast bacilli (AFB). Pumped breast milk could be fed to the infant to maintain milk supply during the isolation period. Isoniazid appears in breast milk, and rifampin colors it red or orange.

Bibliography

Bedinghaus JM, Melnikow J: Promoting successful breastfeeding skills. Am Fam Physician 1992;45:1309–1318.

Committee on Drugs: The transfer of drugs and other chemicals into human milk. Pediatrics 1994;93:137–150.

Goldfarb J: Breastfeeding: AIDS and other infectious diseases. Clin Perinatol 1993;20:225–243.

Goldfarb J, Tibbetts E: Breastfeeding Handbook. Hillside, NJ, Enslow Publishers, 1980.

Lawrence R: Breastfeeding: A Guide for the Medical Profession, 3d ed. St Louis, CV Mosby, 1989.

An educational video: Smith LJ: A Healthier Baby by Breastfeeding. Television Innovation Company, 8349 N. Arrowridge Blvd., Charlotte, NC 28273.

116 Preterm Labor

Scott Corliss

Etiology

1. Chorioamnionitis, 20 to 30 per cent; often associated with preterm rupture of membranes
2. Extrauterine infection, 5 to 10 per cent
   a. Urinary tract infection (UTI) most common; may be as high as 25 per cent of patients with preterm labor (PTL)
   b. Vaginal *Trichomonas* or *Gardnerella* also commonly associated with PTL
   c. Some association also seen with severe respiratory infection
3. Uterine overdistention
   a. Multiple gestation
   b. Macrosomia
   c. Polyhydramnios
4. Other
   a. Uterine or cervical anomalies, such as leiomyomata, incompetent cervix
   b. Placental anomalies or insufficiency, such as placenta previa, marginal cord insertion
   c. Fetal anomalies, such as neural tube defects
5. Unknown causes, 20 to 30 per cent (may be as high as 50 per cent)

Symptoms

1. Menstrual-like cramping; may be constant or intermittent
2. Uterine contractions every 10 minutes or closer. Women with uterine overdistention may have difficulty perceiving contractions.
3. Increase or change in vaginal discharge; may represent vaginal infection
4. Leakage of amniotic fluid, premature rupture of membranes (PROM)
5. Backache, usually described as dull and in the lower back; may come and go
6. Pelvic pressure; may feel like baby is pushing into the pelvis
7. Generalized abdominal cramping

Key Symptoms

- Uterine contractions
- Menstrual cramping
- Backache
- Pelvic pressure
- Abdominal cramping
- Fluid leakage
- Increased or changes in vaginal discharge

Clinical Findings

1. Cervical dilatation or effacement in a preterm patient is a warning sign.
   a. Nulliparous cervix less than 2 cm in length or open early in pregnancy signifies increased risk.
   b. Multiparous cervix greater than 2 to 3 cm dilated at 28 weeks signifies increased risk.
   c. Sonographic evidence for cervical change may be helpful.
2. Diagnosis of active preterm labor depends on the presence of abnormal uterine activity and ruptured membranes or cervical change, significant dilatation, or effacement with intact membranes.
   a. Uterine contractions: 4 in 20 minutes or 8 in 60 minutes
   b. Cervical changes should be documented by a single examiner.
   c. Greater than 2 cm or 75 per cent effacement associated with active contractions should be considered as established preterm labor.
3. Some preterm patients have indications for delivery, and preterm labor should not be stopped in these cases.
   a. Evidence for chorioamnionitis; uterine tenderness, fever, fetal tachycardia, resistance to tocolysis
   b. Advanced labor: greater than 5 cm dilated, 100 per cent effaced with bulging membranes
   c. Fetal growth retardation
   d. Congenital anomalies that are either lethal or better managed outside the uterus

Key Signs

- Early cervical dilatation or effacement
- Uterine contractions, 4 in 20 minutes or 8 in 60 minutes
- Cervical change associated with uterine contractions

Laboratory Tests

1. Testing for extrauterine infections
   a. Urinalysis and culture
   b. Vaginal culture for *Chlamydia* and group B streptococcus
   c. Vaginal wet prep for *Trichomonas* or clue cells (evidence of *Gardnerella*)
2. Vaginal fluid should be tested for evidence of premature rupture of membranes.

491

a. Nitrazine positive indicates rupture.

b. Positive ferning indicates rupture.

3. Amniocentesis may be considered to evaluate for fetal lung maturity (FLM).

a. Lecithin/sphingomyelin (L/S) ratio of more than 2.3 indicates probable lung maturity.

b. Hyaline membrane disease (HMD) will not develop if phosphatidylglycerol (PG) is present with a mature L/S ratio.

4. Amniocentesis also may be used to evaluate for intrauterine infection.

a. Gram's stain with any bacteria, spun or unspun, indicates infection.

b. Aerobic and anaerobic cultures

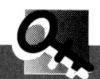

Key Tests

- Urinalysis and culture
- Screen for *Chlamydia*
- Nitrazine and fern test
- Culture for group B streptococcus
- Vaginal wet prep
- Consider amniocentesis

Differential Diagnosis

1. Preterm labor, that is, uterine contractions associated with documented cervical change.

2. Uterine activity not associated with cervical change. Caution should be used when this occurs because it has been shown that a uterus that increases its usual contraction frequency may progress in some cases to delivery in 24 to 48 hours.

Treatment

A. Prevention of early preterm labor

Medication

1. Aggressive antibiotic treatment of cervical, vaginal, or urinary infection.

a. UTI—amoxicillin, 500 mg orally t.i.d. for 10 to 14 days; cephalosporins possible second choice, culture may be needed.

b. Group B streptococcus—oral penicillin effective

c. *Gardnerella* or *Trichomonas*—metronidazole, 500 mg orally b.i.d. for 7 days (safe after 12 weeks of gestation); amoxicillin, 500 mg t.i.d. for 7 days alternative

d. *Chlamydia*—erythromycin, 250 to 500 mg q.i.d. for 7 days; alternative TMP/SMX 160/ 800 mg b.i.d. for 7 days

2. Prophylactic antibiotic treatment for patients with warning signs of preterm labor remains controversial. In patients with PROM, antibiotics have been shown to prolong the onset of preterm labor.

Combinations of erythromycin and clindamycin will adequately cover most potential pathogens.

3. Prophylactic oral tocolytics are also controversial in patients with warning signs due to a lack of proof of their efficacy.

a. Terbutaline, 2.5 mg orally q 6 hr, may be increased to 5 mg q 6 hr; alternative is ritodrine, 20 mg orally q 6 hr.

b. Nifedipine, 10 mg orally q 6 hr; may be increased to 20 mg q 4 hr, but this has a high incidence of side effects.

c. Magnesium gluconate, 1 gm q 4–6 hr; magnesium oxide, 200 mg q 3–4 hr

Diet

1. No special recommendations

2. Possible benefit from supplementation with 2 grams of elemental calcium per day

Activity

1. Reduce workload

a. Less than 8 hr/day and less than 5 days per week recommended for those at risk

b. Reduce long hours of standing

2. Bed rest recommended for increased warning signs

3. Coital abstinence recommended

Patient Education

1. Patients should be taught to recognize the signs and symptoms of preterm labor.

2. If any symptoms should occur, patients need to report them immediately.

3. Symptoms should not be "written off" as round ligament pain or Braxton Hicks contractions.

B. Treatment of established preterm labor

1. Hydration and sedation have been used traditionally, but there is no good proof of efficacy.

2. Prior to initiating tocolytic therapy, the patient should be evaluated for any of the signs indicating a need to proceed with delivery, such as chorioamnionitis, advanced labor, or fetal distress.

Medication

1. Tocolytic agents are widely used and remain the usual first line of therapy. Conclusive proof of an improvement in perinatal outcome, however, is lacking.

a. β agonists—terbutaline (ritodrine as alternative)

(1) 10 mg terbutaline in 500 milliliters of D_5W

(2) Begin infusion at 30 cc/hr (10 μg/min).

(3) Increase 15 ml/hr (5 μg/min) q 15 min until contractions have stopped or to maximum dose of 150 ml/hr (50 μg/min).

(4) After 60 minutes, titrate dose down 15 ml/hr (5 μg/min) q 30 min until minimum effective dose is reached, and maintain for 8 hours.

(5) Wean by decreasing as above until off treat-

ment; 30 minutes before stopping treatment, give 0.25 mg terbutaline subcutaneously and continue this q 4 hr for 24 hours.

(6) After 24 hours of subcutaneous terbutaline, convert to 5 mg orally q 6 hr.

(7) Watch for maternal tachycardia of greater than 120, significant fetal tachycardia, hyperglycemia, hypokalemia, and respiratory distress or pulmonary edema.

b. Magnesium sulfate

(1) Loading dose of 4 to 6 gm intravenously over 20 to 30 minutes

(2) Maintenance dose of 2 to 4 gm/hr

(3) Monitor urine output and total fluid to avoid fluid overload; maximum recommended fluid is 3000 ml/24 hr.

(4) Serum magnesium levels to keep in therapeutic range (5.5 to 7.5 mEq/L)

(5) Maintain on intravenous magnesium for 24 to 48 hours before attempting to wean to oral agents.

c. Other agents—used with some caution—consider perinatology consult.

(1) Calcium channel blockers—nifedipine

(2) Indomethacin

2. Glucocorticoids are recommended for accelerating fetal lung maturation in infants born prior to 34 weeks' gestation. Ideal time of delivery is more than 24 hours and less than 8 days after dosing. Chorioamnionitis is the most significant contraindication.

a. Betamethasone, 12 mg intramuscularly q 24 hr for 2 doses

b. Alternative drug is dexamethasone, 6 mg intramuscularly q 6 hr for 4 doses

c. Consider repeat therapy if delivery is delayed longer than 7 days.

3. Prophylaxis against intraventricular hemorrhage is supported in some studies.

a. Phenobarbital, 10 mg/kg of maternal weight, 500 mg minimum and 700 mg maximum, given intravenously over 30 minutes

b. Vitamin K, 10 mg intramuscularly, followed by 20 mg orally daily

4. Antibiotics are controversial in the management of active preterm labor. If labor is stopped and there is no evidence of chorioamnionitis, they may be effective in prolonging pregnancy. Further study is needed to confirm the efficacy and safety of this therapy.

Diet

1. No special recommendations; monitor fluid intake if on β agonists.

Activity

1. Bed rest

2. If labor is stopped, recommend generally reduced activity and no strenuous activity.

Patient Education

1. Review warning signs of preterm labor.

2. Insist on early reporting of symptoms of recurrence of preterm contractions.

3. Review side effects of oral tocolytic therapy.

Key Treatment	
Drugs of Choice	**Alternative Drugs**
• Tocolytics—terbutaline	• Ritodrine
• Glucocorticoids—betamethasone	• Dexamethasone

Follow-Up

A. Early preterm labor

1. Weekly prenatal visit and cervical examinations beginning at 22 weeks for high-risk patients

a. Assess cervical length, dilatation and development of lower uterine segment

b. May want to consider examination at 28 weeks in all patients regardless of risk status

2. Sonogram every 4 weeks for high-risk patients beginning at 16 weeks

a. Assess fetal growth and placental function

b. Assess cervical length and dilatation

c. Twice-weekly fluid volume assessments for women with PROM

3. Home uterine activity monitoring

a. Controversial; frequent nursing contact may be of equal benefit

b. Does seem to have some established efficacy for multiple gestations and polyhydramnios

B. Established preterm labor

1. Weekly office visits for fetal assessment and cervical evaluation

2. Consider home monitoring, particularly for multiple gestation or patients with difficulty perceiving contractions

Bibliography

Arias F: Preterm labor, in Arias F (ed): Practical Guide to High-Risk Pregnancy and Delivery, 2nd ed. St. Louis, Mosby–Year Book, 1993, pp 71–99.

Gjerdingen D: Premature labor: I. Risk assessment, etiologic factors, and diagnosis. J Am Board Fam Pract 1992;5(5):495–509.

Gjerdingen D: Premature labor: II. Management. J Am Board Fam Pract 1992;5(6):601–615.

LeFevre M, Hueston W: Preterm birth. Primary Care Clin 1993;20(3):639–653.

Leonardi M, Hankins G: What's new in tocolytics. Clin Perinatol 1992;19(2):367–384.

117 First Trimester Bleeding

Scott T. Henderson

Etiology

1. One fourth of all pregnant women experience vaginal bleeding in early pregnancy. In one half of these women spontaneous abortion will occur.
2. Various other causes such as ectopic pregnancy, trophoblastic disease, and cervical and vaginal lesions have been identified.
3. In a number of cases no apparent cause for the bleeding can be identified.

Symptoms

1. Vaginal bleeding—ranging from a scant pinkish or brownish discharge to massive hemorrhage
2. Pelvic or suprapubic pain
3. Uterine cramping
4. Gastrointestinal symptoms—abdominal pain and cramping, nausea and vomiting, and urge to defecate
5. Dizziness and syncope
6. Symptoms of pregnancy

Key Symptoms	
• Vaginal bleeding	• Abdominal pain
• Pelvic pain	• Uterine cramping

Clinical Findings

Clinical findings will vary depending on the cause of the bleeding.

1. Cervical dilatation (inevitable or incomplete abortion)
2. Rupture of membranes (inevitable abortion)
3. Passage of products of conception (incomplete abortion)
4. Soft and involuted uterus (ectopic)
5. Cervical motion tenderness (ectopic)
6. Abdominal tenderness (ectopic)
7. Adnexal/pelvic mass (ectopic)
8. Fever
9. Shock

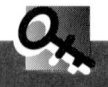

Key Signs	
• Cervical dilatation	• Rupture of membranes
• Passage of tissue	• Adnexal/pelvic mass

Laboratory Tests

1. Pelvic and/or transvaginal ultrasound—to determine the location of the pregnancy or products of conception and assess fetal viability

2. Culdocentesis—Assess for hemoperitoneum if the diagnosis of ectopic pregnancy is in question.
2. Complete blood count (CBC) and differential
3. Blood type and Rh factor
4. Clotting studies and platelet count if history of coagulation disorder or if missed or septic abortion is present.
5. Qualitative serum β-human chorionic gonadotropin (β-hCG) level—Decreasing or abnormally low levels are predictive of problems.
6. Serum progesterone level—Levels less than 25 ng/ml may indicate ectopic or spontaneous abortion.
7. Type and cross-match
8. Vaginal wet prep and cultures for gonorrhea, *Chlamydia*, and group B *Streptococcus*

Key Tests	
• Pelvic or transvaginal ultrasound	• Blood type and Rh factor
• Complete blood count	• Serum β-hCG

Differential Diagnosis

1. Abortion
   a. Threatened—uterine bleeding occurring during the first half of pregnancy
   b. Inevitable—rupture of the membranes with cervical dilatation
   c. Incomplete—part of the conceptus/placenta expelled but part retained
   d. Missed—conceptus dies but the products retained in utero for 8 or more weeks
2. Gestational trophoblastic disease—ranges from benign hydatidiform mole to invasive mole or gestational choriocarcinoma
3. Ectopic pregnancy—The fertilized ovum implants elsewhere than the endometrial cavity of the uterus. Vaginal bleeding occurs in 50 to 94 per cent of patients with ectopic pregnancy.
4. Subchorionic bleeding—can be due to excessive physical activity, gastrointestinal illness with vomiting or diarrhea, placenta previa, or the early stages of spontaneous abortion
5. Lesions—including adenomas, uterine leiomyomas, cervical or uterine polyps, cervical erosions/ulcerations, and neoplasm
6. Genital trauma
7. Infections—vaginitis, cervicitis, or pelvic inflammatory disease

494

8. Implantation bleeding—slight bleeding occurring when the ovum burrows and implants into the uterus. This usually occurs near the time of the first missed menstrual period.

9. Incorrect menstrual dating—Bleeding may actually be a normal period.

10. Maternal disease—including coagulopathies, blood dysplasias, or leukemia

Treatment

The treatment of first trimester bleeding depends on the etiology. If life-threatening conditions, such as shock, are present, management must include appropriate advanced life-support measures.

1. Abortion: If less than 6 to 8 weeks' gestation, the patient may be able to pass the tissue without medical or surgical intervention. An ultrasound may be necessary to assess for any residual tissue. If the bleeding is excessive or the pregnancy is past 8 weeks, the contents of the uterus need to be evacuated with a dilatation and curettage (D&C).

2. Gestational trophoblastic disease: Once the problem is diagnosed, the uterus must be evacuated immediately. D&C under general anesthesia is the preferred procedure. Oxytocin should be given during the procedure to help control bleeding. All patients should have β-hCG determinations followed for evidence of malignant disease.

3. Ectopic pregnancy: Surgical intervention by laparotomy or laparoscopy is required in the majority of cases. If an unruptured tubal pregnancy is less than 4 centimeters in diameter, it may be treated conservatively with methotrexate.

4. Subchorionic bleeds: No specific intervention is indicated, but activity should be limited and the patient put at pelvic rest. Additionally, bleeding should be followed up with an ultrasound examination in 4 to 8 weeks.

Medication
A. Drugs of choice

1. Rh$_o$(D) immune globulin (Rho Gam): if patient is Rh negative, an intramuscular injection should be given within 72 hours of the fetomaternal hemorrhage. Rh$_o$(D) immune globulin is supplied in two different unit doses, standard and microdose. Generally only a single injection is needed to provide protection. The microdose should be used only if the gestation is less than 12 weeks.

2. Oxytocin: intravenous (10 units at a rate of 20 to 100 milliunits per minute) or intramuscular (10 units) route to control uterine bleeding following operative procedure such as D&C. To prepare an intravenous solution, add 10 to 40 units of oxytocin to 1000 ml of a nonhydrating diluent resulting in a final solution concentration of 10 to 40 milliunits per ml.

B. Alternative drugs: Ergots—intramuscular or oral agents such as methlyergonovine maleate (Methergine) may be used in place of oxytocin. Usual oral dosage is 0.2 or 0.4 mg two to four times daily, usually for 2 days. Intramuscular dosage is 0.2 mg (1 ml) and may be repeated in 2 to 4 hours if bleeding is severe.

Diet
Variable

Activity
1. Bed rest until resolution, if appropriate
2. Pelvic rest—no coitus, tampons, or douching

Patient Education
Inform the patient that there is an increased risk of abortion and fetal loss in subsequent pregnancies in women who experience first trimester bleeding.

Follow-Up

1. If the patient proceeds to have an abortion, the products of conception must be identified to confirm diagnosis.

2. If the patient goes on to have an abortion or if the ectopic pregnancy is managed conservatively, the β-hCG level must be followed until it returns to normal.

3. If the patient has gestational trophoblastic disease, the β-hCG levels should be followed for evidence of malignant disease.

4. Psychological support to the woman and her partner is necessary.

5. If the pregnancy is lost, the patient should be advised to use some form of birth control and not attempt another pregnancy until she has had at least two to three normal menstrual cycles.

6. If the patient continues to carry the pregnancy, there may be an increased risk of low birth weight, preterm delivery, and neonatal death. Close obstetric follow-up care is indicated.

Bibliography

For more information on first trimester bleeding, see
Pernoll ML, Garmel SH: Early pregnancy risks. *In* DeCherney AH, Pernoll ML (eds): Current Obstetric and Gynecologic Diagnosis and Treatment, 8th ed. Norwalk, Conn, Appleton and Lange, 1994, pp 306–330.
Chamberlain G: Vaginal bleeding in early pregnancy, part I. Br Med J 1991;302:1141–1143.
Chamberlain G: Vaginal bleeding in early pregnancy, part II. Br Med J 1991;302:1195–1203.
For more information on abortion, see
Cunningham FG, MacDonald PC, Gant NF, et al: Abortion. *In* Williams' Obstetrics, 19th ed. E Norwalk, Conn, Appleton & Lange, 1993, pp 661–690.
For more information on ectopic pregnancy, see
Cunningham FG, MacDonald PC, Gant NF, et al: Ectopic pregnancy. *In* Williams' Obstetrics, 19th ed. E Norwalk, Conn, Appleton & Lange, 1993, pp 691–719.
Hammond CB, Bachus KE: Ectopic pregnancy. *In* Scott JR, Disaia PJ, Hammond CB, Spellacy WM (eds): Danforth's Obstetrics and Gynecology, 7th ed. Philadelphia, JB Lippincott, 1994, pp 187–200.

Bleeding from the genital area in later pregnancy (after fetal viability, 23 to 24 weeks) occurs in 2 to 5 per cent of all pregnancies. Most serious bleeding episodes arise from placental or uterine pathology, but multiple sources have been described. In reported series, up to 50 per cent of cases with third trimester bleeding *do not* have serious pathology.

Placenta Previa

Etiology

1. Prior uterine surgery
   a. Cesarean section: If placenta previa is present and patient has had prior cesarean section, there is an increased risk of placenta accreta.
   b. Dilatation and curettage (D&C), elective abortion
2. Risk increases with age of patient.
3. Risk increases with increasing parity.

Symptoms

1. Vaginal bleeding, frequently painless. There may be no history of trauma, or bleeding may occur after coitus or pelvic examination or with onset of contractions.
2. Crampy lower abdominal pain can occur with bleeding in up to 25 per cent of cases.

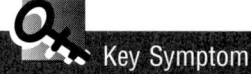

Key Symptom

- Vaginal bleeding

Clinical Findings

> **WARNING**
>
> **The initial history and physical examination will usually reveal the source of bleeding. However, although it depends on the level of expertise of the examiner, internal vaginal examination (digitally or by speculum) should be deferred in most cases until placenta previa has been ruled out.**

1. Breech or transverse lie on abdominal examination is seen in about one third of cases. If vertex lie, vertex palpates well above pelvic brim.
2. Uterine contractions are present in up to 25 per cent of cases.

3. Uterine tenderness is seen in up to 10 per cent of cases due to coexisting abruption.
4. If blood loss is large enough, signs of hypovolemia can be present.
5. If hypovolemia is present, signs of fetal distress can be seen on heart monitor.
6. *If speculum examination is done,* bleeding from cervical os is noted.

Key Signs

- Vaginal bleeding
- Abnormal lie or nonengaged vertex
- Signs of hypovolemia
- Fetal distress

Laboratory Tests

1. Ultrasound of uterus: Area of cervix is viewed with patient's bladder full and then empty. Recently, vaginal probe ultrasound, carefully done, has been shown to resolve some questions when abdominal ultrasound is unclear (e.g., with posterior placenta previa). *Ultrasound examination has up to a 7 per cent false-negative rate.*
2. Complete blood count
3. Type and cross-match at least 2 units of packed red blood cells. ·
4. Magnetic resonance imaging (MRI): Recent studies show that MRI can image cervix better and can be useful if ultrasound findings are unclear. Risk to the fetus is thought to be minimal, but adequate studies are not yet done.

Key Tests

- Ultrasound of uterus
- Type and cross-match 2 units
- Complete blood count

Differential Diagnosis

1. Abruptio placentae: In up to 10 per cent of cases of placenta previa there is coexisting abruption.
2. Vasa praevia: If bleeding is from this source, signs of fetal distress will be seen on heart monitor after relatively little blood loss.
3. Ruptured uterus at site of cesarean section scar. If prior vertical uterine incision, one third of those that do rupture do so before labor. If prior horizontal

uterine incision, rupture, if it occurs, is almost always with labor.

4. Bleeding from other genital site

Treatment

1. Stabilize patient with volume replacement and transfusion as necessary. If bleeding is sufficient to endanger mother or fetus, delivery should be by immediate cesarean section regardless of gestational age.
2. If pregnancy is confidently known to be term, deliver by cesarean section.
3. If pregnancy is of unclear gestational age or less than 36 to 37 weeks and patient is stable, hospitalize at bed rest. Perform weekly amniocentesis and deliver when fetal lungs mature.
4. In certain circumstances, after initial hospitalization with stable patient, expectant management can be done on outpatient basis.

Follow-Up

1. Postpartum hemorrhage is more common.
2. Risk of recurrence with subsequent pregnancy is 4 to 8 per cent.

Abruptio Placentae

Etiology

1. Maternal hypertension: In one study, almost 50 per cent of severe abruptions were in hypertensive patients.
2. Trauma
3. Uterine anomaly or tumor
4. Cocaine use
5. Sudden uterine decompression (e.g., after rupture of membranes or after birth of first twin)

Symptoms

1. Vaginal bleeding
2. Abdominal or low back pain, crampy or continuous in nature
3. Decreased or absent perceived fetal movement

WARNING

Placental abruption, even severe, can occur silently without pain or bleeding.

Key Symptoms

- Vaginal bleeding
- Decreased perceived fetal movement
- Abdominal or low back pain

Clinical Findings

1. Uterine tenderness
2. Bleeding from cervical os
3. Uterine contractions, frequently with uterine "irritability" (mild contractions of short duration with a frequency of 1 to 2 minutes)
4. Fetal distress on fetal heart monitor
5. Labor (uterine contractions with progressive cervical changes)
6. Fetal death
7. Shock: Can occur without excessive external blood loss due to occult collection of blood within the uterus
8. Consumptive coagulopathy: When this accompanies abruption, there is almost always fetal demise.

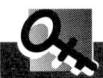

Key Signs

- Bleeding from cervix
- Uterine tenderness
- Uterine irritability
- Fetal distress

Laboratory Tests

1. Ultrasound of uterus
2. Complete blood count
3. Coagulation studies
4. Type and cross-match at least 2 units packed red cells.

WARNING

A normal ultrasound does not rule out abruption.

Key Tests

- Ultrasound
- Uterine and fetal monitoring
- Type and cross-match 2 units
- Coagulation studies
- Complete blood count

Differential Diagnosis

1. Placenta previa
2. Vasa praevia
3. Uterine rupture
4. Normal labor with "bloody show"
5. Bleeding from other genital site

Treatment

1. If the fetus is alive and abruption is mild in a term pregnancy, expeditious delivery should be accomplished by rupture of membranes, with oxytocin as needed.

2. With mild abruption and immature fetus, a judgment must be made as to whether intrauterine environment or intensive-care nursery is safer for fetus.

3. If abruption is more severe (fetal distress, maternal hypovolemia), delivery may need to be by cesarean section if vaginal birth is judged not to be imminent.

4. With abruption and fetal demise, one should expedite labor and perform cesarean section only when either labor is contraindicated or blood loss is excessive and labor is progressing too slowly.

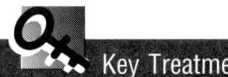

Key Treatment

- Delivery
- Volume and blood replacement

Follow-Up

1. Increased incidence of postpartum bleeding
2. Recurrence risk of 10 per cent for subsequent pregnancy

Vasa Praevia

Etiology

Velamentous insertion of umbilical cord with cord vessels surrounded only by membranes in front of presenting fetal part. It is more common with multiple gestations.

Symptoms

Vaginal bleeding onset with rupture of membranes

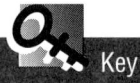

Key Symptom

- Vaginal bleeding onset with rupture of membranes

Clinical Findings

1. Bleeding from cervical os
2. Palpable vessels in membranes felt at internal os of cervix
3. Variable decelerations in fetal heart rate
4. Onset of persistent fetal distress with membrane rupture and bleeding

Key Signs

- Bleeding from cervical os
- Palpable vessels in membranes
- Onset fetal distress with membrane rupture and bleeding

Laboratory Tests

1. Rapid test for fetal hemoglobin on blood from vagina (e.g., Apt test, Kleihauer-Bethke smear)
2. Recent articles suggest that vasa praevia can sometimes be visualized by abdominal or vaginal ultrasound.

Key Test

- Rapid test for fetal hemoglobin

Differential Diagnosis

1. Placenta previa
2. Abruptio placentae
3. Uterine rupture
4. Bleeding from other genital site

Treatment

Rapid delivery, almost always by cesarean section.

Bibliography

Crane S, Chun B, Acker D: Treatment of obstetric hemorrhagic emergencies. *In* Current Opinion in Obstetric and Gynecology, vol 5, no 5. Philadelphia, Current Science Publication, 1993, pp 675–682.

Cunningham FG, MacDonald PC, Leveno KJ, et al (eds): Williams' Obstetrics, 19th ed. E Norwalk, Conn, Appleton & Lange, 1993, pp 819–843.

Green JR: Placenta previa and abruptio placentae. *In* Creasy RK, Resnik R (eds): Maternal-Fetal Medicine: Principles and Practice, 2d ed. Philadelphia, WB Saunders, 1989, pp 592–612.

Lowe TW, Cunningham FG: Placental abruption, and Laury JP: Placenta previa. *In* Levenko KJ (ed): Clinics in Obstetrics and Gynecology, vol 33, no 3. Philadelphia, JB Lippincott, 1990, pp 406–421.

Scott JR, Disia PG, Hammond LB, Spellacy WN (eds): Williams' Obstetrics and Gynecology, 7th ed. Philadelphia, JB Lippincott, 1994, pp 489–500.

119 Postpartum Hemorrhage

Michael S. Wolkomir

Etiology

A. Early postpartum hemorrhage (immediate to 24 hours after birth)

1. Uterine atony

   a. Rapid *or* prolonged labor

   b. Overdistended uterus (twins, macrosomia, polyhydramnios)

   c. High parity or history of previous atonic bleeding

   d. Induction or augmentation of labor

   e. Chorioamnionitis

2. Lower genital tract trauma

   a. Episiotomy (average loss = 200 cubic centimeters)

   b. Vulvar lacerations and hematomas (generally secondary to uncontrolled delivery of head)

   c. Vaginal vault laceration and hematoma

      (1) Forceps can produce vault tears, especially over ischial spines.

      (2) Vacuum can cause avulsion of vaginal mucosa.

   d. Cervical laceration

      (1) Rapid first stage of labor

      (2) Pushing against undilated cervix; manual dilatation or vacuum before complete dilatation of cervix

      (3) Usually occurs at 3:00 and 9:00 positions

      (4) Can extend beyond vault to broad ligament, producing life-threatening intra-abdominal bleeding

   e. Other rare events:

      (1) Uterine rupture—associated with previous uterine surgery, including classic cesarean section (VBACs show no increased risk)

      (2) Uterine inversion—associated with mismanagement of third stage of labor

---

WARNING

Never attempt to separate the placenta by pulling on the cord!

---

3. Retained placenta or membranes (more common with previous cesarean section)

   a. Retained cotyledon or accessory lobe of placenta

   b. Abnormality of implantation (accreta, increta, percreta)

4. Coagulopathies (rare). Obstetric causes include pre-eclampsia, abruptio placentae, amniotic fluid embolism, and dead fetus syndrome.

B. Late postpartum hemorrhage (more than 24 hours)

1. Late recognition of *any* of the causes of early postpartum hemorrhage (PPH)

2. Failure of the placental bed to involute normally

3. Retained products of conception

4. Infection—chorioamnionitis

5. Consider especially coagulopathies.

Symptoms

A. Early PPH. May be none (physiologic adaptations include increase of 40 per cent or more blood volume, and patient may be supine).

B. Late PPH

1. Nurse's or experienced mother's report of excessive lochia.

2. Dizziness or lightheadedness on standing, syncope.

Key Symptoms

- Early: Mental status changes or frank shock.
- Late: Dizziness or syncope.

Clinical Findings

A. Early PPH

1. Obvious vaginal bleeding in excess of your experience. Average blood loss is 500 cubic centimeters. *Triple your "gut" estimate!*

2. Occult bleeding: Large amounts of blood can be lost slowly and easily hidden by drapes.

3. Classic symptoms of impending shock appear *late in the process*—tachypnea, tachycardia, hypotension, mental status changes.

WARNING

Pre-eclamptic mothers are exquisitely sensitive to blood loss (shock) and to its treatment (CHF and pulmonary edema).

B. Late PPH

1. Orthostatic hypotension, tachycardia

499

2. Hemoglobin level fall of 1.5 gm = 1 unit of blood.
3. Low urine output (<30 cc/hr)
4. Signs of puerperal infection
5. Bleeding from other sites (e.g., venipuncture) suggests coagulopathy.

WARNING

Signs of acute anemia without visible external bleeding, especially with expanding abdominal girth, may represent broad ligament hematoma and constitute a surgical emergency.

 Key Signs

- Early: Visible hemorrhage
  Signs of shock
- Late: Orthostatic hypotension
  Laboratory signs of anemia out of proportion to expected loss

Laboratory Tests

1. All mothers should have a preadmission hemoglobin and hematocrit (H&H) for comparison.
2. At first sign of excessive bleeding:
   a. Repeat complete blood count (CBC) with platelet count.
   b. Cross and type 4 units of packed red cells and keep 4 units on hand.
   c. Disseminated intravascular coagulation (DIC) screen including prothrombin time/partial thromboplastin time (PT/PTT), fibrinogen, fibrin split products, and antithrombin III if available. (Do early before transfusions confuse the issue.)
   d. Qualitative clot retraction is easy to do but detects only platelet disorders.
3. For late PPH
   a. CBC with differential. Repeat as necessary to follow, at least daily.
   b. Cultures of lochia and blood as clinically indicated
   c. Coagulation screen as above
   d. Ultrasound may be useful in identifying retained products of conception or hematomas.

 Key Laboratory Tests

- Early: Cross and type packed red cells in sufficient quantity
  Coagulation screening
- Late PPH: Infection workup
  Ultrasound of pelvis

Treatment

A. General principles: PPH is a rapidly evolving emergency!
   1. Get obstetric consultation and treat blood loss and shock *early.*
   2. Treat for *atony* while looking for any other causes.
   3. Start fluid replacement with two large-bore intravenous needles (18 or larger), lactated Ringer's, 1000-ml challenge, then 250 cc/hr. (Reduce rate in pre-eclamptics to prevent fluid overload.)
   4. Administer O_2, 2 to 6 L/min.
   5. Replace other components with reference to the patient's laboratory values. If this is not possible, consider 1 unit fresh frozen plasma for each 3 units of packed red blood cells.
   6. Use intravenous analgesia if necessary to do an adequate pelvic examination.
B. Specific causes
   1. Atony: Vigorous bimanual massage, tamponade. Keep one hand in the vagina, the other on the abdomen, and squeeze/massage the uterus between.

WARNING

Packing the uterus is *almost never* justified.

---

   2. Birth trauma: *These tissues are friable. Avoid synthetic suture materials. Be gentle!*
      a. Vulvar trauma
         (1) Perineal laceration: Close like episiotomy if bleeding.
         (2) Periurethral: Place a catheter before starting to sew.
            (a) Interrupted or "figure-of-8" sutures of 5-0 chromic *only if bleeding*
            (b) Clitoral region is very vascular. Be careful; use minimum suture.
         (3) Hematomas
            (a) If less than 3 cm and stable, observe, ice packs, and compression.
            (b) If more than 3 cm or enlarging, consider exploration and identification of specific bleeding sites. Can be oversewn with 3-0 or 4-0 chromic.
      b. Vault lacerations: *Good visualization is the key!* Use assistants for retraction.
         (1) If secondary to forceps, assume these are *bilateral!*
         (2) Look in hidden places (fornix, posterior vault).
         (3) Make sure you start sutures *above* the apex of laceration.

(4) Close with one or two layers of "figure-of-8" or running 3-0 chromic suture.

c. Cervical laceration

(1) Look at 3:00 and 9:00 positions.

(2) Grasp upper and lower lip of cervix with ring forceps, and visualize apex of laceration.

(3) Close with running lock suture of 3-0 chromic suture, beginning *above* the apex.

3. Retained placenta or membranes

a. If undelivered by 30 minutes, infuse 10 International Units of pitocin in 20 cubic centimeters of normal saline into umbilical vein.

b. Manual exploration, removal: Sedation may be necessary.

(1) Insert hand into uterus and sweep hypothenar ridge under the cleavage plane of the placenta, sweep the uterine wall, and remove the products.

(2) If plane does not develop, consider placenta accreta.

c. Carefully inspect placenta for missing cotyledon or vessels coursing off membranes, indicating an accessory lobe.

d. If not controlled, consider surgical evacuation.

(1) Use suction curettage or a large "banjo" curette.

(2) Very gentle touch is necessary to prevent Asherman's syndrome or perforation.

e. Cover with antibiotics for infection and pitocin for atony.

4. Rare traumatic events

a. Uterine rupture—discovered on manual exploration. If bleeding, requires laparotomy.

b. Uterine prolapse—requires *immediate* reinsertion. *Don't wait for a consultant!*

(1) May require a tocolytic: Be prepared for massive bleeding and shock.

(2) Leave placenta attached.

(3) With one hand on the abdomen and the other in the vagina, revert the uterus like turning a sock inside out.

5. Coagulopathies (manage as described in Chapter 154)

6. Surgical management: In the event of failure of conservative management, several procedures are available. The purpose of these is to reduce the pulse pressure and allow hemostasis to occur.

a. Ligation of hypogastric uterine or ovarian arteries

b. Selective catheter embolization of the iliac or hypogastric arteries (still investigational)

c. If all else fails, hysterectomy may be necessary.

C. Late PPH

1. Subinvolution is usually self-limited. D&C is rarely indicated.

2. Intramuscular methylergonovine is a good therapy in the absense of hypertension.

3. Consider ultrasound to aid in the diagnosis of retained products before electing D&C.

4. Cover with antibiotics for endometritis, as described in Chapter 107.

Diet

After recovery, encourage balanced diet high in iron and protein to aid recovery.

Activity

1. Increase activity as tolerated.

2. Avoid intercourse until all healing has occurred (usually after the 6-week check).

Patient Education

1. Recurrence risk depends on the specific cause. The physician should review the current literature before discussing this with the patient.

2. Make sure patient is educated in the signs and symptoms of recurrent bleeding, acute anemia, and infection.

Key Treatment

Drugs of Choice

- Oxytocin (Pitocin), 20 to 40 IU/L rapid intravenous infusion (intravenous bolus can cause circulatory collapse)

- Methylergonovine, 0.2 mg intramuscularly only

- Prostaglandin (Hemabate), very effective, 0.25 to 1 mg q 15–60 min p.r.n. to maximum of 12 mg

  1. Give intramuscularly or transabdominally into uterine fundus.
  2. Asthma is a contraindication.

Follow-Up

1. Make sure the patient feels free to call if there are any problems.

2. Consider seeing her early. An ideal time is when seeing the baby for a 2-week check.

 ## Bibliography

American College of Obstetricians and Gynecologists: Diagnosis and management of postpartum hemorrhage. ACOG Tech Bull 143, July 1990.

Cunningham FG, MacDonald PC, Leveno KJ, et al: Abnormalities of the third stage of labor. *In* Williams' Obstetrics, 19th ed. E Norwalk, Conn, Appleton & Lange 1994, pp 615–625.

Smith D: Third stage emergencies. *In* Damos J, Beasley J, Byrd J (eds): Advanced Life Support in Obstetrics, draft 3, Madison, Wisc, University of Wisconsin, Department of Family Medicine, 1993, pp 151–163.

Watson P: Postpartum hemorrhage and shock. Clin Obstet Gynecol 1980;23:985.

Watson P, Besch N, Bowes WA Jr: Management of acute and subacute puerperal inversion of the uterus. Obstet Gynecol 1980;55:12.

120 Induction of Labor

Michael L. Sparacino

Definition

The initiation of uterine contractions of sufficient intensity to cause cervical dilatation before the spontaneous onset of labor.

Background

The induction of labor can be categorized as either elective or indicated. Elective induction implies labor induction for the convenience of the patient, her family, or the physician. In general, elective labor induction should be reserved for extraordinary circumstances. The induction of labor is indicated when, in the opinion of the treating physician, the risks of delivery to the mother or fetus or both are less than the risks of continuing the pregnancy. In cases of coexistent maternal and/or fetal medical illness, the decision to induce labor should be individualized, ideally with the consultation of a physician well trained in high-risk obstetric care. Labor inductions under these circumstances are referred to as "inductions of obligation" and imply that delivery should take place within 24 hours of the start of the induction, operatively if necessary.

A common scenario of indicated labor induction is that of impending postdatism. After carefully reviewing the fetus' gestational age, indicated induction should be scheduled to take place by 42 weeks' gestation. In cases where the cervix is not ripe (see below), several methods to induce cervical ripening are available. These include the intracervical use of a prostaglandin E analogue such as Prepidil gel (dinoprostone cervical gel 0.5 mg), insertion of a 30-ml Foley catheter into the cervical os (provided the membranes are unruptured), or use of a low-flow intravenous pitocin infusion the night before the scheduled induction. These methods of cervical ripening should take place on the labor and delivery ward where adequate surveillance techniques are available for the mother and her fetus.

Indications

1. Pregnancy-induced hypertension
2. Premature rupture of the membranes
3. Chorioamnionitis
4. Suspected fetal stress (based on objective fetal surveillance methods)
5. Maternal medical problems
6. Fetal demise
7. Logistical considerations (distance from hospital, weather, and so on)
8. Post-term gestation

Relative Contraindications

1. Placenta previa or vasa praevia
2. Abnormal fetal presentation
3. Suspected umbilical cord prolapse
4. Nonengagement
5. History of prior classic uterine incision
6. Active genital herpes
7. Anatomic pelvic deformity
8. Invasive cervical cancer

Preparation

1. Document indications for labor induction.

WARNING

A physician with privileges to perform cesarean section should be made aware that induction is taking place.

---

2. Document cervical inducibility. The Bishop score can be helpful in cervical assessment (Table 120–1). The score is easily calculated by assigning a numeric value from 0 to 3 to each of five clinically measurable cervical parameters. These parameters include dilatation (in centimeters), effacement (as a percentage of overall cervical shortening), station (measured in thirds above or below the level of the ischial spines), consistency, and cervical position. These values are then added. A score of 8 or more indicates adequate cervical inducibility and predicts a successful delivery within 12 hours after induction. Bishop scores also can be used to grade cervical change in cases of cervical incompetence or preterm labor.

TABLE 120–1. THE BISHOP SCORING SYSTEM

Score	Dilation (cm)	Effacement (%)	Station	Consistency	Cervical Position
0	Closed	0–30	−3	Firm	Posterior
1	1–2	40–50	−2	Medium	Midposition
2	3–4	60–70	−1, 0	Soft	Anterior
3	>4	>70	+1, +2	—	—

Method

Surgical Induction

1. Stripping of membranes. Manual separation of membranes from surrounding endocervix produces localized release of natural prostaglandins, which may help to induce labor. Some physicians believe that membrane stripping only occasionally induces labor, yet is associated with a higher incidence of chorioamnionitis.

2. Amniotomy. Amniotomy should be carried out only if the vertex is engaged. Amniotomy should take place in the labor and delivery area where close monitoring can be accomplished. In cases where the forebag is bulging, gradual decompression by needle amniotomy while monitoring fetal heart rate decreases the possibility of umbilical cord prolapse.

Medical Induction

1. A well-functioning intravenous line should be established to allow free flow of a balanced electrolyte solution.

2. Mix 10 units of oxytocin in 1000 ml of D_5W, and connect this secondary line as near as possible to the insertion of the primary intravenous line.

3. Begin an initial infusion of 0.5 mU/min. Increase this initial rate by 1 milliunit every 30 minutes until the desired contraction pattern is seen or until the infusion rate reaches 40 mU/min (90 per cent of patients will respond to less than 16 mU/min).

4. Once labor has progressed to 5 to 6 cm cervical dilatation, the oxytocin may be decreased similarly, although the infusion may have to be continued in order to maintain labor.

5. Fetal heart rate and uterine activity should be continuously monitored.

> **WARNING**
>
> **In the event of uterine hyperactivity or fetal stress, the oxytocin infusion should be discontinued immediately, and oxygen should be given to the mother, who should be placed in a semilateral recumbent position.**

Augmentation of Labor

If the orderly progressive dilatation of the cervix with accompanying descent of the fetus has ceased and cephalopelvic disproportion and fetal macrosomia have been ruled out, amniotomy should be carried out if not already done according to guidelines mentioned above. An intrauterine pressure catheter should be inserted and calibrated at this time as well. If no improvement in labor progression occurs and there is no fetal stress, labor may be augmented with oxytocin as described above. Because the uterus is often very sensitive to oxytocin at this time, it is recommended that a low initial infusion rate of 0.5 mU/min be used.

 Bibliography

American College of Obstetricians and Gynecologists: Technical Bulletin, number 110, page 2, November 1987.

Laube D, Zlatnik FJ, Pitkin RM, et al: Preinduction cervical ripening with prostaglandin E_2 intracervical gel. Obstet Gynecol 1986;68(1):54–57.

Romero R, Baumann P, Gomez R, et al: The relationship between spontaneous rupture of the amniotic cavity and amniotic fluid concentrations of prostaglandins and thromboxane B_2 in term pregnancy. Am J Obstet Gynecol 1993;168(6, part 1):1654–1664.

Seitchik J, Amico JR, Castillo M, et al: Oxytocin augmentation of dysfunctional labor. Am J Obstet Gynecol 1982;144(8):899–905.

Valenzuela GJ, Germain A, Foster TC, et al: Physiology of uterine activity in pregnancy. Curr Opin Obstet Gynecol 1993;5(5):640–646.

121 Pregnancy-Induced Hypertension *Lisa A. Gleason*

Etiology

1. Although the etiology of pregnancy-induced hypertension (PIH) or pre-eclampsia is not entirely understood, placental insufficiency appears fundamental. Recent data support the possibility of an abnormality in the circulation on the fetal side of the placenta as the initiating event.

2. An imbalance in the ratio of thromboxane A_2, a potent vasoconstrictor, to prostacyclin I_2, a potent vasodilator, may be responsible for the maternal vascular hyperreactivity to angiotensin II that is seen in pre-eclampsia.

3. Eventually, vasospasm and thrombosis in a variety of maternal vascular beds cause end-organ damage and lead to the signs and symptoms of PIH.

Symptoms

1. Persistent headaches and neurologic symptoms can be manifestations of intracerebral ischemia, hemorrhage, or edema.

2. Visual disturbances may be secondary to cerebral ischemia, retinal hemorrhage, or papilledema.

3. Epigastric or right upper quadrant pain can result from hepatic congestion, ischemia, or capsular swelling.

4. Vaginal bleeding may be secondary to placental abruption, disseminated intravascular coagulation (DIC), or thrombocytopenia.

5. Oliguria results from decreased renal perfusion.

Key Symptoms

- Headache
- Visual disturbances
- Abdominal pain

Clinical Findings

1. Hypertension is defined as a blood pressure (BP) of 140/90 or greater or an increase in systolic of 30 or diastolic of 15 mm Hg. Hypertension is severe if it is 160/110 or greater.

2. Proteinuria is defined as mild if 300 to 5000 mg/day or severe if greater than 5 gm per day.

3. Edema, common in pregnancy, is pathologic if rapid in onset or generalized.

4. Patients with pre-eclampsia are at risk for seizures, hypertensive encephalopathy, oliguria of less than 500 ml/day, pulmonary edema, coagulopathy, abruptio placentae, HELLP syndrome (hemolytic anemia, ele-

vated liver enzymes, and low platelets), or intrauterine growth retardation.

5. Risk factors for PIH include primigravida, family history of pre-eclampsia, extremes of childbearing age, polyhydramnios, multigestation, erythroblastosis fetalis, hydatidiform mole, diabetes mellitus, chronic hypertension, renal insufficiency, vascular disease, connective tissue disease, and pheochromocytoma. These patients should be closely followed.

Key Signs

- Systolic BP > 140 mm Hg or diastolic > 90 mm Hg
- Proteinuria
- Rapidly worsening edema

Laboratory Tests

1. Laboratory evaluation is more useful in the management of PIH than in its diagnosis. No currently available test is specific or sensitive enough to be a useful screening tool in predicting the development of PIH. A low 24-hour urinary calcium excretion may prove useful in differentiating pre-eclampsia from chronic hypertension, but further studies are needed.

2. Initial evaluation should include a hematocrit, uric acid, urinalysis, urine culture, creatinine, platelet count, and liver function tests. Abnormalities would be supportive of more severe PIH.

3. Twenty-four-hour urine testing for creatinine clearance and protein should be done each trimester in patients with PIH or patients at high risk for PIH.

4. If hyperglycemia or wide pressure swings with palpitations are noted, a 24-hour urine test for vanillylmandelic acid (VMA) and metanephrines should be ordered to rule out pheochromocytoma.

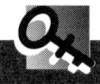

Key Tests

- Complete blood count
- Uric acid
- Urinalysis
- Creatinine
- Aspartate aminotransferase (AST)/ alanine aminotransferase (ALT)

Differential Diagnosis

1. Pre-eclampsia is characterized by hypertension, proteinuria, and generalized edema onset after 20 weeks

of gestation. Eclampsia includes the addition of seizures. Severe pre-eclampsia can exist without severe hypertension.

2. Chronic hypertension is the most likely cause of hypertension in the first or second trimester and persistence of hypertension postpartum.

3. Chronic hypertension with superimposed pre-eclampsia is manifested by a rise in blood pressure, new onset of marked proteinuria, increase in uric acid, or a decrease in platelets. This is associated with significant risk to the mother and fetus.

4. Transient hypertension of pregnancy is merely an increase in blood pressure near term without other evidence of pre-eclampsia. Postpartum resolution is rapid. Recurrence in later pregnancies is common and may be a harbinger for the development of chronic hypertension.

Treatment

Patients with mild chronic hypertension can have their medications discontinued and be followed closely. Their prognosis is similar to that of normotensive patients. Patients with moderate to severe hypertension should receive antihypertensive therapy. They are at high risk for complications from severe hypertension and pre-eclampsia. Patients with pre-eclampsia should be hospitalized, preferably in a tertiary care center with an experienced perinatologist. In cases of severe pre-eclampsia–eclampsia, delivery of the fetus is always right for the mother but may not be right for the fetus. Decisions will have to be individualized.

Medication

1. Methyldopa is the most extensively studied antihypertensive in pregnancy and is very safe. A small inconsequential drop in blood pressure in the neonate resolves within 5 days of delivery. Long-term follow-up shows no developmental abnormalities. Methyldopa is given in divided doses up to 4 gm/day either intravenously or orally.

2. Hydralazine is often considered the drug of choice for acutely lowering blood pressure. A few cases of fetal distress have been noted with loading doses causing precipitous falls in blood pressure. Side effects include headache, tachycardia, tremor, flushing, nausea, and vomiting, which can be confused with pre-eclampsia. A usual dose is a 5-mg intravenous load followed by 5 to 10 mg every 20 to 30 minutes or use of a constant infusion.

3. Diazoxide can be used as a second-line agent to control acute severe hypertension. Small miniboluses must be used to prevent uncontrolled hypotension precipitating cerebral ischemia, fetal distress, and maternal or fetal death. Diazoxide is given as 30- to 150-mg boluses every 2 to 5 minutes or by constant infusion.

4. Beta blockers are controversial. Concerns include decreased uteroplacental blood flow, decreased fetal response to hypoxia, as well as neonatal respiratory distress syndrome, bradycardia, and hypoglycemia. Studies do not show an increase in perinatal or fetal death. Labetalol has been used in several trials and may soon be considered the second-line agent above diazoxide for acute hypertension. It is likely that beta blockers are safe for prolonged use in pregnancy; however, with its long track record, methyldopa remains a more popular drug for mild to moderate hypertension.

5. Calcium channel blockers, nifedipine (Procardia) in particular, show promising results. They are potent antihypertensive agents and have been used effectively as tocolytics. There is, however, a lack of long-term studies at this time. Magnesium can potentiate their effect and precipitate hypotension when used together. Nifedipine is given in doses of 30 to 120 mg/day divided into 3 to 4 doses or daily as an extended-release tablet.

6. Nitroprusside is a last resort. Keep doses less than 4 μg/kg/min, and watch carefully for fetal cyanide toxicity.

7. Prazosin (Minipress) is used in pregnant patients with pheochromocytoma; otherwise, this drug has not been studied extensively in pregnancy.

8. Diuretics evoke mixed opinions. They decrease the normal volume expansion in pregnancy, posing a theoretical concern. Although it is difficult to show benefit in perinatal outcome, a large amount of data show no harm to the fetus. Diuretics can be used in patients with salt-sensitive hypertension who are unresponsive to other agents.

9. Angiotensin-converting enzyme (ACE) inhibitors should not be used in pregnancy. They are associated with neonatal anuria, acute renal failure, oligohydramnios, congenital abnormalities, and intrauterine growth retardation.

10. Magnesium sulfate is used to prevent seizures in the setting of pre-eclampsia. A loading dose of 4 to 6 gm is given slowly followed by a continuous infusion of 2 to 3 gm/hr to maintain a serum level of 4 to 7 mEq/dl. Conventional anticonvulsants are good alternatives.

11. Judicious use of fluid in pre-eclampsia maintains kidney perfusion without causing pulmonary or cerebral edema.

12. Low-dose aspirin, 60 mg/day starting in the twelfth week of pregnancy, has been used to selectively inhibit thromboxane A_2 and prevent pre-eclampsia in high-risk patients. Large multicenter prospective trials are now in progress to evaluate efficacy, but some smaller trials have shown promising results. Several other drugs are currently under investigation for the prevention of PIH.

Diet

Calcium supplementation of 1 to 2 gm/day has been suggested by some to prevent pre-eclampsia. No conclusive information is available presently to substantiate this.

Activity

Patients with severe hypertension or pre-eclampsia should be hospitalized and placed at bed rest.

Patient Education

1. Patients should be educated about the potentially harmful side effects of their antihypertensives, preferably prior to becoming pregnant.
2. Patients also should be educated about signs and symptoms of pre-eclampsia and instructed to seek medical attention immediately.

Key Treatment

Treatment of Choice	Alternative Treatment
• Delivery	• Diazoxide
• Methyldopa	• Beta blockers
• Hydralazine	• Calcium channel blockers
• MgSO$_4$	• Anticonvulsants

Follow-Up

1. Patients with hypertension should be followed every 2 weeks in the first two trimesters and then weekly in the last trimester.

2. Laboratory tests should be obtained at presentation, each trimester, and as otherwise indicated in patients with PIH or patients at high risk for PIH.

3. The fetus should be monitored with serial ultrasounds for evidence of fetal growth retardation. Weekly nonstress tests should be performed after the twenty-sixth week in severe hypertension and after the thirty-fourth week in mild hypertension.

4. Patients should have their blood pressure checked several weeks postpartum to look for evidence of chronic hypertension and to determine the need for continued therapy.

Bibliography

Conde-Agudelo A, Lede R, Belizan J: Evaluation of methods used in the prediction of hypertensive disorders of pregnancy. Obstet Gynecol Surv 1994;49(3):210–222.

Lindheimer MD, Cunningham FG: Hypertension and pregnancy: Impact of the working group report. Am J Kidney Dis 1993;21(5 suppl 2):29–36.

Magness RR, Gant NF: Control of vascular reactivity in pregnancy: The basis for therapeutic approaches to prevent pregnancy-induced hypertension. Semin Perinatol 1994;18(2):45–69.

Probst BD: Hypertensive disorders of pregnancy. Emerg Med Clin North Am 1994;12(1):73–89.

Sibai BM: Hypertension in pregnancy. Obstet Gynecol Clin North Am 1992;19(4):615–632.

122 Gestational Hyperglycemia/Diabetes

Kimberle J. Vore

Etiology

1. Gestational diabetes mellitus (GDM) is hyperglycemia first recognized during pregnancy.
   a. Glucose intolerance resulting in postprandial hyperglycemia occurring later in pregnancy that is thought to be due to the influence of placental hormones causing insulin resistance; usually resolves after delivery
   b. Diabetes that existed prior to pregnancy but was unrecognized
2. Diabetes mellitus (DM) recognized as existing prior to pregnancy (see Chapters 159 and 160)

Symptoms

1. GDM patients are usually asymptomatic.
2. Patients with pre-existing DM may have symptoms of hyperglycemia (polyuria, polydipsia, polyphagia).
3. Both types are prone to infections, especially urinary tract infections (UTIs) and vaginal candidiasis, and may have symptoms associated with these diseases —frequency, urgency, dysuria; vaginal itching and discharge.

Clinical Findings

1. Infants of diabetic mothers
   a. Hyperglycemia during pregnancy puts infants at increased risk of morbidity and mortality.
      (1) There is a threefold increase in congenital malformations if DM is uncontrolled in the first trimester.
      (2) Metabolic derangements can occur at birth, including hypoglycemia, hypocalcemia, hypomagnesemia, polycythemia, and hyperbilirubinemia.
      (3) Fetal macrosomia leading to possible birth trauma
      (4) Stillbirth
      (5) Increased risk of respiratory distress syndrome if born premature
   b. These infants inherit a predisposition to diabetes.
2. Pregestational diabetic mothers
   a. Increased incidence of pre-eclampsia–eclampsia
   b. Increased risk of operative delivery or traumatic vaginal delivery
   c. Greater incidence of polyhydramnios
   d. Greater risk of infections
3. Gestational diabetic mothers
   a. Up to 50 per cent of women diagnosed with GDM will have no identifiable risk factors.
   b. The risk factors listed under Key Signs are associated with GDM.

Key Signs

- Age older than 30 years
- Obesity
- Family history of DM
- Parity more than 5
- Glycosuria in current pregnancy
- Previous pregnancy with GDM
  fetal macrosomia
  prematurity
  stillbirth

Laboratory Tests

1. Glucola screening is recommended for all women between weeks 24 and 28. A 50-gm oral glucose load is given without regard to meals. A venous plasma glucose drawn 1 hour after administration that is 140 mg/dl or greater indicates the need for 3-hour diagnostic oral glucose tolerance test.
2. The diagnostic test for GDM is a 100-gm oral glucose load administered after obtaining a fasting plasma glucose; then hourly plasma glucose tests are drawn for the next 3 hours, during which time the patient should not eat, drink, or smoke. In preparation for the test, the patient should have unrestricted diet and exercise for 2 to 3 days before test and then fast 8 to 12 hours (overnight). Two or more abnormal values indicate a positive test.
3. Once a diagnosis of GDM is made, periodic fasting and 2-hour postprandial plasma glucose measurements are obtained to monitor treatment. Ideal levels are fasting blood glucose (FBG) levels below 105 mg/dl and 2-hour postprandial (pp) levels below 120 mg/dl.

Key Tests

	Abnormal test
Screening 50-gm oral glucose test	≥140 mg/dl
Diagnostic 100-gm oral glucose tolerance test*	
Fasting	≥105 mg/dl
1-hour	≥190 mg/dl
2-hour	≥165 mg/dl
3-hour	≥145 mg/dl

*Requires two abnormal levels.

Based on criteria from National Diabetes Data Group.

Differential Diagnosis

Pre-existing DM should be diagnosed prior to pregnancy to allow for strict control of glucose before pregnancy.

Treatment

1. In patients with pre-existing DM, strict control of blood glucose needs to be maintained before and during pregnancy to prevent complications.

2. Ultrasound screening for congenital defects and to date pregnancy should be done at 16 to 18 weeks of gestation.

3. Maintenance of glucose control (FBG < 105 mg/dl and 2-hour pp < 120 mg/dl) in patients with GDM is initially attempted through diet and exercise, but when these levels are consistently elevated, then insulin therapy is initiated.

4. Monitoring of fetal well-being with weekly nonstress testing is initiated from 30 to 34 weeks of gestation.

5. Delivery is accomplished at or near term unless deterioration of fetal well-being indicates need for earlier delivery.

Medication

1. Human insulin is drug of choice to maintain glucose control.

2. Insulin requirements vary throughout pregnancy and require frequent monitoring and adjustment of insulin dosages.

3. Oral hypoglycemic agents should not be used during pregnancy because they cross the placenta, leading to possible fetal teratogenesis and prolonged serious neonatal hypoglycemia.

Diet

1. American Diabetes Association diet that provides 30 to 35 kcal/kg of ideal body weight on a daily basis

2. If the patient loses weight on this diet, calories may need to be increased.

Activity

Moderate aerobic exercise of 20 to 30 minutes three times a week will help to maintain normal glucose levels. Walking and swimming are ideal exercises.

Patient Education

1. All patients with glucose intolerance or overt diabetes need to visit a dietician for dietary counseling.

2. If insulin is initiated during pregnancy, the patient will need instruction in self-administration of insulin and how to monitor blood glucose levels with a glucometer.

3. Preconception counseling about risks of congenital defects, risks during pregnancy, and need for strict glucose control should be done with all young diabetics considering pregnancy.

Key Treatment

Drug of Choice

• Insulin

Follow-Up

1. Once the infant is delivered, the mother's blood glucose level should be monitored because insulin requirements for diabetics vary for several days, and gestation diabetics who required insulin during pregnancy often no longer need it.

2. Testing of patients with GDM at the 6-week postpartum examination is recommended. Fasting levels greater than 140 mg/dl or a 2-hour value greater than 200 mg/dl after a 75-gm oral glucose load indicates underlying diabetes. If initial testing is normal, yearly follow-up testing should be done due to high incidence of developing diabetes in women with GDM.

3. All women should be counseled in contraceptive use. Estrogen-progestin oral contraceptives and intrauterine devices should be avoided in women with overt diabetes.

 Bibliography

Cunningham FG, MacDonald PC, Gant NF, et al (eds): Endocrine disorders. *In* Williams Obstetrics, 19th ed. E Norwalk, CT, Appleton & Lange, 1993, pp 1201–1212.

Hollingsworth DR, Moor TR: Diabetes and pregnancy. *In* Creasy RK, Resnik R (eds): Maternal Fetal Medicine: Principles and Practice, 2nd ed. Philadelphia, WB Saunders, 1989, pp 925–988.

Langer O: Diabetes in pregnancy. *In* Cherry SH, Merkatz IR (eds): Complications of Pregnancy: Medical, Surgical, Gynecologic, Psychosocial, and Perinatal, 4th ed. Baltimore, Williams & Wilkins, 1991, pp 979–993.

O'Sullivan MJ, Skylar JS, Raimer KA: Diabetes and pregnancy. *In* Gleicher N (ed): Principles and Practice of Medical Therapy in Pregnancy, 2nd ed. E Norwalk, CT, Appleton & Lange, 1992, pp 357–378.

123 Epididymitis

Brian M. Lott

Etiology

Epididymitis has two major forms—bacterial and sexually transmitted. There is a slight association with physical straining and reflux of urine (occasionally sterile). The acute stage begins with cellular inflammation leading to epididymal swelling and induration, with progression from the lower to the upper pole. The tunica vaginalis then secretes a serous fluid (an inflammatory hydrocele) that becomes purulent, the spermatic cord thickens, and the testis becomes swollen from passive congestion, although it is not involved primarily.

1. Sexually transmitted (usually <35 years of age)

   a. *Chlamydia trachomatis*

   b. *Neisseria gonorrhoeae*

   c. *Ureaplasma urealyticum* (not seen on gonococcal or *Chlamydia* DNA probe)

   d. Gram-negative rods (if associated with anogenital intercourse—can be seen with gay men)

2. Bacterial (seen with anatomic abnormalities): Enterobacteriaceae (primarily *Escherichia coli*) and *Pseudomonas*

   a. Older than age 35—associated with postprostatectomy, prostatitis, and benign prostatic hypertrophy (obstruction leads to higher voiding bladder pressures causing reflux)

   b. Children—pathologic connections from the gastrointestinal or urinary tract to the genital duct system. Anomalies usually present early in life, including myelomeningocele, imperforate anus, and VATER syndrome (*v*ertebral defects, *a*nal atresia, *TE* fistula, *r*enal dysplasia).

3. Amiodarone—usually associated with bilateral epididymitis

Symptoms

1. Tenderness over the epididymis—approximately equal occurrence between right and left sides

2. Gradual onset of scrotal pain radiating to the spermatic cord and flank (may be sudden)

3. Inguinal pain—more common in *Chlamydia* than coliform

4. Swelling is usually gradual; however, it may be rapid—doubling the size of the testis in 3 to 4 hours

5. Dysuria is seen in a third of patients, suggesting an initiating cystitis or prostatitis.

6. Discharge is seen with gonorrhea, usually with *Chlamydia,* and can be seen with coliform infection. The sexual act may have been 30 days before symptom onset.

Key Symptoms

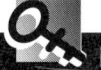

- Scrotal pain
- Scrotal swelling
- Dysuria
- Urethral discharge
- Abdominal pain

Clinical Findings

1. Tenderness over the spermatic cord or over the abdomen on the affected side

2. Enlarged scrotum with overlying erythema

3. Abscess usually has overlying dry, flaky, thinned skin

4. Difficult to distinguish the testis and epididymis after a few hours

5. Urethral discharge—does not have to be present to make diagnosis

6. Fever (possibly up to 104°F)

7. Boggy prostate on rectal examination if prostatitis is present

> **WARNING**
>
> **Massaging prostate may exacerbate epididymitis.**

Key Signs

- Epididymal tenderness and swelling
- Scrotal erythema and edema
- Fever
- Urethral discharge

Laboratory Tests

1. Complete blood count (CBC) may show increased white blood cell (WBC) count with left shift (in patients who appear systemically ill).

2. Gonorrhea and *Chlamydia* culture (or DNA probe) from urethra

3. Urethral smear

   a. Intracellular gram-negative diplococci correlate with gonorrhea

   b. WBCs alone correlate with nonspecific gonococcal urethritis which is *Chlamydia* in two-thirds (greater than 4 WBCs per high-power field suggests urethritis).

   c. Perform smear and culture *before* collecting urine, since this may wash discharge out of urethra.

509

4. Midstream urinalysis, culture, and Gram's stain
   a. Greater than 1 gram-negative rod per high-power field with oil immersion on uncentrifuged urine correlates with 100,000 coliforms per milliliter of midstream urine
   b. A positive urine culture suggests an abnormality that should be evaluated by intravenous pyelogram (IVP) or, especially in prepubertal patients, by voiding cystourethrogram (VCUG). Cystoscopy is also a consideration. Patients older than 11 years with a negative urine culture do not necessarily need a VCUG.
5. Ultrasound of scrotum—very important. May include Doppler flow studies (which are operator-dependent in that they must compress the testicular artery at the external ring to decrease the pulse from inflamed scrotal vessels and should show increased blood flow to the involved side)
6. Radionuclide scanning—considered the best diagnostic tool because it is not operator-dependent

Key Tests

• Ultrasound	• GC/*Chlamydia*
• Urinalysis and culture	• Urethral smear

Differential Diagnosis

1. Torsion of spermatic cord (1 in 4000 males, usually 9 to 15 years old)
   a. Early torsion—epididymis palpable anterior to the retracted testicle
   b. Prehn's sign (helpful, not reliable). Gently lift scrotum onto symphysis pubis.
      (1) Pain is decreased in epididymitis.
      (2) Pain is increased in torsion.

WARNING

A suspected torsion should have immediate surgical exploration. **Testicular loss can occur 2 to 12 hours after torsion, and ultrasound and radionuclide studies should not delay surgical correction in a suspected torsion.**

---

2. Torsion of testicular appendage—Look for the blue dot sign (a blue discoloration seen on the testicle through the skin).
3. Incarcerated inguinal hernia
4. Testicular trauma
5. Testicular tumor—usually painless swelling (acute hemorrhage within the tumor may distend the tunica albuginea causing pain)
6. Mumps orchitis—Check for parotid swelling.

7. Secondary syphilis—8 to 10 years after initial infection
8. Tuberculous epididymitis
   a. Seldom associated with pain or significant fever
   b. Epididymis is distinguishable from testis
   c. May see beading of vas deferens
   d. Prostatic induration and thickened ipsilateral seminal vesicle
9. *Cryptococcus, Brucella*

Treatment

1. *Chlamydia*
   a. Ofloxacin (Floxin), 300 mg orally b.i.d. for 10 days or
   b. doxycycline (Vibramycin), 100 mg orally b.i.d. for 10 days or
   c. erythromycin base, 500 mg orally q.i.d. for 10 days
   d. Treatment should be extended beyond 10 days until clinically asymptomatic if needed.
2. Gonorrhea
   a. Ceftriaxone (Rocephin), 250 mg intramuscularly or
   b. ampicillin, 500 mg orally q.i.d. for 10 days

WARNING

Treat the partners for sexually transmitted diseases (STDs), and look for other STDs.

---

3. Bacterial
   a. Ciprofloxacin (Cipro), 500 mg orally b.i.d. for 10 days or
   b. trimethoprim-sulfamethoxazole (Bactrim, Septra), 160/800 mg orally b.i.d. for 10 days or,
   c. if systematically ill, an intravenous aminoglycoside
   d. *Do not* initially use tetracycline, ampicillin, or a sulfa drug alone in suspected bacterial infection.
   e. If swelling and pain continue, extend treatment.
4. General measures
   a. Oral nonsteroidal anti-inflammatory drug (NSAID) (prednisone is without benefit)
   b. Bed rest for 3 to 4 days with scrotal elevation (with a towel) until pain is gone
   c. *Roomy* athletic supporter
   d. Local injection of 20 cc of 1% lidocaine into the spermatic cord at the pubic tubercle (just above the testicle) over the external ring can provide pain relief (may need it every day for several days).
   e. Ice in early phase, heat in later phase
   f. Avoid sexual activity and physical strain
   g. Patient education—complications

(1) Testicular atrophy occurs in two-thirds of men with epididymitis—possibly secondary to partial vascular thrombosis of the testicular artery.

(2) Infertility—Unilateral incidence is unknown; bilateral possibly 50 per cent.

(3) Abscess and infarction—5 per cent of cases

(4) Chronic epididymitis—irreversible end stage of severe acute epididymitis with extensive scarring and commonly tubular occlusion presenting as chronic pain without swelling (there is an increased risk of infertility).

Key Treatment

- If unsure of etiology, treat with ceftriaxone and doxycycline while awaiting culture results.

Follow-Up

Follow up over the next several weeks until nontender and swelling is gone. With treatment, pain decreases over 2 weeks, and swelling decreases over 4 weeks.

Bibliography

Ball TP: Epididymitis and orchitis. *In* Seidmon JE, Hanno PM (eds): Current Urologic Therapy, 3rd ed. Philadelphia, WB Saunders, 1994, pp 485–489.

Berger RE: Acute epididymitis: Etiology and therapy. Semin Urol 1991;9:28–31.

Berger RE: Epididymitis. *In* Walsh PC, et al (eds): Campbell's Urology, 6th ed. Philadelphia, WB Saunders, 1992, pp 830–832.

Kaver I, Matzkin H, Braf Z: Epididymo-orchitis: A retrospective study of 121 patients. J Fam Pract 1990;30(5):548–552.

Meares E: Nonspecific infections of the epididymis. *In* Tanagho EA, McAninch JW (eds): Smith's General Urology, 13th ed. E Norwalk, CT, Appleton & Lange, 1992, pp 228–231.

124 Varicocele

E. Robert Schwartz

Definition

An abnormal degree of venous dilatation in the pampiniform vascular plexus of the scrotum.

Etiology

1. The exact causes of varicocele are not clearly known, but a possible cause is vascular dilatation caused by valvular incompetence in the internal spermatic veins.
2. Another possible cause is elevated hydrostatic pressure in the left renal vein, inferior vena cava, and internal spermatic veins. Because the left spermatic vein empties into the left renal vein, while the right spermatic vein empties into the inferior vena cava, varicoceles almost always occur on the left.
3. Varicocele also may be caused by the effect of mechanical pressure from the superior mesenteric artery.

Symptoms

1. The patient is often asymptomatic.
2. The patient may experience heaviness in the scrotum and/or rarely a dull ache.
3. There may be concern on the part of the patient about the physical findings associated with varicocele (i.e., many dilated and engorged veins in the scrotum).

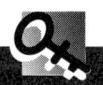

Key Symptoms

- Asymptomatic
- Heaviness or dull ache

Clinical Findings

1. Patients should in general be examined while standing in order to accentuate the dilated veins.
2. The Valsalva maneuver or coughing may help identify the veins.
3. Greater than 90 per cent of varicoceles occur on the left.
4. On palpation, a varicocele often feels like a "bag of worms."
5. The dilated veins are found most often superior to the testis and above the epididymis and slightly posterior.
6. There is a grading system for varicocele:
   a. Grade I: palpable only while the patient performs a Valsalva maneuver.
   b. Grade II: palpable on physical examination while standing.
   c. Grade III: visual inspection of the scrotum reveals varicocele.

7. There is a significant incidence of infertility associated with varicocele.

Key Signs

- Palpable veins in scrotum
- Greater incidence on the left than on the right

WARNING

If sudden appearance of a right-sided varicocele, rule out obstruction of right spermatic vein due to retroperitoneal neoplasm.

Laboratory Tests

1. Noninvasive
   a. Ultrasound
   b. Labeled blood-pool scintigraphy
   c. Thermography
   d. Echo-Doppler
2. Invasive: phlebography, internal spermatic vein

Key Tests

- Scrotal ultrasonography
- Spermatic venography "gold standard"

Differential Diagnosis

1. Hernia
2. Epididymitis
3. Hydrocele
4. Spermatocele
5. Testicular tumor

Treatment

1. Surgical ligation
2. Laparoscopic varicocelectomy
3. Percutaneous varicocele occlusion
4. Guidewire-directed detachable balloon for embolization technique

Medication
None

Diet
None

Activity

1. If patient is asymptomatic, no restrictions are indicated.
2. If patient has scrotal heaviness or discomfort, an athletic supporter may be helpful.

Patient Education

1. Patient reassurance that varicocele is a common problem and that there is no evidence that it is a precursor to malignancy.
2. If infertility is a cause of concern, explanation of the possible association with spermatogenesis and potential improvement of fertility with surgical correction.
3. Clinical course of varicocele is unpredictable.

Key Treatment

- Surgical ligation
- Laparoscopic varicocelectomy
- Percutaneous varicocele occlusion
- Guidewire-directed detachable balloon for embolization technique

Follow-Up

1. In adolescents, there is strong evidence that close follow-up and early treatment may improve long-term fertility.
2. In asymptomatic patients without a history of infertility, no clear guidelines have been established. Yearly physical examination would seem prudent.
3. Good evidence exists that, for men with proven infertility, treatment is beneficial, but periodic physical examinations are necessary in order to diagnose recurrence and/or development of posttreatment complications.

Bibliography

Demas B, Hricak H, McClure RD: Varicoceles—Radiologic diagnosis and treatment. Radiol Clin North Am 1991;29: 619–627.

Geatti O, Gasparini D, Shapiro B: A comparison of scintigraphy, thermography, ultrasound and phlebography in grading of clinical varicocele. J Nucl Med 1991;32(11):2092–2097.

Jarow J, Assimos D, Pittaway D: Effectiveness of laparoscopic varicocelectomy. Urology 1993;42(5):544–547.

Laven JS, Haans LC, Mali WP, et al: Effects of varicocele treatment in adolescents: A randomized study. Fertil Steril 1992;58(4):756–762.

Witt M, Lipshultz L: Varicocele: A progressive or static lesion? Urology 1993;42(5):541–543.

125 Hydrocele/Spermatocele

Grant C. Fowler

Etiology

1. Hydrocele is a cystic fluid accumulation in the tunica or processus vaginalis
   a. Communicating hydrocele—usually congenital, persistent communication between what is normally a potential space (processus vaginalis) and the peritoneal cavity. This allows fluid to descend from the peritoneal cavity and fill the processus vaginalis.
   b. Noncommunicating—possibilities include epididymitis, orchitis, filariasis (due to lymphatic obstruction), germ cell testicular tumors, testicular trauma, renal transplantation with ligation of the spermatic cord, radiation therapy, or unknown etiology
2. Spermatocele: Cause is not certain. They probably arise from cystic structures on the upper pole of the testis or epididymis or from the tubules (ductule efferentes) that connect the rete testis to the head of the epididymides.

Symptoms

Both are usually painless. Occasionally, either can be of sufficient size to cause pain and warrant surgical exploration or correction. Symptoms are usually described as a heaviness in the scrotum or pain in the inguinal area or lower back. Trauma may result in symptoms from hemorrhage into a hydrocele. Pain also may occur in association with epididymitis or if a hydrocele or spermatocele becomes infected. Rarely, torsion of a spermatocele has been described and can cause symptoms.

Key Symptom

- None, or "heaviness" in the scrotum

Clinical Findings

1. Hydrocele
   a. Usually nontender, rounded (unless enclosed in the spermatic cord and fusiform) scrotal mass that transilluminates. They are usually more prominent anteriorly and may surround the testis.
   b. Mass may be soft and cystic or large and tense. In a young boy with a communicating hydrocele, it may be small and soft in the morning, becoming larger and more tense at night.
   c. May be associated with a hernia. Auscultation of a hydrocele should not reveal bowel sounds. Hydroceles usually do not vary in size with respiration or Valsalva maneuver.
2. Spermatocele

   a. Nontender, round scrotal mass that transilluminates. They may be freely movable. They are separate from and usually superior and posterior to the testis.
   b. May be solitary or multiple. Most are less than 1 centimeter in size. Spermatoceles do not vary in size with respiration or Valsalva maneuver.

Key Sign

- Soft, nontender scrotal mass that transilluminates

Laboratory/Diagnostic Tests

1. Aspiration may result in infection requiring surgical repair and should be avoided if possible. However, aspiration of a hydrocele usually results in clear, yellow fluid, whereas aspiration of a spermatocele may result in thin, white, cloudy fluid with dead sperm on microscopic examination.
2. High-frequency (7.5 to 10 megahertz) ultrasound should be performed if the diagnosis is uncertain or if the mass prevents thorough examination of the entire contents of the scrotum. This is especially important in a young male with a newly developed hydrocele and no apparent cause (to exclude tuberculosis or cancer).

Key Tests

- Aspiration of fluid
- Ultrasound

Differential Diagnosis

1. Varicocele
2. Hernia
3. Tumor

WARNING

- **An intratesticular mass or a mass adherent to the testicle is cancer until proven otherwise.**
- **If a hydrocele develops spontaneously between the ages of 18 and 35, careful evaluation should be made to exclude cancer.**

Treatment

1. Hydrocele
   a. In infants, spontaneous closure may occur. Surgical repair is indicated, however, if the presence of bowel is suspected. If a hydrocele persists beyond 1 year of age, spontaneous closure is unlikely.

b. Very tense, large hydroceles that might compromise circulation to the testicle or that are uncomfortable or perhaps cosmetically unsightly may need surgical repair. Infected hydroceles require surgical repair. Otherwise, active therapy is not required. An athletic supporter may relieve symptoms.

2. Spermatocele—same as 1b. above.

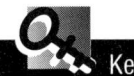

Key Treatment

- Surgical repair

Bibliography

Derkson DJ, Smith AY: Benign conditions of the external genitalia. Primary Care 1989;16:981–995.

Hanno PM, Wein AJ (eds): Clinical Manual of Urology, 2d ed. New York, McGraw-Hill, 1994, pp 67–71.

Pfenninger JL, Fowler GC, James RE: Selected disorders of the genitourinary system. *In* Taylor RB (ed): Family Medicine, Principles and Practice, 4th ed. New York, Springer-Verlag, 1994, pp 785–795.

Disorders of the spermatic cord. *In* Tanagho EA, McAninch JW (eds): Smith's General Urology, 13th ed. E Norwalk, CT, Appleton & Lange, 1992, pp 620–621.

Walsh PC, Retik AB, Stamey TA, Vaughan ED (eds): Campbell's Urology, 6th ed. Philadelphia, WB Saunders, 1992, pp 3132–3145.

126 Undescended Testicle

Timothy P. Daaleman

Etiology

1. Undescended testes (UDT), or cryptorchidism, is a frequent disorder of the male infant. The term "cryptorchidism" is taken from the Greek *kryptos* and *orchis,* which means "hidden testes."

2. The incidence of UDT is correlated with fetal maturity.

   a. In full-term male infants, the incidence of cryptorchidism is 3 per cent. This diminishes to 1 per cent at age 1 due to spontaneous descent.

   b. In preterm males who weigh more than 1500 grams, the incidence of UDT is 21 per cent, but it rises to 60 to 70 per cent among infants weighing less than 1500 gm.

3. Cryptorchidism has been demonstrated in up to 4 per cent of siblings and 6 per cent of fathers of cryptorchid children, which suggests a genetic influence.

4. UDT is seen more frequently in infant males with endocrine disorders, genetic abnormalities, or genitourinary anatomic anomalies.

5. There is no single unified cause of cryptorchidism. A mix of hormonal, neural, and mechanical factors that play a role in normal testicular descent has been implicated.

Symptoms

Cryptorchid males are asymptomatic.

Clinical Findings

1. The physical examination is critical in establishing the diagnosis and classification of UDT. The examination should be performed in a warm and nonthreatening environment and in a systematic manner.

2. For an optimal examination, the patient should be comfortably seated in a crosslegged position, which allows most retractile testes to descend spontaneously, due to relaxation of the cremasteric muscles.

3. After warming his or her hands, the examiner should begin by evaluating the genitalia with attention directed toward the scrotum. The overall size of the sac, as well as any discrepancies between the left and right sides, should be documented. In addition, any hernias, hydroceles, or evidence of hypospadias should be noted.

4. If an empty scrotum is found, liquid soap or KY jelly on the examiners fingers is helpful prior to palpating along the inguinal canal. Begin at the inguinal ring and move medially toward the pubic bone. One helpful technique is to slide the second and third fingers over the canal while using the index finger of the opposite hand in a brushing motion preceding the sliding fingers. When a testis is palpated, an attempt should be made to manipulate it into the scrotum.

5. Undescended testes are generally classified as palpable or nonpalpable.

   a. In patients with nonpalpable testes, atrophy or agenesis should be considered. Most nonpalpable testes have an intra-abdominal location or an intra-canalicular position that may be transient.

   b. Palpable testes may be either ectopic, retractile, or arrested in their normal descent.

      (1) Ectopic testes are usually perineal but may be located at the base of the penis, in the thigh or above the pubic bone, or in the opposite scrotal sac.

      (2) Testes may be retractile secondary to poor scrotal attachment or due to an overactive cremasteric reflex. Retractile testes are usually bilateral and are most commonly identified in preschool boys, although they may be present until puberty.

      (3) Testes that arrest along their normal descent generally reside superior to the external ring and superficial to the external oblique muscle.

Key Signs

- Nonpalpable testes
- Hydrocele
- Penile, pubic, inguinal, thigh, or perineal mass
- Hernia
- Asymmetric or empty scrotum
- Hypospadias

Laboratory Tests

1. When both testes are nonpalpable, baseline assays of luteinizing hormone (LH), follicle-stimulating hormone (FSH), and testosterone can be helpful in evaluating possible anorchidism. Elevated FSH and LH levels and a low baseline testosterone level suggest anorchidism. The presence or absence of testicular tissue also can be determined by human chorionic gonadotropin (hCG) stimulation (2000 IU/square meter for 3 days). The lack of a several-fold rise in testosterone levels in hCG-stimulated males supports the diagnosis of cryptorchidism.

2. A variety of imaging techniques are useful in the diagnosis of the cryptorchid testes.

   a. The use of ultrasound is an optimal diagnostic technique for testes along the inguinal canal, although there are limitations in its ability to identify intra-abdominal testes. Its low cost, noninvasiveness, and lack of radiation make it an attractive first-line technique.

b. Computed tomography (CT) and magnetic resonance imaging (MRI) are superior to sonography in localization and evaluation of the testes and cord structures. The risks associated with radiation exposure (CT) and the need for sedation in a pediatric population must be considered with these modalities.

c. Selective gonadal venography is an infrequently used procedure because it is technically difficult, invasive, and radiation-exposing.

3. The use of laparoscopy continues to be a definitive modality in the localization and management of UDT. It allows direct visualization of the intra-abdominal testes. No other study is as sensitive or specific for localizing undescended testes.

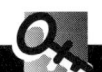

Key Tests

- FSH, LH, and testosterone levels
- hCG stimulation test
- Ultrasound
- CT
- MRI
- Laparoscopy

Differential Diagnosis

Undescended testes are associated with a variety of endocrine disorders, genetic abnormalities, and anatomic variations.

1. Endocrine disorders: hypopituitarism, Kallmann's syndrome, testicular feminization disorder, anencephaly, 5α-reductase deficiency, congenital LH secretory failure

2. Genetic abnormalities: trisomy 13 and 18, Aarskog's, Laurence-Moon-Biedl, Freeman-Sheldon, prune belly, Prader-Willi, Cornelia de Lange's, Noonan's, Beckwith-Wiedemann, and Kleinfelter's syndromes

3. Anatomic variations: gastroschisis, omphalocele, extrophy of the bladder, prune belly syndrome

Treatment

1. Consultation with a pediatric urologist or surgeon familar with the diagnosis and treatment of cryptorchidism is advised.

2. Surgical treatment (orchidopexy and/or laparoscopy) is recommended after the age of 6 months and before 18 months of age for males with palpable or nonpalpable testes. Prepubertal males with retractile testes should be followed with yearly examinations. If the testis does not descend by puberty, orchidopexy is recommended.

3. Due to the increased risk of testicular cancer, postpubertal men younger than 32 years should be considered for orchiectomy. Men older than 32 years of age should be observed with frequent examinations.

4. The use of hormonal therapy (hCG, gonadotropin-releasing hormone, or both) has shown little or no benefit in the treatment of true cryptorchidism. Hormonal treatment may have a role in differentiating the retractile testes from the undescended testes.

Key Treatment

- Surgery: orchidopexy and/or laparoscopy

Follow-Up

1. The maintenance of fertility is the most important consideration in the cryptorchid male. Since there is histologic evidence of testicular germ cell damage by age 2, early identification and appropriate management of UDT are critical.

2. Testicular malignancies occur more frequently in cryptorchid males than in those with normal testicular position. In unilateral UDT, the contralateral, normally placed testicle has an increased risk of having a malignancy. Early orchidopexy (prior to age 6) appears to diminish the chances of developing a malignancy.

3. In patients who have undergone surgical intervention and in those who have followed hormonal or expectant management (retractile testes), the importance of annual physical examinations and monthly testicular self-examinations cannot be overstated.

Bibliography

Cilento BG, Najjar SS, Atala A: Cryptorchidism and testicular torsion. Pediatr Clin North Am 1993;40(6):1133–1149.

Ellis DG: Undescended testes. *In* Ashcraft KW (ed): Pediatric Urology, 1st ed. Philadelphia, WB Saunders, 1990, pp 415–427.

Gandhi K, Maizels M: Management of the undescended testis. Compr Ther 1993;19(1):5–9.

Hadziselimovic F: Cryptorchidism. *In* Gillenwater JY (ed): Adult and Pediatric Urology, 2d ed, vol 2. St. Louis, Mosby–Year Book, 1991, pp 2217–2228.

Palmer JM: The undescended testicle. Endocrinol Metab Clin North Am 1991;20(1):231–240.

127 Common Urinary Symptoms

Symptom **Hematuria**   *Linda E. Kanarvogel*

Hematuria is a perplexing problem due to the wide array of diagnostic possibilities, the difficulty in determining an etiology, and the invasive nature of the workup. The definition of hematuria is controversial. If one erythrocyte per high-power field (HPF) is considered abnormal, then 13 per cent of the general medical population would have hematuria, and yet only 2 per cent of these patients would have significant disease. Therefore, most physicians accept three erythrocytes per HPF as the upper limit of normal.

Differential Diagnosis

1. Infection—cystitis, pyelonephritis, urethritis, and prostatitis
2. Benign prostatic hypertrophy
3. Nephrolithiasis
4. Urologic neoplasms—bladder, renal, prostate, or ureteral
5. Renal parenchymal disease—poststreptococcal glomerulonephritis (GN), Berger's disease, Henoch-Schönlein purpura, lupus, Goodpasture's syndrome, membranous GN, benign familial hematuria, proliferative GN, Alport's syndrome, and multiple myeloma
6. Nonglomerular renal disease—hypertensive nephrosclerosis, runner's hematuria, drug-induced hematuria, papillary necrosis, polycystic kidney disease, renal infarct, medullary sponge kidney, obstructive or reflux nephropathy, tuberculosis, and renal vein thrombosis
7. Coagulopathy
8. Trauma—Foley catheter, meatal ulceration
9. Endometriosis
10. False-positive result from foods such as beets and blackberries, vaginal bleeding, myoglobin, drugs, and factitious sources

---

Refer to Ch. 106, Endometriosis; Ch. 128, Urinary Stones; Hypercalciuria; Ch. 131, Glomerulonephritis; Ch. 132, Pyelonephritis; Ch. 133, Acute Urinary Tract Infection in Adults; Ch. 136, Prostatitis; Ch. 137, Benign Prostatic Hyperplasia; Ch. 138, Prostate Cancer; Ch. 139, Kidney Cancer; and Ch. 140, Bladder Cancer.

History

1. Characterize the bleeding.
   a. Clots usually indicate lower urinary tract bleeding.

b. Association with menses may suggest endometriosis.
c. Relationship to exercise may indicate runner's hematuria.
d. Association with flank pain suggests infection, calculus, or obstruction, whereas painless bleeding is associated with cancer or GN.
e. Association with hesitancy, frequency, or decreased force of stream is suggestive of prostatic hypertrophy.
2. Rule out systemic disease.
   a. Constitutional symptoms such as fatigue, weight loss, or anorexia may indicate cancer.
   b. Presence of rash, arthralgias, or photosensitivity suggests GN secondary to collagen vascular disease.
   c. Tendency toward bleeding may indicate a coagulopathy.
   d. Hypertension (HTN) may indicate nephrosclerosis.
   e. Atrial fibrillation or endocarditis suggests emboli.
3. Rule out infection.
   a. Symptoms of dysuria, fever, nausea, vomiting, urgency, or frequency suggest urinary tract infection (UTI).
   b. Pulmonary symptoms may suggest tuberculosis.
   c. Complaints of vaginal or penile discharge may indicate presence of a sexually transmitted disease (STD).
   d. Recent upper respiratory tract infection may precede poststreptococcal GN, Berger's disease, or Henoch-Schönlein purpura.
   e. Travel abroad may indicate schistosomiasis.
4. Screen for risk factors of urologic cancer, which include age greater than 50 years, tobacco use, pelvic irradiation, and use of analgesics or cyclophosphamide.
5. Medication history
   a. Many drugs can turn urine red, such as rifampin, phenytoin, or ibuprofen.
   b. Others can cause GN, such as penicillamine or gold, or cause interstitial nephritis, such as analgesics.
   c. Anticoagulants often cause hematuria.
6. Screen for family history of sickle cell disease, polycystic kidney disease, Alport's syndrome, benign familial hematuria, or coagulopathy.

Clinical Findings

1. Vital signs: Fever may suggest infection; HTN may either be secondary to GN or cause nephrosclerosis.
2. Cardiac: Auscultate for endocarditis or atrial fibrillation.
3. Back: Examine for costovertebral angle tenderness.
4. Abdomen: Palpate to rule out any masses suggestive of cancer or polycystic kidneys and to rule out tenderness.
5. Genitourinary: Examine the urethral orifice and external genitalia for evidence of condylomata, ulceration, or stenosis. Examine the prostate to rule out the presence of prostatic hypertrophy, nodules, or pain and bogginess.
6. Skin: Examine for ecchymosis suggestive of coagulopathy.

Tests

1. Microscopic urinalysis: Heavy proteinuria is evidence of glomerular disease and should be quantitated with a 24-hour urine protein measurement. Red blood cell (RBC) casts are again suggestive of renal disease, whereas pyuria suggests infection and should be followed by urine culture.
2. Screening laboratory tests: A standard full battery of tests would have low yield and therefore should be guided by the history, physical examination, and urinalysis. These might include an antinuclear antibodies (ANA), complement level, antistreptolysin O (ASO antibody), rapid plasma reagin (RPR) test, urine protein electrophoresis (UPEP), prothrombin time, partial thromboplastin time, serum electrolytes, complete blood count (CBC), hemoglobin electrophoresis, tuberculin skin test (PPD), urine for acid-fast bacilli, and prostate specific antigen (PSA).
3. Urine cytology: Can detect lower urinary tract malignancies and should be obtained in patients younger than age 50 and when suspicion of malignancy is high. False-positive results can occur with infection or nephrolithiasis.
4. Abdominal roentgenogram: Used for evaluating younger patients who have an increased incidence of nephrolithiasis. The results are limited to the proportion of calculi that are opaque and the presence of phleboliths.
5. Intravenous pyelogram (IVP): Provides good evaluation of anatomy and thus can detect silent stones, renal tumors, and hydronephrosis. It is less sensitive for bladder tumors.
6. Renal sonogram: Used if patient is allergic to dye or if a cyst is suspected. It provides a good look at anatomy but is less sensitive than IVP for detecting ureteral stones or collecting system tumors.
7. Cytoscopy: Permits visualization of urethra, bladder, and ureteral orifices. However, in situ carcinomas and sessile or small tumors can be missed.

Management

Management will depend on the diagnosis.

1. Medications that cause hematuria should be avoided.
2. Appropriate dietary recommendations should be made if the patient has HTN, renal failure, or a calculus.
3. If an infection is diagnosed, antibiotics should be instituted.
4. If bladder cancer is found, treatment with chemotherapy or surgery should be guided by a urologist.
5. If there is prostatic hypertrophy, α-adrenergic blockers, 5α-reductase inhibitors, or surgery may be instituted.
6. If nephrolithiasis is found, oral hydration, external wall lithotripsy, or surgery may be needed.

Follow-Up

In many patients, despite a thorough investigation, the cause remains obscure. Fortunately, studies of 5-year follow-up of patients who have undergone a previously negative workup have shown that the future incidence of serious disease is low.

1. Those greater than age 50 or with risk factors for urologic cancer should have a urine cytology every 6 months and yearly cystoscopy and IVP for 3 years.
2. Those under age 50 who are asymptomatic and have no risk factors only require observation.

PEARLS

- Asymptomatic hematuria occurs commonly in the general medical population.

- In patients younger than age 50 with no risk factors for bladder cancer and normal physical examination, the incidence of serious disease is low, and workup can be limited to abdominal x-ray, blood urea nitrogen, creatinine, and microscopic urinalysis.

- Patients greater than age 50 require a full investigation because risk of serious disease is greater.

Bibliography

Connelly JE: Microscopic hematuria. *In* Panzer RJ, Black ER, Grines PF (eds): Diagnostic Strategies for Common Medical Problems. Philadelphia, American College of Physicians, 1991, pp 412–419.

Schaeffer AJ, Del Greco F: Other renal diseases of urologic significance. *In* Walsh PC, Retik AB, Stamey TA, Vaughan ED (eds): Campbell's Urology, 6th ed. Philadelphia, W.B. Saunders, 1992, pp 2065–2072.

Sparwasser C, Cimniak HU, Treiber U, Pust A: Significance of the evaluation of asymptomatic microscopic haematuria in young men. Br J Urol 1994;74:723–729.

Sutton JM: Evaluation of hematuria in adults. JAMA 1990;263:2475–2480.

Yasumasu T, Koikawa Y, Uozumi J, Ueda T, Kumazawa J: Clinical study of asymptomatic microscopic haematuria. Int Urol Nephrol 1994;26:1–6.

Symptom **Proteinuria**

Joseph J. Lieber

The finding of protein by dipstick in a patient's urine is one of the key signs in nephrology. Proteinuria implies finding greater than 50 to 100 mg of protein in a 24-hour urine collection. Naturally, the amount of protein may vary with greater quantities often implying more severe disease. Further, the type of protein may vary as well. Always, a thorough history, physical examination, and key laboratory tests should be performed to help define the nature of the proteinuria, and its causes and possible treatments, if any.

Differential Diagnosis

1. *Glomerular* proteinuria is a manifestation of primary or secondary glomerular disease. It is usually composed of albumin with, at times, globulins and other proteins. When the amount of protein is greater than 3.5 grams in 24 hours, we say the patient has nephrotic range proteinuria. The specific glomerulopathies that cause proteinuria are quite varied and include minimal change disease, membranous nephropathy, diabetic nephropathy, focal sclerosis, amyloidosis, postinfectious glomerulonephritis, IgA nephropathy, and membranoproliferative glomerulopathy.

2. Tubular proteinura normally is less than 1.5 gm in 24 hours. It is composed mostly of B_2 microglobulin and Tamm-Horsfall protein. It is caused by tubular cell damage with inability to resorb these proteins. This is usually seen with tubulointerstitial injury.

3. *Overflow* proteinuria is usually composed of light chain proteins and is caused by a plasma cell dyscrasia with the finding of a paraprotein in the urine. The usual causes are multiple myeloma, amyloidosis, Waldenström's macroglobulinemia, and light chain nephropathy. Such patients may have secondary glomerular changes with glomerular proteinuria as well. Because the urine dipstick will detect only albumin, a large quantity of protein in a 24-hour sample with a trace dipstick reading should suggest a nonglomerular protein, often a light chain.

4. *Transient* proteinuria and orthostatic proteinuria are usually self-limited, although they may cause the patient some concern. Febrile illness, elevation in blood pressure or exercise may lead to mild proteinuria that will usually remit in the near future. Other patients have persistent proteinuria, but the bulk of the protein is associated with ambulation. The prognosis is quite good.

> Refer to Chs. 129 and 130, Acute and Chronic Renal Failure; Ch. 131, Glomerulonephritis; and Chs. 159 and 160, Diabetes Mellitus.

History

1. A family history of kidney disease in the patient with proteinuria suggests a familial nephropathy.

2. A long-standing history of diabetes mellitus suggests diabetic nephropathy.

3. Recent pharyngitis, gross hematuria, arthritis, skin rash, or use of medications (including over-the-counter agents) should be questioned. Finding symptoms of a systemic disease such as fever, weight loss, or myalgias may suggest vasculitis or a secondary amyloid nephropathy. Furthermore, deep visceral infections, endocarditis, or hepatitis can have an associated glomerulopathy with proteinuria.

4. Careful assessment of risk factors for human immunodeficiency virus (HIV) are mandatory, as HIV is associated with glomerular disease. In fact, abuse of illicit drugs such as heroin can cause a chronic glomerulopathy; "skin poppers" are at increased risk for amyloid.

5. Glomerular disease may rarely be a manifestation of an underlying solid tumor or hematological malignancy; evidence for these should be considered in smokers and in patients with weight loss, diffuse symptoms, fevers, bleeding, and severe pain.

6. Many tubulointerstitial diseases are a result of toxins, abuse of analgesics, or exposure to industrial products. A good history will help determine if the patient is at risk for any of these. When asking about analgesic use, attempts to quantify doses are important because chronic injury is usually seen only with large amounts of these agents.

Clinical Findings

1. Assessment of blood pressure is crucial because hypertension may be a clue to fixed renal disease.

2. Edema and anasarca often imply more severe proteinuria, often in the nephrotic range.

3. A thorough eye examination to inspect for diabetic retinopathy is crucial. This will correlate with diabetic nephropathy. Other eye findings may include uveitis or episcleritis, which may suggest vasculitis.

4. A skin examination for a malar rash, erythema nodosum, or palpable purpura may again indicate a vasculitis or systemic lupus erythematosus. Amyloid may be associated with upper extremity purpura. Needle track marks are a clue to drug abuse.

5. Always assess for pericardial or pleural rubs that might be seen with lupus, or, less likely, a systemic infection.

6. The findings of hepatomegaly and splenomegaly may be seen with amyloid, lymphoma, hepatitis, malignancy, or endocarditis. All of these may be associated with glomerular proteinuria.

7. The finding of active arthritis may be seen with lupus, vasculitis, and endocarditis. Clubbing may be a sign

of neoplasia that could have an associated glomerulopathy.

8. Findings on ear, nose, and throat examination of ulcers, masses, and nodules may indicate Wegener's vasculitis.

9. Lymph nodes should be thoroughly palpated and followed to assess for lymphoma, metastatic cancer, or infection that may be associated with glomerular disease.

Tests

1. It is mandatory to quantify the proteinuria in a 24-hour sample to determine the degree of proteinuria. One might wish to quantify the proteinuria in a split collection, with the urine in one container obtained while the patient is ambulating and the other obtained while recumbent to confirm benign orthostatic proteinuria.

2. A urine protein electrophoresis and a urine sample for Bence Jones will determine the nature of the proteinuria. This should be done following a thorough microscopic examination of the urine. This may be crucial to help define the type of renal disease.

3. A renal sonogram assesses the size of the kidneys, determines chronicity of disease, and rules out obstruction. This will also be important if a renal biopsy is contemplated.

4. Serologic studies may include antinuclear antibodies (ANA), antiglomerular basement membrane (anti-GBM), complement (C3 and C4), serum protein electrophoresis (SPEP), cryoglobulins, streptozyme, hepatitis profile, and antineutrophil cytoplasmic antibody. These may be helpful, especially in patients with more severe glomerular proteinuria, azotemia, rash, evidence of a systemic disease, and arthritis. Complement levels are often helpful because usually only lupus nephritis, membranoproliferative glomerulonephritis (GN), poststreptococcal GN, and proliferative GN due to endocarditis, hepatitis, or cryoglobulinemia lower complement levels. ANA testing may be helpful to diagnose lupus nephritis and some related conditions. An SPEP with a monoclonal spike is very suggestive of a plasma cell dyscrasia or amyloid. The anti-GBM and antineutrophil cytoplasmic antibody may be examined in patients with rapidly progressive azotemia and proteinuria often associated with findings in the lungs, skin, and sinuses. Because many of these tests are expensive and may be diagnostic of less common entities, one should order only those tests that are of clinical value in that specific patient.

5. A renal biopsy may be indicated to specifically define the clinical entity. This is a relatively safe procedure and will give diagnostic as well as prognostic information. It is less crucial in patients with under 1 gram of proteinuria in 24 hours. Patients with greater amounts of proteinuria—especially in the nephrotic range—should undergo a biopsy unless the diagnosis is otherwise clear-cut. Patients with azotemia, normal size kidneys, abnormal serologic studies, and severe proteinuria should also undergo biopsy. Patients with tubular proteinuria and orthostatic proteinuria are usually not helped by biopsy. If the renal sonogram reveals small kidneys, a biopsy is best deferred because this indicates chronic scarring and fibrosis.

Management

The management depends on the degree of proteinuria and its cause.

1. Patients with overflow proteinuria in whom the protein is a light chain should undergo a full assessment for myeloma and other plasma cell dyscrasias and be treated for the primary disease. Amyloidosis may be treated with regimens used to manage myeloma or the patient may be tried on colchicine.

2. Tubular proteinuria is usually not treated. The underlying nephropathies are usually not responsive to steroids or immunomodulating agents.

3. Transient proteinuria and benign orthostatic proteinuria are usually not treated.

4. Glomerulopathies with severe proteinuria should be treated based on pathologic and serologic findings.

   (1) Steroids are usually the mainstay of therapy, with different lesions responding at varying degrees. Minimal change disease is quite steroid-responsive, whereas focal glomerulosclerosis is quite resistant. Cyclophosphamide (Cytoxan), azathioprine (Imuran), cyclosporine (Sandimmune), and chlorambucil (Leukeran) have been used as steroid-sparing agents and for their own immune effects. Lupus nephritis is often quite responsive to steroids and cyclophosphamide, as is Wegener's vasculitis and other vasculitides.

   (2) General measures have been used to lessen the degree of proteinuria and attempt to preserve renal function. Angiotensin-converting enzyme inhibitors will lower intraglomerular pressure and lessen protein excretion, especially in diabetic patients. Nonsteroidal anti-inflammatory agents may be used to decrease proteinuria in severe cases. These should be used with caution. Low doses of aspirin and other antiplatelet agents have been used with some glomerulopathies to help reduce sclerosis.

   (3) Restricted protein diets may also lessen proteinuria. In patients with edema, sodium may need to be restricted as well. Patients with proteinuria and advanced renal insufficiency may need to limit their potassium intake.

   (4) It is crucial to recognize that stable patients with proteinuria need not always be treated. Such conditions as azotemia, nephrotic syndrome, and hypertension indicate aggressive therapy if such therapy exists. Many of these regimens can cause considerable toxicity; this must be assessed when

deciding on therapy. Patients are less likely to benefit from aggressive immunosuppressive therapy if signs and symptoms are mild.

    (5) Activity need not be restricted in patients with proteinuria.

- Orthostatic proteinuria and transient proteinuria have a good prognosis. Consider renal biopsy if kidneys are normal size with severe proteinuria if diagnosis is not otherwise clear-cut. Azotemia and abnormal serologies may also add to the urgency of a biopsy.

PEARLS

- Diagnose proteinuria by dipstick. Always repeat the test at a later time if taken during stress, fever, or exercise.

- Always quantify the degree of proteinuria and identify types of protein.

- Assess renal function, blood pressure, and examine the urine for formed elements.

- Search for clues of a systemic disease.

- Obtain appropriate serologies and sonography.

Bibliography

Carlson JA, Harrington JT: Laboratory evaluation of renal function. *In* Schrier RW, Gottschalk CW (eds): Diseases of the Kidney, 5th ed, vol. 1. Boston, Little, Brown, 1993, pp 380–392.

Henry JB: Examination of urine. *In* Clinical Diagnosis and Management by Laboratory Methods, 18th ed. Philadelphia, WB Saunders, 1991.

Larson TS: Evaluation of proteinuria. Mayo Clin Proc 1994;69:1154–1158.

Levey AS, et al: *In* Brenner B, Rector F (eds): The Kidney, 5th ed, vol. 1. Philadelphia, WB Saunders, 1991, pp 940–942.

Rosenberg ME, Hostetter TH: *In* Seldin D, Giebisch G (eds): The Kidney: Physiology and Pathophysiology, 2nd ed, vol. 3. New York, Raven Press, 1992, pp 3054–3055.

Symptom **Dysuria**
Cheri L. Olson

Dysuria is painful or difficult urination. It is usually related to inflammation of the lower genitourinary tract. Dysuria is especially common among women. Most common causes of dysuria can be detected easily in a primary care physician's office with a thorough history, a complete genitourinary examination, and a few simple office laboratory tests.

Differential Diagnosis

1. Urinary tract infection (UTI)
2. Vulvovaginitis
3. Sexually transmitted disease (STD), usually urethritis
4. Mechanical/chemical irritation
5. Allergic reaction
6. Prostatitis
7. Urinary obstruction (calculus)
8. Tumor
9. Postmenopausal atrophic vaginitis
10. Sexual abuse
11. Reiter's syndrome

By far the most common cause of dysuria is UTI. UTIs affect 10 to 20 per cent of women in the United States each year. It is important, however, not to forget other causes of dysuria, particularly vulvovaginitis and STDs. In

> Refer to Ch. 102, Vaginitis; Ch. 105, Sexually Transmitted Diseases; Ch. 133, Acute Urinary Tract Infection in Adults; Ch. 135, Nongonococcal Urethritis; Ch. 136, Prostatitis; Ch. 138, Prostate Cancer; and Ch. 140, Bladder Cancer.

men, prostatic disease, calculus, and tumors become more important diagnostic considerations.

History: Key Questions to Ask

1. What is the nature of the dysuria? Internal? External?
2. When was the onset? How rapid?
3. Any associated symptoms of frequency, urgency, or incomplete voiding?
4. Any blood in urine?
5. Any vaginal discharge, vaginal odor, or external genital pruritus?
6. What is the previous history of urinary and genital infections?
7. Are there new or multiple sexual partners?
8. Any use of chemical irritants, such as bubble baths, feminine hygiene products, or contraceptive gels and foams?
9. Any fever, chills, or other systemic symptoms?

"Internal" dysuria feels like the pain is inside the urethra and is commonly due to UTIs or STDs. "External" dysuria feels like a burning sensation of urine passing over inflamed labia and is commonly due to vaginitis.

Clinical Findings

1. Evaluate temperature.
2. Suprapubic pain or tenderness may be present.
3. Costovertebral angle tenderness should be assessed.
4. The urethral meatus should be examined for discharge, irritability, erythema, and/or lesions.
5. Vaginal discharge, vaginal odor, or labial irritation may be present.

Tests

1. Urinalysis; assess pyuria, hematuria; consider leukocyte esterase and nitrite dipstick testing.
2. Urine culture and sensitivities
3. Vaginal secretion microscopic examination: "wet prep" and potassium hydroxide staining
4. Tests for STDs, particularly *Chlamydia trachomatis, Neisseria gonorrhoeae,* and herpes simplex.

If the diagnosis of uncomplicated cystitis (UTI) is clear from history and urinalysis, a urine culture is not necessary. However, urine culture should be performed when the history is unclear, when systemic symptoms are present, when relapse occurs, and following recent hospitalization or invasive urinary procedures. Dipstick tests for leukocyte esterase and nitrites may substitute for microscopic urinalysis if interpreted correctly. Blood tests such as a complete blood count (CBC) or renal function tests are unnecessary in the majority of cases of dysuria.

Management

Medication

1. Antibiotics for UTIs are indicated. Trimethoprim-sulfamethoxazole (Bactrim, Septra) is the preferred drug. The standard dose is one double-strength tablet every 12 hours for 3 days. Alternatives include cephalosporins, quinolones, and nitrofurantoin.
2. Urinary analgesics such as pyridium may provide rapid symptomatic relief.
3. Treatment of vulvovaginitis should be based on results of "wet prep" and potassium hydroxide staining, except for atrophic vaginitis.

Diet

1. Fluid intake should be at least 8 to 10 glasses of water a day.
2. Some patients benefit from increasing intake of acidic beverages such as cranberry juice or orange juice.
3. Some patients benefit from ingesting yogurt once a day.

Patient Education

1. Patients should report lack of clinical improvement after 3 to 5 days.
2. The entire course of medication needs to be completed.
3. Empty bladder frequently.
4. Avoid or discontinue diaphragm use.
5. Void after intercourse.

6. Discuss risk of STD transmission and long-term sequelae if pertinent.

The length of treatment for uncomplicated UTI is controversial. The best outcome seems to be with a 3-day course of a quinolone. This length of time maximizes therapy while minimizing cost, compliance issues, and side effects. Pyridium can be very helpful for short-term use as a urinary analgesic. It will turn the urine orange and stain clothes and contact lenses. More complicated infections, such as upper tract involvement or relapses, should have a pretreatment urine culture and be treated for 10 to 14 days. Empirical treatment of vulvovaginitis with triple-antibiotic creams should be avoided. Treatment should be based on results of "wet prep" and potassium hydroxide staining of vaginal secretions.

Follow-Up

1. For uncomplicated UTI, STDs, and vulvovaginitis, follow-up may be based on clinical symptoms.
2. Full completion of prescribed treatment is vital.
3. For recurrent, relapsing, or complicated cases, a follow-up urine culture with sensitivities is necessary after completion of antibiotic.

PEARLS

- History of a new sexual partner and a gradual onset of dysuria suggests urethritis.
- Colony counts as low as 10^2 may be significant for UTI in symptomatic patients.
- Pyuria is the most reliable indicator of infection.

Bibliography

Johnson CC: Definitions, classifications and clinical presentation of urinary tract infections. Med Clin North Am 1991;75:241–252.

Johnson MG: Urinary tract infections in women. Am Fam Physician 1990;41:565–571.

Johnson LW: Urinary tract infections. *In* Taylor RB (ed): Family Medicine Principles and Practice, 4th ed. New York, Springer-Verlag, 1994, pp 743–748.

Pappas PG: Laboratory in the diagnosis and management of urinary tract infections. Med Clin North Am 1991;75:313–325.

Powers RD: New directions in the diagnosis and therapy of urinary tract infections. Am J Obstet Gynecol 1991;164:1387.

| Symptom | **Oliguria/Anuria** | | *Mary Ann Kuzma* |

"Oliguria" is defined as a urine output less than 400 ml/day in an adult. Urine flows less than this are insufficient to excrete the daily osmolar load. In the infant and child, oliguria is a urine output less than 240 ml/day and less than 15 to 20 ml/kg/day in the neonate.

"Anuria" is the absence of urine production, defined clinically as a urine output of less than 75 ml/day in an adult (zero urine output in a child). It rarely occurs in adults with normal renal vessels and a normal urinary tract and often indicates a postrenal obstruction.

Differential Diagnosis

1. Prerenal causes
   a. Decreased actual arterial blood volume: hemorrhage, gastrointestinal losses, or renal losses (diuretics)
   b. Decreased "effective" arterial volume
      (1) Vasodilation secondary to drugs, sepsis, anaphylaxis
      (2) Sequestration of extracellular fluid "third spacing"
         (a) Burns, abdominal surgery, peritonitis, or pancreatitis
         (b) Congestive heart failure or cardiogenic shock
         (c) Hepatorenal syndrome
         (d) Hypoalbuminemia
2. Renal causes in order of likelihood
   a. Acute tubular necrosis (ATN) related to
      (1) Ischemia—hypotension, sepsis
      (2) Nephrotoxin—aminoglycosides, contrast material
      (3) Rhabdomyolysis
      (4) Pregnancy-related—eclampsia
   b. Vascular diseases
      (1) Arterial and/or venous occlusion. Consider renal vein thrombosis in infant of diabetic mother.
      (2) Renal vasculitis
      (3) Malignant hypertension
   c. Bilateral cortical necrosis
   d. End-stage renal disease
   e. Acute glomerulonephritis (GN)
   f. Hemolytic-uremic syndrome
   g. Acute interstitial nephritis (AIN)
   h. Hypercalcemia
   i. Paraprotein or crystalline-mediated disease
3. Postrenal causes—rare in pediatric population
   a. Bilateral ureteral obstruction
      (1) Extrinsic compression from retroperitoneal fibrosis, tumor, lymph nodes
      (2) Intrinsic occlusion from calculus or tumor
   b. Bladder outlet obstruction
      (1) Neurogenic bladder retention
      (2) Calculus or tumor
      (3) Posterior urethral valves—newborn male
   c. Urethral obstruction
      (1) Prostatic enlargement
      (2) Stricture
      (3) Trauma
   d. Congenital malformation of the kidney(s)—seen in pediatric patients

Refer to the common cardiovascular symptom shock; Ch. 60, Chronic Heart Failure; Ch. 129, Acute Renal Failure; Ch. 130, Chronic Renal Failure; Ch. 131, Glomerulonephritis; Ch. 137, Benign Prostatic Hyperplasia; and Ch. 140, Bladder Cancer.

History

1. Detailed medical history
   a. Identify previous or concurrent cardiac, hepatic, pelvic, vascular, or neurologic illness.
   b. Identify previous or present history of kidney disease.
   c. Check for family history of renal disease.
   d. Estimate or measure recent urine output.
   e. Identify changes in gross appearance of the urine.
2. Inquire about
   a. Recent or past trauma or surgical procedures.
   b. Recent radiologic procedures.
   c. Recent history of fever, rash, vomiting, diarrhea, blood loss, weight loss, or travel.
   d. Past and present medications.

Clinical Findings

1. Assess blood volume status; look for evidence of volume depletion or overload.
2. Hypertension—funduscopic evidence of malignant retinopathy
3. Cardiopulmonary evidence of congestive heart failure
4. Abdominal mass, prostatic enlargement, or pelvic disease
5. Altered mental status

Tests

1. Urinalysis
   a. Urine volume measurement over 24 hours
   b. Gross examination—presence of bleeding
   c. Dipstick evaluation
      (1) Proteinuria—1 and 2+ proteins suggest ATN; larger amounts suggest GN or malignant hypertension.
      (2) Hematuria—GN, vasculitis, renal arterial emboli, ATN, rhabdomyolysis
   d. Microscopic examination
      (1) Tubular epithelial cell—ATN, AIN
      (2) Red blood cells (RBCs)—GN, vasculitis, renal arterial emboli, ATN, AIN
      (3) RBC casts—GN, vasculitis
      (4) White blood cell (WBC) casts—AIN
      (5) Other casts—ATN, rhabdomyolysis
   e. Urinary indices

Urinary Indices	Prerenal	Renal
Urinary sodium	< 20 mEq/L	>30 mEq/L
Urine osmolality	> 600 mOsm/kg	<350 mOsm/kg
Urine/plasma osmolality	>2:1	<1.5:1
Urine/plasma creatinine	>20:1	<20:1
Fractional excretion of Na	<1	>1
Renal failure index	<1	>1

Fractional excretion of Na =

$$\frac{[urine/serum\ Na]}{[urine/serum\ creatinine]} \times 100$$

Renal failure index =

$$\frac{[urine\ Na \times serum\ creatinine]}{[urine\ creatinine]} \times 100$$

2. Catheterize bladder. If catheterization is difficult to perform, exclude urethral obstruction. If there is no urine, exclude obstruction in or above ureters and renal vascular occlusion.

   (a) Renal ultrasound. Only useful if evidence of obstruction/bilateral hydronephrosis.

   (b) Cystoscopy and retrograde pyelogram

   (c) Renal flow scan

   (d) If above three are normal, proceed with urinalysis.

3. In oliguric patients, a fluid challenge with isotonic saline (500 to 750 ml in an adult or 20 ml/kg in a child) should be done over 1 hour. If there is no improvement in urine volume, renal disease should be assumed.

4. To identify the site of obstruction in pediatric patients:

   a. Ultrasonography

   b. Intravenous pyelogram, voiding cystourethrogram

   c. Cystoscopy, retropyelography

5. Serial measurements of serum creatinine and urine nitrogen

6. Blood chemistries, including sodium, potassium, CO_2, phosphorus, and magnesium, are not usually helpful in establishing the cause of oliguria/anuria but are followed serially to detect electrolyte abnormalities as a consequence of oliguria.

7. Complete blood count (CBC). Absence of anemia in an adult points away from complete renal failure as cause. Hemolytic anemia and thrombocytopenia are hallmarks of hemolytic-uremic syndrome.

Management

1. Correct reversible causes. Relieve obstruction, if present; discontinue nephrotoxic drugs.

2. Optimize arterial blood volume and cardiac status if patient is thought to have prerenal factors contributing to oliguria.

3. Manage electrolyte, acid-base abnormalities.

4. Restrict salt and water intake if caused by cardiac or renal disease.

5. Treat hypertension aggressively in a monitored setting if malignant hypertension is the suspected cause.

6. Measure daily all oral and intravenous intake and output.

7. Maintain urine output once hemodynamics and arterial blood volumes have been optimized. Loop diuretics and low-dose dopamine are agents of choice.

8. Hemodialyze if volume overload or electrolyte (hyperkalemia) or acid-base disturbances are life-threatening.

PEARLS

- Edema and/or ascites does not exclude the presence of volume contraction as the cause of oliguria.

- Anuria should not be attributed to primary renal disease without an evaluation of the bladder, ureters, urethra, renal veins, and arteries. It is unusual for the onset of urination to occur after 24 hours in the newborn.

 Bibliography

For more information on oliguria/anuria in the pediatric patient, see

Bricker NS, Kirschenbaum MA, Fine RN: The Kidney: Diagnosis and Management. New York, Wiley, Sons, 1984, pp 467–470.

For more information on the use of urinalysis and urinary indices in the diagnosis of oliguria, see

Preuss HG, Zelman SJ, Vertuno LL: Management of Common Problems in Renal Disease. New York, Macmillan, 1988, pp 97–99.

Penile discharge is seen fairly frequently in the family physician's office. The cause can be secondary to infectious organisms, trauma, or ectopic tissue. For purposes of discussion, penile discharges will be categorized into those noted for the gross appearance of blood and those purulent, mucoid, or watery in nature.

Purulent/Mucoid Penile Discharges

Differential Diagnosis

1. *Neisseria gonorrhoeae*
2. *Chlamydia trachomatis*
3. *Ureaplasma urealyticus*
4. Group A β-hemolytic *Streptococcus*
5. Reiter's syndrome

N. gonorrhoeae and *C. trachomatis* are the two most frequently encountered infectious pathogens of penile discharge, especially for young men under age 35.

Clinical suspicion of either pathogen should always be confirmed by laboratory testing. Between 20 and 50 per cent of nongonococcal urethritis is attributable to *U. urealyticus*.

Consider group A β-hemolytic streptococcal infection in the case of the prepubertal, uncircumcised male with purulent discharge and a positive history of a recent group A β-hemolytic streptococcal infection.

> Refer to Ch. 105, Sexually Transmitted Diseases; and Ch. 135, Nongonococcal Urethritis.

History

1. Age of patient
2. Length of time symptoms present
3. Associated symptoms of urinary frequency, urgency, dysuria, nocturia, acute epididymitis, fever, chills, night sweats, weight loss, bone/joint pain or effusion, rectal pain, conjunctivitis, skin lesions, terminal hematuria, suprapubic pain or discomfort relieved somewhat by urination, and meatal itching
4. Sexual history to include sexual preference, modes of intercourse, number of partners, and previous sexually transmitted diseases (STDs)
5. Similar illness in sexual partner or diagnosed STD in sexual partner
6. Prior occurrence of similar symptoms

The usual incubation period for *N. gonorrhoeae* is 3 to 10 days but may be 12 hours to 13 months. *Chlamydia* has an incubation period of 7 to 21 days. *U. urealyticus* has a higher incidence in men with a history of three to five sexual partners. A rare complication of chlamydial epididymitis in heterosexual men under age 35 is Reiter's syndrome—urethritis, conjunctivitis, arthritis, and characteristic mucocutaneous lesions occurring with an increased frequency in populations positive for HLA–B27 haplotype. Disseminated *N. gonorrhoeae* infection may cause arthritis or tenosynovitis. Knee joints are most commonly affected. Fever and leukocytosis are generally uncommon. A painless, nontender enlargement of the epididymis suggest tuberculosis.

Chronic urethral discharge in men older than age 35 may be due to chronic prostatitis, with Enterobacteriaceae as an additional pathogen to consider.

Clinical Findings

1. Scant purulent/mucoid urethral discharge
2. Meatal edema or erythema
3. ± Joint involvement (i.e., effusion, tenderness, erythema)
4. ± Adenopathy
5. ± Tender epididymis, prostate

Tests

1. Gram's stain
2. Culture for *N. gonorrhoeae* and *C. trachomatis*
3. Urinalysis and culture
4. Synovial fluid in presence of effusion

Patient should be examined at least 1 hour after last void, preferably 4 hours after voiding, for urethral specimen collection. Using a calcium alginate swab, inserted 2 to 3 centimeters into the urethral opening, rotate gently. The swab should first be rolled on a slide in preparation for Gram's staining and then placed in transport media for *N. gonorrhoeae* and *Chlamydia* cultures. In populations with a high incidence of resistant organisms, *N. gonorrhoeae* culture should be obtained to determine antibiotic sensitivities. There are no known chlamydial resistances to tetracycline at the present time. The specificity of a gram-stained specimen in gonococcal urethritis is 95 per cent. Sensitivity is nearly 100 per cent. The positive gonococcal endourethral smear has four or more polymorphonuclear neutrophils per high-power field with gram-negative diplococci located within the neutrophils. If, in the presence of inflammatory cells, there is an absence of gram-negative diplococci in the neutrophils, treatment should proceed for chlamydial infection. Both *Chlamydia* and tuberculosis will produce inflammatory cells without bacteria. Cystoscopy is usually not indicated unless the diagnosis cannot be found and tuberculosis is suspected.

For a positive history of oral intercourse, pharyngeal swabs for *N. gonorrhoeae* should be taken. For a positive rectal intercourse history, take swabs of the anal epithelium by anoscope. In cases of joint involvement, the synovial fluid is positive for *N. gonorrhoeae* by culture, and leukocytes are greater than 800,000 per microliter.

Management

Medication

1. *N. gonorrhoeae:* Ceftriaxone (Rocephin), 250 mg intramuscularly once, *or* cefixime (Suprax), 400 mg orally once, *or* ciprofloxacin (Cipro), 500 mg orally once, *or* ofloxacin (Floxin), 400 mg orally once. Since 50 per cent of patients with urethritis have concomitant *C. trachomatis* infection, it is recommended at present to also treat for chlamydial infection. *N. gonorrhoeae* joint involvement may require open drainage and irrigation.

2. *Chlamydia:* Doxycycline (Vibramycin), 100 mg orally b.i.d. for 7 days, *or* azithromycin (Zithromax), 1 gm orally once, *or* ofloxacin (Floxin), 300 mg orally b.i.d. for 7 days, *or* erythromycin base, 500 mg orally q.i.d. for 7 days, *or* erythromycin ethylsuccinate, 800 mg orally q.i.d. for 7 days. Between 6 and 7 per cent of ureaplasma are resistant to tetracycline, so if the doxycycline regimen fails, treat with azithromycin, 1 gm single dose.

3. *Trichomonas:* Metronidazole (Flagyl), 2 gm given as a single dose.

Diet

Be sure to warn patients about possible Antabuse-like reaction occurring with metronidazole and alcohol consumption.

Activity

In the case of sexually transmitted disease:
1. VDRL and HIV testing of the patient.
2. Treatment of sexual partners.
3. Knowledge of state/local health department reporting requirements.

Patient Education

In cases of sexually transmitted disease, encourage use of latex condoms with nonoxynal-9 and water-soluble lubricants.

Follow-Up

Repeat laboratory examination after treatment for "test of cure." Arrangement should be made for follow-up of HIV testing, if warranted.

Bloody Penile Discharge

Differential Diagnosis

1. Posterior/anterior urethral injury/urethral contusion
2. Urethral condylomata acuminata (venereal warts)
3. Ectopic prostate tissue

History

1. Bloody urethral discharge
2. Straddle-type fall or penile trauma
3. Self-instrumentation or iatrogenic instrumentation
4. Lower abdominal pain and inability to urinate
5. Sudden edema in the groin or abdomen after voiding
6. Lesions on the skin of the penis or scrotum
7. Urinary symptoms of dysuria, gross hematuria, hemospermia

Urethral injury should be suspected in any patient complaining of bloody discharge and a history of trauma, straddle falls, penile instrumentation (self or iatrogenically induced), or penile fracture. In the case of posterior urethral injury, the patient may complain of lower abdominal pain and the inability to urinate. With injuries to the anterior urethra, bleeding is present with local pain. If voiding has occurred, a sudden swelling may be noted by the patient in the area of extravasation.

Urethral warts are uncommon in the urethra but are always preceded by skin lesions. Although they may be sexually transmitted, nonsexual transmission is possible. With urethral warts, the patient will note bloody spotting from the urethra with occasional dysuria and urethral discharge. Ectopic prostatic tissue, a rare condition, presents with a history of recurrent gross hematuria and intermittent bloody urethral discharge accompanied by symptoms of dysuria, frequency, and hematospermia.

Clinical Findings

1. Blood at meatal opening
2. Suprapubic tenderness
3. Perineal or suprapubic contusion
4. Presence of a palpable, developing pelvic hematoma
5. Prostate normal or displaced superiorly
6. Presence of condyloma acuminata skin lesions

In the presence of a posterior urethral injury, the examination may reveal suprapubic tenderness and presence of a pelvic fracture. A perineal or suprapubic contusion may be visible with a palpable pelvic hematoma. The prostate in posterior urethral injury is displaced superiorly, while in anterior urethral injury it is normal. In the case of the urethral condylomata, 90 per cent of the lesions are in the distal urethra, with other skin lesions evident.

Tests

1. Urethrogram—in presence of trauma
2. Cystourethroscopic examination
3. Complete blood count (CBC)

In the presence of bloody urethral discharge with a history of trauma, a urethrogram should be secured before bladder catheterization is attempted. While the CBC may reflect anemia in the case of posterior urethral injury, an elevated white blood cell count is more often observed in anterior urethral injury secondary to a propensity toward infection and sepsis in the presence of a delayed diagnosis.

If the diagnosis of condylomata acuminata or ectopic prostate tissue is suspected, a complete cystourethroscopic examination must be performed.

Management

1. In presence of trauma:
   a. Control of shock and hemorrhage

b. Treatment of infection

c. Surgical correction

2. Nontraumatic etiologies—chemical, electrical, or surgical resection of lesion

---

PEARL

- Do not catheterize a bloody meatus without initial radiographic evaluation.

Bibliography

Congleton L, Thomason WB, McMullan DT, Worsham GF: Painless hematuria and urethral discharge secondary to ectopic prostate. J Urol 1989;142:1554–1555.

Hoosen AA, O'Farrell N, Ende J: Microbiology of acute epididymitis in a developing community. Genitourinary Med 1993;69:361–363.

Rothenberg R, Judson FN: The clinical diagnosis of urethral discharge. Sex Transm Dis 1993;24:28.

Sanford JP: Guide to Antimicrobial Therapy. Dallas, Texas, Antimicrobial Therapy, Inc., 1993, pp 12–16.

Tanagho EA, McAninch JW (eds): Smith's General Urology, 13th ed. E Norwalk, CT, Appleton & Lange, 1992, pp 246–247, 257–261, 320–325, 602, 605.

Symptom   Urinary Incontinence   *Susan C. Brunsell*

Urinary incontinence is defined as the involuntary loss of urine, so severe as to have social and hygienic consequences. It affects approximately 30 per cent of the elderly in the community and over 50 per cent of nursing home populations. Despite its prevalence, urinary incontinence is under-reported due to lack of physician recognition, patient embarrassment, and the myth that incontinence is a normal part of aging.

Differential Diagnosis

1. Reversible incontinence: causes can be remembered using DRIP (Table 127–1) acronym
2. Stress incontinence
   a. Common among women under age 75
   b. Small amounts of urine lost during activities that increase intra-abdominal pressure (laughing, sneezing); occurs when intravesicular pressure exceeds urethral sphincter pressure
3. Urge incontinence
   a. Common in men and women over age 75
   b. Uninhibited detrusor contractions overcome urethral resistance resulting in the sudden urge to void and the leakage of moderate to large amounts of urine
   c. May be related to chronic cystitis, infiltrative diseases of the bladder, or CNS lesions
4. Overflow incontinence
   a. Occurs when the bladder, unable to empty normally, becomes overdistended, leading to frequent or constant urinary leakage
   b. Most common cause is outlet obstruction from conditions such as benign prostatic hypertrophy
5. Functional incontinence
   a. Incontinence despite a normally functioning urinary tract

---

Refer to Ch. 133, Urinary Tract Infection; Ch. 137, Benign Prostatic Hyperplasia; Ch. 140, Bladder Cancer; Chs. 159 and 160, Diabetes Mellitus; Ch. 283, Stroke; Ch. 299, Multiple Sclerosis; and Ch. 313, Depression.

History

1. *Medical history*: endocrinologic or neurologic conditions, malignancies, pelvic surgery or irradiation, parity
2. *Medications*: prescription and over-the-counter
3. *Pattern of voiding*: frequency, timing, amount, precipitants, character of stream
4. *Other new symptoms*: polydipsia, fever, weight gain/loss, change in bowel habits or sexual function, sensorimotor symptoms
5. *Voiding record*: The patient or caregiver records the timing amount and related symptoms for each void or episode of incontinence over a period of time

Clinical Findings

1. *Mental status*: signs of dementia or delirium
2. *Neurologic*: assess nerve roots S_{2-4} (bulbocavernosus reflex, perineal sensation)
3. *Abdominal*: palpable bladder
4. *Pelvic*: evidence of estrogen deprivation, pelvic relaxation, pelvic masses; observe for urine loss with Valsalva maneuver

---

TABLE 127–1.   REVERSIBLE FACTORS THAT MAY CONTRIBUTE TO URINARY INCONTINENCE

D	Delirium, dementia, depression
R	Restricted mobility, retention
I	Infection, inflammation (atrophic vaginitis), impaction
P	Pharmaceuticals, polyuria (glucosuria, CHF)

From Ouslander JG: Geriatric Urinary Incontinence. Disease-a-Month 1992;38(2):95.

5. *Rectal*: sphincter tone, presence of impaction, prostate size and nodularity. (Note: Prostate size on digital rectal examination has been shown to correlate poorly with resected weights.)

Tests

1. Postvoid residual (PVR)
2. Urinalysis and urine culture
3. Blood urea nitrogen (BUN), creatinine, electrolytes, serum glucose
4. Urine cytology (if microscopic hematuria present)

To determine the PVR, the patient is catheterized after voiding without straining. A residual volume of greater than 100 mL suggests either bladder weakness or outlet obstruction. The urine sample obtained can be used for the urinalysis and culture. Further testing or referral to a urologist or gynecologist should be pursued if indicated by the history, physical, or simple testing. Further testing would include radiographic studies, such as an intravenous pyelogram, ultrasonography or CT scan, or complex urodynamics

Management

1. All reversible factors (Table 127–1) should be identified and treated if possible.
2. Try the intervention that is least invasive and with the fewest side effects first.
3. Further treatment is dictated by the type of incontinence. Many of the medications used in treating incontinence can, if prescribed in the wrong clinical setting, make the incontinence worse.
4. Medications used to treat incontinence are outlined in Table 127–2.

Stress Incontinence

1. Pelvic floor exercises (Kegel exercises): taught by instructing the patient to interrupt voiding or stop a bowel movement. A typical regimen includes 10 to 20 contractions 3 to 4 times a day. The exercises are continued indefinitely to maintain benefit.
2. Medications
   a. Alpha agonists (phenylpropanolamine, pseudoephedrine) increase smooth muscle tone at the bladder outlet.
   b. Tricyclic antidepressants (imipramine, doxepin) decrease detrusor contractility and increase outlet resistance.
   c. Topical estrogen creams may be helpful in postmenopausal women by improving bladder outlet tone.
3. Surgery may be indicated in women who exhibit pelvic prolapse. Procedures available include bladder neck suspension and urethral sling procedures.

Urge Incontinence

1. Scheduling regimens: In bladder retraining the patient gradually lengthens the time between voidings.

TABLE 127–2. PHARMACOLOGY OF URINARY INCONTINENCE

Alpha agonists	
Phenylpropanolamine (Dimetapp)	25–50 mg q 6–8 hrs
Pseudoephedrine (Sudafed)	30–60 mg q 6–8 hrs
Tricyclic antidepressants	
Imipramine (Tofranil)	25–100 mg q h.s.
Doxepin (Sinequan)	25–100 mg q h.s.
Hormonal therapy	
Estrogen vaginal creme (Premarin)	2–4 gm q.i.d. for 1–2 wk then 1 gm 1–3 times/wk
Oral estrogen (Premarin) (cycled with progesterone)	0.3–1.25 mg q.i.d.
Finasteride (Proscar)	5 mg q.i.d.
Anticholinergics	
Propantheline (Pro-Banthine)	15 mg q.i.d.
Imipramine (Tofranil)	25–100 mg q h.s.
Smooth muscle relaxants	
Oxybutynin (Ditropan)	2.5–5 mg b.i.d.–t.i.d.
Flavoxate (Urispas)	100–200 mg t.i.d.–q.i.d.
Dicyclomine (Bentyl)	20 mg q.i.d.
Calcium antagonists	
Nifedipine (Procardia)	10 mg t.i.d.
Alpha blockers	
Prazosin (Minipress)	1–5 mg t.i.d.
Terazosin (Hytrin)	1–5 mg q h.s.
Cholinergics	
Bethanechol (Urecholine)	10–50 mg t.i.d.–q.i.d.

Prompted voiding is used for mobility or cognitively impaired individuals. The patient is asked at regular intervals about the need to void.

2. Medications
   a. Anticholinergic agents (propantheline, imipramine) inhibit involuntary detrusor contractions.
   b. Smooth muscle relaxants (oxybutynin, flavoxate, dicyclomine) are direct-acting smooth muscle depressants.
   c. Calcium antagonists (nifedipine) inhibit bladder contractions. Although efficacy has not been proven, this may be an option for patients being treated simultaneously for hypertension or heart disease.
   d. Estrogen replacement therapy (oral, transdermal, or intravaginal) alleviates the sensory problems of urgency, frequency, dysuria, and nocturia in postmenopausal women. Women with an intact uterus should be cycled with progesterone.
3. Surgery has little role in urge incontinence. Denervation procedures and augmentation cystoplasty are done at tertiary care centers and are reserved for the most difficult cases.

Overflow Incontinence

1. A Credé maneuver (suprapubic external compression) or Valsalva maneuver may facilitate bladder emptying.
2. Medications
   a. Alpha adrenergic blockers (prazosin, terazosin) reduce sphincter resistance.

b. Cholinergic agents (bethanecol) improve detrusor contractility.

c. Hormonal therapy (finasteride) causes regression of hyperplastic prostate tissue through androgen suppression. Two to six months of therapy are required before improvement may become evident.

3. Surgery: transurethral resection of the prostate (TURP) is the procedure of choice in men with overflow due to BPH. Newer approaches include transurethral incision of the prostate (TUIP) and transurethral ultrasound-guided laser-induced prostatectomy (TULIP).

Pharmacologic therapy should be used in conjunction with the nonpharmacologic interventions mentioned. Many of these drugs have significant side effects, which may be magnified in the elderly. Therefore, the lowest possible dosage should be used. Catheterization may be necessary in patients with an inoperable obstruction or an acontractile bladder. Chronic indwelling catheters are associated with significant risks and should be used only on a temporary basis. Clean intermittent catheterization is an option for patients with appropriate manual dexterity and motivation. Candidates for surgery should be selected carefully, weighing the risks and benefits. In high-risk patients, all nonsurgical interventions should be maximized first.

PEARLS

- Recognizing incontinence is the first and most important step in management.
- Search for reversible causes of incontinence.
- Try the least invasive treatments first.
- Catheterization is not a cure for incontinence.

 Bibliography

Nygaard I: Nonsurgical therapy for SUI. Contemp OB/GYN 1993;38:79–94.

Ouslander JG: Geriatric urinary incontinence. Disease-a-Month 1992;38:95.

Rousseau P, Fuentevilla-Clifton A: Urinary incontinence in the aged (Parts I and II). Geriatrics 1992;47(6):22–45.

Urinary Incontinence Guideline Panel. Urinary Incontinence in Adults: Clinical Practice Guidelines. AHCPR Pub. No. 92-0038. Rockville, MD: Agency for Health Care Policy and Research, Public Health Service, U.S. Department of Health and Human Services. March 1992.

Young S, Pingeton D: A practical approach to perimenopausal and postmenopausal urinary incontinence. Obstet Gynecol Clin North Am 1994;21:357–379.

| Symptom | **Enuresis** | *Marc Ringel* |

Enuresis is involuntary voiding of urine. The term is usually reserved for children. (It is called urinary incontinence in adults.) Most children obtain bladder control between 2 and 4 years of age. By age 5, 20 per cent will still be enuretic, gradually decreasing to an incidence of 1 per cent at 18 years. Boys with this problem predominate over girls 2 or 3 to 1. Though the prognosis for spontaneous "cure" is excellent, it can be a source of embarrassment for the child and of conflict within the family. There are quite effective treatments.

Differential Diagnosis

1. Idiopathic (familial, developmental)
2. Urinary tract infection (UTI)
3. Polyuria secondary to excessive fluid intake
4. Sexual abuse
5. Fecal withholding, encopresis
6. Diabetes mellitus
7. Chronic renal failure
8. Diabetes insipidus
9. Renal tubular acidosis
10. Ectopic ureter
11. Sickle cell disease (dilute urine secondary to renal microinfarcts)

Enuresis is almost always developmental in cause and self-limited. Unless there are reasons to suspect psychosocial disturbance or systemic illness, the workup routinely can be quite brief.

Refer to Ch. 129, Acute Renal Failure; Ch. 130, Chronic Renal Failure; Ch. 134, Acute Urinary Tract Infection in Children; Ch. 145, Sickle Cell Anemia; Ch. 159, Diabetes Mellitus, Type I; and Ch. 160, Diabetes Mellitus, Type II.

History: Key Questions to Ask

1. Was either parent enuretic?
2. Is the enuresis at night (nocturnal) or day (diurnal) or both?
3. Has the child never been dry (primary enuresis) or have there previously been 6 months of dryness in a row (secondary enuresis)?
4. Does the child have diabetes, renal disease, sickle cell anemia, or other systemic illness?
5. Have growth and developmental milestones been normal?
6. Is there reason to suspect sexual abuse?

7. Have there been problems with constipation or encopresis (stool incontinence)?

8. How frequently does the child urinate? During the day? At night?

9. Does the child complain of urinary pain or urgency?

10. Is the incontinence sporadic, or is there constant dribbling?

11. What attempts have been made to treat the enuresis thus far?

12. Have family conflicts arisen as a result of this problem?

13. Has enuresis become a social embarrassment to the child? In what situations?

Questions about the social and familial context of enuresis are at least as important as the strictly medical aspects of the history. Family history is the best predictor of functional enuresis. If both parents were enuretic, for example, it is likely that their children will be. Factors that suggest an organic cause are daytime enuresis, secondary enuresis, UTI symptoms (frequency, dysuria, urgency), history of systemic illness or developmental delays, and associated bowel problems.

Clinical Findings

1. Developmental delay
2. Tense family
3. Growth retardation
4. Perineal leak (ectopic ureter)
5. Distended bladder (urine withholding or neurogenic bladder)
6. Distended colon (fecal withholding)
7. Genital trauma, infection (sexual abuse)

The office visit is as much an opportunity to observe parent-child interaction as to examine the child. Look for signs of serious systemic disease and developmental delay.

Tests

1. Urinalysis
2. Bladder capacity (measure total urine volume in a single void after the child has held urine as long as possible)
3. Urinary tract imaging (intravenous pyelogram, voiding cystourethrogram, renal ultrasound)
4. Urine flow studies
5. Chemistry panel, complete blood count (to screen for systemic disease)
6. Developmental testing

For most cases of enuresis—particularly with a positive family history, nocturnal pattern, and unremarkable history and physical examination—a urinalysis to rule out UTI is all the laboratory workup that need be done.

Management

1. Treat UTI, diabetes, encopresis, and any other physical contributor to this problem.

2. Nighttime wetness alarm (best ones fit in underpants)
3. Individual or family counseling
4. Hypnosis

Medication
1. Placebo pills
2. Imipramine, 10 to 75 mg h.s., gradually increasing until minimum effective dose is reached
3. Desmopressin (DDAVP) nasal spray, 20 to 40 µg (2 to 4 sprays) q.h.s.

Diet
1. Limit evening fluid intake.
2. High-fiber diet (for stool withholders)

Activity
1. Behavioral modification with "star chart" (stickers accumulated on a calendar for dry nights, resulting in an agreed-on reward for achieving dryness goals)
2. Nighttime awakening and trips to the toilet (best if done by the child with own alarm clock). These activities also may be monitored on the "star chart."
3. Bladder stretching (holding urine as long as possible during the day)

Patient Education
1. Question about and educate parents on "normal" toilet training as part of routine health maintenance. Usually the child will let them know when ready.
2. Reassurance of parent and child that this is a problem that is almost always outgrown.

PEARLS

- Enuresis almost always resolves, with or without treatment.

- There is a strong familial component to this problem.

- Daytime wetness is more often attributable to an underlying cause than is nighttime wetness.

- Secondary enuresis is more likely to have an underlying cause than primary.

- A urinalysis is the only laboratory test that usually needs to be done in working up this problem.

- Behavioral methods are most effective.

- Unless there are strong social reasons to treat this problem, defer treatment until age 7, by which time 90 per cent of children will be dry.

- Use drug therapy to treat enuresis only if patient age, social situation, or previous treatment failures are factors.

- Always consider the possibility of sexual abuse, especially in secondary enuresis.

3. Discourage punitive attitudes by caretakers and self-blame by child.

4. Encourage giving child as much control as possible (e.g., pick out own stickers and calendar, set own alarm clock, change own sheets).

Simple reassurance, patience, and unintrusive behavioral interventions are all the treatment that is usually needed. Wetness alarms, used correctly, achieve dryness up to 70 per cent of the time in nocturnal enuretics. Unless clear-cut psychopathology is found, psychological counseling is rarely warranted. Use medications when all else has failed. Imipramine works well in the short term. Its best use is intermittently, to avoid embarrassment at a slumber party, for example. DDAVP appears to work well with minimal side effects but is expensive. Relapse when either drug is discontinued is common. Enuresis is one of the few situations in which placebo pills may be effective.

Follow-Up

1. Frequent follow-up and reinforcement for the smallest success are crucial at the beginning of a behavioral regimen.

2. A long-term trusting relationship with a health care professional is most important to lasting success in treating this problem.

Bibliography

For more information on enuresis, see
Rushton HG: Evaluation of the enuretic child. Clin pediatrics 1993; special edition: 14–18.

For more information on enuresis, see
Cohen M: Enuresis. In Hoekelman RA (ed): Primary Pediatric Care, 2nd ed. St. Louis, Mosby-Year Book, 1992, pp 700–703.

For more information on behavioral treatment of enuresis, see
Scott M, Barclay D, Houts A: Childhood enuresis: Etiology, assessment, and current behavioral treatment. Prog Behav Mod 1992;28:83–117 and Miller K: Concomitant nonpharmacologic therapy in the treatment of primary nocturnal enuresis. Clin Pediat 1993; special edition: 32–37.

For more information on drug treatment of enuresis, see
Miller K, Atkin B, Moody M: Drug therapy and nocturnal enuresis, current treatment recommendations. Drugs 1992; 1:47–56.

For more information on nocturnal enuresis, see
Djurhuus J, Norgaard J, Hjalmas K, Wille S: Nocturnal enuresis, a new strategy for treatment against a physiological background. Scand J Urol Nephrol 1992;143:3–29.

128 Urinary Stones; Hypercalciuria
Karl R. Herwig

Etiology
1. Definition: Urinary calculi are concretions of crystals in the urinary tract. They may be composed of calcium oxalate, calcium phosphate, uric acid, or cystine.
2. Epidemiology: In the United States, up to 10 per cent of people will develop urinary calculi during their lifetime. In certain areas of the country, the rate is higher, possibly due to environmental conditions.
3. Predisposing factors
   a. General: Dehydration can predispose to crystal precipitation. The stress of life also increases stone formation.
   b. Supersaturation of urine with crystal enhances stone formation.
   c. Urine contains inhibitors to crystal precipitation and formation. Among the known inhibitors are pH, citrates, pyrophosphates, and magnesium. Changes in these factors can lead to stone formation.
   d. Stasis of urine from obstruction allows crystals to accumulate and form stones. When associated with infection from urea-splitting organisms, ammonio-magnesium phosphate stones (struvite) form.

Symptoms
1. Pain in the flank or costovertebral area is usually the first indication of a stone. It can be acute and debilitating and associated with nausea, vomiting, and acute colic, or can be dull and persistent. Acute colic is one of the most intense pains suffered by humans.
2. Fever and/or persistent urinary tract infection can suggest a stone, especially struvite calculi.

Key Symptoms
- Acute flank pain
- Nausea and vomiting
- Pain not relieved by position

Clinical Findings
1. Hematuria, either gross or microscopic, is usually present in patients with calculi.
2. Costovertebral angle tenderness or flank tenderness usually accompanies acute renal or ureteral colic.

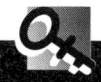

Key Sign
- CVA tenderness

Diagnosis
1. History and physical findings usually strongly suggest the presence of a stone.
2. To confirm a stone and its position in the urinary tract, radiographic studies are required. A plain film of the abdomen will demonstrate opaque calculi.
3. Nonopaque calculi, such as uric acid calculi, can be seen on ultrasonography.
4. An excretory or retrograde pyelogram allows exact definition of calculi and shows the presence or absence of obstruction.

Laboratory Tests
1. Urine analysis usually shows blood.
2. Increased white blood cell counts occur with injection or acute colic.
3. Serum calcium will suggest hypercalcemic states.
4. Urine culture identifies possible urea-splitting organisms such as *Proteus*.

Key Tests
- Plain abdominal film
- Urography

Differential Diagnosis
1. Any causes for an acute abdomen such as cholecystitis, appendicitis, or diverticulitis can mimic acute renal colic.
2. Persistent infections occur with calculi and can be caused by anatomic restrictions such as congenital hydronephrosis.
3. Hematuria may represent a urinary tract tumor. Also, tumors have been seen in patients with renal calculi.

Treatment
1. Acute colic requires immediate relief of pain, nausea, and vomiting. Strong narcotics in adequate doses usually relieve the pain. Rehydration with parenteral fluids may be necessary.
2. The stone, regardless of its composition, should be removed or spontaneously passed if possible. For small stones in the ureter less than 5 to 6 mm in size, spontaneous passage usually occurs, and expectant therapy alone will allow the stone to pass. Larger stones require an operative approach such as ureteroscopy, lithotripsy, percutaneous nephroscopic removal, or even open surgery. When obstruction is present it should be corrected and appropriate antibiotics used

533

for any infection. Failure to treat infection promptly and provide adequate urinary drainage can lead to septicemia.

3. The second goal of therapy is stone prevention. This is based upon analysis of the crystal composition of the calculus. Measurement of urinary crystal and inhibitor content (stone profile) helps in the selection of preventive measures that may reduce recurrence of stones.

Prevention

1. All programs of stone prevention have as their base adequate fluid intake, and this should be over 2 liters during a 24-hour period.

2. Dietary change with reduced animal protein (especially red meat) and increased vegetable fiber have been shown to reduce stone recurrence. Dairy products, when not in excess, should not be prohibited. Common table salt intake should be reduced.

3. Adjusting the pH to above 7 increases the solubility of uric acid; at a pH above 8, cystine crystals dissolve.

Medication

1. Thiazide diuretics reduce the excretion of calcium in the urine and are important in the treatment of hypercalciuria.

2. When inhibitor substances are reduced or lacking, replacement will increase crystal suspension and reduce stone formation. Some of the inhibitors available are potassium citrate, pyrophosphate, and magnesium oxide.

3. Allopurinol, a xanthine oxidase inhibitor, reduces uric acid production and helps to prevent uric acid stones.

4. Antibiotics are indicated when infection is present, especially with urea-splitting organisms.

Key Treatment

- Relieve pain
- Recover stone
- Correct metabolic abnormalities

Follow-Up

Once someone suffers from a stone, there is a 20 to 50 per cent risk of recurrence. Attention to fluid intake, diet, and medication needs repeated emphasis at regular intervals.

 Bibliography

Pak CVC, Skurla C, Harvey J: Graphic display of urinary risk factors for renal stone formation. J Urol 1985;134:867–887.

Pak CVC: Medical management of nephrolithiasis. J Urol 1982;128:1157–1164.

Preminger GM: Is there a need for medical evaluation and treatment of nephrolithiasis in the ''age of lithotripsy''? Semin Urol 1944;12:51–64.

129 Acute Renal Failure

Cynthia L. Short

Definition

1. *Acute renal failure* (ARF): acute onset of complete or partial impairment in renal excretion of solute and/or fluid, resulting in a rise in serum creatinine of 0.5 to 2.0 mg/dl/day as well as urea nitrogen (*azotemia*). Since multiple factors can affect the rate of rise of blood urea nitrogen (BUN), such as a catabolic state, upper gastrointestinal (GI) bleed, increased protein intake, and steroid use, the rate of rise of BUN is not as indicative of the degree of renal failure as the serum creatinine.

> • It is important to remember that the rate of rise of creatinine is only about 1.0 mg/dl/day even in the face of complete renal failure. Therefore, if the serum creatinine is 2.0 mg/dl today but was 1.0 mg/dl yesterday, the creatinine clearance is considered to be less than 10 ml/min. This is important in dosing drugs that are renally metabolized.

2. *Oliguric:* urine output less than 400 ml/day or less than 20 ml/hr
3. *Nonoliguric:* rising BUN and creatinine but maintenance of urine output (fluid removal without solute clearance)
4. *Anuric:* no urine output

Etiology

1. *Prerenal:* decreased renal perfusion
   a. Volume depletion (GI losses, insensible losses, blood loss, poor oral intake)
   b. Decreased effective circulating volume (sepsis, congestive heart failure, cirrhosis)
   c. Vasospasm (ischemia)
   d. Bilateral renal artery occlusion
2. *Renal:* direct damage to the renal parenchyma (interstitium)
   a. Acute tubular necrosis
   b. Drug/toxin (aminoglycosides, amphotericin B, contrast dye, myoglobinuria/hemoglobinuria, acute interstitial nephritis secondary to medication, cholesterol emboli syndrome)

> • After an angiogram, there are two major causes of renal failure: contrast nephropathy (onset within first 24 hours, rapid resolution) and cholesterol emboli (slower onset, other peripheral manifestations of emboli such as livedo reticularis, purple toes, retinal changes, cerebrovascular accident, poor prognosis for renal recovery).

   c. *Intrinsic renal disease* (glomerular): rapidly progressive glomerulonephritis, a clinical syndrome of rapidly progressive renal failure, often associated with crescent formation on renal biopsy. Includes HIV-associated nephropathy.
3. *Postrenal:* obstruction interrupting urine outflow and eventually leading to renal damage
   a. Bladder outlet (prostatic enlargement)
   b. Bilateral ureteral obstruction (stones)
   c. Bilateral renal vein occlusion

> • In evaluating a patient for obstruction or vascular events, it is crucial to know if there are one or two kidneys present. Obstruction of one kidney has little or no effect on renal function if a second, normally functioning kidney is present. In the case of the single kidney, however, unilateral obstruction can lead to renal failure.

Symptoms

Most often *nonspecific.* The degree of symptomatology is often related to the rapidity of onset of renal failure.

1. *Central nervous system:* malaise, cognitive slowing, confusion, seizure, coma
2. *GI:* anorexia, nausea, vomiting, diarrhea, constipation, metallic taste
3. *Cardiovascular:* shortness of breath, dyspnea on exertion, pericarditis (chest pain), lower extremity and periorbital edema
4. *Hematologic:* easing bruising or bleeding (gingival), fatigue secondary to anemia
5. *Genitourinary:* decreased urine output, flank pain, hematuria, foamy urine

Key Symptoms

• Most are nonspecific.

Laboratory Tests

1. Electrolytes (BUN, creatinine, K^+, HCO_3^-)
2. Complete blood count (CBC): white blood cells (WBC), hematocrit (anemia due to decreased erythropoietin production or hemoconcentration if dry)
3. Urinalysis (specific gravity, presence or absence of hematuria, proteinuria, granular, WBC count, RBC casts)
4. Urine electrolytes and fractional excretion of sodium (FENA) to elucidate renal versus prerenal in oliguric acute renal failure:

535

	PRERENAL	**RENAL**
Urine Na	<20	>40

$$FENA = \frac{\text{excreted Na}}{\text{filtered Na}}$$

$$= \frac{U_{Na} \times P_{Cr}}{P_{Na} \times U_{Cr}} \times 100\%$$

| | <1% | >15 |

5. Creatinine kinase, urine myoglobin
6. Ultrasound: Especially helpful in ruling out obstruction, ruling out solitary kidney, checking renal size (patients with chronic renal failure often have smaller, shrunken kidneys).

> • Ultrasound may not show evidence of hydronephrosis early on (within 24 to 48 hours) or in patients with retroperitoneal fibrosis, in whom the collecting system does not dilate. Anterograde and/or retrograde pyelogram is the "gold standard" for ruling out obstruction and should be considered in all patients at high risk for obstruction.

7. Renal flow scan
8. Serologic tests: complement, antinuclear antibody (ANA), antistreptolysin O (ASO) titer, antiglomerular basement membrane (anti GBM) titer, serum and urine protein electrophoresis, antineutrophilic cytoplasmic antibody (ANCA)
9. If creatinine is stable, 24-hour urine for creatinine clearance, total protein
10. Renal biopsy

Key Tests

- Serum electrolytes, BUN, creatinine
- Urinalysis
- Renal ultrasound
- Complete blood count

Differential Diagnosis

1. *Prerenal*
   a. *Volume depletion:* Accurate volume assessment is essential in evaluating any patient with renal failure. This includes the estimation of both total-body volume and actual or effective intravascular volume (how much blood is actually perfusing the kidney). This is assessed by history, physical examination, laboratory values, and Swan-Ganz catheter readings if available.
      (1) Vital signs and orthostatic blood pressures, neck veins flat and at 45 degrees
      (2) Skin turgor
      (3) Intake and output, weight changes
   b. Decreased effective circulating volume
      (1) Sepsis

   (2) Poor cardiac output
   (3) Cirrhosis
   (4) Vasospasm (ischemia, cyclosporine, malignant hypertension, pre-eclampsia)
   (5) Bilateral renal artery stenosis or occlusion

2. *Renal*
   a. Nephritic (hypertension, hematuria, low-grade proteinuria, RBC casts, edema)
   b. Nephrotic (>3.5 grams of protein per 24-hour urine, hypoalbuminemia, edema, hypercholesterolemia)
   c. These are only broad classifications of renal disease, and there is often overlap between the two syndromes in a single patient. They can, however, guide you, since some diseases (e.g., poststreptococcal glomerulonephrosis) tend to be more nephritic, while others (e.g., aggressive focal sclerosis) are more nephrotic.

3. *Postrenal:* obstruction
   a. Bladder outlet
      (1) Prostatic enlargement
      (2) Tumor
      (3) Neurogenic bladder
      (4) Clot
   b. Bilateral ureteral
      (1) Stones
      (2) Tumor
      (3) Sloughed papillae (papillary necrosis)
      (4) Retroperitoneal fibrosis
   c. Bilateral renal vein thrombosis

Treatment

1. Maintain optimal intravascular volume.
   a. Diuretics (loop or thiazide/loop combination) if volume overloaded
   b. Volume expansion (normal saline, blood, albumin, etc.) if volume depleted
2. Optimize cardiac output.
3. Avoid further renal insults.
4. Treat hyperkalemia with resin binders and diuretics.
5. Treat underlying condition (e.g., antibiotics for sepsis, immunosuppressant agents for glomerulonephrosis, relieve obstruction).
6. Fluid restriction if euvolemic or volume overloaded (1 to 1.5 L/day)
7. Dialysis
   a. Intermittent hemodialysis
   b. Acute peritoneal dialysis
   c. Continuous replacement therapies: continuous venovenous hemofiltration (CVVH), continuous arteriovenous hemofiltration (CAVH). Treatment of choice in patients who are hemodynamically

unstable and unable to tolerate standard hemodialysis.

Diet
1. Consider protein restriction for control of uremic symptoms, but remember to adjust to energy needs of catabolic patients.
2. Sodium restriction (2 to 4 gm/day)
3. Potassium restriction (2 to 3 gm/day)

Activity
As tolerated by the patient.

Patient Education
1. Allay fears regarding dialysis and outline limitations.
2. For most forms of ARF, the long-term prognosis is very difficult to predict at time of presentation, and the patient should be aware of this.

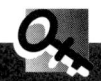

Key Treatment
- Maintain optimal intravascular volume.
- Optimize cardiac output.

Follow-Up
1. Resolving ATN: Increase in urine output usually seen before drop in serum creatinine. Post-ATN diuresis may occur, and it is important to avoid volume depletion.
2. Chronic dialysis or transplant.
3. Termination of dialysis if the prognosis is poor and the patient/family agree.

Bibliography

Better OS, Stein JH: Early management of shock and prophylaxis of acute renal failure in traumatic rhabdomyolysis. N Engl J Med 1990;322:825–829.

Grantham JJ: Acute renal failure. *In* Wyngaarden JB, Smith LH, Bennett JC (eds): Cecil's Textbook of Medicine. Philadelphia, WB Saunders, 1992.

Hou SH, Bushinsky DA, Wish JB, et al: Hospital-acquired renal insufficiency: A prospective study. Am J Med 1983;74:243–248.

Kellen ML, Aronson S, Roizen MF, et al: Predictive and diagnostic tests of renal failure: A review. Anesth Analg 1994;78:134–142.

Lazarus JM, Brenner BM (eds): Acute Renal Failure. New York, Churchill Livingstone, 1993.

130 Chronic Renal Failure

Robert L. Benz

Etiology

1. Chronic renal failure (CRF) describes reduced kidney function that is characteristically prolonged (> 3 months in duration), irreversible, and progressive in nature. These features differentiate it from acute renal failure. The presence of anemia and renal osteodystrophy favors the diagnosis of CRF, as does small kidney size.

2. Mild CRF may be referred to as "renal insufficiency," whereas "end-stage renal disease" (ESRD) refers to the development of symptoms or pathophysiologic alterations that require dialytic intervention or renal transplantation to preserve life.

3. The major categories leading to CRF include glomerulopathies (primary and secondary), hypertensive nephrosclerosis, chronic tubulointerstitial diseases, and obstructive uropathy. Diabetic nephropathy and hypertension represent the two leading causes of ESRD in the United States. Myeloma nephropathy may be diagnosed by finding light chains in the urine.

Symptoms

1. Symptoms of uremia typically develop when advanced CRF has been reached (creatinine clearance < 30 ml/min). The earliest symptom is often nocturia or polyuria due to loss of the concentrating mechanism.

2. Symptoms may be due to the anemia of CRF or neuromuscular sequelae (peripheral, autonomic, or central nervous system).

3. Other symptoms may stem from specific chemical disturbances related to phosphate, calcium, and parathyroid hormonal imbalance.

4. Bleeding-related symptoms may stem from platelet dysfunction or primary gastrointestinal (GI) problems that are increased in CRF patients, such as arteriovenous malformations.

Key Symptoms

• Fatigue	• Pruritus
• Nausea	• Insomnia
• Anorexia	• Confusion
• Nocturia	• Dysgeusia

Clinical Findings

1. Clinical findings, like symptoms, do not usually manifest themselves until CRF is advanced (creatinine clearance < 30 ml/min).

2. Salt and water retention in CRF may be manifested by the following cardiovascular sequelae of volume overload: peripheral edema, new or worsening rise in blood pressure, ascites, congestive heart failure (CHF), pericardial effusion.

3. Neurologic manifestations may include
   a. Central nervous system: asterixis, confusion, lethargy, or coma
   b. Autonomic nervous system: orthostatic disturbances in blood pressure and pulse, gastroparesis
   c. Peripheral nervous system (typically sensory rather than motor): diminished vibratory sensation, hypoesthesia, diminished deep tendon reflexes

Key Signs

• Edema	• Pallor
• Hypertension	• Altered mental state
• Asterixis	• Dyspnea

Laboratory Tests

1. The necessary tests to diagnose CRF include markers of the retention of nitrogen waste products normally excreted by kidneys. In addition to tests that determine the level of kidney function directly are studies to detect sequelae of CRF that have occurred.

2. Tests:
   a. Kidney status: serum creatinine and blood urea nitrogen (BUN), 24-hour urine for protein and creatinine clearance, renal ultrasound for renal size and to rule out obstruction, urinalysis
   b. Tests for metabolic, hematologic, and nutritional sequelae: calcium, phosphorus, albumin, hematocrit, bleeding time (if undergoing surgery), electrolytes, cholesterol, and glucose (if diabetic)

Key Tests

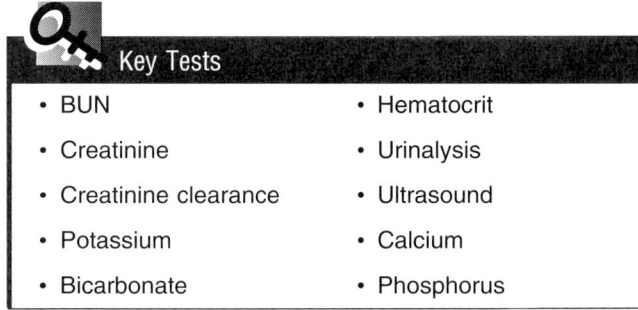

• BUN	• Hematocrit
• Creatinine	• Urinalysis
• Creatinine clearance	• Ultrasound
• Potassium	• Calcium
• Bicarbonate	• Phosphorus

Differential Diagnosis

1. The differential diagnosis for CRF is based on ruling out some degree of acute renal failure (ARF) superimposed on more modest underlying CRF.

2. Because ARF will typically resolve, whereas CRF will persist or progress, one should
   a. Check serial BUN and creatinine values over time.
   b. Try to correct any abnormalities that may be affecting renal function tests, such as medications, hypoperfusion, or obstruction.

Treatment

1. By definition, there is no treatment known to reproducibly correct CRF.

2. In general, the goal of therapy is to retard the rate of progression of CRF and limit the influence of its sequelae on the patient.

Medication

1. Treating the anemia of CRF can be achieved by ensuring adequate iron stores and then initiating recombinant human erythropoietin (rHu-EPO) subcutaneously.

2. Angiotensin-converting enzyme (ACE) inhibitors may preserve renal function by limiting hyperfiltration. Some fall in glomerular filtration rate may occur. Hyperkalemia must be watched for.

3. Control of renal osteodystrophy will require phosphate binders with meals (e.g., calcium acetate or $CaCO_3$) and active vitamin D (1,25-dihydroxycholecalciferol).

4. Diuretics may be necessary to control edema, potassium, and hypertension.

5. Bicarbonate replacement will neutralize associated metabolic acidosis.

6. Ultimately dialysis (hemodialysis or peritoneal) or transplantation will be required once CRF reaches ESRD.

Diet

1. Anecdotal studies indicated that protein-restricted diets might retard CRF, but a recent multicenter study could not confirm this benefit.

2. It is best to ensure adequate nutrition and calories (35 kcal/kg/day).

3. Limit sodium and potassium to 2 grams daily while restricting phosphorus intake if phosphate levels are elevated.

4. Fluids should be restricted if edema, CHF, or hypertension is present.

Activity

Activity restrictions are few and mostly limited to trying to avoid exhausting activities that lead to hyperkalemia and acidosis.

Patient Education

1. Much education is necessary for the patient (and family), considering the serious nature of CRF and given its progressive course.

2. Once the patient reaches ESRD, dialytic intervention makes education that much more imperative.

3. The education generally requires a team that includes the nephrologist, nutritionist, social worker, dialysis nurse, and surgeon (once patient requires access to dialysis or transplantation).

Key Treatment

- Antihypertensives (especially loop diuretics)
- rHu-EPO
- ACE inhibitors
- Salt and potassium restriction
- Dialysis
- Transplantation

Follow-Up

1. Patients with CRF should be referred to nephrologists early on. The nephrologist and primary care physician should work together to closely monitor the patient's blood work, blood pressure, and progression.

2. As patients approach ESRD, frequent office visits and blood work will be necessary.

3. Counseling about eventual dialysis/transplantation is essential.

4. When creatinine clearance is less than 15 ml/min, the patient should have surgical consultation for access placement.

Bibliography

Brenner BM, Rector FC: The Kidney. Philadelphia, WB Saunders, 1991, pp 1997–2036.

Jacobson HR, Striker GE, Klahr S: The Principles and Practice of Nephrology. Philadelphia, BC Decker, 1991, pp 678–708.

Nissenson AR, Fine NR, Gentile DE: Clinical Dialysis. East Norwalk, CT, Appleton & Lange, 1990, pp 1–44, 391–408.

Schrier RW, Gottschaulk CW: Diseases of the Kidney. Boston, Little, Brown, 1993, pp 2703–2878.

Suki WN, Massry SA: Therapy of Renal Diseases and Related Disorders. Boston, Martinus Nijhoff, 1989, pp 459–514.

131 Glomerulonephritis

Michael Allon

Etiology

1. Glomerulonephritis (GN) may be either secondary (associated with a systemic disease) or idiopathic (due to primary kidney disease).
2. Types of idiopathic GN
   a. Membranoproliferative GN
   b. Idiopathic crescentic GN
   c. IgA nephropathy
3. Secondary GN
   a. Infectious, such as poststreptococcal GN, endocarditis, visceral abscess
   b. Collagen vascular disease, such as lupus nephritis
   c. Vasculitis, such as Wegener's granulomatosis, polyarteritis nodosa
   d. Cryoglobulinemia
   e. Goodpasture's syndrome
   f. Henoch-Schönlein purpura

Symptoms

1. Shortness of breath, leg or facial edema
2. Dark urine ("Coke-colored")
3. Symptoms suggesting secondary GN
   a. Pharyngitis or skin infection 2 to 3 weeks earlier (suggests poststreptococcal GN)
   b. Joint pain (suggests lupus nephritis, cryoglobulinemia, or polyarteritis nodosa)
   c. Hemoptysis (suggests Wegener's granulomatosis, Goodpasture's syndrome)
   d. Sinusitis (suggests Wegener's granulomatosis)
   e. Fever (suggests endocarditis, lupus nephritis)

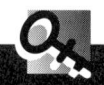

Key Symptoms

• Edema	• Dyspnea
• Dark urine	• Joint pain

Clinical Findings

1. Edema (periorbital, peripheral, or pulmonary)
2. Hypertension
3. Arthritis, malar rash, oral ulcers (suggests lupus nephritis)

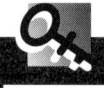

Key Signs

• Periorbital edema

• Peripheral edema

• Hypertension

4. Heart murmur (suggests endocarditis)
5. Palpable purpura (suggests Henoch-Schönlein purpura or cryoglobulinemia)

Laboratory Tests

1. Hematuria, especially red blood cell (RBC) casts
2. Proteinuria by dipstick
3. Serum blood urea nitrogen (BUN), creatinine: Glomerulonephritis frequently causes renal failure.
4. Complete blood count (CBC)
   a. Anemia seen in many cases of GN
   b. Thrombocytopenia (suggests lupus nephritis)
5. 24-Hour urine for creatinine clearance and protein: Protein excretion is usually less than 3 gm, but a minority of patients may be nephrotic.
6. Blood cultures—to screen for endocarditis
7. Antistreptolysin O (ASO) titer, streptozyme titer: If elevated, suggests poststreptoccal GN.
8. Serum antinuclear antibody (ANA)—positive at high titer in lupus nephritis
9. Serum complement (C3, C4, CH50)
   a. Low in poststreptococcal GN, endocarditis-associated GN, lupus nephritis, membranoproliferative GN, cryoglobulinemia
   b. Normal in vasculitis, IgA nephropathy, idiopathic crescentic GN
10. Hepatitis B and C serologies—may be associated with cryoglobulinemia, polyarteritis nodosa, and membranoproliferative GN.
11. ANCA (antineutrophil cytoplasmic antibody)—positive in Wegener's granulomatosis, polyarteritis nodosa, and idiopathic crescentic GN
12. Antiglomerular basement membrane (anti-GBM) antibody—positive in Goodpasture's syndrome
13. Serum cryoglobulin—elevated in cryoglobulinemia
14. Chest radiograph—may see pulmonary edema, pleural effusions, or evidence of pulmonary hemorrhage. Cavitary lesions would suggest Wegener's granulomatosis.
15. Echocardiogram—to screen for valvular vegetations, pericardial effusion
16. Kidney biopsy—helps to define the etiology. Immunofluorescence is especially helpful.
    a. Granular pattern is seen in poststreptococcal GN, lupus GN, and endocarditis.
    b. Linear pattern is seen in Goodpasture's syndrome.
    c. Negative immunofluorescence suggests Wegener's granulomatosis, polyarteritis nodosa, or idiopathic crescentic GN.

d. Idiopathic crescentic GN can have any one of the three patterns.

17. Open lung biopsy may be useful in the diagnosis of suspected Wegener's granulomatosis.

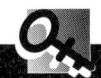

Key Tests

- Urinalysis (hematuria, proteinuria)
- CBC
- ASO titer
- ANA

Differential Diagnosis

1. Low serum complement
   a. Lupus nephritis
   b. Endocarditis
   c. Cryoglobulinemia
   d. Poststreptococcal GN
   e. Membranoproliferative GN
2. Normal serum complement
   a. Polyarteritis nodosa
   b. Wegener's granulomatosis
   c. Goodpasture's syndrome
   d. Henoch-Schönlein purpura
   e. Other vasculitides
   f. Visceral abscess
   g. IgA nephropathy
   h. Idiopathic crescentic GN (idiopathic rapidly progressive GN)

Treatment

Medication

1. No specific medical therapy is indicated for poststreptococcal GN.
2. Appropriate antibiotic therapy is required in endocarditis, based on sensitivities of organisms grown in blood cultures.
3. Glomerulonephritis with visceral abscess requires appropriate antibiotics as well as surgical drainage.
4. Lupus nephritis, Wegener's granulomatosis, polyarteritis nodosa, and idiopathic crescentic GN require prolonged treatment with corticosteroids and cyclophosphamide.
5. Diuretics are frequently required to treat the volume overload and hypertension.
6. Dialysis may be required in patients with GN accompanied by severe renal failure.

Diet

1. Dietary sodium restriction (2 gm/day) to prevent volume overload and hypertension
2. If the patient is hyperkalemic, potassium restriction is also indicated.

Activity

As tolerated

Patient Education

1. In cases of poststreptococcal GN, the patient can be reassured that the prognosis for recovery is excellent. Short-term emphasis is on dietary sodium restriction.

2. In patients with lupus nephritis, Wegener's granulomatosis, or polyarteritis nodosa, the patient must understand the chronic nature of the disease, the systemic manifestations, the need for long-term therapy, the need for close medical follow-up, and the potential adverse drug effects.

Key Treatment

- None for poststreptococcal GN
- Appropriate antibiotic therapy for endocarditis

Follow-Up

1. Most of the patients require close, long-term follow-up as outpatients. Outpatient management falls into two major categories: adjustment of medications to produce and maintain a clinical remission and monitoring for medication side effects.
2. Follow-up of parameters of disease activity
   a. Urinalysis—check for protein and RBCs.
   b. Serum BUN, creatinine, and electrolytes
   c. Serum complement: Low serum complement associated with poststreptococcal GN, endocarditis, and lupus nephritis will return to normal with remission of the systemic disease.
   d. Follow clinical manifestations of systemic diseases, such as pulmonary manifestations, arthralgias, skin rash
3. Complications of corticosteroids
   a. Immunosuppression. Monitor for fever, sore throat, cough, dysuria
   b. Diabetes. Monitor serum glucose.
   c. Hypertension. Monitor blood pressure.
   d. Osteoporosis. Consider estrogen in postmenopausal women.
   e. Cataracts
   f. Cushingoid facies
4. Complications of cyclophosphamide
   a. Immunosuppression
   b. Leukopenia (less commonly, anemia and thrombocytopenia). Need to monitor CBC frequently.
   c. Hemorrhagic cystitis—characterized by urinary tract infection symptoms, hematuria, and negative urine cultures. Immediately discontinue drug.

Bibliography

Falk RJ: ANCA-associated renal disease. Kidney Int 1990; 38:998–1010.

Johnson RJ, Gretch DR, Yamabe II, et al: Membranoproliferative glomerulonephritis associated with hepatitis C virus infection. N Engl J Med 1993;328:465–470.

Kallenberg CGM, Brouwer E, Weening JJ, Tervaert JWC: Antineutrophil cytoplasmic antibodies: Current diagnostic and pathophysiologic potential. Kidney Int 1994;46:1–15.

Kashgarian M: Lupus nephritis: Lessons from the path lab. Kidney Int 1994;45:928–938.

Madaio MP, Harrington JT: The diagnosis of acute glomerulonephritis. N Engl J Med 1983;309:1299–1302.

132 Pyelonephritis

Andy Pinson

Etiology

1. Acute pyelonephritis (APN) is an acute infection of the upper urinary tract. In the adult, chronic pyelonephritis does not generally develop unless there is a major underlying functional or anatomic abnormality.
2. APN usually occurs when colonic bacteria ascend through the urinary tract to invade the renal parenchyma.
3. The short length and the positioning of the female urethra in the vulvar area make it susceptible to contamination with bowel flora, and thus urinary tract infections (UTIs) including APN are seen more frequently in women than in men.
4. Some women have an increased susceptibility to colonization by uropathogenic bacteria.
5. *Escherichia coli* is responsible for most episodes of APN, with other common pathogens including *Proteus, Klebsiella, Staphylococcus saprophyticus,* and *Enterococcus.*
6. Some strains of bacteria possess virulence factors that make them more likely to cause APN.

Symptoms

1. Symptoms of APN usually include one or more of the following:
   a. Fever
   b. Chills
   c. Back or flank pain
   d. Nausea or vomiting
2. Symptoms of cystitis (dysuria, frequency, urgency) are often, but not always, present.
3. One-third of patients who have only symptoms of cystitis have an unrecognized infection of the upper urinary tract.
4. APN in the elderly may present atypically (altered mental status or vague abdominal pain being predominant).

Key Symptoms

- Fever
- Chills
- Dysuria, frequency, or urgency
- Back or flank pain
- Nausea or vomiting

Clinical Findings

1. The presence of fever in the setting of symptoms of cystitis is suggestive of upper UTI.
2. Costovertebral angle tenderness is often present and may represent renal parenchymal inflammation.

3. A pelvic examination can help rule out other causes, such as pelvic inflammatory disease (PID).

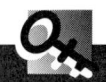

Key Signs

- Fever
- Costovertebral angle tenderness

Laboratory Tests

1. Clean catch or in-and-out catheterization urinalysis
   a. Perform a urinalysis in all cases of suspected APN.
   b. In APN, an uncontaminated spun specimen should show five or more leukocytes per high-power field.
   c. A Gram stain can be useful to help determine if gram-positive cocci are present (which can influence therapy).
2. Urine culture
   a. Should be obtained in all cases of suspected APN so that bacteriuria can be documented and the sensitivity pattern of the infecting organism can be obtained.
   b. A urine culture generally shows 100,000 or more colony-forming units per milliliter in APN, although lower colony counts are possible.
3. Blood cultures
   a. Should be obtained if the patient appears particularly ill.
   b. Are more likely to be positive in older patients.
4. Bilateral ureteral catheterization and the bladder washout technique can be used to more definitively diagnose upper UTI, but these techniques are invasive and impractical for routine clinical use.

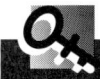

Key Tests

- Urinalysis
- Urine culture

Differential Diagnosis

1. Conditions that can be confused with APN include
   a. Pelvic inflammatory disease
   b. Acute appendicitis
   c. Acute cholecystitis
   d. Nephrolithiasis
2. A careful history, physical examination, and review of a spun urine specimen should help to rule out other diagnoses.

3. The absence of pyuria or an abnormal pelvic examination can be a clue that another diagnosis is present.

Treatment

1. The examining physician must determine if hospitalization is required or if outpatient therapy is possible.

2. Factors favoring hospitalization include
   a. Geriatric age group
   b. Underlying medical condition such as diabetes or pregnancy
   c. Male gender (higher frequency of anatomic abnormality)
   d. Known genitourinary tract abnormality
   e. Uncontrolled nausea and vomiting
   f. Signs of possible sepsis (hypotension, altered mentation)

3. Consider outpatient management for otherwise healthy young females who are reliable and who are tolerating oral intake.

4. Emergency room observation units can allow
   a. Hydration with intravenous fluids for 8 to 12 hours
   b. Administration of antiemetics
   c. Administration of one to two doses of parenteral antibiotics
   d. Reassessment of the patient by a physician to determine whether or not admission will be required

Medication

1. If hospitalization is required, numerous intravenous antibiotic regimens can be effective. Switch to an oral antibiotic after the patient has improved clinically.
   a. Ampicillin (1 gm q 6 hr) and gentamicin (1.5 mg/kg q 8 hr)—traditional regimen and still effective, especially if *Enterococcus* is suspected based on a Gram's stain of urine showing gram-positive cocci.
   b. Ceftriaxone (Rocephin), 1 to 2 gm q 24 hr
   c. Trimethoprim-sulfamethoxazole (Bactrim, Septra), 160 mg/800 mg q 12 hr
   d. Other intravenous antibiotics with gram-negative coverage

2. For outpatient oral antibiotic therapy, choices include
   a. Trimethoprim-sulfamethoxazole, 160 mg/800 mg q 12 hr—inexpensive and effective, but rash sometimes develops.
   b. Fluoroquinolones such as ciprofloxacin (Cipro), 250 mg q 12 hr, or norfloxacin (Noroxin), 400 mg q 12 hr
   c. Amoxicillin-clavulanate (Augmentin), 250 to 500 mg q 8 hr

3. Total duration of antibiotic therapy—10 days (in less ill patients) to 14 days (in more ill or pregnant patients).

Diet
Instruct patients to stay well hydrated.

Activity
Resume normal daily activities within a few days.

Patient Education

1. If outpatient therapy is chosen, the patient should be instructed to call or return for worsening symptoms.
2. Patients often improve markedly after 2 or 3 days of therapy but should be told to complete the entire antibiotic course.
3. Voiding after sexual intercourse can decrease the frequency of UTIs in some women.

Key Treatment (for Inpatients)

Drugs of Choice	Alternative Drugs
• Ampicillin + gentamicin or • Ceftriaxone or • Trimethoprim-sulfamethoxazole	• Other intravenous antibiotics with gram-negative coverage

Key Treatment (for Outpatients)

Drug of Choice	Alternative Drugs
• Trimethoprim-sulfamethoxazole	• Fluoroquinolones • Amoxicillin-clavulanate

Follow-Up

1. For outpatients, a brief follow-up visit (or at least telephone follow-up) is recommended after 1 to 2 days to document clinical improvement.

2. Failure to improve or worsening symptoms after 48 to 72 hours may represent obstruction or abscess, so consider imaging studies such as an ultrasound or an intravenous pyelogram. If such a patient is being managed on oral antibiotics, consider hospitalization and intravenous antibiotics.

3. A "test of cure" urine culture should be obtained approximately 2 weeks after the completion of antibiotic therapy.

4. If a second episode of APN subsequently occurs, a urologic consultation or workup (ultrasound or intravenous pyelogram and possibly cystoscopy) should be considered. In men, a single episode of pyelonephritis justifies a urologic workup.

Bibliography

Johnson JR, Stamm WE: Urinary tract infections in women: Diagnosis and treatment. Ann Intern Med 1989;111:906–917.

Meyrier A, Guibert J: Diagnosis and drug treatment of acute pyelonephritis. Drugs 1992;44(3):356–367.

Pinson AG, Philbrick JT, Lindbeck GH, Schorling JB: Oral antibiotic therapy for acute pyelonephritis: A methodologic review of the literature. J Gen Intern Med 1992;7:544–553.

Pinson AG, Philbrick JT, Lindbeck GH, Schorling JB: ED management of acute pyelonephritis in women: A cohort study. Am J Emerg Med 1994;12(3):271–278.

Stamm WE, Hooton TM: Management of urinary tract infections in adults. N Engl J Med 1993;329:1328–1334.

133 Acute Urinary Tract Infection in Adults

Steven K. Swedlund

Etiology

1. Urinary tract infections (UTIs) are largely a disease of sexually active females.
2. The female-to-male incidence ratio of UTI is 2 to 1 after age 60.
3. Urinary tract infections are the most common bacterial infection in the elderly and are a common source for bacteremia.
4. Gram-negative coliforms are responsible for the majority of bacterial infections, with *Escherichia coli* predominating.

Symptoms

1. Dysuria is a very common symptom, often accompanied by frequency, nocturia, incontinence, and suprapubic pain.
2. Malodorous urine and gross hematuria also may be present.
3. Flank pain and fever are generally considered symptoms of upper UTI.
4. Elderly patients also may display a septic syndrome with altered mental status, tachycardia, and tachypnea; an occasional patient may demonstrate hypothermia.
5. For some patients, gastrointestinal symptoms such as nausea, vomiting, and abdominal tenderness may falsely direct the clinician away from the urinary tract.

Key Symptoms

Lower Urinary Tract	Upper Urinary Tract
• Dysuria	• Flank pain
• Frequency	• Fever
• Nocturia	• Nausea and vomiting
• Suprapubic pain	• Mental changes (in the elderly)
• Hematuria	
• Malodorous urine	
• Incontinence	

Clinical Findings

1. For acute bacterial lower UTIs, the only positive physical finding may be suprapubic tenderness.

2. In addition, upper UTI may be associated with loin or flank tenderness, fever, tachypnea, tachycardia, and mental status changes (particularly in the elderly).

Key Signs

Lower UTI	Upper UTI
• Suprapubic tenderness	• Flank tenderness
	• Fever
	• Tachypnea
	• Tachycardia
	• Mental status changes (in the elderly)
	• Vomiting

Laboratory Tests

1. Microscopic examination and culture of clean midstream urine specimens are the primary laboratory tests for suspected UTI.
2. "Pyuria" is defined as 10 or more leukocytes per milliliter, as measured on a fresh uncentrifuged specimen of urine by microscopy in a hemocytometer chamber.
3. In the absence of a positive midstream urine culture (less than 100 uropathogens per milliliter), pyuria suggests infection by *Chlamydia* or *Neisseria gonorrhoeae,* or tuberculosis.
4. Microscopic or gross hematuria may be observed in UTI but is nonspecific.
5. White blood cell (WBC) casts noted on microscopy strongly suggest pyelonephritis in patients with symptoms of UTI.
6. Between 15 and 30 per cent of patients with acute pyelonephritis may be bacteremic with positive cultures. Elderly patients, diabetics, and individuals with urinary tract obstruction appear to have an increased risk of bacteremia.
7. Four biochemical screening tests for UTI have been devised: the glucose oxidase, catalase, nitrite reduction, and leukocyte esterase tests. Screening methods, in general, are insensitive at bacterial counts less than 10^5 colony-forming units per milliliter.

Key Tests

- Urine microscopy

- Pyuria (greater than 10 leukocytes per milliliter in uncentrifuged urine)

- WBC casts (indicate upper UTI)

- Leukocyte esterase test

- Clean catch midstream urine culture

- Blood culture (in toxic or elderly patients with signs of upper UTI)

Differential Diagnosis

1. Acute bacterial lower UTIs in females may be mimicked by urethritis caused by *C. trachomatis, N. gonorrhoeae,* and herpes simplex virus.

2. Vaginitis from *Candida albicans* and *Trichomonas vaginalis* or bacterial vaginosis also may cause dysuria.

3. Acute upper UTI can be mimicked by diverticulitis, appendicitis, pneumonia, intestinal obstruction, and nephrolithiasis.

Treatment

1. Therapeutic standards have not been defined for many forms of acute bacterial UTIs. However, standards do exist for women with uncomplicated infections.

   a. For acute bacterial uncomplicated lower UTIs in females, 3 to 5 days of oral outpatient therapy is frequently effective.

   b. Treatment of uncomplicated bacterial upper UTIs in females and males includes 14 days of oral or parenteral antibiotics and may necessitate hospitalization.

2. The therapy of uncomplicated bacterial lower UTI in males can be approached in a similar fashion as for uncomplicated upper UTI.

3. Factors that would designate a UTI as complicated include age greater than 65 years, indwelling catheter, recent genitourinary instrumentation, urinary calculi, renal impairment, prostatic involvement, diabetes mellitus, renal transplant, neutropenia, recent antibiotic therapy, recurrent UTI, pregnancy, steroid therapy, immunocompromising disease, and known structural or functional impairment.

4. The presence of obstructing urinary calculi and acute bacterial upper UTI should be considered a surgical emergency and consultation obtained.

5. The physician is limited in treating lower UTI in pregnant females because quinolones cannot be used during pregnancy or sulfonamides near the delivery date. Cephalexin is a reasonable first choice.

6. Antibiotic selection for all other complicated UTIs will be dictated by the clinical situation. Duration of therapy is unknown in these situations. The clinician should consider treating for 14 days and reculture to investigate for structural or functional impairment if there is recurrence.

Medication

A. Oral

- Trimethoprim-sulfamethoxazole (Bactrim DS, [double strength tablet], Septra DS), 160 mg/800 mg q 12 hr

- Trimethoprim, 200 mg q 12 hr

- Norfloxacin (Noroxin), 400 mg q 12 hr

- Ciprofloxacin (Cipro), 500 to 750 mg q 12 hr

- Nitrofurantoin (Furadantin), 5 to 7 mg/kg/day q 6 hr

- Macrocrystalline nitrofurantoin (Macrobid), 100 mg q 12 hr

- Doxycycline, 100 mg orally q 12 hr on day 1; then 100 to 200 mg/day

- Sulfisoxazole, 120 to 150 mg/kg/day, q 6 hr

- Amoxicillin-clavulanate (Augmentin), 250 to 500 mg q 6 hr

- Cephalexin (Keflex), 250 to 500 mg q 6 hr

- Ampicillin, 250 to 500 mg q 6 hr

B. Intravenous

- Ticarcillin-clavulanate (Timentin), 3.1 gm q 4–6 hr

- Ampicillin-clavulanate, 1.5 to 3.0 gm q 6 hr

- Cefazolin (Ancef, Kefzol), 0.25 to 1.5 gm q 6 hr

- Cephalothin (Keflin), 0.5 grams q 6 hr to 2.0 gm q 4 hr

- Ceftazidime (Fortaz), 1.0 to 2.0 gm q 6–12 hr

- Ceftriaxone (Rocephin), 1.0 to 2.0 gm q 12 hr

- Gentamicin (Garamycin), 3 to 5 mg/kg/day, give q 8 hr

Patient Education

1. Educate the patient to stay well hydrated.

2. In the female patient, discuss voiding after intercourse for prophylaxis.

3. Encourage patient to rest if toxic.

4. Discuss alternate contraception if recurrent UTI is associated with use of diaphragm.

5. Consider chemoprophylaxis with recurrent lower UTI.

Key Treatment

Uncomplicated Lower UTI, Female

3 to 5 days of oral therapy:

Primary
- Trimethoprim-sulfamethoxazole
- Norfloxacin or other fluoroquinolone

Alternatives
- Trimethoprim
- Cephalexin
- Nitrofurantoin or macrocrystalline nitrofurantoin
- Doxycycline
- Sulfonamide
- Amoxicillin-clavulanate
- Ampicillin

Uncomplicated Upper UTI in Females and Males and Uncomplicated Lower UTI in Males

14 days of:

Primary
- Trimethoprim-sulfamethoxazole
- Ciprofloxacin
- Norfloxacin

or parenterally
- Ampicillin and gentamicin
- Third-generation cephalosporin
- Ampicillin sulbactam
- Ticarcillin clavulanate, until initial cultures return; then adjust therapy based on culture

Alternatives
- Amoxicillin-clavulanate
- Oral cephalosporin
- Trimethoprim-sulfamethoxazole intravenously

Follow-Up

1. Uncomplicated lower UTI in females does not always require initial midstream culture and does not require follow-up culture; consider urinalysis to document resolution of pyuria.

2. UTI in men and complicated UTI require initial midstream culture, as well as culture after completion of therapy.

3. UTI in men requires thorough genitourinary (GU) examination.

4. Recurrent and complicated UTIs in females require GU examination.

5. Utilize history and GU examination to tailor workup to find functional or structural GU abnormality.

6. Simply assessing postvoid residual urine volume by catheterization may uncover functional bladder outlet obstruction.

7. Medical imaging techniques (ultrasonography, intravenous pyelography, CT scan, MRI scan, nuclear scan) may assist in diagnosis of structural abnormalities such as calculi in the GU tract, renal abscess, bladder diverticula, fistulas, GU tumors, and congenital defects.

8. Urology consultation also may be indicated to evaluate for structural or functional GU deficit.

Bibliography

Gleckman RA: Urinary tract infection. Clin Geriatr Med 1992;8(4):793–803.

Morgan MG, McKenzie H: Controversies in the laboratory diagnosis of community acquired urinary tract infection. Eur J Clin Microbiol Infect Dis 1993;12:491–504.

Ronald AR, Nicolle LE: Infections of the upper urinary tract. *In* Schrier RW, Gottschalk CW (eds): Diseases of the Kidney, 5th ed, vol 1. Boston, Little, Brown, 1993, pp 973–1027.

Ronald AR, Nicolle LE, Harding GKM: Standards of therapy for urinary tract infections in adults. Infection 1992;20:S164–S167.

134 Acute Urinary Tract Infection in Children

Syed M. Ahmed

Etiology

1. Urinary tract infection (UTI) occurs in about 1 to 2 per cent of male children and about 5 per cent of female children.

2. In the neonatal age group there is a male predominance, whereas female predominance occurs afterward.

3. *Escherichia coli* is the most common infecting pathogen, accounting for 80 per cent of the cases.

4. Other pathogens include *Klebsiella pneumoniae, Proteus mirabilis, Pseudomonas aeruginosa, Enterobacter* species, *Staphylococcus aureus, Streptococcus viridans, Enterococcus* species, and *Candida albicans.*

Symptoms

1. Both history and physical examination are of limited value in detecting UTI in pediatric patients because symptoms are not specific and are seldom localized to the urinary tract.

2. Neonates with UTI may present with fever, vomiting, hypothermia, diarrhea, abdominal distention, lethargy, irritability, failure to thrive, convulsions, and bacteremia.

3. Older infants may have feeding problems, vomiting, fever, malodorous urine, and failure to thrive.

4. Older children can present with common symptoms of UTI, such as dysuria, frequency, hesitancy, enuresis, and suprapubic discomfort.

5. Children with pyelonephritis may present with flank pain, high fever, and toxic appearance.

Key Symptoms

• Fever	• Frequency
• Vomiting	• Flank pain
• Dysuria	• Enuresis

Clinical Findings

1. Common signs include abdominal and suprapubic tenderness, pallor, lethargy, and palpable kidneys.

2. Patients with costovertebral tenderness and fever are usually assumed to have pyelonephritis until proven otherwise.

3. In case of a possible UTI, physical examination should exclude hypertension, abnormal genitalia, an abdominal mass, and neurologic deficits.

Key Signs

• Abdominal tenderness	• Fever
• Suprapubic tenderness	• Toxic appearance
• Lethargy	• Costovertebral tenderness

Laboratory Tests

1. A properly collected clean-catch midstream urine specimen is useful for diagnosis of UTI. In infants and children from whom it is difficult to obtain satisfactory clean-catch urine, suprapubic aspiration or bladder catheterization may be necessary.

2. "Dip and read" tests

   a. There are several different kinds of rapid, inexpensive tests available that determine the presence of leukocyte esterase and nitrite concentrations.

   b. False-negative and false-positive tests are common, occurring in 15 to 30 per cent of cases, and they are not sufficiently sensitive to determine the need for urine culture.

   c. Hematuria and proteinuria, assessed by dipstick, may occur with UTI but are not diagnostic.

3. Microscopic examination of urine

   a. Bacteria: The presence of one or more bacteria per oil-immersion field of uncentrifuged urine or greater than 10 organisms per oil-immersion field on a centrifuged unstained sediment correlates well with positive cultures.

   b. Pyuria: The presence of more than 10 white blood cells (WBCs) per high-power field in centrifuged urine has a high sensitivity for UTI. However, UTI can occur without pyuria.

   c. Gram's stain: The presence of one or more bacteria in an oil-immersion field of unspun urine correlates well with the finding of 10^5 colony-forming units (CFUs) or more bacteria per milliliter of urine.

   d. Urine culture: A reliably collected urine culture is the mainstay in the diagnosis of UTI.

      (1) A clean-catch midstream urine specimen with greater than 10^5 organisms and a catheterized urine specimen with greater than 10^4 organisms indicate UTI.

      (2) One positive culture associated with symptoms or two concurrent positive cultures in an asymptomatic child indicate UTI.

547

(3) Most UTIs are caused by a single organism; the presence of two or more organisms usually suggests contamination.

(4) A urine culture is not mandatory in adolescent females, particularly with a first episode. With recurrent episodes, episodes that fail therapy, in females with pyuria without bacteriuria, or in males, a culture is recommended.

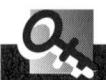
Key Test

• Positive urine culture is the definitive test.

Differential Diagnosis

1. In females, the differential diagnosis includes vulvovaginitis, gonococcal or chlamydial urethritis, acute urethral syndrome, and genital herpes infection. Local dermatitis from using contraceptive agents, foams, feminine hygiene products, soap, or other chemicals can present with UTI symptoms, such as dysuria.

2. In males, the differential diagnosis includes irritation from chemicals such as spermicidal foam, prostatitis, and gonococcal and nongonococcal urethritis. Physicians should consider torsion of testis and epididymitis when diagnosing a child with UTI.

Treatment

1. Outpatient treatment. The initial antibiotic therapy should be based on clinical severity, age, location of infection, presence of structural abnormalities, allergy to certain antibiotics, and cost of alternative antibiotics.

2. Reasonable choices for initial outpatient oral and inpatient antibiotic therapy are shown in Table 134–1. Based on the results of the urine culture and sensitivity, antibiotic therapy may require change.

3. The duration of treatment is controversial. There are studies reporting successful treatment of uncomplicated UTI with short-course therapy (e.g., a single dose of amoxicillin or a 3-day course of various antibiotics), though conventional therapy is for 7 to 10 days.

4. There is also controversy regarding the need for antibiotic treatment of asymptomatic bacteriuria, with reports showing no effects on the emergence of symptoms, kidney function, or kidney scars. Also, questions have been raised about whether treating organisms of low virulence can precipitate acute pyelonephritis by more virulent organisms. Some experts suggest treatment of asymptomatic bacteriuria if children are less than 5 years old or if they have a urinary tract structural abnormality.

TABLE 134–1. ANTIMICROBIAL DRUGS USED IN THE TREATMENT OF UTI IN CHILDREN

DRUG	DOSAGE
Oral therapy	
Amoxicillin	10–15 mg/kg/dose t.i.d.
Amoxicillin-clavulanate (Augmentin)	10–15 mg/kg/dose t.i.d.
Cephalexin (Keflex)	10–15 mg/kg/dose q.i.d.
Nitrofurantoin (avoid in newborns or patients with renal insufficiency)	1.25–1.75 mg/kg/dose q.i.d.
Sulfisoxazole (Gantrisin)	30–40 mg/kg/dose q.i.d.
Trimethoprim-sulfamethoxazole (Bactrim, Septra) (use cautiously during the first month of life because of risk of jaundice)	5 mg (trimethoprim)/kg/dose b.i.d.
Parenteral therapy	
Cefotaxime (Claforan)	50 mg/kg/dose q 8 hr
Ceftriaxone (Rocephin)	50 mg/kg/dose q 12–24 hr
Gentamicin	2.5 mg/kg/dose q 8 hr (neonates q 12 hr)

5. Hospitalization is suggested for symptomatic young infants (less than 3 months), children with clinical evidence of acute pyelonephritis, or children suspected of having upper UTI (toxic appearance, high fever, flank pain). An aminoglycoside in combination with ampicillin or a first-generation cephalosporin is the initial therapy of choice pending urine culture and sensitivity. A third-generation cephalosporin (ceftriaxone or cefotaxime) is also a safe choice, especially for neonates and patients with renal insufficiency. Intravenous therapy is continued until clinical signs (fever, pain, or signs of sepsis) resolve; then oral antibiotics should be taken for 2 to 3 weeks.

6. Ultrasonography is done to rule out obstruction. Though voiding cystourethrogram (VCUG) is usually deferred for 3 weeks to allow for resolution of changes, it can be done as soon as fever has resolved and the urine is sterile.

7. Prophylaxis is recommended for all children younger than age 5 with vesicoureteral reflux of certain grades or other structural urinary tract abnormalities and children with three documented UTIs in a year. With careful monitoring for side effects, prophylaxis can be obtained by a single nightly dose of nitrofurantoin (1 to 2 mg/kg/day) or trimethoprim-sulfamethoxazole (10 mg/kg/day) or sulfamethoxazole for 3 to 6 months or longer. Longer prophylaxis of several years is suggested in selected patients with persistent vesicoureteral reflux.

Patient Education

1. Avoidance or treatment of constipation is a recommended preventive measure against infection.

2. Good hygiene including front-to-back wiping of the anus, especially in female children, is suggested.

3. The use of chemical irritants, bubble baths, and tight clothing should be avoided.

Key Treatment

Outpatient
• Antibiotics as in Table 134–1

Inpatient
• Aminoglycoside + ampicillin or a first-generation cephalosporin

Prophylaxis
• Trimethoprim-sulfamethoxazole or nitrofurantoin

Follow-Up

1. *Urine culture.* A urine culture should be done 3 to 7 days after completion of treatment to exclude relapse.

2. *Urologic evaluation.* For children less than 5 years of age, after the first UTI, renal ultrasonography and cystography (voiding cystourethrogram [VCUG] or radionuclide cystogram [RCG]) are recommended. Fluoroscopic VCUG is recommended in males to rule out posterior urethral valves. Initial evaluation in females may be accomplished by RCG because obstruction within urethra is rare. An RCG is a sensitive indicator of reflux. The VCUG can demonstrate obstruction, residual urine, reflux, or neuropathic bladder changes. A renal ultrasonogram can demonstrate abnormalities of position, number, duplication, hydronephrosis, scarring, dysplasia, stones, or cysts. If both renal sonography and cystography are normal, no further evaluation is indicated. If reflux or morphologic changes are identified, further evaluation with renal scintigraphy or intravenous urography is recommended, though renal cortical scintigraphy has become the standard for the detection of pyelonephritis and renal scarring.

3. For children with recurrent infections and asymptomatic bacteriuria, a full workup including ultrasonography and cystography is recommended.

4. *Urodynamics.* Urodynamic studies may prove useful for children with neurogenic bladder or uninhibited bladder, especially if associated with reflux or hydronephrosis.

5. *Surgical intervention.* Vesicoureteral reflux, which is found in 30 to 50 per cent of children with UTI, is a risk factor for renal scarring. Mild to moderate reflux usually disappears with increasing age and can be monitored by serial imaging. Surgical intervention may be indicated for severe reflux, though some recent studies reported no difference in breakthrough UTI, renal scarring, and renal functions when medical and surgical treatment were compared.

Bibliography

For more information on UTI in children younger than 5 years of age, see
Schlager TA, Lohr JA: Urinary tract infection in outpatient febrile infants and children younger than 5 years of age. Pediatr Ann 1993;22:8.

For more information on workup of recurrent UTI, see
Johnson HW, Lirenman DS, Anderson JD, Nielsen WR: Recurrent urinary tract infections in children. Can Fam Physician 1993;39:1623–1631.

For an excellent review of pediatric UTI, see
Zelikovic I, Adelman RD, Nancarrow PA: Urinary tract infections in children. West J Med 1992;157:554–561.

For current concepts on management of pediatric UTI, see
Hellerstein S: Evolving concepts in the evaluation of the child with a urinary tract infection (editorial). J Pediatr 1994;124(4):513–519.

For evaluating the relation of vesicoureteral reflux and acute pyelonephritis, see
Ditchfield MR, De Campo JF, Cook DJ, et al: Vesicoureteral reflux: An accurate predictor of acute pyelonephritis in childhood urinary tract infection. Radiology 1994;190(2):413–415.

Procedure | BLADDER TAP

Shellie Russell

Indications

1. To obtain a sterile urine sample, especially in infants
2. Release of acute urinary retention

Contraindications

1. Known genitourinary tract anomalies
2. Cellulitis over the site of entry
3. Coagulopathy
4. Previous abdominal surgery (may need ultrasonographic guidance)
5. Bladder tumor
6. Gross hematuria

Preparation

1. The bladder must be distended.
2. Check diaper to ascertain that there was no urinary output 30 minutes prior to procedure. Try to palpate bladder.

Equipment

1. Antiseptic solution
2. Sterile 22-gauge needle attached to a sterile syringe

Anesthesia

None necessary in young infants. Older children or adults may need a local anesthetic.

Technique

1. Restrain patient in supine position, frog-leg position,

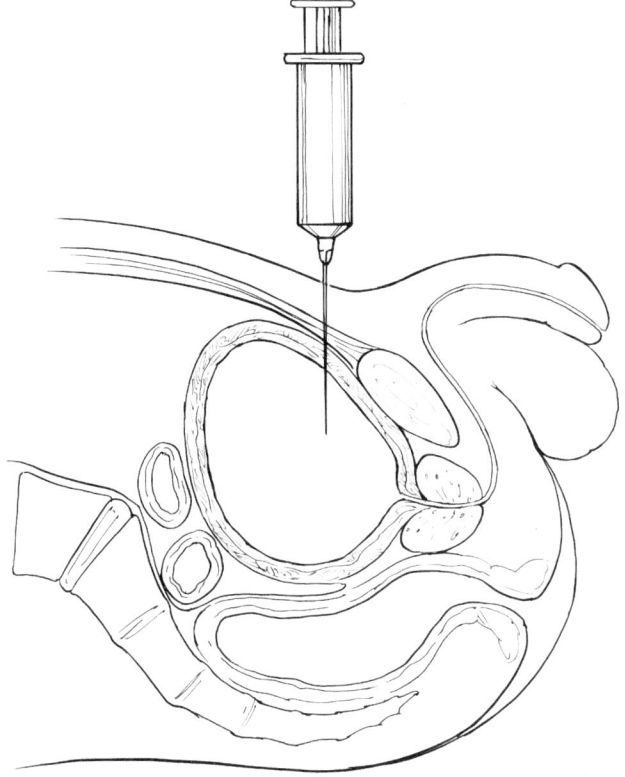

Bladder

or with thighs and hips together. To prevent urination during procedure, anterior rectal pressure in females or penile pressure in males may be used.

2. Clean lower abdominal area with antiseptic solution.
3. Insert 22-gauge needle 1 to 2 cm above the symphysis pubis in the midline, either perpendicular or 10 to 20 degrees to the perpendicular, aiming slightly caudal.

4. Exert slight negative pressure as the needle is advanced until urine enters the syringe.

5. Cover the area with a small dressing after withdrawing the needle.

6. If in doubt, ultrasonographic guidance may be used to locate the bladder.

Follow-Up

1. Complications are uncommon.

2. Transient hematuria, usually less than 24 hours

3. Penetration of bowel. Although this is a documented complication, none of the patients suffered ill effects.

Bibliography

Buys H, et al: Suprapubic aspiration under ultrasound guidance in children with fever of undiagnosed cause. Br Med J 1994; 308:690.

Gotlin R, Durmowicz A: Diagnostic and therapeutic procedures. *In* Hathaway W, et al (eds): Current Pediatric Diagnosis and Treatment, 11th ed. E Norwalk, CT, Appleton & Lange, 1993, p 1120.

Nelson J: Suprapubic aspiration of urine in premature and term infants. Pediatrics 1965;36:132.

Pryles C: Percutaneous bladder aspiration and other methods of urine collection for bacteriologic study. Pediatrics 1965; 36:128.

Shortliffe L, Stamey T: Suprapubic aspiration of the bladder. *In* Alken C, et al (eds): Urology. Chicago, Year Book Medical Publishers, 1982, p 747.

Torchia M (ed): Procedures. *In* Greene M (ed): The Harriet Lane Handbook, 12th ed. St. Louis, Mosby-Year Book, 1991, p 29.

135 Nongonococcal Urethritis

Rose A. Recco

Etiology

Nongonococcal urethritis (NGU) is an inflammation of the urethra not caused by *Neisseria gonorrhoeae.* In the United States and many other developed countries, the incidence of NGU far exceeds that of gonococcal urethritis.

1. Common causes
   a. *Chlamydia trachomatis*
   b. *Ureaplasma urealyticum*
2. Infrequent causes: may be bacterial, viral, fungal, or parasitic.
   a. Bacterial—coliforms, genital mycoplasmas
   b. Viral—herpes simplex, condylomata acuminata
   c. Fungal—*Candida, Rhinosporidium*
   d. Parasitic—*Trichomonas vaginalis,* schistosomes
3. No cause found. No infectious etiology is found in as many as 20 to 30 per cent of cases.

Symptoms

The symptoms in NGU overlap with gonococcal urethritis but are generally considered milder and the incubation period longer than for gonococcal urethritis. NGU may be asymptomatic.

1. Urethral discharge: This is variable. It may be described as scant, profuse, clear, or colored brown, yellow, white, or green.
2. Dysuria or burning on urination
3. Itch in the urethra
4. Incubation period 1 to 5 weeks, peak 2 to 3 weeks

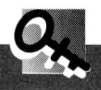

Key Symptoms

- Urethral discharge
- Dysuria
- Urethral itch

Clinical Findings

A. Typical findings
   1. Discharge: This may be spontaneous or expressed and may be mucoid or mucopurulent (i.e., thin cloudy fluid). (It is usually less florid than *N. gonorrhoeae.*)
   2. Crusting at meatus
   3. Redness around meatus
   4. Urethral tenderness
B. Unusual findings
   1. Conjunctivitis (*C. trachomatis*)
   2. Reiter's syndrome (*C. trachomatis*)
   3. Epididymitis (*C. trachomatis*)

4. Regional lymphadenopathy and constitutional symptoms (HSV)

> **WARNING**
>
> **Differentiation of NGU from gonococcal and other forms of urethritis cannot be made on clinical findings alone.**

Key Signs

- Mucopurulent discharge
- Meatal crusting and redness
- Urethral tenderness

Laboratory Tests

The diagnosis of NGU requires a determination of the presence of urethritis in the absence of urethral gonorrhea.

1. Determining the presence of urethritis
   a. Gram's stain of urethral discharge or endourethral swab (five or more polymorphonuclear leukocytes in five oil-immersion fields with no evidence of gram-negative diplococci)
   b. Examine urine sediment of the first 10 to 15 ml of urine (20 or more polymorphonuclear leukocytes in two or more of five high-power fields)
2. Establish the absence of urethral *N. gonorrhoeae* by Gram's stain and appropriate cultures.

> **WARNING**
>
> **Gram's stain may *not* be used to make a diagnosis of simultaneous NGU in the presence of urethral gonorrhea.**

3. Test for *Chlamydia*
   a. Cultures: Isolation in cell culture is the "gold standard."
   b. Nonculture tests: These are primarily based on antigen detection or nucleic acid hybridization methods and may be used on urine and genital swabs.
4. Culture for *U. urealyticum* and other pathogens.

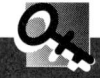

Key Test

- Culture is the definitive test.

552

Differential Diagnosis

The differential diagnosis of NGU includes gonococcal urethritis and noninfectious forms of urethritis.

1. Gonococcal urethritis: Smears and cultures needed for diagnosis
2. Noninfectious urethritis
   a. Urethral foreign body or calculi: Foreign bodies occasionally may be palpated and may produce bloody discharge. Calculi may produce large amounts of crystals in urine that may be visible on urine sediment. Pain is usually intermittent.
   b. A manifestation of systemic diseases
      (1) Stevens-Johnson syndrome
      (2) Wegener's granulomatosis
      (3) Tumors
   c. Chemical irritation of the urethra, as with bath products, shampoos. History of use of such products is essential to the diagnosis.
   d. Congenital anomalies

Treatment

After the exclusion or treatment of gonococcal urethritis, the treatment of NGU is aimed at *C. trachomatis* and *U. urealyticum.* Any one of the following medications is appropriate.

A. Drug of choice
   1. Doxycycline, 100 mg orally b.i.d. for 7 days
   2. Tetracycline, 500 mg orally q.i.d. for 7 days
   3. Azithromycin (Zithromax), 1 gram orally, single dose
B. Other choices
   1. Ofloxacin (Floxin), 300 mg orally b.i.d. for 7 days
   2. Erythromycin, 500 mg orally q.i.d. for 7 days
   3. Amoxicillin, 500 mg orally t.i.d. for 10 days
   4. Clindamycin, 450 mg orally q.i.d. for 10 days
   5. Sulfisoxazole, 500 mg orally q.i.d. for 10 days

WARNING

- **Tetracycline, quinolines, and erythromycin estolate are contraindicated in pregnancy.**
- **Sulfisoxazole may be used in the first and second trimesters but *not* at term.**
- **Ofloxacin (Floxin) is the quinoline of choice; other available quinolines may not be effective.**

Activity

Patients undergoing treatment for NGU should refrain from sexual intercourse until after treatment.

Patient Education

1. Since NGU is sexually transmitted and may be asymptomatic, patients should be cautioned to avoid promiscuity, use barrier contraceptives, and refer sex partners for treatment.
2. *C. trachomatis* and *U. urealyticum* rarely cause serious physical consequences or infertility in males. In contrast, women with *C. trachomatis* genital infection may face future infertility due to tubal occlusion, ectopic pregnancy, and chronic pelvic pain. Infection at term may be transmitted to the infant, causing conjunctivitis and pneumonitis.

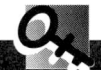

Key Treatment

- A tetracyline or azithromycin
- Other choices depend on clinical situations (see text).

Follow-Up

Evaluation for cure is difficult because NGU may resolve without treatment and urethritis may persist despite microbiologic cure of *C. trachomatis* and *U. urealyticum.*

1. Patients asymptomatic following full course of appropriate antibiotics
   a. Rule out inflammation.
   b. A test of cure for *C. trachomatis* should be done about 3 weeks after completion of therapy. Tests done before this may be falsely negative.
2. Urethritis present after one course of antibiotics
   a. Clinical and microbiologic re-evaluation including cultures for *C. trachomatis* and *U. urealyticum:* If a specific cause is found, it should be treated.
   b. Compliant patients in whom no specific cause is found or in whom cultures are not available should be empirically retreated. Erythromycin or ofloxacin may be given if initial treatment was with tetracycline. Add a single oral dose of 2 gm of metronidazole for *T. vaginalis* if laboratory evaluation is not available.
3. Urethritis present after two courses of antibiotics
   a. Careful clinical and microbiologic re-evaluation to rule out re-exposure and compliance with medications. If no cause is found and urethritis is mild, no further antibiotics are needed.
   b. If florid discharge is present and the patient is symptomatic and no cause is determined, consider a 3-week course of erythromycin.
4. If persistent or recurrent urethritis is present despite prolonged antibiotics or with unusual features, refer the patient for thorough urologic evaluation.

 ## Bibliography

Bowie WR: Urethritis in males. *In* Holmes KK, et al (eds): Sexually Transmitted Diseases, 2nd ed. New York, McGraw-Hill, 1990, pp 627–639.

Drugs for sexually transmitted diseases. Med Lett 1994; 36(913):1–6.

Jones RB: Chlamydial diseases. *In* Mandell GL, Bennett JE, Dolin R (eds): Principles and Practices of Infectious Diseases, 4th ed. New York, Churchill Livingstone, 1994, pp 1676–1701.

McCormack WM, Rein MF: Urethritis. *In* Mandell GL, Bennett JE, Dolin R (eds): Principles and Practices of Infectious Diseases, 4th ed. New York, Churchill Livingstone, 1994, pp 1063–1074.

Stamm WE: Toward control of sexually transmitted chlamydial infections. Ann Intern Med 1993;119:432–434.

136 Prostatitis

Michael O. Kirkpatrick

Etiology

Prostatitis is one of the most common and important causes of urinary tract infection (UTI) in adult males. *Acute prostatitis* is fairly uncommon yet potentially serious in nature. *Chronic prostatitis* is more common and may cause persistent and frustrating symptoms. Both require proper recognition and appropriate therapy. Both acute and chronic prostatitis originate from ascending urethral infection, reflux of infected urine, rectal infection extension, or hematogenous spread. The most common causative agents include

1. Gram-negative bacilli (*Escherichia coli*)
2. Enterococci
3. *Chlamydia*
4. *Ureaplasma* (this may be a causative agent in "nonbacterial prostatitis")

Symptoms

A. *Acute bacterial prostatitis*
   1. Constitutional—fever, chills, malaise, myalgias
   2. Local—decreased urine flow, dysuria, perineal and back pain, nocturia, urinary outlet flow obstruction

B. *Chronic prostatitis:* exhibits a variable clinical presentation. The most common symptoms are associated with urinary outflow obstruction/infection and include
   1. Dysuria
   2. Decreased flow
   3. Hesitancy
   4. Dribbling
   5. Low-grade fever (possibly)

C. *Nonbacterial prostatitis*
   1. Characterized by a clinical presentation similar to chronic prostatitis, yet has no evidence of UTI despite the presence of leukocytes in prostatic secretions. Cultures of both urine and prostatic secretions yield no growth.
   2. *Prostadynia,* otherwise known as prostatosis, is also clinically similar to chronic prostatitis yet shows no inflammatory cells in prostatic secretions.

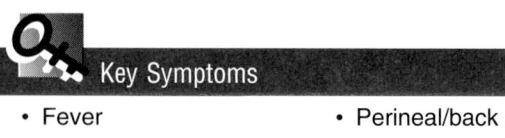

Key Symptoms

- Fever
- Dysuria
- Perineal/back pain
- Decreased flow

Clinical Findings

Gentle rectal examination (do not massage the gland) reveals a swollen, exquisitely tender, and boggy prostate gland, and often bladder distention is noted on abdominal examination.

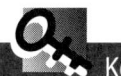

Key Signs

- Fever
- Tender, swollen prostate on rectal examination

Laboratory Tests

1. Expressed prostatic secretions should be examined when diagnosis is in doubt, and bacterial cultures should be obtained when necessary.
2. Care should be taken in patients suspected of having acute bacterial prostatitis because of the possibility of bacteremia.
3. Older patients with negative cultures should be evaluated for neoplastic disease, and cystoscopy and possible prostatic biopsy should be considered, especially if laboratory data such as an elevated prostate specific antigen (PSA) are present.
4. In order to accurately isolate the organism causing a chronic prostatic infection, a fractional urine specimen, along with expressed prostatic secretions, can be of benefit.

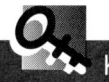

Key Tests

- Urinalysis
- Expressed prostatic secretions
- Urine and blood cultures if needed

Differential Diagnosis

The differential diagnosis of acute prostatitis is straightforward and readily evident with the findings of fever, dysuria, and tender prostate. Chronic prostatitis, on the other hand, may be more difficult and should include

1. Benign prostatic hyperplasia
2. Prostatic carcinoma
3. Urethral stricture
4. Bladder carcinoma
5. Neurogenic bladder
6. Interstitial cystitis

Treatment

Treatment of acute prostatitis, with its diffuse, intense inflammation, allows for many antibiotics to be used.

1. If a patient is hospitalized, intravenous antibiotics may be used initially. Protocols include

   a. Ampicillin/aminoglycosides (gentamicin or tobramycin)

   b. Intravenous cephalosporin with aminoglycoside

2. Once a patient is converted to an oral antibiotic, or if an oral agent is instituted initially, the following regimens may be used:

   a. Trimethoprim-sulfamethoxazole (Bactrim DS), 160 mg/800 mg (double strength) twice a day, is the preferred regimen.

   b. Ampicillin, 500 mg four times a day

   c. Tetracycline, 500 mg four times a day

   d. Doxycycline (Vibramycin), 100 mg twice a day

   e. Carbenicillin (Geocillin), 1 gm four times a day

   f. Ciprofloxacin (Cipro), 500 mg twice a day. Some studies indicate that fluoroquinolones may have better cure rates in chronic prostatitis.

3. All the preceding should be continued for at least 3 to 4 weeks to ensure resolution, and some authors suggest suppression therapy to last approximately 3 months. Regimens include but are not limited to

   a. Trimethoprim-sulfamethoxazole, 160 mg/180 mg once a day

   b. Ciprofloxacin, 500 mg once a day

   c. Doxycycline, 100 mg once a day

Diet

Diet may be altered to help patients avoid irritative urinary outlet symptoms.

1. Caffeine should be avoided, and over-the-counter decongestants should be discontinued.

2. Spicy foods should be avoided only if they cause an exacerbation of symptoms.

Activity

1. Activity usually is not restricted, and patients are encouraged to have a normal level of sexual activity.

2. If a patient has difficulty voiding, warm sitz baths may be of benefit.

Patient Education

1. Patient education includes a full discussion of the particular type of prostatitis and the understanding that prostatitis is *not* the equal of loss of sexual ability.

2. Patients also should be counseled that prostatitis is not the equal of prostate cancer.

3. Side effects of all medications used also should be discussed.

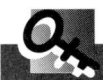

Key Treatment

- Antibiotic regimens and possible suppression therapy

Follow-Up

1. Patients with acute prostatitis should be re-evaluated 48 to 72 hours after the initial evaluation or after discharge from the hospital.

2. Subsequent follow-up evaluations would then be in 2 to 3 weeks and then 1 month after discontinuing antibiotics.

3. Follow-up of other types of prostatitis should be individualized to each patient. If symptoms persist, referral to a urologist may be warranted.

Bibliography

Cox CE, Childs SJ: Treatment of chronic bacterial prostatitis with temafloxacin. Am J Med 1991;91:1345–1393.

de la Rosette JJ, Hubrentse MR, Meuleman EJ, et al: Diagnosis and treatment of 409 patients with prostatitis syndromes. Urology 1993;97:301–307.

Meares EM Jr: Prostatitis. Med Clin North Am 1991;75(2):405–425.

Schwager EJ: Treatment of bacterial prostatitis. Am Fam Physician 1991;44:2137–2141.

Weidner W, Schiefer HG, Brahler E, et al: Refractory chronic bacterial prostatitis: A re-evaluation of ciprofloxacin treatment after a median follow-up of 30 months. J Urol 1991;146:350–352.

137 Benign Prostatic Hyperplasia

Neil K. Hall

Etiology

1. Exact cause is unknown.
2. Probably is prostate response to androgen hormones over time
   a. Does not occur in the absence of testes or androgen
   b. Begins in most men in their forties and tends to become symptomatic in their sixties
3. Fat in diet also may play a role.

Symptoms

1. Obstructive symptoms from pressure on urethra from surrounding prostate tissue impeding urine flow
   a. "Dynamic" component caused by α-adrenergic tone in muscle fibers in prostate gland and capsule and in bladder neck, contraction of muscle fibers causing increased pressure on urethra
   b. "Static" component caused by glandular mass impinging on urethra
2. Irritative symptoms mostly from involuntary bladder muscle contractions and possibly bladder wall hypersensitivity

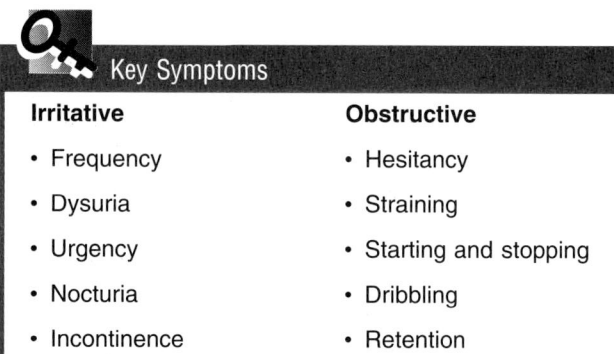

Key Symptoms	
Irritative	**Obstructive**
• Frequency	• Hesitancy
• Dysuria	• Straining
• Urgency	• Starting and stopping
• Nocturia	• Dribbling
• Incontinence	• Retention

Clinical Findings

1. Prostate examination
   a. May be enlarged, but size may appear normal despite symptoms, because rectal examination detects enlargement of peripheral zone of prostate, but symptoms come from periurethral zone, which is not palpable
   b. Consistency usually rubbery and surface smooth. Nodules and areas of increased firmness must be considered possibly malignant.
2. Enlarged bladder may be palpable in severe obstruction.

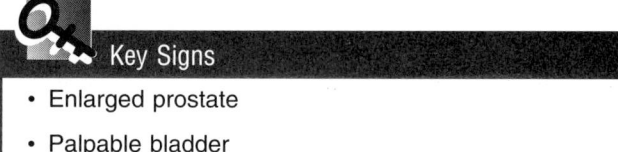

Key Signs
• Enlarged prostate
• Palpable bladder

Laboratory Tests

1. Urinalysis
   a. Pyuria suggests infection
   b. Hematuria may be a sign of malignancy
2. Urine culture to rule out urinary tract infection (UTI) if there are irritative symptoms or positive urinalysis
3. Blood urea nitrogen (BUN) and creatinine determinations to look for renal insufficiency
4. Prostate-specific antigen (PSA)
   a. Recommended by some to screen for malignancy
   b. Values above 10 ng/ml suggest prostate cancer
5. If retention suspected, abdominal ultrasound
   a. To detect hydronephrosis and other abnormalities of the upper urinary tract
   b. To check postvoid residual in bladder
6. Intravenous pyelogram (IVP) not generally recommended, because ultrasound is much safer and gives adequate information in most cases
7. Transrectal ultrasound
   a. If palpable nodule or elevated PSA
   b. Used by some urologists to estimate prostate size

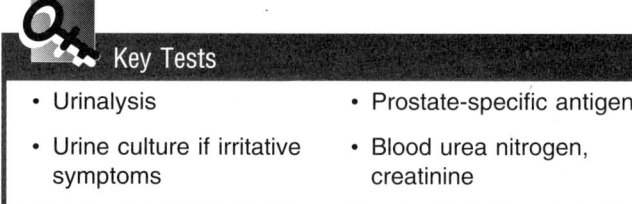

Key Tests	
• Urinalysis	• Prostate-specific antigen
• Urine culture if irritative symptoms	• Blood urea nitrogen, creatinine

Differential Diagnosis

1. Prostatitis, acute or chronic
   a. May cause irritative and obstructive symptoms
   b. Usually has a softer, more boggy gland, which may be tender, particularly if acute inflammation
   c. Positive urine culture common, except in nonbacterial prostatitis
2. Prostate cancer suggested by some signs
   a. Hard nodule or area on examination
   b. Hematuria, microscopic or gross
   c. Elevated PSA

Treatment

A. Mild symptoms

1. If not bothering patient greatly, consider no treatment, because many patients get better spontaneously over time.

2. Avoid medicines that can worsen symptoms.

   a. Decongestants and other sympathomimetics act on α-receptors to increase prostate muscle tone, increasing dynamic obstruction.

   b. Anticholinergics, such as antihistamines, bowel antispasmodics, tricyclic antidepressants, and antipsychotics, decrease bladder muscle contraction, increasing retention.

B. Mild to moderate symptoms

1. α-Blockers relax muscle fibers in the prostate gland and capsule and in the internal urethral sphincter, thus facilitating emptying.

   a. Terazosin (Hytrin) starting at 1 mg at bedtime (first dose may give dizziness or syncope if not taken at bedtime), increasing up to 10 mg at bedtime as needed and tolerated

   b. Prazosin (Minipress) and doxazosin (Cardura) also are used.

   c. Hypotension main side effect

2. Hormonal manipulation

   a. Finasteride (Proscar), 5 mg daily, is best, because of its effectiveness and lack of side effects.

   b. Other hormonal manipulations (estrogens, antiandrogens, gonadotropin-releasing hormone [GnRH] analogues) can be used, but only if finasteride is not tolerated because of adverse effects.

3. May use hormonal and α-blocker treatment together

4. Avoid medicines that increase obstructive symptoms (noted above).

C. Severe or intolerable symptoms

1. Surgery usually is required if significant urinary retention exists. Be sure to remove all drugs that might be contributing to retention before recommending surgery.

2. Type of surgical procedure used is quite variable.

   a. Transurethral resection of the prostate is most common, very effective, has few side effects, but may need to be repeated years later.

   b. Open prostatectomy is also often used; it has a higher risk but there is less need for repeat surgery.

   c. Transurethral incision of prostate, transurethral laser resection, and thermotherapy are still being evaluated for efficacy. Balloon dilatation is out of favor because of high recurrence of symptoms.

3. Urethral stent may be inserted if the patient is not a candidate for standard surgery.

   a. Can be placed under local anesthesia

   b. Preferable to chronic urethral catheterization or suprapubic cystostomy

4. Chronic catheter placement should be avoided because of risk of UTI and sepsis.

Diet

No dietary modification is usually needed.

1. Avoid caffeine and any foods that the patient finds exacerbate symptoms.

2. Despite possible role of dietary fat in etiology, effect of reducing fat is unknown.

Activity

No changes required.

Patient Education

1. Avoid drugs that can exacerbate symptoms or increase retention.

   a. Over-the-counter cold and allergy remedies

   b. Sedatives and over-the-counter sleeping pills

   c. Alcohol

2. Report any blood in the urine, UTI symptoms, and worsening of retention symptoms.

Follow-Up

1. If α-blockers used, check sitting and standing blood pressures weekly while titrating dose.

2. Evaluate symptoms and side effects every 6 months or so when treated with medications.

3. Annual rectal examination, as generally recommended for regular cancer screening (even open prostatectomy does not eliminate prostate cancer risk), with annual PSA recommended by most

4. Annual urinalysis

 ## Bibliography

For more information on medical treatment with finasteride (Proscar), see

Rittmaster RS: Finasteride. N Engl J Med 1994;330:120–125.

For more information on alpha blockers, see

Lowe FC, Stark E: The use of α-blockers in the management of benign prostatic hyperplasia. NY State J Med 1993;93:169–173.

For more information on the various surgical techniques, see

Petrovich Z, Ameye F, Baert L, et al: New trends in the treatment of benign prostatic hyperplasia and carcinoma of the prostate. Am J Clin Oncol 1993;16:187–200.

For a good overview of BPH treatment, see

Alexander W: New guidelines—and many options–for BPH. Patient Care June 15, 1994:18–27. *Note that this is a summary of* Benign Prostatic Hyperplasia: Diagnosis and Treatment. Clinical Practice Guideline No. 8. AHCPR publication no. 94–0582. Rockville, Md, Agency for Health Care Policy and Research, Public Health Service, U.S. Department of Health and Human Services, February 1994. Free copy available; (800) 358–9295.

138 Prostate Cancer

Timothy J. Wilt

Etiology and Epidemiology

1. Unknown etiology
2. Most common nonskin malignancy (incidence = 240,000 per year)
3. Second most common cause of cancer mortality in men (40,000 per year)
4. High prevalence of autopsy-detected asymptomatic cancer (30 to 40 per cent in men ≥ 50)
5. Mean age at diagnosis = 72 years
6. 10-year disease-specific survival for localized disease = 80 to 90 per cent
7. Risk factors: family history, age, black race, possibly vasectomy, and dietary fat
8. Generally slow growing. Poorly differentiated or large-volume tumors may grow rapidly.

Early Detection

1. Not yet demonstrated to reduce prostate cancer mortality and morbidity
2. ACS/AUA recommend annual digital rectal examination (DRE) and prostate-specific antigen (PSA) for all men over age 50 and high-risk men over age 40.
3. U.S. Preventive Task Force Services, National Cancer Institute, and the American College of Physicians state that there is insufficient evidence to recommend for or against early detection (see Table 138–1 for staging).

Symptoms

1. Usually asymptomatic: detected by DRE, PSA testing, or incidentally during transurethral resection of prostate for symptoms due to benign prostatic hyperplasia
2. Local symptoms: due to urinary tract obstruction; nocturia, urgency, frequency, hesitancy. May have more rapid onset than benign causes
3. Regional symptoms: lower extremity edema, hematuria
4. Systemic symptoms: back pain due to spinal metastasis, weakness, weight loss

Key Symptoms

- Asymptomatic
- Rapid onset of urinary obstruction
- Back pain

Clinical Findings

1. DRE: prostatic nodule, induration, enlargement, or asymmetry. Can be normal
2. May rarely present with hydronephrosis, adenopathy, back pain due to bony metastasis, or biopsy revealing "adenocarcinoma of unknown primary"

Key Sign

- Abnormal prostate on digital rectal examination

Laboratory Tests

1. Prostate-specific antigen greater than 4 ng/ml abnormal (can be elevated in benign prostatic hypertrophy or prostatitis). Normal PSA in approximately 40 per cent of prostate cancer.
2. Prostatic acid phosphatase (PAP) may be useful to evaluate for nonlocalized disease.
3. Bone scans generally not indicated in patient with PSA < 10 and no bone pain
4. Transrectal ultrasound: Evaluate hypoechoic areas of prostate for biopsy.
5. Transrectal biopsy or aspiration: Biopsy required for diagnosis

TABLE 138–1. TNM STAGING SYSTEM FOR PROSTATE CANCER

STAGE	DESCRIPTION
T1a	Incidentally detected tumor, ≤5% of resected tissue
T1b	Incidentally detected tumor, ≥5% of resected tissue
T1c	Impalpable tumor, detected by needle biopsy (usually because of elevated prostate-specific antigen level)
T2a	Tumor confined to prostate, <50% of lobe involved
T2b	Tumor confined to prostate, >50% of lobe involved but not both lobes
T2c	Tumor confined to prostate, involves both lobes
T3a	Unilateral extension through prostate capsule
T3b	Bilateral extension through prostate capsule
T3c	Tumor invades seminal vesicle(s)
T4a	Tumor invades bladder neck, external sphincter, or rectum
T4b	Tumor invades levator muscles and/or fixed to pelvic wall
N1	Metastasis to lymph node, ≤2 cm in greatest diameter
N2	Metastasis to lymph node, >2 cm but ≤5 cm in greatest diameter
N3	Metastasis to lymph node(s), >5 cm in greatest diameter

From Thompson IM, Teague JL: Genitourinary tumors. *In* Rakel RE (ed): Conn's Current Therapy. Philadelphia, WB Saunders, 1994, p 680.

Key Tests

- Biopsy and fine-needle aspiration of prostate are the only definitive tests.

Differential Diagnosis

Benign urologic diseases (prostatitis or benign prostatic hypertrophy)

Treatment

1. Clinically localized prostate cancer
    a. Watchful waiting: palliative therapy for symptomatic/metastatic progression
    b. Radical prostatectomy reserved for patients with life expectancy greater than 10 years.
    c. Radiation therapy: poor surgical candidates, high-grade malignancy
    d. Cryotherapy: new procedure; no long-term results available
    e. a to c appear to provide equivalent long-term survival. Recommended therapy should include treatment risks, benefits, comorbidities, and patient preferences.
2. Regional or metastatic prostate cancer: Therapy is palliative.
    a. Mechanical interventions
        (1) Transurethral resection/incision of the prostate (TURP/TUIP)
        (2) Stents
    b. Hormonal therapy (see Table 138–2)
        (1) Bilateral orchiectomy
        (2) Medical orchiectomy: diethylstilbestrol, antiandrogens, LHRH analogues
        (3) Maximum androgen blockade: combination LHRH analogue and antiandrogen
    c. Radiation therapy
    d. Chemotherapy

Key Treatment (Clinically Localized Disease)

- Watchful waiting
- Radical prostatectomy
- Radiation

Follow-Up

1. At 3- to 6-month intervals with digital rectal examination and PSA

TABLE 138–2. OPTIONS FOR HORMONAL TREATMENT OF PROSTATE CANCER

Treatment	Advantage	Disadvantage
Bilateral orchiectomy	Inexpensive 100% compliance Minimal morbidity	Hot flashes Psychological effect Decreased libido/erections
Estrogens (oral)	Inexpensive	High risk of cardiovascular/thromboembolic complications Gynecomastia Hot flashes Decreased libido/erections
Luteinizing hormone-releasing hormone agonists	Convenient (q month dosing)	Very expensive Flare phenomenon Decreased libido/erections
Antiandrogens	Maintenance of potency	Very expensive Elevated testosterone
Combined androgen blockade	Possibly improved survival	Extremely expensive Combines complications of antiandrogen and either LHRH agonist or orchiectomy

From Thompson IM, Teague JL: Genitourinary tumors. *In* Rakel RE (ed): Conn's Current Therapy. Philadelphia, WB Saunders, 1994, p 680.

2. Annual bone scan; less frequent if patient stable
3. Hemoglobin, PAP, liver function tests if suspicious for metastatic disease
4. Evaluate for complications of prostatectomy or radiation (impotence/incontinence)

 ## Bibliography

Chodak GW, Thisted RA, Gerber GS, et al: Results of conservative management of clinically localized prostate cancer. N Engl J Med 1994;330:242–248.

Fleming C, Wasson JH, Albertsen PC, et al: A decision analysis of alternative treatment strategies for clinically localized prostate cancer. JAMA 1993;269:2650–2658.

Garnick MB: Prostate cancer: Screening, diagnosis, and management. Ann Intern Med 1993;118:804–818.

Pienta KJ, Esper PS: Risk factors for prostate cancer. Ann Intern Med 1993;118:793–803.

Wasson JH, Cushman CC, Bruskewitz RC, et al: A structured literature review of treatment for localized prostate cancer. Arch Fam Med 1993;2:487–493.

Wilt TJ, Brawer MK: The Prostate Cancer Intervention versus Observation Trial: A randomized trial comparing radical prostatectomy versus expectant management for the treatment of clinically localized prostate cancer. J Urol 1994;152:1910–1914.

139 Kidney Cancer

Joseph O'Gorman

Etiology

1. Aberration of the short arm of chromosome three.

   a. Found in nearly all sporadic renal cell tumors when sought by polymerase chain reaction.

   b. Near to the locus of von Hippel–Lindau disease, which has renal cell carcinoma as one of its defining features.

   c. Hereditary renal cell carcinoma was the first disease shown to be co-inherited with a definite genotypic abnormality; this abnormality involves a translocation about the short arm of chromosome three.

2. Weak but definite association with tobacco use, male sex, and cadmium exposure.

3. Arises from the proximal tubule.

4. Adenoma to carcinoma progression strongly suspected but not proven.

5. The loci for Wilms' tumor types 1 and 2 also have been mapped. They have recently been sequenced.

Symptoms

1. Unfortunately, remains asymptomatic until late stages in many cases. Often found incidentally during radiologic workup of unrelated medical problem.

2. Macroscopic hematuria is the most common presenting symptom. Unless etiology is clear and renal cell carcinoma unlikely, always work up hematuria. Never ignore hematuria in the anticoagulated patient.

3. Fever, which varies from low grade to hectic.

4. Flank pain, which is usually dull and constant. It can be severe if bleeding or infarction of the tumor has occurred.

5. Weight loss

6. A strong family history in those with the rare diseases of von Hippel–Lindau or hereditary renal cell carcinoma.

Clinical Findings

1. Acute varicocele in up to 11 per cent of cases. Usually left-sided and does not reduce in the recumbent position. The association is common enough that the onset of a new varicocele should prompt the search for a renal mass.

2. The kidney is difficult to palpate in adults, and the signs are mainly confined to confirming the patient's symptoms or the discovery of an unsuspected mass on routine physical examination.

3. Microscopic hematuria

4. Rubor with polycythemia, hypertension, and other paraneoplastic phenomena can be seen, and rarely, amyloidosis. Most of the paraneoplastic phenomena are causes of laboratory abnormalities, as will be noted below.

Laboratory Tests

Diagnosis is done by roentgenographic means.

1. Renal ultrasound is a sensitive and specific screen to evaluate suspected renal masses. If strict criteria for a simple cyst are met, then the evaluation is complete. However, do not accept simple cysts as causes of hematuria.

2. All other masses should be evaluated by computed tomography (CT) with intravenous contrast enhancement of the abdomen and pelvis.

3. Vena cavography has been almost wholly supplanted by magnetic resonance imaging (MRI), and arteriography is necessary only rarely to define a suspected aberrant blood supply prior to surgery.

4. Cyst puncture is a controversial but reasonable procedure to evaluate those cysts which do not meet strict criteria for a simple cyst such as those with slight debris that settles with gravity or a singular delicate septation. Most clinicians elect to simply follow these patients with repeat imaging at defined future times such as 1, 6, and 12 months. Complex cysts should not be punctured.

5. MRI may not be adequate to define the extent of abdominal and pelvic disease but is complementary to other imaging procedures because of its superior visualization of the renal vein and inferior vena cava.

6. Metastatic survey

   a. Technetium-99m bone scan

   b. Whole-lung tomography or lung CT

Staging

- I: within capsule

- II: within Gerota's fascia

- III: regional lymph node, renal vein, or inferior vena cava involvement

- IV: distant metastases other than ipsilateral adrenal gland

---

c. Head CT or other studies only as clinically indicated

7. Staging is also done by roentgenographic means.

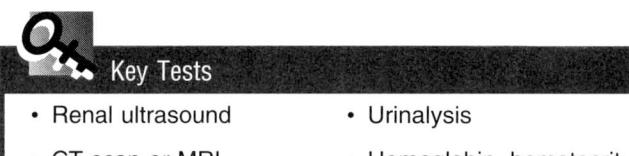

Key Tests

• Renal ultrasound	• Urinalysis
• CT scan or MRI	• Hemoglobin, hematocrit

Laboratory Findings

A. Common
   1. Elevated sedimentation rate
   2. Anemia
   3. Abnormal liver function tests, even in absence of metastatic disease
   4. Microscopic hematuria when the tumor has encroached the collecting system

B. Uncommon
   1. Polycythemia
   2. Hypercalcemia
   3. Increased cortisol

Differential Diagnosis

1. Renal abscess
2. Xanthogranulomatous pyelonephritis
3. Renal cyst
4. Angiomyolipoma
5. Distorted kidney from prior infection, infarction, or congenital anomaly
6. Granuloma
7. Metastasis to the kidney
   a. More common than primary tumors
   b. Rarely clinically significant
8. Numerous types of rare benign and malignant tumors. See Bibliography.
   a. Oncocytoma is only benign tumor seen with any regularity. Difficult to differentiate on clinical grounds and is usually diagnosed at nephrectomy.
   b. There is an adult form of Wilms' tumor. It should be treated with combined surgical, radiation, and drug therapy as in children, although the prognosis is worse in adults. It is relatively rare.

Treatment

1. Every effort should be made to treat surgically all but stage IV tumors with radical nephrectomy and regional lymphadenectomy. The 2-year survival for disseminated disease is less than 5 per cent with or without adjuvant treatment.
2. Renal cell carcinoma is relatively radioresistant. Radiation has not been shown to affect survival but improves local recurrence rate and can often give palliation of bone pain. Rarely, it can halt or reverse neurologic deficits secondary to distant or local metastases.
3. Chemotherapy
   a. Vinblastine is most effective single agent and is included in most regimens.
   b. Chemotherapy trials to date have been disappointing.
   c. Most patients should be followed in clinical trials.
4. Immunotherapy
   a. Both interferon-α and interleukin-2 are modestly effective. Other cytokines show promise. Complete and durable remissions have occasionally been achieved, and survival is improved. Dose-finding trials, combination regimens, and use of lymphocyte-activated killer cells are all being actively investigated at this time.
   b. Xenogeneic immune RNA and bacillus Calmette-Guérin (BCG) vaccines have been under investigation for some time and show slight promise.
   c. Use of nephrectomy to induce regression of metastases, the "mother-daughter" phenomenon, is limited to case reports. It has not been seen in several large series. Although a real occurrence, this phenomenon is sufficiently rare that it should not be offered to patients. The mortality of nephrectomy is as high as 5 per cent in some series. If done at all, it should be done in conjunction with passive or active immunotherapy.
5. Hormonal therapy is of limited effectiveness. Newer trials do not bear out the 5 to 17 per cent response rates seen in studies prior to 1976.
6. Solitary metastases
   a. Surgical removal dramatically improves survival.
   b. Pulmonary metastasis and long duration of time between original diagnosis and finding of metastasis favorably alter prognosis.
7. Bilateral disease or tumor in a solitary kidney can be treated by partial nephrectomy or workbench surgery and autotransplantation. Results approach those of radical nephrectomy. Some argue that the reason for the poorer results of the less aggressive approach is that at least some of these cases represent stage IV disease with spread from one kidney to the other. Asynchronous bilateral disease worsens the prognosis.

Patient Education
1. Necessity of follow-up and compliance
2. Cessation of tobacco use
3. Community resources
4. Rare need for pedigree analysis and family screening

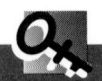

Key Treatment

Stage IV Tumors

- Radical nephrectomy

- Regional lymphadenectomy

Follow-Up

Different centers use different protocols.

1. Imaging and examination at 1 or 2 months and then every 6 months for 2 to 5 years.

2. For diffusely metastatic disease or prohibitive surgical risk, follow-up dictated by treatment protocol or doctor-patient agreement.

3. Lifelong clinical follow-up.

The opinions and assertions contained herein are the private views of the author and are not to be construed as the official policy or position of the U.S. government, the Department of Defense, or the Department of the Air Force.

Bibliography

Angland P, Tory K, Brauch H, et al: Molecular analysis of genetic changes in the origin and development of renal cell carcinoma. Cancer 1991;51:1071–1077.

Cohen AJ, Li FP, Berg S, et al: Hereditary renal cell carcinoma associated with a chromosomal translocation. N Engl J Med 1979;301:592–595.

deKernion JB, Belldegrun A: Renal tumors. *In* Walsh PC, Retik AB, Stamey TA, Vaughan ED (eds): Campbell's Urology, 6th ed, vol 2. Philadelphia, WB Saunders, 1992, pp 1053–1093.

Garnick MB, Richie JP: Primary neoplasms of the kidney and renal pelvis. *In* Schrier RW, Gottschalk CW (eds): Diseases of the Kidney, 5th ed, vol 1. Boston, Little, Brown, 1993, pp 785–809.

140 Bladder Cancer

David L. Hall

Etiology

1. Approximately 50,000 cases of bladder cancer are diagnosed annually, and bladder cancer accounts for about 3 per cent of all cancer deaths in the United States.

2. Among males, it is the fourth most common cause of cancer after lung, colorectal, and prostate.

3. Among females, it is the eighth most common form of cancer.

4. It occurs most often after the fifth decade of life; median age of diagnosis is 67 to 70.

5. Two to three times more common in men, it is more common in industrialized nations and urban areas.

6. Risk factors

   a. Occupational exposures account for one fourth to one third of all cases. Primarily related to aromatic amines used in synthesis of dyes in textiles, printing, plastic, rubber, and cable industries. Those at risk include automobile workers, painters, truck drivers, machinists, and workers in textile and paper manufacturing.

   b. Smoking accounts for about one third of all cases. Fourfold higher incidence of bladder cancer among smokers versus nonsmokers; risk correlates with the number of cigarettes smoked and the number of years the individual has smoked.

   c. Analgesics—Increased incidence of bladder cancer is seen in patients who ingest large amounts of analgesics containing phenacetin.

   d. Long-term use of cyclophosphamide

   e. Recurrent nephrolithiasis

   f. Recurrent urinary tract infections (UTIs), particularly associated with *Schistosoma haematobium* infections. This is a common infection in the Middle East; 10 to 40 per cent of malignant tumors in Egypt are associated with *Schistosoma*.

   g. Caffeine has been implicated in some studies; others show no increased risk.

   h. Artificial sweeteners and excess alcohol use have been proposed as risk factors, but this is controversial.

   i. Endogenous tryptophan metabolites—Some studies have shown increased urinary tryptophan metabolite levels in bladder cancer patients; however, current studies suggest that tryptophan metabolites are not a factor in bladder cancer. The role of endogenous metabolites in bladder cancer is controversial.

Symptoms

1. Hematuria (especially painless hematuria)—seen in 75 per cent of patients

2. Signs of bladder irritability

   a. Dysuria—in 25 per cent of patients

   b. Urinary frequency—in 25 per cent of patients

   c. Urgency—in 25 per cent of patients

3. Ureteral obstruction and pelvic pain seen in a minority of patients

4. Patients may occasionally present with symptoms of advanced disease, such as weight loss and abdominal or bone pain.

Key Symptoms

• Painless hematuria

• Signs of bladder irritability

Clinical Findings

1. Physical examination is often unremarkable.

2. Hematuria on urinalysis

3. Urinary cytology; cystoscopy with biopsies needed for diagnosis

4. Cell types

   a. Transitional cell cancer—about 90 per cent of cases

   b. Squamous cell cancer—about 5 per cent of cases

   c. Mixed cell cancer—about 5 per cent of cases

   d. Adenocarcinoma—very rare

   e. Transitional cell has best prognosis.

Key Sign

• Hematuria

Laboratory and Other Tests

1. Urine cytology

2. Cystoscopy with multiple biopsies

3. Intravenous pyelogram (IVP)—unilateral or bilateral ureteral obstruction, hydronephrosis, filling defects, or lack of bladder distensibility suggests cancer

4. Serum chemistries, chest radiogram, and computed tomographic (CT) scan of abdomen and pelvis needed for staging

5. In general, magnetic resonance imaging (MRI) is not more helpful than CT for staging.

563

Key Tests

- IVP
- Urine cytology
- Cystoscopy with biopsies

Differential Diagnosis

1. Renal pelvic tumors
   a. Also present with painless gross hematuria
   b. Pain and/or ureteral obstruction can occur but is rare
   c. Diagnosis suggested by IVP, which may show obstructed or nonvisualized kidney or filling defects in visualized kidney
   d. Cystoscopy will generally establish nature and location of tumor.
2. Nephrolithiasis
   a. Hematuria often present but rarely painless
   b. Signs of bladder irritability also can occur.
   c. IVP usually confirms diagnosis.
3. Urinary tract infection—Diagnosis is based on presence of pyuria and by positive urine culture.

Treatment

1. Depends on stage
2. Staging is based on Jewett-Strong-Marshall (JSM) classification of 1952 or the tumor, node, and metastases (TNM) system (Table 140–1).
3. Superficial (CIS, stage O and A)
   a. Endoscopic resection
   b. Between 50 and 70 per cent of patients have superficial recurrences within 3 years of initial diagnosis.
   c. Recurrences sometimes treated with intravesical therapy such as doxorubicin, mitomycin, interferons, or bacillus Calmette-Guérin (BCG).

TABLE 140–1. STAGING OF BLADDER CANCER

TUMOR INVOLVEMENT	JSM*	TNM
Does not invade mucosa	—	CIS
Invades mucosa only	O	Ta
Invades submucosa	A	T1
Invades muscularis	B1	T2
Extends over almost entire muscularis	B2	T3a
Extends into perivesical fat	C	T3b
Extends to prostate	D1	T4a
Extends to uterus or vagina	D1	T4b
Positive nodes below aortic bifurcation	D1	TxN + MO −
Positive nodes below aortic bifurcation or bone or soft tissue involvement	D2	TxN + M +

*Jewett-Strong-Marshall classsification of 1952.

d. Laser surgery has been used to treat some superficial bladder tumors and also in high-risk patients with muscle invasive tumors; however, laser surgery has not been adopted for general use.
e. About 12 per cent develop invasive or metastatic disease.
4. Invasive disease (stage B1,2, stage C, stage T2,3a or T3b)
   a. Radical or simple cystectomy most common treatment. Radical cystectomy in males usually accompanied by removal of prostate and seminal vesicles. In females, radical cystectomy usually accompanied by removal of uterus, fallopian tubes, ovaries, and part of vaginal vault.
   b. Radiation
   c. Cystectomy with preoperative radiation may be used, but studies have shown little added benefit of radiation therapy prior to surgery.
   d. Chemotherapy and radiation
   e. The 5-year survival rate is 40 to 50 per cent regardless of mode of therapy.
   f. Surgical techniques to improve quality of life in patients with radical cystectomy include Kock's pouch, Indiana pouch, and Mainz pouch. All these procedures are intended to allow urinary diversion by utilizing portions of small bowel as bladder reservoir
5. Metastatic disease (stage D2,TxN + M +)
   a. Chemotherapy: cisplatin, methotrexate, doxorubicin, cyclophosphamide, vinblastine, or combination therapy
   b. Erythropoietin sometimes given to ameliorate myelosuppression, which is often seen in patients undergoing chemotherapy
   c. Between 30 and 70 per cent of patients show initial response to therapy, but effects rarely last more than 6 months.
   d. Most patients with metastatic disease die within 2 years.

Key Treatment

- Superficial disease—endoscopic resection
- Invasive disease—cystectomy and/or radiation
- Metastatic disease—chemotherapy

Follow-Up

1. Superficial disease—cystoscopy every 3 months for 2 years, then every 6 months for 2 years, and then once a year
2. Invasive and metastatic disease—Follow-up varies

with invasiveness of disease and type of treatment used.

Screening

1. Urine cytology as a screening method has been done in workers exposed to industrial carcinogens, but this is not cost-effective for the general population.

2. Dipstick urinalysis for hematuria was utilized as a screening test in one study.

   a. Advantages—Test was inexpensive, and compliance of subjects was good (2356 out of a possible 3152 subjects responded).

   b. Disadvantages—Sensitivity of dipstick hematuria as a screening test is unknown. Also, specificity of hematuria as a primary screening test is low.

Bibliography

Catalona WJ: Urothelial tumors of the urinary tract. *In* Walsh PC, Retik AB (eds): Campbell's Urology, 6th ed. vol 2. Philadelphia, WB Saunders, 1992, pp 1094–1120.

Droller MJ: Cancer of genitourinary system. *In* Niederhuber JE (ed): Current Treatment in Oncology. St. Louis, Mosby-Year Book, 1993, pp 458–461.

Frazier HA, Paulson DF: Bladder carcinoma and uroepithelial carcinomas. *In* Schrier RW, Gottschalk CW (eds): Diseases of the Kidney, 5th ed., vol 1. Boston, Little, Brown, 1993, pp 811–834.

Garnick MB, Brenner BM: Tumors of the urinary tract. *In* Isselbacher KJ, Braunwald E (eds): Harrison's Principles of Internal Medicine, 13th ed. vol 2. New York, McGraw-Hill, 1994, pp 1338–1339.

Shipley WU, Kaufman DS, Griffin PP, et al: Radiochemotherapy for invasive carcinoma of the bladder. *In* Ackerman R, Diehl V (eds): Malignancies of the Genitourinary Tract. Berlin, Springer-Verlag, 1993, pp 207–216.

Procedure **CIRCUMCISION: GOMCO** *Timothy Ramer*

Indications
1. Nonmedical
   a. Parental preference
   b. Religious tradition
2. Medical
   a. Prevention of conditions requiring circumcision later in life; phimosis, paraphimosis, balanitis
   b. Some studies have shown a decrease in urinary tract infections, penile cancer, and sexually transmitted diseases in circumcised males.

Contraindications
1. Congenital anomaly of the genitourinary system which might be repaired by using the foreskin: hypospadias, megalourethra, webbed penis
2. Other major anomaly that may require major surgery
3. Any signs or symptoms indicating an unstable medical condition or bleeding disorder
4. Prematurity—Circumcision is delayed until discharge.

Preparation
1. Avoid feeding the infant for one hour prior to the procedure.
2. Perform dorsal penile nerve block (see Anesthesia).
3. Swaddle the infant's arms and torso with a blanket.
4. Immobilize infant's legs on circumcision board.
5. Scrub the surgical field with Betadine or other antiseptic solution.
6. Drape infant with fenestrated drape.
7. Inspect equipment tray to ensure that all necessary instruments are in working order.

Equipment
1. Gomco clamp with appropriately sized cone; 1.1 or 1.3 size cones are usually a good fit for term infants.
2. Curved mosquito hemostats (2)
3. Straight hemostat (1)
4. Blunt-tipped probe (1)
5. Tissue scissors
6. Sterile safety pin
7. Scalpel with No. 10 blade.
8. 4 × 4 sterile gauze (4)
9. Warm sterile water
10. Petroleum gauze dressing

Anesthesia: Dorsal Penile Nerve Block
1. Have an assistant restrain the infant with the knees flexed and the hips externally rotated and cleanse the injection site with a topical antiseptic.
2. Draw 0.8 ml of lidocaine without epinephrine into a 1.0-ml tuberculin syringe.
3. Identify by palpation the symphysis pubis and corpora cavernosa at the penile root.
4. Stabilize the penis with one hand and position the needle at the 10 o'clock position, 0.5 to 1.0 cm distal to the point where the penile root passes under the pubic arch.
5. Pierce the skin and fascia with the needle at an acute angle, directed slightly posteromedially. The depth of injection should be about 2 to 5 mm.
6. The needle tip should be freely mobile. Aspirate to avoid intravascular injection.
7. Slowly inject 0.4 ml of lidocaine.
8. Repeat the injection at the 2 o'clock position.
9. Allow 3 to 5 minutes to take effect.

Precautions
Remember that circumcision is usually an elective procedure and so should not be performed if there is the concern regarding a possible contraindication.

Technique
1. Inspect the external anatomy of the penis to identify landmarks, specifically the slight bulge in the foreskin caused by the underlying edge of the corona.
2. Grasp the rim of the foreskin at the 10 o'clock and 2 o'clock positions with the curved mosquito hemostats.

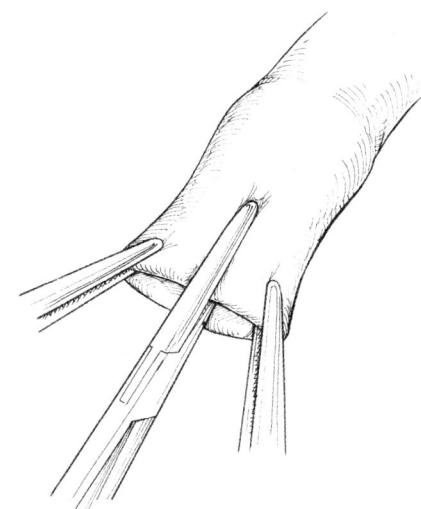

3. Insert the blunt-tipped probe just under the foreskin at the 12 o'clock position up to the corona. Sweep the probe over the glans penis, freeing the prepuce from the glans. Insert the straight hemostat in the closed position, open it and gently withdraw. This procedure assists in breaking down adhesions between the glans and the prepuce.

4. Make a crush line for the dorsal slit by inserting one blade of the straight hemostat under the foreskin at the 12 o'clock position to within a few millimeters of the corona. Close the hemostat and remove after a few seconds (see above figure).

5. Cut the dorsal slit along the crush line with the scissors. Make sure that the incision is confined to the crushed tissue.

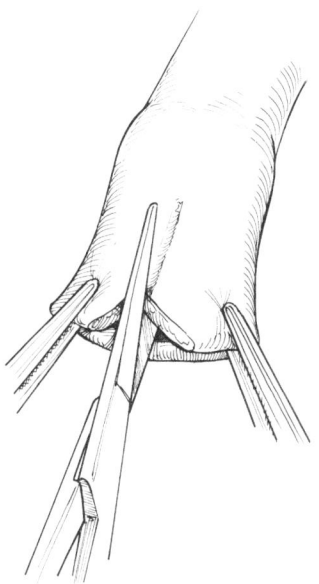

6. Inspect the glans to make sure that the urethral meatus is in the normal position. If you detect hypospadias that was hidden by the foreskin, stop the procedure and consult a pediatric urologist.

7. Retract the foreskin to expose the entire glans to the sulcus just proximal to the corona. Take down any adhesions with the blunt probe or by brushing with the 4 × 4 gauze. Be gentle while freeing adhesions on the inferior aspect of the glans because this is a common site of excessive bleeding.

8. Insert the cone of the Gomco clamp over the glans.

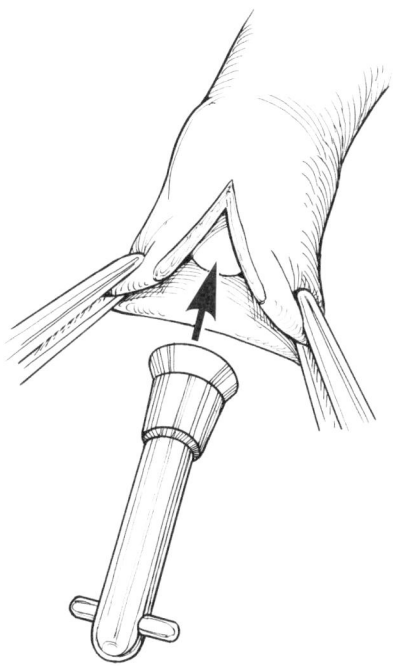

9. Draw the foreskin back over the cone, approximate the two edges of the dorsal slit and secure with the sterile safety pin. Remove the hemostats.

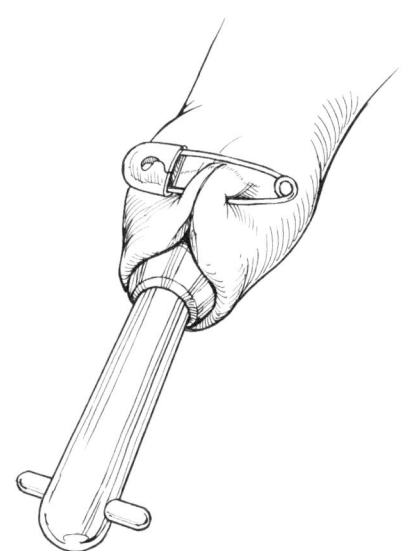

10. Twist the safety pin 90 degrees so that it is parallel to the shaft of the cone, then insert both through the hole in the base plate.

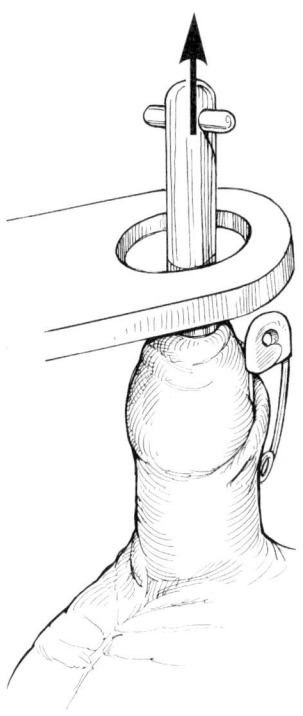

The curved hemostat may also be used to approximate edges of the dorsal slit and guide the prepuce through the base plate.

11. The top plate is hooked under the arms of the cone and slipped into place on the base plate. Inspect to be sure that a symmetrical rim of foreskin now lies above the base plate and that the entire length of the dorsal slit is visible above the base plate.

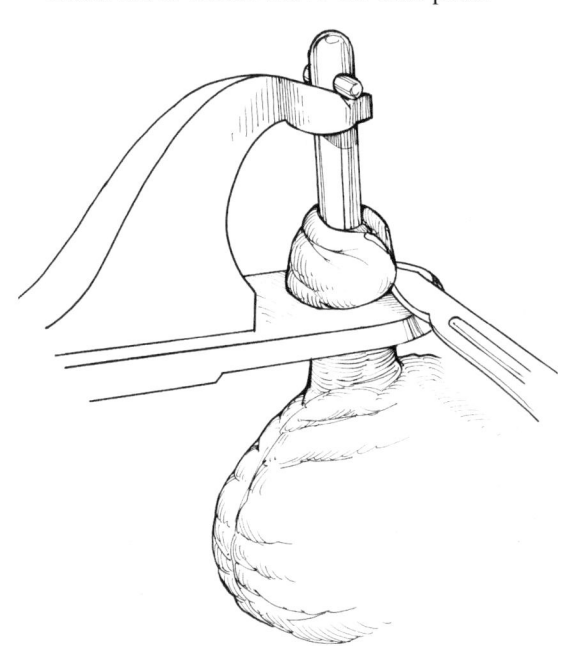

12. Attach the nut to the bolt on the base plate and tighten firmly. Trim off the foreskin just above the base plate, holding the scalpel nearly parallel to the base plate. Many authorities recommend that the clamp be left in place for 5 minutes to allow for hemostasis.

13. Unfasten the nut and remove the upper and lower plates. Gently brush the skin line off the cone with a 4 × 4 gauze.

14. Dress the area with petroleum jelly dressing. Extra gauze can be placed in the infant's diaper to supply additional compression.

Follow-Up

1. The infant should be observed for an hour to ensure that hemostasis has been achieved.

2. The parents should be instructed on how to gently clean the glans with water and to apply petroleum jelly to prevent adherence to the diaper.

3. Complications are rare but include hemorrhage, infection, urinary retention, urethrocutaneous fistula, foreskin adhesions, chordee, meatitis, and meatal ulcer.

4. Parents should be informed that in 1 to 2 days the healing glans will be covered with a yellowish membrane. This should not be confused with infection, which presents with redness and swelling of the glans. A fever, of course, may be a sign of a serious infection and warrants immediate attention.

 Bibliography

Fontaine P: Technique of neonatal circumcision. Personal communication, 1994.

Fontaine P, Toffler W: Dorsal penile nerve block for newborn circumcision. Am Family Physician 1991;43(5):1327–1333.

Hughes WT, Buescher ES, (eds): Pediatric Procedures, 2nd ed. Philadelphia, WB Saunders Company, 1980, pp 292–297.

Kunz H: Circumcision and meatotomy. Primary Care 1986; 13(3):513–525.

Schoen EJ, Anderson G, Bohon C, et al: Report of the Task Force on Circumcision. Am Acad Pediatr News 1989; 5(3):7–8.

Circumcision is one of the oldest surgical procedures known; it has been practiced as long as recorded history. While both the Gomco clamp and the Plastibell are used on newborn infants, the Plastibell can also be used to circumcise children up to 10 years of age.

Indications

Although there is no absolute medical indication for routine circumcision of the newborn, the procedure is performed on 80 to 98 per cent of newborns in the United States.

1. Promotes good penile hygiene (possible without circumcision)
2. Social custom or religious tradition
3. Prevention of:
   a. Phimosis—inability to retract the foreskin
   b. Paraphimosis—entrapment of the foreskin behind the corona
   c. Balanitis—inflammation of the glans penis
   d. Posthitis—inflammation of the foreskin
   e. Carcinoma of the penis (rare)

Contraindications

1. Genitourinary anomaly such as hypospadias, epispadias, congenital megalourethra, webbed penis
2. Sick or premature infant
3. Bleeding disorder
4. Imperforate anus, myelomeningocele

Preparation

1. Physical examination to rule out congenital abnormality
2. Sterile technique including gloves, drapes, instruments, and liberal use of Betadine or other antiseptic solution

Equipment

1. Plastibell (with ligature)—sizes 1.1, 1.2, 1.3 (most common), 1.5, 1.7 cm
2. Small curved mosquito clamps (2)
3. Small straight mosquito clamp
4. Blunt malleable probe
5. Straight tissue scissors
6. Scalpel (No. 11 or No. 15 blade) or small curved scissors

Anesthesia

1. Dorsal penile nerve block (optional)
2. Inject 0.3 to 0.4 ml of 1% lidocaine *without* epinephrine subcutaneously at the base of the penile shaft at the 10 o'clock and 2 o'clock positions, 1 cm distal to the pubic bone. Avoid injecting deeper than the subcutaneous tissue. Allow 3 minutes for anesthesia to take effect.

Precautions

Avoid performing a circumcision if there is any anatomic abnormality of the penis.

Technique

1. Grasp the distal edge of the foreskin at 10 o'clock and 2 o'clock with small curved clamps, being sure to catch both mucosa and skin. Pull gently while using the blunt probe to break any adhesions between the foreskin and the glans, taking care to avoid injury to the frenulum at 6 o'clock.
2. Place the small straight clamp between the two curved clamps at 12 o'clock.

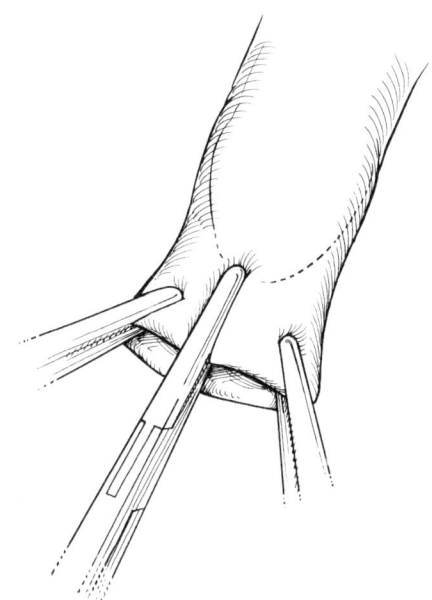

The length of the foreskin to be crushed should be approximately the same as the width of the glans. Making sure the clamp is not in the urethra, close it to achieve crush hemostasis and leave for approximately 10 seconds; then remove and use the scissors to cut down the center of the crushed area making a dorsal slit.

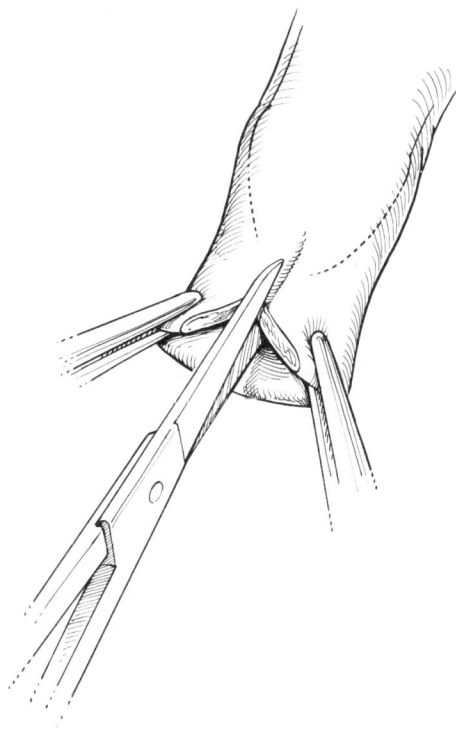

Do not cut beyond the crushed area to avoid bleeding. If the slit is too short it can always be extended, but it is difficult to retrieve one that is made too long.

> **Note**
> The dorsal slit for the Plastibell technique is shorter than for the Gomco so that the foreskin can hold the Plastibell in place while the ligature is tied.

3. Using the two curved clamps, retract the foreskin proximally to expose the corona and sulcus. Under direct visualization use the blunt probe to remove any remaining adhesions, again avoiding injury to the frenulum.

4. Select the proper size of Plastibell. The base should reach the corona without undue pressure on the glans and should not be so large that it extends beyond the corona, allowing the entire glans to slip through. If the bell is too small it may injure the glans and if too large it may slip over the corona onto the shaft. The apex of the dorsal slit should be distal to the bell's groove. The slit will usually be longer than shown in the next two illustrations. There should be approximately 1.0 cm between the sulcus and the groove of the bell where the ligature will be tied. A hemostat may be used to close the slit in order to hold the bell in place while tying the ligature.

5. Place the ligature around the base of the glans using a loose knot to hold it in place. With light pressure on the handle of the Plastibell, position the ligature in the bell's groove and inspect to ensure proper alignment and symmetry so that an even amount of foreskin is included around the entire circumference. Once appropriate positioning is confirmed, draw the ligature *tight* and tie with a surgeon's knot. Use the scissors to cut off excess ligature.

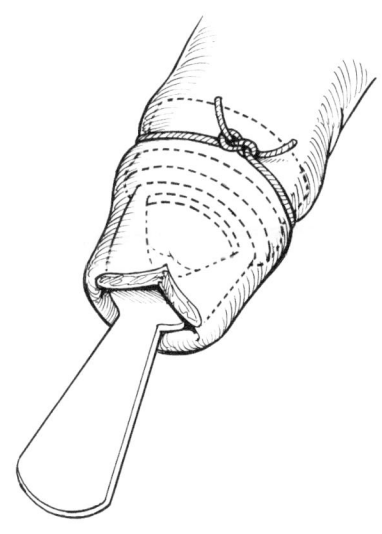

The tight ligature provides adequate hemostasis almost immediately.

6. Use the scalpel or small curved scissors to trim off the foreskin, with the outer ridge of the bell as a cutting guide.

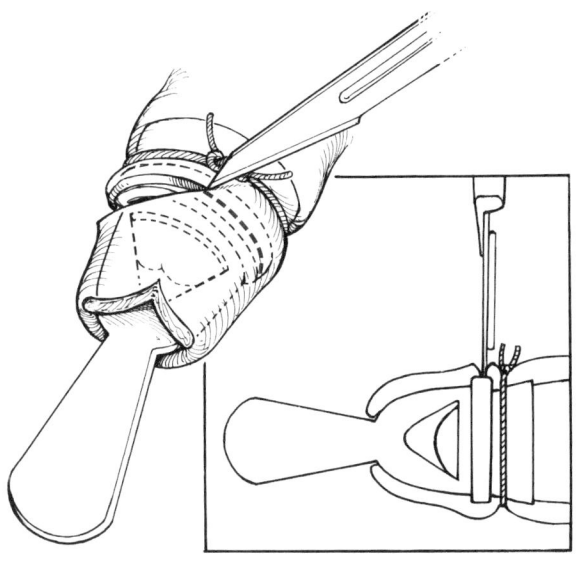

Maintaining slight traction on the foreskin while cutting will reduce the amount of remaining necrotic tissue, leaving a 1- to 2-mm cuff distal to the ligature.

7. Remove the handle by using a gauze pad to grasp the bell in one hand and use the other hand to break off the plastic handle.

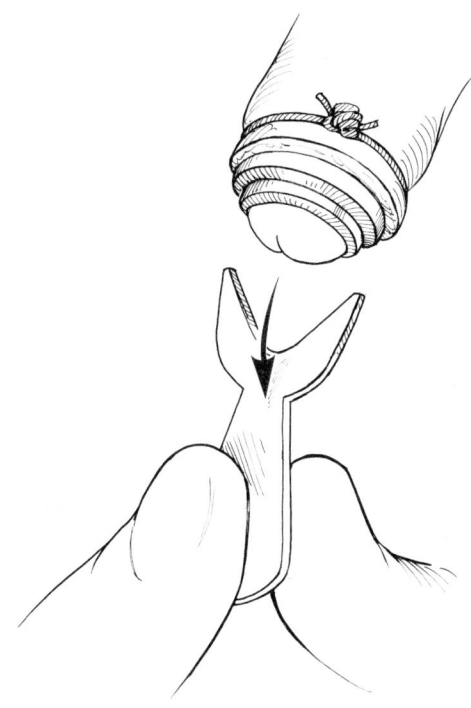

The handle is discarded. No dressing is necessary.

Follow-Up

1. Give the parents the follow-up instructions *Now That Your Baby Has Been Circumcised* that come with the Plastibell. This will avoid unnecessary concern and telephone calls before the next office visit. The bell will separate in 5 to 8 days, leaving a clean, healed line of incision. Remove the bell if it does not come off within 10 days.

2. Parents should confirm voiding over the next 24 hours and be instructed to keep the area clean by washing gently when bathing to avoid infection.

3. Complications
   a. Bleeding is much more common with the Gomco clamp and occurs with the Plastibell only if the ligature is tied too loosely or if the wrong size bell is used.
   b. Edema of the glans can occur if the bell is too small or if it is too large and migrates proximally, causing paraphimosis.
   c. Other complications are rare and consist of urinary retention, ulceration of the meatus, foreskin adhesions, necrotizing fasciitis, and urethrocutaneous fistulas. A rare but potentially serious complication of dorsal penile nerve block is methemoglobinemia, which can be induced by a variety of local anesthetics.

B Bibliography

Fontaine P, Dittberner D, Scheltema KE: The safety of dorsal penile nerve block for neonatal circumcision. J Fam Pract 1994;39:243–248.

Izzidien Al-Samarrai AY, Mofti AB, Crankson SJ, et al: A review of the Plastibell device in neonatal circumcision in 2000 instances. Surg Gynecol Obstet 1988;167:341–343.

Kunz HV: Circumcision and meatotomy. Prim Care 1986; 13:513–525.

Sorensen SM, Sorensen MR: Circumcision with the Plastibell device: a long-term follow-up. Int Urol Nephrol 1988; 20(2):159–166.

Sprinkle RH: Care of the newborn. *In* Rakel RE (ed): Textbook of Family Practice, 5th ed. Philadelphia, WB Saunders, 1995, pp 589–591.

141 Anemia Workup

Dominick Memoli

Etiology

1. Definition: reduction below normal of the number of erythrocytes, quantity of hemoglobin, or the volume of packed red blood cells (RBCs) in the blood

2. Mechanism: results from one or more combinations of three basic factors: blood loss, decreased RBC production, or increased RBC destruction (hemolysis)

Classification

The anemias can be broadly categorized into three major classifications according to the size or mean corpuscular volume (MCV) of the erythrocytes.

A. Microcytosis (decreased MCV)

1. Iron deficiency anemia

2. Alpha or beta thalassemias: inherited disorder, Asian and African varieties

3. Anemia of chronic diseases: chronic inflammation or infection

4. Sideroblastic anemias: acquired (anti-tuberculosis drugs, lead) or congenital

B. Normocytosis (normal MCV)

1. Normal variant: diagnosis of exclusion

2. Anemia of chronic disease (see above)

3. Acute hemorrhage

4. Endocrinopathies: For example, myxedema, Addison's disease, eunuchoidism, panhypopituitarism

5. HIV-related anemia

6. Dilutional: overhydration of patients or rehydration of a dehydrated patient

7. Sports anemia: runners, etc.; multifactorial (hemolysis, plasma volume expansion, gastrointestinal blood loss)

8. Mixed anemias: the presence of two or more causes for anemia, such as iron deficiency anemia and B_{12}/folate deficiency

9. Myelophthisic anemias: replacement of the normal marrow cells by leukemic, myeloma, or metastatic cancer cells or by myelofibrosis. Peripheral smear shows a leukoerythroblastic picture with teardrop RBCs, nucleated RBCs, and immature granulocytes (WBCs). Thrombocytopenia and leukopenia also may be present

10. Liver disease, such as hepatitis or cirrhosis; marked variability of RBC size and shape as well as color

11. Uremia: history of renal dysfunction; burr and spur RBCs on peripheral smear.

12. Hemoglobinopathies: For example, sickle cell anemia, hemoglobin C disease

C. Macrocytosis (increased MCV)

1. Pure red cell aplasia: drug-induced (gold salts, diphenylhydantoin), underlying malignancies (thymoma, lymphoma), viruses (parvovirus B19)

2. Alcoholism: unrelated to liver disease or B_{12}/folate deficiency. Bone marrow reveals vacuolization of erythroid precursors.

3. Aplastic anemia: bone marrow failure resulting from a variety of causes, such as drugs (chloramphenicol), radiation, viral infections, hereditary (Fanconi's anemia). Characterized by stem cell destruction or suppression leading to pancytopenia in the peripheral smear. Paroxysmal nocturnal hemoglobinuria (PNH) is an uncommon cause of aplastic anemia characterized by a defect in the RBC membrane that increases sensitivity to hemolysis by complement. Sucrose hemolysis and Ham acid tests are positive.

4. Myelodysplastic syndromes: anemia of the elderly characterized by peripheral blood cytopenias, bone marrow abnormalities with or without an excess of marrow blasts, and hypercellularity; megaloblastoid changes in the erythroid precursors; B_{12}/folate levels normal (see Bibliography).

5. Megaloblastic anemias: B_{12} or folate deficiency, hypersegmented neutrophils on peripheral smears, pancytopenia if deficiency severe.

6. Hemolytic anemias: variety of disorders characterized by reticulocytosis, erythroid hyperplasia in the marrow, increased levels of serum bilirubin, hemoglobinemia, hemoglobinuria, hemosiderinuria, decreased serum haptoglobin, and increased serum lactate dehydrogenase (LDH). The direct Coombs' test may or may not be positive depending on the type of hemolytic anemia. The hemolytic anemias may be divided into the following:

a. Extrinsic

(1) Antibody-mediated: immunohemolytic anemias (drug-induced)

(2) Microangiopathic hemolytic anemias: thrombotic thrombocytopenic purpura (TTP), disseminated intravascular coagu-

lation (DIC), hemolytic-uremic syndrome (HUS)

   (3) Toxins, malaria

 b. Intrinsic

   (1) RBC membrane defects: hereditary spherocytosis or elliptocytosis PNH

   (2) Hemoglobinopathies: sickle cell disease, thalassemias

   (3) Enzymopathies: G6PD deficiency, pyruvate kinase deficiency

Symptoms

1. Result from tissue hypoxia
2. Severe anemia can produce weakness, headaches, dizziness, and fatigue.
3. If the anemia developed slowly, the patient may be asymptomatic.

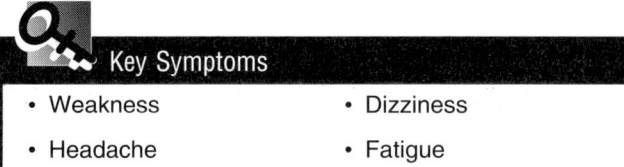

Key Symptoms

- Weakness
- Headache
- Dizziness
- Fatigue

Clinical Findings

1. On physical examination, orthostatic hypotension, tachycardia, and tachypnea may be present.
2. Jaundice and hepatosplenomegaly may be present (i.e., hemolytic anemias).
3. Neurologic manifestations, such as loss of vibratory or positional sensation, may be seen in B_{12} deficiency.
4. Evidence of underlying disease as cause for the anemia

Key Signs

- Orthostatic hypotension, tachycardia, and tachypnea on physical examination
- Jaundice and hepatosplenomegaly
- Neurologic manifestations

Laboratory Tests

1. Microcytic anemia: serum iron, total iron-binding capacity (TIBC), and serum ferritin; transferrin saturation; hemoglobin electrophoresis to identify thalassemias. Less commonly, free erythrocyte protoporphyrin (FEP) can be used to differentiate iron deficiency anemia from other causes of microcytic anemia (FEP) in increased MCV. Check feces for occult blood (see Table 141–1 for key tests and findings).

2. Normocytic anemia: evidence of underlying disease states with symptoms and signs of same, such as specific tests for a particular endocrinopathy based on clinical findings. Hemoglobin electrophoresis to identify hemoglobinopathies

3. Macrocytic anemia: serum B_{12} and folate levels, thyroid function tests. Hemolytic anemias (see under Etiology)

4. General: complete blood count (CBC) with differential and platelet count, reticulocyte count, peripheral smear, and bone marrow biopsy and/or aspirate in most cases

5. Most anemias can be diagnosed by history, clinical findings, and physical examination; for example, pica for clay (geophagia) or ice (pagophagia) is a very common manifestation in iron deficiency anemia.

TABLE 141–1. KEY TESTS AND FINDINGS

	Serum Iron	TIBC	Serum Ferritin	Peripheral Smear	Hemoglobin Electrophoresis	Bone Marrow	Other
Iron deficiency anemia	Decreased	Increased	Decreased	Hypochromia	Normal	Erythroid hyperplasia; No stainable iron	Increased free erythrocyte protoporphyrin (FEP); History of blood loss
α thalassemia	Increased	Normal or increased	Normal or increased	Basophilic stippling, target cells, nucleated RBCs, normochromia	Normal	Erythroid hyperplasia; Increased stainable iron	Diagnosis of exclusion; Asian type: more severe; African type: less severe
β thalassemia	As above	As above	As above	As above	Increased Hemoglobin A₂ Minor: 3–7% Major: 7–90%	As above	Mediterranean ethnic groups; Minor: mild symptoms and hemolysis; Major: more severe; iron overload
Sideroblastic anemias	Increased	Normal or decreased	Increased	Dimorphism: microcytic and normocytic RBCs, basophilic stippling	Normal	Erythroid hyperplasia; Increased stainable iron; Increased number of ringed sideroblasts, vacuolated RBCs	FEP increased
Anemia of chronic diseases	Decreased	Decreased	Increased	Hypochromia or normochromia	Normal	Increased stainable iron	Underlying chronic inflammation, malignancy

Treatment

1. General: blood transfusion support in patients (particularly the elderly) who are symptomatic from their anemia, that is, orthostatic, short of breath, having anginal-type chest pain

2. Microcytic anemia: iron supplementation in iron deficiency anemia, blood transfusions in chronic diseases or thalassemias (watch for iron overload)

3. Normocytic anemia: treatment of the underlying disease; in the case of uremic patients, administration of erythropoietin usually beneficial, transfusion support in the hemoglobinopathies

4. Macrocytic anemia: removal of toxic agents (drugs, alcohol, chemotherapeutic agents); in the megaloblastic anemias, the administration of B_{12} and/or folate will correct the anemia. In the extrinisic hemolytic anemias, the anemia resolves with treatment of the underlying disease, whereas in the intrinsic type, avoidance of inciting drugs in G6PD or PK deficiency and splenectomy in hereditary spherocytosis or elliptocytosis.

Key Treatment

- Blood transfusion (general)
- Iron supplementation (microcytic)
- Treat underlying disease (normocytic)
- Removal of toxic agent (macrocytic)

Bibliography

Bennett JM: The classification of the acute leukemias: Cytochemical and morphologic considerations, *In* Wiernick PH, Caniellos GP, Kyle RA, Schiffer CA (eds): Neoplastic Diseases of the Blood, vol 1. New York, Churchill Livingstone 1985, pp 201–217.

Lee RG: Iron deficiency and iron deficiency anemia. *In* Wintrobe's Clinical Hematology, 9th ed, vol 1. Philadelphia, Lea & Febiger, 1993, pp 745–839, 885–910.

Williams WJ, Bentler E, Earsley AJ, Lichtman MA (eds): Hematology, 4th ed. New York, McGraw-Hill, 1990, pp 175–187, 558–581.

142 Iron Deficiency Anemia

Thomas C. Lee

Etiology

1. Dietary iron deficiency commonly occurs in infants from unsupplemented milk diets and in adolescents.
2. Blood losses from gastrointestinal (GI) and genitourinary (GU) systems such as peptic ulcer disease, malignancy, or menstrual bleeding commonly occur in adults. Iron loss with each menstrual period is about 20 mg and in a pregnancy is about 500 to 1000 mg.
3. Previous gastric or small bowel surgery without adequate iron supplementation can cause anemia from poor iron absorption due to bypassing duodenum (the site of iron absorption), achlorhydria, and high intestinal transit time.
4. Other causes include blood donation (each unit of whole blood contains 250 mg of iron), phlebotomy, pregnancy, lactation, malabsorption syndrome such as celiac disease, intravascular hemolysis, parasitism by hookworms, and pulmonary losses from idiopathic pulmonary hemosiderosis or chronic hemoptysis.

Symptoms

1. Most patients are asymptomatic. Common symptoms attributable to progressively severe anemia are fatigue, exercise intolerance, headache, dizziness, faintness, exertional dyspnea, angina pectoris, palpitation, and claudication.
2. When the anemia develops over a prolonged period, these symptoms do not occur until the hemoglobin falls below 7 gm/dl unless there are coexisting pulmonary or cardiovascular disorders.
3. Pica, compulsive consumption of clay, is associated with severe iron deficiency, as is consumption of ice and other non-nutritive substances.

Key Symptoms

- Fatigue
- Dizziness
- Exertional dyspneas
- Exercise intolerance

Clinical Findings

1. Common features on examination are skin or conjunctival pallor, cheilosis, glossitis, brittle, ridged, or spoon nails, tachycardia, or evidence of congestive heart failure.
2. Esophageal web (Plummer-Vinson syndrome) on upper GI endoscopy and splenomegaly are infrequent findings.

Key Sign

- Skin or conjunctival pallor

Laboratory Tests

1. Peripheral smear is one of the most important tests. In early iron deficiency, the smear may be normal. Microcytosis, poikilocytosis, and hypochromia appear as iron deficiency worsens.
2. The diagnosis of iron deficiency is ultimately based on demonstrating decreased or absent iron stores, which may be estimated by measuring serum iron, total iron-binding capacity, and ferritin. When these tests are inconclusive, bone marrow biopsy is required to directly assess iron stores.
   a. Mean corpuscular volume (MCV) may be normal during early blood loss when iron stores are adequate, in mild iron deficiency anemia, in patients with liver disease, or in combined iron and B_{12} or folate deficiencies.
   b. Low serum iron also occurs in acute and chronic inflammation, malignancy, and infection.
3. Total iron-binding capacity (TIBC) is a measure of transferrin in terms of amount of iron it can bind. It is usually elevated (>300 μg/dl) in iron deficiency but may be normal or low in inflammation, infection, or malignancy.
4. A low level of serum ferritin (<12 μg/dl) indicates iron deficiency anemia. However, a normal or high level does not rule out iron deficiency because it is elevated in infectious, inflammatory, hepatic, or malignant disorders as well as chronic renal failure.
5. Transferrin saturation, measured by Fe/TIBC, less than 9 per cent indicates iron deficiency and more than 15 per cent indicates anemia of chronic disease. If transferrin saturation is between 9 and 15 per cent, bone marrow iron stain is required to further differentiate these two entities.
6. In iron deficiency, the reticulocyte index is inappropriately low for the degree of anemia.
7. Bone marrow iron stain is the "gold standard" test for iron stores. Decreased or absent stainable iron indicates iron deficiency. Adequate iron stores in the bone marrow rule out iron deficiency unless the patient has been treated recently with iron supplementation or transfusion.

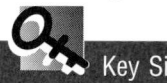

Key Tests

- Peripheral smear
- Serum Fe, ferritin, and TIBC
- Bone marrow biopsy

Differential Diagnosis

1. Iron deficiency anemia accounts for the majority of all hypochromic microcytic anemias.

2. Other causes of hypochromic microcytic anemias include thalassemic syndromes, hemoglobinopathies, anemia of chronic disease, and sideroblastic anemia, in particular, secondary sideroblastic anemia from intoxication of lead, isoniazid, and pyrazinamide.

Parameters from the complete blood count (CBC) provide clues to differentiate these entities. In thalassemia, the red blood cell (RBC) count is greater than 5.0×10^{12} per liter and the red cell distribution width (RDW) is less than 16; however, in iron deficiency, the RBC count is less than 5.0×10^{12} per liter and the RDW is greater than 16. As stated above, a high transferrin saturation indicates anemia of chronic disease. Another helpful test is serum free erythrocyte protoporphyrin (FEP), which is increased in iron deficiency anemia, anemia of chronic disease, and heavy metal exposure and normal in thalassemic syndromes and primary sideroblastic anemia.

Treatment

1. The optimal treatment includes not only treating the symptoms of anemia but also finding and treating the underlying disorder.

2. Transfusion of packed red blood cells is indicated if the patient has symptomatic anemia or if anemia threatens to damage the brain, heart, or other vital organs.

3. Oral iron supplementation is preferred to parenteral therapy to correct the anemia. Gastrointestinal side effects from oral iron therapy including nausea, constipation, diarrhea, and abdominal cramping occur in 20 to 25 per cent of patients.

4. Parenteral iron therapy is reserved for patients with poor tolerance, noncompliance to oral iron preparation, malabsorption of iron, or iron requirement in excess of replacement by oral supplement. The total amount of iron required is calculated from the following formula: milligrams of iron = (normal Hb − patient's Hb) × weight (kg) × 2.21 + 1000. The addition of 1000 mg is the amount of iron required to replenish iron stores.

5. The maximal reticulocyte response and rising hematocrit will occur 7 to 10 days after the initiation of oral iron therapy. Failure of the anemia to respond to the therapy within 5 to 8 weeks indicates ongoing blood loss, noncompliance, impaired absorption from gastric or small bowel pathology, or an incorrect initial diagnosis.

Medication

1. FeSO$_4$, 300 mg (60 mg elemental iron) t.i.d. on an empty stomach orally for at least 6 months, is needed to correct both the anemia and the depleted body iron stores. For patients with significant GI side effects from oral iron therapy, once or twice a day treatment for a year may be considered. Other ferrous salts such as gluconate and fumarate do not cause as many GI side effects. Sustained-release or enteric-coated iron preparations dissolve poorly in gastric and duodenal secretions; therefore, they are not recommended. The addition of ascorbic acid may aid iron absorption.

2. Iron dextran (Imferon) contains 50 mg of iron per milliliter and can be administered intramuscularly or intravenously. Intramuscular injections are painful, may stain the skin, and should be given in large muscles of the buttocks. No more than 1 ml on each side of buttocks should be given per day. Intravenous injections may cause phlebitis, and the dose should not exceed 2 ml/day. The rate of intravenous administration should not exceed 1 ml/min. Because anaphylactic shock occurs in 1 per cent of patients receiving intramuscular or intravenous administration, a test dose of 0.5 ml should be given before initiation of therapy, and epinephrine and diphenhydramine should be readily available. Fever, arthralgias, myalgias, malaise, lymphadenopathy, and splenomegaly may be seen 4 to 10 days after the injection.

WARNING

Rarely, anaphylaxis may occur with parenteral iron therapy.

Diet

Foods containing large amounts of iron include liver, red meat, and legumes.

Activity

In general, activity should be tailored to the patient's physical well-being and symptoms.

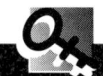 Key Treatment

• Ferrous sulfate, 300 or 325 mg t.i.d. for 6 months

Follow-Up

Patients should be followed in 6 to 8 weeks after initiating therapy with a CBC for observing the response to the treatment. Hemoglobin concentration should normalize by the end of 2 months of therapy. However, treatment should be continued for 6 months until iron stores are replenished.

 Bibliography

Cook JD, Skikne BS: Iron deficiency: Definition and diagnosis. J Intern Med 1989;226:349.

Fairbanks VF, Beutler E: Iron deficiency. In Beutler E, Lichtman MA, Coller BS, et al (eds): Williams Hematology, 5th ed. New York, McGraw-Hill, 1995, pp 490–511.

Green R: Disorders of inadequate iron. Hosp Pract 1991;26(3):25–29.

Massey AC: Microcytic anemia: Differential diagnosis and management of iron deficiency anemia. Med Clin North Am 1992;76(3):549–566.

Mohler ER Jr: Iron deficiency and anemia of chronic disease: Clues to differentiating these conditions. Postgrad Med 1992;92(4):123–128.

143 Megaloblastic Anemia

Wayne A. Bottner

Etiology

1. All megaloblastic states share a common pathophysiologic mechanism, interference with DNA synthesis.
2. Folic acid plays a crucial role in purine and pyrimidine synthesis. Cobalamin (vitamin B_{12}) is required for the proper metabolism of folate. Deficiency of either can ultimately lead to defective DNA metabolism and megaloblastosis.
3. Drugs may induce megaloblastosis by directly interfering with DNA synthesis (hydroxyurea) or by interfering with folate metabolism (methotrexate).

Symptoms

Three areas of involvement
1. Hematologic: anemia with resulting fatigue, pallor, intolerance of exertion
2. Epithelial (less common): atrophy of mucosal surfaces most commonly manifested by tongue or mouth pain
3. Neurologic (cobalamin deficiency only): paresthesias, weakness, gait disturbance, personality change, intellectual decline

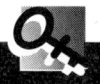

Key Symptoms

- Fatigue, pallor, mouth/tongue pain
- Cobalamin deficiency only
  —Paresthesias, gait disturbance, weakness, intellectual/personality change

Clinical Findings

1. Signs reflect areas of involvement
   a. Patients may be profoundly anemic at presentation.
   b. Pallor and mild hyperbilirubinemia can impart a characteristic "lemon yellow" hue to the skin in severely anemic patients.
   c. Tongue may be smooth as a result of papillary atrophy.
   d. Folate-deficient patients may show signs of malnutrition.

WARNING

Patients with cobalamin deficiency may have no hematologic abnormalities and present with neurologic signs only.

Key Signs

- Pallor (lemon yellow)
- Smooth tongue
- Malnutrition (folate deficient only)
- Cobalamin-deficient only
  —Diminished proprioception and vibratory sense
  —Spasticity
  —Dementia

Laboratory Tests

1. Identification of true tissue deficiency of cobalamin or folate is crucial for precise diagnosis and selection of appropriate therapy.
2. Evaluation should be carried out in two steps
   a. Establish deficiency of cobalamin or folate (or both).
   b. Determine underlying cause.
3. Serum levels alone may not accurately reflect conditions at the tissue level.
4. Peripheral blood findings are similar regardless of cause.
   a. Any or all cell lines may be affected.
      (1) Hypoproliferative anemia
      (2) Leukopenia and thrombocytopenia may be severe.
   b. High mean corpuscular volume (may be masked by coexisting Fe deficiency), with oval macrocytes on smear
   c. Hypersegmented neutrophils
5. Hypercellular bone marrow reflects ineffective erythropoiesis. Presence of megaloblasts is pathognomonic.
6. Elevation of lactate dehydrogenase (LDH) level may be striking.
7. Bilirubin usually is mildly high.
8. *Proving cobalamin deficiency and its cause*
   a. Serum cobalamin level has a relatively low sensitivity and specificity for tissue deficiency.
      (1) Serum or urine methylmalonic acid levels have been shown to be more sensitive than cobalamin levels. Availability may limit use.
      (2) Holotranscobalamin II level can also detect early cobalamin deficiency and may become the screening test of choice because of ease of performance. Availability may limit use.

b. The Schilling test should only be used to determine the cause of cobalamin deficiency, not to prove its existence. Incomplete urine collection or renal functional impairment can affect the results.

c. Anti-intrinsic factor antibodies have a high specificity for pernicious anemia, but only a 50 to 60 per cent sensitivity.

9. *Proving folate deficiency:* Serum folate rises and falls rapidly in response to fluctuations in dietary intake. Red blood cell folate is a better reflector of tissue levels.

Key Tests

- MCV
- Reticulocyte count
- Blood smear
- LDH
- Bilirubin
- Serum B$_{12}$ level
- Serum/red blood cell folate
- Methylmalonic acid
- Holotranscobalamin II
- Schilling test

Differential Diagnosis

1. Cobalamin deficiency
   a. Dietary: vegans
   b. Autoimmune: pernicious anemia
   c. Post-surgical: gastrectomy or ileal resection
   d. Inflammatory: Crohn's disease
   e. Infectious: bacterial overgrowth/parasitic
2. Folate deficiency
   a. Dietary: alcoholics/elderly
   b. Malabsorptive: sprue
   c. Drug: anticonvulsant
   d. Increased utilization: pregnancy/hemolysis
3. Chemotherapy: methotrexate/hydroxyurea/alkylating agents/cytarabine
4. Hereditary

Treatment

1. Cobalamin deficiency
   a. Intramuscular therapy essential except in vegans with dietary deficiency
   b. Cyanocobalamin (vitamin B$_{12}$) used most often: 1000 μg intramuscularly daily for one week, weekly for one month, then monthly, or at more frequent intervals if deemed necessary
2. Folate deficiency
   a. Oral folic acid will adequately treat all except those with malabsorption.
   b. An oral or parenteral dose of 1 mg daily is sufficient.

WARNING

Folic acid will correct the hematologic but *NOT* the neurologic manifestations of cobalamin deficiency. Accurate diagnosis is essential to prevent the erroneous use of folic acid in cobalamin-deficient patients.

Diet

1. Meat-based and vegetarian diets are generally rich in both cobalamin and folate.
2. Vegans should supplement their diet with oral cobalamin.

Patient Education

1. Emphasis on the importance of lifelong therapy will help to prevent relapse in those whose cause is not reversible.
2. Many patients can be taught to administer cobalamin at home to reduce cost and unnecessary clinic visits.

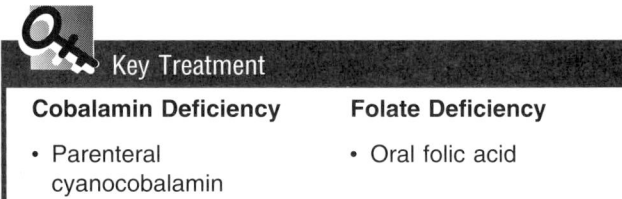
Key Treatment

Cobalamin Deficiency	Folate Deficiency
• Parenteral cyanocobalamin	• Oral folic acid

Follow-Up

1. Early follow-up is important to document response to therapy and rule out coexisting conditions (e.g., iron deficiency) that may interfere with response.
2. Periodic follow-up in patients on lifelong therapy may help to prevent relapse.
3. Pernicious anemia is associated with the development of gastric cancer. The ideal schedule for follow-up and the importance of early detection have not been established.

Bibliography

Babior BM, Stossel TP: DNA replication and hematopoiesis: Megaloblastic anemias. *In* Babior BM, Stossel TP: Hematology: A Pathophysiological Approach, 2nd ed. New York, Churchill Livingstone, 1990, pp 73–91.

Beck WS: Diagnosis of megaloblastic anemia. Annu Rev Med 1991;42:311–322.

Carmel R: Clinical aspects of megaloblastic anemia. *In* Bick RL (ed): Hematology: Clinical and Laboratory Practice, vol 1. St. Louis, CV Mosby, 1993, pp 437–457.

Lindenbaum J, et al: Diagnosis of cobalamin deficiency: II. Relative sensitivities of serum cobalamin, methylmalonic acid, and total homocysteine concentrations. Am J Hematol 1990;34:99–107.

Savage DG, Lindenbaum J, Stabler SP, Allen RH: Sensitivity of serum methylmalonic acid and total homocysteine determinations for diagnosing cobalamin and folate deficiencies. Am J Med 1994;96(3):239–246.

144 Hemolytic Anemia

Vincent A. Rella

Hemolytic anemia is defined as the premature destruction of red cells either within the intravascular space or extravascularly secondary to a variety of congenital and acquired defects.

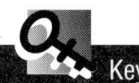

Key

*Denotes intravascular hemolysis
†Denotes extravascular hemolysis
‡Denotes primary red cell hemoglobin abnormality

Etiology

A. Acquired hemolytic disorders
  1. Hypersplenism
  2. Immunohemolytic anemia
     a. Warm antibody-mediated—IgG majority (†)
     b. Cold antibody-mediated—IgM/complement majority (*)
     c. Drug-induced—IgG versus IgM/complement mediated (* versus †)
     d. Alloimmuno—blood transfusion/fetal hemoglobin transfusion
  3. Paroxysmal nocturnal hemoglobinuria (*)
  4. Toxin and metabolic disorders (*)
     a. Arsenic- and copper-induced
     b. Bacteria-induced—*Clostridium welchii, Escherichia coli*
     c. Snake and spider bite—brown recluse
     d. Hypophosphatemia
     e. Spur cell hemolytic anemia (Zieve syndrome)
  5. Parasitic infection–induced (*)
     a. Malaria
     b. Babesiosis
     c. Bartonellosis
  6. Red cell trauma (*)
     a. Secondary to cardiac valvular disease
     b. Disseminated intravascular coagulation
     c. Thrombotic thrombocytopenic purpura
     d. Hemolytic uremic syndrome
B. Hereditary hemolytic disorders
  1. Membrane defects
     a. Hereditary spherocytosis (†)
     b. Hereditary elliptocytosis (†)—seen only in situations of splenic enlargement
  2. Enzyme defects
     a. Embden-Meyerhof pathway (*)

b. Hexose monophosphate shunt (*)—glucose-6-phosphate dehydrogenase deficiency
     c. Defects in glycolysis—pyruvate kinase deficiency (†)
     d. Thalassemia (‡)
     e. Hemoglobinopathies (‡)

Symptoms

1. Fatigue
2. Dyspnea on exertion
3. Worsening of pre-existing angina
4. Heart failure—high-output type
5. Postural dizziness
6. Left upper quadrant pain/fullness secondary to enlarged spleen
7. Palpitations
8. Right upper quadrant pain secondary to gallstones

Key Symptoms

• Fatigue

• Dyspnea on exertion

• Worsening of pre-existing angina

• Heart failure

Clinical Findings

1. Jaundice (*)
2. Pallor
3. Cholelithiasis (*)
4. Splenomegaly (†)
5. Positive family history for hemoglobinopathies or congenital anemia
6. Positive medical history for associated disease—systemic lupus, lymphoma

Key Signs

• Pallor

• Jaundice

• Positive medical history or family history

Laboratory Tests

A. Intravascular hemolysis
  1. Decreased haptoglobin
  2. Increased lactate dehydrogenase (LDH)

3. Increased indirect bilirubin

4. Hemosiderinuria

5. Complement-positive Coombs' antibody

B. Extravascular hemolysis

1. Normal haptoglobin, LDH, indirect bilirubin

2. Increased number of spherocytes

3. No evidence of hemosiderinuria

4. IgG-positive Coombs' antibody

C. General

1. Reticulocyte count—evidence of bone marrow response to anemia

2. Positive blood culture—evidence of gram-negative sepsis

3. Red blood cell morphology

Key Tests

- Coombs' antibody

- Reticulocyte count

- Peripheral blood smear analysis

Differential Diagnosis

1. Distinction between intravascular and extravascular hemolysis

2. Bleeding diathesis

3. Bone marrow failure/primary abnormality

4. Decreased bone marrow stimulant—decreased erythropoietin in renal failure

5. Laboratory error

Treatment

1. Supportive treatment

    a. Bed rest

    b. Oxygen

    c. Packed red blood cell transfusions to treat symptoms, not level of hemoglobin

    d. Folic acid, B_{12} if levels low

2. Specific treatment. Treatment in this regard depends on the underlying cause.

Key Treatment

- Make correct diagnosis of cause

- Aggressive relief of cardiac/end-organ hypoperfusion or ischemia

Follow-Up

There is no generally accepted follow-up schedule. Instead, follow-up should be on an individual basis according to the underlying cause and the patient's physical condition.

 Bibliography

Cooper RA, Bunn HF: Hemolytic anemias. *In* Wilson JD, et al (eds): Harrison's Principles of Internal Medicine, 12th ed. New York, McGraw-Hill, 1991, chap 294, pp 1531–43.

Lux SE: Hereditary defects in the membrane or metabolism of the red cell. *In* Bennett JC, Plum F (eds): Cecil's Textbook of Medicine, 20th ed. Philadelphia, WB Saunders, 1996.

Nathan DC: Hemolytic disorders: Introduction. *In* Bennett JC, Plum F (eds): Cecil's Textbook of Medicine, 20th ed. Philadelphia, WB Saunders, 1996.

Schreiber AD: Acquired hemolytic disorders. *In* Bennett JC, Plum F (eds): Cecil's Textbook of Medicine, 20th ed. Philadelphia, WB Saunders, 1996.

145 Sickle Cell Anemia

Loretta Bobo-Mosley

Epidemiology

1. Sickle cell disease is the most prevalent and serious hemoglobinopathy. It is a genetic disorder characterized by the production of hemoglobin S, an anemia secondary to shortened erythrocyte survival, microvascular occlusion by sickle-shaped erythrocytes, and increased susceptibility to certain infections.

2. In the United States, African-Americans are primarily affected.

3. Persons of African, Mediterranean, Southeast Asian, Caribbean, South and Central American, and East Indian origin also may be affected.

4. Hemoglobin S is transmitted by a Mendelian autosomal recessive gene. Hemoglobin S is designated β6 Glu → Val, indicating that glutamic acid has been replaced by valine at the sixth amino acid position from the N-terminal of the beta chain on chromosome 11. Hemoglobin variants are inherited as autosomal codominants. The thalassemias result from deletions or alterations of the alpha genes located on chromosome 16.

5. There is significant morbidity and shortened life expectancy associated with sickle cell disease.

6. The sickle syndromes' prevalence in African-Americans live births:

   a. Sickle cell disease

      (1) Hemoglobin SS disease (sickle cell anemia), the severest form of the disease, is seen in approximately 1 in 375.

      (2) Hemoglobin SC in approximately 1 in 835

      (3) Hemoglobin S–beta thalassemia in approximately 1 in 1667

      (4) Other variants: HbSO Arab, HbSD Los Angeles, and Hb SE occur with less frequency.

   b. Sickle cell trait, Hb AS, is found in 1 in 12 African-Americans.

      (1) Sickle cell trait is not a part of the sickle cell disease syndrome. The life expectancy of persons with sickle cell trait is the same as the general population. Persons with the trait should not have general restrictions regarding occupations, avocations, and participation in athletic endeavors.

      (2) There is convincing evidence of an association of the trait with the following: splenic infarctions at high altitudes greater than 15,000 feet, bacteriuria in women, hyposthenuria, hematuria, bacteriuria and pyelonephritis in pregnancy, and glaucoma due to anterior chamber hemorrhage.

      (3) The presence of the trait has been associated with otherwise unexplained rare risk for sudden deaths in military recruits. The U.S. military policy has no occupational restrictions for trait-positive recruits.

      (4) The sickle cell trait confers a protective effect against *Plasmodium falciparum* malaria and improves the quality of life by 20 per cent for the first 5 years of life for children living in tropical regions.

Diagnosis

1. Universal screening of all newborns for sickle cell disease is recommended regardless of racial or ethnic background.

2. Screening can be done in the prenatal, neonatal, and postnatal period. It is essential that the earliest possible diagnosis be made so that implementation of medical prophylaxis and appropriate medical access are ensured.

3. Diagnosis can be confirmed by one or more of the following mechanisms:

   a. Hemoglobin electrophoresis using cellulose acetate and citrate agar gel electrophoretic techniques. Hemoglobins F (fetal) and A$_2$ should be specifically requested to assist in identifying hemoglobin variants.

   b. Thin-layer isoelectric focusing on polyacrylamide gel, high-performance liquid chromatography, and globin DNA analysis are more expensive but offer superior resolution of variant hemoglobins.

   c. Sodium metabisulfite sickle cell preparations (sickle cell preps) and Hb AS solubility testing are not acceptable screening methods for newborns because the trait is not differentiated from the disease status.

   d. Abnormality of the peripheral blood smear and complete blood count (CBC) should increase the suspicion of a hemoglobinopathy in a newborn.

Key Symptoms

- Generalized pain in long bones, joints
- Abdominal pain, nausea, vomiting, decreased appetite
- Swelling in hands, feet, joints
- Fever, fatigue, malaise

Clinical Findings

1. Sickle cell disease is characterized by chronic hemolytic anemia, painful episodes, susceptibility to infections, and periodic acute anemic episodes. Virtually no organ is spared from complications of sickle cell disease, and there are tremendous variations among patient manifestations.

2. Chronic hemolytic anemia and other hematologic findings:

   a. Anemia occurs within first 3 to 6 months of life.

   b. Average blood hemoglobin level is 8 ± 2 gm/dl. Average white blood cell (WBC) count is 16,000/mm³.

   c. Peripheral blood smear may reveal sickled red blood cells (RBCs), target cells, hypochromia, poikilocytosis, leukocytosis, reticulocytosis, and thrombocytosis.

3. Acute anemic events. Acute decreases from the steady-state hemoglobin occur. Decreases greater than 20 to 30 per cent may be life-threatening and can require critical monitoring, blood transfusions, and occasionally surgery. Major etiologies:

   a. Hyperhemolysis—decreased hemoglobin and increased reticulocyte count secondary to increased rate of RBC destruction, febrile illness

   b. Marrow or aplastic event—rapid, severe decrease in hemoglobin and reticulocyte count, bone marrow hypoplasia associated with parvovirus B19, febrile illness, folate deficiency

   c. Splenic sequestration—rapid, progressive splenomegaly secondary to sequestration of large blood volume resulting in a decreased hemoglobin and increased reticulocyte count; seen mostly in children prior to splenic atrophy and in adults with hemoglobin SC and hemoglobin S–beta thalassemia

4. Acute vaso-occlusive syndromes (painful episodes or pain crises) occur as a result of RBC sickling, erythrostasis, and vascular obstruction. Factors that promote pain events: fever, dehydration, hyperthermia, hypothermia, strenuous exercise, regional hypoxia, mechanical trauma, acidosis, drug therapy, emotional stress, menstruation. May be multifactorial or unidentifiable cause.

   a. Lifelong suffering begins in infancy.

   b. Severe bouts about four times per year, but may have many mild episodes. There is tremendous variability in frequency, intensity, and debilitation related to individual factors. Pain may persist for 3 to 10 days.

   c. Hand-foot syndrome (dactylitis)—usually the first manifestation of sickle cell disease, seen as early as 3 months of age and persisting sporadically to age 5. Typically characterized by the triad of fever, pallor, and symmetrical pain and swelling of the hands and feet.

5. Other major consequences of sickle cell disease include:

   a. Musculoskeletal and skin complications

      (1) Marrow infarction of the femur, humerus, tibia

      (2) Avascular necrosis of the femoral, humeral heads resulting in limb girdle deformities

      (3) *Salmonella* osteomyelitis

      (4) Fishmouthing of vertebral bodies

      (5) Leg ulcers, particularly on the malleoli

      (6) "Hair-on-end" skull and frontal "bossing" on radiography

      (7) Septic, gouty, and rheumatoid arthritis

   b. Neurologic complications

      (1) Cerebrovascular accidents, transient ischemic attacks

      (2) Seizures, headaches

      (3) Altered mental status

   c. Pulmonary complications

      (1) Multiple lung infarctions secondary to thromboemboli and embolic particles of necrotic fat and marrow

      (2) Acute chest syndrome, which is characterized by the presence of pulmonary infiltrate, pleuritic chest pain, fever, and chest wall tenderness, interstitial lung disease

      (3) Frequent pulmonary infections from *Streptococcus pneumoniae*, *Staphylococcus aureus*, *Mycoplasma pneumoniae*, *Chlamydia pneumoniae*, viruses

   d. Cardiovascular complications

      (1) Cardiomegaly, heart failure rare

      (2) Cardiomyopathy, myocardial infarction

   e. Gastrointestinal

      (1) Visceral mucosal infarctions, paralytic ileus

      (2) Pigmented gallstones, cholecystitis

      (3) Right upper quadrant (RUQ) syndrome (hepatomegaly, RUQ pain), extreme hyperbilirubinemia, chronic jaundice, hepatitis, coagulopathy

      (4) Splenic infarction and sequestration syndrome

   f. Genitourinary

      (1) Isosthenuria, nocturnal enuresis, hematuria, papillary necrosis

      (2) Proteinuria, glomerulopathy, progressive renal insufficiency

      (3) Priapism, impotence

   g. Pregnancy

      (1) Increased frequency of vaso-occlusive painful episodes

      (2) Increased frequency of urinary and respiratory infections

      (3) Maternal mortality less than 2 per cent

(4) Oral contraceptives can be used safely in selected patients.

(5) Intrauterine growth retardation, premature labor and delivery

h. Eye, ear, dental

   (1) Hyphema, retinopathy, blindness, cataracts, arteriovenous anastomoses, icterus

   (2) Otalgia, sensorineural hearing loss

   (3) Mandibular infarction, dental abscesses

i. Endocrine

   (1) Hypogonadism, delayed sexual maturation

   (2) Somatic growth delay

j. Infections—increased because of splenic dysfunction, decreased serum opsonic activity

   (1) *S. pneumoniae* septicemia and meningitis are the most common causes of early childhood morbidity and mortality.

   (2) Pneumonias from *Mycoplasma, Chlamydia, Haemophilus influenzae*

   (3) Viral hepatitis A, B, and C; parvovirus B19

   (4) *Salmonella* osteomyelitis is most common cause of bone, joint infections.

Key Signs

- Chronic hemolytic anemia, tachycardia, fever, tachypnea
- Abdominal distention, jaundice, pallor
- Splenomegaly, hepatomegaly, cardiomegaly

Laboratory Tests

1. The hemoglobin genotype should be confirmed by cellulose acetate and citrate agar gel electrophoresis. The percentage of hemoglobins A_2 and F is helpful in determining the presence of thalassemia.

2. Interpretation of laboratory data is complex in sickle cell disease. Laboratory results vary by hemoglobin genotypes, age, gender, and presence of organ insufficiency (e.g., renal, hepatic).

3. There are significant variations in the complete blood count, RBC indices. Elevated WBCs do not necessarily indicate infection.

4. Platelet counts may be moderately elevated.

5. Increased indirect bilirubin, serum transaminases, alkaline phosphatase

6. Increased factor VIII activity, von Willebrand's factor antigen, thrombin

7. Decreased protein C, protein S

Key Test

- Confirm hemoglobin genotype by cellulose acetate and citrate agar gel electrophoresis

Differential Diagnosis

1. Sickle cell disease may resemble

   a. Thalassemias

   b. Iron deficiency anemia

   c. Other severe anemias, hemoglobinopathies, leukemia

2. Any acute or chronic organ insufficiency in a person with sickle cell disease may confound the diagnosis.

   a. Rheumatic fever, pericarditis

   b. Infectious hepatitis, meningitis, osteomyelitis

   c. Nephropathies, acute abdomen syndromes

Treatment

1. Vaso-occlusive (painful crises) episodes can be excruciating and debilitating for the patient. Therapeutic management of the pain can be difficult and a source of conflict between physician and patient/family. There are no objective laboratory findings to confirm the presence of pain, so a good relationship between physician and patient is essential.

2. Certain signs and symptoms require aggressive evaluation and management:

   a. Fever (oral temperature > 101° F or 38.5° C) requires evaluation for potential source of sepsis.

   b. Any illness or fever in an infant with sickle cell disease may result in a life-threatening medical emergency.

   c. Severe abdominal pain or acute pulmonary complaints

   d. Acute neurologic events

   e. Priapism

   f. Intractable pain unrelieved by oral medications

3. The general approach to pain management includes hydration:

   a. Maintenance oral fluids of 3 to 4 L/day

   b. Intravenous fluids for dehydration, acute illness

   c. Avoid iatrogenic fluid overload, particularly in patients with renal, cardiac, or hepatic insufficiency.

Medication

1. Drugs of choice:

   a. Non-narcotic analgesics: nonsteroidal anti-inflammatory drugs, acetaminophen

   b. Narcotic analgesics: morphine, meperidine, codeine, oxycodone, propoxyphene

2. Alternative drugs are usually given in combination with analgesics.

   a. Antihistamines (diphenhydramine, hydroxyzine)

   b. Tricyclic antidepressants

   c. Phenothiazines for nausea and vomiting

   d. Folic acid—helpful for most anemic sickle cell patients; increases hematopoiesis. Can reduce the role of blood transfusions and help patient recover from aplastic events.

e. Iron supplements indicated only for documented iron deficiency.

f. Oxygen is indicated for hypoxemic patients with Pao$_2$ less than 60 to 70 mm Hg. Use humidified oxygen, 40%. Oxygen can predispose to absorption atelectasis, damage pneumocytes and endothelial cells, cause an adult respiratory distress syndrome (ARDS) picture. Long-term exposure can cause pulmonary fibrosis.

g. Aliphatic butyrate salts and hydroxyurea are used to increase hemoglobin F.

h. Allogeneic bone marrow transplants and stem cell transplants result in cure, but not usually a treatment option.

Blood Transfusions

Essential in management of sickle disease complications.

1. Cerebrovascular accidents. Long-term exchange transfusions to keep hemoglobin S below 30 per cent.

2. Life-threatening illnesses

   a. Acute anemic events

   b. Acute chest syndrome with progressive respiratory failure

   c. Severe intractable pain

3. Complicated by

   a. Transfusional iron overload: Deferoxamine is treatment of choice.

   b. Acute and delayed hemolytic transfusion reactions

Diet

1. Ensure adequate caloric intake and nutrients to meet the increased demands for proteins and carbohydrates.

2. Multivitamins and minerals are beneficial (folate, zinc, vitamins E and C).

Activity

1. Patients with hemoglobin SS (sickle cell anemia) should be advised to avoid physical overexertion. When an active lifestyle is desired, such as participation in athletics or involvement in a physically demanding vocation, patients should be advised to tailor activities to their individual tolerance.

2. Avoid extremes of environmental exposure to heat and cold.

3. Maintain as normal a lifestyle and socialization as possible.

Patient Education

1. Patient education initiatives should be presented in a culturally sensitive manner.

2. Patient and family should understand the difference between sickle cell trait and sickle cell disease.

3. Patient and family should be knowledgeable of the disease course and be aware of key clinical signs and symptoms, particularly those that are potentially and swiftly life-threatening.

4. General counseling on travel, exercise, and healthy lifestyle habits should be provided.

5. Patient and family should receive genetic counseling and understand the transmission of sickle cell disease.

6. Effort should be devoted to psychosocial support

584

structures including self-help programs, development and maintenance of social skills (involving school teachers and others to assist with maintaining and achieving academic goals), and employment and vocation endeavors.

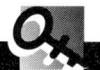
Key Treatment

Drugs of Choice

- Non-narcotic analgesics: nonsteroidal anti-inflammatory drugs, acetaminophen

- Narcotic analgesics: morphine, meperidine, codeine, oxycodone, propoxyphene

Alternative Drugs

- Usually given in combination with analgesics: antihistamines, tricyclic antidepressants

Follow-Up

1. Patients should have access to a physician or provider 24 hours a day.

2. Infants should be seen monthly for the first year of life and quarterly during the second year of life.

   a. All patients with sickle cell disease should receive the standard immunizations, including polio, diphtheria, tetanus, measles, mumps, rubella, hepatitis, *Haemophilus influenzae* type b (Hib), and the polyvalent pneumococcal vaccine.

   b. Prophylaxis against pneumococcal infections with twice-daily oral penicillin should begin no later than 2 months of age (even if the disease has not been confirmed) and continue for at least 5 years. *This cannot be overemphasized.*

3. Adults should be seen at least two or three times a year, but this is dictated by the status of their illness.

4. Health maintenance, disease prevention. Annual assessments dictated by age, gender, and disease status may include Papanicolaou smears, mammography, radiographs and abdominal ultrasounds, and pulmonary function.

Bibliography

Charache S, Lubin B, Reid CD: Management and Therapy of Sickle Cell Disease. Washington, U.S. Department of Health and Human Services, Public Health Service, National Institutes of Health, NIH Publication No. 91-2117, August 1991.

Embury SH, Hebbel RP, Mohandas N, Steinberg MH (eds): Sickle Cell Disease: Basic Principles and Clinical Practice. New York, Raven Press, 1994.

Mankad VN, Moore RB (eds): Sickle Cell Disease: Pathophysiology, Diagnosis, and Management. Westport, CT, Praeger, 1992.

Rodgers GP, Dover GJ, Uyesaka N, et al: Augmentation by erythropoietin of the fetal hemoglobin response to hydroxyurea in sickle cell disease. N Engl J Med 1993;328:78–80.

Sickle Cell Disease Guideline Panel: Sickle Cell Disease: Screening, Diagnosis, Management, and Counseling in Newborns and Infants. Clinical Practice Guideline No. 6. AHCPR Pub. No. 93-0562. Rockville, MD, Agency for Health Care Policy and Research, Public Health Service, U.S. Department of Health and Human Services, April 1993.

146 Thalassemia Syndromes

Vipul N. Mankad

Etiology

1. Definition: Thalassemias are inherited disorders characterized by hypochromic, microcytic anemia caused by decreased synthesis of one of the globin chains.

2. Historical aspects: In 1925, Cooley described a group of children with severe anemia, striking skeletal and facial abnormalities and splenomegaly, bizarre morphology of red blood cells, and circulating nucleated red cells. The term *Cooley's anemia* is frequently used to describe this condition. Early observation that these children were of Italian or Greek ancestry led to the term *thalassemia* (the sea in the blood).

3. Malarial hypothesis: Although severe forms of the disease (e.g., homozygous β-thalassemia) were invariably fatal in the first 2 years of life and therefore could not contribute to propagation of the gene, autosomal recessive thalassemia genes were maintained in certain populations because of the protection conferred against malaria in individuals with the trait.

4. Geographic distribution: Various forms of thalassemia are prevalent in Italy, Greece, Arabian peninsula, Turkey, Iran, India, Southeastern Asia including Thailand, Cambodia, and southern China, and in United States populations with ancestry from those areas; also in Africans and African-Americans.

5. Pathophysiology: The adult hemoglobin (Hb A) molecule is a tetramer of two α globin and two β globin polypeptide chains. When the synthesis of α or β globin chain is decreased as a result of one of the variety of mutations in the globin genes, imbalance in the synthesis of globin chains occurs. Excess globin chains precipitate in the red blood cells, aggregate into protein inclusions (Heinz bodies), and cause membrane changes resulting in hemolysis. Profound deficiency in synthesis of α or β globin chains results in marked reduction in synthesis of hemoglobin A and ineffective erythropoiesis.

6. Genetics:
   a. There are many mutations that account for β-thalassemia syndromes. Thalassemia major (Cooley's anemia), or "homozygous" β-thalassemia, is a clinically severe disease due to the presence of two identical or dissimilar mutations causing decreased β globin chain synthesis. The hypochromic anemia in these patients is so severe that dependency on blood transfusions is established at an early age because the hemoglobin levels decrease below 4 gm/dl. Thalassemia intermedia is characterized as a moderate disorder, usually due to two β-thal mutations, not associated with transfusion dependence. These patients have hemoglo-

bin levels over 7 gm/dl and have splenomegaly. Thalassemia minor is due to the presence of a single β-thal mutation and is characterized by microcytosis, hypochromia, and mild anemia; therefore, it is often misdiagnosed as iron deficiency anemia.

   b. The α globin synthesis is under control of two pairs of α globin genes (total of four genes). Four α-thalassemias are
      (1) α-thalassemia-2 trait or asymptomatic, silent carrier state
      (2) α-thalassemia-1 trait resulting from deletion or malfunctioning of two α globin genes and associated with mild, microcytic, hypochromic anemia
      (3) three loci of α globin genes affected as in hemoglobin H disease (a tetramer of β globin chains) associated with moderately severe hemolytic anemia, usually not requiring chronic transfusions
      (4) all four loci deleted or nonfunctional, which causes formation of hemoglobin Bart's (tetramer of gamma globin chains) and hydrops fetalis.

The α-thalassemia-1 trait (i.e., deletion of two α globin genes) can occur due to either removal of both loci from the same chromosome (*cis* deletion) or removal of one locus each from two chromosomes (*trans* deletion). *Cis* deletion is found in Asian and Mediterranean populations, and therefore hydrops fetalis, deletion of four α globin genes, or homozygous occurrence of *cis* deletions is found in these populations. African American populations are likely to have the *trans* deletion type of α-thalassemia-1 trait and therefore are not as likely to have hydrops fetalis as are Asian and Mediterranean people.

Symptoms and Clinical Findings

1. Hematologic: The child is not anemic at birth because fetal hemoglobin containing gamma globin chains predominates normally. Within the first few months of life, severe microcytic, hypochromic anemia develops when β globin chains fail to replace gamma globin chains. The hemoglobin level is usually 3 to 4 gm/dl. Fetal hemoglobin predominates (10 to 90 per cent) on electrophoresis. Hemoglobin A_2 level may be elevated. Serum bilirubin, SGOT, and SGPT are frequently increased. Low levels of serum zinc and biochemical evidence of folic acid deficiency are found. Increased iron level (serum ferritin) is found due to transfusional iron overload and/or increased absorption of iron from the gastrointestinal tract.

2. Skeletal abnormalities: Hypertrophy and expansion of

585

erythroid marrow results in skeletal deformities. The skull radiograph shows classic hair-on-end appearance due to bony trabeculae and widened diploic spaces. The maxilla is markedly overgrown resulting in malocclusion of teeth. These changes cause the typical facial appearance called *Cooley's anemia facies*. Marked osteoporosis and cortical thinning may predispose to pathologic fractures of long bones and vertebrae which may cause cord compression.

3. Hepatic changes: The liver is enlarged due to extramedullary hematopoiesis, cirrhosis and nodular regeneration, and iron deposition. Gallstones are present in more than 15 per cent of patients over age 15.

4. Cardiopulmonary abnormalities: Cardiac dilatation and congestive cardiac failure secondary to severe anemia would be expected in untransfused thalassemia major patients. Blood transfusion therapy prevents this complication, but in patients who are not on intensive chelation therapy, myocardial hemosiderosis occurs by the second decade. Increased PR interval, first-degree heart block, and premature atrial or ventricular contractions and depression of ST segment are noted. Echocardiography provides a noninvasive assessment of cardiac function. Sterile pericarditis, friction rub, and pericardial effusion are not uncommon. Pulmonary problems are few, but restrictive or obstructive defects may be found.

5. Other organs: The kidneys are frequently enlarged. Massive splenomegaly is unusual in transfused thalassemia major patients. However, splenectomy may help in lengthening the interval between transfusion therapy. Growth retardation, delayed or absent adolescent growth spurt, delayed menarche, oligomenorrhea or amenorrhea, poor development of secondary sexual characteristics, and hypogonadism are common.

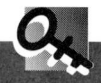 **Key Symptoms**

- Pallor
- Fatigue
- Dark urine

 Key Signs

- Anemia, jaundice
- Hepatosplenomegaly
- Cooley's anemia facies
- Cardiac failure/dilation

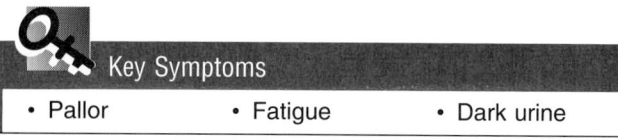 **Key Tests**

- CBC, reticulocyte count, and peripheral blood smear
- Hemoglobin electrophoresis
- Globin biosynthetic studies

Treatment

Improved blood transfusion support and iron chelation therapy have transformed thalassemia major from a fatal disease to a chronic disease with prolonged survival and near-normal quality of life. Bone marrow transplantation is available to

586

some patients, and future prospects of gene therapy have improved. Aggressive programs of prenatal screening and diagnosis can reduce the frequency of birth of patients with thalassemia major. However, these benefits have not accrued to patients in poor, less industrialized countries.

1. Blood transfusion and iron chelation
   a. Patients transfused to levels of hemoglobin adequate to suppress endogenous hematopoiesis (i.e., never permitted to fall below 10 gm/dl) do not develop skeletal malformations and cardiomegaly. Higher baseline level of hemoglobin would be more physiologic but would cause a greater iron overload. Ten ml/kg of packed leukocyte-poor red cells (achieved by using leukocyte filters) should be transfused every 2 to 3 weeks at a rate not to exceed 4 ml/kg/hour. Diuretics may be necessary for patients with potential cardiac decompensation. When requirements of blood exceed 200 ml/kg/year, splenectomy may be performed to reduce the transfusion needs. Such patients should receive a pneumococcal vaccine and be watched for serious infections.
   b. Iron chelation is achieved by subcutaneous administration of deferoxamine at a dose of 40 mg/kg during 8 to 10 hours with a limit of 2 gm during 8 hours daily. Higher intravenous doses can be given for selected patients. There are several candidate compounds for oral chelation under investigation.

2. Bone marrow transplantation and gene therapy
   a. The ultimate therapy would be to remove patients' bone marrow cells, replace the abnormal gene or insert a normal β globin gene, and reinfuse the marrow. Currently, this is not possible. However, several outstanding investigators around the world are attempting to achieve a genetic cure.
   b. Bone marrow transplantation from a histocompatible donor is an alternative. Best results are achieved in patients who are young and are in good clinical condition. Lucarelli's group in Pesaro demonstrated that hepatomegaly and portal fibrosis were the two most important risk factors. The event-free survival varied from 94 per cent in class I patients (neither complication), 80 per cent for class II (one risk factor), and 61 per cent for class III (both risk factors). The decision rests on weighing the risks described above and the benefits of cure with good quality of life.

 Bibliography

Berg PE, Schechter AN: Impact of molecular biology on the diagnosis of hemoglobin disorders. Molecular Genet Med 1992;2:1–38.

Cohen A: Current status of iron chelation therapy with desperrioxamine. Semin Hematol 1990;27:86–90.

Giardina PJ, Hilgartner MW: Update on thalassemia (review). Pediatr in Rev 1992;13:55–62.

Lucarelli G, Galimberti M, Polchi P, et al: Bone marrow transplantation in patients with thalassemia. N Engl J Med 1990;322:417–421.

Piomelli S, Loew T: Management of thalassemia major (Cooley's anemia). Hematol Oncol Clin North Am 1991;5:557–569.

147 Neutropenia

Russell Patrick Gollard

Etiology

1. Neutropenia is the most frequent cause of leukopenia. Neutropenia is termed severe if there are fewer than 500 neutrophils (polymorphonuclear leukocytes and band leukocytes) per microliter, moderate if there are between 500 and 1000 neutrophils per microliter, and mild if there are 1000 to 2000 cells per microliter.

2. Neutropenia may arise from either decreased production, increased destruction, or peripheral margination.

3. Virtually all cytotoxic drugs (chemotherapeutic agents) cause a profound transient neutropenia 10 to 14 days after therapy.
   a. Noncytotoxic drugs such as antibiotics (chloramphenicol, penicillin, and sulfa drugs), antiviral drugs (zidovudine, gancyclovir), phenothiazines, some diuretics, antithyroid drugs, anti-inflammatory agents (gold salts, phenylbutazone), H_2 blocking agents (ranitidine), and numerous other prescription drugs and toxic chemicals (benzene) can cause frank neutropenia or aplastic states of which neutropenia is a part.
   b. Drugs such as aminopyrine, α-methyldopa, phenylbutazone, mercurial diuretics, and some phenothiazines can cause peripheral destruction.

4. Hematologic diseases such as aplastic anemia, leukemia (lymphoid and myeloid), lymphomas (Hodgkin's and non-Hodgkin's), metastatic solid tumors, myelodysplasia, and myelofibrosis can cause neutropenia. In addition, genetic syndromes such as congenital hypoplastic neutropenia (Kostmann's syndrome) and cyclic neutropenia are known causes of neutropenia.

5. Chronic idiopathic neutropenia is characterized by a mild neutropenia of unknown cause. Patients with subpopulations of suppressor T lymphocytes that suppress granulopoiesis through a humoral factor have been described. These syndromes are more common in African-Americans and may have a genetic basis. Vitamin B_{12} and folate are well established causes of neutropenia, particularly in alcoholics. Neutropenia also may occur in individuals with eating disorders (bulimia, anorexia nervosa).

6. The infectious causes of neutropenia are many and include human immunodeficiency virus (HIV) infection, bunyaviruses, arboviruses, phleboviruses, measles, infectious mononucleosis, viral hepatitis, and cytomegalovirus. Other infectious causes include tuberculosis, typhoid fever, brucellosis, tularemia, malaria, histoplasmosis, and leishmaniasis.

7. Neutrophils may be destroyed peripherally in individuals with Felty's syndrome or systemic lupus erythematosus.
   a. Antineutrophil antibodies also cause peripheral destruction, and in cirrhotic individuals or those with Gaucher's disease, neutrophils may be trapped in the spleen.
   b. An overwhelming bacterial infection (sepsis syndrome), hemodialysis, and cardiopulmonary bypass all can cause peripheral margination.

Symptoms

1. Mild and moderate neutropenias may be clinically asymptomatic. When the neutrophil count falls below 1000 cells per microliter, there is a progressively increasing susceptibility to infections with bacterial and fungal pathogens. Infections are uncommon in patients with absolute neutrophil counts greater than 500.

2. Symptoms are usually associated with infection. Common localizing signs of inflammation may be absent.

3. Common pathogens include gram-negative bacilli, *Staphylococcus aureus, S. epidermidis, Candida* species, and *Aspergillus* species.

4. The most likely source of bacteremia in a neutropenic patient with a fever and without an indwelling line is endogenous flora of the mouth and gut.

Key Symptoms

- Fever
- Odynophagia
- Painful defecation
- Respiratory distress
- Inflammation
- Lethargy
- Skin lesions

WARNING

Fever in a neutropenic patient is a medical emergency.

Clinical Findings

1. Findings frequently depend on the duration and severity of neutropenia.

2. Severely neutropenic patients frequently have oral thrush (postchemotherapy neutropenia and prolonged neutropenia) and perianal erythema or perirectal abscesses.

3. In addition, these patients frequently are found to have dullness to percussion and auscultation on lung

examination. Hepatomegaly and splenomegaly also can be seen. Frequent findings in long-term neutropenic individuals include multiple poorly healed skin abscesses.

4. Patients may present with any combination of signs of the sepsis syndrome, including fever, tachycardia, cool clammy skin, hyperventilation, and postural hypotension.

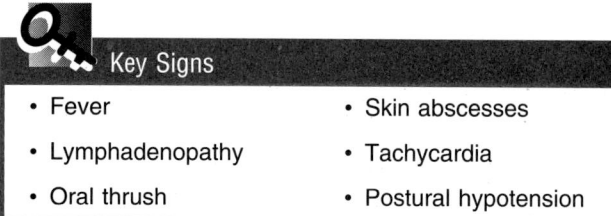

Key Signs

- Fever
- Skin abscesses
- Lymphadenopathy
- Tachycardia
- Oral thrush
- Postural hypotension

WARNING

Digital rectal examinations are strongly contraindicated in neutropenic patients.

Laboratory Tests

1. The peripheral smear is important. A left-shifted differential (>10 per cent bands), toxic granulation, and the presence of Dohle bodies indicate a high likelihood of infection or a marrow in the recovery phase after a toxic insult. A paucity of immature forms, on the other hand, suggests a toxic process.

2. Serial determinations of the complete blood count (CBC) may be most useful in documenting the course of a mild neutropenia rather than other more invasive, expensive, or esoteric tests. (The normal range of white blood cells in African-Americans and Yemenite Jews is somewhat less than average, and neutropenias in these populations are defined as less than 1.5×10^9 cells per liter.)

3. The bone marrow is the "gold standard" for assessment of neutrophil production.

   a. Marrow infiltration (myelophthisis) may be seen in hematologic neoplasms (leukemia, lymphoma) and metastatic solid tumors or in certain infectious processes (presence of granulomas, organisms).

   b. When neutropenia is caused by a toxic insult, near absence of immature forms will be seen.

   c. When neutrophils are destroyed peripherally or marginated (autoimmune processes, sepsis), immature granulocytes are abundant.

4. Macrocytosis (mean corpuscular volume > 100) and nuclear/cytoplasm dyssynchrony suggest vitamin B_{12} and/or folate deficiency. Chronically ill individuals and alcoholics are particularly at risk, but patients receiving chemotherapy or suffering from myelodysplasia also can develop macrocytosis. Strict vegetarians need B_{12} supplementation. Vitamin B_{12} (normally

250 to 1100 pg/ml) and folate levels (2.8 to 15.6 ng/ml) may be drawn to assess stores in such individuals. Vitamin B_{12} deficiency may be masked by prior administration of this drug.

5. The antigranulocyte antibody may be positive in autoimmune disorders and in such disorders as Felty's syndrome and systemic lupus erythematosus (SLE).

6. Chromosomal studies can be useful in differentiating myelodysplasia from drug- or toxin-induced suppression.

7. Blood cultures are mandatory in patients with neutropenia and fevers. Urine, sputum, or other body fluid cultures are suggested if clinically indicated.

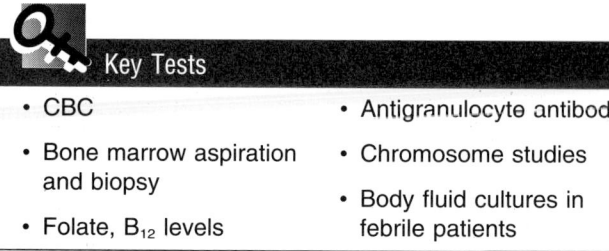

Key Tests

- CBC
- Antigranulocyte antibody
- Bone marrow aspiration and biopsy
- Chromosome studies
- Folate, B_{12} levels
- Body fluid cultures in febrile patients

Differential Diagnosis

1. Decreased production: drug or toxic effect, infection, hematologic neoplasm, metastatic disease, miscellaneous (chronic idiopathic neutropenia, cyclic neutropenia)

2. Peripheral destruction/margination: drug effect, autoimmune phenomena, splenic sequestration, sepsis, cardiopulmonary bypass, hemodialysis

Treatment

1. First, determine the underlying pathogenesis (drug, toxin, infection, neoplasm, vitamin deficiency). All possible drugs should be stopped immediately.

2. Folate is available in many forms and in deficiency states should be administered at a dose of 1.0 mg orally daily. Vitamin B_{12} can be administered intramuscularly or subcutaneously in deficient states, 100 µg daily for 5 to 10 days and then 100 to 200 µg monthly.

3. Granulocyte colony stimulating factor (G-CSF filgrastim [Neupogen]) and granulocyte-macrophage colony stimulating factor (GM-CSF, sargramostim [Leukine, Prokine]) are commercially available genetically engineered cytokines useful in the treatment of severe neutropenia, especially in the postchemotherapy nadir period. Because of their expense and potential side effects or toxicities, it is suggested that they be given only under supervision of a hematologist or oncologist, at least initially. G-CSF and GM-CSF are given daily subcutaneously at a dosage of 5 µg/kg and 250 µg/m², respectively. G-CSF or GM-CSF should never be given concomitantly during the administration of chemotherapy or 24 hours thereafter,

nor should either drug be given in patients with acute leukemia before induction chemotherapy.

4. Febrile neutropenia is a medical emergency and demands hospitalization, culturing of body fluids, and intravenous antibiotics. Prophylactic antibiotic therapy is a controversial issue.

Diet

A low-bacteria diet is necessary in patients with prolonged neutropenia.

Activity

Patients should avoid individuals with known communicable diseases in the home and in the workplace. Most hospitals have infection-control departments and have specific requirements for the care of neutropenic patients.

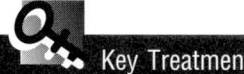

Key Treatment

- Folate
- Vitamin B_{12}
- G-CSF and GM-CSF

Bibliography

For a more detailed look at neutropenia in general, see
Bagby GC Jr: Leukopenia. *In* Bennett JC, Plum F (eds): Cecil Textbook of Medicine. Philadelphia, WB Saunders, 1996.

For a look at the use of colony stimulating factors in patients with neutropenic fever, see
Beveridge RA, Miller JA: Impact of colony stimulating factors on the practice of oncology. Oncology 1993;7(suppl):43–48.

For a general overview of leukopenia, see
Gallin JI: Quantitative and qualitative disorders of phagocytes. *In* Isselbacher KJ, Braunwald E, Wilson JD, et al (eds): Harrison's Principles of Internal Medicine, 13th ed. New York, McGraw-Hill, 1994, pp 329–337.

For a detailed look at the treatment of infections in immunocompromised patients, see
Pizzo PA, Meyers J, Freifeld AG, Walsh T: Infections in the cancer patient. *In* DeVita VT Jr, Hellman S, Rosenberg SA (eds): Cancer: Principles and Practice of Oncology, 4th ed. Philadelphia, JB Lippincott, 1993, pp 2292–2337.

For a general overview of neutropenia, with special emphasis on drug-related causes, see
Rapaport SI: Introduction to Hematology, 2nd ed. Philadelphia, JB Lippincott, 1987, pp 409–412, 426–429.

For more information on low bacteria diets, see
Remington JS, Schimpff SC: Please don't eat the salads. N Engl J Med 1981;304:433–435.

148 Thrombocytopenia

John J. McCarthy

Etiology

1. Platelet structure and function
   a. Platelets circulate as anucleate, discoid corpuscles derived from megakaryocyte cytoplasm and usually measure about 1 μm in diameter. Important in the "second phase" of coagulation, platelets are composed of phospholipid membrane that surrounds cytoplasm, metabolite containing α granules, and delta granules that store adhesion, coagulation, and growth factor proteins. The cell membrane itself is complex, having an array of metabolite and protein receptors as well as an intricate system of invaginating canaliculi.
   b. The normal platelet count ranges between 150,000 and 440,000 per microliter. The life span of platelets in normal individuals is 5 to 7 days; this is considerably shortened during some illnesses. Platelets function by undergoing local adhesion, degranulation, and shape change to plug vascular defects when platelet membrane receptors are first activated.
   c. Thrombocytopenia is defined as a platelet count of less than 150,000 per microliter. Though abnormalities in platelet function also may contribute to bleeding symptoms, here we discuss diagnosis and treatment of quantitative platelet deficiencies.

2. Causes: These can be grouped as *diagnoses present at birth* (including in utero and hereditary etiologies), the *syndrome of diminished platelet production,* and the *syndrome of increased platelet consumption* (see Table 148–1).
   a. Immune thrombocytopenia can be present at birth, have onset during childhood, or begin during adulthood. Though *autoimmune* thrombocytopenia rarely can be found in the neonate, more commonly *isoimmune* thrombocytopenia is seen when maternal antiplatelet antibodies cross the placenta, fix to the infant's platelet membrane antigens, and cause immune clearance by the reticuloendothelial system. These antibodies originating in the mother may actually be *autoimmune* against her own platelet antigens or *alloimmune* against fetal platelet antigens that she became exposed to during pregnancies or via previous transfusion. Isoimmune thrombocytopenia usually resolves within days, but occasionally it persists for weeks.
   b. Childhood *immune thrombocytopenic purpura* (ITP) is usually preceded by a viral-like prodrome and is self-limited, resolving in weeks to months. The adult form of ITP is less often preceded by a viral picture and is seldom self-limited. Relapse, after initial corticosteroid treatment response, is the norm in adults (80 per cent). Approximately 10 per cent of adult ITP cases are resistant to all therapies. Females are affected with ITP more often than males. Pregnancy is a common setting for ITP—estrogens may play an etiologic or aggravational role.
   c. Angioedemic *allergic reactions,* specific *infections* (viral, protozoan, rickettsial), *collagen-vascular diseases,* general *bacterial sepsis* without disseminated intravascular coagulation, *lymphoproliferative diseases,* and *drugs* also are known to precipitate thrombocytopenia by antibody-mediated mechanisms. Human immunodeficiency virus (HIV) is the most common viral association, thought to be mediated via an immune-complex mechanism. β-Lactam antibiotics, H_2-receptor blocking drugs, quinine derivatives, and heparin are common causative agents among the myriad of drug-induced thrombocytopenias. Heparin-related antiplatelet antibodies are commonly associated with both thrombocytopenia and paradoxical mor-

TABLE 148–1. CAUSES OF THROMBOCYTOPENIA

I. Diagnoses at birth
   A. In utero forms (immune thrombocytopenia, viremia, bacteremia, other infections, drugs, thrombocytopenia with absent radius syndrome, vascular malformations)
   B. Hereditary forms (isolated familial thrombocytopenia, Wiskott-Aldrich syndrome, Fanconi syndrome, Alport's syndrome, Bernard-Soulier disease, thrombasthenia, platelet-type von Willebrand's disease, May-Heglin anomaly, Chédiak-Higashi anomaly)
II. Syndrome of diminished platelet production
   A. Metabolite deficiency (B_{12}, folate)
   B. Drugs/physical agents (chemotherapy, x-radiation, chlorthiazides, alcohol, estrogens, many other drugs)
   C. Myelophthisis (granuloma, tumor, fibrosis)
   D. Infection (CMV, HIV, others)
   E. Diminished/defective megakaryocyte precursor cells (myelodysplastic syndrome, myeloproliferative disease, aplastic anemia, paroxysmal nocturnal hemoglobinuria, collagen-vascular disease, thrombocytopenia with decreased megakaryocytes, graft-versus-host disease)
III. Syndrome of increased platelet consumption
   A. Immune (ITP and related autoimmune syndromes, drug-induced, alloimmune, general bacterial sepsis without disseminated intravascular coagulation, specific infections, nonspecific systemic allergic events)
   B. Microangiopathic (disseminated intravascular coagulation, eclampsia, malignant hypertension, thrombotic thrombocytopenic purpura, hemolytic uremic syndrome, renal allograft rejection, intravascular foreign bodies, vascular malformations, burns)
   C. Hypersplenism
   D. Massive transfusion
   E. Hypothermia
IV. Pseudothrombocytopenia

bid thrombotic events due to the precipitation of platelet thrombi (''white clots'').

d. In adults, alloimmunity against foreign platelet HLA antigens frequently occurs in multiparous women but is most common in heavily transfused patients. This can pose a major impediment to platelet transfusion therapy. *Post-transfusion purpura* is a rare severe form of alloimmune thrombocytopenia occurring in some patients lacking the P1-A-1 platelet antigen. It remains unclear why patients in this setting destroy both their own and transfused platelets some 2 to 7 days after blood and/or platelet transfusion.

e. *In utero thrombocytopenia* rarely can be due to nonimmune etiologies such as marrow-suppressive drugs taken by the mother (chlorthiazide, alcohol), developmental aberrations (cavernous hemangioma, thrombocytopenia, and absent radius syndrome), specific infections (rubella, many others), and hereditary disorders. The *hereditary forms of thrombocytopenia* may be isolated, associated with clinical syndromes (Wiskott-Aldrich, Fanconi, Alport's), associated with platelet function defects (Bernard Soulier, thrombasthenia, platelet-type von Willebrand's disease), or associated with morphologic aberrations of white blood cells (WBCs) (May-Heglin, Chédiak-Higashi).

f. There are a number of *nonimmune thrombocytopenias* acquired later in life. *Metabolite deficiency* (B_{12}, folic acid), *physical agents* (x-irradiation), *chemotherapeutic agents* (especially anthracyclines, alkylating agents, and antimetabolites), *myelophthisic disease* (most commonly metastatic adenocarcinoma and primary hematopoietic neoplasia), and specific *infections* (most commonly HIV and cytomegalovirus) can be causes of either isolated megakaryocytic hypoplasia or panmyeloid depression of the bone marrow. *Myeloproliferative* and *myelodysplastic* defects of stem cells can result in depressed megakaryocyte numbers or ineffective platelet production with abnormal megakaryocyte morphology. Karyotypic abnormalities of chromosomes are frequently found in the marrow tissue of the latter two groups, as well as in marrows injured by physical and chemical agents. Dyspoietic morphology can be seen in marrows of all these categories. *Aplastic anemia, collagen diseases,* and *graft-versus-host disease* frequently have features of dysregulatory cellular immune function as a mechanism of the megakaryocyte and marrow depression. The rare syndrome of *thrombocytopenia with decreased megakaryocytes* frequently evolves into more ominous aplastic or leukemia states, as does the instance of thrombocytopenia due to *paroxysmal nocturnal hemoglobinuria* (PNH). The latter is an acquired genetic defect of the marrow resulting, in part, in defective membrane phosphatidyl inositol linkages to complement regulatory proteins. In addition to low platelet numbers, PNH also is associated with thrombotic events, including the Budd-Chiari syndrome.

g. *Nonimmune consumptive thrombopathies* include *microangiopathic states.* These feature red blood cell (RBC) trauma along with platelet consumption. The most common entity in this group is *disseminated intravascular coagulation* (DIC), which can be seen due to a wide variety of obstetric catastrophes, vascular injuries (burns, shock), bacterial sepsis, tissue injuries (brain trauma), and carcinomas (Trousseau's syndrome). *Vascular malformations* (hemangiomas, arteriovenous fistulas), renal allograft rejection, and vascular pathway foreign-body surfaces (artificial valve, Dacron graft, pump-oxygenator membrane, intra-aortic balloon pump, and artificial heart device) also can give rise to increased platelet consumption and RBC microangiopathy. *Thrombotic thrombocytopenic purpura* (TTP) and *hemolytic uremic syndrome* (HUS), as well as *malignant hypertension* and *eclampsia,* affect platelet consumption and RBC trauma via microvascular damage. In TTP, ultra-large von Willebrand's proteins are frequently a marker for the underlying microvascular defect.

h. In patients undergoing *massive transfusion* (vascular surgery) and in patients suffering *hypothermia,* dilution factors (in the former) and intravascular redistribution to hepatic and splenic storage sites (in the latter) may combine with hyperconsumption to cause thrombocytopenia that can last for days. *Splenic enlargement* of any type (congenital or acquired) can cause sequestration resulting in increased destruction of platelets. Usually, these latter situations are not associated with severe thrombocytopenia.

i. *Pseudothrombocytopenia* may result from undercounting of platelets by automated cell counters. This is due to an in vitro platelet clumping phenomenon that is occasionally caused by EDTA and other routinely used in vitro decoagulants.

Symptoms

1. Platelet counts between 100,000 and 150,000 per microliter constitute *mild* thrombocytopenia; between 50,000 and 100,000, *moderate;* and less than 50,000, *severe.* Mild thrombocytopenia is usually asymptomatic; moderate, attended with easy bruisability and excessive bleeding at times of surgery or trauma; and severe, attended with high risk of excessive bleeding. At platelet counts of less than 20,000 per microliter there is a progressive risk of spontaneous hemorrhage. Most notable is intracranial bleeding, which can be fatal. Wound bleeding due to thrombocyto-

penia tends to be "immediate" rather than the delayed pattern seen with some coagulation protein deficiencies.

2. A history of small *bruises* of skin and *mucosal bleeding* is not specific, but these symptoms are most typical of thrombopathy. The timing of these phenomena (especially in association with trauma, hemostatic challenges such as surgery, fever, rheumatic symptoms, drug taking, radiation exposure, and constitutional symptoms) should be scrutinized. Ancillary information pertaining to family patterns of bleeding phenomena, diet, liver disease, transfusion history, and "unrelated" medical diagnoses also should be sought.

Key Symptoms

- Hematoma formation, ecchymoses, large purpura, and organ bleeding do not distinguish thrombocytopenia as a cause of hemorrhage from other vascular and coagulation protein defects.

- Spontaneous mucosal bleeding and bleeding that occurs immediately after skin or membrane trauma are suggestive of (but not specific of) thrombocytopenia.

- Headache in a setting of a patient with known severe thrombocytopenia should always be taken seriously and investigated as a possible spontaneous intracranial bleeding.

Clinical Findings

1. Although *petechiae* can be seen as a manifestation of rare vasculopathies, they are more often the "signature" finding of thrombopathy. These "pinhead-sized" purpura are most frequent on gravitationally impacted skin surfaces and on mucous membranes.

2. Diffuse purpura and retinal hemorrhage can be seen in moderate and severe thrombocytopenia cases, respectively.

3. Life-threatening bleeding is seen rarely without prior skin and mucous membrane manifestations.

4. Correlative examination for aberrant vital signs, signs of infection, rash, signs of rheumatic disease, hepatosplenomegaly, jaundice, lymphadenopathy, vascular bruits, features of neoplasms, and congenital anatomic defects can add focus to the differential diagnosis.

Key Signs

- Petechiae are much more often a sign of platelet disorders than a sign of microvascular disease.

- Hemorrhagic petechiae or bullae on mucous membranes portend a significantly higher risk of clinical bleeding.

Laboratory Tests

1. The initial tests in cases of thrombocytopenia should include a review of the peripheral blood smear (PBS), complete blood count (CBC), platelet count, prothrombin time (PT), partial thromboplastin time (PTT), and fibrin split product (FSP) assay. The PBS and CBC are critical in determining whether platelets alone are affected versus whether thrombocytopenia is part of a broader hematologic picture manifesting aberrations of RBC and WBC morphologies. A high mean platelet volume (MPV) measurement on the CBC indices suggests that the marrow is capable of actively making platelets. Nevertheless, a bone marrow aspirate and biopsy are often required to clarify this issue or to rule out a myelophthisic process. The PT, PTT, and FSP (or D-dimer) levels will assist in deciding if DIC is present.

2. Follow-up testing with liver function tests, fibrinogen level, collagen-vascular serologies, protein electrophoresis, HIV serology, antiphospholipid antibody levels, heparin-related antiplatelet-antibody screen, and others can be done if the findings of the history, physical examination, and initial laboratory tests warrant. The bleeding time and platelet-associated IgG test are not usually helpful or definitive, respectively.

Key Tests

- Peripheral blood smear
- Partial thromboplastin time
- Prothrombin time
- Complete blood count with platelet count
- Fibrin split products

Differential Diagnosis

In the absence of petechiae, it is usually difficult to distinguish thrombocytopenia as a cause of bleeding manifestations from the other major categories of bleeding—such as vasculopathy, procoagulant factor deficiency, and qualitative disorders of platelet function. A review of the peripheral blood smear and/or the platelet count defines whether thrombocytopenia is an element of a patient's bleeding disorder.

Treatment

Platelet transfusion is the primary treatment to *prophylax* against bleeding in instances of *transient* severe thrombocytopenia (counts less than 10,000 to 20,000 per microliter), prepare patients having moderate to severe thrombocytopenia for surgical procedures, and treat acute hemorrhage. *Important exceptions* to this dictum are the diagnoses of post-transfusion purpura (where transfusions prolonged thrombocytopenia), ITP (where transfusions seldom increment the platelet count significantly), and TTP/HUS syndromes (where platelet transfusions have been reported to precipitate morbid or even fatal thrombotic events). Platelet transfusions are used only for life-threatening hemorrhage in these latter clinical diagnoses. No "platelet crossmatch" is done, since this is technically imprecise. In patients who have *chronic severe thrombocytopenia,* platelet transfusions are not used prophylactically because many patients develop alloimmune platelet refractoriness after just a few weeks or months. Rather, platelet transfusions are used only to "trouble shoot" when the patient has bleeding. In aplastic anemia, unnecessary platelet transfusions may alloimmunize against success of later marrow transplantation. *Premedication* before each transfusion with hydrocortisone, diphenhydramine, or acetaminophen is the rule in order to avoid febrile and protein allergy transfusion reactions.

Medication

1. The pharmacologic therapies of thrombocytopenias vary with etiology. In ITP, a common adult malady, there is interestingly a *menu* of treatment approaches to the therapy that produce response rates of 40 to 80 per cent. This menu includes corticosteroids, danocrine, splenectomy, and immunosuppressive drugs (cytoxan, azathioprine, cyclosporine A, others), as well as plasmapheresis with staphylococcal protein A adsorption. Additionally, certain agents can produce temporary responses at times of urgency such as during surgery or acute bleeding. These latter agents include high-dose intravenous immunoglobulin and vincristine.

2. *Diet* and other *drug treatments* of thrombocytopenia remain somewhat diagnosis-specific (e.g., B_{12} therapy in pernicious anemia). *General measures* to be taken in thrombocytopenic patients include avoidance of high bleeding risks (such as head trauma), nonsteroidal anti-inflammatory drugs, and intramuscular injections. Since drug-induced thrombocytopenia is a common consideration, *all* but life-sustaining drugs should be discontinued or substituted for in cases where the etiology of thrombocytopenia is in question. This is especially true of heparin as a possible cause. Discontinuing *all* heparin sources will help eliminate comorbid thrombosis when heparin is the cause of thrombocytopenia.

Key Treatment

- In the absence of TTP, HUS, and post-transfusion purpura, platelet transfusions (with premedication to avoid transfusion reactions) are front-line treatment of severe thrombocytopenia and/or bleeding.

- Menus of treatment are available for specific causes of thrombocytopenia, such as ITP.

Follow-Up

The pace and length of follow-up of thrombocytopenic patients are dictated by the underlying diagnosis and clinical manifestations. For instance, a patient hemorrhaging from DIC may need platelet transfusions more than once daily, while a patient with ITP responding to danazol may need to be seen only as an outpatient once every 3 months while on the drug. The general measures previously mentioned apply to outpatients as well as inpatients. In cases of persistent severe thrombocytopenia, patients should be trained to come to the hospital for platelet transfusion in the event of any significant bleeding or onset of atypical headache.

PEARLS

- The "bleeding time" test, which is so useful in screening for microvasculopathy and qualitative platelet disorders, is usually not useful in the diagnosis or treatment of moderate and severe thrombocytopenia. This is so because the "bleeding time" is usually abnormal in platelet counts below 100,000.

- Severely thrombocytopenic patients with no skin or mucous membrane manifestations are at less risk of bleeding than otherwise expected.

- Hemorrhagic vesicles or bullae on mucosal surfaces suggest the patient is at very high risk of bleeding; therefore, more aggressive treatment of thrombocytopenia is usually warranted.

- Assigning a 20,000 per microliter estimated count to each platelet as seen on a high-power, oil microscopic field (in the "feathered edge" of the PBS) will give a close estimate of the patient's actual platelet count and can sometimes save hours of time in the decision-making process in urgent clinical settings.

- In the absence of hemorrhage and "consumptive" thrombocytopenia, each unit of random donor platelets should increment the platelet count some 5000 to 10,000 per microliter.

B Bibliography

Bithell TC: Thrombocytopenia. *In* Lee GR, Bithell TC, Foerster J, et al (eds): Wintrobe's Clinical Hematology, 9th ed, vol 2. Philadelphia, Lea and Febiger, 1993, pp 1325–1373.

Bussel JB, Schrieber AD, Moake JL, et al: Disorders of platelet number. *In* Hoffman R, Berry EJ, Jr, Shattil SJ, et al (eds): Hematology—Basic Principles and Practice. New York, Churchill Livingstone, 1991, pp 1485–1501.

Gardner FH, Bessman JD, Harlan JM and McMillan R: Quantitative disorders of platelets. *In* Harker LA, Zimmerman TS (eds): Clinics in Haematology: Platelet Disorders, vol 12:1. Philadelphia, WB Saunders, 1983, pp 23–88.

Miyato T, et al: Abnormalities of PIG-A transcripts in granulocytes from patients with paroxysmal nocturnal hemoglobinuria. N Engl J Med 1994;330:249–255.

149 Leukemia

Marc J. Chernoff

Leukemia is characterized by abnormal differentiation and proliferation of the lymphopoietic and hematopoietic stem cells. This disorder of normal cellular development and progression leads to accumulation of leukemic cells that respond poorly to normal regulatory cellular mechanisms, expand at the expense of normal lymphoid and myeloid cell lines, and infiltrate organs causing dysfunction.

Classification

For purposes of identification, prognosis, and treatment, the leukemias are divided into both acute and chronic forms.

A. Acute leukemia
1. Acute myeloid leukemia (AML; acute non-lymphocytic leukemia, ANLL). This class is further divided into
   a. AML-M1
   b. AML-M2
   c. AML-M3 (acute promyelocytic)
   d. AML-M4 (acute myelomonocytic)
   e. AML-M5 (acute monocytic)
   f. AML-M6 (erythroleukemia)
   g. AML-M7 (megakaryocytic)
2. Acute lymphocytic leukemia (ALL). This class is further divided into
   a. ALL-L1
   b. ALL-L2
   c. ALL-L3 (Burkitt type)
3. Acute mixed lineage leukemia (AMLL)
4. Acute undifferentiated leukemia (AUL)

B. Chronic leukemia
1. Chronic myelogenous leukemia (CML)
2. Chronic lymphocytic leukemia (CLL)
3. CLL variants
   a. Hairy cell leukemia
   b. T-cell chronic lymphocytic leukemia
   c. T-cell leukemia lymphoma
   d. Prolymphocytic leukemia
4. The exact causes of leukemia are unknown, but there are associations with the following:
   a. Hereditary factors, as in high-risk families
   b. Congenital disorders
      (1) Down syndrome
      (2) Bloom's syndrome
      (3) Fanconi's anemia
      (4) Kleinfelter's syndrome
      (5) Ataxia telangiectasia
      (6) Osteogenesis imperfecta
      (7) Wiskott-Aldrich syndrome
   c. Underlying hematologic disorders
      (1) Chronic myeloproliferative disorders (CML, agnogenic myeloid metaplasia, polycythemia vera, primary thrombocythemia)
      (2) Preleukemic states/myelodysplastic syndromes
   d. Irradiation
   e. Chemical exposures (benzene, toluene)
   f. Multiagent cytotoxic chemotherapy. Acute leukemia, predominantly myeloid, is a complication in patients treated with alkylators or immunosuppressive therapy in
      (1) Hodgkin's lymphoma (especially those treated with MOPP)
      (2) Non-Hodgkin's lymphoma
      (3) Breast, ovary, lung, gastrointestinal (GI) tract, brain, ALL, myeloma
      (4) Rheumatoid arthritis, Wegener's granulomatosis, histiocytosis X, polycythemia vera, Behçet's syndrome, Crohn's disease

Key Symptoms

- Fatigue, weakness
- Weight loss
- Bleeding (skin, gums, mucous membranes, genitourinary or gastrointestinal tract)
- Infection (skin, throat, sinus, gums, respiratory or urinary tract)
- Headache, nausea, vomiting, blurred vision, cranial nerve involvement
- Bone pain
- Abdominal distention and anorexia
- Lymphadenopathy
- Oliguria
- Obstipation
- Mental status alterations

Clinical Findings

1. The findings on examination also will parallel many of the symptoms.

2. There are also a number of "unusual" presentations of leukemia that may occur:

   a. Hyperleucocytosis

   b. Disseminated intravascular coagulopathy (DIC)

   c. Granulocytic sarcoma (tumors composed of myeloid cells, chloromas)

   d. Central nervous system leukemia

   e. Leukemia cutis (leukemic skin infiltrates)

   f. Sweet's syndrome (fever, neutrophilia, and painful, erythematous skin lesions)

   g. Pyoderma gangrenosum (ulcerating, painful skin lesions)

   h. Acute leukemia diagnosed during pregnancy

Key Signs

- Pallor, lethargy, and weakness

- Weight loss

- Purpura, petechiae, gingival hypertrophy or oozing, hematuria, melena

- Fever, chills, tissue infiltrates, pyoderma gangrenosum

- Papilledema, cranial nerve palsies, meningeal signs

- Bone tenderness

- Hepatosplenomegaly and abdominal tenderness

- Lymphadenopathy

Laboratory and Other Tests

1. Tests that may be useful:

   a. Leukocyte alkaline phosphatase (LAP): decreased in CML

   b. Vitamin B_{12}: elevated in CML

   c. Urine and serum lysozyme (muramidase): seen in some forms of AML

   d. Serum protein electrophoresis: hypogammaglobulinemia seen in CLL

   e. Coombs' test: hemolytic anemias associated with leukemia

   f. Transfusion evaluation studies

   g. HLA typing for potential bone marrow transplant candidates

   h. HIV screen

2. Appropriate radiographic tests:

   a. Chest radiograph

   b. Abdominal series

   c. Computed tomographic scan

   d. Bone scan

   e. Sinus films

   f. Magnetic resonance imaging (especially in cases of suspected cord compression, dural, epidural, or meningeal involvement)

3. Biopsy of infiltrated organs

4. Review the peripheral smear because there may be clues to help categorize the type of leukemia:

   a. Auer rods

   b. Hairy cells

   c. Smudge cells

   d. Platelet morphology

   e. Rouleaux formation

   f. Red cell morphology

Key Tests

- Complete blood count with differential

- Platelet count

- Electrolytes, including calcium, magnesium, PO_4, uric acid

- Liver function profile and renal function profile

- Coagulation studies (prothrombin time, international normalized ratio (INR), partial thromboplastin time) and also a DIC panel (fibrinogen and fibrin split products)

- Blood cultures when appropriate (aerobic, anaerobic, viral, fungal)

- Bone marrow aspirate and core biopsy (histochemical, cytochemical, and immunologic staining and phenotyping, flow cytometry, and karyotypic analysis)

- Analysis of the cerebrospinal fluid (cytology, cultures, and routine studies)

Differential Diagnosis

1. Other considerations in the differential diagnosis include

   a. Distinction between marrow failure from AML/ALL and other entities such as aplastic anemia

   b. Marrow infiltration with nonhematopoietic tumors that may mimic clinical or laboratory features of ALL:

      (1) In children, neuroblastoma or rhabdomyosarcoma

      (2) In adolescents and adults, Ewing's sarcoma or small cell lung carcinoma

   c. When there is the presence of lymphadenopathy and/or splenomegaly, the following also should be considered:

      (1) Infectious causes: viral, bacterial, chlamydial, protozoan, mycotic, rickettsial, mycobacterial, HIV

      (2) Autoimmune causes: rheumatoid arthritis, lupus, dermatomyositis, mixed connective tissue disease, and Sjögren's syndrome

      (3) Iatrogenic hypersensitivity: serum sickness, drug hypersensitivity

(4) Potentially malignant entities: angioimmunoblastic lymphadenopathy and Castleman's disease (angiofollicular lymph node hyperplasia)

(5) Hodgkin's or non-Hodgkin's lymphoma

Treatment/Chemotherapy

A. AML: Treatment is divided into induction, consolidative, and maintenance therapy.

1. Induction therapy consists of daunorubicin (Cerubidine) for 3 days and cytarabine (Cytosar) for 7 days, the so-called 7 + 3 regimen.

2. Idarubicin (Idamycin), a synthetic anthracycline analogue, is also a potentially efficacious substitute for daunorubicin.

3. High-dose cytarabine (ARA-C) (HiDAC) is commonly used in patients with relapsed, refractory, or therapy-related AML.

4. High-dose ARA-C, 1 to 3 gm/m² of body surface area twice daily, is preferred regimen for consolidation and maintenance therapy, and bone marrow transplant is usually reserved for "salvage" therapy.

5. Treatment of the M3 subtype of AML is initiated by using all-*trans* retinoic acid, and further consolidation and maintenance with traditional agents.

B. ALL

1. The most often used drugs in the induction of ALL are prednisone, vincristine (Oncovin), an anthracycline (e.g., daunorubicin), and asparaginase (Elspar).

2. Consolidation therapy consists of regimens including agents such as VM26 (teniposide [Vumon]), VP16 (etoposide [VePesid]), HiDAC; combination VM26 and ARA-C is promising.

3. Maintenance therapy consists of mercaptopurine (Purinethol) and methotrexate.

4. CNS prophylaxis: cranial irradiation, intrathecal methotrexate, administration of methotrexate, ARA-C, and hydrocortisone via intraventricular reservoir, or high-dose systemic chemotherapy.

C. CML, chronic phase

1. Busulfan (Myleran) and hydroxyurea (Hydrea) are agents of choice.

2. Bone marrow transplant is also used in this phase.

D. CLL

1. The major therapeutic modalities for CLL include chemotherapy and radiation therapy; splenectomy is also done.

2. Commonly used agents are

a. Chlorambucil (Leukeran)

b. Cyclophosphamide (Cytoxan)

c. Fludarabine (Fludara)

d. 2-Chlorodeoxyadenosine (cladribine [Leustatin])

e. Deoxycoformycin (Nipent)

E. Hairy cell leukemia. Promising results with 2-chlorodeoxyadenosine with or without interferon-alfa-2b (Intron A)

Bibliography

DeVita T Jr, Hellman S, Rosenberg S: Cancer Principles and Practice of Oncology, 4th ed. Philadelphia, JB Lippincott, 1993.

Hematology/Oncology Clinics of North America. Philadelphia, WB Saunders, April 1990: Chronic Leukemias; February 1993: Management of Acute Leukemia; April 1993: Therapy Related Secondary Malignancies.

Hollard F, Frei E: Cancer Medicine, 3d ed. Philadelphia, Lea & Febiger, 1993.

Holleb I, Fink D, Murphy G: American Cancer Society Textbook of Clinical Oncology. Atlanta, American Cancer Society, 1991.

Lee GR, Bithell T: Wintrobe's Clinical Hematology, 9th ed. Philadelphia, Lea & Febiger, 1993.

Procedure BONE MARROW ASPIRATION AND BIOPSY
Robert M. Heiligman

Indications
1. Evaluate cytopenias (single or multiple cell line).
2. Determine marrow iron stores.
3. Evaluate leukocytosis (consider flow cytometric and cytogenetic studies).
4. Diagnose suspected leukemias (consider flow cytometric and cytogenetic studies).
5. Diagnose suspected myelodysplastic syndromes (consider cytogenetic studies).
6. Diagnose suspected myeloproliferative disorders (consider cytogenetic studies).
7. Diagnose suspected dysproteinemias.
8. Stage lymphomas/solid tumors.
9. Evaluate fever of unknown origin (consider bacterial, fungal, AFB culture).
10. Assess result of therapy for leukemia or lymphoma.

Contraindications
1. Overlying skin infection
2. Local osteomyelitis
3. Major coagulopathy, including severe inherited factor deficiency, active disseminated intravascular coagulation (DIC), profound liver disease, or therapeutic anticoagulation with prothrombin/partial thromboplastin times (PT/PTT) above or at upper limits of therapeutic range
4. Thrombocytopenia, no matter how severe, is *not* a contraindication.
5. Prior therapeutic irradiation may result in a "dry tap" and nondiagnostic biopsy if procedure is performed in the same area.

Preparation
1. Obtain informed consent.
2. Obtain a complete blood count (CBC) with differential on the day of the procedure.
3. Arrange for an assistant from the hematology section of the clinical laboratory to be present. The assistant should be able to prepare several bone marrow smears from a portion of the aspirate and to utilize the remainder to prepare a bone marrow clot (for fixation and histologic evaluation).

Equipment
1. Chux
2. Sterile drape
3. Betadine swabs (three)
4. Sterile 4 × 4 gauze (several packages)
5. Sterile gloves
6. Xylocaine 2% with epinephrine (inquire regarding history of allergic reaction)
7. Sterile disposable needles (25 gauge, 5/8 inch; 22 gauge, 1½ inch; 18-gauge)
8. Sterile disposable Luer-tip syringes (3, 6, and 12 cc)
9. Sterile No. 11 blade (handle not needed)
10. Sterile Jamshidi needle (11 gauge for most routine use, 8 and 13 gauge also available). A spare needle is recommended in case the original becomes contaminated prior to the end of the procedure.
11. Adhesive bandage
12. Sandbag (required only for prolonged tamponade of oozing site)

Anesthesia
1. Premedicate (*after* obtaining informed consent) with intravenous diazepam (or alternative benzodiazepine) and meperidine (or alternative narcotic) in dosages appropriate for age, body size, and coexisting medical conditions (e.g., chronic pulmonary disease). Inquire regarding history of allergic reaction.
2. Raise skin bleb with xylocaine-epinephrine solution (start with 25-gauge needle/6-cc syringe). Infiltrate through skin bleb, distributing remaining several cubic centimeters of local anesthetic partly into subcutaneous tissues but *primarily* into periosteal surface (switch to 22-gauge needle). Inject several sites on periosteal surface, covering an area of at least 1 cm in diameter. (In obese patients, a spinal needle may be required for this step.)

Precautions
1. The posterosuperior iliac spine (PSIS) is the preferred site for both aspiration and biopsy.
2. The sternum (second or third intercostal space) and tibia (upper third) are alternative sites for aspiration. These sites are for experienced operators only. *Never attempt bone marrow biopsy at these sites.*

Technique
1. Position patient in lateral decubitus position with knees drawn up partly to the chest. Use left lateral decubitus position if target is right PSIS (for right-hand-dominant operator) or vice versa (for left-hand-dominant operator) (see figure below).
2. Administer intravenous premedication as discussed above.
3. Place a Chux underneath dependent buttock (to catch Betadine, blood)
4. Locate the PSIS by palpation. If this is difficult, follow the iliac crest anteriorly to posteriorly, searching for the large prominence on the medial

border, several centimeters below the top of the crest.

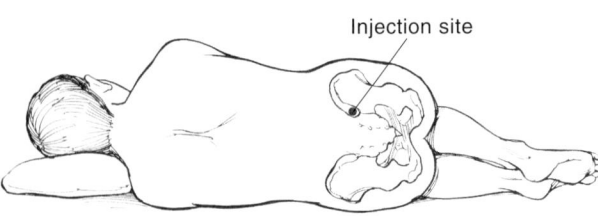

Injection site

5. Use a marker (e.g., the nontipped end of an office-type pen) to make an impression over the PSIS.

6. Prep the skin using Betadine over a wide area (diameter of at least 6 inches) centered on the PSIS. Drape the patient so that the anterosuperior iliac spine (ASIS) can be palpated through the sterile drape.

7. Administer local anesthetic as discussed above.

8. Make an incision at the previously marked site into the subcutaneous tissues with the No. 11 blade using a stabbing motion (see above).

9. While waiting for the anesthetic to take effect, examine the Jamshidi needle, ascertaining that it is complete with needle, stylette, screw cap, and probe.

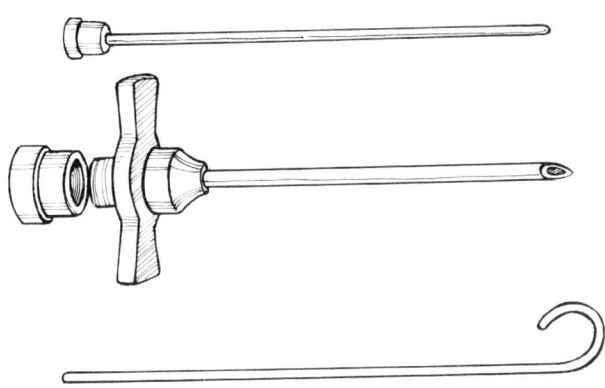

10. Grasp the handle of the reassembled Jamshidi needle with the dominant hand (the needle itself fitting between the third and fourth digits). Insert the needle into the incision site, and use the first and second digits of the nondominant hand to guide the needle down to the periosteum of the PSIS.

11. While stabilizing the needle at the skin using the first and second digits of the nondominant hand, introduce the needle into the PSIS using firm pressure and a rotatory motion with back and forth arcs of 180 degrees. Avoid the natural tendency for the needle to slide medially into the dorsal sacroiliac ligament by angling (pointing) the needle approximately 10 degrees *superior to the horizontal plane, or toward the ASIS.* The pressure required is vari-

able depending on the mineralization of the iliac bone.

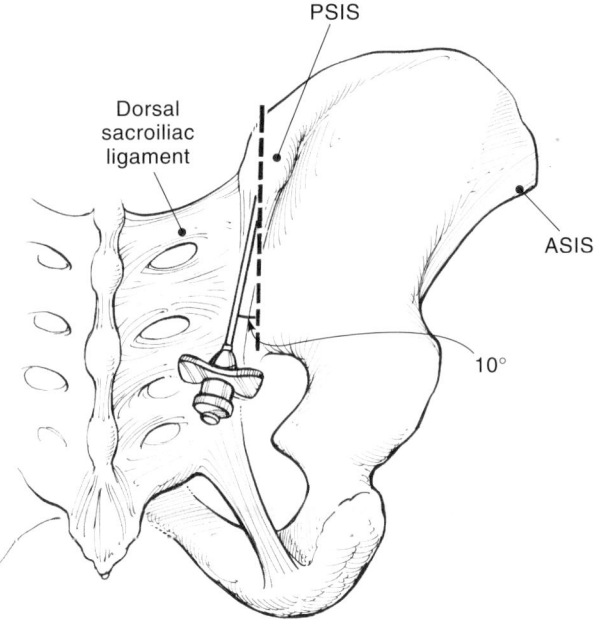

PSIS

Dorsal sacroiliac ligament

ASIS

10°

12. Check for solid placement of the needle by moving it parallel to the plane of the bed. The patient's entire pelvis should move with the needle. A "give" may be appreciated when the marrow cavity is entered, but this sensation is variable.

13. Verify that your assistant is ready to receive the aspirate specimen. If so, unscrew the needle cap and remove the stylette (but keep these sterile). Take a 12-cc syringe, aspirate and expel air through it once, and attach it firmly to the Jamshidi needle.

14. Warn the patient that this next step may be painful. Rapidly pull the plunger of the syringe back nearly all the way. Allow *no more* than 0.5 cc of marrow to enter the syringe. Immediately release all negative pressure on the plunger, detach the syringe, and hand it to the assistant. *This step should be accomplished as rapidly as possible (preferably within 3 seconds) to prevent clotting.* Place the stylette partly into the needle to decrease external bleeding.

15. Wait to see if the assistant finds bone marrow spicules in the specimen. If so, the aspiration is completed. If not, reinsert the stylette, reattach the screw cap, and withdraw the entire needle back to the subcutaneous tissue level. Repeat steps 11 through 14 at an adjacent periosteal site.

16. After the aspiration has been completed successfully, one may obtain (if indicated) additional marrow for culture and/or cytogenetics. A specimen of 10 cc of marrow (inoculated at the bedside into standard blood culture bottles) is recommended for culture; a specimen of 2 cc (collected in a heparinized syringe) is required for cytogenetics.

17. Failure of marrow to enter the syringe after step 14 (i.e., a dry tap) indicates either that the needle is not yet in the marrow cavity or that a pathologic condition (e.g., myelofibrosis, marrow replacement by

tumor) is present. Advance the needle using the same rotatory motion about 1 to 2 cm and try aspirating again.

18. After completing the aspiration or establishing the presence of a dry tap, proceed to bone marrow biopsy. Withdraw the Jamshidi needle to the subcutaneous level, and replace the stylette and screw cap. Reintroduce the needle at a periosteal site 1 cm removed from where the aspirate was done by repeating steps 11 and 12 above. Remove the screw cap and stylette. Fold a 4 × 4 gauze over the proximal end, and advance the needle in its existing direction using the same grip, pressure, and hand motion described previously. Use the first and second digits of the nondominant hand at the skin line to ascertain that the needle has been advanced for another 2 to 3 cm.

19. When the needle has been advanced, it should contain a core specimen. Rotate the needle at least 360 degrees in each direction several times. Tilt the needle to the side in each of four quadrants to help break off the core specimen from surrounding bone. Withdraw the needle *in a controlled manner* while wobbling it from side to side. The core specimen may or may not be visible in the tip of the needle.

20. Use the probe to push the specimen from the *distal* to the *proximal* end of the needle (i.e., "backward"). If aspiration was successful, the biopsy specimen may be dropped directly into a fixative solution. If aspiration was not successful, the biopsy should first be placed on glass slides, where it may be rolled to obtain a cell touch prep, which is useful for evaluating cellular morphology and also can be used for cytochemical stains.

21. Fold the 4 × 4 gauze and tape firmly over the procedure site using the adhesive bandage. If there is much oozing, compress this area by hand for 10 minutes, and ask the patient to lie with the PSIS on the sandbag thereafter.

22. Properly dispose of all needles and sharp equipment. Write a procedure note.

Follow-Up

1. No special patient follow-up is normally required other than as dictated by the underlying disease. Acetaminophen should suffice for postprocedure pain.

2. Rare complications of the procedure include retroperitoneal hemorrhage and fracture of the iliac bone (for the PSIS) as well as perforation into the mediastinum and sternomanubrial separation (for the sternum).

 ## Bibliography

Douglas DD, Risdell RJ: Bone marrow biopsy technic: Artifact induced by aspiration. Am J Clin Pathol 1984;82:92–94.

Hyun BH, Gulati GL, Ashton JK: Bone marrow examination: Techniques and interpretation. Hematol Oncol Clin North Am 1988;2:513–523.

Jamshidi K, Windschitl HE, Swaim WR: A new biopsy needle for bone marrow. Scand J Haematol 1971;8:69–71.

Rothstein G: Origin and development of the blood and blood forming tissues. *In* Lee GR, et al (eds): Wintrobe's Clinical Hematology, vol 1, 9th ed. Philadelphia, Lea & Febiger, 1993, pp 59–75.

Wolff SN, Katzenstein A, Phillips GL, et al: Aspiration does not influence interpretation of bone marrow biopsy cellularity. Am J Clin Pathol 1983;80:60–62.

150 Polycythemia

Khaled Al-Asad

Etiology

1. *Definition: Erythrocytosis* is an increase in the red cell mass secondary to a known stimulus, whereas *polycythemia* is simply the increase in red cell mass. *Polycythemia vera,* on the other hand, is a primary disease of the pluripotent stem cell (PPSC) leading to excessive production of multiple cell lineages as well as extramedullary hematopoiesis. The increase in red cell mass can be detected by ^{15}Cr-labeled red blood cells (RBCs); a concomitant increase in blood volume is usually observed utilizing ^{131}I-albumin fraction.

2. *Classification:* After assessing the blood volume, state of hydration, hemoglobin, and hematocrit, polycythemia can be classified as either relative or absolute. A simplistic approach or classification is shown in Figure 150–1.

3. *Pathogenesis:* Absolute polycythemia is a product of an interaction between the PPSC and erythropoietin (a glycoprotein produced by the peritubular cells of the kidney in response to decreased oxygen delivery). Table 150–1 shows the relation between the hormone level and different types of polycythemia. An inappropriately high level of erythropoietin is observed in certain "autonomous" cases, such as neoplasms (kidney, ovary, liver), cerebellar hemangioblastoma, pheochromocytoma, large fibroid, cystic diseases of the kidney, and after transplants. Testosterone and adrenal steroids are known to increase red blood cell production. Polycythemia rubra vera (PRV) is characterized by abnormal clone at the level of PPSC, and so it is independent of erythropoietin level.

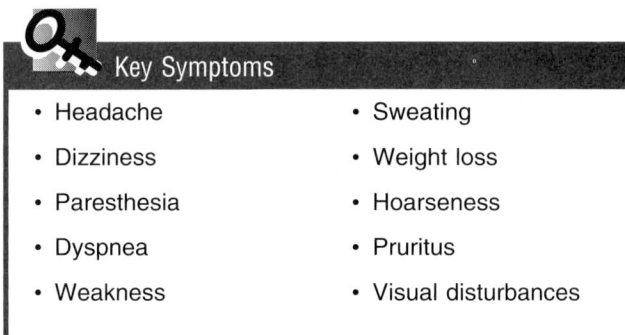

Key Symptoms

- Headache
- Dizziness
- Paresthesia
- Dyspnea
- Weakness

- Sweating
- Weight loss
- Hoarseness
- Pruritus
- Visual disturbances

(Many of these symptoms are related to hyperviscosity syndrome.)

Clinical Findings

Hyperviscosity and hypervolemia are known sequelae of increased red cell mass. Thrombotic events and stagnation form the major underlying mechanism for the clinical presentations. Rubor and erythromelalgia are quite specific presentations. Pruritus after a warm bath has been described with uncertain pathogenesis. Presence of hepatomegaly/splenomegaly is strong evidence of PRV.

Key Sign

- Thrombosis

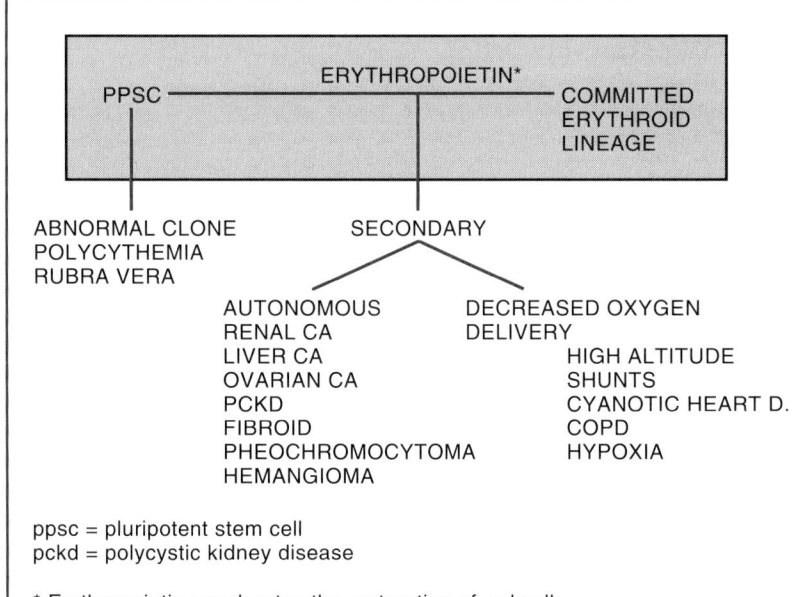

Figure 150–1 Schematic presentation of classification of polycythemia.

ppsc = pluripotent stem cell
pckd = polycystic kidney disease

* Erythropoietin accelerates the maturation of red cells.

TABLE 150–1. RELATIONSHIP BETWEEN VARIOUS CLINICAL CONDITIONS AND BLOOD ERYTHROPOIETIN LEVELS

DISEASE PROCESS	ERYTHROPOIETIN LEVEL
Anemia	Increased
Erythrocytosis	Increased
Polycythemia vera	Decreased

Laboratory Tests

Laboratory tests may be helpful in assessing the hydration status (blood urea nitrogen [BUN], creatinine). An increase in platelet count and white blood cell (WBC) count is seen in PRV. Blood smear in a patient with that disorder reveals a microcytic hypochromic morphology secondary to overconsumption of iron. In case of ineffective erythropoiesis, the lactate dehydrogenase (LDH) and bilirubin will be elevated. The hallmark of the disease is increased hematocrit, RBC count, and hemoglobin.

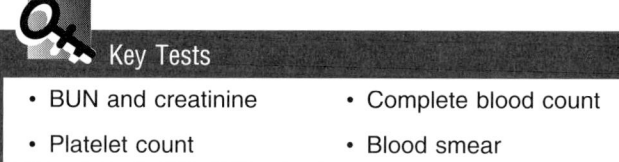

Key Tests

- BUN and creatinine
- Complete blood count
- Platelet count
- Blood smear

Differential Diagnosis

1. Assess volume status and state of hydration. Then do a rational workup to differentiate secondary from primary disease. An easy first step is to obtain an oxygen saturation. A low value directs a physician toward shunts, chronic obstructive pulmonary disease (COPD), and obesity. With a normal saturation, an erythropoietin level is very helpful. A high value is consistent with inappropriate secretion, whereas a low value raises the suspicion of PRV. Supportive evidence toward PRV would be an increased WBC or platelet count. Bone marrow reveals hypercellularity, especially megakaryocytes. A normal oxygen saturation, splenomegaly, and increased red cell mass are sufficient evidence for PRV. Otherwise, any two of the preceding with any two of the following would be another alternative:
   a. WBC count > 12,000
   b. Platelet count > 400,000
   c. Leukocyte alkaline phosphatase (LAP) > 100
   d. Serum vitamin B_{12} > 900 pg/ml
2. Traditionally, PRV has been divided into the following stages:
   a. Proliferative stage: The marrow is producing large numbers of red cells with or without platelet or WBC overproduction. Physical examination commonly reveals a palpable spleen. This is the stage of effective erythropoiesis.
   b. Spent stage: Once the marrow is consumed, inef-

fective erythropoiesis supervenes. Anemia, thrombocytopenia, and leukopenia are common. Extramedullary erythropoiesis takes place involving the spleen (massive enlargement), lymph nodes, and kidneys.
   c. Myeloid metaplasia: In this stage, the main characteristic is the development of acute leukemia.

Treatment

1. Once relative polycythemia has been ruled out, the first step in secondary polycythemia, in the presence of hyperviscosity syndrome, is phlebotomy. It is cheap and simple and almost devoid of any side effects. The aim is to achieve a hematocrit of below 45 per cent.
2. The second step is to identify the underlying disease process. In polycythemia vera, the main problems are related to a high platelet count and thrombosis. It is customary to give such patients aspirin to inhibit platelet aggregation, although such patients have a high incidence of bleeding (minor and major). The chance of acquiring a thrombotic event depends on the presence of a previous event, age above 70, an active disease, and one that has been treated with phlebotomy alone. In the presence of acute process, phlebotomy is indicated at that time, with 200 to 500 ml of blood daily initially and then every other day or three times a week. The treatment of chronic PRV depends on age, symptoms, stage, and risk benefit. The major three options (Fig. 150–2) are:
   a. Phlebotomy, as described above. Most probably this is accompanied by an increased risk for thrombotic events.
   b. Chemotherapy. Hydroxyurea has been the most popular drug because of its short half-life, although no clear evidence is present regarding increased incidence of leukemogenic effect. Alkylating agents have been used also, such as busulfan,

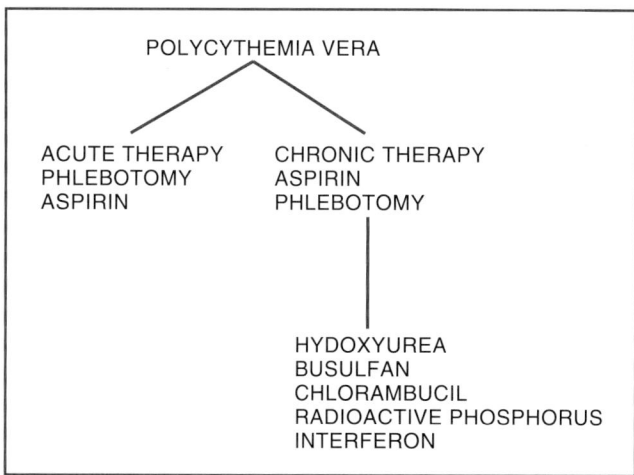

Figure 150–2 Therapeutic options in polycythemia vera.

but they have more side effects, especially the leukemogenic effect.

   c. Radioactive phosphorus. In this therapy, suppression of the marrow takes about 2 to 3 months. It is convenient in noncompliant patients, but an increased risk of leukemia has been observed. The new mode of therapy for active disease is interferon, which has no leukemogenic effect, but it has many side effects, as well as the need to be given subcutaneously.

Most people with this disease live for about a median of 10 years. This, as described earlier, is influenced by the mode of therapy introduced. (Phlebotomy has higher thrombotic events; busulfan and chlorambucil have higher incidences of leukemia.) The development of this "myeloid metaplasia" carries a poor prognosis, because the majority of patients are elderly and have low hematocrits and platelet counts.

Bibliography

Athens J: Polycythemia vera. *In* Lee GR, Bithel TC, Foerster J, et al: Wintrobe's Clinical Hematology, 9th ed. Philadelphia, Lea & Febiger, 1993.

Berk P: Erythrocytosis and polycythemia. *In* Wyngaarden JB, Smith LH, Bennett JC: Cecil's Textbook of Medicine, 19th ed. Philadelphia, WB Saunders, 1992.

Berlin NI: Polycythemia vera: An update. Part 1. Semin Hematol 1986;23(2):131–165. Part 2. Semin Hematol 1986;23(3):167–187.

Donovan PB, Kaplan ME, Goldberg JD: Treatment of polycythemia vera with hydroxyurea. Am J Hematol 1984;17:329.

Erslev AJ: Erythropoietin. N Engl J Med 1991;324(19):1339–1344.

151 Lymphadenopathy

Jacqueline Ewing

Etiology

1. Infection and inflammation cause node enlargement due to proliferation of lymphocytes after antigen exposure. They also cause hyperplasia of nonlymphoid cells. Nodal structure remains intact while size increases.
2. Malignancy causes a change in nodal structure. Lymph nodes capture and provide a place for continued growth of tumor cells in metastatic disease.

Symptoms

1. Node enlargement may be constant or wax and wane.
2. Associated symptoms depend on diagnosis and may commonly include
   a. Cough
   b. Fever
   c. Weight loss
   d. Night sweats
   e. Pruritus
   f. Fatigue
   g. Arthralgias
   h. Myalgias

Clinical Findings

1. Location and consistency of node enlargement are important. A node is considered enlarged if it is greater than 1 cm.
   a. Infection: Nodes often are tender, asymmetric, matted, and superficial and may have inflamed or tender overlying skin.
   b. Lymphoma: Nodes may be large, symmetric, firm, mobile, nontender, and rubbery.
   c. Metastatic tumor: Nodes are fixed, hard, discrete, and nontender.
2. Direct examination is done for signs of infection or abdominal masses, especially splenomegaly and hepatomegaly.

Key Sign

• Nodal enlargement greater than 1 cm

Laboratory Tests

1. If infection is suspected, consider the following: complete blood count with differential and platelet count, sedimentation rate, tuberculin skin test (PPD), chest film, serum protein electrophoresis, heterophil antibodies, transaminases, antibodies to *Toxoplasma gondii.*
2. If malignancy is suspected, excision biopsy with node analysis should be done.

   a. Histologic examination
   b. Culture of node
   c. Antigenic typing
   d. Chromosome analysis
   e. Molecular studies discussed with pathologist
3. To further examine deep nodes: radiography, ultrasonography or CT scan

Key Test

• Biopsy is the only definitive test

Differential Diagnosis

1. The differential diagnosis (Table 151–1) may be approached by first determining whether adenopathy is isolated, regional, or generalized.

TABLE 151–1. DIFFERENTIAL DIAGNOSIS ACCORDING TO LOCATION OF ADENOPATHY

Suboccipital	Scalp infections, mononucleosis, toxoplasmosis, tick bites, lymphoma
Auricular	
Anterior	Ocular infections, cat-scratch fever
Posterior	Rubella
Cervical	Head or neck cancer or infection, mononucleosis, Epstein-Barr virus, cytomegalovirus, toxoplasmosis, rubella, tuberculosis, lymphoma, metastatic disease
Submandibular/ submental	Tumors of mouth or larynx, dental disease, thyroid cancer
Supraclavicular	Lymphoma, cancer of breast, lung, or GI system, infection of lung or retroperitoneal space (Virchow's node is a large left supraclavicular node found with GI metastasis)
Axillary	Infection, trauma, or insect bites of arm/hand, cat-scratch fever, breast cancer, lymphoma, melanoma, brucellosis
Epitrochlear	Hand infection, lymphoma, sarcoidosis, tularemia, secondary syphilis, rheumatoid arthritis
Mediastinal/hilar/ thoracic	Lymphoma, lung infection or cancer, sarcoidosis, mononucleosis, tuberculosis, histoplasmosis
Retroperitoneal	Hodgkin's and non-Hodgkin's lymphoma, tuberculosis, germ cell tumors, seminoma, prostate cancer, and other cancers
Inguinal	Lymphoma, pelvic cancers, sexually transmitted diseases, *Pasteurella pestis,* infection and trauma of legs/feet (with femoral or external iliac adenopathy, malignancy more common)
Generalized (>2 sites)	Infection: Epstein-Barr virus, cytomegalovirus, toxoplasmosis, tuberculosis, hepatitis, syphilis, HIV/AIDS, histoplasmosis, measles, rubella, varicella
	Malignancy: lymphoma, leukemia
Uncommon causes	Amyloidosis, sarcoidosis, mucocutaneous lymph node syndrome (Kawasaki's syndrome), lymphomatoid granulomatosis, angioimmunoblastic lymphadenopathy
Iatrogenic	Serum sickness, drug reaction, silicone, graft-versus-host disease

2. Consider node versus cyst or abscess.

Treatment

1. Observation for 15 to 30 days after appropriate treatment in cases of suspected infection, with care to document location and node size in two dimensions

2. May include empiric treatment with an antibiotic for no more than 1 to 2 weeks with close follow-up evaluation

3. Directed toward specific diagnosis

Follow-Up

1. Fifty per cent of node biopsies are nondiagnostic. Twenty-five per cent of patients with nondiagnostic biopsies develop disease within one year, making repeat examination and biopsy necessary if enlargement persists or recurs.

2. Re-examine 4 weeks after infection is resolved to ensure normalization of affected nodes.

Bibliography

Chesney PJ: Cervical adenopathy. Pediatr Rev 1994;15:276–285.

Faller DV: Diseases of the lymph nodes and spleen. *In* Wyngaarden JB, et al: Cecil Textbook of Medicine, 19th ed. Philadelphia, WB Saunders, 1992, pp 978–981.

Grossman M, Shiramizu B: Evaluation of lymphadenopathy in children. Curr Opin Pediatrics 1994;6:68–76.

Longo DL, et al: Lymphocytic lymphomas. *In* Devita VT, et al (eds): Cancer Principles and Practice of Oncology, 4th ed. Philadelphia, JB Lippincott, 1993, pp 1882–1884.

Pangalis GA, et al: Clinical approach to lymphadenopathy. Semin Oncol 1993;20:570–582.

152 Lymphoma

Barry R. Meisenberg

Etiology and Epidemiology

1. The non-Hodgkin's lymphomas (NHL) are a diverse group of diseases that have in common malignant transformation of lymphocytes or lymphocyte precursors. Despite their common lineage, these diseases are quite heterogeneous with respect to their immunology, biology, natural history, and response to treatment.

2. Over 40,000 NHLs occur annually, equally split between aggressive and indolent forms. The average age of patients is in the early forties. Ten to 20 per cent of NHLs arise outside the lymph nodes or spleen from lymphoid tissue in other organs. Predisposing conditions that have been associated with lymphomas include

   a. Immune suppression related to inherited or acquired conditions (especially the acquired immune deficiency syndrome)

   b. Viruses such as Epstein-Barr virus (EBV) and HTLV-1

   c. Toxins such as herbicides or radiation

3. Most patients with NHL, however, do not have any recognized risk factor or predisposing condition.

Histologic Classification

Histologic classification is very complex, and competing systems exist. The International Working Class Formulation recently has attempted to bring some order to classification. In this system, NHL can be loosely grouped into three classes (Table 152–1).

Clinical Findings

1. Seventy-five per cent of patients present with palpable peripheral lymphadenopathy.

2. Most patients are asymptomatic, although 20 to 30 per cent have fevers, night sweats, or unexplained weight loss, the so-called B symptoms.

3. Other findings depend on the location of the lymphoma.

TABLE 152–1. NHL GROUPING, INTERNATIONAL WORKING CLASS FORMULATION

Low Grade	Intermediate Grade
Small lymphocytic	Follicular large cell
Follicular small cleaved cell	Diffuse cleaved cell
Follicular mixed small and large cell	Diffuse mixed small and large cell
	Diffuse large cell
High Grade	
Large cell immunoblastic	
Lymphoblastic	
Small noncleaved cell	

Key Symptoms

B Symptoms Associated with NHL

- Fever >101.5° F
- Night sweats
- Unexplained weight loss of more than 10 per cent of total body weight

Key Signs

- Nodes may enlarge and decrease apparently spontaneously over several months
- Involved lymph nodes are typically nontender, movable, and feel firm but not rock hard to the touch

Laboratory Tests

1. Laboratory studies are used to confirm the diagnosis of lymphoma and aid in staging, which in turn helps make treatment decisions. Useful laboratory tests include

   a. Complete blood count (CBC) with sedimentation rate (ESR may be useful in following the clinical course)

   b. A chemistry panel including lactate dehydrogenase (LDH) (the LDH is a useful marker for disease activity and correlates with tumor bulk)

   c. Radiographic studies (CT scans of the chest and abdomen to aid in staging)

   d. Bone marrow biopsy for staging

   e. Additional studies as indicated

2. The most important test is an adequate surgical biopsy specimen, which should be reviewed by an experienced pathologist. A needle aspiration of a suspicious lymph node does not allow determination of the nodal architecture and is not acceptable for initial diagnosis of a suspicious lesion. Needle aspiration may be useful in patients with known lymphoma who develop a recurrence but should not be performed to exclude lymphoma in a suspicious node.

Key Tests

- Surgical biopsy is the only definitive test.
- Do not rely on needle aspiration for diagnosis.
- Biopsy the largest lymph node that is accessible to avoid misdiagnosis.

TABLE 152–2. STAGING OF LYMPHOMA, ANN ARBOR CLASSIFICATION

Stage I:	Single lymph node region; for single, extralymphatic organ (1E)
Stage II:	Two or more lymph node regions on the same side of the diaphragm
Stage III:	Lymph node regions on both sides of the diaphragm
Stage IV:	Diffuse involvement of extralymphatic organs not affected by direct spread such as lung, bone marrow, liver

If B symptoms are present (see Key Symptoms), the classification changes to IB, IIB, IIIB, or IVB.

Differential Diagnosis

1. Differential diagnosis of lymphadenopathy is extensive (see Chapter 151). Clinical judgment is required in determining whether a patient is at high risk for another diagnosis. For example:

   a. Isolated cervical adenopathy in a chronic smoker could be due to nasopharyngeal carcinoma.

   b. Isolated unilateral axillary adenopathy in a middle-aged woman suggests breast cancer.

Staging of Lymphoma

1. Staging of lymphoma follows the Ann Arbor Classification (Table 152–2).

2. Eighty per cent of indolent lymphomas present as stage IV disease (usually bone marrow involvement), whereas the more aggressive intermediate- or high-grade lymphomas are sometimes confined to one or more lymph node areas.

Treatment

1. The treatment of lymphoma is determined primarily by the histologic type as well as other factors, such as the age and underlying condition of the patient. Treatment relies primarily on chemotherapy with or without radiation therapy. The timing of treatment, drugs to be used, and therapeutic goals vary with the individual patient.

Key Treatment

Low-Grade Lymphoma

• Patients are older and often have stage IV disease.

• Indolent natural history with a 6- to 10-year average survival

• Chemotherapy leads to remission but not cure.

• Indications for treatment: symptomatic or bulky adenopathy, constitutional symptoms related to lymphoma, dangerous compressions of other vital structures by bulky nodes

2. Low-grade lymphoma is usually treated with one or more chemotherapy drugs such as cyclophosphamide (Cytoxan) or chlorambucil (Leukeran) along with prednisone. Vincristine (Oncovin) may be added. Remissions may be partial or complete and last several years, but adenopathy almost always returns. Additional treatment can be given but becomes progressively less successful.

3. Maintaining full-dose intensity is important. Patients who cannot receive full doses because of age or underlying disease have a poorer prognosis.

Key Treatment

Intermediate-Grade and High-Grade Lymphomas

• More aggressive biologically but with the potential for cure with aggressive chemotherapy.

• Standard treatment is combination CHOP (cyclophosphamide [Cytoxan], doxorubicin [Adriamycin], vincristine [Oncovin], and prednisone) given for six cycles.

• Durable complete remissions occur in 30 to 50 per cent.

• Important prognostic factors include age, bulk of disease, and histologic subtype.

• Lymphoblastic lymphoma is often treated like ALL (see Chapter 149).

• Small noncleaved lymphoma is treated with high-dose cyclophosphamide in addition to methotrexate.

Bibliography

For information on the classification of lymphomas, see
Harris NL, Jaffe ES, Stein H, et al: A revised European-American classification of lymphoid neoplasms: A proposal from the International Lymphoma Study Group. Blood 1994; 84:1361–1392.

For more information on the staging of non-Hodgkin's lymphomas, see
Moormeier JA, Williams SF, Golomb HM: The staging of non-Hodgkin's lymphomas. Semin Oncol 1990;17:43–50.

For information on the treatment of low-grade lymphomas, see
Horning SJ: Treatment approaches to the low-grade lymphomas. Blood 1994;83:881–884.

For more information on the treatment of intermediate- and high-grade lymphomas, see
Armitage JO: Treatment of non-Hodgkin's lymphoma. N Engl J Med 1993;328:1023–1030.

For information regarding the special considerations of lymphoma in patients with AIDS, see
Levine AM: Acquired immunodeficiency syndrome–related lymphoma. Blood 1992;80:8–20.

153 Hodgkin's Disease

A. Steven Fleisher

Etiology

1. Definition: Hodgkin's disease (HD) is a unique malignant disorder most often characterized by the presence of the Reed-Sternberg (R-S) giant cell. It arises in lymph nodes and predictably spreads to contiguous lymph node groups.

2. A specific cause remains unknown. There is evidence to support the involvement of both genetic and environmental factors. Postulated pathogenic processes include infection, genomic alterations, growth factor gene deregulation, and immune defects.
   a. Genetic factors are implicated by an association with certain human leukocyte antigens (HLA) and an increased risk in siblings.
   b. Among environmental factors, evidence for Epstein-Barr virus (EBV) as the etiologic agent is the strongest and lies in the demonstration of clonal EBV DNA in the neoplastic R-S cells.

Epidemiology

1. There is a bimodal disease distribution in the United States; the first peak occurs in young adults (15 to 35 years), and the second peak is seen after age 50.

2. The prevalence is higher in whites and higher socioeconomic groups.

3. The disease is predominant in males, with the predominance being more pronounced in younger individuals (in childhood HD, over 80 per cent are males).

Symptoms

1. Most patients are asymptomatic at the time of presentation.

2. Approximately one third of patients have constitutional symptoms, called B symptoms, which negatively affect prognosis. These are fever, night sweats, and weight loss of greater than 10 per cent in less than 6 months. Constitutional symptoms that do not affect prognosis include generalized pruritus, weakness, malaise, and alcohol-induced lymph node pain.

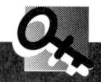

Key Symptoms

- Fever
- Night sweats
- Weight loss

Clinical Findings

1. Most patients present with painless, nontender cervical lymphadenopathy.

2. At the time of presentation, approximately half the patients have mediastinal adenopathy, often detected on routine chest radiograph. More than 90 per cent have neck and/or mediastinal disease.

3. Disseminated disease at the time of presentation is now rare. Nonetheless, patients do sometimes present with
   a. Spinal cord compression
   b. Superior vena cava syndrome

4. Unlike non-Hodgkin's lymphoma, CNS or gastrointestinal tract involvement is unusual.

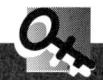

Key Sign

- Painless nontender cervical lymphadenopathy

Laboratory Tests

1. Diagnosis
   a. Biopsy of sufficient involved tissue for an accurate histologic diagnosis is imperative. Needle aspirations or needle biopsies are not adequate for diagnostic purposes.
   b. The diagnosis invariably relies on the presence of the R-S cell (a large cell with a bilobed nucleus and two or more nucleoli), within a setting of benign inflammatory cells and/or fibrosis.
   c. The RYE classification of HD is based on the ratio of R-S cells to the proliferative cellular and/or fibrotic background (Table 153–1).
   d. Helpful adjuncts that aid in the distinction between HD and non-Hodgkin's lymphoma include expression of CD30 and CD15 cell surface antigens by the R-S cell.

2. Routine laboratory evaluation is generally unrevealing, but the following may be demonstrated
   a. Normochromic normocytic anemia of chronic disease
   b. A positive Coombs' test (This sometimes antedates the diagnosis of HD by several months.)
   c. Eosinophilia (especially in patients with pruritus)
   d. An elevated ESR

3. Immunologic abnormalities
   a. T lymphocyte defects that include anergy to routine skin tests, lymphopenia, and/or reversal of the CD4:CD8 ratio, and the development of localized or disseminated herpes zoster following radiotherapy
   b. B lymphocyte defects that usually occur in ad-

607

TABLE 153–1. RYE HISTOLOGIC CLASSIFICATION OF HODGKIN'S DISEASE

| | | PATHOLOGY | | |
	FREQUENCY (%)	R-S Cells	Reactive Component	PROGNOSIS
Lymphocyte predominant	5	Rare	Abundant	Excellent
Nodular sclerosis	60	Rare	Abundant	Excellent
Mixed cellularity	30	Moderate	Moderate	Good
Lymphocyte depleted	5	Many	Minimal	Poor

vanced disease and affect antibody production as well as humoral immunity

  c. Clinical immunologic disorders that include monoclonal protein spikes, idiopathic thrombocytopenic purpura (ITP), which tends to be less responsive to therapy than ITP in other settings, and rarely, autoimmune neutropenia

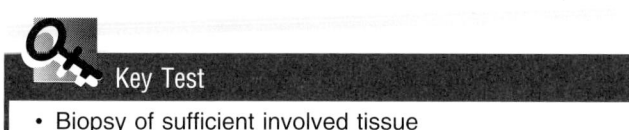

Key Test

- Biopsy of sufficient involved tissue

Differential Diagnosis

1. Reactive adenopathy
2. Metastatic neoplasms
3. Tuberculous adenopathy
4. A variety of non-Hodgkin's lymphomas

Treatment

1. Staging (Table 153–2): This determines treatment and prognosis.
   a. Clinical stage (CS) is defined by the extent of disease apparent after physical examination, chest radiograph, and routine laboratory tests.

   b. Pathologic stage (PS) usually indicates that a laparotomy has been performed.

   c. Procedures required for adequate staging are outlined in Table 153–3.

2. Staging laparotomy:
   a. This includes splenectomy, multiple liver biopsies, biopsies of left and right para-aortic and iliac nodes, and removal of all involved nodes as determined by lymphangiography.

   b. It is usually performed in CS stage I and II patients and its justification is based on the dictum that if it alters stage, it will also alter therapy, necessitating the use of combination chemotherapy rather than radiation therapy for CS I or II that is proved to be PS III or IV disease.

   c. Two subgroups of patients with CS I and II disease, however, do not require staging laparotomy.
      (1) Those with a large mediastinal mass: These patients should receive combined modality treatment.
      (2) Those with CS I who are highly unlikely to have abdominal disease (i.e., male patients with high neck disease and "nodular sclerosing" or "lymphocyte predominant" histology; all females with supradiaphragmatic disease). These patients receive radiation therapy alone.

TABLE 153–2. THE ANN ARBOR STAGING CLASSIFICATION WITH COTSWOLD'S MODIFICATIONS

Stage I	Involvement of single lymph node region or lymphoid structure (e.g., spleen, thymus, Waldeyer's ring)
Stage II	Involvement of two or more lymph node regions on the same side of the diaphragm (the mediastinum is a single site, hilar lymph nodes are lateralized); the number of anatomic sites should be indicated by a suffix (e.g., II3)
Stage III	Involvement of lymph node regions or structures on both sides of the diaphragm III1: With or without splenic hilar, celiac, or portal nodes III2: With para-aortic iliac, mesenteric nodes
Stage IV	Involvement of extranodal site(s) beyond that designated "E"

Modifying characteristics
  A: No symptoms
  B: Fever, drenching sweats, weight loss
  X: Bulky disease: >⅓ widening of mediastinum or >10 cm maximum dimension of nodal mass on chest film
  E: Involvement of a single extranodal site contiguous or proximal to known nodal site
  CS: Clinical stage
  PS: Pathologic stage

TABLE 153–3. RECOMMENDED PROCEDURES FOR STAGING PATIENTS WITH HODGKIN'S DISEASE

History and examination	Documentation of "B" symptoms Physical examination
Radiographic procedures	Plain chest radiograph CT thorax and abdomen Bipedal lymphangiogram
Hematology	Complete blood count Erythrocyte sedimentation rate Bone marrow biopsy, bilateral
Biochemistry	Renal function tests Uric acid Tests of liver function Albumin, lactate dehydrogenase, calcium Erythrocyte sedimentation rate
Under special circumstances	Laparotomy Gallium scans Magnetic resonance imaging Technetium bone scans

d. Stage is advanced in as many as one third of patients.

3. Therapy: It is recommended that HD be treated by a multidisciplinary team, consisting of an experienced medical oncologist, a surgeon, and a radiation oncologist.

   a. Radiotherapy is the treatment of choice for PS I and II disease.

   b. Patients with advanced HD (stage III or IV) should be treated with one of the standard programs of combination chemotherapy: mechlorethamine, vincristine, procarbazine, prednisone (MOPP) or doxorubicin, bleomycin, vinblastine, dacarbazine (ABVD), or MOPP alternating with ABVD. Other chemotherapy regimens include hybrids between MOPP and ABVD as well as experimental regimens.

   c. Combined-modality therapy (radiotherapy and chemotherapy) is indicated only in those adults with massive mediastinal involvement.

4. Complications of therapy: Treatment regimens have improved and many young adults are now being cured. Attention is therefore being focused on minimizing complications of therapy.

   a. Chemotherapy can result in infertility, especially when MOPP is used.

   b. Radiation therapy can result in thyroid dysfunction and an increased risk of thyroid malignancies, accelerated coronary atherosclerosis, second malignancy, and radiation pneumonitis.

   c. Combined-modality treatment can result in

      (1) An enhanced risk of developing secondary acute leukemia with the use of MOPP and radiation therapy

      (2) An increased risk of pulmonary fibrosis and restrictive lung disease with the use of ABVD and radiotherapy

Key Treatment

- Adequate clinical staging
- Consider need for staging laparotomy
- Radiotherapy or chemotherapy

Follow-Up

1. Patients in whom treatment with radiation therapy fails should be treated with combination chemotherapy.

2. Patients who received chemotherapy and in whom remission lasted more than a year should be re-treated with the same chemotherapeutic induction regimen.

3. Patients who received chemotherapy but whose remission lasted less than a year should receive experimental therapy, which is currently marrow transplantation after high-dose chemotherapy.

Bibliography

Bartlett NL, Horning SJ: Hodgkin's disease. *In* Foley JF, Vose JM, Armitage JO (eds): Current Therapy in Cancer. Philadelphia, WB Saunders, 1994, pp 241–250.

DeVita VT, Hubbard SM: Hodgkin's disease. N Engl J Med 1993;328:560–565.

Longo DL, DeVita VT, et al: Treatment of advanced-stage massive mediastinal Hodgkin's disease: The case for combined-modality treatment. J Clin Onc 1991;9:227–235.

Urba WL, Long DL: Hodgkin's disease. N Engl J Med 1992;326:678–687.

Weinshel EL, Peterson BA: Hodgkin's disease. CA Cancer J Clin 1993;43:327–346.

154 Bleeding Disorders

Steven J. Jubelirer

Etiology

1. Type of bleeding
   a. Mucocutaneous (petechiae): suggests platelet disorder
   b. Delayed, recurrent oozing: hematoma (especially soft tissue) or hemarthrosis; suggests plasma coagulation disorder
   c. Menorrhagia or gastrointestinal bleeding possible in either type of disorder
2. Duration of bleeding
   a. Lifelong: suggestive of congenital defect, usually of a single factor
   b. Recent onset: suggests an acquired disorder, usually defects of multiple factors; confirm by history of no bleeding with prior trauma, surgery, tooth extraction, or menses
3. Systemic illnesses associated with bleeding
   a. Liver disease
   b. Malignancy
   c. Uremia
   d. Collagen vascular disease
   e. Gastrointestinal reflux disease
4. Use of medications
   a. Aspirin/nonsteroidal anti-inflammatory drugs (NSAIDs)
   b. Oral anticoagulants: cause vitamin K deficiency
   c. Quinidine, sulfonamides, heparin, gold salts, thiazide diuretics, alcohol, chemotherapy agents: cause thrombocytopenia

---

FAMILY HISTORY

Helpful if positive, but a negative history does not exclude a congenital clotting disorder.

Clinical Findings

1. Skin
   a. Petechiae: thrombocytopenia
   b. Ecchymoses, hematomas: platelet dysfunction
   c. Telangiectasias (blanch with pressure)
2. Joints
   a. Hemarthroses (prominent in large weight-bearing joints): severe plasma coagulation factor deficiency
3. Organomegaly
   a. Hepatomegaly: possible cause of coagulopathy of cirrhosis
   b. Splenomegaly due to a systemic disorder: possible etiology of thrombocytopenia

Key Signs

- Petechiae
- Ecchymosis
- Hemarthrosis

Laboratory Tests

1. Prothrombin time (PT)
2. Activated partial thromboplastin time (APTT)
3. Thrombin time (TT)
4. Fibrinogen level
5. Platelet count
6. Peripheral blood smear (if thrombocytopenic)
7. Bleeding time
8. Factor levels

Differential Diagnosis

1. Isolated prolongation of PT
   a. Early vitamin K deficiency due to malnutrition or chronic use of broad-spectrum antibiotics
   b. Moderately severe liver disease
   c. Oral anticoagulants (first 24 hours)
   d. Congenital factor VII deficiency
2. Isolated prolongation of partial thromboplastin time (PTT)
   a. Mixing study (1:1 normal plasma + patient's plasma) corrects
      (1) Clinical bleeding
         (a) Factor VIII deficiency: hemophilia A
         (b) Factor IX deficiency: hemophilia B
         (c) Factor XI deficiency
      (2) No clinical bleeding—Deficiency of factor XII, prekallikrein, or high-molecular-weight kininogen
   b. Mixing study does not correct the prolonged PTT or prolongs it with 1- to 4-hour incubation.
      (1) Clinical bleeding—acquired inhibitor + factor VIII
      (2) No clinical bleeding—lupus anticoagulant
3. Isolated prolongation of the PT and PTT (normal TT, fibrinogen platelet count, and bleeding time)
   a. Acquired deficiency
      (1) Vitamin K deficiency
      (2) Oral anticoagulants

610

(3) Moderate-to-severe liver disease

(4) Acquired factor X deficiency due to amyloidosis

b. Congenital deficiency

(1) Congenital deficiency of factor II, V, or X

4. Prolongation of thrombin time

a. Heparin administration or contamination (i.e., when blood is drawn through an arterial line)

b. Elevation of fibrin split products

c. Hypofibrinogenemia (especially if less than 100 mg/dl)

d. Dysfibrinogenemia (time and markedly prolonged)

(1) Acquired: due to severe reptilase time, liver disease, or hepatoma

(2) Congenital

e. Inhibitor of fibrin polymerization

(1) Paraprotein in myeloma or Waldenström's macroglobulinemia

(2) Heparinoid or heparin-like inhibitor

5. Prolongation of PT, PTT, thrombin time, and hypofibrinogenemia

a. Thrombocytopenia present

(1) Disseminated intravascular coagulation (DIC)

(2) End-stage liver disease

(3) Coagulation factor washout due to massive transfusion (>10 units blood)

b. Thrombocytopenia not present

(1) Hypo/dysfibrinogenemia, congenital

(2) Thrombolytic agents

6. Thrombocytopenia

a. Pseudothrombocytopenia (i.e., platelet clumping on peripheral blood smear due to EDTA-dependent platelet agglutinin)

b. Thrombocytopenia due to decreased platelet production

(1) Infiltrative process (e.g., leukemia, lymphoma, metastatic cancer)

(2) Aplastic anemia

(3) Alcohol ingestion (excessive)

(4) Drugs (e.g., thiazide diuretics, chemotherapeutic agents)

c. Thrombocytopenia due to increased platelet destruction

(1) Microangiopathic changes on peripheral smear (i.e., fragmented red cells, helmet cells)

(a) Disseminated intravascular coagulation

(b) Thrombotic thrombocytopenic purpura (TTP) (i.e., neurologic signs, hemolysis/fever, renal insufficiency)

(c) Widespread metastatic cancer

(d) Leaking aortic aneurysm

(e) Malignant hypertension

(f) Vasculitis

(2) No microangiopathic changes on smear

(a) Idiopathic thrombocytopenic purpura

(b) Sepsis

(c) Drugs (e.g., quinidine sulfate, sulfonamides, heparin, gold salts)

(d) Massive transfusion

(e) Hypersplenism

7. Prolongation of bleeding time (longer than 9 minutes)

a. Rule out thrombocytopenia

(1) Harker formula:
$$\text{bleeding time} = 30.5 - \left(\frac{\text{patient's platelet count}}{3850}\right)$$

b. If platelet count is normal, consider platelet dysfunction

(1) Acquired causes

(a) Drugs (e.g., aspirin, NSAIDs)

(b) Uremia

(c) Myeloproliferative disorder

(d) Dysproteinemia (e.g., myeloma)

(e) Pump oxygenator (for coronary artery bypass graft procedure)

(2) Congenital causes

(a) von Willebrand's disease

8. Causes of abnormal bleeding not detected by PT, PTT, thrombin time, fibrinogen, platelet count, or bleeding time.

a. Poor fibrin polymer cross-linking

(1) Factor XIII deficiency (congenital)

(2) Inhibitor + factor XIII due + INH therapy

(3) Abnormal fibrinogen

b. Abnormal or excessive fibrinolysis

(1) α_2-Antiplasmin deficiency

c. Mild hemophilia A and B (20 to 25 per cent)

d. von Willebrand's disease (VWD) variant

e. Vascular purpura; defect lies in abnormal vascular fragility

(1) Scurvy

(2) Amyloidosis

(3) Senile purpura

(4) Cryoglobulinemia due to vasculitis, dysproteinemia

(5) Congenital connective tissue disorders (e.g., Marfan's syndrome, Ehlers-Danlos syndrome)

Treatment

1. Vitamin K deficiency

a. Vitamin K, 5 to 10 mg intravenously or intramuscularly; repeat PT and PTT in 24 hours

b. Fresh frozen plasma if active bleeding

2. Isolated prolongation of PTT

   a. Hemophilia A and B: treatment with monoclonal or recombinant F VIII or IX concentrates if active bleeding or if preoperative

   b. Factor XI deficiency: fresh frozen plasma if active bleeding

   c. Factor XII deficiency: no treatment required

   d. Desmopressin (DDAVP), 0.3 mg/kg in 50 cc normal saline over 30 minutes for mild hemophilia A

3. Bleeding due to heparin

   a. Stop heparin

   b. Protamine sulfate, 10 mg intravenously; repeat PTT in 15 minutes to see if PTT corrected

4. Thrombocytopenia

   a. Exclude pseudothrombocytopenia on smear

   b. Stop potentially offending drugs (e.g., heparin, sulfonamides)

   c. Treat sepsis if present; if no improvement in platelet count in 5 to 7 days, consider bone marrow examination

   d. Platelet transfusion if patient has active bleeding or if platelet count is less than 50,000 and patient is undergoing surgery

   e. ITP (immune thrombocytopenia)

     (1) No treatment if platelet count 20,000 or more

     (2) Corticosteroids if platelet count is less than 20,000; splenectomy for steroid-refractory patients

     (3) Platelet transfusion and/or intravenous IgG if there is active bleeding

   f. TTP: plasmapheresis ± aspirin/Persantine

5. Platelet dysfunction

   a. Platelet transfusion for platelet dysfunction due to aspirin or nonsteroidal anti-inflammatory drugs; membrane oxygenator if patient is actively bleeding

   b. Dialysis for uremic bleeding. Consider DDAVP (0.3 mg/kg in 50 cc normal saline over 30 minutes), cryoprecipitate, or intravenous or oral estrogens if bleeding occurs despite dialysis

   c. Plasmapheresis if active bleeding from dysproteinemia

   d. Cryoprecipitate or Humate P if bleeding from VWD; DDAVP for mild bleeding episodes

Bibliography

Development Task Force of the College of American Pathologists: Practice parameters for the use of fresh-frozen plasma, cryoprecipitate, and platelets. JAMA 1994;271(10):777–781.

Ratnoff OD: Some therapeutic agents influencing hemostasis. *In* Coleman RW, Hirsch ED, Marder VJ, Salzman EW (eds): Hemostasis and Thrombosis: Basic Principles and Clinical Practice. Philadelphia, JB Lippincott, 1994.

Roberts HR, Lozier JN: New perspectives on the coagulation cascade. Hosp Pract 1992;27(1):97–110.

Santoro SA, Eby CS: Laboratory evaluation of hemostatic disorders. *In* Hoffman R, Benz EJ, Shattil SJ, et al (eds): Hematology: Basic Principles and Practice, 2nd ed. New York, Churchill Livingstone, 1995, pp 1622–1632.

White GC, Marder VJ, Coleman RW, et al: Approach to the bleeding patient. *In* Coleman RW, Hirsch ED, Marder VJ, Salzman EW (eds): Hemostasis and Thrombosis: Basic Principles and Clinical Practice. Philadelphia, JB Lippincott, 1994.

155 Use of Blood Products

William A. Ghali

Early reports of blood transfusion date back to the 17th century. Unfortunately, these early transfusions often led to catastrophic results, and it was only after the discovery of ABO blood groups by Landsteiner in 1900 that blood transfusion became a relatively safe and valuable form of therapy in modern medicine. Transfusion of blood products is extremely common in a variety of medical settings, but overuse of these products is widespread. It is thus essential for clinicians to become familiar with the indications for transfusion to avoid unnecessary risks. Use of whole blood is now uncommon. Instead, blood is usually transfused by component, as indicated by specific requirements. Transfusable blood components include red blood cells, platelets, and plasma products.

Red Blood Cell Transfusion

1. *Characteristics of component:* Packed red blood cells are separated from plasma by centrifugation of whole blood. This removes approximately 200 ml of plasma from each unit of whole blood and leaves 300 ml of red blood cells. The hematocrit of packed red blood cells is 70 to 80 per cent.

2. *Indications*
   a. Acute anemia associated with signs and symptoms of hypovolemia that do not respond to treatment with crystalloid alone
   b. Chronic anemia associated with significant symptoms (e.g., angina, cerebral ischemia, or dyspnea) which are attributable to the anemia. Chronic anemia usually should be managed by treatment of the underlying cause for anemia (e.g., iron replacement therapy for iron deficiency anemia).
   c. Use of a "transfusion trigger" (a hematocrit at which all patients are transfused regardless of symptoms) is discouraged.

3. *Technical aspects of use*
   a. Before transfusion, patient's blood must be drawn for blood grouping (ABO and Rh typing) and screening for the presence of antibodies against common red blood cell antigens. A crossmatch test between patient serum and donor blood is then performed immediately prior to transfusion to ensure compatibility.
   b. Packed red blood cells must be stored in a refrigerator and removed from cold storage a maximum of 30 minutes before use.
   c. Before transfusion, careful identification checks must be performed to ensure that compatible blood is transfused.
   d. Normal saline can be infused with red blood cells. Glucose (5%) and Ringer's solutions should *not* be used because these solutions cause cell damage or coagulation.
   e. The intravenous infusion catheter should be 20 gauge or larger.
   f. Vital signs should be checked every 15 minutes for the first hour of transfusion and every 30 minutes thereafter. Transfusion should be stopped if vital signs change (e.g., fever, hypotension, tachypnea)—this may indicate transfusion reaction.
   g. A hemoglobin rise of about 1 gm/dl can be expected from transfusion of 1 unit of packed red blood cells.

4. *Special situations*
   a. Leukocyte-free red blood cells can be used in patients who have a history of two or more febrile transfusion reactions. Administration of leukocyte-depleted red blood cells is achieved by transfusion through microaggregate filters.
   b. Washed red blood cells, which are free of plasma proteins, can be used to avoid anaphylactic reactions in patients with antibodies to IgA.
   c. Whole blood is occasionally used in patients who have acute ongoing blood loss with significant hypovolemia.
   d. Human recombinant erythropoietin is a potential substitute for transfusion in the treatment of anemia caused by chronic renal failure or AZT therapy.

Platelet Transfusion

1. *Characteristics of component:* Each platelet unit contains approximately 5.5×10^{10} platelets, along with a small amount of plasma, leukocytes, and red blood cells.

2. *Indications:* Platelets are transfused in patients who have thrombocytopenia related to decreased platelet production, sequestration, or abnormal platelet function. Platelets are generally *not* transfused in thrombocytopenia caused by platelet destruction (e.g., idiopathic thrombocytopenic purpura, thrombotic thrombocytopenic purpura, disseminated intravascular coagulation). Appropriate situations for platelet use are
   a. Platelet count less than 5000 to 10,000 per microliter, with or without active bleeding
   b. Platelet count less than 20,000 per microliter, with active bleeding
   c. Platelet count less than 50,000 per microliter in patients undergoing major surgery

613

d. Platelet count less than 100,000 per microliter and/or prolonged bleeding time in postcardiopulmonary bypass patients with active bleeding.

3. *Technical aspects of use*

   a. Platelets are stored at room temperature and have a shelf life of only 5 days.

   b. The standard dose for platelet transfusion is 1 unit of platelets for each 10 kilograms of body weight (i.e., a 70-kg patient should receive 7 units of platelets).

   c. Platelet count should be checked immediately after transfusion to ensure that there has been an increase of at least 10,000 platelets per microliter.

4. *Special situations*

   a. Single-donor platelets are indicated in alloimmunized patients who are refractory (i.e., platelet count does not increase) to pooled-donor platelet transfusions.

   b. Vasopressin (DDAVP) may be an alternative to platelet transfusion when platelet dysfunction contributes to bleeding (e.g., uremia or postcardiopulmonary bypass).

Plasma Products

1. *Fresh frozen plasma*

   a. Preparation and storage: Plasma is separated from the cellular components of whole blood and subsequently stored frozen for up to 1 year.

   b. Indications: Fresh frozen plasma may be used for the treatment of blood coagulation abnormalities caused by multiple clotting factor deficiencies (e.g., severe liver disease with prothrombin time greater than 1.5 times normal). Warfarin-induced factor deficiencies also can be rapidly reversed with fresh frozen plasma, although vitamin K can be used when instant reversal of warfarin anticoagulation is not essential.

   c. Contraindications: Fresh frozen plasma should *not* be used for isolated factor VIII, factor IX, or fibrinogen deficiencies because specific plasma components are available for treatment of these deficiencies. Plasma also should not be used as a simple volume expander because saline and albumin solutions are safer.

   d. Dose: When needed, fresh frozen plasma should be given at a "dose" of 10 ml/kg of body weight. Each unit of fresh frozen plasma is approximately 200 ml (i.e., an 80-kg patient therefore needs 4 units of fresh frozen plasma).

2. *Cryoprecipitate*

   a. Preparation and storage: Cryoprecipitate is prepared by slowly thawing fresh frozen plasma at 4 to 6° C. This leads to the deposition of a precipitate, which is recovered and refrozen for storage. This cryoprecipitate contains high concentrations of factor VIII, fibrinogen, and von Willebrand's factor.

   b. Indications

      (1) Active bleeding in von Willebrand's disease

      (2) Hemophilia A (but factor VIII concentrate is better)

      (3) Hypofibrinogenemia (primary and secondary)

   c. Dose: Each unit of cryoprecipitate contains 200 to 250 mg fibrinogen and 80 to 120 units of factor VIII. Units of cryoprecipitate are usually pooled for use (e.g., 10 units).

3. *Other plasma products*

   a. Factor VIII:C concentrate: hemophilia A

   b. Factor IX complex: hemophilia B

   c. Albumin (5% and 25%): blood volume expansion and treatment of hypovolemia

   d. Immune globulin (IM or IV): treatment of immunodeficiency diseases and certain autoimmune diseases (e.g., immune thrombocytopenic purpura)

Risks of Blood Product Transfusion

1. *Noninfectious complications*

   a. Acute or delayed hemolytic transfusion reaction

   b. Febrile nonhemolytic transfusion reaction (common)

   c. Anaphylactic reaction (occurs in IgA-deficient patients)

   d. Noncardiogenic pulmonary edema

   e. Graft-versus-host disease

   f. Possible immunosuppressive effects

   g. Circulatory overload

2. *Infectious complications*

   a. HIV infection (risk approximately 1 in 225,000)

   b. Hepatitis B, C, and non-A non-B (risk now <1 in 3000 for hepatitis C and 1 in 25,000 for hepatitis B)

   c. Other viruses: cytomegalovirus, Epstein-Barr virus, HTLV-1 and 2, parvovirus B19.

   d. Syphilis (rare)

   e. Parasitic infection: malaria, babesiosis, others

   f. Bacterial sepsis due to blood contamination

 Bibliography

For a detailed textbook on transfusion medicine, see
Mollison PL, Engelfriet CP, Contreras M: Blood transfusion. *In* Clinical Medicine, 9th ed. Oxford, Blackwell Scientific, 1993.

For a practical handbook on transfusion medicine, see
Westphal RG: Handbook of Transfusion Medicine. Washington, American Red Cross, 1990.

For a review of recent literature in transfusion medicine, see
Summers SH, Smith DM, Agranenko VA: Transfusion Therapy: Guidelines for Practice. Arlington, VA, American Association of Blood Banks, 1990.

For a review of perioperative blood component therapy, see
Irving CA: Perioperative blood and blood component therapy. Can J Anesth 1992;39(10):1105–1115.

For recent red blood cell transfusion guidelines, see
American College of Physicians: Practice strategies for elective red blood cell transfusion. Ann Intern Med 1992; 116(5):403–406.

156 Adverse Reactions to Blood Transfusions

David H. Yawn

Immediate Immunologic Transfusion Reactions

1. Acute intravascular hemolysis (ABO-incompatible red cells or plasma)
   a. Caused by naturally occurring complement-fixing IgM and IgG antibodies to group A and B red cells
   b. Fever, pain at infusion site, hypotension, acute renal failure, hemoglobinemia, hemoglobinuria
   c. Occurs in less than 1 in 50,000 transfusions
   d. Prevented by transfusing ABO-compatible red cells and plasma

> **WARNING**
>
> **Clerical errors (misidentification of patient or crossmatch sample) cause most fatal hemolytic reactions.**

2. Urticarial reactions
   a. Patient sensitized to plasma proteins and/or other antigens
   b. Rapid onset of hives after or during transfusion
   c. 1 to 3 per cent of all transfusions
   d. Prevented by the use of washed red cells or by premedication with antihistamines
3. Anaphylaxis
   a. Anti-IgA in IgA-deficient recipients (rarely caused by antibodies to HLA or platelet antigens)
   b. Sudden hypotension and respiratory distress during transfusion
   c. Expected in less than 1 in 1000 transfusions
   d. Prevented by recognition of IgA-deficient patients or by use of washed red cells or provision of blood components from IgA-deficient donors
4. Febrile nonhemolytic reactions
   a. Passive transfer of donor leukocytes to patients who have produced leukoagglutinins
   b. Rapid onset of fever and chills, rarely pulmonary distress
   c. 1 to 3 per cent of transfusions, more common in multiply transfused or multiparous recipients
   d. Prevented by use of leukocyte depletion filters
5. Adverse reactions caused by platelet alloantibodies
   a. HLA- or platelet antigen-specific antibodies (such as anti-PLA-1) in the recipient
   b. Fever, pulmonary edema, and failure to achieve increments after platelet transfusions. Antibodies to PLA-1 (a high-frequency platelet antigen): petechiae, associated with purpura and severe thrombocytopenia within days after transfusion (posttransfusion purpura)
   c. High frequency of platelet alloantibodies in multiply transfused recipients
   d. Prevention of alloimmunization (due primarily to the stimulating effect of HLA antigens on transfused leukocytes) by the use of leukocyte depletion filters for all cellular blood components
6. Transfusion-related acute lung injury
   a. Etiology uncertain. Volume overload and/or immunologic factors, leukoagglutinins in donor plasma
   b. High-protein noncardiogenic pulmonary edema
   c. Very rare but life-threatening
   d. Avoid donors with plasma leukoagglutinins; use leukocyte depletion filters or washed red cells.

Immediate Nonimmunologic Reactions

1. Volume overload
   a. Rapid infusion of excess volume
   b. Right and left ventricular heart failure, pulmonary and peripheral edema
   c. Very common, frequently unrecognized
   d. Careful attention to cardiovascular function and volume status of the patient during transfusion therapy. Diuretics for selected patients
2. Citrate toxicity
   a. Sudden lowering of ionized calcium
   b. Hypotension and cardiac dysfunction
   c. Rare except during rapid and massive blood transfusion (adult: 12 units of blood per hour)
   d. Treated with intravenous calcium gluconate or calcium chloride. Washed red cells for neonates or small recipients
3. Air embolism
   a. Accidental infusion of air contained in blood component bags
   b. Loss of consciousness, vascular collapse, rapid heart rate, chest tightness, pain, and dyspnea
   c. An extremely rare complication (current risk greatest with intraoperative blood salvage systems)
   d. Prevention by awareness. Treatment: Place the patient on the left side in a head-down, feet-up position (reduction of pumping of air in the right ventricle into the pulmonary arteries).
4. Potassium overload
   a. Elevated potassium in older or irradiated packed cells or whole blood
   b. Hyperkalemia in massively transfused or small patients
   c. Very rare unless patient has pre-existing renal dysfunction or acidosis

d. Prevented by the use of washed red cell components, especially important for neonates and small transfusion recipients

Delayed Transfusion Complications

1. Delayed immune hemolysis

    a. Sensitization to red cell antigens (especially Rh, Kidd, Duffy, MNS antigens) due to remote pregnancies or transfusions. Anamnestic production of non-complement-fixing IgG antibodies a few days after a recent blood transfusion. Extravascular removal of antibody-coated cells

    b. Anemia, fever, arthralgia, mild hyperbilirubinemia. Positive direct antiglobulin test. Renal dysfunction usually mild (rarely severe)

    c. 1 in 5000 transfusions (previously transfused or multiparous recipients)

    d. Patient education. Wallet card identifying the offending antibodies. Transfusion from donors lacking the red cell antigen(s) to which the patient is sensitized

2. Graft-versus-host disease

    a. Proliferation of transfused HLA-incompatible lymphocytes. Immune-suppressed recipients or immune-competent recipients who receive blood components from relatives

    b. Dermatitis, gastrointestinal and liver dysfunction, and immune suppression. High mortality rate

    c. Occurs in less than 1 in 1000 transfusions

    d. Irradiate (at least 2500 rads) all blood components donated by family members or if transfusing immune-suppressed patients; absolutely required for bone marrow transplant recipients

3. Transfusion-related immune suppression

    a. Mechanism unknown

    b. Increased risk for bacterial infections and cancer progression

    c. Common, subclinical, frequently unrecognized

    d. Prevention by reducing homologous blood exposure. Increase use of autologous blood components.

4. Iron overload (transfusion hemosiderosis)

    a. 1 mg of iron in 1 cc of red cells

    b. Chronically transfused patients at great risk with deposition of iron in liver, heart, and lungs and marrow

    c. Common in chronically transfused patients

    d. Minimize unnecessary transfusion. Iron chelation therapy. Reduce transfusions with recombinant erythropoietin therapy.

Infections Transmitted by Transfusion

1. Deadly viruses

    a. Failure to recognize asymptomatic donors infected with immunodeficiency viruses (HIV 1 or 2), human T-cell lymphotrophic viruses (HTLV-I or -II), hepatitis viruses, cytomegaloviruses (CMV), and others

    b. Clinical features related to virus transmitted. Long latency period common with HIV and HTLV-I viruses. CMV not important unless recipient is immune suppressed.

    c. Risk per component transfused: HIV, hepatitis B: fewer than 1 in 200,000; hepatitis C: fewer than 1 in 3000; HTLV-I/II: fewer than 1 in 60,000; CMV: 50 to 100 per cent of donors infected

    d. Reduce risk with careful donor screening and serologic testing. Leukocyte filters to remove strictly cell-associated viruses (HTLV-I/II and CMV). Donors negative for antibodies to CMV less likely to transmit CMV. (Immune-compromised patients and premature neonates are candidates for CMV seronegative donors and leukocyte-reduced blood components.)

2. Transmission of bacteria and endotoxins

    a. Unrecognized bacteremia in the donor or bacterial contamination during processing. Cryophilic organisms (*Escherichia coli* and *Pseudomonas*) associated with refrigerated blood components. *Yersinia, Serratia,* and *Salmonella* implicated with room temperature–stored blood components (platelets)

    b. High mortality rate. Shock and disseminated intravascular coagulation

    c. Cause of death in less than 1 in 500,000 transfusions. As viral transmission risk decreases, the risk of bacterial contamination becomes relatively more important

    d. Prevention with correct cleaning of the donor phlebotomy skin area, good manufacturing practices, deferring donors with febrile illnesses, and the use of leukocyte-depleted blood components

3. Parasitic agents

    a. Donors infected with parasites (e.g., malaria or trypanosome causing Chagas' disease)

    b. Clinical problems of the specific parasitic infection

    c. Rare in United States. Chagas' disease endemic in Central and South America. Increased risk of Chagas' disease by transfusion is a current growing concern in the United States.

    d. Prevention by donor screening and development of appropriate serologic tests

B Bibliography

Dodd RY: Adverse consequences of blood transfusion: Quantitative risk estimates. *In* Nance ST (ed): Blood Supply: Risks, Perceptions, and Prospects for the Future. Bethesda, MD, American Association of Blood Banks, 1994, pp 1–24.

Lundberg GD (ed): Practice parameter for the use of fresh frozen plasma, cryoprecipitate, and platelets. JAMA 1994; 271(10):777–781.

McCullough J: The nation's changing blood supply system. JAMA 1993;269:2239–2245.

Mollison PL, Engelfriet CP, Contreras M: Blood Transfusion in Clinical Medicine, 9th ed. Oxford, Blackwell Scientific Publications, 1993, pp 677–709.

Walker RH: Special report: Transfusion risks. Am J Clin Pathol 1987;88:374–378.

157 Disseminated Intravascular Coagulation

Timothy P. Daaleman

Etiology

1. Disseminated intravascular coagulation (DIC) is an acquired thromboembolic disorder that virtually always occurs in the presence of a concomitant disease or clinical state.
2. DIC results from the activation of the coagulation and fibrinolytic systems and can be an acute or chronic event.
   a. Acute DIC is an uncompensated hemorrhagic and thrombotic disorder that involves both laboratory and clinical evidence of pathology.
   b. Chronic DIC is a compensated hematologic state with mild, protracted, or often subclinical disease manifested by laboratory abnormalities.
3. The causes of DIC are listed in Table 157–1.

Symptoms

1. Bleeding is the predominant clinical symptom.
2. Other symptoms (fever, tachycardia) are nonspecific and not diagnostically helpful.
3. Patients display the signs and symptoms of the concomitant primary disease rather than those of DIC.

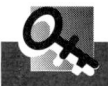

Key Symptom

- Bleeding

TABLE 157–1. CAUSES OF DISSEMINATED INTRAVASCULAR COAGULATION

Obstetric	**Infectious**
Amniotic fluid embolism	Gram-negative/positive/anaerobic
Abruptio placentae	Mycobacterial
Eclampsia	Viral (cytomegalovirus, varicella
Uterine rupture	zoster virus, hepatitis)
Retained dead fetus	Rickettsial (Rocky Mountain spotted
Septic or missed abortion	fever)
	Fungal *(Aspergillus, Candida,*
Tissue Injury	*Histoplasma)*
Trauma (head or crush injury)	Protozoal (malaria)
Burns	
Extensive surgery	**Malignancy**
Hypo- or hyperthermia	Leukemia
Anoxia/asphyxia	Solid tumors
Ischemia/infarction	
	Cardiovascular
Immunologic	Giant hemangioma
Anaphylaxis	Aortic aneurysm
Hemolytic transfusion	Aortic balloon pump
reaction	Acute myocardial infarction
Adverse drug reaction	Vascular surgery
Autoimmune vasculitis	Peripheral vascular disease
Pulmonary	**Miscellaneous**
Adult respiratory distress	Acute or chronic liver disease
syndrome (ARDS)	Envenomation
Pulmonary embolism	Fat embolism
Pulmonary infarction	Amyloidosis

Clinical Findings

1. In the appropriate clinical settings, the following signs should warn the clinician of the possibility of acute DIC:
   a. Petechiae
   b. Ecchymoses
   c. Hemorrhagic bullae
   d. Wound-site bleeding
   e. Gangrene
   f. Gingival bleeding
   g. Vascular access site oozing
   h. Purpura
   i. Acral cyanosis
   j. Hematuria
   k. Epistaxis
   l. Purpura fulminans
2. Patients with chronic DIC present with bleeding that is problematic (i.e., epistaxis, gingival bleeding) but not life-threatening, in addition to diffuse thromboses.

Key Signs

• Petechiae	• Purpura
• Ecchymoses	• Acral cyanosis
• Hemorrhagic bullae	• Hematuria
• Wound-site bleeding	• Epistaxis
• Gangrene	• Purpura fulminans
• Gingival bleeding	• Thromboses (chronic)
• Vascular access site oozing	

Laboratory Tests

1. There is no consensus regarding laboratory criteria that confirm a diagnosis of DIC. All laboratory values must be interpreted in the appropriate clinical setting.
2. The following laboratory tests support the diagnosis of DIC:
   a. Thrombocytopenia (generally less than 60,000 per microliter)
   b. Prolonged prothrombin time (PT) and/or partial thromboplastin time (PTT)
   c. Elevated fibrin(ogen) degradation products (FDPs)
   d. Low or falling fibrinogen levels
   e. Schistocytosis (fragmented red blood cells) on peripheral smear

f. Elevated D dimer

g. Microangiopathic anemia

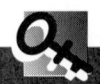

Key Tests

- Complete blood count with peripheral smear
- Fibrinogen level
- Fibrin(ogen) degradation products (FDPs)
- PT and PTT
- Single tube clot retraction and clotting time

Differential Diagnosis

Several diseases resemble DIC; however, they can be ruled out on clinical grounds.

1. Vitamin K deficiency
2. Renal failure
3. Dysfibrinogenemias
4. Systemic lupus erythematosus
5. Thrombotic thrombocytopenic purpura
6. Liver disease
7. Sickle cell crisis
8. Sepsis

Treatment

1. In acute DIC, identifying and treating the underlying disease process remain the cornerstones of treatment.

   a. Aggressive treatment of the primary disease (i.e., antibiotics, evacuate uterus) in addition to appropriate supportive measures to correct or prevent shock, hypoxemia, and acidosis often will be sufficient.

   b. The use of blood products should be guided by the clinical picture.

   (1) Fresh frozen plasma (FFP) provides volume replacement and clotting factors. The dosage of FFP is 10 to 15 cc/kg. The clinician should look to achieve a prothrombin time within 2 to 3 seconds of control.

   (2) Cryoprecipitate should be reserved for hypofibrinogen states. The dosage is 0.2 bag/kg (a 70-kg patient requires 12 to 15 bags).

   (3) Platelet transfusion is appropriate if the platelet count is less than 10,000 to 20,000 per microliter or if major bleeding is present with a count less than 50,000 per microliter.

   c. There is no clear consensus regarding the use of heparin in acute DIC. Heparin is probably indicated in the following clinical situations: amniotic fluid embolism, aortic aneurysm, evidence of thrombosis (in sepsis or malignancy), and severe transfusion reaction.

   (1) Heparin is contraindicated in patients with CNS injury, fulminant liver failure, and most obstetric accidents.

   (2) Two dosing regimens are 80 to 100 units/kg subcutaneously every 4 to 6 hours or 5 to 10 units/kg by continuous intravenous drip. Improvement should be noted by decreasing FDPs and increasing fibrinogen levels.

2. Treatment of the underlying disease process is the initial therapy in chronic DIC.

   a. Anticoagulant therapy with low-dose subcutaneous heparin may be indicated.

   b. Combination antiplatelet agents also have been useful:

   (1) ASA, 600 mg b.i.d. with 30 cc liquid antacid plus dipyridamole, 50 mg q.i.d.

   (2) Sulfinpyrazone, 200 mg b.i.d. with 30 cc liquid antacid plus dipyridamole, 50 mg q.i.d.

Bibliography

Bick, RL: Disseminated intravascular coagulation and related syndromes. *In* Bick, RL (ed): Hematology: Clinical and Laboratory Practice, 1st ed, vol 2, St. Louis, Mosby, 1993, pp 1463–1499.

Gilbert JA, Scalzi RP: Disseminated intravascular coagulation. Emerg Med Clin North Am 1993;11(2):465–480.

Giles AR: Disseminated intravascular coagulation. *In* Bloom AL, et al (eds): Haemostasis and Thrombosis, 3rd ed, vol 2. Edinburgh, Churchill Livingstone, 1994, pp 969–986.

Marder VJ, Feinstein DI, Francis CW, Colman RW: Consumptive thrombohemorrhagic disorders. *In* Colman RW, Hirsh J, Marder VJ, Salzman EW (eds): Hemostasis and Thrombosis: Basic Principles and Clinical Practice, 3rd ed. Philadelphia, JB Lippincott, 1994, pp 1023–1063.

Williams EC, Mosher DF: Disseminated intravascular coagulation. *In* Hoffman R, Benz EJ, Shattil SJ (eds): Hematology: Basic Principles and Practice, 1st ed. New York, Churchill Livingstone, 1991, pp 1394–1405.

158   Common Endocrine Symptoms

1. Excessive growth of body hair in women is called hirsutism. This is an androgen-dependent condition associated with an increase in terminal hair. The distribution of this hair follows a male pattern of hair growth.

2. Hypertrichosis is a condition that is associated with a general increase in body hair of both the vellus and the terminal type of hair growth and is not an androgen-mediated phenomenon.

3. Terminal hair is pigmented, coarse, greater in diameter, and normally found on the scalp, eyebrows, mons pubis, and axillary region. Vellus hair is soft, fine, and downy, and is found on most areas of the body. There are no hair follicles on palms and soles, and hence no hair is found in these areas.

4. Genetic and racial factors influence hair growth. Asian people and Native Americans have less hair than people of Occidental and Mediterranean origins.

5. Age also influences the nature of hair growth. With onset of puberty, pubic hair growth is seen (adrenarche), and hair loss is noticed with menopause. Aging is associated with increased facial hair. There is an increase in body hair in the first trimester of pregnancy.

6. The pilosebaceous unit is composed of the hair follicle with its dermal papillae and the sebaceous gland. There are three phases of hair growth: anagen, catagen and telogen. The active anagenic phase and the change from vellus to terminal hair are under the influence of androgens, specifically the influence of dihydrotestosterone (DHT), which is mainly derived from the conversion of testosterone by the enzyme 5α-reductase. The level of 5-α reductase activity may be significantly higher in hirsute women than in normal women.

7. One sees a continuum of symptoms based on the level of the circulating androgens. Hirsutism, with its increase in facial, chest, lower abdomen, inner thigh, and lower back terminal hair, progresses to disturbance in menstrual cycles and ovulation, to acne, and to frank virilization with increased muscle mass, deepening of the voice, temporal recession of hair, and clitorimegaly (>35 mm^2). Levels of testosterone >150 ng/dl should raise the question of ovarian or adrenal tumor. The same should be suspected if a rapid evolution of hirsutism occurs.

Differential Diagnosis

In women, the endogenous androgens are from two sources: ovarian and adrenal glands. The differential diagnoses are listed in Tables 158–1 and 158–2. It is useful to differentiate hypertrichosis from hirsutism.

TABLE 158–1.   HYPERTRICHOSIS (NONANDROGENIC PHENOMENON)

Drug-induced
    Dilantin N (Phenytoin Na)
    Minoxidil
    Cyclosporine
    Penicillamine
    Phenothiazines
    Acetazolamide
    Psoralens
Congenital (genetic disorders)
    Edwards' syndrome (trisomy 18)
    Hurler's syndrome
    Cornelia de Lange's syndrome
    Congenital hypertrichosis
    Seckel's dwarfism
    Turner's syndrome (gonadal dysgenesis)
Metabolic
    Anorexia nervosa
    Hypertrichosis lanuginosa
    Juvenile hypothyroidism
    Porphyria

TABLE 158–2.   HIRSUTISM (ANDROGEN-DEPENDENT)

Idiopathic
Polycystic ovarian disease (PCOD)
Hyperandrogenism with insulin resistance with acanthosis nigricans (HAIR AN)
Late-onset adrenal hyperplasia
21 hydroxylase deficiency
11 hydroxylase deficiency
Cushing's syndrome
Adrenal neoplasm (adenoma; carcinoma)
Ovarian neoplasia
Arrhenoblastoma (Sertoli-Leydig cell tumors)
Gynandroblastoma
Thecoma
Brunner's tumor
Lipid cell tumor
Gonadoblastoma
Drug-induced
    Testosterone creams
    Anabolic steroids
    Danazol; halotestin
    Progesterone-dominant oral contraceptives

History

1. History should include the time of onset, duration of increased hair growth, menstrual and gestational history, drug and medication use, and finally any history of diabetes mellitus, hypertension, or emotional difficulties.

2. Physical examination should include assessment of terminal hair and the appearance of the skin. The skin might exhibit thinning, easy bruisability, or the presence of purple stria, which would suggest, in the presence of hypertension and obesity, Cushing's syndrome. The skin lesion of acanthosis nigricans, in the presence of hirsutism, would point to polycystic ovarian disease (PCOD) with insulin resistance. The presence of galactorrhea concurrent with menstrual irregularity would indicate an underlying hyperprolactinemia.

Clinical Findings

1. Two objective ways to assess the growth of terminal hair are the Ferriman and Gallwey scoring system and the vellus index, as described by Madames and Novotny. The grading system of Ferriman and Gallwey assesses the growth of terminal hair at 11 different sites: upper lip, chin, chest, upper back, lower back, upper abdomen, lower abdomen, arms, forearms, thighs, and legs—grades 0 to 4 at each site. Another recent assessment includes vellus index. The index of 55 separates normal women from those with hirsutism.

2. The most common causes are probably familial hirsutism and idiopathic hirsutism, followed by the syndrome of polycystic ovarian disease. The former two are associated with regular menstrual cycles and the onset of hirsutism at puberty. The latter has menstrual irregularity with the onset of puberty. Hirsutism associated with late-onset congenital adrenal hyperplasia may or may not be familial, but the onset is at puberty and may be associated with menstrual irregularity. A sudden onset of a progressive form of hirsutism with defeminization and virilization should raise the question of adrenal or ovarian neoplasia, which would require a careful abdominal and pelvic examination and check for clitorimegaly.

Tests

1. Laboratory testing is based on history and physical examination.

2. Preliminary tests should include testosterone (T 0.2 to 0.7 ng/ml or <3.5 nmol/L), dehydroepiandrosterone sulfate (DHEAS 400 to 3200 ng/ml), androstenedione (A 0.5 to 2.5 ng/dl), luteinizing hormone (LH 5 to 25 mIU/ml), follicle-stimulating hormone (FSH 5 to 20 IU/L; 5 to 20 mIU/ml), and prolactin (PRL 5 to 15 µg/L; 2 to 15 ng/ml).

3. Further testing may require fasting blood glucose, serum electrolytes, morning cortisol, 17-hydroxy-progesterone (follicular phase 0.6 to 3 nmol/L; 0.20 to 1 µL; luteal phase 1.5 to 10.6 nmol/L; 0.5 to 3.5 µL), thyroid stimulating hormone (TSH 0.4 to 5 µ/L; 0.4 to 5 µU/ml), and thyroxine (T$_4$ 154 nmol/L; 5 to 12 mg/dl).

Management

1. Patients should be encouraged to use cosmetic methods of depilation. Shaving is the least costly method and, contrary to common notion, does not increase hair growth. Other methods, such as electrolysis and waxing, are more costly and also painful.

2. Medical treatment of hirsutism is based on reducing the androgens from the ovaries and the adrenals and also reducing the effects of the androgens on the pilosebaceous units. In PCOD testosterone, androstenedione, and LH are increased, and the LH/FSH ratio exceeds 2 to 1. The levels go down with the use of oral contraceptives, which suppress gonadotropins and also increase the sex hormone binding globulin, thereby decreasing the free testosterone levels. Oral contraceptives combined with spironolactone (Aldactone) in doses of 50 to 200 mg, which is primarily an antiandrogen, are effective both in reduction of hirsutism and in re-establishing menstrual regularity. The control of obesity may have an added advantage in reducing insulin resistance in PCOD.

3. With adrenal causes of hirsutism, an increase in cortisol, DHEAS, or 17-hydroxyprogesterone may be observed. Based on the general principles of endocrine testing, to reveal a deficiency, stimulation testing is required, and to demonstrate an excess of hormone production, suppression is required. In late-onset adrenal hyperplasia (21-hydroxylase deficiency), the level of 17-hydroxyprogesterone is 200 ng/dl and a measurement of 17-HP 30 minutes after IV or IM ACTH 1-24 in a dosage of 250 µg will increase the value above 1200 ng/dl of 17-HP. Treatment in this case would be 5 mg of prednisone per day or 0.5 mg of dexamethasone per day. It should be borne in mind that five days of dexamethasone therapy should lead to complete suppression of the androgen excess, whereas in the presence of an adrenal tumor there is no suppression or incomplete suppression of DHEAS.

4. In Cushing's syndrome the morning cortisol is increased and fails to suppress to less than 5 µg with 1 mg of dexamethasone given at 11 at night.

5. A marked increase in testosterone (>150 ng/dl) should raise the question of adrenal and ovarian tumors, and a thorough search for such a lesion with pelvic ultrasonography and adrenal MRI should be undertaken.

6. In future the use of drugs like GnRH agonist and opiate antagonist may prove useful in the treatment of PCOD, and hyperandrogenic disorders evolving out of the adrenal gland may be treated with such drugs as ketoconazole (Nizoral), cyproterone acetate

(Androcur), and flutamide (Eulexin). The 5α-reductase inhibitor finasteride (Proscar) and drugs of this class will also be included in the treatment of hirsutism in the future.

PEARLS

- Hirsutism may be a sign of adrenal or ovarian tumor.

- The majority of cases of hirsutism are due to benign conditions such as idiopathic hirsutism, PCOD, or late-onset congenital hyperplasia.

- Treatment, which is directed toward reducing androgenic effects on the pilosebaceous unit, requires a combination of cosmetic and pharmacologic methods.

- It is important for the patient to understand that resolution of hirsutism will take 9 to 12 months.

 Bibliography

Ehrmann AD, Rosenfield RL: Clinical review 10. An endocrinologic approach to the patient with hirsutism. J Clin Endocrinol Metab 1990;71:1–4.

Fruzzetti F, De Lorenso D, Rerrini D, Ricci C: Effects of finasteride, a 5-alpha reductase inhibitor, on circulating androgens and gonadotropin secretion in hirsute women. J Clin Endocrinol Metab 1993;79(3):831–835.

McKenna TJ: Screening for sinister causes of hirsutism. N Engl J Med 1994;331(15):1015–1016. (Editorial Comment)

Rittmaster RS: Hirsutism. In Bennett JC, Plum F (eds): Cecil Textbook of Medicine, 20th ed. Philadelphia, WB Saunders, 1996.

Rittmaster RS: Treating hirsutism. The Endocrinologist 1993; 3:211–218.

| Symptom | **Gynecomastia** | *Marlene Goldwein* |

Gynecomastia is an enlargement of the male breast secondary to proliferation of both the fibroblastic stroma and the ductal system. In all causes of gynecomastia, physiologic as well as pathologic, increased growth of breast tissue is secondary to a change in the estrogen-to-androgen ratio, either in absolute plasma levels or in its local effects on breast tissue.

Differential Diagnosis

1. Physiologic gynecomastia of puberty
2. Drugs: estrogens, digitalis, cimetidine, spironolactone, methyldopa, calcium channel blockers, enalapril, captopril, ketoconazole, isoniazid, metronidazole, omeprazole, reserpine, tricyclic antidepressants, phenothiazines, nadolol, diazepam, phenytoin, marijuana, amphetamines, heroin, alcohol
3. Cirrhosis
4. Physiologic gynecomastia of aging
5. Hyperthyroidism
6. Radiation or chemotherapy
7. Renal failure
8. Hypogonadism
9. Starvation/refeeding
10. Physiologic gynecomastia of the newborn period
11. Testicular tumors
12. Other tumors: bronchial, gastric, pancreatic, adrenal, hepatic

It is important to differentiate gynecomastia from other forms of breast enlargement, such as breast cancer, neurofibromas, hematomas, and lipomas. Gynecomastia also must be differentiated from pseudogynecomastia or lipomastia, which is fatty enlargement of the breast. Once it is determined that true gynecomastia is present, it should then be determined whether there is a physiologic or pathologic cause.

Refer to Ch. 3, Growth and Developmental Guidelines; Ch. 90, Cirrhosis; Ch. 130, Chronic Renal Failure; and Ch. 163, Hyperthyroidism.

History

1. Age of onset
2. Duration
3. Presence of nipple discharge
4. Presence of tenderness
5. Symptoms of hypogonadism: changes in libido, testicles, skin, voice, hair
6. Medication and drug history
7. Symptoms of hyperthyroidism: anxiety, heat intolerance
8. Symptoms of liver failure
9. Alcoholism
10. Renal failure
11. Starvation/weight loss
12. Headaches or visual field disturbances

Clinical Findings

1. Palpable breast glandular tissue, usually bilateral, may be asymmetric or unilateral
2. Tenderness
3. Firm or rubbery texture
4. Mobile

5. Symmetric mound around nipple

6. Signs of hypogonadism

7. Signs of Cushing's syndrome: central obesity, striae

8. Signs of thyroid disease: goiter, exophthalmos, increased heart rate

9. Testicular examination for atrophy or nodules

10. Abdominal examination for adrenal tumor

11. Signs of hepatocellular failure: jaundice, spider angiomas

12. Arm span greater than height in Klinefelter's syndrome

The first five items in the physical examination differentiate gynecomastia from other causes of breast enlargement, such as tumors and lipomastia. The remainder of the clinical findings help differentiate secondary causes of gynecomastia.

Tests

1. Thyroid function tests

2. Liver function tests

3. Serum chorionic gonadotropin levels

4. Testosterone, estradiol, luteinizing hormone

5. Mammogram and/or biopsy if breast cancer suspected

6. Chromosomal karyotype if Klinefelter's syndrome suspected

In the vast majority of cases, tests are unnecessary because the diagnosis can be discerned readily from the history and physical examination alone.

Management

1. Management is not needed in most cases. There is frequently spontaneous regression.

2. Removal of the offending agent if possible

3. Correction of the underlying cause when possible

4. Treat only if pain or embarrassment

5. Medication will not be effective if fibrosis has replaced original ductal hypoplasia; dihydrotestosterone, danazole, and tamoxifen all have been used.

6. Surgical removal of breast tissue usually by subcutaneous mastectomy

Patient Education

If no pathologic cause is found, patient should be informed of the following:

1. Gynecomastia frequently resolves on its own.

2. Gynecomastia is not associated with feminization or loss of virility.

PEARLS

- Gynecomastia has a high prevalence in the pubertal and adult population.

- In the majority of cases, gynecomastia is physiologic and needs no treatment other than reassurance.

- A careful drug and medication history frequently reveals the cause of gynecomastia.

Bibliography

Braunstein GD: Gynecomastia. N Engl J Med 1993;328(7): 490–495.

Hands LJ, Greenall MJ: Gynaecomastia. Br J Surg 1991; 78(8):907–911.

Harman SM: Common problems in reproductive endocrinology. *In* Berker LR, et al (eds): Principles of Ambulatory Medicine, 3rd ed. Baltimore, Williams & Wilkins, 1991, pp 1049–1050.

Mahoney CP: Adolescent gynecomastia. Pediatr Clin North Am 1990;37(6):1389–1403.

Wilson JD: Endocrine disorders of the breast. *In* Isselbacher EJ, Braunwald E, Wilson JD, et al (eds): Harrison's Principles of Internal Medicine, 13th ed. New York, McGraw-Hill, 1994, pp 2036–2039.

| Symptom | **Goiter** | *Isaac Kleinman* |

A goiter is any visible or palpable thyroid gland. (It may not be visible or palpable if located substernally.) It may be diffuse or nodular, toxic or nontoxic, endemic or sporadic, malignant or nonmalignant, congenital (rare) or acquired. The normal gland weighs about 20 grams. Clinical goiter affects 200 million persons worldwide (7 per cent of the world population [World Health Organization, 1958]; 3 to 4 per cent of the United States population [Framingham Study]; and 15 per cent of the German population). Iodine deficiency is the most common cause worldwide (especially in Germany, Fiji, New Guinea, and the Himalayas). Thyroiditis is the most common cause in the United States. By postmortem examination in the United States, goiters or nodules are found in 50 per cent of the population.

Types

Congenital

1. Type I: associated with defects in iodine transport

2. Type II: associated with defects in organification of iodine

3. Type III: associated with defects in dehalogenase

4. Type IV: associated with defects in thyroglobulin synthesis

Acquired

1. Benign

   a. Nontoxic

      (1) Endemic (colloid) goiter: most common type of goiter; associated with puberty, menopause,

and pregnancy. In addition to iodine deficiency, it may be caused by goitrogens such as turnips, aminosalicylic acid, and lithium: goitrogens block thyroxine formation, which leads to increased TSH (thyroid-stimulating hormone) secretion from the pituitary, which in turn induces gland hyperplasia. (This does not explain nodularity, a circumstance in which only parts of the gland undergo hyperplasia.) Colloid goiter patients may be euthyroid or hyperthyroid.

   (2) Hashimoto's thyroiditis (autoimmune thyroiditis)

      (a) Chronic; characterized by lymphocytic infiltrates

      (b) Most common cause of primary hypothyroidism

      (c) Frequently associated with autoimmune disorders and other endocrine disorders

      (d) Painless and nontender

  b. Toxic

    (1) Granulomatous thyroiditis (subacute, giant cell)

      (a) Acute, inflammatory type

      (b) Sudden onset

      (c) Fever

      (d) Neck pain

      (e) Tenderness

    (2) Silent thyroiditis

      (a) Mainly postpartum women

      (b) Nontender; transient hyperthyroid phase followed by a limited period of hypothyroidism

      (c) Probably autoimmune

2. Malignant

  a. Papillary: most common (50 to 70 per cent); F/M = 2.5 to 1; lymphatic spread

  b. Follicular: 15 per cent; hematogenous spread

  c. Mixed

  d. Medullary: may be associated with other endocrine disorders; metastasizes via lymphatics to cervical and mediastinal nodes, to lungs, and to bone; may be associated with ectopic production of other hormones; produces excessive calcitonin, which can lower calcium and phosphorus

Differential Diagnosis of Anterior Neck Masses

1. Cystic hygroma (will usually transilluminate)
2. Thyroglossal duct cyst (may transilluminate)
3. Malignancy, metastatic
4. Lymphadenopathy and lymphoma
5. Goiter, toxic and nontoxic, benign and malignant

History may reveal symptoms of hypo- or hyperthyroidism or other endocrinopathies; note mechanical symptoms and history of irradiation. Inquire about goitrogens.

Environmental Goitrogens

- Iodine deficiency
- Iodine process
- Radiation
- Chemicals: sulfonyl ureas, thiocyanate, lithium, propylthiouracil, resorcinol, cobalt, aminoglutethimide, fluoride, calcium, cassava, soya beans, turnips (contain thiouracil-like antithyroid substances)

Although most goiters are asymptomatic and present as a simple swelling in the neck, they themselves may produce symptoms that are

Mechanical

1. Dysphasia, dyspnea, sensation of constriction in chest or throat
2. Hoarseness, increased phlegm in the throat
3. Symptoms of superior vena caval obstruction (substernal goiter); positive Pemberton's sign (see below)

Hormonal

1. Hyperthyroidism

  a. Cardiac rhythm irregularities, tremor, nervousness, heat intolerance

  b. Tachycardia, increased appetite, frequent bowel movements, increased pulse pressure

  c. Muscle weakness, eye signs (proptosis, lid lag, lid retraction, stare, conjunctival injection)

  d. Weight loss

  e. Thyroid storm (confusion, psychosis, coma, cardiovascular collapse)

2. Hypothyroidism

  a. Hair loss, periorbital puffiness, drooping eyelids

  b. Dry skin, macroglossia, bradycardia, menstrual disturbances

  c. Mental sluggisness, myxedema coma (rare), change in personality, psychosis (rare)

Clinical Findings

Physical examination should first define the extent and character of the enlargement: diffuse or nodular, firm or soft, symmetric or asymmetric, associated lymphadenopathy. Check for Pemberton's sign (increased heart rate, usually with distention of the cervical veins, when the arms are abducted). Assess metabolic status and levels of thyroid hormone; look for associated endocrine changes or autoimmune disorders. General findings may include

1. Thyroid enlargement and/or nodularity
2. Tenderness (thyroiditis)

3. Symptoms and/or signs of thyrotoxicosis (see above)
4. Cardiac irregularity
5. Congestive heart failure
6. Muscle wasting and weakness
7. Displacement of trachea or esophagus
8. Superior vena caval obstruction (substernal goiter)
9. Symptoms and/or signs of hypothyroidism (see above)

Findings Suggestive of Malignancy

1. Young age
2. Male
3. Solitary nodule (multinodular goiters are 99 per cent benign)
4. Cold nodules on scan (20 per cent are malignant; "hot" nodules are rarely malignant)
5. History of radiation to head or neck
6. Stippled calcification on radiograph
7. Recent or rapid enlargement
8. Stony hard consistency
9. Nodule with adjacent lymphadenopathy
10. Nodule with ipsilateral vocal cord paralysis

Tests

Laboratory tests are done to assess metabolic status and thyroid hormone levels and to search for associated endocrine disorders.

1. T_3, T_4, TSH, reverse T_3, free thyroxine, TRH test, ^{131}I uptake, and TBG (thyroid-binding globulin): to assess thyroid function.
2. Thyroid scans: to search for metastases (often not visible on radiograph)
3. Radiography, magnetic resonance imaging: to evaluate large tumors, substernal tumors
4. Calcitonin assay: in suspected medullary cancer
5. Ultrasound: to document size and follow growth or shrinkage; to determine if mass is solid or cystic; to document unilateral agenesis of a thyroid lobe
6. Laryngoscopy: to evaluate hoarseness (possible laryngeal nerve paralysis)
7. Needle biopsy: one of the most useful tests; potentially the most direct approach to diagnosis, short of open surgery. There are four categories of biopsy reports
   a. Cancer: In the case of medullary cancer, patients should be evaluated for other endocrinopathies, especially pheochromocytoma.
   b. Suspicious: occurs in 20 per cent of biopsies, usually follicular or Hürthle cell tumors. Twenty per cent of "suspicious" specimens ultimately prove to be malignant.
   c. Benign
   d. Inadequate specimen: self-explanatory

Needle biopsy is not recommended in patients with a history of neck irradiation because 40 per cent of previously irradiated patients will have cancer in some other area of the gland than the nodule undergoing biopsy. Open biopsy should be used if biopsy is indicated in these patients.

Management

1. None required in asymptomatic euthyroid goiter. Iodine deficiency should be corrected and goitrogens discontinued if found. Surgical removal may be desirable for cosmetic reasons.
2. ^{131}I therapy: for thyrotoxicosis, especially in poor surgical risks
3. Surgery: indications
   a. Suspicion of malignancy (cold nodules, follicular neoplasia, signs of invasion such as tracheal traction, lateral distortion or hoarseness, rapid growth, rock hard gland)
   b. Compressive symptoms
   c. Cosmesis
   d. Presence of autonomously functioning thyroid tissue
4. Medical
   a. Nontoxic goiter: two-thirds of diffuse goiter and small nodular goiter will decrease in size on 150 to 200 μg/day levothyroxine. Change in size can be followed and documented by ultrasonography. Hashimoto's thyroiditis, pubescent goiter, and nontoxic goiter in younger patients respond best.
   b. Toxic goiter: Propylthiouracil (100 to 150 mg every 8 hours orally to start) and methimazole (10 to 15 mg every 8 hours to start) are the mainstays of treatment. They work by impairing organification of iodine. When control of symptoms is achieved, the dose is reduced to the lowest level that maintains it (usually 100 to 150 mg/day of propylthiouracil or 10 to 15 mg of methimazole in divided doses b.i.d. or t.i.d.).

Classification of Goiter

- Stage 0A: no goiter
- Stage 0B: detectable by palpation but not visible even with the neck fully extended
- Stage I: palpable and visible only with the neck fully extended
- Stage II: visible with the neck in normal position
- Stage III: large goiter visible at a distance

PEARLS

- Thyroid disease in the elderly may be occult. Clues include cardiac irregularity, unexplained cardiac hypertrophy, occult congestive failure, and change in mental status.

- Thyroid hormone promotes bone mineral loss in postmenopausal women who are not receiving estrogen replacement therapy and may increase estrogen requirements.

- Avoid radiation treatment and hypothyroid status if possible during pregnancy.

- Avoid radiation treatment in the young patient.

Bibliography

Clark O: Nontoxic goiter. *In* Cameron JL: Current Surgical Therapy—3. Philadelphia, BC Decker, 1989, pp 446–453.

Foley TP Jr: Goiter in adolescents. Endocrinol Metab Clin North Am 1993;22:593–606.

Rakel R: Conn's Current Therapy. Philadelphia WB Saunders, 1994.

Roher H-D, Goretzki PE: Management of goiter and thyroid nodules in an area of endemic goiter. Surg Clin North Am 1987;67(2):233–249; and Brunt M, Wells SA Jr: Advances in the diagnosis and treatment of medullary thyroid carcinoma. Surg Clin North Am 1987;67(2):263–277.

Schneider D, Barett-Conner E, Morton DJ: Thyroid hormone use and bone mineral density in elderly women. JAMA 1994;271:1245–1249.

159 Diabetes Mellitus, Type I

Stephen A. Brietzke

Etiology

1. Genetic susceptibility plus an environmental "trigger" (viral infection or toxin exposure) initiate an autoimmune cascade.
2. Autoimmune-mediated destruction of pancreatic islet B cells causes progressive and ultimately absolute insulin deficiency.
3. Absolute insulin deficiency results in hyperglycemia for two cardinal reasons:
   a. *Increased hepatic production of glucose* via accelerated glycogenolysis and gluconeogenesis
   b. *Decreased peripheral utilization of glucose* by insulin-responsive tissues such as skeletal muscle

Symptoms

1. Increased renal excretion of glucose, osmotic diuresis, and obligate water loss produce symptoms of *polyuria, polydipsia,* and *orthostasis.*
2. Insulin deficiency produces a starvation-like catabolic state, resulting in *weight loss* and *polyphagia.*
3. Accumulation of glucose and/or polyols in lens and neural tissue produces functional alteration resulting in *blurred vision* and *pedal paresthesias* and/or *hypesthesia.*
4. Metabolic derangement nonspecifically causes *pruritus, nausea and vomiting, abdominal pain* (mimicking acute abdomen), and *altered sensorium* (obtundation to coma).

Key Symptoms

- Polyuria
- Polydipsia
- Polyphagia
- Weight loss
- Blurred vision
- Foot paresthesias
- Pruritus
- Abdominal pain
- Orthostasis

Clinical Findings

1. Physical examination may be entirely normal.
2. Orthostatic hypotension and/or tachycardia, decreased skin turgor, and flat neck veins (in supine position) reflect dehydration.
3. Loose skin folds and poorly fitting clothing may suggest recent weight loss.
4. Decreased visual acuity, decreased peripheral nerve vibratory/position threshhold, and eruptive xanthomas (due to marked hypertriglyceridemia) may suggest significant hyperglycemia and/or insulin deficiency.

5. Vitiligo, goiter, and early menopause (less than age 40) are signs of other autoimmune diseases sometimes associated with type I diabetes.

Laboratory Tests

1. Urinalysis: Glucose and ketones are usually strongly positive in the newly recognized, untreated diabetic.
2. Serum glucose is greater than 140 mg/dl in the untreated, newly recognized patient and is usually greater than 200 mg/dl in the symptomatic patient.
3. Hemoglobin A1c is the nonenzymatically glycosylated fraction of hemoglobin reflecting ambient glycemia over a 45- to 60-day period. It is invaluable as an objective measure of glycemic control.

Key Tests

- Plasma glucose > 140 mg/dl (fasting) or > 200 mg/dl (random)
- Nonfasting ketonuria
- Serum islet cell antibodies (ICAs) positive
- Serum C-peptide low

Differential Diagnosis

1. The principal distinction that must be made is between insulin-dependent diabetes mellitus (IDDM) and non-insulin-dependent diabetes mellitus. Clues to diagnosis of IDDM are as follows:
   a. Age less than 35 at onset
   b. Lean body habitus (at or below ideal body weight)
   c. "Ketosis-prone": recurrent ketoacidosis by history *or* fasting ketonuria that does not clear postprandially (i.e., nonfasting ketonuria)
2. Definitive laboratory diagnosis of IDDM:
   a. Islet cell autoantibodies (ICAs): positive in 80 per cent of new-onset IDDM patients
   b. Serum C-peptide (marker of endogenous insulin) less than detectable lower limit 5 minutes following intravenous stimulation with 1 mg glucagon

Treatment

Medication

1. Conventional insulin therapy (Table 159–1) has principal goals of eliminating symptoms of diabetes and preventing major metabolic derangements (ketoacidosis and hypoglycemia)

TABLE 159–1. HUMAN INSULIN PREPARATIONS

TYPE OF INSULIN*	PEAK EFFECT (hrs)	DURATION (hrs)
Regular (R)	2–4	6–8
NPH (N)	6–12	18–24+
Lente (L)	6–12	18–24+
Ultralente (U)	8–20	24–30+

*Brand names: Humulin (Eli Lilly); Novolin (Squibb-Novo).

    a. Initial dose 0.5 to 1.0 units/kg/day

    b. Divide total daily dose: two thirds before breakfast, one third before supper

    c. Breakfast dose: two thirds intermediate-acting insulin (NPH or Lente) plus one third short-acting insulin (regular)

    d. Supper dose: one half intermediate-acting plus one half short-acting insulin

2. Intensified insulin therapy has the principal goal of achieving a near-euglycemic state in hopes of preventing chronic complications of diabetes.

    a. Initial dose 0.5 to 1.0 units/kg/day (adolescents may require 1.0 to 1.5 units/kg/day).

    b. Total daily dose: one quarter, 30 minutes before each meal (as regular insulin) t.i.d. and one quarter NPH (or Lente) at bedtime.

    c. Mealtime insulin dose adjusted as needed by patient according to a dosing algorithm (see Key Treatment) using fingerstick capillary glucose testing as the data source.

    d. Programmed insulin dose at mealtimes and NPH/Lente at bedtime can be adjusted by ±10 per cent of total daily dose based on established 3-day trends.

Diet

1. Total calories roughly 25 times desirable body weight (in kilograms)

2. Total fat less than 30 per cent and saturated fat less than 10 per cent of total calories

3. Cholesterol less than 300 mg/day

4. Distribution of calories: 20 per cent breakfast, 20 per cent lunch, 30 per cent supper, 10 per cent midmorning snack, 10 per cent midafternoon snack, and 10 per cent bedtime snack

5. Desirable foods include slowly absorbed carbohydrates such as pasta, lentils, and beans.

Activity

1. Regular aerobic exercise of 30 to 60 minutes' duration three to five times weekly attenuates the tendency toward weight gain, reduces coronary heart disease/peripheral vascular disease risk by favorably altering serum lipids, and improves stamina and general sense of well-being.

2. Patient precautions for exercise

    a. Treadmill exercise test if older than age 35

    b. Check Fasting Plasma Glucose (FPG) prior to vigorous exercise.

    c. Ingest rapidly absorbed carbohydrate (glucose gel or Lifesavers) prior to extended period of exercise if FPG is low or normal.

    d. Avoid exercise if FPG is extremely high.

    e. Avoid exercising within 4 hours after administration of regular insulin.

Patient Education

1. Basic skills and knowledge

    a. Insulin injection technique

    b. Fingerstick capillary glucose testing technique

    c. Factors that raise and lower glucose

2. Hypoglycemia

    a. Warning symptoms, such as sweating, apprehension, tremulousness, hunger, and confusion

    b. Test FPG STAT for hypoglycemic symptoms.

    c. Family members and close companions should be taught how to administer glucagon, 1 mg intramuscularly, for unresponsiveness.

3. "Sick day" management

    a. Insulin requirement increases with minor illness, even if appetite and food intake reduced.

    b. Self-aid includes frequent FPG testing (at least four times daily) and urine ketone testing for FPG >250 mg/dl.

    c. May augment usual insulin dosing with up to 50 per cent dose increase at time of each FPG measurement.

    d. Consult physician/nurse if FPG is persistently greater than 250 mg/dl, ketonuria greater than trace positive, or if nausea/vomiting prevent oral food intake.

4. Foot care

    a. Inspect feet daily

    b. Use moisturizer cream daily after bath, if skin dry.

    c. Avoid going barefoot.

    d. Wear professionally fitted shoes.

    e. *Do not smoke!*

Key Treatment

Insulin Dosing Algorithm

Capillary blood glucose (fingerstick) (mg/dl)	Regular insulin dose (units)
<60	Programmed dose −4
61–90	Programmed dose −2
91–120	Programmed dose
121–150	Programmed dose +1
151–180	Programmed dose +2
181–240	Programmed dose +3
241–300	Programmed dose +4
>300	Programmed dose +6

Follow-Up

1. Assess control
   a. Ask frequency and severity of hypoglycemic symptoms
   b. Review FPG daily
   c. Measure hemoglobin A1c (frequency: 2- to 3-month intervals)
2. Assess compliance
   a. Ask frequency and results of FPG testing.
   b. Discuss attitudes toward diabetes, food, and weight.
3. Assess/screen for complications
   a. Retinopathy: Perform funduscopic examination at 6- to 12-month intervals, and refer for ophthalmologic evaluation after 5 years' duration of diabetes (or sooner if visual symptoms occur).
   b. Peripheral neuropathy and peripheral vascular disease
      (1) Inspect feet for deformity, ulceration, and vascular sufficiency at 3- to 6-month intervals.
      (2) Measure deep tendon reflex at ankles.
      (3) Measure vibratory and light pressure sensory thresholds in feet.
   c. Nephropathy
      (1) Measure blood pressure each visit.
      (2) Measure quantitative urinary protein (preferentially, a microalbuminuria assay) and creatinine clearance annually.
      (3) Consider treatment of "hypertension" when microalbuminuria or azotemia is identified.
   d. Coronary heart disease
      (1) Measure triglycerides, HDL, and LDL cholesterol annually.
      (2) Optimize glycemic control first if undesirable levels of TG/HDL/LDL identified.
      (3) Consider pharmacologic therapy of high-risk lipid profiles if abnormalities persist after trial of intensified glycemic control.
4. Assess adequacy of diabetes-specific education:
   a. Ask about meal planning and calorie plan.
   b. Inquire about "sick day" management.
   c. Ask to describe hypoglycemic symptoms.
   d. Ask about factors that raise and lower glucose.

The opinions and assertions contained herein are the private views of the author and are not to be construed as the official policy or position of the U.S. Government, the Department of Defense, or the Department of the Air Force.

 Bibliography

American Diabetes Association: Clinical practice recommendations (1992–1993). Diabetes Care 1993;16(suppl 2).

Boulton AJM: The diabetic foot. Med Clin North Am 1988;72:1513–1530.

Diabetes Control and Complications Trial Research Group: The effect of intensive treatment of diabetes on the development and progression of long-term complications in insulin-dependent diabetes mellitus. N Engl J Med 1993;329:977–986.

Nolte MS: Insulin therapy in insulin-dependent (type I) diabetes mellitus. Endocrinol Metab Clin North Am 1992;21:281–312.

Thai AC, Eisenbarth GS: Natural history of insulin-dependent diabetes mellitus. Diabetes Rev 1993;1:1–14.

160 Diabetes Mellitus, Type II

Bruce E. Wilson

Etiology

1. Type II diabetes mellitus, also known as non-insulin-dependent diabetes mellitus (NIDDM), comprises a heterogeneous group of disorders in adults, and it accounts for the vast majority of cases of diabetes mellitus. Type II diabetes mellitus is caused by both a degree of insulin resistance in peripheral tissues and an abnormality in insulin secretion. In most instances, insensitivity to insulin is produced via a postreceptor mechanism. Type II diabetes mellitus is accompanied by obesity in about 80 per cent of cases.

2. Heredity plays a significant role in the pathogenesis of type II diabetes mellitus; there is greater than a 90 per cent concordance between monozygotic twins. Some patients with maturity-onset diabetes of the young (MODY) have a mutation in the glucokinase gene.

Symptoms

The cardinal symptoms of diabetes mellitus, type II, are similar to those of diabetes mellitus, type I, but are generally more insidious in onset. Many patients may have clinical diabetes for many years prior to the diagnosis.

Key Symptoms

- Polyuria
- Polydipsia
- Fatigue
- Chronic cutaneous infections
- Yeast vaginitis
- Blurred vision
- Paresthesias

Clinical Findings

1. Patients with type II diabetes mellitus may have complaints due to hyperglycemia or may present in a nonketotic hyperosmolar state. In times of extreme physiologic stress, these patients may develop ketoacidosis.

2. Greater than 80 per cent of patients with type II diabetes mellitus have obesity, usually central (android) obesity. Hypertension is common.

3. Diabetes mellitus, type II, may be a component of a larger group of patients with hyperglycemia, insulin resistance, dyslipidemia, and hypertension (syndrome X).

Key Signs

- Obesity

- Family history of adult-onset diabetes mellitus

- In long-standing untreated diabetes mellitus, patients may present with complications of diabetes, including nephropathy with proteinuria, retinopathy, vitreous hemorrhage, glaucoma, neuropathic lower extremity lesions, or signs or symptoms of coronary artery disease or peripheral vascular disease.

- Delivery of large infants

Laboratory Tests

1. The diagnosis of diabetes mellitus can be made by demonstrating a fasting plasma glucose (FPG) level of greater than or equal to 140 mg/dl on two separate occasions.

2. If a patient has an FPG of 120 to 139 mg/dl, an oral glucose tolerance test can be performed. After 3 days of a normal diet including at least 150 grams of carbohydrate, this test is performed by giving the patient 75 gm of glucose in aqueous solution orally after a 16-hour fast. Samples for glucose are obtained at 30, 60, 90, and 120 minutes. The test is normal if the FPG is less than 115 mg/dl, the 120-minute value is below 140 mg/dl, and no value in between is 200 mg/dl or more. If the 120-minute sample and any other sample is 200 mg/dl or more, the test is diagnostic of diabetes mellitus. Patients are diagnosed with "impaired glucose tolerance" if values exceed normal but are not high enough for a definitive diagnosis of diabetes mellitus.

3. Glycosuria occurs when the plasma glucose level is greater than the renal threshold, about 175 mg/dl. The renal threshold may be much higher (250 to 300 mg/dl) in diabetics.

4. Glycosylated serum proteins: The level of glycosylation of hemoglobin is indicative of the glycemic control over the prior 8 weeks. Fructosamine also can be employed to monitor glycemic control. Because fructosamine has a shorter half-life, its level is indicative of the glycemic control over the prior 1 to 3 weeks.

5. Proteinuria: Individuals with normal renal function will excrete less than 100 mg protein every 24 hours, albumin being about 10 per cent of this total. Elevations in urinary protein excretion may be the first sign

of diabetic nephropathy. Any patient with urinary protein noted on dipstick should be evaluated with a 24-hour urine collection for quantitation of urinary protein/albumin excretion and creatinine clearance. Patients with diabetic nephropathy will have a disproportionately high percentage of albumin excretion. More convenient measures of urinary albumin include a timed overnight urine collection for albumin. Normal values for albumin excretion are less than 15 μg/min. Microalbuminuria may be an early indication of diabetic nephropathy. Uncontrolled hypertension also will increase microalbuminuria. Patients with microalbuminuria or proteinuria may benefit from treatment with angiotensin converting enzyme inhibitors, blood pressure control, low-protein (0.6 gm/kg/day) diets, and tight glycemic control.

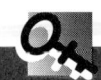 **Key Test**

• Fasting plasma glucose ≥140 mg/dl on two separate occasions

Differential Diagnosis

1. Drug toxicity: Many pharmacologic agents act by interfering with insulin secretion, including beta-adrenergic blocking agents, thiazides, phenytoin, and possibly calcium channel blockers and clonidine. Others, such as glucocorticoids, estrogen, and nicotinic acid, may induce significant insulin resistance. Pentamidine is directly toxic to islet B cells. Cyclosporine also may affect glucose tolerance by various mechanisms.

2. Endocrine disorders: Endocrine disorders or autonomous counterregulatory hormone overproduction in Cushing's syndrome, glucagonoma, acromegaly, and pheochromocytoma may induce clinical diabetes.

3. Long-standing pancreatic disease or pancreatectomy

4. Severe insulin resistance with acanthosis nigricans

5. Type II diabetes mellitus is rarely associated with ataxia-telangiectasia, myotonic dystrophy, leprechaunism, or genetic abnormalities in the insulin or proinsulin molecules.

6. Diabetes mellitus, type I, in remission

Treatment

Diet

Diet is the most important aspect of the treatment of type II diabetes mellitus. Weight loss may significantly diminish glucose intolerance. Behavioral modification and caloric restriction are essential elements of weight loss and weight maintenance. It is extremely important to limit refined sugars, ethanol, and saturated fats in the diet.

Exercise

Exercise enhances insulin sensitivity and aids weight loss. The physician must make realistic recommendations

based on the ability of the patient. Simple goals such as walking for 20 minutes three times weekly are adequate initially; however, one must strive for exercise at 60 to 70 per cent of maximal heart rate for 1 to 2 hours weekly.

Medication

1. *Sulfonylureas:* Sulfonylureas enhance insulin secretion and insulin sensitivity at target tissues. Second-generation sulfonylureas (glyburide, glipizide) are most commonly prescribed initially for patients with type II diabetes mellitus. First-generation sulfonylureas are not commonly used due to significant side-effect profiles. Glipizide (Glucatrol) has a duration of action of 12 to 24 hours, and glyburide has a duration of action of 16 to 24 hours. Glipizide is usually administered in one or two daily doses (5 to 40 mg daily). Dosage ranges of glyburide (Micronase) are 1.25 to 20 mg daily administered as one daily dose. Both agents are excreted in the bile and kidney; thus these agents are contraindicated in patients with significant renal or hepatic disease. Because of its long duration of action, glyburide is contraindicated in elderly patients susceptible to hypoglycemia. Sulfonylureas should not be used in gestational diabetes mellitus.

2. *Insulin:* Many type II diabetic patients will not have adequate glycemic control with sulfonylurea medications and will require insulin. Human insulin should be used. One can start therapy with a single injection of intermediate-acting insulin (NPH or Lente) daily (0.2 to 0.5 units/kg); however, most patients will require at least two injections daily. If postprandial glucose remains elevated for several hours after meals, regular insulin should be added to the intermediate- or long-acting insulin before meals. Premixed insulin preparations (e.g., Novolin 70/30) are convenient for patients who have difficulty mixing insulin. These preparations contain 70% NPH and 30% regular insulin.

3. *Sulfonylureas and insulin:* Occasional patients can maintain adequate glycemic control with intermediate- or long-acting insulin (e.g., Ultralente) administered at bedtime in addition to sulfonylurea therapy. Bedtime insulin diminishes fasting hyperglycemia in the early morning, whereas sulfonylureas enhance insulin secretion with meals.

4. *Acarbose:* This agent inhibits α-glucosidase in the gut and blocks the digestion of starch, sucrose, and maltose. Acarbose may improve glycemic control when combined with a sulfonylurea.

5. Investigational drugs include the biguanide *metformin,* which has been used effectively for treatment of hyperglycemia in type II diabetes mellitus in Europe and is now available in the U.S. as Glucophage, and *pioglitazone,* which may diminish insulin resistance at the insulin receptor level.

Patient Education

1. Self-monitoring of glucose: All diabetic patients must

be instructed in the use of a glucometer for self-monitoring of glucose levels and the symptoms and treatment of hypo- and hyperglycemia. The benefits of tight glycemic control also should be taught to diabetic patients; however, elderly patients or those with chronic complications of diabetes may not benefit from tight glycemic control. In fact, tight control may produce significant morbidity from hypoglycemia in elderly patients.

2. Foot and skin care: It is essential that all diabetics maintain skin integrity to avoid infections. Patients with peripheral vascular disease or neuropathy are especially at risk for life- or limb-threatening foot infections.

3. Infections and sick days: Infections and other illnesses increase counterregulatory hormone levels, which antagonize insulin effects. Insulin requirements may increase, and patients treated with only oral medications may require insulin. Adequate fluid intake and frequent blood sugar monitoring are essential during any intercurrent illness.

4. Diet and exercise: It is essential that each diabetic understands the benefits of dietary compliance, exercise, and weight loss.

Key Treatment

Drugs of Choice

- Sulfonylureas (glipizide, glyburide)

Alternative Drugs

- Insulin

- Metformin

- Acarbose

Follow-Up

1. Patients should seek follow-up at least every 6 months.

2. Annually, a complete physical examination should be performed, including weight, blood pressure, cardiovascular evaluation, skin integrity, peripheral neural function, and funduscopic examination. This visit should also re-emphasize dietary measures, weight loss if relevant, and exercise.

3. Laboratory testing
   a. Glycosylated hemoglobin: This should be checked at least twice yearly with the goal of maintaining a normal value.
   b. Urine protein excretion: In any patient who has had diabetes for 5 years, an evaluation of total albumin excretion and creatinine clearance should be performed annually.
   c. Fasting lipid levels: Type II diabetic patients commonly have a combined hyperlipidemia that should be treated aggressively.

4. Blood pressure control is essential to decrease the future morbidity of atherosclerotic cardiovascular disease and microvascular disease, especially nephropathy. The initial drug of choice for diabetic patients with hypertension should be an ACE inhibitor unless contraindications exist.

5. Patients with diabetes of greater than 5 years' duration should have a retinal examination performed by an ophthalmologist at least every other year and more often if significant diabetic retinopathy is present.

Bibliography

American Diabetes Association: Nutritional recommendations and principles for individuals with diabetes: 1986. Diabetes Care 1987;10:126–132.

Gerich JE: Oral hypoglycemic agents. N Engl J Med 1989;321:1231–1242.

Lewis EJ, Hunsicker LG, Bain RP, Rohde RD: The effect of angiotensin-converting-enzyme inhibition on diabetic nephropathy. N Engl J Med 1993;329:1456–1462.

Pandit MK, Burke J, Gustafson AB, et al: Drug-induced disorders of glucose tolerance. Ann Intern Med 1993;118:529–539.

Weir GC, Leahy JL: Pathogenesis of non-insulin dependent diabetes mellitus. In Kahn CR, Weir GC (eds): Joslin's Diabetes Mellitus, 13th ed. Philadelphia, Lea and Febiger, 1994, pp 240–264.

161 Ketoacidosis

Van B. Hayne

Etiology

1. Ketoacidosis occurs due to a relative or absolute deficiency of insulin as well as an increase in glucagon and other counterregulatory hormones such as cortisol, growth hormone, and catecholamines that affect glucose and lipid metabolism leading to ketosis and a widened anion gap (AG) metabolic acidosis.

2. Clinical ketoacidosis is primarily caused by diabetic ketoacidosis (DKA) and alcoholic ketoacidosis (AKA).

   a. DKA can develop in the following situations:

      (1) New-onset type I diabetes mellitus

      (2) Inappropriate use of insulin by a type I diabetic

      (3) Type I diabetic with systemic infection

      (4) Type I diabetic with acute myocardial infarction or other acute vascular event

      (5) Trauma in type I diabetes

      (6) The use of steroids, adrenergic agonists, hyperthyroidism, or pheochromocytoma in type I diabetics

   b. AKA may occur in the alcoholic with poor nutrition who has been drinking ethanol and who stops with developing anorexia, nausea, and vomiting.

   c. A diabetic with alcohol abuse may present with both conditions above.

Symptoms

1. Nausea
2. Vomiting
3. Anorexia
4. Abdominal pain
5. Fatigue
6. Weight loss
7. Shortness of breath
8. Muscle cramps
9. Dizziness
10. Thirst

Key Symptoms

- Nausea
- Vomiting
- Abdominal pain
- Anorexia

Clinical Findings

1. Tachycardia with pulse greater than 100 per minute

2. Tachypnea with respiratory rate greater than 20 per minute

3. Abdominal tenderness by examination that may mimic an acute abdomen

4. Hypotension with orthostasis (systolic blood pressure <100)

5. Hypothermia

   a. Presence of fever strongly suggests possibility of infection.

   b. Infection may need to be ruled out even with hypothermia.

6. Ketotic breath

7. Altered mental status or coma

Key Signs

- Tachycardia
- Tachypnea
- Abdominal tenderness (may mimic acute abdomen)
- Ketotic breath

Laboratory Tests

1. Blood or serum glucose
2. Plasma ketones using test strips or tablets

> **REMEMBER**
>
> **Nitroprusside reaction from test strips or tablets that are clinically widely available measure only acetoacetate and acetone, not β-hydroxybutyrate.**

   a. Acetone, which causes the ketotic breath, is not an organic acid and does not cause ketoacidosis.

   b. In ketoacidosis, some patients may have extremely high concentrations of β-hydroxybutyrate with little acetoacetate, making plasma ketone measurements by the nitroprusside test spuriously low.

3. Other necessary tests

   a. Plasma blood urea nitrogen (BUN) and creatinine

   b. Plasma electrolytes

      (1) A widened anion gap is present and can be calculated: anion gap (AG) = $(Na^+) - (Cl^- + HCO_3^-)$ = 12 + 4 mEq/L.

      (2) Hyponatremia/hypernatremia may be present.

      (3) When hyperglycemia is present with ketoacidosis,

$$\text{corrected serum Na}^+ = \text{measured serum Na}^+ + \left(\frac{\text{plasma glucose} - 100}{100}\right)(1.6 \text{ mEq Na}^+/\text{L})$$

    (4) Hypokalemia/hyperkalemia may be present, although all patients have total body potassium deficits.

  c. Arterial blood gases to measure pH, P_{CO_2}, and P_{O_2}

  d. Serum osmolarity

  e. Complete blood count (CBC) including white blood cell count, hemoglobin, and differential.

REMEMBER

- **Leukocytosis may occur without infection being present.**
- **Anemia and thrombocytopenia may occur secondary to gastrointestinal blood loss, inadequate nutrition, and ethanol abuse.**

---

  f. Cultures including blood, urine, throat, sputum, cerebrospinal fluid, and others when appropriate

  g. ECG

    (1) To monitor for significant hyperkalemia or hypokalemia

    (2) To rule out acute myocardial infarction and arrhythmias

  h. Chest radiograph and other radiographs, including CT scan of the head when indicated

  i. Hemoccult stool testing for suspected gastrointestinal blood loss

  j. Serum amylase and serum lipase in suspected pancreatitis

---

REMEMBER

Elevations in serum amylase may not represent pancreatitis.

 Key Tests

- Plasma glucose
- Plasma ketones
- Serum electrolytes to calculate AG
- Arterial blood gases

Differential Diagnosis

1. Ketoacidosis is a widened anion gap metabolic acidosis.

  a. Diabetic ketoacidosis—glucose >250; pH <7.35; HCO_3^- <15; positive serum ketones

  b. Alcoholic ketoacidosis—pH <7.35; HCO_3^- <15; positive serum ketones

  c. Starvation ketoacidosis

  d. Uncommon heritable disorders of branched-chain amino acid metabolism

  e. Uncommon heritable short-chain organic acidemias of amino acid metabolism

2. Other causes of widened anion gap acidosis

  a. Lactic acidosis

  b. Renal failure with glomerular filtration rate below 20 ml/min

  c. Salicylate intoxication

  d. Methanol ingestion

  e. Ethylene glycol ingestion

  f. Paraldehyde ingestion

  g. Formaldehyde ingestion

  h. Toluene ingestion

Treatment

1. The objective is to reverse the metabolic acidosis and replace fluid and electrolyte losses.

2. Fluid replacement

  a. Normal saline (NS)—15 ml/kg/hr for 1 hour; then 7.5 ml/kg/hr for 2 to 4 hours; then 3.75 ml/kg/hr for 24 to 36 hours until fluid losses are corrected

  b. If serum Na^+ >145, use one half NS at similar rates as for NS.

3. Insulin therapy (for those with DKA)

  a. 0.15 units/kg human regular insulin by intravenous bolus

  b. Then 0.1 unit/kg/hr of human regular insulin by intravenous infusion adjusted to maintain glucose in the 100 to 200 range.

  c. Change to subcutaneous insulin and long-acting insulin when ketoacidosis has cleared and patient is eating.

  d. Insulin is rarely needed in AKA.

4. Glucose replacement

  a. D_5 fluids added to fluid replacement immediately in AKA

  b. D_5 fluids added to fluid replacement in DKA when plasma glucose = 250 mg/dl

5. Potassium replacement

  a. If serum K^+ <3, add 0.5 mEq/kg/hr in intravenous fluids.

  b. If serum K^+ 3 to 4, add 0.4 mEq/kg/hr in intravenous fluids.

  c. If serum K^+ 4 to 5, add 0.3 mEq/kg/hr in intravenous fluids.

  d. Electrolytes including serum K^+ must be followed initially and every 2 to 3 hours during treatment, allowing for adjustments in K^+ replacement.

6. Neither HCO_3^- nor phosphate replacement has been shown to improve recovery or mortality in ketoacidosis.

7. Oral/intravenous magnesium therapy for magnesium deficiency

8. Thiamine replacement with alcoholic ketoacidosis to prevent Wernicke's encephalopathy

9. Subcutaneous heparin therapy for patients at increased risk of venous thrombosis

10. Assess for precipitating factors
    a. Acute myocardial infarction or other vascular event
    b. Systemic infection
    c. Acute pancreatitis
    d. Imbibition of other drugs, chemicals, or alcohols

11. Diet
    a. Initially nothing by mouth until ketoacidosis and nausea/vomiting resolve
    b. Appropriate diet, nutrition, and vitamins
    c. Intake and output monitoring

12. Activity
    a. Patients at bed rest for close monitoring until improved
    b. Once improved, patient can resume normal activities.

13. Patient education (see under Follow-Up)

Key Treatment

- Intravenous fluids: NS or ½ NS
- Glucose in intravenous fluids (see under Treatment)
- Potassium replacement
- Thiamine (see under Treatment)
- Regular insulin in DKA
- Close monitoring (see under Treatment)
- Precipitating factors (see under Treatment)

Follow-Up

1. Ketoacidosis is a life-threatening but reversible condition with proper treatment.

2. Patients with AKA need follow-up of other associated medical problems and treatment of alcoholism with the help of physicians and support groups.

3. Patients with DKA need
    a. Education regarding diabetic therapy during sick days
    b. Treatment of underlying diabetic complications
    c. Education regarding drugs that affect diabetic control
    d. Treatment of any associated or chronic nondiabetic medical problem.

Bibliography

For more information on diabetic ketoacidosis, see
Kitabchi AE, Fisher JN, Murphy MB, et al: Diabetic ketoacidosis and the hyperglycemic, hyperosmolar nonketotic state. *In* Kahn CR, Weir GC (eds): Joslin's Diabetes Mellitus, 13th ed. Malvern, PA, Lea & Febiger, 1994, pp 738–770.

For more information on diabetic ketoacidosis treatment in childhood, see
Davidson JK: Diabetic ketoacidosis and the hyperglycemic hyperosmolar state. *In* Davidson, JK (ed): Clinical Diabetes Mellitus: A Problem-Oriented Approach, 2d ed. New York, Thieme Medical Publishers, 1991, pp 394–413.
Kecskes SA: Diabetic ketoacidosis. Pediatr Clin North Am 1993;40:355–363.

For more information on alcoholic ketoacidosis, see
Adams SL: Alcoholic ketoacidosis. Emerg Med Clin North Am 1990;8:749–760.
Fulup M: Alcoholic ketoacidosis. Endocrinol Metab Clin North Am 1993;22:209–219.

For more information on heritable diseases of animo acids causing ketoacidosis, see
Finkelstein JD, Gohl WA: Heritable disease of amino acid metabolism. *In* Becker KL, et al (eds): Principles and Practice of Endocrinology and Metabolism, 1st ed. Philadelphia, JB Lippincott, 1990, pp 1422–1430.

162 Hypothyroidism

Ronald S. Watts

Etiology

Hypothyroidism is a clinical disease characterized by decreased thyroid gland production of free thyroxin (T_4). The disease may be a primary thyroid disorder or a central pituitary disorder. Central hypothyroidism is due to a decrease in thyrotropin (thyroid-stimulating hormone [TSH]) secretion from the pituitary (secondary hypothyroidism) or to a decrease in thyrotropin-releasing hormone (TRH) secretion or transport to the pituitary (tertiary hypothyroidism). Primary hypothyroidism is more common in women between the ages of 40 and 60 years.

Primary Hypothyroidism (Thyroprivic Hypothyroidism)

1. Autoimmune thyroid disease: most common cause of primary hypothyroidism
   a. Hashimoto's thyroiditis: chronic lymphocytic thyroiditis is most common cause of goitrous or atrophic hypothyroidism
   b. Idiopathic hypothyroidism: TSH receptor blocking antibodies
   c. Graves' disease remission: without prior radioiodine (^{131}I) therapy or surgery
   d. Polyglandular failure: rare syndrome of adrenal failure, type I diabetes mellitus, pernicious anemia, hypoparathyroidism, ovarian failure, and hypophysitis
2. Postablative hypothyroidism
   a. Following radioactive iodine (^{131}I) treatment for Graves' disease or thyroid carcinoma
   b. Following external irradiation to neck for lymphoma
   c. Following thyroidectomy for treatment of Graves' disease or thyroid carcinoma
3. Thyroiditis: subacute, silent, or postpartum; may have transient or permanent hypothyroidism
4. Drugs
   a. Antithyroid drugs: propylthiouracil (PTU) and methimazole (MMI); may cause goiter and/or hypothyroidism
   b. Iodine excess: goiter and/or hypothyroidism
      (1) Underlying thyroid disease and chronic use of iodine-containing cough medicine or amiodarone
      (2) Iodine goiter without hypothyroidism endemic in areas where seaweed (kelp) is consumed in large quantities
      (3) Iodine administration to pregnant mothers commonly causes goiter and hypothyroidism at birth, and possibly death from neonatal asphyxia.

   c. Lithium: Chronic administration can cause goiters and/or hypothyroidism.
5. Rare causes of hypothyroidism
   a. Sporadic cretinism: developmental defect of the thyroid causing severe hypothyroidism in infancy resulting in retardation of mental and physical development
   b. Iodine deficiency: world-wide problem, but rare in North America
      (1) Endemic goiter: Some may develop hypothyroidism if iodine deficiency is severe, but most are euthyroid.
      (2) Endemic cretinism: Both parents usually have endemic goiters and developmental disorder in addition to the clinical signs of cretinism. Thyroid is goitrous or atrophic.
   c. Genetic defects in hormone biosynthesis: Goiters are present at birth or appear later in life.
      (1) Iodide transport defect, organification defect, iodotyrosine coupling defect, iodotyrosine dehalogenase defect, and abnormal secretion of iodoproteins
   d. Infiltrative disorders: scleroderma, amyloidosis, hemochromatosis, sarcoidosis, Riedel's thyroiditis

Central Hypothyroidism (Trophoprivic Hypothyroidism)

1. Thyrotropin (TSH) deficiency, secondary hypothyroidism, rarely occurs alone without other pituitary hormone deficiency (panhypopituitarism). There is also deficiency of growth hormone, gonadotropins (LH, FSH), adrenocorticotropin (ACTH), or vasopressin.
   a. Pituitary macroadenomas, Sheehan's syndrome, craniopharyngiomas, infiltrative disorders of the pituitary, hypophysitis, or after severe head trauma with basal skull fracture
2. TRH deficiency: Tertiary hypothyroidism due to hypothalamic disease is rare.

Symptoms

1. Clinical symptoms are listed below; subclinical disease is asymptomatic.
2. History of symptoms in multiple organ systems: general fatigue, lethargy, cold intolerance, *mild weight gain,* dry rough skin, hair loss, brittle nails, puffy face, memory or concentration problems, personality disturbances, weakness, muscle stiffness or cramps, arthralgia, nausea, constipation, decreased exercise tolerance, decreased libido, decreased fertility, and menstrual abnormalities. Severity of symptoms may

be related to duration of onset of hypothyroidism; a rapid onset of hypothyroidism is associated with more symptoms than is gradual onset.

3. Many of the symptoms are common complaints, which are not specific by themselves but together make up a constellation of symptoms and signs of clinical hypothyroidism.

Key Symptoms

• Fatigue	• Lethargy
• Cold intolerance	• Weight gain
• Constipation	• Dry skin
• Mental impairment	• Hair loss
• Menstrual abnormalities	• Paresthesias

Clinical Findings

1. Physical examination may reveal typical puffy facies, periorbital edema, dry coarse thick skin and hair, brittle nails, hypersomnolence, slow speech, bradykinesia, hoarseness, large tongue, bradycardia, mild diastolic hypertension, psychological disorders, cerebellar ataxia, carpal tunnel syndrome, hyporeflexia, delayed relaxation phase of reflexes, or seizures.

2. Thyroid may be nonpalpable (atrophic) or goitrous. Goiter may be smooth or nodular.

3. Myxedema is characterized by clinical signs of pallor, carotenemia, nonpitting edema of hands, face, and ankles, secondary to dermal infiltration with mucopolysaccharides. The patient may also have ascites, pleural effusion, and pericardial effusion.

4. Myxedema coma is severe hypothyroidism presenting with altered mental status (lethargic to comatose), hypothermia, bradycardia, hypoventilation, hypoglycemia, adrenal insufficiency, and usually a precipitating factor such as noncompliance with levothyroxine, infection, or stress.

Key Signs

• Bradycardia	• Nonpitting edema (myxedema)
• Bradykinesia	
• Hyporeflexia	• Delayed relaxation phase of reflexes
• Muscle weakness	
• Dry coarse thick skin	• Goiter

Laboratory Tests

1. Laboratory tests consistent with primary hypothyroidism confirm clinical suspicion.

   a. Low free T_4 by radioimmunoassay (RIA) and elevated TSH

   b. Low total T_4, T_3 resin uptake, and free thyroxine index

   c. Free T_3 by RIA usually normal, or may be mildly decreased in primary hypothyroidism; not necessary to measure free T_3 in evaluation of primary hypothyroidism

   d. Transient TSH elevation common during recovery from subacute or silent thyroiditis

   e. Transient TSH elevation common during recovery from postpartum thyroiditis, but greater risk of eventual hypothyroidism because of underlying autoimmune thyroiditis

   f. High titer of antimicrosomal antibody usually indicates permanent hypothyroidism.

2. Low free T_4 and free T_3 by RIA; and low, normal, or mildly elevated TSH.

   a. Central hypothyroidism: TSH is usually very low or normal; rarely mildly elevated.

   b. Nonthyroidal illness (sick euthyroid syndrome): marked decrease in free T_3 in nonthyroidal illness, "low T_3 syndrome"; TSH usually normal, or mildly increased. Reverse T_3 will be increased in nonthyroidal illness.

3. Normal free T_4 and mildly increased TSH (5 to 15 μU/ml).

   a. Subclinical hypothyroidism

   b. Recovery from subacute, silent, or postpartum thyroiditis

   c. Recovery from nonthyroidal illness

4. Thyroid antibodies

   a. Antimicrosomal antibody: thyroid peroxidase antibody inhibiting the enzyme activity

      (1) Diagnostic for Hashimoto's thyroiditis when present in high titers ($>$1:400)

      (2) Degree of elevation correlates with clinical hypothyroidism.

      (3) Antibody titers tend to fall when hypothyroidism is present for a long time.

   b. Antithyroglobulin antibody not as specific for Hashimoto's thyroiditis, but also increased.

   c. If no antibodies are detected at time of diagnosis, it is idiopathic hypothyroidism, which may still be a form of autoimmune thyroiditis.

   d. It is not always necessary to check for antibodies if it is not going to make a difference in a decision to treat or not.

5. Other laboratory abnormalities: elevated creatinine kinase, normochromic normocytic anemia, hyperlipoproteinemia, hyponatremia, hyperprolactinemia, hyperlipoproteinemia, and abnormal electrocardiogram with nonspecific ST and T wave abnormalities, or low voltage of QRS complexes

6. Radioactive iodine scan and uptake are not necessary

in the evaluation of hypothyroidism, but are indicated only in the evaluation of a single nodule or to confirm multinodular goiter.

7. Euthyroid hypothyroxinemia: low total T_4, increased T_3 resin uptake, normal or mildly decreased free T_4 index, and normal TSH due to decreased thyroid binding globulin. Free T_4 and TSH are usually normal as these patients are euthyroid.

Key Tests

- Thyrotropin (thyroid-stimulating hormone [TSH])
- Free thyroxine (T_4) or free T_4 index (FTI)
- Antimicrosomal antibody

Differential Diagnosis

1. Nonthyroidal illness is often associated with decreased free triiodothyronine (T_3) and/or decreased free thyroxine (T_4) without clinical hypothyroidism. Usually the TSH is normal or could be mildly increased during recovery from nonthyroidal illness.

2. Euthyroid hypothyroxinemia: euthyroid with decreased T_4 due to decreased thyroid binding globulin concentration caused by nephrotic syndrome, exogenous testosterone, or high-dose steroids. Also, total T_4 may be decreased by drugs that inhibit T_4 binding, such as phenytoin, phenobarbital, and salicylates.

Treatment

Medication

1. Levothyroxine (e.g., Synthroid): synthetic preparation of thyroxine (T_4)

   a. Dose: 1.6 to 1.8 μg/kg of ideal body weight. Healthy patients can be started on a full replacement dose. Patients who are elderly or have coronary artery disease need to start on 25 μg by mouth daily (or 12.5 μg daily) and increase gradually by 25 μg daily (or 12.5 μg daily) every 4 to 6 weeks. If angina occurs during levothyroxine replacement, the dose should be decreased and cardiac evaluation and treatment done before continuing to increase the levothyroxine.

   b. Lower dose could be given in the treatment of subclinical hypothyroidism (0.5 to 1.0 μg/kg).

   c. If diagnosis of hypothyroidism is uncertain in a patient already on levothyroxine, the dose can be reduced by half and the free T_4 and TSH reassessed in 6 to 8 weeks. If the TSH is increasing, resume the previous dose. If the TSH is normal, discontinue the levothyroxine and check the TSH again in 6 to 8 weeks for any increase.

   d. The goal of TSH replacement in primary hypothyroidism is to normalize, not suppress, the TSH. Suppressed TSH causes decreased bone mineral density over several years.

   e. The replacement goal in central hypothyroidism is to normalize the free T_4 since TSH is not reliable.

   f. TSH suppression is indicated only for those with a history of thyroid carcinoma, nontoxic simple goiter, or benign thyroid nodule.

   g. Drugs that commonly interfere with absorption include cholestyramine and ferrous sulfate.

2. Treatment of myxedema coma: ventilatory support if indicated, treatment of hypothermia, and intravenous levothyroxine, 300 to 500 μg daily to restore thyroxine concentrations to normal quickly.

Key Treatment

- Levothyroxine

WARNING

- **In treating myxedema coma, T_4 replacement can precipitate adrenal crisis in a patient with borderline ACTH reserve; therefore, during acute therapy, administer high-dose (stress) steroids concomitantly.**

Follow-Up

1. After therapy has been initiated with levothyroxine, the laboratory should check levothyroxine levels in six to eight weeks to determine whether adjustment of the levothyroxine dose is necessary. Increasing the levothyroxine dose more often than six- to eight-week intervals will probably lead to overreplacement.

2. Once a stable dose of levothyroxine has been obtained, the TSH level in primary hypothyroidism or the free T_4 level in central hypothyroidism can be checked biannually or annually.

Bibliography

For more information on the thyroid gland, see
Larsen PR, Ingbar SH: The thyroid gland. *In* Wilson JD, Foster DW (eds): Williams Textbook of Endocrinology, 8th ed. Philadelphia, WB Saunders, 1992, pp 414–445.

For more information on autoimune thyroiditis, see
Volpe R: Autoimmune thyrioditis. *In* Braverman LE, Utiger RD (eds): Werner and Ingbar's The Thyroid, A Fundamental and Clinical Text, 6th ed. Philadelphia, JB Lippincott, 1991, pp 921–933.

For more information on levothyroxine therapy, see
Mandel SJ, Brent GA, Larsen RD: Levothyroxine therapy in patients with thyroid disease. Review. Ann Intern Med 1993;119:492–499.

For more information on practical approach to the treatment of hypothyroidism, see
Wolf PG, Meek JC: Practical approach to the treatment of hypothyroidism. Am Fam Physician 1992;45(2):722–731.

163 Hyperthyroidism

Ronald S. Watts

Etiology

Thyrotoxicosis is defined as elevated concentration of free thyroxine (T_4) and/or free triiodothyronine (T_3). Thyrotoxicosis may be due to hyperthyroidism, which is an increase in thyroid hormone synthesis and release, but thyrotoxicosis may also be due to increased T_4 and/or T_3 concentrations without hyperthyroidism (increase in thyroid hormone synthesis). It is more common in young women.

Thyrotoxicosis and Hyperthyroidism: Increased Thyroid Radioactive Iodine Uptake (RAIU)

1. Graves' disease: most common cause of thyrotoxicosis
2. Toxic multinodular goiter (MNG): multiple autonomous functioning thyroid nodules
3. Toxic adenoma (Plummer's disease): solitary large autonomous functioning thyroid nodule
4. Hashitoxicosis: coexistent Hashimoto's thyroiditis and Graves' disease
5. Pituitary (thyrotroph) adenoma: thyrotropin-secreting (thyroid-stimulating hormone [TSH]) adenoma
6. Selective pituitary resistance to thyroxine: hypersecretion of TSH without adenoma
7. Trophoblastic tumor: human chorionic gonadotropin (hCG) secreting tumor
8. Exogenous iodine excess: only cause of hyperthyroidism with low RAIU—due to iodine-containing drugs such as cough medicine, amiodarone, contrast agents, or kelp (seaweed)

Thyrotoxicosis Not Due to Hyperthyroidism: Decreased Thyroid RAIU

1. Subacute thyroiditis: inflammatory response causing increase in thyroxine release
2. Silent thyroiditis: inflammatory response causing increase in thyroxine release
3. Postpartum thyroiditis: inflammatory response two to six months postpartum
4. Surreptitious exogenous thyroid hormone use: typically the health care professional
5. Struma ovarii: ectopic thyroid tissue
6. Functioning metastatic thyroid cancer: ectopic thyroid tissue

Pathogenesis of Common Causes of Thyrotoxicosis

1. Graves' disease: thyroid-stimulating immunoglobulins (TSI) bind TSH receptors stimulating T_4 synthesis.
2. Subacute thyroiditis: antecedent viral infection causes a subsequent inflammatory infiltrate of neutrophils, lymphocytes, histiocytes, and multinucleated giant cells.

3. Silent thyroiditis: may be a variant of lymphocytic thyroiditis; focal or diffuse acute lymphocytic infiltration that appears like chronic lymphocytic thyroiditis
4. Postpartum thyroiditis: underlying chronic autoimmune thyroiditis
5. Toxic adenoma and toxic MNG: gradual growth of autonomous functioning nodule(s)
6. Exogenous iodine excess: causes hyperthyroidism with underlying subclinical thyroid disease, but the thyroid RAIU will be low instead of high

Symptoms

Symptoms of common causes of thyrotoxicosis
1. Graves' disease: symptoms of ophthalmopathy such as dry eyes, excessive tearing, proptosis, diplopia, impaired visual acuity, or field defects
2. Subacute thyroiditis: preceded by 1 to 2 weeks by a viral syndrome and presents with thyroid or neck pain, which may radiate to jaw or ear
3. Silent and postpartum thyroiditis: mildly symptomatic or asymptomatic
4. Toxic MNG and toxic adenoma: insidious onset, few symptoms, and more common in the elderly

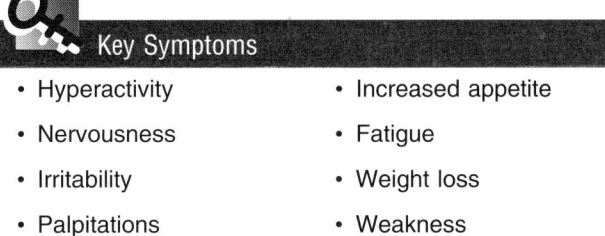

Key Symptoms	
• Hyperactivity	• Increased appetite
• Nervousness	• Fatigue
• Irritability	• Weight loss
• Palpitations	• Weakness
• Heat intolerance	• Frequent defecation
• Sweating	• Menstrual abnormalities

Clinical Findings

1. Thyrotoxicosis usually causes clinical disease, but can present with subclinical disease.
   a. General: hyperactivity, nervousness, anxiety, and warm moist smooth skin
   b. Eyes: lid retraction, lid lag, and stare
   c. Thyroid: firm smooth or nodular goiter present in most causes of thyrotoxicosis
   d. Cardiac: sinus tachycardia, paroxysmal supraventricular tachycardia, atrial fibrillation, hyperactive precordium, systolic flow murmurs, congestive heart failure, and angina
   e. Neurologic: fine tremor of hands, tongue, or closed eyelids, hyperreflexia, proximal muscle weakness,

myopathy, emotional lability, and psychiatric manifestations

2. Clinical signs in specific causes of thyrotoxicosis
   a. Graves' disease: degree of thyrotoxicosis varies from mild to severe
      (1) Diffuse firm thyroid enlargement which may have bruit
      (2) Infiltrative ophthalmopathy
         (a) Bilateral proptosis defined as exophthalmometer measurements exceeding 20 mm
         (b) Lid retraction, corneal ulcers, keratitis, conjunctivitis, periorbital edema
         (c) Diplopia with upward and lateral extremes of gaze, or may be constant
         (d) Papilledema, or impairment of vision due to involvement of optic nerve
      (3) Rarely, localized myxedema, or thyroid acropachy (thickening of extremity)
      (4) Coexistent Hashimoto's thyroiditis with a lobular thyroid consistency
      (5) Thyroid storm: severe thyrotoxicosis with hyperpyrexia, tachyarrhythmias, shock, and acute metabolic encephalopathy. Look for precipitating factor such as infection, noncompliance with antithyroid drugs, trauma, iodine, or parturition.
   b. Subacute thyroiditis: thyroid pain and tenderness the predominant problem in a firm goiter mild to moderate in size and mild thyrotoxicosis
   c. Silent and postpartum thyroiditis: painless with mild thyrotoxicosis or subclinical disease
   d. Toxic multinodular goiter and toxic adenoma
      (1) Usually appears in elderly with prior history of goiter for several years
      (2) In elderly, may have only cardiac signs, or weight loss
      (3) May occur in young patients with progressively enlarging goiter
      (4) Toxic adenoma usually more than 3.0 cm
   e. Surreptitious exogenous T_4 or T_3 use: suspect whenever thyrotoxicosis is present without a goiter. The only cause of low thyroglobulin concentration in thyrotoxicosis.

Key Signs

• Restlessness	• Stare
• Tachycardia or arrhythmia	• Eyelid retraction
	• Goiter
• Systolic hypertension	
	• Muscle weakness
• Hyperreflexia	
	• Warm, moist, smooth skin
• Tremor	

Laboratory Tests

1. Thyroid function tests consistent with chemical thyrotoxicosis confirm clinical suspicion.
   a. Elevated free T_4 and/or T_3 concentrations by radioimmunoassay (RIA)
   b. Elevated total T_4, T_3 resin uptake, and free thyroxine index (FTI)
   c. Suppressed TSH (<0.1 µU/ml) utilizing a sensitive TSH assay. Exception: TSH is not suppressed in TSH-secreting pituitary adenoma or pituitary resistance to thyroxine.
   d. Serum thyroglobulin is suppressed only in surreptitious thyroxine or triiodothyronine use.
2. Other tests
   a. Erythrocyte sedimentation rate increased in subacute or silent thyroiditis
   b. Thyroid-stimulating immunoglobulins (TSI) confirm Graves' disease, but not necessary for diagnosis and usually an expensive test.
   c. Antimicrosomal antibodies: high titer in postpartum thyroiditis and hashitoxicosis
   d. Molar ratio of alpha subunit to TSH >1.0 only in pituitary TSH-secreting adenoma
   e. May have hypercalcemia, anemia, hypokalemia, osteoporosis
3. RAIU is required in all evaluations of thyrotoxicosis.
   a. Increased thyroid RAIU in hyperthyroidism
      (1) Graves' disease, hashitoxicosis, toxic multinodular goiter, and toxic adenoma
      (2) Pituitary (TSH-secreting) adenoma, selective pituitary resistance to thyroxine, and trophoblastic (HCG-secreting) tumor are all rare causes of hyperthyoidism.

WARNING

If TSH is not suppressed (>0.1 µU/ml) and RAIU is increased, evaluate the pituitary by CT or MRI for either TSH-secreting pituitary adenoma or selective pituitary resistance to thyroxine if imaging of the pituitary is normal.

---

   b. Decreased thyroid RAIU in other causes of thyrotoxicosis
      (1) Thyroiditis: subacute, silent, and postpartum
      (2) Exogenous thyroid hormone use and exogenous iodine excess
      (3) Struma ovarii, and functioning metastatic thyroid cancer are rare
   c. Thyroid radioiodine scan is not always necessary in evaluating thyrotoxicosis.
      (1) Diffuse homogeneous uptake confirms Graves' disease, but is probably unnecessary in a pa-

tient with a diffusely enlarged goiter on examination.

   (2) Useful test if there is a concern about a palpable thyroid nodule(s) in a thyrotoxic patient; may reveal heterogeneous uptake (toxic multinodular goiter), or a single hot nodule (toxic adenoma), or a cold nodule (coexistent neoplasm)

4. Euthyroid hyperthyroxinemia: elevated total T_4, decreased T_3 resin uptake, normal or mildly elevated free T_4 index, or normal mildly increased free T_4 by RIA; commonly due to increase in thyroid-binding globulin or, rarely, to nonthyroid illness, generalized resistance to thyroid hormone

Key Tests

- Free T_4, free T_3 by RIA, or free T_4 index (FTI)
- Thyrotropin (thyroid-secreting hormone [TSH])
- Thyroid radioactive iodine uptake (RAIU)
- Thyroid radioiodine scan—necessary only if palpable nodule(s)

Differential Diagnosis

1. Laboratory tests confirm chemical thyrotoxicosis. The specific cause of thyrotoxicosis may be determined clinically and by the thyroid RAIU (explained above).

2. If euthyroid findings exclude thyrotoxicosis, consider disorders associated with hypermetabolism such as anxiety disorder, diabetes mellitus, pheochromocytoma, myeloproliferative disorder, cirrhosis, and chronic obstructive pulmonary disease.

3. Euthyroid hyperthyroxinemia: euthyroid with increased T_4 due to increase in thyroid-binding globulin concentration commonly caused by estrogens or hepatitis; rarely due to nonthyroidal illness, familial dysalbuminemia (increased albumin-binding T_4), or increased T_4 binding to thyroid-binding pre-albumin (TBPA) and anti-T_4 antibodies

Treatment

Medication

1. β-Blockers

   a. Mechanism: decrease the beta adrenergic mediated effects of thyrotoxicosis, and decrease the peripheral conversion of T_4 to T_3

   b. Drugs: propranolol, 10 to 80 mg by mouth q.i.d.; atenolol, 50 to 100 mg by mouth daily; nadolol; or metoprolol

   c. Indication: all forms of thyrotoxicosis; titrate dose according to heart rate

   d. Side effects: bronchospasm, bradycardia, decreased cardiac output, depression

2. Antithyroid drugs: propylthiouracil (PTU), and methimazole (MMI) (Tapazole)

   a. Mechanism: both PTU and MMI inhibit T_4 synthesis. Only PTU inhibits peripheral conversion of T_4 to T_3. Possible immunosuppressive effect

   b. Dose: PTU, 50 to 300 mg by mouth every 6 to 8 hours, or MMI, 5 to 20 mg by mouth every 12 hours

      (1) Treatment is usually required for 1 to 2 years for a possible remission to occur.

      (2) If not in remission by 2 years, should consider ^{131}I or surgery.

      (3) Remission is more likely if goiter is small or decreasing in size, or if mild thyrotoxicosis is controlled with minimal dose of antithyroid drugs.

      (4) Recurrence after remission is possible.

   c. Indications: hyperthyroidism (increased RAIU)

      (1) Drugs of choice for treating pregnant Graves' patient, or children

      (2) Before and/or after radioiodine (^{131}I) therapy to help control severe hyperthyroidism

   d. Contraindicated in low RAIU thyrotoxicosis

   e. Side effects

      (1) Common (<5 per cent): rash, transient leukopenia, and drug fever

      (2) Rare (<0.5 per cent): agranulocytosis, aplastic anemia, thrombocytopenia, lupus-like syndrome, hepatitis, cholestasis, gastrointestinal symptoms, abnormal taste, and arthralgia

   f. Check neutrophil count and liver enzymes before and periodically during therapy.

WARNING

Patients should be instructed, if temperature >101° F, to discontinue antithyroid drugs until neutrophil count is checked to exclude agranulocytosis.

---

3. Anti-inflammatory and immunosuppressive drugs

   a. Acetylsalicylic acid in moderate doses, or nonsteroidal anti-inflammatory drugs indicated for treatment of subacute silent thyroiditis. If no improvement, switch to steroids.

   b. Steroids

      (1) Prednisone, 40 to 60 mg by mouth daily, tapered over 4 weeks for subacute thyroiditis

      (2) Decreased T_4 secretion and T_4 to T_3 peripheral conversion in severe hyperthyroidism

      (3) Temporary therapy for severe Graves' ophthalmopathy until surgery or irradiation

4. Radioactive iodine-131 (^{131}I): therapy of choice for Graves' disease

 a. Mechanism: inflammation and radiation destroy the thyroid gland.

 b. Indication: hyperthyroidism (increased RAIU); contraindicated if RAIU is low

 c. Contraindication: pregnancy, therefore, must check serum HCG before treatment

 d. Dose: one treatment of 10 to 20 mCi of ^{131}I is effective in 75 per cent of patients, and 10 to 20 per cent of patients will require more than one treatment with ^{131}I.

 e. In toxic MNG or toxic adenoma, more than 20 mCi of ^{131}I usually required.

 f. Side effects: pain in neck, radiation thyroiditis, and increase in T_4 release

 g. Very safe without increased risk of cancer or gonad chromosomal abnormalities

 h. Hypothyroidism is expected, and free T_4 and TSH level should be monitored after therapy.

5. Iodine-containing compounds: potassium iodide (SSKI), Lugol's solution, ipodate sodium

 a. Mechanism: acutely decreases T_4 release and decreases T_4 to T_3 peripheral conversion

 b. Indication: adjunctive therapy after ^{131}I treatment, preparation for surgery, or management of severe hyperthyroidism, or "thyroid storm"

 c. Contraindication: pregnancy—must check serum hCG before treating

 d. Dose: SSKI or Lugol's solution, 3 to 5 drops q.i.d. by mouth or IV

 e. Comments: Begin only after one dose of antithyroid drug has already been given to block T_4 synthesis. One treatment will decrease RAIU and prevent effective treatment with radioactive ^{131}I for several months.

6. Therapy of thyroid storm: fluid resuscitation, treatment of hyperpyrexia, high dose of β-blockers, high dose of antithyroid drugs, "cold" iodides (SSKI, Lugol's solution, or ipodate), and high-dose (stress) steroids.

Surgery

1. Indications

 a. Severe thyrotoxicosis during pregnancy when antithyroid drugs have been unsuccessful

 b. Suspicion of malignancy: palpable thyroid nodule, lymphadenopathy, hoarseness, and rapid growth of goiter

 c. Toxic adenoma or toxic MNG in a good surgical candidate

2. Preparation: patient should be rendered euthyroid with an antithyroid drug and "cold" iodide (SSKI, or Lugol's solution) before surgery.

3. Procedure: near-total thyroidectomy should be done only by an experienced surgeon.

4. Complications: recurrent laryngeal nerve damage, hypocalcemia, bleeding, infection, and expected hypothyroidism.

Key Treatment

- β-Blockers: propranolol, nadolol, or metoprolol
- Antithyroid drugs: propylthiouracil and methimazole
- Anti-inflammatory and immunosuppressive drugs— Only indicated for thyroiditis: ASA, NSAIDs, steroids
- ^{131}I

Follow-Up

1. Hypothyroidism

 a. Expected after treatment of Graves' disease with surgery, or ^{131}I, or antithyroid drugs

 b. Recovery from thyroiditis (subacute, silent, or postpartum) may cause transient hypothyroidism, but most patients eventually become euthyroid. Thyroxine therapy should be withheld unless the patient has many symptoms of hypothyroidism or TSH elevation persists for a long time. If treatment is started for symptoms, titrate dose according to symptoms and not to completely normalize the TSH.

2. Recurrent thyrotoxicosis possible with Graves' disease or thyroiditis

3. Thyroxine replacement: L-thyroxine $\sim$ 1.6 to 1.8 μg/kg by mouth daily to normalize TSH

Bibliography

For more information on the thyroid gland, see
Larsen PR, Ingbar SH: The thyroid gland. *In* Wilson JD, Foster DW (eds): Williams Textbook of Endocrinology, 8th ed. Philadelphia, WB Saunders, 1992, pp 414–445.

For more information on treatment of thyrotoxicosis, see
Burch HB, Wartofsky L: Life-threatening thyrotoxicosis thyroid storm. Endocrinol Metabol Clin North Am 1993;22:263–275.
Cooper DS: Treatment of thyrotoxicosis. *In* Braverman LE, Utiger RD (eds): Werner and Ingbar's The Thyroid, A Fundamental and Clinical Text, 6th ed. Philadelphia, JB Lippincott, 1991, pp 887–916.

For more information on Graves' disease, see
Volpe R: Graves' disease. *In* Braverman LE, Utiger RD (eds): Werner and Ingbar's The Thyroid, A Fundamental and Clinical Text, 6th ed. Philadelphia, JB Lippincott, 1991, pp 648–680.

For more information on hyperthyroidism, see
Klein I, et al: Treatment of hyperthyroid disease. Ann Intern Med 1994;121:281–288.

164 Thyroid Nodule; Thyroid Carcinoma

Harold V. Werner

Etiology

1. Thyroid nodules are very common; 50 per cent prevalence by autopsy or ultrasound but less than 1 in 10 are palpable; about 5 per cent of palpable nodules harbor malignancy, but very few cause death. Do not do scans or ultrasound studies to *screen* for cancer, since extremely high false-positive results are seen.

2. Very little is known of specific causes of nodules.

3. Presence of palpable nodules, however, is influenced by

   a. Age

      (1) Prevalence of nodules increases linearly with age.

      (2) Palpable nodules are present in more than 5 per cent of people over 60 years of age.

      (3) Multinodular goiters start to appear ages 30 to 50; malignancy potential of a dominant nodule probably equals that of a solitary nodule.

      (4) Nodule in a child less than 14 years old demands surgery; high malignancy potential.

   b. Sex

      (1) Five to six times more nodules in women; thus most cancers are in women.

      (2) Malignant potential, however, probably is higher in nodules in men.

   c. Family or personal history suggesting multiple endocrine neoplasia type II

      (1) Hypercalcemia, that is, hyperparathyroidism

      (2) Hypertension, that is, pheochromocytoma

      (3) Medullary carcinoma of the thyroid

   d. History of neck irradiation

      (1) Ascertain by history or records that irradiation did occur.

      (2) Incidence of nodules increases linearly with 50 to 2000 rads.

      (3) Twenty-seven per cent of all irradiated patients get nodules (16.5 per cent by examination, 11 per cent more by scan).

      (4) One third of nodules are malignant by histology, but not more aggressive.

Symptoms

1. Often the patient or a family member discovers the nodule accidentally.

2. Ascertain at once that there are no obstructive symptoms, such as inspiratory stridor. Then the only goal is to exclude malignancy of the thyroid nodule safely and at lowest cost.

3. No symptom or combination of symptoms can positively identify malignancy.

4. Nevertheless, it may sometimes be helpful, as in using the results of fine-needle aspiration biopsy (FNAB) of the nodule, to find symptoms suggestive of malignancy:

   a. History of external neck irradiation

   b. Rapidly enlarging nodule

   c. Unexplained hoarseness

   d. Nodule discovered at less than 14 or greater than 65 years of age

   e. Family history of medullary thyroid cancer or multiple endocrine neoplasia

Clinical Findings

1. At other times the nodule is found by the physician palpating during screening physical examination or in response to pain, mass, or tenderness in the neck.

2. Again, no signs on physical examination can identify malignancy, but characteristics consistent with malignancy should be sought:

   a. Very firm or hard nodule

   b. Nodule or thyroid "fixed" to adjacent tissues

   c. Ipsilateral neck lymph node enlargement

Laboratory Tests

1. The following positive tests are, like symptoms and clinical findings noted above, of some aid only in estimating the likelihood that the patient has a thyroid malignancy:

   a. Vocal cord paralysis by laryngoscopy

   b. Distant metastases to lung (chest film) or to bone (scan)

   c. Solitary or dominant nodule hypofunctioning ("cold") on thyroid scan

   d. Cystic nodule greater than 4 cm or complex cyst on ultrasound

2. Only rarely will you have done any of the preceding tests. Instead, you have found either a solitary nodule or a dominant nodule in a multinodular gland on physical examination.

3. Gradually over the last 10 years has evolved the following approach to *all* nodules:

   a. If there has been a history of external ionizing irradiation in childhood, usually surgery is performed immediately.

   b. If no history of irradiation, an FNAB is done in the office.

      (1) The person doing the aspiration must be expe-

rienced and *currently* performing a significant number monthly. The cytopathologist reading the biopsy also should be *currently* reading a significant number monthly. Major false-negatives occur if *either* of these criteria is not met.

(2) If the FNAB is read as "malignant," surgery is performed.

(3) If the FNAB is read as "benign," the patient is followed carefully.

(4) If the FNAB is "suspicious," [123]I scan was done by some in the past:

    (a) If the nodule is "cold," surgery is done.

    (b) If "hot," one observes and follows the patient.

    (c) Most do surgery on all "suspicious" nodules because

        i. Only 5 per cent of solitary nodules are "hot"; thus high cost just to identify this low percentage of nodules.

        ii. Previously, a "hot" nodule by definition was thought to exclude a malignancy, but in recent studies 30 to 50 per cent of "hot" nodules were read as "suspicious," operated and histologically diagnosed as "follicular adenoma." But even on whole-gland histology, pathologists disagree 26 per cent of the time between follicular adenoma and follicular cancer.

(5) Because of the preceding results, thyroid scans no longer are done routinely.

(6) If the FNAB is "inadequate sample" or "nondiagnostic," FNAB is repeated until an adequate sample is obtained, even an ultrasound-guided FNAB.

Key Tests

- Werner's maneuver is done first to find and then to define nodule characteristics.

- FNAB is performed on all nodules (contraindicated if patient anticoagulated). It is not a definitive test but a very important adjunct to management.

Differential Diagnosis

1. Modern diagnosis of thyroid cancer depends completely on your confident palpation of the thyroid to identify a nodule in the first place.

2. Is the neck mass truly thyroid gland?

    a. Locate the notch of the thyroid cartilage, then the lower border of the thyroid cartilage, and the cricoid cartilage immediately below it (Fig. 164–1).

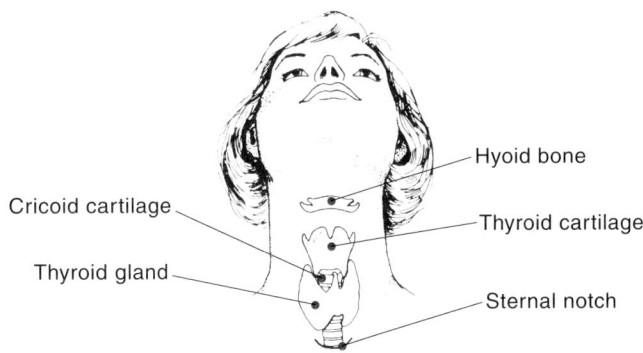

Figure 164–1 Landmarks for the anatomic location of the thyroid gland. (From Becker KL [ed]: Principles and Practice of Endocrinology and Metabolism. Philadelphia, JB Lippincott, 1990, p 264; used with permission.)

    b. The gland almost always will be between the cricoid and the sternal notch.

    c. Move your finger midline downward from the cricoid, sensing for the thyroid isthmus (usually 4 to 8 mm wide).

    d. Palpate each lobe in turn using Werner's maneuver. Stand behind the seated patient. With the patient's head slightly flexed forward, to palpate the left lobe, turn the patient's head 15 to 20 degrees to the left to relax the left sternocleidomastoid muscle. Immobilize the trachea with your right hand at the same time you palpate the left lobe with your left hand. Next, retract the relaxed muscle with the fingers of your left hand, and palpate thoroughly the left lobe with your right hand. Frequently, I will perform the same palpation with the patient supine because this relaxes the muscle even more. Do the reverse procedure for the right lobe.

    e. Once you have located the gland or mass in each position, have the patient swallow. If the nodule or mass moves upward with swallowing, it is likely thyroid-related. If it does not rise with swallowing, it probably is not a thyroid nodule.

3. If the mass (nodule) is thyroid, then perform FNAB and proceed as outlined above.

4. If the neck mass is not thyroid:

    a. If it is midline, it may be

      (1) Thyroglossal duct cyst

        (a) A 1- to 2-cm remnant of pyramidal lobe, thus located above isthmus

        (b) Usually adjacent and inferior to hyoid bone

        (c) May rise on deglutition too but also rises with maximal tongue protrusion

      (2) Epidermoid cyst

        (a) Usually nontender

        (b) Located submental, infrahyoid region

b. If mass is not midline, think

  (1) Laryngocele

    (a) Expands with Valsalva maneuver but not pulsatile (Valsalva may cause a vascular anomaly to enlarge but it often is pulsatile)

    (b) May be bilateral (Dizzie Gillespie)

    (c) May be seen with chronic obstructive pulmonary disease

  (2) Branchial cleft cyst

    (a) 1 to 2 cm in size

    (b) Located along anterior aspect sternocleidomastoid muscle

5. Nonthyroid neck masses in adult—"80 per cent rule"

  a. 80 per cent neoplastic, 80 per cent malignant, and 80 per cent of these are metastatic to the neck.

  b. 80 per cent of primary tumors arise above the clavicles and are metastatic to neck nodes.

Treatment

1. If the FNAB is either "malignant" or "benign," the issue is clear.

2. If "malignant," surgery is indicated (surgery usually also is done with a confirmed history of external irradiation alone). Only the extent of surgery is controversial.

  a. Near-total thyroidectomy probably is indicated in all except less than 1 cm differentiated carcinoma or minimally invasive follicular carcinoma. Get your best surgeon!

  b. In differentiated cancers, occult multifocal cancer occurs in 30 per cent, and occult lymph node metastases are found in 50 per cent. Extensive surgery still is not needed, and only involved lymph nodes found at surgery need be removed before ablation treatment.

  c. Lymph node spread, however, is a more serious prognostic finding in anaplastic, lymphoma, medullary, or less differentiated papillary or follicular cancers. Expect more aggressive behavior in these, so treat vigorously.

  d. Dictating more aggressive postoperative ablation therapy are: age less than 20 or greater than 45, invasion outside thyroid capsule, size greater than 4 cm, male, intraglandular invasion of follicular cancer, tall cell variant of papillary, markedly multicentric cancer.

  e. Postoperative ^{131}I ablation therapy (in all except solitary less than 1 cm papillary or minimally invasive follicular cancer). Patient may desire ablation therapy even for these latter cancers, so I offer it to them, since there is some evidence of benefit.

    (1) Want TSH greater than 30 before ^{131}I. Thus always stop L-T$_4$ therapy (0.1 mg/day) 6 weeks

before ^{131}I; then give L-T$_3$ maintenance dose (Cytomel, 25 μg t.i.d.) for the next 4 weeks; for last 2 weeks before ^{131}I, stop L-T$_3$ and have the patient eat a low-iodine diet.

    (2) In "low-risk" patients, low dose (30 mCi) ^{131}I. If needed, a second low dose is given 6 months later. If determined by whole-body ^{131}I scan and serum thyroglobulin levels that further ablation is needed, 100 mCi is given. Above preparation to get TSH above 30 always is done before ^{131}I ablation.

    (3) In "high-risk" (see above) patients, use the same procedure except treat with 100 mCi ^{131}I initially and repeat same dose if needed (in 6 months).

3. If the nodule by FNAB is "benign," medical therapy or careful follow-up is done.

  a. Until recently, all nodules would have been treated with suppressive doses of L-thyroxine either to decrease the size or stop further growth of the nodule.

  b. Today, suppressive therapy either should not be done or the length of time a therapeutic trial is done should be limited strictly because

    (1) Double-blind, placebo-controlled study showed no effect in reducing size of nodules over 6 months' suppression (but may be subgroup with good response).

    (2) Suppressive doses of L-thyroxine accelerate osteoporosis.

4. If the nodule is "suspicious" by FNAB, cancer still is found in 10 to 20 per cent.

  a. Favoring surgery would be the presence of risk factors noted above or patient's emotional preference, but most do surgery in all with "suspicious" FNAB.

  b. If surgery is refused and no risk factors, such as woman 20 to 60 years and small nodule, you could try thyroid hormone suppression (keep TSH suppressed but not less than 0.05), and repeat FNAB in 6 months, but vigorous clinical follow-up is dictated.

5. Do surgery even if "benign" FNAB, such as rapid-growth solid mass, hard or fixed nodule, obstructive symptoms, palpable lymph nodes, or vocal cord paralysis.

Key Treatment

- If FNAB is "malignant," surgery is indicated.
- If FNAB is "benign," medical therapy is indicated.

Follow-Up

1. In a patient with a "benign" nodule by FNAB, thor-

ough palpation of the thyroid as well as regional lymph nodes is performed carefully at *all* future examinations. Appearance of *any* of the above: rapid growth, nodule hardens, obstructive symptoms, etc. dictates immediate surgery.

2. Patient having thyroid cancer already operated is ablated with ^{131}I until total-body ^{131}I scan and serum thyroglobulin are both negative (tested 6 and 12 months later).

3. Total-body ^{131}I scans are done then about every 5 years in "low-risk" patients and every 2 years in "high-risk" patients, or more frequently if serum thyroglobulin levels increase. The latter are done every 6 months at first after ablative therapy and later every 1 to 2 years.

 Bibliography

For more information on FNAB, see
Gharib H: FNAB of thyroid nodules. Mayo Clin Proc 1994;69:44–49.

For more information on risk factors for malignancy in nodules, see
Hamming JF, Goslings BM, van Steenis GJ, et al: Value of FNAB in patients with nodular thyroid disease divided into groups of suspicion of malignant neoplasms on clinical grounds. Arch Intern Med 1990;150:113–116.

For more information on suppression by levothyroxine, see
LaRosa GL, Lupo L, Giuffrida D, et al: Levothyroxine and iodine are both effective for treating benign solitary solid cold nodules of the thyroid. Ann Intern Med 1995;122:1–8.
Gharib H, James EM, Charboneau JW, et al: Suppressive therapy with levothyroxine for solitary thyroid nodules. N Engl J Med 1987;317:70–75.

For more information on levothyroxine and osteoporosis risk, see
Paul TL, Kerrigan J, Marie Kelly A, et al: Long-term L-thyroxine therapy is associated with decreased hip bone density in premenopausal women. JAMA 1988;259:3137–3141.

For more information on management of thyroid nodules, see
Robbins J: Thyroid nodules and thyroid cancer, in Syllabus of the Endocrinology Board Review Course. Washington, Endocrine Fellows Foundation, 1993, pp 491–498.

165 Thyroiditis

Edward J. Gurza

Thyroiditis, the most common thyroid abnormality encountered in clinical practice, encompasses a heterogeneous group of inflammatory diseases of the thyroid. They may be classified into five major categories:

1. Acute thyroiditis (suppurative)
2. Subacute granulomatous
3. Subacute lymphocytic
4. Chronic lymphocytic (Hashimoto's)
5. Invasive fibrous (Riedel's)

Table 165–1 summarizes the etiology, signs and symptoms, and treatment of these five categories of thyroiditis.

Etiology

1. *Acute:* This rare form occurs more commonly in women 20 to 40 years old, with more than 50 to 60 per cent of patients having pre-existing thyroid disease and 70 per cent having concurrent upper respiratory symptoms. The cause is bacterial in 68 per cent, fungal in 15 per cent, and parasitic in less than 1 per cent.

2. *Subacute granulomatous:* A relatively common form that is the most frequent cause of "painful thyroid"
   a. Seasonal (summer/fall), often preceded by upper respiratory infection (URI), suggesting a viral etiology
   b. The association with HLA-Bw35 in two-thirds of patients suggests a genetic predisposition.

3. *Subacute lymphocytic*
   a. "Painless thyroiditis" occurs in two forms: sporadic (90 per cent) and postpartum (10 per cent).
   b. Thyroid microsomal antibodies are present in about 10 per cent of postpartum patients, and the association with other autoimmune disorders suggests an autoimmune cause. A viral etiology has been suggested for the sporadic form.

4. *Chronic lymphocytic*
   a. This is the most common thyroiditis and is responsible for a significant amount of hypothyroidism in patients over age 65 (found histologically in 2 per cent of women incidentally at autopsy).
   b. Clearly an autoimmune etiology, although probably more than one mechanism is involved. A strong genetic predisposition is related to the inheritance of HLA-B8 and DR5 antigens.

5. *Invasive fibrous*
   a. The rarest form of inflammatory thyroid disease, it is characterized by replacement of the thyroid parenchyma by dense fibrous tissue and affecting woman (3:1) 30 to 60 years of age.
   b. The cause is as yet unknown.

Key Symptoms

Acute
- Neck pain
- Fever
- Dysphagia

Subacute Granulomatous
- Viral prodrome
- Neck pain → ear

Subacute Lymphocytic
- Painless
- Abrupt hyperthyroidism (rare)

Chronic Lymphocytic
- Asymptomatic neck fullness or thyroid nodule

Invasive Fibrous
- Painless neck enlargement, vocal cord paralysis

Symptoms

1. *Acute*
   a. An abrupt onset of illness (which may be preceded by an upper respiratory infection) characterized by anterior neck pain (100 per cent), fever (92 per cent), and dysphagia (91 per cent)
   b. Four phases occurring over 4 to 6 months:
      (1) Initial acute phase (3 to 6 weeks) with hyperthyroidism
      (2) Euthyroidism
      (3) Hypothyroidism (several weeks to months)
      (4) Asymptomatic recovery phase

2. *Subacute granulomatous*
   a. Eighty per cent occurring in women 20 to 50 years old
   b. Viral prodrome followed by an abrupt onset of significant anterior neck pain that is usually unilateral and, in a third, radiating to the ear. Symptoms of coexisting hyperthyroidism also may be present.

3. *Subacute lymphocytic*
   a. Clinical course is similar to subacute granulomatous.
   b. Relatively abrupt onset of hyperthyroidism

4. *Chronic lymphocytic*
   a. Ninety-five per cent in women 30 to 50 years old
   b. Most patients are asymptomatic with a painless, gradually enlarging thyroid usually found incidentally. Late in the course the gland becomes small and undetectable.
   c. Occasional mechanical compression symptoms

d. At the time of presentation, symptoms of hypothyroidism were found in 20 per cent, hyperthyroidism in 5 per cent ("hashitoxicosis"), and euthyroidism or relative thyroid insufficiency in 75 per cent.

e. It is the most common cause of primary hypothyroidism, and it may be associated with the polyglandular failure syndrome (versus multiple endocrine failure).

5. *Invasive fibrous*

a. Characteristically, the initial symptom is the recent enlargement of a pre-existing goiter, typically painless, which may progress gradually to produce symptoms of pressure.

b. Associated with other focal sclerosing syndromes (retroperitoneal, cholangitis, orbital, mediastinal), which are found in 12 of 37 patients with Riedel's thyroiditis.

Signs

1. *Acute:* Typical findings include neck tenderness in a febrile patient.

2. *Subacute granulomatous*

a. Exquisitely tender thyroid in a thyrotoxic patient.

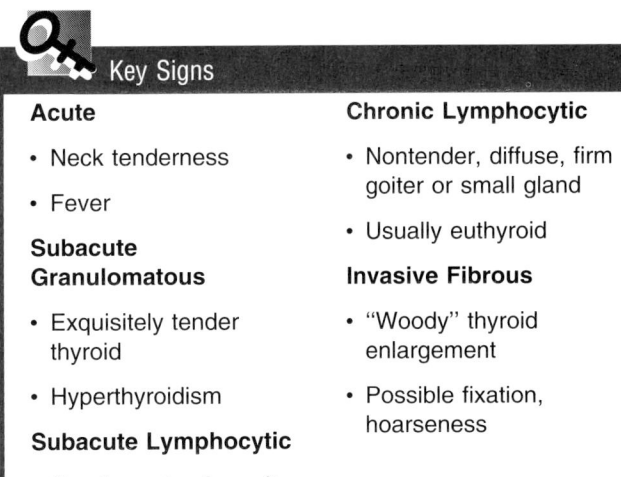

Key Signs

Acute
- Neck tenderness
- Fever

Subacute Granulomatous
- Exquisitely tender thyroid
- Hyperthyroidism

Subacute Lymphocytic
- Small, nontender goiter
- Hyperthyroidism

Chronic Lymphocytic
- Nontender, diffuse, firm goiter or small gland
- Usually euthyroid

Invasive Fibrous
- "Woody" thyroid enlargement
- Possible fixation, hoarseness

b. There is only slight to moderate, usually unilateral, swelling; however, the clinical picture may vary considerably.

3. *Subacute lymphocytic*

a. Physical findings are limited to a nontender goiter in about 50 per cent of patients.

b. Findings of thyrotoxicosis found in 5 to 23 per cent.

TABLE 165–1. THYROIDITIS

Type	Frequency	Etiology	Signs/Symptoms	Laboratory Signs	Differential Diagnosis	Treatment, Follow-Up
Acute	Rare Female 20–40 years old	(Rare) bacterial (70%)	Abrupt onset; concurrent infection; pain, fever; 4 phases	↑ WBC, C&S	Hemorrhage into cyst or adenoma malignancy	Parenteral antibiotics Surgical drainage of fluct abscess
Subacute granulomatous	Female 20–50 years old	Common cause of painful thyroid Probably viral Associated with HLA-Bw35	Viral prodrome followed by abrupt onset of pain, exquisitely tender thyroid	↑ ESR (>50) ↑ T₄ (50%) Triphasic pattern ↓ RAIU	As above	NSAIDs Corticosteroids β-blockers (hyperthyroid phase) L-thyroxine (permanent hypothyroid <5%)
Subacute lymphocytic ("Painless thyroiditis")	Painless	Sporadic (90%)? Viral Postpartum (10%), autoimmune	Abrupt onset of hyperthyroidism Clinical course similar to SAG	↑ T₄/T₃, ↓ RAIU ESR *not* significantly increased Positive AMA in postpartum form	Graves' disease	β-blockers L-T₄ if hypothyroid 6% perm. hypothyroid
Chronic lymphocytic (Hashimoto's)	Painless Most common Female 30–50 years old	Autoimmune with genetic predisposition	Asymptomatic thyroid enlargement Most euthyroid on presentation Associated polyglandular failure	Positive thyroid AB's (hallmark) TFTs variable	↑ risk of 1° thyroid, lymphoma	No Rx in many L-T₄ (hypothyroid 5%/year)
Invasive fibrous (Riedel's)	Rarest Etiology unknown		Painless enlargement of pre-existing goiter "Woody" thyroid mass Fixation/pressure Associated sclerosing syndromes	Open Bx for Dx Hypothyroid and hypoparathyroid rare	Malignancy Fibrosing Hashimoto's	Surgical Recurrences rare

4. *Chronic lymphocytic*

 a. Diffuse, firm goiter, eventually shrinking to a small, lobulated, very firm gland

 b. Findings consistent with euthyroid, hypothyroid, or rarely, hyperthyroid

5. *Invasive fibrous*

 a. Classically presents as diffuse enlargement or an extremely hard, ''woody'' thyroid mass.

 b. Characteristic fixation to surrounding tissues

 c. Findings related to extracervical fibrosclerosis

Laboratory Tests

1. *Acute*

 a. High white blood cell (WBC) count in more than 70 per cent

 b. Fine-needle aspiration (Gram's stain and culture of material) can confirm diagnosis.

 c. T_4 and radioactive iodide uptake (RAIU) are usually normal. Antibodies are absent.

 d. Ultrasonography to exclude a cervical abscess

2. *Subacute granulomatous*

 a. High erythrocyte sedimentation rate (ESR) (usually greater than 50 and often greater than 100 mm per hour). A normal test virtually excludes the diagnosis.

 b. High T_4 in approximately 50 per cent

 c. Low RAIU. An uptake greater than 5 per cent makes diagnosis unlikely.

 d. Elevated thyroglobulin

 e. Mild normocytic anemia with normal or slightly increased WBC count

3. *Subacute lymphocytic*

 a. Elevated T_4/T_3 with decreased RAIU

 b. ESR normal or mildly elevated

 c. The antimicrosomal antibody (AMA) test may be positive in the postpartum form; otherwise, thyroid antibodies are usually undetectable by ordinary serologic techniques.

4. *Chronic lymphocytic*

 a. Antibodies are the hallmark of the disorder. Antimicrosomal antibodies are present in 90 per cent of cases; titers of 1:2500 or greater are virtually diagnostic.

 b. T_4, T_3 or T_3U or T_3RU, and TSH values are related to the clinical stage of the disease. These should be done to rule out ''subclinical hypothyroidism'' (normal T_4 and increased TSH).

 c. RAIU is variable and of little help.

5. *Invasive fibrous*

 a. No typical laboratory findings

 b. Biopsy is essential to establish diagnosis and to rule out carcinoma.

c. T_4 is generally normal. It declines proportionate to the fibrous replacement.

Key Tests

Acute	**Chronic Lymphocytic**
• Leukocytosis	• ↑ Thyroid antibodies
• Culture and sensitivity	**Invasive Fibrous**
Subacute Granulomatous	• Biopsy
• ↑ ESR	
• ↑ T_4/T_3, ↓ RAIU	
Subacute Lymphocytic	
• ↑ T_4/T_3, ↓ RAIU	

Differential Diagnosis

1. *Acute* and *subacute granulomatous:* The other painful thyroid disorders that should be clinically excluded are

 a. Subacute granulomatous—usually less painful

 b. Hemorrhage into an adenoma or carcinoma

 c. A malignant neoplasia of the thyroid that grows fast may develop focal necrosis and mimic a primary pyogenic infection. Rarely, it also may cause hyperthyroidism due to release of colloid-stored thyroxine.

 d. Subacute granulomatous thyroiditis and hemorrhage into an adenoma account for 90 per cent.

2. *Subacute lymphocytic*

 a. Painless thyroiditis with hyperthyroidism should be differentiated from Graves' disease, which may be impossible to differentiate on clinical grounds alone.

 b. Postpartum thyroiditis can present with hyper- or hypothyroidism.

3. *Chronic lymphocytic*

 a. Early on, the differential involves that of a painless goiter, which would include simple goiter, colloid goiter, Hashimoto's, use of goitrogens, iodine deficiency, lymphoma. Later, hypothyroidism develops in most.

 b. Thyroid carcinoma must be ruled out in any patient who presents with a dominant nodule, as can occur in some patients with Hashimoto's.

 c. Primary thyroid lymphoma has been associated with this entity and is a possibility, especially in the elderly patient with rapid enlargement or tracheal compression.

4. *Invasive fibrous*

 a. Fine-needle aspiration will reveal the typical histologic features of dense fibrosis and generally exclude carcinoma or lymphoma, which also may present this way.

b. Other major clinical entities that must be distinguished include the fibrosing variant of chronic lymphocytic and subacute granulomatous thyroiditis.

Treatment

1. *Acute*

   a. Medication

      (1) Parenteral antibiotics

      (2) Anti-inflammatory drugs (ASAs, NSAIDs)

   b. Surgical: drainage of any large abscess

   c. Activity: rest and local heat

2. *Subacute granulomatous:* medications

   a. NSAIDs are the "first-line agents" for pain relief

   b. Prednisone, 20 to 40 mg daily, is the treatment of choice in severe cases not responding to other therapy. It can provide dramatic relief and can be tapered after 1 week and discontinued within 2 to 4 weeks. Restart if pain recurs (in about 20 per cent of cases).

   c. β-Blockers for symptoms of hyperthyroidism

3. *Subacute lymphocytic*

   a. Medication: Treatment often can be limited to reassurance and observation.

      (1) Symptoms of hyperthyroidism can be treated with β blockade (e.g., propranolol, 20 to 40 mg q.i.d.).

      (2) Glucocorticoids are used only for severe symptoms.

      (3) Thyroid replacement (0.05 to 0.15 mg daily) when the patient presents with hypothyroidism

   b. Surgical: Thyroidectomy occasionally has been performed in rare instances where recurrent, disabling episodes occur.

4. *Chronic lymphocytic*

   a. Medications: Some patients require no therapy.

      (1) Chronic replacement therapy with sodium L-thyroxine when hypothyroidism exists with the goal to normalize the T_4 and TSH.

      (2) Subclinical hypothyroidism also should be treated with replacement.

      (3) L-Thyroxine also may be indicated in euthyroid patients with symptomatic thyroid enlargement. Reduction in size has been seen, especially in young patients.

   b. Surgery rarely may be necessary to relieve symptoms of compression.

5. *Invasive fibrosing*

   a. Medications: none

   b. Surgical: Surgical therapy is generally considered the only useful therapeutic approach. It is necessary in order to establish the diagnosis and/or relieve pressure symptoms.

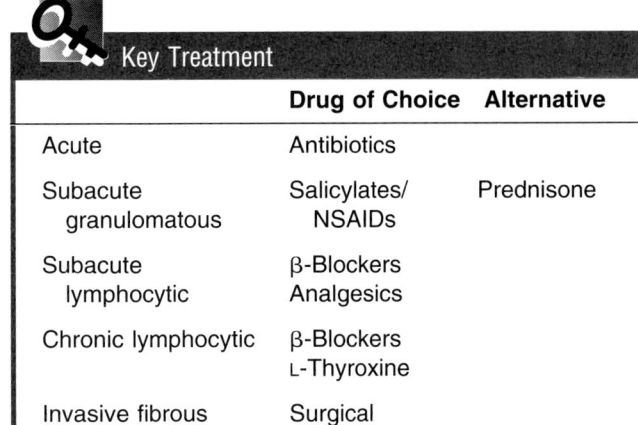

Key Treatment	Drug of Choice	Alternative
Acute	Antibiotics	
Subacute granulomatous	Salicylates/ NSAIDs	Prednisone
Subacute lymphocytic	β-Blockers Analgesics	
Chronic lymphocytic	β-Blockers L-Thyroxine	
Invasive fibrous	Surgical	

Follow-Up

> **WARNING**
>
> • **Caution should be exercised in giving thyroid replacement to patients over age 65 and to those patients with coronary artery disease.**
>
> • **In patients with associated polyglandular disease and borderline adrenal function, thyroid replacement may precipitate adrenal insufficiency.**

1. *Acute*

   a. Permanent sequelae are rare. Hypothyroidism may occur if destruction of the gland has been complete.

   b. Recurrences suggest an undiagnosed anatomic abnormality, such as persistent thyroglossal duct or fistula.

2. *Subacute granulomatous*

   a. The clinical course is variable; however, the average duration for the typical form is approximately 2 to 5 months; 20 per cent have recurrence that prolongs the course.

   b. Persistent abnormalities are considered uncommon.

      (1) Permanent hypothyroidism is reported in less than 5 per cent.

      (2) Continued observation is necessary because there is some suggestion that a persistent thyroid abnormality may occur.

3. *Subacute lymphocytic*

   a. The clinical course is similar to that of subacute granulomatous except the outcome is different; 54 per cent of patients will have a persistent thyroid abnormality.

b. The presence of positive AMAs in the postpartum period is thought to predict the increased occurrence of postpartum thyroid dysfunction. If antibody-positive thyroiditis does occur, rapid recovery can be expected over a 2- to 4-month period.

c. Patients with postpartum thyroiditis should be observed for the development of hypothyroidism.

d. The following patients should be advised to have antibody screening after successive pregnancies:

   (1) Those with a prior history of postpartum thyroiditis

   (2) Those with a prior history of Graves' or Hashimoto's disease

   (3) Those with a family history of autoimmune thyroid disorders

4. *Chronic lymphocytic*

a. Left untreated, patients with subclinical hypothyroidism will develop overt hypothyroidism at a rate of 5 per cent per year.

b. Long-term follow-up is mandatory for the following reasons:

   (1) To pick up the patients with hypothyroidism

   (2) To adjust the dose of thyroid replacement in treated cases

   (3) To observe for possible associated polyendocrine insufficiencies, pernicious anemia, vitiligo

5. *Invasive fibrous*

a. Recurrences after surgical resection are rare.

b. Left untreated, the course is slowly progressive.

c. Complications of the neck disease are rare (hypothyroidism and hypoparathyroidism).

d. In those cases associated with extracervical fibrosclerosis, the prognosis will depend on the extracervical disease rather than the neck mass.

Bibliography

Amino N, Mori H, Iwatani Y, et al: High prevalence of transient post-partum thyrotoxicosis and hypothyroidism. N Engl J Med 1982;306:14–49.

DeGrott W, Quintans J: The causes of autoimmune thyroid disease. Endocr Rev 1989;20:537.

Hay I: Thyroiditis: A clinical update. Mayo Clin Proc 1985;60:836–843.

Levin SN: Current concepts of thyroiditis. Arch Intern Med 1983;143:1952–1956.

Singer P: Thyroiditis. Acute, subacute and chronic. Med Clin North Am 1991;75(1):61–77.

Tunbridge WM, Brewis M, French J, et al: Natural history of autoimmune thyroiditis. Br Med J 1981;282:258–262.

Tunbridge WM, Evered DC, Hall R, et al: The spectrum of thyroid disease in a community: The Whickham Survey. Clin Endocrinol 1977;7:481.

Volpe R: Sub-acute thyroiditis. Prog Clin Biol Res 1981;74:115.

166 Cushing's Syndrome/Disease

Andrew J. Norton

Etiology

1. Endocrinologic syndrome of persistent inappropriate hypercortisolemia
2. Two etiologic categories determined by presence or absence of the stimulatory hormone adrenocorticotropic hormone (ACTH) at the time of measured hypercortisolemia
   a. ACTH-dependent
      (1) Pituitary neoplasm (Cushing's disease): 65 per cent of total
      (2) Nonpituitary neoplasm (ectopic): 15 per cent of total
      (3) Hypothalamic or ectopic corticotropin-releasing hormone (CRH)–producing tumors: rare
   b. ACTH-independent
      (1) Adrenal neoplasm (adenoma or carcinoma): 15 per cent of total
      (2) Nodular adrenal hyperplasia: 5 per cent of total
         (a) Primary pigmented nodular adrenal disease
         (b) Macronodular adrenal hyperplasia
      (3) Iatrogenic: common
      (4) Factitious: uncommon
3. ACTH-dependent Cushing's syndrome is most commonly associated with a pituitary adenoma secreting ACTH (classic Cushing's disease).
   a. Female/male ratio 8:1
   b. Usual onset age 20 to 40 years
4. Ectopic ACTH-dependent Cushing's syndrome
   a. Most commonly caused by tumors of the APUD system
      (1) Small cell carcinoma of the lung
      (2) Medullary carcinoma of the thyroid
      (3) Carcinoid
         (a) Bronchial
         (b) Thymic
      (4) Pheochromocytoma
      (5) Islet cell tumors
   b. Female/male ratio 1:1

Symptoms

1. General
   a. Weight gain—usually central (truncal)
   b. Weakness/fatigue
2. Dermatologic
   a. Easy bruisibility
   b. Excessive hair growth in women
   c. Poor wound healing
3. Neuropsychiatric
   a. Depression
   b. Insomnia
4. Gonadal
   a. Menstrual disturbances/amenorrhea
   b. Impotence
   c. Decreased libido
5. Musculoskeletal
   a. Back pain
   b. Muscular weakness
6. Metabolic
   a. Polyuria
   b. Ureteral colic

Key Symptoms

- Weakness/fatigue
- Weight gain
- Dermatologic changes
- Depression
- Gonadal dysfunction

Clinical Findings

1. General
   a. Obesity and fat redistribution
      (1) Central obesity, particularly facial rounding and supraclavicular fullness
      (2) Generalized weight gain may occur.
   b. Hypertension
2. Dermatologic
   a. Hirsutism, particularly increased facial lanugo hair growth
   b. Acne and facial plethora
   c. Wide-based purple striae on the abdomen
   d. Skin/subcutaneous thinning with ecchymosis
   e. Superficial fungal infections
3. Neuropsychiatric: depression
4. Musculoskeletal
   a. Osteopenia/osteoporosis with pathologic fractures (vertebral, rib)
   b. Proximal muscle weakness
5. Metabolic
   a. Impaired glucose tolerance or diabetes mellitus
   b. Kidney stone formation

Key Signs

- Central obesity with supraclavicular fullness
- Facial rounding with plethora
- Hypertension
- Proximal muscular weakness
- Hirsutism and acne
- Glucose intolerance

Laboratory Tests

1. Basic laboratory studies are usually normal.
2. Leukocytosis, lymphopenia, polycythemia, hyperglycemia, and hypokalemia may be seen. Hypokalemia is commonly found (60 per cent) in ectopic ACTH production but is unusual in pituitary Cushing's syndrome (10 per cent).
3. Dexamethasone suppression test
   a. Screening test for Cushing's syndrome
   b. 1 mg dexamethasone orally in the late evening (2300 hours) with early morning serum cortisol determination in nonstressed ambulatory individual
   c. Normal values less than 3 µg/dl
   d. False-positive results with physiologic stress, renal failure, estrogen and anticonvulsant drug therapy, and endogenous depression
4. Urine free cortisol
   a. Best test for confirmation and when initial clinical suspicion is high
   b. 24-hour urine collection for free cortisol and creatinine
   c. False-positive result uncommonly seen in physiologic stress, alcoholism, endogenous depression, and exogenous steroid use
   d. False-negative result seen in intermittent cortisol secretion syndromes (uncommon)

Key Tests

- Overnight dexamethasone suppression test
- 24-hour urine free cortisol determination

Differential Diagnosis

1. Diagnostic confirmation of Cushing's syndrome and determination of its cause should be done with the collaboration of an experienced endocrinologist.
2. Determine plasma ACTH level by immunoradiometric assay (IRMA) technique to distinguish ACTH-dependent from ACTH-independent Cushing's syndrome.
3. If ACTH-dependent (>10 pg/ml)
   a. High-dose overnight dexamethasone suppression test
      (1) 8 mg dexamethasone in the late evening (2300 hours) with early morning cortisol
      (2) In pituitary-dependent ACTH Cushing's syndrome, the morning cortisol is usually less than 50 per cent of baseline. In ectopic ACTH or ACTH-independent Cushing's syndrome, the cortisol level usually does not suppress.
   b. MRI scan of the pituitary
   c. Referral for bilateral inferior petrosal sinus sampling for ACTH to definitively ascertain the source of ACTH production (pituitary or ectopic)
4. If ACTH independent (<5 pg/ml), abdominal computed tomographic scan for adrenal neoplasm

Treatment

1. Surgery
   a. Transsphenoidal pituitary microsurgery is the treatment of choice for pituitary ACTH-secreting adenoma and should be done by an experienced neurosurgeon.
   b. Adrenalectomy (unilateral or bilateral) for adrenal adenoma or hyperplasia and for persistent or recurrent pituitary Cushing's syndrome after pituitary microsurgery.
2. Radiotherapy is adjunctive therapy for pituitary Cushing's syndrome.
3. Medical management of Cushing's syndrome employs drugs that inhibit adrenal hormone biosynthesis. Drugs used include
   a. Ketoconazole (Nizoral)
   b. Metyrapone (Metopirone)
   c. Aminoglutethimide (Cytadren)
   d. Mitotane (Lysodren)

Bibliography

For general information, see

Tyrrell JB: Cushing's syndrome. *In* Wyngaarden JB, Smith LH, Bennett JC (eds): Cecil Textbook of Medicine, 19th ed. Philadelphia, WB Saunders, 1992, pp 1284–1288.

For more detailed information, see

Nieman N, Cutler GB: Endocrinology, 3d ed. Philadelphia, WB Saunders, 1995, pp 1741–1769.

For a review of the diagnostic workup, see

Meikle AW: A diagnostic approach to Cushing's syndrome. Endocrinologist 1993;3(5):311–320.

For a review of ectopic ACTH syndromes, see

Findling JW, Raff H: Ectopic ACTH. *In* Mazzaferri EL, Samaan NA (eds): Endocrine Tumors. Cambridge, England, Blackwell Scientific Publications, 1993, pp 554–566.

167 Adrenal Insufficiency

James K. Rone

Etiology

A. Primary adrenal insufficiency (PAI)
1. Autoimmune adrenalitis (often part of a polyglandular autoimmune syndrome)
2. Infections
   a. Tuberculous (adrenal function may return after early treatment)
   b. Fungal
   c. AIDS-associated (cytomegalovirus, *Mycobacterium avium,* cryptococcus, primary HIV)
3. Vascular
   a. Hemorrhage (sepsis, anticoagulation, or coagulopathy)
   b. Infarction (hypoperfusion or thrombosis)
4. Metastatic disease (lymphoma, leukemia, lung, breast)
5. Bilateral adrenalectomy
6. Drugs
   a. Steroidogenesis inhibitors (ketoconazole, adrenolytic agents, etomidate)
   b. Inducers of cortisol metabolism (rifampin, phenytoin, phenobarbital)
7. Other (sarcoidosis, amyloidosis, hemochromatosis, adrenoleukodystrophy)

B. Secondary adrenal insufficiency (SAI)
1. Suppression of the hypothalamic-pituitary-adrenal (HPA) axis
   a. Exogenous glucocorticoids or ACTH
   b. Following surgical treatment of Cushing's syndrome
2. Any lesion of the pituitary or hypothalamus resulting in ACTH deficiency
   a. Tumors (pituitary adenoma, craniopharyngioma, metastatic disease)
   b. Surgery or trauma
   d. Infarction (Sheehan's syndrome)
   e. Other (sarcoidosis, infectious or autoimmune adenohypophysitis)

Symptoms

1. The clinical presentation of adrenal insufficiency is highly variable.
   a. Acute versus chronic
      (1) Acute adrenal insufficiency (Addisonian crisis) is a medical emergency presenting with shock and perhaps mimicking an acute abdomen.
      (2) Chronic disease may present with vague "neurotic" complaints and go undiagnosed for a prolonged period.
   b. Primary versus secondary
      (1) PAI results in loss of all adrenocortical hormones (glucocorticoids, mineralocorticoids, and adrenal androgens).
      (2) SAI affects only glucocorticoids. The renin-angiotensin-aldosterone axis remains intact.
2. Symptoms (in approximate order of frequency)
   a. Fatigue and weakness
   b. Anorexia or frank revulsion to food
   c. Nausea and vomiting
   d. Other gastrointestinal complaints (abdominal pain, diarrhea)
   e. Psychiatric symptoms (depression, apathy, confusion, psychosis, paranoia)
   f. Amenorrhea and decreased libido in women
   g. Salt craving, caused by mineralocorticoid loss (PAI only)
   h. Postural dizziness or syncope (usually PAI)
   i. Diffuse musculoskeletal pain
   j. Hypoglycemic symptoms

Key Symptoms

- Weakness and fatigue
- Anorexia
- Nausea and vomiting
- Abdominal pain
- Salt craving
- Postural dizziness

Clinical Findings

1. Weight loss
2. Hyperpigmentation (PAI only), due to increased melanocyte-stimulating activity, which parallels ACTH secretion. Prominent over elbows, knees, knuckles, palmar creases, gingival margins, buccal mucosa, lips, scars, and areas of chronic mild trauma (belts, bra straps).
3. Hypotension or shock (both PAI and SAI), due to decreased cardiac output, decreased vascular resistance, and inhibition of catecholamine action.
4. Loss of body hair in women, due to loss of primary androgen source
5. Auricular calcifications
6. Vitiligo (rare, but if present suggests autoimmune etiology)

Key Signs

- Weight loss
- Hypotension
- Hyperpigmentation

Laboratory Tests

A. General findings

1. Hyponatremia

    a. Glucocorticoid deficiency results in decreased stroke volume, which increases heart rate and stimulates vasopressin release, promoting increased free water retention.

    b. Mineralocorticoid deficiency causes increased urinary sodium loss.

2. Hyperkalemia, due to loss of mineralocorticoid-induced potassium excretion

3. Hypercalcemia (usually mild to moderate but occasionally life-threatening)

4. Normocytic normochromic anemia, neutropenia, eosinophilia, and lymphocytosis

5. Hyperchloremic metabolic acidosis

6. Azotemia

7. Fasting hypoglycemia

B. Screening and diagnostic testing

1. Serum cortisol

    a. Random cortisol levels are not generally adequate for screening, since levels vary with time of day and physiologic stress in normal subjects. However, in the presence of severe physiologic stress, a level less than 20 μg/dl is strongly suggestive of adrenal insufficiency.

    b. At a minimum, blood should be drawn for a cortisol level prior to treating suspected acute adrenal insufficiency. Treatment must not be delayed while waiting for results, however.

2. ACTH stimulation test

    a. Procedure: Inject 0.25 mg ACTH (Cortrosyn) intravenously or intramuscularly, and measure serum cortisol at 0, 30, and 60 minutes. A peak cortisol greater than 20 μg/dl is considered a normal response.

    b. Test of choice for diagnosis of adrenal insufficiency in most settings

    c. Can be performed in suspected acute adrenal insufficiency if dexamethasone, which does not interfere with cortisol measurement, is used for initial treatment. Therapy must not be delayed for diagnostic testing.

    d. Evaluates the entire HPA axis and will be abnormal in most cases of PAI and SAI. Results may be normal in early, partial PAI, or ACTH deficiency resulting from recent pitu-

itary surgery or resection of an ACTH-secreting tumor.

3. Insulin tolerance test (ITT)

    a. Procedure: Induce symptomatic hypoglycemia (glucose less than 40 mg/dl) with regular insulin, 0.1 to 0.15 unit/kg body weight intravenous bolus. Draw serum glucose and cortisol at 0, 30, 60, and 90 minutes. A peak cortisol greater than 20 μg/dl is considered normal.

    b. A physician must be present during this test. Fatal hypoglycemia may occur, and testing is contraindicated in patients with seizures or ischemic heart disease.

    c. The ITT is the "gold standard" for assessment of the HPA axis but is rarely needed. It offers no advantage over ACTH stimulation testing, except in the first few days after acute ACTH deprivation.

C. Localization (primary versus secondary)

1. Serum ACTH

    a. Markedly elevated in PAI

    b. Low or inappropriately normal in SAI

2. Aldosterone response to ACTH stimulation—Peak levels less than 4 ng/ml suggest PAI.

D. Other tests. If the cause of the adrenal disorder is not obvious, consider a chest radiograph, PPD testing, and adrenal or pituitary imaging as appropriate.

Key Tests

- ACTH stimulation test
- Serum ACTH

Differential Diagnosis

1. Acute adrenal insufficiency should be considered in all cases of unexplained hypotension or shock, especially if associated conditions are present or the patient has been on glucocorticoid therapy in the past year. May mimic acute abdomen, sepsis, and hypovolemic shock.

2. Chronic adrenal insufficiency

    a. The onset is often insidious with nonspecific complaints, making diagnosis difficult. Consider in any patient with chronic fatigue, especially if associated with weight loss, gastrointestinal symptoms, or hyperpigmentation.

    b. The differential diagnosis is broad but may include

    (1) Major depression

    (2) Mild thyrotoxicosis, especially in the elderly ("apathetic hyperthyroidism")

    (3) Gastrointestinal malignancy

    (4) Chronic infection

(5) Insulinoma, in which hypoglycemia is associated with increased appetite and weight gain

(6) Other hyperpigmented conditions (racial pigmentation, pregnancy, hemochromatosis, drug or heavy metal toxicity, Peutz-Jeghers syndrome)

(7) Ectopic ACTH secretion by some malignancies may present with weight loss, fatigue, hyperpigmentation, and elevated ACTH levels. Unlike Addison's disease, these patients have hypertension, hyperglycemia, hypercortisolemia, and hypokalemic metabolic alkalosis.

Treatment
Medication
A. Acute adrenal insufficiency

1. Hydrocortisone, 100 mg intravenously every 6 to 8 hours. This dose is rapidly tapered, typically to a total of 100 to 150 mg on the second day, 50 to 75 mg the third day, and maintenance starting the fourth day. Taper patients with other serious illnesses more slowly.

2. Alternatives include methylprednisolone or dexamethasone in equivalent doses, though hydrocortisone is preferred because of its greater mineralocorticoid activity. Dexamethasone is often used for the first dose while ACTH stimulation testing is accomplished.

3. Additional mineralocorticoids are not needed if high-dose hydrocortisone is used.

4. Boluses of normal saline with 5% dextrose must be given to correct volume depletion, hyponatremia, and hypoglycemia.

B. Chronic therapy

1. Maintenance

a. Hydrocortisone in the lowest effective dose is preferred. Prednisone and dexamethasone should be avoided because longer half-lives may increase the risk of Cushing's syndrome and osteoporosis. Some authorities, however, recommend prednisone, citing better symptom control and lower cost.

b. Hydrocortisone dose: 12 to 15 mg/m² orally daily.

(1) Usually two thirds of the total daily dose is given in the morning and one third in the evening (typically 20 and 10 mg, respectively). Single daily dosing may increase compliance and minimize side effects.

(2) Some authorities recommend determining the lowest effective dose by tapering the daily dose until evidence of deficiency (fatigue, gastrointestinal symptoms, hyponatremia) appears. The dose is then increased just enough to correct the abnormalities.

(3) Another approach is to treat in three divided doses (i.e., 10 mg t.i.d.) in order to maintain hormone levels throughout the day. This might be considered in patients who have persistent symptoms on more standard regimens.

c. Prednisone dose: 3 to 4 mg/m² daily (4 to 5 mg every morning and 1 to 2.5 mg at 3 P.M.).

d. Mineralocorticoid replacement (only needed in PAI): fludrocortisone (Florinef), 0.05 mg every other day to 0.2 mg daily. A typical dose is 0.1 mg/day. Higher doses are needed if a glucocorticoid other than hydrocortisone is used.

2. Stress coverage

a. Minor stress (fever >100° F, flu-like illness, nausea): double maintenance dose. Parenteral therapy needed if patient is unable to tolerate oral intake.

b. Major stress (severe trauma, illness, or surgery): as for acute adrenal insufficiency

Diet
High sodium intake beneficial in PAI

Activity
As tolerated

Patient Education
1. Patients and families must understand the need for stress coverage. They must know how to make appropriate dosage adjustments when a physician is not available.

2. Patients should wear identification jewelry, such as a Medic-Alert bracelet.

3. Patients should have in their possession and know how to use parenteral glucocorticoids in case of emergency (especially if traveling in remote areas).

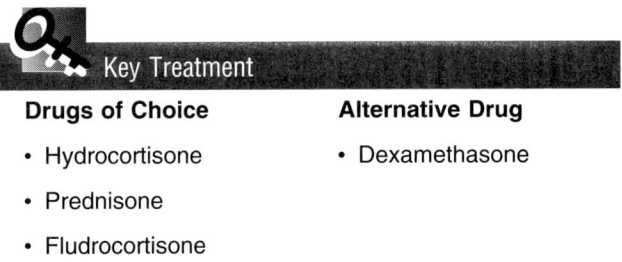

Key Treatment

Drugs of Choice	Alternative Drug
• Hydrocortisone	• Dexamethasone
• Prednisone	
• Fludrocortisone	

Follow-Up
1. Monitoring glucocorticoid replacement

a. The best indicators to follow are clinical findings (appetite, well-being, body weight) and serum electrolytes. ACTH and cortisol levels do not reflect clinical status and need not be followed.

b. Signs of Cushing's syndrome suggest overreplacement.

c. Bone mineral density measurements should be performed periodically.

2. Monitoring mineralocorticoid replacement

a. Plasma renin activity is the best indicator of plasma volume and should be titrated to the upper normal range. Serum potassium levels also should be normal.

b. The blood pressure should be checked. Dangerous hypertension may occur in patients taking fludrocortisone, especially when recumbent.

Bibliography

Chodosh LA, Daniels GH: Addison's disease. Endocrinologist 1993;3:166–181.

Grinspoon SK, Biller BMK: Laboratory assessment of adrenal insufficiency. J Clin Endocrinol 1994;79:923–931.

Orth DN, Kovacs WJ, DeBold CR: The adrenal cortex. *In* Wilson JD, Foster DW (eds): Williams' Textbook of Endocrinology. Philadelphia, WB Saunders, 1992, pp 489–620.

Stoffer SS: Addison's disease: How to improve patient's quality of life. Postgrad Med 1993;93:265–278.

Werbel SS, Ober KP: Acute adrenal insufficiency. Endocrinol Metab Clin North Am 1993;22:303–328.

168 Pheochromocytoma

Anderson Spickard, III

Etiology

1. Pheochromocytomas are rare tumors of chromaffin cells in the adrenal medulla and extra-adrenal sympathetic ganglia that secrete catecholamines causing hypertension and other symptoms and clinical findings.

2. Cause is unknown. Between 5 and 10 per cent of cases are inherited in an autosomal dominant fashion in families as isolated tumors or tumors associated with the multiple endocrine neoplasia type II (MEN II) or MEN III syndromes, von Hippel–Lindau disease (VHLD), or neurofibromatosis (NF).

3. Most tumors secrete predominantly norepinephrine (NE) with or without epinephrine (E); very few tumors secrete E alone.

4. Ten per cent of pheochromocytomas are malignant. In extra-adrenal familial tumors, the incidence of malignancy is 30 per cent.

Symptoms

1. Patients typically have paroxysms of headache, diaphoresis, or palpitations. At least one of these symptoms is present in 90 per cent of cases, and two symptoms are present in 70 per cent of cases. The presence of all three symptoms strongly suggests pheochromocytoma; only 6 per cent of patients with essential hypertension have the triad symptom complex.

2. Paroxysms have variable duration (minutes to hours) and frequency (monthly to 20 times per day).

Key Symptoms

- Headache
- Diaphoresis
- Palpitations
- Others: pallor, anxiety, tremor, nausea, vomiting, abdominal or chest pain, weight loss, constipation, flushing, fatigue

Clinical Findings

1. Eighty-five per cent of patients are hypertensive; 15 per cent are normotensive despite abnormal levels of catecholamines. Hypertension is sustained with episodic exacerbations or purely paroxysmal with normal blood pressure between attacks.

2. Severe pressor responses, hypotension, and even collapse can occur with anesthesia induction, certain medications, and labor onset.

3. Orthostatic hypotension results from blunted constriction reflexes.

4. Episodic hypotension may indicate the less common epinephrine-secreting tumor, which has powerful β-adrenergic effects.

5. Other features are hyperglycemia, weight loss, tachyarrhythmias, heart failure, and cholelithiasis.

Key Signs

- Hypertension with paroxysmal symptoms (see Key Symptoms)
- Hypertension with orthostasis
- Unexplained episodic hypotension
- Shock or pressor response to anesthesia, antihypertensives, or parturition
- Positive family history of pheochromocytoma, MEN II, MEN III, VHLD, or NF
- Hypertension in children
- Labile or resistant hypertension

Laboratory Tests

A. Biochemical testing

1. Due to low prevalence of disease (0.1 per cent of all hypertensive patients), only patients with the key signs above are tested for pheochromocytoma.

2. The clinician can diagnose 95 per cent of cases using one of three equally effective tests: 24-hour urine catecholamines, 24-hour urine metanephrines (a catecholamine metabolite), or plasma catecholamines.

   a. Patient convenience and ease of laboratory handling favor urine over plasma sampling in most situations.

   b. Note that the 24-hour urine vanillylmandelic acid (VMA) test is insensitive and is no longer recommended for diagnosis of pheochromocytoma.

3. NE and E values greater than twice the normal limit are diagnostic of pheochromocytoma; borderline values are repeated. Persistent equivocal results necessitate additional considerations and testing.

   a. Before testing, medications that can affect catecholamine levels should be discontinued (see Differential Diagnosis for list of medications).

   b. NE to dihydroxyphenylglycol (DHPG) ratio: A ratio greater than 1 is specific for NE-secreting pheochromocytomas (Duncan).

   c. Clonidine suppression or glucagon stimulation:

657

In patients with pheochromocytoma, plasma NE levels fail to suppress 3 hours after 0.3 mg of oral clonidine; NE levels rise 3-fold or more 2 minutes after 1 mg of intravenous glucagon (Grossman).

B. Anatomic localization

1. Localization of tumor for surgical planning follows biochemical confirmation of pheochromocytoma. The majority of tumors (>95 per cent) reside in the abdomen and are readily identified by abdominal CT or MRI.

2. Pelvis, chest, and neck views are reserved for the patient with high catecholamine levels and a negative abdominal imaging study or the patient with known abdominal disease who is at increased risk for extra-abdominal disease (familial-associated tumors, metastatic tumors).

3. Tumor invasion of adjacent structures or distant metastasis defines malignant pheochromocytoma.

4. M-iodobenzylguanidine (MIBG) scintigraphy can detect tumors that are widespread, functional, and small. Despite these advantages, its use is limited by expense, lack of availability, and suitable performance of MRI.

5. Selective percutaneous venous blood sampling for catecholamines is used for difficult cases.

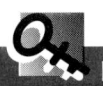

Key Tests

Diagnosis	Anatomic Localization
• 24-hour urine catecholamines or	• Abdominal CT or MRI
• 24-hour urine metanephrines or	
• Plasma catecholamines	

Differential Diagnosis

1. Conditions with similar presentations as pheochromocytoma

   a. Normal catecholamines: essential hypertension, panic attacks, hyperthyroidism, menopause, migraine headaches

   b. Potentially high catecholamines: subarachnoid hemorrhage, brain tumor, diencephalic epilepsy, posterior fossa lesions, acute porphyria, hypoglycemia, carcinoid, eclampsia, clonidine withdrawal

2. Medications reported to increase catecholamine levels: β-blockers, tricyclic antidepressants, sympathomimetics (Ephedrine), α-blockers (prazosin, terazosin), vasodilators (hydralazine), methyldopa, theophylline, chlorpromazine, tetracycline, and trifluoperazine

Treatment

1. Surgical resection is definitive therapy. For benign disease, cure rates approach 85 per cent, and 5-year survival rates average 96 per cent.

2. α-Blockers, phenoxybenzamine (Dibenzyline), 20 to 150 mg/d, or prazosin (Minipress), 3 to 20 mg/d, are used for 7 to 10 days before surgery to restore extracellular volume and stabilize symptoms and hypertension. Gradually increased dosing prevents orthostasis and reflex tachycardia with these drugs. Of note, alpha blockers may cause severe hypotension in tumors that secrete large amounts of epinephrine.

3. β-Blockers are used for preoperative tachycardia (heart rate >110) only after alpha blockade has been established to counter the NE-mediated vasoconstriction uncontested by β vasodilation.

4. Metyrosine (Demser), an inhibitor of NE synthesis, provides symptomatic relief; however, severe CNS side effects limit its use to patients who fail standard therapy.

5. Radiation and combination chemotherapy yield only transient success in treating malignant pheochromocytoma.

Key Treatment

Surgical resection

Drugs of Choice	Alternative Drug	Hypertensive Crisis
• Phenoxybenzamine	• Metyrosine	• Nitroprusside
• Prazosin		• Phentolamine

Follow-Up

1. Because 5 to 10 per cent of pheochromocytomas recur, urine or plasma catecholamines should be obtained 2 to 3 months after surgery and thereafter once a year for 2 to 5 years.

2. All first-degree relatives with hypertension or typical pheochromocytoma symptoms should have urine or plasma catecholamines sampled. In familial cases, asymptomatic family members, even with normal catecholamine levels, may need to be tested with CT or MRI (Neumann).

Bibliography

Duncan MW, Compton P, Lazarus L, Smythe GA: Measurement of norepinephrine and 3,4-dihydroxyphenylglycol in urine and plasma for the diagnosis of pheochromocytoma. N Engl J Med 1988;319:136–142.

Gilford RW Jr, Manger WM, Bravo, EL: Pheochromocytoma. Endocrinol Metab Clin North Am 1994;23(2):387–404.

Grossman E, Goldstein DS, Hoffman A, Keiser HR: Glucagon and clonidine testing in the diagnosis of pheochromocytoma. Hypertension 1991;17:733–741.

Neumann HPH, Berger DP, Sigmund G, et al: Pheochromocytomas, multiple endocrine neoplasia type 2, and von Hippel-Lindau disease. N Engl J Med 1993;329:1531–1538.

Stein PP, Black HR: A simplified diagnostic approach to pheochromocytoma: A review of the literature and report of one institution's experience. Medicine 1991;70:46–66.

169 Hyperprolactinemia

Geoffrey R. Swain

Etiology

Hyperprolactinemia can be caused by many factors.

1. Physiologic (pregnancy and up to 6 months after delivery or after stopping breast-feeding)
2. Prolactin-producing pituitary adenoma
3. Medications (e.g., opioids, tricyclics, metaclopramide, verapamil, phenothiazines, alphamethyldopa, isoniazid, estrogens, cocaine, reserpine, butyrophenones)
4. Hypothyroidism
5. Chest wall conditions (e.g., herpes zoster, post-thoracotomy, fibrocystic changes, breast stimulation)
6. Hypothalamic disease
7. Postoperative state (any major surgery but especially oophorectomy)
8. Idiopathic
9. Miscellaneous causes (e.g., sarcoid, renal failure, Cushing's disease, acromegaly, cirrhosis, and head or spinal cord trauma)

Symptoms

1. The most common presenting symptoms of hyperprolactinemia are galactorrhea, oligomenorrhea, amenorrhea, infertility, or impotence in men.
2. Patients also may have symptoms of other underlying etiologic processes (e.g., hypothyroidism, Cushing's disease, acromegaly, fibrocystic breast disease).
3. Patients also may have signs and symptoms of pituitary enlargement (e.g., headache, visual field loss).

Key Symptoms

- Galactorrhea
- Oligomenorrhea/ amenorrhea
- Infertility
- Impotence (in men)

Clinical Findings

1. Generally speaking, patients with hyperprolactinemia have few clinical findings.
2. A milky nipple discharge may be expressible on physical examination.
3. Patients may have findings stereotypical of other underlying etiologic processes (e.g., hypothyroidism, Cushing's disease, acromegaly, fibrocystic breast disease).

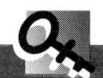

Key Sign

- Galactorrhea

Laboratory Tests

1. Thyroid function should be checked in all hyperprolactinemic patients.
2. Check follicle-stimulating hormone (FSH) and luteinizing hormone (LH) *if* the patient is also amenorrheic.
3. Check growth hormone and adrenal steroids *if* there is clinical suspicion of acromegaly or Cushing's disease.
4. Pituitary CT or MRI scanning should be done on all patients with significant hyperprolactinemia to rule out a pituitary tumor. Plain films, tomograms, or coned-down sellar radiographs are *not* sufficient.
5. Formal visual field testing should be performed if a pituitary adenoma is suspected.

Key Tests

- Thyroid function
- Pituitary CT or MRI scan

Differential Diagnosis

Since hyperprolactinemia is diagnosed by laboratory measurement of prolactin levels, differential diagnosis is not an issue, except for the possibility of laboratory error.

Treatment

1. Treatment is on an outpatient basis unless pituitary resection is needed (very rare). Treat underlying causes/diseases as indicated. Discontinue offending medications, if any.
2. Other reasons to treat include symptom management (if symptoms such as galactorrhea cause patient anxiety): fertility restoration, to cause growth retardation or regression of a pituitary adenoma, or to prevent osteoporosis (if the patient is estrogen-deficient).
3. "Watchful waiting" is often the most appropriate strategy. Most cases of idiopathic hyperprolactinemia resolve spontaneously, and many small pituitary adenomas do not continue to grow.
4. Large adenomas may be treated with x-ray therapy (variable success, 50 per cent risk of panhyperpituitarism at 5 years) or transsphenoidal adenoma removal (90 per cent success, 5 per cent major complications).

Medication

1. Drug of choice: bromocriptine (Parlodel). Start at 2.5 mg daily and then increase as tolerated over several weeks to 2.5 mg t.i.d. Contraindications include uncontrolled hypertension, sensitivity to any ergot alkaloids, and pre-eclampsia. Precautions include nausea,

orthostasis, drowsiness, lightheadedness and syncope, hypertension (rare), and seizures (rare).

2. Alternative drugs

  a. Bromocriptine is available in a long-acting form and in an intravaginal form as well.

  b. Several other new dopamine agonists (e.g., quinagolide, carbegoline) will become available in the United States in the future.

Diet

There is no special diet generally recommended for hyperprolactinemic patients.

Activity

There are no special activities or restrictions generally recommended for hyperprolactinemic patients.

Patient Education

1. Patients should be informed of treatment rationale and risks.

2. Patients with pituitary adenomas should be educated about symptoms of complications of growing pituitary adenoma (e.g., central headache, visual field loss).

Follow-Up

1. Follow-up depends on the underlying etiology. In general, check prolactin level every 6 to 12 months,

Key Treatment

- Discontinue offending medications
- Bromocriptine
- Watchful waiting

formal visual field testing yearly, and MRI every 2 to 5 years, depending on clinical course.

2. The expected course and prognosis depend on the underlying cause. Symptoms tend to recur after discontinuation of bromocriptine. Note that adenomas can grow dramatically during pregnancy.

Bibliography

Katz E, Adashi EY: Hyperprolactinemic disorders. Clin Obstet Gynecol 1990;33(3):622–639.

Molitch ME: Pathologic hyperprolactinemia. Endocrinol Metab Clin North Am 1992;21(4):877–901.

Sarapura V, Schlaff WD: Recent advances in the understanding of the pathophysiology and treatment of hyperprolactinemia. Curr Opin Obstet Gynecol 1993;5:360–367.

Swain GR: Hyperprolactinemia. *In* Dambro MR (ed): The 5-Minute Clinical Consult, 3rd ed. Philadelphia, Lea & Febiger, 1995, pp 514–515.

170 Hyperparathyroidism

S. Shekar Chakravarthi

Parathyroid hormone (PTH), secreted by the four parathyroid glands located behind the upper and lower poles of the thyroid gland, is important for maintaining calcium-phosphorus homeostasis. PTH release is stimulated by a fall in serum calcium or a rise in serum phosphate. PTH increases the calcium level by reducing urinary calcium excretion, stimulating bone resorption, and increasing the gastrointestinal absorption of calcium. It is also phosphaturic. In primary hyperparathyroidism, one or more adenomatous or hyperplastic parathyroid glands secrete excess PTH.

Etiology

1. Eighty per cent of primary hyperparathyroidism is due to a hyperfunctioning parathyroid adenoma. About 15 per cent of patients have parathyroid hyperplasia; various causes, including parathyroid malignancies or multiple parathyroid adenomas, account for the remaining few per cent.
2. Primary hyperparathyroidism occurs in a familial pattern in 10 to 15 per cent of cases. These patients may harbor multiple adenomas resulting from an autosomal dominant trait with variable penetrance. Classically, the multiple endocrine neoplasia (MEN) syndromes are divided into two major types.
   a. In MEN type I, the major associated abnormalities are adenomas of the pituitary and the pancreas.
   b. In MEN type IIA, parathyroid abnormalities may occur with medullary carcinoma of the thyroid and pheochromocytomas. In MEN type IIB, the additional findings include cutaneous neuromas and marfanoid habitus.

Symptoms

Although hyperparathyroidism is detected in asymptomatic patients by routine laboratory screening, patients may occasionally present with symptoms of hypercalcemia and kidney disease, specifically nephrolithiasis.

1. Symptoms of hyperparathyroidism are often subtle and may consist of fatigue, weakness, lethargy, and difficulty concentrating.

Key Symptoms

- General: weakness, fatigue
- Musculoskeletal: bone pain, arthralgia
- Neurologic: confusion, depression
- Gastrointestinal: nausea, vomiting, constipation, ulcers
- Genitourinary: renal colic, polyuria

2. Vague gastrointestinal complaints such as nausea, abdominal discomfort, and constipation can occur (see Chapter 171, Hypercalcemia).
3. Bone symptoms such as pain, tenderness, arthralgia, gout, pseudogout, osteoporosis, and pathologic fractures may be seen.

Clinical Findings

The physical examination in most patients with hyperparathyroidism (with the exception of MEN IIB) is unremarkable.

1. Possible findings are changes in muscle strength, altered mental status, bone tenderness, loosened teeth, and soft tissue calcification.
2. Sometimes patients with prolonged hypercalcemia have corneal calcifications, which are found on slit-lamp examination.

Key Signs

- Musculoskeletal: weakness, bony tenderness, joint effusion
- Neurologic: confusion, hyperreflexia, coma
- Gastrointestinal: tenderness, obstipation
- Cardiovascular: hypertension
- Ophthalmologic: corneal bands

Laboratory Tests

After confirming hypercalcemia, measuring the immunoreactive parathyroid hormone (iPTH) in a reliable laboratory is critical. An elevated fasting iPTH in the presence of hypercalcemia confirms hyperparathyroidism. Because an elevated calcium should suppress PTH secretion, a high-normal or mildly elevated level may indicate hyperparathyroidism in hypercalcemic patients.

1. Other biochemical abnormalities associated with hyperparathyroidism include a mild hyperchloremic acidosis and a low serum phosphorus. The chloride-to-phosphate ratio generally is greater than 33:1. Enhanced bone resorption can elevate the alkaline phosphatase level.
2. Routine radiographs are rarely helpful. Subperiosteal bone resorption of the digits and at the sternoclavicular joints may be evident. Additional findings include bone cysts, renal calcifications, pathologic fractures, and a rare "brown tumor."
3. Imaging procedures to localize the parathyroid glands are usually necessary only when hyperparathyroidism recurs and a reoperation is required. Ultrasound is

cost-effective and accurate but lacks sensitivity. Other noninvasive imaging methods include computed tomography, magnetic resonance imaging, and thallium scan.

4. In rare cases where the initial exploration was negative or hyperparathyroidism persists, arteriography and selective venous catheterization with iPTH measurements are needed to identify the parathyroid glands.

Key Tests

- Serum calcium and phosphorus
- Fasting immunoreactive parathyroid hormone (iPTH)

Differential Diagnosis

The differential diagnosis consists of other causes of hypercalcemia (see Chapter 171, Hypercalcemia). Hyperparathyroidism may be primary, secondary, or tertiary.

1. Primary hyperparathyroidism is the idiopathic, abnormally regulated secretion of PTH by the parathyroid gland(s). It is two to four times more common in women and increases in incidence over age 50.

2. Secondary hyperparathyroidism results from disease in another organ system, usually the kidneys. Renal failure is associated with a high phosphate and a low calcium and stimulates parathyroid hyperplasia.

3. Tertiary hyperparathyroidism occurs in renal failure, when PTH secretion becomes independent of the serum calcium.

4. Familial hypocalciuric hypercalcemia may be confused with primary hyperparathyroidism. Although PTH levels usually are normal, a limited number of patients show mild elevations, but the urinary calcium is extremely low.

Treatment

Management of primary hyperparathyroidism can be surgical or medical. In general, the higher the serum calcium level, the more likely patients will develop symptoms requiring surgical interventions.

1. Although surgery is curative, mild and uncomplicated asymptomatic cases of primary hyperparathyroidism may be followed medically. These patients should have a serum calcium less than 11.5 mg/dl and must be compliant with regular follow-up visits. Bone den-

sity should be normal, and there must be no evidence of renal insufficiency. Medical management also may be considered when contraindications to surgery exist and in some very frail elderly patients. Patients need semiannual checkups to follow blood pressure, serum calcium concentration, and bone mass. Patients should avoid dehydration, immobilization, and thiazide diuretics. Hypertension should be treated aggressively. Some clinicians use estrogen therapy for postmenopausal women.

2. Surgery is the treatment of choice. Exploration requires identification of all parathyroid glands. Single or multiple adenomas are removed. In four-gland hyperplasia, three glands are removed, and portions of the fourth are implanted in the forearm. An experienced surgeon is highly desirable, since the normal glands are very small and may be aberrant in location. The initial surgical success rate is about 90 per cent. Complications include vocal cord paralysis, hypocalcemia, and hematoma formation.

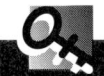
Key Treatment

- Surgery

Follow-Up

Perioperatively, patients need observation for hypocalcemia and tetany. Flare-ups of gout, pseudogout, and decreased renal function may occur. Monitoring clinical symptoms and serum calcium is essential, and some patients may require calcium and vitamin D supplementation to avoid hypocalcemia and prevent bone demineralization. In familial forms of hyperparathyroidism, family members require periodic monitoring. Genetic screening is now available for MEN syndromes.

Bibliography

Deftos LJ, Parthemore JG, Stabile BE: Management of primary hyperparathyroidism. Annu Rev Med 1993;44:19–26.

Diagnosis and management of asymptomatic primary hyperparathyroidism: Consensus development conference statement. Ann Intern Med 1991;114:593–597.

Mallette LE: Management of hyperparathyroidism in the multiple endocrine neoplasia syndromes and other familial endocrinopathies. Endocrinol Metab Clin North Am 1994;23(1):19–36.

Petti G: Hyperparathyroidism. Otolaryngol Clin North Am 1990;23(2):339–355.

Bennett JC, Plum F (eds): Cecil Textbook of Medicine, 20th ed. Philadelphia, WB Saunders, 1996.

171 Hypercalcemia

Martin S. Lipsky

Hypercalcemia is defined as a serum calcium level greater than 10.5 mg/dl. Since only the free or non–protein-bound calcium is biologically active, it is necessary to either measure the free calcium directly or estimate it based on the albumin level. To calculate the corrected calcium, add 0.8 mg/dl to the serum calcium for each 1.0 gm/dl decrease in the normal serum albumin. Malignancies and hyperparathyroidism account for over 90 per cent of hypercalcemic patients.

Symptoms

1. Frequently, hypercalcemia is mild and asymptomatic. It may first be detected by routine blood testing. A medication history is essential because many common drugs can cause hypercalcemia.

2. Asking about general symptoms suggestive of cancer, such as weight loss, anorexia, previously diagnosed cancers, or specific symptoms connected to the common cancers that cause hypercalcemia is appropriate.

3. Also important are questions about symptoms associated with an elevated calcium level, such as constipation, polyuria, confusion, abdominal pain, kidney stones, and peptic ulcers.

4. A family history of hypercalcemia raises the possibility of a familial disorder.

Key Questions

- Do symptoms suggest malignancy?
- Are symptoms of hypercalcemia present?
- Family history, diet, and medication history?

Clinical Findings

1. The presence and severity of clinical findings are related to the calcium level and its duration, the patient's age, and the rate of rise in serum calcium.

2. Many patients are asymptomatic; others can present in a coma.

3. General findings may include weight loss, cachexia, dehydration, and vomiting.

4. Mental status changes are common.

5. Pruritus, constipation, and bradycardia are sometimes attributed to hypercalcemia.

6. Sometimes physical findings, such as a breast mass, provide important clues to the cause of hypercalcemia.

Key Signs

- Abnormal mental status
- Signs of dehydration
- Palpable neck nodule/breast mass

Tests

Hypercalcemia should be confirmed with repeat testing. Frequently, the history and physical examination combined with a chemistry profile, complete blood count (CBC), and chest radiograph will suggest the cause of a patient's hypercalcemia.

1. Hypercalcemia associated with a low serum phosphate, an elevated alkaline phosphatase, an elevated serum chloride, and a low serum bicarbonate suggests hyperparathyroidism. An elevated immunoreactive parathyroid hormone level confirms most cases.

2. Generally, a history and physical examination along with studies such as a mammogram, urinalysis, stool for occult blood, serum protein electrophoresis, and in selected individuals a bone scan are adequate to exclude a neoplasm.

3. An abnormal chest film may suggest a granulomatous disease, such as sarcoidosis or an occult carcinoma.

4. An anemia, increased plasma cells on a blood smear, or an abnormal serum protein electrophoresis raises the possibility of multiple myeloma.

5. Familial hypocalciuric hypercalcemia is characterized mild hypercalcemia, an increased magnesium level, decreased urinary calcium, and a normal to low parathyroid level. Thyroid studies can rule out hyperthyroidism.

6. Electrocardiographic findings include a shortened QT interval, a prolonged PR interval and QRS complex, T-wave flattening, and varying degrees of atrioventricular block.

Key Tests

- Chemistry profile
- Chest radiograph

Differential Diagnosis

1. In hospitalized patients, malignancies are the most common cause for hypercalcemia. Breast cancer and squamous cell carcinoma of the lung account for the majority of cases. Other malignancies frequently

associated with hypercalcemia include squamous cell carcinoma of the head and neck, renal cell carcinoma, lymphomas, and multiple myeloma. Most cases of malignancy-associated hypercalcemia occur in patients with previously diagnosed cancers. One important exception is multiple myeloma, which may first present with hypercalcemia.

2. In ambulatory patients, hyperparathyroidism is the most common cause of hypercalcemia (see Ch. 170, Hyperparathyroidism). Other endocrinologic disorders that can cause hypercalcemia are hyperthyroidism, adrenal insufficiency, and pheochromocytoma.

3. Medications can either cause or contribute to hypercalcemia. Examples are thiazide diuretics, which cause mild hypercalcemia, and milk-alkali syndrome, seen in patients who ingest large amounts of calcium-containing antacids. Other drugs associated with hypercalcemia include vitamin D intoxication, vitamin A, lithium, and tamoxifen.

4. Granulomatous diseases associated with hypercalcemia are sarcoidosis and less frequently tuberculosis, berylliosis, coccidioidomycosis, and leprosy.

5. Immobilized elderly patients, particularly those with Paget's disease, and children with total-body casts can exhibit hypercalcemia.

6. Familial hypocalciuric hypercalcemia and idiopathic hypercalcemia of infancy are rare.

Treatment

Whenever possible, the treatment of hypercalcemia should always be directed at the underlying cause (see Ch. 170, Hyperparathyroidism). Until the diagnosis is established, treatment directed at lowering the calcium level depends on the level and the presence of symptoms. Treatment goals are to increase the urinary excretion of calcium, reduce the intestinal absorption, and inhibit the bone resorption.

1. Mild hypercalcemia ($<$11.5 mg/dl) may require only careful follow-up. When possible, avoid medications that elevate calcium. Increasing fluid intake to maintain a urine output of 2500 cc/day promotes calcium diuresis and prevents dehydration. A regular exercise program and estrogen in postmenopausal women inhibit bone resorption.

2. The treatment of moderate hypercalcemia (11.5 to 12.9 mg/dl) is based on the severity of symptoms.

3. Severe hypercalcemia ($>$13.0 mg/dl) requires urgent treatment. Due to the dehydration that accompanies hypercalcemia, initial therapy with intravenous saline is indicated for volume replacement and to promote calcium diuresis. Large volumes, up to 4 to 6 L/day, may be required with careful monitoring to avoid fluid overload. Once the patient is adequately hydrated, furosemide (Lasix) in doses of 20 to 40 mg up to every 2 hours maintains the diuresis and promotes calcium excretion. Careful monitoring of fluid balance, electrolytes, calcium, magnesium, and phosphate levels is essential. Calcium levels typically fall by 1 to 3 mg/dl within 24 hours.

4. Calcitonin (Calcimar, Miacalcin) acts by inhibiting osteoclastic activity and renal tubular absorption of calcium. Some authorities recommend a test dose to avoid the possibility of an anaphylactic reaction. A typical dose is 100 units subcutaneously every 8 hours, which usually acts within 12 to 24 hours and may lower the serum calcium by 2 to 3 mg/dl. Unfortunately, patients can develop tachyphylaxis within 2 to 3 days.

5. Biphosphonates inhibit osteoclasts. Etidronate disodium (Didronel) in a dose of 7.5 mg/kg given in 250 ml of normal saline over 2 hours lowers calcium levels in 50 to 75 per cent of patients. This dosage may be repeated daily for up to 3 days. Pamidronate disodium (Aredia), a new biphosphonate, may be administered intravenously in a dose of 30 to 90 mg in 1 L of normal saline infused over 24 hours. Although it works slower than etidronate, the effect lasts 10 to 14 days. Hypocalcemia, hypomagnesemia, and hypophosphatemia are potential complications.

6. Mithramycin (Mithracin) is a cytotoxic agent that inhibits osteoclastic activity and is usually reserved for patients with hypercalcemia resulting from malignancy. A single infusion of 15 to 25 μg/kg acts within 1 to 2 days and lasts up to 7 to 10 days. After 48 hours, a repeat dose may be given if needed. Side effects include renal toxicity, liver toxicity, and thrombocytopenia, particularly with repeated doses.

7. Steroids (prednisone, 40 to 80 mg/day) may be helpful in hypercalcemia from sarcoidosis, vitamin D intoxication, and hematologic malignancies. Since long-term use has serious complications, steroids should be discontinued as soon as possible or discontinued if there is no response within 2 weeks.

8. Cancer patients with hypercalcemia have a poor prognosis and usually die within a few months. Although treating hypercalcemia does not improve survival, it usually improves the quality of life.

Key Treatment

- Mild hypercalcemia: careful follow-up

- Severe hypercalcemia: intravenous saline, then furosemide

Bibliography

Bilezikian JP: Management of hypercalcemia. J Clin Endocrinol Metab 1993;77(6):1445–1449.

Kinirons MT: Newer agents for the treatment of malignant hypercalcemia. Am J Med Sci 1993;305(6):403–406.

Mundy GR: Evaluation and treatment of hypercalcemia. Hosp Pract 1994;29(6):79–86.

Nussbaum SR: Pathophysiology and management of severe hypercalcemia. Endocrinol Metab Clin North Am 1993;22:343–362.

Bennett JC, Plum F (eds): Cecil's Textbook of Medicine, 20th ed. Philadelphia, WB Saunders, 1996, pp 1414–1418.

172 Hypocalcemia

Leland Graves, III

Etiology

1. Hypoalbuminemia is the most common cause of a low total serum calcium.

   a. In the circulation, calcium is present, bound to protein (45 per cent), in the free ionized form (45 per cent), and complexed to anions (10 per cent).

   b. Free calcium ion is the form of calcium important for the neuromuscular, enzymatic, and secretory functions of calcium. If free ionized calcium is normal, the patient does not have a hypocalcemic disorder. Free ionized calcium can be measured directly; however, many clinical laboratories do not have this capability.

   c. Total serum calcium can be corrected for hypoalbuminemia by adding 0.8 mg/dl to the serum calcium for every decrease of 1 gm/dl in serum albumin.

   d. The percentage of calcium bound to albumin varies in the critically ill patient, particularly in extremes of pH and osmolality. In these situations the correction formula may not accurately reflect ionized calcium.

2. Decreased parathyroid hormone (PTH) activity resulting from decreased PTH secretion or peripheral resistance to PTH activity will result in hypocalcemia. Normally, PTH acts to raise serum calcium by increasing calcium resorption from bone, increasing calcitriol production, and increasing renal calcium reabsorption.

   a. Hypoparathyroidism (inadequate PTH secretion by the parathyroid glands) may result following surgical removal, autoimmune destruction (isolated or associated with other hormone resistance syndromes), or irradiation. Severe hypomagnesemia and, less commonly, infiltrative and genetic disorders may also cause hypoparathyroidism.

   b. Resistance to PTH action peripherally occurs with chronic renal failure, magnesium deficiency, vitamin D deficiency, and pseudohypoparathyroidism.

3. Vitamin D deficiency may be a consequence of inadequate intake and sun exposure, malabsorption, anticonvulsant therapy, hepatobiliary disease, and rarely vitamin D–resistant states.

4. Calcium sequestration (soft tissue deposition, increased bone deposition, or chelation) is a common cause of hypocalcemia in the critically ill patient.

   a. Acute pancreatitis may cause saponification of calcium by free fatty acids.

   b. Hyperphosphatemic disorders such as chronic renal failure, rhabdomyolysis, and tumor lysis syndrome may cause the calcium/phosphorus product to exceed 60. This predisposes calcium/phosphorus complex deposition in soft tissues.

   c. Citrate, present as the anticoagulant in transfused blood, may chelate calcium, resulting in hypocalcemia in patients requiring multiple blood transfusions.

   d. Increased influx of calcium into bone may occur following surgical correction of hyperparathyroidism—"hungry bone syndrome." Osteoblastic metastasis may also result in hypocalcemia.

5. Sepsis syndrome may produce hypocalcemia; the mechanism is multifactorial.

6. Medications

   a. Anticalcemic agents used to treat Paget's disease or hypercalcemia, including bisphosphonates, calcitonin, plicamycin, and phosphate, may cause hypocalcemia.

   b. Antineoplastic agents such as doxorubicin, cytosine arabinoside, and cisplatin may cause hypocalcemia directly or by causing hypomagnesemia.

Note

Correct calcium for hypoalbuminemia

Corrected serum calcium = 0.8 (4 − serum albumin) + serum calcium

---

Symptoms

1. Neuromuscular symptoms result from neuromuscular excitability induced by hypocalcemia. Symptoms are related to the degree and the rate of drop of ionized calcium. Mild symptoms include perioral numbness and paresthesia in the extremities. Symptoms progress with muscle cramping, carpopedal spasm, tetany, and laryngospasm.

2. Central nervous system manifestations include lethargy, depression, psychosis, hyperirritability, and seizures.

Key Symptoms

- Paresthesias
- Muscle cramp, carpopedal spasm
- Tetany, laryngospasm
- Lethargy, confusion, psychosis
- Seizures
- Symptoms of heart failure, hypotension, and bradycardia

Clinical Findings

1. Signs of neuromuscular excitability resulting from hypocalcemia may be present spontaneously or may be induced with maneuvers during the physical examination.

   a. Chvostek's sign is contraction of the facial muscles produced by tapping over the facial nerve just anterior to the ear. This may be present in hypocalcemia or hypomagnesemia but is also present in 10 per cent of normal individuals.

   b. Trousseau's sign is demonstrated by inflation of the blood pressure cuff to the level of the systolic blood pressure for 3 to 5 min. In hypocalcemia, ensuing mild ischemia induces neuromuscular excitability, and carpal spasm occurs.

2. Cardiovascular manifestations result from impaired contractility, vasodilatation, and conduction abnormalities. Hypocalcemia may present with hypotension, congestive heart failure, prolonged QT interval, and arrhythmia.

3. Chronic hypocalcemic conditions may be associated with the presence of subcapsular cataracts, dry skin, brittle nails, intracranial calcification, papilledema, and parkinsonian type movement disorders.

Key Signs

• Chvostek's sign	• Hypotension
• Trousseau's sign	• Tetany
• Prolonged QT interval	• Seizure
• Congestive heart failure	

Laboratory Tests

1. Free ionized calcium should be determined. Serum albumin can be used to calculate corrected serum calcium, or ionized calcium can be measured directly.

2. Laboratory tests should assess parathyroid function, renal function, magnesium, vitamin D levels, and possible causes of sequestration.

3. Cardiovascular effects and stability should be assessed by electrocardiography (ECG), and continuous monitoring may be indicated.

Key Tests

• Albumin	• ECG
• Phosphorus	• Creatinine
• PTH	• Magnesium
• Vitamin D	

Differential Diagnosis

Hypomagnesemia may cause hypocalcemia or may produce many of the same clinical manifestations as hypocalcemia.

Treatment

1. Emergency management: Patients with symptomatic hypocalcemia should receive calcium replacement to a level at which the patient is no longer symptomatic or at risk of complications of hypocalcemia. Therapy for tetany, seizures, or cardiovascular manifestations of hypocalcemia should include

   a. Intravenous calcium gluconate 10 per cent, 10 to 20 ml (93 mg elemental calcium/10-ml vial) infused over 10 minutes

   b. In situations of persistent hypocalcemia (e.g., post-parathyroidectomy), a continuous infusion may be necessary and may be given at 10 to 15 mg/kg over 8 to 10 hours. This could be expected to raise the serum calcium by 2 to 3 mg/dl.

   c. Calcium should be monitored closely, every 4 to 6 hours. The calcium infusate should be as dilute as possible. Extravasation may cause soft tissue injury and necrosis.

WARNING

Phosphorus and bicarbonate are not compatible in the same IV line with calcium.
Patients taking digitalis should be monitored closely if intravenous calcium is required as calcium potentiates digitalis toxicity.

---

2. Management of chronic hypocalcemia: Disorders such as hypoparathyroidism causing chronic hypocalcemia require a combination of oral calcium and vitamin D supplementation.

   a. Oral calcium supplementation should be started using 1 to 3 gm elemental calcium daily in a t.i.d. dose. Calcium carbonate is the least expensive and most widely used. If calcium carbonate is not tolerated, other forms of calcium such as calcium lactate or calcium citrate are available.

   b. Vitamin D is usually required in chronic hypocalcemic disorders such as hypoparathyroidism. Vitamin D is most frequently given in the form of ergocalciferol or calcitriol.

      (1) Ergocalciferol (vitamin D_2) should be given in an initial dose of 50,000 units (1.25 mg/capsule) daily. The onset of action is two to four weeks. If toxicity (hypercalcemia) occurs, the effects of ergocalciferol may persist for two to eight weeks.

      (2) Calcitriol (1,25-$(OH)_2$ vit D) is the active form of vitamin D. The onset of action is one to

three days. If hypercalcemia occurs, the time to reverse toxicity is 3 to 10 days. Initial dosage is 0.25 to 0.5 μg daily with the usual dose range of 0.5 to 2.0 μg/day. Dosage may be increased as indicated at 2- to 4-week intervals. Ergocalciferol is the least expensive preparation; however, the onset of action and the shorter half-life in cases of toxicity make calcitriol the agent of choice in many cases.

Follow-Up

The goal of therapy is to alleviate symptoms of hypocalcemia and avoid the toxicity of hypercalcemia and hypercalciuria.

1. Serum calcium should be restored to the low normal range (8 to 8.5 mg/dl). At that time urinary calcium should be determined. If hypercalciuria (>250 mg/24 hours) is present, vitamin D dosage should be decreased.

2. If hypercalcemia develops, vitamin D and calcium should be discontinued and serum calcium monitored frequently until hypercalcemia resolves. In cases of symptomatic hypercalcemia, prednisone may be beneficial.

3. While calcium and vitamin D dosages are being adjusted, serum calcium should be monitored once or twice weekly. After maintenance dose has been reached, serum calcium and 24-hour urinary calcium should be monitored every 3 months.

 Bibliography

Aurbach GD, Marx SJ, Spiegel AM: Parathyroid hormone, calcitonin, and the calciferols. *In* Wilson JD, Foster, DW (eds): Williams Textbook of Endocrinology, 8th ed. Philadelphia, WB Saunders, 1992.

Rude RK: Magnesium metabolism and deficiency. Endocrinol Metab Clin North Am 1993;22:377–395.

Tohme JF, Bilezikian JP: Hypocalcemic emergencies. Endocrinol Metab Clin North Am 1993;22:363–375.

Zaloga GP: Hypocalcemia in critically ill patients. Crit Care Med 1992;20:251–262.

Zaloga GP, Chernow B: Hypocalcemia in critical illness. JAMA 1986;256:1924–1929.

173 Hypoglycemia

Harris C. Taylor

Etiology

1. Hypoglycemia is either *reactive* (within the first 5 hours after eating) or *fasting* (more than 5 hours after eating). Contrary to common belief, reactive hypoglycemia is infrequent. The typical office presentation of a young (often female) patient with postprandial "spells" and the self-diagnosis of hypoglycemia is infrequently confirmed by serum glucose measurement while symptomatic. These patients usually have pseudohypoglycemia, the cause of which is unclear. True postprandial hypoglycemia may be caused by
   a. Gastrointestinal surgery such as vagotomy and pyloroplasty, gastrectomy, or gastrojejunostomy
   b. Early diabetes mellitus (unusual)
   c. True idiopathic "functional" hypoglycemia (unusual)
2. Among true hypoglycemic patients, the large majority have the fasting type. The following are the causes of fasting hypoglycemia in approximate declining order of frequency in emergency room and hospitalized patients. Keep in mind that underlying malnutrition or even missed meals, together with chronic liver and/or renal disease, accentuate the hypoglycemia.
   a. Drugs
      (1) Insulin and sulfonylureas (therapeutic or factitious use)
      (2) Alcohol, with or without another drug (impairs gluconeogenesis)
      (3) Propranolol (more often in patients on hemodialysis)
      (4) Salicylates (mostly in children)
      (5) Quinine (intravenously for cerebral malaria)
      (6) Pentamidine (usually in undernourished AIDS patients)
      (7) Disopyramide (Norpace) (usually in elderly nondiabetics with liver or renal disease)
   b. Renal insufficiency
   c. Substrate deficiency
      (1) Severe malnutrition (in the United States in nursing home patients)
      (2) In pregnancy, where it is usually asymptomatic
   d. Liver disease with hepatic failure or severe heart failure; cirrhosis, especially when accompanied by sepsis
   e. Septicemia
   f. Insulinoma
      (1) May be benign or malignant
      (2) Nesidioblastosis (diffuse growth of insulin-producing cells from pancreatic ductules), usually in children
   g. Hormone deficiency
      (1) Adrenal insufficiency primary and secondary (more common in children).
      (2) Growth hormone deficiency
      (3) Thyroxine, catecholamine, and glucagon deficiency (unusual)
   h. Mesenchymal tumor, generally very large and located in the abdomen, pelvis, or thorax; also may be seen with adrenal, renal, and gastrointestinal carcinomas and hepatoma; detectable by physical examination, plain radiograph, or computed tomographic scan. Insulin-like growth factor 2 (IGF-2) may cause hypoglycemia.
   i. Glycogen storage disease (rare and begins in childhood)
   j. Systemic carnitine deficiency (rare)
   k. Artifactual hypoglycemia may be seen in leukemia if red stopper tubes are used. Employ gray stopper tubes instead.
   l. Autoimmune insulin syndrome and anti-insulin receptor antibody

Symptoms

Plasma glucose values of less than 50 mg/dl usually, but not always, produce symptoms. Fasted young healthy women may have plasma glucose levels well under 50 mg/dl without symptoms. Conversely, poorly controlled diabetics may experience symptoms of hypoglycemia with serum glucose levels of 70 mg/dl and above. Symptoms are subdivided into adrenergic and neuroglycopenic.

1. Frequent adrenergic symptoms are anxiety, tremulousness, hunger, sweating, irritability, and palpitations.
2. Frequent neuroglycopenic symptoms are headache and visual, cognitive, and behavioral (aggressive and abusive) changes. Patients may, however, manifest more severe symptoms, including hemiparesis, aphasia, coma, and convulsions.

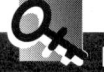 **Key Symptoms**

Adrenergic	Neuroglycopenic
• Anxiety, hunger	• Headache; behavioral, cognitive, and/or visual changes
• Sweating, palpitations	
	• Seizures, coma

Clinical Findings

1. Adrenergic signs: tachycardia, diaphoresis, hypo- and hyperthermia

668

2. Neuroglycopenic signs: seizures (more often in children), coma, aphasia, hemiparesis, and extensor plantar reflexes

Key Signs

Adrenergic	Neuroglycopenic
• Tachycardia ± PVCs	• Convulsions, aphasia
• Diaphoresis, hypothermia, or hyperthermia	• Coma, Babinski's sign

Laboratory Tests

1. Hypoglycemia may be arbitrarily defined as a laboratory (not a portable monitor) plasma or serum glucose of less than 50 mg/dl.

2. In a known diabetic who experiences hypoglycemia, clinical circumstances may suggest serum alcohol and cortisol level, liver function tests, blood urea nitrogen (BUN), and creatinine.

3. In a nondiabetic, when hypoglycemic, obtain preceding plus

   a. Total insulin with insulin antibodies and C-peptide. If insulin antibodies are present, obtain free insulin.

   b. If total (free) insulin and C-peptide are inappropriately increased for the hypoglycemia (greater than 6 microunits/ml insulin), obtain a sulfonylurea level.

   c. If total insulin is increased, no insulin antibodies are present and C-peptide is normal or low, obtain anti-insulin receptor antibodies.

4. If drugs, alcohol, liver or renal disease, malnutrition, sepsis, and previous gastrointestinal (GI) surgery are not identified as causes of hypoglycemia on first evaluation, endogenous hyperinsulinemia is more likely. If the initial hypoglycemic serum does not demonstrate inappropriately increased levels of insulin and C-peptide, perform a 72-hour fast. Occurrence of hypoglycemia with increased insulin and C-peptide levels in the absence of insulin antibodies and sulfonylureas makes the diagnosis of insulin-producing tumor. If anti-insulin antibodies are present, the auto-immune insulin syndrome or surreptitious injection of insulin must be ruled out.

Key Tests

(Initial hypoglycemic serum [preferred] or later 72-hour fast)

• Glucose, BUN, creatinine	• Insulin, C-peptide, and insulin antibodies
• Alcohol and cortisol level	• Sulfonylurea level if insulin increased
• Liver function tests	

> **WARNING**
>
> **Five-hour glucose tolerance test is rarely used to diagnose hypoglycemia. Unless insulinoma is diagnosed biochemically or there is a high suspicion of a large mesenchymal tumor, computed tomographic scanning of the pancreas and/or abdomen is not routinely indicated.**

Differential Diagnosis

1. Office patients (without past GI surgery) presenting with the self-diagnosis of hypoglycemia occurring several hours after meals usually are found to have pseudohypoglycemia. Other disorders to be considered in this setting where complaints are similar to the adrenergic symptoms of hypoglycemia are

   a. Generalized anxiety disorder

   b. Panic attacks

   c. Hyperventilation

   d. Pheochromocytoma

2. Neuroglycopenic symptoms of hypoglycemia usually, though not always, encountered in inpatients or in the emergency room. Consider

   a. Seizure disorder

   b. Psychosis

   c. Drug or alcohol intoxication

   d. Transient ischemic attack or cerebrovascular accident

   e. Multiple causes of coma

Treatment

Therapy of hypoglycemia is divided into the acute phase (where treatment is the same independent of cause) and chronic phase (where therapy does depend on the underlying cause).

1. Acute therapy: 6 to 12 ounces of juice or nondiet soda if the patient is responsive. If unresponsive, give 50 cc of 50% glucose intravenously, followed by continuous drip of 10% to 20% D/W until the patient is able to eat. Remember, any cause of hypoglycemia may produce prolonged and/or recurrent depression of the serum glucose level, and continued intravenous therapy and/or repeat boluses of 50% glucose may be required.

2. After treatment of the acute episode and availability of diagnostic tests, the underlying disorder can be treated.

   a. Patients with pseudohypoglycemia often do well on a six-feeding high-protein, low-carbohydrate diet.

   b. Alcohol must be discontinued if implicated.

   c. Sulfonylurea doses should be decreased and/or discontinued and/or metformin (Glucophage) or shorter-acting glipizide (Glucotrol) substituted for longer-acting glyburide (Micronase) and chlorpropamide (Diabinese).

d. Decrease and adjust insulin doses; adjust diet; accept poorer control in diabetics with neuroglycopenia.

e. If other drugs at fault, consider substitutes.

f. Patients with renal failure not on dialysis require increased amounts of carbohydrate in their diet and/or more frequent feedings; those on dialysis may benefit from a decrease in the dialysis glucose concentration.

g. Patients with severe hepatic failure require continuous intravenous glucose administration until recovery has begun.

h. Malnutrition requires implementation of adequate nourishment; nasogastric tube feeding or percutaneous enteral gastrostomy tube may be necessary.

i. Cortisol replacement for adrenal insufficiency

j. Insulinomas and mesenchymal tumors require endocrine consultation and expert surgical resection. Nonoperable insulinomas can be managed with diazoxide and thiazide.

Follow-Up

Observe for recurrence of original symptoms. If present, obtain serum glucose.

Key Treatment

Drug of Choice

• Glucose

Alternative Drug

• Fructose

Other Treatment

• D/C or change doses of offending drugs

• Diet for pseudohypoglycemia, malnutrition, or renal failure

• Surgery for insulinoma or large mesenchymal tumor

Bibliography

Comi RJ: Approach to acute hypoglycemia. Endocrinol Metab Clin North Am, 1993;22:247–262.

Field JB (ed): Hypoglycemia. Endocrinol Metab Clin North Am 1989;18:1–252.

Marks V, Teale JD: Hypoglycemia in the adult. *In* Gregory JW, Aynsley-Green A (eds): Bailliere's Clinical Endocrinology and Metabolism, vol 7. London, Bailliere Tindall, 1993, pp 705–730.

Palardy J, Havrankova J, Leparge R, et al: Blood glucose measurements during symptomatic episodes in patients with suspected post prandial hypoglycemia. N Engl J Med 1989; 321:1421–1425.

Service FJ: Hypoglycemias. J Clin Endocrinol Metab 1993; 76:269–272.

174 Hyperkalemia

John P. Speck

1. Hyperkalemia is often encountered in patients with disturbed renal function, among those taking medications that alter potassium homeostasis, and in those subjected to a massive influx of potassium. Hyperkalemia is often multifactorial, and its incidence increases with aging.

2. The kidneys play a pivotal role in potassium homeostasis. However, it takes hours for the kidneys to change urinary potassium excretion. The body's acute defense against rises in the serum potassium consists of insulin and probably catecholamine release. In response to acute rises in the plasma potassium, insulin is released, which then drives potassium as well as glucose into cells. Diabetics are at increased risk of developing hyperkalemia due to their impaired insulin release. Another probable defense mechanism against hyperkalemia involves the acute release of catecholamines. The overall effect of released norepinephrine and epinephrine is to relocate plasma potassium intracellularly.

3. In a slower but powerful way, the kidneys protect against hyperkalemia. Potassium is freely filtered by the glomerulus into the tubular fluid. In a complex manner, it is then completely reabsorbed, with the potassium appearing in the urine, having been actively secreted by the collecting tubule under the influence of aldosterone. The kidneys have a remarkable ability to vary potassium excretion into the urine from less than 5 mEq/L to 100 mEq/L. Factors that favor potassium excretion include increased plasma aldosterone, increased tubular sodium flow, diuretics, and bicarbonate appearing in the urine.

Etiology

Table 174–1 summarizes the causes of hyperkalemia.

1. Pseudohyperkalemia: This is a fairly frequent occurrence and results from

   a. Excessively long tourniquet application before phlebotomy, causing potassium egress from muscle cells distal to the tourniquet

   b. Hemolysis, during or after phlebotomy: For hemolysis to raise serum potassium more than 0.5 mEq/L above the baseline, gross hemolysis should be evident to the naked eye.

   c. Thrombocytosis and/or leukocytosis: If the platelet count is more than 1 million or the white cell count is over 100,000, the normal process of clot formation and retraction causes lysis of some of the platelets or WBCs with attendant release of their rich intracellular potassium into the serum. If this condition is suspected, one should obtain a plasma potassium determination: the blood is drawn into an anticoagulated tube and spun down. Normal serum potassium is only 0.1 to 0.2 mEq/L more than plasma potassium. If the plasma potassium is normal in the face of an elevated serum potassium, the diagnosis is made and no treatment is needed.

2. Massive influx of potassium into the plasma: This can occur in several ways. There can be release of the high intracellular potassium into the plasma from tissue destruction such as hemolysis or rhabdomyolysis, or from resorption of a hematoma. Exuberant oral intake of high potassium foods (such as citrus fruits and potassium salt substitutes), and intravenous potassium supplements can cause hyperkalemia, especially if other causes of hyperkalemia are present.

3. Redistribution of potassium from within cells into the plasma: Multiple medications can cause at least mild hyperkalemia by inhibiting potassium movement into cells. These include digoxin (at toxic levels), succinylcholine, β-blockers, α-agonists, arginine, and lysine (often used in hyperalimentation). Hyperosmolar states, as from hyperglycemia, can cause hyperkalemia, probably due to intracellular flux of water into the plasma, which drags potassium with it. Normal anion gap (but not large anion gap) metabolic acidosis causes intracellular potassium to translocate into the plasma. A drop in pH of 0.1 here raises the serum potassium up to 0.6 mEq/L. Large anion gap metabolic acidosis from organic acidoses such as lactic acidosis or ketoacidosis and respiratory acidosis has little effect on the plasma potassium. A rare disorder, periodic paralysis, can cause hyper- and/or hypokalemia.

4. Inadequate renal potassium excretion

   a. Adrenal disorders such as Addison's disease and

TABLE 174–1. CAUSES OF HYPERKALEMIA

1. Pseudohyperkalemia
2. Massive potassium influx into the plasma
   Oral or intravenous potassium salts; dietary indiscretions; salt substitutes; hemolysis; rhabdomyolysis
3. Redistribution from within cells into plasma
   Medications (digoxin toxicity, succinylcholine, β-blockers, α-agonists, arginine, and lysine); hyperosmolar states; hyperkalemic periodic paralysis; normal anion gap metabolic acidosis
4. Inadequate renal potassium excretion
   Adrenal disorders (hyporenin hypoaldosteronism, Addison's disease); tubular secretory defects (systemic lupus erythematosus, obstructive uropathy, sickle cell disease, renal transplant); renal failure; medications (potassium-sparing diuretics, nonsteroidal anti-inflammatory drugs, angiotensin-converting enzyme inhibitors, cyclosporine A); diminished effective circulating plasma volume

hyporenin hypoaldosteronism (renal tubular acidosis) can cause hyperkalemia via diminished aldosterone-mediated tubular potassium secretion.

b. Hyporenin hypoaldosteronism is a fairly common cause of hyperkalemia. It occurs in middle-aged to elderly patients who have mild to moderate renal insufficiency that is not of itself severe enough to cause hyperkalemia. Half are diabetic. Glucocorticoid function is normal, and most patients have low-normal or low plasma renin and aldosterone levels. If efforts are made to stimulate plasma renin and aldosterone release (as by salt deprivation or furosemide administration), the plasma renin and aldosterone levels are definitely low. Some of these patients have normal renin studies but low aldosterone levels.

c. When renal failure has progressed to a creatinine clearance or less than 5 cc/min, renal potassium excretion is inadequate and hyperkalemia often occurs.

d. Medications such as potassium-sparing diuretics (spironolactone, triamterene, amiloride) may cause hyperkalemia. Nonsteroidal anti-inflammatory drugs, heparin, and angiotensin-converting enzyme inhibitors each may cause at least some degree of hyperkalemia by blocking aldosterone release.

e. Diminished effective plasma volume, which causes diminished sodium delivery to the distal tubule, can cause mild hyperkalemia.

Diagnosis

1. A finding of hyperkalemia should be confirmed with at least one other measurement of serum potassium, with particular attention to nontraumatic phlebotomy and proper blood handling.

2. Hyperkalemia is often multifactorial, with several mild disorders combining to cause severe hyperkalemia. An example would be the patient with mild chronic renal failure who is taking a nonsteroidal anti-inflammatory drug and a potassium salt substitute. The diagnosis of pseudohyperkalemia is outlined above. Adrenal insufficiency can be diagnosed by doing a cosyntropin stimulation test. Hyporenin hypoaldosteronism should be suspected by the finding of otherwise unexplained hyperkalemia in a middle-aged patient with mild renal failure. Baseline and stimulated plasma renin and aldosterone levels are confirmatory tests.

Symptoms and Clinical Findings

The signs and symptoms of hyperkalemia are muscle weakness and perioral paresthesias. These findings are inconsistently present and are not to be relied upon.

Key Signs and Symptoms

- Muscle weakness (inconsistently present)
- Perioral paresthesias (inconsistently present)

Tests

The life-threatening danger of hyperkalemia arises from its depolarizing effect on the myocardium. With progressive rises in the plasma potassium, there is peaking of the T waves on ECG, especially in the precordial leads (inverted T waves become shorter), prolongation of the PR interval, and loss of the P wave. The QT interval does not become prolonged. As hyperkalemia worsens, the QRS complex widens and then degenerates into a sine wave and the patient arrests. Prior to cardiac arrest, these ECG changes can be reversed within minutes or seconds by prompt efforts to stabilize the myocardium and lower the plasma potassium (Fig. 174–1).

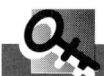
Key Test

- Electrocardiogram (ECG)

Treatment

1. If the serum potassium is less then 6.5 mEq/L and either no ECG changes are present or there is at most T wave peaking, treatment can usually consist of prompt efforts to identify and correct the cause of hyperkalemia. For example, if the patient is taking potassium salts or NSAIDs, these medications should be stopped and the serum potassium rechecked.

2. If the patient has hyperkalemia from advanced renal failure, tubular defects, or hyporenin hypoaldosteronism, loop diuretics may augment potassium excretion. Additionally, in hyporenin hypoaldosteronism, fludrocortisone (Florinef) may be used, starting at a dose of 0.1 mg daily. Loop diuretics may cause dehydration and Florinef can worsen hypertension and edema.

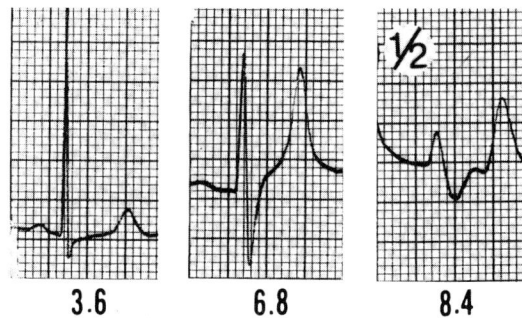

Figure 174–1 ECG changes with hyperkalemia. When serum potassium[+] is 6.8, there is prolongation of the PR and QRS intervals. When K[+] is 8.4, the P wave is difficult to identify and QRS is further widened. (From Braunwald E [ed]: Heart Disease: A Textbook of Cardiovascular Medicine, 3rd ed. Philadelphia, WB Saunders, 1984, p 236.)

A sodium-potassium exchange resin, sodium polystyrene sulfonate (Kayexalate), mixed with 1 ml 70% sorbitol per gram Kayexalate, may also be used. A starting dose of 15 gm Kayexalate orally on alternate days is reasonable.

WARNING

If serum potassium ≥8 mEq/L *or* if ECG changes beyond peaked T waves are present, emergency therapy is needed.

---

3. Emergency therapy: An intravenous line must be placed immediately with continuous ECG monitoring; 10 to 30 ml of a 10% solution of calcium gluconate should be given immediately by IV push. This does not change the plasma potassium level but transiently stabilizes myocardial cells. Calcium begins to work within minutes but lasts for only a half hour. As soon as calcium has been given, the IV line should be cleared and IV glucose and insulin and/or sodium bicarbonate should be given: 200 to 500 ml of 10% dextrose with 1 ampul of sodium bicarbonate should be infused over 30 minutes with regular insulin, 10 units intravenously or subcutaneously, given concurrently. This combination may be repeated several times. The glucose/insulin and bicarbonate both cause potassium to move from the plasma into cells. Plasma potassium begins to drop in 30 minutes. The effect lasts several hours. More long-lasting lowering can be achieved with Kayexalate, 25 to 50 gm given with sorbitol (see above), administered as an oral solution or as a one-hour retention enema. It takes hours to begin to work, and peak effect is seen at 4 hours. Hemodialysis lowers plasma potassium efficiently; peritoneal dialysis removes potassium slowly.

4. When there is suspicion of continuing influx of potassium into the plasma (from ongoing tissue necrosis), treatment of hyperkalemia must be extremely aggressive.

 Bibliography

DeFronzo RA: Hyperkalemia and hyporeninemic hypoaldosteronism. Kidney Int 1980;17:118.

Grem AS: Disorders of potassium homeostasis. Pediatr Clin North Am 1990;37:419.

Kupin WL, Narins RG: The hyperkalemia of renal failure: Pathophysiology, diagnosis, and therapy. Contrib Nephrol 1993;102:1.

McClure RJ: Treatment of hyperkalemia using intravenous and nebulized salbutamol. Arch Dis Childh 1994;70:126.

Michael MF: Hyperkalemia in the elderly. Am J Kidney Dis 1990;16:296.

175 Hypokalemia

Abbas Y. El-Khatib

Hypokalemia is a plasma potassium concentration less than 3.5 mmol/L.

Physiology

The total body content of potassium is between 2500 and 3000 mmol.

1. Most of this is intracellular (98 per cent), with a concentration of 160 mmol/L intracellularly compared to 4 mmol/L in extracellular fluid. Therefore potassium is the main intracellular cation. This potassium gradient across the cell membrane is maintained by an active transport system mediated by Na^+, K^+-stimulated ATPase in cell membranes. Although extracellular potassium is a small fraction of the total body potassium, it has a greater effect on neuromuscular function than the intracellular potassium.

2. Extracellular potassium concentration is controlled by several mechanisms (Table 175–1).

   a. Renal mechanism: Most of the filtered potassium is reabsorbed by proximal convoluted tubules and the loop of Henle. The potassium in the urine is usually secreted by the distal part of the nephron. Factors that increase secretion of potassium include

      (1) Increased urine flow to the distal part of the nephron

      (2) Increased sodium concentration in the distal part of the nephron

      (3) Increased aldosterone. This will increase secretion of potassium from the distal part of the nephron

   b. Extrarenal mechanism

      (1) Insulin: Insulin promotes influx of potassium from outside to inside the cells by stimulating Na^+,K^+-ATPase.

      (2) Catecholamines: B_2 catecholamines increase cellular uptake of potassium by stimulating Na^+,K^+-ATPase.

      (3) Aldosterone: Aldosterone also can increase secretion of potassium in the gastrointestinal tract.

      (4) Glucocorticoids: These hormones have some mineralocorticoid effect, which increases potassium secretion by the kidneys.

      (5) Acid-base balance: Acidosis tends to shift potassium out of cells causing hyperkalemia, but alkalosis favors movement from extracellular fluid into cells, which may lead to hypokalemia.

Etiology

The principal causes of hypokalemia can be categorized into

1. Renal

   a. Diuretics: the most common cause of hypokalemia

   b. Osmotic diuresis, as in diabetes mellitus

   c. Nonreabsorbable anion (e.g., bicarbonate) or penicillin, especially carbenicillin

   d. Drugs: amphotericin B and gentamicin

   e. Excessive mineralocorticoid effects

      (1) Primary hyperaldosteronism (Conn's syndrome)

      (2) Secondary hyperaldosteronism (e.g., renal artery stenosis and Bartter's syndrome)

      (3) Glucocorticoid excess (Cushing's disease, exogenous steroids, or ectopic ACTH production)

      (4) Licorice ingestion

2. Gastrointestinal

   a. Decreased dietary intake

   b. Gastrointestinal loss of potassium (e.g., vomiting, diarrhea, villous adenoma, fistula, and laxative abuse)

3. Transcellular distribution of potassium (no potassium depletion)

   a. Metabolic alkalosis

   b. Hormones: insulin and β-adrenergic agonists

   c. Familial hypokalemic periodic paralysis. This is an autosomal dominant condition with higher penetrance in males.

   d. Drugs: salbutamol, ritodrine, and theophylline

Clinical Findings

Signs and symptoms of hypokalemia are more likely to be seen with acute changes in extracellular potassium ion concentration than with chronic changes.

1. The most important feature is muscle weakness. Severe cases may lead to total paralysis or rhabdomyolysis.

2. Patients may have paralytic ileus.

TABLE 175–1. REGULATORY MECHANISMS OF POTASSIUM

1. Renal
   a. Urine flow rate
   b. Sodium concentration in distal part of nephron
   c. Aldosterone
2. Nonrenal
   a. Insulin
   b. B_2 catecholamines
   c. Aldosterone (gastrointestinal effect)
   d. Glucocorticoids
   e. Acid-base balance

---

3. Hypokalemia may cause renal tubular dysfunction with decreased concentration abilities of the kidney, which causes polyuria and polydipsia.

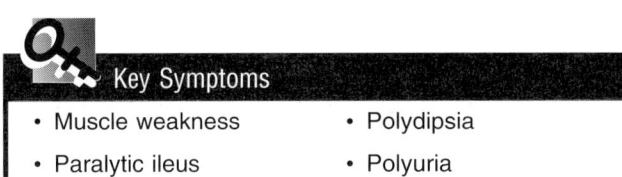

Key Symptoms

• Muscle weakness	• Polydipsia
• Paralytic ileus	• Polyuria

4. On physical examination, patient may have decreased tendon reflexes in addition to decreased motor strength. Patient may also have signs of paralytic ileus, and in severe cases, some patients may have cardiac arrhythmias.

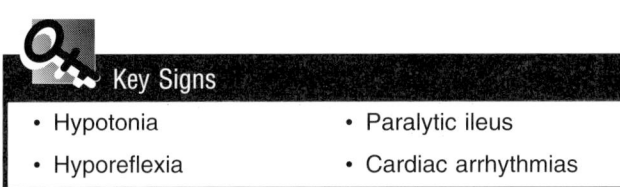

Key Signs

• Hypotonia	• Paralytic ileus
• Hyporeflexia	• Cardiac arrhythmias

Laboratory Tests

1. Serum potassium: below 3.5 mmol/L

2. Electrocardiogram: may show flattening of T wave and increased prominence of U wave. In severe cases, ventricular arrhythmias may be noted.

3. Blood sugar: may be high secondary to glucose intolerance because hypokalemia has been shown to impair insulin secretion

---

WARNING

Fatal cardiac arrhythmia may occur in patients taking digoxin, even if the hypokalemia is mild.

Differential Diagnosis

The cause of hypokalemia is usually evident from the history.

TABLE 175–2. ORAL PREPARATIONS OF POTASSIUM

PREPARATION	POTASSIUM CONTENT
K + 8	Each tablet contains 8 mEq potassium
K + 10	Each tablet contains 10 mEq potassium
K + Care 20 mEq powder	Each powder contains 20 mEq potassium
K + Care ET 25 mEq (potassium carbonate effervescent tablets)	Each tablet contains 25 mEq potassium
K-DUR 20	Each tablet contains 20 mEq potassium
K-DUR 10	Each tablet contains 10 mEq potassium
K-LOR powder packets	Each packet contains 20 mEq potassium
SLOW-K	Each tablet contains 8 mEq potassium
TEN-K	Each tablet contains 10 mEq potassium
KAOCHLOR 10% liquid	Each 15 ml contains 20 mEq potassium
KAOCHLOR S-F 10% liquid sugar free	Each 15 ml contains 20 mEq potassium
KAON-CL 10 tablet	Each tablet contains 10 mEq potassium
KAON-CL 6.7 tablet	Each tablet contains 6.7 mEq potassium
KAON-CL 20% liquid	Each 15 ml contains 40 mEq potassium
KAON-Grape elixir	Each 15 ml contains 20 mEq potassium
Klor-Con 8	Each tablet contains 8 mEq potassium
Klor-Con 10	Each tablet contains 10 mEq potassium
Klor-Con powder	Each packet contains 20 mEq potassium
Klor-Con/25 powder	Each packet contains 25 mEq potassium
Klor-Con Ef 25 mEq	Each tablet contains 25 mEq potassium
Klor Vess granules	Each packet contains 20 mEq potassium
Klor Vess tablets	Each tablet contains 20 mEq potassium
Klor Vess 10% liquid	Each 15 ml contains 20 mEq potassium
Kay CIEL	Each tablet contains 20 mEq potassium
Kay CIEL powder	Each packet contains 20 mEq potassium
Micro-K	8 mEq & 10 mEq potassium tablets
Micro-K LS	Each packet contains 20 mEq potassium
K-Lyte/cl 50 effervescent tablets	Each tablet contains 50 mEq potassium
K-Lytes effervescent tablets	Each tablet contains 25 mEq potassium
K-Lyte/cl tablets	Each tablet contains 25 mEq potassium
K-Lytes DS effervescent tablets	Each tablet contains 50 mEq potassium
Klotrix-slow release tablets	10 mEq potassium
K-Norm capsules	Each capsule contains 10 mEq potassium
K-phos M F tablets (potassium phosphate tablet)	Each tablet contains 44.5 mEq potassium and 125 mEq phosphorus
K-phos Neutral tablets	Each tablet contains 250 mEq phosphorus and 1.1 mEq potassium
K-phos No. 2 tablets	Each tablet contains 88 mEq potassium & 250 mEq phosphorus
K-phos Original	Each tablet contains 114 mEq phosphorus & 3.7 mEq potassium

1. Patients may have diarrhea or vomiting or they may be taking diuretics.
2. The presence of hypertension may be a sign of hyperaldosteronism or Cushing's syndrome.
3. Measuring urinary potassium excretion is important. If it is more than 20 mmol/L per day, the most likely cause of hypokalemia is renal in origin; however, if it is less than 20 mmol/L per day, it is usually secondary to an extrarenal cause.
4. Measurement of blood pH will help to diagnose conditions like metabolic alkalosis or renal tubular acidosis.

WARNING

Patients with hypokalemia and hypertension should be investigated for primary hyperaldosteronism (Conn's syndrome) or Cushing's syndrome.

Treatment

1. Correction of hypokalemia can be achieved by oral supplements in most cases (see Table 175–2). Potassium chloride is the preferred salt, especially in alkalotic patients.
2. Intravenous supplements may be required in patients with gastrointestinal problems who cannot take oral medications or when the potassium deficiency is severe. Concentration of potassium in intravenous solution should not exceed 40 mmol/L. The rate of infusion should not exceed 20 mmol/hr. Patients should be monitored by electrocardiogram during rapid infusion of potassium to avoid cardiac toxicity.
3. If the hypokalemia is secondary to diuretics, a potassium-sparing diuretic may be used such as triamterene, amiloride, or aldosterone antagonist (spironolactone).
4. Every attempt should be made to treat the underlying cause of hypokalemia.

 Bibliography

Brem AS: Disorder of potassium homeostasis. Pediatr Clin North Am 1990;37:419.

Brenner BM, Rector FC: The Kidney, 5th ed. Philadelphia, WB Saunders, 1995.

Krishna GG: Hypokalemia states: Current clinical issues. Semin Nephrol 1990;10:515–524.

Schrier RW, Gottschalk CW (eds): Diseases of the Kidney, 4th ed. Boston, Little, Brown, 1988.

176 Hypernatremia

Steven Thompson

Etiology

1. *Excessive free water loss* is the most significant cause of hypernatremia in adults and must be accompanied by inability to obtain or adequately replace lost water due to physical or mental limitations. Causes of free water loss include

    a. Insensible losses associated with fever

    b. Diarrhea

    c. Use of diuretics together with fluid restriction

    d. Osmotic diuresis (glucose, urea, mannitol)

    e. Diabetes insipidus

    f. Loss of renal concentrating ability due to polyuric phase of acute tubular necrosis, postobstructive uropathy, hypercalcemia, or hypokalemia

2. *Excessive sodium intake* is seen more often in infants than in adults. Causes include

    a. Incorrect reconstitution of infant formula

    b. High osmolar enteral feedings

    c. Use of $NaHCO_3$ in cardiopulmonary resuscitation

    d. Hypertonic dialysate

    e. Table salt ingestion

3. *Hypothalamic dysfunction* can lead to impaired thirst and result in hypernatremia. This condition is seen especially with congenital lesions but can occur with neoplasms, with granulomatous disease, or after trauma.

4. *Shifts of hypotonic water* from the intravascular space can occur after intensive exercise or seizures. Clinically significant hypernatremia does not occur generally.

5. *Adrenal hyperfunction* in Cushing's syndrome or primary hyperaldosteronism can cause mild hypernatremia.

Symptoms

1. Central nervous system dysfunction causes the principal symptoms seen with hypernatremia. These symptoms include

    a. Lethargy

    b. Muscle weakness

    c. Seizures in infants

    d. Coma

    e. Death

2. Thirst sensation may not be verbalized owing to decreased consciousness.

3. Symptoms are related more to the *rate* of change than to the absolute degree of change.

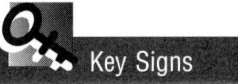

Key Symptoms

- Lethargy
- Confusion
- Muscle weakness
- Coma

Clinical Findings

1. Acute hypertonicity leads to brain shrinkage and produces more clinical effects than are seen in the chronic process. These include somnolence, coma, and even death.

2. During chronic hypernatremia, the brain adapts by increasing brain cell osmolarity via the uptake of sodium and potassium as well as the manufacture of idiopathic iso-osmoles. As a result, brain volume is restored to normal.

3. Signs of dehydration such as poor skin turgor and sunken eyes may not be recognized in elderly patients.

4. Infants often show irritability and have a high-pitched cry.

5. Intracerebral or subarachnoid bleeding can occur due to rupture of cerebral veins as a result of changes in brain volume.

6. Adults and children usually have an associated systemic disorder and may have related findings.

Key Signs

- Decreased level of consciousness
- Evidence of dehydration including weight loss, hypotension, tachycardia

Laboratory Tests

1. Plasma electrolytes need to be monitored frequently to assess response to therapy. The etiology of the hypernatremia will often be evident from the clinical setting.

2. Most patients have an underlying systemic disease such as infection or stroke, and appropriate tests should be done to address these problems.

3. The estimated water deficit should be calculated using the measured serum sodium concentration and the patient's weight. This calculation will be used as a guide for initial therapy.

    a. Water deficit = total body water $\times$ (measured $[Na^+]/140 - 1$)

677

b. Total body water = 0.6 × body weight in kilograms

4. If a lumbar puncture is performed, an elevated CSF protein will be present without a pleocytosis.

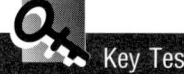

Key Test

- Serum sodium

Differential Diagnosis

1. Hypernatremia should be considered in the differential diagnosis of patients with altered mental status.

2. Because an associated illness is often present which contributed to the development of hypernatremia, the etiology of the hypernatremia and related medical conditions present should be identified. These related conditions include

   a. Renal insufficiency
   b. Dementia
   c. Ischemic heart disease
   d. Pneumonia
   e. Sepsis
   f. Cardiac dysrhythmia
   g. Anemia
   h. Hypertension
   i. Congestive heart failure
   j. Stroke

Treatment

1. The desired rate of correction of hypernatremia is no more than 0.5 mEq/L reduction per hour.

2. Calculation of the "water deficit" should be used to guide treatment.

3. The fluid volume to be delivered (the water deficit) should be administered over the necessary time period to meet the 0.5 mEq/L/hr goal. This time period is calculated by dividing the difference between measured and desired serum [Na$^+$] by 0.5.

Example

A 70-year-old woman, a nursing home resident, is found to have serum [Na$^+$] 168 mEq/L while being evaluated for altered mental status. She weighs 60 kg. The calculated water deficit is $(0.6 \times 60) \times (168/140 - 1) = 7.2$ liters water deficit. The desired reduction in [Na$^+$], 168 to 140, is 28 mEq/L. At a rate of correction of 0.5 mEq/L/hr, the correction should occur over 56 hours (28/0.5); 7.2 liters free water delivered over 56 hours would equal 130 ml/hr D$_5$W.

---

4. Ideally, if the patient is awake, replacement of the fluid deficit can be done orally. Typically, these patients have decreased alertness and need IV fluid therapy.

5. If the patient is hypotensive and tachycardic, normal saline or other isotonic fluid may be used initially. When the patient is hemodynamically stable, hypotonic fluids such as D$_5$W or half normal saline should be used. Remember that the presence of sodium or potassium in the IV fluids decreases the amount of free water delivered.

6. Frequent electrolyte measurements are necessary to determine the response to therapy.

7. Seizures can occur with over-rapid correction of hypernatremia.

Key Treatment

- Water replacement
- If conscious, give water by mouth
- If hypotensive and tachycardic, give isotonic fluids (normal saline, lactated ringers)
- If hemodynamically stable, give hypotonic fluids (D$_5$W, half normal saline)

Follow-Up

1. If underlying conditions that led to the development of hypernatremia have been identified, these conditions should be treated together with the hypernatremia. Mortality is high and is often related to the underlying problems.

2. Survivors often show neurologic sequelae.

3. When the hypernatremia has developed secondary to inability to obtain water, the factors that prevented access should be identified and corrected. In nursing home patients, hypernatremia may suggest neglect.

 ## Bibliography

Alvis R, Geheb M, Cox M: Hypo- and hyperosmolar states: Diagnostic approaches. *In* Arieff AI, DeFronzo RA (eds): Fluid, Electrolyte, and Acid-Base Disorders. New York, Churchill Livingstone, 1985, vol 1, pp 200–207 and vol 2, pp 1007–1014.

Gullans SR, Verbalis JG: Control of brain volume during hyperosmolar and hypoosmolar conditions. Ann Rev Med 1993; 44:289–301.

Oh MS, Carroll HJ: Disorders of sodium metabolism: Hypernatremia and hyponatremia. Crit Care Med 1992;20(1):94–103.

Ross EJ, Christie SBM: Hypernatremia. Medicine 1969;43:441–473.

Snyder NA, Feigel DW, Arieff AI: Hypernatremia in elderly patients. Ann Intern Med 1987;107:309–319.

177 Hyponatremia

Steven Thompson

Etiology

1. The causes of hyponatremia with hypotonicity can be broken into three clinical states—volume depletion, normal extracellular fluid volume, and edema-forming states. Identification of the etiology should be the initial step in evaluation of hyponatremia.

2. Hyponatremia seen in *edema-forming states* occurs despite an excessive body sodium content. In these conditions, although the extracellular fluid volume is increased, a decreased effective arterial blood volume leads to sodium and water retention by the kidney. Diseases in this category include
   a. Congestive heart failure (CHF)
   b. Nephrotic syndrome
   c. Hepatic cirrhosis
   d. Acute or chronic renal failure

3. Hyponatremia associated with *volume depletion* is seen with either renal or extrarenal salt loss, which is followed by replacement with hypotonic fluid. Volume depletion in this setting stimulates ADH release despite the presence of hypotonicity. Causes of this form of hyponatremia include
   a. Diuretic use
   b. Addison's disease
   c. Third space loss due to peritonitis and pancreatitis
   d. Salt-losing nephritis
   e. Osmotic diuresis
   f. Gastrointestinal loss from vomiting or diarrhea

4. Hyponatremia with *normal extracellular fluid volume* is seen in the following disorders
   a. Syndrome of inappropriate antidiuretic hormone (SIADH) is characterized by ongoing ADH release despite the presence of hypotonicity. Causes include
      (1) Malignancies including carcinomas of lung and pancreas, lymphoma, thymoma, and mesothelioma
      (2) Central nervous system diseases including infection, trauma, and tumors
      (3) Pulmonary disorders including tuberculosis, pneumonia, pulmonary abscess, and positive pressure ventilation
      (4) Medications including chlorpropamide, vincristine, and cyclophosphamide
   b. Postoperative hyponatremia can occur when patients receive hypotonic fluids following surgery.
   c. Severe hypothyroidism can cause hyponatremia.
   d. Primary polydipsia is seen in psychiatric patients who ingest large volumes of water at a rate faster than the kidneys can excrete.

5. Causes of hyponatremia with normo- or hypertonicity include the following
   a. *Pseudohyponatremia* is seen when hyperlipidemia or hyperproteinemia produces a falsely decreased measurement of the serum [Na+].
   b. *Hyponatremia with hypertonicity* occurs when hyperglycemia or the presence of other osmotically active solutes causes the shifting of water from the intracellular to extracellular space.

Symptoms

1. Symptoms are related to both the degree of hyponatremia and the rate at which the serum sodium concentration changed. Symptoms usually are not seen until the serum [Na+] has fallen below 125 mEq/L suddenly or even lower if the condition develops slowly.

2. Neuropsychiatric symptoms predominate
   a. Lethargy, apathy
   b. Headache
   c. Disorientation
   d. Agitation
   e. Nausea, vomiting

Key Symptoms	
• Weakness	• Disorientation
• Lethargy	• Nausea, vomiting

Clinical Findings

1. Neurologic signs are present which correlate with the degree and rapidity of development of hyponatremia.
   a. Decreased deep tendon reflexes
   b. Focal signs including weakness, hemiparesis, ataxia, and a Babinski sign
   c. Muscle twitching
   d. Grand mal seizures
   e. Cognitive impairment

2. Cheyne-Stokes respirations may be present.

3. The fluid volume status of the patient should be assessed. The patient should be categorized as normo-, hypo-, or hypervolemic.

4. Underlying illnesses should be identified and treated since the mortality associated with hyponatremia is often due to these.

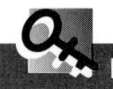

Key Signs

* Decreased level of consciousness
* Seizures

Laboratory Tests

1. Serum osmolality should be checked as the initial step to exclude the presence of pseudohyponatremia and osmotically active solutes (e.g., glucose, mannitol). If the serum osmolality is normal or increased, these conditions should be considered.
2. Once the presence of hyponatremia with hypotonicity has been established, the following tests should be ordered
   a. Serum electrolytes, glucose, blood urea nitrogen (BUN), and creatinine
   b. Urinary sodium concentration
   c. Serum and urine osmolalities
   d. Serum uric acid
3. Tests of thyroid or adrenal function should be checked if clinically indicated.

Key Tests

* Serum sodium, glucose, BUN, osmolality
* Urine sodium, osmolality

Differential Diagnosis

1. Hyponatremia should be considered in the differential diagnosis of patients who have altered mental status (Table 177–1).
2. A careful history and physical examination will establish the volume status of many hyponatremic patients and identify underlying illnesses. The presence of obvious causes of hyponatremia such as hyperglycemia, water intoxication, or postoperative hyponatremia can be quickly established.
3. When a volume contracted state is present due to extrarenal losses (such as gastrointestinal loss), the urinary [Na$^+$] is reduced (less than 10 to 15 mEq/L). Hyperuricemia is often present.

TABLE 177–1. DIFFERENTIAL DIAGNOSIS

	SERUM OSMOLALITY	URINE [NA$^+$]	URINE OSMOLALITY
Hyperglycemia	Increased		
Primary polydipsia	Decreased		Decreased
Edematous disorders			
Cirrhosis, CHF, nephrotic syndrome	Decreased	Low	Increased
Renal failure	Decreased	High	Increased
Hypovolemic states			
Renal causes	Decreased	High	Increased
Extrarenal causes	Decreased	Low	Increased
SIADH	Decreased	High	Increased

4. If the volume contracted state is due to renal salt wasting, the urinary [Na$^+$] is high (greater than 30 mEq/L). In this case, if the volume status is not apparent by examination, a trial of water restriction will be useful. Salt wasting will continue and the hyponatremia will not correct if renal salt wasting is present.
5. SIADH is characterized by hyponatremia with high urinary [Na$^+$] (greater than 30 mEq/L), high urine osmolality, normal or reduced serum creatinine, and hypouricemia. A trial of fluid restriction will produce correction of the hyponatremia and reduction of the urinary [Na$^+$] over a few days.
6. Diseases producing the edematous states are usually clinically apparent. Urinary [Na$^+$] is low (usually less than 10 to 15 mEq/L). Urine osmolality is increased.
7. If primary polydipsia is present, urine osmolality will be low (less than 100 mOsm).

Treatment

1. The first step in treating hyponatremia is to establish whether the condition requires urgent treatment. The dangers of acute severe hyponatremia are brain swelling leading to herniation and uncontrolled seizures. Unless hyponatremia is of acute onset or the patient is comatose or having seizures, the patient's treatment should be intended to produce a slower increase in the serum [Na$^+$] (less than 0.5 mEq/L/hr increase).
2. If the situation is emergent, hypertonic saline (3 or 5%) can be given. The serum [Na$^+$] should be increased at a rate of no more than 2 mEq/L per hour. The total increase should be no more than 20 mEq/L in the first 24 hours. If volume overload is a concern, IV furosemide can be given.
3. The optimal rate of correcting hyponatremia is controversial. A reasonable conclusion, however, is that rapid correction should be saved for true emergencies.
4. A recognized danger of over-rapid correction of hyponatremia is a demyelinating condition of the brain, central pontine myelinolysis. This condition is characterized by quadriplegia, impaired swallowing, and pseudobulbar signs.
5. If a hyponatremic patient is asymptomatic or the hyponatremia is subacute or chronic in onset, the initial step should be water restriction (800 to 1000 cc/day) unless the patient is volume contracted. In SIADH, if free water restriction alone is not successful, demeclocycline can be used.
6. Underlying disease processes in hyponatremia need to be addressed. In the edematous states such as CHF and cirrhosis, water and salt restriction may be necessary.
7. Postoperative hyponatremia can usually be avoided by not using hypotonic fluids in the postoperative patient.

Key Treatment

- If emergent, give hypertonic saline
- SIADH: fluid restriction, consider demeclocycline
- Edematous states: treat underlying disorder
- Hypovolemic states: give normal saline

Follow-Up

1. In treatment of acute hyponatremia, ongoing monitoring of serum electrolytes is important. These patients often need to be monitored in the intensive care unit.

2. If a treatable condition has led to the hyponatremia, management of this problem is important.

3. In conditions with chronic hyponatremia, such as SIADH, periodic ongoing monitoring of serum electrolytes should be performed.

Bibliography

For more information on hyponatremia, see
Alvis R, Geheb M, Cox M: Hypo- and hyperosmolar states: Diagnostic approaches. *In* Arieff AI, DeFronzo RA (eds): Fluid, Electrolyte, and Acid-Base Disorders. New York, Churchill Livingstone, 1985, vol 1, pp 207–214 and vol 2, pp 992–1007.
Arieff AI: Management of hyponatremia. Br Med J 1993; 307:305–308.
Berl T, Schrier RW: Disorders of water metabolism. *In* Schrier RW (ed): Renal and Electrolyte Disorders, 4th ed. Boston, Little, Brown, 1992, pp 50–71.

For more information on SIADH, see
Schwartz WB, Bennett W, Curelop S, Bartter FC: A syndrome of renal sodium loss and hyponatremia probably resulting from inappropriate secretion of antidiuretic hormone. Am J Med 1957;23:529–542.

For more information on brain damage related to hyponatremia, see
Arieff AI: Hyponatremia associated with permanent brain damage. Adv Intern Med 1987;32:325–344.

178 Fluid Balance

Diane S. Voss

1. Sodium is the principal osmotic ion in the extracellular space. Total body sodium content is determined by net salt intake and losses (mainly gastrointestinal [GI] and renal) and dictates the fluid balance of a patient. Water passively follows ions and equilibrates among all body compartments (Fig. 178–1).

2. A common mistake is an attempt to derive the fluid status of a patient from measurement of serum sodium. The serum sodium concentration indicates only the *ratio* of total body sodium (solute) to total body water (solvent); it gives no information about actual total body salt because salt and water are independently regulated.

3. Unfortunately, there is no formula to accurately estimate total body salt in the evaluation of fluid deficit or overload. The clinical assessment (physical examination and history) is the most important indicator of the fluid status of a patient.

Volume Depletion (Extracellular Volume Depletion)

Etiology

1. Vascular: acute hemorrhage
2. Skin: profuse diaphoresis, large burns, extensive dermatitis
3. Interstitial fluid shifts "third space": crush injury, pancreatitis, peritonitis, bowel obstruction, bowel necrosis, rhabdomyolysis, noncardiac pulmonary edema
4. GI: vomiting, nasogastric suction, GI fistulas, diarrhea
5. Renal:
   a. Solute diuresis: diuretics, urea, ketones, glucosuria, sodium chloride, bicarbonaturia (renal tubular acidosis), hypoaldosteronism (adrenal insufficiency, interstitial nephritis)
   b. Water diuresis: diabetes insipidus, ethanol, mannitol, postobstructive diuresis
6. Increased vascular capacitance: septic shock, autonomic dysfunction, medications

---

> **WARNING**
>
> **Rule out causes of ↓ cardiac output such as congestive heart failure, cardiac tamponade, or tension pneumothorax.**

Clinical Findings

1. Total body sodium depletion is detected clinically by history and physical examination findings of extracellular volume (ECV) contraction (Table 178–1).
2. Since true fluid depletion and poor cardiac output are treated differently, clinical differentiation is imperative. If your clinical assessment is equivocal, consider invasive hemodynamic evaluation.

Key Findings

Tachycardia, orthostatic changes, urine electrolytes, osmolality, and specific gravity are the most reliable signs of volume depletion. The sensitivity of such parameters may vary depending on the rate of fluid loss, age, and renal and cardiac function.

Differential Diagnosis

If the history and physical examination are not conclusive, the following steps may help define the etiology of volume depletion.

1. Check serial hematocrits if there is a history of trauma or bleeding.
2. Check urinary Na^+ and pH; and serum K^+ and HCO_3^- (Fig. 178–2).
3. Patients with metabolic alkalosis have obligatory sodium loss due to bicarbonaturia. High urinary sodium in this setting will be misleading in the face of nonrenal hypovolemia. Therefore, if the urinary pH exceeds

---

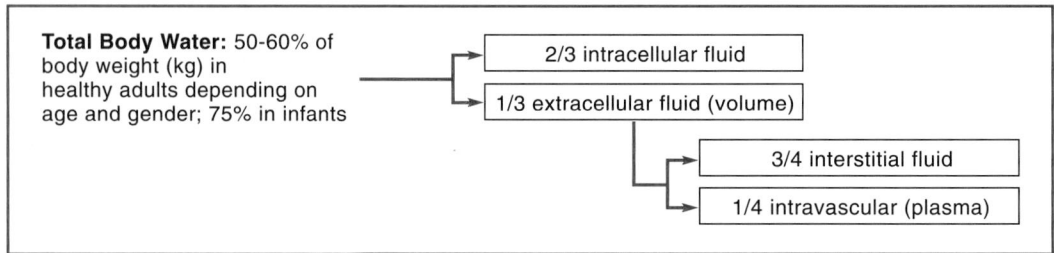

Figure 178–1 Body fluid compartments.

TABLE 178–1. CLINICAL EVALUATION AND KEY FINDINGS OF VOLUME DEPLETION

SEVERITY	KEY SYMPTOMS	KEY SIGNS	KEY LABORATORY FINDINGS
Mild (<5%) 1–2 L*	Thirst, fatigue	Dry mucosa; concentrated urine	Urine osm >500, ↑ urine sp gr Hemoconcentration (↑ HCT, ↑ protein)
Moderate (5–10%) 2–4 L*	Anorexia, nausea, cramps, cry sans tears, no axillary sweat, near-syncope	↑ Resting heart rate, ↓ urine output, ↓ weight, flat neck veins Orthostatic changes: ↑ HR >20 ↓ BP sys >20 ↓ BP dias >10 associated with symptoms	↑ BUN, BUN/Cr ratio >20, hyperuricemia, ↑ phosphate, ↑ systemic vascular resistance
Severe (>10%) 4–6 L*	Lethargy, confusion	Sunken eyes, hypotension, hypothermia	↑ Creatinine
Moribund (>20%) 8 L*	Cool extremities	Vasoconstriction, shock, coma	

*In a 70-kg person.

TABLE 178–2. ESTIMATED ELECTROLYTE LOSSES/LITER OF COMMON BODY FLUIDS AND RECOMMENDED IV FLUID REPLACEMENT

FLUID LOST	Na mEq/L	K mEq/L	Cl mEq/L	HCO3 mEq/L	RECOMMENDED REPLACEMENT
Urine	10–60	20–40	90	—	1/2 NS + 20 mEq KCl
Gastric	40–110*	10	120	—	NS
Small bowel	130	10	110	30	NS
Colon	120	30	90	50	1/2 NS + KCl + NaHCO₃‡
Skin–insensible	10	—	—	—	D₅W
Skin–active loss	20–70†	—	—	—	1/2 NS

*Low at low pH, high at high pH, †burns, extensive dermatitis, profuse sweating, ‡ each amp of NaHCO₃ has 45 mEq of Na
Abbreviations: NS = normal saline; D₅W = 5% dextrose in water.

7, you should measure the urinary Cl⁻ as in Figure 178–2 instead of urinary Na⁺. Laboratory values for Cl⁻ are the same as those for Na⁺.

4. From a clinical standpoint you can predict volume status and electrolyte loss based on the type of fluid being lost, and anticipate replacement needs (Table 178–2).

Treatment

1. Restore the intravascular volume. Give sodium (normal saline or an osmotic equivalent such as lactated Ringer's) as rapidly as possible until the patient is hemodynamically stable.

2. Administer packed red blood cells or other plasma expanders to replace blood loss.

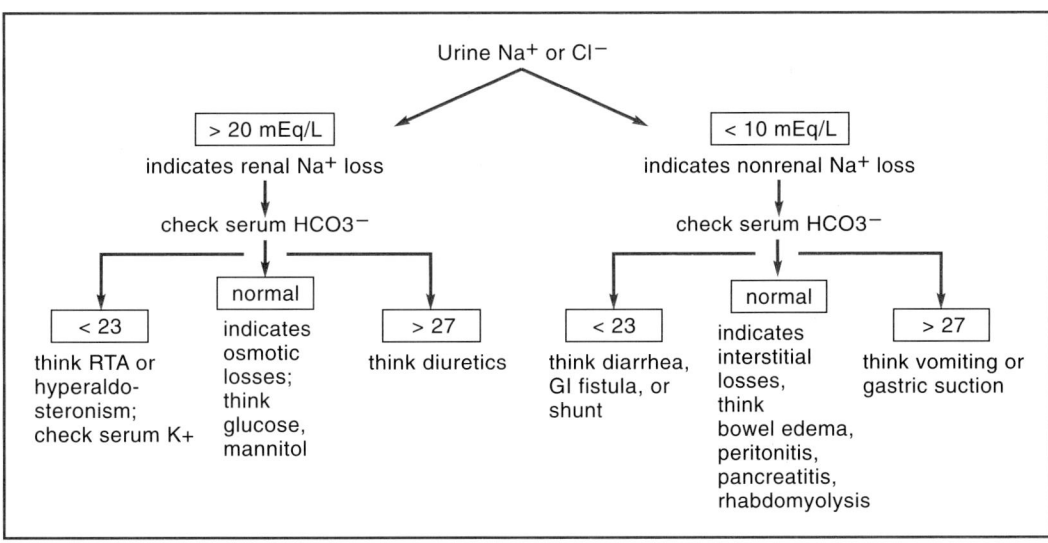

Figure 178–2 Differential diagnosis of extracellular volume depletion.

3. Stop or reverse medications that may contribute to the problem (diuretics, antihypertensives, sedatives). Remember to remove transdermal medications (clonidine and nitrate patches).

4. Reassess the volume status of the patient every one to eight hours depending on presentation, and adjust your therapeutic plan as indicated by response to therapy (vital signs, symptoms, examination and laboratory data).

5. The ratio of total body sodium and water can then be therapeutically adjusted as indicated by the type of fluid being lost and the serum sodium concentration when the patient is hemodynamically stable. Remember to monitor electrolytes and replace as anticipated and needed.

6. Mild volume depletion in the stable patient may be replaced orally with 2 to 4 L of water/day and a 10- to 20-gm Na diet, or with approximately isotonic oral fluids.

7. Evaluate and treat the underlying cause of the volume depletion when the patient is hemodynamically stable. *Volume depletion is a consequence, not a primary pathologic process.*

WARNING

The most common mistakes are
(1) Inadequate rate and volume of saline replacement
(2) Neglecting to re-evaluate the patient's status and laboratory findings frequently enough
(3) Failure to anticipate changes in fluid and electrolyte status

---

Volume (Total Body Sodium) Overload

Etiology

1. Sodium retention
   a. Renal failure: acute and chronic
   b. Hormonal: hyperaldosteronism, syndrome of inappropriate antidiuretic hormone, Cushing's syndrome (these are generally not associated with edema)

2. Decreased effective circulating volume
   a. Decreased cardiac output: acute myocardial infarction, cardiomyopathy, hypertensive emergency, cor pulmonale
   b. Cirrhosis
   c. Nephrotic syndrome

WARNING

Rule out underlying infection as a cause of decompensation.

---

3. Iatrogenic excess intake (intravascular fluid, total parenteral nutrition, medication [e.g., sodium-containing penicillins])

Clinical Findings

See Table 178–3.

Key Finding

Weight gain is the most sensitive and consistent sign of fluid overload. Weight should be obtained daily to assess the response to therapy. Edema and other clinical signs are often not evident until there is an excess of 2 to 4 L of fluid (300 to 600 mEq of sodium and its requisite free water).

Differential Diagnosis

Rule out the diagnoses of pericardial tamponade, venous lymphatic obstruction, venous thrombosis, and idiopathic lymphedema (Table 178–4).

Treatment

1. Sodium restriction (regardless of serum sodium): acutely as little as 1 gm/day. Realistically it is difficult to consume less than 2 gm/day long term.

2. Water restriction: less than 1.5 L/day (orally and intravenously combined)

3. Diuresis (*except pericardial tamponade or right ventricular infarction*): Generally, cor pulmonale can be aggressively treated with loop diuretics. Unless the patient has pulmonary edema, volume overload can be treated less aggressively (0.5 to 1 kg/day) to avoid intravascular volume depletion. In patients with ascites but no peripheral edema, the diuretic dose must be adjusted to provide a more gentle diuresis of about 0.25 kg/day. Spironolactone is the diuretic of choice because it does not need to be filtered by the kidney to exert its effect. The use of diuretics should be re-evaluated in patients with a rising creatinine level.

TABLE 178–3. CLINICAL EVALUATION AND KEY FINDINGS OF FLUID OVERLOAD

Symptoms	Signs	Laboratory Tests
Fatigue, extremity swelling, ↑ girth, exertional dyspnea, paroxysmal nocturnal dyspnea, resting dyspnea, early satiety	Tachypnea, tachycardia, crackles, S$_3$, ↑ weight, dependent edema, jugular venous distention, hepatojugular reflux, tender hepatomegaly, ascites, pleural effusion, subungual edema	Chest radiograph, BUN/creatinine, urine specific gravity, fractional excretion of Na$^+$ or Cl$^-$, hemodynamic monitoring, echocardiogram, abdominal ultrasonography

TABLE 178–4. DIFFERENTIAL DIAGNOSIS OF VOLUME OVERLOAD: KEY FINDINGS

DISEASE	KEY SYMPTOMS	KEY SIGNS	KEY LABORATORY FINDINGS
Nephrotic syndrome	Anasarca	Periorbital edema	Urine protein >3.5 gm/day $\downarrow$ S. albumin, $\uparrow$ Chol, normal BUN, creatinine
Renal failure	Nausea, vomiting; anorexia	Uremic fetor	$\uparrow\uparrow$ BUN, creatinine
Hyperaldosteronism	Few symptoms	Hypertension	$\downarrow$ Serum K^+
Cirrhosis	$\uparrow$ Abdominal girth	Spider angiomas, palmar erythema, gynecomastia, asterixis, ascites, no jugular venous distention	$\uparrow$ Bilirubin
Left ventricular failure	Dyspnea, paroxysmal nocturnal dyspnea, orthopnea	Rales, S_3, $\uparrow$ pulse and respiratory rate	Pulmonary edema on chest film, $\uparrow$ PCWP
Right ventricular failure	Dependent edema with clear lungs	Jugular venous distention, hepatojugular reflex, hepatic congestion	$\uparrow$ Central venous pressure

PCWP = pulmonary capillary wedge pressure

> **WARNING**
>
> **Avoid inducing intravascular volume depletion in the edematous patient.**

4. Discontinue drugs that may interfere with renal sodium excretion or cardiac performance, such as nonsteroidal anti-inflammatory drugs and negative inotropes.

5. Mechanical removal of fluid if indicated (paracentesis, thoracentesis, hemodialysis) may provide temporary relief for the patient and diagnostic information.

6. Treatment of pulmonary edema and the associated symptoms and hypoxia may be augmented with nitrates or morphine in the acute setting to reduce vascular pressure.

7. Bed rest, the safest diuretic, may be helpful in mobilizing fluid in the patient with decreased effective circulating volume.

8. Treat the underlying problem when the patient is hemodynamically stable. *Fluid overload is a consequence, not a primary pathologic process.* See the appropriate chapters for the evaluation of cirrhosis, chronic heart failure, and nephrosis.

Key Treatment

- Sodium restriction
- Water restriction
- Diuresis

Bibliography

Muther RS: Clinical disorders of sodium balance. *In* Muther RS, et al (eds): Manual of Nephrology. Philadelphia, BC Decker, 1990, pp 187–209.

O'Shea MH: Fluid and electrolyte management. *In* Woodley M, Whelan A (eds): Manual of Medical Therapeutics, 27th ed. Boston, Little, Brown, 1992.

Pemberton B: Treatment of Water, Electrolyte, and Acid-Base Disorders in the Surgical Patient. New York, McGraw-Hill, 1994.

179 Common Nutritional Symptoms

| Symptom | Loss of Appetite | *John B. Coombs* |

Just as the body's control of appetite is multifactorial and intertwined, so are both the internal and external factors that influence appetite. With loss of appetite, the physician's recognition of which of the basic phases of appetite are affected will assist in the efficient identification of the most likely cause. These phases include the desire to eat, hunger, satiety, prospective anticipation, and the pleasure of eating.

Loss of appetite is most often temporary and of no medical concern. Given that in most people's minds a robust appetite is closely associated with well-being, if loss persists for more than 10 to 14 days, the patient and/or the family become anxious, fearing cancer or a serious illness. An organized, efficient approach by the physician toward persistent loss of appetite avoids unnecessary testing and expense and, perhaps of greatest importance, helps to put the patient's mind at ease. The presence or absence of objective weight loss is pivotal when considering the source of loss of appetite. In the absence of weight loss, a physiologic or iatrogenic cause predominates, with a change in mood next in line. Given weight loss and loss of appetite, somatic/organic illness or more severe forms of those conditions leading to loss of appetite without weight loss factor more prominently into the differential diagnoses.

Differential Diagnosis

All the listed conditions may be seen either with or without associated weight loss.

1. *Loss of appetite most often without weight loss*
   a. Physiologic causes (those causes associated with normal fluctuations within the life cycle)
      (1) The "picky eater" of childhood
      (2) Adolescent poor eating habits
      (3) Anorexia in the elderly (decreased taste; smell, vision; decreased feeding drive)
      (4) Pregnancy
      (5) Food aversion
   b. Iatrogenic causes
      (1) Drug effect (antidepressants, smoking, excessive alcohol, chemotherapy, digoxin, nonsteroidal anti-inflammatory drugs)
      (2) Food faddism/self-imposed dietary habits
      (3) Poor attention to oral health
   c. Changes in mood
      (1) Depression/melancholia
      (2) Stress, fear, anxiety

2. *Loss of appetite most often with weight loss*
   a. Preceding conditions with more pronounced presentations
   b. Somatic illness
      (1) Cancer, malignancy
      (2) Psychiatric conditions (anorexia nervosa, severe depression, psychosis)
      (3) Gastrointestinal disturbances (chronic liver disease, lactose intolerance, esophageal dysfunction, gallstones, gastroparesis)
      (4) Diabetes mellitus
      (5) Infection, AIDS
      (6) Renal dysfunction/failure

Appetite varies in all of us at different stages of the life cycle. The physician's first consideration should be directed toward these cyclic changes. Likewise, many drugs affect taste sensation (potassium preparations, antibiotics), mouth moisture (antidepressants), suppression of appetite (antineoplastics), and sense of smell (antihistamines and bronchodilators)—all of which can change appetite.

In the presence of otherwise unexplained weight loss, somatic illness should strongly be considered. Most often, attention to a complete history (including the dietary and psychosocial components) and physical examination allows the physician to focus concern. Historical attention to the phase of appetite that is or is not affected sharpens the physician's diagnostic acumen (Table 179–1).

History: Key Questions to Ask

1. Dietary history
   a. Desire to eat?
   b. Hunger?
   c. Satiety?
   d. Prospective anticipation?
   e. Pleasure of eating?
2. Psychosocial history

TABLE 179–1. HOW VARIOUS CONDITIONS AFFECT SELECTED PHASES OF APPETITE

| | PHASE OF APPETITE | | |
CONDITION	Hunger/Desire to Eat	Satiety	Pleasure of Eating
Physiologic (elderly)	↓ or Normal	↑	↓
Depression	↓	↑	↓
Somatic illness	↓	Normal	Normal

a. Does patient live alone? eat alone?

b. Have there been recent sad events/changes in lifestyle?

c. Are there adequate resources (money, time to shop) to support good nutrition?

d. Has the patient noticed a change in sleeping habits?

3. Weight loss

a. Has the patient noticed a loss of weight?

b. If so, how has this been recognized?

c. Has this occurred before?

4. System review: A complete review of systems, especially in light of weight loss, allows the examiner to focus on specific somatic/system-specific complaints.

The length of symptoms, nature of onset, and associated changes/symptoms are crucial in directing the investigation. Likewise, in the absence of findings and persistence of symptoms, follow-up history in 4 to 6 weeks or if the patient/family notices change is important.

Clinical Findings

1. Anthropometric measurements

a. Is there weight loss? evidence of malnutrition? (The use of a body mass index nomogram or growth chart using weight and height can be helpful.)

b. Skin fold measurement may be of use in determining nutritional status.

c. Trended measurements are very useful and essential to map progress or future relative change.

2. General appearance: Sad? Anxious? Well-nourished? Well-kept? Chronically ill? Well cared for (in the case of children)?

3. Sensory dysfunction: Signs of conditions that might interfere with sensory input (taste, smell, vision) or oral health (mouth lesions, poor dentition, jaw dysfunction)

4. Focal signs on physical examination: Associated findings with specific organic disease conditions

Measuring height and weight and applying the body mass index nomogram assist in assessing nutritional status and, over time, the impact of weight loss/gain. The finding of an abdominal mass, an enlarged liver, or an abnormal psychometric screen influences the physician's concern for the presence of organic disease.

Tests

The use of tests in the absence of specific findings on history or physical examination is not recommended. As an example, less than 1 per cent of tests in children with apparent poor appetite and failure to thrive proved to be of diagnostic value when ordered without some degree of suspicion created by history or physical examination.

With persistent weight loss and no specific findings, the physician should consider

1. Complete blood count (CBC), chemistry profile (liver, renal, and thyroid function), and urinalysis

2. Chest radiograph

Management

1. Following establishment of a working diagnosis, management should be directed toward the root cause. All therapeutic management plans should include provisions for patient education, dietary alteration (if indicated), and ongoing surveillance and follow-up.

2. Physiologic cause: In the absence of weight loss, explanation alone followed by surveillance for weight loss and new symptoms/signs is recommended. Given documented weight loss or poor nutritional status, dietary change or nutritional supplementation discussed below should be followed. Often this may require the consultative expertise of a registered dietitian.

3. Somatic/organic cause: Therapy directed toward the root condition and education/nutritional intervention as outlined below in the presence of weight loss or malnutrition. If medications are causative, either change in dose, medication type, or patient education as to source followed by an ongoing trial is indicated.

Diet

1. Dry mouth: Add liquid (gravy/sauces) or butter/margarine to meals; casseroles are more acceptable.

2. Early satiety: Small, frequent meals—emphasis on a breakfast rich in calories and protein

3. Altered taste and smell: Experiment with seasonings; enhance or minimize food odors. Serve food at room temperature; eliminate offensive foods.

4. Nausea: Bland foods; eat when less nauseated; coordinate meals with an antiemetic

5. Malnutrition: Supplemental nutritional products may be required.

Patient Education

1. Explain working diagnosis (key points); allay fear by explaining what the condition is not; anticipate individual concerns.

2. Create a therapeutic alliance. Lay out a therapeutic course and approach to ongoing surveillance. "Red flags" prompting early return also should be provided to the patient and/or family.

3. At follow-up, reassess and then reinforce or adjust the outlined approach.

Obviously, treatment of a symptom such as loss of appetite relies on addressing the underlying cause. When loss of weight or malnutrition exists, good nutritional principles should be applied to remedy the identified condition. Most often, loss of appetite can be addressed by a simple adjustment of diet, good patient education, and sound, timely surveillance. When it is the harbinger of a more serious condition, loss of appetite should be managed aggressively with the assistance of a registered dietitian and the modalities of dietary adjustment, nutritional support, and ongoing evaluation so as to maintain or restore good nutritional health.

PEARLS

- Loss of appetite
  Think of:
  - Life cycle–associated change
  - Drug-related
  - Mood-related

- Loss of appetite with weight loss

- Look carefully and sequentially, if needed, for focal historical or physical clues.

- Limited laboratory image screen indicated unless associated symptom or sign directed

Bibliography

Bray GA: Body mass index: Obesity. Med J Aust 1985; 142:52–58.

DeWys W: Anorexia as a general effect of cancer. Cancer 1979; May(suppl):2013–2019.

Hill AJ, Blundell JE: Nutrients and behavior: Research strategies for the investigation of taste characteristics, food preferences, hunger sensations and eating patterns in man. J Psychiatr Res 1982/83;17(2):203–212.

Kazes M, Danion JM, Grange D, et al: The loss of appetite during depression with melancholia: A qualitative and quantitative analysis. Int Clin Psychopharmacol 1993;8:55–59.

Morley JE, Silver AJ: Anorexia in the elderly. Neurobiol Aging 1988;9:9–16.

Rabinovitz M, Pitlik S, Leifer M, et al: Unintentional weight loss. Arch Intern Med 1986;146:186–187.

Symptom | Weight Loss   *Lawrence G. Smith*

Weight loss is a common presenting complaint to primary care physicians. This complaint frequently triggers extensive medical workups in search of organic causes of the weight loss. These workups often prove unrewarding. Key to the understanding and successful management of weight loss is the fact that severe underlying organic illnesses rarely present with only weight loss.

Differential Diagnosis

1. Psychiatric conditions are the most common causes of weight loss, accounting for over 20 per cent of patients.
2. Malignancy accounts for an additional 20 per cent of patients with involuntary weight loss.
3. A gastrointestinal (GI) disease accounts for approximately 10 per cent.
4. An additional 10 per cent have a variety of disorders, such as drug reactions, endocrine problems such as hyperthyroidism and diabetes, and other severe systemic illnesses.
5. Fully 25 per cent of all patients presenting with weight loss have no cause discovered, even after an extensive evaluation.

Major Causes of Weight Loss (In Order of Frequency)

1. Psychiatric disease
2. Malignancy
3. GI disease
4. Severe systemic illness
5. Hyperthyroidism
6. Medication side affect

History

1. Essential to this evaluation is the assessment of the extent of actual weight loss. Over half of all patients complaining of weight loss to primary care physicians do not have that weight loss verified. Thus, verification of weight loss is essential before any evaluation takes place.
2. One must be certain that the patient has not engaged in voluntary weight loss and simply does not offer that as an explanation. One should look for clues, such as lack of concern over weight loss or distorted body image, that may signify a primary eating disorder such as anorexia nervosa.
3. A dietary history and assessment of appetite, as well as a careful review of systems, must be carried out, searching in detail for systemic illness, especially malignancy and GI disorders.
4. Most important, throughout the history taking the physician must be attuned to the presence of psychiatric disorders, specifically depression.
5. One key concept to remember while taking the history is that weight loss with increased appetite causes one to think of diagnoses such as hyperthyroidism, malabsorption, diabetes, and certain hypermetabolic states associated with malignancy, whereas weight loss with associated anorexia would draw one's attention toward depression and other systemic illnesses and gastrointestinal disorders that would decrease appetite. Separating weight loss early in history taking to these two broad categories is extremely helpful.
6. Questions concerning the social state of the patient and his or her ability to carry out activities of daily living must be asked. This is specifically important

with elderly patients, whose ability to purchase or prepare food may be important in the etiology of the weight loss. Weight loss due to a combination of depression and social situation is particularly common when there has been a recent change in the social support structure of the patient, such as the death or institutionalization of a spouse. These are particularly vulnerable periods when the ensuing weight loss may be the only sign that brings the patient to the attention of the health care system.

Clinical Findings

1. Physical signs of significant weight loss. Weight loss should not be considered significant unless there has been a 5 per cent loss of body weight over 6 months, without significant voluntary reduction in the caloric intake or the institution of diuretic therapy for an edematous state. Clues to significant weight loss would be changes in clothing size, general appearance of the patient, and testimony from observers, such as family members.

2. Following verification of significant weight loss, the remainder of the physical examination should focus on the presence or absence of overt psychiatric disorders, as well as severe systemic disease.

3. It is most important to note that a systemic illness rarely presents without other signs and symptoms at the time that significant weight loss exists.

Tests

There is much controversy regarding the extent of medical evaluation for weight loss. It seems clear from the medical literature that extensive evaluations, including computed tomographic scans, without specific symptoms to guide the evaluation are not fruitful. A suggested initial screen for weight loss would be

1. Complete blood count
2. SMA12
3. Urinalysis
4. Chest radiograph
5. Stool for occult blood
6. Upper GI series if upper abdominal symptoms are present
7. Thyroid testing, only if signs and symptoms are suggestive, or in elderly patients, in whom apathetic hyperthyroidism may exist

Testing directed at confirming a specific diagnosis because other clues are present in the history or physical examination should be done when appropriate. When no diagnosis is evident, long-term follow-up with appropriate evaluation, depending on subsequent pattern of illness, should be planned.

Management

1. The management of involuntary weight loss focuses on the underlying problem. If there is a primary eating disorder, referral to an appropriate specialized center needs to be made, as these conditions can become life threatening.

2. Otherwise, a focus on the presence or absence of other psychiatric conditions, underlying severe systemic disease, GI disorders, or hormonal disorders is needed.

3. Specific attempts at forced feeding without correction of the underlying problem have been universally unsuccessful.

PEARLS

- Weight loss should be verified before an extensive evaluation is performed.

- Psychiatric conditions dominate the outpatient setting.

- Systemic diseases, such as malignancy, rarely present only with weight loss.

- Extensive evaluations without the presence of signs or symptoms rarely produce a diagnosis.

 Bibliography

Chapman KM, Nelson RA: Loss of appetite: Managing unwanted weight loss in the older patient. Geriatrics 1994; 49(3):54–59.

Garfinkel PE, et al: Differential diagnosis of emotional disorders that cause weight loss. Can Med Assoc J 1983;129:939–945.

Martin KI, Sox HC, Krupp JR: Involuntary weight loss: Diagnosis and prognostic significance. Ann Intern Med 1981;95:568–574.

Rabinovitz M, et al: Unintentional weight loss: A retrospective analysis of 154 cases. Arch Intern Med 1986;146:186–187.

Thompson MP, Morris LK: Unexplained weight loss in the ambulatory elderly. J Am Geriat Soc, 1991;39:497–500.

180 Nutritional Assessment in Clinical Practice

Hilary I. Hertan

Malnutrition occurs when nutritional requirements are not met by dietary intake. This is discovered by means of a nutritional assessment, which includes clinical and dietary history, physical examination, body composition analysis, biochemical tests, and evaluation of immune competence.

Etiology

1. Dietary: frequency, types, consistency of meals; changes in diet
2. Gastrointestinal and other disease states: ulcers, malabsorption, bowel obstruction, inflammatory bowel disease, liver and pancreatic disease, malignancy, diabetes, renal failure
3. Other conditions: surgery, trauma, burns, pregnancy, lactation, infections, AIDS, neurologic disorders
4. Drugs: antibiotics, analgesics, chemotherapy
5. Socioeconomic factors: marital status, age, poverty
6. Habits: alcohol, smoking, drug abuse, food fads

Key Symptoms

- Weight loss: extent and rate are important
- Anorexia
- Nausea
- Vomiting
- Diarrhea
- Steatorrhea
- Constipation
- Dysphagia
- Early satiety
- Fatigue

Clinical Findings

1. In protein-calorie deficiency
   a. Muscle and fat wasting
   b. Edema
   c. Liver and parotid enlargement
2. In vitamin and mineral deficiency
   a. Poor dentition
   b. Glossitis
   c. Stomatitis
3. In zinc deficiency: dermatitis
4. In B_{12}, iron, and folate deficiency: pallor due to anemia

Key Signs

- Muscle and fat wasting
- Peripheral edema
- Stomatitis, glossitis

Laboratory Tests

Protein and calorie deficiency is more common than individual vitamin or mineral deficiency.

1. Body composition analysis; anthropometric measurements: estimate fat and protein stores
   a. Body weight
      (1) Body weight compared with usual weight
         (a) 85 to 95 per cent usual weight—mild malnutrition
         (b) 75 to 85 per cent usual weight—moderate malnutrition
         (c) Less than 75 per cent usual weight—severe malnutrition
      (2) Percentage of ideal body weight (IBW): based on Metropolitan Life tables (which list ideal weights for a given sex, height, and body frame)
         (a) 80 to 90 per cent IBW—mild malnutrition
         (b) 70 to 80 per cent IBW—moderate malnutrition
         (c) Less than 70 per cent IBW—severe malnutrition
   b. Fat stores: 20 per cent of body weight for a healthy male adult; measured by multiple skinfold thickness based on assumption that 50 per cent of body fat is subcutaneous
   c. Triceps skinfold (TSF): most commonly used; measured midway between acromial and olecranon processes of upper arm in millimeters. When compared with age and sex-specific standards, the following relationships between TSF percentile and nutritional status are accepted.
      (1) 35 to 45 per cent of predicted—mild malnutrition
      (2) 25 to 35 per cent of predicted—moderate malnutrition
      (3) Less than 35 per cent of predicted—severe malnutrition
   d. Muscle mass represents 4 to 6 kg of the body's 10 to 12 kg of protein. It is the main protein source in starvation and stress.
   e. Mid-arm circumference (MAC) and mid-arm muscle circumference (MAMC): estimates somatic protein mass; measured at same level as TSF in centimeters with a tape measure and compared with normal values for given sex and age. The following relationships between the percentile of MAC and MAMC and nutritional status are accepted.

(1) 35th to 45th percentile—mild malnutrition

(2) 25th to 35th percentile—moderate malnutrition

(3) Less than 25th percentile—severe malnutrition

MAMC is derived from the TSF and the MAC by the following equation

$$MAMC = MAC - (0.314 \times TSF)$$

Problems with using these parameters include interobserver variation and uneven muscle and fat distribution; these measurements are helpful in following a patient's progress over weeks to months.

2. Biochemical measurements

a. Somatic protein mass

(1) 24-hour urinary creatinine: Creatine from muscle is metabolized to creatinine, which cannot be utilized and is excreted. This is a good reflection of muscle mass.

(2) Creatinine-height index (CHI): determined by comparing patient's 24-hour creatinine excretion with expected creatinine excretion for adults of the same sex and height. Decreased CHI indicates somatic protein depletion.

(a) CHI 60 to 80 per cent predicted—moderate protein loss

(b) CHI less than 60 per cent predicted—severe protein loss

b. Visceral protein mass: measurement of circulating transport proteins synthesized in the liver; decreased in malnutrition, catabolism, and liver disease

(1) Albumin: the major protein synthesized by the liver. Decreased levels indicate decreased intake, or stress. Half-life is 18 to 20 days. Drops rapidly in catabolic states such as severe acute pancreatitis. Falsely low in overhydration and elevated in dehydration. Albumin parallels visceral protein depletion.

(a) Greater than 3.5 gm/dl—normal

(b) 2.8 to 3.5 gm/dl—mild depletion

(c) 2.1 to 2.8 gm/dl—moderate depletion

(d) Less than 2.1 gm/dl—severe depletion

(2) Transferrin: reflects acute changes in protein stores. Half-life is 8 days. Falsely elevated by iron deficiency. Transferrin is related to the total iron-binding capacity (TIBC) as follows:

$$Transferrin = 0.8 \times TIBC - 43$$

Transferrin parallels protein stores

(a) Greater than 200 mg/dl—normal

(b) 150 to 200 mg/dl—mild protein deficiency

(c) 100 to 150 mg/dl—moderate protein deficiency

(d) Less than 100 mg/dl—severe protein deficiency

3. Immune competence: Malnutrition affects cellular and humoral immunity.

a. Total lymphocyte count (TLC) = Total white blood count × % Lymphocytes

A gross assessment of immune competence, predicts postoperative sepsis. Affected by radiation, chemotherapy, drugs, infections. TLC relates to malnutrition as follows:

(1) Greater than 2000—normal

(2) Less than 2000—mild malnutrition

(3) Less than 1200—moderate malnutrition

(4) Less than 800—severe malnutrition

b. T cell function; delayed hypersensitivity: Common skin test antigens (tuberculin, *Candida*) are administered intradermally on patient's forearm. Induration greater than 5 mm at 48 hours is a positive skin test. If 0/3 skin tests is positive, patient is anergic, which is associated with increased morbidity and mortality.

In summary, anthropometric measurements and laboratory tests are readily available and provide the necessary tools to assess nutritional status. The most useful tests are body weight compared with usual weight, total lymphocyte count, and albumin level (Table 180–1).

TABLE 180–1. PARAMETERS FOR NUTRITION ASSESSMENT

Measurement	Mild	Moderate	Severe
Anthropometric			
% ideal body wt	80–90%	70–80%	<70%
% usual wt	85–95%	75–85%	<75%
TSF (percentile)	35–45%	25–35%	<25%
MAC, MAMC (percentile)	35–45%	25–35%	<25%
Biochemical			
Serum albumin	2.8–3.5 gm/dl	2.1–2.8 gm/dl	<2.1 gm/dl
Transferrin	150–200 mg/dl	100–150 mg/dl	<100 mg/dl
Total lymphocyte count	1200–2000	800–1200	<800
Creatinine-height index		60–80%	<60%

Treatment

1. *Calculate Caloric Requirements — Harris-Benedict Equation Determines Basal Energy Expenditure (BEE)* (in kilocalories/day)

    Males: $66 + (13.8 \times weight) + (5 \times height) - (6.8 \times age)$

    Females: $655 + (9.6 \times weight) + (1.8 \times height) - (4.7 \times age)$

    (Weight in kg; height in cm; age in years)
    BEE is multiplied by a stress factor and an activity factor to determine total caloric need (in Kcal/day).

    Total Caloric Need = BEE × stress factor × activity factor

    a. Stress factors

        (1) 1.3—mild stress

        (2) 1.5—trauma, sepsis

    b. Activity factors

        (1) 1.2—in bed

        (2) 1.3—ambulatory

2. Calculate protein requirements (gm/day)

    a. Wt in kg × 0.8 gm/kg—normal person

    b. Wt in kg × 1.0 gm/kg—mild to moderate stress

    c. Wt in kg × 1.5 gm/kg—severe stress

Based on these data, adequate protein and calories are administered in the form of regular food, enteral feedings, or parenteral feedings. Different preparations have different protein concentration and caloric density.

Bibliography

Bistrian BR, Blackburn GL: Assessment of protein-calorie malnutrition in the hospitalized patient. *In* Schneider HA, Anderson CE, Coursin DB (eds): Nutritional Support of Medical Practice. Harper and Row, Philadelphia, 1983, pp 128–139.

Lukakski HC: Methods for the assessment of human body composition: Traditional and new. Am J Clin Nutr 1987;46:537–556.

Mullen JL, Smith LE: Nutritional assessment and indications for nutritional support. Surg Clin North Am 1991;71(3):449–457.

Rolandelli RH, Ulrich JR: Nutritional support of the frail elderly surgical patient. Surg Clin North Am 1994;74(1):79–92.

Wright RA, Heymsfield S: Nutritional Assessment. Boston, Blackwell, 1984.

181 Obesity

Lawrence G. Smith

Etiology

1. Definition: Obesity is defined as an excess of body fat.
   a. Several methods exist for estimating total body fat. However, due to limited availability and high cost, body composition studies are seldom performed in routine clinical practice.
   b. Simple anthropometric measurements such as body mass index (calculated by dividing body weight in kilograms by square of the height in meters) and relative weight (calculated by dividing actual weight by desirable body weight) are used clinically to define and classify obesity (Table 181–1).
2. Epidemiology: An estimated 24 per cent of adult males and 27 per cent of adult nonpregnant women are overweight in the United States.
   a. Obesity is associated with various health risks (Table 181–2).
   b. Studies have shown that obesity-related medical problems including mortality correlate positively with the severity of obesity.
3. Causes: The final common pathway for weight gain requires an energy intake in excess of energy expended over a prolonged period of time.
   a. Idiopathic or essential obesity accounts for a vast majority of obese patients. Various poorly understood genetic, metabolic, cultural, social, and psychological factors are implicated in the pathogenesis of idiopathic obesity.
   b. Secondary causes of obesity are rare and may be broadly classified into three categories as follows:
      (1) Endocrine disorders such as Cushing's syndrome, hypothyroidism, hypothalamic diseases, polycystic ovary disease, and insulinoma
      (2) Genetic disorders such as Prader-Willi syndrome, Laurence-Moon-Biedl syndrome, and Alström syndrome
      (3) Drugs such as glucocorticoids, tricyclic antidepressants, phenothiazines, and cyproheptadine

Symptoms

1. Patient's main reason for seeking medical help may be other than obesity. Therefore, the history should always begin with chief complaint.
2. Common symptoms include fatigue, lack of energy, weakness, joint pain, and shortness of breath. Patients with obstructive sleep apnea secondary to obesity complain of excessive daytime sleepiness.
3. A careful history may reveal low self-esteem and underlying depression.
4. A detailed lifetime weight history including age of onset, previous attempts at losing weight, and results and complications of such therapies often provides useful information for the future therapeutic plan.

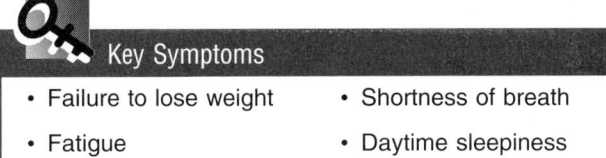

Key Symptoms	
• Failure to lose weight	• Shortness of breath
• Fatigue	• Daytime sleepiness

TABLE 181–1. CLASSIFICATION OF SEVERITY OF OBESITY

CLASS	BODY MASS INDEX	PERCENTAGE OVERWEIGHT
Mild	27–30	20–40
Moderate	30.1–35	41–100
Severe	>35	>100

TABLE 181–2. HEALTH RISKS OF OBESITY

Cardiovascular: hypertension, coronary artery disease, congestive heart failure
Pulmonary: restrictive defects, obstructive sleep apnea, obesity-hypoventilation
Endocrine and metabolic: diabetes mellitus, hyperlipidemia, gout
Gastrointestinal: cholelithiasis, fatty liver
Renal: focal and segmental glomerulopathy
Joint: osteoarthritis
Others: varicose veins, chronic venous insufficiency, increased risk of cancer

Clinical Findings

1. Examination reveals excessive adiposity, measured by body mass index. The pattern of regional fat distribution provides useful clinical information. Waist-to-hip ratio greater than 1 in men and 0.8 in women indicates upper body obesity, which places an obese individual at a significantly greater cardiovascular risk.
2. Physical examination may also disclose obesity-related health problems such as hypertension, congestive heart failure, pedal edema, varicose veins, and degenerative joint disease.
3. Proximal myopathy, easy bruising, hirsutism, purple striae, buffalo hump, supraclavicular fat pad, and central obesity should prompt a workup for Cushing's syndrome. Bradycardia, dry skin, loss of lateral eyebrows, hoarseness, myxedematous skin changes, and delayed relaxation of tendon reflexes suggest hypo-

thyroidism. Genetic causes of obesity are commonly associated with mental retardation and hypogonadism.

Key Signs

- High body mass index (>27 kg/m^2)
- Hypertension

Laboratory Tests

1. Laboratory tests are not required for establishing the diagnosis of obesity. However, before initiating a strict diet program, complete blood count, blood glucose, serum electrolytes including magnesium and calcium, uric acid, liver function tests, and fasting lipid profile should be performed. A baseline electrocardiogram with careful attention to QT$_c$ interval is also recommended.

2. Screening tests for hypothyroid state and Cushing's syndrome should be performed whenever clinically warranted. In the absence of clinical clues, an extensive workup to rule out an underlying endocrine disorder should be avoided.

3. Other laboratory tests are required for evaluating obesity-related medical problems such as coronary artery disease. Patients with suspected sleep apnea should be referred for polysomnography.

Key Tests

- Blood glucose
- Lipid profile
- Electrocardiogram

Differential Diagnosis

1. Establishing the diagnosis of obesity does not require more than a quick look and measurement of simple anthropometric parameters. It is of greater importance to identify a small subset of patients with secondary obesity for whom further laboratory testing is needed.

2. Because marked obesity may limit performance and interpretation of physical examination and diagnostic tests, an accurate assessment of obesity-related medical problems requires considerable experience.

Treatment

1. The therapy of obesity is difficult and often frustrating for both physician and patient. It is important to discuss various therapeutic options and set a reasonable goal weight before initiating the therapy.

2. It is often encouraging for the patient to know that even a modest weight loss may lead to significant improvement in the medical problems aggravated by obesity.

Medication

1. Amphetamine analogues (e.g., methamphetamine and diethylpropion) and central serotonergic drugs such as fenfluramine have modest appetite suppressant action and have been shown to produce weight loss in short-term studies.

2. Although these drugs may be used as an adjunct to therapy in selected patients, anorectic drugs have no role in the routine management of obesity due to addiction potential and a high incidence of adverse effects.

Diet

1. Dietary therapy remains the mainstay of obesity treatment. Dietary management should start with a balanced low-calorie diet (LCD) providing about 1200 kcal/day. Such a therapeutic regimen is useful for mildly obese patients and does not require close medical supervision.

2. Very low-calorie diet (VLCD) should be prescribed only for patients who are a minimum of 30 per cent overweight and have failed more conservative approaches.

   a. Commonly, commercially available powdered protein formula diets are used; they provide about 800 kcal/day, 60 to 90 gm of protein with high biological value, and 100 per cent of essential vitamins and minerals. Similar dietary goals may be achieved by protein-sparing modified fast (PSMF), in which dietary protein is provided by lean meat, fish, or fowl.

   b. A typical course of VLCD starts with a one- to four-week introductory phase in which a balanced low-calorie diet is consumed. This is followed by VLCD for the next 12 to 16 weeks. Conventional foods are gradually reintroduced over the next four to eight weeks. This is followed by a prolonged weight maintenance phase which involves healthy eating habits, behavioral modification, and exercise.

   c. Initiation of VLCD should be preceded by a detailed medical evaluation. Adequate fluid and mineral and vitamin supplementation should be ensured. The patient should be seen at least weekly, and close monitoring for electrolyte imbalance such as hypokalemia and hypomagnesemia, hyperuricemia, prolongation of QT$_c$ interval, and cardiac arrhythmia is essential.

   d. Use of VLCD is contraindicated in patients with cardiac arrhythmia, unstable angina, pregnancy, lactation, hepatic or renal insufficiency, type I diabetes, and gout.

Activity

1. Because exercise expends calories and reduces cardiovascular risk, increasing physical activity is an important aspect of obesity treatment. However, it is important to emphasize that exercise alone is not sufficient to produce sustained weight loss.

2. Studies suggest that persistent commitment and adherence to a simple exercise program are useful predictors of weight loss maintenance.

Surgery

1. Morbidly obese patients who are at least 100 lb overweight and have failed to achieve a reasonable goal weight should be evaluated for obesity surgery.

2. Currently, vertical-banded gastroplasty and gastric bypass are the two most commonly performed operations for the treatment of obesity. Intestinal bypass procedure has largely been abandoned due to the high incidence of complications.

Patient Education

1. The most important component of patient education in the treatment of obesity is behavioral therapy aimed at accomplishing two basic goals: decrease food intake and increase physical exercise.

2. Self-monitoring, record keeping, and stimulus-controlling techniques help to reduce overeating.

3. It is useful to instruct the patient regarding the actual act of eating. Advice regarding slowing the pace of eating and avoiding activities associated with excessive eating (such as watching television) are very helpful.

Key Treatment	
• Diet	• Behavioral therapy
• Exercise	• Obesity surgery

Follow-Up

1. Conservative therapy with LCD, behavioral therapy, and exercise will lead to 8 to 9 kg of weight loss in 15 to 20 weeks. Moderately obese individuals treated with VLCD may lose up to 20 kg in 12 to 16 weeks. Unfortunately, attrition is a common problem, and a majority of patients regain most of the weight over the next few years.

2. Obesity surgery gives the best long-term results in carefully selected morbidly obese patients. An impressive 40 to 60 per cent of excess weight loss with an attendant improvement in diabetes, hypertension, hyperlipidemia, and sleep apnea is encouraging. Up to 50 per cent of patients maintain a reduction of greater than 50 per cent of excess body weight over five years.

 ## Bibliography

Karl JG: Surgical treatment of obesity. Med Clin North Am 1989;73:251–264.

Pi-Sunyer FX: Medical hazards of obesity. Ann Intern Med 1993;119:655–670.

Wadden TA: The treatment of obesity: An overview. *In* Stunkard AJ, Wadden TA (eds): Obesity: Theory and Therapy. New York, Raven Press, 1993, pp 197–217.

Wadden TA, Bartlett SJ: Very low calorie diets: An overview and appraisal. *In* Wadden TA, Van Itallie TB (eds): Treatment of the Seriously Obese Patient. New York, Guilford Press, 1992, pp 44–79.

Williamson DF: Descriptive epidemiology of body weight and weight change in U.S. adults. Ann Intern Med 1993;119:646–654.

182 Malnutrition

Diana S. Dark

1. Undernutrition is widespread in the developing countries of the world. It is estimated that 400 million persons world-wide suffer from serious nutritional deficiencies. Although severe malnutrition is not widespread in the United States, it does exist. In this country, cases of severe undernutrition are the result of ignorance, extreme poverty, neglect, mental illness, or unusual environmental conditions.

2. Malnutrition is a condition in which there is an actual nutritional deficiency or potential alteration in the dietary or nutritional requirements, which may lead to an abnormality in body mass or composition. Although this definition includes both obesity and undernutrition, this chapter will focus on protein-energy malnutrition.

3. Major forms of protein-energy malnutrition (PEM) are

   a. Marasmus: deficiency primarily of energy-providing foods

   b. Kwashiorkor: characterized by protein deficiency

   c. Marasmic kwashiorkor: deficiencies of both energy and protein

4. The patient may also have a deficiency of a specific nutrient. Isolated vitamin and mineral deficiencies can occur even in the face of apparent good nutrition.

Etiology

1. Protein-energy malnutrition occurs when there is/are

   a. Insufficient energy or protein available to meet metabolic demands

   b. Increased metabolic demands due to disease

   c. Increased nutrient losses

2. Protein deficiency may also arise in the face of adequate protein intake if the dietary protein is of poor quality.

3. Protein nutrition is also influenced by the intake of energy relative to the intake of protein because the efficient utilization of dietary protein requires energy from nonprotein calories.

Symptoms

1. Body weight is the most commonly used indicator of caloric status. A decrease of more than 10 per cent of the usual body weight, particularly when the rate of loss is greater than 3 to 6 per cent per month, is a good indicator of PEM.

2. The patient may complain of listlessness, loss of energy, and fatigue.

Key Symptoms

- Weight loss

- Loss of energy and fatigue

Clinical Findings

1. Reduction in subcutaneous fat together with weight loss constitutes the most obvious and constant physical features of PEM in adults.

2. Significant reduction in fat mass can be overlooked unless quantitative criteria are assessed.

3. Decreased muscle mass can be recognized on physical examination although mild malnutrition is usually underestimated.

4. Changes in hair, skin, eyes, lips, teeth, and tongue are common.

5. Many organ systems may be affected, including the cardiovascular system, gastrointestinal system, and the nervous system, particularly if malnutrition is severe.

Key Signs

- Weight loss, evidence of pronounced wasting of subcutaneous fat

- Dry, wire-like, easily plucked hair

- Scaling skin, dependent edema, pallor

- Cheilosis, glossitis

Tests

Laboratory Tests

Biochemical tests: No single biochemical indicator is diagnostic. The combined use of several indicators provides a much better measure of status.

1. Measures of plasma protein compartment

   a. Measurement of serum albumin is usually done routinely. However, the validity of serum albumin as a reflection of the status of the visceral protein compartment is poor in the setting of acute or critical illness. The long half-life of albumin (20 days), the fact that it is distributed extensively in the extravascular as well as intravascular compartment, and the fact that its synthesis is influenced by the presence of circulating inflammatory mediators and by liver function all limit its value as a measure of nutrition.

   b. Serum proteins with shorter half-lives—such as

transferrin, prealbumin, and retinol-binding protein—are better indicators than albumin in this circumstance.

2. Measures of immune system integrity: anergy

a. Malnutrition is associated with depressed immune competence manifested by decreased lymphocyte count. Total lymphocyte count can be affected by an acute stress response or by the presence of a large wound.

b. Additionally, skin testing to common recall antigens (mumps, *Candida*) may be done, and the presence of one positive test indicates intact immunity. However, a wide variety of medical treatments and metabolic abnormalities (e.g., trauma, sepsis, malignancy, and edema) can interfere with the skin reactions.

Other Tests

1. Anthropometric measurements (body size and composition)

a. Height, weight, and skinfold thickness are measurements frequently used.

b. Skinfold thickness measurements provide information about fatness and leanness. The width of the fat layer that lies directly beneath the skin is measured in various places on the body by means of a caliper. Skinfold thickness measurements obtained are then compared with averages for persons of the same age and sex.

2. A thorough diet history can signal the possibility of malnutrition, can serve as a check on the findings of the physical examination and laboratory tests, and can provide a basis for making changes in food habits should this be necessary.

Key Tests

- Measurement of serum proteins, including serum albumin, prealbumin, and transferrin
- Measurement of total lymphocyte count or measure of delayed hypersensitivity
- Anthropometric measurements
- Diet history

Treatment

1. The etiology of malnutrition should be vigorously pursued to rule out other disease processes such as pancreatic insufficiency, malabsorption, malignancy, or AIDS. There also may be socioeconomic factors that should be discussed with the patient. In the face of terminal disease, the patient may prefer to withhold supplemental nutrition.

2. Nutritional assessment should be done to estimate the protein and energy needs of the patient.

a. Basal energy expenditure (BEE) represents the resting basal metabolic rate. It is dependent on the size of lean tissue mass and is influenced by metabolic demands, fever, ambient temperature, and activity. Although there are more than 150 formulas for estimating energy expenditure, the most widely used is the Harris-Benedict equation (see Chapter 180, Nutritional Assessment and Chapter 184, Parenteral Nutrition). Indirect calorimetry also can be used but is labor-intensive, requires expensive equipment, and may be inaccurate unless a steady state is reached. The BEE obtained is then usually increased by the addition of a stress/activity factor, depending on severity of illness and patient activity.

b. Protein needs should be estimated, depending on severity of illness. The majority of calories will be delivered by carbohydrates and fats, both of which are required for adequate nutritional support.

3. Alteration of diet or oral supplementation is always the preferable method for correcting dietary inadequacies.

4. If oral intake is inadequate, and oral supplementation not feasible, the patient may need nutritional supplementation either enterally or parenterally.

Enteral Nutrition

1. Enteral nutrition has significant advantages over parenteral nutrition. Feeding the patient with an enteral formulation is the simplest, least expensive, least invasive, and most physiologic means for supplementation.

2. Feedings can be done by way of a nasally introduced soft-bore tube into either the stomach or the small bowel.

3. For patients who will need supplementation long term, a semipermanent enteral feeding tube can be placed percutaneously using endoscopic guidance (percutaneous endoscopic gastrostomy [PEG]) or surgically (gastrostomy tube, jejunostomy tube).

4. There are a number of enteral formulations available for use. Specialty formulas are available for a number of disease states including diabetes, severe renal disease, and severe hepatic disease.

Parenteral Nutrition

Parenteral nutrition (TPN) may be delivered by either peripheral or central intravenous access.

1. Peripheral nutrition uses a lipid-based solution with lower osmolality. It is designed for short-term use ($\leq$10 days) because of potential difficulty with continued peripheral access; fluid volume required to deliver adequate calories is usually higher than with central TPN.

2. Central TPN requires central intravenous access. The solution can be concentrated if fluid restriction is necessary and can be given long term, even on an outpatient basis if semipermanent access is placed.

The solution can be tailored to the patient's specific needs and either delivered continuously or cycled to be delivered only during the night. There is a significant risk of line sepsis, particularly in a hospital setting.

Patient Education

Both the patient and the family need to be instructed as to the importance of proper nutrition.

Key Treatment

- Oral supplementation is preferred.

- If oral intake is not adequate, enteral alimentation should be used.

- Parenteral nutrition can be given either peripherally or via a central line.

Follow-Up

1. Follow-up should include determination of nitrogen balance. It is a measure of the extent of protein utilization. Daily nitrogen intake is measured and nitrogen excretion is calculated using a 24-hour urine urea nitrogen collection with additional insensible loss estimated.

2. Plasma proteins (prealbumin, albumin, transferrin) should be followed to document improvement in nutritional status and ensure adequacy of nutritional support.

3. Routine tests of hepatic and renal function should also be followed as well as other tests such as hematocrit, serum chemistries, and electrolytes in order to avert complications related to nutritional supplementation.

Patients will need long-term follow-up to ensure that nutrition remains adequate and that nutritional state continues to improve. Periodic weights and nutritional assessment are needed to prevent malnutrition from recurring or worsening.

Bibliography

Cahill GF: Starvation in man. N Engl J Med 1970;282:668–675.

Mahan LK, Arlin MT: Food, Nutrition and Diet Therapy. 8th ed. Philadelphia, WB Saunders, 1992.

Spiekerman AM: Proteins used in nutritional assessment. Clin Lab Med 1993;13:353–369.

Williams SR: Nutrition and Diet Therapy, 5th ed. St. Louis, CV Mosby, 1985, pp 327–349.

183 Anorexia and Bulimia Nervosa *Dawn M. Grinenko*

Etiology

1. Anorexia nervosa and bulimia nervosa are believed to be primarily psychiatric in origin although both have significant medical sequelae.

2. The mean age of onset for anorexia nervosa is 13.5 years with a bimodal distribution, occurring in early adolescence associated with puberty and in later adolescence associated with college. Bulimia typically occurs in later adolescence through adulthood.

3. The etiology of eating disorders is unknown but is believed to be multifactorial.

   a. Biologic: hypothalamic, opiate receptor theories

   b. Psychological: deficits in the individual's self-identity/autonomy

   c. Familial: interactions that discourage development of independence and autonomy (enmeshment, overprotectiveness, rigidity, a lack of conflict resolution)

   d. Sociocultural: societal emphasis on diet and thinness

Symptoms

1. Presenting symptoms in anorexia nervosa are nonspecific and include weight loss, amenorrhea, abdominal pain, bloating, vomiting, constipation, cold intolerance, and dizziness.

2. Common behavioral symptoms include increased exercise, obsessive behavior, and sleep disturbance. Denial is typical.

3. Bulimics usually present with more symptoms of depression and a sense of loss of control, despair, or anxiety. Common complaints include fatigue, swelling, bloating, diarrhea, polyuria, and weakness. Bulimics tend to have more insight into the possibility that they have an eating disorder.

4. Patients with anorexia nervosa may present with some bulimic behaviors, especially self-induced vomiting.

Key Symptoms

Anorexia Nervosa	Bulimia Nervosa
• Weight loss	• Bloating
• Amenorrhea	• Swelling
• Constipation	• Depression
• Cold intolerance	• Fatigue
• Hyperactivity	• Diarrhea

Clinical Findings

1. Anorexia nervosa often presents with severe weight loss with emaciation. The patients often wear baggy clothing to conceal their body habitus.

2. Other physical findings in anorexia nervosa include

   a. Bradycardia, hypotension

   b. Hypothermia

   c. Bradypnea

   d. Yellow, dry-appearing skin, increased lanugo, hair loss

   e. Edema of the lower extremities

   f. Active, restless, fidgety

3. Physical findings in bulimia nervosa include normal or slightly increased weight, parotid gland swelling, dental enamel erosion from gastric acid, and excoriation or bruising of the pharynx or the dorsum of the hand from mechanical induction of vomiting.

4. Ominous findings in either disorder include those of metabolic derangement such as

   a. Dehydration evidenced by orthostasis

   b. Hypokalemia manifested through muscle cramping or cardiac arrhythmias

   c. Metabolic acidosis or alkalosis presenting with syncope or seizures

   d. Lethargy in an anorexic heralds physiologic decompensation.

Key Signs

Anorexia Nervosa	Bulimia Nervosa
• Weight loss/cachexia	• Bruised/excoriated pharynx or fingers
• Hyperactivity	• Edema
• Scaly, yellow skin	• Dental erosions
• Hypothermia	• Parotid swelling
• Bradycardia	

Laboratory Tests

1. In general, laboratory and radiographic evaluations are more useful in excluding organic disorders and medical complications than in making the diagnosis of an eating disorder.

2. Useful laboratory tests may include

   a. Electrolytes, including phosphorus, calcium, and magnesium

   b. Urinalysis, including urine electrolytes

   c. Complete blood count

699

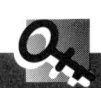

Key Laboratory Tests

Diagnostic Test	Purpose
• Electrolytes	• Exclude ↓ K, phosphorus, acidosis, alkalosis
• Urinalysis	• Evaluate diuretic use
• Thyroid function tests	• Exclude thyrotoxicosis; in anorexia ↓ T_3, ↑ rT_3, nl T_4, and TSH
• Cholesterol	• Usually normal or elevated in acute anorexia
• Carotene	• Exclude malabsorption; ↑ in anorexia
• Erythrocyte sedimentation rate	• Exclude inflammatory bowel disease; ↓ in anorexia
• Albumin, total protein	• Usually normal in anorexia
• Exercise tolerance testing	• Helpful in convincing patients of severity of disease
• Gastric emptying study	• Excludes achalasia, but often abnormal in anorexia

d. Thyroid function tests

e. Electrocardiogram

f. Cholesterol

g. Carotene

h. Erythrocyte sedimentation rate

i. Albumin, total protein, prealbumin

j. Exercise tolerance test

k. Gastric emptying study/upper gastrointestinal (GI) radiography

3. Diagnostic testing should be used prudently, as unnecessary testing may augment, encourage, or exacerbate the patient's denial.

Diagnostic Criteria

1. Anorexia nervosa

   a. Morbid fear of gaining weight

Figure 183–1 Weight criteria for anorexia nervosa (15% below ideal body weight for height).

b. Refusal to maintain minimal normal weight for age and height (Fig. 183–1)

c. Disturbance in body image with denial of seriousness of low weight

d. Amenorrhea of at least three months' duration

2. Bulimia nervosa

   a. Recurrent episodes of binge eating characterized by consuming a larger amount of food than most people would consume in a discrete time period

   b. Fear of inability to stop eating during a binge episode

   c. Recurrent inappropriate compensatory behavior (regular self-induced vomiting and laxative or diuretic use)

   d. Minimum of two binge episodes per week for 3 months

   e. Self-esteem unduly influenced by body shape and weight

Differential Diagnosis

1. GI disorders are the most frequently encountered organic disorders to consider in the differential diagnosis.

   a. Inflammatory bowel disease (regional enteritis, ulcerative colitis)

   b. Acid peptic disease

   c. Malabsorption syndromes (sprue, protein-losing enteropathy)

   d. Hepatitis

   e. Irritable bowel syndrome

2. Chronic infection with intestinal parasites, tuberculosis, Epstein-Barr virus, and human immunodeficiency virus should be considered.

3. Psychiatric disorders to consider in the diagnosis include schizophrenia and major depressive disorders. The main difference between major depression and the eating disorders is that appetite is suppressed in depression but normal or increased in eating disorders.

4. Endocrine disorders to consider include

   a. Thyrotoxicosis

   b. Insulin-dependent diabetes mellitus

   c. Addison's disease

5. Malignancy may present with weight loss, but usually the history and examination are not consistent with an eating disorder.

6. Very rare conditions to consider include

   a. Diencephalic (hypothalamic) tumors

   b. Cystic fibrosis variants

   c. Juvenile rheumatoid arthritis

   d. Systemic lupus erythematosus

Treatment

1. Establish the seriousness of the condition with the patient and the family.

2. Evaluate and replenish metabolic and nutritional deficits.

   a. In hypokalemic alkalosis, correct hypomagnesemia along with potassium supplementation.

   b. When refeeding, be aware of the possibility of hypophosphatemia.

   c. When supporting nutritional plans, the goal should be to increase the caloric intake by 200 kcal per day, with care to limit weight gain to no more than a half pound or 200 gm per day.

3. Coordinate treatment team activities. Team members should include the patient, family, primary care physician, psychiatrist, and optimally, a nutritionist, psychotherapist, and physical therapist. Behavior modification is a crucial component of treatment.

4. Criteria for acute hospitalization

   a. Severe bradycardia or dysrhythmia

   b. Hypotension or hypovolemia

   c. Marked emaciation/severe caloric restriction ($<$500 kcal/day)

   d. Hypokalemia

   e. Neurologic deficits/listlessness in anorexia

   f. Inability to gain weight with outpatient regimen

   g. Adverse home environment

5. Provide patient and family education.

Key Treatment

- Establish seriousness of condition with patient and family.

- Evaluate and replenish metabolic and nutritional deficits.

- Behavior modification is a critical component of treatment.

Follow-Up

1. Communication with treatment team members, especially psychiatric members, is crucial for both disorders.

2. The mortality rate in anorexia nervosa is 2 to 8 per cent and is attributable to starvation and suicide.

   a. 30 to 40 per cent recover

   b. 25 to 30 per cent improve

   c. 15 to 20 per cent are chronically affected and do not improve

   d. 2 to 8 per cent die

3. Frequently encountered problems in anorexics after treatment include a change to bulimic behavior patterns, irritable bowel syndrome, peptic ulcer disease, and constipation.

4. In bulimia nervosa, roughly 50 per cent may be cured through appropriate intervention. Again suicide contributes significantly to morbidity.

5. The primary care physician should remain involved in a sensitive, supportive role even if the greater part of treatment is provided by a psychiatrist.

Bibliography

Comerci G: Eating disorders in adolescents. Pediatr Ann 1992;21:707–774.

Comerci G: Medical complications of anorexia nervosa and bulimia nervosa. Med Clin North Am 1990;74:1293–1310.

McClain CJ, Humphries LL, Hill KK, Nickl NJ: Gastrointestinal and nutritional aspects of eating disorders. J Am Coll Nutrition 1993;12:466–474.

Powers PS: Anorexia nervosa: Evaluation and treatment. Compr Ther 1990;16(12):24–34.

Task Force on DSM IV, American Psychiatric Association: Diagnostic and Statistical Manual of Mental Disorders, 4th ed. Washington, DC, American Psychiatric Association, 1994, pp 539–550.

184 Parenteral Nutrition

David J. Cooper

Etiology

1. *Definition:* Malnutrition results from depletion of essential nutrients secondary to inadequate intake or abnormalities in digestion, absorption, metabolism, or excretion.

2. *Epidemiology:* It has been reported that malnutrition could be identified in 30 to 50 per cent of hospitalized patients.

3. *Risk factors:* Malnutrition can occur over long periods of time, such as chronic disease states, or suddenly, in response to stress (e.g., infection, fever, catabolic illness) or injury. This leads to depletion of the body's energy reserve and total-body proteins, so-called *protein-energy (protein-calorie) malnutrition.*

Symptoms

1. Most patients do not present with symptoms or a chief complaint except decreased energy reserve and easy fatigability. This accounts for the large number of hospitalized patients who are never diagnosed with malnutrition.

2. It is the secondary symptoms of malnutrition that alert most clinicians to its presence. Left untreated, patients develop depressed immune function, a higher likelihood of infection, and decreased wound healing.

Key Symptom

- None except for a complaint of decreased energy and fatigue

Clinical Findings

1. Weight loss is the most useful indicator of risk for malnutrition. The largest determinant of basal metabolic rate or energy reserve is lean body mass. Decreases in this body compartment lead to malnutrition and inadequate nutritional reserves to combat acute stress or injury.

   a. The most commonly accepted value is a 10 per cent weight loss from either usual body weight or "pre-illness" weight or over a short time period (3 months).

   b. If patients are more than 15 per cent below ideal body weight, they are also at risk for malnutrition with decreased lean body mass and energy stores.

2. Although not specific for malnutrition, there is a decrease in immune function with anergy to common skin antigen tests. A normal response is restored with repletion of nutrients.

3. Methods of analyzing body composition including anthropometric measurements such as triceps skin fold and mid-arm circumference have fallen from favor due to their low sensitivity, low specificity, and examiner-dependent variability. Bioimpedance devices may be more reliable.

Key Signs

Primary Signs	Secondary Signs
• 10 per cent weight loss (most reliable)	• Infection
	• Depressed immunity
• 15 per cent below ideal body weight	• Decreased wound healing

Laboratory Tests

1. The most useful indicator for malnutrition is serum albumin, because it reflects hepatic protein synthesis and the body's protein stores.

   a. The serum albumin level, however, can be falsely lower in fluid overload states and in sepsis due to redistribution of serum proteins.

   b. In addition, the half-life of albumin is approximately 2 weeks; therefore, levels obtained on hospitalization may reflect protein stores from 2 weeks before.

2. Prealbumin or transferrin have shorter half-lives; however, they are more expensive to follow and can rise as acute-phase reactants.

3. Decreased nutrient intake leads to a selective lymphopenia and ultimately to anemia.

4. Other tests available but used less frequently are 24-hour urinary creatinine determination with calculation of the creatinine/height index (CHI), 24-hour urine for nitrogen balance, and total-body nitrogen isotope studies.

Key Tests

- Serum albumin (most useful)
- Lymphocyte count and CBC
- Anergy to common skin antigens

Differential Diagnosis

A previously healthy individual can show signs of nutritional deficits with semistarvation or reduced caloric intake after 2 weeks. During the first 48 to 72 hours of starvation, an individual with normal reserves suffers only water and glycogen losses. This normal response to decreased nutrient intake should be distinguished from that of the hospitalized patient, who may be catabolic secondary to disease or nutritional stresses that require nutritional support.

WARNING

After 7 days of minimal or no nutrient intake, almost all hospitalized patients require nutritional support—sooner if they are nutritionally stressed with fever, infection, or catabolic disease or elderly with reduced lean body mass.

Treatment

1. Total parenteral nutrition (TPN) is widely prescribed in the hospital setting and even in the home. As much care and deliberation should go into deciding and prescribing TPN as for other interventions such as dialysis or chemotherapy.

2. Only patients with either a nonfunctioning (e.g., malabsorption) or inaccessible (e.g., esophageal carcinoma, coagulopathy) gastrointestinal tract in whom use of a feeding tube is not possible should be considered for TPN.

   a. If the patient meets the definition of protein-energy malnutrition, is a candidate for TPN, and requires nutritional support secondary to nutritional stress, then the patient's daily caloric needs must be calculated and nutrients prescribed.

   b. Calculating daily caloric needs

      (1) **Method One:** Calculate patient's basal energy expenditure (BEE) using the Harris-Benedict equation, which takes into account height (H, in cm), weight (W, in kg), age (A, in years), and sex:

      Women: BEE = 655.10 + 9.56W
      $$+ 1.85H - 4.68A$$
      Men: BEE = 66.47 + 13.75W + 5.00H
      $$- 6.76A$$

      Then multiply BEE times a stress factor (0.85 for mild starvation to 1.55 for severe infection or trauma) times an activity factor (1.25 if patient is ambulatory or 1.0 if paralyzed or on a ventilator). Result will be in kilocalories (kcal).

      (2) **Method Two:** "Rough rule of thumb." Multiply 30 kcal times the patient's weight in kilograms (try to use ideal body weight or average of actual and ideal if large discrepancy). This will deliver sufficient calories in 90 per cent of hospitalized patients and possibly overfeed 10 per cent.

3. TPN prescription: After the daily caloric requirements are determined by either method one or method two, individual nutrients are prescribed as follows:

   a. Protein requirements: 0.8 to 1.0 gm/kg per day in normal adults and 1.5 gm/kg if nutritionally stressed.

   b. Carbohydrate: 2.0 to 5.0 mg/kg/min. Use 3.5 mg/kg/min and adjust down for brittle diabetic or carbon dioxide retainer and upward for severely catabolic, such as a burn patient.

   c. Only protein and carbohydrates are required. Intralipids are used to "fill in calories" to meet daily needs and to prevent fatty acid deficiency.

   d. Add electrolytes: sodium, potassium, chloride, phosphorus, calcium, magnesium, and acetate (as needed for electron neutrality).

   e. Add 10 ml of multivitamins and 3 ml of trace elements per day in TPN.

   f. Add 1 unit of heparin per 1 ml of TPN to prevent thrombus formation at catheter tip.

   g. Insulin and other TPN-compatible drugs can be added as needed.

4. Calculating nutrient calories and volume (Table 184–1)

   a. Protein (the amino acid mix) is 4 calories per gram and currently available in an 8.5%, 10%, or 15% solution.

   b. Carbohydrate or dextrose is 3.4 calories per gram (glucose is 4 calories per gram), and a 70% (D70) solution is used.

   c. The intralipid is a 20% solution and contains 2 calories per milliliter.

TABLE 184–1. CALCULATION OF TPN

Example: A 5-foot, 10-inch 70-kg man is admitted to the hospital for exacerbation of Crohn's disease and has not eaten in 7 days. He is febrile and thought to be catabolic; TPN is requested.

CALCULATION

Step 1: Total daily caloric needs equal 70 (kg) × 30 (kcal/day) = 2100 kcal/day

Step 2: Calculate required *protein* calories: 70 kg × 1.5 gm/kg = 105 grams; then 105 gm/day × 4 kcal = 420 protein kcal/day
Calculate required *carbohydrate* calories: 70 kg × 3.5 mg/kg × 1440 minutes/day divided by 1000 mg/gm = 353 gm/day; then 353 gm/day × 3.4 kcal/gm = 1200 kcal/day
Calculate remaining caloric needs and provide lipid calories: 2100 kcal/day − 420 protein kcal/day − 1200 carbohydrate kcal/day = 480 kcal/day
Intralipids are 2 kcal/ml, so 240 ml (480 divided by 2) of 20% intralipid will be added to the TPN.

Step 3: Calculate volume and rate of TPN:
   a. Protein: using an 8.5% amino acid solution will require 105 gm/day divided by 0.085 gm/ml = 1235 ml/day
   b. Carbohydrate: using a 70% dextrose solution will require 353 gm/day divided by 0.70 gm/ml = 504 ml/day
   c. 1235 ml of amino acids + 504 ml of carbohydrate + 240 ml of intralipid = 1979 ml/day (abc). The rate would be 1979 ml/day divided by 24 hours/day = 82 ml/hr.

Step 4: Add electrolytes, 10 ml of multivitamins, and 3 ml of trace elements as well as 2000 units of heparin (1 unit/ml) to TPN.

> **WARNING**
>
> **The TPN formulation must be adjusted in certain disease states. Protein should be reduced in liver or renal failure, as well as potassium, phosphorus, magnesium, and fluid concentration. Salt and fluid concentration should be restricted in congestive heart failure and carbohydrates reduced in diabetes or chronic obstructive pulmonary disease. TPN is highly osmolar and must be administered via a central line.**

Follow-Up

1. Initially, daily electrolytes must be followed and strict fluid intake and output monitored. Platelet counts must be followed to rule out thrombocytopenia secondary to heparin or the need to restrict lipids (lipids may interfere with platelet quantity and function). When fluid and electrolytes are stabilized, can reduce to twice-weekly blood tests.

2. Must watch for signs of catheter sepsis or wound infection.

3. Patient's weight should be followed at least weekly. A 24-hour urinary nitrogen balance should be obtained weekly to assess sufficient protein calories.

4. Gastrointestinal activities should be monitored for bowel sounds and function. Oral intake should be resumed as soon as possible with calorie counts to guide cessation of TPN.

5. Patients who may require TPN for prolonged periods of time should be assessed and counseled for home TPN.

Bibliography

For more information on nutritional support, see
ASPEN Board of Directors: Guidelines for the use of parenteral and enteral nutrition in adult and pediatric patients. JPEN 1993;17(4):1SA–26SA.
Nehme A: Nutritional support of the hospitalized patient. JAMA 1980;243:1906–1908.
Wilmore DW, van Woert JH: Enteral and parenteral nutrition in hospital patients. *In* Rubenstein E, Federman D (eds): Scientific American. sec 4. New York, Library of Congress, 1992, chap 14, pp 1–21.
For more information on complications of TPN, see
Wolfe BM, Ryder MA, Nishikawa RA, et al: Complications of parenteral nutrition. Am J Surg 1986;152:93–99.
For more information on home TPN, see
Position of the American Dietetic Association: nutrition monitoring of the home parenteral and enteral patient. J Am Diet Assoc 1994;6:664–666.

185 Common Bone Symptoms

Symptom **Bone Pain and Swelling**   *Sandesh R. Patil*

Bone pain and swelling have a wide variety of causes that range from fractures to primary biliary cirrhosis. To adequately care for the patient with these symptoms requires diligence in history taking and physical examination to narrow the focus. Early diagnosis and intervention are imperative to correct potentially reversible devastating diseases.

Differential Diagnosis

1. Trauma
2. Infectious
   a. Tuberculosis
   b. Syphilis
   c. Osteomyelitis
3. Hematologic/bone marrow disorders
   a. Leukemia
   b. Lymphomas
   c. Sickle cell disease
   d. Granulocyte colony-stimulating factor (GCSF) therapy
4. Metastatic disease
   a. Prostate cancer
   b. Thyroid cancer
   c. Breast cancer
   d. Lung cancer
   e. Renal cell cancer
5. Renal failure
6. Electrolyte disorders
7. Primary biliary cirrhosis
8. Gaucher's disease
9. Vitamin D disorders
10. Cystic fibrosis
11. Bone tumors
    a. Benign: osteochondroma, giant cell tumor, aneurysmal bone cyst
    b. Malignant: multiple myeloma, osteosarcoma, fibrosarcoma
12. Neurofibromatosis
13. Hyperthyroidism

The differential diagnosis of bone pain and swelling, as noted above, is diverse, trauma being the most common cause. The "great masqueraders," tuberculosis and syphilis, must be remembered in the differential. A wide variety of hematologic malignancies commonly cause bone pain. Recently, GCSF used to stimulate bone marrow recovery in the post-chemotherapy phase has been noted to cause bone pain. Patients are often rightly concerned that bone pain may represent some form of cancer, either primary bone tumor or a form of metastatic disease. Renal failure—with its accompanying derangements in calcium, phosphorus, and vitamin D metabolism—leads to bone pain. Rarely, Gaucher's disease, primary disorders of vitamin D metabolism, or cystic fibrosis may cause bone pain.

History

1. History of presenting illness
   a. Duration
   b. Nature and character of pain
   c. Aggravating and relieving factors
   d. Location of the pain
   e. Referred pain
   f. Setting in which pain occurred
2. Medical history
   a. Recent trauma
   b. Sickle cell disease
   c. Underlying malignancy
   d. Renal disease
   e. Exposure to venereal disease or tuberculosis
   f. Steatorrhea
   g. Muscle cramps, weakness, pruritus
   h. Lung infections
3. Family history
   a. Sickle cell disease
   b. Malignancy, especially leukemias, breast cancer
   c. Cirrhosis
   d. Renal failure
   e. Hyperthyroidism
4. Review of symptoms
   a. Weakness, fatigue, weight loss
   b. Fever
   c. Breast mass
   d. Urinary complaints

A complete and detailed history assumes paramount importance in the diagnosis of disease processes for bone pain and swelling. The history of presenting illness, as with most symptoms, is often the harbinger. Duration of symptoms often points to benign versus malignant etiologies, especially if a tumor is found. A deep boring pain that awakes patients at night often points to a malignant process. An understanding of the setting in which the pain occurs allows the physician to make prudent decisions regarding laboratory tests and radiologic procedures.

Physical Examination

1. General appearance
   a. State of nutrition
   b. Complexion
2. Hand, eye, ear, nose, and throat
   a. Lymphadenopathy
   b. Thyroid nodules
3. Breast
4. Abdominal
   a. Hepatosplenomegaly
   b. Prostate
   c. Color of stools
5. Extremities
   a. Clubbing
   b. Excoriation (signs of pruritus)
   c. Short fourth metacarpal
6. Bone
   a. Inspection
   b. Size of swelling if any
   c. Tenderness
   d. Mobility
   e. Consistency

The physical examination can render important clues to the diagnosis. A detailed examination can bring to light a thyroid nodule suggesting metastatic disease. If a swelling is present, the local examination can guide the examiner. Large tumors, hard consistency, and fixture to underlying structures point to probable malignant etiologies.

Tests

1. Routine
   a. Complete blood count, peripheral blood smear, and erythrocyte sedimentation rate
   b. Chemistry profile to include creatinine, calcium, phosphorus, potassium, alkaline phosphatase, liver function tests
   c. Urinalysis
   d. Chest radiograph
   e. Radiologic examination of affected area
2. Specialized
   a. Bone marrow biopsy
   b. Antimitochondrial antibody
   c. Venereal Disease Research Laboratories (VDRL), rapid plasma reagin test (RPR)
   d. Purified protein derivative, sputum for acid-fast bacillus
   e. Magnetic resonance imaging (MRI) scan of affected extremity
   f. Thyroid biopsy
   g. Serum parathyroid hormone (PTH) by radioimmunoassay, nephrogenic cyclic AMP
   h. Serum protein electrophoresis
   i. Mammogram
   j. Prostate-specific antigen (PSA)

Definitive diagnosis is done by the use of tests. A peripheral blood smear can be used to diagnose leukemias. Chemistries can aid in diagnosing renal failure or vitamin D disorders. A radiologic examination is necessary to rule out possible malignancies; when deemed necessary, specialized tests can be ordered. Tests for syphilis, tuberculosis, primary biliary cirrhosis, and multiple myeloma are readily available. MRI of the extremities is becoming a useful tool for differentiating tumors of the bone from less benign causes.

Management

1. Analgesics are the mainstay of treatment.
2. Patient's fears and concerns should be respected.

PEARLS

- Bone marrow biopsy is imperative in undiagnosed cases.

- Local examination of bone swelling is rewarding.

- Remember to test for tuberculosis and syphilis.

B | ## Bibliography

Aichroth P: Bone, swelling on. *In* Hart D (ed): French's Index of Differential Diagnosis, 12 ed. Bristol, England, Wright Company, 1985, pp 88–103.

McRae R: Clinical Orthopaedic Examination, 3rd ed. New York, Churchill Livingstone, 1990, pp 1–9.

Negendank W, Soulen R: Magnetic resonance imaging in patients with bone marrow disorders. Leuk Lymph 1993; 10(4–5):287–298.

Wilkins R, Sim F: Evaluation of bone and soft tissue tumors. *In* D'Ambrosia R (ed): Musculoskeletal Disorders. Philadelphia, JB Lippincott, 1986, pp 189–217.

186 Osteoporosis

Cheryl A. Oncken

Etiology and Epidemiology

1. Responsible for 1.3 million fractures each year
2. Most common metabolic bone disorder
3. Defined as a loss of bone mass that increases susceptibility to fracture
4. Predisposes to fractures of the hip, vertebrae, distal forearm, and humerus, although may occur at other sites as well
5. Occurs as a primary disorder that includes idiopathic osteoporosis and involutional osteoporosis (postmenopausal and age-related)
6. Postmenopausal osteoporosis
   a. Usually affects women 15 to 20 years after menopause
   b. Rate of trabecular bone loss is markedly increased
   c. Predisposes vertebral bodies and radius to fractures but may occur in other sites as well
   d. Related to decrease of endogenous estrogen at menopause
7. Age-related or "senile" osteoporosis
   a. Affects men and women 70 years of age or older
   b. Usually hip and vertebral fractures
   c. Proportionate loss of trabecular and cortical bone
   d. Osteoporosis is believed to be secondary to age-related bone loss.
8. Risk factors for osteoporosis in women: positive family history, white or Asian descent, low calcium intake, smoking, heavy alcohol use, inactivity, leanness
9. Other secondary causes of osteoporosis include
   a. Endocrine conditions (hyperthyroidism, glucocorticoid excess, hyperparathyroidism, hypogonadism)
   b. Gastrointestinal (malabsorbtion syndromes, primary biliary cirrhosis, gastric or small bowel resection)
   c. Malignancies (multiple myeloma, disseminated carcinoma)
   d. Connective tissue disorders
   e. Drugs (anticonvulsants, steroids, long-term heparin therapy)
   f. Other (immobilization, congestive obstructive pulmonary disease, alcoholism)

Symptoms

1. Major clinical manifestations result from fractures of the vertebrae, wrist, hip, and humerus.
2. Generalized skeletal pain is uncommon.
3. Vertebral fractures
   a. Pain usually results from collapse of the vertebrae.
   b. Fracture may occur spontaneously or with minimal trauma (lifting, coughing, or sneezing).
   c. Symptoms range from asymptomatic to severe pain.
   d. Pain is usually acute and is exacerbated with movement.
   e. Symptoms should resolve within three months.
   f. Multiple fractures may lead to chronic back pain.
4. Hip fractures
   a. Usually a result of moderate trauma (fall from standing height or less)
   b. Pain mild to severe
   c. Impaired ability to walk
   d. Most serious of fractures—high morbidity/mortality (20 per cent death rate in 6 months; 30 per cent nursing home placement; 30 per cent disabled and unable to walk without assistance)
5. Distal forearm fracture
   a. May result when trying to break a fall
   b. Pain in affected area
   c. Long-term morbidity rare

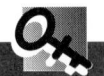

Key Symptom

- Pain at fracture site

Clinical Findings

1. Multiple collapsed vertebral bodies in the lower dorsal and lumbar regions may result in a "dowager's hump."
2. Loss of height (1 cm on average for each compression fracture)
3. Point tenderness and possible deformity if there is acute fracture

Key Signs

- Dowager's hump
- Loss of height

Laboratory Tests

1. Useful in differentiating primary from secondary osteoporosis
   a. Complete blood count, calcium, phosphorus, alkaline phosphatase, thyroid-stimulating hormone, sedimentation rate, and urinalysis are usually normal in persons with primary osteoporosis.

b. Alkaline phosphatase may be elevated after a fracture.

2. Special procedures

a. Routine radiograph

(1) Osteopenia and vertebral abnormalities are neither sensitive nor specific for osteoporosis.

(2) Baseline radiograph may be useful in evaluating subsequent episodes of back pain.

(3) Bone density measurements should be done if radiograph is suggestive of osteoporosis.

b. Bone density measurements (BDM)

(1) These are helpful in diagnosis and prevention of osteoporosis, as historical risk factors and physical findings are not accurate predictors of bone mass.

(2) Measurements are different at various skeletal sites due to differing amounts of cortical and trabecular bone.

(3) Techniques for measurement of bone mass: single-photon absorptiometry (SPA), dual-photon absorptiometry (DPA), quantitative computed tomography (QCT), and dual energy x-ray absorptiometry (DEXA)

c. SPA

(1) Measures density of appendicular bone (i.e., radius, calcaneus)

(2) Examination time is short (10 to 20 minutes).

(3) Radiation exposure (5 mrem)

(4) Cost ($35 to $120)

d. DPA

(1) Measures density of axial bone (i.e., spine, hip)

(2) Examination time is long (20 to 60 minutes).

(3) Radiation exposure (5 to 15 mrem)

(4) Cost ($100)

e. QCT

(1) Used mostly for spinal area

(2) Examination time is short (10 to 20 minutes)

(3) Significantly more radiation exposure (>200 mrem)

(4) Cost high ($100 to $400)

(5) Less reproducible and less accurate than other techniques

f. DEXA

(1) State of the art technique

(2) Can measure density at spine, hip, wrist, total skeleton

(3) Accurate and precise

(4) Examination time low (10 minutes)

(5) Radiation low (1 to 3 mrem)

(6) Cost ($120 to $225)

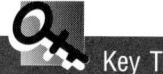

Key Test

• Bone density measurement

Differential Diagnosis

1. Osteomalacia

2. Paget's disease

3. Secondary causes of osteoporosis (see Etiology), especially

a. Malignancies

b. Hyperparathyroidism

Treatment

1. Prevention of osteoporosis

a. Maximization of peak bone mass (adequate calcium and vitamin D intake, avoidance of smoking and heavy alcohol use, regular exercise)

b. Minimizing bone loss as a consequence of menopause

(1) Estrogen replacement therapy (ERT)

(a) Prevention against accelerated bone loss that occurs during menopause

(b) Decreases risk of subsequent osteoporotic fractures by 50 per cent

(c) Should be considered in all women if no contraindications

(d) Encourage in menopausal or postmenopausal women whose BDM is <1 SD below the mean

(e) In order to be effective, needs to be continued long term

(2) Intake of 1000 mg to 1500 mg of calcium as well as adequate vitamin D

(3) Weight-bearing exercise should be encouraged.

2. Treatment of established osteoporosis

a. Ensure adequate calcium (1200 mg to 1500 mg) and vitamin D intake (400 to 800 IU)

b. ERT should be instituted in women if no contraindications

c. Calcitonin (50 U/day) is an acceptable substitute for women unwilling or unable to take estrogen or for men

(1) Limited by expense, need for injections, and side effects

(2) May have intrinsic analgesic properties

d. Sodium fluoride, bisphosphonates, anabolic steroids, and parathyroid hormone should be considered investigational in the treatment of osteoporosis.

e. Nonsteroidal anti-inflammatory drugs (NSAID) or other analgesic therapy as needed for pain

f. Patients with vertebral fractures may benefit from physical therapy or orthopedic garment for back support.

Medication

1. Conjugated estrogen, 0.625 mg per day or equivalent dosage in women
2. Addition of progestin (i.e., 2.5 mg medroxyprogesterone daily or 10 mg on days 1 to 14 of calendar month) if uterus is present
3. Ensure adequate elemental calcium (1200 mg to 1500 mg daily) and vitamin D intake (400 to 800 IU daily)
4. Calcitonin (50 U daily) is an alternative to ERT
5. NSAID for chronic pain management

Diet

The diet should contain adequate calcium and vitamin D, as discussed above.

Activity

1. Encourage weight-bearing activity.
2. Avoid periods of immobilization.

Patient Education

1. Encourage adequate diet of calcium and vitamin D.

2. Avoid smoking and heavy alcohol use.
3. Counsel risks/benefits of ERT.

Key Treatment

• Estrogen replacement therapy

Follow-Up

Frequency should be individualized to patient symptomatology.

Bibliography

Christiansen C: Prevention and treatment of osteoporosis: A review of current modalities. Bone 1992;13:S35–39.

Cummings SR, et al: Epidemiology of osteoporosis and osteoporotic fractures. Epidemiol Rev 1985;7:178–208.

Fleming LA: Osteoporosis: Clinical features and prevention and treatment. J Gen Intern Med 1992;7:554–562.

Lindsay R: Hormone replacement therapy for prevention and treatment of osteoporosis. Am J Med 1993;95(5A):375–395.

Riggs BL, Melton LJ III: The prevention and treatment of osteoporosis. N Engl J Med 1992;327:620–627.

187 Paget's Disease of Bone

Mark E. Hroncich

Etiology

1. Paget's disease is caused by hyperactivity of multinucleated osteoclasts with intact bone formation. The resultant lamellar bone is formed in a disordered mosaic pattern. The cause of the osteoclast activation is unknown.
2. Paget's disease may be caused by a slow virus.
   a. Paramyxovirus-like particles have been found in pagetic bones by structural studies and immunohistochemistry.
   b. The long latency period is similar to that of other slow virus diseases.
   c. Polymerase chain reaction techniques do not confirm a viral presence.
3. There is a hereditary component of Paget's disease.
   a. Twelve per cent of cases have a family history of the disease.
   b. Paget's disease is very common in England, the United States, Australia, New Zealand, and Western Europe.
   c. HLA-DQw1 antigen is common.
4. An immune cause or effect of Paget's disease is possible, because a low CD4/CD8 ratio is present.

Symptoms

1. Eighty to 90 per cent of Paget's disease is asymptomatic. It is incidentally discovered as an elevated alkaline phosphatase or an abnormal radiograph.
2. Paget's disease has multiple osseous manifestations.
   a. Painful bones are present, worse on weight bearing. The following bones are affected in decreasing order of frequency:
      (1) Pelvis
      (2) Lumbar spine
      (3) Femur
      (4) Skull
      (5) Other bones
   b. Bone deformities
   c. Loss of height
   d. Deafness (due to cranial nerve entrapment)
   e. Visual loss (due to cranial nerve entrapment)
   f. Headache (due to skull involvement)
   g. Increased hat size (due to cranial thickening)

Clinical Findings

1. Warmth over affected bones due to the increased blood supply that is present.

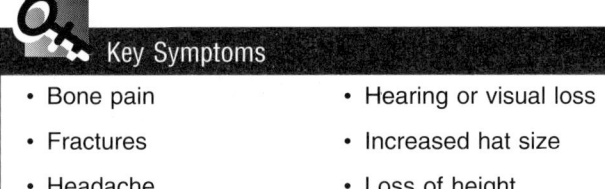

Key Symptoms

- Bone pain
- Fractures
- Headache
- Hearing or visual loss
- Increased hat size
- Loss of height

2. The weight-bearing bones become bowed with a genu varum pattern.
3. Fractures are common.
4. Skull thickening is common. The most severe form of this is platybasia. Patients present with paraparesis. The cranium compresses the spinal cord, brain stem, and its blood supply.
5. Cranial nerves I, II, V, VII, and VIII can become compressed.
   a. Deafness
   b. Blindness
6. Spinal cord compression
7. Radiculopathies
8. High-output congestive heart failure
9. Bruit over affected areas
10. Osteosarcomas (<1 per cent), fibrosarcomas, benign giant cell tumors

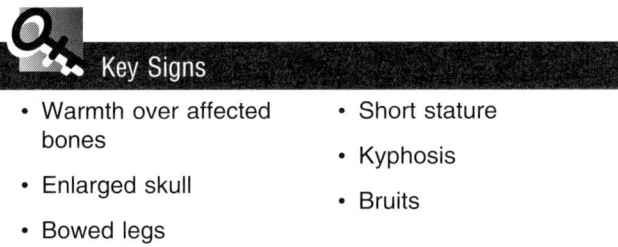

Key Signs

- Warmth over affected bones
- Enlarged skull
- Bowed legs
- Short stature
- Kyphosis
- Bruits

Laboratory Tests

1. A universal feature of Paget's disease is an elevation of serum alkaline phosphatase and urinary hydroxyproline. These tests are useful for diagnosing the disease as well as the following treatment responses.
   a. Laboratory tests that increase with disease activity
      (1) Alkaline phosphatase
      (2) Urinary hydroxyproline
      (3) Osteocalcin
      (4) β-2 microglobulin
      (5) Calcium (only if immobilized)
   b. Laboratory tests that decrease with disease activity: 24,25-(OH)$_2$ vitamin D$_3$ level

c. Laboratory tests that do not change with Paget's disease
   (1) Calcium (ambulatory)
   (2) Phosphorus
   (3) Parathyroid hormone
   (4) 25-OH vitamin D_3
   (5) 1,25-$(OH)_2$ vitamin D_3

2. Radiologic studies are extremely helpful in the diagnosis and treatment of Paget's disease. Plain roentgenograms show a characteristic fluffy appearance with expansion and cortical thickening. Lytic lesions also occur. The characteristic lesions of Paget's disease advance in untreated bones at a rate of 1 cm/year. The nuclear medicine bone scan is very sensitive at detecting pagetic lesions and may help determine prognosis. Magnetic resonance image scan is useful in diagnosing nerve entrapments.

3. Biopsy of pagetic bone shows a very characteristic pattern of giant multinucleated osteoclasts. These are on a background of disorganized lamellar bone called a "mosaic pattern."

Key Tests

• Alkaline phosphatase	• Plain roentgenograms
• Urinary hydroxyproline	• Bone scan

Differential Diagnosis

1. The combination of elevated urinary hydroxyproline and serum alkaline phosphatase, along with the characteristic radiographic appearance, is usually sufficient to diagnose the disease. Prostate cancer can give a similar radiologic appearance but can be detected with an elevated prostate-specific antigen. Both diseases are common, and occasionally, a bone biopsy may be necessary to distinguish between the two or confirm the presence of both. Myeloma also can give a similar radiologic appearance along with other metastatic tumors. Osteogenic sarcoma and benign giant cell tumors rarely occur in pagetic bones and are detected on MRI scans. Definitive diagnosis requires biopsy.

2. Degenerative disease and Paget's disease frequently coexist. Both diseases affect the same populations. It can be difficult to determine the source of a patient's pain. A therapeutic trial of anti-Paget therapy can be very helpful in this situation.

Treatment

Many patients require no treatment. Nonsteroidal anti-inflammatories (NSAIDs) are frequently enough for pain control. Reasons to use specific anti-Paget therapy would be

1. Neurologic complications

2. Impending fractures or bone surgery
3. Hypercalcemia
4. Hypercalciuria

Medication

1. Calcitonin
   a. Salmon calcitonin (Calcimar) is effective for acute disease and much stronger than the human form. Side effects include nausea, flushing, and allergic reactions. The response is short lived. Nasal preparations are sometimes used. Relapses are common. The dosage is 50 to 100 IU subcutaneously or intramuscularly daily or every other day.
   b. Human calcitonin (Cibacalcin) is reserved for use in patients allergic to salmon calcitonin. The dosage is 0.5 mg subcutaneously three times weekly.

2. Biphosphonates
   a. Etidronate (Didronel) is the only oral medication approved by the FDA for treating Paget's disease. The drug causes long remissions of the disease but may cause abnormal bone mineralization and cannot be given continuously. The chief side effect is gastrointestinal upset. The dosage is 5 mg/kg daily for no greater than 6 months continuously.
   b. Pamidronate (Aredia) is a new biphosphonate that is given in an intravenous form. Its side effects are an elevated temperature and lymphopenia. It does not cause abnormal mineralization. A solution of 30 mg in 500 ml of normal saline is infused over 4 hours.

3. Plicamycin (Mithracin) works well for Paget's disease. It is usually reserved for refractory cases because it causes significant bone marrow toxicity.

4. Gallium nitrate (Ganite) is administered in the nuclear medicine department. The agent works quickly to destroy osteoclast function but is only used in refractory cases.

Diet

There is no specific dietary therapy for Paget's disease.

Activity

Exercise that avoids undue stress to affected bones is encouraged.

Patient Education

The Paget Foundation [(800) 23-PAGET] is an excellent source of information and support for patients.

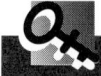

Key Treatment

Drugs of Choice	**Alternative Drugs**
• Salmon calcitonin	• Pamidronate
• Disodium etidronate	• Plicamycin
	• Gallium nitrate
	• New investigational biphosphonates

Follow-Up

1. A minimum of annual physical examination and alkaline phosphatase level is recommended.

2. Disease activity can be followed with urinary hydroxyproline levels.

3. There is no satisfactory system of tumor surveillance.

Bibliography

Bone HG, Kleerekoper M: Clinical review 39: Paget's disease of bone. J Clin Endocrinol Metab 1992;75:1179–1182.

Gallacher SJ: Paget's disease of bone. Curr Opin Rheumatol 1993;5:351–356.

Nunziata V, Giannattasio R, DiGiovanni G, et al: Vitamin D status in Paget's bone disease. Clin Orthop 1993;293:366–371.

Siris ES: Paget's disease of bone. *In* Favus MJ (ed): Primer on the Metabolic Bone Diseases and Disorders of Mineral Metabolism, 1st ed. Kelseyville, American Society for Bone and Mineral Research, 1990, pp 253–259.

Siris ES, Ottman R, Flaster E, Kelsey JL: Familial aggregation of Paget's disease of bone. J Bone Miner Res 1991;6:495–500.

188 Osteomyelitis

Thomas B. Golemon

Etiology

1. Osteomyelitis occurs by hematogenous spread of bacteria (20 per cent), contiguous contact of bone with an infected wound (45 per cent), and in association with peripheral vascular disease (35 per cent).

2. Hematogenous spread

   a. Infants and children: metaphyses of long bones. *Staphyloccocus aureus* most common isolate; group B streptococcus and *Escherichia coli* common in the age group 12 months and under. For the age group 1 to 16 years, *Staphylococcus, Streptococcus,* and *Haemophilus influenzae* are most common. *Salmonella* species are seen with sickle cell disease.

   b. In adults, hematogenous spread less common. Occurs in vertebrae; *S. aureus* or aerobic gram-negative rods. Immunosuppressed: tuberculosis, *Monilia,* or *Cryptococcus.*

3. Contiguous spread

   a. Contaminated wounds, postoperative infections, and open fractures

   b. Dental, foot, intra-abdominal, sinuses, human bites, and decubiti: polymicrobial and anerobic

4. Associated peripheral vascular disease

   a. Diabetes and atherosclerotic disease predispose. Bacteriology diverse, *S. aureus* and *S. epidermidis* leaders. Various streptococci, gram-negative rods, and *Pseudomonas* species are seen.

   b. Unrecognized trauma, fissures, chronic ulcers as portals of entry

Symptoms

1. Pain: varies in severity depending on age and mechanism of infection

   a. Hematogenous spread in children: half with vague pain for 1 to 3 months; may refuse to walk or bear weight. Can mimic septic joint. In adults, dull, constant pain over vertebral body with focal pain on percussion. Paravertebral spasm and ache common.

   b. Contiguous spread: Sensory neuropathy will diminish symptoms.

2. Fever: variable

   a. Hematogenous spread in pediatric patients: 50 per cent present with abrupt fever and lethargy, as with classic septicemia. Other children and most adults have low-grade or absent fevers.

   b. Contiguous spread: often without fever

3. Chronically draining sinuses

Key Symptoms

- Fever
- Draining sores
- Pain

Clinical Findings

1. Local pain and tenderness
2. Erythema (may be minimal or absent)
3. Draining sinuses connecting skin with infected bone site
4. Fever, especially with hematogenous disease
5. Chronic skin ulcers in setting of vascular disease

Key Signs

• Pain	• Fever
• Erythema	• Draining sinuses
• Skin ulcers	

Laboratory Tests

1. Blood and bone cultures (percutaneous or at surgery). Cultures of sinus tracts unreliable (exception: *S. aureus*)

2. White blood cell (WBC) count: greater than 15,000 (most reliable in children)

3. Erythrocyte sedimentation rate (ESR): frequently in the 50 to 100 mm/hr range

4. Imaging tests

   a. Radiographs: periosteal elevation or cortical erosion specific but not sensitive; occurs late

   b. Bone scan: more sensitive, but not specific

   c. Computed tomography (CT) scan: relatively high sensitivity

   d. Magnetic resonance imaging (MRI) scan: highest sensitivity, good specificity, allows differentiation from soft tissue infection; most accurate but most expensive

   e. Radionuclide studies: technetium, gallium, and indium-111–labeled leukocytes; less accurate but less expensive

5. Doppler studies: important in patients with peripheral vascular disease to determine vascular adequacy

713

Key Tests

• Blood cultures	• Bone cultures
• WBC count	• ESR
• Plain radiographs	• MRI or CT scans
• Dopplers	• Radionuclide imaging

Differential Diagnosis

1. Hematogenous spread—children
   a. Septicemia
   b. Meningitis
   c. Septic arthritis
2. Hematogenous spread—adults (uncommon)
   a. Arthritis of spine
   b. Back strain and/or spasm
   c. Compression fracture of spine
   d. Metastatic or primary tumor of vertebral body
3. Contiguous spread
   a. Cellulitis
   b. Chronic skin ulcer/decubitus

Treatment

1. Intravenous antibiotics: 4 to 6 weeks, followed in many cases by oral antibiotics for another 2 months. Time course individualized with other components of therapy. Home intravenous therapy ideal in this disease.
2. Surgical débridement with obliteration of dead space
3. Partial amputation or suppressive antibiotics: best choice in critically or terminally ill
4. Balloon angioplasty may be helpful prior to surgery.

Medication

1. *S. aureus:* A penicillinase-resistant penicillin (oxacillin [Prostaphilin], nafcillin [Nafcil], methicillin [Staphcillin], cloxacillin [Tegopen]) is drug of choice. Alternatives: first-generation cephalosporins. Vancomycin (Vancocin) for methicillin-resistant staphylo-cocci. Add rifampin (Rifadin) in chronic staphyloccal infections.

2. *H. influenzae:* Use cefuroxime (Ceftin) or a third-generation cephalosporin.

3. *Pseudomonas:* May use ticarcillin-clavulanic acid (Timentin), a third-generation cephalosporin, or a quinolone. Fluoroquinolones also active against most gram-negative organisms; may offer less costly alternative to intravenous drugs but have not yet attained the same level of confidence. Watch use in pediatric age groups (cartilage).

Diet

Usually unchanged; may need higher protein content.

Activity

1. As tolerated. Individualize for pain and postoperative needs

2. Home treatment: offers greater freedom in rehabilitation phase

Patient Education

1. Must understand need for long-term antibiotic therapy for compliance

2. Home therapy: requires teaching on care of intravenous access lines

Follow-Up

1. Home therapy: nursing visits for care of intravenous lines and/or wounds and compliance on antibiotic regimen

2. Physician visits (home or office): biweekly, weekly, or bimonthly, as required by severity and availability of physician extenders

Bibliography

Bamberger DM: Osteomyelitis. Postgrad Med 1993;94(5):177–183.

Mackowiak PA, Jones SR, Smith JW: Diagnostic value of sinus-tract cultures in chronic osteomyelitis. JAMA 1978; 239: 2772–2775.

Sanford J: Guide to Antibiotic Therapy. Dallas, Antimicrobial, Inc., 1993.

Weinstein D, Wang A, Chambers R, Stewart CA: Evaluation of magnetic resonance imaging in the diagnosis of osteomyelitis in diabetic foot infections. Foot Ankle 1993;14(1):18–22.

189 Common Immune Symptoms

Patients with significant immunodeficiencies usually present in infancy with recurrent severe infections. Normal children have six to twelve, and adults two to four respiratory infections yearly and do not require further evaluation. Patients with recurrent biliary and urinary tract infections should be evaluated for obstruction. Immunodeficiency is rare in the setting of recurrent colds, sore throats, superficial skin infections, or sinusitis without otitis media. Occasionally, cystic fibrosis presents as recurrent infection later in life. Many infections, malignancies, drugs, and systemic illnesses can cause an acquired immunodeficiency manifested by recurrent infections. HIV infection is perhaps the most severe example.

Differential Diagnosis in Order of Likelihood

1. Antibody-deficient syndromes

   a. Selective IgA deficiency is common and can be autosomal recessive (AR) or dominant (AD). Most patients are asymptomatic, but some may manifest recurrent sinopulmonary infections, atopy, gastrointestinal tract disease, systemic lupus erythematosus (SLE), rheumatoid arthritis (RA), pernicious anemia, malignancies, and anaphylactic reactions to transfused IgA.

   b. X-linked (XL) agammaglobulinemia (congenital hypogammaglobulinemia) presents in infancy or later in childhood. Patients produce almost no immunoglobulin.

   c. Transient hypogammaglobulinemia of infancy begins at 5 to 6 months of age and represents a delay in the infant's own ability to produce antibodies.

   d. Immunodeficiency with increased IgM (XL): Patients are deficient in IgG and IgA, and manifest recurrent pyogenic infections.

   e. Common variable immunodeficiency (CVID) (AR or AD) becomes apparent by 15 to 35 years of age with recurrent pyogenic infections, a predisposition to autoimmune disease, chronic bacterial conjunctivitis, malabsorption, ITP, dermatomyositis, hemolytic anemia, lymphadenopathy, and splenomegaly. Patients often have a family history of IgA deficiency. Ig levels can be depressed. B cells are detectable, but plasma cells are absent in lymphoid tissue.

   f. IgG subclass deficiency (AR) can exist in the setting of normal IgG levels. Recurrent pyogenic infections can be seen with deficiency of IgG1, IgG2, or IgG4.

2. Combined antibody and cell-mediated deficiency syndromes

   a. Severe combined immunodeficiency (SCID) includes adenosine deaminase deficiency (AR) and XL SCID. Patients have absence of all or almost all intrinsic immune function.

   b. Immunodeficiency with ataxia telangiectasia (AR) is characterized by variable deficiencies of IgG, IgA, or IgE; cerebellar ataxia; oculocutaneous telangiectasia; chronic sinopulmonary disease; and increased frequency of malignancies.

   c. Wiskott-Aldrich syndrome (XL) is characterized by thrombocytopenia, chronic eczematoid dermatitis, normal numbers of T and B cells, low normal immunoglobulin levels, and a poor response to polysaccharide antigens. *Pneumococcus, Pneumocystis carinii,* and herpesviruses are common infecting agents.

3. Phagocyte dysfunction

   a. Neutropenia

      (1) Infant genetic agranulocytosis presents with severe infections and death early in infancy.

      (2) Cyclic neutropenia can last 5 to 8 days and occurs every 2 to 5 weeks. It manifests as aphthous stomatitis, fever, malaise, and cutaneous infections during neutropenia.

   b. Chronic granulomatous disease (XL or AR) is manifested by recurrent infections with *Staphylococcus, Salmonella, Pseudomonas aeruginosa, Serratia marcescens, Nocardia asteroides,* and *Aspergillus.* Neutrophils are unable to produce H_2O_2 or superoxide secondary to a variety of defects. Patients may have pyogenic dermatitis, suppurative adenitis, recurrent pneumonia, failure to thrive, idiopathic pulmonary fibrosis, and discoid lupus erythematosus.

   c. Leukocyte adhesion deficiency syndrome manifests as recurrent pyogenic infections, delayed separation of the umbilical cord, omphalitis, and necrotic infections of soft tissue and mucosa.

   d. Hyper IgE syndrome, or "Job's syndrome," (AD) is manifested by eczema; recurrent "cold" staphylococcal infections; pneumonia; mucocutaneous candidiasis; normal IgG, IgA, and IgM levels; and eosinophilia.

715

e. Chédiak-Higashi syndrome (AR) manifests as generalized dysfunction of granule-containing cells. Patients have partial oculocutaneous albinism, rotatory nystagmus, peripheral neuropathy, neutropenia, and recurrent staphylococcal and gram-negative infections.

4. Cell-mediated deficiencies

a. Congenital thymic aplasia or hypoplasia (DiGeorge syndrome) is characterized by severe hypocalcemia and tetany in the neonatal period; lymphopenia; and increased susceptibility to herpes viruses, *Candida albicans,* and *Pneumocystis carinii.*

b. Chronic mucocutaneous candidiasis (AR) involves a selective defect in T cell immunity to *Candida.* Patients often have endocrinopathies.

c. Nezelof syndrome includes purine nucleoside phosphorylase deficiency (AR) and manifests in infancy with recurrent pulmonary infections, failure to thrive, candidiasis, chronic diarrhea, gram-negative sepsis, and varicella.

5. Complement deficiencies (AR)

a. Deficiency of either C1q, C1r, C1s, C2, C3, C4, or factors H or I leading to C3 deficiency can manifest as recurrent pneumonia, meningitis, and peritonitis, particularly with *Pneumococcus.* Occasionally these patients have autoimmune disease.

b. Deficiency of C5, C6, C7, C8, or C9—the membrane attack complex; factor B; factor D; or factor P (properdin) leads to a high frequency of *Neisseria* infections.

6. Secondary immunodeficiencies

a. Acquired humoral deficiency is seen in B cell malignancies, severe burns, protein-losing enteropathies, nephrotic syndrome, and asplenia.

b. Acquired deficiency of cell-mediated immunity can be found in many bacterial, viral, fungal, and mycobacterial infections. HIV infection is the most notable. Hodgkin's disease, lymphomas, cyclophosphamide, methotrexate, corticosteroids, radiation therapy, cyclosporin A, uremia, diabetes mellitus, surgery, anesthesia, sarcoidosis, cystic fibrosis, prolonged zinc deficiency, chronic protein-calorie malnutrition, SLE, RA, psoriasis, and old age can all contribute to cell-mediated immune dysfunction.

History: Key Questions to Ask

1. Onset and duration of symptoms?
2. Family history of immunodeficiency or autoimmune disorders?
3. Location and severity of infection, as well as infecting organisms?
4. Presence of systemic illnesses causing an acquired immunodeficiency?
5. Risk factors for AIDS (e.g., IV drug abuse, unprotected intercourse especially in the setting of ulcerative sexually transmitted diseases, and transfusion prior to 1985)?

Clinical Findings

1. Antibody deficiencies most often manifest themselves by recurrent sinopulmonary tract infections and chronic otitis media secondary to encapsulated organisms. Viral, fungal, and parasitic infections are rarely a problem, with the occasional exceptions of *P. carinii, Giardia,* and enterovirus.

2. Cell-mediated deficiency causes increased frequency or severity of infection due to intracellular organisms, viruses, fungi, and protozoa; lymphopenia; absent delayed type hypersensitivity; growth retardation; wasting; diarrhea; susceptibility to graft-versus-host disease; and a high incidence of malignancy.

3. Phagocyte dysfunction manifests as recurrent staphylococcal, gram-negative, and fungal infections that are slow to respond to treatment.

Tests

Tests most useful to rule in or exclude diagnosis

1. Initial evaluation for immunodeficiency should include

a. Complete blood count with differential can rule out congenital or acquired neutropenia or lymphopenia, the abnormal granules of Chédiak-Higashi, the thrombocytopenia of Wiskott-Aldrich, and the neutrophilia of leukocyte adhesion deficiency.

b. A sedimentation rate is elevated in patients with recurrent infections.

2. If one suspects an immunoglobulin deficiency, functional assays are most useful.

a. Measure antibody levels before and 2 to 3 weeks after immunization with a protein antigen (tetanus toxoid) and a polysaccharide antigen (pneumococcal vaccine). A rise in both of these antibody levels makes it unlikely that serious B cell abnormalities exist.

b. Measure quantitative immunoglobulin levels to exclude hyper IgE syndrome, selective IgA or IgM deficiency, SCID, XL agammaglobulinemia, CVID, and hyper IgM. IgG subtyping is rarely beneficial.

3. T cell abnormalities can be evaluated with delayed type hypersensitivity testing: Normal skin testing with mumps, tetanus, *Candida,* or *Trichophyton* indicates an intact cell-mediated immunity.

4. Phagocyte function should be assessed: Quantitative nitro blue tetrazolium test rules out chronic granulomatous disease or G6PD deficiency.

5. Complement function should be assessed: Total hemolytic complement function (CH50), if normal, rules out significant component deficiency. If reduced, individual components can be studied.

6. HIV testing should be ordered in all patients with evidence of T cell dysfunction.

7. If all of the above tests are normal and suspicion of immunodeficiency is still high, the patient should be referred to a specialty center.

Management

1. Intravenous immunoglobulin is administered monthly at doses of 200 to 500 mg/kg in patients with XL agammaglobulinemia, CVID, hyper IgM with IgG deficiency, IgG subclass deficiency, Wiskott-Aldrich, and SCID. IvIg is not useful in selective IgA or IgM deficiency.

2. Bone marrow transplantation is useful in treating Wiskott-Aldrich, LAD, and SCID. Thymic transplantation may be useful in DiGeorge syndrome.

3. Prophylactic antibiotics and/or antifungals are beneficial in hyper IgE, chronic mucocutaneous candidiasis, agammaglobulinemia, and CVID.

PEARLS

- A normal ESR essentially rules out chronic bacterial infections.

- Immunization with live vaccines (BCG, vaccinia, measles, rubella, and mumps) should not be used in patients with cellular immunodeficiencies.

Bibliography

Buckley RH: Immunodeficiency diseases. JAMA 1992; 268(20):2797–2806.

Buckley RH: Breakthroughs in the understanding and therapy of primary immunodeficiency. Pediatr Clin North Am 1994; 41(4):665–690.

Iseki M, Heiner DC: Immunodeficiency disorders. Pediatr Rev 1993;14(6):226–236.

Lopez M, Fleisher T, deShazo RD: Use and interpretation of diagnostic immunologic laboratory tests. JAMA 1992; 268(20):2970–2990.

Rotrosen D, Gallin JI: Evaluation of the patient with suspected immunodeficiency. *In* Mandell GL, Douglas RG, Bennett JE (eds): Principles and Practice of Infectious Diseases. 3rd ed, vol 1. New York, Churchill Livingstone, 1990, pp 139–147.

190 Asymptomatic HIV Infection

Nancy O. Tatum

Etiology

1. Human immunodeficiency virus (HIV), a human retrovirus, has been known since 1983 to be the etiologic agent for acquired immune deficiency syndrome (AIDS).

2. By coding for the enzyme reverse transcriptase, this virus inserts itself into the cellular genome and causes persistent and latent infection.

3. Although the virus may be found in all body fluids, only blood, semen, and vaginal secretions have been implicated in transmission.

4. While there are no overt symptoms during the asymptomatic phase, the virus continues to replicate, infects more host cells, and progressively destroys cellular immunity.

5. There are three known routes of transmission.
   a. Sexual transmission (anal, oral, or vaginal intercourse)
   b. Blood or blood products (transfusions, infected needles)
   c. Perinatal transmission (in utero, at delivery, or via breast-feeding)

6. In the United States there are more than 400,000 cases of AIDS and an estimated 1.5 million people infected with HIV who are asymptomatic.

7. The World Health Organization estimates that over 10 million people world-wide are HIV infected.

8. While homosexual men and IV drug users account for the majority of HIV/AIDS cases in the United States, AIDS is expected to be a predominantly heterosexual disease by the end of the 1990s.

Symptoms and Clinical Findings

1. Asymptomatic HIV patients must have had no previous signs or symptoms attributable to HIV infection.

2. History may be suggestive of an acute mononucleosis or influenza-like syndrome with or without aseptic meningitis.

Laboratory Tests

1. A positive enzyme-linked immunosorbent assay (ELISA) test followed by a positive Western blot test confirms HIV infection.

2. After confirmation of HIV seropositive status, CD4 and CD8 (T4 helper and T8 suppressor) lymphocyte subsets are used to stage HIV infection.

3. Other initial laboratory evaluations should include complete blood count, rapid plasma reagin, hepatitis B profile, *Toxoplasma gondii* and *Cytomegalovirus* titers, tuberculin skin test, and β human chorionic gonadotropin (women).

Key Tests

- ELISA (enzyme-linked immunosorbent assay) for HIV antibodies
- Western blot test
- CD4 and CD8 lymphocyte counts

Differential Diagnosis

1. The acute primary infection phase of HIV may be confused with mononucleosis, influenza, or a number of acute self-limited viral illnesses that have associated fever, myalgias, sore throat, and generalized skin rash.

2. Only a high index of suspicion of HIV exposure would suggest HIV infection; clinical findings in the asymptomatic stage are completely lacking.

Treatment

1. Treatment of asymptomatic HIV patients is indicated in the presence of laboratory evidence of immune dysfunction.
   a. Acute viral phase: symptomatic treatment only
   b. CD4 cell count exceeding 500: none
   c. CD4 cell count 200 to 500: zidovudine (AZT, Retrovir), 100 mg five times a day or 200 mg every 8 hrs
   d. CD4 cell count < 200: *Pneumocystis carinii* pneumonia prophylaxis with TMP/SMZ (Bactrim, Septra) DS three times a week

2. Prophylaxis for *Cryptococcus,* toxoplasmosis, esophageal candidiasis, and *Mycobacterium avium–intracellulare* complex is sometimes recommended when CD4 cell count exceeds 100.

3. Consideration should be given to alternative treatment protocols when there is evidence of rapid decline in CD4 cell counts, clinical progression to symptomatic disease, or intolerance to zidovudine (e.g., zalcitabine [ddC], 0.75 mg q8h, or didanosine [ddI], 125 to 300 mg b.i.d.).

Diet

1. Patients with asymptomatic HIV infection should follow good general nutrition principles, choosing foods from all major food groups daily. Multivitamin supplementation is recommended.

2. Care must be taken to prevent possible exposures to potentially deadly gastrointestinal pathogens (particularly *Campylobacter, Listeria,* and *Salmonella*). Avoid nonpasteurized milk products and rare or undercooked meats.

Activity
1. Regular aerobic exercise, in moderation only, is encouraged because of its beneficial effects on immune function.
2. Extreme exercise regimens (e.g., marathon racing) may damage the immune system and are generally discouraged.

Patient Education
1. Education of patients with HIV and those people at risk for HIV exposure has proved to be the only effective means of prevention.
2. Patients should be cautioned to use "safer sex" practices.
3. Consistent use of latex condoms, preferably with non-oxynol-9, a viricidal spermacide, is recommended to prevent sexual transmission of HIV. Petroleum-based lubricants should be avoided because they increase the risk of condom rupture.
4. Sexual partner notification of risk of HIV exposure is essential to prevent transmission.

Key Treatment (Asymptomatic)

CD4 cell count	
>500	No treatment
200–500	Zidovudine (AZT) or no treatment
<200	Zidovudine (AZT) 200 mg q 8 h or 100 mg 5 times a day

Follow-Up
1. Follow-up intervals depend on changes in clinical and laboratory parameters.
   a. For CD4 cell count exceeding 750, patients should be re-evaluated every 6 to 12 months with history, physical examination, and repeat CD4 counts.
   b. For CD4 cell count of 500 to 750, follow-up should be every 6 months.
   c. For CD4 cell count under 500, repeat for confirmation and begin antiretroviral therapy with zidovudine.
   d. For CD4 cell count of 200 to 500, follow-up should be every 3 months.
   e. Patients with CD4 cell count under 200 should begin *Pneumocystis carinii* pneumonia prophylaxis and follow-up should be every 1 to 2 months.
2. For patients with rapidly declining CD4 counts or the onset of symptoms (e.g., persistent generalized lymphadenopathy, oral candidiasis, herpes zoster), more frequent follow-up is indicated.
3. Recommended routine immunizations include Td, MMR, HbCV, pneumococcal, influenza, HBV, and eIPV. Avoid live attenuated vaccines except MMR. More frequent boosters are often indicated.
4. Visits for psychosocial evaluation may also be indicated due to the incidence of family dysfunction, depression, and suicide associated with HIV infection.

Bibliography

Horn J, Yamaguchi E, Chaisson RE: Ambulatory care for the HIV-infected patient. *In* Barker LR, Burton JR, Zieve PD (eds): Principles of Ambulatory Medicine, 3rd ed. Baltimore, Williams & Wilkins, 1991, pp 375–383.

Hughes MP, Stein DS, Gundacher HM, et al: Within-subject variation in the CD4 lymphocyte count in asymptomatic human immunodeficiency virus infection: Implications for patient monitoring. J Infect Dis 1994; 169(1):28–36.

Landerking WR, Gelber RD, Cotton DJ, et al for the AIDS Clinical Trial Group: Evaluation of the quality of life associated with zidovudine treatment in asymptomatic human immunodeficiency virus infection. N Engl J Med 1994; 330(11):738–743.

Saag MS: Natural history of HIV-1 disease. *In* Broder S, Merigan TC, Bolognesi D (eds): Textbook of AIDS Medicine. Baltimore, Williams & Wilkins, 1994, pp 45–54.

Sanford JP, Sande MA, Gilbert DN, Geberding JL: The Sanford Guide to HIV/AIDS Therapy 1992. Dallas, TX, Antimicrobial Therapy, Inc., 1992, pp 5–7, 31–32, 58.

191 Early Symptomatic HIV Infection *Linda L. Krishna*

Etiology

1. Human immunodeficiency virus (HIV) is spread via contact with parenteral/bodily fluids.
2. HIV binds to CD4 protein receptors on T-helper lymphocytes as well as monocytes, macrophages, and other cells.
3. With disease progression, CD4 lymphocyte counts decrease. Below 200 cells/mm^3, there is increased risk of opportunistic infections. Also, immune complexes may lead to renal disease, vasculitis, myalgias, arthralgias, and thrombocytopenias.
4. Early symptomatic HIV infection usually occurs when CD4 counts begin to decrease and the CD4/CD8 ratio inverts.

Symptoms

1. Weight loss
2. Night sweats
3. Fever/chills
4. Fatigue/malaise
5. Lymphadenopathy
6. Changes in cognition
7. Personality change
8. Cough, shortness of breath
9. Myalgia/arthralgia
10. Paresthesias
11. Oral lesions/ulcers
12. Abdominal discomfort
13. Diarrhea
14. Vesicular skin lesions
15. Skin rashes

Key Symptoms

• Weight loss	• Oral ulcers/lesions
• Fever, chills, sweats	• Skin rashes/lesions
• Diarrhea	• Fatigue/malaise
• Lymphadenopathy	• Myalgias/arthralgias

Clinical Findings

1. Generalized wasting
2. Hairy leukoplakia
3. Oral candidiasis
4. Periodontal disease
5. Oral herpes
6. Aphthous ulcers
7. Cotton wool spots
8. Lymphadenopathy
9. Hepatosplenomegaly
10. Herpes zoster
11. Tinea infections
12. Seborrheic dermatitis
13. Folliculitis/acne
14. Rashes
15. Myopathy
16. Neuropathy
17. Genital lesions
18. Ataxia
19. Decreased cognition
20. Depression

Key Signs

• Generalized wasting	• Skin rashes
• Hairy leukoplakia	• Tinea infections
• Oral candidiasis	• Decreased cognition
• Lymphadenopathy	• Myopathy
	• Neuropathy

Laboratory Tests

1. HIV diagnosis: Seroconversion is nearly always within 3 to 6 months of HIV exposure.
   a. HIV enzyme-linked immunosorbent assay (ELISA)
   b. Western blot for confirmation
2. Follow up with periodic CD4 counts
3. Complete blood count (CBC) with differential
4. Chemistry panel (SMA-20)
5. Stool studies, if indicated (ovum and parasites, routine culture, fecal leukocytes, *Clostridium difficile* toxin, colon biopsy if other tests are negative)
6. Purified protein derivative (PPD) with control
7. Pap smears
8. Serologic tests for syphilis (RPR/VDRL)
9. Biopsies of uncertain skin and mucous membrane lesions
10. Sputum for culture, acid-fast, *Pneumocystis carinii* smear, if indicated
11. Iron studies, B$_{12}$, folate
12. Cerebrospinal fluid (CSF) studies if indicated
13. Antinuclear antibodies (ANA), sedimentation rate

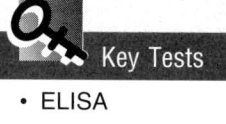

Key Tests

• ELISA	• CBC with differential
• Western blot	• Stool studies
• CD4 count	• Sputum studies

Differential Diagnosis

1. Lymphoma
2. Leukemia
3. Other cancers
4. Tuberculosis
5. Malabsorption syndromes
6. Fungal/viral infections
7. Pneumonias
8. Mononucleosis
9. Systemic lupus erythematosus (SLE)/rheumatologic disorders
10. Subacute bacterial endocarditis

Treatment

Medication

1. Antiretroviral medications (CD4 count < 500 cells/μL or symptomatic)
   a. Zidovudine (AZT) (Retrovir): 100 mg 5 times a day or 200 mg orally t.i.d.
   b. Didanosine (ddI) (Videx): <60 kg: 100 mg orally b.i.d.; >60 kg: 200 mg orally b.i.d.
   c. Zalcitabine (ddC) (Hivid): <45 kg: 0.375 mg orally t.i.d.; >45 kg: 0.750 mg orally t.i.d.
2. *P. carinii* pneumonia (PCP) prophylaxis (CD4 count < 200 cells/μL, prior episode PCP, other HIV-related symptoms/signs)
   a. TMP-SMZ (Bactrim, Septra): one DS tablet orally 3 times per week or every day
   b. Pentamidine (NebuPent): 300 mg inhaled solution via breathing treatment every 4 weeks
   c. Dapsone: 25 to 50 mg orally b.i.d. or 50 to 100 mg orally every day or 200 mg orally every week
   d. Dapsone plus pyrimethamine, 75 mg orally every day, or TMP-SMZ, 15 mg/kg per day
   e. Clindamycin (Cleocin), 450 to 600 mg orally b.i.d.–t.i.d., plus primaquine, 15 mg orally every day
   f. Atovaquone (Mepron), 750 mg orally every day or b.i.d. with or without pyrimethamine
3. Tuberculosis prophylaxis: PPD+ without positive chest radiograph, anergic patients in high-risk areas: isoniazid (INH), 300 mg orally every day or 900 mg orally 2 days per week for 12 months
4. *Candida albicans* (oral)
   a. Ketoconazole (Nizoral), 400 mg orally every day for 14 days, then 200 mg orally every day or 7 consecutive days every month
   b. Fluconazole (Diflucan), 100 to 200 mg orally every day for 14 days, then 100 to 200 mg orally every week or 50 to 100 mg orally every day
   c. Clotrimazole (Mycelex) troches, 10 mg dissolved in the mouth 5 times a day
   d. Nystatin swish/swallow, 5 ml orally q.i.d.
5. Diarrhea (symptomatic treatment)
   a. Imodium, 4 mg orally, then 2 mg orally every 6 hours or p.r.n.
   b. Lomotil, 2.5 to 5 mg orally 3 to 6 times per day, then t.i.d. or p.r.n.
   c. Paregoric (0.4 mg morphine/ml), 5 to 10 ml orally every day q.i.d. or p.r.n.
   d. Octreotide (Sandostatin), 100 μg subcutaneously t.i.d., then increase for a maximum of 500 μg subcutaneously q.i.d.
6. Weight loss
   a. Megestrol (Megace), 80 mg orally t.i.d. (max. 800 mg orally daily)
   b. Dronabinol (Tetrahydrocannabinol, Marinol), 2.5 mg orally b.i.d. before meals

Diet

High protein, calories, vitamins, minerals, with small, frequent meals and generous fluids

Activity

As tolerated. Increased physical activity has not been shown to increase HIV progression.

Patient Education

1. Explain natural course of HIV and manifestations.
2. Explain safe sex/abstinence and encourage patient to inform appropriate others to be tested for HIV.
3. Educate/assist with housing, financial assistance, counseling.
4. Inform patient of the state's HIV reporting requirements.
5. Educate about laboratory tests and follow-up, medications, and oral/skin care.

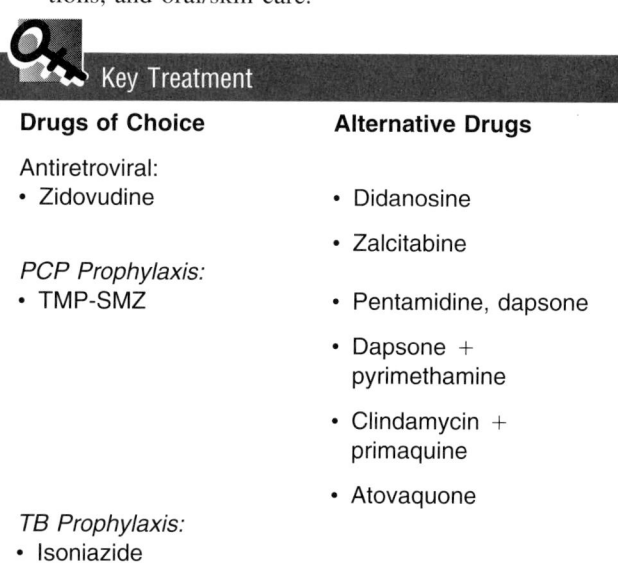

Key Treatment

Drugs of Choice	Alternative Drugs
Antiretroviral:	
• Zidovudine	• Didanosine
	• Zalcitabine
PCP Prophylaxis:	
• TMP-SMZ	• Pentamidine, dapsone
	• Dapsone + pyrimethamine
	• Clindamycin + primaquine
	• Atovaquone
TB Prophylaxis:	
• Isoniazide	

Follow-Up

1. CD4 count: every 6 months for CD4 > 600, every 3 months for CD4 count > 200 and < 600, every 3 months for CD4 < 200 to assess antiretroviral therapy's effect

2. High risk: regular PPD, chest radiograph

3. VDRL or RPR every year or less if indicated. If patient had syphilis in past, follow up with nontreponemal serologies at 1, 2, 3, 6, 9, and 12 months after treatment and annually afterward.

4. Regular oral, funduscopic, dental, physical, and pelvic examinations

Bibliography

DeVita VT, Hellman S, Rosenberg SA: AIDS: Etiology, Diagnosis, Therapy, and Prevention. Philadelphia: JB Lippincott, 1988, pp 107–120, 155–184.

Early HIV Infection Guideline Panel (Wafaa El-Sadr, et al): Managing early HIV infection. Am Fam Physician 1994(4):801–814.

Goldschmidt RH, Dong BJ: Treatment of AIDS and HIV-related conditions—1994, J Am Bd Fam Pract 1994;7(2):155–175.

Rakel RE: Conn's Current Therapy—1994. Philadelphia, WB Saunders, 1994; pp 33–40.

Wyngaarden JB, Smith LH, Bennett JC: Cecil Textbook of Medicine. Philadelphia, WB Saunders, 1992; pp 1908–1909, 1928–1949.

192 Late Symptomatic HIV Infection

Philip C. Johnson

Etiology

1. Definition: CD4 count less than 300/mm³
2. Progressive destruction of CD4 cells by HIV infection places the person at risk for
   a. Opportunistic infections and routine infections
   b. Malignancies (e.g., Kaposi's sarcoma, B cell lymphoma)
   c. Sequelae related to immune imbalance
      (1) Drug allergies and sinusitis
      (2) Wasting syndrome

Symptoms

1. Depend on reactivation of previous infectious diseases or exposures to new infections
2. Fever invariably seen with infectious diseases
3. Other symptoms depend on the organ systems affected
4. Headache: may be associated with fever
5. Seizures
6. Blindness and blurred vision
7. Dyspnea
8. Diarrhea
9. Weight loss
   a. Febrile illnesses
   b. Odynophagia and dysphagia
   c. *Mycobacterium avium* complex
      (1) Presents with abdominal complaints and fever
      (2) CD4 less than 100/mm³

Key Symptoms

- Headache
- Seizures
- Blindness and blurred vision
- Dyspnea
- Diarrhea
- Weight loss

Clinical Findings

1. Tachypnea
   a. Best early indication of a pulmonary process
   b. May be seen in septic shock
   c. Pulse oximetry not useful because most patients maintain adequate oxygen saturation by increasing their respiratory rate
2. Oral lesions
   a. Candidiasis: reddened satellite lesions or cottage cheese–like plaques
   b. Herpes simplex: shallow-based ulcers
3. Retinitis and papilledema
4. Dullness on chest percussion
   a. Pleural effusions unlikely in *Pneumocystis carinii* pneumonia (PCP)
   b. Can be seen with other pulmonary processes
5. Hepatomegaly, splenomegaly, and lymphadenopathy
6. Cranial nerve palsies

Key Signs

- Tachypnea
- Oral lesions
- Retinitis and papilledema
- Dullness on chest percussion
- Hepatomegaly, splenomegaly, and lymphadenopathy
- Cranial nerve palsies

Laboratory Tests

1. CD4 count is main indicator, but it can vary widely.
2. p24 antigenemia is present in late-stage infection.
3. Tests for specific diseases
   a. Aphthous ulcers: exclude herpes simplex and cytomegalovirus (CMV)
   b. Candidiasis: smear and culture in difficult cases
   c. *Coccidioides immitis*
      (1) Culture
      (2) Spherule found in bronchial secretions or sputum
      (3) Serology is useful
      (4) Skin testing invariably negative
   d. Community-acquired pneumonia
      (1) Lobular infiltrate on chest roentgenogram
      (2) Gram's stain with bacterial organisms
      (3) Resident oral flora influenced by antibiotics
   e. Cryptococcal meningitis
      (1) Cryptococcal antigen in serum or cerebrospinal fluid (CSF) positive in 97 per cent
      (2) India ink test of CSF positive in 75 per cent
      (3) Fungal culture
   f. CMV
      (1) Viral culture with determination of CMV early antigen
      (2) CMV IgM serology
      (3) Pathology: frequently negative

g. Diarrhea
   (1) Fecal leukocytes indicate diffuse colonic inflammation.
   (2) Bacterial, acid-fast bacilli (AFB) culture
   (3) Parasite examination including *Cryptosporidium parvum*
   (4) *Clostridium difficile* toxin assay
h. Kaposi's sarcoma of the lung
   (1) Bronchoscopy
i. *Mycobacterium avium* complex
   (1) Lysis centrifugation blood culture
   (2) Bone marrow culture and smear
   (3) Stool culture
j. *Pneumocystis carinii* pneumonia
   (1) Interstitial infiltrates on chest roentgenogram
   (2) Elevated lactate dehydrogenase (LDH)
   (3) Increased A-a gradient on arterial blood gas analysis
   (4) Sputum or pulmonary secretions show organism after Giemsa staining.
   (5) Atypical presentations for people taking aerosolized pentamidine prophylaxis
k. Progressive disseminated histoplasmosis
   (1) Histoplasma antigen by RIA of urine or serum
   (2) Lysis centrifugation blood culture
   (3) Bone marrow examination or peripheral smear shows yeast
   (4) Biopsy of skin lesions
   (5) Elevated LDH, ferritin
l. Progressive multifocal leukoencephalopathy
   (1) Fluffy or diffuse non–contrast-enhancing subcortical white matter lesions on computed tomography (CT) of brain
   (2) Brain biopsy
   (3) No treatment, and so empiric treatment of toxoplasmosis is usually tried first
m. Toxoplasmosis
   (1) Multiple spherical ring-enhancing lesions with mass effect on CT of brain
   (2) Toxoplasma serology helpful if there is a seroconversion
   (3) Toxoplasma IgM-positive
   (4) Response to empiric therapy establishes the diagnosis. It usually takes 2 weeks.
n. Tuberculosis
   (1) AFB smear and culture
   (2) Knowledge about PPD status or exposures
   (3) Diagnosis of tuberculous meningitis is difficult—CSF sugar normal or low, CSF protein modest increase, lymphocytic pleocytosis

Key Tests

- CD4 count
- Fecal leukocytes
- Chest roentgenogram
- Cryptococcal antigen
- Lumbar puncture with opening pressure
- Lysis centrifugation blood culture
- Fiberoptic bronchoscopy
- Histoplasma antigen by RIA
- Automated chemistry
- Arterial blood gases
- CT of brain

Differential Diagnosis

1. Side effects from medications
2. Other infectious disease processes or multiple infections
   a. Cryptococcal meningitis
      (1) Cranial nerve palsies
      (2) Nuchal rigidity
      (3) Headache that improves after spinal tap and relief of increased intracranial pressure
      (4) Blurred vision and papilledema
   b. Toxoplasmosis
   c. Progressive multifocal leukoencephalopathy
   d. B cell lymphoma
   e. Tuberculosis
   f. Cytomegalovirus retinitis
   g. *Pneumocystis carinii* pneumonia
   h. Progressive disseminated histoplasmosis
   i. *Coccidioides immitis*
   j. Kaposi's sarcoma of the lung
   k. Community-acquired pneumonia
   l. Mucocutaneous candidiasis
   m. Oral herpes
   n. Aphthous ulcers
   o. Malabsorption
   p. Hepatitis B or C
   q. *Mycobacterium avium* complex
   r. Syphilis

Treatment

Primary Therapy for HIV

1. Most people have already started zidovudine by this time.
2. Resistance to zidovudine occurs more quickly in patients with advanced disease, within 9 months in persons with CD4 under 300/mm³.
3. At this point zalcitabine, in addition to zidovudine, is indicated.

4. Patients with new opportunistic infections on zidovudine are switched to didanosine, or zalcitabine is added to zidovudine.

5. Zidovudine and didanosine combination is under study.

Prophylaxis

1. Candidiasis

   a. Clotrimazole (Mycelex) troches t.i.d.

   b. Nystatin swish and swallow t.i.d.

   c. Ketoconazole (Nizoral) 200 mg orally daily on an empty stomach with citrus juice

2. Herpes simplex: acyclovir (Zovirax), 200 mg orally t.i.d.

3. Influenza: yearly vaccination

4. *Mycobacterium avium* complex: Rifabutin (Mycobutin), 300 mg orally daily when CD4 $<100/mm^3$

5. *Pneumocystis carinii* pneumonia

   a. Use when CD4 $<200/mm^3$ or CD4 <20 per cent.

   b. Trimethoprim/sulfamethoxazole (Bactrim, Septra), one double strength tablet orally every Monday, Wednesday, and Friday

   c. Dapsone, 100 mg every Monday, Wednesday, and Friday

   d. Aerosolized pentamidine, 300 mg via Respirgard nebulizer

6. Pneumococcal pneumonia: vaccination once in a lifetime

7. Tuberculosis: isoniazid, 300 mg orally daily for 1 year if PPD-positive or at high risk

8. Varicella zoster: acyclovir, 800 mg b.i.d.

Treatment of Opportunistic Infections

1. Aphthous ulcers

   a. Symptomatic therapy

   b. Trial therapy for CMV if lesions severe

2. Candidiasis

   a. Clotrimazole (Mycelex) troches q 4 hr

   b. Ketoconazole (Nizoral), 200 mg orally daily, taken on empty stomach with citrus juice

   c. Fluconazole (Diflucan), 200 mg orally daily (most expensive option)

3. *Coccidioides immitis*

   a. Amphotericin B, 2.5 gm total dose

   b. Suppression therapy with fluconazole, 400 mg orally daily

4. Community-acquired pneumonia

   a. Cefotaxime (Claforan), 2 gm intravenously q 8 hr, and erythromycin, 500 mg intravenously q 6 hr

5. Cryptococcal meningitis

   a. Amphotericin B, 0.7 mg/kg intravenously for 14 days, then fluconazole, 400 mg orally daily for suppression; if flucytosine used with amphotericin B, 100 mg/kg q 6 hr.

b. Control of intracranial pressure is vital to prevent complications.

   (1) Measure opening pressure initially.

   (2) If more than 18 cm H_2O, remove enough CSF to decrease pressure.

   (3) Retap with symptoms of headache, meningismus, or cranial nerve palsies.

   (4) Some patients require a lumboperitoneal shunt.

   (5) Increased intracranial pressure can occur after successful treatment is started.

   (6) Risk of herniation even with very high pressures is extremely small.

WARNING

Permanent complications of cryptococcal meningitis result from increased intracranial pressure. The infection attacks the subarachnoid villi that reabsorb produced CSF. Increased pressures can occur even after appropriate antifungal therapy has started. *Measure opening pressures and remove CSF if necessary.*

---

6. Cytomegalovirus

   a. Ganciclovir (Cytovene), 5.0 mg/kg intravenously q 12 hr for two weeks, then 6.0 mg/kg intravenously daily for 5 days each week

   b. Foscarnet (Foscavir), 60 mg/kg intravenously (infuse over 2 hours) q 8 hr for 2 to 3 weeks, then 90 to 120 mg/kg intravenously daily

7. Diarrhea

   a. Trial of ciprofloxacin (Cipro), 500 mg orally q 12 hr for 5 days, and metronidazole (Flagyl), 250 mg orally q 8 hr for 7 days unless specific pathogen is known

   b. Symptomatic treatment with loperamide, 2 mg orally q 6 hr in the absence of dysentery

8. Kaposi's sarcoma of the lung

   a. Vincristine (Oncovin), 0.05 to 0.1 mg/kg/week intravenously

   b. Do not give next dose until white cell count exceeds $4000/mm^3$.

9. *Mycobacterium avium* complex

   a. All regimens have clarithromycin, 500 to 1000 mg orally q 12 hr (azithromycin is a second-line agent.)

   b. In addition one or more of the following drugs

      (1) Ciprofloxacin, 500 mg orally q 12 hr

      (2) Rifampin, 600 mg orally daily

      (3) Ethambutol, 15 mg/kg orally daily

      (4) Amikacin (Amikin), 7.5 mg/kg intravenously daily

10. *Pneumocystis carinii* pneumonia

    a. Trimethoprim/sulfamethoxazole (Bactrim, Septra), 2 double-strength tablets q 6 hr for 21 days or TMP/SMX IV (equivalent of TMP 5 mg/kg daily intravenously q 6 hr) for 21 days

    b. Atovaquone (Mepron), 750 mg orally q 8 hr

       (1) Take with food; food increases absorption.

       (2) Mild cases only

    c. Dapsone, 100 mg orally daily and trimethoprim, 5 mg/kg orally q 6 hr for 21 days

    d. Pentamidine isethionate

       (1) 4 mg/kg intravenously daily

       (2) Aerosolized 600 mg via Respirgard nebulizer daily for 14 days

    e. Prednisone, 40 mg orally q 12 hr (or equivalent) for 5 days; then 40 mg orally daily for 5 days, then 20 mg orally daily for remainder of PCP therapy if

       (1) PCP documented

       (2) Po_2 under 60 mm Hg on room air

11. Progressive disseminated histoplasmosis

    a. Amphotericin, 0.7 mg/kg IV daily until stable, then itraconazole, 200 mg orally q 12 hr

    b. Itraconazole (Sporanox) 200 mg orally q 12 hr if patient is stable

12. Progressive multifocal leukoencephalopathy

    a. Empiric treatment for toxoplasmosis usually tried for 2 weeks

    b. High-dose AZT and cytarabine experimental treatment

13. Toxoplasmosis

    a. Pyrimethamine, 50 to 75 mg orally daily, and clindamycin, 450 mg orally q 8 hr (or 600 mg intravenously q 6 hr) plus folinic acid, 10 mg orally daily

    b. Sulfisoxazole can be added if patient is allergic to pyrimethamine or clindamycin.

    c. Steroids are needed if there is brain edema on CT.

14. Tuberculosis—combination therapy

    a. Isoniazid, 300 mg orally daily, with pyridoxine, 25 mg orally daily

    b. Rifampin, 600 mg orally daily

    c. Pyrazinamide, 15 to 25 mg/kg/day

    d. Ethambutol, 15 mg/kg/day

    e. Can simplify regimen when susceptibility is known

Key Treatment

- Primary therapy for HIV: zidovudine plus zalcitabine or didanosine

Follow-Up

1. All infections and malignancies are likely to be chronic and recurrent at this stage.

2. Resistance to treatment can develop.

Bibliography

Bartlett JG: Antiretroviral therapy in HIV-infected patients: Update. Infect Dis in Clin Pract 1994;3:340–344.

Cohen PT, Sande MA, Volberding PA (eds): The AIDS Knowledge Base. 2nd ed. Boston, Little, Brown, 1994.

Hammer SM, Kessler HA, Saag MS: Issues in combination antiretroviral therapy: A review. JAIDS 1994;7 (suppl 2):524–537.

Hirsch MS, D'Aquila RT: Therapy for human immunodeficiency virus infection. N Engl J Med 1993;328:1686–1695.

Sanford JP, Sande MA, et al: The Sanford Guide to HIV/AIDS Therapy. Dallas, Texas, Antimicrobial Therapy, Inc., 1993–1994.

193 Drug Allergy

David L. Smith

Etiology

1. False history of drug reaction: This may be suspected with a detailed, accurate history.

   a. Specific drug allergies cannot be inherited. Patients may believe they are allergic to a drug because an ancestor was allergic to it.

   b. Vague reactions occurring in early childhood are usually irreproducible in adult life.

   c. Side effects may be mistaken for allergy, for example, nausea from codeine or coincidence such as weight gain. Symptoms of overdosage despite usual dose administration may occur due to drug interactions or decreased metabolism, as in the elderly.

   d. If an allergic reaction has not actually occurred, the patient should be instructed and the medical record corrected.

2. Reactions associated with particular drug classes

   a. β-lactams are the drugs most frequently associated with allergic skin reactions.

      (1) Reactions may be Coombs' and Gell class I (IgE-mediated, anaphylactic), class III (serum sickness), or less well defined, such as maculopapular rashes.

      (2) Cephalosporins produce reactions in 5 to 15 per cent of penicillin-sensitive patients, with third-generation cephalosporins perhaps less likely to react than first-generation ones. Imipenem also may cross-react, but aztreonam does not.

      (3) Cefaclor may be particularly likely to cause serum sickness–like reactions; allergy to cefaclor does not usually predict allergy to other cephalosporins.

   b. Sulfonamides are associated with frequent class I and maculopapular rashes and drug fevers and are the most frequent cause of Stevens-Johnson syndrome (SJS) and toxic epidermal necrolysis (TEN) reactions. Cross-reactions may occur with other sulfa-containing compounds such as thiazides.

   c. The cause of most reactions to vancomycin ("red man" syndrome) is unclear. Patients will often respond to slowing the infusion rate and have been desensitized successfully. The role of H_1 antagonists in treatment is also unclear.

   d. Nonsteroidal anti-inflammatory drugs (NSAIDs) are associated with urticaria and aspirin-sensitive asthma, probably by excess leukotriene production; the latter may be benefited by desensitization.

Asthmatics without a history of aspirin sensitivity should not be denied the benefit of NSAIDs for other conditions.

   e. Angiotensin-converting enzyme (ACE) inhibitors are associated with chronic cough and angioedema. Life-threatening angioedema may occur months to years after starting treatment. ACE inhibitors should not be given to patients with any prior history of angioedema.

   f. β-blockers can precipitate asthma in patients with underlying bronchial hyperreactivity and should not be given to patients who are at risk for anaphylaxis, such as those on allergy immunotherapy, because they block the action of epinephrine.

   g. Anticonvulsants are frequent causes of maculopapular rashes and serum sickness and have been associated with hepatic necrosis and aplastic anemia.

   h. Local anesthetic reactions are seldom reproducible and may be most frequently due to vasovagal syncope, anxiety, or inadvertent systemic injection, particularly if epinephrine is present in the preparation.

   i. Radiocontrast media (RCM) and opioids cause mast cell histamine release by non–IgE-mediated mechanisms. Repeat reactions to RCM occur in only 20 to 30 per cent of cases, even without premedication, but are unpredictable. These have nothing to do with seafood allergy; allergy to iodine has not been described.

   j. Unexpected reactions may be due to agents other than the "active ingredient." Excipients, preservatives, and even latex in intravenous tubing may on occasion cause true allergic reactions.

   k. Hemolytic anemia and drug-induced lupus may be due to autoimmune antibodies stimulated by a drug, such as methyldopa or penicillamine. Drug withdrawal will almost always bring about rapid cessation of symptoms.

Drugs Frequently Causing Allergic-Like Reactions

• β-lactams	• Sulfonamides
• Other antibiotics	• NSAIDs
• ACE inhibitors	• β-blockers

Diagnosis

1. The nature of the reaction frequently will reveal the likely causative drug and the likelihood of a repeat reaction. Most allergic reactions have skin manifestations.

a. Urticaria, angioedema, and anaphylactoid manifestations: These imply mast cell degranulation. This is not always by an IgE-mediated mechanism, but if it is, a repeat reaction is likely.

b. Morbilliform eruptions: These are poorly understood. They may represent a coincident viral infection (e.g., roseola) or be immunologically mediated but are often not reproducible. Progression to Stevens-Johnson syndrome (SJS) or toxic epidermal necrolysis (TEN) is rare.

c. Photodermatitis: This may be a toxic or immunologically mediated phenomenon.

d. Contact dermatitis and fixed drug eruptions: These are delayed hypersensitivity responses and are not amenable to desensitization or suppression other than by potent medications such as oral corticosteroids.

e. SJS and TEN: The etiology of these is unknown; an immunologic mechanism is presumed. Although sulfonamides are most often implicated, many other drugs as well as viral infections may be responsible.

f. Reactions involving other organ systems

(1) Hematologic: Coombs-positive hemolytic anemia, thrombocytopenia, and neutropenia are immunologically mediated and may be mild or severe. Peripheral eosinophilia is rarely accompanied by eosinophilic infiltration of heart, lung, or other tissues.

(2) Hepatic reactions may be hepatocellular with liver function abnormalities and possible hepatic necrosis, cholestatic with reversible jaundice, or granulomatous.

(3) Renal reactions may be nephrotic (edema, proteinuria), nephritic (hematuria), or mixed.

(4) Serum sickness (rash, fever, malaise) may be due to IgE- and IgG-mediated (immune complex) mechanisms. Drug fever may be due to interleukin-1 (IL-1) release from macrophages.

Key Signs and Symptoms

• Urticaria/angioedema	• Hemolytic anemia
• Morbilliform rash	• Liver/kidney dysfunction
• Eczematoid rash	• Fever

2. Diagnostic testing

a. Allergy skin testing: This is useful for predicting IgE-mediated reactions to polypeptides and proteins such as heterologous serums (but not to predict serum sickness), local anesthetics, and neuromuscular blockers. A negative skin test for β-lactam allergy (which is due to metabolites

rather than the parent drug) will be reliable only when a wide variety of metabolites ("minor determinants") become commercially available.

b. Skin and in vitro testing for IgE to other agents must still be considered as a research procedure.

c. Certain metabolic phenotypes predispose to drug reaction; for instance, the slow acetylator is more likely to react to sulfonamides. Monitoring and appropriate adjustment of serum levels may reduce the frequency or severity of reactions. Some reactions, such as hydralazine-induced lupus, are HLA-linked.

d. Patch and phototesting may reveal the etiology of contact or photodermatitis.

e. If an anaphylactic reaction seems unlikely and alternative drugs are unavailable, it may be rational to give the patient a full challenge dose, preferably orally, of the drug. The patient must be observed inhouse for at least an hour and by telephone overnight, and medical personnel must be prepared to treat anaphylaxis.

f. Drug package inserts are usually helpful in determining the frequency with which hematologic, hepatic, and renal systems should be monitored.

Key Tests

• Allergy and patch skin testing

• Serum level and hepatic/renal monitoring

• Challenge dosing

Treatment

1. Treatment of ongoing drug reactions

a. Withdrawal of the drug may be the only treatment required.

b. Rapid but sometimes temporary relief from urticaria/angioedema can be produced by 1:1000 epinephrine, 0.3 to 0.5 ml subcutaneously, which can be repeated every 20 minutes. This may be followed by oral or intravenous antihistamines (e.g., Benadryl, 25 to 50 mg) and prednisone stat and then every 6 hours for 4 doses in an effort to prevent a prolonged or biphasic course. Wheezing may be treated with inhaled bronchodilators. More serious anaphylactoid reactions are covered in Chapter 195.

c. Symptomatic treatment of morbilliform rashes and serum sickness may require 1 to 2 weeks of treatment with antihistamines, and/or systemic corticosteroids.

d. The use of corticosteroids in SJS is controversial. TEN is treated as a burn; prognosis depends on the amount of skin loss.

e. Patients may sometimes be treated through a reaction. A sulfonamide-induced maculopapular rash in HIV-positive patients will often resolve spontaneously, as will symptomatically treated urticarial reactions to β-lactams. However, any suggestion of SJS/TEN requires immediate discontinuation.

2. Prevention of drug reactions

a. An alternative drug of a different class should be used whenever possible.

b. Premedication may be successful for non-IgE-mediated (anaphylactoid) reactions such as to RCM but will *not* prevent true IgE-mediated reactions. It consists of

   (1) Prednisone, 50 mg 13, 7, and 1 hour prior to RCM

   (2) Diphenhydramine, 1 mg/kg 1 hour prior

   (3) Some authorities recommend cimetidine, 4 mg/kg (or equivalent), and/or ephedrine, 25 mg, 1 hour prior.

   (4) The use of a low-osmolar agent

c. Desensitization to antimicrobials, allopurinol, and polypeptides (e.g., insulin) is frequently successful but temporary; if therapy is interrupted, allergic manifestations will appear again. Desensitization should be attempted only under the supervision of an experienced allergist.

Follow-Up

1. Patients with bona fide drug allergy should be educated in reference to drugs that are likely or not likely to cause problems. A written list may be helpful.

Key Treatment

- Discontinue drug
- Antihistamines, corticosteroids for prolonged reactions
- Premedication or desensitization
- Epinephrine for urticaria/anaphylaxis
- Use of alternative drugs

2. Unnecessary medications should always be avoided. For instance, antibiotics should only be prescribed when a bacterial infection is highly likely.

3. Patients with a history of life-threatening reactions may best be given a medical warning bracelet and epinephrine injection kit.

Bibliography

Bayard PJ, Berger TG, Jacobson MA: Drug hypersensitivity reactions and human immunodeficiency virus disease. J Acquired Immune Deficiency Syndromes 1992;5:1237–1257.

Bigby M, Jick S, Jick H, Arndt K: Drug-induced cutaneous reactions. JAMA 1986;256:3358–3363.

Deswarte JR: Drug allergy. *In* Patterson R (ed): Allergic Diseases: Diagnosis and Management, 4th ed. Philadelphia, JB Lippincott, 1993, pp 395–552.

Petz LD: Immunologic cross-reactivity between penicillins and cephalosporins: A review. J Infect Dis 1978;137(S):S74–79.

Sullivan TJ: Drug allergy. *In* Middleton E, Reed CE, Ellis EF, et al (eds): Allergy: Principles and Practice, 4th ed, vol 2. St Louis, Mosby–Year Book, 1993, pp 1726–1746.

194 Food Allergy

W. Anderson Nish

General

1. Adverse food reaction—any untoward reaction after the ingestion of a food
   a. "Food intolerances" account for most reactions and are not immunologically mediated.
   b. "Food allergies" refer to those which are immunologically mediated.
2. Estimated incidence of food allergy is 4 per cent in children and 1 per cent in adults, although studies vary, and up to 40 per cent of adults report adverse food reactions.
3. The role of food allergy has been well established in some patients with diseases such as atopic dermatitis, anaphylaxis, chronic urticaria, food protein gastroenteropathy, and eosinophilic gastroenteritis but is unproven in others such as migraine, chronic asthma or rhinitis, irritable bowel syndrome, or inflammatory bowel disease.

Etiology

1. Children—cow's milk, egg, soy, peanut, wheat
2. Adults—peanut, true nuts, fish, shellfish
3. Oral allergy syndrome—fresh fruits, vegetables
4. Food-associated exercise-induced anaphylaxis—wheat, celery, shellfish
5. Increased incidence of food allergy in young children and atopic individuals

Symptoms

1. Oral allergy syndrome—pruritus, tingling, and edema of oral mucosa, lips, tongue, and pharynx
2. Generalized reactions
   a. Cutaneous—pruritus, urticaria/angioedema, increased eczema
   b. Respiratory—shortness of breath, chest tightness, cough, hoarseness, rhinitis
   c. Gastrointestinal—cramping, diarrhea, nausea, emesis
   d. General—syncope, feeling of impending doom
   e. Genitourinary—uterine cramping, incontinence

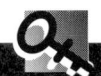

Key Symptoms

• Pruritus	• Urticaria/angioedema
• Increased eczema	• Chest tightness
• Shortness of breath	• Abdominal cramping
• Diarrhea	

Clinical Findings

1. Cutaneous—urticaria/angioedema, eczematous lesions, flushing
2. Respiratory—wheezing, rhinorrhea, stridor
3. Cardiovascular—hypotension, tachycardia
4. Ocular—conjunctivitis

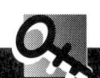

Key Signs

• Urticaria/angioedema	• Flushing
• Wheezing	• Oropharyngeal edema
• Hypotension	• Tachycardia

Laboratory Tests

1. Elimination diet followed by reintroduction, for chronic symptoms only
2. Prick skin tests with appropriate extracts
   a. Sensitive for IgE-mediated allergy
   b. Not specific; must be correlated with history
3. Radioallergosorbent testing (RAST)
   a. Also detects IgE antibody
   b. Less sensitive than skin testing
   c. Consider if cannot skin test because of medicines or concern about anaphylaxis in a very food-sensitive patient or one with extensive skin disease
4. Double-blind, placebo-controlled food challenge
   a. "Gold standard" for confirming food allergy
   b. Must be done under carefully controlled conditions
5. No role for leukocytotoxic testing or provocation/neutralization

Key Tests

• Prick skin tests
• Double-blind, placebo-controlled food challenge

Differential Diagnosis

1. Reactions to food additives
   a. Monosodium glutamate—Chinese restaurant syndrome (in some cases may be caused by histamine in foods)
   b. Sulfites—may trigger asthma
2. Food toxicity
   a. Bacterial—*Salmonella, Shigella, Escherichia coli*
   b. Toxins—*Vibrio,* botulism, ciguatera, scombroid

3. Pharmacologic effects
   a. Alcohol—vasodilatation and flushing
   b. Tyramine in wine and cheese headache
4. Enzyme deficiencies
   a. Disaccharidase deficiency—lactose intolerance
   b. Galactosemia
5. Gastrointestinal disease
   a. Gastroesophageal reflux
   b. Inflammatory bowel disease
6. Functional/psychological

Treatment

1. The only appropriate treatment for food allergy at present is avoidance.
2. There is no current role for food immunotherapy.

Medication

1. Patients with suspected or proven food anaphylaxis must be given an epinephrine kit.
2. Proper instruction for use of epinephrine kit is essential.
   a. Patient must have it available at all times.
   b. Patient and caretakers/family members must know how to use it.
   c. Administer for reaction that is initially severe or with any progressive symptoms; then seek care at an emergency room.

Diet

1. Elimination diet trial for chronic symptoms.
2. Strict avoidance for foods causing anaphylaxis.
3. For food allergy prophylaxis, breast-feeding and/or use of hypoallergenic formulas during the first 6 months of life combined with delaying introduction of the most allergenic foods may at least delay the onset of food allergy in atopy-prone infants.

Patient Education

1. Instruct in proactive avoidance of food(s) causing allergy.
2. Instruct about special caution at day care, school, parties, and restaurants.
3. Explain ubiquitous nature of some allergens such as peanuts.

4. Patients with exercise-induced anaphylaxis should not eat implicated foods for at least 4 to 6 hours prior to exercise.
5. Medic-Alert bracelet stating food allergy

Key Treatment

- Food avoidance
- Epinephrine kit

Follow-Up

1. Periodic follow-up to reinforce education and renew epinephrine kit if necessary
2. Particularly in children, cow's milk, soy, and egg may be tolerated after a period of time.
3. Allergy to peanuts, true nuts, fish, and shellfish is likely to persist.
4. Follow growth of patients on a restricted diet.
5. Egg-allergic patients need further evaluation prior to receiving measles-mumps-rubella, influenza, or yellow fever vaccines.

Bibliography

For more information on the general approach to diagnosis of food allergy, see

Burks AW, Sampson HA: Diagnostic approaches to the patient with suspected food allergies. J Pediatr 1992;121:564–571.

For more information on double-blind, placebo-controlled food challenge, see

Bock SA, Sampson HA, Atkins FM, et al: Double-blind, placebo-controlled food challenge as an office procedure: a manual. J Allergy Clin Immunol 1988;82:986–997.

For more information on severe allergic reactions to foods, see

Sampson HA, Mendelson L, Rosen JP: Fatal and near-fatal anaphylactic reactions to food in children and adolescents. N Engl J Med 1992;327:380–384.

For more information on reactions to food additives, see

Weber RW: Food additives and allergy. Ann Allergy 1993; 70:183–190.

For more information on recent advances in food allergy, see

Anderson JA: Milestones marking the knowledge of adverse reactions to foods in the decade of the 1980s. Ann Allergy 1994;72:143–154.

195 Anaphylaxis

James K. Buck II

Etiology

1. Anaphylaxis is a clinical syndrome of systemic allergic response to any of a number of potential inciting agents. Through one of several initial pathways, these agents cause the release of mediators from mast cells and basophils throughout the body. These mediators include histamine, platelet-activating factor, leukotrienes LTC_4, LTD_4, and LTE_4 (slow-reacting substance of anaphylaxis), and others. They act on blood vessels, airways, and other tissues and are responsible for the physiologic effects that comprise the syndrome.

2. Virtually any substance from a number of types might induce anaphylaxis in a given susceptible individual. An exhaustive list of inciting agents is beyond the scope of this text. Some of the more common causes of anaphylaxis are

   a. Antibiotics
      (1) Penicillins
      (2) Cephalosporins
      (3) Sulfonamides
      (4) Ciprofloxacin
      (5) Vancomycin
      (6) Amphotericin B

   b. Other drugs and therapeutic agents
      (1) Insulin
      (2) Protamine
      (3) Allergen extracts
      (4) Vaccines
      (5) Opiates
      (6) Radiocontrast media
      (7) Aspirin and nonsteroidal anti-inflammatory drugs (NSAIDs)
      (8) Streptokinase

   c. Foods and food additives
      (1) Nuts
      (2) Fish
      (3) Shellfish
      (4) Legumes
      (5) Egg whites
      (6) Dairy products (especially milk)
      (7) Fruits and berries
      (8) Metabisulfites

   d. Blood products
      (1) Whole blood
      (2) Plasma
      (3) Immunoglobulin
      (4) Cryoprecipitate

   e. Venoms
      (1) Fire ant venom
      (2) Hymenoptera venom (beesting)
      (3) Snake venom

   f. Miscellaneous
      (1) Latex
      (2) Exercise

Symptoms

1. Anaphylactic reactions are generally rapid, and initial symptoms are typically noticed seconds to minutes after exposure. The vast majority of these reactions occur within 1 hour of antigen exposure.

2. Individual patients' symptoms may vary widely in scope and severity. A given patient may present with any subset or combination of the following:

   a. General: Warmth, flushing, and generalized pruritus (as well as nasal, palatal, and ocular pruritus in particular) may be seen. Other general complaints may include a feeling of faintness and a sense of impending doom.

   b. Respiratory: Initial symptoms may include sneezing, cough, rhinorrhea, hoarseness, or "a lump in the throat" and may progress quickly to shortness of breath and dyspnea.

   c. Cardiovascular: Palpitations or a sensation of faintness may be present.

   d. Gastrointestinal: Symptoms may include a peculiar taste (possibly metallic), dysphagia, nausea, bloating, and/or abdominal cramping.

3. Pulmonary and/or cardiovascular symptoms and signs are the most potentially troublesome, since pulmonary complications account for the large majority of anaphylactic deaths, followed by cardiovascular complications.

Key Symptoms

• Pruritus	• Sneezing
• Lump in throat	• Abdominal cramping
• Hoarseness	• Nausea
• Shortness of breath	• Palpitations
• Cough	• Faintness

Clinical Findings

1. Clinical signs also may vary widely from patient to patient. In the patient with profound anaphylactic

shock, there may be few or no distinguishing clinical features present.

2. Possible clinical findings include

a. Dermatologic: Classic skin manifestations include *urticaria,* usually pruritic and more prominent on the trunk and proximal limbs, and *angioedema,* usually seen as periorbital and circumoral edema. Generalized flushing also may be seen.

b. Respiratory: Early signs may include sneezing, cough, and/or rhinorrhea. These may progress rapidly to include wheezing, stridor, tachypnea, use of accessory muscles, and cyanosis, possibly leading to complete asphyxia.

c. Cardiovascular: Patients may manifest hypotension, shock, syncope, tachycardia, conduction defects, and dysrhythmias. Myocardial infarction may complicate anaphylaxis or its treatment in some patients.

d. Gastrointestinal: Signs may include vomiting, diarrhea, and/or bloating.

Key Signs

• Urticaria	• Stridor
• Angioedema	• Hypotension
• Flushing	• Shock
• Rhinorrhea	• Syncope
• Wheezing	• Tachycardia
• Tachypnea	• Vomiting

Laboratory Tests

1. The diagnosis of anaphylaxis is a clinical one, and laboratory studies are generally not helpful in making the diagnosis acutely.

2. General laboratory studies (electrocardiogram [ECG], arterial blood gases [ABGs]), are helpful in some patients in the acute setting for evaluating specific complications such as hypoxemia, cardiac dysrhythmias, and acid-base disruptions and in monitoring the response of these same areas to therapeutic measures.

3. Consider ECG, ABGs and the like in individual cases as signs, symptoms, and circumstances dictate.

Differential Diagnosis

1. In a patient who has collapsed or cannot give a history and who may lack urticaria or angioedema, the differential diagnosis may be extensive. One should consider

a. Other conditions associated with sudden loss of consciousness (e.g., acute myocardial infarction, arrhythmias, seizure disorders, vasovagal syncope)

b. Other conditions manifesting acute respiratory compromise (e.g., epiglottitis, status asthmaticus, foreign body aspiration, pulmonary embolus)

c. Other conditions with similar skin or respiratory findings (e.g., carcinoid syndrome, hereditary angioedema, mastocytosis)

2. Vasovagal syncope may be the most common similar syndrome but usually may be differentiated by the presence of bradycardia (as opposed to tachycardia in anaphylaxis) with diaphoresis and maintenance of blood pressure, as well as pale appearance (as opposed to generalized flushing) and lack of pruritus or true respiratory difficulty.

Treatment

1. The treatment of acute anaphylaxis must begin with prompt evaluation and recognition, since complications and death may occur within minutes. As in other medical emergencies, the initial management is aimed at establishing an effective airway and circulatory system.

2. General measures include establishing intravenous access and the administering of intravenous fluids (i.e., saline) and supplemental oxygen (by cannula, mask, or endotracheal tube, if necessary). Cardiac monitoring should be instituted.

Medication

1. *Epinephrine* is the initial drug of choice in treating acute anaphylactic reactions. Epinephrine is routinely administered as a subcutaneous or intramuscular injection of 0.01 ml/kg of aqueous epinephrine 1:1000 (maximum adult dose 0.3 to 0.5 ml). The dose may be repeated approximately every 5 to 10 minutes if symptoms persist or recur. For patients in profound circulatory collapse, continuous intravenous infusion of epinephrine may be necessary but should be used with extreme caution. An epinephrine drip may be started with 2 ml of 1:1000 solution added to 500 ml of saline at a rate of 2 to 20 μg/min.

2. Both H_1 and H_2 antihistamines are recommended for treatment of anaphylaxis. A suggested regimen would include diphenhydramine, 25 to 50 mg intravenously or intramuscularly, and ranitidine (Zantac), 50 mg intravenously. In the absence of hypotension, the use of an H_2 antihistamine is optional. Patients generally should be maintained on H_1 antihistamines orally every 6 hours for 48 hours after the initial attack to help protect against rebound and/or relapse.

3. Corticosteroids are too slow in onset of action to be efficacious in acute episodes of anaphylaxis; it is recommended that they be used early, primarily to prevent late-phase reactions or recurrences. Higher doses (i.e., hydrocortisone, 5 mg/kg intravenously) are given initially and are often followed by a quickly tapered oral regimen.

4. Other medications to consider in specific circumstances are
   a. Aerosolized β agonists (i.e., albuterol) to further combat bronchospasm (also may consider aminophylline)
   b. Atropine or isoproterenol for refractory bradycardia
   c. Dopamine or levarterenol for refractory hypotension (give adequate intravenous fluids for volume expansion first).
   d. Glucagon may be useful in patients on β-blocking drugs (which may make them refractory to epinephrine treatment).

Diet
1. The patient should be kept to nothing by mouth (NPO) until the acute episode is under control.
2. No other dietary restrictions apply, unless one or more foods are suspected as causative agents (in which case they should be avoided).

Activity
1. Patients with moderate systemic anaphylactic reactions should be monitored for at least 8 to 12 hours prior to discharge.
2. Those with severe, life-threatening reactions should be admitted to a hospital for continued evaluation and treatment.
3. There are no other specific limitations on activity once the acute event has been stabilized.

Patient Education
1. The patient should be counseled on the nature of his/her illness and the steps to take to avoid the offending agent(s) if possible.
2. Patients should be prescribed an emergency epinephrine kit (Ana-Kit, EpiPen) and instructed in its use in case of recurrent anaphylactic episodes.

Key Treatment

Drugs of Choice	Alternative Drugs
• Epinephrine (1:1000), 0.01 ml/kg subcutaneously or intramuscularly	• None (to epinephrine)
	• Hydroxyzine and others
• Diphenhydramine, 25 to 50 mg intramuscularly or intravenously	• Cimetidine and others
	• Methylprednisolone and others
• Ranitidine, 50 mg intravenously	
• Hydrocortisone, 5 mg/kg intravenously	

Follow-Up

All patients who experience significant anaphylactic reactions should be referred to a specialist in allergy and immunology for further evaluation, testing, counseling, and/or preventive therapy as specifically indicated.

Bibliography

Atkinson TP, Kaliner MA: Anaphylaxis. Med Clin North Am 1992;76:841–855.

Kyle JM: Exercise-induced pulmonary syndromes. Med Clin North Am 1994;78:413–421.

Lieberman P: The use of antihistamines in the prevention and treatment of anaphylaxis and anaphylactoid reactions. J Allergy Clin Immunol 1990;86:684–686.

Marquardt DL, Wasserman SI: Anaphylaxis. *In* Middleton E, Reed CE, Ellis EF (eds): Allergy Principles and Practice, 4th ed, vol 2. St. Louis, Mosby–Year Book, 1993, pp 1525–1536.

Reisman RE, Lieberman P (eds): Anaphylaxis and anaphylactoid reactions. Immunol Allergy Clin North Am 1992;12:501–690.

196 Common Musculoskeletal Symptoms

| Symptom | Neck Pain | *Kevin M. McKown* |

Neck pain is a very common problem in adults. Prior incidences of 35 per cent or more and prevalences of 10 per cent have been reported. The pain is usually self-limited, with 70 per cent of episodes resolving within 1 month. Once unusual and potentially serious causes of neck pain are excluded, treatment is conservative in almost all instances.

Differential Diagnosis

1. Cervical spondylosis
2. Neck strain/sprain
3. Radiculopathy
4. Cervical myelopathy
5. Trauma
6. Chronic pain syndrome
7. Rheumatoid arthritis (RA)
8. Torticollis
9. Neoplasm
10. Vertebral osteomyelitis
11. Referred pain—especially from the shoulder, diagraphm, apical lung, heart, and aorta
    a. Temporomandibular joint pain
    b. Bursitis, tendinitis, or arthritis of the shoulder
    c. Reflex sympathetic dystrophy
    d. Thoracic outlet syndrome
    e. Bronchogenic carcinoma
    f. Coronary artery disease
    g. Aortic dissection
    h. Peptic ulcer disease
    i. Pancreatitis
    j. Cholecystitis
12. Ankylosing spondylitis (AS) or other spondyloarthropathies
13. Giant cell arteritis, polymyalgia rheumatica
14. Paget's disease
15. Fibromyalgia
16. Meningitis

In most patients, a definite cause of neck pain cannot (and need not) be established, and the pain is attributed to neck strain or cervical spondylosis. Cervical spondylosis describes degenerative changes in disks, ligaments, and joints of the cervical vertebral column (which are ubiquitous with aging). Psychologic factors are important predictors of chronic, unexplained neck pain. History and physical examination will identify other causes of neck pain.

Refer to Ch. 188, Osteomyelitis; Ch. 201, TMJ Syndrome; Ch. 202, Osteoarthritis; Ch. 203, Rheumatoid Arthritis; Ch. 206, Myofascial Syndromes; and Ch. 295, Reflex Sympathetic Dystrophy.

History: Key Questions to Ask

1. Duration, onset, and course of pain?
2. Trauma?
3. Radiation of pain?
4. Character of pain and any radiation?
5. Better or worse with certain activities, movements?
6. Relieved by rest?
7. Numbness or weakness?
8. Loss of bowel or bladder control?
9. Fever, weight loss, other active problems?
10. Cancer, other past medical history?

Most neck pain lasts days to a few weeks, is nonradiating, and is influenced by movement and position. Cervical spondylosis pain may radiate short distances in a fairly constant, achy, nondermatomal fashion. Radiculopathy pain is intermittent, sharp, dermatomal, and can be associated with numbness and weakness. Pain improved by activity suggests a spondyloarthropathy. Pain *not* relieved by rest or which is progressive suggests infection or neoplasm. Bowel or bladder dysfunction or lower extremity numbness, weakness, or ataxia suggests myelopathy. Systemic complaints and past history may suggest infection, neoplasm, or referred pain. Patients with RA are prone to instability. Patients with AS are prone to fracture with trivial trauma. Psychosocial factors may be important in chronic cervical spondylosis pain.

Clinical Findings

1. Tenderness, loss of motion of neck, shoulders
2. Numbness or weakness of upper or lower extremities
3. Hypo- or hyperreflexia
4. General physical examination if *any* suspicious history

Neck pain *without* neck tenderness, loss of neck motion, or pain with neck motion suggests a referred cause. Nuchal rigidity suggests meningitis. Polyradiculopathy suggests neoplasm, infection, or widespread spondylosis. Lower extremity ataxia, hyperreflexia, or hypertonicity suggests myelopathy. A general physical examination should be done with any suggestion of an unusual source of neck pain.

WARNING

Never force a neck when evaluating range of motion.

Tests

1. Cervical radiographs (AP and lateral)
2. Magnetic resonance imaging (MRI) or computed tomography (CT)
3. Bone scan
4. Electromyography/nerve conduction velocity studies (EMG/NCVs)
5. Laboratory studies as indicated

Cervical radiographs can demonstrate evidence of neoplasm, osteomyelitis, fracture, or traumatic subluxation. In trauma or RA, add odontoid view. Gentle flexion-extension views may show instability in RA. Radiographs may be omitted in young patients with a straightforward, nontraumatic history and examination. Bone scans can demonstrate early osteomyelitis or neoplasm. MRI is superior to CT for soft tissue imaging; both are used for preoperative imaging. They should not be obtained routinely—many asymptomatic individuals have disk degeneration, herniated disks, or foraminal stenosis by MRI. EMG/NCV may be helpful preoperatively or in differentiating neurologic problems.

Management

1. Pain relief with relative rest, medications, physical modalities
2. Exercises—once there is improvement in pain
3. Surgery—occasionally indicated

Medication

1. Analgesics—acetaminophen, aspirin, nonsteroidal anti-inflammatory drugs (NSAIDs), mild narcotics
2. "Muscle relaxants"—benzodiazepines, cyclobenzaprine, methocarbamol

Activity

1. Relative rest. May use cervical pillow, soft cervical collar, traction

2. Physical modalities—such as hot, cold, ultrasound—may give relief.
3. Isometric exercises—once pain lessens

Patient Education

1. Reassurance as to self-limited nature of problem
2. Instruction on proper body positioning during daily activities

No treatment has been shown to alter the natural history of mechanical neck pain. Management is directed at patient comfort and the hope of secondary prevention by improving posture and muscle strength. Manipulation by skilled physicians should be used cautiously, if at all; neurologic catastrophes can result. Trigger point and epidural injections may give additional relief in skilled hands. Surgery is indicated for myelopathic symptoms; instability with neurologic abnormalities or severe pain, and severe radicular pain from a definable lesion not resolving after weeks to months of conservative therapy.

Follow-Up

1. Return in 2 to 4 weeks to reassess clinically for improvement.
2. Encourage patients to call for systemic or neurologic symptoms or unremitting pain.

PEARLS

- Unremitting pain suggests neoplasm, infection.
- Cervical myelopathy presents with lower extremity corticospinal tract signs.

B **Bibliography**

Bland JH: Disorders of the Cervical Spine, 2d ed. Philadelphia: WB Saunders, 1994.

Ellenberg MR, Monet JC, Treanor WJ: Cervical radiculopathy. Arch Phys Med Rehabil 1994; 75:342–352.

Mathews JA: Neck pain. *In* JM Klippel, PA Dieppe (eds): Rheumatology. London, Mosby–Year Book Europe, 1994, pp 5.5.1–14.

Nakano KK: Neck pain. *In* WN Kelley et al (eds): Textbook of Rheumatology. Philadelphia, WB Saunders, 1993, pp 397–416.

Thorn RP, Curd JG: A systemic approach to disorders of the cervical spine. Hosp Pract 1993;28:49–58.

Symptom **Whiplash**   *David C. Agerter*

"Whiplash" of the neck is a controversial term. Symptoms attributed to this syndrome are often vaguely described. Often the mechanisms of injuries are not fully understood. Many authorities would argue that "whiplash" should be used in historical terms only. However, the word is so well ingrained among practitioners that it still is used currently.

It would be best to describe the method of injury in terms of deceleration or acceleration forces. This would more accurately describe the mechanics of the force being hyperflexion or hyperextension.

The cervical spine and head may be subjected to six general types of injuries:

1. *Pure flexion injury* may result in posterior ligamentous injury with possible stable wedge fracture of a vertebral body.

2. *Flexion with a rotation injury* may cause posterior ligaments to rupture.

3. *Hyperextension injuries* may cause the possibility of vertebral fracturing. Hyperextension loading may cause rupturing of the disk and involvement of the anterior longitudinal ligament. If sufficient force is applied, there may be resultant spinal cord paralysis.

4. *Hyperextension with rotation* may be associated with fractures and dislocations.

5. *Vertical compression* is often seen with diving accidents. The vertical load shatters vertebral endplates and forces the nucleus of the disk into the vertebral body causing it to explode.

6. *Lateral flexion injuries* often occur from playing football. This may be associated with brachial plexus injuries, with or without compression fracture.

Differential Diagnosis

Whenever there is a head injury, one must always rule out any associated cervical spine involvement.

1. Myofascial sprain: An injury involving tearing of the muscle ligamentous components of the neck.

2. Herniated disk (also called "slipped disk"): The nucleus pulposus is extruded through a tear and annulus fibrosis with resulting nerve root irritation or compression.

3. Spinal stenosis: A narrowing of the cervical spinal canal that may predispose the patient to spinal cord or nerve injury with relatively minor trauma.

4. Cervical instability: Occurs after ligamentous injury. This may or may not be associated with cervical fractures.

5. Fractures: There is injury to the bony components of the spine, usually resulting in compression of vertebral bodies. These may be classified as stable, where the integrity of the spine is still preserved, or unstable, where excess movement between adjacent osseous elements is occurring.

Refer to later parts of Ch. 196 on Shoulder Pain, Elbow Pain, and Wrist and Hand Pain; Ch. 202, Osteoarthritis; and Ch. 203, Rheumatoid Arthritis.

History

1. Whenever a patient has a suspected "whiplash" injury or neck pain, it is important to obtain the exact mechanism of injury in the patient's own words. If it is a result of a motor vehicle accident, it is important to get the specifics of the accident and to ascertain whether the patient was wearing a seatbelt or not.

2. It is extremely important to determine if the patient has had any previous injury to the head or neck. Previous injuries to the cervical spine predisposes the patient to a new injury that is likely to be more disabling.

3. As with all chief complaints of pain, it is important to determine factors that aggravate or alleviate the pain; are there any associated symptoms to include involvement of upper extremities?

4. It is also important to determine if Valsalva maneuvers accentuate the neck pain.

Clinical Findings

1. All patients who present to the family physician's office with chief complaint of "whiplash" should be immobilized.

2. It is best to obtain a lateral cervical spine film to be certain there is no evidence of an underlying unstable fracture.

3. Once this has been established, one should check cervical range of motion and then palpate for evidence of paraspinous muscle spasm and localized tenderness that may be present.

4. One also should check for neurologic deficits, including weakness and reflex changes (Table 196–1).

Tests

1. Although most cervical spine film findings are normal, it is important to obtain these radiographs in patients with acute trauma to their cervical spine. In order to properly evaluate the cervical spine, the following views should be obtained:

   a. Dontoid view

   b. Anteroposterior view

   c. Lateral view

   d. Right oblique view

2. It is extremely important to be certain that all seven cervical vertebrae are visualized. Often C7 is not well delineated. It is then important to depress the shoulders by gentle but firm downward traction of

TABLE 196–1. NEUROLOGIC DEFICITS WITH CERVICAL OR NERVE ROOT INJURIES

Disk Space	Nerve Root Affected	Distribution of Motor Deficit	Sensory Abnormalities (Usually Numbness)	Reflex Abnormalities
C4	C5	Deltoid	Lateral aspect of shoulder	None
C5–6	C6	Biceps	Thumb	Biceps
C6–7	C7	Triceps	Middle finger	Triceps

the arms. If this is not possible, a so-called swimmer's view may be obtained. This view is done when the patient lies in a prone and oblique position with the higher tube-side arm above the head and the lower table-side arm beside the body.

3. MRI, CT scanning, or myelography should be used only in those patients who do not respond according to the usual treatment or who have definite suspected spinal cord injury or nerve root compressions.

Management

1. Hospitalization is rarely indicated in the absence of a fracture-dislocation. Antispasmodics or muscle relaxants may be helpful but should be used for short periods of time only, such as 5 to 7 days. Analgesics such as nonsteroidal anti-inflammatory drugs (NSAIDs) may be of benefit to the patient.

2. A soft collar that is properly fitted and correctly used is of significant benefit for many patients. The flexed position for the collar is advocated, since this position separates the facets and opens the foramina. It is preferred that a soft collar be used over a more rigid collar. Duration for wearing a collar will vary widely. Most authorities would now indicate that brief splinting and early mobilization have the best outcome. Brief splinting implies approximately 7 to 10 days. The collar is also best worn during the nighttime. Once the patient's pain is markedly reduced, gentle range-of-motion exercises should be begun. Heat applied before exercising may be of benefit.

3. The use of cervical traction is not uniformly accepted at this time. It is often used based on the physician's personal preference. It may best be reserved for the patient who does not show good improvement within 2 to 3 weeks after the initial injury.

4. It has been clearly documented in the medical literature that whiplash injuries are often slow to resolve because of impending litigation.

PEARLS

- Suspect cervical spine injury in all cases of head injuries.

- Always visualize C7.

- Early mobilization is the key to avoid long-term disability for most patients.

Bibliography

Bring G, Westman G: Chronic posttraumatic syndrome after whiplash injury. Scand J Primary Health Care 1992;9(2):135–141.

Bruno LA, Gennarelli TA, Torg JS: Management guidelines for head injuries in athletics. Clin Sports Med Head Neck Injuries 1987;6(1):17.

Callet, R: Whiplash: Neck and Arm Pain. Philadelphia, FA Davis, 1982, pp 60–85.

Carroll PG: Acute neck strain—The value of judicious early mobilization. Aust Fam Physician 1992;21(3):275–276.

Rockwood CA Jr, Green DP, Bucholz RW: Rockwood and Green's Fractures in Adult, vol 3. Philadelphia, JB Lippincott, 1991, pp 1309–1356.

Watkins RG, Dillin WH, Maxwell J: Cervical spine injuries in football players. Spine State Art Rev 1990;4:391–408.

Symptom   Shoulder Pain   *Jerry Ryan*

Patients of all ages are affected by both acute and chronic shoulder pathology. Many causes of shoulder pain are resistant to treatment and require patience on the part of both physician and patient. The judicious use of surgery is helpful in selected cases. Timely diagnosis and initiation of appropriate care afford the best chance of a favorable outcome for those afflicted with shoulder pain.

Differential Diagnosis

The differential diagnosis can be grouped depending on a history of prior trauma.

1. Prior trauma
   a. Rotator cuff tear—more common in the elderly
   b. Dislocation (90 per cent are anterior dislocations)
   c. Fractures (clavicle, humerus, rarely scapula)
   d. Acromioclavicular joint or sternoclavicular joint injury

2. No prior trauma
   a. Rotator cuff inflammation
   b. Bursitis (subacromial, subdeltoid)
   c. Adhesive capsulitis (frozen shoulder)
   d. Biceps tendinitis or rupture
   e. Arthritis (glenohumeral, acromioclavicular, sternoclavicular)
   f. Glenohumeral instability
   g. Neurologic disorders (cervical spine, brachial plexus)
   h. Neoplastic process (primary or metastatic)
   i. Infection

Refer to Ch. 198, Bursitis; Ch. 199, Tendinitis; Ch. 202 and 203, on Arthritis; Ch. 206, Myofascial Syndromes; and Ch. 217, Shoulder Dislocations.

History

1. Prior trauma: Increases likelihood of fracture, acute rotator cuff tear, clavicle injury, or dislocation.

2. Age: Adhesive capsulitis, bursitis, and tendinitis common in elderly.

3. Work-related activities: Patients in occupations requiring repetitive movement of the arms are at high risk for bursitis and rotator cuff tendinitis (e.g., carpenters, painters, assembly-line workers).

4. Recreational activities: Overhand-throwing athletes and swimmers are at high risk for rotator cuff impingement and tears as well as glenohumeral instability and labrum tears (e.g., pitcher, quarterback, tennis and volleyball players).

5. Night pain: Pain due to bursitis and rotator cuff inflammation is often worse at night.

6. Sensation of slipping or instability of the head of the humerus: Suggestive of prior dislocation.

7. Crepitations or popping with movement—common with calcific tendinitis.

8. Weakness of distal extremity: Suggests cervical spine or axillary nerve injuries.

9. Constitutional symptoms may suggest infectious or neoplastic process.

Clinical Findings

1. Inspection: The shoulder should be carefully inspected for any signs of swelling, warmth, or deformity. Atrophy of the muscles of the shoulder, in particular the deltoid, which overlies the head of the humerus, points toward a neurologic injury. A depression above the humeral head (sulcus sign) is suggestive of glenohumeral instability and ligamentous laxity.

2. Palpation: The clavicle, acromioclavicular (AC) joint, and the sternoclavicular joint are palpated. Deformities of these structures or pain with palpation points to an underlying injury. Anterior shoulder pain is found in a recently dislocated shoulder. The axilla and supraclavicular area are examined for lymphadenopathy.

3. Range-of-motion testing: Decreased range of motion (ROM) is often the first indication of underlying rotator cuff difficulties, adhesive capsulitis, or bursitis. Limits to abduction and internal or external rotation should be searched for carefully.

   a. Passive ROM limitations—indicative of adhesive capsulitis

   b. Active ROM limitations—indicative of rotator cuff inflammation

   c. Method of testing

      (1) Abduction: Patient standing, arm is raised out from side with elbow extended. Normal 0 degrees (arm at side) to 180 degrees (arm straight up)

      (2) Flexion: Patient standing, arm is raised forward with elbow extended. Normal 0 degrees (arm at side) to 180 degrees (arm straight up)

      (3) Rotation: Patient supine, arm abducted 90 degrees, elbow flexed 90 degrees, and forearm perpendicular to table surface (reference position). Normal internal and external rotation is approximately 90 degrees from reference position.

4. Resistive testing: Patient's arm is placed in position to isolate each of the tendons of the rotator cuff. Inflammation of the rotator cuff will produce pain and/or weakness when patient raises arm against examiner's resistance.

   a. Supraspinatus—abduction; usually first tendon to be affected

      (1) Patient standing

      (2) Arm abducted to approximately 90 degrees

      (3) Elbow extended and arm in 30 degrees of forward flexion

      (4) Arm internally rotated and the thumb pointed to the floor

      (5) Arm pushed upward against the examiner

   b. Subscapularis—internal rotation

      (1) Elbow flexed to 90 degrees and held at patient's side

      (2) Arm rotated internally against resistance of examiner

   c. Teres minor and infraspinatus—external rotation

      (1) Arm in same position as for subscapularis testing

      (2) Arm rotated externally against examiner resistance

   d. Biceps—resisted flexion of elbow

5. Apprehension testing

   a. Evaluates glenohumeral instability

   b. Positive in patients with anterior dislocation and glenoid labrum tear

   c. Method of testing

      (1) Patient supine with arm abducted 90 degrees, elbow flexed to 90 degrees, and arm externally rotated until limit of rotation or patient feels discomfort

      (2) Upper arm is pulled forward (anteriorly). If instability present, the discomfort is worsened with this anterior pressure (positive apprehension sign).

6. Impingement testing: Forces rotator cuff against coracoacromial ligament, worsening pain if inflammation or tear or rotator cuff abnormality is present. Testing done with patient supine.

   a. Impingement I: Elbow extended, arm internally rotated, arm flexed forward, holding arm close to patient's head

   b. Impingement II: Upper arm held perpendicular to table, elbow flexed to 90 degrees, arm rotated internally until limit of rotation or pain produced

c. Impingement III: Elbow extended, arm brought across front of patient's chest

7. Neurologic testing: Evaluates for cervical or axillary nerve injury.

   a. Biceps and triceps deep tendon reflexes

   b. Light touch. Careful attention should be paid to decreased sensation of deltoid area at point of shoulder, which may be the only sign of nerve root injury.

   c. Grip strength and intrinsic muscle strength of hand

Tests

1. Plain film radiographs: Useful to evaluate for following:

   a. Fractures of clavicle, humerus, or rarely, scapula

   b. Calcification of rotator cuff tendons (indicates chronic inflammation)

   c. Widening or calcifications of AC or sternoclavicular joint

   d. Lytic or sclerotic bone lesions

   e. Dislocation of humerus

2. MRI: Best to evaluate for rotator cuff tear or inflammation

3. CT arthrogram: Test of choice to find glenoid labrum tear

4. Nerve conduction studies (EMG): To evaluate for nerve root injuries

5. CT or MRI of cervical spine if indicated by EMG

Management

1. Fractures

   a. Clavicle: Careful observation or figure-of-8 splint; surgery is rarely indicated.

   b. Humerus: Sling and swath initially, and begin physical therapy as soon as possible; prolonged immobilization should be avoided.

   c. Scapula: Physical therapy for ROM and strengthening as soon as pain subsides

2. Rotator cuff inflammation and tears, subacromial bursitis

   a. Nonsteroidal anti-inflammatories and aggressive physical therapy to increase ROM and strength; immobilization should be avoided.

   b. Corticosteroid injection of subacromial bursa if physical therapy not helpful

   c. Arthroscopic surgery for rotator cuff tears if not helped by therapy or injections: should not be first-line treatment.

3. Dislocations

   a. Patients under age 20 have 90 per cent chance of subsequent dislocation and should have surgical repair after initial dislocation.

   b. Patients over 40 have low risk of subsequent dislocation and should begin physical therapy as soon as symptoms permit.

   c. Choice of surgery versus physical therapy for patients between 20 and 40 depends on frequency of subsequent dislocations and/or the physical activity of the patient.

4. Acromioclavicular and sternoclavicular inflammation and injury

   a. Symptomatic treatment for pain

   b. Corticosteroid injection for persistent pain

   c. Resection of distal clavicle for recalcitrant pain of AC joint

5. Cervical nerve root or axillary nerve abnormalities: Surgical decompression if indicated.

6. Lytic bone lesions: Search for underlying cause.

Bibliography

Macnab I, McCulloch J: Neck Ache and Shoulder Pain. Baltimore, Williams & Wilkins, 1994, pp 252–488.

Matsen FA, Lippitt SB, Sidles JA, Harryman DT: Practical Evaluation and Management of the Shoulder. Philadelphia, WB Saunders, 1994.

Morris MB, Walsh WM, Shelton GL: The Team Physician. Philadelphia, Hanley & Belfus, 1990, pp 313–333.

Zuckerman JD, Mirabello SC, Newman D, et al: The painful shoulder: I. Extrinsic disorders. Am Fam Physician 1991;43:119–128.

Zuckerman JD, Mirabello SC, Newman D, et al: The painful shoulder: II. Intrinsic disorders and impingement syndrome. Am Fam Physician 1991;43:497–512.

Symptom **Elbow Pain**

Francis G. O'Connor

Elbow injuries are among the most challenging that face the primary care physician. The central positioning of the elbow in the upper extremity predisposes to overuse microtrauma, as well as referred pain from the neck, shoulder, and wrist.

Differential Diagnosis

A. Overuse injuries

   1. Anterior

      a. Biceps tendinitis

      b. Pronator teres syndrome—median nerve entrapment

   2. Posterior

      a. Triceps tendinitis

      b. Olecranon impingement syndrome

      c. Olecranon bursitis

   3. Lateral

a. Tennis elbow—lateral epicondylitis

b. Posterior interosseous nerve entrapment

c. Osteochondritis dissecans

4. Medial

a. Golfer's elbow—medial epicondylitis

b. Ulnar collateral ligament strain

c. Cubital tunnel—ulnar nerve entrapment

B. Traumatic injuries

1. Fractures

2. Dislocations

3. Compartment syndromes

4. Apophyseal disorders

Overuse injuries represent the predominate form of musculoskeletal injury seen by physicians. Tennis elbow is the most common overuse injury involving the elbow, occurring nearly twice as often as medial epicondylitis. Little League elbow occurs frequently in young throwing athletes and involves a constellation of injuries, including a medial apophyseal stress lesion, lateral osteochrondritis dissecans of the capitellum, and olecranon apophysitis.

Refer to Ch. 198, Bursitis; Ch. 199, Tendinitis; Ch. 200, Epicondylitis; Ch. 206, Myofascial Syndromes; and Ch. 212, on Nerve Entrapments.

History

1. The character of the pain should be clearly established.

a. Onset—traumatic versus overuse

b. Quality

(1) Aching pain: tendon overuse

(2) Burning pain and tingling: nerve entrapment

c. Frequency and duration

d. Activities that exacerbate or relieve the pain

2. History of injury

a. Prior elbow fracture or dislocation

b. Prior elbow overuse injury

c. History of cervical radiculopathy or carpal tunnel syndrome

3. Occupational and sports history

a. Racquet and throwing sports predispose to overuse injuries.

b. Occupations requiring repetitive wrist motion predispose to injury (e.g., carpenters, typists, auto mechanics).

The history is the key to a good pathoanatomic diagnosis. The physician's inquiry should search to identify a recent period of transition, such as a vigorous tennis weekend, a new racquet, increased typing, or the start of Little League baseball.

Clinical Findings

1. A careful examination includes inspection, palpation, range-of-motion testing, special tests, and neuromuscular testing of the entire upper extremity.

2. Normal carrying angles measure 5 degrees of valgus in males and 10 to 15 degrees in females.

3. Passive limitation of extension—mechanical blockade or a muscular flexion contracture. Pain with forced extension—olecranon impingement syndrome

4. Palpation should include all four quadrants through a full range of motion.

a. The point of maximal tenderness for tennis elbow is at the insertion of the wrist extensors at the lateral epicondyle.

b. The point of maximal tenderness for golfer's elbow is at the flexor origin at the medial epicondyle.

c. A Tinel's test should be performed at the cubital tunnel, where the ulnar nerve crosses the elbow.

5. Both varus and valgus instability should be assessed at 0 and 30 degrees of elbow flexion and compared with the other extremity.

6. Resisted dorsiflexion, palmar flexion, pronation, and supination should be performed to identify musculoskeletal dysfunction.

Pain with resisted dorsiflexion with the elbow in full extension suggests a better prognosis than with the elbow in 90 degrees of flexion. Classic signs of Little League elbow include tenderness over the medial epicondyle and pain with resisted flexion and/or pronation. Findings that suggest more advanced involvement include tenderness over the lateral condyle, swelling, and a limitation of elbow motion.

Tests

1. Standard radiographs include anteroposterior and lateral views. Special views include oblique, axial, radial head, and stress views.

2. CT arthrography and MRI can be used to evaluate for loose bodies, soft tissue mechanical blockade, and osteochondritis.

3. EMG and NCV can be used to evaluate for ulnar nerve dysfunction, median nerve entrapment with the pronator syndrome, and posterior interosseous nerve entrapment.

In the young patient with open growth plates, radiographs of both elbows should be ordered. Fat pad signs are frequently helpful in diagnosing subtle fractures. Posterior fat pads are always considered abnormal and suggestive of elbow fracture. Anterior fat pads are frequently present normally. When a fracture is present, the anterior fat pad can elevate, indicating the classic "sail sign."

Management

1. Pathoanatomic diagnosis: Successful treatment begins with an accurate diagnosis.

2. Control of inflammation

a. Medication

(1) A 7- to 10-day course of an NSAID frequently helps to control pain and inflammation, such as Naproxen, 375 mg twice a day for 7 days.

(2) Corticosteroid injections: Short-term relief, but corticosteroid can cause tissue degeneration.

b. Modalities: High-voltage pulsed galvanic stimulation, iontophoresis, and phonophoresis can all be of assistance in managing elbow overuse pain.

c. Protection: Elbow immobilization is used only in select cases because stiffness and atrophy are not infrequent complications.

3. Promotion of healing: The promotion of healing only occurs through rehabilitative exercise and cardiovascular conditioning.

a. Exercise progresses from isometrics to isotonics, with emphasis on wrist flexors and extensors.

b. The entire upper extremity should be rehabilitated to include the shoulder and scapular stabilizers.

c. Home isoflex (surgical tubing) exercises are very effective.

4. Control abuse

a. Control of force loads: Re-education of proper sports and/or occupational technique and control of intensity and duration of activity

b. Counterforce bracing: Helpful in rehabilitation and in early return to sport

c. Proper equipment is important to avoid overuse injury.

5. Patient education

a. Ongoing maintenance rehabilitation is necessary to avoid recurrent injury.

b. Progression should be gradual.

c. Patients should never play or participate through the pain.

d. Premedicating with pain medication before athletic or occupational activity should be avoided.

Rest from abusive activity should be relative and not complete. Surgery for elbow overuse injuries is indicated only after failure of a quality rehabilitative program (3 to 6 months), persistent pain at rest or with activities of daily living, and an unacceptable quality of life.

PEARLS

- When tennis elbow fails to improve, posterior interosseous nerve entrapment should be ruled out.

- The patient with an elbow overuse injury frequently has associated rotator cuff tendinitis.

- Cervical radiculopathy and carpal tunnel syndrome not uncommonly produce referred pain patterns involving the elbow.

B **Bibliography**

Foley AE: Tennis elbow. Am Fam Physician 1993;48:281–288.

Morrey BF: The Elbow and Its Disorders. Philadelphia, WB Saunders, 1985.

Morrey BF, Regan WD: Tendinopathies about the elbow. In De Lee JC, Drez D (eds): Orthopaedic Sports Medicine: Principles and Practice. Philadelphia, WB Saunders, 1994, pp 860–881.

Nirshl RP: Soft tissue injuries about the elbow. Clin Sports Med 1986;5:637–652.

O'Connor FG, Ollivierre CO, Nirchl RP: Elbow and forearm injuries. In Lillegard WA, Rucker KS (eds): Handbook of Sports Medicine. Boston, Andover Medical Publishers, 1993, pp 99–110.

| Symptom | **Wrist and Hand Pain** | *Douglas G. Browning* |

Hand and/or wrist pain is a common presenting complaint, and finding the correct diagnosis may sometimes be difficult due to the large number of anatomic structures confined within this small space. Following a structured history and examination for these problems may help make the challenge of narrowing the differential diagnosis a much easier task.

Differential Diagnosis

1. Tendinitis (see also Chapter 199)

a. de Quervain's tenosynovitis (stenosing tenosynovitis of the first dorsal compartment of the wrist)

b. Wrist/finger extensor

c. Wrist/finger flexors

d. Intersection syndrome—tendinitis between first and second dorsal compartments on the dorsum of the forearm ≈ 2 to 3 finger breadths proximal to the wrist joint

2. Peripheral nerve entrapments (see also Chapter 212)

a. Median nerve entrapments

(1) Carpal tunnel syndrome (may have both motor and sensory involvement)

(2) Pronator teres entrapment (usually with sensory involvement only)

(3) Anterior interosseous syndrome (motor syndrome)

b. Ulnar nerve entrapments

(1) Ulnar nerve entrapment at the wrist (Guyon's canal)—motor, sensory, or mixed

(2) Ulnar nerve entrapment at the elbow

3. Ganglion cyst(s)

4. Sprain

a. Ligamentous injuries to the carpal bones

b. Triangular fibrocartilaginous complex

c. Radioulnar ligament sprain

d. Carpometacarpal sprain

5. Fractures (see also Chapters 221 and 222)

   a. Carpal navicular/scaphoid

   b. Distal radius

   c. Ulnar styloid

   d. Other carpal bones

6. Osteonecrosis (avascular necrosis)

7. Arthritic conditions

   a. Rheumatoid arthritis

   b. Gout

   c. Pseudogout

   d. Connective tissue diseases (systemic lupus erythematosus, scleroderma)

   e. Psoriatic arthritis

   f. Septic arthritis

   g. Osteoarthritis

Determining whether the pain is trauma-related or not often will quickly narrow the list of possible diagnoses. Osteoarthritis often occurs in the fingers distally but is unusual in the wrist and hand without a history of trauma. When it does occur, the carpometacarpal joint of the thumb is the most common area of involvement. Avascular necrosis usually involves the scaphoid or lunate and may or may not have an associated history of trauma and fracture.

> Refer to Ch. 199, Tendinitis; Ch. 202, Osteoarthritis; Ch. 203, Rheumatoid Arthritis; Ch. 204, Gout; Ch. 207, Systemic Lupus Erythematosus; Ch. 208, Scleroderma; Ch. 212, Carpal Tunnel and Other Nerve Entrapments; Ch. 221, Wrist Fractures; and Ch. 222, Finger Fractures.

History: Key Questions to Ask

1. Did you injure the area? If so, how?

2. When did the pain start?

3. Where is the pain located?

4. Describe the pain.

5. Does it swell?

6. Does it make any noise?

To narrow the differential diagnosis, it should be determined if the onset of pain was gradual or sudden, insidious or occurred after trauma. Determining the mechanism of injury by asking about a history of trauma and occupational and recreational activities may help in identifying the source of the problem. Asking about a history of other similar musculoskeletal pains or problems is also useful. The nature of the pain and whether it is sharp and stabbing or a dull ache, whether it is constant or intermittent, will help in guiding your diagnostic workup. A history of paresthesias (numbness, tingling), particularly at night, may point toward a nerve entrapment as the culprit, in which case associated retrograde pain to the elbow or even to the shoulder is not uncommon. Associated "squeaking" with movement may indicate inflammation in a tendon, while

"popping" or "clicking" might indicate a cartilage tear or ligamentous laxity. A "grinding" sensation may occur with arthritic degeneration.

Clinical Findings

1. Edema

2. Ecchymosis

3. Tenderness

4. Deformity or atrophy

5. Loss of motion

6. Loss of strength

7. Loss of sensation

8. Crepitus

Comparison with the uninvolved side on initial examination is important to establish physiologic laxity and to determine any previous injury causing similar physical findings and may prevent unnecessary testing and expense. Ecchymosis may coincide with a traumatic origin of symptoms. Active and passive range of motion in all directions should be documented (including flexion, extension, radial deviation, ulnar deviation, pronation, and supination). Strength and sensation should be tested in the wrist, hand, and fingers and in the median, ulnar, and radial distributions. Atrophy of the thenar or hypothenar eminence may indicate involvement of the median or ulnar nerve, respectively.

Tests

1. Tinel's sign: percussion (tapping) of the median nerve at the carpal tunnel reproduces paresthesias

2. Phalen's sign: forced volar flexion of the wrist to 90 degrees for up to 60 seconds reproduces paresthesias.

3. Finkelstein's test: pain over the distal radius with tucking the thumb inside the other fingers and moving the wrist into ulnar deviation suggests stenosing (de Quervain's) tenosynovitis.

4. Radiographs

5. Electromyography/peripheral nerve conduction velocities

6. Aspiration (arthrocentesis)/synovial fluid analysis (with cell count, crystal analysis, Gram's stain and culture)

7. ^{99m}Tc bone scan

8. Magnetic resonance imaging

9. Arthrography

10. Complete blood count

11. Erythrocyte sedimentation rate (? rheumatoid factor and antinuclear antibody)

Joint aspiration is best performed with a 22-gauge needle from the dorsal aspect of the wrist or hand to prevent injury to arteries or nerves. Routine laboratory tests are not generally indicated when a patient presents with wrist pain occurring secondary to trauma. Plain radiographs may be the most useful and cost-effective way to rule out fracture or dislocation whenever pain from injury persists for more than 48 to 72 hours, swelling is present, or joint motion is limited. Internal and external oblique views may be required, in addition to standard anteroposterior and lateral views, to identify carpal fractures. If symptoms persist, repeat radiographs in 2 to 8 weeks may be indicated to rule out a navicular or other carpal fracture or osteonecrosis, since this is often not evident on initial films. A bone scan may confirm an occult carpal fracture, while magnetic resonance imaging is sometimes useful in demonstrating ligamentous tears. Electromyography and nerve conduction velocity testing are sometimes diagnostic when nerve injury or entrapment is suspected. If a systemic disease or inflammatory origin is suspected, full physical and routine screening laboratory tests are useful.

Management

1. Nonsteroidal anti-inflammatory drugs (NSAIDs) may help in reducing inflammation and symptoms.

2. Corticosteroid injections may be useful in some situations initially (e.g., ganglion cyst) or as a second line of therapy. *Do not inject directly into nerves or tendons.*

3. Tetanus toxoid status should be checked with any penetrating wound.

4. Surgical referral and intervention

Diet

1. Dietary restriction of purine-rich foods (as well as alcohol) may be appropriate for gout.

2. Adequate calcium and vitamin D intake may help in maintaining bone density and promoting bone healing after injury.

Activity

1. Restriction/avoidance of specific painful activities

2. Immobilization with a splint, brace, or cast may be indicated.

Patient Education

Retraining of problematic techniques (particularly for occupationally related overuse syndromes)

Rehabilitation

1. Stretching the involved area

2. Strengthening the involved muscles and tendons

3. Physical or occupational therapy

Rehabilitation exercises should begin with range-of-motion and stretching exercises, followed by strengthening the involved area with light-resistance (<5 lb), high-repetition exercises (30 to 50 per set). Modalities that also may prove to be helpful include ice, heat, ultrasound and phonophoresis, and/or iontophoresis.

Follow-Up

Regular follow-up of wrist or hand pain or both is useful until the correct diagnosis and treatment is ensured.

PEARLS

- In looking for injuries to the carpal bones on radiographs, internal and external oblique views are often helpful in addition to the standard AP and lateral views. Repeat radiographs may be needed in 2 to 8 weeks if symptoms persist, since carpal fractures or osteonecrosis may not be evident on initial films.

- Ice/cryotherapy is often useful in helping the initial symptoms of wrist and hand pain.

- Many problems involving wrist and hand pain may be rehabilitated by initial range of motion and gentle stretching, followed by low-weight, high-repetition strengthening of the involved muscles and tendons.

- Consider early referral of carpal fractures due to their slow healing and relatively high risk of osteonecrosis.

 Bibliography

For more information on examination of the wrist and hand, see
Hoppenfeld S: Physical Examination of the Spine and Extremities. East Norwalk, Conn, Appleton & Lange, 1976, pp 59–104.
For more information on wrist and hand pain, see
Wade JP, Bell JG: Wrist pain. *In* MH Liang (ed): Primary Care Clinics in Office Practice: Musculoskeletal Pain Syndromes, vol 15, no 4. Philadelphia, WB Saunders, 1988, pp 737–749.
For more information on wrist and hand pain, see
American Society for Surgery of the Hand: The Hand: Primary Care for Common Problems. New York, Churchill Livingstone, 1985.
For more information on wrist and hand pain, see
Ferlic TP: Hand and wrist injuries. *In* Mellion MB, Walsh WM, Shelton GL (eds): The Team Physician's Handbook. Philadelphia, Hanley & Belfus, 1990, pp 346–364.
For more information on rehabilitation of the wrist and hand, see
Hunter JM, Schneider LH, Mackin EJ, Callahan AD: Rehabilitation of the Hand, 3d ed. St. Louis, CV Mosby, 1989.

| Symptom | **Back Pain** | *Sarah S. Marlowe* |

The syndrome of low back pain (LBP) is ubiquitous, afflicting up to 90 per cent of people over their life span. Most LBP resolves with conservative management, but physicians are commonly vexed in their management of these patients because the pathophysiology of LBP is poorly understood and a precise diagnosis is found in fewer than 10 per cent of patients. The cause of pain may evolve during the course of illness (e.g., diskogenic pain may be superseded by muscle pain) or involve several structures simultaneously (e.g., disks and facets). Pain from the spine is poorly localized, and pain from visceral structures of the chest, abdomen, or pelvis may refer dorsally. This discussion focuses on musculoskeletal pain syndromes of the back.

Differential Diagnosis

1. Myofascial: muscle strain or insertion tendinitis
2. Diskogenic: herniated nucleus pulposus (HNP) or degenerative disk
3. Osteoarthritis, including facet joints
4. Spondylolisthesis (spondylolysis controversial as cause of pain)
5. Spinal stenosis, congenital or acquired
6. Fractures: traumatic or pathologic
7. Inflammatory or rheumatologic diseases
8. Infiltrative diseases: infection, malignancy, Paget's disease

The likelihood of diagnosis is age-related. Disk disease and myofascial pain are most common in adults age 50 and younger, with spondylolysis and inflammatory diseases occurring less commonly. Spinal stenosis, malignancies, and Paget's disease preferentially affect adults over age 50.

> Refer to Ch. 187, Paget's Disease of Bone; Ch. 202, Osteoarthritis; and Ch. 206, Myofascial Syndromes.

History

1. Pain descriptors: acuity of onset, duration, location and radiation of pain, precipitating factors, positional variance (flexion versus extension), and history of LBP
2. Occupational history: especially presence of heavy lifting, repetitive twisting, and operating heavy equipment (4 to 6 Hz vibration)
3. Neurologic symptoms, including pain, numbness or paresthesia in either radicular or myofascial referral patterns, motor weakness (e.g., foot drop), neurogenic claudication, and pelvic visceral dysfunction
4. Psychosocial factors, including job satisfaction, perception of disability, and secondary gain (e.g., worker's compensation, litigation, avoidance of responsibilities)

As with any disease, the history is of paramount importance in the diagnosis of LBP and also commonly directs therapy. Positive motor symptoms mandate further examination and diagnostic testing. However, the psychosocial history is most predictive of eventual outcome.

Clinical Findings

1. Neurologic examination: gait abnormalities (try toe walking, heel walking), muscle strength, tendon reflexes, and perianal sensation
2. Posture, range of motion, hamstring flexibility
3. Point tenderness: spine, muscles, tendon insertions, sacroiliac joints
4. Pelvic stress tests: Patrick or Faber maneuvers

Perianal sensory loss with pelvic visceral dysfunction or loss of anal tone implies cauda equina syndrome, which is rare but requires urgent surgical referral. Straight-leg testing is widely used but has poor predictive value. Posture is often very revealing, with acute HNP patients preferring to stand and myofascial pain patients preferring to sit or recline.

Tests

1. Radiographs can reveal fractures, lytic lesions, spondylolysis, and degeneration and, with the neurologic examination, will exclude most serious causes of LBP. Recommended in all trauma patients, adolescents, and adults over age 50 years
2. Bone scans reveal inflammatory and infiltrative processes, occult fractures, and active spondylolysis. Highly sensitive for ruling out serious pathology
3. Computed tomography (CT) and magnetic resonance imaging (MRI) are usually reserved for patients who may require surgery. T_2-weighted MRIs give myelogram-like information.
4. Myelogram: Not recommended unless MRI is not available.
5. Electromyelography tests peripheral nerve function.
6. Blood tests: Erythrocyte sedimentation rate screens for inflammation and chronic infection; other serologic tests can screen for specific rheumatologic disorders.

Most patients with LBP are managed clinically. Testing should be reserved for trauma, patients with known cancer, those with abnormal neurologic examinations or systemic illness, or those with symptoms that worsen or do not improve despite 6 weeks of appropriate therapy. Symptoms and functional disability generally correlate poorly with objective anatomic tests.

Management
Medication
1. Nonsteroidal anti-inflammatory drugs (e.g., ibuprofen)

2. Tricyclic antidepressants or related compounds

3. Other analgesic agents (e.g., acetaminophen)

4. Oral or intrathecal steroids for HNP

Physical Modalities

1. Ice, heat, ultrasound

2. Osteopathic or chiropractic manipulation

3. Lumbosacral corset or thoracolumbosacral orthosis: diskogenic pain, spinal stenosis, spondylolisthesis, sacroiliac pain

4. See also Chapter 206, Myofascial Syndromes.

Activity

1. Relative rest with early return to activity

2. Aerobic exercise

3. Trunk muscle exercises (see Procedure on Low Back Pain Exercises)

Diet

1. Weight loss

2. Tobacco cessation

Patient Education

1. Reassurance: Avoid overdiagnosis, overtesting.

2. Modified workplace ergonomics

3. Avoidance of biomechanical stresses of disks (back school)

4. Resolution of psychosocial stressors

5. Lifelong fitness

Patients should be encouraged to play an active role in their rehabilitation. Passive modalities such as traction and massage are not only ineffective but encourage inactivity. Bed rest greater than 48 hours promotes deconditioning and should be discouraged.

Follow-Up

1. Should be aggressive to promote early return to activity

2. Consider referral to physical therapy early in course if not improving.

3. Surgical consultation: any patients with progressive neurologic findings or cauda equina syndrome. Consider in patients whose pain has not improved within six weeks.

PEARLS

• Observation of the patient's gait, posture, and affect often yields the diagnosis.

• In the absence of hard neurologic findings, there is usually more danger in too much rest than in too much exercise.

Bibliography

For more information on lumbar disk disease, see
Gilmer HS, Papadopoulos SM, Tuite GF: Lumbar disk disease: Pathophysiology, management and prevention. Am Fam Physician 1993;47:1141–1152.

For more information on low back pain, see
Nachemson AL: Newest knowledge of low back pain: A critical look. Clin Orthop 1992;279:8–19; and Weinstein JN, Wiesel SW (eds): The Lumbar Spine. Philadelphia, WB Saunders, 1990.

For more information on radiologic diagnosis of back pain, see
Practice parameters: Magnetic resonance imaging in the evaluation of low back syndrome (summary statement). Report of the Quality Standards Subcommittee of the American Academy of Neurology. Neurology 1994;44:767–770.

For more information on myofascial low back pain, see
King JC, Goddard MJ: Pain rehabilitation: 2. Chronic pain syndrome and myofascial pain. Arch Phys Med Rehabil 1994;75:S9–14.

| Symptom | **Hip Pain** | *Thurayya Arayssi* |

The hip joint serves a crucial function in locomotion and weight bearing. It may be subject to extreme stresses or trauma, and diseases that affect it may cause severe disability. Much of this disability is secondary to the pain associated with these processes.

Of all the symptoms of hip disease, hip pain is the most common. Though often manifest as groin pain, it may also be felt in the thigh or buttocks; moreover, pain felt about the proximal femur or more superior pelvis is often also described by patients as "hip pain." The structures that underlie these complaints must also be considered in the diagnosis and management of hip pain.

Hip pain in children and adolescents presents a diagnostic dilemma that may be distinct from that encountered in adults. At the same time, diseases of the hip that begin in childhood may lead to pain and disability in adulthood.

Differential Diagnosis

Groin, Anterior Thigh, and Medial Thigh Pain

1. Osteoarthritis (OA)

2. Transient synovitis

3. Hip fracture

4. Rheumatoid arthritis (RA)

5. Idiopathic avascular necrosis

6. Polymyalgia rheumatica (PMR)

7. Septic arthritis/osteomyelitis

8. Ankylosing spondylitis (AS)

9. Pigmented villonodular synovitis

10. Referred pain (e.g., from testicular torsion)

11. Adductor/quadriceps muscle strain

12. Iliopectineal or iliopsoas bursitis

With specific relation to children and adolescents

1. Slipped upper femoral epiphysis
2. Juvenile RA
3. Perthes' disease
4. Sickle cell disease
5. Hemophilia
6. Acute leukemia

Lateral Hip and Thigh Pain

1. Trochanteric bursitis
2. Fascia lata syndrome
3. Abductor, gluteus muscle strain

Posterior Hip and Thigh Pain

1. Radiculopathy
2. Tumors
3. Diskitis
4. Spondylolisthesis
5. Ischial bursitis
6. Sacroiliitis

The most common cause of hip pain in adults is degenerative joint disease or osteoarthritis. Other rheumatic conditions, such as PMR and RA, as well as bursitis, fractures, and avascular necrosis, make up the majority of the remaining etiologies. More rarely, conditions such as AS, pigmented villonodular synovitis, and septic arthritis are found to be the cause. Referred pain from structures outside the hip joint itself must also be considered. Lumbar spinal problems and disorders of the pelvic cavity may refer pain to the hip.

In children, acute septic arthritis and osteomyelitis of the proximal femur/greater trochanter must be given more attention in the differential diagnosis. Other causes of acute hip pain include traumatic injuries, the sequelae of acute systemic illnesses, and the entity known as "irritable hip." Conditions that lead to more chronic hip pain in children include chronic slipped upper femoral epiphysis and Perthes' disease, both of which may lead to osteoarthritis in adulthood.

History: Key Questions to Ask

1. Where is the pain located? ("Point with one finger to the area where you are having pain.")
2. Does the pain move or radiate from its primary location?
3. What were you doing when the pain came on? Was there any trauma?
4. Did the pain come on suddenly or more gradually?
5. What things make the pain better or worse (specifically with regard to activity)?
6. Is there pain in any other distinct location or joint?
7. Is there stiffness in the joint (i.e., pain with movement) in the morning? If so, how long does it last?
8. Do your medications include steroid drugs? How do you use alcohol?
9. Do you have a fever or feel feverish?

The effect of activity on the hip pain is particularly important. For example, hip stiffness may improve with activity in RA but will worsen with OA. Also, bilateral pain that comes on with walking and is relieved by rest may point more specifically to vascular or neurogenic claudications. As outlined above, the location of the pain may be important in eliciting the correct diagnosis and treatment plan. Associated trauma or injury also helps to narrow the differential diagnosis. More general questions regarding systemic symptoms and medication/substance use may bring diagnoses such as infection and avascular necrosis, respectively, to the fore.

Clinical Findings

1. Gait abnormalities including adductor lurch, antalgic gait, and Trendelenburg gait (pelvis on side opposite the affected side drops during the stance phase).
2. Muscle atrophy in quadriceps denotes severe disease in the hip joint.
3. Positive Trendelenburg sign (non–weight-bearing side of pelvis drops when the patient is asked to stand on the affected leg/hip) is suggestive of hip abductor weakness.
4. The presence of ecchymosis or abrasions is suggestive of trauma.
5. Tenderness to palpation along the lateral aspect of the hip and the greater trochanter points toward trochanteric bursitis.
6. Abnormalities in range-of-motion testing, mainly limitation of abduction and internal rotation, are common with intra-articular hip disease.
7. Pain on hip extension suggests sacroiliac pain, lumbar spine disease, or articular hip pain.
8. Sensory and motor neurologic examination abnormalities are suggestive of radiculopathy.

Tests

1. Radiographic examination is done of both hips with weight-bearing films.
2. Complete blood count, sedimentation rate, and serum uric acid level are essential to differentiate inflammatory from noninflammatory causes of hip pain.
3. Aspiration of the hip joint for Gram's stain and culture if septic arthritis is a concern.

The interpretation of the above tests should be done in the context of the history and the physical examination. Special attention should be paid to findings on x-ray film which do not always correlate with pathology; for example, the presence of osteophytes in a patient with hip pain does not necessarily mean that the patient has OA as a cause of his symptoms.

Management

Management includes the use of medications, surgery, physical therapy, and patient education to relieve pain and maintain function.

Pharmacologic Therapy

1. Nonsteroidal anti-inflammatory medications can be helpful in reducing hip pain of noninfectious etiology. The choice of the medication depends on the response of the patient.
2. Acetaminophen can reduce pain if used on a regular basis.
3. Depot corticosteroids injected locally can be helpful in treating trochanteric bursitis.
4. Low-dose tricyclic antidepressants may be useful for chronic hip pain.
5. Topical medications such as capsaicin may provide some relief.
6. Short-term use of narcotics may be necessary for severe acute pain.

Nonpharmacologic Therapy

1. Local heat and ultrasound therapy can reduce symptoms secondary to bursitis and muscular strain.
2. Physical therapy referral is advised to maintain range of motion and strengthen target muscle groups when pain is adequately controlled.
3. Weight loss is recommended.
4. Femoral osteotomy or hip replacement surgery may be indicated for specific causes of articular hip pain unresponsive to more conservative therapy.

IMPORTANT

The treatment of hip pain caused by infection (osteomyelitis or septic arthritis) deviates from the general scheme outlined above. In this case, prompt antibiotic therapy based on culture data is essential to the prevention of irreversible joint destruction. Surgical debridement and drainage may also be indicated.

Activity

1. Activity and weight bearing are restricted in the acute phase.
2. Graduated increase in activity and weight bearing is soon recommended.
3. Assistive devices such as cane or crutches can be helpful to unload the affected hip.

Patient Education

Education for weight loss is recommended in obese patients, especially those with OA of the hip.

PEARLS

- Osteoarthritis is the most common cause of hip pain in adults over 50 years of age.

- If infection is suspected, prompt diagnosis and antibiotic treatment, preferably based on specific culture data, are essential.

- Palpation over the proximal lateral thigh and/or greater trochanter which reproduces or exacerbates the patient's pain is highly suggestive of trochanteric bursitis.

- Findings on plain radiographs consistent with osteoarthritis do not necessarily rule out other etiologies for hip pain.

 Bibliography

Boyd RJ: Evaluation of hip pain. *In* Goroll AH, et al (eds): Primary Care Medicine, 3rd ed. Philadelphia, JB Lippincott, 1995, pp 762–765.

Hill RA, Fixsen JA: Investigation and management of the painful hip in childhood. Br J Hosp Med 1994;51(6):270–274.

Hodges DL, McGuire TJ: Hip pain in children: An anatomic approach. Orthopaed Rev 1988;xvii(3):251–256.

Roberts WN, Williams RB: Hip pain. Primary Care 1988;15(4):783–793.

Schon L, Zuckerman JD: Hip pain in the elderly: Evaluation and diagnosis. Geriatrics 1988;43(1):48–62.

| Symptom | **Knee Pain** | *Craig C. Young* |

Knee pain is a common complaint. The etiology of the pain varies with age, illness, and mechanism of injury. Correct diagnosis of the cause will determine the appropriate treatment of the patient.

Differential Diagnosis

A. Acute knee pain—traumatic injury
   1. Very common cause: medial collateral ligament (MCL) sprain
   2. Common causes
      a. Anterior cruciate ligament (ACL) sprain
      b. Medial meniscus tear
      c. Subluxed or dislocated patella
      d. Contusions
      e. Traumatic bursitis
   3. Uncommon causes
      a. Lateral collateral ligament sprain, fracture, traumatic patellofemoral pain syndrome (PFPS), posterior cruciate ligament (PCL) sprain
      b. Muscle strain: includes quadriceps, hamstrings, gastrocnemius, soleus

4. Rare cause: muscle rupture—includes plantaris, quadriceps, hamstrings

B. Acute knee pain—nontraumatic injury

1. Common causes

a. Arthritis

b. Gout

c. Calcium pyrophosphate dihydrate (CPPD) crystal deposition disease

d. Referred pain

(1) In adults includes herniated disk, muscle strain, and hip injury

(2) In children, hip pathology commonly refers pain to the knee.

2. Uncommon causes: septic knee, ruptured Baker's cyst

3. Rare cause: popliteal aneurysm rupture

C. Chronic knee pain

1. Very common causes

a. Arthritis

b. Patellofemoral pain syndrome (PFPS)

2. Common causes

a. Patellar tendinitis, "jumper's knee"

b. Iliotibial band syndrome, "runner's knee"

c. Meniscal tears

d. Pes anserine bursitis

e. Osgood-Schlatter disease (common in adolescents)

f. Quadriceps tendinitis

3. Uncommon causes

a. Baker's cyst, plica syndrome, recurrent patellar subluxation

b. Loose bodies, "joint mice": chondral fracture, osteochondral fracture, osteochondritis dissecans (OCD)

4. Rare causes: osteochondritis dissecans, neoplasm, popliteal aneurysm

Refer to Ch.198, Bursitis; Ch. 199, Tendinitis; Chs. 202 and 203, on Arthritis; Ch. 211, Osteochondritis (Osgood-Schlatter Disease); and Ch. 214, Runner's Injuries.

History

1. Onset of injury

a. Sudden versus gradual onset

b. Associated change in training pattern, intensity, or activities

c. Ability to continue activities after injury

2. Mechanism of injury

a. Varus or valgus contact—ligament sprains, patellar subluxation, meniscal tear, fracture

b. Direct blow—patellofemoral joint injuries, PCL sprain, fracture

c. Hyperextension injury—ACL sprain, PCL sprain, posterior capsule injuries

d. Deceleration injury—ACL sprain

e. Rotational injury—meniscal injury, ligament injuries, osteochondral fracture, patellar dislocation or subluxation

f. Dashboard injury—fracture, ligament and capsular injuries

g. Other important factors: weight-bearing or non–weight-bearing; direct or indirect force

3. Pop or snap—may indicate rupture of ligament, tendon, or muscle or a fracture

4. Swelling—how quickly the swelling occurred; bloody effusion immediately after injury indicates a high probability of ACL rupture.

5. Pain—location, radiation pattern, and type

a. Sharp, stabbing pain more likely to be associated with mechanical problems

b. Dull, aching pain more likely to be associated with degenerative and overuse problems

6. Buckling—Does the knee give way?

a. Which activities cause it to give way—changing directions, pivoting, walking, or running?

b. Buckling is associated with anterior cruciate ligament injury.

7. Pseudobuckling—a feeling of giving way but without actually giving way of knee; associated with anterior cruciate ligament injury, patellofemoral pain syndrome, arthritis

8. Locking—knee getting caught in specific positions; associated with meniscal injury, loose bodies, OCD, patellar dislocation

9. Pseudolocking—knee feels like it catches without actually locking; associated with patellofemoral pain syndrome, arthritis, patellar subluxation

10. Other important factors: stiffness, level of function, previous injury

Clinical Findings

1. Observation

a. Effusions, quadriceps atrophy, standing position, gait

b. Anatomic malalignment

(1) Anatomic variances are frequently associated with overuse injuries.

(2) Common malalignments: Q-angle, patellar position, tibial torsion

2. Palpation—effusion, patellar facets, tendons, joint line

3. Range of motion (ROM)—passive, active, resisted, patellar tracking

4. Ligament stability
   a. Lachman—evaluates ACL integrity
   b. Varus and valgus stress testing—evaluates collateral ligament integrity
   c. Posterior drawer—evaluates PCL integrity
   d. Sag test—evaluates PCL integrity
5. Grind test—evaluates patellofemoral pain syndrome
6. Apprehension test—evaluates patella subluxation and dislocation
7. McMurray test (circumduction tests)—evaluates meniscus
8. Functional tests—walking (forward and backward), squatting, bounce squat, stairs, running, figure-8's, jumping

Tests

1. Joint aspiration
   a. Bloody effusion—traumatic injury (especially ACL sprain), Charcot joint, tumor, sickle cell joint. Fat droplets indicate intra-articular fracture.
   b. Purulent effusion—septic joint (bacterial, tuberculosis, fungal) is more than 80,000 WBC/mm^3, 90 per cent polymorphonuclear leukocytes (PMNs), very low glucose
   c. Inflammatory effusion—rheumatoid arthritis, gout, CPPD, viral arthritis is 1000 to 50,000 WBC/mm^3, 30 to 50 per cent lymphocytes, 50 to 70 per cent PMNs
   d. Crystal examination—gout—rods or needles—negatively birefringent (yellow). CPPD—rods, rectangles, or rhomboids—weakly positive birefringent (blue)
2. Radiographs—Use to evaluate possible fractures and injuries that are not responding to treatment. Standard series: AP weight bearing (to evaluate joint space), lateral, notch, Merchant (or other tangential/skyline view).
3. Magnetic resonance imaging—especially useful for evaluation of ligaments, menisci, bone bruises
4. Computed tomography—especially good for evaluation of OCD and other bony pathology
5. Bone scan—useful for evaluation of overuse injuries, infection, and tumors

6. Arthrography—useful for evaluation of menisci and plica

Management

1. Arthritis: See Chapters 202, 203, and 204.
2. Acute treatment (goals: control pain, minimize swelling, minimize tissue damage): protection, rest, ice, compression, elevation
3. Short-term treatment (goals: control pain, maintain ROM): protection, relative rest, ice, painless ROM, nonsteroidal anti-inflammatory drugs (NSAIDs)
4. Intermediate-term treatment (goals: prepare for return to normal activities): NSAIDs, strengthening (start with isometric strengthening; advance to eccentric and concentric strengthening), stretching, cardiovascular conditioning, functional drills, full ROM exercises
5. Long-term treatment (goals: prevention of future injury): strengthening and stretching

---

PEARLS

- Bags of poly-wrapped frozen corn kernels make a good reusable substitute for crushed ice.

- Artificial ice substitutes are colder than ice and thus place the body at greater risk for frostbite. Always wrap artificial ice in towels before placing against skin.

 ## Bibliography

For more information on physical assessment, see
Magee D: Orthopedic Physical Assessment, 2nd ed. Philadelphia, WB Saunders, 1992, pp 372–447.
For more information on assessment and treatment, see
Ferrari DA: Knee. In Steinberg GG, Akins CM, Baran DT (eds): Ramamurti's Orthopaedics in Primary Care, 2nd ed. Baltimore, Williams & Wilkins, 1992, pp 194–230.
Fulkerson JP: Patellofemoral pain disorders: Evaluation and management. J Am Acad Orth Surg 1994;2:124–132.
Johnson DL, Warner JJP: Diagnosis for anterior cruciate ligament surgery. Clin Sports Med 1993;12(4):671–684.
Silbey MB, Fu FH: Knee injuries. In FH Fu, DA Stone (eds): Sports Injuries: Mechanisms, Prevention and Treatment. Baltimore, Williams & Wilkins, 1994, pp 949–976.

| Symptom | **Ankle and Foot Pain** | *James R. Barrett* |

A recent Gallup poll showed that three quarters of United States citizens over age 18 complained that their feet hurt. Amazingly, nearly two thirds thought that their feet were supposed to hurt. Foot and ankle pain are common problems that are often seen by primary care physicians. Although rarely life-threatening, these complaints do cause significant discomfort and disability due to the importance of ambulation for work and leisure.

Ankle Pain

Differential Diagnosis

1. Ankle sprain
2. Fracture (tibia, fibula, osteochondral, fifth metatarsal)
3. Peroneal tendinitis, subluxation, dislocation
4. Arthritides
5. Anterior/posterior impingement
6. Reflex sympathetic dystrophy (RSD)
7. Osteochondritis dissecans

> Refer to Ch. 202 and 203, on Arthritis; Ch. 214, Runner's Injuries; Ch. 223, Ankle Fractures; and Ch. 224, Foot Fractures.

History: Key Questions to Ask

1. Description of the pain: exact location, quality, timing, relieving or aggravating features, referral to other areas, associated symptoms?
   a. Acute onset pain with no trauma? Early morning stiffness (arthritis)?
   b. Pain with extreme dorsi- or plantar flexion (anterior/posterior impingement)?
   c. Pain out of proportion to injury? Vasomotor disturbances and/or edema (RSD)?
2. Mechanism of injury (if injured)?
3. Previous foot or ankle injury?
4. Occupational or athletic history?
5. Family history of arthritis, cancer, hypertension, or cardiovascular disease?
6. Can the patient ambulate?
7. Swelling or ecchymosis?
8. Mechanical symptoms: Popping or snapping noticed (peroneal tendon dysfunction)? Locking or instability of ankle (osteochondritis dissecans)?

Clinical Findings

1. Skin appearance, including swelling, ecchymosis, erythema, mottled appearance
2. Range of motion (ROM)

3. Palpable tenderness over bones, ligaments, and tendons
4. Neurovascular examination
5. Anterior drawer, talar tilt, compression test of tibia and fibula

Tests

1. Radiograph of ankle (AP, lateral, and oblique) if fracture suspected; consider radiograph of *entire* tibia/fibula (especially medial sprains) or foot (fifth metatarsal tenderness)
2. Bone scan for suspected stress fracture
3. Tomography or CT for suspected osteochondral lesion
4. MRI for soft tissue pathology or osteochondral lesion

Management

1. Management of acute injury is based on RICED mnemonic:
   a. *R*est from pain-producing activities
   b. *I*ce for 20 minutes several times a day while area is swollen
   c. *C*ompression with padding and a wrap
   d. *E*levation above level of heart to reduce edema
   e. Nonsteroidal anti-inflammatory *d*rugs for pain and inflammation if not contraindicated
2. Physical therapy (PT) aimed at improving motion, strength, flexibility, and proprioception. Non–weight-bearing exercises early until protected weight bearing is tolerated (pain as a guideline) and inflammatory phase subsides.
3. Peroneal tendon dysfunction—peroneal tendon stretching, lateral heel wedge, ankle brace, PT, occasionally surgery
4. RSD—pain relief with anti-inflammatories or mild narcotics, early ROM, PT, occasional referral to anesthesia for sympathetic blocks

Heel Pain

Differential Diagnosis

> **Inferior**
> • Plantar fasciitis or fascial rupture
> • Arthritides
> • Calcaneal fracture
> • Nerve entrapment
> • Lumbar radiculopathy (S1)

Posterior

• Achilles tendinitis* or rupture

• Haglund deformity ("pump bump")

• Bursitis

Medial

• Posterior tibial tendinitis

• Tarsal tunnel

• Nerve entrapment

*Calcaneal apophysitis (Sever's disease) in children

History: Key Questions to Ask

1. Description of the pain (see ankle section)
   a. Pain when first step down after sleeping or sitting (plantar fasciitis)?
   b. Pain activity related? History of increased activity (tendinitis or stress fracture)?
   c. Burning or tingling sensation/pain at night (neurologic origin)?
2. Occupational or athletic history
3. History of low back pain or injury (radiculopathy)?

Clinical Findings

1. Palpable tenderness over bone, tendon, plantar fascia, soft tissue
2. Pain with medial and lateral compression of calcaneus (stress fracture); active inversion (posterior tibialis tendinitis); percussion (fracture)?
3. Lumbar back examination including straight leg raise (S1 radiculopathy)
4. Positive Tinel's sign (tarsal tunnel)
5. Palpable gap in Achilles tendon; positive Thompson test: squeeze calf—no plantar flexion noted (Achilles tendon rupture)
6. Foot type—cavus or pronated (associated with plantar fasciitis)

Tests

1. Radiograph—calcaneus
2. Laboratory:ESR, HLA-B27, rheumatoid factor if arthritis is suspected
3. Electromyogram and nerve conduction velocity test (EMG/NCV) for neurologic abnormalities

Management

1. RICED (see above)
2. Supportive footwear with a firm heel counter and arch support, lace-up shoes
3. Plantar fasciitis—heel pad or wedge, stretching exercises for plantar fascia, PT, low dye taping, orthotics, steroid injection, night splints, surgery
4. Posterior tibialis tendinitis—medial arch support or wedge, PT

5. Haglund deformity, Achilles tendinitis, bursitis—¼ inch heel wedge, calf stretching, PT
6. Achilles tendon rupture—surgical consultation (debated in literature whether casting or primary repair results in better outcome)

Forefoot Pain

Differential Diagnosis

First Metatarsal Pain

• Bunion/hallux valgus

• Hallux limitus/rigidus

• Sesamoiditis

• Arthritides

• Diabetic neuropathy

• Infection

Forefoot Pain (Metatarsalgia)

• Interdigital neuroma

• Sprain

• Calluses/warts

• Stress fracture

• Nerve entrapment—posterior tibial

• Diabetic neuropathy

• Infection

History: Key Questions to Ask

1. Description of the pain (see above)
   a. Pain better with shoe off? Better with massage of foot? Burning or sharp pain with weight bearing? "Electric shock" (neuroma)?
   b. Numbness or tingling into the toes (neurologic origin)?
   c. Great toe pain when toeing off, on tiptoeing (hallux rigidus or sesamoiditis)?
   d. Atraumatic hot, swollen first toe? Gnawing or throbbing pain (gout/infection)?
   e. Stocking distribution to pain (diabetic neuropathy)?
   f. Pain only with activity? During standing or weight bearing (stress fracture)?
2. Frequent wearing of high-heeled shoes with narrow toe box?

Clinical Findings

1. Evaluation of footwear: Does it fit correctly? Wear pattern? Wide or narrow toe box? Is heel counter firm? Height of heel?

2. Palpable tenderness: on metatarsal head, metatarsal body, between metatarsal heads, at ball of foot, over sesamoids?

3. Warmth/swelling

4. Foot type

5. Decreased plantar/dorsiflexion at first MTP (hallux rigidus/limitus)

6. Any visual deformities of the foot; protuberance medially or laterally (bunion)

7. Hyperesthesia in web space (neurologic origin)

8. Palpable mass on plantar aspect; positive Mulder's sign—pain on compressing forefoot from side to side while squeezing the tissue between met heads with fingertip (neuroma)

Tests

1. Radiograph of foot

2. Joint aspiration if gout, pseudogout, or joint infection is suspected

3. EMG/NCV for suspected neurologic problem

Management

1. RICED (see above)

2. Avoid constrictive footwear—Use wide toe box, low heel, and supportive arch.

3. Neuroma—metatarsal pad, corticosteroid injection, PT, surgery

4. Hallux limitus/rigidus—padding to shift weight laterally, hard-soled shoe, joint injection with steroid/anesthetic, surgery

5. Hallux valgus—Trim hyperkeratosis area, bunion shield/pad medial side, orthotics, surgery for severe deformity or pain unresponsive to conservative measures.

6. Sesamoiditis—crescent-shaped pad, stiff-soled shoe, orthotics, PT, rarely surgery

7. Calluses—Remove hyperkeratosis area with scapel or pumice stone, insoles or orthotics to relieve friction.

8. Warts—keratolytic agent (TCA, salicylic acid), cryosurgery, electrodesiccation

---

PEARLS

* Urgent referral to orthopedic surgeon if acute neurovascular impairment.

* Referral or consultation for displaced ankle fracture, Jones fracture, peroneal tendon dislocation, or osteochondritis dissecans.

* Warts can be distinguished from calluses by interruption of skin lines, blood vessels in the core, and tenderness on squeezing.

* Stress fractures are common in the foot and frequently do not show up on radiographs; maintain a high index of suspicion.

Bibliography

Birrer R, DellaCorte M, Grisafi P: Common Foot Problems in Primary Care. Philadelphia, Hanley & Belfus, 1992.

Calliet R: Foot and Ankle Pain. Philadelphia, FA Davis, 1983.

Garrick J, Webb D: Sports Injuries: Diagnosis and Management. Philadelphia, WB Saunders, 1990, pp 279–320.

Kwong P (ed): Foot and Ankle Injuries, vol 13, no 4. Philadelphia, WB Saunders, 1994.

McBryde AM Jr: Disorders of the ankle and foot. In Grana WA, Kalenak A (eds): Clinical Sports Medicine. Philadelphia, WB Saunders, 1991, pp 466–489.

Procedure LOCAL AND REGIONAL ANESTHESIA OF THE UPPER EXTREMITY   *Jack R. Woodside, Jr.*

Indications

Surgical procedures in the distribution of nerves blocked, such as paronychia, wound repair, nail removal, or foreign body removal

Contraindications

1. Hypersensitivity to local anesthetic. Reactions are usually to epinephrine or preservatives. Hypersensitivity to the amide-type local (e.g., lidocaine, bupivacaine) anesthetics is rare.
2. Injection through areas of infection may spread infection to deeper structures. Often the nerve may be blocked successfully at a site more proximal to the infection.

Equipment

1. Local anesthetic solution
2. Antiseptic solution
3. Syringe with 23- to 27-gauge 1½-inch needle

Precautions

1. *Do not exceed toxic dose of local anesthetic (e.g., 7 mg/kg for lidocaine and 3 mg/kg for bupivacaine).*
2. No epinephrine in areas of terminal circulation (e.g., fingers, toes, nose, ear, penis)
3. Severe pain during the injection suggests that the needle bevel lies within the nerve bundle, and the injection should be halted and the needle repositioned slightly.

WARNING

Aspirate before injecting large doses of local anesthetic in the vicinity of blood vessels.

Wrist Block

Technique

1. Review the three nerves supplying the hand, and determine the nerve(s) that supply the surgical field.

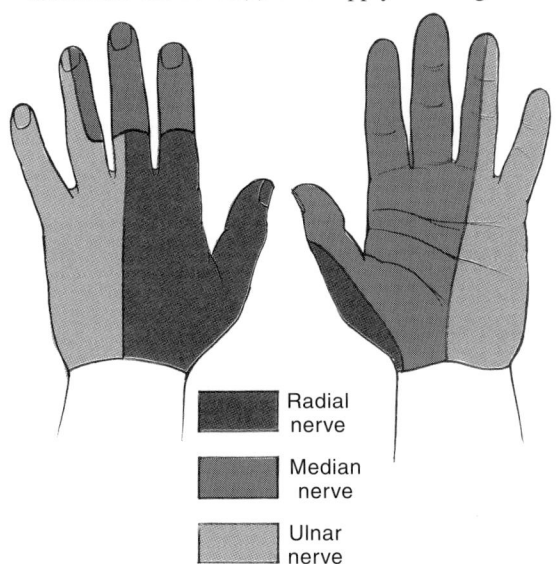

Radial nerve

Median nerve

Ulnar nerve

2. The ulnar nerve is most easily located and blocked in the ulnar notch at the elbow. The needle is placed in the ulnar notch, and 3 to 5 ml of local anesthetic is injected. If a paresthesia is elicited, 1 to 2 ml will be sufficient.
3. The median nerve is located between the palmaris longus tendon and the flexor carpi radialis tendon at the level of the proximal volar crease of the wrist.

The needle is introduced, and 3 to 5 ml of local anesthetic is infiltrated into the space between the tendons.

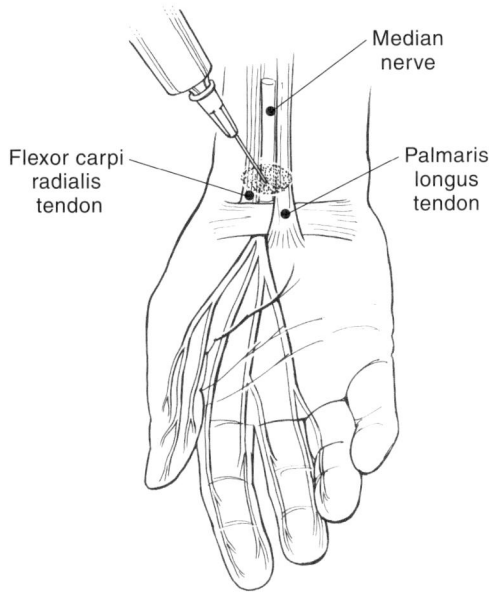

Median nerve

Flexor carpi radialis tendon

Palmaris longus tendon

If a paresthesia is elicited, then 2 ml of solution is injected at that location.

4. The radial nerve is represented by several subcutaneous branches at the level of the wrist which supply the dorsal aspect of the hand on the radial side. The location of these branches is variable and is blocked with a continuous subcutaneous cuff of local anesthetic.

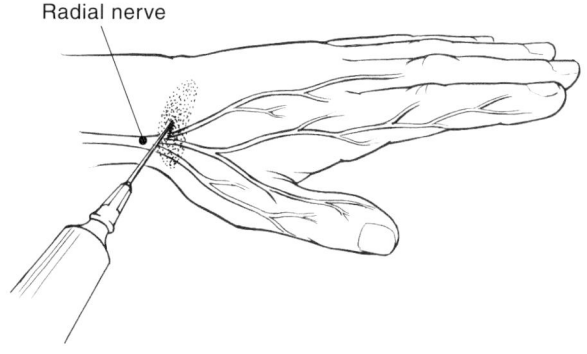

Radial nerve

5. It is crucial to allow 10 to 15 minutes for the anesthetic to diffuse and the block to become complete. This time can be spent preparing the skin, draping, and organizing the instruments.

Digital Block

Technique

1. The principal nerves innervating the digit lie on either side of the phalanx toward the palmar (plantar) surface located at the 5 and 7 o'clock positions as seen in cross section.

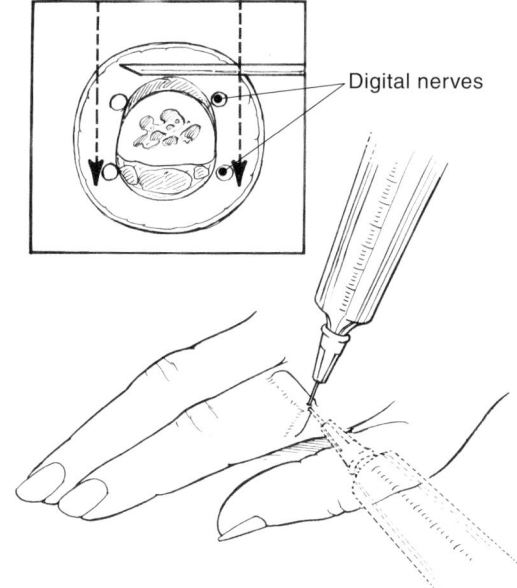

Digital nerves

The dorsal aspect of the digit is innervated by smaller dorsal branches at 10 and 2 o'clock.

2. A fine-gauge (25 to 27 gauge) needle is introduced at the base of the proximal phalanx at a point dorsal and lateral. The needle is advanced until the point lies at the estimated position of the palmar digital nerve, and 1.0 ml of local anesthetic is injected.

3. The needle is withdrawn to just beneath the skin while injecting a subcutaneous wheal of local anesthetic.

4. The needle is redirected 90 degrees, and a subcutaneous wheal is placed across the dorsum of the digit (see illustration).

5. The needle can be introduced on the opposite side of the digit through this dorsal wheal, sparing the patient the pain of a second needle stick. The block is completed by injecting 1.0 ml at the location of the remaining palmar digital nerve and placing a subcutaneous wheal along the lateral aspect.

6. The total volume injected should not exceed 4 ml, since large volumes can compress the digital vessels and produce ischemia. For the same reason, vasoconstrictors (epinephrine) should never be used.

7. It is crucial to allow 5 to 10 minutes for the anesthetic to diffuse and the block to become complete. This time can be spent preparing the skin, draping, and organizing the instruments.

Bibliography

Adriani J: Labat's Regional Anesthesia, 4th ed. St Louis, MO, Warren H Green, 1985, pp 524–526.

Eriksson E (ed): Illustrated Handbook in Local Anesthesia, 2nd ed. Philadelphia, WB Saunders, 1979, pp 86–92.

Ferrera PC, Chandler R: Anesthesia in the emergency setting: I. Hand and foot injuries. Am Fam Physician 1994;50:569–573.

Moore DC: Regional Block, 1st ed. Springfield, Ill, Charles C Thomas, 1953, pp 189–230.

Procedure **LOW BACK PAIN EXERCISES** *Roslyn D. Taylor*

Goals in Prescribing Exercises for Low Back Pain Patients

1. Decreasing pain
2. Increasing strength
3. Stretching contracted muscles
4. Improving posture
5. Decreasing mechanical stress
6. Improving general fitness
7. Stabilizing hypermobile segments
8. Improving mobility

Types of Exercises Used with Low Back Pain Patients

1. Mobility and strengthening exercises
2. Lumbar flexion exercises (Williams)
3. Hyperextension exercises (McKenzie method)

There are no good data to favor the utility of one method over another.

Indications

1. Acute low back pain after some response to conservative therapy
2. Low back pain associated with postural factors
3. Fibrositis or fibromyalgia syndrome
4. As a part of general rehabilitation and to maintain flexibility
5. Chronic low back pain

Contraindications

1. Signs and symptoms of systemic illness such as fever, weight loss, and so on
2. Acute trauma
3. The young and elderly who have not had sufficient workup
4. Cauda equina syndrome. This is the only surgical emergency with acute low back pain.
5. Radiculopathy and muscle atrophy without adequate workup

Preparation

1. Patient's pain should have partially responded to rest, nonsteroidal anti-inflammatory drugs (NSAIDs), and/or muscle relaxants.
2. Patient should be in athletic or nonbinding clothes.
3. Physical therapist or physician should instruct the patient and check progress.

Equipment

Exercise pad on the floor or examining table and a pillow

Precautions

1. Flexion exercises should not be done if
   a. There is acute disk prolapse.
   b. Exercise is to begin immediately after prolonged bed rest, because hyperhydrated disks are susceptible to injury.
   c. Back pain is postural due to flexion or lateral trunk list.
2. Extension exercises may cause an increase in symptoms in patients who
   a. Have acute disk prolapse.
   b. Have had multiple back operations.
   c. Have limited flexion due to paraspinous scarring.
   d. Have spinal stenosis.
   e. Have facet syndrome.

Technique

A. Mobility and strengthening exercises
   1. Low back stretch
      a. Lie supine on the floor with the legs extended.
      b. With the right hand, pull the left leg over the right leg.
      c. Shoulders should remain on the floor; turn the head to the left.
      d. Pull up the left thigh to stretch the lower back and buttocks.
      e. Repeat from the other side.
   2. Full spinal stretch
      a. Lie supine flat on the floor with the knees bent.
      b. Place hands on the back of the thighs and bring the thighs to the abdomen.
      c. Curl the head up toward the knees; uncurl; repeat.
   3. Heel cord stretch
      a. Stand facing a solid wall.
      b. Place one foot about 18 inches from the wall and the other behind about 8 to 12 inches.
      c. Keep the rear foot flat and place hands shoulder high against the wall.
      d. Bend the forward leg and move the chest toward the wall and feel the stretch in the calf; change the anterior and posterior feet, and repeat.
   4. Hamstring stretching
      a. Sit with one leg flexed and one leg straight.
      b. Reach toward the toes and stretch gently.
      c. Change the position of the legs so that the opposite hamstring is stretched.
   5. Hip flexor stretching
      a. Lie supine with one leg straight and one flexed.
      b. Take the flexed thigh and pull toward the chest.

c. Prevent the extended leg from elevating; repeat by changing legs.

6. Back rotation
   a. Lie supine with both knees flexed.
   b. Keep shoulders flat and swing the knees from side to side to tolerance.

B. Flexion exercises (Williams exercises)

All flexion exercises should begin with the pelvic tilt as illustrated to decrease lumbar lordosis. The lower back should be flat against the floor.

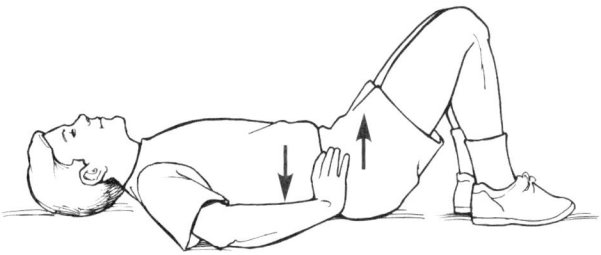

1. Knee to chest
   a. Begin by lying on the back with the knees flexed.
   b. Place the hands on the knees and pull to chest.
   c. Alternative method: can do one leg at a time.
   d. Raising head slightly will stretch neck and other paraspinal muscles.

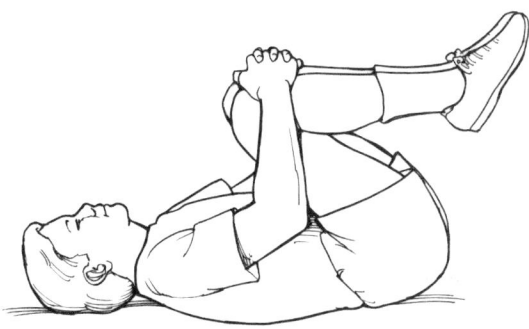

2. Curl-up—strengthens the abdominal muscles
   a. Lie supine with knees flexed and feet on floor.
   b. Place hands on chest; pelvic tilt.
   c. Bring head and shoulders off the floor and hold for count of three.
   d. Relax by uncurling.

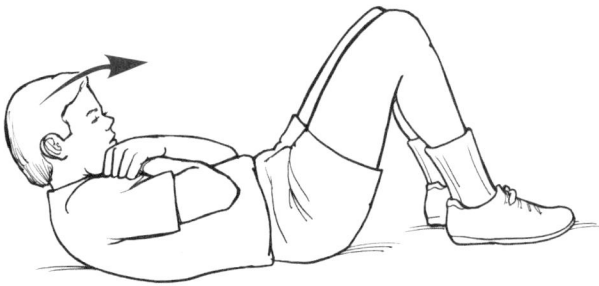

C. Extension exercises (McKenzie technique)

1. Lying exercises
   a. Lie prone, face to one side, arms to side, relax. Pain should lessen or move toward the lower back.
   b. Lie prone and then place forearms under shoulders and lift the chest off the floor; hold and then repeat.
   c. Lie prone, place hands under shoulders, and push up lifting chest, straighten elbows to tolerance, eventually get elbows straight and chest and part of the abdomen off the floor.

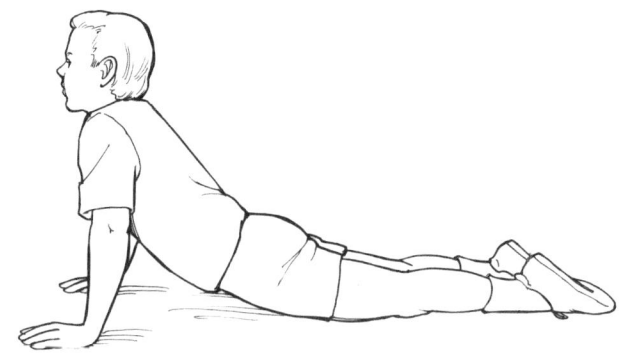

2. Extension in standing
   a. Stand with feet apart, hands on hips with fingers toward the small of the back or hands clasped in small of the back.
   b. Bend the trunk backward at the waist as far as possible, keeping the knees straight.

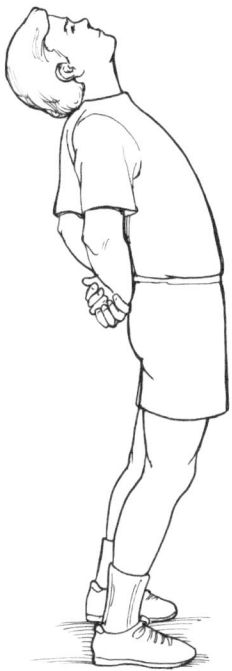

c. Repeat after holding a second or two, trying to extend a little farther each time.

Follow-Up

When using the McKenzie method exercises, after the acute pain has resolved, flexion exercises should then be followed by extension exercises to prevent recurrence. These exercises also can be used in chronic back pain to maintain flexibility and to strengthen and balance the muscles used in maintaining an erect posture. These exercises are also helpful in the conservative treatment of some herniated disks without neurologic signs.

Bibliography

Borenstein DG, Wiesel SW: Low Back Pain: Medical Diagnosis and Comprehensive Management. Philadelphia, WB Saunders, 1989, pp 467–475.

Caillet R: Low Back Pain Syndrome. Philadelphia, FA Davis, 1977, pp 58–77.

McKenzie R: Treat Your Own Back, 4th ed. London, Spinal Publications, 1991, pp 40–49.

Nwuga G, Nwuga V: Relative therapeutic efficacy of the Williams and McKenzie protocols in back pain management. Physio Ther Pract 1985;1:99–104.

Swezey RL: Conservative care for low back pain: The what and how of it. J Musculoskeletal Med 1989;6:57–72.

| Procedure | **LOCAL AND REGIONAL ANESTHESIA OF THE LOWER EXTREMITY** | *Mark Byler* |

Types of Regional Anesthetic Blocks

1. Specific nerve block (peripheral block). Placed to anesthetize a specific area by blocking a specific nerve.
   a. *Advantage:* No distortion of surgical area
   b. *Disadvantage:* Requires precise knowledge of anatomy
2. Infiltrative nerve block: Anesthetic is injected in area of procedure.
   a. *Advantage:* Simplicity
   b. *Disadvantages:*
      (1) Larger amounts of anesthetic agent usually needed
      (2) Possible tissue distention and distortion of surgical field
      (3) Tissue distention may interfere with vascular supply.
      (4) Painful
      (5) Multiple injections may be needed.

Indications for Regional Anesthesia

1. Local and regional anesthesia makes office procedures possible.
2. Patient has medical condition that increases risk for general anesthesia.
3. Postoperative anesthesia

Precautions

1. Vascular insufficiency to extremity
2. Peripheral neuropathies
3. Allergy to local anesthetic
4. Skin infections near site of injection
5. Maximum dose of lidocaine over 90 minutes
   a. With epinephrine, 7 mg/kg
   b. Without epinephrine, 4.5 mg/kg
   c. 1% solution = 10 mg/ml

Complications from Local Anesthesia

1. Central nervous system
   a. Stimulation—seizures, restlessness, disorientation
   b. Depression—unconsciousness, lethargy, dysphasia
2. Cardiovascular
   a. Anaphylactic shock
   b. Bradycardia
   c. Hypotension
   d. Arrhythmia

Preparation for Complications

1. Intubation equipment

2. ECG monitoring capabilities
3. Defibrillator
4. Intravenous equipment available
5. Drugs available
   a. Ephedrine to treat hypotension
   b. Atropine to treat bradycardia

Specific Nerve Blocks to Lower Extremity

1. Common peroneal nerve at the knee
   a. Anatomy: Exits the popliteal fossa laterally passing posterior to the head of the fibula coursing lateral to the neck of the fibula, entering the head of the peroneus longus muscle and dividing into the superficial and

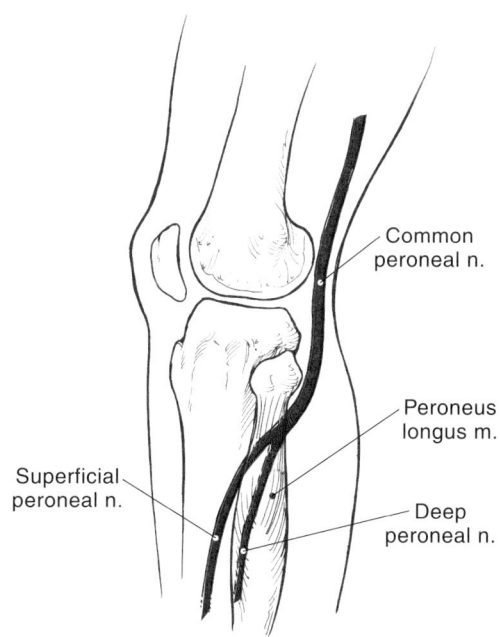

   deep peroneal nerves.
   b. Area of anesthesia: lateral calf, ankle, and dorsal foot
   c. **Technique**
      (1) Identify landmarks: head and neck of fibula.
      (2) Prepare skin with antiseptic.
      (3) Raise skin wheal 2 cm posterior to head of fibula.
      (4) Advance needle, attempt aspiration, inject 5 ml of local anesthetic posterior to head of fibula.
2. Tibial nerve at ankle
   a. Anatomy: At the ankle the tibial nerve passes medially between the Achilles tendon and the flexor digitorum longus tendon posterior to the medial malleolus.

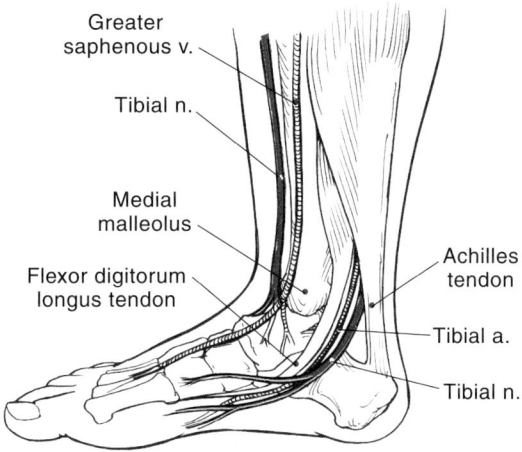

b. Area of anesthesia: planter surface of the foot

c. **Technique**

   (1) Identify landmarks: palpation of posterior tibial artery posterior to medial malleolus.

   (2) Inject 2 to 3 ml of anesthetic just posterior to artery at depth of 1 to 2 cm.

   (3) To avoid vascular injection, always aspirate, since the posterior tibial vein is between the artery and nerve.

3. Sural nerve

   a. Anatomy: Passes 1 to 1.5 cm posterior to the lateral malleolus.

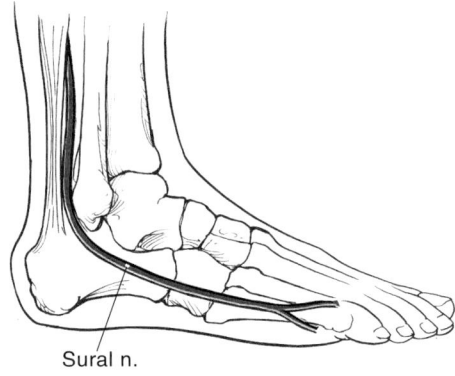

b. Area of anesthesia: lateral fifth metatarsal area

c. **Technique (two options)**

   (1) Specific block

      (a) Identify landmark: lateral malleolus.

      (b) Infiltrate subcutaneous tissue 0.5 to 2 cm posterior to lateral malleolus with 3 to 5 ml of anesthetic.

   (2) Infiltrative block: 5 to 6 cm proximal to lateral malleolus, inject subcutaneous tissue from lateral edge of tibia to Achilles tendon.

4. Saphenous nerve

   a. Anatomy: courses in the superficial fascia in the distal anterior medial foreleg, just medial to the greater saphenous vein and lateral to the medial malleolus.

b. Area of anesthesia: distal anterior medial foreleg including medial malleolus area

c. **Technique (two options)**

   (1) Specific block

      (a) Identify landmark: medial malleolus.

      (b) Palpate nerve just anterior and lateral to medial malleolus at ankle. Inject 1 to 2 ml of anesthetic medial to greater saphenous vein.

   (2) Infiltrative block: 5 to 6 cm proximal to malleolus, inject subcutaneous tissue from medial edge of tibia to medial edge of Achilles.

5. Digital block

   a. Anatomy: Each toe has four sensory nerves, two running medially and two laterally along the dorsal and planter surface. The nerves are *subcutaneous,* close to the dermis.

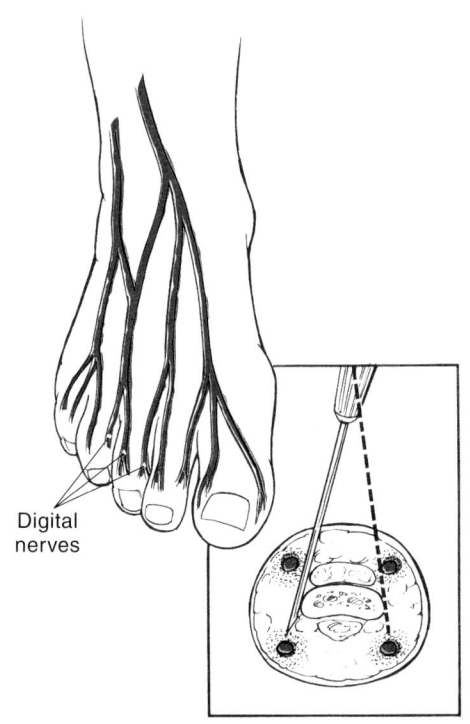

b. **Technique:** Two wheals of anesthetic agent are injected on the lateral-dorsal and medial-dorsal surfaces in the proximal digit. The needle is then advanced dorsally to the dermis on the planter surface. Then 1 ml of local anesthetic is injected both laterally and medially.

Bibliography

McGlamry ED: Fundamentals of Foot Surgery. Baltimore, Williams & Wilkins, 1987.

Yale JF: Yale's Podiatric Medicine, 3d ed. Baltimore, Williams & Wilkins, 1986.

Zenz M, Panhams C, Niesel H, et al (eds): Regional Anesthesia. Chicago, Year Book Medical Publishers, 1987.

197 Ankle Sprain

Ben L. Glaspey

Etiology

1. Inversion and plantar flexion: injury to lateral ligaments (anterior and posterior talofibular, calcaneofibular). Anterior talofibular usually injured first.
2. Eversion: injury to medial ligaments (deltoid, anteroinferior tibiofibular, interosseous membrane)

Symptoms

1. Aid in determining grade or severity of sprain. Classified as grades 1, 2, and 3 (Table 197–1)
2. One or more of the following should be present: pain, inability to bear weight (especially with grades 2 and 3), swelling (immediate with grades 2 and 3, hours later with grade 1), decreased range of motion.

Clinical Findings

1. In conjunction with symptoms, used to determine grade or severity of injury
2. One or more of the following should be present: swelling, ecchymosis, point tenderness over ligament or insertion point, diffuse tenderness, laxity when ligaments stressed (only with grades 2 and 3).

> ### WARNING
>
> **Severe ankle sprains (especially grade 3) can be associated with either fractures of adjacent bones or sprains in other areas (e.g., knee). As with all significant orthopedic injuries, palpate adjacent joints and bones to screen for associated injuries.**

Laboratory Tests

1. Ottawa ankle rules: Determine necessity of ankle and foot radiographs (see Fig. 197–1 legend for guidelines). Note: A 28 per cent decrease in numbers of radiographs ordered (foot and ankle) with no "significant" fractures missed.
2. Stress radiographs or arthrograms: Differentiate grades 2 and 3 by widening of the ankle mortise. Grade 3 injury shows widening of anterior tibial tubercle–fibula interval more than 5 mm.
3. If septic joint or inflammatory arthritis is suspected, do arthrocentesis, joint fluid analysis.

Differential Diagnosis

1. Fracture of the lateral malleolus, medial malleolus, dome of talus, tarsal navicular, or proximal fifth metatarsal. Note: Proximal fifth metatarsal fractures are often missed because the area is not palpated.
2. Growth plate injury: In children, the ligaments and joint capsules are two to five times stronger than the physis; therefore, growth plate injuries are more common than sprains.
3. Syndesmosis sprains (i.e., sprains of the tibiofibular ligament)
4. Arthritis (e.g., gout, septic joint): Onset may coincide with or be triggered by trauma.
5. Myositis ossificans: extraskeletal ossification that can be confused with sarcoma

> ### PEARL
>
> Myositis ossificans usually involves the diaphysis, pain, and mass decrease with time, and radiographs demonstrate an intact underlying cortex. This is a contraindication to early mobilization.

6. Compartment syndrome of the leg

Treatment

PRINCE:

1. *P*rotection. Determination by grade, symptoms, and activity level (grade 1 = Ace wrap; grade 2 = aircast, soft brace, posterior splint, or Unna boot; grade 3 = cast or refer)
2. *R*est. Crutches with grades 2 or 3. Start rehabilitation early.
3. *I*ce. First 24 to 72 hours. Apply ice bag for 10 to 20 minutes every 1 to 2 hours during the day.
4. *N*SAIDs. Use nonsteroidal anti-inflammatory drugs (NSAIDs) around-the-clock *not* as needed (p.r.n.) for first couple of days.
5. *C*ompression. Elastic bandage with or without contoured pad around the malleolus. The wrap should be snug around foot and slightly loose as you wrap

TABLE 197–1. CLASSIFICATION OF LIGAMENT INJURIES

GRADE	AMOUNT OF TEAR	ABLE TO CONTINUE ACTIVITY?	SWELLING	LAXITY
1	<25%	Yes	Hours later	None
2	25–75%	No	Within minutes	Mild (firm end point)
3	75%–complete	No	Within minutes	Yes (soft end point, "clink")

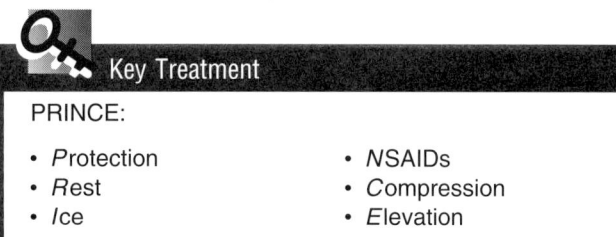

A) Posterior edge or tip of Lateral Malleous

Malleolar Zone

Midfoot Zone

6 cm

6 cm

B) Posterior edge or tip of Medial Malleolus

C) Base of Fifth Metatarsal

D) Navicular

Lateral View

Medial View

Figure 197–1 Ottawa ankle rules. An ankle radiologic series needed with malleolar pain and tenderness at A, B, C, or D, or inability to bear weight both immediately and in emergency department. (Modified from Stiell IG, Greenberg GH, McKnight RD, et al: Decision rules for the use of radiography in acute ankle injuries: Refinement and prospective validation. JAMA 1994;271:827–832.)

toward calf. Swelling is the enemy. The sooner it resolves, the sooner activity can be advanced.

6. *Elevation.* Ideally, above the heart for 24 to 48 hours

Medication

1. NSAIDs. Ibuprofen is inexpensive and effective. Use every 6 hours around the clock for 24 to 48 hours and then as needed.

2. Narcotic analgesics in conjunction for grades 2 and 3 as needed

Key Treatment

PRINCE:

- *Protection*
- *Rest*
- *Ice*
- *NSAIDs*
- *Compression*
- *Elevation*

Follow-Up

1. Ankle rehabilitation

   a. Passive range-of-motion exercises early: flexion/extension with towel under ball of foot, toe circles, heel walk, toe walk. May use water exercises in pool.

   b. Wobble board: especially for athletes; helps regain proprioception.

   c. Athletes: Progress through stages and advance when activity no longer hurts. Stages: walk, run in straight line, run in wide circles, run in figure-

of-8. Rule of thumb: Football player can practice when can run tight (20 yards long) figure-of-8 with little or no pain. (Return to previous stage if pain or disability increases.)

   d. Chronic unstable ankles: 3-mm lateral heel and sole wedge to prevent inversion

   e. If swelling persists for 3 to 7 days, use contrast baths

   f. If healing is delayed, repeat radiographs at 3 to 4 weeks. Keep high level of suspicion for talar dome fractures.

   g. Follow-up appointment in 3 to 4 weeks

2. Avoid reinjury

   a. Tape ankle after first injury.

   b. Braces for chronic or recurrent sprains (lace-up, air splints). Consider underlying cause of recurrent sprains.

   c. High-top, lace-up shoes/sneakers

Bibliography

Gillette RD: Using the Ottawa Ankle Rules. Fam Pract Management 1994;July/Aug:21–23.

Meisterling RC, Johnson RJ: Recurrent lateral ankle sprains. Physician Sportsmed 1993;21:123–132.

Shea MP, Manoli A: Recognizing talar dome lesions. Physician Sportsmed 1993;21:109–121.

Stiell IG, McKnight RD: Implementation of the Ottawa ankle rules. JAMA 1994;271:827–832.

Taylor DC, Bassett FH: Syndesmosis ankle sprains. Physician Sportsmed 1993;21:39–46.

198 Bursitis

Christopher L. Hays

Etiology

1. Definition: Bursae are sac-like structures that are lined by synovial-type cells. They serve to reduce friction that arises from motion between fascial planes.

2. Location: Over 100 bursae are found within the human body. They tend to overlie bony prominences where muscle or tendons pass. Bursae are generally identified by the structures with which they are associated. Some of the more commonly involved bursae are: subacromial, olecranon, prepatellar, trochanteric, pes anserine, retrocalcaneal, ischial, and iliopectineal.

3. Causative factors

   a. Repetitive motion activities: Bursitis most commonly arises from overuse activity.

   b. Repetitive microtrauma: Areas that are exposed to constant pressure and rubbing may develop a chronically thickened and low-grade bursitis. The prepatellar bursae, the olecranon bursae, and the retrocalcaneal bursae are commonly involved.

   c. Acute trauma: An acute traumatic event such as a direct blow or fall may precipitate a hemorrhagic bursitis.

   d. Overlying skin abnormalities: Septic bursitis has been reported as a result of an overlying cellulitis or skin breakdown. Direct puncture wounds and lacerations may also introduce infection to the bursae. Septic bursitis may also arise as a result of hematogenous spread.

   e. Gout/pseudogout: A crystal-induced bursitis can arise in association with these disorders.

   f. Autoimmune disease: Bursitis is seen in association with rheumatoid arthritis.

Symptoms

1. The typical presenting complaint of a patient with bursitis is an insidious onset of an aching type of pain. The pain tends to be localized to the affected region; rarely will bursitis cause a radiating pain.

2. Intensity of pain from bursitis is generally of a low to moderate degree; however, a septic bursitis can be extremely painful.

3. Repetitive activity exacerbates the pain; rest tends to relieve the pain.

Key Symptom

Pain
- Aching type: mild to moderate intensity

- Well localized: exacerbated by activity

Clinical Findings

1. The clinical findings of bursitis are specific to each site affected. The classic sign universally present is localized tenderness to palpation over the affected bursae.

2. Swelling is usually present but may be difficult to detect if the bursa lies deep or if overlying tissues contain large amounts of muscle or fat.

3. Erythema and warmth may be present with classic bursitis but should raise the suspicion of an infectious etiology.

4. Joint range of motion is generally not reduced.

Key Signs

- Localized tenderness to palpatation
- Soft tissue swelling

Common Sites

Several of the more commonly encountered types of bursitis are described below.

1. Olecranon bursitis: commonly seen in contact sports such as football. May present with acute swelling up to 10 cm or more as a result of hemorrhage into the bursa overlying the tip of the elbow. If evaluated acutely, a compression wrap may help to limit amount of swelling. Protective padding is used to prevent reinjury. Septic bursitis may be encountered at this site.

2. Prepatellar bursitis: often referred to as "housemaid's knee" and commonly seen in wrestlers. Symptoms are exacerbated by kneeling. Large prepatellar swelling may develop, causing limitation in flexion. Septic bursitis is commonly seen at this site. Aspiration as a means of treatment should be avoided as the risk of introducing infection is significant.

3. Retrocalcaneal bursitis: pain with both passive and active ankle dorsiflexion. There is localized tenderness deep to the Achilles tendon. Achilles tendon should be assessed to ensure integrity.

4. Pes anserine bursitis: usually a history of change in activity level or overuse; more common in overweight women. Stair climbing may exacerbate symptoms. Tenderness is localized along the insertion of the sartorius, gracilis, and semitendinosis tendons, which overlie the anteromedial tibia inferior to the joint line. Symptoms will be exacerbated when the knee and hip are flexed to 90 degrees and the femur is internally rotated against resistance.

5. Trochanteric bursitis: affects bursa overlying the

greater trochanter of the femur. Patients usually complain of hip pain or thigh pain but may present with referred pain to the knee. Symptoms are exacerbated when patient lies on the affected side. Tenderness to palpation is usually localized over the posterior aspect of the greater trochanter. A provocative maneuver places the patient's unaffected side down and the affected leg is abducted against the examiner's resistance. Local injection is often effective in relieving symptoms.

6. Subacromial bursitis: pain with overhead activities. Symptoms may radiate to the lateral deltoid region. Tenderness should localize to the lateral edge of the acromion. Signs of muscle atrophy or weakness should raise suspicion of rotator cuff disease.

7. Iliopectineal bursitis: usually a history of overuse activity; may present with acute pain in the anterior hip region. Patients may hold the hip in slight flexion and external rotation to alleviate symptoms. Tenderness is localized to the lateral border of the femoral triangle under the inguinal ligament. Hip flexion against resistance should exacerbate the symptoms.

Laboratory Tests

1. Most types of bursitis require no laboratory testing to establish the diagnosis.

2. In cases in which infection is suspected, the bursa should be aspirated and fluid obtained for culture and Gram's stain. If gout or pseudogout is suspected, fluid should be sent for crystal analysis. Normal bursal fluid is typified by a low white blood cell count with a predominance of monocytes. Septic bursitis does not typically produce the high white cell response seen in septic joint fluid aspirates, and therefore treatment should rely more upon the result of culture and Gram's stain. The most common pathogen seen with septic bursitis is *Staphyloccocus.*

3. Radiographs are not routinely ordered. Chronic bursitis may reveal subcutaneous thickening, soft tissue calcifications, or bone spur formation.

Differential Diagnosis

1. Consider infectious etiology.

2. Soft tissue swelling must be distinguished from intra-articular effusion. If intra-articular effusion is identified, bursitis is an unlikely cause.

3. Stress fracture, pathologic fracture, or degenerative joint disease must be ruled out.

4. Systemic illnesses such as gout, pseudogout, and rheumatoid arthritis should be considered.

Treatment

1. The goal of treatment is to alleviate the pain and restore function. This is best done by removing the offending agent, which is often an overuse or repetitive activity. In cases of microtrauma, a protective pad over the site may be helpful.

2. Most cases of bursitis respond to conservative man-

agement consisting of one or a combination of the following

a. Activity modification

b. Ice massage

c. Compression wrap to reduce the acute swelling seen with hemorrhagic bursitis

d. NSAIDs. Best results are obtained by utilizing a full anti-inflammatory dose regimen such as

(1) Ibuprofen, 600 to 800 mg orally t.i.d. *or*

(2) Indomethacin, 25 to 50 mg orally t.i.d.

e. Site-specific stretching exercises

f. Physical therapy modalities such as ultrasound or phonophoresis

3. For refractory symptoms

a. Further activity restriction and/or splinting

b. Intrabursal injection at the site of maximal tenderness with a long-acting corticosteroid/local anesthetic combination such as

(1) Hydrocortisone acetate, 25 mg/ml or 50 mg/ml, 25 to 50 mg with 1 to 2 ml 1% lidocaine *or*

(2) Methylprednisolone acetate, 40 mg/ml, 40 mg with 1 to 2 ml 1% lidocaine

4. Chronic cases with soft tissue thickening and calcification may require surgical excision.

5. Septic bursitis

a. Empiric antibiotic therapy with a β-lactamase–resistant antibiotic such as

(1) Dicloxacillin, 250 mg orally q.i.d. *or*

(2) Cephalexin, 500 mg orally q.i.d.

b. Severe cases may require surgical drainage with intravenous antibiotic therapy.

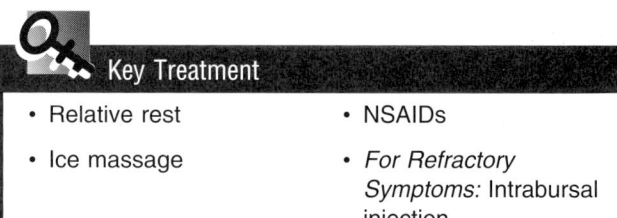

Key Treatment

- Relative rest
- Ice massage

- NSAIDs
- *For Refractory Symptoms:* Intrabursal injection

Bibliography

Antonelli MAS, Vater RL: Nonarticular pain syndromes: Differentiating generalized, regional and localized disorders. Postgrad Med 1992;91(2):95–104.

Bolin AL, Deland JT: Sports medicine. *In* Kelley WN (ed): Textbook of Rheumatology, 4th ed. Philadelphia, WB Saunders, 1993, pp 1695–1696.

Hazelman BL: Principles of joint aspiration and steroid injection. *In* Doherty M, Hazelman BL, Hutton CW, Maddison PJ, Perry JD (eds): Rheumatology Examination and Injection Techniques. Philadelphia, WB Saunders, 1992, pp 121–124.

Steinfeld R, Rock MG, Younge DA, Cofield RH: Massive subacromial bursitis with rice bodies. Report of three cases, one of which was bilateral. Clin Orthop 1994;301:185–190.

Stephens MM: Haglund's deformity and retrocalcaneal bursitis. Orthop Clin North Am 1994;25(1):41–46.

199 Tendinitis

Daniel T. Davison

Introduction and Definitions

1. Tendon injuries often occur by traumatic means or overuse during sporting activity, work, or day-to-day activities.
2. Certain inflammatory arthropathies may present as tendinitis.
   a. Rheumatoid arthritis
   b. Systemic lupus erythematosus
3. Macrotrauma: traumatic tendinitis
   a. An acute traumatic injury resulting from an excessive compression force (contusion) or sudden overstretching (strain).
   b. Macrotrauma is an event, not a process.
4. Microtrauma: overuse, overload
   a. An injury that occurs to a particular anatomic structure that cannot adapt to the cumulative stress of a repetitively applied force
   b. Overuse is a process, not an event; repetitive microtrauma accumulates over time and results in local tissue injury.
   c. Tendon injuries are likely the most common overuse conditions encountered in sports.
   d. Two locations within the tendon are particularly prone to overuse injury: the tendon body and the bony site of insertion (insertional tendinitis).
   e. There is good evidence that the insidious process of chronic tendon degeneration is quite distinct from the acute traumatic response (i.e., the term ''tendinosis'' is used to describe the noninflammatory degeneration frequently seen).

Etiology

A. Traumatic tendinitis
   1. Strain
      a. Strains result from excessive tensile forces on the musculotendinous junction causing overstretching and tearing.
      b. Contributing factors: lack of sufficient flexibility, inadequate warmup, following local corticosteroid injection, fatigue, deconditioning, recent injury
   2. Contusions
      a. Result from high-velocity compressive forces
      b. The more contracted the muscle at the time of injury, the more severe is the injury.
B. Overuse tendinitis/tendinosis
   1. Excessive pressure on the tendon: acromial clavicular arthritis causing rotator cuff impingement.
   2. Friction between soft tissue planes: iliotibial band syndrome resulting from friction of the iliotibial band as it passes over the lateral knee.
   3. Tissue overload, as in patellar tendinitis
   4. The sheath of tendons that overlies a joint may be a bursa, which may become inflamed from friction of the tendon as it moves under a rigid arch, as in subacromial bursitis secondary to shoulder impingement syndrome.
   5. Bursitis may result as a secondary effect of the proximity of the bursae to the inflamed tendon, as in retrocalcaneal bursitis secondary to Achilles tendinitis.
   6. Extrinsic risk factors
      a. Training: The amount, intensity, and frequency of the activity (i.e., exercise) are major factors in the evolution of overuse; too much, too fast, too soon.
      b. Playing/work surfaces: hard (concrete versus asphalt), soft (dirt versus grass), canted (track versus road)
      c. Equipment/footwear
      d. The biomechanics of the sport or activity involved usually dictates the body part/tissue at risk.
   7. Intrinsic risk factors
      a. Anatomic malalignment: excessive femoral neck anteversion, foot pronation/supination, tibial torsion, bow legs (genu varum), knock knees (genu valgum)
      b. Leg length discrepancy
      c. Muscle imbalance: very important in all levels of athletes
      d. Muscle weakness: more important in lesser-trained athletes
      e. Flexibility/inflexibility
      f. Excessive joint laxity
      g. Associated disease states (i.e., rheumatoid arthritis, hypothyroidism, diabetes mellitus)
      h. Previous injury *not* treated properly
      i. Growth cartilage: sites of injury
         (1) Physeal (growth) plate injuries, as in microfractures of the proximal humeral physeal plate—''Little League shoulder''
         (2) Epiphysis: articular cartilage, as in osteochondritis dissecans
         (3) Apophyses: traction apophysitis, as in tibial apophysitis—Osgood-Schlatter disease
      j. Growth process

(1) Growth spurt: longitudinal bone growth, relative muscle-tendon tightness

(2) Loss of flexibility: overuse injury risk, as in traction apophysitis

Symptoms

A. Traumatic tendinitis

1. Mechanism of injury: An accurate description of the injury mechanism frequently leads to the correct diagnosis.

2. Recent injury: One of the more common causes of a reinjury is a previous injury that was misdiagnosed or was diagnosed properly but improperly rehabilitated.

3. An audible "pop" or "snap" indicates significant muscle-tendon tearing.

4. Patients frequently report that they thought they were struck by a bat or stick or were kicked.

5. Initially, there is frequently very little pain and disability, and patients may report that they could return to the activity.

6. Swelling, pain, and disability progress over several hours and are maximal the day following the injury.

7. Referred/radicular pain

   a. Hamstring pain from lumbar disk herniation

   b. Shoulder pain from carpal tunnel syndrome

B. Overuse tendinitis

1. Athletic training/work errors: too much, too fast, too soon, too often, too long

2. Alteration in athletic training/work routine

   a. Interval training, hill-running

   b. A normally sedentary individual who suddenly performs physical work

3. Improper technique

4. Inappropriate equipment and shoes

5. Grading of overuse injuries

   a. The degree of pain in overuse injuries provides a prognostic measure.

   b. Grade 1: Symptoms are present for less than 2 weeks.

      (1) "Soreness" after the aggravating activity

      (2) Pain resolves quickly, usually hours

      (3) No functional impairment

   c. Grade 2: Symptoms persist for 2 to 3 weeks (true overuse).

      (1) Pain during the latter phase of the aggravating activity

      (2) Pain persists after the activity is completed.

      (3) No functional impairment

   d. Grade 3: Symptoms present for 3 to 4 weeks

      (1) Pain during most of the aggravating activ-

ity and continues after the activity is completed

      (2) Performance is affected.

   e. Grade 4: Symptoms are present for more than 4 weeks.

      (1) Pain is continuous, present before, during, and after the aggravating activity.

      (2) Performance is definitely affected and frequently prevented by the injury.

      (3) Activities of daily living frequently impaired

Clinical Findings (Table 199–1)

A. Traumatic and overuse tendinitis

1. Always compare affected side with its opposite.

2. Skin: warmth/coolness

3. Always assess circulatory, motor, and sensory status.

   a. Weakness without reproduction of pain indicates a nerve injury.

   b. A compartment syndrome may occur in virtually any extremity injury, and one should always consider it.

B. Strains/contusions

1. In general, early on, the pain from a traumatic muscle-tendon injury is increased by active resisted motion testing.

2. Grading of traumatic muscle-tendon injuries

   a. A mild, or first-degree, strain is a "pulled" muscle; it is an overstretching of the muscle-tendon unit with no palpable defect and mild inflammatory changes.

   b. A moderate, or second-degree, strain consists of a more significant disruption (10 to 90 per cent tearing) of the musculotendinous unit resulting in a palpable defect with surrounding intact tissue and more significant inflammatory changes.

   c. A severe, or third-degree, strain is a complete rupture of the muscle-tendon unit resulting in a large, palpable defect with a proximal contracted ball of torn tissue.

   d. When soft tissue swelling is severe, be wary of a developing compartment syndrome.

C. Overuse tendinitis

1. Palpation of the involved portion of the tendon frequently elicits a tender, palpable nodule and reproduces the patient's pain.

2. Resisted active contraction of the involved tendon generally reproduces the patient's pain.

Differential Diagnosis/Complications

1. Vascular: Compartment syndrome: suspect in cases of overuse tendinitis in which pain occurs early in the activity.

TABLE 199–1. CLINICAL FINDINGS

INJURY	ETIOLOGY/MECHANISMS	SYMPTOMS	SIGNS
Traumatic Tendinitis			
Acute Achilles tendon strain	Rapid, unexpected plantar flexion as in stepping into a hole Following long-standing Achilles tendinitis	"Feeling like someone kicked my Achilles"	Defect palpable 3 to 6 cm proximal to calcaneus; + Thompson's sign (lack of plantar response with passive calf squeeze)
Adolescent Overuse Tendinitis			
Patellar apophysitis (Osgood-Schlatter's disease)	Rapid growth Traction apophysitis of patellar tendon	Usual age 10 to 15 years Painful prominence of tibial tubercle	Pain with palpation of tibial tubercle Tight hamstrings and quadriceps
Calcaneal apophysitis (Sever's disease)	Rapid growth Fraction apophysitis of Achilles tendon	Usual age 10 to 11 years Pain in heel typically following sports	Focal pain with palpation of calcaneal apophysis Tight calf muscles
Overuse Tendinitis/Tendinosis			
Rotator cuff tendinitis (RCT)	Activities that require repetitive overhead motion	Several-week history of shoulder pain usually anterior, lateral; exacerbated by activity	± Supraspinatus sign ± Infraspinatus sign
RCT secondary to impingement	Narrowing of subacromial space (i.e., AC joint arthritis)	As with RCT	As with RCT ± Neer sign (the shoulder is passively forward flexed and internally rotated) ± Hawkins sign (pain with active resistance of the shoulder placed at 90 degrees of forward flexion and internally rotated)
RCT secondary to shoulder instability	Hypermobility of the shoulder leading to instability	As with RCT "Feeling that my shoulder slips out of joint"	± Apprehension sign Painful click with resisted internal and external rotation, indicative of tear

2. Neurologic
   a. Nerve injuries with a radicular pattern may mimic traumatic or overuse tendinitis.
   b. Distal nerve compression injuries may present with proximal symptoms; that is, carpal tunnel syndrome may present as shoulder or upper thoracic pain.
3. Collagen-vascular disorders may present as overuse tendinitis or be complicated with acute tendon rupture.
4. Steroid abuse: Suspect steroid abuse in cases of tendon rupture at unusual sites, that is, patellar tendon rupture.
5. Myositis ossificans: an abnormal formation of cartilage or bone following an acutely strained or contused muscle
6. Coagulation disorders: Numerous contusions in an individual, especially after mild trauma, should cause one to suspect an underlying coagulation disorder (i.e., hemophilia).
7. Stress fracture

Laboratory Tests

1. Radiographs
   a. Radiographs are not generally necessary when the diagnosis is tendinitis.
   b. Soft tissue radiographs should be obtained when myositis ossificans is suspected (repeat radiographs may be necessary in 2 to 3 weeks to prove the diagnosis).
   c. Radiographs for suspected stress fractures may be

"normal" for extended periods, that is, 6 to 8 weeks or more.
2. Bone scan: "gold standard" for stress fracture diagnosis
3. Coagulation laboratory tests: bleeding time, factor VIII assay
4. Rheumatologic conditions should be screened with an erythrocyte sedimentation rate (ESR), C-reactive protein (CRP), antinuclear antibodies (ANA), and rheumatoid factor.
5. Compartment pressures: Normal pressures are frequently found even following exercise in chronic compartment syndrome.

Treatment

A. Traumatic tendinitis
   1. RICED: *r*est, *i*ce, *c*ompression, *e*levation, nonsteroidal anti-inflammatory *d*rugs
   2. Jones dressing: two alternating layers of cast padding and Ace wrap applied from distal to proximal
   3. Nonsteroidal anti-inflammatory drugs (NSAIDs) for pain relief
   4. Painless range of motion
   5. Strengthening exercises after swelling has subsided and range of motion is pain-free and complete
   6. Aerobic conditioning as tolerated using pain as limit
   7. Return to sports when pain-free, equal range of motion, and able to complete functional testing

(i.e., running and cutting 100 yards following lower extremity injury rehabilitation)

B. Overuse tendinitis

1. Grade 1: ice; reduce/adjust training regimen

2. Grade 2: ice; reduce/adjust training program 25 to 50 per cent; NSAIDs for 7 to 10 days; specific flexibility and strengthening exercises; kinetic chain exercises

3. Grade 3: Same as grade 2 except
   a. Rest from aggravating activity until able to perform without pain
   b. May perform nonaggravating aerobic exercises (i.e., bicycling generally permissible with running-induced injuries)
   c. NSAIDs for 10 to 14 days
   d. Physical therapy modalities (i.e., phonophoresis with 10% hydrocortisone, interferential current, H-wave current)

4. Grade 4: Same as for grade 3 except rest from aggravating activity until pain-free for 1 to 2 weeks.

Follow-Up

A. Traumatic tendinitis

1. Re-evaluate grade 2 and 3 injuries within 7 to 10 days.

2. Evaluate adolescent patients before return to activity, especially in adolescent athletes.

3. NSAIDs should not be continued to permit return to activity.

B. Overuse tendinitis

1. Re-evaluate grades 2, 3, and 4 injuries every 2 to 4 weeks.

2. Follow-up all grade 3 and 4 injuries prior to return to activity.

3. Discontinue NSAIDs prior to return to activity.

4. Consider referring injuries that do not improve in 2 to 3 months.

Bibliography

Giffin JR, Stanish WD: Overuse tendinitis and rehabilitation. Can Fam Physician 1993;39:1762–1769.

Hess GP, Cappiello WL: Prevention and treatment of overuse tendon injuries. Sports Med 1989;8:371–384.

Meister K, Clancy WG: Overuse and inflammatory conditions: Etiology and pathophysiology. Sports Med Update 1992; 7(3):4–7.

Scioli MW: Achilles tendinitis. Orthopedic Clin North Am 1994; 25:177–182.

Young JL, Laskowski ER: Thigh injuries in athletes. Mayo Clin Proc 1993;68:1099–1106.

Zarins B, Ciullo JV: Acute muscle and tendon injuries in athletes. Clin Sports Med 1982;2:167–182.

200 Epicondylitis

Aaron Rubin

Etiology

1. Definition
   a. Lateral epicondylitis (tennis elbow)
      (1) Pain at the lateral epicondyle of the elbow. The wrist extensors originate at the lateral elbow. Condition may be due to tendinitis or, in more chronic cases, tendinosis.
      (2) Most commonly involved are the origin of the extensor carpi radialis brevis followed by the extensor digitorum communis and the extensor carpi radialis longus.
   b. Medial epicondylitis (medial tennis elbow, golfer's elbow)
      (1) Pain near the medial epicondyle of the elbow. The wrist flexors and forearm pronators originate at the medial epicondyle.
      (2) Most often involved are the pronator teres, flexor carpi radialis, and palmaris longus, but the flexor carpi ulnaris and flexor sublimis may also be involved.
2. Cause
   a. Overuse: repetitive eccentric extensor muscle overload for lateral epicondylitis and eccentric flexor/pronator overload for medial epicondylitis. *Eccentric* means contraction of a muscle while an applied force is causing it to lengthen.
   b. In the younger group the cause is sports-related injury; in the much larger group of older individuals, the cause is workplace overuse injury.
   c. Typical characteristics
      (1) Patients 30 to 50 years old
      (2) High-repetition activity level
      (3) Symptoms for 3 to 6 weeks (usually chronic condition when reported)
      (4) In tennis consider improper grip size, strings too tight, metal racquet, practice longer than 2 hours per day, improper backhand technique (snapping wrist). More advanced players may get medial epicondylitis from repeated flexion during serve or imparting topspin on forehand strokes
      (5) In golf, consider evaluating proper swing mechanics.

Symptoms

1. Lateral epicondylitis
   a. Pain over lateral elbow, worsened with activities that cause resisted extension of wrist. This may include lifting objects with wrists in extension.
   b. Often able to lift only with elbow flexed and adducted and forearm supinated

2. Medial epicondylitis: pain over medial epicondyle, worsened by resisted wrist flexion or forearm pronation.

Key Symptoms

Lateral Epicondylitis

- Pain over lateral elbow and muscle mass

Medial Epicondylitis

- Pain over medial elbow and muscle mass

Clinical Findings

History should include questions of recent and remote injuries to elbow, upper extremity, and neck. One should also question type of work, sport, and other activity, eliciting information about repetitious motions and biomechanics of activities.

1. Lateral epicondylitis
   a. Tender over lateral epicondyle and conjoined tendon of the common extensors
      (1) Tenderness more posterior suggests posterior interosseous nerve entrapment (see Differential Diagnosis, next page).
      (2) Lack of tenderness with paresthesia suggests cervical radiculopathy.
   b. May note diminished grip strength when tested.
   c. Increased pain with resisted extension at wrist as well as third finger MCP
   d. Motion loss of 10 degrees compared with unaffected side is noted with more chronic process.
2. Medial epicondylitis
   a. Tenderness at the medial epicondyle
      (1) Tenderness more anterior or pain with application of valgus stress suggests collateral ligament injury
      (2) Tenderness over cubital tunnel (posterior to medial epicondyle) and positive Tinel's sign are suggestive of ulnar nerve entrapment.
   b. Motion may be absent with chronic problem.

Key Signs

Lateral Epicondylitis

- Tenderness over lateral epicondyle and lateral proximal muscle mass

Medial Epicondylitis

- Tenderness at the medial epicondyle and medial proximal muscle mass

Laboratory Tests

Radiographs are necessary in cases of trauma and to narrow differential. Look for calcifications or exostosis in extensor or flexor area, although they are of little known prognostic significance.

Differential Diagnosis

1. Lateral elbow pain
   a. Radial nerve irritation
      (1) Radial tunnel syndrome with paresthesia, a positive Tinel's over the nerve, tenderness to palpation 4 cm distal to the lateral epicondyle, pain with resisted supination with elbow extended, weakness of full finger extension
      (2) Posterior interosseous nerve (deep branch of radial nerve) can become entrapped within the supinator muscle, producing small finger extensor weakness.
   b. Radial head fracture
   c. Lateral epicondyle avulsion fracture
   d. Radiculopathy of C6 nerve root
2. Medial elbow pain
   a. Medial collateral ligament injury
   b. Valgus extension overload
   c. Ulnar nerve entrapment
   d. T1 nerve root radiculopathy
3. Medial or lateral pain
   a. Rheumatoid, gouty, or degenerative arthritis
   b. Loose bodies
   c. Referred pain from shoulder arthritis, carpal tunnel syndrome, angina pectoris
   d. Joint space infection
   e. Primary or metastatic tumor

Refer to procedure on Joint Aspiration and Injection (after Ch. 203)

Treatment

1. Acute phase
   a. Relative rest: Eliminate the activity that causes pain. May return to activity (e.g., golf or tennis) when symptoms have decreased, generally in 1 to 2 weeks.
   b. Continue passive then active range of motion through pain-free range.
   c. Cryotherapy: Cold reduces swelling, edema, and pain. Ice bag should be placed over area for 20 minutes three times a day or ice massage applied to area for 5 minutes three times a day. No excessive use of area should occur soon after icing. Cryotherapy is contraindicated in patients with Raynaud's disease and similar cold-induced disease. Relative contraindications include history of

frostbite, cold hypersensitivity, peripheral vascular disease, impaired sensation, and fragile skin.
   d. Counterforce (tennis elbow) brace
   e. Wrist splint in 20-degree extension may be used. It relieves tension on the extensor mass in lateral epicondylitis and prevents pronation in medial epicondylitis.
   f. Ultrasound may increase rate of tissue healing, reduce interstitial edema, and increase elasticity of tendons: It is generally recommended for 2 to 4 minutes three times per week. Caution is advised in possible infected joint, over open growth plates, and during pregnancy.
   g. High-voltage galvanic stimulation may increase healing rate.
   h. Nonsteroidal anti-inflammatory drugs (NSAIDs) (see below)
   i. Consider injection with corticosteroids (see below).
2. Improvement phase
   a. Normal range of motion is present with no pain. There may be some discomfort at extremes of range.
   b. Continue stretching wrist in extension and flexion.
   c. Begin active resistance exercise, initially isometrically, then with light weights (a hammer works very well) or surgical tubing: Begin with elbow flexed, then progress elbow extension until the following are done with the elbow fully extended.
      (1) Wrist flexion
      (2) Wrist extension
      (3) Radial and ulnar deviation
      (4) Forearm pronation and supination
3. Return to sport/activity phase
   a. Continued work on strength
      (1) Isometric and higher resistance exercise to build strength
      (2) High-repetition exercise to build endurance
      (3) Sports-specific activity
   b. Gradual return to sports activity with close attention to causative factors

Medication

1. NSAIDs: may be helpful for lateral and medial epicondylitis. Be cautious about side effects. Patient should undergo one or two courses, 2 to 3 weeks each.
2. Local medications
   a. Lateral epicondyle
      (1) Careful injection of corticosteroid with local anesthetic deep in area of lateral epicondyle has been helpful in reducing pain and inflammation in area and found superior to anesthetic alone.

(2) Injection with local anesthetic prior to steroid helps to localize the area for the steroid injection.

(3) Side effects include tendon weakening and rupture if injected directly into tendon (but this is generally not a major problem in this area), flair-up of pain for several days (which may be reduced by application of cryotherapy), local dimpling or discoloration of skin (occurs in too-superficial injection).

(4) Technique

(a) Prepare syringe with anesthetic (1% lidocaine plain [without epinephrine]). This may be mixed with 0.25% bupivacaine for longer-lasting results. Mix, or prepare separate syringe with triamcinolone suspension, 20 mg/ml, or triamcinolone, 25 mg/ml (or physician's corticosteroid of choice), with small-gauge needle. A second syringe may be used with local anesthetic for local infiltration of the skin.

(b) Area is prepped.

(c) Area of tenderness is palpated and sprayed with Fluori-Methane spray or ethyl chloride spray, then injected with local anesthetic followed by deeper injection with the steroid/anesthetic combination. Injection should be deep to the extensor carpi radialis brevis tendon, approximately 2 to 5 mm anterior and distal to the lateral epicondyle. Injection may be repeated three times over several months.

(d) Controversy exists about return to activity. Some recommend 2 to 3 weeks off strenuous activity. Studies have shown that full tendon strength has returned by this time. One should certainly wait until local anesthetic has worn off.

b. Medial epicondyle: Same preparation as above may be used—with extreme caution due to proximity of ulnar nerve.

c. Phonophoresis (use of ultrasound) with fluocinonide (Lidex) gel 0.05% for 2 to 5 minutes two to three times per week for 3 weeks is an alternative method of treatment with corticosteroid. Efficacy is uncertain.

Activity

1. The athlete should be closely observed for recurrence of symptoms and given early treatment and activity modification as well as appropriate coaching changes to prevent problems.

2. The worker should avoid repetitive overuse. Modification of length of time, position, and equipment should be considered. The worker should be instructed in a rehabilitation program.

Special thanks to David Anderson, M.D., for assistance in preparing this chapter.

 Bibliography

Amundson M: Golf. *In* Mellion MB, Walsh WM, Shelton GL (eds): The Team Physician's Handbook. Philadelphia, Hanley & Belfus, 1990, pp 628–629; and Nicola TL: Tennis. *In* Mellion MB, Walsh WM, Shelton GL (eds): The Team Physician's Handbook. Philadelphia, Hanley and Belfus, 1990, pp 646–648.

Foley AE: Tennis elbow. Amer Fam Phys 1993;48(2):281–288.

Galloway M, DeMaio M, Mangine R: Rehabilitative techniques in the treatment of medial and lateral epicondylitis. Orthopedics 1992;15(9):1089–1096.

Gelman H: Tennis elbow (lateral epicondylitis). Orthop Clin North Am 1992;23(1):75–82.

Nirschl RP: Elbow tendinosis/tennis elbow. Clin Sports Med 1992;11(4):851–870.

201 Temporomandibular Joint (TMJ) Syndrome

T. K. Cumarasamy

Etiology

1. Definition: The term *temporomandibular (TMJ) syndrome* may be used to describe the presence of the following collection of symptoms of TMJ dysfunction, given in general order of appearance:

   a. Pain in and around the TMJs—occurs early

   b. Tenderness/spasm of the muscles of mastication and head and neck—occurs early with or without joint pain

   c. Joint noises—occur late

   d. Limited mandibular movement—occurs later, usually with joint noises

   When the first two symptoms mentioned are the only or predominant ones with zero to minimal presence of the other two, the term *myofascial pain dysfunction (MPD) syndrome* is used, indicating fatigue or spasm of the muscles of mastication and of the head and neck. This primarily comes from muscle overuse or tension. Prolonged muscle dysfunction can contribute to intra-articular dysfunction. The term *TMJ syndrome* describes the presence of all the preceding symptoms, indicating intra-articular dysfunction due to either traumatic injury of joint structures secondary to abnormal forces arising from malfunction or pathology due to disease of the joint. Malfunction is seen more frequently than pathology.

   Persistent malfunction of the TMJ gradually causes derangement of the intra-articular disk, resulting in displacement, deformity, and eventually perforation of the disk, concurrent meniscitis, synovitis, capsulitis, and in later stages bone-to-bone contact, all of which cause pain, tenderness, or spasm in the related regional muscles, noises in the joint due to disk derangement, and limited mandibular movement.

2. Epidemiology: May be seen in all after the first decade of life but more commonly in white women in the second to fourth decades. The TMJ syndrome with clinically detectable signs may be present in over 50 per cent of the population, but only about half may be aware of the problem and only about another half of that number need treatment. Patients who have signs but are symptom-free when TMJ dysfunction is discovered during routine examinations should be evaluated for the presence of risk factors, which are frequently subtle.

3. Risk factors: Risk factors that predispose the TMJs to traumatic injury and thus malfunction include

   a. Fatigue and spasm of regional muscles (MPD syndrome) due to

      (1) Stress and tension for various reasons

      (2) Parafunctional habits (bruxism, clenching of teeth, excessive gum chewing) with or without stress

   b. Malocclusion of teeth, as well as missing teeth and malfitting dentures

   c. Excessive and prolonged opening of the mouth

   d. Maxillary/mandibular malalignment

   While major trauma is easily recognized, minute trauma to the intra-articular structures due to the preceding risk factors is not and thus escapes the attention of the patient and physician until the cumulative effect has caused irreversible damage and associated symptoms.

   e. Pathologic causes of TMJ dysfunction include

      (1) Inflammatory and degenerative joint diseases (rheumatoid arthritis, degenerative joint disease, gout)

      (2) Infectious arthritis

      (3) Tumors of the joint structures and surrounding areas

      (4) Developmental joint anomalies

Symptoms

1. Joint and regional pain—dull to sharp pain aggravated by jaw movement with possible radiation to the ear, eye, head, and face and tenderness in the muscles of mastication and of the head and neck. Patients may thus complain of earache, headache, facial pain, neck pain, anxiety, and stress.

2. Joint sounds—clicking, grinding, and grating sounds audible to the patient and if loud enough also to those in close proximity to the patient. Patients may have already started to avoid opening wide to bite into a hamburger or apple, started to cut food into smaller than usual pieces, and also changed to a softer texture.

3. Limited jaw movement/stiffness—occurs due to inflammation and displacement of the disk. Patients may find the jaw locking during the opening or closing movement resulting in decreased opening, deviated movements, and having to do wiggling actions to unlock.

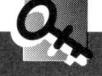

Key Symptoms	
• Joint pain	• Joint noises
• Joint stiffness	• Limited jaw movement

Clinical Findings

1. A normal to very tense patient

2. Tender muscles of mastication and of the head and

772

neck with or without spasm—Palpate regional muscles.

3. Joint sounds such as clicking, grinding, or grating —Auscultate over joint with stethoscope during movement.

4. Limitation or deviation in opening and closing movements of the jaw (normal interincisal opening for adults is 40 to 50 mm, and dental midline lateral deviation is 8 to 10 mm)

5. The presence of risk factors mentioned above. Unless quite obvious, these risk factors will require a TMJ specialist to detect as well as eliminate.

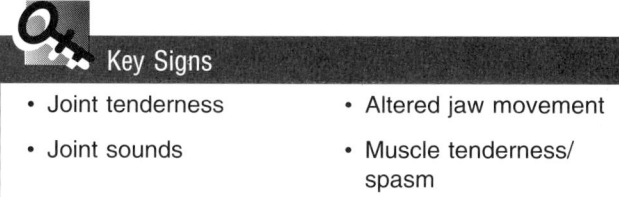

Key Signs

- Joint tenderness
- Joint sounds
- Altered jaw movement
- Muscle tenderness/ spasm

Diagnostic Tests

1. TMJ radiographs. These consist of panoramic, reversed Towne's, and transcranial views and can be used as a screening measure. Bony changes can be seen in advanced cases.

2. Computed tomography (CT) scans may be used to identify bony changes over plain radiographs or plain tomograms. Early changes can be seen better with CT scans.

3. Magnetic resonance imaging (MRI) scans are very good to see soft tissue pathology in the disk, synovium, and capsule.

4. TMJ arthrography will demonstrate disk deformity, abnormal motion, and perforation. Although MRI scans show more detail in the soft tissue changes, arthrography is a popular technique to evaluate joint dynamics.

5. Arthroscopy of the TMJ is done for both diagnostic and therapeutic reasons.

6. Injection of local anesthetic solution into the joint or trigger points in the muscles confirms the source of pain.

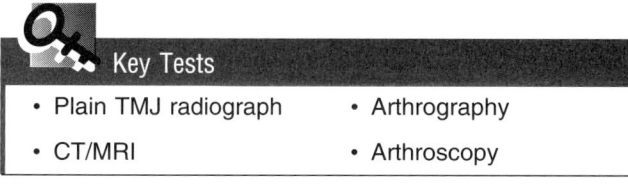

Key Tests

- Plain TMJ radiograph
- CT/MRI
- Arthrography
- Arthroscopy

Differential Diagnosis

Otitis media, neuralgia, sinusitis, arthritis (RA, DJD, gout, psoriatic, septic), tooth pain, parotid gland pathology, tumors of the brain, tumors of the head and neck, and muscular and neurologic conditions can all cause pain and/ or limitation of jaw movement.

Treatment

1. *Initially:* Mandibular rest, softer diet, and local application of heat with use of NSAIDs (ibuprofen, naproxen) control symptoms. Anxiolytics and muscle relaxants may be of value in individual cases. Use of intra-articular or systemic steroids is not common now. Narcotic analgesics should almost always be avoided due to the protracted nature of the condition. The preceding conservative management for 2 to 4 weeks may provide relief for an extended period of time.

2. *Later:* Referral to a *TMJ specialist* is prudent after remission of symptoms for further investigation of risk factors. Behavior modification to eliminate stress and parafunctional habits as needed includes use of occlusal bite guards, occlusal repositioning appliances, biofeedback, hypnosis, and psychological counseling, usually performed by the TMJ specialist and his or her team.

3. *Surgery:* Advanced internal derangement of the joints requires surgical management, usually carried out by the oral and maxillofacial surgeon with view to improve symptoms. Arthroscopic surgery is now widely performed in appropriate situations.

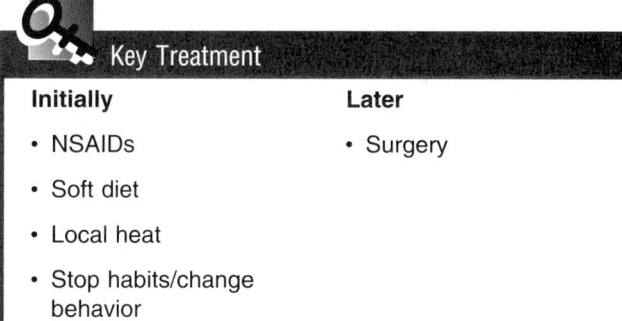

Key Treatment

Initially	Later
• NSAIDs	• Surgery
• Soft diet	
• Local heat	
• Stop habits/change behavior	

Follow-Up

During acute symptoms, a biweekly follow-up helps to reassure the patient and reinforce conservative measures. Since long periods of remission from symptoms do occur, the patient may neglect to undertake further evaluation. Patients should thus be motivated to see the TMJ specialist earlier in the disease rather than later.

Bibliography

Dolwick MF, Sanders B: TMJ Internal Derangements and Arthrosis. St Louis, CV Mosby, 1985.

Parameters of care for oral and maxillofacial surgery. J Oral Maxillofac Surg 1992;50(7)(suppl 2):122–143.

Peterson LJ: Principles of Oral and Maxillofacial Surgery. Philadelphia, JB Lippincott, 1992.

Sarnat BG, Laskin DM: The Temporomandibular Joint: A Biological Basis for Clinical Practice. Philadelphia, WB Saunders, 1992.

Waite DE: Textbook of Practical Oral Surgery. Philadelphia, Lea & Febiger, 1987.

202 Osteoarthritis

Wolfe Blotzer

Etiology

1. Primary (cause unknown—may be genetic)
2. Hereditary (collagen gene defects)
3. Secondary
   a. Previous cartilage damage
      (1) Trauma (meniscal tear, and so on)
      (2) Any *inactive antecedent* inflammatory arthritis
      (3) Noninflammatory joint disease (neuroarthropathy, and the like)
      (4) Bone disorders (osteonecrosis, and the like)
   b. Congenital (congenital dislocation of the hip, bone dysplasias)
   c. Metabolic (obesity [knee], hemochromatosis, CPPD [calcium pyrophosphate dihydrate disease], ochronosis, and so on)
   d. Endocrine (acromegaly)

Symptoms

1. Dull, aching joint pain
2. Pain worsened by activity and relieved by rest; pain typically worsens as the day progresses.
3. *Generalized* morning stiffness absent. Local morning joint stiffness usually less than ½ hour in duration.
4. Joint crepitus, "cracking," and loss of joint range of motion

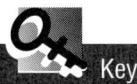

Key Symptoms

• Aching joint pain	• Relieved with rest
• Accentuated by activity	• Brief morning stiffness

Clinical Findings

Osteoarthritis (primary) typically involves the distal interphalangeal (DIP), proximal interphalangeal (PIP), first carpal metacarpal (CMC) joints, the spinal facet joints, the hips, knees, and the first metatarsophalangeal joints (MTPs) and spares the metacarpophalangeal joints (MCPs), wrists, elbows, etc.

1. Joint enlargement usually due to bony overgrowth—*Heberden's and Bouchard's nodes are pathognomonic for osteoarthritis.* Occasionally, effusions (usually in the knees) produce enlargement.
2. Joint tenderness
3. Joint crepitus
4. Joint pain on passive range of motion
5. Joint limitation of motion, contractures, deformities
6. Joint-specific features

   a. Finger DIP joints—Heberden's nodes, dorsal mucinous cysts
   b. Finger PIP joints—Bouchard's nodes
   c. First CMC joints (base of the thumb)—"squaring," "shelf sign"
   d. First MTP joint—osteoarthritic bunion
   g. Knee—medial compartment involvement, varus deformity (bowleg); lateral compartment involvement, valgus deformity (knock-knee)
7. *Erosive osteoarthritis* involves DIP and PIP joints and is more often associated with joint instability and occasionally ankylosis.

Key Signs

• Heberden's and Bouchard's nodes are pathognomonic for osteoarthritis.

Laboratory Tests

1. In primary osteoarthritis, the erythrocyte sedimentation rate (ESR) and blood and urine tests are normal and are useful only in excluding other diagnoses.
2. The synovial fluid is "noninflammatory"—200 to 2000 WBCs/mm³, occasionally up to 3500 WBCs; PMNs <25%.
3. Imaging. Osteoarthritis is diagnosed on clinical and radiologic grounds.
   a. The radiologic features of osteoarthritis are joint space loss, subchondral increase in bone density —"sclerosis/eburnation," osteophyte formation, subchondral cysts
   b. The variant *erosive osteoarthritis* is marked by subchondral erosive changes leading to "gull's wing" appearance in some cases.

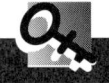

Key Test

• Radiograph

Differential Diagnosis

Osteoarthritis is relatively distinct. It is in the differential diagnosis of *chronic monarthritis* (osteonecrosis, osteochondritis dessicans, synovial osteochondromatosis, pigmented villonodular synovitis, joint neoplasms, mechanical internal derangements, sarcoidosis, and mycobacterial and fungal infections) and *chronic polyarthritis* (rheumatoid arthritis, psoriatic arthritis, sarcoidosis, systemic lupus erythematosus, chronic gout), but can be differentiated by the characteristic hand distribution, normal ESR, absence of systemic features, noninflammatory synovial fluid, and radiographic features.

WARNING

Osteoarthritis is ubiquitous. Radiographic changes of osteoarthritis are common in asymptomatic older patients. *Beware a new onset inflammatory arthritis* **(such as rheumatoid arthritis)** *superimposed on pre-existing osteoarthritis.*

Treatment

Patient Education

1. This is the cornerstone of treatment. Emphasize that to the best of current knowledge medications do not change the natural history of osteoarthritis.

2. Emphasize that the goals of therapy are reduction of stress on the involved joints, maintenance of function, and pain reduction.

3. Arthritis Foundation patient education pamphlets are very useful.

Activity

1. Protect involved weight-bearing joints—weight loss, cane/crutch, modify activities of daily living.

2. Physical therapy to improve/maintain range of motion and muscle strengthening to maintain stability of weight-bearing joints

3. Occupational therapy to cope with and prevent functional disability

Medication

1. Acetaminophen, 1.0 gm q.i.d.

2. Capsaicin cream (Zostrix)

3. Nonsteroidal anti-inflammatory drugs (NSAIDs)

4. Intra-articular glucocorticoid injections (no more than once every 6 months)

Orthopedic Surgery

For intractable pain, orthopedic surgery is indicated for pain relief (and mobility).

Key Treatment

Drug of Choice

• None—There is no known drug that changes the natural history of osteoarthritis.

• Patient education

• Unloading afflicted weight-bearing joints

• Analgesia (see above)

Follow-Up

1. First follow-up within 4 weeks to address questions on diagnosis, management, and issues raised from reading educational materials.

2. Subsequent follow-up every 3 to 6 months if stable. Assessment of response to analgesic/NSAID medications can be done per telephone 2 to 3 weeks after a therapy is initiated.

 ## Bibliography

Bradley JD, Brandt KD, Katz BP, et al: Comparison of an antiinflammatory dose of ibuprofen, an analgesic dose of ibuprofen, and acetaminophen in the treatment of patients with osteoarthritis of the knee. N Engl J Med 1991;325:87–91.

Brandt KD: Management of osteoarthritis. *In* Kelley WN, Harris ED Jr, Ruddy S, Sledge CB (eds): Textbook of Rheumatology, 4th ed, vol 2. Philadelphia, WB Saunders, 1993, pp 1385–1399.

Brittberg M, et al: Treatment of deep cartilage defects in the knee with autologous chondrocyte transplantation. N Engl J Med 1994;331:889–895.

Felson DT: The course of osteoarthritis and factors that affect it. Rheum Dis Clin North Am 1993;19:607–616.

Mankin HJ: Clinical features of osteoarthritis. *In* Kelley WN, Harris ED Jr, Ruddy S, Sledge CB (eds): Textbook of Rheumatology, 4th ed, vol 2. Philadelphia, WB Saunders, 1993, pp 1374–1384.

203 Rheumatoid Arthritis

Raymond H. Feierabend, Jr.

Etiology

1. Chronic inflammatory disease of uncertain etiology
2. Genetic predisposition appears to be important.
3. Cellular and immune mechanisms result in destructive inflammatory process, primarily involving the synovium.
4. Inciting factor suspected to be infectious, although no specific agent has been identified.

Symptoms

1. Course
   a. Affects women three times more commonly than men
   b. Begins insidiously in most cases but may be abrupt in onset (10 per cent of cases)
   c. Usually progressive but often with exacerbations and remissions (incomplete)
2. Musculoskeletal symptoms
   a. Multiple painful and tender joints; typically symmetrical distribution
      (1) Proximal interphalangeal (PIP), metacarpophalangeal (MCP) and wrist joints typically involved.
      (2) Metatarsophalangeal (MTP), ankle, knee, and elbow joints and cervical spine also commonly involved.
      (3) Hip, shoulder, and temporomandibular joints (TMJ) are less commonly involved.
      (4) Distal interphalangeal (DIP) joints and thoracic and lumbar spine are typically spared.
   b. Characteristic morning stiffness lasting more than 1 hour, improving with activity
3. Constitutional symptoms
   a. Malaise
   b. Easy fatiguability
   c. Muscle weakness
   d. Anorexia
   e. Weight loss
   f. Low-grade fever
4. Symptoms may be associated with extra-articular manifestations, including pleural effusions, pulmonary nodules, pulmonary fibrosis, pericarditis, cardiac rheumatoid nodules, vasculitis, compression neuropathies, mononeuritis multiplex, Sjögren's syndrome, scleritis, and episcleritis.

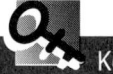

Key Symptoms

- Morning stiffness
- Painful, swollen joints
- Malaise, easy fatigue, weakness
- Symmetrical joint involvement
- PIPs, MCPs, wrists
- MTPs, ankles, knees

Clinical Findings

1. Musculoskeletal
   a. Swelling (typically "boggy" to feel), warmth, tenderness, and decreased range of motion of affected joints; typical fusiform shaped swelling of PIP joints
   b. Effusions of larger affected joints
   c. Effects of joint destruction, including subluxations, dislocations, and ankylosis
2. Rheumatoid nodules (25 per cent of patients): subcutaneous nodules over extensor surfaces and juxta-articular regions
3. Signs associated with extra-articular manifestations noted above

Key Signs

- Symmetrical joint findings
- Tenderness
- Warmth
- Boggy swelling
- Effusion
- Decreased motion
- Rheumatoid nodules
- Joint deformities

Laboratory Tests

1. Blood
   a. Rheumatoid factor: single most useful test
      (1) Helps to confirm the diagnosis if positive in a patient with history and clinical findings consistent with rheumatoid arthritis (RA). Positive in about 80 per cent of RA patients
      (2) Does not establish the diagnosis if clinical findings are not present. False-positive results

occur in other systemic diseases and in about 1 per cent of normal population (especially older women).

(3) Does not exclude the diagnosis if negative.

(a) Negative in up to 20 per cent of RA patients

(b) Often negative during the first several months of clinical disease

b. Anemia of chronic disease commonly present

c. Erythrocyte sedimentation rate (ESR) typically elevated. Nonspecific but may be helpful in monitoring severity of disease

d. Antinuclear antibodies (ANA) positive with high titers in up to 30 per cent of RA patients, usually with diffuse immunofluorescence pattern

e. Hypergammaglobulinemia with polyclonal gammopathy often present

2. Synovial fluid: Inflammatory fluid: White blood cell (WBC) count 2000 to 50,000 per cubic millimeter; usually 10,000 to 30,000 per cubic millimeter

3. Radiologic

a. Periarticular soft tissue swelling

b. Juxta-articular osteoporosis

c. Juxta-articular erosions characteristic in RA

d. Joint space narrowing

Key Tests

- Rheumatoid factor
- Sedimentation rate
- Joint fluid analysis
- Radiographs, especially of hands

Differential Diagnosis

1. Osteoarthritis
2. Spondyloarthropathies
   a. Ankylosing spondylitis
   b. Psoriatic arthritis
   c. Reiter's syndrome
   d. Colitic arthritis
3. Systemic lupus erythematosus
4. Systemic sclerosis
5. Lyme disease
6. Crystal-induced arthritis
   a. Gout
   b. Pseudogout

Treatment

1. No curative therapy
2. Integrated approach is necessary, including patient education, physical and occupational therapy, pharmacotherapy, and surgery.
3. Pharmacotherapy is rapidly changing; must be individualized.

Medication

1. Nonsteroidal anti-inflammatory drugs (NSAIDs)
   a. Useful as sole or initial agents in mild disease and as adjunctive therapy when other agents are needed
   b. Aspirin most economical
   c. Other NSAIDs
2. Corticosteroids
   a. Limited role because of serious toxicity
   b. Intra-articular injection useful for acutely inflamed joints
   c. Low-dose oral therapy may have some role.
3. Slow-acting drugs, some of which may modify the disease course
   a. Gold salts. Parenteral preparations more effective but less well tolerated
   b. Methotrexate. Generally effective and well tolerated, but serious toxicity may occur. Liver biopsy recommended after several years of therapy
   c. Penicillamine, hydroxychloroquine, and sulfasalazine are useful in selected patients; preferred agents according to some rheumatologists.

Surgery

Useful in patients with more severe disease with joint erosions/destruction

1. Synovectomy
2. Joint fusion
3. Arthroplasty

Diet

No specific role other than maintenance of overall good nutrition.

Activity

1. Balance between rest and activity is essential.
   a. Adequate physical rest, up to 10 hours of bed rest per 24 hours
   b. Prolonged immobilization may be counterproductive.
2. Physical therapy is of major importance. Regular exercise program to include
   a. Aerobic exercise to maintain overall physical conditioning
   b. Passive and active range-of-motion exercises to prevent contractures and maintain function
   c. Isometric and isotonic exercises to develop and maintain muscle strength
   d. Immobilization of specific joints with splinting may be useful.
   e. Heat modalities such as hot packs and paraffin baths

Patient Education

Essential for the patient's overall well being

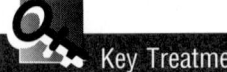

Key Treatment

- **Medications**
  - Aspirin and other NSAIDs
  - Gold salts
  - Methotrexate
- **Surgery for more advanced disease**

- **Physical Therapy Modalities**
  - Heat
  - Splinting
  - Exercises

Follow-Up

Regular re-evaluation and appropriate alteration of management are essential.

Bibliography

Bhardwaj N, Paget SA: Rheumatoid arthritis. *In* Paget SA, Fields TR (eds): Rheumatic Disorders. Boston, Andover Medical Publishers, 1992, pp 19–78.

Borenstein DG, Silver G, Jenkins E: Approach to initial medical treatment of rheumatoid arthritis. Arch Fam Med 1993;2:545–551.

Cash JM, Klippel JH: Second-line drug therapy for rheumatoid arthritis. N Engl J Med 1994;330:1368–1375.

Krane SM, Simon LS: Rheumatic arthritis: Clinical features and pathogenetic mechanisms. Med Clin North Am 1986;70:263–284.

Pincus T: A pragmatic approach to cost-effective use of laboratory tests and imaging procedures in patients with musculoskeletal symptoms. Primary Care 1993;20:795–814.

| Procedure | **JOINT ASPIRATION AND INJECTION** | *Jon Divine* |

Indications
1. Pain relief
   a. Aspiration of tense hemearthrosis or joint effusion
   b. Injection of bursitis, tendinitis, arthritis
2. Diagnostic
   a. Nontraumatic history
      (1) Septic arthritis
      (2) Crystal-induced arthritis
      (3) Rheumatic arthritis
   b. Traumatic or activity-related
      (1) Intra–articular fracture
      (2) Ligamentous tear
      (3) Synovial/capsular tear

Contraindications
1. Absolute
   a. Localized abscess or cellulitis at injection site
   b. Active herpes simplex virus (HSV) or tuberculosis (TB) infections
   c. Previous hypersensitivity to injectable anesthetic
2. Relative
   a. Bleeding diatheses
   b. Anticoagulant therapy
   c. Bacteremia
   d. Partial tendon rupture at injection site
   e. Joint prosthesis

Preparation
1. Obtain informed consent.
2. Ensure proper, comfortable patient position.
3. Identify landmarks; mark sight of insertion with a scratch, sterile marking pen, or skin indentation.
4. Wide-field skin cleaning/sterilization with povidone-iodine
5. Assemble materials while solution is drying on skin.
6. Apply sterile drape.
7. Always use sterile gloves; mask and gown optional.

Equipment
1. Iodine (Betadine) solution, alcohol wipes
2. Sterile 4 × 4 gauze
3. Sterile gloves, drape; mask and gown optional
4. 18- and 20-gauge needles for aspirations; 22- and 25-gauge needles for injections
5. 6-cc syringe, two 12-cc and two 35-cc syringes
6. Lidocaine 1% (single-dose vials are ideal)
7. Injectable corticosteroids
8. Sterile dressings and Ace wrap(s), purple (EDTA containing) and red top tubes
9. Appropriate culture medium
10. Glass microscope slides/cover slips

Anesthesia
Local anesthesia (aspirations only): Lidocaine 1% with 25- to 30-gauge needle. Apply localized skin wheal, and then redirect toward joint. Apply liberal amount at joint capsule. Continuously aspirate while directing the needle.

> ### REMEMBER
> **Joint fluid will flow easily when the joint capsule is penetrated.**

Precautions
1. When using anesthetic agents, have intravenous diazepam ready in case seizures occur.
2. Appropriate clotting factors should be given to patients with bleeding diatheses prior to arthrocentesis.
3. When redirecting needle, always withdraw to subcutaneous tissue prior to redirecting needle.
4. Avoid removing needle completely from skin and re-injecting.
5. Localized cutaneous atrophy can be avoided by not allowing injectable steroids to leak out into near-surface (<5 mm) tissues.
6. Postprocedural compression and ice will reduce subcutaneous swelling and pain.
7. Practice sterile technique (postprocedural infection rate 1 in 10,000). Always use unopened vials of injectable solutions or single-dose vials.
8. Avoid tendons to avoid tendon damage.
9. Postinjection steroid "flairs" (pain developing 6 to 12 hours after injection) can be relieved with nonsteriodal anti-inflammatory drugs (NSAIDs) and ice.

Technique

A. Shoulder
   1. Injection for subacromial bursitis
      a. Patient position: sitting, with arm at side, humeral head detracted distally as far as possible
      b. Locate: Palpate superiorly along spine of scapula to posterolateral portion of the acromion (aromial angle), superior to humeral head.
      c. Insert 4-cm, 25-gauge needle 1 cm below acromial angle. Direct anteromedially, staying close to inferior border of acromion; insert approximately 2.5 cm. Avoid rotator cuff tendon inferiorly.

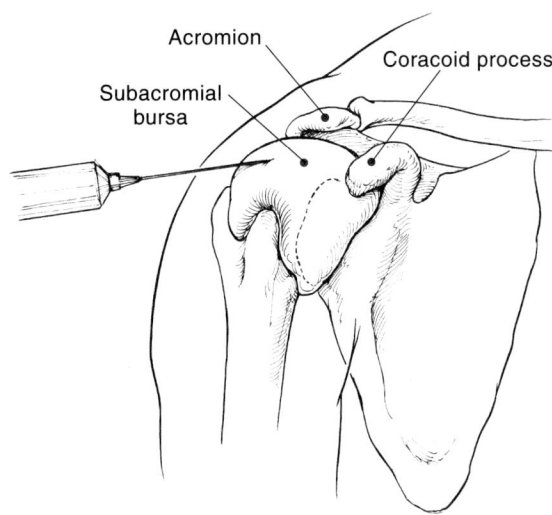

d. Inject anesthetic (lidocaine 1%, 5 to 10 cc) and corticosteroid. Move the joint through full range of motion to distribute mixture. To avoid potential tendon damage, the patient should avoid strenuous activity for 1 week. Note: The injection of corticosteroids in patients younger than 40 years of age is controversial.

2. Glenohumeral joint aspiration
   a. Patient position: sitting forward with arm in lap
   b. Locate inferolateral border of coracoid process, the anterolateral border of the acromion, and the medial border of humeral head.
   c. Insert 4-cm, 22-gauge needle in space between inferolateral border of coracoid and humeral head. Direct posteriorly toward glenoid rim.

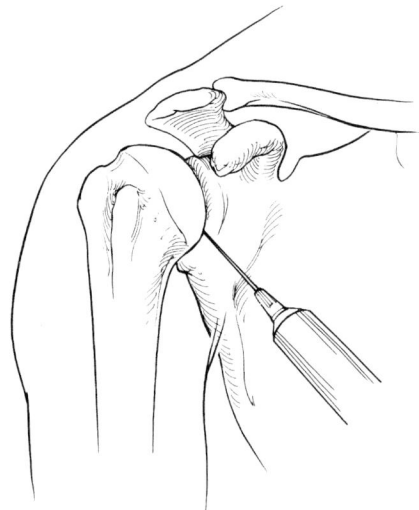

Aspirate fluid for studies.

B. Elbow
   1. Injection for lateral epicondylitis
      a. Patient position: sitting with shoulder abducted

to allow for the forearm to rest on a side table, elbow flexed 90 degrees with hand pronated
   b. Locate point of maximum tenderness near lateral epicondyle. The patient may extend wrist with a clenched fist to increase localized tenderness.
   c. Insert 1-cm, 25-gauge needle into point of maximum tenderness, parallel to the tendon direction.

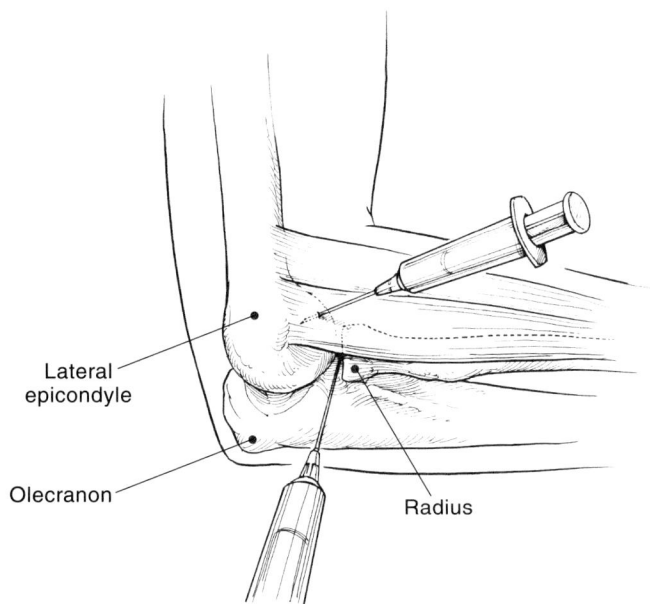

d. Inject a mixture of anesthetic (lidocaine 1%, 0.5 cc) and corticosteroid, bathing the tendon sheath.

2. Radiohumeral joint aspiration
   a. Patient position: same as above
   b. Locate space between distal lateral epicondyle and proximal tip of olecranon process of radial head.
   c. Insert 4-cm, 22-gauge needle at a 90-degree angle to skin. Direct medially and posterior. Aspirate fluid for studies.

C. Knee: aspiration of joint fluid
   1. Patient position: supine, with leg extended
   2. Locate (lateral approach) space between the superolateral border of the patella and the lateral femoral epicondyle.
   3. Insert 4-cm, 20-gauge needle (for septic joint, use 18-gauge) parallel to floor in space 1 cm lateral to patella border.

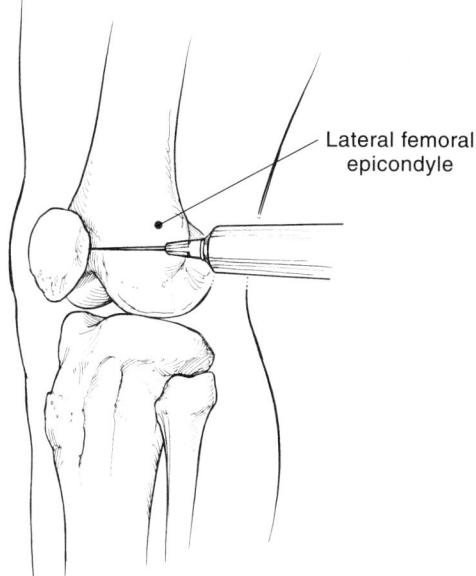

Lateral femoral epicondyle

Direct toward undersurface of patella, with the quads relaxed. The patella may be lifted to ease insertion. The knee is capable of having 50 to 70 cc of interarticular fluid: have two 35-cc syringes ready to aspirate joint fluid/effusion.

D. Ankle

1. Aspiration of tibiotalar joint

a. Patient position: supine with leg fully extented, foot partially plantar flexed

b. Locate the joint line, 1 cm superior to the line joining the inferior borders of the malleoli, and bordered medially by the tibialis anterior tendon. Also locate the points where the anterior tibial artery and the extensor hallicus longus tendon cross the joint line.

c. Insert a 4-cm, 22-gauge needle anywhere along the joint line, avoiding the artery and tendon. Direct the needle superiorly 2 to 3 cm into the joint space.

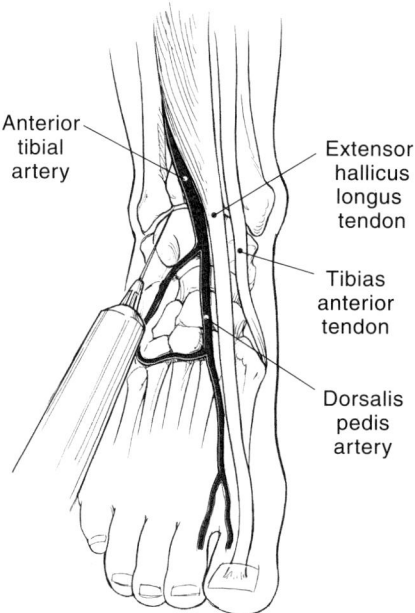

Anterior tibial artery

Extensor hallicus longus tendon

Tibias anterior tendon

Dorsalis pedis artery

Aspirate fluid for analysis.

Joint Aspirate Studies

1. Cell count and differential (EDTA tube)
2. Gram's stain, culture, and sensitivity
3. Crystal analysis under polarized light
   a. Urate: needle-shaped, negative bifringence
   b. Calcium pyrophosphate: rhomboid-shaped, positive bifringence
4. Glucose (compare with serum glucose)
5. String test: Normal fluid when gently pushed from a syringe will form a 5- to 10-cm "string." With infection, the string will be shorter.

Bibliography

Bach BR, Bush-Joseph C: Subacromial space injections. A tool for evaluating shoulder pain. Phys Sports Med 1992; 20(2):93–97.

Kobernick M: Arthrocentesis. In Roberts JR, Hedges JR (eds): Clinical Procedures in Emergency Medicine, 1st ed. Philadelphia, WB Saunders, 1985, pp 687–697.

Neustadt DH: Injection therapy of bursitis and tendinitis. In Roberts JR, Hedges JR (eds): Clinical Procedures in Emergency Medicine, 1st ed. Philadelphia, WB Saunders, 1985, pp 661–674.

Pfenninger JL: Injections of joints and soft tissue (part I). Am Fam Physician 1991;44(4):1196–1202; (part II) Am Fam Physician 1991;44(5):1690–1701.

Warner WC: Infectious arthritis. In Crenshaw AH (ed): Campbell's Operative Orthopaedics, 8th ed, vol 1. St. Louis, Mosby–Year Book, 1992, pp 152–175.

Zarins B: Arthrocentesis: ankle, knee. In Wilkins EW (ed): Emergency Medicine, 3d ed. Baltimore, Williams & Wilkins, 1989, pp 1048–1051.

204 Gout

Thomas Harder

Gout is best known as an acutely painful recurrent inflammatory arthritis that only sometimes becomes chronic and disabling. The precursor to gout is hyperuricemia. *Hyperuricemia* is defined as a uric acid level 2 standard deviations above the mean of a random population or as the supersaturation of uric acid in the plasma (≥7 mg/dl). Four stages characterize the natural history of gout: asymptomatic hyperuricemia, acute gouty arthritis, intercritical gout, and chronic tophaceous gout.

Etiology

1. Monosodium urate crystal deposits in connective tissue lead to gout.
2. Polymorphonuclear cells (PMNs) initiate the inflammatory response when they ingest the crystals.
3. Hyperuricemia is the most important risk factor for gout, resulting from
   a. Undersecretion by the kidneys (80 to 90 per cent of patients with gout)
   b. Metabolic overproduction (10 to 15 per cent of patients with gout)
   c. A combination of both of the above
4. Additional risk factors for gout and hyperuricemia
   a. Male gender (most common inflammatory joint disorder in men over age 40)
   b. Alcohol abuse
   c. Obesity
   d. Age—at highest risk are middle-aged men and postmenopausal women
   e. Family history of gout
   g. Drugs—includes diuretics, salicylates (low-dose), and cyclosporine
   h. Other—renal insufficiency, hypertension, hematologic malignancy
5. Provocative factors that can trigger an acute attack
   a. Repetitive joint trauma
   b. Surgical stress
   c. Drugs—diuretics in the elderly and initiation of antihyperuricemics
   d. Binge on alcohol or "rich" foods

Symptoms

1. Stage I: Asymptomatic hyperuricemia—no symptoms
2. Stage II: Acute gouty arthritis
   a. Attacks are often sudden, occurring at night in a lower extremity joint.
   b. Joint symptoms: Within hours of slight discomfort the joint becomes

(1) Excruciatingly painful, sensitive even to light touch
(2) Throbbing
(3) Swollen
(4) Hot
   c. Systemic symptoms include anorexia, malaise, headache, and mild chills.
3. Stage III: Intercritical gout—defines the asymptomatic intervals between attacks
4. Stage IV: Chronic tophaceous gout—Recurrent attacks may damage joints or lead to the deposition of tophi. Tophi are deposits of urate in connective tissue.
   a. Joint damage leads to chronic pain, stiffness, and loss of joint function.
   b. Tophi become symptomatic if they ulcerate and become infected or if they enlarge and subsequently restrict movement.

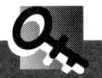
Key Symptom

- Acute severe throbbing joint pain

Clinical Findings

1. Stage I: Asymptomatic hyperuricemia—no clinical signs
2. Stage II: Acute gouty arthritis
   a. Affected sites show signs of inflammation:
      (1) Warmth
      (2) Redness
      (3) Swelling
      (4) Tenderness
   b. Acute attacks are usually monarticular:
      (1) Podagra (acute arthritis of first metatarsophalangeal joint) is experienced during the course of the disease by 90 per cent of patients.
      (2) Less common initially involved joints include, in decreasing order of frequency, the instep, ankles, heels, knees, wrists, fingers, and elbows.
      (3) Spine articulations are rarely involved.
   c. Skin may peel and desquamate as the inflammation subsides.
   d. Fever is more likely if polyarticular or when a large joint is involved.
3. Stage III: Intercritical gout—no signs as a general rule
4. Stage IV: Chronic tophaceous gout—defined by tophi

and disabling arthritis. Tophi are firm and movable; overlying skin can be thin and red. Tophi form first in cooler body parts (areas of decreased uric acid solubility) such as the pinnae, the olecranon tips, and the distal joints in the hands and feet.

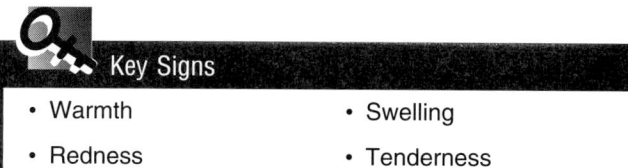

Key Signs

- Warmth
- Redness
- Swelling
- Tenderness

Laboratory Tests

1. Synovial fluid or tophaceous aspiration is the "gold standard."
   a. Aspirate is usually turbid.
   b. Polarized microscopy reveals classic intracellular needle- or rod-shaped crystals that are strongly negatively birefringent (bright yellow when parallel to the plane of slow vibration of light; blue when perpendicular).
   c. Wet mount may reveal the pathognomonic needle-shaped crystals.
   d. White blood cell (WBC) count is typically 10,000 to 30,000 per microliter (occasionally up to 100,000).
   e. Gram's stain and culture (crystals do not rule out septic arthritis)
2. Serum uric acid is usually always elevated but can be within normal limits.
3. Radiographs (changes are not always specific)
   a. Early stages: effusions and soft-tissue swelling
   b. Chronic stages
      (1) Tophi appear as cloudlike increases in density; may be calcified.
      (2) Gouty erosions have a punched-out appearance with overhanging edges, usually eccentrically located in juxta-articular bone.
   c. Latest stages: demineralization and loss of articular structures
4. 24-hour excretion of uric acid has therapeutic implications (please see below under Treatment).
5. Peripheral WBC count is usually normal; occasionally it may be elevated to 15,000 per microliter.

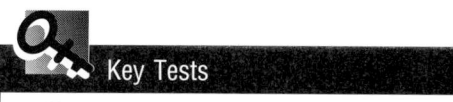

Key Tests

- Serum uric acid
- Synovial fluid analysis

Differential Diagnosis

1. Differential diagnosis for acute gouty arthritis
   a. Infection—septic arthritis or cellulitis
   b. Rheumatoid arthritis
   c. Calcium pyrophosphate dihydrate deposition disease (CPPD)
   d. Bursitis (usually prepatellar or olecranon)
   e. Acute trauma
   f. B27-associated diseases (includes Reiter's syndrome and reactive arthritis)
   g. Other—lipid crystal and intra-articular steroid-induced inflammation
2. Differential diagnosis for a tophus
   a. Rheumatoid nodule
   b. Benign nodule
   c. Other—neoplasm, granuloma annulare, xanthomatosis, leprosy, sarcoidosis

Treatment

Medication

Goals of medical therapy are to terminate the acute attack, prevent recurrent attacks, and normalize the hyperuricemia.

1. *Terminate the acute attack*—begin treatment immediately. Medications include nonsteroidal anti-inflammatory drugs (NSAIDs), colchicine, and corticosteroids.
   a. NSAIDs—initial drugs of choice (most NSAIDs are effective)
      (1) Indomethacin, 50 to 75 mg orally, and then 50 mg orally every 8 hours, or naproxen, 750 mg orally, and then 250 mg orally every 8 hours.
      (2) After attack resolves, taper medications over 24 to 48 hours.
      (3) Side effects: gastrointestinal (GI) bleed, GI ulcer, nausea, rash, fluid retention, and in less than 1 per cent either renal or hepatic impairment.
   b. Colchicine: oral or intravenous (effective if given within 48 hours of onset)
      (1) *Oral:* 0.5 to 0.6 mg every hour until attack resolves or toxicity develops; use limited by side effects of nausea, vomiting, diarrhea, and abdominal pain; do not exceed total of 5 to 6 mg.
      (2) *Intravenous:* 1 to 2 mg in 20 ml of normal saline infused slowly over 20 minutes; rarely used because of low benefit/toxicity ratio; if used, do not give additional oral or intravenous colchicine for 7 days.
   c. Corticosteroids: oral, intramuscular, intra-articular, or ACTH preparations
      (1) *Oral or intramuscular:* Prednisone, 30 mg orally b.i.d., tapered quickly over 5 to 7 days, or triamcinolone acetonide, 60 mg intramuscularly, may be effective.
      (2) *Intra-articular injection or ACTH subcutane-*

ously or intramuscularly: Both are options in patients with contraindications or resistance to other medications.

2. *Prevent recurrent attacks*

   a. Avoid prophylaxis until after second or third acute attack.

   b. Medication options for prophylaxis include

      (1) Colchicine, 0.5 to 2.0 mg orally daily (given in one or two doses)

      (2) NSAIDs: One example is indomethacin, 25 mg orally b.i.d.

   c. Consider concomitant therapy for hyperuricemia (see 3 below).

   d. May discontinue if attack-free for 6 to 12 months.

3. *Normalize the hyperuricemia*

   a. Patients with asymptomatic hyperuricemia

      (1) First treat risk factors and attempt to correct the underlying cause.

      (2) If that does not work, consider medical therapy for either

         (a) Patients with a serum uric acid greater than 13 mg/dl or

         (b) Patients who excrete more than 1100 mg uric acid per 24 hours.

   b. Antihyperuricemic therapy is indicated in patients with gout and progressive tophi, joint erosions, or uric acid kidney stones.

   c. Medication options to lower uric acid

      (1) Uricosuric agent: Drug of choice in "under-secreter" who is less than 60 years old, has good renal function, and has no history of kidney stones.

         (a) Before using uricosuric, measure 24-hour uric acid excretion: Greater than 1000 mg per 24 hours is abnormal; 800 to 1000 mg per 24 hours is borderline.

         (b) Probenecid is the uricosuric of choice; start with 500 mg orally b.i.d.; maximum daily dose is 1500 mg orally b.i.d. Probenecid is a safe drug; side effects include skin rash and GI upset.

      (2) Allopurinol—to decrease uric acid production: Used in "overproducer" or "undersecreter" who does not meet requirements for probenecid; with allopurinol, there is no need to check 24-hour uric acid excretion; side effects can be severe: GI upset, headache, rash, marrow suppression, fever, liver or kidney failure, vasculitis, alopecia, lymphadenopathy. Start with

300 mg orally once daily; up to 600 or 800 mg daily is occasionally necessary to reduce the serum uric acid to an acceptable level.

      (3) Adjust medications initially on response after 2 to 6 months. The goal of antihyperuricemic therapy is to reduce serum uric acid to ≤6 mg/dl.

Diet

Instruct patients to modify dietary and alcohol-use patterns. Purine restriction is difficult to follow and of uncertain benefit.

Activity

Restrictions apply to patients with chronic arthritis; instruct these patients in activities that limit stress on the joints.

Patient Education

1. Teach patients that gout is a "symptom" of the disease hyperuricemia.

2. Teach patients the causes of gout and hyperuricemia.

3. Teach patients the indications for and the side effects of their medications.

Key Treatment

- NSAIDs

- Colchicine

- Corticosteroids

Follow-Up

1. Follow-up in 1 to 2 weeks after acute attack to review therapy, laboratory results, and medication side effects and to plan antihyperuricemic therapy.

2. See patient again in 4 to 6 weeks to adjust medications and to review treatment goals.

3. Eventually, the well-managed patient can be followed yearly.

Bibliography

Crystal-induced joint disease. Sci Am Med 1992;15(9):1–14.

Kelley WN, Schumacher HR Jr: Gout. *In* Kelley WN, Harris ED, Ruddy S, Sledge CB (eds): Textbook of Rheumatology, 4th ed, vol 2. Philadelphia, WB Saunders, 1993, pp 1291–1336.

Tan N, Lertratanakul Y, Barr WG: Acute gouty arthritis. Postgrad Med 1993;94(2):73–87.

Tate G, Schumacher HR: Gout—Clinical features. *In* Schumacher HR, Klippel JH, Robinson DR (eds): Primer on the Rheumatic Diseases, 9th ed. Atlanta, Arthritis Foundation, 1988, pp 198–202.

Tiliakous NA: Gout. *In* Hurst JW (ed in chief): Medicine for the Practicing Physician, 3d ed. Boston, Butterworth-Heinemann, 1992, pp 202–206.

205 Costochondritis

Val Gene Iven

Etiology

1. Inflammation in the costal cartilages of costochondral or chondrosternal junction of unknown etiology
2. Often used synonymously with Tietze's syndrome. Tietze's syndrome, however, is more specifically described as distinct swelling most commonly of an isolated single lesion at the second and third costal cartilages in the absence of another definitive diagnosis.

Symptoms

1. Pain in the parasternal area of sudden or gradual onset
2. Possible radiation of pain to arms, shoulders, or entire chest
3. Pain potentially aggravated by sneezing, coughing, deep inspiration, twisting motion, or reaching, especially overhead
4. Differentiated from Tietze's syndrome by absence of swelling and likelihood of multiple sites of involvement

Key Symptom

- Parasternal, costochondral pain

Clinical Findings

1. Pain to palpation of anterior chest wall with localized tenderness over one or more costochondral junctions
2. Erythema of overlying skin
3. Absence of visible swelling
4. Often multiple sites of involvement
5. Most commonly left-sided anterior chest wall

Key Signs

- Erythema
- Tender to palpation
- Absence of swelling or crepitus

Laboratory Tests

1. Chest radiograph to rule out other diseases
2. Erythrocyte sedimentation rate (ESR) and complete blood count (CBC) are of little value.
3. Computed tomography not useful
4. Echocardiography best delineates Tietze's syndrome.
5. ^{99m}Tc phosphate bone scintigraphy especially if suspect infectious cause (intravenous drug abuse)

6. ^{67}Ga imaging most commonly for associated soft-tissue inflammation and monitoring response to antibiotic therapy

Key Tests

- None—Diagnosis is by clinical examination

Differential Diagnosis

1. Ankylosing spondylitis
2. Bone metastases
3. Contusion
4. Coronary artery ischemia
5. Costochondral cartilage separation
6. Herpes zoster
7. Infectious lesions
8. Lipoma
9. Muscle spasm
10. Neoplasm
11. Rib fracture
12. Reiter's syndrome
13. Rheumatoid arthritis
14. Septic arthritis
15. Slipping rib syndrome
16. Sternalis syndrome
17. Xiphoidalgia

> **WARNING**
>
> **Costochondritis may coexist with atherosclerotic heart disease.**

Treatment

A. Medical
   1. Nonsteroidal anti-inflammatory drugs (NSAIDs, e.g., naproxen [Naprosyn], 500 mg b.i.d. with meals, etodolac [Lodine], 300 mg t.i.d. with meals)
   2. Analgesics (e.g., acetaminophen [Tylenol])
   3. Salicylates
   4. Injection of lidocaine/corticosteroid preparation into joints (e.g., 1 to 2 ml 1% lidocaine combined with 20 mg methylprednisolone acetate (Depo-Medrol)
   5. Local heat
B. Surgical: Resection of involved cartilages in severe/refractory cases

Diet

No restrictions

Activity

1. Refrain from aggravating maneuvers or misuse of pectoralis major muscles during repetitive activity.

2. Modify improper posture.

3. Stretching exercises—particularly pectoralis major —and continued for at least 3 weeks after improvement of symptoms.

Patient Education

1. With reassurance, improvement usually occurs in 3 to 6 weeks (self-limited)

2. Occasionally symptoms last months and can recur.

3. Emphasize smoking discontinuation.

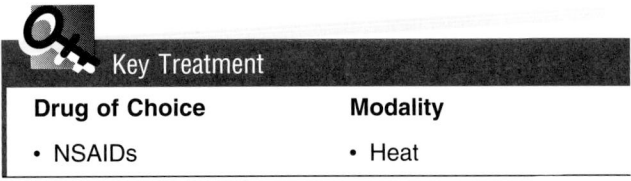

Key Treatment	
Drug of Choice	**Modality**
• NSAIDs	• Heat

Follow-Up

1. Routine visits until clinical diagnosis is made; then regular follow-up to ensure treatment success or further workup as necessary.

2. Awareness that costochondritis may coexist with other disease processes, particularly atherosclerotic heart disease.

Bibliography

For more information on echocardiographic study of Tietze's syndrome, see

Martino F, D'Amore M, Angelelli G, et al: Echographic study of Tietze's syndrome. Clin Rheumatol 1991;10:2–4.

For more information on Tietze's syndrome, see

Aeschlimann A, Kahn MI: Tietze's syndrome: a critical review. Clin Exp Rheumatol 1990;8:408–412.

For more information on differential diagnosis of chest pain, see

Semble E, Wise C: Musculoskeletal chest wall syndrome in patients with noncardiac chest pain: A study of 100 patients. South Med J 1988;81:64–68.

For more information on bone scintigraphy and costochondritis, see

Massie J, Sebes J, Cowles S: Bone scintigraphy and costochondritis. J Thorac Imaging 1993;8:137–142.

For more information on differential diagnosis of noncardiac chest pain, see

Coluccielo S: Chest pain that isn't cardiac. Emerg Med 1994; July:71–79.

206 Myofascial Syndromes (Fibromyalgia and Myofascial Trigger Points)

Jimmy H. Hara

Etiology

1. *Fibromyalgia* (or *fibrositis*) is a chronic rheumatologic syndrome seen in 4 to 11 per cent of the population, more common in women. Etiology unknown

2. *Myofascial trigger points* are seen in up to 50 per cent of the normal healthy population, equally common in men and women, representing tender foci of muscle hyperirritability with specific reference zone pain radiation caused by muscular strain. Muscular strain is often a product of

   a. Mechanical stresses, such as structural asymmetry (leg-length discrepancy, pelvic asymmetry, short humerus), poor posture, or prolonged immobilization

   b. Nutritional deficiency (especially B and C vitamins)

   c. Metabolic endocrine inadequacies (especially thyroid)

   d. Emotional stress/distress and sleep disturbance

Symptoms

1. In fibromyalgia, patients complain of "total body" pain and fatigue, sleep disturbance, and various psychophysiologic symptoms (especially irritable bowel).

2. Patients suffering from myofascial trigger points (or tension myalgia) complain of pain and dysfunction specific to the affected muscle(s).

   a. The pain of a specific myofascial trigger point is in the distribution of the reference zone pain pattern (areas where pain radiates when pressure is applied to the trigger points) for that specific muscle. Frequently, multiple myofascial trigger points occur in the same patient.

   b. Some myofascial trigger points (such as the sternomastoid) have associated autonomic epiphenomena (such as lacrimation and rhinorrhea).

3. Commonly encountered myofascial trigger points and their specific reference zone pain patterns include

   a. The upper trapezius trigger located along the superior margin of the trapezius and referring up the neck, behind the ear, and over the ear to the angle of the jaw

   b. The levator scapular trigger at the superomedial angle of the scapula and referring up the neck, laterally across the shoulder, and down the back

   c. The posterior cervical trigger located a few centimeters below the nuchal ridge and referring up to the occiput

Key Symptoms

Fibromyalgia
- Total-body pain
- Sleep disturbance
- Psychophysiologic symptoms

Myofascial Trigger Points
- Pain in reference zone pattern
- Dysfunction of affected muscle
- Autonomic epiphenomena possible

Clinical Findings

1. In fibromyalgia, a patient must have 11 of 18 tender points on digital examination (with 4 kg of pressure).

   a. Eight of the tender points (four pairs) are those of tendinitis or bursitis: lateral epicondylitis, anserine bursitis, supraspinatus impingement tendinitis, and trochanteric bursitis.

   b. Two of the tender points are those of costochondritis.

   c. Eight of the tender points are true myofascial trigger point pairs (upper and middle trapezius, posterior cervical, and quadratus lumborum).

2. Myofascial trigger points are identified by the finding of the trigger point specific for the affected muscle, which reproduces the reference zone pain pattern when palpated with firm digital pressure.

Key Signs

- Tender points in fibromyalgia
- True trigger points in myofascial syndrome

Laboratory Tests

1. There are no specific diagnostic laboratory tests recommended (complete blood count and erythrocyte sedimentation rate are typically normal).

2. Specialized immunologic testing may reveal an increased CD4/CD8 level (helper/suppressor ratio) in fibromyalgia.

3. Sleep electroencephalogram may reveal an alpha/delta pattern.

Differential Diagnosis

1. The differential diagnosis of fibromyalgia includes depression, metabolic imbalance, hypothyroidism, polymyalgia rheumatica, and polymyositis.

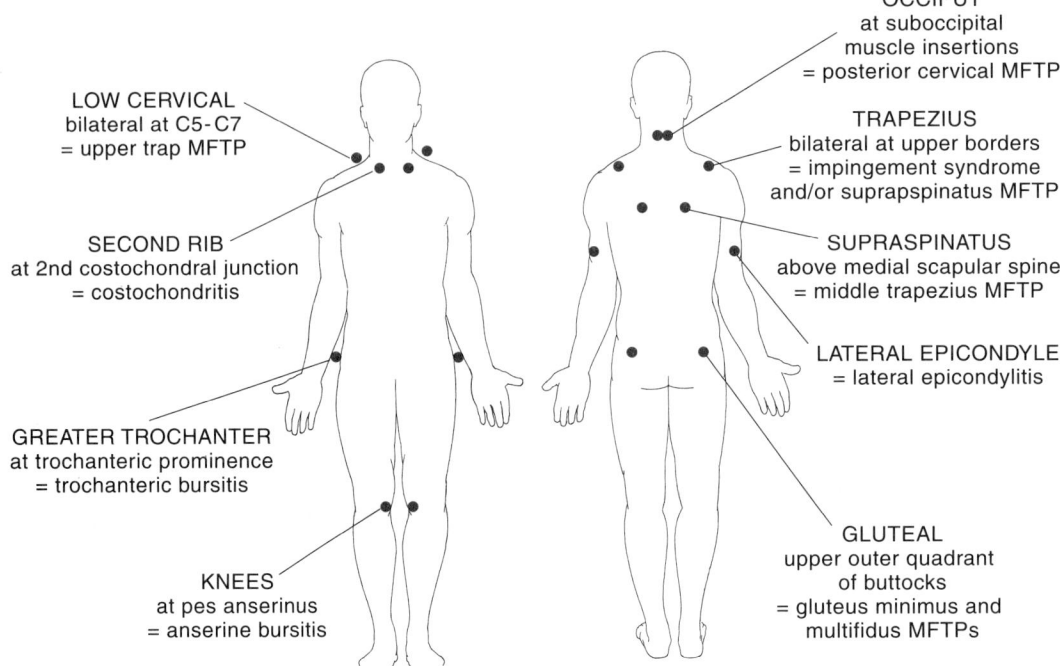

Figure 206-1 Occipital/suboccipital corresponds to posterior cervical myofascial trigger point (MFTP). Low cervical corresponds to the upper trapezius myofascial trigger point. Trapezius corresponds to the lesser trapezius myofascial triggers and the supraspinatus peritendinitis/impingement syndrome tender points. Supraspinatus corresponds to the middle trapezius myofascial trigger point. Lateral epicondyle corresponds to lateral epicondylitis tendinosis/enthesitis. Gluteal corresponds to gluteus minimus and multifidus myofascial triggers. Second rib corresponds to costochondritis tender points. Knees correspond to tender points of the anserine bursitis.

2. The differential diagnosis of specific myofascial trigger point syndromes includes any cause of pain or dysfunction in the involved anatomic site (Fig. 206–1).

Treatment

1. Pharmacotherapy for fibromyalgia includes low-dose selective serotonin reuptake inhibitor (SSRI) antidepressants (fluoxetine [Prozac], sertraline [Zoloft], paroxetine [Paxil]), low-dose heterocyclic antidepressants (trazodone [Desyrel], bupropion [Wellbutrin], venlafaxine [Effexor], and cyclobenzaprine [Flexoril]).

2. Tendinitis, bursitis, and costochondritis tender points may be injected with xylocaine and steroid.

3. Anesthetic injection of trigger points with 0.5% procaine (patient should experience pain/warmth in reference zone pain pattern as anesthetic is infused)

4. Stretch and intermittent cold therapy (vapocoolant stretch and spray) may be applied to specific myofascial trigger point muscle.

5. Other stretching modalities may be applied, such as the Lewit technique, strain-counterstrain, or proprioceptive neuromuscular facilitation (PNF).

6. Ischemic compression may be applied for approximately 3 minutes to extinguish trigger point pain. Shiatsu and acupressure may be effective as ischemic compression techniques

Diet
1. Basic nutritionally sound diet
2. Ensure adequate water-soluble vitamins.
Activity
1. Advise exercise as tolerated.

2. Focus on adequate stretching of involved muscles.
Patient Education
1. Explain chronic nature of fibromyalgia.

2. Prevent precipitating factors if identified (poor body mechanics, compensations for body asymmetry, poor diet).

3. Encourage stretching of involved muscles.

Key Treatment

For Fibromyalgia	**For Trigger Points**
• Low-dose SSRI or heterocyclic antidepressant	• Injection with procaine
	• Stretching modalities
• Injection with xylocaine/steroid	• Ischemic compression

Follow-Up

1. Fibromyalgia patients require periodic follow-ups to treat symptomatic tender points and titrate drugs.

2. Patients with chronic and recurrent myofascial trigger

points may need periodic revisits for injections or stretch and intermittent cold therapy.

3. Patients with acute or episodic myofascial trigger point syndromes do not typically require follow-up.

 Bibliography

McCain, GA: Treatment of fibromyalgia and myofascial pain syndrome. *In* Rachlin, ES (ed): Myofascial Pain and Fibromyalgia. St Louis, Mosby-Year Book, 1994, pp 31–44.

Thompson J: Tension myalgia as a diagnosis at the Mayo Clinic and its relationship to fibrositis, fibromyalgia, and myofascial pain syndrome. Mayo Clin Proc 1990;65:1237–1248.

Travell J, Simons DG: Myofascial Pain and Dysfunction: The Trigger Point Manual, vol 2. Baltimore, Williams & Wilkins, 1991, pp 8–22.

Yunus MB: Fibromyalgia syndrome and myofascial pain syndrome: Clinical features, laboratory tests, diagnosis, and pathophysiologic mechanisms. *In* Rachlin, ES (ed): Myofascial Pain and Fibromyalgia. St Louis, Mosby-Year Book, 1994, pp 3–29.

207 Systemic Lupus Erythematosus

Laura Carbone

Etiology

Specific cause is unknown, multifactorial.

1. Genetic factors
   a. Increased frequency of both systemic lupus erythematosus (SLE) and immunologic abnormalities in relatives of patients with SLE, with especially high concordance rate among monozygotic twins
   b. Association with complement deficiencies C2 and C4 as well as HLA-DR, DR3, and deletion of C4A gene (in whites)
   c. Increased prevalence of SLE among certain ethnic groups including African Americans, Puerto Ricans, Asians, and Polynesians

2. Hormonal factors
   a. In young adults SLE is 10 to 13 times more common in females than in males.
   b. Both males and females with SLE have increased hydroxylation of estrone to 16 hydroxyestrone, a potent estrogenic hormone.
   c. Males with Kleinfelter's disease are prone to develop SLE.

3. Environmental factors
   a. Increased frequency of autoantibodies in laboratory workers who handle blood of patients with SLE.
   b. Certain medications such as hydralazine and procainamide can trigger SLE or SLE-like syndromes.

Symptoms

The course of SLE is fluctuating, with many exacerbations and remissions in multiple systems.

1. Fatigue: common
2. Raynaud's phenomenon: in approximately one third of cases
3. Cardiac manifestations
   a. Pericarditis
      (1) Most common cardiac manifestation: anterior chest pain
      (2) Rarely can progress to constrictive pericarditis or tamponade with dyspnea and pedal edema
   b. Coronary atherosclerosis: high incidence of coronary artery disease in SLE patients treated with steroids
   c. Myocarditis: suspect with unexplained tachycardia or congestive heart failure
4. Pulmonary involvement
   a. Pleurisy and pleural effusions most common
   b. Dyspnea and cough suggest pulmonary fibrosis or pneumonitis

5. Neurologic manifestations
   a. Grand mal seizures develop in approximately 20 per cent, but it is important to exclude secondary causes such as infection, drug reaction, uremia, and uncontrolled hypertension; may progress to coma.
   b. Psychosis
   c. Hemiplegia, transverse myelitis and chorea: important to assess for presence of antiphospholipid antibody or anticardiolipin antibody
   d. Guillain-Barré syndrome, peripheral neuropathy, and mononeuritis multiplex are uncommon, but may present with motor or sensory symptoms.
   e. When neurologic disease occurs in SLE patients, it is important to assess for activity of disease in other organ systems.
6. Nephrologic manifestations
   a. Renal disease occurs in approximately 50 per cent.
   b. The timing of biopsy remains controversial. However, renal biopsy will provide information on severity, chronicity, and type of lesion.
7. Arthralgia with or without joint swelling is present in 90 per cent of patients at some time during disease course.
8. Oral ulcers, often painful
9. Sicca symptoms are not uncommon, with dry eyes and dry mouth.

Signs

1. Fever: imperative to exclude infection
2. Arthritis
   a. Polyarticular, nonerosive, mostly nondeforming symmetric arthritis
   b. When deformities occur, they are usually secondary to tenosynovitis.
   c. Proximal interphalangeal and knee joints are most commonly affected.
   d. Spontaneous tendon rupture, especially of Achilles and patellar tendons, may rarely occur.
3. Rashes: very common, many types
   a. Malar rash: "butterfly rash," sparing nasolabial folds
   b. Discoid lesions
      (1) Occur on face, neck, scalp, and external ears
      (2) Central scarring with atrophy
   c. Subacute cutaneous SLE
      (1) Occurs on upper torso
      (2) Association with HLA DR3 and Ro antibody

(3) Unlike discoid lesions, scarring does not occur and telangiectasias are common.

4. Alopecia

a. Usually diffuse, nonscarring

b. Can be first sign of disease activity

c. When associated with discoid lesions, may scar

5. Lymphadenopathy and splenomegaly

Laboratory Tests

1. Anemia

a. Anemia of chronic disease with suppressed erythropoiesis

b. Iron deficiency anemia secondary to gastrointestinal blood loss

c. Hemolytic anemia; however, positive Coombs' test is not always associated with hemolysis

2. Leukopenia with lymphocytopenia

3. Thrombocytopenia

a. May be secondary to antiplatelet antibodies

b. The first manifestation of SLE may be immune thrombocytopenia purpura (ITP), and obtaining an antinuclear antibody test should be considered in all patients with ITP.

4. Lupus anticoagulant

a. Antiphospholipid antibody that causes a prolonged partial thromboplastin time not corrected by addition of normal plasma

b. Associated with thrombosis

c. May occur without SLE

5. Antinuclear antibody (ANA)

a. Positive in more than 95 per cent of patients with SLE

b. Not all patients with positive ANA have SLE (associated with aging, medications, no disease state, other connective tissue diseases).

c. Course not used to follow activity of disease

d. Four patterns

(1) Rim: correlates with renal disease

(2) Speckled

(3) Homogeneous

(4) Nucleolar: sometimes associated with scleroderma

6. AntidsDNA

a. Correlates with renal disease

b. Used to follow activity of SLE, especially renal disease, with rising levels indicating active disease

7. Complements (C3, C4, CH50): In absence of congenital complement deficiency, falling levels are usually associated with active disease, especially renal disease.

Criteria for SLE Classification (4 of these must be present or positive for diagnosis)*

1. Malar rash

2. Discoid rash

3. Oral or nasal ulcers

4. Arthritis

5. Photosensitivity

6. Serositis

a. Pleurisy

b. Pericarditis

7. Neurologic disorder

a. Seizures

b. Psychosis

8. Renal disease

a. Proteinuria greater than 0.5 gm/day or 3+ on dipstick

b. Cellular casts

9. Hematologic disorder

a. Hemolytic anemia with reticulocytosis

b. Leukopenia (less than 4000/mm^3)

c. Lymphopenia (less than 1500/mm^3)

d. Thrombocytopenia (less than 100,000/mm^3)

10. Immunologic disorder

a. Positive LE preparation

b. Positive antidsDNA

c. Positive anti Sm

d. False-positive test for syphilis

11. ANA

Differential Diagnosis

1. Infection

a. Subacute bacterial endocarditis

b. HIV (False-positive test for HIV can occur in SLE.)

2. Malignancy—especially lymphomas

3. Other connective tissue disease

a. Mixed connective tissue disease

b. Rheumatoid arthritis (RA) (with features of both RA and SLE often called ''rhupus'')

c. Vasculitis

Treatment

1. Hydroxychloroquine sulfate (Plaquenil)

a. Indications for usage

(1) Rashes

(2) Serositis

(3) Arthritis

b. Dosage: 200 to 400 mg daily

---

*Tom EM, Cohen AS, Fries JF, et al: The 1982 revised criteria for the classification of SLE. Arthritis Rheum 1982;25:1271–1277.

c. Side effects
   (1) Retinal toxicity, although rare, is major serious complication.
   (2) Rashes, gastrointestinal (GI) intolerance, bone marrow suppression are rare complications.
   d. Monitoring: ophthalmologic examination before therapy and every 6 months

2. Nonsteroidal anti-inflammatory drugs (NSAIDs) (Avoid ibuprofen, sulindac, and tolmetin because they can be associated with aseptic meningitis.)
   a. Indications for usage
      (1) Arthritis
      (2) Serositis
   b. Dosage: standard dosages for treatment of arthritis as per PDR for individual NSAID
   c. Side effects
      (1) GI intolerance
      (2) Renal and hepatic insufficiency
      (3) Bone marrow depression
   d. Monitoring: baseline complete blood count (CBC) with differential, and chemistry profile; then every 3 to 6 months

3. Steroids
   a. Indications for usage
      (1) Arthritis (uncontrolled by 1,2)
      (2) Serositis
      (3) Hematologic, nephrologic, or CNS complications
   b. Dosage (prednisone equivalents)
      (1) Low dosage (10 to 20 mg/day) for short period for arthritis, serositis
      (2) Higher doses (1 mg/kg/day) may be needed for hematologic, CNS, or nephrologic complications.
   c. Side effects: multiple, including bruising, osteoporosis, aseptic necrosis, cataracts, glaucoma, hypertension, weight gain, diabetes, acne, depression or psychosis, GI intolerance, accelerated atherogenesis, opportunistic infections
   d. Monitoring
      (1) Ophthalmologic examination for those on long-term steroids
      (2) Serial blood pressure checks
      (3) Monitor glucose levels

4. Cyclophosphamide (Cytoxan)
   a. Indications for usage: certain nephrologic problems (diffuse proliferative nephritis), CNS or refractory hematologic conditions
   b. Dosage: intermittent intravenous (0.5 to 1 gm/m² body surface area) every 4 to 6 weeks
   c. Side effects
      (1) Hemorrhagic cystitis and bladder carcinoma
      (2) Opportunistic infections
      (3) Suppression of gonadal function

   (4) Bone marrow depression
   (5) Increased incidence of lymphoma and other hematologic malignancies
   d. Monitoring
      (1) Baseline CBC with differential, chemistry profile, and urinalysis
      (2) Monitor CBC with differential closely during treatment
      (3) Urinalysis and urine cytology in those requiring long-term treatment
      (4) Repeat urinalysis and obtain urine cytology if there are any bladder symptoms.
      (5) Cytoscopy if hematuria is present or if there is abnormal urine cytology

Diet
1. Strict control of hypertension with low-sodium diet and weight loss as appropriate
2. Control of hyperlipidemia with weight loss and low cholesterol, triglyceride diet as appropriate

Activity
1. Adequate rest
2. Sufficient exercise

Patient Education
1. Regular medical follow-up and adhere to medical regimen.
2. Avoid sunlight; use sunscreens with high SPF (>30) and long-sleeved clothing with hats when unable to avoid sun
3. Early treatment of infections
4. Immunizations with influenza and pneumoccocal vaccines if no contraindications
5. Avoidance of pregnancy at times of disease activity
6. Preferably use of barrier contraception; if oral contraceptives used, use lowest dose of estrogen available.

Follow-Up
1. Review patient's history for any suggestion of disease flare (e.g., rash, oral ulcers, alopecia).
2. Regular monitoring of CBC and urinalysis and consider ordering antidsDNA, C3, C4 if there is suspicion of increased disease activity, especially renal disease.
3. Quantify degree of proteinuria if present.
4. Strict control of hypertension

Bibliography

Gladman D, Vrowitz M: Systemic lupus erythematosus. *In* Schumacher R (ed): Primer on the Rheumatic Diseases. 10th ed. Atlanta, Arthritis Foundation, 1993, pp 106–111.

Isenberg D, Horsfall AC: Systemic lupus erythematosus—adult onset. *In* Maddison PJ, Isenberg D, Woo P, Glass D (eds): Oxford Textbook of Rheumatology, vol 2. New York, Oxford University Press, 1993, pp 733–756.

Rothfield N: Systemic lupus erythematosus. *In* McCarty D, Koopman W (eds): Arthritis and Allied Conditions. 12th ed, vol 2. Philadelphia, Lea & Febiger, 1993, pp 1155–1177.

Schur P: Clinical features of SLE. *In* Kelley W, Harris E, Ruddy S, Sledge C (eds): Textbook of Rheumatology. 4th ed, vol 2. Philadelphia, WB Saunders, 1993, pp 1017–1042.

208 Scleroderma (Systemic Sclerosis)

Carlos M. Swanger

Etiology

1. The cause of systemic sclerosis is unknown.
2. Theories of pathogenesis
   a. Genetic predisposition—haplotype HLA A1, B8, DR3
   b. Connective tissue—excessive deposition of tissue matrix proteins, primarily collagen
   c. Vascular—microvascular and endothelial injury
   d. Immunologic—the association of specific antinuclear antibodies (ANAs) and the presence of mononuclear cell infiltrates
   e. Epidemiology
      (1) Incidence 4 to 12 cases per million, increasing with age
      (2) The disease is three to four times more common in women, particularly young black females.

Symptoms

1. Raynaud's phenomenon—episodic digital ischemia
   a. Presents as pallor followed by cyanosis and rubor. Pallor is the most reliable component of this triad.
   b. Syndrome occurs in 90 to 98 per cent of patients with systemic sclerosis; it is the first symptom in 70 per cent of cases.
2. Skin
   a. Skin thickening
      (1) Often begins with hands
      (2) Development of taut facial skin that may lead to restriction of mouth opening
      (3) Areas of hyper- or hypopigmentation
   b. Edema
      (1) Swelling mainly of hands
      (2) May also be present on trunk, proximal arms, and face
3. Musculoskeletal
   a. Morning stiffness and arthralgias. Arthritis occurs as the initial symptom in up to 66 per cent of patients.
   b. Limitation of joint function and movement
   c. Muscle weakness secondary to disuse atrophy and/or myositis
4. Gastrointestinal
   a. Intermittent heartburn and regurgitation secondary to esophageal involvement
   b. Dysphagia and odynophagia
   c. Early satiety

d. Telangiectasias may cause symptoms of both upper and lower gastrointestinal (GI) bleeding.
   e. Persistent vomiting from functional gastric outlet obstruction
   f. Acute and chronic diarrhea
   g. Symptoms associated with small bowel obstruction
5. Pulmonary
   a. Worsening dyspnea on exertion
   b. Nonproductive cough
   c. Less commonly, there may be chest pain, pleurisy, or productive cough.
6. Cardiac
   a. Palpitations from atrial or ventricular arrhythmias
   b. Congestive heart failure (CHF) manifest as dyspnea or edema
   c. Chest pain—such as that associated with pericarditis
7. Renal: symptoms associated with severe hypertension:
   a. Headaches
   b. Visual disturbances
   c. Symptoms of acute left ventricular failure
8. Other
   a. Sicca syndrome—dry eyes, dry mouth
   b. Numbness, paresthesias, and weakness associated with entrapment neuropathies and facial nerve palsies

Key Symptoms

- Raynaud's phenomenon
- Edema
- Skin thickening
- Arthralgias/arthritis
- "Heartburn"
- Dysphagia/odynophagia
- Hematemesis, melena
- Dyspnea, nonproductive cough
- Headaches
- Visual disturbances
- Sicca syndrome

Clinical Findings

1. Vascular: Nailfold capillary microscopy shows a dropout of capillary loops.
2. Skin and musculoskeletal
   a. Shiny and taut appearance

b. Skin thickening—involving forearms, hands, and face in limited scleroderma (LSS)

c. Skin thickening extends proximally in diffuse scleroderma (DSS).

d. Palpable tendinous friction rubs—wrists, ankles, knees

e. Subcutaneous calcinosis of fingers and distal extensor surfaces occurs in 40 per cent of patients with LSS

3. Gastrointestinal: There is impaired function of the lower esophageal sphincter and impaired peristalsis of the lower two thirds of the esophagus.

4. Pulmonary

a. Reduced lung volumes and diffusing capacity lead to hypoxemia.

b. Pulmonary hypertension, more common in LSS, leads to signs of right ventricular overload and failure.

5. Renal: scleroderma renal crisis

a. Signs of malignant hypertension and rapidly progressive renal insufficiency, which may be accompanied by microangiopathic hemolytic anemia

b. Often associated with rapid progression of skin involvement

6. Cardiac

a. Atrial, nodal, and ventricular arrhythmias

b. Signs of left ventricular failure

Key Signs

• Skin thickening

• Tendinous friction rubs

• Subcutaneous calcinosis

• Inspiratory rales

• Signs of pulmonary hypertension

• Arrhythmias

• Left ventricular gallops

• Accelerated/malignant hypertension

Laboratory Tests

Antinuclear antibodies—present in 90 per cent of patients

1. Scl-70 (Topoisomerase I). Sensitivity approximately 75 per cent and specificity 99 per cent for diffuse scleroderma

2. Centromere/kinetochore

a. More commonly seen in LSS—Sensitivity is between 50 and 96 per cent in various studies.

b. Present in less than 10 per cent of individuals with DSS

Key Tests

• Antinuclear antibodies

• Anti-Scl-70

• Anticentromere

Differential Diagnosis

1. Disorders characterized by or associated with skin thickening on the fingers and hands:

a. Acrodermatitis chronica atrophicans

b. Adult celiac disease

c. Vibration disease

d. Bleomycin-induced scleroderma

e. Reflex sympathetic dystrophy

f. Amyloidosis

g. Vinyl chloride disease

h. Mycosis fungoides

i. Digital sclerosis of DM

2. Disorders characterized by or associated with generalized skin thickening but typically sparing the fingers and hands:

a. Scleroderma adultorum of Buschke

b. Scleromyxedema

c. Eosinophilic fasciitis

d. Eosinophilic-myalgia syndrome

e. Generalized subcutaneous morphea

f. Human adjuvant disease

g. Amyloidosis

h. Porphyria cutanea tarda

i. Graft-versus-host disease

j. Pentazocine-induced disease

3. Disorders characterized by asymmetric skin change:

a. Morphea

b. Linear scleroderma

c. Coup de sabre

4. Disorders characterized by similar internal organ involvement:

a. Primary pulmonary hypertension

b. Primary biliary cirrhosis

c. Intestinal pseudo-obstruction

d. Idiopathic pulmonary fibrosis

e. Infiltrative cardiomyopathy

f. Collagenous colitis

5. Disorders characterized by Raynaud's phenomenon

Treatment
Medication

1. D-Penicillamine

a. May lead to improvement of cutaneous manifestations

b. Decreases incidence of new visceral involvement

c. Initial dose is 250 mg/day, with the goal being 750 to 1500 mg/day.

2. Corticosteroids

a. Do not slow disease progression

b. Can be helpful in inflammatory myositis, arthralgias/myalgias, and some cases of interstitial lung disease

c. Can precipitate normotensive renal crisis at doses ≥30 mg/day of prednisone or the equivalent

d. Low doses (<30 mg/day prednisone) preferred for palliative effects

3. Calcium channel blockers

a. May produce subjective relief of Raynaud's phenomenon

b. Available doses of long-acting calcium channel blockers include nifedipine (Adalat, Procardia) 30 to 90 mg q.d., diltiazem (Cardizem) 120 to 300 mg/day, verapamil (Calan, Isoptin) up to 480 mg/day.

4. ACE inhibitors

a. Control hypertension

b. May slow progression of renal insufficiency

c. Captopril (Capoten) in doses up to 50 mg t.i.d. and enalapril (Vasotec) in doses up to 20 mg b.i.d. are the agents of choice for renal crisis

5. H$_2$ blockers, ranitidine (Zantac) up to 150 mg q.i.d., omeprazole (Prilosec) 20 to 40 mg q.d., metoclopramide (Reglan) 5 to 10 mg q.i.d., cisapride (Propulsid) 10 to 20 mg q.i.d. for the treatment of esophageal disease

6. Other/experimental: immunosuppressive agents, ketotifen, iloprost, pentoxifylline, and apheresis

Patient Education

1. Avoid cold temperatures; wear layered clothing.

2. Abstain from smoking.

3. Use skin lubrication.

4. Use range-of-motion exercises.

5. Elevate head of bed.

6. Avoid large meals.

7. Frequent blood pressure monitoring

B Bibliography

Fritzler MJ: Autoantibodies in scleroderma. J Dermatol 1993;20:257–268.

Medsger TA: Treatment of systemic sclerosis. Ann Rheum Dis 1991;50:877–886.

Seibold JR: Scleroderma. In Kelley WN, Edwards ED, Ruddy S, Sledge CB (eds): Textbook of Rheumatology, 4th ed, vol 2. Philadelphia, WB Saunders, 1993, pp 1113–1134.

Silver RM: Clinical aspects of systemic sclerosis (scleroderma). Ann Rheum Dis 1991;50:854–861.

Steen V, Medsger TA: Epidemiology and natural history of systemic sclerosis. Rheum Dis Clin North Am 1990;16(1): 1–10.

209 Polymyalgia Rheumatica

John Meyerhoff

Etiology

The etiology of polymyalgia rheumatica (PMR) is unknown. Many theories have been suggested, but none has held up. While it is clearly inflammatory, joint and muscle biopsies are negative in PMR patients.

Symptoms

1. Onset of symptoms over age 50
2. Bilateral shoulder pain
3. Stiffness (or gelling) in the proximal shoulder (more often than hip girdles) with inactivity, usually longer than 1 hour in the morning
4. May be felt to be "just getting old" by patients
5. Often associated with mild weight loss and/or depression
6. May be associated with symptoms of temporal arteritis (see below)

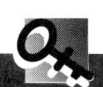

Key Symptoms

- Shoulder pain
- Depression
- Morning stiffness
- Weight loss

Clinical Findings

1. Pain on range of motion of the shoulder joints
2. True weakness not present, but patients frequently report pain in the shoulder muscles on muscle strength testing.
3. Muscle tenderness, in distinction to joint tenderness, is common in PMR but is rare in other rheumatologic diseases involving the shoulder.
4. Osteoarthritis frequently found in these patients; inflammatory arthritis rarely
5. Findings of temporal arteritis also may be seen (see below).

Key Sign

- Pain in the shoulder with range-of-motion testing, muscle strength testing, and palpation of the muscles

Laboratory Tests

1. Anemia of chronic disease often present if symptoms have been present long enough
2. Erythrocyte sedimentation rate (ESR) is frequently very elevated.
3. PMR can occur with a normal hemoglobin and a normal ESR, and neither should be used to rule out the disease.
4. Muscle enzymes (creatine phosphokinase [CPK] or aldolase) must be normal.
5. Muscle, joint, and other biopsies (other than temporal artery) are uniformly normal and should not be done.
6. Bone scans may be abnormal but are not helpful.

Key Tests

- CBC
- ESR
- CPK

Differential Diagnosis

1. Painful muscle syndromes are most likely to be confused with PMR.
   a. Fibromyalgia is more diffuse and associated with tiredness (nonrestorative sleep) and pain in the morning more than stiffness. May be associated with tender points that are not found in PMR and occurs below age 50.
   b. Myalgias due to viral infections may be similar but rarely last more than 4 weeks.
2. Joint disease may be confused with PMR.
   a. Rheumatoid arthritis (RA) often will give morning stiffness greater than 1 hour in duration, pain on motion of the shoulders, anemia, and an elevated ESR. RA usually does not give tenderness of the shoulder muscles, and PMR does not usually give a peripheral arthritis.
   b. Osteoarthritis may give morning stiffness, but it usually rarely lasts more than 10 to 15 minutes. These patients also may have pain on motion of the shoulders, but they also usually do not have muscle tenderness either. Anemia is rare, and ESR should be normal.
3. Bursitis and tendinitis of the shoulder gives pain on motion and tenderness and occasionally morning stiffness, but it is rarely symmetrical.
4. Polymyositis will give true muscle weakness and is painless and affects distal as well as proximal symptoms.
5. Neoplastic disease may present similarly to PMR, and patients with known primary neoplastic disease, lack of response to corticosteroids, or symptoms suggestive of neoplasia should be screened carefully for primary or secondary neoplasia.

6. Depression may present with the muscle pain, morning stiffness, and fatigue. These patients should not have anemia or an elevated ESR and often will appear depressed.

Treatment

Medication

1. Corticosteroids are the treatment of choice.

   a. Response is dramatic, with improvement overnight and almost complete resolution within 48 hours.

   b. Failure to respond this dramatically is usually due to one of the following:

      (1) Incorrect diagnosis, particularly depression or neoplasia-related

      (2) Underlying or coexisting condition such as bursitis, tendinitis, osteoarthritis, or rheumatoid arthritis, which will improve more slowly

   c. Low doses of prednisone with rapid taper to replacement doses are often effective in many patients as follows: 15 mg/day for 3 to 5 days, 10 mg/day for 1 to 2 weeks, 5 mg/day for 12 months, then taper by 1 mg/day per month afterward.

   d. If patients have a flare, symptoms are easily controlled by resuming previous dose (or 5 mg/day if on less) for 1 to 2 weeks with taper afterward.

   e. Patients may have recurrent, consistent flares of PMR or coexisting osteoarthritis as prednisone is tapered below 5 mg/day and may need to be kept on 1 to 4 mg/day of prednisone for a prolonged period of time.

   f. Consider rheumatologic consultation for use of an alternative schedule in patients in whom prednisone cannot be tapered or for the use of other drugs such as steroid-sparing agents in patients who are having steroid side effects and whose dosage cannot be tapered.

2. Nonsteroidal anti-inflammatory drugs (NSAIDs) are rarely effective.

Patient Education

1. Patients should be instructed in the signs and symptoms of temporal arteritis (see below) and should be told to take 60 mg prednisone immediately if they develop any of these findings and then to call their physician.

2. Patients should be instructed in the treatment and follow-up schedule because they will be seeing their doctor for an asymptomatic condition.

Key Treatment

- Low-dose prednisone
- Regular follow-up
- Surveillance for giant cell arteritis

Follow-Up

1. Patients should keep in touch over the first several weeks to ensure that they have the expected response to steroids.

2. The initial follow-up visit should be scheduled at 4 to 6 weeks after the initial visit and then at 2- to 4-month intervals for the first year depending on the patient's compliance.

3. At each visit patients should be asked about symptoms of PMR and GCA with emphasis on what they should do if they develop symptoms of GCA.

4. Visits should be every 1 to 2 months as prednisone is being tapered from 5 mg.

Bibliography

Bird HA, Esselinckx W, Dixon AStJ, et al: An evaluation or criteria for polymyalgia rheumatica. Ann Rheum Dis 1979;38:434–439.

Cimmino MA, Moggiana G, Montecucco C, et al: Long-term treatment of polymyalgia rheumatica with deflazacort. Ann Rheum Dis 1994;53:331–333.

Ellis ME, Ralston S: The ESR in the diagnosis and management of the polymyalgia rheumatica/giant cell arteritis syndrome. Ann Rheum Dis 1983;42:168–170.

Hellmann DB: Immunopathogenesis, diagnosis, and treatment of giant cell arteritis, temporal arteritits, polymyalgia rheumatica, and Takayasu's arteritis. Curr Opin Rheumatol 1993;5:25–32.

Kyle V, Hazelman BL: The clinical and laboratory course of polymyalgia rheumatica/giant cell arteritis after the first two months. Ann Rheum Dis 1993;52:847–850.

210 Temporal Arteritis

Michael Lewko

Etiology

1. Temporal arteritis (TA), or giant cell arteritis, is a disease of the elderly, rarely found in those under age 50. It is more common in females and is rare in blacks.
2. TA: vasculitis of unknown etiology
   a. Possible pathogenic factors: genetic, infectious, immunologic
   b. May be etiologically related to polymyalgia rheumatica
3. TA affects medium- to large-sized arteries with internal elastic lamina.
   a. Preferential sites of involvement: branches of internal and external carotid arteries, particularly temporal artery
   b. Typically inflammation consists of mononuclear cells, infiltrative granuloma, usually with giant cells, and disruption of the internal elastic membrane

Symptoms

1. Onset may be abrupt or insidious.
2. Classic symptoms: headache, jaw claudication, visual changes, polymyalgia rheumatica
3. Loss of vision is the most serious complication, frequently preceded by diplopia or amaurosis fugax.
4. Atypical presentations: fever of unknown origin, weight loss, failure to thrive in elderly

Key Symptoms

- New headache
- Jaw claudication
- Visual symptoms
- Proximal myalgias
- Weight loss
- Malaise
- Fever

Clinical Findings

1. Localized temporal artery tenderness, redness, decreased pulsation, induration, or even scalp necrosis. Temporal arteries are normal in one third of patients.
   a. Ophthalmologic findings: ophthalmoplegia, visual loss
   b. Funduscopic abnormalities
      (1) Pallor and swelling of optic disks (early)
      (2) Optic atrophy (late)
2. Systemic manifestations usually result from ischemia of affected arteries or inflammation related to giant cell arteritis.

   a. Bruits in head and neck
   b. Absent upper extremities pulses
   c. Neurologic deficits: mononeuritis, progressive dementia, delirium, stroke, transient ischemic attacks (TIAs)
   d. Inflammatory signs: synovitis, pericarditis, breast masses

Key Signs

- Temporal artery tenderness or decreased pulsation
- Ophthalmoplegia
- Visual field cuts
- Ptosis
- Retinal or optic disk ischemia
- Neurologic deficits
- Bruits, head and neck
- Diminished or absent pulses in upper extremities

Laboratory Findings

1. Erythrocyte sedimentation rate (ESR) by Westergren method
   a. Almost always increased
   b. Usually greater than or equal to 50 mm/hr
   c. May be normal in 15 per cent of patients
2. Diagnostic temporal artery biopsy is recommended in patients with suspected TA. A negative biopsy does not always rule it out.
3. To increase the biopsy yield
   a. Biopsy segment should be greater than 5 cm.
   b. Biopsy should be bilateral if frozen sections of initial biopsy are negative.
   c. Pathologists should evaluate in detail multiple sections of biopsied segment.
   d. Upon initiation of steroid therapy, biopsy should be done within 2 to 5 days at the latest.
4. Other laboratory findings include
   a. Elevated C-reactive protein
   b. Normocytic, normochromic anemia
   c. Abnormal liver function test—elevated alkaline phosphatase
   d. Elevated globulin fraction in serum electrophoresis
   e. Elevated Von Willebrand factor

Key Tests

- Erythrocyte sedimentation rate (ESR)
- Temporal artery biopsy

Differential Diagnosis

1. Temporal arteritis is distinguishable from other forms of vasculitis by differences in organ involvement, histopathology, clinical manifestations, age, and affected population.
2. The differential diagnosis consists of Takayasu's arteritis, Wegener's granulomatosis, polyarteritis nodosa, hypersensitivity, and vasculitis.
3. Other possibilities include arteriosclerotic disease, malignancy, infection, primary amyloidosis, other causes of fever, headache, blindness, arthralgias, and myalgias.

> **WARNING**
>
> **The most common dreaded complication is vision loss resulting from untimely diagnosis and inadequate treatment.**

Treatment

1. The treatment for temporal arteritis is high-dose corticosteroids.
   a. Prednisone, 40 to 60 mg/day in two to four divided doses *or*
   b. Equivalent dosage of another corticosteroid (Medrol) *or*
   c. Intravenous pulse Solu-Medrol in patients with recent blindness, less than 24 to 36 hours
2. High-dose corticosteroids should be initiated promptly when the suspicion is high and when visual symptoms are present.
   a. Only high-dose corticosteroids will prevent blindness.
   b. Alternate-day regimens are not effective in the initial treatment.
   c. The decision to continue treatment or initiate treatment will depend on the results of the temporal artery biopsy, the clinical presentation, and laboratory tests.
3. Clinical response to treatment is usually
   a. Rapid and dramatic—within 3 to 7 days
   b. The ESR normalizes in 2 to 4 weeks.
   c. Reversal of blindness is rare.

Medication

1. Treatment with prednisone
   a. Initial dose is 40 to 60 mg/day in two to four divided doses.
   b. Consolidate total dose to one single morning dose once response has occurred.
   c. Initiate reduction of daily dose when symptoms have resolved and the ESR has normalized.
2. Reduction of prednisone is
   a. Empirical
   b. Gauged by symptoms and ESR
   c. Gradual to prevent exacerbations
3. An approach to reduction
   a. Reduce the dose by 10 per cent every 2 to 4 weeks down to a total dose of 15 to 30 mg, and maintain at this dose for several months.
   b. Follow this by 2.5-mg decrements every 2 to 4 weeks down to a total dose of 5 to 7.5 mg, and maintain at this dose for several months.
   c. Follow by 1-mg decrements every 1 to 3 months until discontinued.
   d. In general, treatment is necessary up to 1 to 2 years or sometimes longer, up to 5 years or more.
4. Corticosteroid toxicity is common and should be anticipated in older patients. It may result in
   a. Cushinoid features
   b. Osteopenia
   c. Hypertension
   d. Impaired wound healing
   e. Fractures
   f. Proximal myopathy
   g. Cataracts
   h. Glucose intolerance
   i. Easy bruisability
   j. Depression
   k. Insomnia
5. Prevention of corticosteroid-induced toxicity
   a. Monitor blood pressure, glucose, and calcium.
   b. Add calcium, 1 to 1.5 gm, with vitamin D, 400 to 800 IU daily, to diet
   c. Switching to alternate-day steroids is not recommended.
   d. Addition of steroid-sparing agents, methotrexate, dapsone, or azathioprine (Imuran) may be appropriate.
   e. Do not treat the ESR; adjust corticosteroid dose mainly on the basis of symptoms.

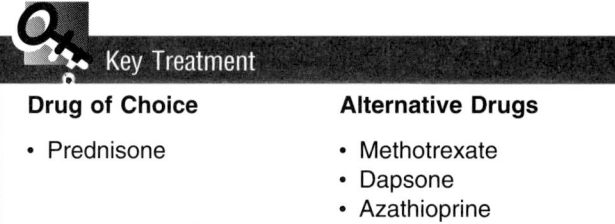

Key Treatment

Drug of Choice	Alternative Drugs
• Prednisone	• Methotrexate
	• Dapsone
	• Azathioprine

Follow-Up

1. Prognosis of treatment is good.
2. In general, there is no difference in survival from rest of the general population.
3. Blindness rarely occurs during treatment.

4. In most cases, remission is maintained after withdrawal of therapy.

Bibliography

Buchbinder R, Detsky AS: Management of suspected giant cell arteritis: A decision analysis. J Rheumatol 1992;19(8):1220–1228.

Fernandez-Herlihey L: Temporal arteritis: Clinical aids to diagnosis. J Rheumatol 1988;328:463–468.

Goodwin SJ: Progress in gerontology: Polymyalgia and temporal arteritis. J Am Geriatr Soc 1992;40:515–525.

Nosher G, Sonnenblick M: Steroid sparing medications in temporal arteritis: Report of three cases and review of 174 reported patients. Clin Rheumatol 1994;8:84–92.

Wind BE: Temporal arteritis: Aggressive treatment prevents visual complications. Postgrad Med 1992;91:337–338, 341–342.

211 Osteochondrosis (Osgood-Schlatter Disease)

Lawrence H. Miller

Etiology

1. Microtearing of the fibers of the quadriceps tendon at its attachment to the anterior tibial tubercle with or without partial separation of the physis

2. Most commonly encountered in Tanner stage 2 or 3 adolescent males (age 11 to 13) (three times more common in males) who are very physically active, particularly in sports requiring torsion at the knee (running, kicking, jumping).

Symptoms

1. Patient presents with activity-related pain localized over the tibial tubercle, aggravated by stair climbing, kneeling.

2. The dominant leg is typically more symptomatic.

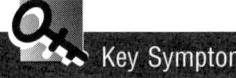

Key Symptom

- Localized pain at proximal tibia

Clinical Findings

1. Patient presents with a limping gait.

2. The tibial tubercle may be swollen, exquisitely tender, and warm to touch.

3. Pain is reproducible by repeated flexion and extension of the knee or by direct pressure on the tubercle.

4. Notably *absent* are synovial thickening and joint effusion.

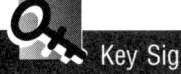

Key Signs

- Tender enlarged tibial tubercle

- Absence of synovial thickenings and effusion

Laboratory Tests

1. Although none are needed, a lateral radiograph of the knee may help exclude other unusual diagnoses.

2. Radiographic findings may not correlate with the clinical presentation but, when positive, may show sclerosis, fragmentation, or separations with overlying soft tissue swelling (Fig. 211–1).

3. Other diagnostic imaging techniques have been used (ultrasound, computed tomography, magnetic resonance imaging) but offer no advantage over plain radiographs and are more costly.

Differential Diagnosis

1. Tumor
2. Infection
3. Bone cyst
4. Stress fracture
5. Arthritis
6. Chondromalacia patellae
7. Osteochondritis dissecans
8. Sinding-Larsen-Johansson syndrome
9. Meniscus injuries
10. Hemophilia

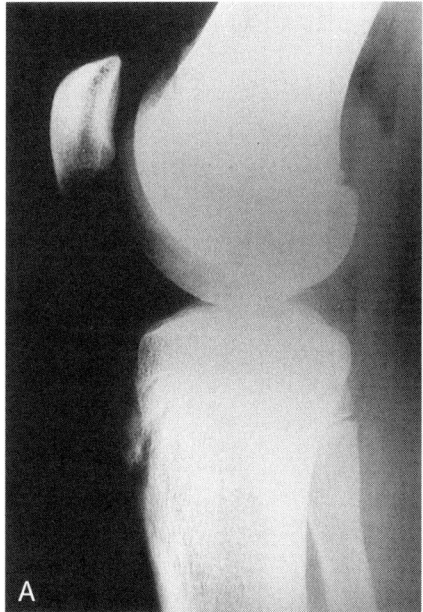

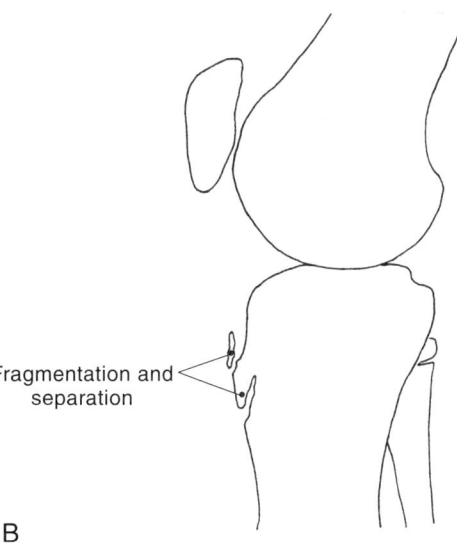

Figure 211–1 *A* and *B*, Fragmentation and separation of the physis.

Tibial tubercle tenderness may be associated with the first four diagnoses, but the knee radiograph will aid in differentiation. Focal patellar or knee joint pain is common with the latter six diagnoses but is not expected with Osgood-Schlatter disease.

Treatment

1. Limitation of activities that cause pain

2. Ice packs to the swollen tubercle

3. Protective padding to the knee during activities where trauma could be a possibility

4. Although nonsteroidal anti-inflammatory drugs (NSAIDs) have been used, their potential benefit has not been shown conclusively.

5. Local corticosteroid injections are contraindicated and could cause increased injury.

6. Patient education, particularly regarding cause and clinical course, is crucial in negotiating appropriate activity restrictions. Overly stringent restrictions may result in

   a. Excessive deconditioning

   b. Muscle wasting

   c. Negative self-image or even depression secondary to a feeling of physical inadequacy

   d. Worsening of the disorder due to noncompliance with physician-imposed excessive limitations

7. Immobilization by cast or splint should be avoided.

Key Treatment

- Limitation of activities causing pain

- Ice packs

- Protective padding

Follow-Up

1. Periodic follow-up should focus on the expected gradual remission of symptoms, which allows a gradual increase in physical activity.

2. This is a self-limited disorder that resolves spontaneously with closure of the proximal tibial growth plate.

3. Very rarely, bony ossicles may fail to unite with the tibia and require surgical excision from the infrapatellar portion of the quadriceps tendon.

Bibliography

Binazzi R, Felli L, Vaccari V, et al: Surgical treatment of unresolved Osgood-Schlatter lesion. Clin Orthop 1993; 289:202–204.

Bloom RA, Felli L, Vaccari V, et al: Ossicles anterior to the proximal tibia. Clin Imag 1993;17(2):137–141.

Carnick JG: Sports injuries and the osteochondroses. In McAnarnay E, et al (eds): Textbook of Adolescent Medicine. Philadelphia, WB Saunders, 1992, pp 759–766.

Krause BL, Williams JP, Catterall A: Natural history of Osgood-Schlatter disease. J Pediatr Orthop 1990;10(1):65–68.

212 Carpal Tunnel Syndrome and Other Nerve Entrapments

Kevin R. Nelson

Carpal Tunnel Syndrome

Etiology

1. The carpal tunnel is bounded by the volar transverse ligament and dorsally by the carpal bones. Coursing through the carpal tunnel are the flexor tendons of the digits and the median nerve. The carpal tunnel is physically confined in a large proportion of otherwise normal individuals. Symptoms of carpal tunnel syndrome (CTS) are produced by increased pressure within the tunnel, leading to nerve ischemia, demyelination, and perhaps axonal injury.

2. Medical conditions associated with CTS include diabetes, pregnancy, rheumatoid arthritis, hypothyroidism, chronic renal failure, multiple myeloma, amyloidosis, and acromegaly.

3. A generalized peripheral neuropathy of any cause often predisposes to CTS and other nerve entrapments.

4. Occupations requiring repetitive wrist movements, the use of vibrating tools, or sustained hand positions involve a higher incidence of CTS.

5. Local infections, fractures, tenosynovitis, aberrant anatomy, or masses of the wrist also may lead to CTS.

6. A congenitally narrow canal increases the risk of nerve compression, particularly in later life when degenerative changes further compromise the space or with the aggravating factors described above.

Symptoms

1. The earliest symptom is often intermittent hand paresthesias or pain, often awaking the patient at night.

2. Digital sensory disturbances may impair fine motor tasks.

3. Pain occurs in the wrist and hand and may radiate up the arm.

4. Symptoms are provoked by repetitive motion and sustained hand positions (e.g., driving).

5. Relief is sometimes obtained by shaking or moving the wrist.

Key Symptoms

- Nocturnal hand paresthesias
- Median sensory disturbance
- Wrist or hand pain

6. Patients may complain of poor grip and often drop objects.

7. Symptoms typically involve the dominant hand and may be bilateral.

Clinical Findings

1. Sensory loss (especially two-point discrimination) occurs in the median nerve distribution (digits I, II, III, and sometimes IV).

2. Weakness of thumb abduction is usually found only after sensory symptoms are well developed.

3. Thenar atrophy occurs late in the course.

4. Flexing the wrist for 1 minute (Phalen maneuver) or tapping over the median nerve at the wrist (Tinel's sign) may provoke symptoms in the hand. Tinel's sign may be found in normal persons, and positive results should be interpreted with caution.

Key Signs

- Sensory loss in the first three digits
- Thenar wasting
- Phalen or Tinel sign

Laboratory Tests

1. Nerve conduction studies (NCS) demonstrate slowed median nerve conduction through the wrist. This will be recorded from the sensory fibers first.

   a. NCS have a high degree of diagnostic sensitivity and specificity. Best laboratory method of establishing the diagnosis of CTS.

   b. NCS also will detect underlying generalized neuropathies.

   c. In mild or acute CTS, the NCS may be normal.

2. Obtain wrist radiographs in patients suspected of having fractures and joint disease.

3. Laboratory studies to evaluate associated diseases (as indicated)

Key Test

- Nerve conduction study is the most definitive test

Differential Diagnosis

1. C6 and C7 radiculopathies may present with sensory symptoms within the median nerve territory. Neck pain, weakness in the muscles proximal to the wrist, and reflex loss may be present.

2. Tenosynovitis and osteoarthritis produce wrist pain worsened by movement.

3. A generalized neuropathy (e.g., diabetic) can manifest as an isolated nerve compression.

4. Proximal median nerve injury (e.g., at elbow)

5. Brachial plexus lesion

Treatment

1. Medical

   a. Avoid activities that flex and extend the wrist.

   b. Splint the wrist in the neutral position. The splint should be worn at night as well as during the day, particularly if the symptoms are nocturnal.

   c. Scheduled nonsteroidal anti-inflammatory agents (NSAIDs) for several weeks.

   d. Steroid injections into canal may provide temporary or long-standing relief. This should be performed by experienced physicians.

      (1) Complications include local infection, inflammation, and permanent nerve injury.

      (2) Multiple injections risk damaging the flexor tendons and predispose them to later rupture.

   e. Thiazide diuretics may be effective for CTS associated with pregnancy, if treatment is needed.

2. Indications for surgical decompression

   a. Symptoms that are sufficient to interfere with work or daily life and are unresponsive to conservative therapy

   b. Persistent or progressive neurologic deficits, particularly motor weakness

   c. Acute CTS with severe pain and weakness (e.g., hemorrhage) may require immediate decompression.

Key Treatment

• NSAIDs	• Wrist splinting
• Surgical release	• Avoid provocative activity

Follow-Up

1. Most patients with mild disease do well with conservative treatment. Improvement may take several months.

2. If a 3- to 6-month trial of medical therapy fails, consider surgery.

3. Patients may report marked improvement shortly after surgical decompression. Continued improvement may be evident over several months.

4. Patients with recurrent symptoms after surgery should be considered for re-exploration. Repeat NCS may be helpful in this instance.

Ulnar Nerve Compression at the Elbow

Etiology

1. Excessive forearm flexion/extension and leaning on the elbow can traumatize the nerve over time. Persons with a shallow condylar groove or a dislocating ulnar nerve are vulnerable to nerve injury.

2. Patients at risk are those who are comatose, anesthetized, or at prolonged bed rest.

3. Elbow fractures (acute or remote), degenerative or rheumatoid arthritis, or masses near the elbow may entrap the nerve.

4. In many patients, no antecedent cause is found. In some, the nerve is compressed by fibrous tissue in the condylar groove or the cubital tunnel (aponeurosis of the flexor digitorum sublimus muscle).

Key Symptoms

• Progressive hand weakness	• Numbness in an ulnar distribution

Clinical Findings

1. Sensory deficits are usually found within the ulnar distribution (digit, IV, V). Sensory loss that splits the ring finger is typical of an ulnar nerve injury and is uncommon with a radiculopathy.

2. Weakness is often prominent and is found in finger abduction, thumb adduction, and other intrinsic hand muscles.

3. Atrophy may be seen in the hypothenar area, over the first web space, and in the dorsum of the hand.

4. "Claw hand" deformity is produced by hypertension of the metacarpophalangeal joints and flexion at the interphalangeal joints of the fourth and fifth digits. This arises from unopposed action of muscles innervated by the median and radial nerves.

5. Pain may be present at the elbow or more diffusely in the arm.

6. Tapping the ulnar nerve at the elbow may elicit paresthesias in the hand (Tinel's sign). The specificity of this sign is poor.

Key Signs

• Ulnar sensory disturbance	• Claw hand
• Shallow condylar groove	• Atrophy of intrinsic hand muscles

Key Tests

• Nerve conduction studies and electromyography

Differential Diagnosis

1. C8/T1 radiculopathy
2. Lower trunk brachial plexopathy
3. Early motor neuron disease (amyotrophic sclerosis)
4. Ulnar entrapment at the wrist or hand

Treatment

1. Avoid activities that can compress the nerve.
2. Protect the nerve with an elbow pad.
3. Scheduled NSAIDs
4. In patients with an elbow mass, a dislocating nerve, or structural deformities of the elbow, surgical transposition should be considered early.

Follow-Up

1. Patients should be given a trial of medical treatment (usually 2 to 3 months).
2. Consider surgery in patients with severe or progressive weakness that is resistant to therapy.

Peroneal Nerve Compression at the Fibular Head

Etiology

Causes include habitual leg crossing, frequent squatting, positioning during anesthesia or coma, weight loss, leg casts, and masses in the knees. The nerve is also subject to injury from fibular fractures, knee dislocations, and blunt injury.

Key Symptom

• Foot drop

Clinical Findings

1. Weakness of ankle and toe dorsiflexion. Often foot eversion is preserved.
2. When walking, the patient lifts the foot high for the toes to clear the ground as the leg swings forward. The leg is then brought abruptly down, slapping the foot (steppage gait).
3. Sensory loss occurs in the peroneal nerve distribution.

Key Signs

• Weak ankle dorsiflexion

• Steppage gait

Key Tests

• Nerve conduction studies and electromyography are the definitive tests.

Differential Diagnosis

1. L5 radiculopathy
2. Lumbosacral plexopathy
3. Sciatic neuropathy
4. Central nervous system cause for footdrop (e.g., stroke)

Treatment

1. Avoid activities that can compress the nerve (see above).
2. Shoes with support above the ankle or an ankle-foot orthosis may assist the patient's gait and reduce tripping.
3. Rarely, acute swelling of the anterior tibial muscle from trauma will compress the nerve (compartment syndrome). This should be surgically decompressed.

Follow-Up

1. The prognosis for pressure palsies is generally good. Time of recovery varies from days to months among patients.
2. Surgical exploration of the peroneal nerve at the fibular head might be considered if weakness persists.

 Bibliography

American Association of Electrodiagnostic Medicine, American Academy of Neurology, American Academy of Physical Medicine and Rehabilitation: Practice parameters for electrodiagnostic studies in carpal tunnel syndrome: Summary statement. Muscle Nerve 1993;16:1390–1391.

Jablecki CK, Andary MT, So YT, et al: Literature review of the usefulness of nerve conduction studies and electromyography for the evaluation of patients with carpal tunnel syndrome. Muscle Nerve 1993;16:1392–1414.

Katz RT: Carpal tunnel syndrome: A practical review. Am Fam Physician 1994;49:1371–1379.

Mumenthaler M, Schliak H: Peripheral Nerve Lesions: Diagnosis and Therapy, 5th ed. New York, Thieme Medical Publishers, 1991.

Rosenbaum RB, Ochoa JL: Carpal Tunnel Syndrome and Other Disorders of the Median Nerve. Boston, Butterworth-Heinemann, 1993.

Stewart JD: Focal Peripheral Neuropathies, 2nd ed. New York, Raven Press, 1993.

213 Swimmer's Injuries

Robert P. Vogt

Shoulder Injuries

Etiology

1. Between 40 and 60 per cent of competitive swimmers develop shoulder problems in their careers, making it the most commonly injured joint. It is caused by repetitive microtrauma and usually becomes symptomatic after 6 to 8 years of swimming. This overuse syndrome may be accelerated in older athletes or those with pre-existing shoulder problems.
2. Both the rotator cuff and bicipital tendon syndromes are caused by impingement of those structures between the humeral head and acromial process. Impingement occurs during swimming strokes with repetitive arm abduction and internal rotation alternating with adduction and external rotation.
3. Impingement is caused by relatively weak rotator cuff muscles, especially the supraspinatus (SSM), compared with the deltoid. The deltoid contraction pulls the humeral head into the underside of the acromion, squeezing the supraspinatus tendon (SST) as the arm is abducted.

Symptoms

1. Pain while swimming, especially during the recovery phase of the arm stroke (bringing the arm forward for the next pull)
2. Pain with abduction or inability to raise the arm(s) above the head without pain (e.g., combing hair)
3. Night pain (may interfere with sleep)

Key Symptom

- Pain with abduction

Clinical Findings

1. Positive impingement maneuver: With the patient upright, have him or her push toward the ceiling against your hand while he or she holds the straightened arm at shoulder level with the hand rotated thumb down toward the floor ("empty can" position). This is done repeatedly in a 90-degree horizontal arc from straight in front of the patient to his or her side. It is positive if it reproduces the pain.
2. Pain with resisted supination
3. Tenderness over the long head of the biceps tendon in the bicipital groove. Examine with the elbow at 90 degrees and the arm externally rotated.
4. Tenderness over the rotator cuff muscles

Key Signs

- Positive impingement maneuver
- Pain with resisted supination

Laboratory Tests

1. Plain radiographs of the shoulder may reveal
   a. Calcific deposits in the supraspinatus tendon (a response to microtrauma, not a cause of the pain)
   b. Inferior aspect of the glenoid fossa should not be below the inferior aspect of the humeral head—if so, denotes laxity of the SSM/rotator cuff muscles.
   c. Degenerative changes of the acromial process causing decreased subacromial space and impinging on the SST
2. Arthrogram or magnetic resonance imaging (MRI) may be required to rule out rotator cuff tear (RCT).

Key Tests

- Plain radiograph of shoulder
- Arthrogram or MRI (to rule out RCT)

Differential Diagnosis

1. RCT—usually associated with inability to abduct the shoulder. Try a subacromial bursa injection with local anesthetic and re-examine. Those patients with a tear still cannot move, but those with impingement syndrome usually can.
2. Biceps tendon rupture
3. Glenohumeral arthritis
4. Acromioclavicular joint arthritis

Treatment

1. *All* treatment must focus on strengthening the rotator cuff, especially the SSM. Shoulder abduction/external rotation exercises done from 0 to 90 degrees with weights or against elastic bands ("fly-aways") are the basis for rehabilitation.
2. Subacromial injection of steroids (with or without local anesthetic) may be needed if the athlete cannot perform exercises because of pain.

Medication

1. Nonsteroidal anti-inflammatory drugs (NSAIDs) for analgesia. Consider using them only after practices, competition, or at night, because continuous use may relieve pain and allow the athlete to overuse the joint without pain to indicate limits to motion.

2. Anatomic abnormalities
   a. Decreased vascularity to the tendon or the peritenon sheath surrounding it
   b. Hyperpronation of the foot
   c. Tight calf muscles

Symptoms

1. The runner may complain of pain and swelling in the distal Achilles tendon near its insertion on the calcaneus.
2. The tendon is tight, making walking difficult.

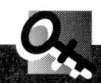

Key Symptoms

- Pain
- Swelling
- Stiffness in the tendon

Clinical Findings

1. Tenderness on palpation and with active motion of the tendon
2. The tendon or the paratenon sheath is frequently swollen and produces palpable crepitus with motion.
3. Most runners exhibit weakness of the calf muscle secondary to tendon pain.
4. Erythema and heat may be present, but their absence does not rule out Achilles tendinitis.
5. In cases of chronic tendinitis, nodules may be palpable in the substance of the tendon.

Key Signs

• Tenderness	• Heat
• Swelling	• Weakness secondary to pain
• Erythema	

Laboratory Tests

Radiographs are frequently normal and of little diagnostic help unless a complete tendon rupture is suspected, which may be present as a soft tissue density.

Key Test

- Radiographs frequently add little diagnostic information.

Differential Diagnosis

1. Retrocalcaneal bursitis
2. Retroachilles bursitis

Treatment

1. NSAIDs for 1 to 2 weeks
2. Ice massage to painful area for 15 minutes several times a day
3. Limited immobilization to allow the inflammation to improve but the tendon needs motion to properly repair the collagen fibers
4. New shoes and possibly orthotics to control pronation
5. When the inflammation is controlled, the Achilles tendon and muscle groups should be strengthened with toe raises in a pain-free range of motion.

 Bibliography

McKeag DB, Dolan CD: Overuse syndromes of the lower extremity. Phys Sportsmed 1989;17(7):108–123.

Paulos LE, Kolowich PA: Patellar instability and pain. *In* Reider B (ed): Sports Medicine: The School-Age Athlete. Philadelphia, WB Saunders, 1991, pp 332–354.

Achilles tendinitis, tibia, plantar fasciitis, patella: *In* Pavlov HP, Torg JS (eds): The Running Athlete: Roentgenograms and Remedies. Chicago, Year Book Medical Publishers, 1987, pp 136–168.

Schon LC, Baxter DE, Canton TO: Chronic exercise-induced leg pain in active people. Phys Sportsmed 1992;20(1):100–114.

Warren BL: Plantar fasciitis in runners: Treatment and prevention. Sports Med 1990;10(5):338–345.

215 Patellofemoral Pain Syndrome

Mark D. Bracker

Etiology

1. Definition
   a. Patellofemoral pain syndrome (PFPS) is a common problem encountered by primary care physicians. A variety of names have been used synonymously for PFPS over the years including chondromalacia patella, anterior knee pain, retropatellar pain syndrome, patellofemoral arthralgia, exterior mechanism disorder, lateral patellar compression syndrome, patellalgia, and patellofemoral dysfunction.
   b. Classically, chondromalacia patella involves degeneration of the articular cartilage and is a surgical or radiographic diagnosis. In most cases of PFPS, fortunately, there is no damage to the articular surface of the patella; no epidemiologic evidence exists that PFPS progresses to chondromalacia if left untreated. Pain most likely originates from irritation of the richly innervated subchondral bone and soft tissues around the patella.

2. Epidemiology: The patella is a sesamoid bone that serves as a fulcrum for the quadriceps tendon proximally and the patellar tendon distally. As such, it serves to improve the efficiency of the quadriceps mechanism in extending the knee. With normal movement the patella must slide (track) within the femoral groove as the knee joint moves through its range of motion. The medial and lateral retinacula keep the patella centered within the femoral groove and oppose the natural tendency toward lateral displacement generated by the pull of the quadriceps muscles.

3. Risk factors: Patellofemoral disorders may be the result of congenital or genetic conditions, developmental anomalies, and acquired conditions resulting from acute trauma or repetitive activity. Patellofemoral pain may result from abnormal patellar mechanics, repetitive injury from overuse, or both. Causes of abnormal patellar tracking include excessive Q angle, shallow intercondylar sulcus, deformed patellar facets, weakness of the vastus medialis obliquus muscle, and abnormalities of the medial or lateral retinaculum. PFPS is frequently encountered in young athletes. Numerous studies show an increased incidence in females and running as a major causative factor.

Symptoms

1. The hallmark of PFPS is insidious onset of vague, dull, achy pain around the knee joint. Patients often locate the site of discomfort medially and retropatellar, but pain may be peripatellar or referred to the popliteal fossa.

2. Frequently the onset of pain is temporally related to a recent increase in activity such as running, descending stairs, hiking, squatting, or kneeling.

3. Once there is inflammation, prolonged sitting with the knees flexed may produce pain with subsequent movement. This has aptly been called the "theater sign."

Key Symptoms

- Vague, dull, achy peripatellar pain
- Referred pain to medial joint line and popliteal fossa
- Pain descending stairs
- Pain after prolonged sitting

Clinical Findings

1. Crepitus during knee flexion and extension is commonly found on examination of asymptomatic knees and alone does not imply pathology. Swelling, locking, or "giving way" sensation usually signifies a more serious condition within the knee joint.

2. Careful physical examination is essential for making an accurate diagnosis of PFPS and excluding other conditions. Three physical findings are commonly encountered. First, and most important, palpation of the medial articular surface reproduces pain. Second, the patella can be forced down into the femoral groove with passive knee flexion to reproduce pain symptoms. Finally, the superior pole of the patella may be resisted during quadriceps muscle contractions. This maneuver may produce apprehension, pain, or inhibition.

3. In addition to these specific tests, the knee should be fully examined for other conditions that may mimic PFPS. Particular attention should be directed to inspection of the patellar tendon, the quadriceps tendon, and exclusion of intra-articular knee pathology. Since biomechanical abnormalities may contribute to the development of PFPS, predisposing factors such as patella alta, leg length discrepancies, quadriceps atrophy, and abnormal Q angles should be noted. Effu-

Key Signs

- Pain on palpation of medial articular surface of patella
- Patellar compression reproduced pain
- Apprehension and/or quadriceps inhibition against resistance

sions, when present, are rare with PFPS, and usually indicate other pathology such as meniscus tear, synovial plica, synovitis, or chondromalacia.

Laboratory Tests

1. Radiographs are usually unremarkable in patients with PFPS. If taken, radiographic views should include anteroposterior, lateral, and axial views. Axial views, also known as sunrise (Hughston's) views or Merchant's views, are helpful in visualizing the undersurface of the patella, the height of the femoral condyles, the depth of the sulcus between the condyles, and the positioning of the patella within the femoral sulcus. A normal sulcus angle should be less than 130°.

2. Additional information that may be gained from standard knee radiographs includes the presence of osteophytes, free-floating calcium deposits, and sclerosis of the articular surface. Advanced diagnostic tests including bone scans, computed tomography, magnetic resonance imaging, and electromyography are not helpful in diagnosis.

Key Tests

- Radiographs usually normal
- Abnormal sulcus angle
- Chrondromalacia in severe cases

Differential Diagnosis

1. Three distinct conditions should be considered in the differential diagnosis of anterior knee pain. These are PFPS, chondromalacia patella, and patellar subluxation.

2. Chondromalacia patella is a degenerative condition of articular cartilage tending to occur in older patients in the setting of knee trauma or severe malalignment.

3. Subluxation implies that the patella moves out of the femoral groove at some point of knee flexion. As a result, patients who suffer from subluxation complain of a sense of "giving way," "popping," or "locking" with knee activity. Patients with subluxation generally have marked lateral patellar mobility with apprehension on physical examination.

Treatment

1. Medical management should be effective and adequate in at least 75 per cent of patients and should be appropriate for the degree of severity of symptoms.

2. The most important aspect of treatment entails a period of relative rest with restriction of the symptom-producing activity. This may take several weeks and should be followed with a gradual return to activity.

Medication

1. Nonsteroidal anti-inflammatory drugs (NSAIDs) relieve pain in acute cases of PFPS but should not be used for more than two weeks on a regular basis.

2. Patients who experience periodic exacerbation of

symptoms can be instructed to use NSAIDs before and after activity only.

Alternative Treatment

1. Physical therapy modalities should be directed toward educating the patient to strengthen the quadriceps musculature (particularly the vastus medialis obliquus) to offset lateral tracking of the patella. Quadriceps strengthening exercises should not increase discomfort if done correctly. Increasing pain may indicate a more serious condition. Biomechanical evaluation is important, and correction of underlying abnormalities is crucial. Patients should be encouraged to warm up slowly and apply ice to the knees for 15 to 20 minutes after activity and as often as every two to three hours thereafter.

2. Knee bracing to correct abnormal patellar tracking has been advocated for management of PFPS; however, well-controlled studies demonstrating benefit are lacking. Commonly used braces consist of neoprene sleeves or air bladders in an attempt to restrain patellar movement.

3. Patellar taping has recently been advocated for the treatment of PFPS and can be applied by the patient or athletic trainer prior to activity.

4. Surgical management should be limited to a very small subset of patients in whom medical management has clearly failed. Conservative management should be continued at least three to six months before surgical referral. Correcting PFPS in the absence of chondromalacia, subluxation, or significant biomechanical abnormality has only limited success. Procedures currently being used include releasing the lateral retinaculum, tightening the medial retinaculum, transposing the vastus medialis obliquus (VMO) tendon, and transferring the patellar tendon to a more medial position. In older patients with chondromalacia, arthroscopic or open debridement may offer relief.

Key Treatment

- Relative rest
- NSAIDs
- Physical therapy
- Knee bracing
- Patellar taping
- Surgery

Bibliography

Davidson K: Patellofemoral pain syndrome. Am Fam Physician 1994;48:1254–1262.

Ghelman B, Hodge JC: Imaging of the patellofemoral joint. Orthoped Clin North Am 1992;23:523–543.

Kelly MA, Insakk JN: Historical perspectives of chondromalacia patellae. Orthoped Clin North Am 1992;23:17–21.

Thabit G, Micheli LJ: Patellofemoral pain in the pediatric patient. Orthoped Clin North Am 1992;23:567–585.

Tria AJ, Palumbro RC, Alicea JA: Conservative care for patellofemoral pain. Orthoped Clin North Am 1992;23:545–554.

216 Plantar Fasciitis

Lee A. Beatty

Etiology

1. The most common causes, often coexisting, as seen in primary care practices
   a. Biomechanical disorders
      (1) The cavus (high-arched and rigid) foot cannot absorb the shock of heel strike and toe-off. Puts more stress on the "bowstring" function of the plantar fascia
      (2) The planovalgus (flat and flexible) foot pronates excessively, further flattening the arch and stretching the plantar fascia.
      (3) Tight gastrocnemius-Achilles complex. A tight "heel cord" is an inefficient shock absorber, thus overloading the plantar fascia during the toe-off phase of gait.
   b. Overweight. A problem especially for people who stand for long periods
   c. Improper footwear. Flimsy or worn-out heel counters accentuate foot pronation and flatten the heel's fat pad, reducing its shock-absorbing capacity.
   d. Heel fat pad atrophy. A problem after age 50
2. Overtraining
   a. The most common contributing factor in runners
   b. A greater than 10 per cent increase in weekly baseline training intensity or duration (the 10 per cent rule) increases the likelihood of developing plantar fasciitis.

Symptoms

1. Inferior heel pain, usually on the medial aspect. Pain described as burning or aching. Usually unilateral, but 20 to 30 per cent of cases are bilateral.
2. Gradual onset, develops over weeks
3. A *hallmark symptom*: The worst pain occurs with the first step upon arising from bed, diminishing with the next few steps. This "first step" phenomenon may occur because the plantar fascia is relatively contracted during rest, lengthening with weight bearing. Thus tension on the inflamed portion of the fascia is maximal with the first step, decreasing somewhat as the fascia stretches. The baseline pain gradually increases as the day continues.
4. Other common symptoms
   a. Climbing hills or stairs and standing on toes stretch the plantar fascia, increasing the pain
   b. Patients describe the plantar surface of the involved foot as "weak."
   c. Patients may complain of nocturnal cramps in the toe plantar flexors.

Key Symptoms

- Inferior heel pain
- Gradual onset
- Worse with climbing
- Foot feels "weak"
- Burning or aching
- "First step" pain
- Worse with toe-walking
- Nocturnal foot cramps

Clinical Findings

1. Point tenderness
   a. Noted at the medial process of the calcaneal tuberosity, where the inflamed plantar fascia originates. The tender point is located medial to the midline of the plantar surface of the heel, just posterior to a vertical line drawn from the tip of the medial malleolus.
   b. Tenderness also may be noted along the proximal plantar fascia, medial side.
2. Other inflammation signs—swelling, redness, and heat—hardly ever seen in plantar fasciitis.
3. Passively dorsiflexing the great toe evokes pain, because that stretches the fascia.
4. Etiologic findings (not necessary for diagnosis but may be contributing factors)
   a. Biomechanical foot disorders.
      (1) Cavus foot: high, rigid arch. Patient's shoe wear pattern shows exclusive lateral wear.
      (2) Planovalgus foot: flat arch and valgus deviation of the heel. Shoes show medial midfoot wear and breakdown of the medial side of the heel counter.
   b. Tight gastrocnemius-Achilles complex (the heel cord)
      (1) Heel cord is tight if patient cannot dorsiflex foot beyond neutral when the leg is extended at the knee.
      (2) Can occur in neurologic disorders, such as cerebral palsy and mild polio
      (3) Can occur in patients with significant leg-length discrepancies
      (4) Associated with overuse of high-heeled shoes

Key Signs

- Point tenderness over origin of plantar fascia
- Passive toe dorsiflexion reproduces the pain.
- Usual absence of other inflammatory signs

Laboratory Tests

1. History and physical examination are enough to establish diagnosis in most cases.
2. Radiographs of foot and calcaneus
   a. Obtain at first visit if
      (1) Symptoms developed or exacerbated acutely (rule out stress fracture).
      (2) Symptoms and signs are atypical (rule out neoplasm, arthritis, or bone cyst).
      (3) The patient is preadolescent (fasciitis rare in that age group).
      (4) The patient is adolescent but still growing (rule out Sever's disease).
   b. Obtain at follow-up visit if symptoms not improving.
   c. Presence of a heel "spur" on radiograph is considered by most experts as an incidental finding not associated with plantar fasciitis.
   d. A bone scan can help distinguish plantar fasciitis from calcaneal stress fracture when radiograph is normal and symptoms are not improving.

Key Tests

- History and physical examination are sufficient in most cases.
- Foot and calcaneus radiographs to rule out other conditions

Differential Diagnosis

Note: The following conditions are unlikely to show the "first step" symptom or passive toe dorsiflexion pain.

1. Stress fracture of calcaneus
   a. Acute or subacute onset, not protracted onset as in fasciitis
   b. Tenderness on medial *and* lateral aspects of heel
   c. Associated with repetitive, high-impact activity, such as running
   d. Radiograph and/or bone scan positive for fracture
2. Tarsal tunnel syndrome
   a. Burning pain extending into plantar aspect of toes.
   b. May have positive Tinel's sign at tarsal tunnel
3. Sever's disease
   a. Apophysitis of growth plate at Achilles insertion
   b. Occurs in adolescents during growth spurt
4. Less common conditions
   a. Neoplasm—both benign and malignant
      (1) Pain often worse or unchanged during rest
      (2) Unlikely to improve significantly with fasciitis treatment
   b. Gout, rheumatoid arthritis (RA) ankylosing spondylitis (AS), Reiter's syndrome

(1) Pain and tenderness more posterior, at Achilles insertion
(2) Joint or bursa swelling is common.
(3) RA, AS, and Reiter's more likely to be bilateral, gout more likely to be acute onset
   c. Arterial insufficiency
      (1) Burning pain that worsens with increasing activity
      (2) Presence of atherosclerosis risk factors
      (3) Diminished or absent pulses on examination

WARNING

- **Always do a thorough neurovascular examination of the lower extremity when evaluating heel pain.**
- **Keep a high index of suspicion for neoplasm.**
- **Swelling and heat suggest arthritis rather than fasciitis.**

Treatment

A. Basic treatment—successful in most cases
   1. Reduction of inflammation
      a. Ice, applied for 20 minutes, three times daily, especially after weight-bearing activity
      b. Nonsteroidal anti-inflammatory drugs (NSAIDs) for 2 to 3 weeks (if no contraindications). Chronic NSAIDs are usually not helpful.
      c. Relative rest
         (1) If problem seems related to weight-bearing exercise, cease that exercise for 1 to 2 weeks and then rebuild slowly over several weeks as symptoms permit.
         (2) Substitute non–weight-bearing exercises during the relative rest period.
   2. Strengthening and stretching of ankle and foot
      a. Strengthen intrinsic foot muscles to support the arch.
         (1) While sitting, use toe flexors to pull a towel, spread flat on the floor, toward the chair. Do two to three repetitions, twice a day.
         (2) Throughout the day, roll a small cylinder, such as a soup can, back and forth with the shoeless foot, curling the toes with each repetition.
      b. Plantar fascia and Achilles tendon stretching program: both legs, three times a day
         (1) Lean forward against a wall, bare feet pointing straight ahead.
         (2) Stretch one leg at a time, keeping the heel flat on the ground.

(3) Lean forward until a gentle stretch, not pain, is felt.

(4) Continue the stretch for 30 seconds, avoiding bobbing or jerking. Apply ice after stretching.

3. Support and cushioning of the heel

   a. Wear shoes with firm heel counters that snugly hold the heel (increases the fat pad's effectiveness).

   b. Tuli heel cup or similar cushioned heel cup insert in *both* shoes for extra cushioning

   c. Lace-up shoes support the heel better than slip-ons.

   d. Wear shoes and heel support *all the time* except during non–weight bearing and stretching.

4. Correction or reduction of contributing factors

   a. Shoes and orthotics

      (1) Custom-made orthotics help reduce hyperpronation of the planovalgus foot. Orthotics much less helpful for the cavus foot.

      (2) Eliminate shoes with worn-out or flimsy heel counters. If patient cannot afford new shoes, try rigid plastic heel cup inserts.

   b. Stretches described above help the tight gastrocnemius-Achilles complex.

   c. Encourage weight loss for overweight patients.

   d. Discourage overtraining. Athletes should follow the "10 per cent rule" described above.

B. Possible treatment for recalcitrant cases

1. Local corticosteroid injection at site of maximal tenderness

   a. Very painful

   b. Has been associated with fat pad atrophy and rupture of plantar fascia

   c. Occasionally beneficial in cases unresponsive to vigorous "conservative" care

2. Posterior short-leg night splint

   a. Several studies report good success for patients who have had symptoms for 6 to 12 months.

   b. Keeps ankle in 5 degrees of dorsiflexion while patient sleeps, gently stretching plantar fascia and Achilles tendon

   c. Patient wears each night for 3 months and then weans off gradually.

3. Surgery (various procedures)

   a. Reserved for those who have long-term pain and disability in activities of daily living or in activities that are considered very important to the patient

   b. Try 6 months of conservative treatment without any improvement before considering surgery.

Key Treatment

- Ice
- Relative rest
- Brief NSAIDs trial
- Plantar fascia and Achilles stretching
- Constant, firm, snug heel support
- Lose weight if necessary
- Address contributing factors
- Night splint

Follow-Up

1. Patient returns 2 to 3 weeks after first visit to review diagnosis and treatment

2. If improving, continue therapy and return in 4 to 8 weeks

   a. Review contributing factors.

   b. Review maintenance therapy (proper footwear and continued stretching).

   c. Return in 8 weeks or p.r.n.

3. If not improving 8 weeks after initial visit, review treatment adherence. Return in 4 to 8 weeks.

4. If not improving 12 to 16 weeks after initial visit

   a. Consider night splint or injection.

   b. Consider referral if no improvement after 6 months of therapy.

 Bibliography

DeMaio M, Paine R, Mangine RE, Drez D Jr: Plantar fasciitis. Sports Med Rehab Series 1993;16:1153–1163.

Schepsis AA, Leach RE, Gorzyca J: Plantar fasciitis. Clin Orthop 1991;266:185–196.

Painful conditions of the heel, *In* R Cailliet (ed): Foot and Ankle Pain, 2nd ed. Philadelphia, FA Davis, 1983, pp 139–147.

Wapner KL, Sharkey PF: The use of night splints for treatment of recalcitrant plantar fasciitis. Foot Ankle 1991;12:135–137.

217 Shoulder Dislocations

Joe E. Himes

Etiology

1. Anterior shoulder dislocation: abduction, external rotation, and extension of arm
2. Posterior shoulder dislocation: adduction, internal rotation, and flexion of arm

Symptoms

1. Anterior and/or posterior shoulder pain
2. Periarticular muscle spasms
3. Possible neurovascular compromise of extremity

Key Symptoms

- Shoulder pain
- Limitation of glenohumeral motion

Clinical Findings

1. Anterior shoulder dislocation
   a. Inability to internally rotate and abduct humerus
   b. Apprehension
2. Posterior shoulder dislocation
   a. Inability to externally rotate and abduct arm
   b. Inability to fully supinate hand with shoulder in forward flexion
   c. Findings subtle and may be missed on initial examination in 60 to 80 per cent of cases

> **WARNING**
>
> **Always evaluate and document the neurovascular status of the entire extremity at the time of injury and after treatment. Compromised neurovascular status constitutes a true medical emergency.**

Laboratory Tests

Roentographic Evaluation

1. Purposes
   a. Identify fracture of humerus, clavicle, and glenoid fossa (Bankart lesion)
   b. Identify Hill-Sachs lesion of humerus
   c. Confirm suspected dislocation
2. Recommended views
   a. True AP of shoulder
   b. True lateral view of scapula (scapular "Y" view)
   c. Axillary view

Differential Diagnosis

1. Fracture of humerus, clavicle, glenoid fossa
2. Combined fracture-dislocation
3. Muscular contusion
4. Brachial plexopathy
5. Acromioclavicular separation

Treatment

1. Anterior shoulder dislocation
   a. Elevation and internal rotation of humerus while applying posterior pressure to anterior humeral head.
   b. Stimson maneuver: Place patient prone on plinth, hanging arm off edge of table. Apply weights to arm to provide traction. May enhance patient relaxation with muscle relaxants, analgesics, or anesthesia (Fig. 217–1).
   c. Double-sheet method: Patient supine on treatment table. One sheet is held around the patient's torso by an assistant. A second sheet around the patient's upper arm provides lateral traction while the physician provides firm, but gentle traction to the arm along the axial plane.
2. Posterior shoulder dislocation
   a. With patient supine, apply lateral traction with internal rotation followed by external rotation.

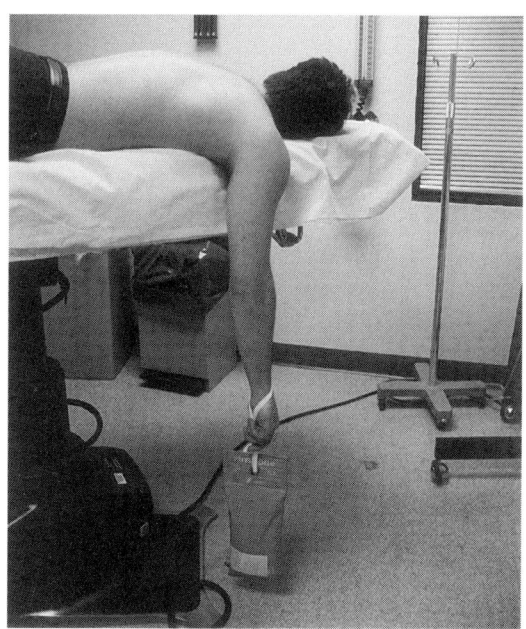

Figure 217–1 Stimson technique for relocation of anterior shoulder dislocation.

Surgery

1. Surgical reduction indicated if conservative approach to reduction unsuccessful.

2. Surgical stabilization following reduction in patients with high risk of recurrence.

   a. Acute anterior shoulder dislocation recurrence

      (1) If patient younger than age 20, greater than 80 per cent

      (2) If patient older than 20, about 25 per cent

   b. Acute posterior shoulder dislocation recurrence

      (1) Less than 40 per cent, with younger patients more likely to suffer

   c. Chronic dislocators

      (1) Attempt to identify voluntary dislocators and educate them

      (2) Much less likely to respond to conservative treatment

---

WARNING

Voluntary subluxors/dislocators are not considered suitable for surgical stabilization as they often continue subluxing/dislocating, thereby lengthening the repair in the early postoperative period.

Medication

Analgesics and anti-inflammatory medications can provide pain relief and minimize soft tissue swelling.

Activity

1. Following reduction of acute, first-time dislocations, arm is immobilized for 2 to 4 weeks, followed by sling for comfort to a total of 6 weeks.

2. Chronic dislocations are likely to recur with less force and less soft tissue damage. Conservative therapy includes relocation with subsequent shoulder stabilization exercises.

Patient Education

1. Educate the patient regarding recurrent dislocations

2. For patients active in sports, educate regarding proper

   a. Strength

   b. Conditioning

   c. Technique

Follow-Up

1. Follow-up roentgenograms to document:

   a. Successful relocation

   b. Bankhart or Hill-Sachs lesions

2. Physical therapy

   a. Control pain and swelling

   b. Restore range of motion

   c. Restore strength and endurance

   d. Relearn proprioceptive and functional reflexes

3. Bracing

   a. Anterior shoulder dislocation: limits abduction and external rotation of shoulder

   b. Posterior shoulder dislocation: no effective bracing available

 Bibliography

Craig EV, Hsu KC: Shoulder problems in the weekend athlete. Orthop Rev 1992;21(2):155–167.

Fields KB, Rasco T, Kramer JS, et al: Rehabilitation exercises for common sports injuries. Am Family Phys 1992; 45(3):1233–1243.

Jobe FW, Pink M: The athlete's shoulder. J Hand Ther 1994;7(2):107–110.

Tibone JE, Bradley JP: The treatment of posterior subluxation in athletes. Clin Orthop 1993;291:124–137.

Yu J: Anterior shoulder dislocations. J Fam Pract 1992; 35(5):567–571, 575–576.

218 Elbow Dislocations

Nina Skattum

The elbow is a hinge joint with three articulations—olecranotrochlear, radiocapitellar, and proximal radioulnar. The trochlear notch of the olecranon articulates with the trochlea of the humerus and provides the primary bony stability of the elbow joint, particularly to varus stress. The medial collateral ligament, specifically the anterior oblique band, is the primary ligamentous stabilizer, resisting valgus stress particularly in flexion. Additional soft tissue support is provided by the anterior capsule, which offers stability in extension, principally against distractional and valgus forces. Despite inherent stability, the elbow follows the shoulder as the second most frequently dislocated joint in the body. The majority of elbow dislocations (90 to 93 per cent) occur posteriorly or posterolaterally, whereas anterior and medial dislocations are rare (0 to 10 per cent).

Etiology

1. The most common mechanism of injury is a fall on an outstretched arm with hyperextension and valgus stress; this usually causes rupture or avulsion of the medial collateral ligament and the anterior capsule with a consequent disengagement of the coronoid process of the ulna from the trochlea of the humerus, resulting in a posterior shift. The radial head often follows the ulnar path, and contraction of the biceps and triceps maintains the dislocated position.

2. In young children, usually under age 4 years, "nursemaid's elbow" (subluxation or dislocation of the imperfectly formed radial head with damage to or unfolding of the immature annular ligament) occurs secondary to the pulling on the extended pronated arm to lift the child. Pain comes from impingement of the annular ligament between the radius and ulna.

3. Dislocations resulting from high-impact trauma, such as motor vehicle and occupational accidents, are less common but warrant specific assessment for fractures and neurovascular injury.

Symptoms

1. Severe pain
2. Limited range of motion; pronation/supination better preserved than flexion/extension
3. Swelling; deformity posteriorly often obvious as well as swelling in antecubital fossa
4. Paresthesias

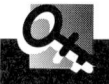
Key Symptoms
- Severe elbow pain and swelling

Clinical Findings

1. Arm held in flexion and forearm pronation in children with "nursemaid's elbow"
2. Deformity/swelling posteriorly; olecranon and radial head palpable posteriorly
3. Child who holds arm with elbow flexed and forearm pronated.
3. Apparent shortening of the forearm
4. Antecubital fossa swelling
5. Palpable indentation of the distal triceps muscle above the olecranon
6. Findings suggestive of neurovascular compromise: decreased radial and ulnar pulses, slow capillary refill, ecchymoses, cyanosis, pallor, temperature changes in skin, decreased (or altered) sensation to pinprick and/or two-point discrimination and motor loss in the distribution of the median and ulnar nerves
7. Forearm and wrist tenderness should be radiographically evaluated to exclude fracture/dislocation of the distal radioulnar joint and carpal bones.

Key Signs
- Arm flexed at elbow with deformity and swelling
- Evidence of neurovascular compromise

Laboratory Tests

1. Radiographs: AP and lateral views are usually sufficient to confirm dislocation and exclude associated fractures. If examination is not suggestive of fracture, reduction can be attempted before radiologic evaluation.
2. In skeletally immature patients it is particularly important to exclude supracondylar fractures.
3. Subtle radiographic findings may be difficult to interpret, and additional films (e.g., comparison views of the contralateral side, gravity stress test views) may be helpful.
4. In nursemaid's elbow with no history of significant trauma, radiographs may not be necessary before or after uncomplicated reduction if there is prompt resolution of symptoms with reduction and examination confirms full active range of motion without pain.
5. Urgent angiography should be performed if there is concern of vascular compromise.
6. Consider nerve conduction studies if neurologic symptoms persist.
7. Radiographs of cervical spine are indicated if history and examination suggest neck involvement.

Key Tests

- Consider radiographs prereduction to exclude fracture.

- Always obtain radiographs postreduction to confirm anatomic alignment.

- Evaluate secondary ossification centers with contralateral films.

Differential Diagnosis

1. Supracondylar fracture: crucial in skeletally immature patients

2. Other fractures (epicondylar, radial head and neck, coronoid, olecranon, capitellum): Evaluate for fracture fragments trapped in the joint, particularly medial epicondylar epiphysis in skeletally immature patients. Radiographs may only show increased medial joint space. Fibrous union of a displaced medial epicondylar fragment may result in functional shortening or lengthening of the medial collateral ligament with consequent flexion contracture or instability.

3. Consider distal radioulnar dissociation.

4. Consider child abuse.

WARNING

Supracondylar fractures in skeletally immature patients are orthopedic emergencies.

Treatment

1. Neurovascular examination is mandatory prior to reduction.

2. Most elbow dislocations can be treated with closed reduction by applying gentle traction along the longitudinal axis of the humerus with the elbow flexed. Use intravenous sedation or general anesthesia as needed. If closed reduction is unsuccessful, the patient should be evaluated for open reduction. Dislocation with associated unstable fractures should be considered for open stabilization. In children with nursemaid's elbow, flex the elbow 90 degrees and gently supinate the forearm with one hand while the thumb of the other applies pressure over the radial head.

3. Adults: Immobilize with long-arm posterior splint at 90 degrees initially. Consider using long-arm cast in patients with associated fractures. Individualize the period of immobilization; patients with uncomplicated dislocations and no significant instability may tolerate discontinuation of the splint within the first few days. Patients with evidence of instability may need radiographic re-evaluation (while in plaster) in a few days and may need a sling or a hinged brace for support when the plaster is removed. Immobiliza-

tion for more than 2 weeks is associated with increased prevalence and severity of flexion contractures and pain.

4. Children: In nursemaid's elbow, goal is to reduce impinged portions of the annular ligament.

5. Early active range-of-motion rehabilitation is essential to prevent loss of extension, flexion, pronation, and supination. Start gentle flexion/extension exercises within the first week, limited by pain and instability.

Activity

1. Aim for gentle active and active-assisted flexion/extension as soon as tolerated and unprotected flexion/extension within 2 weeks. Use a single-axis orthosis if there is valgus/varus instability. Also, start wrist flexion/extension stretches and strengthening as tolerated. Avoid forced passive extension as this increases risk of flexion contracture.

2. Start progressive resisted exercises as soon as possible.

3. Allow a gradual return to activity when motion is functional and pain-free.

Patient Education

1. After initial reduction, patients should be aware of the warning signs of neurovascular compromise and know how to reach their provider.

2. Stress the importance of early and continued range-of-motion rehabilitation. Explain that flexion contracture and pain are the most common complications of elbow dislocations, that recurrent dislocations are rare, and that a shorter period of immobilization and early motion significantly improves outcome.

3. Outline the expected course of rehabilitation and the need for follow-up, particularly if the patient experiences difficulties or is not improving as expected. Some patients note improvement in range of motion for several months.

4. Discuss the possibility of residual range-of-motion loss, particularly flexion contracture secondary to adhesions and fibrosis of the anterior capsule, shortening of the medial collateral ligament, scarring of the brachialis muscle, and/or proliferative fibrofatty tissue intra-articularly. Normal range of motion is 150 degrees flexion, -10 to 0 degrees extension, and 80 to 90 degrees supination/pronation, but most activities of daily living require only 30 to 130 degrees extension/flexion and 50 to 50 degrees supination/pronation. Throwing athletes, however, need full range of motion.

Key Treatment

- Closed reduction and early mobilization

- Neurovascular examination prereduction and postreduction

Follow-Up

1. Careful evaluation of range of motion. Use standard goniometry to measure flexion, extension, pronation, and supination compared to the uninjured side.

2. Assess degree of motion, discomfort, pain, instability, neurovascular deficit, and function. Consider radiography for evaluation of missed fractures and heterotopic ossification.

3. Consider further evaluation by an orthopedic consultant and formal physical therapy for patients who are not improving as expected.

Bibliography

Hoffman DF: Elbow dislocations: Avoiding complications. Phys Sportsmed 1993;21(11):56–67.

Melhoff TL, Noble PC, Bennett JB, et al: Simple dislocation of the elbow in the adult. J Bone Joint Surg 1988;70A:244–249.

Morrey BF, An KN: Articular and ligamentous contributions to the stability of the elbow joint. Am J Sports Med 1983;11(5):315–319.

Schwab GH, Bennett JB, Woods GV, et al: Biomechanics of elbow instability: The role of the medial collateral ligament. Clin Orthop 1980;146:42–52.

Timmerman LA, Andrews JR: Arthroscopic treatment of post-traumatic elbow stiffness. Am J Sports Med 1994;22(2):230–235.

219 Finger Dislocations

Ellen T. Geminiani

Distal Interphalangeal (DIP) Joint

Etiology: Mechanism of Injury

1. Dislocation is usually the result of hyperextension —uncommon injury.
2. Ligament and tendon injuries are more common at DIP joint.

Symptoms

1. Pain, swelling, or inability to flex or extend at DIP joint
2. Complaint of obvious deformity—may have been reduced already

Clinical Findings

1. Deformity of distal phalanx position
   a. Displaced dorsally or laterally—most common (see Fig. 219–1 for normal anatomy)
   b. Volar dislocations are rare.
2. *Careful* inspection for an open wound

Radiographic Findings

1. Anteroposterior (AP) and lateral views of individual digits for clear view

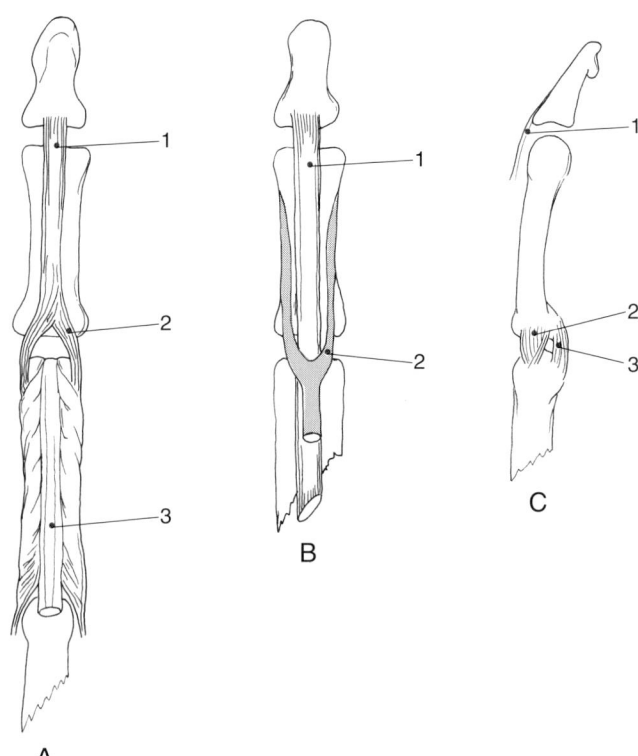

Figure 219–1 Normal anatomy. *A,* Dorsal (1) extensor tendon, (2) central slip, (3) extensor digitorum; *B,* palmar (1) flexor digitorum profundus, (2) flexor digitorum superficialis; *C,* lateral (1) extensor tendon, (2) collateral ligament, (3) volar plate.

2. Evaluate for avulsion fracture
3. Refer to hand surgeon if fracture greater than 25 per cent of articular surface

Associated Ligament Injuries (Compare Injured with Uninjured Side)

1. Collateral ligament sprains—Assess with varus and valgus stress in extension and 10 to 15 degrees of flexion.
2. Volar plate injuries—Assess with hyperextension stress at DIP.

Associated Tendon Injuries (Compare Injured with Uninjured Side)

1. Extensor tendon rupture—"baseball" or "mallet" finger
   a. Result of forced flexion during active extension
   b. Assess active and resisted extension at DIP joint.
2. Flexor digitorum profundus tendon (FDP) rupture— Jersey finger
   a. Result of forced hyperextension during active flexion
   b. Test for active and resisted flexion at DIP and with other digits held in extension to isolate FDP tendon.

Treatment

1. DIP dorsal dislocations/volar plate and collateral ligament injury
   a. Open dislocations should be referred to hand surgeon.
   b. Digital block should produce adequate anesthesia.
   c. Apply gentle traction in line with digit and pressure on dorsal aspect of distal phalanx until relocated.
   d. Evaluate for associated ligament/tendon injuries and repeat radiographs to rule out articular fracture after reduction.
   e. Dorsal splint for 3 weeks with DIP in 10 to 15 degrees of flexion
2. Tendon injuries
   a. Extensor tendon rupture with or without associated avulsion fracture—Splint DIP in full extension for 6 to 8 weeks.
   b. FDP rupture—Splint in slight flexion and refer to hand surgeon; requires surgical repair.

Activity/Follow-Up

1. DIP dorsal dislocations/volar plate and collateral ligament injury
   a. Continue usual activities with splint for initial 3 weeks.

b. For athlete, splint for additional 6 to 8 weeks.

2. Tendon injuries
   a. Continue usual activity with splint for 6 to 8 weeks and then only for sports for additional 6 to 8 weeks.
   b. FDP injury—per hand surgeon based on severity of injury

Proximal Interphalangeal (PIP) Joint

Etiology/Mechanism of Injury

Dorsal dislocation due to axial loading and hyperextension

Symptoms

1. Pain and swelling at PIP joint
2. Complaint of previous deformity—may have already been reduced

Clinical Findings

1. Deformity of middle phalanx in relation to proximal phalanx
   a. Dorsal dislocation most common—involves volar plate tear
   b. Volar dislocation—rare injury—disrupts extensor mechanism
2. Location of tenderness suggests structures involved.

Radiographic Findings

AP and lateral views of individual digit for unobstructed view

1. Evaluate for articular surface or avulsion fracture.
2. If fracture greater than 25 per cent of articular surface, refer.

Associated Ligament Injuries (Compare Injured with Uninjured Side)

1. Volar plate tear—can occur with or without dorsal dislocation.
   a. Pain on volar surface of PIP joint
   b. Laxity and pain with hyperextension of PIP
2. Collateral ligament injury—jammed or "stoved" finger
   a. May occur alone or with other injuries
   b. Detected by laxity with varus and valgus stress at PIP

Associated Tendon Injury: Central Slip Injury

1. Results from blunt trauma, lacerations, or forced hyperflexion
2. Inability to extend at PIP actively or with resistance
3. Failure to treat leads to boutonniere deformity

Treatment

1. Dorsal dislocations—Digital block may be used for anesthesia.
   a. Relocate by accentuating deformity, apply *gentle* traction, and flex finger to normal position.
   b. Radiograph after reduction to rule out articular fracture.
   c. Assess for associated injuries—volar plate usually torn.
   d. Splint PIP in 25 to 30 degrees of flexion for 2 to 3 weeks.
2. Volar plate tears splinted in 20 to 30 degrees of flexion for 2 to 3 weeks
3. Collateral ligament injuries
   a. Buddy tape in slight flexion until pain-free (about 4 to 6 weeks)
   b. Complete tears may require surgical correction.
4. Central slip tears—splint PIP in extension for 5 to 6 weeks.

Activity/Follow-Up

1. Encourage early motion with protection.
2. Dorsal dislocation—buddy tape until pain-free motion
3. Volar plate tears—Continue usual activities with splint for initial 2 to 3 weeks, then extension block splint until pain-free, and then buddy tape with sports activities.
4. Collateral ligament injury—buddy tape until pain-free
5. Central slip injury—initial treatment for 5 to 6 weeks
   a. Protective splint/buddy tape for additional 6 to 8 weeks
   b. Surgical repair for boutonniere deformity

Metacarpophalangeal (MP) Joint (Including Thumb)

Etiology/Mechanism of Injury

1. Dorsal dislocation results from forced hyperextension
2. Second or fifth digit most commonly involved
3. Lateral and volar dislocations much less common

Symptoms

1. Pain and disability in flexion at MP joint
2. Deformity of proximal phalanx at MP joint

Clinical Findings

1. Dorsal dislocation may be simple or complex.
   a. Simple dislocation presents with the proximal phalanx in 60 to 90 degrees of hyperextension on dorsum of metacarpal head—articular surfaces remain in contact.
   b. Complex dislocation shows only slight hyperextension and a characteristic dimple of palmar skin.
2. Lateral dislocation associated with collateral ligament injury
   a. Tenderness over involved collateral ligament

b. Swelling in the space between the metacarpal heads

c. Laxity with varus and valgus stress with MP in full flexion

d. Thumb requires specific evaluation (see below).

Radiologic Findings

1. Simple dorsal dislocations show articular surfaces in contact.

2. Complex dorsal dislocation (pathognomonic sign) sesamoid within joint space

Associated Ligament Injuries

1. Volar plate is torn from insertion on neck of metacarpal.

   a. Complex dislocation results from entrapment of volar plate between base of proximal phalanx and metacarpal head.

   b. Simple dislocation can become complex when closed reduction is done incorrectly.

2. Collateral ligament injury with lateral dislocation

Associated Tendon Injury: Rupture of Extensor Hood

1. Results in tendon subluxation between metacarpal heads

2. Decreased extension at MP joint with weakness

Treatment

1. Simple dorsal dislocation—Traction may cause complex dislocation.

   a. Anesthesia—wrist or metacarpal block

   b. Wrist and IP joints flexed to relax tendons

   c. Proximal phalanx hyperextended to approximately 90 degrees—*no traction*

   d. Push base of proximal phalanx across articular surface.

   e. Flex gently to confirm positioning.

   f. Splint in 50 to 70 degrees of flexion for 7 to 10 days.

2. Complex dislocation—refer to hand surgeon for open reduction.

3. Collateral ligament injury with lateral dislocation

   a. Without fracture—splint in 50 to 70 degrees of flexion for 3 weeks.

   b. Unstable joint or avulsion fracture—refer to hand surgeon.

Activity/Follow-Up

1. Simple and complex dislocation—early active motion with buddy tape until pain-free

2. Collateral ligament injury—buddy tape for an additional 4 weeks

Thumb-Ulnar Collateral Ligament Injuries

Etiology/Mechanism of Injury

1. Sudden valgus (abduction) stress with hyperextension

2. Commonly called "gamekeeper's" or "skier's" thumb.

Symptoms

1. Pain and swelling at MP joint

2. Point of greatest pain localizes to ulnar aspect of MP joint

Clinical Findings

1. Tenderness at ulnar aspect of MP joint

2. Assess degree of laxity—partial or complete tear

   a. Test in both flexion and extension

   b. Compare injured and uninjured thumb

3. Stener lesion develops when adductor aponeurosis lies between ends of torn ligament

Radiographic Findings

Avulsion fracture of proximal phalanx or articular surface

Treatment

1. Partial tears—thumb spica cast for 3 to 6 weeks

2. Complete tear—operative repair, refer to hand surgeon

3. Avulsion fractures

   a. Nondisplaced—thumb spica cast for 3 to 6 weeks

   b. Displaced greater than 5 mm or greater than 25 per cent articular surface—refer

Activity/Follow-Up

1. Partial tears and nondisplaced fractures, continue usual activities with appropriate splint for 3 to 6 weeks, then activity as tolerated

2. Operative repair—activities with cast for 4 weeks

   a. Removable splint for 2 to 3 weeks after casting

   b. Activity without splint *not* allowed until 10 to 12 weeks

B | Bibliography

Duay GJ, Eaton RG: Dislocations and ligament injuries in the digits. *In* Green DP (ed): Operative Hand Surgery, 3rd ed. New York, Churchill Livingstone, 1993, pp 767–791.

Green DP, Strickland JW: Hand and wrist: section B: The hand. *In* DeLee JC, Drez D Jr (eds): Orthopedic Sports Medicine: Principles and Practice, vol 1. Philadelphia, WB Saunders, 1994, pp 945–983.

Hoffman DF, Schaffer TC: Management of common finger injuries. Am Fam Physician 1991;43(5):1594–1607.

Kahler DM, McCue FC III: Metacarpophalangeal and proximal interphalangeal joint injuries of the hand, including the thumb. Clin Sports Med 1992;11(1):57–76.

Rettig AC: Closed tendon injuries of the hand and wrist in the athlete. Clin Sports Med 1992;11(1):77–99.

220 Patellar Dislocations

Jan Fronek

Etiology

1. The classification is based on the clinical factors contributing to the episode.
   a. Acute dislocation is usually observed immediately after the traumatic event.
   b. Recurrent instability: With repetitive trauma, the patient may experience recurrent, repeated patellar dislocations.
   c. Missed, unreduced dislocation: If the treatment is delayed due to missed diagnosis or poor patient compliance, the patella may remain chronically unreduced.
   d. Congenital (developmental) dislocation presenting in infants and children is one of the less common etiologies of patellar dislocations.
   e. Postoperative dislocation may be present following patellar realignment or knee replacement surgery.
2. The mechanism responsible for patellar dislocation may be classified as internal, external, or a combination of both.
   a. The internal application of forces is due to the powerful quadriceps contraction while the patient pivots on a fixed surface.
   b. The external mechanism is due to direct trauma or a blow to the patella resulting in dislocation.
   c. The propensity for the patella to dislocate is further enhanced by predisposing factors that include genu valgum, genu recurvatum, increased ligamentous laxity, and external tibial torsion with a laterally inserted patellar tendon.

Symptoms

The patient will describe a pivoting or twisting injury to the knee or occasionally will remember direct trauma or impact to the knee. The individual may state that the "knee cap went out" or "popped out" once or twice. Often the first sensation is due to the dislocation and the second "pop" is noted with spontaneous reduction as the knee is extended. Within a few minutes to hours, the patient may notice significant swelling (hemarthrosis) or inability to extend or flex (often due to the hemarthrosis as well as possible osteochondral fracture, which may block motion).

Clinical Findings

1. Patella dislocated: The patella remains in a laterally displaced, painful position and may be visibly tenting the skin. Any motion of the knee, particularly flexion, will be associated with increased pain. The associated findings may include a hemarthrosis and skin abrasions at the site of impact.
2. Patella reduced: If spontaneous reduction took place, the patient presents with a hemarthrosis and pain. Pain is usually retropatellar or at the medial joint line of the patella. With palpation, the medial peripatellar region (medial retinaculum) is tender and a defect may be present. The positive Fairbank's test may be elicited by pushing the patella laterally. This elicits resistance, panic, or apprehension by the patient.

Key Signs

Patella dislocated

- Patella is laterally displaced.
- Skin trauma at site of impact
- Locked knee: Patient is unable to flex or extend the knee joint.

Examination following spontaneous reduction

- Fairbank's apprehension test +

Laboratory Tests

1. Initial radiographs should include the anteroposterior (AP), lateral, and oblique views. These views allow for evaluation of any post-traumatic changes such as avulsion fractures, osteophytes, or loose bodies.
2. Merchant's (tangential) view is important for the assessment of the patellofemoral articulation.

Key Symptoms

- Hemarthrosis
- Knee cap "pops out" once or twice (initially with dislocation; second "pop" is noted w/ spontaneous reduction as the knee is extended)
- Pain: usually retropatellar, may be at medial joint line of the patella

Key Tests

Initial radiographs

- AP, lateral, and oblique views
- Merchant's (tangential) view

Postreduction radiographic views (same as above)

- Check for osteochondral fragments

825

3. After satisfactory reduction, AP, lateral, and Merchant's views should be obtained. These films will provide information about any residual patellar subluxation or tilt and presence of osteochondral fragments.

Differential Diagnosis

1. The differential diagnosis of patellar dislocation includes
   a. Meniscus tear
   b. Anterior cruciate ligament tear
   c. Knee (femoral/tibial) dislocation
   d. Patellar fracture
   e. Osteochondral fracture
   f. Osteochondritis dissecans/avascular necrosis
   g. Loose body, intra-articular
   h. Patellar or quadriceps tendon tear (partial or complete)

2. In addition to patellar dislocation, the patient may have an associated injury involving the structures noted in the list directly above.

Treatment

1. Acute reduction is managed with gentle extension of the knee and pressure on the lateral border of the patella directed medially. Rarely, closed reduction under general anesthesia or open reduction is necessary. A knee immobilizer or cylinder cast is applied, immobilizing the knee in extension. During the first 24 to 48 hours after injury, ice, elevation, and compression are particularly valuable.
   a. Nonathlete / first dislocation / no defect in medial retinaculum
      (1) Immobilization for 3 weeks
      (2) Rehabilitation program aimed at quadriceps strengthening and regaining normal range of motion of the knee
   b. Competitive athlete: first dislocation
      (1) Operative arthroscopy may be considered.
      (2) Medial retinaculum repair if significant palpable defect is noted
      (3) Rehabilitation program aimed at quadriceps strengthening and regaining normal range of motion of the knee
   c. Osteochondral fracture present
      (1) Operative arthroscopy and the osteochondral

fragment repaired (if large) or removed (if small)
      (2) Rehabilitation program aimed at quadriceps strengthening and regaining normal range of motion of the knee
   d. Intra-articular dislocation
      (1) Prompt open reduction if closed reduction cannot be accomplished easily
      (2) Immobilization for 4 to 6 weeks

2. Recurrent patellar instability management is determined by the patient's response to the nonsurgical program and overall disability.
   a. Nonsurgical modalities most commonly include
      (1) Quadriceps strengthening
      (2) Patellar bracing
      (3) McConnell taping of the patella
   b. Symptomatic recurrent patellar instability, refractory to nonsurgical treatment: surgical treatment is based on surgical pathology and may include
      (1) Operative arthroscopy and lateral retinacular release
      (2) Possible proximal and distal realignment

3. Chronic unreduced dislocation is rare. Usually an open procedure is required to achieve reduction of the patellofemoral joint.

4. Congenital, developmental dislocation often represents a complex malformation of the patellofemoral joint. Generally, proximal and distal surgical realignment is necessary to avoid significant functional disability

Medication

1. Salicylates
2. Nonsteroidal anti-inflammatory drugs (NSAIDs)
3. Analgesics

B Bibliography

Frymoyer JW (ed): Orthopaedic Knowledge Update, 4th ed. Rosemont, IL, American Academy of Orthopaedic Surgeons, 1993.

Fulkerson JP: Patellofemoral pain disorders: Evaluation and management. J Am Acad Orthopaed Surg 1994;2:124–132.

Rockwood CA, Green DP (eds): Fractures in Adults, 3rd ed. Philadelphia, JB Lippincott, 1992.

Scott WN (ed): Ligament and Extensor Mechanism Injuries of the Knee. St. Louis. Mosby-Year Book, 1991.

Shea KP: Clinical evaluation of patellofemoral pain and instability. Op Tech Sports Med 1994;2:248–255.

221 Wrist Fractures

Reid B. Blackwelder

Etiology

1. One of the most common fractures
2. Usually occur due to a fall on an outstretched hand

Symptoms

1. Painful, swollen distal forearm and wrist and a history of a fall
2. Serious complication may be damage to an associated nerve, most commonly the median nerve; sensory deficits in the distribution of this nerve may be found.
3. As for any trauma, be aware of associated symptoms unrelated to the wrist injury that may be important to address, such as syncope, seizures, and so on.
4. A thorough history is essential in approaching a wrist injury.
   a. Ask about mechanism of injury, specifically about dorsi- or volar-flexion, supination or pronation of forearm, point of contact, and activity (fall or blow).
   b. Ask about motor and sensory function.
   c. Document which hand is dominant.

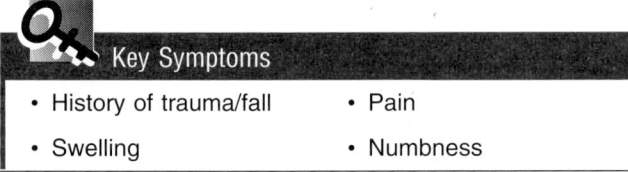

Key Symptoms	
• History of trauma/fall	• Pain
• Swelling	• Numbness

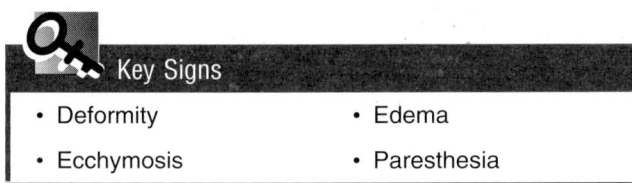

Key Signs	
• Deformity	• Edema
• Ecchymosis	• Paresthesia

Anatomy

1. Knowledge of the anatomy of the wrist is essential; missed diagnoses can lead to difficult management problems and instability in the long run.
2. Wrist starts 3 cm proximal to the radiocarpal joint and extends to the carpometacarpal joints.
3. Bony components
   a. Distal end of the radius, the articular disk and the articulations with the proximal carpal row (scaphoid, lunate, and triquetral); this inherently unstable joint is strengthened by several groups of strong ligaments.
   b. Ulna has no direct bony articulations.
   c. Scaphoid, or navicular bone, serves a critical function as the stabilizer of the wrist complex during motion.

4. Muscular components
   a. No muscles originate or insert in the wrist.
   b. Extrinsic muscles arise on the forearm and insert at the base of the metacarpals, except for the flexor carpi ulnaris, which inserts on the pisiform; this arrangement causes motion to be translated across the rows of carpal bones and emphasizes the importance of the stability the scaphoid provides for the carpal bones.
5. Neurovascular components
   a. Radial and ulnar arteries cross the wrist to enter the palm with superficial and deep branches forming arches.
   b. Ulnar nerve provides motor enervation to almost all the intrinsics and sensation to entire ulnar 1½ fingers.
   c. Radial nerve does not supply any motor function to intrinsic muscles but does provide sensation to the dorsum of the hand and the dorsum of the radial 3½ fingers and motor function of the extrinsic wrist and finger extensors.
   d. Median nerve travels in the carpal tunnel and supplies sensation to the palmar aspect and the dorsal fingertips of the radial 3½ fingers and motor function to the thenar muscles.

Tests

1. Examination
   a. Completely expose the injured arm, and remove all rings, bracelets, etc.; often helpful to compare it with the uninjured side.
   b. Observe hand in relaxed position—should see slight flexion, with normal curve of digits.
   c. Inspect both dorsal and volar surfaces for deformity, laceration, swelling, and discoloration.
   d. Palpate gently to try and localize the site of maximal pain; pay particular attention to the anatomic "snuffbox" located between the tendons of the extensor pollicus longus and the extensor pollicus brevis; pain in this area suggests a fracture of the scaphoid.
   e. Assess vascular function by checking radial and ulnar pulses, performing Allen's test, and checking capillary refill. Be concerned about a pulsatile swelling, which may indicate an arterial injury.
   f. Assess neurologic function by performing a complete sensory examination of the hand; deficits may be created by direct nerve damage, associated vascular injury, or compression.
      (1) Checking light touch is not sufficient.

(2) Use a pin for sharp and dull and a paper clip for two-point discrimination (>4 mm is suspicious for injury); check at each side of the finger pulp.

(3) Distribution of the sensory changes points to the nerve involved; as stated previously, median nerve injuries are the most common with wrist fractures.

(4) Realize the value of serial neurovascular checks, especially if a reduction is planned; signs of ischemia from compression may be slow to develop.

(5) Any symptoms suggesting nerve damage warrant immediate attention and, if not transient, referral to an orthopedist.

g. Assess motor function, including strength of muscle groups and range of motion of the wrist and fingers, specifically flexion, extension, and pronation-supination.

2. Radiographs

a. Radiographs are crucial in the evaluation of wrist injuries.

b. Obtain anteroposterior (AP; some texts say PA) and true lateral views with wrist in neutral position (no ulnar-radial deviation or palmar dorsiflexion of hand or wrist), and obliques with 45 degrees each of supination and pronation.

c. May need scaphoid view if a carpal fracture is suspected

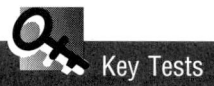

Key Tests

- Complete vascular examination
- Complete neurologic examination
- Wrist radiographs

Differential Diagnosis

1. Colles' fracture

a. The most common type, which presents with the classic "silver (dinner) fork" deformity

b. Distal radius is fractured and displaced dorsally, often with shortening and radial deviation of the distal fragment; sometimes associated ulnar styloid or ulnar collateral ligament injury.

2. Smith's fracture (reverse Colles'): Results from fall with forearm supinated and hand extended, or after throwing a punch, or after sustaining a direct blow to the dorsum of the wrist with hand flexed and forearm pronated

3. Barton's fracture: Involves an oblique dorsal rim fracture-dislocation through the articular surface of the distal radius

4. Pediatric wrist fractures

a. Epiphyseal fracture-separation (pediatric Colles')

(1) Diagnosis may be difficult if nondisplaced; remember wrist sprains are uncommon in children because the ligamentous complexes are stronger than the epiphyseal plate.

(2) Tenderness over epiphysis strongly suggests fracture.

b. Torus fractures

(1) Occur approximately 2.5 cm proximal to wrist

(2) No displacement occurs; radius "buckles"

5. Scaphoid fracture

a. Most commonly encountered carpal bone fracture; must be considered in differential diagnosis of wrist fractures

b. Complication is avascular necrosis, although 90 per cent heal without complication.

c. Clinical examination will reveal pain at the wrist but particularly in the anatomic snuffbox.

Treatment

Reduction of Fractures

1. General points

a. If seen within a few hours, usually can reduce under local anesthesia (hematoma block)

b. Reduction involves reversing the forces causing the injury.

c. Always repeat a neurovascular examination after any reduction.

2. Colles' fracture

a. Disimpact the distal fragment with longitudinal traction and thumb pressure to reduce the dorsal angulation.

b. Provide ulnar deviation with thumb pressure to reduce the radial displacement.

c. Apply upward pressure with wrist slightly flexed and ulnarly deviated to maintain reduction until a cast is placed, usually a sugar-tong splint for 3 to 7 days.

d. Elevate with ice for 48 to 72 hours, with active motion of the fingers.

e. Repeat radiograph within 7 to 10 days; occasional loss of reduction may occur when the swelling subsides—may be acceptable in older patients.

f. Immobilize with sugar-tong or short-arm cast for 6 weeks.

3. Smith's fracture

a. If no involvement of the articular surface, may be treated as Colles', except the wrist is immobilized in supination

b. If the articular surface is involved, refer for treatment.

4. Barton's fracture: refer in all cases, since often requires open reduction and fixation
5. Pediatric fractures
   a. Epiphyseal fracture-dislocation
      (1) With presence of tenderness, consider placing a short-arm cast or sugar-tong even if the radiographs are normal.
      (2) Repeat radiograph in 2 weeks—if callous, continue cast 2 more weeks; if none, can remove cast and sprain has been treated.
      (3) Important to discuss the possibility of growth plate injury with parents; risk of premature closure and shortening of the limb exists
      (4) Consider referral to orthopedic surgeon; definitely refer for displacement with angulation.
   b. Torus fracture: Treat with short-arm cast for 3 to 4 weeks.
6. Scaphoid fracture
   a. Since fractures are often not initially seen on radiograph, may treat as fracture with immobilization for 2 weeks and repeat film; if study is still inconclusive and the clinical picture is still suspicious, get bone scan.
   b. Good reduction is necessary—put palmar to dorsal pressure on the distal fragment to reduce volar flexion.
   c. Place in short-arm spica thumb cast to the tip of the thumb; may require up to 12 to 24 weeks.
   d. Refer for greater than 1 mm displacement.

Medications
1. Unless contraindicated, nonsteroidal anti-inflammatory drugs (NSAIDs) are often helpful.
2. Appropriate analgesia is always beneficial—broken bones hurt!
3. Consider mild sedation prior to reduction of fractures.

Patient Education
1. Elevate wrist for 24 to 48 hours after treatment.

2. Ice may be applied, but keep cast dry; limit icing to 20 minutes an hour.
3. If sugar-tong placed, provide a sling.
4. Discuss signs and symptoms of ischemia and need to contact you immediately if numbness, cyanosis, or severe pain occurs.

 Key Treatment

- Definitive treatment depends on type of fracture.
- Initial treatment is reduction, if needed, or referral.
- Rest, ice, compression, elevation, nonsteroidal anti-inflammatory drugs (RICED)
- Splint/immobilize
- Repeat radiograph if reduced and splinted/casted
- Analgesia

Follow-Up
1. See patient in 3 to 4 days to evaluate cast.
2. If necessary, radiographs may be taken with the cast on to check on adequacy of reduction.
3. Once the appropriate time has passed, usually 6 weeks, remove the cast and repeat radiograph.
4. Initiate rehabilitation exercises for hand and wrist.

 Bibliography

Mellion MB: Office Management of Sports Injuries and Athletic Problems. Philadelphia, Henley & Belfus, 1988, p 197.
Mercier LR: Practical Orthopedics, 3rd ed. St Louis, Mosby–Year Book, 1991, pp 119–124.
Schwartz GR, Cayten CG, Mangelsen MA, et al (eds): Principles and Practice of Emergency Medicine, 3rd ed, vol 1. Philadelphia, Lea & Febiger, 1992, pp 1104–1105.
Steinberg GG, Akins CM, Baran DT, et al (eds): Ramamurti's Orthopaedics in Primary Care, 2nd ed. Baltimore, Williams & Wilkins, 1992, pp 88–93.
Tolo VT, Wood B: Pediatric Orthopaedics in Primary Care. Baltimore, Williams & Wilkins, 1993, pp 55–61.

222 Finger Fractures

Kenneth L. Taylor-Butler

Because finger function is crucial to so many activities of daily living, it is important to have a clear understanding of the anatomy of the finger and hand in order to develop a system for proper injury evaluation, treatment, and referral. In order to prevent long-term disability, the supporting ligaments and tendons of the metacarpophalangeal and proximal interphalangeal joints must be evaluated and treated quickly. It is easy to assume that the inability to move a joint is a result of the pain and swelling of the injury. However, soft tissue injuries are a major source of instability with functional impairment. Therefore, the assumption that as swelling dissipates, function will return, is not always valid. Further, fractures may be occult with patients having performed "on the field" reduction of the finger returning it to normal appearance. For that reason the fate of the injured hand will be determined by the judgment of the physician who first sees the patient.

In evaluating the finger, it is important to understand first the normal biomechanics and second the mechanism of injury. The most frequently seen fractures in the body are those of the metacarpals and phalanges. Phalangeal fractures are commonly seen in ball sports. The etiology of finger fractures is often age dependent: sports being the leading cause among those 10 to 29 years of age, whereas falls predominate in those over 70 years of age. Common fractures, such as the mallet/baseball finger, can be diagnosed readily based on the disability and mechanism of injury. Unusual injuries such as the Jersey finger will require a high index of clinical suspicion in order to make the diagnosis. Because the distal hand is most readily exposed to trauma, it is understandable that the long finger is injured twice as often as the next most injured digit, the thumb.

Tests

1. Inspect for maximum tenderness and swelling.
2. Test neurologic function (two-point discrimination, strength).
3. Assess vascular status (capillary refill).
4. Evaluate individual joint range of motion.
5. Look for signs of instability: rotation or angulation.

PEARL

Since there is wide variability of laxity in individuals, always compare the uninjured side. During stress testing flex the joint at 30 degrees in order to reduce the stabilizing effects of the volar plate.

---

6. Perform stress testing of anatomic structures involved.
7. Three radiographic views (posteroanterior, lateral, and oblique) are necessary in order to completely evaluate any swollen digit.

Complications

1. Malunion: malrotation, volar or lateral angulation, shortening
2. Loss of motion
3. Infection
4. Post-traumatic arthritis

Clinical Findings

Is there articular surface disruption? Fractures that involve more than 25 per cent of the articular surface are considered unstable and require surgical intervention in order to prevent long-term disability with stiffness, deformity, and pain.

1. Rotation is disruption of the fracture around the center of the longitudinal axis of the digit. When alignment is correct, the tubercle of the scaphoid is the focus of all fingers (Fig. 222–1).
2. Angulation is disruption of the longitudinal axis of the digit with the fracture fragment falling out of alignment.

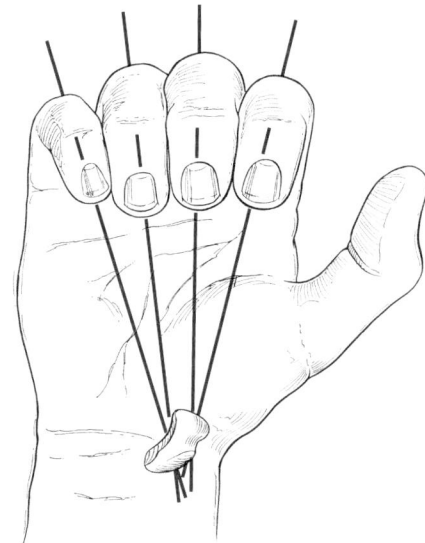

Figure 222–1 With correct alignment, tubercle of the scaphoid is the focus of all fingers. (Copyright Joan M. Beck, Beck Visual Communications, Inc., Minneapolis, MN. Used with permission.)

Differential Diagnosis/Treatment

1. Fractures of the distal phalanx
   a. Extra-articular: longitudinal, comminuted, transverse

Treatment
- Splint the DIP joint for 4 weeks.
- Treat soft tissue; evacuate hematoma

   b. Intra-articular
      (1) Dorsal avulsion (mallet finger): hyperflexion at the distal interphalangeal (DIP) joint. Extensor tendon may be stretched, ruptured, or avulsed from its attachment to the distal phalange.

Treatment
- Immobilize in extension with dorsal splint for 4 weeks.

      (2) Flexor digitorum profundus avulsion (Jersey finger): hyperextension of the DIP joint while the flexor tendon is contracting

Treatment
- Requires early referral to a hand surgeon since the tendon tends to retract into the palm

2. Fractures of the middle and proximal phalanx: crush injuries with force perpendicular to the long axis of the digit

Treatment
- Stable (no angulation, rotation, or displacement); dynamic splinting (buddy taping); early range of motion
- Unstable: early surgical reduction with immobilization

3. Volar plate disruption: hyperextension of the proximal interphalangeal (PIP) joint often with dislocation (Fig. 222–2).

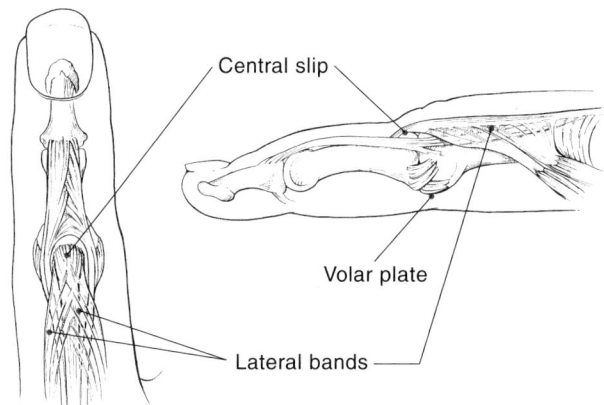

Figure 222–2 Injury to central clip with volar subluxation of lateral bands. (Copyright Joan M. Beck, Beck Visual Communications, Inc., Minneapolis, MN. Used with permission.)

   a. Swan neck deformity: distal disruption of the volar plate
   b. Pseudoboutonniere deformity: proximal disruption of the volar plate

Treatment
- Immobilization or dynamic splinting of the PIP joint for 4 weeks

4. Boutonniere deformity: injury to central slip (Fig. 222–2) with volar subluxation of lateral bands
   a. Direct dorsal trauma over the joint
   b. Forced flexion of the PIP joint
   c. The post-injury volar position of the lateral bands makes them extensors of the DIP joint.

Treatment
- Splint the PIP joint in extension for 4 to 6 weeks
- Dynamic splinting with range-of-motion exercises

5. Thumb injuries
   a. Ulnar collateral ligament strain (gamekeeper's thumb): abduction stress with the MP joint in extension

      Stener lesion: The adductor pollicis longus aponeurosis folds back on itself and becomes interposed between the ends of the ligament, preventing healing.

Treatment
- Since Stener lesion occurs frequently, it is recommended that gamekeeper's thumb injuries be treated surgically in order to prevent chronic instability.

---

b. Carpometacarpal joint of the thumb (Bennett's fracture): a fracture/subluxation at the base of the first metacarpal. It occurs when the thumb metacarpal is axially loaded and partially flexed. The abductor pollicis longus is the deforming force pulling the metacarpal fragment radially, proximally, and dorsally.

Treatment
- Nondisplaced: long-arm thumb spica cast for three weeks; followed by three weeks in a short-arm thumb spica cast

- Displaced: internal fixation required

- An active exercise program in order to obtain full range of motion in both nondisplaced and displaced treatment

---

Bibliography

Bowman SH, Simon RR: Metacarpal and phalangeal fractures. Emerg Med Clin North Am 1993;11:671–702.

Culver JE, Anderson TE: Fractures of the hand and wrist in the athlete. Clin Sports Med 1992;11:101–128.

DeJonge JJ, Kingma J: Phalangeal fractures of the hand. Br J Hand Surg 1994;198(2):168–170.

Hoffman DF, Schaffer TC: Management of common finger injuries. Am Fam Physician 1991;43:1594–1607.

Stern PJ: Fractures of the metacarpals and phalanges. *In* Green DP (ed): Operative Hand Surgery. New York, Churchill Livingstone, 1993, pp 695–758.

223 Ankle Fractures

David O. Hough

Etiology

1. Definition: Ankle fractures involve a combination of ligamentous rupture or avulsion and abnormal talus motion resulting in fracture to surrounding bony structures.

2. Mechanism of injury: Less than 15 per cent of patients with blunt ankle trauma present to the emergency department with clinically significant fractures.

   a. Ankle fracture injury depends on the following factors: activity being performed, age of the patient, quality of the bone, and position of foot at the time of injury.

   b. Most ankle fractures are related to the position of the foot, which contributes to the direction of deforming forces that occur.

   c. Common deforming forces on the ankle include adduction, abduction, external rotation, and vertical loading.

   d. Adduction and abduction are deforming forces resulting in rotation of the talus around the long axis of the tibia.

   e. Internal and external rotation occur around the vertical access of the tibia.

Diagnosis

1. Diagnosis of ankle injuries is based on the history and physical findings at the initial examination. The clinical appropriateness of radiography in acute ankle injuries has been validated (see Fig. 197–1, p. 762).

2. Radiographic studies should be performed in the following situations.

   a. Inability to bear weight both immediately after the injury and in the emergency department

   b. Bony tenderness at the posterior edge or tip of the lateral malleolus

   c. Bony tenderness at the posterior edge or tip of the medial malleolus

3. Any of the above findings are believed to be statistically significant in predicting a fracture.

4. Significant swelling and ecchymosis are not statistically significant in predicting ankle fractures.

5. Physical findings of obvious deformity or ankle joint dislocation are evident and require no further decision making in regard to further work-up. These injuries should be reviewed by an orthopedic surgeon.

6. Physical examination should also include anterior drawer testing for anterior ligament instability and talar tilt testing for lateral instability of the calcaneofibular and posterior talar fibular ligaments; in addition, a complete neurovascular examination should be performed.

7. Classification of injury

   a. Based on the mechanism of injury and radiographic findings, ankle fractures can be placed into a number of different classification systems.

   b. Classification systems by Lauge-Hansen, Danis-Weber, and the AO System have been utilized.

   c. Today, a combination of these systems has made classification of ankle injuries far simpler. Approximately 95 per cent of all ankle injuries can be placed into one of four groupings, and the system is based on the position of the foot at the time of injury and the direction of the deforming force.

   d. The Danis-Weber system, in combination with the AO Classification, is based on the level of fracture of the fibula. The more proximal the fracture line is along the fibula, the greater the risk of injury to the syndesmosis and the future instability of the ankle joint. This classification system is simple and emphasizes the lateral aspect of the ankle when planning conservative or surgical treatment. This classification system will lead to proper management of most ankle fractures.

      (1) Type A injury involves the fibular fracture below the level of the tibial plafond. These involve evulsion fractures resulting from supination of the foot.

      (2) Type B injury is an oblique or spiral fracture caused by external rotation.

      (3) Type C injury is a fracture of the fibula above the syndesmosis which is disrupted and associated with injury to the medial aspect of the ankle.

Radiographic Evaluation

1. Standard views of the ankle include anteroposterior (AP), lateral, and mortise views.

2. AP views should include the entire fibula if there is lateral tenderness above the joint line.

3. AP views are useful in evaluating fractures of the medial or lateral malleolus, anterolateral tibia, and proximal fibula. AP views also will spot osteochondral fractures of the distal tibia or talus.

4. A lateral view is useful in evaluating asymmetry of the articular space or anterior widening, which may suggest ankle instability.

5. The mortise view evaluates the clear space (articular space) between the talus and medial malleolus, distal

tibia, and lateral malleolus. This space should be equal throughout the ankle joint.

6. Specialized evaluation of the ankle may include inversion stress films to confirm ankle instability from ligamentous injury. Stress views of the opposite ankle are utilized for comparison and should result in less than five degrees of talar tilt in a normal ankle.

7. The anterior drawer test can also be done under stress views on a lateral radiograph and can reveal subluxation of the talus. An anterior shift of greater than 8 to 10 millimeters compared to the uninjured ankle indicates a tear of the anterior talar fibular ligament.

Treatment

1. General principles
    a. Treatment options involve consideration of whether a fracture requires surgical intervention.
    b. Nonoperative treatment consists of casting and immobilization.
    c. Stable ankle fractures may allow for early weight-bearing, but controversy exists regarding this recommendation.
    d. Unfamiliarity with certain types of fractures warrants referral to an orthopedic surgeon.
    e. Knowledge of what constitutes an unstable fracture based on examination and radiographic findings requires orthopedic surgery referral and initial splinting in a posterior Jones-type splint.
    f. Many stable fractures or fractures with minimum displacement can be successfully cared for by the primary care physician with proper immobilization and casting. Posterior splinting using an Ace wrap and Jones-type dressing will allow for swelling to expand after the initial injury.
    g. A full circumferential cast can be applied after seven to ten days.
    h. Stable fractures can be treated with a walking cast, fracture brace, or protected weight-bearing.
    i. Analgesic medication can be utilized initially for pain reduction and anti-inflammatory medication should be withheld for 24 to 36 hours until initial bleeding has slowed.
    j. Patient's activity level is advanced as healing progresses.
    k. Bracing can then be combined with rehabilitation exercises until functional return is completed.
    l. Icing during the initial stages of the rehabilitation process is critical for inflammation reduction.
    m. Orthopedic consultation should be obtained at any time during the management course that the primary care physician is uncertain of the patient's management.

2. Points to remember
    a. Reduction should be accomplished within six to eight hours.
    b. Reconstitution of joint surfaces must be precise.
    c. Maintenance of the reduction during the healing period is essential.
    d. Mobilization of the joint as soon as possible yields the best prognosis.
    e. The integrity of the ankle joint is primarily dependent on
        (1) Correct length of the fibula
        (2) Integrity of the tibiofibular ligaments
    f. The lateral malleolus is the key to ankle joint stability.
    g. Minimal displacement of the talus in the ankle mortise will result in destruction and degenerative joint disease of the ankle. Recommendations for surgery (open reduction and internal fixation [ORIF]) are as follows
        (1) 1 mm or less of shortening or widening requires no ORIF
        (2) 2 mm or greater of shortening or widening requires ORIF
        (3) Between 1 and 2 mm: ORIF depends on age and activity level of the patient.
    h. The higher the fibular fracture, the greater the damage to the syndesmosis and the greater the instability of the ankle joint.

Bibliography

Amedola A: Controversies in diagnosis and management of syndesmosis injuries of the ankle. Foot Ankle 1992;13:44–50.

Harper MC: Ankle fracture classifications systems: A case for integration of the Lauge-Hansen and AO-Danis-Weber schemes. Foot Ankle 1992;13:404–407.

Michelson J, Curtis M, Magid D: Controversies in ankle fractures. Foot Ankle 1993;14:170–174.

Ryd L, Bengtsson S: Isolated fracture of the lateral malleolus requires no treatment: Forty-nine prospective cases of supination-eversion type II ankle fractures. Acta Orthop Scand 1992;63:443–446.

Stiell IG, Greenberg GH, McKnight RD, et al: Decision rules for the use of radiography in acute ankle injuries: Refinement and prospective validation. JAMA 1993;26:1127–1132.

Indications
1. Fractures of the extremities
2. Ligament sprains and tears
3. Overuse injuries

Contraindications
1. Unstable or irreducible fractures
2. Avoid circumferential casting for an acute injury with soft tissue swelling; splint instead.

Preparation
1. Size and position of cast or splint
   a. Each injury is unique (see Bibliography for discussion of the types of cast/splint for a particular injury).
   b. Immobilize joint above and below the fracture.
   c. Immobilize forearm and hand injuries in position of function (wrist extension 30 degrees, hand like it is holding a half tennis ball).
   d. Keep foot in neutral or slight dorsiflexion for lower leg and foot injuries.
2. Determine type of material.
   a. Plaster—inexpensive and easy to form but falls apart when wet and may impede radiographic evaluation.
   b. Fiber glass—strong, lightweight, waterproof, and radiolucent. However, harder to mold and expensive.
   c. Thermoplastics—used for splints, expensive.
   d. Be familiar with package insert of the material.
3. Select appropriate width of material.
   a. Circumferential casts
      (1) 5- to 6-inch rolls for the upper leg
      (2) 4- to 5-inch rolls for the lower leg
      (3) 2- to 4-inch rolls for the hand, wrist, and lower arm
   b. Splints are one-half the circumference of the extremity.
4. Remove jewelry from injured extremity (e.g., rings).
5. Assistant to control the extremity

Equipment
1. Casting or splinting material
2. Sink with plaster trap
3. Soap and water
4. Stockinette
5. Thick cotton padding (Webril)
6. Heavy-duty scissors
7. Elastic wrap for splints
8. Gloves for handling material
9. Cast shoe, sling, or crutches

Anesthesia
Local or digital block with Xylocaine for some closed reductions

Precautions
1. Avoid cast that is too tight and does not allow for soft tissue swelling.
2. Avoid pressure over bony prominences and superficial neurovascular bundles; pad liberally.
3. Cast or splint should not be too loose or poor stabilization of joint or fracture will result.

WARNING

- **Be vigilant for any patient complaints in the first 24 to 48 hours after cast application**
  1. **Increasing pain, especially with passive movement of digits**
  2. **Paralysis**
  3. **Paresthesia**
  4. **Pallor**
  5. **Pulselessness**
- **To treat, bivalve the cast, cotton padding, and stockinette.**
- **If problem persists, suspect compartment syndrome, and obtain urgent orthopedic consultation.**

Technique

1. Measure the material needed over the patient's uninjured side.
2. For casting, stockinette should be 3 inches longer than needed on each end. Gently slide this over the injured extremity, and avoid bunching the material.
3. Wrap thick cotton padding (Webril) over the stockinette. Start distally and work proximally, overlapping the rolls 50 per cent. Apply extra padding over bony prominences and superficial neurovascular bundles.
4. When handling plaster or fiber glass, wear gloves. Hold the edge of the roll between the index finger and thumb so that the beginning of the roll is not lost as it is immersed in water. Immerse plaster roll in tepid water (77 to 95° F) until bubbles stop rising

from the roll. Remove from water and gently compress the ends of the roll inward to remove excess water from the plaster.

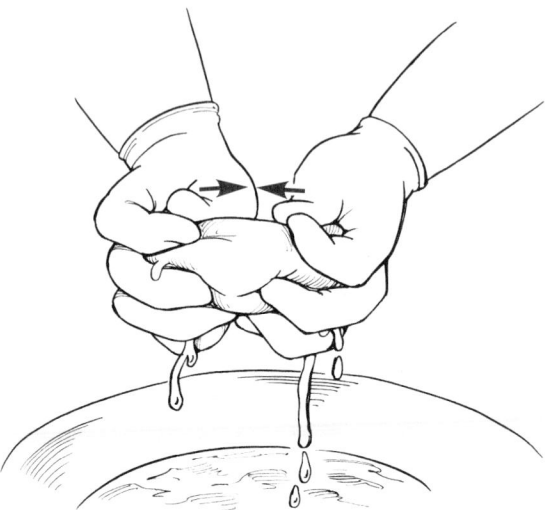

For fiber glass, immerse in cool water (68° F) and squeeze the roll several times. Remove and shake excess water off the fiber glass roll before application. Keep in mind, the warmer the water, the faster the material sets.

5. Follow the direction of the cotton padding, and apply the rolls of casting material to the extremity, overlapping each roll by 50 per cent. Do not pull or stretch the material; simply lay it down. Tuck and smooth excess material with the palms.

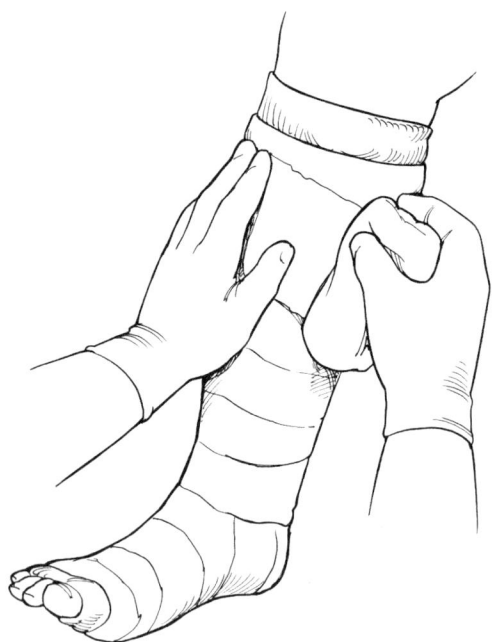

Use three layers on upper extremity casts and four layers for the lower extremity. Thicken weight-bearing areas and incorporate longitudinal splints into the cast to give extra support where needed, especially when using plaster.

6. Be careful not to indent plaster with the fingertips. Trim rough edges, and fold stockinette over the ends of the cast.

7. Splinting requires 12 strips of plaster measured slightly longer than the injured extremity. Three to four strips of fiber glass achieve the same purpose. The splinting material is immersed in water, squeezed out in an accordian fashion, laid flat, and gently massaged into a uniform slab. Apply a cover of four layers of cotton padding on both sides of the splint, and wrap the padded splint on the extremity with elastic wrap.

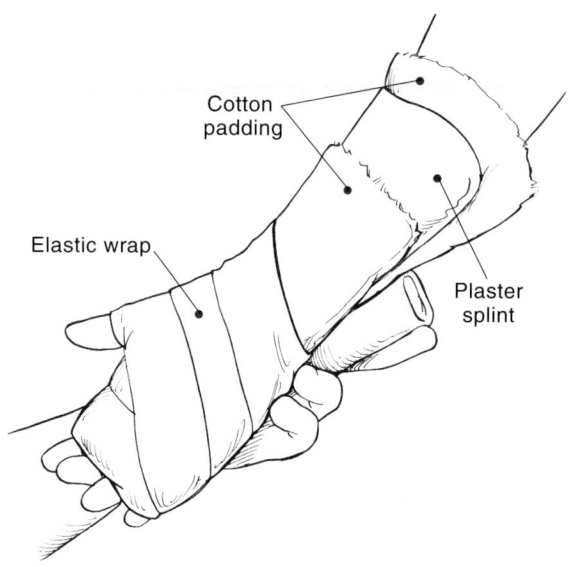

Cotton padding

Elastic wrap

Plaster splint

As an alternative, preformed splinting material may be used.

8. Plaster will set within 5 to 10 minutes and completely harden within 48 hours. Fiber glass also sets in 5 minutes and hardens for weight bearing in 20 minutes. Avoid manipulation of the cast after it has set.

9. Use a cast shoe to protect the lower extremity cast. A rubber walking platform can be incorporated into the bottom of the cast for weight-bearing patients.

Follow-Up

1. Repeat radiograph after casting if fracture is unstable.
2. Care of the extremity
   a. Keep elevated for 24 to 48 hours.
   b. Move muscles and joints that are free.
   c. Watch for danger signs of compression.
   d. Avoid getting cast and padding wet (synthetic stockinette and padding required if fiber glass cast expected to get wet).
3. Re-evaluate patient in 1 to 2 weeks.
4. Cast removal
   a. Brace hand when using cast saw.

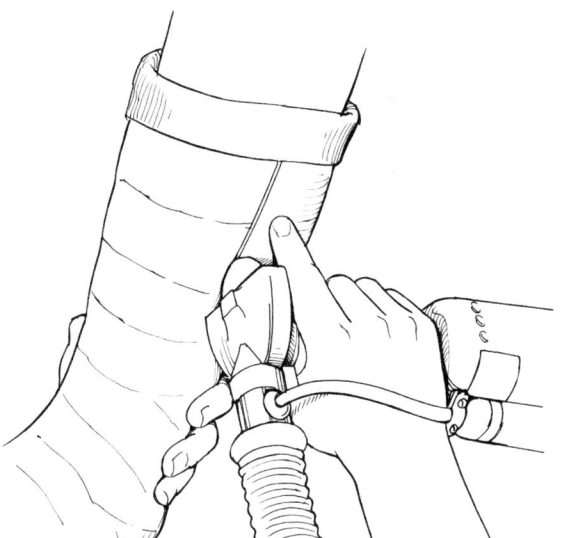

b. Bivalve cast; then use cast separator.

Bibliography

Billotti JD, McKeag DB, Menkes JS: Fast splinting techniques for fractures. Patient Care 1993;148–180.

Connolly J: The Management of Fractures and Dislocations, 3d ed. Philadelphia, WB Saunders, 1981, pp 115–120.

Dvorkin ML: Office Orthopaedics. Norwalk, Conn, Appleton & Lange, 1993, pp 1–296.

Monahan JJ: Mechanical therapeutics (casts, splints, traction). *In* Steinberg GG, Akins CM, Baran DT (eds): Ramamurti's Orthopedics in Primary Care, 2d ed. Baltimore, Williams & Wilkins, 1992, pp 290–315.

Morrill CE: Casting. *In* Mayhew HE, Rodgers LA (eds): Basic Procedures in Family Practice. Bethany, Conn, Fleschner, 1984, pp 122–127.

224 Foot Fractures

Robert L. Hatch

Tarsal Fractures

There are two broad classes of tarsal fractures, with differing etiologies and management.

Tarsal Avulsion Fractures

Etiology
Twisting injury (usually)

Symptoms
Localized pain following injury

Clinical Findings
Point tender at fracture site, mild to moderate swelling

Differential Diagnosis
1. Sprain (examination may be identical, but radiograph should be normal with a sprain)
2. Accessory ossicle or old fracture. Radiographically, these generally appear rounded, are well corticated on all sides, and are usually nontender. Acute avulsion fractures are more irregular, lack cortical thickening along the inside edge, and are point tender.

WARNING

Beware of chip fractures that involve articular surfaces (the dome of the talus is a common site). These injuries often lead to severe degenerative joint disease. Referral of such fractures is strongly recommended (management differs from below). Suspect these when a sprain is slow to heal.

Treatment and Follow-Up
1. Recommend consultation or referral if tender on both sides of foot (possible subluxation) or if fragment displaced more than 2 mm.
2. Nondisplaced or minimally displaced (i.e., less than 2 mm)
   a. Following initial management (Tables 224–1 and 224–2), apply short-leg walking cast (SLWC). Some avulsions are best managed without casting.
   b. Re-evaluate every 2 to 3 weeks.
   c. Special considerations
      (1) Consider referral if fragment becomes more distracted
      (2) Healing may occur without development of obvious callus, so base further treatment deci-

sions less on follow-up radiographs and more on symptoms such as pain and tenderness.

Fractures Through the Body of a Tarsal Bone

Etiology
High-energy blows (e.g., crush or a fall from a great height), twisting injuries

Symptoms
Swelling and pain, which may be marked

Clinical Findings
Swelling, tenderness, ecchymosis (later)

Differential Diagnosis
1. Dislocation (comparison view of other foot or reference to radiographic anatomy text may facilitate recognition of a dislocation, particularly in children).

TABLE 224–1. INITIAL MANAGEMENT OF AN ACUTE FRACTURE

1. Rule out complications that require emergent referral/consultation: neurovascular injury, significant soft tissue injury, open fracture, and compartment syndrome.
2. Splint, ice, elevation, pain control. If must apply cast acutely (e.g., fracture unstable), strongly recommend splitting cast to avoid iatrogenic compartment syndrome.
3. Give instructions about warning signs of vascular compromise.

TABLE 224–2. FOLLOW-UP OF FOOT FRACTURES: GENERAL GUIDELINES

1. Apply cast when no further swelling is expected (preferably after most swelling has resolved), i.e., 2 to 5 days after injury.
2. Consider cast check in 12 to 24 hours to be sure cast is comfortable and to rule out iatrogenic compartment syndrome (especially if compliance with elevation questionable or high risk for more swelling).
3. If fracture stable (i.e., unlikely to lose position), examine out of plaster in 3 to 6 weeks (varies by fracture).
   a. Discontinue cast if radiographic and clinical evidence of healing is present (i.e., callus seen on radiograph and resolution of all but minimal point tenderness at the fracture site).
   b. If not yet healed, replace cast and re-evaluate every 1 to 2 weeks until healed or until benefits of continued casting are outweighed by drawbacks (such as permanent decreased range of motion due to prolonged immobilization); consultation beneficial if unsure.
   c. After removal of cast, begin range-of-motion (ROM) exercises and gradual resumption of activity; re-evaluate 2 to 4 weeks after cast removal to assess progress, and consider referral to physical therapist if ROM/normal function slow to return.
4. If fracture unstable or potentially unstable, repeat radiographs *in plaster* (i.e., do not remove cast) before callus expected (i.e., 8 to 10 days after fracture for an adult). If fracture has lost position, refer it then while it is relatively easy to reposition. If position maintained, obtain later radiographs in plaster when possible.

2. Navicular fractures often mistaken for a sprain (similar mechanism of injury, fracture may only be seen on lateral view).

> ### WARNING
>
> **Due to the mechanism of injury, patients with calcaneus fractures frequently have associated thoracic or lumbar spine fractures. Strongly consider radiographs of these regions.**

Treatment

1. Consultation or referral recommended
   a. May require inpatient observation
   b. Talus may develop avascular necrosis.
   c. If fracture extends to a joint surface, there is a high risk of future degenerative joint disease (DJD) even if position anatomic.
2. Some primary care physicians manage selected calcaneal fractures (if nondisplaced and no extension to joint surface) (see McRae R: Practical Fracture Management, pp 307–11, for discussion of management).

Metatarsal Fractures

Multiple Metatarsal Fractures

1. Compared with fractures of a single metatarsal (MT), these fractures
   a. Have a higher risk of associated dislocation or vascular compromise (which may be delayed, i.e., compartment syndrome)
   b. Often have significant displacement (may require fixation)
2. Consider referral unless experienced in the management of these fractures; management similar to that outlined below (first MT)

Avulsion Fracture of Proximal Fifth Metatarsal (Fracture of Styloid)

Probably the most common fracture of the lower extremity

Etiology
Inversion of ankle.

Symptoms
Acute lateral foot pain following inversion injury

Clinical Findings
Local swelling and point tenderness

Radiographic Findings
Transverse or oblique lucency less than 1.5 cm from proximal tip of fifth MT

> ### Key Test
>
> • Palpate proximal fifth MT of all patients who sustain ankle inversion injuries to avoid missing this fracture.

Differential Diagnosis

1. Jones' fracture (see below)
2. Apophysis (growth center seen in older children and adolescents). Lucency of apophysis lies *parallel* to long axis of fifth MT, fracture usually transverse. If apophysis is tender,
   a. Obtain comparison view of other foot to rule out avulsion of apophysis.
   b. Consider referring or treating like a Salter I fracture even if radiograph is normal.
3. Sesamoid bone (os peroneum or os vesalianum)

Treatment

1. Consider consultation or referral if displaced more than 2 to 3 mm (unusual).
2. If displacement is less than 2 to 3 mm
   a. Generally require only a firm-soled, comfortable shoe for 4 to 8 weeks, plus initial ice and elevation.
   b. If patient is very symptomatic despite above, SLWC may help (for 4 to 7 weeks).

Follow-Up

1. Follow up every 2 to 4 weeks until patient has resumed most normal activities.
2. Switch patient to normal shoes when symptoms allow.
3. Patient occasionally may need physical therapy (PT) (more likely if cast used).

Jones' Fracture

Etiology

1. Acute variety: sudden force under distal fifth MT
2. Chronic (stress) variety: chronic overloading (especially pivoting), usually in young male athletes

Symptoms

1. Acute: sudden pain following injury
2. Chronic: pain for weeks, often with sudden worsening

Clinical Findings

Point tenderness over proximal fifth MT *diaphysis*

Radiologic Findings

1. Transverse lucency through proximal diaphysis *at least 1.5 cm from the proximal tip* of the fifth MT.

2. If chronic, radiograph often negative initially but may show periosteal reaction, narrowing of medullary canal, or faint lucency. Diagnosis may require bone scan.

Differential Diagnosis
1. Avulsion fracture
2. Apophysis

Treatment and Follow-Up

> **WARNING**
>
> **Jones' fractures have a high risk of delayed union or nonunion. Consider referral for early internal fixation, especially in young athletes.**

Conservative treatment used most often in patients who are less active, prefer to avoid surgery, or have the acute variety.
1. Short-leg non–weight-bearing cast for 2 to 6 months
2. Follow every 3 to 4 weeks until radiographic evidence of healing
3. Consider referral for possible open reduction and internal fixation (ORIF) if healing has not occurred by 3 to 4 months.

Proximal Metatarsal Fractures (Other than Fifth)

High incidence of associated tarsometatarsal joint (Lisfranc) injuries, which may be subtle, disabling, and difficult to manage. Recommend referral of proximal fractures, especially if multiple.

Midshaft or Distal Fracture of a *Single* Metatarsal (Second to Fifth)

Etiology
1. Direct blow or twist with toes fixed
2. Common site of stress fractures, which usually occur after a sudden increase in activity (e.g., athletes and new military recruits, i.e., "march" fracture).

Symptoms
1. Dorsal forefoot pain, increased with weight bearing.
2. With stress fracture, onset gradual.

Clinical Findings
1. Point tenderness, usually with swelling and ecchymosis
2. Pain with axial compression

Radiographic Findings
Fracture usually spiral or oblique, generally with little or no displacement (if adjacent metatarsals are intact, they "splint" the fracture). Consider referral if
1. Fracture involves a joint surface (high risk of future DJD even if anatomic position).
2. Significant dorsal or ventral (more common) angulation of metatarsal head (develop abnormal forefoot biomechanics and chronic keratosis if not corrected).

Key Test

A full foot series (anteroposterior, oblique, and lateral) is necessary to assess all potential metatarsal fractures. Due to overlying shadows on lateral view, it is necessary to carefully follow the cortex of each metatarsal to determine the position of the fracture. Undetected angulation can lead to significant long-term sequelae.

Treatment and Follow-Up
If displaced 2 mm or less and no significant angulation: usual initial care and follow-up (see Tables 224–1 and 224–2), using SLWC for 2 to 3 weeks, followed by early ambulation in well-padded shoe

First Metatarsal

Etiology
Usually a high-energy crushing injury

> **WARNING**
>
> **Crush injuries (particularly of the foot) are prone to extensive soft tissue damage, which may be more problematic than the fracture itself. Consider early referral/consultation if suspected.**

Symptoms/Findings
Similar to those of midshaft or distal fracture of a single metatarsal (above)

Treatment
1. Vast majority should probably be referred.
   a. May require overnight observation of vascular status
   b. Anatomic position more important because of its important weight-bearing function
   c. Associated dislocation possible if fracture is proximal
2. For selected patients with nondisplaced, stable fracture:
   a. Initial care as in Table 224–1 (special emphasis

on immediate return if signs of vascular compromise develop)

   b. Follow-up as in Table 224–2, including recheck at 12 to 24 hours and repeat films at 8 to 10 days to check position. Use a short leg non–weight-bearing cast until healing, with re-evaluation every 2 weeks.

Toes

First Toe (Great Toe)

Etiology

Usually a direct blow (falling object or stubbing injury)

Symptoms

Pain (patient often presents days after injury)

Findings

1. Point tenderness
2. Swelling
3. Ecchymosis
4. Subungual hematoma (especially first toe)

Differential Diagnosis

1. Sprain
2. Contusion
3. Dislocation

Treatment and Follow-Up

1. Important weight-bearing function, so consider referral if displaced (especially proximal phalanx) or if intra-articular (especially MTP joint).
2. Nondisplaced
   a. Buddy tape (i.e., tape to adjacent toe with padding between them)

   b. Firm-soled shoe

   c. Crutches with partial weight bearing for 2 to 3 weeks

   d. If pain control not adequate, use SLWC with toe platform for 2 weeks, followed by above; see also Tables 224–1 and 224–2

Lesser Toes

Etiology, symptoms, findings, and differential diagnosis as in first toe (great toe) above

Treatment and Follow-Up

1. Rarely need referral unless open fracture is present.
2. Nondisplaced
   a. Buddy tape for comfort
   b. Re-evaluate in 2 to 4 weeks.
   c. Rarely require follow-up radiographs; see also Tables 224–1 and 224–2.
3. Displaced
   a. Following local anesthesia (achieved with ice for 5 to 10 minutes or occasionally with digital block) reduce using gentle traction.
   b. Buddy tape to hold position.
   c. Same follow-up as for nondisplaced toe fracture

Bibliography

Byrd T: Jones fracture: Relearning an old injury. South Med J 1992;85(7):748–750.

Connolly F: DePalma's The Management of Fractures and Dislocations, 3rd ed, vol. 2. Philadelphia, WB Saunders, 1981, pp 1952–2078.

Holubec KD, Karlin JM, Scurran BL: Retrospective study of fifth metatarsal fractures. J Am Pod Med Assoc 1993; 83(4):215–222.

McRae R: Practical Fracture Treatment. 2nd ed. New York, Churchill Livingstone, 1989.

Shea MP, Manoli II A: Recognizing talar dome lesions. Physician Sports Med 1993;21(32):109–121.

225 **Common Infectious Disease Symptoms**

Body temperature is determined by the balance between heat production and heat loss. This balance is under control of the nervous system and regulated by the hypothalamus to maintain a set body temperature. Fever results from a resetting of the hypothalamus, so that heat production and loss are balanced to maintain a higher body temperature. The hypothalamus can be reset by

1. Circulating substances (termed pyrogens): The most common mechanism that elicits fever is the elaboration of endogenous pyrogens by stimulated circulating monocytes and tissue macrophages.

2. Damage from hemorrhage, infarction, or compression: Due to individual and diurnal variations, there is no well-established discrete body temperature that defines fever. Simplifying the complex issues of clinical thermometry, an oral temperature greater than 38° C in an adult will be defined as a fever. Although some individuals without recognizable illnesses may have body temperatures above 38° C, this definition will be sensitive enough to detect almost all of those patients with significant disorders that produce fever. Chills are a secondary symptom associated with fever, resulting from the need for muscular activity to increase heat production and raise body temperature to the level desired by the reset hypothalamus. Thus, chills are most often seen while the body temperature is rising. Fever is a common presenting symptom: approximately 2 to 6 per cent of unselected adults presenting to hospital emergency departments or ambulatory walk-in clinics have a fever or history of fever.

Differential Diagnosis

1. Fever can be due to
   a. Infection: essentially all causes, whether bacterial, viral, or parasitic. The potential causes depend on the patient's age, underlying host factors, and epidemiologic associations. For example, an acute undifferentiated fever in Southeast Asia is often due to malaria, whereas a similar presentation in rural areas of the mid-Atlantic United States during the spring and summer is possibly Rocky Mountain spotted fever.
   b. Immunologic disorders: associated with an inflammatory reaction, such as acute inflammatory arthritis, serum sickness, immune hemolytic anemia
   c. Neoplastic disorders: sometimes seen with solid

tumors and often seen with reticuloendothelial tumors
   d. Vascular thrombosis or infarction: acute myocardial infarction, deep venous thrombosis, pulmonary emboli, cerebrovascular accidents
   e. Trauma: usually involves significant skeletal muscle injury from a crushing mechanism
   f. Miscellaneous: acute gout, acute porphyria, acute adrenal insufficiency, hyperthyroidism, tonic-clonic seizures
   g. Drug-induced: drugs most often reported include methyldopa, quinidine, procainamide, phenytoin, carbamazepine, penicillin, cephalothin, tetracycline, sulfonamide, isoniazid, bleomycin

2. Acute bacterial infection is the etiology for which timely diagnosis and treatment is most important. The initial diagnostic approach to evaluating an adult with an acute fever usually involves detecting a treatable infection (most often bacterial) or excluding such an infection to a reasonable degree of clinical certainty. Patients without a diagnosis on initial evaluation can usually be followed expectantly.

History

1. Fever: onset, duration, maximal value, chronologic pattern (although of little diagnostic value)
2. Secondary symptoms: chills, sweats, malaise, and myalgias
3. Localizing symptoms: most otherwise healthy adults with the acute onset of fever also report localizing symptoms (e.g., sore throat, cough, dysuria) caused by the specific illness producing the fever.
4. Medical history: underlying disorders that reduce resistance or predispose to infection, especially diabetes, malignancy, AIDS, sickle cell anemia, alcoholism, intravenous drug use
5. Current medications: especially antipyretics or leftover antibiotics
6. Epidemiologic factors: others ill at home with fever, recent travel, unusual exposures

Clinical Findings

1. An oral temperature above 38° C should be considered a fever and should prompt a search for a definable cause. Because of age, diurnal variation, or antipyretic use, patients may report a history of fever but will not have an oral temperature above 38° C at presentation.

2. Secondary clinical findings: chills, sweats, and malaise

3. Tachypnea, tachycardia, or hypotension with fever may represent the systemic "septic" response and is associated with a 37 to 47 per cent incidence of bacteremia.

4. Observe general condition: Does patient appear acutely ill (or "toxic") or to tolerate fever without obvious effects?

5. The following clinical findings suggest a focal disorder or infection
   a. Altered mental status: lethargy, confusion, stupor, or coma
   b. Head and neck: inflamed tympanic membranes, pharyngeal erythema or exudate, sinus tenderness, nasal exudate or congestion, cervical adenopathy
   c. Chest: localized rales, rhonchi, or evidence of consolidation
   d. Heart: regurgitant valvular murmur
   e. Abdomen: focal tenderness, guarding, or rebound
   f. Genitourinary: flank or kidney tenderness, exudate from cervical os, cervical motion, or adnexal tenderness
   g. Rectum: focal anal tenderness or swelling, exudate
   h. Extremities: focal erythema, tenderness, or swelling; monoarticular joint effusion
   i. Skin: petechial, pustular, or other rashes

6. Using the combination of symptoms and clinical findings, the clinician can categorize the patient into a general syndrome. For example
   a. Upper respiratory infection (URI): nasal congestion, earache, sore throat, postnasal drip
   b. Lower respiratory infection (LRI): cough, rales, evidence of consolidation
   c. Acute gastroenteritis: nausea, vomiting, diarrhea
   d. Urinary: dysuria, frequency, urgency, costovertebral angle (CVA) or flank tenderness

Tests

1. Laboratory tests are most useful when the results will alter diagnosis, treatment, or disposition and are least useful (possibly not necessary) when results will not change decisions.

2. For febrile adults with localizing symptoms or findings, specific laboratory tests are chosen based upon the clinical syndrome; there is little need for "shotgun" testing. Examples include
   a. Streptococcal screen for patients with exudative pharyngitis
   b. Urinalysis for patients with urinary symptoms
   c. Chest radiograph for patients with a productive cough

3. For febrile adults, laboratory tests—such as the white blood cell count, urinalysis, chest radiograph, and blood culture—to detect occult bacterial infection have some value. They are helpful in
   a. Febrile adults without localizing symptoms or findings: approximately a 30 per cent incidence of occult bacterial infection and 15 per cent incidence of bacteremia
   b. Febrile neutropenic patients
   c. Febrile adults with systemic immunodeficiencies

4. White blood cell count: The WBC has little utility when used indiscriminately but has a modest predictive value for bacterial infection or bacteremia when "abnormal" in
   a. Febrile adults without localizing symptoms or findings: WBC >15,000/mm³ associated with approximately a 50 per cent incidence of bacterial infection and 30 per cent incidence of bacteremia
   b. Febrile patients when the history suggests the possibility of neutropenia: neutrophil count <1000/mm³
   c. The febrile elderly patient: WBC >14,000/mm³ associated with about a 50 per cent incidence of bacterial infection

5. White cell differential: The white cell differential also has modest predictive value in detecting bacterial infection or bacteremia in
   a. Febrile adults without localizing symptoms or findings: neutrophil band count >1500/mm³ associated with about a 50 per cent incidence of bacterial infection and 20 per cent incidence of bacteremia
   b. The febrile elderly patient: neutrophil band >6 per cent associated with about 70 per cent incidence of bacterial infection

6. Urinalysis: The urinalysis is useful in
   a. Febrile adults with urinary symptoms: internal dysuria, frequency, urgency, flank or abdominal pain. Upper urinary tract infections in otherwise healthy adults are almost always associated with pyuria with WBC >5/hpf. The absence of pyuria essentially excludes this diagnosis, except in neutropenic patients.
   b. Febrile adults without localizing symptoms or findings: about 10 to 15 per cent incidence of occult urinary tract infection
   c. Febrile elderly patients

7. Urine culture: The large majority of otherwise healthy adults with pyelonephritis respond to empiric antibiotic selection, and so culture and determination of sensitivity, although commonly performed, do not influence treatment. Urine culture is recommended when bacteriologic diagnosis is important.
   a. Febrile neutropenic or immunocompromised patients

b. Febrile patients with urinary tract obstruction

8. Chest radiographs: The clinical examination lacks accuracy in detecting pulmonary consolidation; the chest radiograph is the most accurate technique to detect pneumonia. Clinically occult infiltrates have been detected by chest radiography in 3 to 4 per cent of

   a. Febrile adults without localizing symptoms or signs

   b. Febrile neutropenic patients without pulmonary symptoms

   c. Febrile adults with a productive cough

9. Blood culture: Indiscriminate use of blood cultures has low utility. Blood cultures are recommended for

   a. Situations in which blood culture is the primary modality for diagnosis (e.g., bacterial endocarditis). Two populations are at special risk: febrile intravenous drug users and patients with prosthetic heart valves.

   b. Febrile adults without localizing symptoms or signs when the WBC is >15,000/mm^3 or the neutrophil band count is >1500/mm^3 have about a 20 to 30 per cent incidence of bacteremia. Conversely, when the WBC is <15,000/mm^3 and the neutrophil band count is 1500/mm^3, the incidence of bacterial infection is 3 per cent and the incidence of bacteremia is less than 1 per cent.

   c. Febrile elderly patients

   d. Febrile neutropenic or immunocompromised patients

Management

1. Specific antibiotic treatment is indicated when a clinical syndrome has a sufficient probability of being caused by bacteria. For example, exudative tonsillitis, fever, and cervical adenopathy in a 20-year-old has up to a 60 per cent likelihood of being due to streptococci, and treatment with penicillin is recommended.

2. Empiric antibiotic therapy is indicated when the clinical syndrome suggests the possibility of a serious, potentially fatal bacterial infection. For example, patients with acute meningitis or septic shock should receive empiric antibiotics before cultures and other ancillary tests are completed. Ideally, such treatment is initiated after appropriate cultures are obtained, but antibiotics should not be unduly delayed.

3. Broad-spectrum antibiotic therapy for undifferentiated febrile illnesses is to be avoided.

4. Antipyretic therapy is appropriate for patient comfort with

   a. Acetaminophen, 10 to 15 mg/kg orally every 4 hours

   b. Ibuprofen, 5 to 10 mg/kg orally every 6 hours

PEARLS

- The patient's general condition—how well the illness is being tolerated—determines the need for hospitalization.

- Febrile adults with serious co-morbid conditions or underlying immunodeficiencies are usually admitted to the hospital for fear of serious complications developing rapidly because of delayed diagnosis or treatment.

- As with the febrile 5-month-old with a ''negative septic workup,'' febrile adults with a nondiagnostic evaluation upon initial contact should be seen again or contacted by phone in 24 hours.

B **Bibliography**

For more information on serious illness in febrile adults, see
Gallagher EJ, Brooks F, Gennis P: Identification of serious illness in febrile adults. Am J Emerg Med 1994;12:129–133.

For more information on manifestations of sepsis, see
Harris RL, Musher DM, Bloom K, et al: Manifestations of sepsis. Arch Intern Med 1987:147:1895–1906.

For more information on normal body temperature, see
Mackpwiak PA, Wasserman SS, Levine MM: A critical appraisal of 98.6°F, the upper limit of the normal body temperature, and other legacies of Carl Reinhold August Wunderlich. JAMA 1992;268:1578–1580.

For more information on the febrile adult without localizing findings, see
Mellors JW, Horwitz RI, Harvey MR, Horwitz SM: A simple index to identify occult bacterial infection in adults with unexplained fever. Arch Intern Med 1987;147:666–671.

For more information on the effects of fever and antipyretic treatment, see
Styrt B, Sugarman B: Antipyresis and fever. Arch Intern Med 1990;150:1589–1597.

226 Fever of Unknown Origin

James E. Svenson

Etiology

1. Classically, fever of unknown origin (FUO) has been defined as a fever of greater than 38.3° C (101° F) measured on several occasions, with an overall duration of fever of more than 2 weeks, without a diagnosis after routine investigations. Some authors have extended the definition to a fever of three weeks' duration, without a diagnosis after at least one week of inpatient observation. With the advent of chemotherapy, prolonged hospitalization of debilitated individuals, and the human immunodeficiency virus (HIV), new definitions and classifications for FUO have been proposed, subdividing patients into those with classic FUO, neutropenic FUO, nosocomial FUO, and HIV-associated FUO. This chapter will focus only on adult patients with classic FUO.

2. Causes of FUO can be classified as infectious, collagen vascular diseases, malignancy, and a variety of miscellaneous disorders, although about 10 per cent remain undiagnosed. The etiologic spectrum seems to have shifted in the 1980s away from infections as being the principal cause of FUO as they were in earlier studies. This shift in the spectrum of diseases causing FUO has been attributed to the early diagnosis of many such disorders by diagnostic modalities, such as ultrasonography and computed tomography (CT), that were not as readily available in early series. Despite this shift, the majority of eventually diagnosed FUOs are caused by infections, collagen vascular diseases, and malignancies.

Symptoms

1. The only common symptom in patients with FUO is their reported fever. Since many patients with FUO often have atypical manifestations of their diseases, many symptoms of the eventually diagnosed cause of the fever may not be present or present only transiently. Nonspecific symptoms such as malaise, myalgia, and weight loss may be due to the fever itself or to the underlying illness.

2. It is important to establish that the patient is having fever. In one series of patients with FUO of longer than six months, 27 per cent had no fever during two to three weeks of inpatient observation. The fever pattern is not helpful in the diagnosis of prolonged fever. Diseases with marked periodicity in fever such as malaria and cyclic neutropenia are the exception. In other diseases, such as familial Mediterranean fever and Hodgkin's disease, the fever may or may not be periodic.

3. Often, more important to the diagnosis of a FUO is a thorough history rather than a specific set of symptoms. The history should focus on the genetic background, travel history, exposure to biologic agents and chemicals, occupational history, and sexual history. History of travel and exposure to certain agents or animals is crucial. For example, a history of travel to a malaria-endemic area, having birds as pets, or exposure to beryllium can help in leading to a diagnosis. A thorough drug exposure history is essential. Prescription medications, recreational drugs, and the adulterants that accompany the use of many recreational drugs can cause fevers. The removal of the offending agent does not always cause rapid defervescence; however, fever persisting one week after the agent is removed makes the diagnosis of drug fever unlikely. A history of transfusions, previous surgery, or implantation of prosthetic devices may be clues to the cause of the patient's fever.

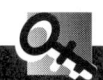

Key History/Symptoms

- Documented fever
- Travel
- Exposure
  Occupation
  Animals/pets
  Drugs
  Transfusions
  Surgery
- Sexual history
- Genetic background

Clinical Findings

1. A complete physical examination, repeated on a regular basis, is an integral part of the evaluation of a patient with FUO. Patients with FUO may develop physical findings at any time during their disease course. Physicians often mistakenly rely on laboratory investigations rather than repeating the physical examination.

2. While the complete examination is important, several areas require particular attention in the patient with an FUO. These include examination of the skin and nail beds, auscultatation of the heart, palpation of the abdomen and lymph nodes, and complete eye examination. Many of the diseases known to cause FUO (e.g., infections, collagen-vascular diseases, and hematologic malignancies) may produce retinal or uveal lesions.

Key Signs

- Lymphadenopathy
- Cardiac murmur
- Skin rash
- Hepatomegaly and/or splenomegaly
- Eye findings
  Uveitis
  Retinal lesions

Laboratory Tests

Routine Tests

1. All patients should have a complete blood count, urinalysis and culture, liver function tests, antinuclear antibody (ANA), and rheumatoid factor.

2. A chest radiograph should be done on all patients.

3. A tuberculin test (PPD) should be done (although a negative test should not preclude a further work-up for miliary TB) and serum tested for HIV.

4. Serologic and immunologic tests have limited diagnostic value, as rising antibody titers to specific pathogens must be requested, but serum samples should be obtained at regular intervals in case such testing is indicated at a later time.

5. Testing for infectious mononucleosis is simple and worthwhile.

6. Repeated blood cultures are important in evaluating the patient with an FUO. Patients with endocarditis are continuously bacteremic, and cultures should be positive regardless of the timing of the culture in relation to the fever. Of more importance is the volume of blood cultured. Recovery of organisms is enhanced by using the maximum amount of blood. The laboratory should be informed that the patient has an FUO and the cultures should be incubated for prolonged periods (at least 3 weeks).

7. Other tests should be done as directed by the history and physical examination (e.g., direct smear for malaria or serum testing for psittacosis in patients with birds).

Noninvasive Procedures

1. The relative role of computed tomography (CT), ultrasonography, and gallium scintigraphy in the evaluation of FUO is unclear. The techniques are complementary, and each has about the same overall sensitivity in detecting the site of inflammation in febrile patients. The major advantage of gallium scanning is its utility in total-body scanning and tracer accumulation for infectious, inflammatory, and some neoplastic diseases. CT scanning is probably superior to ultrasonography in the visualization of intra-abdominal or pelvic abscesses.

2. The gastrointestinal tract should be evaluated by upper gastrointestinal radiography with small-bowel follow-through, and with colonoscopy or barium enema, because of the possibility of colon cancer and Crohn's disease.

3. Technetium-99m sulfur scans can be helpful in the early diagnosis of osteomyelitis, but these lesions are also localized by gallium scan.

4. Indium-labeled leukocyte imaging has been shown to be relatively insensitive in the evaluation of patients with FUO, particularly in subacute and chronic infections, in which the procedure may be negative, and in noninfectious causes of FUO, in which there is no localization of white cell uptake.

5. The role of magnetic resonance imaging (MRI) in the diagnostic evaluation of patients with FUO has yet to be evaluated.

Invasive Procedures

1. Biopsy of the bone marrow with bone marrow cultures is indicated if the above studies are nondiagnostic.

2. Biopsy of the liver can often reveal the diagnosis even in the absence of hepatomegaly or liver function abnormalities on blood chemistries.

3. Prior to the advent of newer diagnostic modalities such as CT and gallium scanning, diagnostic laparotomy or laparoscopy was performed on many patients with FUO. Studies before the use of these noninvasive tests showed a success rate of 26 to 85 per cent. These procedures are now of limited value in patients with FUO and are only indicated if there are abdominal signs and symptoms, if the diagnosis is uncertain after noninvasive imaging, and if the benefits of a diagnosis outweigh the risks from the procedure.

4. More directed biopsy of tissues such as skin, pleura, lymph nodes, intestine, kidney, or blood vessels should be directed by the physical examination and noninvasive scanning.

Key Tests

Routine Laboratory Tests

- Blood culture
- HIV
- ANA, Rheumatoid factor
- PPD

Noninvasive Imaging

- Gallium scintigraphy
- Abdominal/total body CT
- Abdominal ultrasonography

Invasive Tests

- Bone marrow biopsy/culture
- Percutaneous liver biopsy

Differential Diagnosis

The differential diagnosis for prolonged fever without other localizing signs is broad; 179 different diseases have been documented as a cause of FUO, and a detailed list is beyond the scope of this review.

1. The majority of cases of FUO are caused by infections, malignancies, or collagen vascular diseases.

2. Most cases are unusual manifestations of common diseases, and these should be evaluated before launching an investigation for other causes.

3. The most common infectious causes of FUO include intra-abdominal abscesses, tuberculosis, endocarditis, and, recently, infection with the HIV.

4. The most common malignancies associated with FUO are lymphomas, leukemias, and renal cell carcinomas.

5. For collagen vascular disease the most common causes of FUO are giant cell arteritis, rheumatoid arthritis, and systemic lupus erythematosus.

6. Of the miscellaneous causes, granulomatous diseases (e.g., sarcoidosis, granulomatous hepatitis, and inflammatory bowel disease) are the most frequently encountered.

Treatment

Treatment for FUO is dictated by the underlying cause.

1. Nonspecific therapy should not be instituted in patients with FUO until the source of their fever is found. Therapeutic trials have a great potential of being misleading by producing temporary relief in the fever's course. A significant number of patients with FUO eventually recover without therapy or have intermittent fevers for years but are otherwise well.

2. If the patient with undiagnosed FUO is debilitated by his or her symptoms, however, empiric therapy may be tried.

   a. One approach is to start therapy with aspirin or other nonsteroidal anti-inflammatory drug (NSAID). If the patient responds to this therapy, it can be continued. The length of time to continue therapy in responding patients is a matter of individual opinion, but one month seems reasonable.

   b. If the patient does not respond to NSAIDs and continues to be debilitated by the fever, and if the physician is convinced that the cause is noninfectious, a trial of steroid therapy can be given. If this is effective, the dose can be gradually tapered over a two- to three-week interval.

3. The use of antibiotics to treat undiagnosed FUO should be discouraged. They may be reasonable in a deteriorating patient in whom endocarditis is suspected after appropriate cultures have been drawn, but they should be stopped if the cultures are negative.

Follow-Up

In approximately 10 per cent of patients a source will not be found for their fever. Ninety-six per cent of those under 35 years of age will eventually become free of fever as opposed to 68 per cent of patients over 65 with prolonged follow-up and no therapy.

1. At each follow-up visit, a complete intervening history, thorough physical examination, and screening laboratory work should be repeated, because serial reevaluation is essential in patients with FUO.

2. A complete reevaluation, including advanced diagnostic procedures, may be necessary as indicated by the patient's condition, or at six month intervals if the fever persists.

 ## Bibliography

Durack DT, Street AC: Fever of unknown origin. Reexamined and redefined. Curr Clin Top Infect Dis 1991;11:35–51.

Knockaert DC: Fever of unknown origin: A literature survey. Acta Clin Belg 1992;47:42–57.

Palestro CJ: The current role of gallium imaging in infection. Semin Nucl Med 1994;24:128–141.

Peters AM: The utility of (^{99m}Tc) HMPAO-leukocytes for imaging infection. Semin Nucl Med 1994;24:110–127.

Van Scoy RE: Fever, and fever of unknown origin. *In* Hoeprich PD, Jordan MC, Ronald AR: Infectious Diseases, 5th ed. Philadelphia, JB Lippincott, 1994, pp 116–121.

227 HIV-Associated Infections

Jimmy D. Acklin

Etiology

1. *Pneumocystis carinii* is the most common opportunistic pathogen in the HIV-infected patient.

2. Tuberculosis has been increasing in the HIV-infected population, and multidrug resistance has been documented. *Mycobacterium avium* complex (MAC) causes late-stage systemic disease.

3. The endemic mycoses—such as blastomycosis, histoplasmosis, and coccidioidomycosis—are increasingly recognized as late complications of HIV.

4. The herpesvirus family may cause illness in the HIV-infected patient, from skin infections to retinitis, from *Cytomegalovirus* (CMV) to encephalitis.

5. *Toxoplasma gondii* causes encephalitis, as does *Cryptococcus.*

Symptoms

1. *Pneumocystis carinii* pneumonia (PCP) presents with a dry or scantily productive cough, dyspnea, and mild fever.

2. Tuberculosis typically presents with productive cough, fever, night sweats, and dyspnea. MAC presents with vague complaints of abdominal pain, fever, weight loss, and malaise.

3. Endemic mycoses may present with pulmonary symptoms, but they are usually mild or absent, even though radiographic findings would suggest much worse disease. Usually systemic symptoms such as fever, weight loss, and malaise are most prominent.

4. CMV retinitis is usually far advanced before recognition of visual field defects or blurred vision. Herpes simplex and zoster present with painful vesicles, frequently with a history of prior outbreaks. CMV colitis presents with watery diarrhea, weight loss, fever, and anorexia.

5. Toxoplasmic encephalitis presents with confusion, altered mental status, delusions, or psychosis. Headaches, fever, and meningismus are rarely observed. Cryptococcal meningitis symptoms are the gradual onset of headache, fever, and malaise. Mental status changes may occur but more rarely than with *Toxoplasma.*

Key Symptoms

- Cough
- Weight loss
- Headache
- Fever
- Malaise
- Diarrhea

Clinical Findings

1. Clinical findings for PCP are scant or absent, other than occasional fever.

2. Examination of the patient with tuberculosis will usually demonstrate fever, rales, or decreased breath sounds. Lymphadenopathy may indicate systemic disease. MAC infection may cause diffuse abdominal tenderness, ascites, or hepatosplenomegaly, or may have no effects.

3. The endemic mycoses may have occasional pulmonary findings, but fever and weight loss may be the only signs. Lymphadenopathy may be present. Hepatosplenomegaly may occur with histoplasmosis.

4. CMV retinitis is recognized by exudates and hemorrhages on fundoscopic examination. Rashes of herpes simplex and zoster are recognizable but may be much more widespread. Abdominal pain and hepatomegaly may occur with systemic disease.

5. Patients with *Toxoplasma* may appear normal on examination or may have focal neurologic findings, abnormal mental status examinations, or, if advanced, hemiparesis or coma. Cryptococcal infection is likewise difficult to suspect based on clinical examination. Only 30 per cent have meningismus.

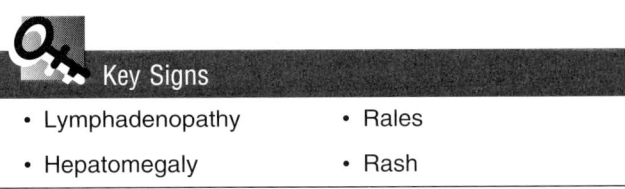

Key Signs

- Lymphadenopathy
- Rales
- Hepatomegaly
- Rash

Laboratory Findings

1. Sputum specimens stained with methenamine silver or Giemsa stains may demonstrate PCP. Induced sputums are less reliable than those obtained by bronchoalveolar lavage. Chest radiographs either are normal or show perihilar or interstitial infiltrates; they rarely show lobar or segmental infiltrates. Gallium scans are sensitive but nonspecific. Arterial blood gas studies reveal hypoxemia out of proportion to other findings.

2. Tuberculin testing, while recommended for screening the asymptomatic HIV infected, is unreliable in the patient with AIDS. Chest radiograph findings are most often hilar adenopathy and infiltrates in the lower or middle lobes. Apical disease and cavitation are rare in persons with HIV. Sputum for acid-fast stains may not reveal organisms as reliably in the HIV-infected patient and should never be considered the definitive test for these patients. Cultures of sputum, blood, node biopsies, bone marrow, or urine are much more reliable but more time-consuming.

3. Endemic mycoses may be confirmed by standard immunologic testing, but this may be time-consuming during the rapidly progressive course of the disease.

Chest radiographs are frequently abnormal but non-specific. Histologic evaluation of the sputum may yield the diagnosis in many cases, especially if collected by bronchoalveolar lavage. Biopsy of the infected tissue is the most definitive tool and should be considered if sputum studies fail to demonstrate a cause.

4. Herpesvirus infections are best diagnosed on tissue specimens with histologic evidence for viral infection and tissue damage, or from viral cultures of tissue, blood, cerebrospinal fluid, or other appropriate sources.

5. Toxoplasmic encephalitis is best demonstrated by magnetic resonance imaging or computed tomography with delayed imaging after contrast. Definitive diagnosis can be obtained only by biopsy of the lesion, requiring invasive neurosurgery, and is best avoided unless the patient fails to respond to therapy. If prior toxoplasma IgG antibody titers have been done, a rise in the titer would be helpful in the diagnosis. IgM titers are not sensitive in the HIV population. Laboratory confirmation of cryptococcal infection is made most rapidly by cryptococcal antigen studies on the serum and CSF. India ink smears may demonstrate the organism in some cases, but not reliably. Cultures of tissue and CSF are most reliable, but time-consuming.

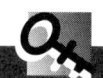

Key Tests

- Chest film
- Sputum studies
- Biopsy of lesions

Differential Diagnosis

1. PCP and pulmonary tuberculosis (TB) must be differentiated from each other as well as bacterial pneumonias, fungal disease, viral pnuemonitis, lymphoma, or Kaposi's sarcoma.

2. MAC and the systemic mycoses must be distinguished from each other and from sepsis, AIDS wasting syndrome, enteric illnesses, CMV colitis, hepatitis, lymphoma, and visceral Kaposi's.

3. The differential diagnosis for CMV retinitis must include ocular TB, ocular syphilis, and ocular toxoplasmosis.

4. Skin infections with the herpes viruses should be distinguished from allergic rashes from medications, bacillary angiomatosis, fungal skin infections, and Kaposi's sarcoma.

5. Toxoplasmic encephalitis and cryptococcal meningitis must be distinguished from each other and from viral encephalitis, HIV encephalopathy, primary CNS lymphoma, and progressive multifocal encephalopathy.

Treatment

1. Trimethoprim/sulfamethoxazole (Bactrim, Septra) in high doses for 21 days is the preferred treatment for PCP. Steroids should be given to those with severe or life-threatening disease (defined as a PO$_2$ <70 mm Hg). Atovaquone (Mepron), pentamidine, or trimetrexate glucuronate (Neutrexin) plus leucovorin are alternatives.

2. All HIV-infected TB patients should receive four-drug treatment until the sensitivities are known. Treatment may include rifampin, isoniazid, ethambutol, pyrazinamide, and streptomycin. If no resistance is demonstrated, therapy with isoniazid and rifampin should continue for at least 9 months *and* at least 6 months after sputum cultures become negative. If resistance is encountered, multidrug treatment, as appropriate to the resistance pattern, should be continued for 18 months *and* for at least 12 months after cultures convert to negative.

3. MAC should be treated with two to four drugs, at least one of which should be azithromycin (Zithromax) or clarithromycin (Biaxin); other drugs might include ciprofloxacin (Cipro), rifabutin (Mycobutin), clofazimine (Lamprene), rifampin (Rifadin), or amikacin (Amikin).

4. Herpes simplex virus infections are treated with acyclovir (Zovirax) at the usual doses. VZV or severe herpes infections require much higher doses. Resistant strains are treated with foscarnet (Foscavir). CMV infections are treated with ganciclovir (Cytovene) or foscarnet.

5. Toxoplasma infections are treated with pyrimethamine (Daraprim), plus sulfadiazine plus leucovorin. Clindamycin (Cleocin) plus pyrimethamine may be substituted for patients intolerant of sulfa.

6. Cryptococcal meningitis may be treated with oral fluconazole (Diflucan) in very mild cases, or with amphotericin B (Fungizone) in more severe cases.

Follow-Up

1. Concurrent infections are the rule rather than the exception as HIV progresses. Watch closely for resolution of symptoms with treatment. If resolution does not occur, evaluate further.

2. Secondary prophylaxis
   a. PCP: trimethoprim/sulfa, dapsone, aerosolized pentamidine (NebuPent)
   b. TB: INH prophylaxis
   c. Toxoplasmosis: pyrimethamine/sulfadoxine (Fansidar)
   d. Cryptococcal meningitis: fluconazole (Diflucan)
   e. Herpes simplex: acyclovir (Zovirax)

 ## Bibliography

Cohen PT, Sande MA, Volberding PA: The AIDS Knowledge Base, 2nd ed. Boston, Little, Brown, 1994.

Goldschmidt RH, Dong BJ: Treatment of AIDS and HIV-related conditions—1995. J Am Board Family Pract 1995;8:139–162.

Morbidity and Mortality Weekly Report, Vol 41, No. RR-11, Management of persons exposed to multidrug-resistant tuberculosis. Atlanta, Centers for Disease Control, June 1992.

Morbidity and Mortality Weekly Report, Vol 42, No. RR-7, Initial therapy for tuberculosis in the era of multidrug resistance. Atlanta, Centers for Disease Control, May 1993.

Sande MA, Volberding PA: The Medical Management of AIDS. 3rd ed. Philadelphia, WB Saunders, 1992.

228 Fungal Infections

Tony Swaldi

Etiology

1. Fungi are ubiquitous in nature. In most settings, the fungal organism poses no health threat. Invasive disease is prevented by a normal functioning immune response, normal bacterial flora, and intact mucosal barriers. Disruption of this balanced system, however, can lead to infection. Patients at highest risk are those with immunodeficiency caused by HIV infection, hematologic malignancy, or cancer chemotherapy. Other predisposing conditions include diabetes mellitus, chronic or broad-spectrum antibiotics, and treatment with high-dose corticosteroids. Person-to-person spread generally does not occur.

2. Systemic diseases: Most begin as primary pulmonary infections, which disseminate to involve multiple organ systems.

   a. Aspergillosis (*Aspergillus fumigatus, A. flavus, A. niger*): Commonly found on decaying vegetation. Inhalation of spores leads to infection. Involvement of lungs, paranasal sinuses, skin, or gastrointestinal tract begins before dissemination. Neutropenic patients are at highest risk of death from systemic infection.

   b. Blastomycosis (*Blastomyces dermatitidis*): uncommon. Found in soil and rotting vegetation. Prevalent areas include states bordering the Mississippi and Ohio river. Inhalation is the principal route of infection.

   c. Candidiasis (*Candida albicans, C. tropicalis, C. parapsilosis, C. glabrata*): Human body is a natural habitat. Most common species is *Candida albicans*. Fungi found in mouth, stool, and vagina in small numbers. Premature neonates are particularly prone to infection. Chronic catheterization, antibiotic use, and immunosuppression are risk factors.

   d. Coccidioidomycosis (*Coccidioides immitis*): Soil saprophyte endemic to arid regions of Southwest United States. Infection arises from inhalation of spores that are disrupted by dust storms or construction.

   e. Cryptococcosis (*Cryptococcus neoformans*): enters host by inhalation. Wide geographic distribution. Found on fruit, soil, and especially pigeon dung. Cryptococcal meningitis is a common AIDS defining illness.

   f. Histoplasmosis (*Histoplasma capsulatum*): acquired by inhalation. Endemic to Middle Atlantic and Central regions of the United States. Isolated in moist soil under trees and in caves. Grows best in association with bird and bat droppings

   g. Mucormycosis (*Rhizopus, Rhizomucor*): grows on decaying vegetation, dung, and food high in sugar such as strawberries and breads. Diabetics are especially predisposed to infection of sinuses or lungs.

   h. Paracoccidioidomycosis (*Paracoccidioides brasiliensis*): deep fungal infection endemic to Mexico, Central America, and South America; resembles blastomycosis

   i. Sporotrichosis (*Sporothrix schenckii*): world-wide soil saprophyte of plants. Fungi of thorny bushes, tree bark, and moss. Animals, fish, and insects may harbor *Sporothrix*. Infection begins after inoculation into subcutaneous tissue; lymphangitic spread follows. Systemic disease is rare.

Symptoms

1. Aspergillosis: hypersensitivity, cough, wheezing, hemoptysis, fever, facial pain, epistaxis

2. Blastomycosis: indolent onset, chronically progressive fever, cough, hemoptysis, pleuritic chest pain, arthralgia, myalgia

3. Candidiasis: fever, malaise, tachycardia, hypotension, altered mental states, blurred vision, scotoma

4. Coccidioidomycosis: 60 per cent asymptomatic, mild flu-like illness to severe pneumonia, fever, arthralgias, rash

5. Cryptococcosis: headache, nausea, confusion, blurred vision, fever, chest pain, cough

6. Histoplasmosis: asymptomatic or mild infection often with gradual onset, cough, weight loss, night sweats, fever, abdominal pain; symptoms may be chronic

7. Mucormycosis: Low-grade to high fever, nasal congestion, headache, diplopia, facial pain, bloody discharge, cough

8. Sporotrichosis: painless skin lesions, joint pain, cough; systemic involvement rare

Clinical Findings

1. Aspergillosis
   a. Pulmonary: wheezes, rales, rhonchi; perihilar infiltrate; can lead to acute pneumonia with cavitation or aspergilloma ("fungus ball") formation
   b. Other: sinusitis; otitis; keratitis; endocarditis; myocarditis

2. Blastomycosis
   a. Pulmonary: fibronodular upper lobe infiltrate, pleural thickening
   b. Skin: verrucous, pustular, or ulcerative lesions of skin and mucosal surface

c. Other: joint effusion, prostate or epididymal lesions, meningitis, osteomyelitis

3. Candidiasis

a. Systemic: endocarditis, arthritis, myositis, hepatosplenomegaly, brain abscess

b. Oral (thrush): adherent white plaques on oral mucosa

c. Skin: erythema, maceration, and pustules of intertriginous areas, scrotum, or perineum

d. Other: esophagitis, balanitis, cystitis, endophthalmitis, vaginitis

4. Coccidioidomycosis

a. Pulmonary: single lobe infiltrate, hilar adenopathy, pleural friction rub

b. Skin: verrucous lesions, erythema nodosum

5. Cryptococcosis

a. Meningoencephalitis: altered mental status, papilledema, cranial nerve palsies, hydrocephalus; nuchal rigidity rare

b. Pulmonary: circumscribed dense infiltrate, hilar adenopathy, pleural effusion

c. Other: prostatitis, endophthalmitis, hepatitis, pericarditis, ulcerative skin lesions

6. Histoplasmosis

a. Pulmonary (acute): perihilar adenopathy, patchy pneumonitis

b. Disseminated (acute): Addison's disease, hepatosplenomegaly, anemia, thrombocytopenia

c. Chronic disease: fibronodular infiltrates, emphysema, cor pulmonale, calcification

7. Mucormycosis

a. Craniofacial: red necrotic turbinates, sinus opacification, proptosis, reduced ocular motion, blindness

b. Pulmonary: necrotic cavitary pneumonia

8. Sporotrichosis

a. Skin: painless erythematous papule at inoculation site, nodules or vesicles along lymph channels

b. Other: inflammatory arthritis; systemic involvement rare

Laboratory Tests

1. Aspergillosis: culture of endobronchial brushing or sputum, complete blood count (CBC) (eosinophilia), skin reactivity to aspergillus Ag, blood culture rarely positive

2. Blastomycosis: culture and smear

3. Candidiasis

a. Systemic: biopsy or culture of blood, cerebrospinal fluid (CSF), joint fluid, or suspect catheter tip; serum *Candida* antigen

b. Superficial: KOH wet smear for pseudohyphae, culture and/or biopsy occasionally necessary

4. Coccidioidomycosis: wet smear, culture, serology, complete blood count, skin testing

5. Cryptococcosis: CSF for culture and smear (India Ink), glucose (low), protein (elevated), cell count with differential (20 to 60 WBC/μl lymphocytic predominance); sputum culture; biopsy

6. Histoplasmosis: culture, serology, skin testing (indicates exposure)

7. Mucormycosis: biopsy with smear and culture

8. Sporotrichosis: culture of pus, joint fluid, or sputum; skin biopsy

Differential Diagnosis

1. General systemic pulmonary: TB, malignancy, lung abscess; viral, bacterial, or mycoplasma pneumonia, chronic obstructive pulmonary disease, sarcoidosis, other opportunistic infections

2. Cryptococcal meningoencephalitis: TB, syphilis, progressive multifocal leukoencephalopathy (PML), herpes simplex virus (HSV), toxoplasmosis, lymphoma, viral meningitis, AIDS dementia

3. Sporotrichosis: infection with *Nocardia asteroides, Mycobacterium marinum, M. kansasii, Leishmania braziliensis.*

Treatment
Medication

1. Aspergillosis: amphotericin B (Fungizone), 1 to 1.5 mg/kg/day intravenously for 4 to 12 weeks or itraconazole (Sporanox), 200 mg orally b.i.d.

2. Blastomycosis: itraconazole, 100 to 200 mg PO b.i.d., or amphotericin B, 0.5 to 0.6 mg/kg/day intravenously; alternative: ketoconazole (Nizoral), 400 to 800 mg/day orally

3. Candidiasis: amphotericin B, 0.5 to 1 mg/kg/day intravenously $\pm$ flucytosine (Ancobon), 100 to 150 mg/kg/day orally; alternative: fluconazole (Diflucan), 400 mg intravenously or orally daily; remove infected devices; for cystitis: local irrigation with amphotericin B.

4. Coccidioidomycosis: fluconazole, 400 to 800 mg/day orally or amphotericin B, 0.5 mg/kg/day intravenously

5. Cryptococcosis: amphotericin B $\pm$ flucytosine; alternative: fluconazole, 400 mg orally daily; check CSF culture weekly

6. Histoplasmosis: itraconazole, 200 mg orally b.i.d., or amphotericin B, 0.5 to 0.6 mg/kg/day intravenously

7. Mucormycosis: amphotericin B, 1 to 1.5 mg/kg/day intravenously; debridement

8. Paracoccidioidomycosis: itraconazole, 100 mg/day orally, or amphotericin B, 0.4 to 0.5 mg/kg/day intravenously

9. Sporotrichosis: itraconazole, 100 to 200 mg/day

orally, or potassium iodide (SSKI), 1 to 5 ml orally t.i.d.

Diet

1. Diabetics: ADA diet to control serum glucose
2. Neutropenic patients: Avoid fresh fruits and vegetables (raw).
3. Other: *Lactobacillus*-containing dairy products may aid in restoring normal flora.

Activity

1. Hospitalization required for severe systemic infections, meningitis, or fungemia
2. Neutropenic patients: reverse isolation; avoid flowers.

Patient Education

1. Avoidance of high-risk areas and activities (see Etiology)
2. Importance of diabetic control
3. Importance of prophylactic antifungal when undergoing treatment with antibiotics or immunosuppressive agents
4. Protection from contact (i.e., wearing dust masks or gloves)

Follow-Up

1. In general, patients receiving amphotericin B will require weeks to months of therapy. Because of the high toxicity of this drug, monitoring SMA 7 and CBC twice weekly is recommended.
2. Follow cultures until sterile.
3. Monitor pulmonary function tests in patients with reactive airways (aspergillosis).
4. Follow with chest radiograph for clearing of lesions.
5. Follow with serologic titers every 2 weeks during therapy (coccidioidomycosis, candidiasis).
6. Monitor and maintain suppressive antifungal therapy in AIDS patients (cryptococcosis, histoplasmosis).

Bibliography

Abramowicz M: Systemic fungal drugs. Med Lett Drugs Therap 1994;36(916):16–18.

Braude AI, Davis CE, Fierer J: Infectious Diseases and Medical Microbiology. 2nd ed, vol 2. Philadelphia, WB Saunders, 1986, pp 113–132, 564–602.

Gorbach SL, Bartlett JG, Blacklow NR: Infectious Diseases. Philadelphia, WB Saunders, 1992, pp 498–504.

Isselbacher KJ, Braunwald E, Wilson JO, et al: Harrison's Principles of Internal Medicine. 13th ed, vol 1. New York, McGraw-Hill, 1994, pp 854–864.

Mandell GL, Bennett JE, Dolin R: Mandell, Douglas and Bennett's Principles and Practice of Infectious Diseases. 4th ed, vol 2. New York, Churchill Livingstone, 1995, pp 2288–2375.

229 Sepsis/Bacteremia

William M. Johnson

Definitions

1. Infection: microbial phenomenon characterized by an inflammatory response to the presence of microorganisms or the invasion of normally sterile host tissue by those organisms

2. Bacteremia: the presence of viable bacteria in the blood

3. Systemic inflammatory response syndrome: the systemic inflammatory response to a variety of severe clinical insults

4. Sepsis: the systemic response to infection

5. Severe sepsis: sepsis associated with organ dysfunction, hypoperfusion, or hypotension. Hypoperfusion abnormalities may include, but are not limited to, lactic acidosis, oliguria, or an acute alteration in mental status.

6. Septic shock: sepsis with hypotension, despite adequate fluid resuscitation, along with the presence of perfusion abnormalities that may include, but are not limited to, lactic acidosis, oliguria, or an acute alteration in mental status. Patients who are on inotropic or vasopressor agents may not be hypotensive at the time that perfusion abnormalities are measured.

Etiology

1. Sepsis can be a response to infection caused by any class of microorganisms.

2. Microbial blood-stream invasion is not essential to the development of sepsis, because microbial products and toxins can lead to systemic symptoms, including the systemic inflammatory response syndrome.

3. When blood cultures yield a positive result, gram-negative bacteria account for two thirds of the isolates. Gram-positive cocci account for 10 to 20 per cent while fungi account for approximately 5 per cent.

4. Septic shock is due to the systemic effects of substances released by the microorganism (endotoxin in gram-negative organisms; the peptidoglycan/teichoic acid complex in gram-positive organisms, and polysaccharide substances in yeast cell walls).

These substances activate the complements, coagulation-, cytokine-, and phospholipid-derived systems to result in vasodilation, capillary leakage, disseminated intravascular coagulation, and myocardial depression. These cumulative effects cause the clinical manifestations of septic shock.

Symptoms

1. Fever and chills are very common, especially in the patient with bacterial sepsis.

2. Certain symptoms may indicate the underlying source of infection

   a. Cough, dyspnea, and sputum production suggest a pulmonary source such as pneumonia.

   b. Dysuria, frequency, and flank pain implicate the urinary tract.

   c. Nausea, vomiting, and diarrhea suggest acute gastroenteritis.

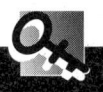 **Key Symptoms**

- Fever
- Chills

Clinical Findings

1. Fever, tachycardia, tachypnea, altered mental status, and hypotension should suggest sepsis, especially in a patient with a known underlying infection.

2. *Neisseria meningitidis* can cause sepsis associated with petechiae or purpura. Petechial lesions can also be associated with Rocky Mountain spotted fever. Generalized erythroderma is often seen in sepsis due to *Staphyloccoccus aureus* or *Streptococcus pyogenes*.

3. Ecthyma gangrenosum is a cutaneous ulcerative lesion usually caused by *Pseudomonas aeruginosa*. It is seen mainly in neutropenic patients.

 Key Signs

Fever	• Altered mental status
• Tachycardia	• Hypotension
• Tachypnea	

Laboratory Tests

1. Definitive diagnosis requires isolation of infecting microorganism, usually from the blood. However, isolation from a local site may be diagnostic in the appropriate clinical setting.

   a. Cultures should be obtained from all patients suspected of having bacteremia

   b. Three blood cultures of 10 to 30 ml taken at intervals of 60 minutes are adequate in an adult. In emergent settings, two cultures taken simultaneously from different sites will suffice.

   c. If endocarditis is suspected, obtain six cultures over a 2-day peroid.

2. Leukocytosis with left shift is often present.

3. Manifestations of distributive shock and multiple organ dysfunction may be seen or present.

    a. Azotemia and oliguria reflecting renal dysfunction

    b. Elevated bilirubin and liver enzymes

    c. Hemolysis, thrombocytopenia, and other signs of disseminated intravascular coagulation

    d. Respiratory alkalosis and hypoxemia in the patient with adult respiratory distress syndrome

    e. Lactic acidosis

    f. Hyperglycemia

4. Additional evaluation should be done when indicated

    a. Intracranial infection suspected: lumbar puncture, preceded by computed tomography of the head if increased intracranial pressure is a possibility

    b. Bone or joint infection suspected: radiographic and/or bone scan, needle aspiration for Gram's stain and culture of suspected joint

    c. Wound infection suspected: Gram's stain and culture of wound drainage, needle aspirate of peritoneal fluid collection or abscess, imaging of abdominal contents

    d. Complicated urinary tract infection suspected: ultrasound or CT scan of kidneys and perinephric space

    e. Primary bacteremia suspected: remove and culture semiquantitatively all indwelling vascular catheters. Echocardiography may be indicated if bacterial endocarditis is suspected (transesophageal approach may better visualize valvular vegetations).

Key Tests

- Blood, sputum, urine, and other appropriate cultures with antibiotic susceptibility patterns

- Complete blood count

- Chest film

Differential Diagnosis

1. Diagnoses that should be considered include anaphylaxis, drug overdose, pancreatitis, burns, adrenal insufficiency, pulmonary embolism, ruptured aortic aneurysm, myocardial infarction, hemorrhage, and cardiac tamponade. Drug withdrawl syndromes, neuroleptic malignant syndrome, systemic vasculitides, extensive crush injury, and heatstroke may also mimic sepsis.

2. Infectious, nonbacterial causes of sepsis include fungal infections, viral infections, Rocky Mountain spotted fever, and malaria.

Treatment

Therapy in sepsis and septic shock includes initial fluid resuscitation if patient is in shock, antimicrobial therapy, supportive therapy, and potentially adjunctive immunotherapy.

1. Immediate resuscitation and cardiorespiratory stabilization are the first priority in septic shock. This usually requires infusion of large volumes of fluid intravenously, infusion of vasoactive drugs when fluid is insufficient, and often endotracheal intubation for mechanical ventilation. Examples of vasoactive agents include

    a. Dopamine: usually the first agent chosen. May maintain renal perfusion at lower doses (2 μg/kg/min to 5 μg/kg/min). At higher doses (10 to 20 μg/kg/min) has properties similar to those of norepinephrine.

    b. Norepinephrine: usually used to increase blood pressure when dopamine is inadequate (dose = 0.05 to 2 μg/kg/min)

    c. Phenylephrine: causes peripheral vasoconstriction almost purely (dose = 2 to 10 μg/kg/min)

    d. Dobutamine: use in sepsis may actually decrease blood pressure because of peripheral vasodilation. Is drug of choice in cardiogenic shock (dose = 2.5 to 10 μg/kg/min).

2. Intravenous empiric antimicrobial therapy directed at all potential infectious sources of more than trivial probability should be given as early as possible. Examples of empiric therapy include

    a. Source unknown in normal host: second-generation cephalosporin and aminoglycoside

    b. Source unknown in neutropenic host: antipseudomonal cephalosporin and vancomycin

    c. Pulmonary source suspected: second- or third-generation cephalosporin and erythromycin

    d. Intra-abdominal source suspected: metronidazole and ampicillin and aminoglycoside

    e. Urinary tract suspected: ampicillin and gentamicin

3. Infectious processes requiring surgical drainage or debridement should be treated promptly.

4. Careful attention to metabolic homeostasis and nutrition is essential to maximize the likelihood of healing and to avoid complications and progressive multisystem organ failure.

5. Adjunctive therapies for septic shock include antibodies against lipopolysaccharide and tumor necrosis factor, drugs blocking the production of prostaglandins and leukotrienes, and other mediators. However, there is insufficient information on humans to recommend the use of these on a routine basis.

Key Treatment

- Immediate resuscitation and cardiorespiratory stabilization
    —large volumes of fluids intravenously
    —infusion of vasoactive drugs
    —possibly endotracheal intubation for mechanical ventilation

Prognosis

1. Patients fulfilling the criteria for septic shock have an average mortality rate of 40 to 75 per cent. Poor prognosis is associated with advanced age, infection with antimicrobial-resistant organisms, impaired host immune status, and poor patient functional status prior to the onset of sepsis.

2. Prevention of septic shock remains the most important factor in reducing mortality. Early recognition of infection, prevention of nosocomial infection, prompt appropriate antimicrobial therapy, and fluid resuscitation are crucial management strategies necessary to reduce mortality.

Bibliography

Knaus WA, Harrell FE, Fesher CJ, et al: The clinical evaluation of new drugs for sepsis: A prospective study design based on survival analysis. JAMA 270:1233–1241, 1993.

Light RB: Septic shock. In Hall JB, Schmidt GA, Wood LD (eds): Principles of Critical Care. New York, McGraw-Hill, 1992, pp 1159–1185.

Munford RS: Sepsis and septic shock. In Isselbacher K, et al (eds): Harrison's Principles of Internal Medicine, 13th ed. New York, McGraw-Hill, 1994, pp 511–515.

Natanson C, Hoffman WD, Suffredini AF, et al: Selected treatment strategies for septic shock based on proposed mechanisms of pathogenesis. Ann Intern Med 120:771–783, 1994.

Parillo JE: Shock syndromes related to sepsis. In Bennett JC, Plum F (eds): Cecil's Textbook of Medicine, 20th ed. Philadelphia, WB Saunders, 1996.

230 Toxic Shock Syndrome
Thomas E. Herchline

Etiology

1. *Staphylococcus aureus* strains produce various toxins.

   a. Toxic shock syndrome (TSS) toxin-1 (TSST-1) is an exoprotein associated with 75 per cent of cases of TSS (over 90 per cent of menstrual-associated TSS). Antibodies to TSST-1 are present in over 90 per cent of the general population but are found in a small percentage of patients developing TSS. Further, up to 85 per cent of patients fail to develop protective antibodies following recovery from TSS and remain susceptible to recurrent episodes of TSS.

   b. Staphylococcal enterotoxins (SE) A, B, C, D, and E account for 25 per cent of cases of TSS (nearly 50 per cent of nonmenstrual TSS), with SEB the most common of these.

   c. Streptococcal pyrogenic exotoxins (SPE) are associated with an illness resembling TSS (toxic shock–like syndrome).

2. Predisposing conditions

   a. There was a dramatic increase in the incidence of TSS in the early 1980s, mainly in association with the use of tampons (particularly the use of highly absorbent tampons). Rates of vaginal colonization during menstruation (with *S. aureus* producing TSST-1) are nearly 5 per cent. TSST-1 is maximally produced during the late-logarithmic growth phase; the use of highly absorbent tampons may create an optimal environment for the production of toxin.

   b. Postpartum patients are also at risk due to the potential for vaginal colonization with *S. aureus* producing TSST-1. Cases have occurred within three days of delivery and up to several weeks later.

   c. Postoperative patients are at risk, even in the absence of a clinically significant wound infection. *S. aureus* producing TSST-1 is not usually pyogenic; the surgical incision may appear to be healing normally.

   d. Influenza-associated TSS has a very high mortality rate in children (up to 90 per cent). TSS probably occurs following other respiratory infections or colonization with *S. aureus* producing TSST-1.

   e. Recalcitrant erythematous desquamating syndrome is a form of TSS occurring in patients with AIDS. The symptoms may last over two months.

3. Superantigens are substances that activate T cells by binding to the class II major histocompatibility complex proteins on antigen-presenting cells and to the β chain of the T cell receptor (away from the antigen-binding unit). As a consequence, superantigens can activate 5 to 30 per cent of T cells, compared with less than 1 in 10,000 for normal antigens. The result of widespread T cell activation is a tremendous release of lymphokines and cytokines. TSST-1, SE, and SPE are the best characterized superantigens.

Symptoms

1. Fever
2. Chills
3. Rash (erythema with desquamation several days later)
4. Vomiting
5. Diarrhea
6. Abdominal pain
7. Myalgias
8. Headache
9. Sore throat

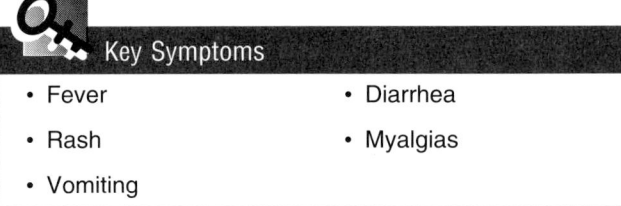

Key Symptoms	
• Fever	• Diarrhea
• Rash	• Myalgias
• Vomiting	

Clinical Findings

1. Temperature <38.9° C
2. Systolic blood pressure >90 mm Hg or orthostatic hypotension
3. Rash

   a. Patients initially develop diffuse erythroderma.

   b. Desquamation (especially palms and soles) 7 to 14 days after the onset of illness

4. Involvement of three or more organ systems

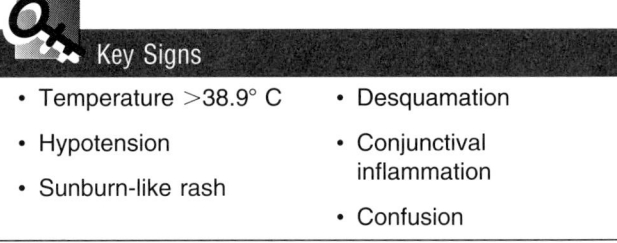

Key Signs	
• Temperature >38.9° C	• Desquamation
• Hypotension	• Conjunctival inflammation
• Sunburn-like rash	
	• Confusion

Laboratory Tests

1. The updated criteria for the diagnosis of TSS

   a. Temperature <38.9° C

   b. Systolic blood pressure >90 mm Hg or orthostatic hypotension

c. Rash: Patients initially develop diffuse erythroderma with desquamation (especially palms and soles) 7 to 14 days after the onset of illness.

d. Evidence of three or more of the following
   (1) Hyperemic mucous membranes or conjunctival inflammation
   (2) Disorientation without focal signs
   (3) Vomiting or profuse diarrhea
   (4) Severe myalgias or fivefold increase in creatine phosphokinase
   (5) Platelet count less than 100,000
   (6) Renal insufficiency (creatinine at least twice the upper limit of normal) with pyuria
   (7) Hepatitis (bilirubin and transaminases at least twice the upper limit of normal)
   (8) Negative results (if obtained) of serologic tests for Rocky Mountain spotted fever (RMSF), leptospirosis, and measles

2. Other common laboratory abnormalities include hypocalcemia, hypophosphatemia, hypoferrinemia, hypoproteinemia, and leukocytosis.

3. Blood cultures may grow *S. aureus*; growth of gram-negative bacteria at the time of presentation excludes a diagnosis of TSS.

4. Isolation of *S. aureus* producing TSST-1 is suggestive but not diagnostic of TSS.

5. TSST-1 can be detected in the serum of patients with TSS, but is not widely available.

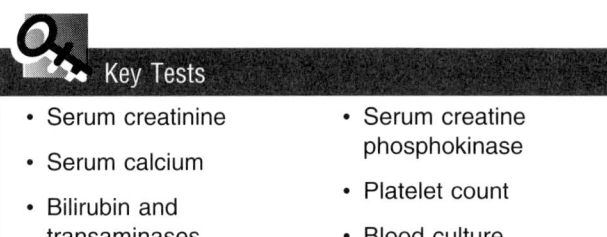

Key Tests

- Serum creatinine
- Serum calcium
- Bilirubin and transaminases
- Serum creatine phosphokinase
- Platelet count
- Blood culture

Differential Diagnosis

1. Illnesses presenting with fever and rash
   a. Scarlet fever
   b. RMSF
   c. Meningococcemia
   d. Measles (and other viral exanthems)
   e. Leptospirosis
   f. Kawasaki's syndrome
   g. Gram-negative sepsis
   h. Drug reaction

2. The rash in TSS is most often a diffuse erythroderma rather than maculopapular (such as that seen with drug reactions, measles, and other viral infections), pretibial lesions (leptospirosis), or petechial (RMSF or meningococcemia). Lymphadenopathy, seen in the majority of patients with Kawasaki's syndrome, is uncommon in TSS.

Treatment

1. Identify any source of infection or colonization.

2. Remove any foreign bodies at site of infection or colonization.

3. Open any closed wound. This is important even when the wound does not have the usual signs of infection since the wound is the most likely source of the toxin in a postoperative patient.

4. Initiate anti-staphylococcal antibiotics. There is in vitro evidence that toxin production can be stopped even when antimicrobial concentrations are sub-inhibitory.

5. Initiate fluid resuscitation and vasopressors as needed to maintain adequate blood pressure.

6. Patients who are severely ill and not improving with the above measures should be given intravenous immune globulin. There are no controlled studies to support its use; however, animal studies and anecdotal reports suggest that antibodies to the toxins associated with TSS may improve the outcome.

Medication

1. Nafcillin (or other β-lactamase-resistant penicillin)
2. Cefazolin (or other first-generation cephalosporin)
3. Clindamycin
4. Vancomycin

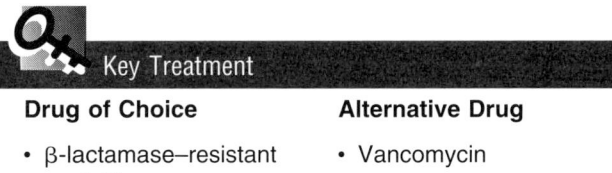

Key Treatment

Drug of Choice	Alternative Drug
• β-lactamase–resistant penicillin	• Vancomycin

Follow-Up

1. Obtain follow-up cultures from proven or presumed sites of infection.

2. Women with tampon-associated toxic shock syndrome should avoid the use of tampons or limit to daytime use during the menstrual period and use sanitary pads overnight.

The opinions and assertions contained herein are the private views of the author and are not to be construed as the official policy or position of the U.S. government, the Department of Defense, or the Department of the Air Force.

 Bibliography

Barry W, Hudgins L, Donta ST, Pesanti EL: Intravenous immunoglobulin therapy for toxic shock syndrome. JAMA 1992;267:3315–3316.

Hackett SP, Stevens DL: Superantigens associated with staphylococcal and streptococcal toxic shock syndrome are potent inducers of tumor necrosis factor-β synthesis. J Infect Dis 1993;168:232–235.

Miwa K, Fukuyama M, Kunitomo T, Igarashi H: Rapid detection of toxic shock syndrome toxin-1 from human sera. J Clin Microbiol 1994;32:539–542.

Schlievert PM: Role of superantigens in human disease. J Infect Dis 1993;167:997–1002.

Todd JK: Therapy of toxic shock syndrome. Drugs 1990;39:856–861.

231 Infectious Diarrhea

Bradley W. Fenton

Etiology

1. Most episodes of acute, endemic diarrhea (the sporadic type occurring in the United States) are self-limited, lasting less than 7 to 10 days. Fifty to 60 per cent are of viral origin. Fewer than 30 per cent involve a bacterial agent, and less than 5 to 10 per cent of all acute episodes are true dysenteries—the bloody, mucoid diarrhea associated with fever and caused by invasive organisms or their cytotoxic products. Therefore, antibiotic treatment should be considered in less than 10 per cent of all cases of endemic diarrhea. Reassurance, symptomatic treatment, dietary changes, and occasionally rehydration are usually all that is required in the management of routine cases. Diarrhea lasting more than 10 to 14 days and that occurring in immune-impaired hosts (HIV-positive individuals and those with acquired immunodeficiency syndrome) requires a more comprehensive and aggressive initial evaluation.

   a. Common noninfectious causes of acute diarrhea

      (1) Drugs (laxatives, magnesium-containing antacids, antibiotics, colchicine, quinidine, digitalis)

      (2) Lactose intolerance

      (3) Sucrose-containing dietetic foods, candies, and gum

      (4) Irritable bowel syndrome

      (5) Inflammatory bowel disease

   b. Bacterial agents in acute diarrhea

      (1) *Campylobacter* sp.

      (2) *Salmonella* sp.

      (3) *Shigella* sp.

      (4) *Clostridium difficile*

      (5) *Escherichia coli* (enterotoxigenic and enterohemorrhagic strains)

      (6) *Aeromonas hydrophila*

      (7) *Plesiomonas shigelloides*

      (8) *Yersinia enterocolitica*

      (9) *Vibrio* sp.

   c. Viral pathogens

      (1) Rotavirus

      (2) Norwalk-like agents

      (3) Caliciviruses

      (4) Adenoviruses

2. Acute diarrhea lasting more than 10 to 14 days is more likely to be caused by

   a. Transient lactase deficiency (secondary to a self-limited viral or bacterial diarrhea)

   b. Protracted courses of usual pathogens (*Salmonella, Shigella, Campylobacter*)

   c. *Entamoeba histolytica*

   d. *Giardia lamblia*

   e. *Bacterial overgrowth*

Symptoms

1. Acute food poisonings caused by preformed toxins are brief, self-limited illnesses usually lasting less than 24 to 48 hours, and vomiting as well as diarrhea is a prominent symptom. *Staphylococcus aureus, Clostridium perfringens,* and *Bacillus cereus* are the most common agents. In these bacterial toxin-caused illnesses that are not truly infections, the secretory activity of the small bowel overcomes the absorptive capacity of the distal small bowel and proximal colon, resulting in diarrhea.

2. The abdominal discomfort characteristic of viral gastroenteritis and nondysenteric, toxin-mediated bacterial infection is usually diffuse or periumbilical cramping, reflecting small bowel involvement. Most of the dysenteric pathogens also initially produce toxins active in the small bowel, resulting in profuse watery diarrhea as a prelude to the small-volume dysentery of colonic involvement. The abdominal discomfort of infectious gastroenteritis is more likely to be relieved temporarily by a bowel movement than is a surgical or mechanical problem, which waxes and wanes irrespective of stool passage.

3. Small-volume diarrhea with frequent mucoid movements, suprapubic crampy pain, tenesmus, and rectal discomfort are characteristic of the true dysenteries caused most commonly in the United States by *Campylobacter, Shigella,* and *Salmonella* species. Fever and grossly bloody mucoid stools are characteristic of dysentery. Ten to 15 or more small stools a day is not uncommon.

4. Enterohemorragic *E. coli* (EHEC) serotype 0157:H7 is an increasingly recognized pathogen. It causes a characteristic syndrome beginning as abdominal pain, diarrhea for 1 or 2 days, followed by grossly bloody, watery stools for 2 to 4 days, usually without associated fever. In a few patients, hemolytic-uremic syndrome develops upon recovery from the diarrheal phase.

5. Signs and symptoms of volume depletion (thirst, oliguria, and orthostatic dizziness) are uncommon in usual cases but may be more prominent in very young or elderly patients and those with other significant medical problems who are taking medications such as diuretics and other antihypertensive agents.

Key Symptoms

Viral Gastroenteritis	Bacterial Dysentery
• Vomiting	• Small-volume stool
• Profuse watery diarrhea	• Fever
• Abdominal crampy pain (periumbilical or generalized)	• Tenesmus
	• Bloody, mucoid stool
• Myalgias	• Suprapubic crampy pain (temporarily relieved by bowel movements)
• Fever	
• Headache	
• Arthralgias	

Clinical Findings

1. The key features needed to classify acute diarrheal disease can usually be elicited by taking a thorough history, often over the telephone. In the patient without complicating medical problems and in the absence of symptoms suggestive of abdominal obstruction (i.e., severe pain, persistent vomiting with feculent vomitus, marked abdominal distention, or the cessation of bowel movements and flatus), significant volume depletion, or clear-cut dysenteric stools, an office visit is not always necessary.

2. A toxic appearance, scleral icterus, fever, and orthostatic signs should be noted on clinical examination. The presence of marked guarding, referred or rebound pain, a quiet abdomen, or high-pitched rushes suggesting obstruction may warrant an evaluation of an acute surgical abdomen with plain films and a surgical consultation.

3. In the female patient, when the clinical picture is unclear and lower abdominal symptoms are present, a pelvic examination should be performed.

4. Rectal examinations with occult blood testing should almost always be done in patients examined for acute abdominal pain and diarrhea. However, occult or gross blood from concurrent hemorrhoidal bleeding can confuse the picture.

Key Signs

Findings consistent with a nonsurgical abdomen
- Mild tenderness
- Soft abdomen
- Hyperactive bowel sounds
- Absence of peritoneal signs

Laboratory Tests

1. For those patients examined, all that is usually necessary as the initial laboratory work-up of acute diarrhea is stool testing for occult blood and fecal white cell smears. Methylene blue–stained fecal smears are positive for white cells in approximately two thirds of invasive or dysenteric diarrheas. The finding of 25 or more white blood cells per high-powered field correlates well with the presence of bacterial pathogens. Alternatively, a Gram's stain of a thin fecal smear can be just as satisfactory for counting cells.

2. In the United States, when a patient is acutely ill with diarrhea, cultures are not generally necessary or cost-effective unless the diarrhea lasts more than 7 to 10 days. Stools for ova and parasite determinations can be delayed for at least the first few weeks of an illness, and then three separate specimens should be evaluated by an experienced, reliable laboratory. Giardia antigen testing on fresh stool is now available and is more sensitive and less expensive than ova and parasite evaluations. A freshly passed specimen for *C. difficile* toxin assay (rather than culture) can be obtained in the appropriate setting. For HIV-positive patients, diarrhea persisting more than five to seven days usually warrants a more comprehensive initial laboratory evaluation, including stool culture for enteric pathogens, ova and parasite determinations, and acid-fast smears that can identify mycobacteria and cryptosporidia.

3. Sigmoidoscopy has no place in the routine office management of acute diarrhea in uncomplicated cases. One exception is diarrhea occurring within four weeks following antibiotic therapy, when antibiotic-associated pseudomembranous colitis can be diagnosed endoscopically by recognizing the characteristic whitish-yellow membranes. Sigmoidoscopy or colonoscopy is indicated in cases of persistent diarrhea in HIV-positive patients whose bacterial cultures, *C. difficile* toxin assays, and ova and parasites determinations have been unrevealing.

Key Test

- Stool white cell smear
A specimen of stool obtained from a rectal swab or freshly passed stool is thinly smeared on a glass slide and flooded with two or three drops of methylene blue and allowed to stain the white cell nuclei for three or four minutes. The polymorphonuclear plus mononuclear cells (nuclei) per high-powered field are counted. More than 25/HPF are consistent with dysentery.

Differential Diagnosis

1. Figure 231–1 outlines a practical approach to the differential diagnosis for the patient presenting with acute diarrhea. Once surgical problems and other non-infectious etiologies have been considered and satisfactorily ruled out, the algorithm helps to direct diagnostic and therapeutic decisions.

2. More than 60 per cent of cases in the United States are due to a viral etiology. Norwalk and related viruses attack older children and adults, often causing outbreaks in the household or workplace. Rotaviruses are the most common cause of watery diarrhea in children and in adults in contact with children.

3. Twenty-five to 30 per cent of the cases of infectious

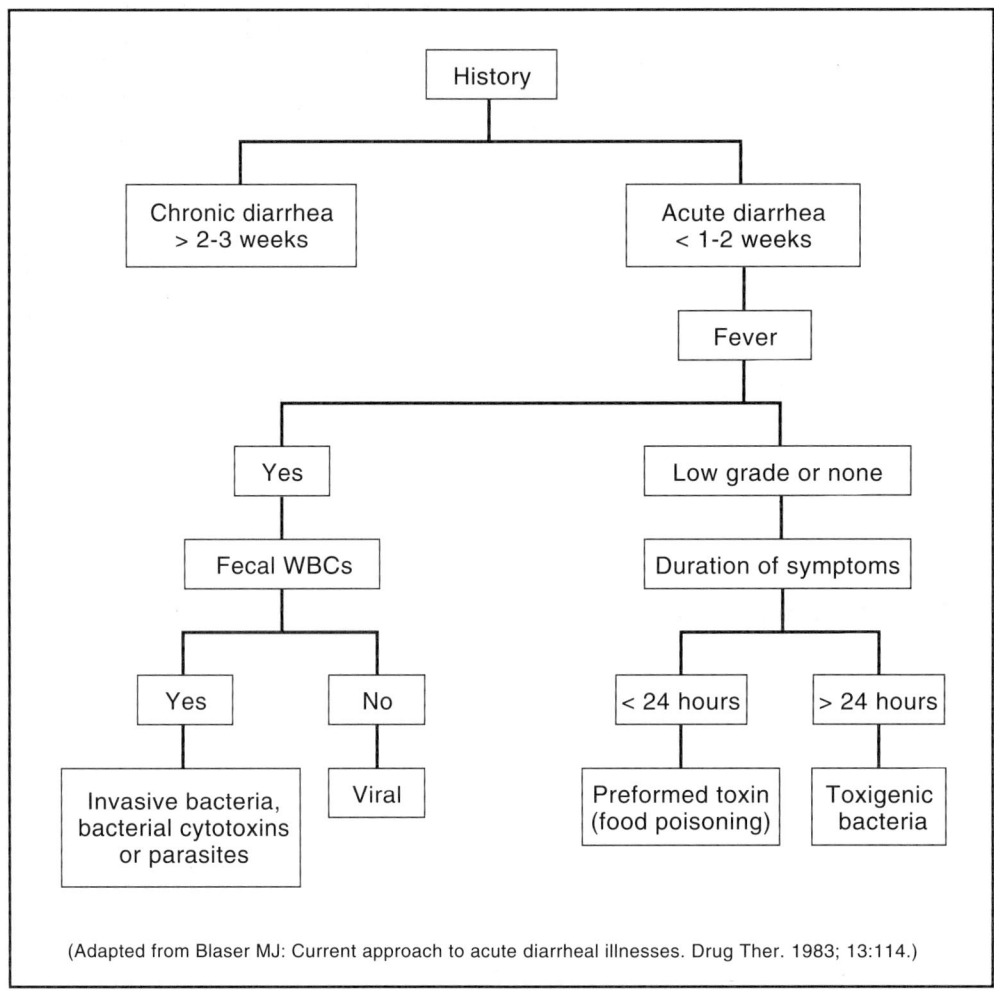

(Adapted from Blaser MJ: Current approach to acute diarrheal illnesses. Drug Ther. 1983; 13:114.)

Figure 231–1 Diagnostic approach to acute diarrheal illnesses. (Adapted from Blaser MJ: Current approach to acute diarrheal illnesses. Drug Ther 1983;13:114.)

diarrhea in patients older than 6 months are caused by the invasive enteropathogens *Campylobacter, Shigella,* and *Salmonella.* Less frequently, *Yersinia enterocolitica,* enterohemorrhagic *E. coli* (serotype 0157), *Aeromonas hydrophila,* and *Plesiomonas* species are isolated. *Vibrio* species are now causing isolated cases in individuals exposed to seafood from the Gulf Coast of the United States.

4. Although many epidemiologic associations (particularly foods) have been documented in texts and medical literature, such information is rarely useful clinically. The incubation period of agents causing acute infectious diarrhea ranges from a few hours to 2 weeks; yet patients tend to associate their illness with foodstuffs eaten just before the onset of symptoms.

Treatment

1. Since the majority of cases of endemic diarrhea will not respond to antibiotic therapy, becoming adept at *treating symptoms* will provide more rapid comfort to patients and minimize absenteeism from work or school and decompensation of underlying medical problems.

   a. *Adsorbents* such as attapulgite (Kaopectate) will firm up stools but do not decrease total stool

volume and so have little to offer from a practical standpoint. Currently they are the only agents available for use by pregnant women.

   b. Bismuth subsalicylate (Pepto-Bismol) is an *antisecretory* agent that also has antibacterial properties. It is useful for reducing the amount of watery diarrhea by about 50 per cent. Co-administration of salicylates should be avoided to prevent salicylism. A black tongue and dark stools usually develop.

   c. The *antiperistaltic agents,* which include codeine, paregoric, and the synthetic opioids loperamide HCL (Imodium) and diphenoxylate HCL with atropine sulfate (Lomotil), are the most active and useful for diminishing abdominal cramps as well as reducing the number of stools. Anticholinergics (e.g., atropine) have no demonstrated role in the treatment of diarrhea and so the safety and side-effect profile makes loperamide currently the agent of first choice. Recent studies in travelers' diarrhea confirm the utility and safety of loperamide even in the presence of bacterial pathogens. Patients with low-grade fever (<101.5° F) and occult blood–positive stool that grew *Shigella* and *Campylobacter* responded well. *Salmonella* carriage may occasionally be prolonged by antiperistaltic agents, but clinical deterioration is rare. These agents should be avoided in toxic-appearing patients with high fevers and grossly bloody stools lest they contribute to the development of a toxic megacolon.

2. The *antibiotics* of choice for empiric therapy in adult patients ill with fever and dysentery are the quinolones: ciprofloxacin HCL (Cipro), norfloxacin (Noroxin—unlabeled use), and ofloxacin (Floxin). Although antibiotic therapy for three days shortens clinical illness in *Campylobacter* and *Shigella* infections and shortens intestinal shedding and communicability in *Shigella* infections, no therapy has a beneficial effect in nontyphoidal *Salmonella* enteritis, and antibiotics may prolong fecal carriage. *Salmonella typhi* infection (typhoid fever) should always be treated, as should patients with bacteremic *Salmonella* infections with nontyphoidal strains, which can occur in 5 per cent of those with gastroenteritis. Those at risk of bacteremic complications include individuals with lymphoproliferative disorders, sickle cell anemia, prosthetic heart valves, aortic aneurysms, and HIV infection. Due to resistance, ampicillin and trimethoprim/sulfamethoxazole are no longer predictably active against *Shigella* and *Salmonella* and are never effective for *Campylobacter.* If cultures and antibiotic sensitivities are available, they can be used to specifically direct therapy for a duration of no more than 3 to 5 days. Antibiotics have no benefit in hemorrhagic colitis caused by EHEC, and there is some concern that they may predispose to the development of the hemolytic-uremic syndrome.

3. In antibiotic-induced pseudomembranous colitis due to *Clostridium difficile* infection, discontinuing the offending antibiotic may be all that is necessary to treat mild episodes. Although bile-acid–binding resins such as cholestyramine (Questran—unlabeled use) and colestipol HCL (Colestid—unlabeled use) may be effective in binding toxin and improving mild cases, metronidazole (Flagyl; Protostat—unlabeled use) or oral vancomycin (Vancocin, Vancoled) is recommended in moderate to severe cases. Metronidazole is much less expensive and currently is the drug of choice.

Diet
1. Avoiding lactose-containing foods (especially milk, cheese, and ice cream) may decrease bloating, flatulence, and diarrhea. Infectious diarrhea can lead to lactase depletion in the intestinal epithelium of the proximal small bowel, lasting for days to weeks.

2. Caffeine stimulates intestinal motility and should also be avoided initially. Coffee, chocolate, nonherbal teas, and caffeinated sodas are included.

3. Hydration with broth, clear juices (containing no pulp), herbal teas, and commercial electrolyte/glucose solutions (Gatorade) is recommended, especially with high fever and profuse diarrhea.

4. Low-residue, carbohydrate-rich foods are the main-

stay of nutrition once vomiting has ceased: noodles, rice, boiled or baked potatoes, and breads.

5. As diarrhea ceases, cooked vegetables, broiled or baked poultry, and fish can be reintroduced.

6. Meats, raw fruit and vegetables, and lastly lactose-containing diary foods are reintroduced as tolerated.

7. Temporarily stopping diuretics may also be necessary.

Activity
Fever, malaise, myalgias, and abdominal discomfort will generally limit the patient's activities, including work. Control of diarrhea and cramping with dietary measures and antiperistaltic agents will allow early return to usual daily activities once a patient is confident that immediate access to the bathroom is not necessary. Food handlers should be culture negative before returning to work after bacterial enteritis has been documented.

Patient Education
1. Avoidance of high-risk foods (unpasteurized dairy products, raw eggs, undercooked poultry and raw seafood from risky sources) may prevent infectious diarrheal illness.

2. Reminding patients of the need for hand washing after bathroom use is important to minimize family and other point source outbreaks.

3. Educating patients about the use of OTC antidiarrheal agents and dietary restrictions may allow them to manage mild, uncomplicated illnesses without physician involvement.

 Key Treatment

Symptomatic Therapy
- Bismuth Subsalicylate (Pepto-Bismol), 30 cc or two tabs q 30 min up to maximum of eight doses
- Loperamide HCl (Imodium), 4 mg initially; 2 mg after each loose stool, not to exceed 16 mg/D

Antibiotic Therapy—Empiric
- Ciprofloxacin HCL, 500 mg PO b.i.d. × 3D
- Norfloxacin HCL, 400 mg PO b.i.d. × 3D
- Ofloxacin, 200 mg PO b.i.d. × 3D
  (Quinolones should not be given to prepubertal children or to pregnant or lactating women.)

Difficile Enterocolitis
- Metronidazole, 250 mg PO b.i.d. for 10 to 14 days
- Vancomycin, 125 mg PO q.i.d. for 10 to 14 days

 Bibliography

Besser RE, et al: An outbreak of diarrhea and hemolytic uremic syndrome from *Escherichia coli* 0157:H7 in fresh-pressed apple cider. JAMA 1993;269(17):2217.

Blaser MJ: Current approach to acute diarrheal illnesses. Drug Ther 1983;13:114.

DuPont HL: Infectious diarrhea: From *E. coli* to *Vibrio.* Patient Care 1991(May) pp 18–43.

Fekety R, Shah AB: Diagnosis and treatment of *Clostridium difficile* colitis. JAMA 1993;269(1):71.

Goodman LJ, et al: Empiric antimicrobial therapy of domestically acquired acute diarrhea in urban adults. Arch Intern Med 1990;150:541.

232 Cellulitis

Carol L. Ellis

Etiology

1. Cellulitis is an acute infection of the skin and subcutaneous tissues. It may arise from
   a. Entry of bacteria through a disruption in the integrity of the skin (i.e., a laceration, puncture wound, or fungal intertrigo)
   b. Extension from a contiguous focus (i.e., an abscess)
   c. Metastatic dissemination from bacteremia (e.g., pneumococcal cellulitis)
2. Cellulitis is a serious disease because of the propensity of infection to spread via the lymphatics and blood stream, especially in patients with chronic edema.
3. Certain conditions appear to predispose to cellulitis including
   a. Prior trauma
   b. An underlying skin lesion
   c. Diabetes
   d. Pedal edema
   e. Venous and lymphatic compromise (e.g., saphenous venectomy for bypass surgery)
4. Causative organisms
   a. Group A β-hemolytic *Streptococcus* and *Staphylococcus aureus* are responsible for the majority of cases. Streptococci of other groups (groups C, G, B) may occasionally be causal.
   b. In immunocompromised or granulocytopenic patients, gram-negative rods (e.g., *Serratia, Proteus, Enterobacter*) and fungi (*Cryptococcus neoformans*) may be the etiologic agents.
   c. In persons handling fish, meat, or poultry, *Erysipelothrix rhusiopathiae* may be the cause of a cellulitis that begins on the hands.
   d. *Aeromonas hydrophila,* a gram-negative bacillus found in lakes, rivers, and soil may cause cellulitis by contaminating an open wound in fresh water; salt water wounds exposed to *Vibrio* (e.g., *V. vulnificus, V. alginolyticus, V. parahaemolyticus*) can progress to cellulitis, necrosis, and bacteremia.

Symptoms

1. Within several days of the inciting trauma, local tenderness, pain, swelling, and erythema develop, rapidly intensify, and spread.
2. Fever, chills, and malaise may be present.

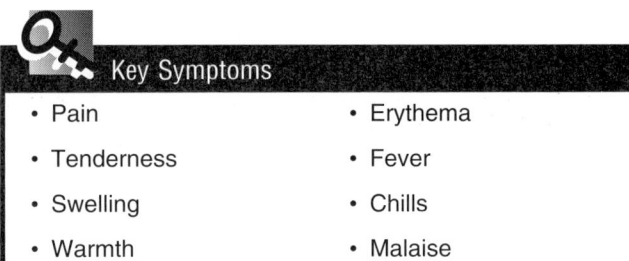

Key Symptoms

• Pain	• Erythema
• Tenderness	• Fever
• Swelling	• Chills
• Warmth	• Malaise

Clinical Findings

1. Erythema with indistinct margins, warmth and tenderness of the skin
2. Regional lymphadenopathy is common; bacteremia can occur, and some patches of overlying skin may necrose.

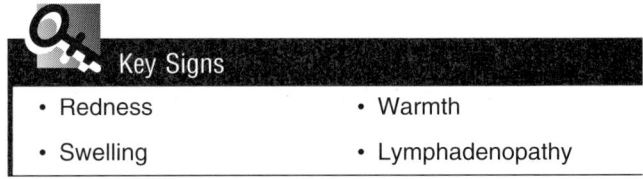

Key Signs

• Redness	• Warmth
• Swelling	• Lymphadenopathy

Laboratory Tests

1. Laboratory tests add little to the management of the typical patient; identification of the infecting organism is usually not obtained and may not be necessary.
2. Blood cultures and skin site cultures may prove helpful in guiding antibiotic therapy in patients who
   a. Fail to respond to standard therapy
   b. Have serious underlying medical problems
   c. Have ulcers or abscesses that could yield microorganisms

Differential Diagnosis

1. Erysipelas is superficial cellulitis involving skin but not soft tissue. It is characterized by bright red color and a raised advancing border and caused by the same pathogens that produce other types of cellulitis.
2. It is important to differentiate cellulitis from skin infections that are rapidly progressive and cause tissue necrosis, such as necrotizing fasciitis or gas gangrene, where drainage and debridement will be required.
3. Cellulitis of the lower extremity in older patients is frequently complicated by deep vein thrombosis.
4. Diffuse inflammatory carcinoma of the breast and cutaneous neoplasms may look like cellulitis.

Treatment

Medication

Presumptive antibiotic therapy to cover streptococci and staphylococci is generally the appropriate choice.

1. Outpatient treatment:

    a. A reasonable option if the cellulitis is limited and if the patient is not seriously ill and is without comorbid conditions.

        (1) A penicillinase-resistant oral penicillin: Dicloxacillin (Dynapen), 500 mg to 1 gm q.i.d., or

        (2) A first-generation cephalosporin: cephalexin (Keflex), 500 mg q.i.d.

    b. For penicillin allergic patients: erythromycin, 500 mg q.i.d.

    c. For sicker patients: ceftriaxone (Rocephin) 1 gm intramuscularly daily for the first few days

    d. Duration of therapy: 10 to 14 days

2. Inpatient treatment:

    a. When intravenous antibiotics are needed

        (1) Nafcillin (Nafcil, Unipen) 1 to 2 gm intravenously q 4 hr

        (2) Cefazolin (Ancef), 2 gm intravenously q 6 hr

    b. For immunocompromised patients:

        (1) Ticarcillin/clavulanate (Timentin), 3.1 gm q 6 hr

        (2) Cefoxitin (Mefoxin), 1 gm q 6 hr

3. Atypical cellulitis

    a. *Erysipelothrix*: penicillin

    b. *Vibrio* species: aminoglycosides and tetracyclines

    c. *Aeromonas hydrophila*: aminoglycosides and chloramphenicol

Activity

1. Immobilization and elevation of an affected limb may be helpful initially.

2. Moist heat may serve to localize the infection.

Patient Education

The goal of education is to prevent recurrences. Use of support stockings, good skin hygiene, and foot care can reduce or eliminate recurrences.

Follow-Up

1. Follow-up is needed to ensure eradication of the infection.

2. *Tinea* skin infection, when present, should be treated with topical antifungal creams such as miconazole.

3. Long-term low-dose daily antibiotic therapy (e.g., penicillin G, 250 to 500 mg orally b.i.d.) may be effective in selected patients with frequent recurrences.

Bibliography

Baddour L: Primary skin infections in primary care: An update. Infect Med 1993;10(9):42–48.

Hanson P, Standridge J, et al: Freshwater wound infection due to *Aeromonas hydrophila.* JAMA 1977;238:10.

Lindbeck G, Powers R: Cellulitis. Hosp Pract 1993;28(suppl 2):10–14.

Swartz M: Cellulitis and superficial infections. *In* Mandel G (ed): Principles and Practice of Infectious Disease. Churchill Livingstone, 1990, pp 796–807.

Weekly CPC: N Engl J Med 1989;321(15):1029–1038.

233 Varicella Infections

Virginia E. Robertson

Etiology

1. Varicella zoster virus (VSV) of Herpesviridae family
2. VSV causes two distinct clinical presentations.
   a. The primary infection is *chickenpox*.
   b. Reactivation causes *herpes zoster* (shingles).
3. Transmission occurs through close contact with a VZV-infected person.
   a. Chickenpox may be acquired by
      (1) Inhalation of aerosolized respiratory droplets
      (2) Direct contact with open shingle lesions
      (3) Maternal-fetal transmission via placenta
   b. VSV becomes latent in dorsal root ganglia after primary infection, re-emerging as shingles when the immune system wanes with age or other disease.

Chickenpox

Epidemiology

The primary infection is commonly a disease of childhood.

1. Equally distributed between genders and races
2. Endemic, with peaks during late winter and early spring
3. Secondary attack rates range between 60 and 90 per cent
4. Incubation is 14 to 15 days (range 10 to 20)
5. Infectious period begins 48 hours before onset of clinical symptoms and persists through the period of new lesion formation (3 to 5 days).

Symptoms

1. A prodrome of low-grade fever and general malaise may precede the defining rash by 1 to 2 days.
2. The classic rash begins as scattered small vesicles with erythematous bases, seen first on the trunk or face.
   a. The lesions spread centrifugally to involve all skin surfaces and possibly mucous membranes (lips, vulva).
   b. The lesions are pruritic; many patients will scratch.
   c. Intact and ruptured vesicles will be present simultaneously; scratching may yield excoriations and superficial skin infections.
3. Constitutional symptoms may occur, especially in older patients, or the patient may be otherwise asymptomatic.
   a. Mild anorexia, listlessness
   b. Low-grade fever, 100° to 103° F
   c. Myalgias or headaches

4. In an older or immunocompromised patient, symptoms present similarly, but expect an increased number of lesions, possible hemorrhagic bases, and more severe constitutional symptoms.

Key Symptoms

- Vesiculopapular rash
- Centrifugal spread of lesions
- Pruritus
- Mild constitutional symptoms

Clinical Findings

1. The classic description of the lesion is a "dewdrop on a rose petal," corresponding to a clear vesicle on erythematous base.
2. As rash spreads, multiple stages of lesions will be present simultaneously in a random, nonclustered pattern.
   a. New clear vesicles, 3 to 5 mm in diameter
   b. Older, cloudy-looking vesicles
   c. Recently ruptured or excoriated lesions
   d. Healing bases
3. Excoriations if scratching is prominent
4. Possible superinfected lesions
5. Evidence of constitutional symptoms
6. New lesions cease appearing within 3 to 5 days (range 3 to 7)
7. In utero infection yields various fetal malformations.

Key Signs

- "Dewdrop" vesicular lesions
- Multiple stages of lesions simultaneously
- Evidence of systemic illness in some patients

Laboratory Tests

1. Diagnosis usually rests on history of exposure, symptoms, and signs.
2. In difficult cases, possible serum studies include
   a. Acute and convalescent varicella serum titers
   b. Enzyme-linked immunosorbent assay, direct fluorescent antibody, or other radioassays
3. Direct skin studies may include
   a. Tzanck smear of unroofed lesion to look for multinucleated giant cells (Wright or Giemsa stains)

b. Tissue culture systems

c. Skin biopsy

d. Gram's stain/bacterial cultures of superinfected lesions

Key Tests

- None usually required

- Consider serum titers, Tzanck smear, or skin biopsy

Differential Diagnosis

1. Atypical measles

2. Impetigo

3. Herpes simplex virus

4. Enteroviral infections, usually group A coxsackieviruses

Complications

1. In adolescent and older patients or those in an immunocompromised state (lymphoreticular cancer, HIV), complications are more common and may necessitate hospitalization and treatment.

2. Complications include

   a. Visceral VZV, especially pneumonia; also nephritis, myocarditis, arthritis

   b. Neurologic VZV or sequelae: meningitis, encephalitis, transverse myelitis, optic neuritis

   c. Superinfections of the skin lesions, with cellulitis

   d. Hematologic complications: thrombotic thrombocytopenic purpura, purpura fulminans

---

WARNING

Reye's syndrome has been associated with aspirin use during varicella infection in children. No aspirin or aspirin-containing product should be used.

Treatment

Symptomatic therapy alone is needed by most patients.

1. Keeping lesions clean is crucial: Use mild soap for bathing, trim fingernails, and wash hands often.

2. Antipruritic measures include

   a. Lukewarm baths with colloidal oatmeal or baking soda

   b. Calamine, oatmeal, other topical anti-itch lotions

   c. Oral antihistamines may be useful

      (1) Diphenhydramine: in children, 5 mg/kg/24 hours given q 6 hr; in adults, 10 to 50 mg t.i.d. or q.i.d.

      (2) Hydroxyzine: in children, 2 mg/kg/24 hours given q 6 hr; in adults, 25 to 200 mg t.i.d. or q.i.d.

3. Control fever with acetaminophen. See warning box.

4. Antiviral therapy should be reserved for those who are at risk for more symptomatic or complicated chickenpox: immunocompromised individuals, older patients, and possibly secondary cases.

   a. In children 2 to 12 years old, acyclovir (Zovirax), 20 mg/kg q.i.d. for 5 days (max 800 mg/day) initiated within 24 hr

   b. In patients older than 12 years, give acyclovir 800 mg orally 5 times a day for 7 days.

   c. Consider intravenous acyclovir in immunocompromised patients.

Activity

Quarantine until all lesions heal to minimize transmission of varicella.

Patient Education

1. Reassurance of generally benign and limited course

2. Emphasize keeping lesions clean.

3. Inform family of expected secondary outbreaks and incubation period for susceptible individuals.

4. Ask about immunocompromised household/close contacts, consider prophylaxis.

5. Warning signs of complications: change in mental status, dyspnea, shortness of breath

6. Avoid use of aspirin.

Key Treatment

- Symptomatic therapy

- Acyclovir in selected populations

Prevention

1. Consider prophylaxis of susceptible high-risk individuals: Varicella zoster immunoglobulin (VZIG) is given up to 96 hours after exposure to prevent or reduce illness.

2. In hospital settings, or for hospital workers, isolation through the potential infectious period is recommended.

3. Varicella immunization (Varivax) is now recommended for all who have not had chickenpox.

   a. Age 1 to 12 years 0.5 ml Varivax subcutaneously

   b. Adults and adolescents ≥13 years old, two 0.5 ml doses 4 to 8 weeks apart

Follow-Up

1. As needed if complications arise

2. Chickenpox is a reportable disease.

Shingles

Epidemiology

Shingles is seen primarily in the elderly or in the immunocompromised, especially those with HIV or lymphoreticular malignancies.

1. Incidence does not vary with gender or race
2. Endemic without periods of epidemicity
3. May be seen in young children whose mothers had chickenpox during pregnancy (early reactivation)

Symptoms

1. Pain typically precedes any skin manifestations by several days.
   a. Pain is sharp or lancinating and often severe.
   b. Dermatomal distribution may or may not be recognized.
   c. Hyperesthesia of the area may be present.
2. The rash begins as erythematous maculopapules which become vesiculated in 12 to 24 hours; linear clustering is evident.
   a. Weeping and subsequent crusting occurs over 10 to 12 days.
   b. Resolution of the crusts, often with scarring, occurs within 2 to 3 weeks.
3. Pain during and after the rash is often remarkable.

Key Symptoms

- Erythematous vesicular rash
- Pain before, during, and after rash
- Dermatomal distribution

Clinical Findings

1. In the absence of the rash, pain and hyperesthesia may not be associated with specific clinical findings.
2. Defining rash: clear vesicles on an erythematous base clustered in a linear region along a unilateral dermatome and associated with pain. The appearance of the lesions may become
   a. Umbilicated and cloudy or frankly pustular
   b. Hemorrhagic
   c. Weeping
3. The rash characteristically stops at the midline.
4. Adjacent dermatomes may be involved.

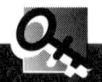

Key Signs

- Erythematous vesicular rash
- Dermatomal distribution
- Unilateral, clustered lesions

Laboratory Tests

1. Diagnosis is usually made on clinical findings.
2. Direct skin tests may include
   a. Tzanck smear of unroofed lesion to examine for multinucleated giant cells (Wright or Giemsa stain)
   b. Skin biopsy

Key Laboratory Tests

- None usually required
- Consider Tzanck smear or skin biopsy

Complications

1. These are more likely in some immunocompromised patients. Patients with HIV, however, do not appear to have more complications, although shingles is common.
2. Complications include
   a. Disseminated shingles
   b. Visceral VZV—pneumonia
   c. Multiple neurologic manifestations can occur
      (1) Cranial nerve palsies
      (2) Motor weakness, transverse myelitis
      (3) Encephalitis, cerebral vasculitis
   d. Superinfections of lesions
   e. Persistent radicular pain after the rash heals, called *postherpetic neuralgia*

Differential Diagnosis

1. Before rash erupts, there may be a wide differential for the pain, given location, severity, and coincident symptoms.
2. The rash may resemble that of herpes simplex.

Treatment

For most patients the major emphasis should be symptomatic relief and prevention of secondary skin infections.

1. Keeping lesions clean is critical, using appropriate measures such as soothing cleansing soaks with Burow's solution.
2. Pain management depends on severity
   a. Simple analgesics such as acetaminophen or ibuprofen
   b. Narcotic analgesics such as Demerol or dilaudid
   c. Radicular nerve blocks
   d. Transcutaneous electrical nerve stimulation (TENS)
   e. Consider consultation for managing pain
3. Antiviral agents may be initiated depending on patient characteristics; the route will depend on severity.
   a. For mild to moderate cases:

(1) Famciclovir (Famvir) 500 mg t.i.d. for 7 days may decrease postherpetic neuralgia

(2) Oral acyclovir (Zovirax), 800 mg five times a day for 7 to 10 days

b. For severe cases:

(1) Intravenous acyclovir, 12.4 mg/kg (1-hr infusion) q 8 hr for 5 to 7 days

(2) Intravenous vidarabine (Vira-A), 10 mg/kg/day (12-hr infusion) for 5 to 7 days

4. Postherpetic neuralgia may be severe and linger over months.

a. Tricyclic antidepressants

b. Ongoing TENS

c. Topical capsaicin cream

Activity

Quarantine until all lesions heal to minimize transmission of varicella.

Patient Education

1. Education and involvement of the patient in pain management issues, especially postherpetic neuralgia, is helpful.

2. Notification of possible transmission of varicella to susceptible contacts (will manifest in secondary cases as chickenpox)

3. Expect scarring.

Key Treatment

- Symptomatic care
- Acyclovir in selected populations

Follow-Up

1. As needed, if complications arise
2. Ongoing pain management when appropriate
3. Consider VZIG prophylaxis of susceptible high-risk contacts.

Bibliography

Enders G, Miller E, et al: Consequences of varicella and herpes zoster in pregnancy: Prospective study of 1739 cases. Lancet 1994;343:1548–1551.

Lieu TA, Cochi SL, et al: Cost-effectiveness of a routine varicella vaccination program for US children. JAMA 1994;271(5):375–381.

Pastuszak AL, Levy M, et al: Outcome after maternal varicella infection in the first 20 weeks of pregnancy. N Engl J Med 1994;330(13):901–905.

Whitley RJ: Varicella-zoster virus. *In* Mandell GL, Douglas RG, and Bennett JE: Principles and Practice of Infectious Diseases, 4th ed. New York, Churchill Livingstone, 1995, pp 1345–1351.

Wood MJ, Johnson RW, et al: A randomized trial of acyclovir for 7 days or 21 days with and without prednisolone for treatment of acute herpes zoster. N Engl J Med 1994;330(13):896–900.

234 Rubella

Joseph V. Connelly

Etiology

1. Rubella (German measles) is caused by the rubella virus. Although it is usually a mild illness, it can cause devastating consequences to the fetus when it is acquired during pregnancy.
2. Humans are the only known host for the virus. There is no vector transmission.
3. Transmission is probably via respiratory droplets. Patients are most contagious when the rash is erupting, but viral shedding occurs from 10 days prior to 15 days after the onset of the rash.
4. Incubation period is 18 ± 3 days.
5. The disease is most commonly seen in the winter and spring.

Symptoms

1. Symptoms, if present at all, are usually mild.
2. Prodromal symptoms, when they occur, precede the rash by one to five days.
3. During the exanthem period there may be mild pruritus from the rash or a low-grade fever. Other symptoms usually disappear after the first day of the rash.

Key Symptoms

- Eye pain
- Sore throat
- Headache
- Malaise
- Upper respiratory complaints

Clinical Findings

Postnatal Infection

1. Lymphadenopathy
   a. Begins 1 to 5 days before the rash
   b. Along with generalized lymphadenopathy, suboccipital and postauricular nodes are characteristically involved.
   c. May be the only sign of infection
2. Rash
   a. Appears first on face then progresses down the body
   b. Maculopapular. Lesions are discrete (not confluent); however, they sometimes coalesce on the trunk.
   c. Lasts 3 to 5 days
   d. Sometimes desquamates during convalescence
3. Occasionally an enanthem, consisting of petechial lesions on the soft palate, occurs at the same time as the exanthem.

4. Mild conjunctivitis
5. Fever
   a. Low-grade or absent
   b. Resolves by first day of rash
6. Complications are rare but may include
   a. Arthritis and arthralgia: more common in adult women
   b. Thrombocytopenia or leukopenia
   c. Encephalitis (very rare)

Key Signs: Postnatal

- Lymphadenopathy (suboccipital and postauricular)
- Maculopapular rash
- Enanthem
- Conjunctivitis
- Low-grade fever

Congenital Infection

1. The manifestations are most severe the earlier in pregnancy the illness occurs.
2. Fetal death, premature delivery, and many congenital abnormalities may result. These include
   a. Nerve deafness (80 to 90 per cent frequency)
   b. Growth retardation (50 to 85 per cent)
   c. Cataracts and/or retinopathy (35 per cent each)
   d. Patent ductus arteriosus (30 per cent)
   e. Pulmonary artery stenosis (25 per cent)
   f. Neurologic abnormalities including mental retardation, meningoencephalitis, and behavior disorders (10 to 20 per cent each)
   g. Hepatosplenomegaly (10 to 20 per cent)
   h. Bone lesions (10 to 20 per cent)
   i. Thrombocytopenic purpura (5 to 10 per cent)

Key Signs: Congenital

- Deafness
- Growth retardation
- Cataracts
- Retinopathy
- Congenital heart disease
- Mental retardation

Laboratory Tests

1. Laboratory testing is generally not useful or recommended in diagnosing the acute disease.
2. Viral isolation from nose, throat, urine, or other body fluid is the definitive test for acute or congenital infection.

3. Elevations in rubella IgM antibody can be measured, but false positives frequently occur.

4. Maternal and infant sera may be measured for IgM antibody. Its presence in the infant is highly suggestive of congenital infection.

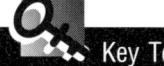
Key Tests

- Usually not necessary for postnatal infection
- Virus isolation for congenital

Differential Diagnosis

1. Enteroviral infections
   a. Shorter incubation period (3 to 7 days)
   b. More common in younger children
   c. Frequently has a higher fever
   d. More common in summer and fall
2. Measles
   a. Frequently has a higher fever
   b. Rash is confluent
3. Scarlet fever
4. Infectious mononucleosis
5. Toxoplasmosis
6. Roseola
7. Erythema infectiosum
8. Drug reactions

Treatment

Symptomatic treatment is given for postnatal infection (e.g., starch baths for pruritus).

Medication

1. Acetaminophen for fever; aspirin for arthralgia
2. Some authors recommend immune globulin for the susceptible pregnant woman with less than 20 weeks gestation who has been exposed within 72 hours.

Diet

No special diet is necessary.

Activity

1. Patients with rubella should not have contact with susceptible persons until 7 days after the onset of the rash.
2. Infants with congenital rubella should be isolated while in the hospital. They should avoid susceptible persons when at home.

Prevention

1. All adults born in 1957 or later should receive one dose of measles, mumps, rubella (MMR) vaccine unless
   a. They can provide proof of one dose of live vaccine having been given on or after their first birthday
   b. They have documentation of physician-diagnosed disease or
   c. They have laboratory evidence of immunity
2. Two doses of MMR vaccine for children
   a. First dose at 15 months of age (12 months for those in high-risk areas).
   b. Second dose prior to school entry
   c. College students, military recruits, and hospital workers born after 1957 should also receive two doses.
   d. Those born in or after 1957 who are traveling to endemic areas should receive two doses.
3. Contraindications to MMR vaccine
   a. Immunocompromised patients (with the exception of HIV patients)
   b. Febrile illness: postpone
   c. Recent reception of blood products or immunoglobulin: postpone for 3 months
   d. Those with a history of anaphylactic reaction after ingestion of eggs or exposure to neomycin should be given the vaccine with extreme caution according to protocols developed for this situation.
   e. Pregnancy
4. All cases should be reported to the appropriate authorities.

Bibliography

Centers for Disease Control and Prevention: Update on Adult Immunization. MMWR 1991;40 (No. RR-12):24–26.

Feigin RD, Cherry JD (eds): Textbook of Pediatric Infectious Disease, 3rd ed. Philadelphia, WB Saunders, 1992, pp 1792–1811.

Krugman S, Katz S: Infectious Diseases of Children, 9th ed. St. Louis, Mosby-Year Book, 1992, pp 381–399.

Mandell GL, Douglas RG Jr, Bennett JE (eds.): Principles and Practice of Infectious Diseases, 4th ed. New York, John Wiley, 1995.

Peter G, et al (eds): 1994 Red Book: Report of the Committee on Infectious Diseases, 23rd ed. Elk Grove Village, Illinois, American Academy of Pediatrics, 1994, pp 406–411.

235 Measles

Joseph V. Connelly

Etiology

1. Measles is caused by the highly contagious rubeola virus.
2. Human beings are the only natural host for the virus.
3. Transmission is by aerosolized respiratory droplets.
4. Incubation period is 10 ± 2 days.
5. Atypical measles characteristically occurs in those previously immunized, particularly with the inactivated (killed) vaccine.

Symptoms

1. Prodromal symptoms of coryza, conjunctivitis, and cough last 2 to 4 days.
2. During the exanthem period, fever peaks on the second or third day of the rash. The conjunctivitis and nasal symptoms decrease as fever defervesces. The cough may persist for several weeks.
3. Atypical measles
   a. High fever
   b. Headache
   c. Abdominal pain
   d. Myalgias
   e. Dry cough
   f. Vomiting
   g. Pleuritic chest pain

Key Symptoms

Prodromal	Exanthem Period
• Coryza	• Fever
• Cough	• Upper respiratory symptoms
• Conjunctivitis	• Cough
• Photophobia	• Sore throat
• General malaise	• Diarrhea
• Fever	• Vomiting
	• Abdominal pain

Clinical Findings

Typical Measles

1. Koplik's spots
   a. Bluish-white papules on a bright red base on the buccal and labial mucosa that appear shortly after the coryza and before the rash
   b. Pathognomonic for measles
2. Rash
   a. Begins at hairline of forehead and behind ears then spreads down the body
   b. Initially erythematous and maculopapular, then becomes confluent in the same progression as the initial spread and resolves in the same manner (from head down)
   c. Begins to fade and turn brown after 3 to 4 days
   d. Duration is 6 to 7 days
3. Other findings may include
   a. Pharyngitis: common
   b. Adenopathy
      (1) Cervical: most common
      (2) Suboccipital and posterior auricular: occasional
   c. Laryngitis
   d. Croup

Atypical Measles

1. Koplik's spots are unusual.
2. Rash
   a. Initially erythematous and maculopapular
   b. First appears on hands and feet, then spreads upward
   c. Particularly prominent on wrists and ankles
3. Pneumonia
4. Pleural effusion
5. Coryza and conjunctivitis are unusual.

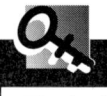

Key Signs

Typical	Atypical
• Koplik's spots	• High fever
• Rash	• Rash
• Pharyngitis	• Pneumonia

Complications

1. Pneumonia
   a. Bronchiolitis in infants
   b. Secondary bacterial infection can occur
2. Otitis media: more common in young children
3. Laryngitis/laryngotracheitis
4. Myocarditis
5. Pericarditis
6. Encephalitis: rare (0.5 to 1 per 1000 cases).
7. Thrombocytopenic purpura
8. Severe, even fatal, complications often occur in the immunocompromised.

9. Not teratogenic, but has been associated with an increased perinatal mortality and spontaneous abortion.

Laboratory Tests

1. Viral culture is the definitive test.
2. The presence of measles-specific IgM antibody is diagnostic.
3. Chest radiograph should be obtained in all cases of atypical measles.
4. Serial antibody titers (HAI or CF) will show a four-fold rise, most dramatically in atypical measles.

Key Test
- Viral culture or antibody titers

Differential Diagnosis

1. Infectious mononucleosis
2. *Mycoplasma pneumoniae* infections
3. Drug eruptions
4. Rocky Mountain spotted fever

Treatment

There is no specific treatment for uncomplicated infection.

Medication

1. Vitamin A, 200,000 IU (60 mg) given on the first 2 days of hospital admission, may reduce morbidity and mortality in children with measles admitted to the hospital for croup, pneumonia, or diarrhea.
2. Acetaminophen for fever, headache, and sore throat
3. Antitussives for cough

Diet

A liberal fluid intake is important.

Activity

1. Should be curtailed while the patient is febrile.
2. Chest radiograph should be used as a guide in determining the level of activity in patients with atypical measles.
3. Patients with measles should not have contact with susceptible persons.

Prevention

1. All adults born in 1957 or later should receive one dose of measles, mumps, and rubella (MMR) vaccine unless

a. They can provide proof of one dose of live vaccine having been given on or after their first birthday.
b. They have documentation of physician-diagnosed disease.
c. They have laboratory evidence of immunity.

2. Two doses of MMR vaccine for children
a. First dose at 15 months of age (12 months for those in high-risk areas)
b. Second dose prior to school entry
c. College students, military recruits, and hospital workers born after 1957 should also receive two doses.
d. Those born in or after 1957 who are traveling to endemic areas should receive two doses.

3. Contraindications
a. Immunocompromised patients (with the exception of HIV patients)
b. Febrile illness: postpone
c. Recent reception of blood products or immunoglobulin: postpone for 3 months
d. Those with a history of anaphylactic reaction after ingestion of eggs or exposure to neomycin should be given the vaccine with extreme caution according to protocols developed for this situation.
e. Pregnancy

4. Immune globulin, 0.25 ml/kg (maximum dose 15 ml), when a susceptible person has a definite exposure.
a. Given within 5 days may prevent infection
b. Given after 5 days will reduce severity
c. Should be administered to HIV-infected children regardless of vaccination status if a definite exposure takes place.

Bibliography

Centers for Disease Control and Prevention: Update on Adult Immunization. MMWR 1991;40 (No. RR-12):19–22.

Feigin RD, Cherry JD (eds): Textbook of Pediatric Infectious Disease, 3rd ed. Philadelphia, WB Saunders, 1992, pp 1591–1605.

Krugman S, Katz S: Infectious Diseases of Children, 9th ed. St. Louis, Mosby-Year Book, 1992, pp 223–244.

Mandell GL, Douglas RG Jr, Bennett JE (eds): Principles and Practice of Infectious Diseases, 4th ed. New York, John Wiley and Sons, 1995.

Peter G, et al (eds): 1994 Red Book: Report of the Committee on Infectious Diseases, 23rd ed. Elk Grove Village, IL, American Academy of Pediatrics, 1994, pp 308–322.

236 Infectious Mononucleosis
William R. Scheibel

Etiology/Epidemiology

A. Most frequently caused by Epstein-Barr virus (EBV)
1. EBV is a double-stranded DNA virus from the herpesvirus family.
2. Humans are the sole source, with transmission by intimate contact.
3. EBV infects epithelial cells of oropharynx, cervix, and resting B lymphocytes, which disseminate throughout the body and proliferate until checked by activated T cells.
   a. Transmission is usually by infected saliva and rarely by blood transfusions or bone marrow transplantation.
   b. Viral excretion occurs for months and asymptomatic carriage is common.
   c. Transmission probably requires repeated and prolonged contact with infected oral secretions, yet few patients can identify a known contact.
4. Incubation period is 3 to 7 weeks.
5. Endemic in children in developing countries; infection delayed until adolescence and adulthood in developed or industrialized countries with high-quality sanitary conditions
6. Reactivation of EBV can occur in transplant or immunocompromised patients only.

B. Infrequent causes (<10 per cent)
1. Cytomegalovirus
2. Human immunodeficiency virus (HIV)
3. *Toxoplasma gondii*
4. Human herpesvirus type 6

Symptoms

1. Wide spectrum of disease from asymptomatic to fulminant infection and even death in immunocompromised patients
   a. Often unrecognized in infants and young children as usually ranges from asymptomatic to a brief febrile illness
   b. Overt illness most common in adolescents and young adults
2. Prodrome of malaise, fatigue, and persistent low-grade headache followed by severe sore throat
   a. Anorexia, myalgias, chills, nausea, abdominal discomfort, cough, or arthralgias may occur.
   b. Acute phase lasts 1 to 3 weeks, with most patients completely recovered by 6 to 8 weeks.

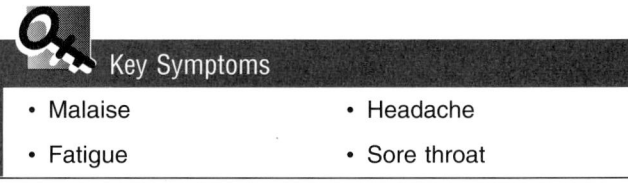

Key Symptoms

• Malaise	• Headache
• Fatigue	• Sore throat

Clinical Findings

1. Severe pharyngitis is the most prominent feature and can be exudative or accompanied by palatine petechiae.
2. Lymphadenopathy more characteristically involves the posterior cervical chain than the anterior cervical chain but can be generalized.
3. Splenomegaly is usually present by the second week.
4. Hepatomegaly, palatal enanthem, rash (usually transient, generalized, and maculopapular), jaundice, and periorbital swelling or palpebral edema may occur.
5. There is little support for EBV now as cause of chronic fatigue syndrome.
6. Complications
   a. Bacterial pharyngitis
   b. Splenic rupture
   c. Upper airway obstruction, pneumonitis
   d. Hematologic with hemolytic anemia, thrombocytopenia or granulocytopenia
   e. Neurologic with seizures, meningoencephalitis, Bell's palsy, Guillain-Barré syndrome, psychosis, and Reye's syndrome
   f. Cardiac with myocarditis or pericarditis
   g. Dermatologic with rash after exposure to ampicillin
   h. Renal with glomerulonephritis
   i. Hepatic with jaundice
   j. Malignant with Burkitt's lymphoma, nasopharyngeal carcinoma, or B lymphoma

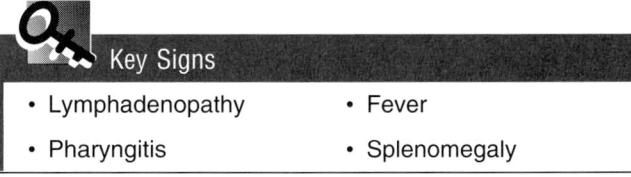

Key Signs

• Lymphadenopathy	• Fever
• Pharyngitis	• Splenomegaly

Laboratory Tests

1. Mild hepatitis with two- to threefold increases of liver enzymes
2. Modest leukocytosis during acute phase
3. Mild reduction of platelet count

4. Positive IgM heterophile antibodies (HA) in 90 per cent of patients by the third week of illness.

5. Other serologic tests are useful when heterophile antibody is absent.

   a. IgM antibodies to EBV viral capsid antigen (anti-VCA) evolve quickly and persist only for weeks to months.

   b. IgG anti-VCA persist lifelong.

   c. IgA anti-VCA are useful in nasopharyngeal carcinoma.

   d. Antibodies to EBV early antigens (anti-EA) are of a diffuse or restricted pattern and appear 2 to 3 weeks after the onset of illness, then peak and gradually decline.

   e. Antibodies to EBV nuclear antigen (anti-EBNA) develop late and persist lifelong.

6. No EBV infection: negative serologic tests

7. Acute EBV infection: positive HA, IgM anti-VCA, IgG anti-VCA, and IgG anti-EA

8. Past EBV infection: positive IgG anti-VCA and anti-EBNA

Key Tests

- Absolute lymphocytosis (>50 per cent)
- Atypical lymphocytes (>10 per cent)
- Presence of heterophile antibodies

Differential Diagnosis

1. Bacterial disease

   a. Exudative pharyngitis with group A β-hemolytic streptococcus

   b. Mycoplasma

   c. Bacteremia

2. Viral infection

   a. *Cytomegalovirus,* toxoplasmosis

   b. Respiratory viruses: influenza, para-influenza, or adenovirus

   c. Viral hepatitis

   d. Rubella, mumps

   e. Human immunodeficiency virus, human herpesvirus type 6

3. Drug reaction

4. Hematologic malignancies: leukemia or lymphoma

Treatment

Medication

1. Uncomplicated acute infectious mononucleosis usually only requires supportive therapy.

   a. Warm salt water or anesthetic (lidocaine 2%, phenol 1.4%) gargles for pharyngitis

   b. Acetaminophen, 650 to 1000 mg every 4 hours for fever or malaise

2. Antibiotic treatment of concomitant group A β-hemolytic *Streptococcus pyogenes*

   a. Penicillin or erythromycin for 10 days are first choices.

   b. Avoid amoxicillin or ampicillin, as they usually produce a morbilliform rash in patients with mononucleosis.

3. Corticosteroids: prednisone, 40 to 80 mg per day and tapering over 5 to 14 days

   a. May shorten duration of fever and pharyngitis in uncomplicated disease

   b. There is concern that corticosteroids may adversely influence long-term immunity to EBV or increase the number of lymphocytes with EBV latent infection.

   c. Can reduce obstructive tonsillar enlargement and may improve autoimmune hemolytic anemia, thrombocytopenia, granulocytopenia, aplastic anemia, encephalitis, or myocarditis

   d. No evidence corticosteroids improve splenomegaly or prevent rupture

4. Acyclovir, ganciclovir, bromovinydecoxyuridine, zidovudine, foscarnet, and human interferon inhibit replication of EBV in vitro.

   a. Acyclovir has little or no clinical benefit in uncomplicated infectious mononucleosis.

   b. Aforementioned agents are used in fulminant infections and immune deficient patients, but benefits may be only transient.

5. Vaccine development with a subunit or inactivated virus vaccine is ongoing.

Activity

1. Limited activity during acute phase, with gradual return to daily activities

2. Restrict strenuous activity to prevent precipitating splenic rupture.

3. No contact sports for 4 weeks, longer if spleen is still palpable or is enlarged on radiologic examination

Patient Education

1. Restricting intimate contact during the acute symptomatic phase may decrease transmission.

2. Isolation is unnecessary, as EBV shedding continues after the acute illness.

3. Acute symptoms usually last 1 to 2 weeks, with resolution of fatigue over 2 to 4 weeks.

Key Treatment

- Uncomplicated acute infectious mononucleosis generally requires only supportive therapy.

- Penicillin or erythromycin is given for concomitant group A β-hemolytic *Streptococcus pyogenes.*

Bibliography

Bailey RE: Diagnosis and treatment of infectious mononucleosis. Am Fam Physician 1994;49(4):879–885.

Chetham MM, Roberts KB: Infectious mononucleosis in adolescents. Pediatr Ann 1991;20:206–213.

Maki DS, Reich RM: Infectious mononucleosis in the athlete. Am J Sports Med 1982;10:162–173.

Straus SE, Cohel JI, Tasato G, Meier J: NIH Conference. Epstein-Barr virus infections: Biology, pathogenesis and management. Ann Intern Med 1993;118:45–58.

Sumaya CV, Ench Y: Epstein-Barr virus infectious mononucleosis in children. I. Clinical and general laboratory findings. II. Heterophile antibody and viral specific responses. Pediatrics 1985;75:1003–1019.

237 Chronic Fatigue Syndrome

Leah B. Kaltman

Historical Information

Historically, chronic fatigue syndrome (CFS) is known by names such as

1. Nervous exhaustion
2. Neurasthenia
3. Icelandic disease
4. Atypical poliomyelitis
5. Acute encephalitis
6. Chronic mononucleosis (chronic Epstein-Barr virus [EBV] infection)

Demographics

1. More than 80 per cent of patients are women.
2. Average age is the late 30s
3. More than 95 per cent of patients are white.

Definition

1. Evolved in the late 1980s
2. Was proposed to describe a symptom complex: a syndrome of unknown cause characterized primarily by chronic fatigue
3. Definition requires both of two major criteria plus eight minor criteria.
   a. Major criteria
      (1) Persistent or relapsing fatigue. Characteristically, the fatigue
         (a) Comes on abruptly, within hours or days
         (b) Frequently follows a virus-like illness
         (c) Reduces daily activity by more than 50 per cent
         (d) Persists for at least 6 months
      (2) Exclusion of other chronic conditions such as
         (a) Malignancy
         (b) Autoimmune disease
         (c) Chronic psychiatric disorders*
         (d) Chronic inflammatory disease
         (e) Chronic infectious states†
         (f) Drug side effects
         (g) Rheumatologic diseases (except fibromyalgia)
         (h) Substance abuse
         (i) Endocrinopathy

   b. Minor criteria: CFS diagnosis requires at least six *symptom* criteria plus at least two *physical* criteria, or at least eight symptom criteria alone.
      (1) Symptom criteria
         (a) Mild fever or chills
         (b) Sore throat
         (c) Painful cervical or axillary adenopathy
         (d) Generalized muscle weakness
         (e) Myalgias
         (f) Prolonged fatigue after previously tolerated physical activity
         (g) Migratory arthralgia without swelling or redness
         (h) Neuropsychologic complaints
         (i) Sleep disturbance
         (j) Generalized headache
         (k) Symptom develops acutely (hours) or subacutely (days)
      (2) Physical criteria
         (a) Low-grade fever
         (b) Nonexudative pharyngitis
         (c) Palpable or tender cervical or axillary lymph nodes

Etiology

Currently the cause is unknown, but suspects include
1. Infection
   a. EBV
   b. Human herpesvirus 6
   c. Enterovirus
   d. Human retrovirus
   e. Other infectious agents
2. Immune dysfunction (attendant, but not known whether cause or effect); reported conditions include
   a. Cellular abnormalities
      (1) Decreased number of natural killer (NK) cells
      (2) Decreased function of NK cells
      (3) Reduced lymphocyte proliferation after mitogen
      (4) Increased production of gamma interferon
      (5) Increased or decreased CD8 suppressor cell population
   b. Humoral abnormalities
      (1) Autoantibodies such as RF, ANA, antithyroid
      (2) Partial hypogammaglobulinemia
      (3) Decreased IgG subclasses

---

*A person can be considered to have CFS if he or she has a diagnosis of *non*psychotic depression, somatization, anxiety disorder, and/or panic disorder.

†Patients with *inadequately* treated Lyme disease should be excluded from diagnosis of CFS; patients with *adequately* treated Lyme disease may be diagnosed with CFS.

  (4) Polyclonal activation of B cells

 c. Other immunologic findings

  (1) History of allergy

  (2) Increased or decreased circulating immune complexes

  (3) Cytokine abnormalities

3. Neurochemical disturbances

Diagnosis

Key Points

- There is no existing laboratory test to confirm CFS.
- Tests should be done solely to exclude other diagnoses as the cause of the patient's syndrome.

1. Routine recommended tests
   a. Urinalysis
   b. Complete blood count with differential
   c. Electrolytes
   d. Thyroid function tests
   e. Erythrocyte sedimentation rate
   f. Antinuclear antibodies
2. Diagnosis as indicated by history and clinical judgment
   a. Digital palpation for tender point sites
   b. Cortrosyn stimulation test
   c. Rheumatoid factor
   d. Immunoglobulin levels
   e. Tuberculin (PPD) test
   f. HIV testing
   g. Lyme serology
   h. Mental health scale

Key Point

- EBV serologic tests are not valid for diagnosis of CFS. There is extensive overlap in antibody levels among patients with CFS, patients with non-EBV disease, and asymptomatic healthy people.

Laboratory Findings

1. Mild leukocytosis or leukopenia
2. Atypical lymphocytosis
3. Relative lymphocytosis
4. Electrolytes usually within the normal range
5. Mild elevation of liver function tests
6. Normal erythrocyte sedimentation rate (ESR) (elevation of ESR suggests other diagnoses)

Differential Diagnosis

1. Autoimmune diseases
2. Malignancies
3. Endocrine diseases (hypothyroidism, Addison's, Cushing's, diabetes mellitus)
4. Chronic inflammatory states (sarcoid, chronic hepatitis B, C, multiple sclerosis)
5. Rheumatologic diseases (Sjögren's syndrome, polymyalgia rheumatica, polymyositis)
6. Chronic psychiatric diseases (major depression, bipolar disorder, schizophrenia)

Treatment

Key Point

- In the absence of therapy proven to be effective for all patients, therapy should be individually tailored and focused on alleviating specific symptoms.

1. Symptomatic treatment

Key Point

- Apparent disturbances in brain neurochemistry may serve as a basis for effectiveness of some antidepressants in some CFS patients. Responses to antidepressants tend to occur at doses lower than those used in major depression.

2. Experimental treatment
   a. Zovirax
   b. Immunoglobulin
   c. Magnesium sulfate therapy
   d. Ampligen
   e. Essential fatty acids
   f. 5-Hydroxytryptophan

Patient Education

1. Support group literature and referral to local support groups
2. Progressive exercise program
3. Nutritional guidance
4. Emphasis on control of symptoms rather than cure

Bibliography

Cho W, Stollerman G: Chronic fatigue syndrome. Hosp Pract 1992;27:221–236.

Klimas N, et al: Immunologic abnormalities in chronic fatigue syndrome. J Clin Microbiol 1990;28(6):1403–1410.

New Jersey Chronic Fatigue Syndrome Center Brochure, Newark, NJ. November 1993.

Schluederberg A, et al: Chronic fatigue syndrome research definition and medical outcome assessment. Ann Intern Med 1992;117(4):325–331.

238 Influenza

John G. Spangler

Etiology

1. Influenza A, B, and C, single-stranded RNA of Orthomyxovirus family; classification based on hemagglutinin and neuraminidase antigens
2. Frequent nuclear rearrangement (antigenic drift and antigenic shift) gives rise to epidemics and pandemic (especially with influenza A)
3. Influenza C is responsible only for mild respiratory illness.

Symptoms

1. Rapid onset of fever and headache
2. Respiratory symptoms such as sore throat, nasal stuffiness, and nonproductive cough (may become productive in setting of bacterial superinfection)
3. Muscle aches and extreme malaise lasting several days

Key Symptoms

- Fever
- Sore throat
- Nasal congestion
- Nonproductive cough
- Muscle aches
- Extreme malaise

Clinical Findings

Uncomplicated Influenza
1. Fever (frequently up to 103° F) for 3 to 5 days
2. Upper respiratory signs including conjunctival injection, nasal discharge, pharyngeal erythema, and cough
3. Mild muscle tenderness to palpation
4. Paucity of pulmonary findings

Primary Influenza Viral Pneumonia
1. Severe, often fatal, disease frequently progressing to adult respiratory distress syndrome (ARDS)
2. Occurs predominantly in younger patients, patients with cardiovascular (especially rheumatic heart) disease, and pregnant women
3. Dyspnea, cyanosis, scant sputum production; occasional crackles

Secondary Bacterial Pneumonia
1. Bacterial superinfection of typical influenza in an elderly or chronically ill patient
2. Purulent sputum production, fever, pleuritic chest pain; localized rales or rhonchi with consolidation

Reye's Syndrome
1. Childhood complication of influenza with cerebral edema, fatty infiltration of the liver, and mental status changes; peak onset at 6 years of age
2. High association with aspirin use during respiratory viral diseases

Key Signs

Uncomplicated Influenza	Secondary Bacterial Pneumonia
• Fever	• Productive cough
• Myalgias	• Localized crackles or rhonchi
• Nonproductive cough	• Pleuritic chest pain
• Few pulmonary findings	
Primary Viral Pneumonia	**Reye's Syndrome**
• Severe dyspnea	• Hepatomegaly (fatty liver)
• Occasional rales	• No jaundice
• Cyanosis	• Mental status changes
• Scant sputum	• Hypoglycemia

Laboratory Tests

1. Viral culture of throat swab or sputum definitive test, but takes 3 to 7 days
2. Rapid test packs available for diagnosis in 10 minutes
3. Serologic diagnosis requires a fourfold rise in complement-fixing antibody titers 2 to 4 weeks after acute illness.
4. Epidemiologic "diagnosis" can be presumed with 85 per cent certainty in setting of documented community outbreak of influenza with presence of fever, cough, and muscle aches
5. Chest radiograph: in primary viral pneumonia, patchy bilateral infiltrates, basilar streaking or ARDS; in secondary bacterial pneumonia, bilateral or unilateral lobar processes
6. Sputum Gram's stain and culture most helpful in secondary bacterial pneumonia, showing *Pneumococcus* and *Staphylococcus* in most cases; *Haemophilus influenzae* and gram-negative rods also common

Key Tests

- Viral culture for definitive diagnosis
- Serology
- Chest film (in complicated influenza)
- Sputum microbiology (in secondary bacterial pneumonia)

Differential Diagnosis

1. Other respiratory viruses (e.g., adenovirus, measles, respiratory syncytial virus)

2. Primary bacterial pneumonias (e.g., *Mycoplasma*, *Pneumococcus*)

3. Rarely, pneumonic forms of *Rickettsia*, plague, or *Hantavirus*

Treatment

Uncomplicated Influenza

1. Bed rest, antipyretics, and cough suppressants

2. Amantadine (Symmetrel) and rimantadine (Flumadine) (both 100 mg b.i.d. for approximately 5 days) can shorten course of influenza A if given within 48 hours of onset of symptoms (renal dosing needed; see Table 238–1)

Complicated Influenza

1. Primary viral pneumonia: intensive care hospitalization to maintain oxygenation

2. Secondary bacterial pneumonia: antibiotic treatment directed at most common organisms (see above)

3. Reye's syndrome: intensive care support to manage hypoglycemia, increased blood ammonia, and cerebral edema

Prevention

Influenza vaccine: goal is to reduce the incidence of lower respiratory tract disease and its complications

1. Inactivated, egg-grown, highly purified vaccine containing two influenza A subtypes and one influenza B subtype; updated annually

2. Contraindicated in anaphylactic egg allergy; patients with acute febrile illnesses should delay vaccination; otherwise, side effects include local pain and swelling, and infrequently fever, malaise, and myalgias

3. Target groups

   a. Persons 65 years old and older

   b. Long-term care facility residents

   c. All persons with cardiopulmonary disease (e.g., valvular heart disease, chronic obstructive lung disease), or chronic metabolic diseases (e.g., diabetes mellitus, sickle cell anemia, Addison's disease)

   d. Children on long-term aspirin (e.g., juvenile rheumatoid arthritis)

   e. Health care workers and others who may transmit influenza to high-risk individuals

   f. Other groups, while not specifically targeted, may also benefit from vaccination including pregnant women (after first trimester), HIV-positive individuals, and foreign travelers.

   g. Except in cases of egg allergy or previous hypersensitivity, the general population may receive vaccination, including children.

   h. Patients unable to tolerate vaccine who are at risk for complicated influenza should be maintained on amantadine prophylaxis (200 mg daily) throughout the influenza season in their community (usually 5 to 6 weeks)

Patient Education

1. Influenza is self-limited in healthy individuals, but its potentially severe consequences must be stressed to elderly or chronically ill patients to ensure their annual vaccination.

2. Patients at risk for severe disease traveling abroad (May to September in Southern Hemisphere; October to April in Northern Hemisphere; year round in tropics) should be vaccinated.

3. Parents must not give aspirin to children during upper respiratory illnesses or chickenpox because of the risk of Reye's syndrome.

Key Treatment

Drug of Choice

• Amantadine or rimantadine (treat only influenza A)

Primary Viral Pneumonia

• Aggressive oxygen support

Secondary Bacterial Pneumonia

• Intravenous antibiotics

Reye's Syndrome

• Maintain euglycemia

• Monitor and treat cerebral edema

TABLE 238–1. AMANTADINE DOSAGE IN RENAL IMPAIRMENT

CREATININE CLEARANCE (ml/minute per 1.73 m²)	MAINTENANCE DOSAGE
≥80	100 mg twice daily
60–79	200 mg/100 mg on alternate days
40–59	100 mg once daily
30–39	200 mg twice weekly
20–29	100 mg 3 times weekly
10–19	200 mg/100 mg alternating every 7 days

From AHFS Drug Information 94, page 395. Copyright American Society of Hospital Pharmacists, Bethesda, MD, 1994. Used with permission.

Follow-Up

Elderly or chronically ill patients require frequent monitoring for prolonged malaise, depression, or pulmonary complications.

Bibliography

For general reference on virology, epidemiology, and clinical aspects of influenza, see

Betts RF: Influenza virus. *In* Mandel GL, Bennett JE, Dolin R (eds): Principles and Practice of Infectious Diseases, 4th ed. New York, Churchill Livingstone, 1995, pp 1546–1567.

For information regarding the use of amantadine, see

American Hospital Formulary Service: Amantadine hydrochloride. *In* AHFS Drug Information 94. Bethesda, MD, American Society of Hospital Pharmacists, 1994, pp 392–395.

For influenza vaccine recommendations, see

Centers for Disease Control and Prevention: Prevention and Control of Influenza. Part I, Vaccines. Recommendations of the Advisory Committee on Immunization Practices (ACIP). MMWR 1994;43:1–13.

For general information regarding Reye's syndrome, see

Quam DA: Recognizing a case of Reye's syndrome. Am Fam Physician 1994;50:1491–1496.

For information on the impact of influenza among the elderly, see

McBean AM, Babish JD, Warren JL: The impact and cost of influenza in the elderly. Arch Intern Med 1993;153:2105–2111.

239 Lyme Disease

Armando Jose Jarquin

Etiology

Lyme disease is caused by the spirochete *Borrelia burgdorferi.*

1. Most common vector-borne disease in the United States
2. Transmitted to human by Ixodes ticks, which are part of the *Ixodes ricinus* complex.
3. White-footed mouse and white-tailed deer are the major animal reservoirs for *B. burgdorferi.*

Symptoms

A. Stage I: early localized infection (1 to 4 weeks after bite)
   1. Erythema migrans (found in 75 per cent of patients)
      a. Mostly asymptomatic; causes burning sensation, itching, or pain in 14 per cent of patients
      b. About one week after bite, lesion appears at the site, which is commonly in the groin or the axilla.
   2. Flu-like symptoms (found in 50 per cent of patients): regional lymphadenopathy, fever, chills, malaise
B. Stage II: early disseminated infection (1 to 6 months)
   1. Persistent malaise and fatigue (most common)
   2. Migratory pain in joints, muscles, and tendons
   3. Intermittent headaches and focal neurologic changes
   4. Occasional palpitations
C. Stage III: late persistent infections (months to years)
   1. Prolonged arthritis and persistent arthralgias (60 per cent of patients)
   2. Joint subluxations or tenderness below lesions of acrodermatitis
   3. Various neurologic changes: ataxic gait, dementia, mood changes, paresthesias

Key Symptoms

- Stage I: fever, chills, malaise
- Stage II: headache, arthralgias, minor neurologic changes
- Stage III: severe fatigue and arthralgias, neurologic deficit

Clinical Findings

A. Stage I manifestations
   1. Erythema migrans: macule or papule enlarging to form annular lesion with red border and central clearing in trunk or extremities
   2. Flu-like symptoms: fever, malaise, myalgia
B. Stage II manifestations
   1. Skin
      a. Worsening erythema migrans (5 to 40 cm in diameter)
      b. Secondary annular skin lesions (17 per cent of patients)
      c. Lymphocytoma (rare, only 1 per cent of patients): red and violet nodule occurring in earlobe or nipple; usually asymptomatic
   2. Musculoskeletal
      a. Fatigue and malaise (most common)
      b. Migratory arthritis
      c. Panniculitis (rare)
   3. Central nervous system (10 to 20 per cent of patients)
      a. Aseptic meningitis, encephalitis
      b. Bell's palsy, peripheral neuropathy
   4. Cardiac (4 to 10 per cent of patients)
      a. First-degree atrioventricular block (PR <0.3 sec)
      b. High-degree atrioventricular block
      c. Myocarditis or, in rare cases, pancarditis
C. Stage III manifestations
   1. Skin
      a. Acrodermatitis chronicum atrophicans (rare): bluish-red discoloration with edema and central areas of atrophy, mostly on lower extremities
      b. Scleroderma-like lesions: sclerotic or fibrotic plaques and subcutaneous nodules around knees and elbows
   2. Musculoskeletal
      a. Prolonged arthritis (associated with HLA DR4 and DR2)
      b. Synovitis, periostitis
      c. Severe fatigue
   3. Central nervous system
      a. Subacute encephalopathy (most common): dementia, sleep disturbance, and mood changes
      b. Axonal polyneuropathy: distal paresthesias and radicular pain

c. Leukoencephalitis (rare): ataxia, cognitive dysfunction, spastic paraparesis, and bladder dysfunction

Key Signs

- Stage I: malaise, expanding macule or papule with central clearing
- Stage II: headache, neuropathies, worsening erythema, palpitations
- Stage III: fatigue, dementia, ataxia, bluish-red lesions with atrophy

Laboratory Tests

1. Detection of specific antibodies to *B. burgdorferi*
   a. Indirect immunofluorescence assay (IFA)
   b. Enzyme-linked immunosorbent assay (ELISA) (in early disease 50 per cent of patients are seronegative; in later stages over 90 per cent are seropositive)
2. Cultures
   a. Blood (about 30 per cent are positive)
   b. CSF (less than 10 per cent are positive)
   c. Erythema migrans biopsy specimens (about 60 per cent are positive)
3. Special silver staining of chronic synovitis shows spirochetes in 33 per cent of patients.

Key Test

- ELISA is preferred, because it is more sensitive and specific. IgM antibody appears first at 2 to 4 weeks after skin lesions, peaks at 6 to 8 weeks, then declines after 4 to 6 months of illness. Persistent IgM suggests recurrent illness. IgG increases later at 6 to 8 weeks of disease, peaks at 4 to 6 months, and remains high indefinitely.

Differential Diagnosis

A. Lyme disease as multisystemic disease
   1. Autoimmune diseases (fibromyalgia, systemic lupus erythematosus, rheumatoid arthritis)
   2. Rocky Mountain spotted fever, rat-bite fever
   3. Chronic fatigue syndrome
   4. Secondary syphilis
B. Dermatologic manifestations
   1. Erythema migrans versus
      a. Insect bites, drug eruptions
      b. Erythema multiforme and tinea corporis
   2. Acrodermatitis chronica atrophicans versus
      a. Venous insufficiency
      b. Arterial insufficiency

c. Stasis dermatitis and scleroderma
   3. Lymphocytoma versus erythema nodosum, rheumatic nodules
C. Neurologic manifestations
   1. Bacterial and viral meningitis
   2. Multiple sclerosis
D. Cardiac manifestations: viral myocarditis

Treatment

Treatment should be given depending on the clinical findings of the disease.

Medication

1. Tetracycline, 500 mg orally q.i.d., or doxycycline, 100 mg orally b.i.d., or amoxicillin, 250 to 500 mg orally t.i.d., or erythromycin, 250 mg orally q.i.d., should be given for
   a. Erythema migrans (10 to 20 days)
   b. First-degree AV block (20 to 30 days)
   c. Arthritis (30 days)
   d. Acrodermatitis atrophicans (30 days)
   e. Bell's palsy (30 days)
2. Ceftriaxone (Rocephin), 2 gm intravenously daily or penicillin G, 20 million units in six divided doses per day intravenously for
   a. Neurologic disease other than Bell's palsy (14 days)
   b. High-degree AV block (14 days)
   c. Persistent arthritis (14 days)

Diet

Unless there is any particular objection, a regular diet should be given. Nasogastric tube feeding may be needed.

Activity

Activity should be undertaken as tolerated. Physical therapy may be needed for arthritis or any neurologic sequelae.

Patient Education

Patient and relatives should be well aware of the nature of this disease and complications.

Key Treatment

Drug of Choice	Alternative Drugs
• Tetracycline, 500 mg PO q 6 hr for 10 to 30 days	• Amoxicillin or erythromycin
	• Nonsteroidal anti-inflammatory drugs should be given for symptoms

Follow-Up

1. Should be individualized depending on the stage of the disease
2. In noncomplicated cases, follow-up as outpatient every week

3. Complicated cases should be hospitalized and seen daily.

 Bibliography

Fitzpatrick TB, Johnson RA, Polano MK, Suurmond D, Wolff K: Color Atlas and Synopsis of Clinical Dermatology, 2nd ed. New York, McGraw-Hill, 1992, pp 360–369.

Rahn DW, Malawista SE: Lyme disease: Recommendations for diagnosis and treatment. Ann Intern Med 1991;114:472–481.

Steere AC: Lyme disease. N Engl J Med 1989; 321:586–595.

Steere AC, Taylor E, McHugh GL, Logigian EL: The overdiagnosis of Lyme disease. JAMA 1993; 269:1812–1816.

Tierney LM Jr, McPhee SJ, Papadakis MA: Current Medical Diagnosis and Treatment. 33rd Annual Revision. East Norwalk, CT, Appleton & Lange, 1994, pp 1176–1179.

240 Salmonellosis

Lisa G. King

Etiology

1. *Salmonella* is a nonencapsulated, gram-negative bacillus.
2. *Salmonella* is transmitted by the fecal-oral route. Poultry, beef, eggs, and milk products are common sources.
3. Those most vulnerable are under 20 or over 70 years of age.

Symptoms

Salmonella infection manifests itself in three clinical syndromes.

1. Gastroenteritis is the most common. "Food poisoning" may be *salmonellosis.* After an incubation period of up to 48 hours, these symptoms begin
   a. An abrupt onset of nausea and vomiting
   b. Crampy abdominal pain
   c. Diarrhea ranging in severity from mild to dysenteric
   d. Self-limited fever

   Healthy adults are symptomatic for 2 to 5 days.
2. Enteric fever (typhoid fever) typically has a 1- to 2-week incubation period during which ingested bacteria penetrate the gut mucosa and travel via the lymphatics into the blood.
   a. The earliest symptoms are headache, malaise, chills, abdominal pain, and a fever, which increases incrementally over a period of days.
   b. After about a week, the fever becomes sustained.
   c. Other manifestations may include constipation or mild diarrhea, anorexia, nausea, vomiting, epistaxis, rose spots, bronchitis, and altered mental status.
3. Bacteremia and focal infections may follow intestinal infection. The symptoms vary with the site of infection, which can be intravascular, skeletal, meningeal,

Key Symptoms

Salmonella Gastroenteritis

- Nausea
- Crampy abdominal pain
- Diarrhea

Enteric Fever

- Fever that increases in a stepwise manner over several days
- A flu-like syndrome

splenic, hepatobiliary, urinary, or pulmonary. Most patients give a history of fever, chills, sweats, and weight loss.

Clinical Findings

1. The gastroenteritis manifests mainly periumbilical or right lower quadrant pain with watery stools that sometimes contain mucus or blood.
2. Enteric fever's primary signs are bradycardia relative to the degree of fever, a musty body odor, and right lower quadrant tenderness. Rose spots are evident on the trunk in over 50 per cent of patients. They appear as erythematous macules up to half a centimeter in diameter, which blanch with pressure.
3. For bacteremia with focal infections, the clinical findings are related to the site of infection.

Key Signs of Enteric Fever

- Prolonged fever
- Relative bradycardia
- Rose spots

Laboratory Tests

1. With gastroenteritis there is usually no leukocytosis, although there may be hemoconcentration. The stool smear will contain leukocytes. By the time a positive stool culture returns, the patient is typically recovering.
2. In enteric fever, blood cultures are usually positive for one to three weeks after symptoms begin. Cultures of stool, urine, and rose spots may increase the diagnostic yield. Bone marrow cultures are the most sensitive; over 90 per cent are positive.
   a. Nonspecific lab abnormalities include anemia, leukopenia to normopenia with relative bandemia, and thrombocytopenia. Bilirubin and aspartate transaminase may be elevated, and disseminated intravascular coagulation may occur. If the patient has diarrhea, the stool may show many leukocytes.
   b. Two thirds of patients have a fourfold or greater elevation in the O or H antibody titers over two to three weeks. This is a positive Widal's test, but it is not diagnostic due to many false positives and negatives.
3. Isolation of *Salmonella* from the blood or site of localized infection confirms the diagnosis in patients with bacteremia and focal infections.

Key Tests

- Diagnosis is based on isolation of organisms from stool, blood, urine, bone marrow, rose spots, or tissue fluid.

Differential Diagnosis

1. For gastroenteritis consider *E. coli, Campylobacter jejuni, Yersinia enterocolitica, Clostridium difficile, Shigella,* viruses, ulcerative colitis, and Crohn's disease.

2. In atypical cases enteric fever may resemble mononucleosis, rickettsiosis, brucellosis, leptospirosis, miliary tuberculosis, *Cytomegalovirus* infection, malaria, viral hepatitis, or lymphoma.

Treatment

Medication

1. Gastroenteritis: Only those who are infants, elderly, immunocompromised, or at increased risk of focal infection should receive antibiotic therapy, because treatment does not alleviate symptoms and may prolong intestinal carriage.

   a. Drug of choice: amoxicillin or ampicillin for 3 to 5 days

   b. Alternative drugs: chloramphenicol or trimethoprim-sulfamethoxazole

2. Enteric fever

   a. Drug of choice: chloramphenicol, 50 mg/kg/day intravenously or orally, in four divided doses for 2 to 4 weeks

   b. Alternative drugs: amoxicillin, also trimethoprim-sulfamethoxazole or ampicillin

3. Systemic infection: Antibiotic therapy must be accompanied by removal of infected tissue.

   a. Drugs of choice: parenteral chloramphenicol or third-generation cephalosporin

   b. Alternative drugs: trimethoprim-sulfamethoxazole or amoxicillin

Diet

The primary treatment of the gastroenteritis is oral fluids.

Patient Education

1. Education on proper handwashing and food preparation techniques can prevent the transmission of *Salmonella.*

2. Advise travelers to developing countries where enteric fever is endemic not to drink untreated water or eat ice, peeled fruit, or other uncooked foods. They may also wish to get the vaccine, which offers 70 per cent protection against serotypes of salmonellae that cause enteric fever.

Key Treatment

Salmonella Gastroenteritis

- Oral fluid replacement

Enteric Fever

Drug of Choice	Alternative Drugs
• Chloramphenicol	• Amoxicillin
	• Trimethoprim-sulfamethoxazole
	• Ampicillin

Follow-Up

1. Complications of enteric fever usually occur 2 to 4 weeks after the initial symptoms and can include intestinal ulcers with hemorrhage or perforation, cholecystitis, hepatitis, meningitis, pneumonia, arthritis, nephritis, myocarditis, osteomyelitis, parotitis, prostatitis, epididymitis, and orchitis.

2. About 10 per cent of patients with enteric fever experience a relapse after 4 to 5 weeks whether or not the initial infection was treated. Relapses are treated in the same manner as a first episode.

3. Three per cent of patients who have had enteric fever and 0.5 per cent of patients exposed to other serotypes of *Salmonella* become chronic fecal carriers. True asymptomatic carriage is diagnosed when *Salmonella* are shed in the stool for a year or more. Chronic carriers are treated with 4 to 6 weeks of ampicillin or amoxicillin plus probenecid. Chronic carriers with gallstones may also require cholecystectomy.

Bibliography

Butler T: Typhoid fever. *In* Bennett JC, Plum F (eds): Cecil Textbook of Medicine, 20th ed. Philadelphia, WB Saunders, 1996.

Hook EW: Salmonella species (including typhoid fever). *In* Mandell GL, Douglas RG Jr, Bennett JE (eds): Principles and Practice of Infectious Disease, 3rd ed. New York, Churchill Livingstone, 1990, pp 1700–1716.

Kaye D: Salmonella infections other than typhoid fever. *In* Bennett JC, Plum F (eds): Cecil Textbook of Medicine, 20th ed. Philadelphia, WB Saunders, 1996.

Keusch GT: Salmonellosis. *In* Isselbacher KJ, Braunwald E, Wilson JD, Martin JB, Fauci AS, Kasper DL (eds): Harrison's Principles of Internal Medicine, 13th ed. New York, McGraw-Hill, 1994, pp 671–676.

Rubin RH, Hopkins CC, O'Hanley PO: Infections due to gram-negative bacilli. *In* Rubenstein E, Federman DD (eds): Scientific American Medicine. New York, Scientific American Inc., 1992, 7-II pp 1–7.

241 Malaria

Gary A. Goforth

Etiology

1. Parasitic agents (*Plasmodium falciparum, Plasmodium vivax, Pityrosporum ovale,* or *Plasmodium malariae*) infect man, the host/reservoir, via the female *Anophales* species mosquito vector.
2. Protective effect against *P. falciparum* infection if sickle cell disease or trait, glucose-6-phosphate dehydrogenase (G6PD) deficiency, or hereditary ovalocytosis. Resistant to *P. vivax* infection if Duffy-negative blood type.

Symptoms

1. Incubation period 9 to 40 days (average 12 days [*P. falciparum*], 13 days [*P. vivax*], 17 days [*P. ovale*], 28 days [*P. malariae*])
2. Initial symptoms: cold stage (rigors, chills); hot stage (fever, seizures); defervescent stage (diaphoresis)
3. Periodicity of fever corresponds to release of merozoites from red blood cells in asexual cycle every 48 hours for *P. falciparum* (malignant tertian malaria), for *P. vivax* (benign tertian malaria), and for *P. ovale* and every 72 hours for *P. malariae* (quartan malaria).
4. Other common symptoms: nonproductive cough, myalgias, postural hypotension, diarrhea, persistent fatigue, marked lethargy (especially cerebral malaria).

Key Symptoms

• Periodic fever	• Chills
• Diaphoresis	• Diarrhea (often bloody)
• Persistent fatigue	• Lethargy/Coma (cerebral malaria)

Clinical Findings

1. Common physical findings: mild jaundice, liver tenderness, hemolysis, splenomegaly (with chronic infection)
2. *P. falciparum* infection: significant parasitemia common with life-threatening complications including acute renal failure (blackwater fever), hemolytic anemia, pulmonary edema
3. *P. malariae* infection: Nephrotic infection occasionally seen in chronic infections

Key Signs

• Hemolytic anemia	• Jaundice
• Liver tenderness	• Splenomegaly (chronic infection)
• Pulmonary edema	
	• Renal failure

Laboratory Tests

1. Thick and thin blood smears standard for diagnosis. If malaria suspected but smear negative, repeat every 12 to 24 hours for 3 consecutive days. (Malaria is unlikely if smears remain negative.)
2. Other useful tests: complete blood count with peripheral smear (hemolytic anemia, leukopenia, thrombocytopenia), liver function tests (alanine aminotransferase [ALT], aspartate aminotransferase [AST], direct and indirect bilirubin elevated), albumin (decreased)
3. Quantitative buffy coat (QBC), DNA probe, and ribosomal RNA probes are under development as diagnostic tests.

Key Tests

- Thick and thin blood smears
- Liver function tests (ALT, AST, direct/indirect bilirubin)
- Complete blood count, peripheral smear

Differential Diagnosis

1. Severe *P. falciparum* infection—dysentery, acute gastroenteritis, viral syndrome, acute hepatitis, acute hemolytic anemia, meningitis, pneumonia, influenza and other febrile illnesses in a tropical environment, cerebrovascular accident
2. Chronic infection: hyperreactive malarial syndrome, differential diagnosis of splenomegaly (infectious, inflammatory, hematologic neoplasms, nonmalignant hematologic disorders, congestive splenomegaly, infiltrative disorders, trauma)

Treatment

Medication—Drugs of Choice

A. P. malariae, P. vivax, P. ovale, *or* P. falciparum *infection in areas with chloroquine sensitivity*

  1. *Oral therapy:* chloroquine phosphate (Aralen)
     a. Adults: 600 mg base (1 gm salt) followed by 300 mg base (500 mg salt) 6 hours later, then 300 mg base daily for 2 days.
     b. Pediatric: 10 mg/kg base (max 600 mg base), followed by 5 mg/kg base 6 hours later, then 5 mg/kg base daily for 2 days.
  2. *Parenteral therapy* (if unable to tolerate oral therapy, parasitemia >5 per cent, or evidence of complications)
     a. Adults: quinidine gluconate, 10 mg/kg salt in 500 ml of normal saline intravenously over 1 to 2 hours, then 0.02 mg/kg/min continuous

infusion until oral therapy can be started (maximum 72 hours). Central venous catheter to monitor fluid balance and cardiac monitoring necessary.

    b. Pediatric: same as adults

B. *P. falciparum infection acquired in areas with chloroquine resistance*

    1. *Oral therapy*

        a. Adult: quinine sulfate, 650 mg salt q 8 hr for 3 to 7 days orally *plus* tetracycline, 250 mg orally q.i.d. for 7 days *or* pyrimethamine sulfadoxine (Fansidar), 3 tablets orally in single dose. If acquired in Thailand, 7-day course of quinine required.

        b. Pediatric: quinine sulfate, 10 mg/kg salt q 8 hr orally for 3 to 7 days *plus* tetracycline, 5 mg/kg q.i.d. for 7 days *or* pyrimethamine sulfadoxine (Fansidar) in single dose [<1 yr—¼ tablet, 1–3 yr—½ tablet, 4–8 yr—1 tablet, 9–14 yr—2 tablets, >14 yr—3 tablets]. The benefit of using tetracycline must be weighted against known adverse events in children under 8 years old.

    2. *Parenteral therapy:* see above under chloroquine-sensitive *P. falciparum* malaria

Medication—Alternative Drugs

1. Mefloquine hydrochloride (Lariam), 15 mg/kg salt orally single dose up to 1250 mg (adult and child)

    a. Treatment dose associated with dose-related increased incidence of neuropsychiatric side effects.

    b. Contraindicated for persons with known hypersensitivity, history of serious psychiatric or seizure disorder, children <15 kg, patients with cardiac conduction abnormalities, and during pregnancy.

2. Halofantrine (Halfan), 6 tablets (250 mg salt each) orally, 2 tablets q 6 hr × three doses. Pediatric dosage 8 mg/kg salt orally q 6 hr × 3 doses.

3. Pregnant patients: quinine (as above) *plus* clindamycin (Cleocin), 450 mg orally q 8 hr × 3 days

4. *Prevention* Use 1 week before arrival (1 to 2 days for doxycycline) and 4 weeks after leaving endemic area

    a. *Chemoprophylaxis against all species except chloroquine-resistant* P. falciparum
    Chloroquine phosphate, 300 mg base (500 mg salt) or 5 mg/kg base (children) once weekly

    b. *Chemoprophylaxis against chloroquine-resistant* P. falciparum

        (1) Mefloquine, 228 mg base (250 mg salt) orally weekly. Children 15–19 kg—¼ tablet, 20–30 kg—½ tablet, 31–45 kg—¾ tablet, >45 kg—1 tablet

        (2) Doxycycline, 100 mg orally daily (children >8 years, 2 mg/kg up to 100 mg/day)

    c. *Prevention of* P. vivax *and* P. ovale *relapse* (start after leaving endemic area)
    Primaquine, 15 mg base (26.3 mg salt) or 0.3 mg/kg base (children) orally daily for 14 days *or* 45 mg base (adults) or 0.9 mg/kg base (children) weekly for 8 weeks.

WARNING

Primaquine can cause hemolytic anemia in G6PD-deficient patients. Avoid during pregnancy.

Diet

No restrictions; oral fluids and feeding as tolerated in severe cases.

Activity

Bed rest with febrile phase. Gradual return to full activities when afebrile.

Patient Education

Emphasize prevention of future disease to include chemoprophylaxis before and after travel to endemic area, use of personal protective measures against mosquito bites (DEET insect repellent, mosquito netting).

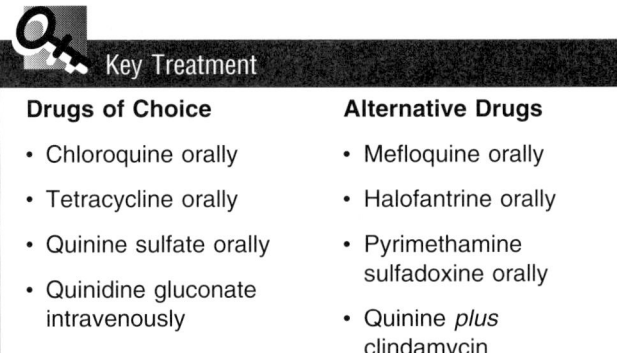

Key Treatment	
Drugs of Choice	**Alternative Drugs**
• Chloroquine orally	• Mefloquine orally
• Tetracycline orally	• Halofantrine orally
• Quinine sulfate orally	• Pyrimethamine sulfadoxine orally
• Quinidine gluconate intravenously	• Quinine *plus* clindamycin

Follow-Up

1. Consult physician if treated for malaria while abroad or if febrile syndrome occurs after return.

2. Because of emerging *P. vivax* chloroquine resistance, recommend follow-up blood smear at 3 and 7 days after chloroquine treatment to assess parasite clearance. Treat as chloroquine-resistant *P. falciparum* if parasitemic within 3 weeks of treatment.

 ## Bibliography

Barry M: Medical considerations for international travel with infants and older children. Infect Dis Clin North Am 1992;6(2):389–404.

McCarthy AE, Keystone JS: Malaria. *In* Rakel RE (ed): Conn's Current Therapy 1994. Philadelphia, WB Saunders, 1994, pp 94–100.

Strickland GT: Malaria. *In* Strickland GT (ed): Hunter's Tropical Medicine, 7th ed. Philadelphia, WB Saunders, 1991, pp 586–614.

Wyler D: Malaria chemoprophylaxis for the traveler. N Engl J Med 1993;329(1):31–37.

Zucker J, Campbell C: Malaria principles of prevention and treatment. Infect Dis Clin North Am 1993;7(3):547–567.

242 Typhoid Fever

Paul J. Jaster

Etiology

1. From Greek "typhos," which means smoke, referring to fever-induced apathy and confusion. An acute usually severe systemic illness caused by *Salmonella typhi* characterized by prolonged fever, prostration, abdominal pain, diarrhea, delirium, rose spots, splenomegaly, hepatomegaly, and occasionally complicated by intestinal perforation and/or bleeding. Synonymous with enteric fever occasionally caused by *S. enteritidis* bioserotype *paratyphi* A or B.

2. The human is the only reservoir for *S. typhi*, a gram-negative flagellated, nonencapsulated, nonsporulating facultative anaerobic bacillus of Enterobacteriaceae family with flagellar (H) antigen, cell wall (O) lipopolysaccharide antigen, and polysaccharide virulence (Vi) antigen located in the cell wall capsule.

3. Occurs mainly in developing countries (Peru, India, Pakistan, Chile, Haiti, southern Europe [Italy, Spain, Greece]). In the United States there are about 500 cases a year, more than half in recently arrived travelers. Sewage workers, medical care personnel, laboratory technicians are at risk also. Median age is 23; in endemic areas the highest incidence is in ages 5 to 20 years.

4. Transmission is fecal-oral through food or water contamination. Anal-oral (homosexual), contaminated endoscopes, or enemas also are possible transmission routes. Mostly affects those with lowered host defenses; decreased gastric acid, intestinal motility disorders, altered normal intestinal flora from antibiotics.

5. *S. typhi* penetrates the terminal ileum by way of Peyer's patches and is phagocytized and carried to mesenteric lymph nodes, then carried by the blood to the thoracic duct or portal circulation to the liver. Bacteremia (demonstrated by fever, chills, hemagglutinating antibody) lasts 1 to 3 weeks with mild symptoms building to prostration. Second stage is inflammatory and involves spleen and liver (>50 per cent diffuse abdominal pain or right lower quadrant over terminal ileum, rare jaundice, occasionally acute cholecystitis, typhoid nodules), bone marrow, rose spots (mononuclear cell vasculitis of the skin; 1- to 5-mm-diameter erythematous macules or papules that blanche with pressure but may become hemorrhagic on shoulders, thorax, abdomen, and rarely extend), Peyer's patches (pain, diarrhea, bleeding, perforation in less than 5 per cent, usually after second week), lung (pneumonia from superinfection), cardiovascular (myocarditis), CNS (delirium, aphonia, "toxic" staring, coma, seizures, meningitis).

Symptoms

1. Bacteremia stage: fever (universal, classically stepwise but can be continuous or intermittent), weakness, anorexia, headache, dizziness, sore throat

2. Inflammatory stage: diffuse abdominal or right lower quadrant pain, nausea and vomiting, constipation or diarrhea, cough, myalgia and arthralgia, confusion, decreased hearing, epistaxis, blood in stool or urine, jaundice

3. Relapse: reappearance of acute disease

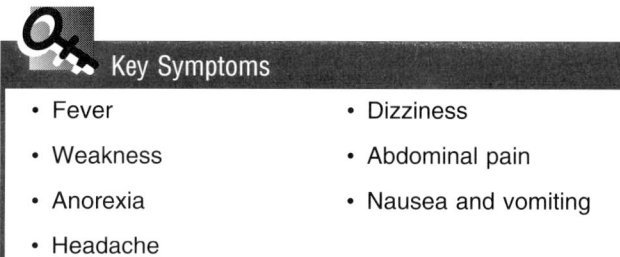

Key Symptoms

- Fever
- Weakness
- Anorexia
- Headache
- Dizziness
- Abdominal pain
- Nausea and vomiting

Clinical Findings

1. Bacteremia stage: fever, relative bradycardia ("classic" but in less than 25 per cent and usually not in children), possible abdominal tenderness, leukopenia

2. Inflammatory stage: rose spots, splenomegaly, hepatomegaly, delirium, aphonia, "toxic" staring, coma, seizures, meningitis

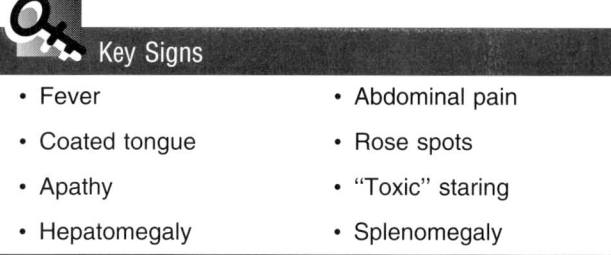

Key Signs

- Fever
- Coated tongue
- Apathy
- Hepatomegaly
- Abdominal pain
- Rose spots
- "Toxic" staring
- Splenomegaly

Laboratory Tests

1. Anemia: white blood count normal or decreased with increased bands, possible thrombocytopenia, increased aminotransferases and bilirubin, possible stool leukocytes.

2. Widal test (for agglutinating antibodies against O and H antigens) is suggestive but not diagnostic (not considered useful); O titer ≥1:80 or fourfold rise.

3. Latex particle agglutination slide test, rapid fluorescence method (MUCAP test), and enzyme-linked immunosorbant assay antibody test available but widespread long-term testing has not been done.

4. Cultures: blood (25 to 42 per cent positive), stool

(26 per cent), urine (30 per cent), bone marrow (75 per cent, usually not recommended initially unless prior antibiotic usage), bile (duodenal string test 86 per cent).

Key Tests

- Complete blood count and differential

- Cultures

- Abdominal radiography showing free air if intestinal perforations are present

Differential Diagnosis

1. Malaria
2. Hepatitis
3. Typhus
4. Amebic liver abscess
5. Shigellosis
6. Nontyphoid salmonellosis
7. Leptospirosis
8. Septicemia from urinary tract infection or gastrointestinal tract
9. Influenza
10. Infectious mononucleosis
11. Meningococcemia
12. Miliary tuberculosis
13. Bacterial endocarditis
14. Any febrile illness of unknown cause exceeding 3 days' duration.

Treatment

Prognosis: With treatment less than 1 per cent of patients die in developed and 12 per cent in developing countries; 2 to 5 per cent become chronic carriers (duration of shedding longer than 12 months). At highest risk for the carrier state are those with gallbladder disease, increased age, and women (affected three times more frequently than men). There is an increased risk of gallbladder carcinoma.

WARNING

- **Profound hypothermia may occur with even small doses of aspirin.**
- **Enteric precautions are needed until three consecutive negative stool cultures have been obtained.**

Medication

Optimal treatment is still controversial.
1. Chloramphenicol: 50 to 75 mg/kg daily orally or intravenously divided q 6 hr × 2 weeks, max 3 gm daily still the drug of choice in developing countries due to cost, but there is risk of bone marrow suppression, aplastic anemia, and treatment does not prevent the chronic carrier state; 10 to 36 per cent relapse rate. (Resistance reported.)

2. Ampicillin: possibly slower to work. Use high doses; 150 to 200 mg/kg daily intravenously divided q 6 hr × 2 weeks, max 8 gm daily.

3. Trimethoprim/sulfamethoxasole (TMP/SMX) (Bactrim, Septra): drug of choice for chloramphenicol or ampicillin resistance (but R factor coding for chloramphenicol resistance also codes for sulfonamide resistance; therefore, with TMP/SMX, only TMP is active). TMP, 10 mg/kg daily + SMX 50 mg/kg daily divided q 12 hr × 2 weeks, max TMP, 160 mg/SMX 800 mg q 12 hr.

4. Fluoroquinolones (not for patients under age 18)
   a. Ofloxin (Floxin), 200 to 300 mg b.i.d. 1 to 2 weeks
   b. Ciprofloxacin (Cipro), 500 mg b.i.d. 10 to 14 days
   c. Norfloxin (Noroxin), 400 mg b.i.d. × 2 weeks (higher relapse rate than ofloxin or cipro); floxacin

5. Cephalosporins with high levels of biliary excretion show 90 to 97 per cent cure rates with shorter courses, less relapsing and mortality than with chloramphenicol.
   a. Cefoperazone (Cefobid), 2 to 4 gm intravenously q 6 to 12 hr × 2 weeks
   b. Cefotaxime (Claforan) (drug of choice if younger than 1 year because of possibility of resistant strains and of CNS disease) 150 mg/kg daily divided q 6 hr × 2 weeks, max 12 gm daily
   c. Ceftriaxone (Rocephin), 100 mg/kg daily × 2 weeks, max 4 gm daily, adult, 1 to 2 gm intravenously q day × 2 weeks (alternate regimen: 3 gm daily × 3).

6. Ampicillin/sulbactam (Unasyn) (defervescence in 3 to 5 days instead of 10 days with chlorampenicol); 1 gm q 6 hr × 7 to 10 days

Additional Drugs/Treatment

1. Laparotomy for suspected perforation.

2. Dexamethasone 3 mg/kg loading dose, then 1 mg/kg q 6 hr × 48 hr for patients with delirium, coma, and/or shock.

3. Chronic carrier state
   a. High-dose ampicillin +/− probenicid (4 to 6 gm daily × 4 to 6 weeks)
   b. TMP/SMX +/− rifampin
   c. Ciprofloxacin (Cipro) (750 mg b.i.d. × 4 weeks) or norfloxin (Noroxin) (400 mg b.i.d. × 4 weeks)

Diet
No restrictions. Adequate oral or intravenous fluids.
Activity
Bed rest while febrile
Patient Education
1. Prevention
    a. Do not consume untreated water, drinks served with ice, fruits you have not peeled yourself, and other food that is not served hot.
    b. Observe strict handwashing before eating or serving food.
    c. Boil water 5 to 10 min or treat with iodine or chlorine.
    d. Breast-feeding lowers incidence in infants.
2. Vaccination
    a. Live-attenuated oral vaccine: Ty21a 1 capsule q.o.d. × 4 doses and repeat primary series every 4 to 5 years. Keep caps refrigerated and avoid concurrent antibiotic use. Separate dose 24 hr from weekly mefloquine antimalarial dose (inhibits in vitro growth of *S. typhi*).
    b. Typhoid vaccine U.S.P. (heat or acetone inactivated [more efficacious]) 0.5 ml subcutaneously (0.25 ml < 10 y/o) × two doses 4 weeks apart with booster every 3 years.
    c. Vi antigen vaccine not yet available. Vaccine efficacy (all) is 50 to 90 per cent. No safety or efficacy data on any vaccines in pregnancy. Do not give live vaccine to HIV or immunocompromised patients.

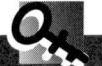

Key Treatment

Drugs of Choice

- Chloramphenicol
- Ampicillin
- TMP/SMX

Alternative Drug

- Dexamethasone

Note that optimal treatment is still controversial.

Follow-Up

Watch for relapse or chronic carrier state (occurs in 1 to 6 per cent of patients).

Bibliography

Butler T: Typhoid fever. *In* Bennett JC, Plum F (eds): Cecil's Textbook of Medicine, 20th ed. Philadelphia, WB Saunders, 1996.

Gorbach SL: Infectious Diseases. Philadelphia, WB Saunders, 1992, pp 585–589.

Hayani KC, Pickering LK: Salmonella infections. *In* Feigin RD (ed): Pediatric Infectious Diseases, 3rd ed. Philadelphia, WB Saunders, 1992, pp 620–636.

Hoffman SL: Typhoid fever. *In* Strickland GT (ed): Hunter's Tropical Medicine, 7th ed. Philadelphia, WB Saunders, 1991, pp 344–359.

Trujillo Z: Fluoroquinolones in the treatment of typhoid fever and the carrier state. Eur J Clin Microbiol Infect Dis 1991;10:334–341.

243 Leprosy

Earle E. Morton

Etiology

1. Causative agent: *Mycobacterium leprae,* in the order Actinomycetales, is a weakly acid-fast bacillus that measures 0.3 to 0.5 by 4 to 7 μm; it was first discovered in 1873.
2. Growth is slow, with a generation time of 11 to 13 days.
3. Transmission is via the nasorespiratory system, skin to skin, and possibly through arthropod vectors. Transfer via lactation and the placenta does occur.
4. Animal reservoirs: leprosy may be a zoonosis; this theory is indicated by the discovery of naturally acquired leprosy in armadillos, chimpanzees, and mahogany monkeys.
5. Incubation period: 2 to 5 years (may be as long as 20 years)

Epidemiology

1. WHO estimates that there are 10 to 12 million cases worldwide, with the highest prevalence in tropical Africa, South America, India, Southeast Asia, and the Philippines.
2. There are 6000 cases in the United States (HI, LA, TX, CA, and FL).
3. Living conditions in many developing countries may contribute to the transmission of leprosy.

Symptoms

These depend on the immune response and subsequent type of leprosy acquired (Table 243–1).

1. Prodromal symptoms are not well established; early manifestations include irregular bouts of fever with occasional sweating, progressive malaise, headache, nasal congestion with frequent epistaxis, peripheral edema, and focal paresthesias.
2. Cutaneous: hypopigmented macules with papulated or vague borders. Nodular thickening of the cooler areas of skin may occur. Sweating and normal hair pattern may be disrupted.
3. Neural: Recurrent or persistent paresthesia, neuralgia, and numbness occurs due to granulomas invading neural structures and appendages; enlarged tender main nerve trunks occur.

Key Symptoms

- Neural symptoms (decreased sweating, enlarged tender peripheral nerves, footdrop)
- Cutaneous lesions
- Deformities
- Trophic changes

Clinical Findings

1. Most clinicians follow the classification schema outlined by Ridley and Jopling (Table 243–1).
2. Indeterminate leprosy (I): Frequently earliest stage; may heal spontaneously, remain unchanged, or progress toward the tuberculoid or lepromatous forms.
3. Tuberculoid leprosy (TT): A single or few macules with papulated edges; leprosy should be suspected with enlarged or tender nerves.
4. Borderline leprosy (BB): An unstable form that contains features of both tuberculoid and lepromatous leprosy.

TABLE 243–1. CLASSIFICATION OF LEPROSY

GROUP	CLINICAL FEATURES	LEPROMIN REACTION	BACILLARY DENSITY
Tuberculoid (TT)	Single or few anesthetic macules or plaques; borders well defined; peripheral nerve involvement common	Strongly positive	Rare
Borderline tuberculoid (BT)	Lesions similar to TT but more numerous; borders less distinct. Satellite lesions sometimes present around larger lesions; peripheral nerve involvement common	Positive	Scanty
Borderline (BB)	More lesions than BT; borders more vague; satellite lesions often seen; peripheral nerve involvement common	Negative or weakly positive	Moderate
Borderline lepromatous (BL)	Lesions numerous and similar to BB; some nerve damage	Negative	Heavy
Lepromatous (LL)	Multiple, nonanesthetic, macular or papular, symmetrically distributed lesions; no neural lesions until late; late complications of madarosis, leonine facies, testicular damage	Negative	Heavy
Indeterminate (I)	Vaguely defined hypopigmented or erythematous macule	Weakly positive or neg	Rare or scanty

5. Lepromatous leprosy (LL): The bacillus multiplies freely and the disease disseminates widely.

   a. Juvenile leprosy: "Prelepromatous leprosy" afflicts children; can progress to disfiguring forms.

   b. Macular lesions: early LL with slight or no sensory changes. Skin smears and biopsy reveal acid-fast bacilli (AFB).

   c. Nodular changes: The early LL forms progress to nodules. Cooler areas (ears, face, extremities, and buttocks) have the heaviest infiltrations. Sensory loss occurs with nerve enlargement in the hands and feet. The testes become atrophic; the corneas, nasal mucosa, and larynx may become involved.

   d. Lucio leprosy: Patients of Latino descent can develop an obstructive vasculitis (Lucio phenomenon).

   e. Neuritic leprosy: One or more major nerve trunks become involved, leaving patients with pain, anesthesia, paresis, or muscular atrophy.

6. Acute reactional episodes are hypersensitivity phenomena that afflict half of all patients.

   a. Reversal reactions are a delayed-type hypersensitivity to *M. leprae* antigens in BB leprosy. Red, edematous lesions are frequently associated with an acute neuritis. Self-healing may occur. Severe sensory loss and paralytic deformities may occur.

   b. Erythema nodosum leprosum (ENL) afflicts LL and BL patients who are predisposed to immune-complex disease.

Key Signs

- Hypopigmented macules
- Enlarged and tender nerves
- Clawing of hands
- Nodular thickening of skin along cool areas

Laboratory Tests

1. Skin smears: for AFB along the edges of macules or plaques, nodules, earlobes, and nasal mucosa.

2. Pre-emptive diagnosis includes lymphocyte transformation test, migration inhibition factor, fluorescent leprosy antibody absorption, radioimmunoassay, counterimmunoelectrophoresis, passive hemagglutination test, and enzyme-linked immunosorbent assay, which are positive for LL and BL disease but are not reliable for TT and BT. Established skin lesions are used for pin prick, histamine test, sweating test, and the thermal tests.

3. Lepromin test: An intradermal injection of killed *M. leprae* may have an early response (Fernandez reactions) at 24 to 48 hours or a late response (Mitsuda reactions) at 3 to 4 weeks. The late reaction correlates with the immunologic status of the patient, being strongly positive in tuberculoid patients, negative in lepromatous patients, and intermediate in borderline patients. It is not useful for diagnosis.

Key Tests

- Clinical history and physical examination
- Serial skin and peripheral nerve biopsies

Differential Diagnosis

1. Macular changes: scars, birthmarks, actinic dermatitis, dermatophytosis, and filariasis.

2. Infiltrative lesions: leishmaniasis, granuloma annulare, granuloma multiforme, lupus erythematosus, psoriasis, pityriasis rosea, sarcoidosis, and neurofibromatosis.

3. Peripheral neuropathies: carpal tunnel syndrome, syringomyelia, lead toxicity, diabetes mellitus, primary amyloidosis, familial hypertrophic neuropathy, and congenital insensitivity to pain

Treatment

1. Medications of choice include

   a. Dapsone: 100 mg/day in adults and 0.9 to 1.4 mg/kg/day in children. The half-life is 28 hours.

   b. Clofazimine (Lamprene): 50 to 100 mg/day in adults and unestablished in children. The half-life is 70 days.

   c. Rifampin (Rifadin): 600 mg/month in adults and 150 to 300 mg (up to age 5) and 300 to 450 mg (up to age 14). The half-life is 3 hours.

2. Alternative drugs

   a. Ethionamide (Trecator-SC) and prothionamide* are alternatives to clofazimine in combined regimens.

   b. Aminoglycosides (streptomycin, kanamycin [Kantrex], and amikacin [Amikin]) as well as diuciphon* and thiacetazone* have limited antileprosy activity.

   c. Fluoroquinolones pefloxacin* and ofloxacin (Floxin), macrolide antibiotics (erythromycin and clarithromycin [Biaxin]), and tetracyclines (minocycline [Minocin]) have strong antileprosy effects.

3. Approaches to leprosy chemotherapy

---

*Not available in the U.S.

a. Monotherapy: not recommended for either PB or MB disease because of steadily rising dapsone resistance

b. WHO multidrug therapy:

  (1) Multibacillary leprosy (BB, BL, and LL): dapsone 100 mg and clofazimine 50 mg daily unsupervised, with clofazimine 300 mg and rifampin 600 mg, supervised, monthly for 2 years or until skin smears are negative.

  (2) Paucibacillary leprosy (BT and TT): dapsone 100 mg daily unsupervised and rifampin 600 mg monthly for 6 months. Continue surveillance every 6 months.

4. Treatment of reactions: These are medical emergencies that are treated with analgesics, high-dose corticosteroids, thalidomide, and clofazimine.

Prognosis

1. Borderline and tuberculoid patients suffer mutilations and may downgrade to the lepromatous form. LL patients can become debilitated. Death may result from laryngeal obstruction or renal failure. With effective treatment, the prognosis is good.

2. Patient education/control: Vaccines containing *M. leprae* or immunologically related nonpathogenic mycobacteria are being used in very large trials. Cell wall complexes are also being utilized as vaccines.

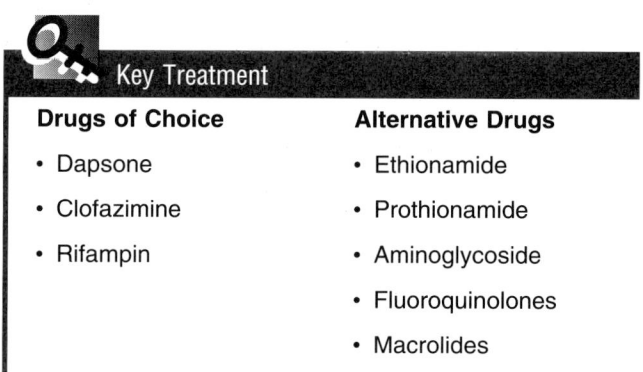

Key Treatment

Drugs of Choice	Alternative Drugs
• Dapsone	• Ethionamide
• Clofazimine	• Prothionamide
• Rifampin	• Aminoglycoside
	• Fluoroquinolones
	• Macrolides
	• Tetracyclines

Follow-Up

Patients should be followed indefinitely after treatment.

Bibliography

Meyers WM: Leprosy. *In* Strickland, GT (ed): Hunter's Tropical Medicine, 7th ed. Philadelphia, WB Saunders, 1991, pp 483–494.

For more information on treatment, see

Becx-Bleumink M: Success of the WHO multidrug therapy? Trop Geogr Med 1994;46(2):61–64.

Meyers WM, Marty AM: Current concepts in the pathogenesis of leprosy. Drugs 1991;41(6):832–856.

Okoro AN: Pre-emptive diagnosis of leprosy. Int J Dermatol 1991;30(11):767–771.

Pattyn SR: Future trends in the treatment of leprosy. Trop Geogr Med 1994; 46(2):85–88.

244 Common Protozoal Disease Symptoms

Anson L. Thaggard

The symptoms of protozoal and helminthic disease are protean and nonspecific. An appropriate index of suspicion for these diseases is particularly important in developed countries where they are less common. Historical questions should be directed toward exposure to infectious agents. The symptoms most commonly encountered are diarrhea, general abdominal discomfort, and passage of the parasites.

Common Symptoms

1. Abdominal pain (*Giardia, Entamoeba,* hookworms, *Strongyloides, Ascaris, Enterobius*)
2. Wheezing or hemoptysis may represent pulmonary migration of larvae (Löffler's syndrome with *Ascaris,* hookworms, *Strongyloides, Toxocara*).
3. Dermatitis (hookworms, *Strongyloides, Toxocara, Cercaria*)
4. Diarrhea (*Entamoeba, Cryptosporidium, Giardia, Isospora, Sarcocystis, Trichinella, Trichuris, Strongyloides*)
5. Dysentery (*Entamoeba, Trichuris*)
6. Pruritus ani (*Enterobius, Taenia, Entamoeba*)
7. Rectal prolapse (*Trichuris*)
8. Steatorrhea (*Cryptosporidium, Giardia*)
9. Passage of parasites (*Ascaris, Enterobius, Taenia* proglottids). Although this may be disconcerting, it makes the diagnosis quite simple.
10. Bowel obstruction (*Taenia, Ascaris*)

Gastrointestinal symptoms are commonly encountered in parasitic disease. Diarrhea of more than 10 days' duration, particularly when accompanied by weight loss, should prompt one to consider *Giardia* or *Cryptosporidium.* Several parasites (*Ascaris, Enterobius, Strongyloides,* and *Entamoeba histolytica*) are known to cause or to mimic appendicitis when they colonize the cecum. *Entamoeba histolytica* causes a classic dysentery, while *Trichuris* may cause a colitis mimicking inflammatory bowel disease.

History

Key elements that raise the index of suspicion for parasitic disease include

1. Travel to underdeveloped or high risk areas
2. Outbreak-associated illness (*Giardia, Trichinella*)
3. Day care exposure (*Giardia, Cryptosporidium*). Toddlers are at higher risk for *Giardia* than are infants. Parents of children involved in day care are also at risk.
4. Homosexual behavior (*Giardia, Entamoeba*)
5. Immunocompromised host (*Cryptosporidium, Entamoeba, Strongyloides, Giardia*)

6. Animal exposure (*Cryptosporidium,* and *Sarcocystis* in cattle, *Giardia* in beaver and house pets)
7. Diet including undercooked or improperly prepared meats

> Refer to specific diseases in this section (Part 16), the gastrointestinal diseases (Part 5), and skin diseases (Part 17).

Clinical Findings

1. Weight loss
2. Meteorism (excess gas) or abdominal distention
3. Hyperperistalsis
4. Perianal inflammation
5. Rectal prolapse
6. Wheezing

Tests

1. Fecal smears: Look for white blood cells (WBC), red blood cells (RBC), Charcot-Leyden crystals, ova, cysts, and parasites.
2. Stool cultures should be considered, since multiple parasitic infections can occur.
3. Complete blood count (CBC): Eosinophilia may be seen with many invasive parasites. Iron deficiency anemia may be seen with hookworm and *Strongyloides* infections.
4. Entero-Test or "string test": A weighted string in a gelatin capsule is swallowed and the free end is secured to the face. After 2 or 3 hrs the capsule dissolves and the string passes into the duodenum. The string is then retrieved and the bile-stained mucus is examined for parasites (*Giardia, Strongyloides*).
5. Graham's test or the "Scotch Tape" test: A length of clear adhesive tape is held adhesive side out on a tongue depressor and used to swab the anus. The tape is then applied to a slide and examined under a microscope. This is most effective when obtained early in the morning before bathing or defecation. It is useful in the diagnosis of pinworms (enterobiasis), but it will occasionally pick up other helminths or eggs of tapeworms.

Management

Medications (Symptomatic Treatment of Diarrhea)

1. Attapulgite (Diasorb, Donnagel, Kaopectate, 600 to 750 mg/5 ml). Adults, 1200 mg initially and then 1200 mg after each loose stool up to 8400 mg/day.

Children aged 6 to 12, half the adult dose. Children aged 3 to 6, one fourth the adult dose.

2. Polycarbophil (Mitrolan, FiberCon, 500-mg tablets). Adults, 4 to 6 gm/day divided t.i.d. or q.i.d. Children aged 6 to 12, 0.5 to 1 gm t.i.d. up to 3 gm/day. Children aged 3 to 6, 0.33 to 0.5 gm t.i.d. up to 1.5 gm/day.

3. Loperamide (Imodium A-D, 2 mg caplets, 1 mg/5 ml). Adults, 2 to 4 mg initially and then 2 mg after each loose stool up to 8 mg/day. Children aged 6 to 11, 1 mg per dose up to 4 mg/day.

4. Bismuth subsalicylate (Pepto-Bismol, 262 mg/15 ml). Adults, 524 mg per dose. Children aged 9 to 12, 262 mg per dose. Children aged 6 to 9, 175 mg per dose. Children aged 3 to 6, 87 mg per dose. One dose every hour up to eight doses per day.

5. Chemotherapeutic agents for each parasite are outlined in subsequent chapters.

Diet

1. Intravenous hydration may be required initially.

2. An oral fluid, preferably a balanced salt solution with glucose to facilitate absorption of the electrolytes, is the best means of rehydration.

3. Avoid dairy products because the parasitosis may cause a transient lactase deficiency.

As with any illness, treatment should be focused on the primary cause. Definitive diagnosis is important so that the appropriate anthelmintic or antiprotozoal agent may be used. Care should be taken not to mask a treatable cause with symptomatic care only.

Often diarrhea has been long-standing before a specific diagnosis is made. Therefore, one must pay close attention to the state of nutrition and hydration. A history of fever and blood in the stool are contraindications to the use of antidiarrheal agents. Again, symptomatic treatment should never be substituted for proper diagnosis and definitive therapy.

PEARLS

- Pepto-Bismol tablets have a calcium binder that may interfere with the absorption of other medications, particularly tetracycline.

- Metals such as bismuth, magnesium, aluminum, and barium may obscure subsequent microscopic examination of stools.

- Bismuth subsalicylate carries the same risks as other salicylates (e.g., salicylate toxicity and Reye's syndrome).

- Giardiasis is an upper gastrointestinal tract parasitosis, and stool examinations are often negative. In patients at high risk for giardiasis, an empirical trial of metronidazole or furazolidone may be warranted.

Bibliography

Beaver PC, Jung RC (eds): Animal Agents and Vectors of Human Disease, 5th ed. Philadelphia, Lea & Febiger, 1985.

Genta RM: Diarrhea in helminthic infections. Clin Infect Dis 1993;16(suppl 2):S122–9.

Guerrant RL, Hughes JM, Lima NL, et al: Diarrhea in developed and developing countries: Magnitude, special settings, and etiologies. Rev Infect Dis 1990;12(suppl 1):S41–50.

Johnson PC, Ericsson CD: Acute diarrhea in developed countries. Am J Med 1990;88(suppl 6A):5S–9S.

Wolfe MS: Acute diarrhea associated with travel. Am J Med 1990;88(suppl 6A):34S–7S.

245 Pinworms

Louis B. Jacques

Etiology

1. *Enterobius vermicularis,* formerly called *Oxyuris vermicularis,* is the most common helminthic parasite in humans, afflicting approximately 15 per cent of the population of the United States. School-age children have the highest prevalence rate.

2. In contrast to the tropical distribution of most other parasites, pinworm infection is more common in temperate climates. Outbreaks may be clustered in schools, day care centers, or other institutional settings.

3. Transmission is largely through the fecal-organ ingestion of *Enterobius* ova that have been deposited in the perianal area by airborne dissemination, and by person-to-person contact. Adult worms inhabit the cecum, appendix, and proximal colon. Reinfection is common.

4. Serious sequelae are rare and usually are related to ectopic worm migration; current opinion is that pinworms do not cause appendicitis.

Symptoms

1. Anal pruritus is common, although many patients are asymptomatic. Patients or their parents may describe seeing an adult worm in the perianal area.

2. Insomnia, irritability, or other nonspecific behavior changes may be present.

3. Almost 50 per cent of infected girls have nocturia, and about 25 per cent are enuretic, but dysuria is no greater than in controls.

Key Symptom
• Anal pruritus

Clinical Findings

1. Perianal irritation from persistent scratching. Cutaneous perineal granulomata may contain adult worm parts.

2. Ectopic migration to the urogenital tract may produce signs of urethritis, vulvovaginitis, or salpingitis, such as pelvic pain and local erythema. Bacteriuria may be noted on urinalysis.

3. Weight loss may be seen in chronic cases.

Key Sign
• Perianal irritation

Laboratory Tests

1. The "Scotch Tape test" is the preferred initial test. The adhesive side of the tape is placed in contact with the perianal skin, then the tape is affixed, adhesive side down, to a glass microscope slide. A drop of toluene applied under the tape allows clearer examination. Subsequent viewing reveals characteristic ovoid 30×50 to 60 micron ova, asymmetrically flattened on one side.

2. A single stool sample may be collected for laboratory screening for ova. A negative test may be repeated if necessary. Digital rectal examination may be used to procure fecal material.

3. Patients or parents may bring in adult worms retrieved from the perianal area. These may be collected in alcohol or adhered to Scotch Tape. Adult female worms, white with tapered ends, average 10 mm in length and may reach 13 mm. Males are similar in appearance but shorter, about one third as long.

4. Eosinophilia is not a characteristic of pinworm infections, as pinworms are not generally invasive.

Key Test
• Scotch Tape test

Differential Diagnosis

1. Pruritus ani of other causes, such as hemorrhoids
2. Other intestinal parasitic infestations (e.g., *Ascaris, Trichuris*)
3. Urinary tract infection
4. Perianal dermatitis from dermatophytes or contact irritants

---

WARNING

Although less likely to cause side effects, mebendazole is not recommended for pregnant patients and should be used cautiously in young children.

Treatment

Treatment of asymptomatic household members is recommended, as coincidental infection is common. Because the medications are effective only against adult worms, infected patients should be re-treated 7 to 14 days later.

Medication
1. Mebendazole (Vermox), 100 mg (adults and children) in a single dose
2. Pyrantel pamoate (Antiminth), 11 mg/kg (max 1000 mg adults and children) in a single dose

Diet
As tolerated

Activity
As tolerated

Patient Education
1. Scrupulous attention to hand washing and personal hygiene is advisable, especially in day care and institutional settings.
2. Shaking out of bed linens should be avoided, as *Enterobius* ova can become airborne.
3. Frequent laundering of underpants and pajamas in hot water with detergent
4. Cleaning of sleeping areas, with caution to avoid raising dust, which may cause ova to become airborne
5. Because the diagnosis of pinworms can be emotionally traumatic, reassurance about the ubiquity of this condition is appropriate.

Key Treatment
- Mebendazole, 100 mg in a single dose
- Pyrantel pamoate, 11 mg/kg (max 1000 mg) in single dose

Follow-Up
Re-evaluate if symptoms persist.

Bibliography

Gokalp A, Gultekin EY, Kirisci MF, Ozdamar S: Relation between *Enterobius vermicularis* infestation and dysuria, nocturia, enuresis nocturna and bacteriuria in primary school girls. Ind Pediatr 1991;28:948–950.

Jones JE: Pinworms. Am Fam Physician 1988;38(3):159–164.

Russell LJ: The pinworm, *Enterobius vermicularis*. Primary Care 1991;18(1):13–24.

Sun T, Schwartz NS, Sewell C, Lieberman P, Gross S: Enterobius egg granuloma of the vulva and peritoneum: Review of the literature. Am J Trop Med Hyg 1991;45(2):249–253.

Wiebe RM: Appendicitis and *Enterobius vermicularis*. Scand J Gastroenterol 1991;26:336–338.

246 Giardiasis

Louis B. Jacques

Etiology

1. *Giardia lamblia,* also known as *G. intestinalis* and *G. duodenalis,* is a flagellated protozoan that exists in cyst and trophozoite forms.

2. Transmission is generally fecal-oral, person-to-person, or through the ingestion of water or food contaminated with *Giardia* cysts. Sexual transmission has been reported.

3. Day care, institutional, and waterborne community-wide outbreaks are not uncommon. Hikers and campers may become infected through inadequate purification of drinking or dishwashing water. Animal reservoirs have been noted; beavers are a classic example.

4. Pathogenesis is related to noninvasive disruption of the normal structure and function of the intestinal brush border/microvillus apparatus.

Symptoms

Severity is variable; many subjects are asymptomatic. Differences in host immune characteristics, virulence of individual strains of *Giardia,* and the general health status of the host have been postulated to explain this variability.

A. Acute
1. Diarrhea, abdominal pain, flatulence, fatigue, abdominal cramping, foul-smelling stool, bloating and other nonspecific abdominal symptoms
2. Incubation period varies from a few days to weeks; 3 to 4 days to 2 weeks is usual. Acute symptoms generally resolve within several weeks.

B. Chronic
1. Flatulence, upper abdominal pain, altered bowel habits, weight loss, mucus or blood in stool
2. Anxiety and nonspecific constitutional symptoms

Key Symptoms

- Diarrhea

- Abdominal pain or cramping

- Flatulence

- Foul-smelling stool

Clinical Findings

Weight loss, childhood failure to thrive, malnutrition, malabsorption syndromes, or low-grade fever may be noted. Blood or mucus in stool is seen uncommonly. Patients may have unremarkable examinations.

Key Sign

- Foul-smelling, bulky stool

Laboratory Tests

1. Identification of the *Giardia* trophozoite or cyst on microscopic examination of one stool specimen has been recommended. If necessary, digital rectal examination may be performed to acquire fecal material. If the initial sample is negative and the patient remains symptomatic, additional samples may be obtained. The trophozoite, which measures approximately 15 μ in body length (about 1.5 × the diameter of a white blood cell) is classically described as having an appearance suggesting a monkey face.

2. The string test is rarely needed, since fecal examination appears to provide equivalent diagnostic power with less inconvenience to the patient. Its use is indicated for patients with repeatedly negative stool samples.

3. Detection of anti-*Giardia* IgM is compatible with acute infection. Serum IgG may be detectable long after the infection has resolved, and is therefore not clinically useful in the diagnosis of symptomatic individuals.

4. Enzyme-linked immunosorbent assay (ELISA) testing for fecal *Giardia* antigen has sensitivity and specificity greater than 90 per cent for acute infection and may be more cost effective than other tests.

5. Duodenoscopy (with biopsy and duodenal fluid sampling) should be reserved for diagnostically difficult cases or when endoscopy is needed to rule out other gastrointestinal pathology.

6. Eosinophilia is not characteristic, since *Giardia* is noninvasive.

Key Tests

- Microscopic identification of *Giardia* cyst or trophozoite in stool

- Fecal antigen detection by ELISA

Differential Diagnosis

1. Irritable bowel syndrome

2. Other protozoan or helminthic infestations (e.g., *Ascaris,* amebiasis)

3. Bacterial infections (e.g., *Salmonella, Shigella, Escherichia coli*)

4. Viral gastroenteritis
5. Malabsorption syndromes
6. Inflammatory bowel disease
7. Peptic disease
8. Cholecystitis

WARNING

Metronidazole is known to cause a disulfiram-like reaction to alcohol, and caution is recommended when treating patients with CNS illness. Quinacrine and furazolidone can cause severe reactions, including hemolysis in G6PD-deficient patients, and a disulfiram-like reaction to alcohol. Quinacrine may cause toxic psychosis. Check prescribing information for full details.

Treatment

Treatment may be started empirically on the basis of symptoms, especially after travel to endemic areas.

Medication

1. Metronidazole (Flagyl, Protostat, Metryl)

   a. Adults: 2 gm orally q.d. × 3 days or 250 mg t.i.d. × 5 to 7 days

   b. Children: 15 mg/kg a day, divided t.i.d. × 5 days

2. Quinacrine HCl (Atabrine)

   a. Adults: 100 mg b.i.d. to t.i.d. after meals × 5 to 7 days

   b. Children: 6 mg/kg a day, divided t.i.d. after meals × 5 days (max 300 mg/day)

3. Furazolidone (Furoxone)

   a. Adults: 100 mg q.i.d. × 7 days

   b. Children: 8 mg/kg a day (max 400 mg a day), divided t.i.d. × 10 days

Diet

As tolerated

Activity

As tolerated

Patient Education

1. Scrupulous attention to handwashing and personal hygiene is advisable, especially in day care and institutional settings.

2. Campers and hikers should use caution when drinking from local water sources. Portable purification systems that filter out *Giardia* are readily available from outdoor supply stores.

Key Treatment

- Metronidazole 2 gm orally q.d. × 3 days

Follow-Up

1. Re-evaluate if symptoms persist.
2. Consider testing close household contacts.

Bibliography

Adam RD: The biology of *Giardia* spp. Microbiol Rev 1991;55(4):706–732.

Addiss DG, Mathews HM, Stewart JM, et al: Evaluation of a commercially available enzyme-linked immunosorbent assay for *Giardia lamblia* antigen in stool. J Clin Microbiol 1991;29(6):1137–1142.

Isaac-Renton JL: Laboratory diagnosis of giardiasis. Clin Lab Med 1991;11(4):811–827.

Jones JE: Giardiasis. Primary Care 1991;18(1):43–52.

Thompson RCA, Reynoldson JA, Mendis AHW: *Giardia* and giardiasis. Adv Parasitol 1993;32:71–160.

247 Amebiasis

Timothy R. Sterling

Etiology

1. Epidemiology of *Entamoeba histolytica*

   a. It is estimated that 10 per cent of the global and 1 to 4 per cent of the United States population is infected. Prevalence of infection approaches 50 per cent in developing countries.

   b. Only 10 per cent of strains (zymodemes) are virulent. Virulent strains, and resultant invasive disease, are more common in developing countries.

2. Life cycle

   a. Cyst

   (1) Fecal-oral transmission: poverty, mental retardation, institutionalization, and male homosexual oral-anal intercourse increase risk of transmission

   (2) Resistant to gastric acid as well as chlorine and possibly iodine water purification and can exist for weeks in a moist environment outside of the body

   (3) Excystation in the small intestine results in release of trophozoites.

   b. Trophozoite

   (1) Grows in the lumen or wall of the colon, requiring bacteria for growth

   (2) Found in stool in severe disease but usually encysts before exiting the colon

3. Pathogenesis of invasive disease

   a. Factors that predispose to tissue invasion: virulent zymodeme, male sex, young age, corticosteroids, malnutrition, pregnancy, immunocompromise (e.g., HIV infection)

   b. Altered colonic mucus and certain bacterial strains allow for tissue lysis and invasion

   c. Cecum and ascending colon involved most often; rectum, sigmoid less frequently

   d. Muscularis mucosa involvement can lead to granulation tissue, ameboma formation

   e. Trophozoites may enter portal venous circulation, leading to periportal fibrosis, hepatic necrosis, and abscess formation

   f. Protective immunity may develop after invasive, noninvasive disease; usually incomplete

Symptoms

1. Intestinal amebiasis

   a. Asymptomatic: due to noninvasive colonic lumen infection, which accounts for more than 90 per cent of amebic infections

   b. Symptomatic: due to either noninvasive luminal or invasive colonic wall infection

   (1) Intermittent diarrhea, lasting months to years; may contain mucus; blood if invasive

   (2) Lower abdominal cramping

   (3) Flatulence

2. Extraintestinal amebiasis

   a. Hepatic

   (1) Amebic hepatitis: fever, right upper quadrant pain, tender hepatomegaly, in the presence of amebic colitis

   (2) Amebic abscess: fever, right upper quadrant pain of acute or subacute onset; referred pain to right shoulder, nonproductive cough, weight loss

   b. Pleuropulmonary: cough, fever, pleuritic pain, expectoration of necrotic material if rupture into bronchus occurs

   c. Pericarditis: chest pain, congestive heart failure after persistent fever and abdominal pain

   d. Peritonitis: severe abdominal pain, fever

Key Symptoms

Intestinal	Hepatic
• Intermittent diarrhea; can be profuse and bloody	• Right upper quadrant pain
• Abdominal cramping	• Right shoulder pain
• Flatulence	• Fever

Clinical Findings

1. Asymptomatic cyst passer

2. Intestinal amebiasis

   a. Noninvasive infection: may be symptomatic or asymptomatic

   b. Invasive infection

   (1) Acute rectocolitis (dysentery): profuse bloody diarrhea, which may be associated with hepatomegaly and high fever

   (2) Fulminant colitis with perforation

   (3) Chronic postdysenteric colitis: follows recurrent severe intestinal amebiasis; mimics inflammatory bowel disease; unresponsive to antiamebic therapy

   (4) Ameboma: cecum and ascending colon most frequent site; intestinal obstruction

(5) Perianal ulceration: ulcerative or condylomatous

3. Extraintestinal amebiasis
   a. Hepatic
      (1) Associated more often with asymptomatic than symptomatic intestinal infection
      (2) Right upper quadrant tenderness; hepatomegaly in more than 50 per cent
      (3) Serous pleural effusion and atelectasis are common but do not indicate disease extension into lung parenchyma
   b. Pleuropulmonary
      (1) Pneumonia or lung abscess due to direct extension from liver in 10 to 20 per cent of patients with hepatic abscess; may also spread hematogenously
      (2) Empyema: associated with 15 to 35 per cent mortality
   c. Pericarditis: due to extension from left hepatic lobe; cardiac tamponade rare
   d. Peritonitis: due to extension from or rupture of hepatic abscess
   e. Brain abscess: rapidly fatal if untreated
   f. Genitourinary disease

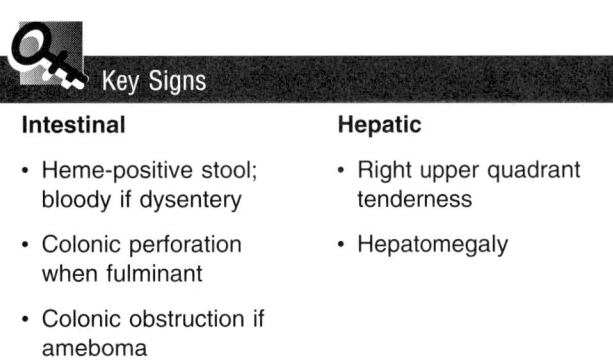

Key Signs

Intestinal	Hepatic
• Heme-positive stool; bloody if dysentery	• Right upper quadrant tenderness
• Colonic perforation when fulminant	• Hepatomegaly
• Colonic obstruction if ameboma	

Laboratory Tests

1. Intestinal amebiasis
   a. Diagnosis established by identifying trophozoites or cysts in stool or tissue
      (1) Liquid and semiformed stool should be immediately examined by wet mount to look for motile trophozoites; more than three specimens, concentrating stool increases yield
      (2) Hematophagous trophozoites or blood seen in invasive infection only; no polymorphonuclear neutrophil leukocytes (PMN)
      (3) Specimens fixed in polyvinyl alcohol required for definitive diagnosis
   b. Serology: indirect hemagglutination (IHA) antiamebic antibody titers remain increased years after invasive disease; counterimmunoelectrophoresis (CIE) becomes negative after cure of invasive

disease; enzyme-linked immunosorbent assay (ELISA) also a very sensitive test. Antibodies present in invasive and noninvasive infection
   c. Sigmoidoscopy: trophozoites on aspirate of typically flask-shaped mucosal lesions, which are present only in invasive infection; yield highest at ulcer edge
   d. Stool culture: for diagnosis of chronic or asymptomatic intestinal infection

2. Extraintestinal amebiasis
   Diagnosis requires combination of clinical presentation, imaging study, and serology.
   a. Organism rarely recovered from stool or tissue
   b. Leukocytosis (without eosinophilia), mild anemia, elevated alkaline phosphatase
   c. Serology: antibodies present in 99 per cent of hepatic amebic abscesses, although may be negative during first week of symptoms
   d. Imaging studies: ultrasonography (US) and computed tomography (CT) scan are both sensitive but not specific for hepatic amebic abscess
   e. Aspiration of abscess (under CT or US guidance): to distinguish between pyogenic and amebic infection when the patient's condition is too unstable to await serology result. Aspirate resembles anchovy paste, contains no PMN or organisms.

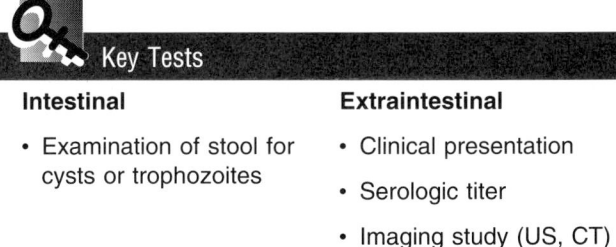

Key Tests

Intestinal	Extraintestinal
• Examination of stool for cysts or trophozoites	• Clinical presentation
	• Serologic titer
	• Imaging study (US, CT)

Differential Diagnosis

1. Intestinal amebiasis
   a. Nondysenteric
      (1) Infection: *G. lamblia,* enterotoxigenic *Escherichia coli, Campylobacter, Salmonella, Cryptosporidia, Isospora*
      (2) Irritable bowel syndrome
      (3) Diverticulitis
      (4) Regional enteritis
      (5) Viral gastroenteritis
      (6) Malabsorption syndrome
   b. Dysentery/acute amebic rectocolitis
      (1) Exacerbation of inflammatory bowel disease; amebiasis must be excluded—corticosteroid therapy will increase severity of amebiasis, cause toxic megacolon
      (2) Infectious colitis: *Salmonella, Shigella, Cam-*

pylobacter, invasive *Vibrio* sp., *Yersinia,* invasive *E. coli,* schistosomiasis

c. Ameboma:

(1) Colon cancer

(2) Lymphoma

(3) Tuberculosis

2. Hepatic abscess

a. Pyogenic abscess

b. Hepatocellular carcinoma

c. Echinococcal cyst

Treatment

Medication

1. Asymptomatic cyst passer: treatment is recommended because subsequent tissue invasion can occur if cysts are not eradicated. Requires agent with intraluminal activity; iodoquinol (Yodoxin), 650 mg t.i.d. × 21 days or paromomycin (Humatin), 25 to 30 mg/kg a day in three doses × 7 days are agents of first choice. Alternatively, could use diloxanide furoate (Furamide), 500 mg t.i.d. × 10 days, but available only from the Centers for Disease Control and Prevention (CDC).

2. Intestinal disease: metronidazole (Flagyl), 750 mg t.i.d. × 10 days preferred for both moderate and severe disease; tinidazole is at least as effective and has fewer adverse effects but is unavailable in the United States. Dehydroemetine (Mebadin), an alternative for severe disease, is available only through CDC. Follow treatment with an intraluminal agent to eradicate cysts, which may be resistant to metronidazole.

3. Hepatic abscess: metronidazole 750 mg t.i.d. × 10 days is the drug of choice; tinidazole is also effective. Dehydroemetine followed by chloroquine is an alternative regimen. Aspiration of abscess unnecessary unless no improvement after 72 hr of therapy or severe liver tenderness, swelling. Must also follow treatment with an intraluminal agent to eradicate cysts

Diet

Avoid fecally contaminated food, water; vegetables grown in endemic areas often contaminated.

Activity

No restrictions

Patient Education

1. Appropriate waste disposal is crucial in preventing spread of amebiasis.

2. Water must be boiled to eradicate infection.

3. Vegetables should be cleaned with a detergent and soaked in vinegar or acetic acid for 10 minutes to eliminate cysts.

4. Peel all fruit.

5. Sexual practices that promote fecal-oral spread of infection must be avoided.

Key Treatment

- For intestinal disease and hepatic abscess, metronidazole is the drug of choice.

Follow-Up

Examination of the stool for cysts after course of therapy is necessary due to lack of a treatment completely effective in eradicating intestinal infection.

The opinions and assertions contained herein are the private views of the author and are not to be construed as the official policy or position of the U.S. government, the Department of Defense, or the Department of the Air Force.

Bibliography

Drugs for parasitic infections. The Medical Letter 1993;35:111–122.

Petri WA Jr., Clark CG, Diamond LS: Host-parasite relationships in amebiasis: conference report. J Infect Dis 1994;169:483–484.

Ravdin JI, Petri WA Jr: Entamoeba histolytica (amebiasis). *In* Mandell GL, Bennett JE, Dolin R (eds): Principles and Practice of Infectious Diseases, 4th ed. New York, Churchill Livingstone, 1995, pp 2395–2408.

Reed SL: Amebiasis: an update. Clin Infect Dis 1992;14:385–393.

Wolfe MS: Amebiasis. *In* Strickland GT (ed): Hunter's Tropical Medicine, 7th ed. Philadelphia, WB Saunders, 1991, pp 550–565.

248 Tapeworm Infections

Gregory Juckett

Broad or Fish Tapeworm (*Diphyllobothrium latum*)

Life Cycle

1. Common in fish-eating mammals (including humans), which serve as the final or definitive hosts.
2. Host feces must enter water, where eggs hatch into a larval *coracidium* that then may be swallowed by a freshwater crustacean or copepod (the first intermediate host).
3. The copepod, now containing a procercoid larva, is in turn swallowed by a fish (the second intermediate host) in whose flesh the organism develops as a *pleurocercoid* or *sparganum.*
4. Larger fish become infected by *pleurocercoids* of any fish they swallow.
5. When raw infected fish is consumed by humans, these larvae survive digestion and grow rapidly into segmented adults.
6. The worms have a lifespan of many years and may reach 10 meters in length.

Epidemiology

1. Especially common in Scandinavia and the Baltic region, although it is also found in the northern Midwest and Alaska as well as parts of the Orient.
2. Raw or undercooked fish transmit the infection.
3. Fish-eating carnivores act as a reservoir for eggs, as does the discharge of untreated sewage into water.

Symptoms

1. Although mild infections may be asymptomatic, anorexia, nausea, abdominal discomfort, loose stools, and weight loss may occur.
2. An interesting megaloblastic anemia resembling pernicious anemia is well known in Finland; this worm competes effectively with its host for vitamin B_{12}.

Diagnosis

1. The appearance of characteristic proglottids (worm segments) in stools or the discovery of eggs leads to the diagnosis.
2. *D. latum* proglottids are known to have a central rosette-shaped egg-filled uterus.
3. The characteristic yellow eggs are 60 to 70 μm long with an operculum at one end and a small knob at the other.

Treatment

Two effective regimens are currently accepted for this (and other) tapeworms.

1. Praziquantel (Biltricide) 5 to 10 mg/kg taken once (adults and children). Side effects: usually well tolerated but malaise, headaches, dizziness, abdominal discomfort, and urticaria may occur as the tapeworm dies
2. Niclosamide (Yomesan or Ni:closide) is effective as a single adult dose of 2 gm (4 tablets) chewed thoroughly. In children: 11 to 34 kg, 2 tablets (1 gm); over 34 kg, 3 tablets (1.5 gm). Side effects: similar to Praziquantel with gastrointestinal upset, headache, and possible rash. Cure is not considered complete for either regimen until stool ova and parasite testing is negative for three months. If found, the scolex, or "head," of the tapeworm should be examined after passage to aid in species identification.

Prevention

Thorough cooking of fish is the most effective method of prevention, although freezing fish for 24 to 48 hours at $-10°$ C ($14°$ F) is also satisfactory.

Pork Tapeworm (*Taenia solium*) and Cysticercosis

Life Cycle

1. *T. solium* is a world-wide tapeworm for which the pig is the intermediate host and the human the final or definitive host.
2. Pigs consume the eggs deposited in human feces; hexacanth larvae then hatch in the intestine and develop into bladder worms or cysticerci in host tissue.
3. Humans contract the infection by consuming inadequately cooked infected (measly) pork.
4. The worm can live in its human host 25 years or more.

Epidemiology

1. Although not as common as the beef tapeworm, the pork tapeworm is far more dangerous because human autoinfection can take place either through the fecal-oral route or rarely by the migration of egg-laden proglottids to the stomach.
2. In such a situation, the bladder worms develop in human tissue (cysticercosis) rather than that of the pig, often with grave consequences. Thus humans may serve as either intermediate or final hosts.
3. Pork tapeworm infection is most common in Central and South America but may be found around the world.

Symptoms

1. *Adult tapeworm:* infection often asymptomatic but may cause vague abdominal discomfort, nausea, malaise, or weight loss.
2. *Cysticercosis*
   a. Symptoms depend on where the cysticerci locate. Most commonly, this is in subcutaneous tissue where symptoms are minimal; however, the eye, brain, muscles, and internal organs may all be involved.
   b. Blindness or sudden onset of seizures may occur from eye or brain involvement; there is even the potential for fatal allergic reactions when a cysticercus dies.

Diagnosis

1. *Adult tapeworm*
   a. Active or passive migration of a proglottid from the anus usually results in a prompt diagnosis.
   b. The pork tapeworm proglottid has 7 to 13 lateral uterine branches as opposed to 15 to 20 in the beef tapeworm, but their eggs appear identical.
2. *Cysticercosis*
   a. Often calcified cysticerci are discovered incidentally on radiographs, on which they may appear as rice grains.
   b. The parasite also may appear on other imaging studies or, in the case of the eye, with direct visualization.
   c. Serologic tests have also been developed.

Treatment

1. *Adult tapeworm:* same as *D. latum.* Purging 2 hours after treatment reduces risk of egg release.
2. *Cysticercosis*
   a. Albendazole (Zentel) 15 mg/kg/day in three doses × 28 days repeated as necessary for adults and children. Side effects similar to mebendazole.
   b. Praziquantel (Biltricide) 50 mg/kg/day in three doses × 15 days; contraindication exists in ocular cysticercosis because destruction of the parasite in the eye (or any sensitive neurologic structure) could cause further injury. Bioavailability is increased with cimetidine.
   c. Surgical excision when possible. Asymptomatic cysticercosis may not require treatment.

Prevention

1. Thorough cooking or freezing of pork kills cysticerci, although pickling and salting do not.
2. Proper disposal of human feces prevents swine infection.
3. Human cysticercosis may be prevented by prompt treatment of the adult worm and by taking measures to avoid fecal-oral contact.

Beef Tapeworm (*Taenia saginata*)

Life Cycle

1. *T. saginata* is an abundant cosmopolitan tapeworm, utilizing humans as the definitive host (harboring sexual stage) and cattle or another grazing animal as the intermediate (nonsexual phase) host.
2. Eggs are passed in human feces and can remain viable on pasture land for at least 4 months.
3. After eggs are consumed by cattle, cysticerci encyst in their muscle and, in turn, infect humans if they ingest this undercooked "measly" beef.
4. This tapeworm takes 10 to 12 weeks to mature in the intestines.

Epidemiology

1. *T. saginata* is one of the most common tapeworms in the world, with a high prevalence in South America, Africa, and Muslim regions.
2. Fortunately, its cysticerci do not develop in people who happen to ingest eggs, and thus it is far less dangerous than the pork tapeworm.

Symptoms

1. Usually there are no symptoms; however, vague abdominal discomfort, decreased appetite, nausea, intestinal obstruction, and weight loss are reported.
2. Surprisingly, increased hunger is not very common.
3. Some symptoms such as headache, dizziness, skin sensitivity, and even delirium may be caused by the absorption of this and other tapeworm's excretions.

Diagnosis

1. Proglottids with 15 to 20 lateral uterine branches are passed in the stool with the eggs or they may actively migrate out.
2. *T. saginata* eggs are more likely to be detected on anal swabs.

Treatment

Same as *D. latum*

Prevention

1. Proper disposal of human feces and the thorough cooking of beef until it is no longer pink inside is very effective.
2. Cysticerci are killed at 56° C or by freezing for 1 week.

Unilocular Hydatid Disease (*Echinococcus granulosus*)

Life Cycle

1. *E. granulosus* is a tiny (3 to 6 mm) tapeworm of dogs (the definitive host), with sheep serving as the usual intermediate host.

2. Dogs are affected by consuming sheep organs that harbor infective cysts.

3. Sylvatic echinococcosis occurs in northern Canada and involves wolves and caribou.

4. Domestic sled dogs may become infected if they have access to caribou meat.

Epidemiology

1. Humans become abnormal intermediate hosts when they ingest the eggs (which are passed in dog feces).

2. The infection is common in sheep-rearing areas worldwide, especially if there is close contact between shepherds and their dogs.

3. The hydatid cyst, as the bladder stage is called, develops slowly with numerous brood capsules forming inside, each containing several larval protoscolices.

4. In some cases, up to 20 years may pass before symptoms appear, and the fluid-filled cyst can become huge if its growth is not restricted by its location.

5. A similar tapeworm, *Taenia (Multiceps) multiceps*, follows a similar life cycle and occasionally causes a CNS infection in humans called coenuriasis.

Symptoms

1. As in cysticercosis, symptoms depend on cyst location; however, these cysts are much larger.

2. Hydatids can cause spontaneous fractures if they grow in bone, biliary colic if in the liver, cough or hemoptysis in the lung, and neurologic symptoms mimicking brain tumor if in the brain.

3. Cyst rupture releases proteinacious fluid, often causing sudden, fatal anaphylaxis.

Diagnosis

1. "Cannonball"-shaped cysts may be noted on radiography or other imaging studies and at times fremitus ("hydatid thrill") may be palpated over a large cyst.

2. Eosinophilia is present in only a minority of cases.

3. In the past, Casoni's test, an intradermal hydatid protein skin test, has been utilized, but it is now being replaced by enzyme-linked immunosorbent assay and other serologic tests.

Treatment

1. Surgical excision of the cyst requires predosing with steroids to prevent anaphylaxis in the event of accidental rupture. A partial cyst aspiration with replacement by hypertonic saline to kill the contents has also been recommended before removal.

2. Albendazole 400 mg b.i.d. × 28 days repeated as necessary (pediatric: 15 mg/kg/day × 28 days). This medication causes cyst regression and is sometimes used in conjunction with surgery.

Prevention

Avoiding dog feces, the regular worming of dogs, and preventing canine consumption of infected sheep are all key interventions.

Alveolar Hydatid Disease (*Echinococcus multilocularis*)

Life Cycle

1. This is another small tapeworm with foxes (or occasionally dogs and cats) as definitive hosts and small rodents serving as intermediate hosts.

2. When hydatids within the rodent are consumed, the carnivore develops tapeworms.

3. The cycle repeats when rodents ingest the eggs passed in fox feces.

Epidemiology

1. Human infection is uncommon but is found in trappers or sled dog owners in the far north (including several states in the northern U.S.).

2. In these regions, pets feeding on infected mice could pass this infection to their owners through their feces.

3. Unlike the single cysts of unilocular hydatid disease, an aggregate of tiny alveolar cysts form in the host; these may infiltrate organs and even metastasize as cancer does.

Symptoms

1. The liver is usually involved and may become honeycombed to the point of cavitation.

2. Hepatomegaly and ascites are frequent manifestations of this chronic disease.

Diagnosis

1. Liver scanning suggests and liver biopsy confirms the diagnosis.

2. Even on gross examination, the affected organ is often thought to have been ravaged by a malignancy.

Treatment

1. Surgical excision is the only reliable option, but this infection must be caught while it is still operable.

2. Albendazole or mebendazole may help as long-term systemic therapy.

Prevention

1. Avoiding close contact with foxes or other host animals is necessary or, in the case of pets, regular worming.

2. Washing wild berries before eating in endemic regions is recommended in case they are contaminated by fox feces.

3. This uncommon but dangerous sylvatic infection is difficult to eradicate because of the wild fox reservoir.

Dwarf Tapeworm (*Hymenolepis [Vampirolepis] nana*) and Rat Tapeworm (*Hymenolepis diminuta*)

Life Cycle

1. *H. nana* is a tiny cosmopolitan tapeworm of mice and rats with an optional arthropod intermediate host (larval fleas or beetles); however, unlike all other known tapeworms, no intermediate host is required, and autoinfection is common.

2. Ingested eggs hatch in the duodenum, develop into tiny cysticercoids in the villi, then emerge within a week as adults in the small intestine.

3. *H. diminuta* is a similar parasite of domestic rats with an obligate intermediate insect host that must be consumed (usually in grain) to cause human infection.

Epidemiology

1. This very common tapeworm infection of children is contracted by fecal-oral contact with infected rodent or human feces.

2. Infected grain beetles or fleas are an alternate source of infection and the only one in the case of *H. diminuta*.

Symptoms

1. Usually asymptomatic, but heavy infections may cause abdominal discomfort, dizziness, pruritus, headaches, and weakness.

2. A host immune response may occur.

Diagnosis

1. *H. nana* has ovoid eggs measuring 30 to 47 μm containing internal polar filaments on the inner membrane.

2. *H. diminuta* eggs are larger (60 to 86 μm) and lack polar filaments.

Treatment

Similar in both infections.

1. Praziquantel 25 mg/kg once (adult and pediatric)

2. Niclosamide

   a. Adult: initial dose of 4 tablets (2 gm) chewed, then 2 tablets daily × 6 days

   b. Pediatric: 11 to 34 kg daily—2 tablets (1 gm) first day then 1 tablet (0.5 gm) daily × 6 days; >35 kg—3 tablets (1.5 gm) then 2 tablets (1 gm) daily × 6 days

Prevention

1. Rodent control and improved grain storage reduce numbers of both tapeworms.

2. Treatment of infected individuals and proper disposal of human feces may be even more important, especially with *H. nana*.

Bibliography

Marx MB: Parasites, Pets, and People. Primary Care 1991; 18(1):153–165.

Schantz PM, McAuley J: Current Status of food-borne parasitic zoonoses in the United States. Southeast Asian J Trop Med Public Health 1991;22 Suppl:65–71.

Schmidt GD, Roberts LS: Tapeworms. *In* Foundations of Parasitology, 4th ed. Boston, Times Mirror/Mosby College Publishing, 1989, pp 346–378.

Tanowitz HB, Wittner M: Cestode Infections. *In* Strickland GT: Hunter's Tropical Medicine, 7th ed. Philadelphia, WB Saunders, 1991, pp 831–859.

The Medical Letter on Drugs and Therapeutics. Drugs for Parasitic Infections 35 (Issue 911) Dec 10, 1993.

249 Ascaris and Hookworm Infection

Mark Byler

Ascaris

Etiology

1. *Ascaris lumbricoides* (roundworm)
2. Distribution is worldwide. It is endemic in southeastern United States. Over one billion are infected worldwide.
3. Morphology: largest intestinal nematode; adult female, 20 to 35 cm; adult male, 15 to 20 cm; ''pencil'' size with tapered blunt ends. Color is white, cream, or pink.
4. Life cycle and transmission: It lives primarily unattached in jejunum of host, where females lay up to 200,000 eggs per day. Eggs can survive for years in shaded soil at 25° C (77° F). Infection is spread by consumption of food or drink exposed to feces-contaminated soil. Eggs hatch in the intestine, the larvae then penetrate blood or lymph vessels and pass to the lungs, perforate the alveoli, and migrate up bronchial passages to the epiglottis and down the esophagus to the small intestine, where maturation occurs. Eggs appear in the stool 2 months after ingestion.

Symptoms/Clinical Findings

Both are dependent upon the parasite load. A few ascaris usually result in no symptoms.

1. Larval stage: During larval migration pneumonitis may develop with cough, fever, pulmonary infiltrate, and eosinophilia (Löffler's syndrome).
2. Adult stage: Adult worms cause no specific pathology except to compete for available ingested food. Symptoms during the adult stage depend primarily on two criteria
   a. The number of adult worms in relation to the size of the host will determine symptoms. If the mass of worms is large enough, intestinal lumen obstruction may occur. In one series of acute abdominal emergencies in Cape Town, South Africa, 10 to 15 per cent were due to ascaris, with children having the peak incidence.
   b. Adult worms are usually confined to the jejunum but may migrate. This migration may lead to obstruction of various ducts resulting in appendicitis,

pancreatitis, cholecystitis, or jaundice. Worms may also migrate up the esophagus to the eustachian tube and paranasal sinuses, emerging from the nose or mouth.

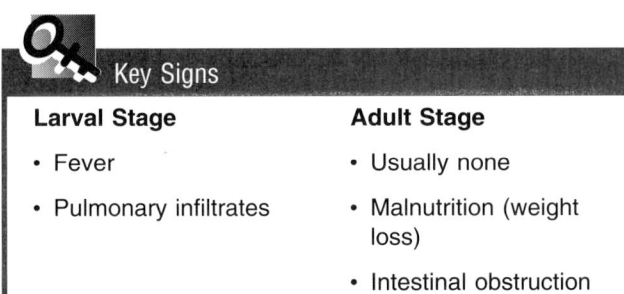

Key Signs	
Larval Stage	**Adult Stage**
• Fever	• Usually none
• Pulmonary infiltrates	• Malnutrition (weight loss)
	• Intestinal obstruction

Laboratory Tests/Diagnosis

1. Definitive diagnosis can only be made by three means
   a. Identify eggs microscopically in feces (most common means).
   b. Identify adult worm in feces, emesis, nares, or at surgery.
   c. Identify larval worm in sputum or tissue sample.
2. Eosinophilia occurs only during the larva's tissue migration, NOT during the adult stage in the jejunum.

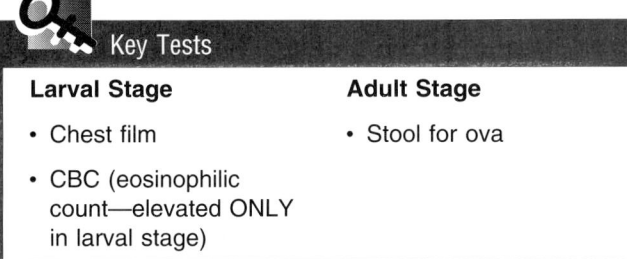

Key Tests	
Larval Stage	**Adult Stage**
• Chest film	• Stool for ova
• CBC (eosinophilic count—elevated ONLY in larval stage)	

Treatment

See treatment for hookworm.

Hookworm

Etiology

1. Two species: *Ancylostoma duodenale* and *Necator americanus*
2. Distribution: subtropics and tropics; the two species overlap in many regions
3. Morphology: pink or white in color; adult male, 8 to 11 mm; adult female, 10 to 13 mm
4. Life cycle and transmission: almost identical for the two species. Adults attach to mucosa of small intestine, where females lay 10,000 to 30,000 eggs per day. Once eggs are released into soil, a larva is

Key Symptoms

Larval Stage	**Adult Stage**
• Cough	• Usually none
• Pneumonitis	• Abdominal pain if obstruction present

hatched within 24 to 48 hours and can survive for months in warm, moist soil. On contact with unprotected human skin, the larva penetrates the epidermis, enters the venous system, and is carried to the lungs. There it penetrates the alveoli and migrates up the bronchial tree to the esophagus and back to the small intestine. Total elimination of the parasite takes 5 to 15 years if reinfection does not occur.

Symptoms/Clinical Findings

1. Larva stage: A dermatitis known as "ground itch" or "coolie itch" may occur at the site of larva penetration of the skin. During migration through the lung, the larvae seldom produce the severe reaction that can be seen with ascaris.
2. Adult stage: Findings depend on parasite load. There are primarily two pathologic features of infection.
   a. Anemia: The severity of the anemia is proportional to the content of iron in the diet, duration of infection, and parasite load. The anemia is classically hypochromic microcytic. In diets low in vitamin B_{12} or folate, the anemia may be normocytic or macrocytic.
   b. Hypoproteinemia: Protein loss is usually in excess of the red blood cell loss. Protein loss is the consequence of plasma loss from ingestion by the worm and traumatized intestinal lumen. The resulting hypoproteinemia and hypoalbuminemia can lead to edema resembling kwashiorkor in children or congestive heart failure in adults.

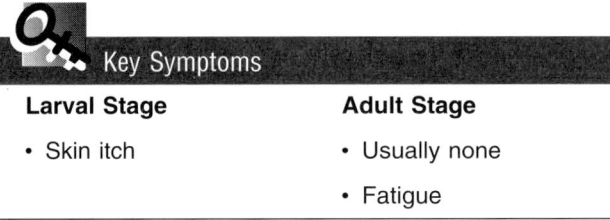

Key Symptoms	
Larval Stage	**Adult Stage**
• Skin itch	• Usually none
	• Fatigue

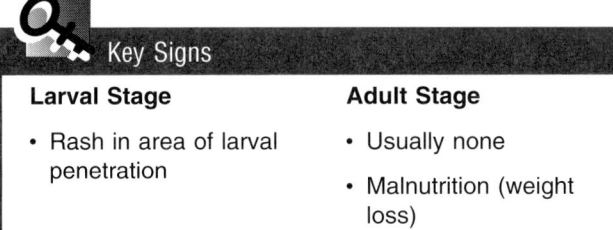

Key Signs	
Larval Stage	**Adult Stage**
• Rash in area of larval penetration	• Usually none
	• Malnutrition (weight loss)

Laboratory Tests

1. Hypochromic microcytic anemia
2. Hypoproteinemia and hypoalbuminemia
3. Eosinophilia, which is usually a mild elevation

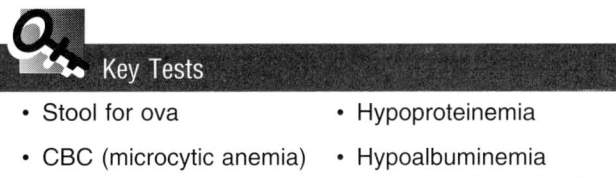

Key Tests	
• Stool for ova	• Hypoproteinemia
• CBC (microcytic anemia)	• Hypoalbuminemia

Diagnosis

Microscopic hookworm eggs found in the fecal sample are diagnostic.

Treatment for Ascaris and Hookworm

1. Treatment of choice is mebendazole (Vermox). Pediatric and adult dosage: 100 mg b.i.d. × 3 days
2. Alternative treatments
   a. Pyrantel pamoate (Antiminth). Pediatric and adult dosage: 11 mg/kg once (max dose 1 gm)
   b. Albendazole (Zentel). Pediatric and adult dosage: 400 mg once

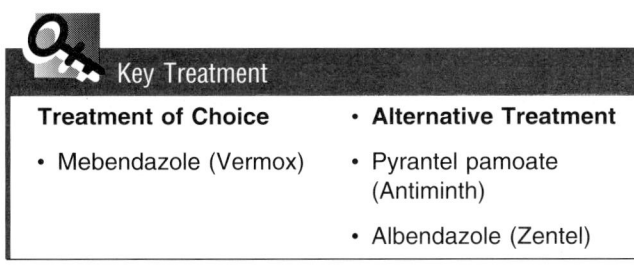

Key Treatment	
Treatment of Choice	**• Alternative Treatment**
• Mebendazole (Vermox)	• Pyrantel pamoate (Antiminth)
	• Albendazole (Zentel)

Bibliography

Drugs for Parasitic Infections. Med Lett Drugs Ther 1993; 35.
Jong EC, McMullen R: The Travel and Tropical Medicine Manual, 2nd ed. Philadelphia, WB Saunders, 1995.
Strickland GT (ed): Hunter's Tropical Medicine, 7th ed. Philadelphia, WB Saunders, 1991.
Warren S, Mahmound Adel AF (eds): Tropical and Geographical Medicine, 2nd ed. New York, McGraw-Hill, 1990.
Wilson ME: World Guide to Infections: Diseases, Distribution, Diagnosis. London, Oxford University Press, 1991.

250 Common Dermatologic Symptoms

Itching, or pruritus, is an unpleasant sensation that provokes the urge to scratch. Causes of itching range from the serious (lymphoma) to the simple (flea bites). Whatever the cause, itching can make life miserable and is worthy of careful evaluation and treatment.

Differential Diagnosis

The diagnostic possibilities for itching are daunting. Fortunately, most itching is caused by a primary dermatologic condition. The challenge is to focus on finding and treating common causes without forgetting that itching is occasionally the presenting symptom of serious systemic disease.

1. Dermatologic causes
   a. Xerosis (dry skin)
   b. Infections (dermatophytosis, folliculitis, *Candida*, varicella, HIV)
   c. Infestations (scabies, lice, pinworms, other parasitic diseases)
   d. Other (atopic dermatitis, contact dermatitis, urticaria, insect bites, seborrheic dermatitis, pityriasis rosea, psoriasis, stasis dermatitis, senile pruritus, dermatitis herpetiformis, lichen planus, pemphigus)
2. Physical causes (sunburn, fiber glass, chemical irritants, overdrying, too-frequent bathing, pressure, low-intensity electrical stimulation, suction)
3. Medication-related causes
   a. Allergy to drug
   b. Idiosyncratic drug reactions
   c. Pruritus-producing drugs (oral contraceptives and other hormones, opiates, barbiturates, aspirin, vitamin B complex, phenothiazines, tolbutamide, quinidine, and many others)
4. Pregnancy-related causes
   a. Nonspecific pruritus of pregnancy
   b. Intrahepatic cholestasis of pregnancy
   c. Pruritic urticarial papules and plaques of pregnancy (PUPPP)
5. Systemic causes
   a. Renal (uremia)
   b. Obstructive biliary disease
   c. Hematologic (iron deficiency anemia, polycythemia vera, systemic mastocytosis)
   d. Endocrine (hyperthyroidism, hypothyroidism, hypercalcemia, carcinoid)
   e. Malignant (lymphoma, multiple myeloma, visceral malignancy)
   f. Neurologic (multiple sclerosis, stroke, brain tumor or abscess, peripheral neuropathy)
6. Psychological (psychogenic itching, neurodermatitis, stress, depression)

> Refer to Ch. 152, Lymphoma; Ch. 193, Drug Allergy; to Urticaria, elsewhere in this chapter (Ch. 250); Ch. 251, Atopic Dermatitis; Ch. 252, Seborrheic Dermatitis; Ch. 253, Contact Dermatitis; Ch. 262, Psoriasis; and Ch. 330, Insects and Spiders.

History: Key Questions to Ask

1. Where is the itching? (localized vs. generalized)
2. How severe is the itching? (interference with work, sleep, or daily activities)
3. When do you get the itching? (onset, duration, morning/night, time of year)
4. What makes the itching worse? (cold air, stress, sun, bathing, clothing)
5. What are you exposed to? (pets, allergens, soaps, irritants, medications including nonprescription, travel, occupational)
6. Is anyone else itching?
7. What have you tried for the itching so far?
8. Do you have any other problems? (weight loss, fever, jaundice, fatigue, night sweats)

Clinical Findings

1. Nonspecific signs of scratching or rubbing
   a. Excoriations (linear arrays of erosions in areas within reach of fingernails)
   b. Lichenification (thickening of skin with prominence of superficial markings)
   c. Hyperpigmentation
2. Signs of skin disease (may be subtle)
   a. Rash suggestive of specific diagnosis
   b. Pattern of rash (localized versus generalized, fingernail-accessible)
   c. Scaling, dryness, cracking (xerosis)
   d. Erythema
   e. Urticaria (hives) or dermatographism (wheal after rubbing skin with blunt object)

f. Interdigital lesions, linear or S-shaped burrows (scabies is often atypical)

g. Lice or nits

3. Signs of underlying disease

a. Jaundice

b. Lymphadenopathy

c. Thyromegaly

d. Hepatosplenomegaly

Tests

Tests are usually not needed for the effective treatment of itching. A careful history and physical often reveal a cause. Often empiric treatment brings relief of symptoms even if the cause is not known. Tests should be reserved for those with significant itching, but without dermatologic disease, who have not responded to nonspecific treatment. Test selection should be guided by clinical judgment.

1. Complete blood count

2. Creatinine, blood urea nitrogen

3. Thyroid function tests

4. Calcium

5. Bilirubin

6. Urinalysis

Consider:

7. Chest radiograph

8. Sedimentation rate

9. Serum protein electrophoresis

10. Liver function tests

11. Stool for occult blood

12. Electrolytes

13. Fasting glucose

14. Stool for ova and parasites

15. HIV test

Management

1. First treat any specific causes of itching (e.g., scabicides for scabies, dialysis for uremia).

2. Skin hydration measures are often the most effective treatment. Use them in addition to any other treatment you try.

Medication

1. Emollients (moisten skin)

a. Use preparations without perfumes or additives. White petroleum jelly is effective and inexpensive.

b. Use especially after washing and before bed.

c. Avoid lotions and creams that may sensitize the skin.

2. Creams with urea or lactic acid (hydration)

3. Camphor/menthol/phenol lotions (soothe by counterirritation)

4. Antihistamines (for histamine-related itching)

a. Hydroxyzine (Atarax), chlorpheniramine, and other alkylamines are a good choice.

b. Nonsedating antihistamines are less effective because the sedation seems to be an important mechanism of action.

c. Use of antihistamines for nonallergic itching is controversial and probably works through sedation.

5. Tricyclic antidepressants (H_1 blockade, sedation, and other mechanisms): Doxepin (Sinequan) is especially useful.

6. Hydrocortisone creams (use for specific indications)

7. Risks of systemic steroids must be considered if used for severe, intractable cases.

8. Specific treatments

a. Phototherapy for itching due to uremia

b. Cholestyramine (Questran) for itching due to cholestasis

9. Calamine lotion is very drying and should only be used on weeping wounds.

10. Topical anesthetics and antihistamines are often ineffective and sensitizing.

11. A number of other therapies for itching have been suggested without definitive studies supporting their usefulness. Transcutaneous electrical nerve stimulation, acupuncture, EMLA cream, H_2 blockers, opiate antagonists, and capsaicin may eventually have a role in the treatment of itch.

Diet

1. Avoid spicy food, alcohol, hot foods, or hot liquids (vasodilatory).

2. Drink lots of fluids.

Activity

1. Use pressure with palm near pruritic area instead of scratching.

2. Apply cool washcloth or ice to area.

3. Trim fingernails short; keep them clean.

4. Hydration measures

a. Minimize bathing, avoid hot baths.

b. Pat dry instead of rubbing.

c. Use bath oils (caution patients about slipping in bathtub).

d. Use superfatted or nonalkaline soaps rather than drying soaps.

5. Avoid rough clothing (e.g., wool).

6. Double rinse clothes; add lotion to rinse cycle.

7. Change one sheet at a time to avoid static electricity.

8. Avoid the sun and sweating.

Patient Education

1. Because many of the interventions require changing long-standing habits, written instructions will help to increase compliance.

2. Increase humidity of the house.

3. Lower stress levels.

4. Have all pets evaluated for fleas and lice.

Follow-Up

1. Repeating a careful history and physical examination at follow-up visits may yield clues to the cause of the itching.

2. Consider scabies, HIV, and psychiatric causes for difficult cases.

3. Consider skin biopsy or dermatology referral.

PEARLS

- Most itching is caused by skin diseases, especially dry skin. Clues may be subtle, such as the fine scaling and cracking of xerosis (dry skin).

- If in doubt, treat dry skin. Even if it is not the cause of the itching, dry skin makes any itching worse.

- Reserve laboratory evaluation for patients with significant itching but no skin disorder who do not respond to empiric treatment.

Bibliography

For a review of the treatment of pruritus, including some experimental treatments, see
Bernhard JD: Pruritus: Advances in treatment. Adv Dermatol 1991:6:57–71.
For an extensive review of pruritus, see
Denman ST: A review of pruritus. J Am Acad Dermatol 1986;14:375–392.
For a practical and compassionate article on psychological causes of itching, see
Fried RG: Evaluation and treatment of "psychogenic" pruritus and self-excoriation. J Am Acad Dermatol 1994;30:993–999.
For more information on pruritus, especially for diagnosis and treatment of localized itching, see
Greco JG, Ende J: An office-based approach to the patient with pruritus. Hosp Pract 1992;27(5A):121–128.
For a review of pathophysiology and treatment of pruritus, see
Greaves MW: New pathophysiological and clinical insights into pruritus. J Dermatol 1993;20:735–740.

Symptom   Urticaria and Angioedema   *Constantine Saadeh*

Urticaria (commonly known as hives) and angioedema are the result of a similar pathophysiologic defect: the release of histamine and other mediators.

1. Urticaria usually involves the epidermis and the upper portions of the dermis, whereas angioedema involves the deeper layers of the dermis and the subcutaneous tissue. The release of mediators leads to dilatation of the blood vessels with extravasation of fluid and edema in the interstitial region. Because urticarial lesions are superficial, the clinical appearance is that of swelling and redness, referred to as wheal and flare respectively, whereas in angioedema the involvement is deeper; the skin may appear normal and only swelling is noted.

2. Angioedema usually occurs in association with urticaria. Approximately 20 per cent of the American population will experience at least one episode of acute urticaria during a lifetime. It usually subsides spontaneously. Acute urticarial episodes are transient and do not last more than 24 to 48 hours; chronic urticaria or angioedema occurs much less frequently, probably in less than 10 per cent of cases.

Etiology and Differential Diagnosis

Urticaria and angioedema can be classified, based on the duration of the lesion, as to whether it is acute or chronic. In chronic urticaria, a known etiologic agent can be identified only about 20 per cent of the time.

1. If angioedema occurs in the absence of urticaria,

suspect hereditary or, rarely, (acquired) C1 esterase inhibitor deficiency.

2. Acute urticaria usually subsides within 24 to 48 hours. The offending agent is probably an ingested substance such as a food item (peanuts, shellfish), drugs (penicillin, aspirin), or insect bite hypersensitivity (Hymenoptera venom) and rarely aeroallergens.

3. Parasitic infestations can also be a cause of chronic urticaria.

4. Intravenous radiocontrast iodinated media can induce urticaria and/or anaphylaxis via direct stimulation of mast cells.

5. Chronic urticaria can be induced by physical factors.

   a. Dermographism (DG) (writing on the skin), which is probably the most common cause of chronic physical urticaria: transient wheal and flare occurring within a few minutes of mechanical stroking of the skin. DG can be present by itself or can accompany other physical urticarial conditions listed below.

   b. Vibratory urticaria, which appears when vibration is the predominant motion, such as a shaking steering wheel

   c. Solar urticaria is of six types and is related to sun exposure.

   d. Cold-induced urticaria is usually acquired and is noted within minutes after cold exposure.

e. Pressure urticaria, which occurs at the site of pressure application, could be of two types: the immediate and the delayed, occurring within 5 to 10 minutes, and 4 to 6 hours following pressure application respectively (e.g., wearing a tight belt). It is to be noted that the delayed reaction can be associated with other systemic symptoms such as fever and elevated sedimentation rate.

f. Cholinergic urticaria is present after a hot shower or exercising in a humid environment. Typically, it appears around the neck area, and the lesions are smaller in size than the usual hives.

6. Chronic urticaria from autoimmune and malignant causes

a. Essential mixed cryoglobulinemia (EMC) can present with urticaria, fever, elevated sedimentation rate with low complement levels (C3 and C4) and cryoglobulins.

b. Similar urticarial rash can occur in association with other autoimmune diseases (lupus erythematosus and rheumatoid arthritis) and malignant conditions (Hodgkin's and non-Hodgkin's lymphomas).

7. If none of the above etiologies has been identified in a particular patient, the diagnosis of chronic *idiopathic* urticaria (CIU) is suspected. CIU, therefore, is defined by

a. The absence of a known etiology of urticaria

b. Lesions appearing either continuously or several days during the week for at least 6 weeks

8. Psychogenic factors and hyperthyroidism can worsen chronic urticarial lesions but by themselves cannot be the sole etiology.

a. Histamine release could be related to immunoglobulin E (IgE)-dependent mechanisms as in food and in the physical urticarias. Direct release of histamine independent of IgE from the mast cell could also occur, as in the case of intravenous radiocontrast dye and opiates.

b. The activation of other mediators as in the leukotriene pathway could be important in aspirin-induced urticaria, although the true mechanism of this phenomenon is not fully understood.

Refer to Ch. 152, Lymphoma; Ch. 153, Hodgkin's Disease; Ch. 163, Hyperthyroidism; Ch. 193, Drug Allergy; Ch. 194, Food Allergy; Ch. 207, Systemic Lupus Erythematosus.

History

The diagnosis of urticaria/angioedema is usually obvious: the lesion is typical, with a wheal and flare type response in urticaria and a swelling in the normally appearing area of the skin in angioedema. Investigation of the cause of the lesion depends on the history, such as the ingestion of certain food items, with peanuts and shellfish being the most commonly incriminated. The patient may have been eating the same type of food or had ingested the same drug earlier, but an allergic response to the same food or the drug based on an IgE-mediated reaction could still develop.

Clinical Findings

Physical examination, such as a search for an underlying lymphoma and palpation of the thyroid gland, could identify subtle causes or exacerbating factors of urticaria/angioedema, respectively.

The key findings of hereditary angioedema include

1. Attacks of angioedema of the extremities, eyelids, lips, larynx, or scrotal areas in early childhood, either spontaneously or in response to exercise or stress

2. The attacks usually last 48 to 72 hours in the absence of itching and urticaria.

Tests

1. Minimum laboratory investigation: a complete blood count to check for increased eosinophils and anemia associated with chronic disease. Stool for ova and parasite in search for helminthic infections.

2. An urticarial eruption 5 minutes following the stroking of the skin gently with a tongue depressor is characteristic of dermographism, and placing a finger in a vortex tube with an immediate urticarial reaction suggests vibratory induced urticaria.

3. A positive satellite response to the subcutaneous application of methacholine is noted in one third of patients with cholinergic urticaria, whereas a giant hive appearing at the site 15 to 20 minutes following the application of an ice cube is diagnostic of cold-induced urticaria. Although a biopsy of an urticarial lesion is generally not necessary, there are two situations in which biopsy is helpful. In patients with EMC, lupus, and other autoimmune conditions, the biopsy will show leukocytoclastic vasculitis; in patients with CIU, an increased number of mast cells that are degranulated and other inflammatory cells such as T lymphocytes, macrophages, neutrophils, and eosinophils, usually in a perivascular location, is noted.

4. Other useful laboratory data include

a. Erythrocyte sedimentation rate (ESR) and antinucleic acid antibodies are elevated in EMC and lupus

b. Thyroid panel: CIU can be exacerbated by hyperthyroidism

c. Complement 4 (C4) is usually suppressed in hereditary angioedema, even between attacks, a fact that makes this test very sensitive. If C4 is low, specific determination of a low C1 esterase inhibitor, either antigenically or functionally, will establish the diagnosis.

Management

1. Avoid the offending agent if known and use epinephrine if a vital organ is involved, such as angioedema of the larynx. In most situations, however, the lesions would subside spontaneously within 24 to 48 hours.

2. If itching is persistent, antihistamines can be used, such as chlorpheniramine or hydroxyzine. Hydroxyzine, classically, has been the drug of choice for chronic idiopathic urticaria and other forms of physical urticarias and should be given in doses of 25 to 50 mg every 4 to 6 hours. The major side effect of these antihistamines is sedation. Many patients can become tolerant to the sedative effect within a few days. In situations in which it cannot be tolerated, one can then resort to the new generation of antihistamines, which are currently approved for the treatment of chronic urticaria/angioedema, including terfenadine (Seldane), astemizole (Hismanal), and loratadine (Claritin). A fourth agent known as cetirizine (Reactin), which also holds promise in the control of the delayed pressure urticaria, is pending FDA approval.

3. In a patient with continued urticaria/angioedema despite the use of the newer antihistamines, an H_2 blocker can be added: the combination of H_1 and H_2 blockers has been shown to be effective in more than 60 per cent of the patients with this condition. Fortunately, most patients with CIU recover within weeks or months.

4. In the rare patient who continues to have problems despite the use of H_1 and H_2 blockers, referral to an allergist is necessary to try other agents, many of which are considered experimental, such as colchicine, dapsone, and methotrexate. Oral or parenteral steroids are usually effective but should be used only on a short-term basis (1 to 2 weeks) in resistant patients.

PEARLS

- Food is the most common cause of acute urticaria.

- Urticaria for more than 6 weeks with no known etiology is labeled chronic idiopathic urticaria.

- Hyperthyroidism can make chronic urticaria worse but is not a cause.

- Tonsillitis and cholecystitis are not causes of urticaria.

- Addition of an H_2 blocker to an H_1 blocker can induce remission in 60 to 80 per cent of patients with CIU.

- Hereditary angioedema does not itch and is not associated with urticaria.

- Eosinophilia with chronic urticaria suggests parasitic infestation.

Bibliography

Huston DP, Bressler R: Urticaria and angioedema. Med Clin North Am 1992;76:805–840.

Kaplan AP: Urticaria and angioedema. *In* Middleton E Jr, Reed C, Ellis E, et al (eds): Allergy Principles and Practice. St Louis, MO, CV Mosby, 1993, pp 1553–1580.

Kaplan AP: Urticaria and angioedema. *In* Frank MM, Austin KF, Claman HN, Unanue E (eds): Samter's Immunological Diseases, 5th ed. Boston, Little Brown, 1995, pp 1329–1343.

Mahmood T: Physical urticarias. Am Fam Physician 1994; 49(6):1411–1414.

Membranous nephropathy associated with hypocomplementemic urticarial vasculitis: report of two cases and a review of the literature. (Editorial) Nephron 1994;66(1):1–7.

Symptom	**Dry Skin**	*Suzanne Bruce*

Synonyms for dry skin include xerosis, asteatosis, winter itch, and eczema craquelé. Xerosis occurs when moisture is lost from the epidermis. This moisture loss results in a stratum corneum that is mechanically less pliable and therefore prone to cracking and scaling. Numerous factors affect the degree of hydration of the epidermis. The main source of moisture for the stratum corneum is diffusion from the underlying cutaneous vasculature and, to a lesser degree, from perspiration produced by sweat glands. The rate of evaporation from the epidermal surface determines the hydration of the skin. Sebum, because of its ability to prevent transepidermal water loss, helps to maintain hydration of the skin. Stratum corneum also contains what has collectively been termed natural moisturizing factors; these are substances such as lactic acid and urea that absorb large quantities of water and help to impart plasticity to the stratum corneum. External factors also have an impact on the development of xerosis. Dryness usually occurs when relative humidity is below 30 to 60 per cent. Excessive bathing and the use of soaps that remove sebum from the surface of the skin can lead to dry skin. The elderly are particularly susceptible to dry skin because of a reduction in the number and activity of sebaceous glands and decreased perspiration.

Differential Diagnosis

1. Atopic eczema
2. Nummular eczema
3. Ichthyosis vulgaris

History: Key Questions to Ask

1. Is there any history of skin disorders, such as atopic dermatitis or ichthyosis?
2. Are you bathing excessively or exposed to drying soaps or detergents?
3. Are you using hot rather than warm water to bathe?
4. Are you using heating pads or sitting in front of an open fire?
5. Do you use a humidifier in the home?
6. Are you exposed to wind and sun?

Clinical Findings

1. The skin surface is rough and flaking or scaly.
2. Dryness commonly occurs on the extremities, especially the shins, but may also affect the trunk and face.
3. Dry skin is exacerbated by cold, dry weather and by the low humidity associated with central heating and air conditioning.
4. Dry skin may be associated with hyperpigmentation in some skin types.
5. Xerotic eczema may occur if the dry skin is severe enough to become inflamed. The dermatitis may be erythematous and fissured.
6. Pruritus frequently accompanies dry skin.

Tests

The diagnosis of dry skin is a clinical one, and there are no laboratory tests that are routinely indicated.

Management

Medication

1. Ammonium lactate lotion is useful for xerosis, but stinging can occur if there are any open fissures. It is available by prescription (Lachydrin Lotion 12%) or over-the-counter (Lachydrin Five Lotion 5%).
2. Moisturizers work by preventing evaporation from skin.
3. Forms of moisturizing products
   a. Ointments: mixtures of water in oil (typically either lanolin or petrolatum) (e.g., Vaseline, Aquaphor)
   b. Creams: mixtures of oil in water (e.g., Eucerin, Moisturel, Pen-Kera)
   c. Lotions: preparations of powder crystals dissolved in water and held in suspension by surface active agents (e.g., Lubriderm, Keri Lotion, Vaseline Intensive Care)
   d. Foams: foamy materials that leave an oily residue
   e. Oils: bath oil, mineral oil, baby oil (e.g., Alpha Keri, Domol)
4. The greasier and more occlusive the emollient, the more effective the lubricating qualities. However, because some patients find ointments such as petrolatum aesthetically unappealing, they may prefer a cream or lotion.

Patient Education

1. Room humidifiers help increase relative humidity.
2. Patients with dry skin should avoid excessive bathing.
3. Only mild cleansers such as Dove or Cetaphil should be used.
4. Moisturizers should be applied daily immediately after bathing to trap moisture in the stratum corneum.
5. Bath oils should be avoided in patients such as the elderly, who are prone to slipping in the tub.

PEARLS

- Petrolatum is an inexpensive, effective moisturizer.
- Always apply moisturizers immediately after bathing.
- Ammonium lactate is an extremely effective treatment for severe xerosis.

 Bibliography

Dotz W, Berman B: The facts about treatment of dry skin. Geriatrics 1983;38:93–100.

Frantz RA, Gardner S: Clinical concerns: Management of dry skin. J Gerontol Nurs 1994;20(9):15–18, 45.

Lazar AP, Lazar P: Dry skin, water, and lubrication. Dermatol Clin 1991;9(1):45–51.

Potts RO, Buras EM Jr, Chrisman DA Jr: Changes with age in the moisture content of human skin. J Invest Dermatol 1984;82:97–100.

Rogers RS, Callen J, Wehr R, Krochmal L: Comparative efficacy of 12% ammonium lactate lotion and 5% lactic acid lotion in the treatment of moderate to severe xerosis. J Am Acad Dermatol 1989;21:714–716.

| Symptom | **Purpura** | | *Edward M. Zimmerman* |

Purpura is a condition characterized by hemorrhage into the skin and/or mucous membranes, resulting in patches of purplish discoloration, petechiae, or ecchymosis. These areas do not blanch, may occur in crops over time, and gradually resolve or leave hyperpigmented hemosiderin deposits. They may be palpable if caused by an inflammatory vasculitis. Nonpalpable purpura is probably caused by a platelet abnormality—quantitative or qualitative—due to autoimmunity, leukemia or some other marrow disorder, or, rarely in North America today, scurvy.

Differential Diagnosis

A. By age

1. Children:

a. Henoch-Schönlein purpura—especially if viral upper respiratory infection within 3 weeks

b. Leukemia

2. Teenagers:

a. Infections: transmitted sexually or through drug abuse

b. Systemic lupus erythematosus in women

c. Hypersensitivity (drug) reactions

3. 30 years and older:

a. Drug reactions

b. Rheumatoid disease

c. Connective tissue vasculitis

4. Older:

a. Drug reactions

b. Mechanical/senile/actinic purpura

c. Infections

d. Malignancies

e. Cryoglobulinemias

B. By causes of vasculitis (palpable purpura)

1. Idiopathic

a. Drug (hypersensitivity) reaction: most are not true allergies and do not involve autoantibodies. Most often caused by commonly used drugs. No one category is more likely than another. No urticaria. One exception: Quinidine can induce production of an antibody that destroys platelets with quinidine on their surface causing a thrombocytopenic purpura.

b. Hepatitis

c. Embolic disease

d. Connective tissue diseases/vasculitis

(1) Systemic lupus erythematosus

(2) Henoch-Schönlein purpura (usually a pediatric disease); unknown cause

e. Systemic diseases: rheumatoid disease

f. Disseminated intravascular coagulation

g. Mixed cryoglobulinemia syndrome

2. Infectious

a. Viral

(1) Atypical measles

(2) Echovirus 9

(3) Toxoplasmosis, rubella, cytomegalovirus, herpesvirus (TORCHS)

b. Rickettsial

(1) Rocky Mountain spotted fever

(2) Epidemic typhus

c. Bacterial

(1) Meningococcemia

(2) Gonococcemia

(3) Staphylococcal sepsis

(4) Pseudomonas sepsis

(5) Subacute bacterial endocarditis

d. HIV

3. Other causes of purpuric lesions

a. Mechanical purpura: Cough, convulsion, or labor increases intercapillary pressure. Usually seen on head, neck, and arms

b. Orthostatic purpura: seen in the lower extremities after prolonged standing

c. Purpura simplex: easy bruising—especially of the legs—in children and middle-aged women; no other symptoms; work-up entirely within normal limits

d. Factitious or self-inflicted purpura: fairly common, more often in women with neurotic or psychotic symptoms

---

Refer to Ch. 88, Hepatitis; Ch. 149, Leukemia; Ch. 157, Disseminated Intravascular Coagulation; Ch. 190 to 192, HIV Infections; Ch. 193, Drug Allergy; Ch. 207, Systemic Lupus Erythematosus.

History: Key Questions to Ask

1. Is it a local or systemic disorder?

2. Is there a familial bleeding disorder?

3. Are lesions palpable? Tender? Where located?

4. Have you started on *any* new prescription or nonprescription drug recently?

5. Do you use chronic or large doses of aspirin or nonsteroidal anti-inflammatory drugs? Warfarin? Heparin? Steroids?

6. Has there been weight loss?

7. Fever?

8. Hematuria?

9. Evidence of infection?

10. Joint symptoms?

11. Do you use recreational drugs?

12. Have you recently had a transfusion?

13. Is there high-risk behavior for sexually transmitted diseases, especially HIV?

14. Do you have a history of miscarriages, gestational hypertension, sun sensitivity, malar rash? (Think SLE.)

Clinical Findings

It may be helpful to bear in mind differences commonly found between disorders of platelets and blood vessels versus disorders of coagulation. Purpura characteristically presents as multiple small, superficial ecchymoses or petechiae, rarely as deep hematomas or hemarthrosis. Bleeding from cuts and scratches may be persistent and sometimes profuse and is rarely delayed. Purpura is found more often in women. Eighty to 90 per cent of hereditary coagulation disorders are found only in men. Look for

1. Palpable purpuric lesions: Note stages of development, found primarily on lower extremities.
2. Evidence of embolic disease
   a. Retinal hemorrhages or exudates
   b. Splinter hemorrhages, Osler's nodes, Janeway lesions
   c. Cardiac murmurs
   d. Liver or spleen enlargement
   e. Petechiae
3. Evidence of systemic disease
   a. Hair loss, sun sensitivity, gestational hypertension, malar rash, scalp lesions, mouth sores suggest SLE.
   b. Telangiectasia could indicate vasculitis.
   c. Splinter hemorrhages: a classic finding in bacterial endocarditis; may be seen in primary systemic vasculitis, too
   d. Swollen, hot, red, or tender joints indicative of arthritis
   e. Tender/trigger points indicative of fibrositis
   f. Purpura tends to be parafollicular in HIV-seropositive patients.
   g. Malnourished: Consider leukemia, lymphoma, scurvy.
   h. Neurologic manifestations may be due to intercranial hemorrhage resulting from thrombocytopenia.
   i. Abdominal pain may be due to hemorrhage into bowel walls. May cause necrosis or intussusception, colic, hematochezia or hematemesis, and mucoid stool
   j. Acute renal failure
4. Distribution and features
   a. Allergic purpura: variable appearance, usually small, +/− palpable, even bullous; symmetric; proximal extremities, usually legs and buttocks; may be pruritic; no generalized bleeding; appears and regresses in crops
   b. Thrombocytopenic purpura: superficial ecchymoses of various sizes and shapes, anywhere, but especially in dependent areas and constriction and pressure points; generalized bleeding from mucosa
   c. Scurvy: petechiae around hair follicles; also ecchymoses and large subcutaneous hematomas; often symmetric ''saddle'' area of thighs and buttocks; lassitude, generalized bleeding; positive tourniquet test; painful periosteal hemorrhage in children

Tests

1. Identify thrombocytopenia due to decreased production, qualitative disorders, destruction, sequestration.
   a. Complete blood count and peripheral smear
   b. Iron deficiency may be secondary to bleeding.
   c. B_{12} and folate deficiency may be secondary to malnutrition or excessive alcohol intake.
2. Erythrocyte sedimentation rate
3. Urinalysis: hematuria +/− proteinuria may indicate vasculitis.
4. Serum automated analysis, including creatinine, liver function, and creatine kinase
5. Coagulation (DIC) profile
6. Capillary fragility (Rumpel-Leede) test
7. Bone marrow biopsy
8. Antiplatelet antibody test
9. If palpable purpura, biopsy. Identify vasculitis, emboli, amyloid, cholesterol crystals.
10. Chest radiograph: Look for infiltrates that may indicate vasculitis.
11. Electrocardiograph: to assess pericarditis or coronary vasculitis
12. Antinuclear antibodies: If positive, consider rheumatoid factor, cryoglobulin, hepatitis panel.
13. Lipid panel
14. Serum protein electrophoresis: Look for monoclonal proteins.
15. Cryoglobulin
16. Serum immunoelectrophoresis
17. Transesophageal echocardiogram if history consistent with embolic cause
18. Stop a new drug if clinical and serologic data have been nondiagnostic. New lesions should stop developing in a few weeks if the drug was the cause. (Weigh the risks/benefits of stopping the drug.)

Management

Treatment depends on identifying the cause of the purpura. Specific treatments are preferable to generalized therapy whenever possible.

1. Extended (4 to 6 weeks of prednisone at 1 to 2 mg/kg/day orally) course of oral steroids with slow taper
2. Stop offending drug(s).
3. Antihistamines for urticarial vasculitis
4. Nonsteroidal anti-inflammatory drugs
5. Tricyclic antidepressants for treatment of fibrositis; doxepin as H_1 and H_2 inhibitor for vasculitis
6. Immunosuppressive agents
7. Danocrine, 200 mg t.i.d. or q.i.d. orally
8. RhoGAM intramuscularly or intravenously
9. Splenectomy (reserved for patients with severe blood loss who cannot tolerate or are not responsive to steroids)
10. α-Interferon
11. Plasmapheresis +/− immunoglobulin G
12. Ascorbic acid or vitamin K as required

13. Platelet transfusions and IV immunoglobulin are only transiently helpful in raising platelet counts

Follow-Up

Follow-up should be carried out as necessary for any systemic illness or disease.

PEARLS

- Probably 50 per cent of purpura is idiopathic and self-limiting.

- Drugs are the primary cause of palpable purpura and should be exhaustively ruled out before undertaking an extensive and expensive work-up if no other obvious cause is uncovered in a thorough history and physical examination.

- Steroid therapy is the treatment of choice while investigation is pending.

- Stop new drugs if possible.

Bibliography

Bithell TC: Bleeding disorders caused by vascular abnormalities. *In* Lee GR, et al (eds): Wintrobe's Clinical Hematology, 9th ed, vol 2. Malvern, PA, Lea & Febiger, 1993, pp 1374–1386.

Lightfoot RW: Palpable purpura: Identifying the cause. Hospital Pract 1992;27(12):39–47.

Rakel RE (ed): Conn's Current Therapy 1994. Philadelphia, WB Saunders, 1994, pp 374–378, 436–437, 756–757.

Wyngaarden JB, et al (eds): Cecil Textbook of Medicine, 19th ed. Philadelphia, WB Saunders, 1992, pp 897, 990, 998–999, 1538–1539, 2303–2304.

Symptom Alopecia   *James W. Haynes*

Hair loss can be psychosocially devastating if it occurs on commonly exposed areas (i.e., scalp, eyelashes, eyebrows), and therefore it is extremely important to recognize normal inherited hair loss, search for reversible causes, and refer when necessary to resource organizations that might help patients cope with their hair loss.

Differential Diagnosis

A. Generalized hair loss
　　1. Telogen effluvium
　　2. Anagen effluvium
　　3. Alopecia totalis/universalis
　　4. Secondary syphilis
B. Localized hair loss
　　1. Androgenic alopecia (male versus female pattern)
　　2. Alopecia areata
　　3. Hirsutism
　　4. Trichotillomania
　　5. Traction
　　6. Scarring alopecia
　　　　a. Hereditary and developmental
　　　　　　(1) Aplasia cutis congenita
　　　　　　(2) Epidermal nevi
　　　　　　(3) Facial hemiatrophy (Romberg's syndrome)
　　　　b. Infection
　　　　　　(1) Fungal
　　　　　　(2) Bacterial (folliculitis)
　　　　　　(3) Viral (herpes zoster)
　　　　　　(4) Protozoan (leishmaniasis)
　　　　c. Neoplasms

　　　　　　(1) Basal cell carcinoma
　　　　　　(2) Squamous cell carcinoma
　　　　　　(3) Lymphomas
　　　　　　(4) Metastatic tumors
　　　　d. Physical/chemical
　　　　　　(1) Burns
　　　　　　(2) Radiation
　　　　　　(3) Acids/alkalis
　　　　　　(4) Drugs
　　　　e. Others
　　　　　　(1) Lupus erythematosus (can be nonscarring)
　　　　　　(2) Lichen planus
　　　　　　(3) Sarcoidosis
　　　　　　(4) Scleroderma
　　　　　　(5) Cicatricial pemphigoid
　　　　　　(6) Graham-Little syndrome
　　　　　　(7) Acne keloidalis

The first determination to be made is whether the hair loss is diffuse or localized and whether or not the underlying skin is normal. Generalized hair loss refers to the area of involvement only.

Telogen effluvium is diffuse hair loss characterized by hair follicles being suddenly thrust into a premature resting state in response to some stress (e.g., pregnancy, physical or emotional trauma) usually 2 to 3 months prior. Full recovery is expected. Anagen effluvium is an abrupt loss of growing stage hairs due to some stressor (e.g., chemotherapeutic agents, radiation). Since 90 per cent of hairs are in the growing phase at any one time, this is diffuse and usually occurs 1 to 4 weeks after the insult. Alopecia totalis (total scalp) and universalis (total body) are the more severe forms of alopecia areata. They are usually preceded by areata, which rapidly progresses to these severe forms. No definitive cause has been found, but an autoimmune etiology is proposed. Spontaneous remissions and exacerbations are the hallmark, and in contrast to telogen effluvium, recovery usually does not occur. Hair loss due to syphilis should present with history or stigmata of secondary or tertiary syphilis.

Androgenic alopecia presents characteristically with appropriate family history. Alopecia areata is a common asymptomatic malady with rapid total loss of hair in a sharply defined area. This form usually occurs in young adults and children, and the skin at the affected site is normal. Hirsutism can present with a characteristic "male pattern baldness" which is slightly different in women, in whom there is central scalp regression with retention of the frontotemporal hairline. A work-up for hirsutism should be instituted in all females with "male pattern baldness." Trichotillomania is characterized by manual extraction of hair, most commonly occurring in young children, adolescents, and women. The affected area is most commonly the frontoparietal region of the scalp, and broken hairs of varying length can be found. Traction alopecia is related to chronic tension on the hair associated with various hairstyles (e.g., corn rows, pony tails, use of rollers) or activities (football helmet, prolonged supine position). This form is usually temporary if the trauma is transient, but it may persist if trauma is prolonged. Most nonscarring causes of alopecia can be diagnosed by history and physical examination. Most scarring forms have characteristic physical findings or may be differentiated with further testing or biopsy.

> Refer to Ch. 50, Sarcoidosis; Ch. 207, Systemic Lupus Erythematosus; Chs. 265 and 266 on Herpes; Ch. 272, Hair Disorders; and Ch. 278, Fungus Infections of the Skin.

History: Key Questions to Ask

1. Was onset sudden or gradual?
2. Have you had a recent physical or emotional stress (e.g., pregnancy, illness)?
3. What is the exposure history (e.g., medication, chemicals, radiation)?
4. Have you had a systemic disease or high fever (e.g., STDs, lupus)?
5. Is there a family history of hair loss?

These questions should help to narrow your investigative focus.

Clinical Findings

1. Pattern of hair loss (diffuse or localized)
2. Scarring versus nonscarring
3. Inflammatory versus noninflammatory
4. Hair density: normal or decreased
5. Skin disease in other areas (LOOK!)

Androgenic alopecia (male-pattern baldness), a common finding in genetically predisposed men, is characterized by increased frontotemporal recession accompanied by midfrontal recession. Hair loss then occurs in a round area on the vertex and then density decreases over the top of the scalp. In females the pattern is slightly different, as discussed above with hirsutism. In telogen effluvium, no more than 50 per cent of the hair is affected in the appropriate setting of an inciting stressor. Anagen effluvium leaves only those hairs in telogen stage, and thus only 10 to 15 per cent of hair remains. Alopecia areata presents as well-circumscribed, round areas of hair loss with only short broken hairs present toward the periphery of the lesion. Trichotillomania-affected areas have irregular angulated borders without complete balding as in alopecia areata. Short broken hairs of varying length are randomly distributed. Secondary or tertiary syphilis can present as a "moth-eaten," scaly scalp alopecia. Lateral eyebrows may be affected as they are in hypothyroidism. Gumma and ulcer formation can occur in tertiary syphilis, resulting in a scarring alopecia. Findings associated with traction alopecia vary depending on the tension site, but inflammatory papules and broken hairs may be seen.

The scarring forms of alopecia vary in appearance, but some have classic presentations. Aplasia cutis congenita usually involves a prominent, permanent hair loss on the vertex. Epidermal nevi are hamartomas of the skin and result in well-circumscribed alopecia, most commonly on the scalp. Romberg's syndrome may be associated with a frontal scalp alopecia due to localized scleroderma.

Infectious agents can lead to scarring alopecia. The most common infection is tinea capitis, which usually occurs in prepubertal children and has a variety of presentations depending on the causative agent. The most common form involves patchy alopecia, fine dry scaling, and no inflammation. Hairs can be broken with short stubs or broken off at the surface (black dot tinea). Another form presents with patchy alopecia, swelling, and a purulent discharge. Kerion formation is a severe inflammatory reaction with boggy induration. Hair loss caused by neoplasms have findings consistent with that type of tumor. Physically or chemically induced alopecia can have a variety of presentations, depending on the inciting agent. History of exposure is the key.

Systemic lupus erythematosus may be accompanied by scaly, erythematous, irregular macules or plaques, which scar without hair. Lichen planus affecting the scalp usually has accompanying bulla formation, which also scars without hair. Sarcoid granulomas can involve the scalp and present as brown or violet papules or plaques when active, but they scar devoid of hair. Scleroderma can have accompanying scalp lesions, which appear as violet or tan macules that develop into firm plaques and ultimately scarring alopecia. Pemphigoid can have subepidermal blisters, which eventually scar without hair. Graham-Little syndrome is a progressive, scarring alopecia of the scalp which can involve the axillae and pubic area. Atrophic scars result on the scalp but not in other affected areas. Acne keloidalis is a long-term pustular eruption, localized to the occiput and posterior neck, which eventually forms keloids devoid of hair.

Tests

1. Hair pluck test
2. Fungal tests (e.g., KOH preps, Wood's lamp, fungal cultures)
3. Hormone studies (e.g., DHEA-S, testosterone)
4. Scalp biopsy

The hair pluck test is the most accurate way to establish an anagen-to-telogen ratio and thus help to diagnose anagen or telogen effluvium. The hairs are obtained by firmly grasping about 50 hairs at the same height with a rubber-tipped needle holder, rotating the needle holder one turn and quickly pulling upward. Cut the excess hair 1 cm from the roots and place on a wet microscope slide and examine under X10 lens. DACA (4-dimethyaminocinnamaldehyde) reacts with an internal root sheath amino acid which can distinguish anagen from telogen hairs. Telogen hairs have small ovoid bulbs that do not stain with DACA due to their lack of a sheath, whereas anagen hairs have elongated, larger bulbs surrounded by the brightly red-stained sheath. Telogen effluvium shows increased counts of telogen hairs from 30 to 60 per cent (normal 10 to 15 per cent). In anagen effluvium only telogen hairs remain, and thus 100 per cent are telogen. Potassium hydroxide (KOH) preparations involve taking easily plucked hairs and suspending them in KOH on a slide. Findings can include a "sack full of marbles" within and upon the hair shaft visible with low power. Furthermore, for *Microsporum canis* and *M. audouinii* species, Wood's light examination may reveal blue-green fluorescence of the hair. Fungal cultures of plucked hair may be helpful if the diagnosis is in question. If female pattern alopecia (FPA) is found, hirsutism must be ruled out. Finally, with scarring alopecia or those in question, scalp biopsies may be taken. The best site for these is the most active area of disease, which is usually the periphery of lesions.

Management

Alopecia can have significant psychological implications and thus an accurate diagnosis is vital before beginning therapy.

1. Inherited disorders of hair loss should be recognized, and some men may decide to forgo treatment. Topical minoxidil (Rogaine), can be applied twice daily, and ideal candidates are men under 30 with less than 5 years of hair loss. It must be used continuously to preserve growth. Surgical procedures to include hair transplants, scalp reduction, and flaps may be options for selected patients.

2. Griseofulvin is the treatment of choice for tinea capitis at 7 to 10 mg/kg/day in daily or b.i.d. dosing. Patients should be examined every 3 to 4 weeks, and if KOH preps or cultures are positive, increase the dose to 15 mg/kg/day. Topical antifungals are generally ineffective and ketoconazole (Nizoral), is usually less effective. Treatment should be continued for 2 weeks after cultures and KOH preparations become negative (total duration usually 6 to 12 weeks). Contaminated objects (e.g., combs) must be cleaned and family members examined.

3. Alopecia areata, if limited in extent, can be treated by observation only as most cases resolve spontaneously, but more extensive or refractory forms require specialized care. Intralesional or topical steroids may be used without significant side effects, but systemic steroids should be avoided. Anthralin creme, applied once daily, has been reported to induce growth but causes a significant visible dermatitis, which may be poorly tolerated. Various other treatments have been proposed to include photochemotherapy, topical allergens, and minoxidil, but they are either poorly tolerated or marginally effective when compared to spontaneous remission rates. Wigs can be obtained if desired.

4. Other infectious etiologies, hirsutism, and systemic causes should respond to the appropriate therapy for that individual disease.

PEARLS

- Look for fungus!
- Recognize androgenic patterns
- National Alopecia Areata Foundation, P.O. Box 150760, San Rafael, CA 94915-0760

 Bibliography

Fitzpatrick TB: Dermatology in General Medicine, 4th ed. New York, McGraw-Hill, 1993, pp 676–689.

Habif TP: Clinical Dermatology: A Color Guide to Diagnosis and Therapy. St. Louis, CV Mosby, 1990, pp 598–614.

Levy ML: Disorders of the hair and scalp in children. Pediatr Clin North Am 1991;38:905–919.

251 Atopic Dermatitis

Mitchell F. Finnie

Etiology

1. Cause is unknown.
2. Inherited tendency to dry, sensitive, pruritic skin with lowered itch threshold resulting in itch-scratch-rash cycle
3. Not an allergic condition, but possible immunologic basis with evidence of altered T-cell function

Symptoms

1. Pruritus is the sine qua non.
2. Infants demonstrate irritability, restlessness, poor sleep.
3. About 70 per cent have family history of asthma, allergic rhinitis, or eczema.
4. Chronic condition exacerbated by heat, dry air, emotional stress

Key Symptoms

- Pruritus
- Family history of atopy
- Dry skin

Clinical Findings

1. No unique skin lesions
2. Chronic, recurring dermatitis
   a. Distribution by age
      (1) Infants: face, cheeks, trunk, extensor surfaces; if generalized, spares diaper area
      (2) Children (2 to 12 years): antecubital and popliteal fossae, neck, wrist, ankles
      (3) Adult: hands, eyelids, genitalia, neck, flexural areas
   b. Morphology by age
      (1) Infants: erythema, scaling, papulovesicular, oozing
      (2) Children: inflammation, coalesced papules, lichenification
      (3) Adults: scaling, erythema, lichenification
3. Secondary infections and associated conditions
   a. Secondary infections
      (1) *Staphylococcus aureus*: weeping, crusted
      (2) Herpes simplex (eczema herpeticum): can be life-threatening
      (3) Molluscum contagiosum
      (4) Dermatophytosis

b. Associated features
   (1) Pigmentary changes including pityriasis alba
   (2) Extra infraorbital eyelid fold (Dennie-Morgan line)
   (3) White dermatographism (white blanch after blunt stroke)
   (4) Dry skin, xerosis, keratosis pilaris, ichthyosis vulgaris
   (5) Facial erythema/pallor, conjunctivitis
   (6) Cataracts (10 per cent), hyperlinear palms, hand dermatitis

Key Signs

- Dry skin and itching
- Erythema, inflammation
- Scaling
- Papules, crusting
- Lichenification

Laboratory Tests

1. No specific laboratory features to confirm diagnosis
2. Elevated serum IgE and positive skin tests are common.

Differential Diagnosis

1. Consider any disorder manifested by dermatitis.
2. Differential depends on age-related morphology and distribution.
   a. Infants: irritant dermatitis, seborrhea, candidiasis
   b. Children: contact dermatitis, scabies, tinea, psoriasis, polymorphous light eruption, HIV dermatitis
   c. Adults: psoriasis, lichen simplex chronicus, drug eruption, nummular eczema, contact dermatitis
3. Rare conditions of infancy
   a. Wiskott-Aldrich syndrome, ataxia-telangiectasia
   b. Phenylketonuria (PKU), acrodermatitis enteropathica
   c. Histiocytosis X (Letterer-Siwe, Hand-Schüller-Christian disease)

> **WARNING**
>
> **Consider immunodeficiency and metabolic disorders if dermatitis appears before 2 months of age.**

Treatment

1. Patients must understand natural history (chronicity) of disease.

919

2. Education is key to effective therapy.

   a. Avoid dry skin, irritants, and allergens.

   b. Eliminate inflammation and secondary infection.

Medication

A. Topical therapy

   1. Topical steroids for inflammation

      a. Low potency for infants, face, intertriginous areas

         (1) Hydrocortisone 1% cream b.i.d.

         (2) Desonide (Tridesilon) 0.05% cream b.i.d.

      b. Moderate potency (ointments) for lichenified areas; may need occlusive therapy for 10 to 14 days

         (1) Triamcinolone 0.1% cream or ointment

         (2) Mometasone furoate (Elocon) 0.1% cream or ointment

      c. Tar ointments (Fototar, T-Derm, Estar Gel 5%) are a safe but slow-acting alternative to topical steroids.

   2. Moisturizers

      a. Use frequently, long term

      b. Petroleum jelly, Moisturel, Eucerin, Keri, Lubriderm

   3. Wet dressings for acute, weeping dermatitis

      a. Plain water or normal saline

      b. Burow's solution

B. Systemic therapy

   1. Antibiotics for secondary infections

      a. Erythromycin, 50 mg/kg/day, or 250 to 500 mg q.i.d.

      b. Dicloxacillin (Dynapen), 40 mg/kg/day or 250 to 500 mg q.i.d.

   2. Antihistamines (at bedtime) for pruritus

      a. Hydroxyzine (Atarax), 0.5 to 1.0 mg/kg/dose or 10 to 25 mg

      b. Diphenhydramine (Benadryl), 1 to 2 mg/kg/dose or 25 to 50 mg

   3. Prednisone for severe cases only

Diet

   1. Dietary restrictions are controversial.

   2. In food-sensitive children (a small percentage), avoid eggs, peanuts, milk, fish, soy, and wheat.

Activity

   1. Avoid sweating, temperature extremes, low humidity, and wool clothing.

   2. Bathing: short, infrequent, tepid water; Cetaphil or mild soaps (Dove, Basis, Tone, Purpose, *not* Ivory)

Patient Education

   1. Control, not cure, is goal of therapy.

   2. Keep skin well hydrated with bath oils and moisturizers.

3. Not an allergy, but avoid known irritants and allergens, including cosmetics, detergents, fabric softeners, dust, and animal dander

4. Not emotional disorder, but exacerbated by stress

Key Treatment

Drug of Choice	Alternative Drugs
• Topical steroids	• Antihistamines
	• Antibiotics
• Skin hydration	
• Avoid drying, irritants	
• Control environment and emotional stress	

Follow-Up

1. Frequency of visits depends on severity of disease.

2. Maintenance therapy

   a. Mild soaps or soap substitute (Cetaphil)

   b. Moisturizer twice daily and immediately after baths

   c. Antihistamines for itching as needed

   d. Topical steroid twice daily for 2 to 3 days for flares

3. Physician evaluation when maintenance therapy fails

4. Watch for complications and associated conditions.

   a. Associated conditions

      (1) Asthma or hayfever will develop in 50 per cent.

      (2) Cataracts in 10 per cent (15- to 25-year-olds)

      (3) Exfoliative erythroderma: life-threatening

   b. Complications

      (1) Secondary infections

      (2) Steroid side effects including striae, atrophy, and dermatitis with chronic use or high-potency corticosteroids

5. Reassurance

   a. Infantile: two-thirds resolve by childhood

   b. Childhood: two-thirds resolve by puberty

Bibliography

Arnold HL Jr, Odom RB, James WD (eds): Andrews' Diseases of the Skin, 8th ed. Philadelphia, WB Saunders, 1990, pp 68–74.

Cohen BA: Atlas of Pediatric Dermatology. London, Wolff Publishing, 1993, pp 3.11–3.19.

Habif TP: Clinical Dermatology: A Color Guide to Diagnosis and Therapy, 2d ed. St Louis, CV Mosby, 1990, pp 74–90.

Leung DYM, Rhodes AR, Geha RS: Atopic dermatitis. *In* Fitzpatrick TM, Eisen AZ, Wolff K, et al (eds): Dermatology in General Medicine, 3d ed. New York, McGraw-Hill, 1987, pp 1385–1408.

Weston WL, Lane AT: Color Textbook of Pediatric Dermatology. St Louis, Mosby–Year Book, 1991, pp. 26–32.

252 Seborrheic Dermatitis

Gregory Bahtiarian

Etiology

1. Despite extensive investigation, the exact cause of seborrheic dermatitis (SD) is still unclear.
2. Although there are many theories as to the cause of SD, most have been thoroughly investigated without producing significant proof.
   a. Excessive sebum production
   b. Epidermal hyperproliferation
   c. Infectious
      (1) Bacterial
      (2) Yeast
3. Recently, attention has been placed on a lipophilic yeast, *Pityrosporum ovale*. The yeast seems to be more abundant in the areas affected by SD, and control of the yeast population appears to correlate with clinical improvement of the disease. However, despite extensive clinical investigation, a direct causative relationship still has not been proved.
4. There are multiple other variables that are associated with SD.
   a. Worse in the fall and winter and improves in the spring and summer
   b. Common in a variety of neurologic diseases, including Parkinson's disease, facial paralysis, and quadriplegia
   c. Appears to be worse in patients who are depressed and with increased emotional stress
   d. Has a high frequency of occurrence in patients infected with HIV
   e. May be more common in alcoholics and in patients with diabetes mellitus
   f. Appears to have a genetic predisposition

Symptoms

1. Scaling of the involved areas is the predominant symptom.
2. Itching is usually present in varying degrees.

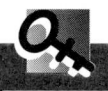

Key Symptoms

- Scaling lesions
- Itching

Clinical Findings

1. A common skin disorder with variable frequency and severity affecting adults and infants
   a. The average prevalence in the general population is about 2 per cent.
   b. Peak incidence is between 20 and 40 years of age.
   c. There is a male predilection.
2. A chronic superficial inflammatory disease of the skin with recurrent exacerbations
3. Classical features include scaling lesions on an erythematous base
   a. Lesions may be scales or crusts.
   b. Gray-white or yellow
   c. Dry or greasy
   d. A variety of sizes and thicknesses
   e. Initially somewhat adherent but become loose and flake with scratching
   f. Scales or crusts may coalesce to involve a large area or may be found in small patches.
4. Affects a variety of areas
   a. Most commonly the scalp, face, and chest
   b. Affects the hair-bearing areas, including the scalp, hairline, eyebrows, beard and mustache areas, and parasternal area
   c. Also affects the paranasal areas, nasolabial folds, glabella, eyelid margins, in and around the ears, and cheeks
   d. Other areas are affected less frequently, including the central back, axilla, inframammary areas, umbilicus, groin, and gluteal cleft.
5. Individual areas are affected differently.
   a. SD of the scalp only causes scaling with minimal or no erythema.
   b. The face, chest, and back are usually affected with scaling on an erythematous base.
   c. The body creases are usually devoid of scales and just have erythema.
6. Pruritus is usually present and can be mild to moderate but may become worse with heat exposure and sweating.
7. Infantile SD is a common skin disorder of infancy.
   a. It usually occurs between 2 weeks and 4 months of life.
   b. Scales or crusts are usually greasy, thick, and yellow and may be on an erythematous base.
   c. The most commonly involved area is the scalp (cradle cap) but the forehead, eyebrows, eyelids, nasal folds, ears, neck, and intertriginous folds also may be involved.
   d. The disease may last for weeks to months but typically undergoes spontaneous remission by 1 year of age with a good prognosis.

e. Rarely it can progress to a severe form called erythroderma desquamativum (Leiner's disease).

(1) This is associated with diffuse inflammation of the skin with severe cracking and thickening.

(2) The infant is usually severely ill with fever, diarrhea, and vomiting and has a poor prognosis.

8. The histopathology of SD is nondiagnositic with nonspecific features that are similar to other low-grade inflammatory diseases such as psoriasis and atopic dermatitis.

Key Signs

- Loose, gray-white scales
- Erythematous base
- Involvement of the scalp, face, chest
- Pruritus

Laboratory Tests

No specific laboratory test is available or necessary.

1. Diagnosis is based on clinical features.

2. Biopsy is very rarely indicated and would be nonspecific and therefore probably not helpful.

Differential Diagnosis

1. The differential diagnosis for SD is limited and varies depending on the extent of the disease; diagnosis made based on the distribution and type of skin lesions as compared with other skin disorders.

2. The most significant problem is to differentiate SD from psoriasis. However, certain elements unique to psoriasis usually distinguish it from SD.

3. Atopic dermatitis is also in the differential, especially with respect to infants. However, atopic dermatitis usually involves the arms and legs.

4. The malar rash commonly seen in lupus can resemble SD of the face.

5. The following skin diseases can all be included in a broad differential:

a. Contact dermatitis

b. Tinea versicolor

c. Tinea corporis

d. Pityriasis rosea

e. Impetigo

Treatment

1. SD is a chronic disease without a cure. The treatment is directed toward reducing the exacerbations and limiting the severity.

2. A variety of treatments are available, mainly medicated shampoos and topical steroids.

3. The majority of treatments have one or more of the following activities:

a. Cytostatic

b. Antimycotic

c. Anti-inflammatory

Medication

1. The mainstay of treatment involves the use of medicated shampoos that can be used on all affected areas (not just the scalp). The frequency of shampooing depends on the severity of the disease, but two times per week is the minimum. A number of shampoos are available and usually include one of the following active agents:

a. Selenium sulfide (Selsun) 1% or 2.5% has cytostatic as well as antimycotic effects and is a very effective treatment.

b. Pyrithione zinc (Head & Shoulders) 1% or 2% also has cytostatic and antimycotic effects and is also very effective.

c. Ketoconazole (Nizoral) 2% has antimycotic effects and is a newer treatment that has been shown to be very effective. Most studies show similar results when compared with selenium sulfide; however, a few studies suggest a lower relapse rate and better tolerance.

d. Sulfur, salicylic acid, and tar derivatives are other ingredients with differing modes of activity. Shampoos with these agents seem less effective.

2. Besides shampoos, a number of creams and lotions are available. They may be more useful in areas without hair but can be used to treat all affected areas. The most popular are the topical steroids, but ketoconazole cream is also effective.

a. Topical steroids offer excellent treatment and can be found as creams, lotions, or solutions.

(1) These can be applied to all affected areas one to three times per day.

(2) The mainstay of the steroid preparations is hydrocortisone 1% cream or lotion.

(3) The more potent steroids such as triamcinolone 0.1% or betamethasone 0.1% also can be used (except for the face) but should be reserved for more severe cases.

(4) The risks of steroid use should always be explained to include steroid dermatitis, steroid atrophy, and steroid rebound, although these side effects are usually minimal, especially when using 1% hydrocortisone.

b. Ketoconazole 2% cream is also very effective and can be applied two times per day to all affected areas. Topical ketoconazole is very safe with minimal side effects.

3. My treatment recommendations are as follows:

a. Selenium sulfide 2.5% shampoo two to three times per week

b. Alternated with zinc pyrithione 2% shampoo two to three times per week

c. Hydrocortisone 1% cream or lotion can be applied to all affected areas one to three times per day depending on the severity of the symptoms. Hydrocortisone 1% solution may be applied to the scalp one to two times per day if needed.

d. If this regimen does not appear to be working after 1 month, then I recommend ketoconazole 2% shampoo to be applied two times per week on all affected areas.

4. Infantile SD should be treated as follows:

a. Remove crusts by shampooing with a mild baby shampoo two to three times per week (other medicated shampoos may be too irritating).

b. Hydrocortisone 1% cream or lotion can be applied to the affected areas one to two times per day.

Diet and Activity
No special diet or restriction of activity

Patient Education

1. Patients need to be aware that SD is a chronic disease with exacerbations and remissions.

2. Patients should be instructed to apply shampoos to all affected areas. When treating the scalp, the shampoo needs to be left in for 3 to 5 minutes so that it can penetrate to the scalp.

3. Personal hygiene may have a small influence on SD.
   a. Patients should use a nondrying moisturizing soap.
   b. Women should avoid cosmetics.
   c. Men should shave regularly.

Follow-Up

1. Because SD is a chronic disease with recurrent exacerbations, follow-up initially should be frequent, every 1 to 2 months, to establish an individual treatment strategy. Once a therapeutic regimen is developed that is acceptable, less frequent follow-up is needed. More frequent follow-up can be arranged if severity or frequency worsen.

2. In more severe, refractory cases, consultation with a dermatologist may be necessary.

The opinions and assertions contained herein are the private views of the author and are not to be construed as the official policy or position of the U.S. government, the Department of Defense, or the Department of the Air Force.

Key Treatment

Drugs of Choice	Alternative Drugs
• Selenium sulfide 2.5% shampoo	• Ketoconazole 2% shampoo
• Pyrithione zinc 2% shampoo	• Ketoconazole 2% cream
• Hydrocortisone 1% cream or lotion	• Other topical steroids

Bibliography

McGrath J, Murphy GM: The control of seborrheic dermatitis and dandruff by antipityrosporal drugs. Drugs 1991;41(2): 178–184.

Plewig G: Seborrheic dermatitis. In Fitzpatrick T, Eisen A, Wolff K, et al: (eds): Dermatology in General Medicine, 3d ed. New York, McGraw-Hill, 1987, pp 978–981.

Rebora A, Rongioletti F: The red face: Seborrheic dermatitis. Clin Dermatol 1993;11:235–242.

Seborrheic dermatitis, psoriasis, recalcitrant palmoplantar eruptions, and erythroderma, In Arnold HL, Odom RB, James WD (eds): Diseases of the Skin: Clinical Dermatology, 8th ed. Philadelphia, WB Saunders, 1990, pp 194–198.

White JW: Localized eczematous disease. In Sams WM, Lynch PJ (eds): Principles and Practice of Dermatology. New York, Churchill-Livingstone, 1990, pp 403–407.

253 Contact Dermatitis

Anne R. Lockett

Etiology

1. Contact dermatitis is a cell-mediated type IV delayed hypersensitivity reaction.
   a. Antigenic substances penetrate the skin and bind to proteins in the epidermis.
   b. Langerhans' cells process the antigen and present it to T lymphocytes in regional lymph nodes.
   c. T lymphocytes start a cascade of events mediated by lymphokines resulting in the observed inflammatory response.
2. Common causes of contact dermatitis are
   a. Plants (e.g., poison ivy and poison sumac)
   b. Nickel (e.g., inexpensive pierced earrings and belt buckles)
   c. Rubber (e.g., sterile gloves and shoes)

Symptoms

1. Pruritus
2. Stinging and burning
3. Pain

Clinical Findings

1. Varies with the patient's susceptibility and the amount of offending substance contacting the skin
2. Lesion often in the shape of the object causing the reaction (e.g., necklace or shoe strap) or the distribution of the application or exposure to the substance (e.g., lower face reacting to shaving lotion or hands reacting to a cleaning solution)
3. Acute lesions: erythematous plaque covered with numerous small vesicles
4. Subacute lesions: scaling, erythematous lesions without clear borders
5. Chronic lesions: thick plaques with accentuated skin lines

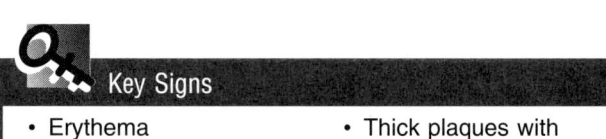

Key Signs

- Erythema
- Vesicles
- Bullae
- Scaling
- Thick plaques with accentuated skin lines
- Shape of lesion same as offending agent

Laboratory Tests

1. Standard patch testing

924

2. Controlled application of the suspected offending agent

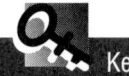

Key Test

- Patch testing is the only available test.

Differential Diagnosis

1. Atopic dermatitis
   a. Tends to start in early childhood
   b. Type I hypersensitivity reaction
   c. May be exacerbated by stress or change in temperature
2. Lichen simplex chronicus
   a. Caused by repeated physical trauma such as scratching
   b. Usually solid plaques with minimal scaling
   c. Characteristic distribution: nuchal area, scalp, lower extremity, and the anogenital region
3. Nummular eczema
   a. Coin-shaped plaques composed of grouped small vesicles on an erythematous base
   b. Random distribution
4. Psoriasis
   a. May be accompanied by constitutional symptoms such as fever and arthritis
   b. Characteristic plaques with scales. The adherent scale is silvery-white and reveals bleeding points when removed (Auspitz's sign).
   c. Can have nail involvement resulting in pitting or onycholysis
5. Seborrheic dermatitis
   a. Usually occurs in areas of high concentration of sebaceous glands, such as the scalp, face, presternal area, and in body folds
   b. Lesions are typically white to yellowish, greasy, scaling macules and papules.
   c. Pruritus is variable.

Treatment

A. General principles
   1. Avoiding contact with the substance. (In the case of a substance that may remain on the skin, copious irrigation to prevent further protein binding is important.)
   2. Cool, wet compresses using plain water or Burow's solution

3. Steroids appropriate to severity of the reaction
   a. Topical steroids may be used for simple erythema two to four times a day.
   b. Oral steroids such as prednisone, 20 mg twice daily for 6 days in widespread inflammation
   c. Intramuscular steroids may be used for severe, systemic reactions.
4. Symptomatic treatment may include
   a. Cool tub baths with colloidal oatmeal
   b. Oral antihistamines such as diphenhydramine
5. Antibiotics for secondary infection

B. Specific therapies
1. Acute
   a. Topical steroids
   b. Symptomatic treatment
2. Subacute
   a. No wet compresses because the lesions are dry
   b. Topical steroids under occlusion
   c. Lubrication 1 to 2 hours after application of the steroid three to four times a day
3. Chronic
   a. Potent topical steroids under occlusion for 1 to 3 weeks.
   b. May consider intralesional steroid administration for resistant lesions

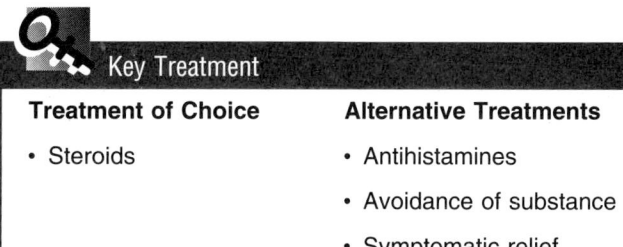

Key Treatment

Treatment of Choice	Alternative Treatments
• Steroids	• Antihistamines
	• Avoidance of substance
	• Symptomatic relief

Follow-Up

1. Lesions should be monitored for signs of secondary infection.
2. Patient should be encouraged to avoid the substance in the future.

 Bibliography

del Savio B, Sheretz EF: Is allergic contact dermatitis being overlooked? Arch Fam Med 1994;3(6):537–543.

Habif TP: Clinical Dermatology: A Color Guide to Diagnosis and Therapy. St Louis, CV Mosby, 1990, pp 28–37, 58–73.

Hogan DJ: The prognosis of occupational contact dermatitis. Occup Med 1994;9(1):53–58.

Klaus MV, Wieselthier JS: Contact dermatitis. Am Fam Physician 1993;48:629–32.

Patil S, Maibach HI: Effect of age and sex on the elicitation of irritant contact dermatitis. Contact Dermatitis 1994;30(5):257–264.

254 Miliaria

Gregory T. Soltner

Etiology

1. Miliaria is caused by blockage of sweat glands at the level of the epidermis or dermis.

2. Subtypes of miliaria are based on the depth at which the blockage occurs.

   a. Miliaria crystallina results from mild damage to the keratin layer of the epidermis. For example, a thermal injury such as sunburn causes keratin to slough off and clog sweat pores at the most superficial portion. When sweating occurs, the classic thin-walled vesicles are seen. Inflammation is minimal. In the newborn, miliaria crystallina may result from immature sweat glands or may be seen after phototherapy.

   b. Miliaria rubra (prickly heat) results from blockage in the mid to lower level of the epidermis. Sodium chloride from dried sweat and thermal injury have been implicated in the pathogenesis. It is very common in hot, humid areas and may also occur in hot, dry areas if pores are blocked by clothing. In addition, greasy topical agents may block sweat glands.

   c. Miliaria profunda is a rare disorder that results from a deeper blockage of sweat ducts in the lower epidermis or dermis. History will reveal prolonged heat exposure in tropical areas while performing heavy physical activity. Exhaustion and heat intolerance may be associated.

Symptoms

1. Miliaria crystallina is asymptomatic and very rarely causes clinical problems.

2. Patients with miliaria rubra have stinging, pruritic lesions mostly confined to the face, neck, and upper trunk. Symptoms are usually worse with the initiation of sweating.

3. Patients with miliaria profunda often describe lesions similar to miliaria rubra as the primary lesion. As heat exposure and physical activity continue, discrete vesicular lesions appear. There is decreased or absent sweating in the area of the lesions. Inability to sweat may lead to heat intolerance and exhaustion.

Key Symptoms

- Crystallina: none

- Rubra: stinging, itching

- Profunda: decreased sweating

Clinical Findings

1. Miliaria crystallina results in the formation of 2- to 3-mm thin-walled vesicles that are easily ruptured. Distribution is often over the face, neck, and upper trunk. The lesions have no associated erythema but may occur in areas of desquamating sunburn.

2. Miliaria rubra is an erythematous papulovesicular rash that usually occurs over clothed (covered) skin. The lesions are pinhead-sized and spare the palms and soles.

3. When miliaria profunda does occur it is often the result of progression from miliaria rubra. Discrete vesicular lesions occur with decreased sweating. Fever and exhaustion may occur.

Key Signs

- Crystallina: thin-walled vesicles, no erythema

- Rubra: papulovesicular lesion with surrounding erythema

- Profunda: vesicles in areas of decreased sweating, fever, fatigue (late)

Laboratory Tests

Laboratory tests are not useful in the diagnosis of the miliarias. Diagnosis is based on history and physical findings.

Differential Diagnosis

1. Miliaria rubra can resemble folliculitis, papular urticaria, and erythema toxicum.

2. Miliaria rubra usually has less associated erythema than papular urticaria and erythema toxicum.

3. Miliaria rubra can be distinguished from folliculitis by its nonfollicular distribution.

Treatment

1. Treatment common to all forms of the miliarias includes moving to a cooler environment, application of cool compresses, wearing light-weight, loose-fitting clothing, and avoidance of greasy topical agents.

2. Afterward, natural desquamation will occur.

Medication

The stinging and itching of miliaria rubra may be relieved with the application of anhydrous lanolin or calamine lotion.

Diet

Assess for signs of dehydration; ensure adequate hydration.

Activity

Rest, along with moving to a cooler environment, is important to decrease sweating.

Patient Education

The disorder is self-limiting once the provoking factors have been eliminated.

Key Treatment

- Cool environment
- Loose clothing
- Natural desquamation
- Anhydrous lanolin or calamine for stinging

Follow-Up

Follow up for re-evaluation if the expected resolution does not occur over several days.

Bibliography

Arnold HL Jr, Odom RB, James WD: Diseases of the Skin: Clinical Dermatology, 8th ed. Philadelphia, WB Saunders, 1990, pp 23–25.

Champion RH: Textbook of Dermatology, 5th ed. Boston, Blackwell Scientific, 1992, pp 1758–1759.

Fitzpatrick TB: Dermatology in General Medicine, 4th ed. New York, McGraw-Hill, 1993, pp 749–750.

Hurwitz S: Clinical Pediatric Dermatology, 2nd ed. Philadelphia, WB Saunders, 1993, pp 156–159.

Zitelli BJ, Davis HW: Atlas of Pediatric Physical Diagnosis, 2nd ed. New York, Gower, 1992, pp 8–18.

255 Hyperhidrosis

David M. Pariser

Etiology

1. Definition: hyperhidrosis is the term used for excessive eccrine sweating. Exactly what constitutes "excessive" may not be precisely definable, because there is a continuum of degrees of sweat production, and the threshold of sweat production that prompts a patient visit varies by the individual. Hyperhidrosis is an end-organ response of many diverse causes and may be divided into two general categories, localized and generalized. It may be both a subjective symptom or a physical finding, but in either case, it evokes a differential diagnosis of etiologies.

2. Clinical presentation: the most common presentation of hyperhidrosis is the localized excess sweating of the palms and/or soles or of the axillae.

   a. *Palmar* hyperhydrosis may be a disability for patients in certain occupations in which the excess moisture impairs the ability to handle instruments, tools, or papers. Evaporative heat loss cools the skin and may further increase sympathetic nerve outflow and increase sweating further. The moisture on the skin may be a contributing factor to development of contact dermatitis, because it may leach out sensitizing chemicals from objects such as gloves.

   b. *Axillary* hyperhidrosis does not necessarily coincide with palmar/plantar hyperhidrosis. In fact, only 25 per cent of patients with axillary hyperhidrosis also have palmar/plantar involvement. Axillary sweating is far more dependent on temperature than palmar/plantar sweating. Axillary odor is independent of eccrine hyperhidrosis. The odor is thought to be more of a function of the apocrine sweat glands, which are not necessarily more active in patients with simple eccrine axillary hyperhidrosis.

   The presence of axillary or palmar/plantar hyperhidrosis often severely affects a patient's quality of life due to social embarrassment, staining of clothing, reduction of self-esteem, and in some cases occupational disability.

3. Risk factors and differential diagnosis of *localized* hyperhidrosis: Localized hyperhidrosis of the hands and/or feet and the axillae may be

   a. Idiopathic

   b. Due to anxiety states

   c. Neurologic

   d. Other forms of localized hyperhidrosis do occur but are uncommon, such as compensatory hyperhidrosis around leg ulcers or isolated patches of hyperhidrosis on glabrous skin.

4. Risk factors and differential diagnosis of *generalized* hyperhidrosis: generalized hyperhidrosis may be caused by

   a. Neurologic disorders, such as spinal cord injuries and certain peripheral neuropathies and CNS lesions

   b. Systemic diseases, such as hyperthyroidism, diabetes mellitus, pheochromocytoma

   c. Menopause

   d. Anxiety states

   e. Drugs, such as certain antidepressants and alcohol intoxication

   f. "Night sweats" (nocturnal diaphoresis) from such causes as carcinoid syndrome, tuberculosis, Hodgkin's disease

   g. Other thermoregulatory conditions such as fevers of any etiology

Key Symptoms

- Excess sweating
- Inability to handle instruments, tools, or papers
- Staining of clothes
- Emotional embarrassment

Clinical Findings

History

A relatively complete medical history may be needed to determine if any of the factors mentioned above in the differential diagnosis pertain to the patient under evaluation. Specific questions to ask would be those designed to determine the severity and duration of the problem, the anatomic location(s) involved in the process, and any other systemic symptoms that might lead to the diagnosis of any of the conditions mentioned in the differential diagnosis.

Examination

Palmar/plantar hyperhidrosis is a physical finding. In severe cases, drops of sweat drip from the fingers. A handshake with the patient may be the only examination technique necessary to detect palmar hyperhidrosis. Axillary hyperhidrosis is evident from clinical inspection of the axillae showing excess moisture present or by inspecting the clothing.

Key Sign

- Excessive moisture on the palms or soles or the axillae

Clinical Tests

There are no objective tests needed to measure hyperhidrosis clinically. There are investigational techniques for measuring and quantifying skin sweating, but these techniques are not used for routine examination or assessment.

Key Tests

- None necessary unless one of the systemic causes is suspected

Treatment

1. Medical treatment: Treatment of axillary or palmar/plantar hyperhidrosis is not uniformly effective, and many patients respond only minimally to any form of treatment.

   a. In some patients, axillary or palmar/plantar hyperhidrosis responds to some degree to topical application of aluminum salts such as Drysol, which is aluminum chloride in a hydroalcoholic vehicle. Usually, this preparation is applied under occlusion, but nonoccluded applications also may be successful.

   b. Systemic anticholinergic agents such as propantheline have been used in a starting dose of 15 mg three times a day, but often doses high enough to suppress either axillary or palmar/plantar sweating (up to 150 mg/day) produce side effects such as dryness of mucosae and visual disturbances due to failure of accommodation and preclude their use, because the side effects may be more bothersome to the patient than the hyperhidrosis.

2. Physical modality: iontophoresis. Tap water iontophoresis is a safe and inexpensive modality that may be more effective than application of aluminum salts for some patients. A relatively inexpensive device may be used for home treatment. Daily treatments for 2 weeks may decrease sweat output.

3. Surgical treatments: For both axillary and palmar/plantar hyperhidrosis, thoracic sympathectomy is a seldom-used last resort. Axillary hyperhidrosis is occasionally managed by excision of axillary skin.

Key Treatment

Treatments of Choice	Alternative Treatments
• None	• Anticholinergics
• Aluminum chloride	• Surgery
• Iontophoresis	

Bibliography

Akins DL, Meisenheimer JL, Dobson RL: Efficacy of the drionic unit in the treatment of hyperhidrosis. J Am Acad Dermatol 1987;16:828–832.

Brandup P, Larson PO: Axillary hyperhidrosis: Local treatment with aluminum chloride hexahydrate 25% in absolute alcohol. Acta Derm Venereol 1978;58:461.

Elgart ML, Fuchs G: Tapwater iontoporesis in the treatment of hyperhidrosis: Use of the Drionic device. Int J Dermatol 1987;26:194–197.

Sato K: Disorders of the eccrine sweat glands. In Fitzpatrick TB et al (eds): Dermatology in General Medicine. New York, McGraw-Hill, 1993.

256 Erysipelas

Joseph R. Masci

Etiology

1. Erysipelas is a specific type of superficial cellulitis accompanied by pronounced lymphedema.
2. Almost all cases are caused by group A β-hemolytic streptococci (*Streptococcus pyogenes*). Other organisms including *Staphylococcus aureus* are occasionally implicated.
3. Erysipelas is seen most commonly in young children and elderly adults. The following may be predisposing conditions:
   a. Pre-existing lymphedema secondary to lymphatic occlusion (e.g., malignancies or postoperative)
   b. Pre-existing breaks in the epidermis (e.g., xerosis, ichthyosis, fungal infections)
   c. Venous stasis

Symptoms

1. Pain and swelling in the involved area
2. Fever and chills are common.
3. Painful swelling in regional lymph nodes may be seen.

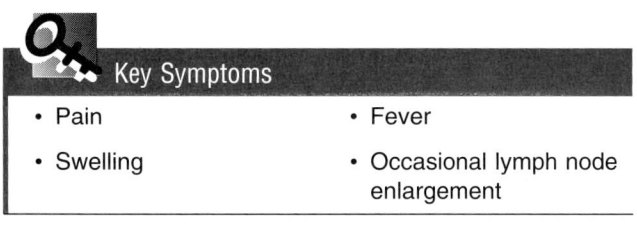

Key Symptoms	
• Pain	• Fever
• Swelling	• Occasional lymph node enlargement

Clinical Findings

1. Most common sites of involvement are the face and the lower extremities.
2. Characteristic features include
   a. Erythema and lymphedema in the involved area
   b. Palpable advancing margin that may progress over hours to days. Formation of bullae may be seen. Multiple sites of involvement are unusual.
3. Systemic signs of infection are often present; these may include
   a. Fever
   b. Peripheral leukocytosis
   c. Lymphangitis and regional tender lymphadenopathy
   d. Approximately 5 per cent of patients have positive blood cultures. Rarely, the sepsis syndrome may be seen with hypotension, systemic acidosis, and disseminated intravascular coagulation.

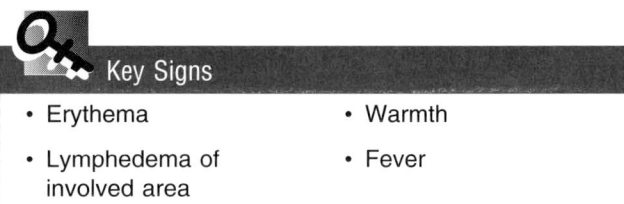

Key Signs	
• Erythema	• Warmth
• Lymphedema of involved area	• Fever

Laboratory Tests

1. Culture and Gram's stain of aspirate from advancing margin of lesion if possible
2. The following blood tests should be considered in severe cases:
   a. Complete blood count
   b. Blood urea nitrogen (BUN), creatinine, electrolytes
   c. Blood cultures

Key Test

• Consider culture of aspirate of involved area in severe cases or when response to therapy is delayed.

Differential Diagnosis

1. Other bacterial soft tissue infections
2. A variety of other disorders may be confused with erysipelas; these include
   a. Seborrheic dermatitis
   b. Erythema chronicum migrans
   c. Early herpes zoster
   d. Contact dermatitis
3. Erysipelas usually may be distinguished from these disorders on the basis of the following criteria:
   a. Soft tissue infections due to other bacteria are less commonly associated with significant lymphedema and a palpable advancing margin.
   b. Other aids in diagnosis include
      (1) Fever rarely occurs in association with seborrheic dermatitis or contact dermatitis but is seen commonly with erysipelas.
      (2) Erythema chronicum migrans should be considered in persons who have recently traveled to areas endemic for Lyme disease.
      (3) Herpes zoster typically occurs in a dermatomal distribution. The appearance of grouped vesicles suggests the diagnosis of herpes zoster.

Treatment

1. Treatment consists of antibiotic therapy, which may be instituted on the basis of characteristic physical findings of erysipelas.

930

2. Local care and bed rest may be beneficial.

Medication

1. Penicillin is the antibiotic of choice. Oral therapy with phenoxymethyl penicillin (7.5 mg/kg four times daily for 7 to 10 days) may be sufficient for mild cases in healthy individuals. Hospitalization and parenteral therapy with penicillin G (1 to 2 million units every 4 hours) may be necessary for more severe cases or in elderly or debilitated hosts.

2. For patients allergic to penicillin, erythromycin (500 mg by mouth four times daily) is the drug of choice for oral therapy. Clindamycin (600 mg intravenously every 8 hours) may be used if parenteral therapy is required.

3. Underlying skin disorders, if present, should be treated

4. Antipyretics and cool and wet dressings as necessary for comfort

Diet

No modification in diet necessary

Activity

1. Bed rest, elevation of involved area

2. Hospitalized patients should be placed on skin precautions.

Patient Education

1. Underlying skin disorders should be treated, if possible.

2. Recurrence of erysipelas may be seen in areas of recurrent breaks in the dermis or of lymphatic or venous occlusion.

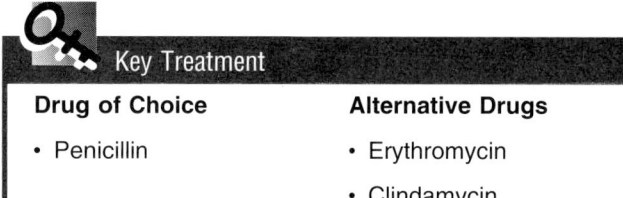

Key Treatment

Drug of Choice	Alternative Drugs
• Penicillin	• Erythromycin
	• Clindamycin

Follow-Up

1. Response to therapy usually occurs within several days.

2. Patient should return if worsening or no improvement occurs within 48 hours.

3. Follow-up evaluation of underlying skin conditions, if present, including

   a. Xerosis, ichthyosis, fungal infections

   b. Venous stasis

Bibliography

Dreizen S: The butterfly rash and the malar flush: What diseases do these signs reflect? Postgrad Med 1991;89:225–228, 233–234.

Feingold DS, Hirschmann JV: Cellulitis. *In* Gorbach SL, Bartlett JG, Blacklow NR (eds): Infectious Diseases. Philadelphia, WB Saunders, 1992, pp 1072–1074.

Kahn RM, Goldstein EJ: Common bacterial skin infections: Diagnostic clues and therapeutic options. Postgrad Med 1993;93:175–182.

Ochs MW, Dolwick MF: Facial erysipelas: Report of a case and review of the literature. J Oral Maxillofac Surg 1991;49:1111–1120.

Sjoblom AC, Bruchfeld J, Eriksson B, et al: Skin concentrations of phenoxymethylpenicillin in patients with erysipelas. Infection 1992;20:30–33.

257 Acne

Jack L. Arbiser

Etiology

1. Acne is an extremely common disorder arising from inflammation of the pilosebaceous unit.

2. Pilosebaceous units are anatomically present over most of the skin surface, and pilosebaceous units containing a relatively large number of sebaceous glands are particular targets for acne. This accounts for the common distribution of acne involving the face, back, and upper chest.

3. Despite its prevalence, its pathogenesis is poorly understood. Many factors affect the incidence and severity of acne and include genetics, use of cosmetics, microflora, endocrine status of patients, drugs, immune status, and occupation. The initial evaluation of the acne patient should include all these factors.

4. Acne is extremely common in teenagers of both sexes but is a significant problem up to the fifth decade of life.

5. The initial insult in acne is thought to be altered keratinization of epithelial cells in the hair follicle infundibulum.

6. The resulting plug, along with free fatty acids liberated by the action of the bacterium *Propionibacter acnes,* elicits inflammation. This initial lesion is termed a comedone.

7. Keratinization is affected by genetic factors, so acne often runs in families.

History

1. Endocrine: irregular menstruation, hirsutism, infertility (virilizing disorders)

2. Medication and cosmetic use (including previous acne therapy)

3. Occupation

Agents Associated with Promotion of Acne

1. Occupational: cutting oils, greases, chlorinated hydrocarbons

2. Endocrine: testosterone, progesterone, glucocorticoids

3. Drugs: lithium, phenytoin, bromides, iodides, isoniazide, thiouracil (The amount of iodide in table salt is insufficient to cause acne.)

4. Diet: No conclusive relationship between diet and acne has been established.

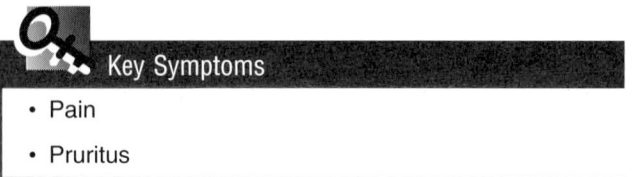

Key Symptoms

- Pain
- Pruritus

Clinical Findings

1. Comedones: small raised erythematous lesions (1 to 4 mm), with either black center (open comedone) or white center (closed comedone)

2. Nodules and cysts: true cysts do not exist in acne, but "cystic lesions" represent advanced lesions that have spilled foreign material and inflammation into the dermis.

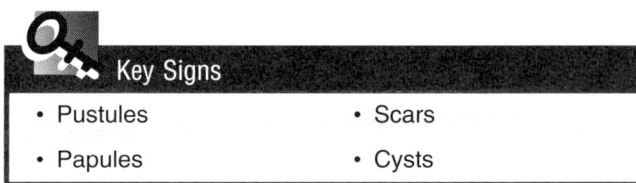

Key Signs

- Pustules
- Papules
- Scars
- Cysts

Laboratory Tests

No laboratory test is diagnostic for acne. Measurement of dehydroepiandrosterone sulfate (DHEAS) may be useful in elucidating a systemic basis.

Differential Diagnosis

1. Staphylococcal pyoderma
2. Gram-negative folliculitis
3. Appendageal and adnexal tumors
4. Basal cell carcinoma
5. Osteoma cutis
6. Epidermal cysts
7. Sebaceous hyperplasia

Treatment

1. Treatment of the patient with acne should be geared toward severity of the disease, compliance of the patient, and cost of therapy.

2. Limited disease and superficial lesions can be treated with topical medication alone.

3. Deeper lesions and acne on the back and chest, which is poorly reached by topical therapy, can be treated with systemic agents, including antibiotics and hormones.

4. Recalcitrant acne is treated with oral isotretinoin (Accutane).

Topical Therapy

1. Benzoyl peroxide: Numerous proprietary formulations of benzoyl peroxide exist, in concentrations of 2.5%, 4%, 5%, and 10%. Many benzoyl peroxide preparations are drying to the skin and, if the patient has dry skin, may be better tolerated if used in conjunction with a moisturizer. Benzoyl peroxide is bactericidal and keratolytic but may be irritating to some patients.

2. Topical antibiotics
   a. Erythromycin: possibly the most commonly used topical antibiotic, available in concentrations of 1.5 to 3% or in combination with benzoyl peroxide (Benzamycin)
   b. Clindamycin: available in 1% concentration in a variety of vehicles. Use of topical clindamycin has been associated rarely with pseudomembranous colitis.
   c. Tetracycline/oxytetracycline: less effective than erythromycin
3. Topical retinoids: A synthetic retinoid, tretinoin (Retin-A), is thought to alter keratinization and thus be of benefit to both existing comedones and for the prevention of new comedones. Topical tretinoin exists in creams as 0.025%, 0.05%, and 0.1%; in gel as 0.01% and 0.025%; and in liquid as 0.05%. There are no generic topical retinoids. This drug is initially drying and irritating; these side effects can be mitigated by initial use every 2 to 3 days, with gradual buildup to once-daily application. Topical retinoids are mild photosensitizers, so sunlight should be avoided. Little topical tretinoin is systemically absorbed, but given the teratogenic potential of oral retinoids, it is prudent to avoid this during pregnancy.

Intralesional Therapy

Injection of 2.5 mg/ml triamcinolone acetonide is effective in reducing the size and inflammation of a limited number of lesions. The major side effect of this therapy is skin atrophy.

Systemic Therapy

1. Antibiotics: Systemic antibiotics are effective in the management of moderate to severe acne. Their effectiveness likely results from inherent anti-inflammatory effects of the antibiotics as well as antibacterial activity. The decision to use an antibiotic should take into account what antibiotics the patient has used previously, a history of allergy, and the cost of the antibiotics. All antibiotics increase the risk of vaginal yeast infections and theoretically decrease absorption of oral contraceptives. The effectiveness of antibiotics should be judged at 2-month intervals.
   a. Tetracycline, 500 mg to 2 gm daily, not with meals, usually given in two divided doses. Side effects: photosensitizing
   b. Erythromycin, 1 gm daily, usually given in two or three divided doses. Side effects: gastrointestinal distress
   c. Doxycycline (Vibramycin), 100 mg twice daily, with water. Side effects: esophagitis, photosensitizing
   d. Minocycline (Minocin), 50 to 100 mg twice daily, most effective and expensive of acne antibiotics. Side effects: dizziness with initial doses, self-resolving, rare blue-gray hyperpigmentation in areas affected by acne
   e. Other antibiotics: Trimethoprim-sulfamethoxazole (Bactrim, Septra), is an effective acne medication, but it is used less because of the higher incidence of skin eruptions and other adverse effects. Ampicillin is sometimes used and may be given to pregnant women, although the use of oral antibiotics for acne in pregnant women should be discouraged.

2. Isotretinoin (Accutane) is a synthetic retinoid (13-*cis*-retinoic acid) that is indicated for acne recalcitrant to antibiotic therapy. This drug, at doses of 0.5 to 1.0 mg/kg/day, over a 16- to 20-week period, leads to long-term and often permanent remissions from acne. Isotretinoin has many side effects. Since it is highly teratogenic, isotretinoin is absolutely contraindicated in pregnancy. Administration to women of childbearing age should be preceded by a pregnancy test, and the woman must use contraception up to 1 month after therapy has ended. Isotretinoin has no teratogenic potential in men.

Common side effects include dry lips, nosebleed, hair loss, hypertriglyceridemia, and muscle pain. Isotretinoin should not be given concurrently with oral antibiotics, since the risk of pseudotumor cerebri is increased. A long-term side effect of uncertain significance is the development of vertebral hyperostoses. Monthly monitoring of liver function tests, blood urea nitrogen, creatinine, serum lipids, and β subunit of human chorionic gonadotropin and clinical assessment of the patient are recommended.

3. Hormonal agents: These are useful in selected cases of acne.
   a. Prednisone is useful in doses of 5 mg daily for the suppression of adrenal androgen.
   b. Androgen antagonists: Spironolactone is sometimes used at doses of 150 to 200 mg daily. Potassium should be monitored.
   c. Oral contraceptives: Estrogens likely act by suppressing adrenal androgens. Progesterone-containing preparations should be avoided. The most frequently used oral contraceptives for acne suppression are Demulin, Ovulen, and Enovid E.

Key Treatment

- Topical antibiotics
- Oral antibiotics
- Accutane

 Bibliography

Arndt KA: Acne. *In* Arndt KA (ed): Manual of Dermatologic Therapeutics, 4th ed. Boston, Little, Brown, 1989, pp 3–13.

Arnold HL, Odom RB, James WD: Andrews' Diseases of the Skin, 8th ed. Philadelphia, WB Saunders, 1990, pp 250–262.

Lucky AW: Hormonal correlates of acne and hirsutism. Am J Med 1995;98:895–945.

Plewig G, Kligman AM: Acne and Rosacea, 2d ed. New York, Springer-Verlag, 1993, pp 479–553.

Taylor MB: Treatment of acne vulgaris: guidelines for primary care physicians. Postgrad Med 1991;89:40–42.

258 Impetigo

Laeth Nasir

Etiology

1. *Staphylococcus aureus*: Coagulase-positive *Staphylococcus* has become the dominant microorganism in all forms of this superficial skin infection. *Staphylococcus* is considered to be the sole cause of bullous impetigo, a manifestation of localized infection with phage group II staphylococci. The severest form of this infection is known as "staphylococcal scalded skin syndrome" (SSSS). *Streptococcus, Staphylococcus,* or mixed *Strep-Staph* infection causes impetigo contagiosa. All forms of impetigo are highly contagious and spread by direct contact, insect vectors, and fomites.

2. *Streptococcus pyogenes* (group A β-hemolytic streptococci): The major consequence of infection with this organism is the nonsuppurative sequelae caused by infection with nephritogenic strains of *Streptococcus*. Scarlet fever and erythema multiforme also may occur. Antibiotic treatment of impetigo has not been demonstrated to reduce the incidence of poststreptococcal glomerulonephritis. Rheumatic fever is not a sequela of skin infection.

Symptoms

1. Impetigo contagiosa: may present with an itching, crusting, often indolent rash. Exposed or traumatized skin are the sites most commonly affected.

2. Bullous impetigo: often a dramatic presentation with rapidly growing blisters in localized areas; may become very large. This condition is most commonly seen in neonates.

Key Symptoms

- Itching
- Crusting
- Blisters

Clinical Findings

1. Impetigo contagiosa: begins as tender papules becoming vesicular and subsequently rupturing, leaving the classic "honey-colored crusts." Removal of this crust reveals superficial weeping erosions. Regional lymphadenopathy is seen in the majority of cases. Constitutional symptoms are absent.

2. Bullous impetigo: begins as a small vesicle, rapidly enlarging to bullae filled with purulent fluid. Spontaneous rupture occurs, leaving red, tender erosive areas. Lymphadenopathy and constitutional symptoms

are absent. Both bullous and nonbullous forms of impetigo heal without scarring.

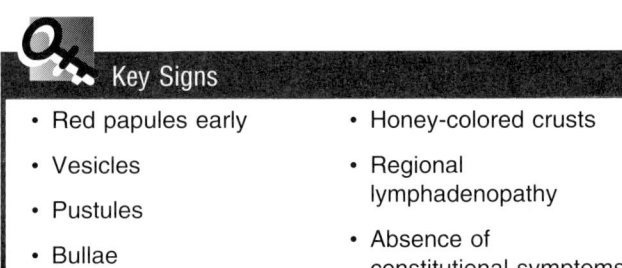

Key Signs

- Red papules early
- Vesicles
- Pustules
- Bullae
- Honey-colored crusts
- Regional lymphadenopathy
- Absence of constitutional symptoms

Laboratory Tests

1. Diagnosis is clinical. Laboratory tests are not performed routinely. However, in special situations, the following tests may be considered:
   a. Gram's stain
   b. Culture and sensitivity
   c. Tzanck's smear to rule out herpes simplex infection
   d. Antihyaluronidase and antideoxyribonuclease B serum titers to rule out or confirm group A β-hemolytic streptococcal infections. Streptolysin O production (by streptococci) is inhibited by lipids in the skin; therefore, ASO titer is not useful in diagnosis.

Differential Diagnosis

1. Ecthyma: considered a "deep" form of impetigo. Lesions often covered with a thicker and more adherent crust than observed in impetigo. Removal of the crust reveals purulent red ulcers with raised margins.

2. Folliculitis: lesions localized to hair follicles with inflammation and central pustules.

3. Eczema: often seen around the nose and mouth in a distribution similar to that observed in impetigo. Additionally, these lesions may become secondarily impetiginized.

4. Herpes simplex: also susceptible to secondary impetigination. Tends to be more painful that impetigo.

Treatment

1. Topical antibiotic therapy. Treatment of localized, easily accessible lesions is best accomplished through topical antibiotic therapy and debridement of lesions as outlined under "Patient education."

2. Systemic antibiotic therapy. Indications for systemic antibiotic therapy are
   a. Widely disseminated or inaccessible lesions

b. Outbreaks of impetigo in multiple family members or others in close contact, such as day care

c. Bullous impetigo

3. Duration of both systemic and topical forms of therapy is 7 to 10 days or until complete resolution occurs.

Medication

A. Drug of choice

1. Topical therapy: Mupirocin (Bactroban) ointment applied t.i.d. to affected areas.

2. Systemic therapy

a. Erythromycin, adult dose, 1 gm/day, divided dose. Pediatric dose (erythromycin estolate, Ilosone), 40 mg/kg/day, every 6 hours.

b. Dicloxacillin (Dynapen) adult dose, 250 mg/q.i.d., 1 hour before or 2 hours after meals. Pediatric dose, 25 mg/kg/day every 6 hours.

B. Alternative drugs

1. Cephalexin (Keflex), adult dose, 250 mg q.i.d. Pediatric dose, 50 mg/kg/day, every 6 hours

2. Clindamycin (Cleocin), 300 mg every 8 hours. Pediatric dose, 20 mg/kg/day, every 6 hours

3. Ciprofloxacin (Cipro), 500 mg b.i.d. (adults only)

Patient Education

1. Debridement of crust with wet soaks for 20 minutes, three times daily, followed by gentle scrubbing with a washcloth

2. Fingernails should be kept short and scratching discouraged to avoid spread of infection.

3. Impetigo is extremely contagious. Use of an antibacterial soap, as well as avoidance of towels and washcloths used by the affected individual, is crucial to avoiding spread of infection.

4. Children should be removed from day care until 24 hours after antibiotic treatment is initiated.

Key Treatment

Drugs of Choice	Alternative Drugs
• Mupirocin	• Cephalexin
• Erythromycin	• Clindamycin
• Dicloxacillin	• Ciprofloxacin

Follow-Up

1. If lesions clear promptly (3 to 5 days), no further follow-up is necessary.

2. Failure to eradicate the lesions within 7 days or acute spread of lesions necessitates prompt re-evaluation of the diagnosis and/or treatment.

3. If a nephritogenic strain of *Streptococcus* is strongly suspected as the causative organism, follow-up with a urinalysis in 2 weeks may be a reasonable precaution.

Bibliography

American Academy of Pediatrics: Children in out-of-home child care. *In* Peter G (ed): 1994 Red Book: Report of the Committee on Infectious Diseases, 23rd ed. Elk Grove Village, IL, American Academy of Pediatrics, 1994, p 82.

Esterly NB: The skin. *In* Behrmann RE (ed): Nelson Textbook of Pediatrics, 14th ed. Philadelphia, WB Saunders, 1992, pp 1427–1429.

Goldstein BG, Goldstein AO: Bacterial diseases. *In* Practical Dermatology, 1st ed. St. Louis, CV Mosby, 1992, pp 65–67.

Parish LC, Witkowski JA: Systemic management of cutaneous bacterial infections. Am J Med 1991;91(6A):106–110.

Rice TD, Duggan AK, DeAngelis C: Cost effectiveness of erythromycin versus mupirocin for the treatment of impetigo in children. Pediatrics 1992;89(2)210–214.

259 Basal and Squamous Cell Carcinoma

Marsha DuPree

Etiology

1. Basal cell carcinoma (BCC) is the most common malignancy in the United States, and squamous cell carcinoma (SCC) is the second most common cutaneous malignancy. Approximately 500,000 new cases of nonmelanoma skin cancer occur yearly, and the incidence is increasing.
2. Definitions
   a. BCC is a malignant tumor arising from basal cell layer of epidermis.
   b. SCC is a malignant tumor arising from keratinizing cells of epidermis.
3. Risk factors
   a. Excessive cumulative sun exposure
   b. Light complexion, light hair, light eyes
   c. History of radiation treatment in area, trauma, or arsenic ingestion
   d. Immunosuppression (SCC seen most commonly)
   e. Genetic syndromes (xeroderma pigmentosa, albinism and basal cell nevus syndrome)

Symptoms

BCC and SCC are generally asymptomatic.

Clinical Findings

A. Basal cell carcinoma
   1. Average age of onset 64 years, more common in males
   2. Common sites
      a. Face, especially nose
      b. Neck, chest, and upper back
      c. Very rare on mucous membranes, hands, and extremities
   3. Clinical presentation
      a. Nodular BCC: white, translucent papule, telangiectasia, with or without ulcer
      b. Superficial BCC: scaly, erythematous macule, telangiectasia, with or without crust
      c. Pigmented BCC: nodular BCC with irregular pigmentation
      d. Morpheaform or sclerosing (rare form approximately 0.1 per cent): waxy, yellow "scarlike" plaque, telangiectasia
      e. Metastasis very rare
B. Squamous cell carcinoma
   1. Average age onset 66.2 years, 3:1 male/female ratio
   2. Common sites
      a. Face
      b. Dorsal hands, lower extremities (chronic ulcers, burns)
      c. Mucous membranes (especially lower lip, glans penis)
   3. Clinical presentation
      a. Early lesions (actinic keratosis, solar keratosis, SCC in situ) scaly, erythematous macule (<5 mm) with telangiectasia
      b. Later lesions firm, scaly plaque or nodule with telangiectasia or ulceration
   4. Metastasis: Increased incidence of metastasis in SCC involving
      a. Eyelid, external ear, scalp, dorsal hand, mucous membranes
      b. Areas of burns, ulcers, and immunocompromised hosts
      c. Recurrent lesions
      d. Large lesions greater than 2 cm
      e. Aggressive histologic pattern (see "Laboratory Tests")

Key Findings

BCC	SCC
• Translucent, white papule	• Scaly erythematous macule or plaque
• Scaly patch with crust	• Firm papule or plaque
• Telangiectasia	• Telangiectasia
• Ulceration centrally	• Central ulceration
• Face and upper back	• Face, dorsal hand, and lower lip

Laboratory Tests

1. The only laboratory procedure for confirming the diagnosis of BCC or SCC is biopsy (shave or punch). Biopsy before treatment because this will help determine treatment. *Always do a punch biopsy if you suspect a skin cancer at the site of a scar.*
2. The histopathology of BCC and SCC is important in determining treatment.
   a. Histopathology of BCC (nodular or superficial): foci or lobules of basaloid cells extending from epidermis
   b. Histologically aggressive variants of BCC

936

(1) Morpheaform or sclerosing BCC

(2) Infiltrating BCC

(3) Metatypical or basosquamous cell carcinoma

(4) Tumors with perineural invasion

c. Histopathology of SCC

(1) Irregular downward proliferation of atypical keratinocytes showing individual cell keratinization, atypical mitosis, and invasion into the dermis

(2) Actinic keratosis shows these features confined to epidermis.

d. Histologically aggressive variants of SCC

(1) Spindle cell SCC

(2) Adenoid SCC

(3) Verrucous carcinoma

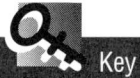
Key Test

- Biopsy (shave or punch)

Differential Diagnosis

1. Clinical mimics easily diagnosed on histology

   a. Pigmented BCC can mimic melanoma.

   b. Keratoacanthoma (rapidly growing, crater-like nodule) mimics SCC.

2. Genetic diseases (important in differential diagnosis of young people with skin cancers)

   a. Basal cell nevus syndrome (autosomal dominant) (see Habif reference): nevus-like lesions (BCC histologically) arising at puberty

   b. Albinism

   c. Xeroderma pigmentosa (see Habif reference)

Treatment

It is important to evaluate the *anatomic site* (area involved), the *histologic type,* whether the lesion is a *recurrence,* and the *age* of patient in choosing treatment. *Appropriate initial treatment offers the best cure rates and best cosmetic results.*

1. *Surgical excision* (recurrence rate approximately 10 per cent)

   a. Best for tumors (BCC or SCC) less than 2 cm with distinct borders

   b. Surgical margins for nonaggressive BCC less than 2 cm is 2 to 4 mm.

   c. Surgical margins for nonaggressive SCC less than 2 cm is 5 to 6 mm.

   d. If surgical margins are positive, then immediate re-excision or Mohs' surgery.

   e. *Contraindications:* recurrences, histologically aggressive tumors

2. *Electrodesiccation and curettage* (recurrence rate approximately 7 per cent)

   a. Simple procedure in skilled hands

   b. Good for small (<2 cm) nodular and superficial BCC

   c. Good for tumors on firm surfaces (chest, forehead, temple, ears)

   d. *Contraindications:* recurrences, histologically aggressive, scalp

3. *Cryosurgery* (recurrence rate 7.5 per cent in experienced hands)

   a. Actinic keratosis, BCC, and nonaggressive SCC

   b. Can be used on larger tumors, patients on anticoagulants or with pacemakers, and on difficult anatomic sites (nasal ala, ears, eyelid)

   c. *Contraindications:* recurrences, lower leg (delayed healing)

4. *Radiotherapy* (recurrence rate 8.7 per cent)

   a. BCC, SCC, recurrences, or residual tumors

   b. Facial areas (where cosmesis and function are important, such as the eyelid)

   c. Larger size (1 to 5 cm), patients on anticoagulants, or keloid formers

   d. Age 40 years or older, because treated areas deteriorate cosmetically with time

   e. *Contraindications:* recurrences treated initially with radiation, scalp

5. *Mohs' micrographic surgery:* procedure where the tumor is excised and frozen sections of the entire cut surgical margin are evaluated until the margins are clear (usually same day). Circumstances best used in

   a. Recurrent tumors

   b. Tumor with aggressive pathology (see "Laboratory Tests")

   c. Large tumors

   d. Tumors where recurrence rate is high (see BCC and SCC recurrence)

   e. *Tissue-sparing* aspect of Mohs' is helpful in functionally and cosmetically difficult areas

   f. *Recurrence rates for primary:* 1 per cent; for recurrent tumors, 5.6 per cent

   g. Disadvantages: expensive and difficult for patients in poor health

6. *Chemotherapy*

   a. Topical 5-fluorouracil (5-FU) (see Bennett reference)

   (1) Extensive actinic keratosis, keratoacanthoma, and superficial BCC

   (2) Patients are often noncompliant because of pain and erosions (temporarily cosmetically disfiguring).

   b. Intralesional interferon-alpha (see Bennett reference)

   (1) Useful in superficial and nodular BCC; has shown an approximate 80 per cent cure

(2) Side effects: some flulike symptom and pain in area

  c. Retinoid (oral)

    (1) Useful in patients with genetic syndromes (see "Differential Diagnosis")

    (2) Numerous severe side effects in long-term use

7. *Photodynamic therapy:* newer treatment combining laser and photoactive drugs

Prevention

1. Education on sunscreens

2. Avoiding exposure to midday sun and burning

3. A 3-inch brim on hats

4. Protect children: *Remember, it is cumulative ultraviolet (UV) radiation.*

Key Treatment

- Surgical excision

- Electrodesiccation, curettage

- Cryosurgery

- Radiotherapy

- Mohs' micrographic surgery

- Chemotherapy

- Photodynamic therapy

Follow-Up

1. First year: every 3 months for recurrence and new BCC or SCC

2. At least yearly for 5 years; some authors believe a lifetime, since more than 50 per cent of patients will develop a *new* BCC or SCC within 4 to 5 years.

Recurrence: BCC
- Areas of common recurrences: nose, ears, lips, periorbital, scalp
- Large size (>2 cm)
- Aggressive histologic variants
- Previously treated lesions

Recurrence: SCC
- Sites of common recurrences: lip, nose, ear, scalp, dorsum of hand
- Occurrence in scar site
- Large size (>2 cm)
- Previously treated lesions
- Immunocompromised host
- Aggressive histologic types

Bibliography

AAD Committee on Guidelines of Care (Lynn A. Drake, chairman): Guidelines of care for cutaneous squamous cell carcinomas. J Am Acad Dermatol 1993;28:628–631.

Arnold HL, Odom RB, James WD: Andrews' Diseases of the Skin, 8th ed. Philadelphia, WB Saunders, 1990, pp 763–786.

Bennett RG: Fundamentals of Cutaneous Surgery. St Louis, CV Mosby, 1988, pp 619–659.

Goldstein AM, Bale SJ, Peck GL, DiGiovanna JJ: Sun exposure and basal cell carcinoma in the nevoid basal cell carcinoma syndrome. J Am Acad Dermatol 1993;29(1):34–41.

Habif TP: Clinical Dermatology: A Color Guide to Diagnosis and Therapy. St Louis, CV Mosby, 1990, pp 519–539.

Procedure **PUNCH AND SHAVE BIOPSY** *Robert M. Howse, Jr.*

Indications

1. Shave biopsy: epidermal lesions such as seborrheic dermatoses, actinic keratoses, warts, skin tags, scabies
2. Punch biopsy: epidermal, intradermal lesions such as carcinoma, infection, nevi, and autoimmune, parasitic, and pyogenic granulomas

Contraindications

1. Highly vascular lesions, such as hemangioma
2. Benign or self-limited lesions, such as strawberry hemangioma
3. Referral and special treatment required, such as cavernous hemangioma, extensive facial basal cell or squamous cell carcinoma

Preparation

Patient history and education about lesion, anesthesia, procedure, risks of bleeding, infection, scarring, benefits, follow-up, signature and witness on informed consent, wound care, cosmetic procedures

1. Bleeding history
   a. *Aspirin:* Prophylactic doses of 325 mg or less a day seldom prevent hemostasis; higher doses may delay hemostasis but can be managed with 10 to 15 minutes of postoperative pressure.
   b. *Coumarin:* If the prothrombin time is within therapeutic range, achieve hemostasis with 10 to 15 minutes of pressure postoperatively.
   c. *Factor deficiency:* Patient must be on therapeutic replacement.
   d. *Thrombocytopenia:* Hemostasis is adequate down to a platelet count of 20,000 unless platelet function is also abnormal (e.g., idiopathic thrombocytopenic purpura).
2. Tetanus status: Document allergies. To prepare sterile field, spiral out from lesion with surgical scrub (isopropyl alcohol is sufficient) and drape.
3. Punch biopsy patients must keep wound clean and dry for 24 hours. After that, keep wound clean and dry except to gently remove crust with warm soap and water twice a day until the suture removal. This minimizes scar width.

Equipment

1. Punches, 1 to 6 mm
2. Scalpel
3. Blades
4. Scissors
5. Forceps
6. Formalin
7. 1% or 2% lidocaine with or without epinephrine
8. Syringes
9. Needles
10. Surgical scrub
11. Drapes
12. Sterile gloves
13. Monofilament suture
14. Electric cautery
15. $AgNO_3$ sticks. For epidermal lesions only. Use in dermis will tattoo.

Anesthesia

1. 1% lidocaine if the patient is not allergic
2. May use epinephrine if not contraindicated by
   a. Site: Avoid use in nose, ears, fingers, toes, and genitalia.
   b. Medical contraindications: coronary artery disease, uncontrolled hypertension, allergy
3. Preoperative acetaminophen (1000 mg) or ibuprofen (400 mg) ½ to 2 hours prior to procedure
4. Postoperative acetaminophen or ibuprofen. Narcotics are rarely necessary.

Precautions

Lesions suspicious for melanoma may be better managed by referral to a physician skilled in managing melanoma.

WARNING

- *Do not* use epinephrine on nose, ears, fingers, toes, or genitals.
- *Do not* use cautery on the plantar surface of the foot.
- *Use* universal precautions.

Technique

Punch Biopsy

1. Select a punch slightly larger than the lesion if complete excision is the goal. Otherwise, plan the punch to be as small as possible and yet obtain adequate tissue for diagnosis.

2. Diagnosis of blistering diseases and keratoacanthoma requires contiguous, normal tissue to be present. Estimate the depth of the lesion by its color and palpation.

3. Put tension on the skin perpendicular to the observed skin tension lines to create an elliptical wound.

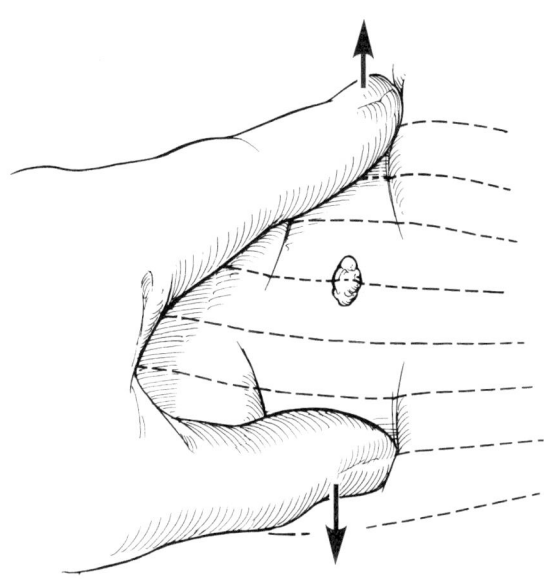

4. Insert the punch with a continuous, clockwise twist to the necessary depth.

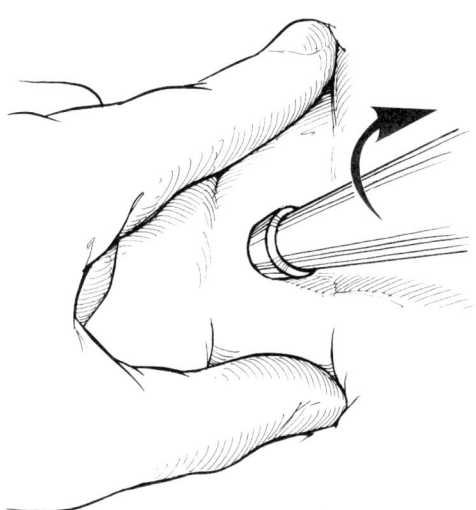

5. *Gently* extract the tissue column with forceps and remove it from the its base in the subepidermal fat with scissors or a scalpel blade.

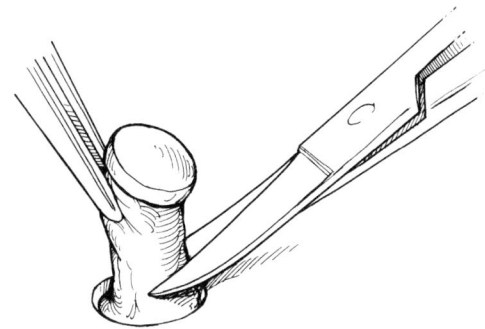

6. Repair with monofilament suture matched to skin type and site. Hide the scar along the skin tension lines; 5- and 6-mm wounds may need two interrupted stitches.

7. Cleanse the wound, apply a dry, nonocclusive dressing without medication, creams, or ointments to enhance re-epithelialization without infection and prevent scar widening from direct cellular toxicity.

Shave Biopsy

1. *Seborrheic keratosis:* Carefully grasp seborrheic keratoses with forceps, and gently remove by gliding the scalpel blade parallel to the skin surface at the level of the epidermis.

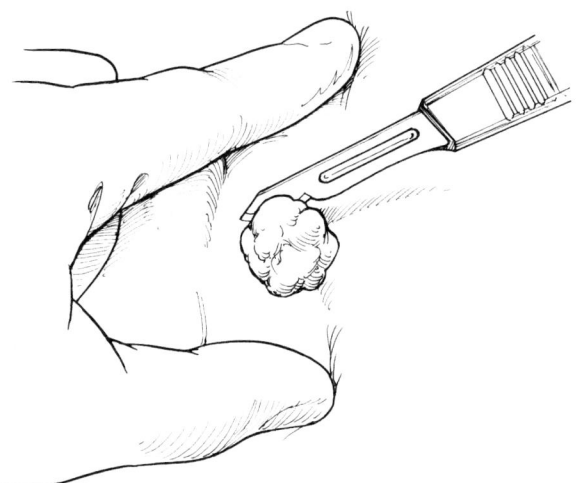

Lightly cauterize.

2. *Verruca (warts)*

   a. Shave verruca and further pare until punctate bleeding appears.

   b. Light cautery followed by scraping out the residual, sticky material will destroy the remaining wart. Do not use cautery on plantar warts because it may induce painful, permanent scarring.

   c. Mild acids or vesicants, such as trichloroacetic acid 10% to 35% or salicylic acid paste or plaster, may be applied and weekly paring continued until the wart is destroyed.

3. *Actinic keratosis*

   a. Remove actinic keratoses by scraping with a blade held perpendicularly to the skin.

   b. Push the buttery material into a specimen container to confirm the diagnosis and rule out basal cell carcinoma. The usual tensile resistance of the underlying normal tissue is felt against the blade when all the actinic tissue has been removed.

  c. Light cautery destroys any remaining abnormal cells and is hemostatic.

  d. After cleansing, apply a dry, nonocclusive dressing without medication, creams, or ointments to allow re-epithelialization without infection and prevent scar widening from cellular toxicity.

Follow-Up

Follow at 5 to 10 days based on the expected time for suture removal or crust resolution.

1. Inspect for infection and tensile strength.

2. Remove sutures; alternate if necessary.

3. Discuss pathology. Malignant lesions minimally require yearly follow-up with a complete body inventory. Refer as needed.

4. Review cosmetic instructions.

5. Rub wound gently with hand cream at least twice a day for 6 weeks and up to 1 year. This alleviates redness and minimizes the thickness and stiffness of the scar.

6. Gently remove crust with warm soap and water to minimize scar width.

7. Protect from ultraviolet (UV) radiation with sunscreen 40 for 1 year until scar repigmentation is complete.

Bibliography

Fitzpatrick TB, Eisen AZ, Wolff K, et al: Dermatology in General Medicine. New York, McGraw-Hill, 1979, pp 35–36.

Fitzpatrick TB, Polano MK, Suurmond D: Color Atlas and Synopsis of Clinical Dermatology. New York, McGraw-Hill, 1983.

Gilman AG, Goodman LS, Gilman A: Goodman and Gilman's The Pharmacological Basis of Therapeutics. New York, Macmillan, 1985, p 951.

Moschella SL, Hurley HJ: Dermatology, vols 1 and 2. Philadelphia, WB Saunders, 1985, pp 2010–2013.

260 Melanoma

Harriet A. Jakob

Etiology

1. *Definition:* A skin cancer arising from the malignant transformation of epidermal melanocytes. There are four classic subtypes of melanoma:

   a. *Superficial spreading melanoma* (70 per cent) occurs more often in young adults on sun-exposed areas such as the lower legs, arms.

   b. *Nodular melanoma* (15 to 30 per cent) occurs more often in young adults on the trunk and sun-exposed areas and tends to grow quickly.

   c. *Lentigo maligna melanoma* (5 to 10 per cent) occurs mainly in older adults, particularly in sites that are continually exposed to the sun, such as the face. Arises from lentigo maligna or melanoma in situ

   d. *Acral lentiginous melanoma* (10 per cent) occurs on the palms, soles, subungual, and mucous membrane areas. This type of melanoma is most often seen in Asians and African Americans and is not related to sun exposure.

2. *Epidemiology:* Melanoma is on the rise in the United States, with an annual incidence of 13 per 100,000, or a lifetime risk of approximately 1 per cent. The incidence of melanoma is increased in populations living close to the equator. The median age at diagnosis is 45 years, with only lentigo maligna melanoma occurring predominantly in the elderly. Approximately 50 per cent of melanoma arises de novo, with the remainder arising from precursor lesions.

3. *Risk factors:* There are many factors that affect an individual's risk

   a. Sun exposure: Both cumulative and episodic intense sunlight exposures (primarily ultraviolet B [UVB] but possibly also ultraviolet A [UVA]) are important risks.

   b. History of three or more blistering sunburns in childhood or adolescence

   c. Skin type: Individuals with green or blue eyes or blonde or red hair are at increased risk.

   d. Personal or family history of melanoma

   e. Large number of moles

   f. Immunosuppression

   g. Precursor lesions of melanoma

      (1) *Lentigo maligna:* also known as "Hutchinson's freckle" or "melanoma in situ," a pigmented macule that arises on the sun-exposed surfaces of elderly patients with actinic damage

      (2) *Congenital melanocytic nevi:* The risk of melanoma is approximately 6 per cent or greater over a lifetime.

      (3) *Dysplastic nevus syndrome*

         (a) Familial: A patient with dysplastic nevi and two or more first-degree relatives with dysplastic nevi and melanoma has a lifetime risk of melanoma that approaches 100 per cent.

         (b) Sporadic: A patient with nonfamilial dysplastic nevi is at increased risk for melanoma, but there is no clear consensus on the magnitude of that risk.

      (4) *Acquired melanocytic nevi:* The risk of melanoma increases with the number of acquired nevi.

Symptoms

1. Changing mole (especially rapid enlargement of the mole or the appearance of raised areas)
2. Bleeding
3. Ulceration or scaling
4. Itching or burning
5. New pigmented lesion

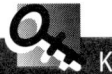

Key Symptoms

- Change in an existing pigmented lesion
- New pigmented lesion

Clinical Findings

The ABCD rules are key warning signs that a lesion may be melanoma:

- A = asymmetry in the shape of a mole
- B = border irregularity (angularity, notching)
- C = color variegation (red, brown, black, white, gray, blue)
- D = diameter greater than 6 mm (the size of a pencil eraser)

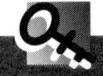

Key Signs

- Asymmetry
- Irregular borders
- Color variegation
- Diameter >6 mm

Laboratory Tests

1. An excisional biopsy (full-thickness) of the lesion is the standard (see Treatment for excision margins).

2. If the lesion is too large for excision, an incisional or punch biopsy is acceptable. If using this approach, it is best to sample from the most deeply pigmented or raised areas of the lesion.

3. Sampling by shaving or curetting may compromise the histology of the lesion and is contraindicated.

Key Tests

- Excisional biopsy is the definitive test.

- Incisional or punch biopsy may be used for very large lesions.

Differential Diagnosis

1. Melanocytic nevus
2. Blue nevus
3. Lentigo simplex
4. Solar lentigo
5. Seborrheic keratosis
6. Pigmented basal cell carcinoma
7. Vascular lesions (Kaposi's sarcoma, hemangioma, pyogenic granuloma)

WARNING

- **Melanoma may be amelanotic.**
- **Clinical findings of asymmetry, irregular borders, color variegation, and diameter do not apply to the nodular melanoma subtype.**

Treatment

Treatment of melanoma is based on stage. *Stage I* melanoma refers to lesions that are confined to the skin, with prognosis related to the Breslow thickness (Table 260–1). *Stage II* melanoma involves nodal metastases and has a 36 per cent 5-year survival. *Stage III* melanoma involves distant metastases and has a 5 per cent 5-year survival (traditional staging system).

1. Early melanoma (in situ melanoma or lesions less than 1 mm thick) may be surgically excised with margins of 0.5 to 1.0 cm without regional lymph node dissection.

2. Thicker lesions should be excised with margins of 3

TABLE 260–1. PROGNOSIS OF STAGE 1 MELANOMA

BRESLOW THICKNESS	FIVE-YEAR SURVIVAL
Less than 0.75 mm	96%
0.76–1.49 mm	87%
1.50–2.49 mm	75%
2.50–3.99 mm	66%
Greater than 4.0 mm	47%

From Koh HK: Cutaneous melanoma. N Engl J Med 1991;325:171–182.

cm; prophylactic lymph node dissection is controversial.

3. *Stage II and III* disease may be treated with surgical excision, lymph node dissection, and adjuvant therapy to prolong disease-free survival. Various adjuvant therapies include chemotherapy, radiotherapy, immunotherapy, and isolated limb perfusion with melphalan and hyperthermia.

Diet

No restrictions

Activity

No restrictions

Patient Education

1. Recognize the importance of cumulative sun exposure and the increased risk associated with blistering sunburns in childhood and adolescence.

2. Avoid strong midday sun.

3. Wear protective clothing and broad-brimmed hats.

4. Liberal use of sunscreens with UVB and UVA protection. The sun protection factor (SPF) of the chosen sunscreen should be appropriate for the intensity of sunlight, the length of exposure, the skin type, and the risk of burning.

5. Perform monthly self skin examinations, and report suspicious lesions to your physician.

Key Treatment

- Recognition of early melanoma (less than 1 mm thick)

- Surgical excision of early melanoma

Follow-Up

1. Patients with a personal history of early melanoma (less than 1 mm thickness) should be followed with skin examinations every 6 months, since their relative risk of a second melanoma is increased five- to eightfold. If there is no evidence of recurrence, skin examinations may then be performed annually.

2. Patients with dysplastic nevi should have skin examinations every 6 to 12 months, with selective excision of suspicious lesions.

3. Patients with small to medium congenital nevi should consider excision of the lesions at puberty.

Bibliography

Austoker J: Melanoma: Prevention and early diagnosis. Br Med J 1994;308:1682–1686.

Early melanoma: NIH Consensus Conference. JAMA 1992; 268:1314–1319.

Evans G, Manson PN: Review and current perspectives of cutaneous malignant melanoma. J Am Coll Surg 1994;178:523–540.

Hoffman S, Yohn J, Robinson W, et al: Melanoma: Clinical characteristics. Hosp Pract 1994;29(6):37–50.

Walton RG: Recognition and importance of precursor lesions in the diagnosis of early cutaneous malignant melanoma. Int J Dermatol 1994;33:302–307.

261 Kaposi's Sarcoma

David M. Amron

Definition

Multicentric cutaneous and extracutaneous vascular tumor characterized by violaceous macules, papules, plaques, and nodules.

Subtypes of Kaposi's Sarcoma (KS)

1. Classic
2. African endemic
3. Iatrogenically immunosuppressed
4. Epidemic: AIDS-related

Epidemiology

A. Classic KS
   1. First described by Kaposi in 1872
   2. Between 0.02 and 0.06 per cent of all malignant tumors in the United States
   3. More common in Jews of Eastern European or Mediterranean descent
   4. Male predominance, peak incidence sixth decade
   5. Chronic course: survival average 10 to 15 years with death usually attributed to other conditions
   6. Increased risk of developing lymphoreticular neoplasms
   7. Specific HLA marker not known

B. African-endemic KS
   1. First noted 1950s in equatorial Africa
   2. Mean age of onset 35 years, with strong male predominance
   3. Usually benign nodular disease but sometimes rapidly progressive and fatal in 5 to 8 years
   4. Fulminant course in children with dissemination to viscera and death in 2 to 3 years

C. Iatrogenically immunosuppressed KS
   1. In organ transplant recipients and others on chronic immunosuppressive therapy
   2. Male predominance
   3. Clinical course usually similar to classic KS, rarely rapidly progressive
   4. Commonly see spontaneous remission once immunosuppressive therapy discontinued

D. Epidemic: AIDS-related KS
   1. Dramatically increased incidence in homosexual/bisexual men and their female partners
   2. Rare in intravenous drug abusers, hemophiliacs, blood transfusion recipients
   3. Implies a sexually transmitted cofactor
   4. Decreasing proportion of HIV-infected patients presenting with AIDS KS

Clinical Manifestations

A. Classic KS
   1. Usually progresses very slowly and runs benign course
   2. Commonly begins as violaceous macule on unilateral distal lower extremity
   3. Papules may coalesce to form large plaques or alternatively become nodules
   4. With advancing disease becomes bilateral and multifocal
   5. Early lesions soft, later ones firm, brownish, and may become hyperkeratotic or ulcerate
   6. Marked edema of surrounding tissues may ensue
   7. May involve mucous membranes, especially gastrointestinal tract

B. African-endemic KS
   1. Four clinicopathologic subtypes
      a. Nodular: benign course resembles classic KS
      b. Aggressive localized cutaneous: nodular variant that may invade subcutaneous tissue or bone
      c. Florid mucocutaneous and visceral disease
      d. Lymphadenopathic: rapidly disseminating to lymph nodes and viscera in children, usually without cutaneous lesions

C. Iatrogenically immunosuppressed KS: clinically like classic KS

D. Epidemic: AIDS-related KS
   1. Five-sixths of patients with CD4+ T-cell counts less than 500 cells/mm³
   2. Commonly multicentric and symmetrical presentation
   3. Extremities usually less severely affected than classic KS
   4. May present as violaceous macules or papules that can progress to large plaques or tumors
   5. Individual lesions may spontaneously involute.
   6. Lesions tend to flare after intercurrent illness.
   7. Predisposed areas: face (especially nose), oral cavity, postauricular area, trunk (follow skin tension lines), penis, legs
   8. Lymphatic involvement common with resultant lymphedema
   9. Between 75 and 80 per cent have some gastrointestinal involvement with possible nausea, bleeding, or perforation but usually asymptomatic
   10. May also involve lungs, bone marrow, heart, urogenital tract, ocular structures, brain

11. Extracutaneous KS accounts for 10 to 20 per cent of deaths in AIDS. However, patients usually die of unrelated causes.

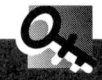

Key Signs

- Violaceous macules, plaques, or nodules on face, oral cavity, trunk, upper and lower extremities

Diagnosis

1. Clinical appearance is suggestive, but diagnosis should be confirmed histologically by skin biopsy (preferably a firm palpable papule or nodule).
2. Lesions are easier to diagnose histologically as they evolve.

Key Test

- Biopsy

Differential Diagnosis

Includes hemangioma, dermatofibroma, bacillary angiomatosis, hemorrhage, postinflammatory hyperpigmentation, melanoma, blue nevus, cutaneous lymphoma, pyogenic granuloma, prurigo nodularis

Histopathology

Three characteristic stages
1. Patch: proliferation of small irregular slits outlined by oval spindle-shaped cells surrounding normal dermal vessels
2. Plaque
   a. Expansion of angulated vascular channels throughout dermis
   b. Usually perivascular mixed inflammatory infiltrate
3. Tumor: sheets and fascicles of spindle cells with trapped erythrocytes in slitlike vascular spaces

Pathogenesis

1. Etiology remains unknown.
2. Possible indirect role of a retrovirus
3. Cell of origin is unclear.

Treatment

May not be indicated unless lesions symptomatic or causing cosmetic disfigurement (especially AIDS-related KS). For AIDS KS, neither systemic nor local therapy has been shown to prolong survival. Therapy for AIDS KS primarily aimed at reducing morbidity.
A. Local therapy
   1. Radiation therapy
      a. Treatment of choice for non-AIDS KS
      b. Best suited for symptoms caused by mass effects such as localized painful lymphadenopathy
      c. About 80 per cent response rate for non-AIDS KS treated with localized or extended-field radiotherapy or total electron beam therapy
      d. Large-volume treatment fields discouraged in AIDS patients because of potential for immunosuppression
   2. Liquid nitrogen cryotherapy: greater than 70 per cent cosmetic improvement probably due to consequence of superficial scarring that camouflages deeper lesion
   3. Surgical excision: acceptable for small lesions
   4. Laser therapy
      a. Pulsed-dye laser: For macular lesions, but tend to recur
      b. Carbon dioxide laser
         (1) For large oral lesions
         (2) Potential exposure to HIV in laser plume
   5. Intralesional therapy
      a. Vinblastine
         (1) 0.1 to 0.2 mg/cm^2 (0.5 ml of a 0.2 mg/ml solution) with a maximum total clinic visit dose of 2.0 mg
         (2) Up to 88 per cent complete or partial response
         (3) Pain for 1 to 2 days most frequent side effect
         (4) Avoid injections next to large peripheral nerves.
      b. Interferon alfa-2b (IFN-α2b)
         (1) Costly and requires frequent treatments
         (2) Currently considered experimental
B. Systemic therapy
   1. Systemic interferon alfa-2b (Intron A)
      a. Higher dosage regimens of IFN-α2b (20 to 50 million U/m^2 body surface for 5 to 7 days/week) gives superior response rates of 20 to 40 per cent.
      b. Gradual dosage increases reduce side effects of fever, chills, and malaise.
      c. Patients with CD4+ counts of more than 400/mm^3 have best response rates. Those with counts less than 200/mm^3 have poorest response rates.
      d. No advantage of IFN-β over IFN-α in terms of response
      e. FDA-approved for AIDS KS but costly
   2. Systemic interferon in combination with zidovudine (AZT) (Retrovir)
      a. Enhanced clinical response rates 30 to 60 per cent for AIDS KS

b. Neutropenia, anemia, thrombocytopenia, hepatotoxicity possible dosage-limiting side effects

c. Granulocyte-macrophage colony-stimulating factor (GM-CSF) increases myelopoiesis in AIDS patients on this regimen.

3. Systemic chemotherapy

a. For patients with rapidly progressive disease (previously used only for classic and African-endemic KS; recent reports of use for AIDS KS)

b. Vinblastine (Velban) and vincristine (Oncovin) accepted as drugs of choice

c. Single-agent regimens have increased cumulative toxicities.

d. Alternate-week administration of vinblastine and vincristine (polychemotherapy) reduces side effects without affecting response rates.

e. Partial or temporary regression common; complete regressions rarely

f. Vinblastine and vincristine have both been used in combination with bleomycin, Adriamycin, actinomycin D, dacarbazine (even with AIDS or immunosuppressed KS).

g. No evidence that systemic chemotherapy increases risk for opportunistic infections in patients treated for AIDS KS

4. Future therapies

a. Directed at developing antiangiogenic drugs (e.g., vitamin D_3 analogues, recombinant human platelet factor 4)

b. Inhibitors of cytokine growth factors

Key Treatment

- May not be indicated unless lesions symptomatic or causing cosmetic disfigurement

- Radiation therapy is treatment of choice for non-AIDS KS.

Bibliography

Armes J: A review of Kaposi's sarcoma. Adv Cancer Res 1989;53:73–87.

Friedman-Kien AE, Saltzman BR: Clinical manifestations of classical, endemic African, and epidemic AIDS-related Kaposi's sarcoma. J Am Acad Dermatol 1990;22(6, pt 2):1237–1250.

Mitsuyasu RT: Clinical aspects of AIDS-related Kaposi's sarcoma. Curr Opin Oncol 1993;5(5):835–844.

Rappersberger K, Wolff K, Stingl G: Kaposi's sarcoma. In Fitzpatrick TB, Eisen AZ, Wolff K et al (eds): Dermatology in General Medicine. New York, McGraw-Hill, 1993, pp 1244–1256.

Tappero JW, Conant MA, Wolfe SF, Berger TG: Kaposi's sarcoma: Epidemiology, pathogenesis, histology, clinical spectrum, staging criteria and therapy. J Am Acad Dermatol 1993;28(3):371–395.

262 Psoriasis

Ellen M. Okun

Etiology

The etiology of psoriasis is unknown. Both environmental and genetic factors are thought to be involved.

1. Environment
   a. Climate has a profound influence on the development and course of psoriasis. Hot weather and sunlight improve symptoms of psoriasis; symptoms tend to worsen in cold weather. The incidence of psoriasis is higher in colder regions of the world.
   b. Stress and anxiety are thought to exacerbate psoriasis.
   c. Trauma to the skin may lead to the development of psoriasis in the affected areas. This is known as the Koebner phenomenon.
   d. Drugs that may exacerbate psoriasis are steroid withdrawal, antimalarials, lithium, β-blockers, and indomethacin.
   e. Infections can cause the onset or flare of psoriasis.
2. Genetics: There often is familial clustering of psoriasis. Many patients with the disease have affected relatives. There is an increased incidence of psoriasis in patients with certain HLA types. The specific mode of inheritance is not known, however.

Symptoms

1. The skin lesions of psoriasis may be pruritic or slightly painful.
2. Psoriatic skin lesions may be of great cosmetic concern to some patients.
3. Thermoregulation, due to increased heat loss via the skin, may be a problem in patients with a large amount of body surface area involved.
4. Patients with psoriatic arthritis may have arthralgias.

Key Symptoms	
• Cosmetic concerns	• Discomfort or pain
• Scaling	• Heat loss
• Pruritus	• Arthralgia

Clinical Findings

1. Epidemiology
   a. Approximately 1 per cent of the population is affected.
   b. Males and females are affected equally.
   c. The onset of psoriasis can occur at any age; most patients develop initial skin lesions in their twenties.

2. Physical examination
   a. Skin involvement is manifested by erythema, silvery micaceous scales, and thickening. These plaques have well-demarcated borders and a symmetrical distribution. There is a wide range in the amount of skin involvement from patient to patient. The removal of scale from psoriasis will cause small areas of bleeding; this is known as the Auspitz sign and is fairly specific for psoriasis.
   b. Nail involvement is seen commonly in patients with psoriasis. There is pitting of the nail plate, onychodystrophy with onycholysis (separation of the nail plate from the nail bed), hyperkeratosis under the nail, and light brown discoloration of the nail (oil spots).
   c. Joint involvement in psoriasis generally occurs after skin involvement but may precede it. There is often involvement of the distal interphalangeal joints. Most patients have an asymmetrical oligoarticular arthritis, sometimes with tendon involvement. Sacroiliitis and spondylitis commonly are associated with the psoriasis. Arthritis mutilans is a very destructive arthritis of the fingers that can occur.

3. Types of psoriasis
   a. Psoriasis vulgaris is the most commonly seen form. It involves predominately extensor surfaces (knees and elbows), lower back, and scalp. The plaques are generally persistent.
   b. Guttate psoriasis appears as multiple small drop-like lesions on the trunk and extremities. Its onset is often preceded by streptococcal pharyngitis.
   c. Pustular psoriasis can be of two forms: It can involve the palms and soles, or it can be generalized (Von Zumbusch).
   d. Psoriatic erythroderma is generalized involvement of the entire body. These patients are very ill.
   e. Human immunodeficiency virus (HIV) infection sometimes precipitates new-onset psoriasis or flares of pre-existing psoriasis.

Key Signs	
• Plaques with well-differentiated borders	• Nail pitting
	• Onycholysis
• Micaceous scale	• Oil spots
• Erythema	• Arthritis
• Auspitz sign	

Laboratory Tests

1. Laboratory tests are generally not used in diagnosing psoriasis. There are some laboratory findings that are often seen in patients with psoriasis: elevated uric acid, anemia, hypoalbuminemia, and elevated erythrocyte sedimentation rate. Psoriatic arthritis is seronegative.
2. Skin biopsy shows thickened stratum corneum, hyperplasia of the epidermis, and little inflammation.

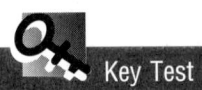

Key Test

- Skin biopsy is diagnostic but not generally necessary.

Differential Diagnosis

Usually the diagnosis is easy to make on clinical grounds. Other diagnoses that may be considered are eczema, tinea, candidiasis, drug eruptions, syphilis, seborrhea, Paget's disease, Bowen's disease, mycosis fungoides, and lichen planus.

Treatment

Medication

1. Topical therapy is the most common form of treatment and is adequate for most patients.
   a. Glucocorticoids are the first-line therapy; these may be used under occlusive dressings to increase their potency. Less potent steroids should be used before the more potent ones. Examples of topical steroids in order of increasing frequency are: hydrocortisone 2.5% cream, lotion, or ointment, triamcinolone acetonide 0.1% cream, lotion, or ointment, and fluocinonide 0.05% cream or ointment. Generally, the ointment is more potent than the cream. The lotion is more convenient for use on the scalp.
   b. Tar, which comes in many different forms, also can be used topically; it is often combined with salicylic acid. Over-the-counter tar-based shampoos may be used.
   c. Anthralin is another topical preparation. It can be used a Drithocreme (0.1%, 0.25%, 0.5%, and 1.0%) and as Dritho-Scalp (0.25% and 0.5%). These can be applied once daily to the skin or scalp respectively and then washed off within an hour. Anthralin can stain the skin.

WARNING

High-potency steroids should not be used on the face or genitals because they cause skin atrophy.

---

2. Phototherapy
   a. Sunbathing will often lead to an improvement in psoriasis.
   b. Ultraviolet B light is often used in conjunction with tar or anthralin.
   c. PUVA therapy (oral psoralen and ultraviolet A light) is useful in refractory disease. Psoralen is a photosensitizing agent.

WARNING

There is an increased incidence of dermatologic malignancy from PUVA.

---

3. Systemic therapy: The agents used in systemic therapy of psoriasis must be used with great care because of their many side effects and contraindications. They are generally used in severe cases after failure of other forms of therapy.
   a. Methotrexate can be used in the treatment of psoriasis and psoriatic arthritis.
   b. Etretinate (Tegison), is a vitamin A analogue. It may be used in conjunction with PUVA.

WARNING

Etretinate is teratogenic and must not be used in pregnant women.

---

   c. Cyclosporine (Sandimmune), and hydroxyurea (Hydrea) also have been used to treat psoriasis.
   d. Zidovudine (AZT [Retrovir]) is useful in clearing lesions in patients with HIV-associated psoriasis.

Diet
There are no dietary restrictions.

Activity
There are no restrictions of activity.

Patient Education
Patients should be aware of factors that can exacerbate psoriasis. They should be instructed not to pick their skin lesions, because this can lead to koebnerization (psoriasis at the site of skin trauma). They also should be aware that their disease has relapses and remissions.

Key Treatment

Drugs of Choice	Alternative Drugs
• Topical glucocorticoids	• Methotrexate
• Phototherapy	• Etretinate
• Coal tar	• Cyclosporine
• Anthralin	• Hydroxyurea

Follow-Up

Follow-up depends on the severity of disease.

 Bibliography

Fitzpatrick TB, Eisen AZ, Wolff K, Freedberg IM, Austen KF, eds: Dermatology in General Medicine, 4th ed, vol. 1. New York, McGraw-Hill, 1993, pp 489–514.

Kelly WN, Harris ED, Ruddy S, Sledge CB, eds: Textbook of Rheumatology, 4th ed, vol 1. Philadelphia, WB Saunders, 1993, pp 974–984.

Menter A, Barker JNWN: Psoriasis in practice. Lancet 1991;338:231–234.

Rubenstein E, Federman DD, eds: Scientific American Medicine, sec 2III. New York, Scientific American Inc., 1994.

Saver GC: Manual of Skin Diseases, 6th ed. Philadelphia, JB Lippincott, 1991, pp 133–139.

263 Pityriasis Rosea

Stephen D. Saglio

Etiology

1. Unknown
   a. Most likely caused by an infectious agent
      (1) Discrete clinical course
      (2) Apparent lifelong immunity after illness
   b. Relatively noncontagious, uncommon case clusters
2. Moderately common
   a. Worldwide distribution
   b. All races affected
   c. Typical spring and autumn peaks in temperate zones
   d. Females affected slightly more than males
   e. Patients usually 10 to 43 years old
3. An increased incidence described with
   a. Atopy
   b. Seborrheic dermatitis
   c. Acne vulgaris
   d. Dandruff
4. Medications reported to cause rashes resembling pityriasis rosea (PR)
   a. Bismuth
   b. Barbiturates
   c. Captopril
   d. D-Penicillamine
   e. Gold
   f. Isotretinoin
   g. Metronidazole
   h. Sulfas

Symptoms

1. Occasionally a mild prodromal syndrome
   a. Malaise
   b. Nausea
   c. Decreased appetite
   d. Fever
   e. Arthralgias
   f. Fatigue
   g. Headache
   h. Sore throat
2. The pruritus of the rash
   a. None (25 per cent of cases)
   b. Mild (50 per cent of cases)
   c. Severe (25 per cent of cases)

Key Symptoms

- Occasional mild "viral syndrome" type prodrome
- Mild pruritus

Clinical Findings

1. A self-limited illness
2. The classic disease progression (80 per cent of cases) is pathognomonic
3. Primary lesion (or "herald patch")
   a. Large, typically 2 to 6 cm in diameter
   b. Located on the torso
   c. Precedes the general rash by 2 to 21 days
4. Secondary lesions
   a. Miniatures of the primary lesion
   b. Appear in crops
   c. 0.5 to 1.5 cm in diameter
   d. Papulosquamous
   e. Erythematous
   f. Oval with central clearing
   g. The border is darker, thin, and scaly.
5. Lesions may continue to appear for 2 to 3 weeks.
6. Complete resolution of the rash by 6 to 8 weeks (may take up to 14 weeks)
7. The distribution of PR is mainly on the torso
   a. Classic "Christmas tree" pattern
   b. May also affect the proximal extremities
8. Recurrences occur in no more than 3 per cent of cases.
9. Involvement of internal organs is never seen.

Key Signs

- "Herald patch"
- "Christmas tree" pattern
- Papulosquamous
- Erythematous
- Central clearing
- Secondary rash in 2 to 21 days
- Truncal distribution
- Oval
- Discrete
- Thin, scaly border

Laboratory Tests

1. None are of diagnostic importance.
2. A syphilis test should be obtained.
3. On biopsy, the pathology is nonspecific.

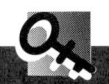

Key Test

• Syphilis serology recommended

Differential Diagnosis

1. Tinea versicolor
   a. The lesions are more brown.
   b. The borders are not as ovoid.
   c. KOH testing is usually positive for hyphae.
2. Drug eruptions
   a. Usually no "herald patch"
   b. History of exposure to suspicious medications
   c. Very resistant to therapy
   d. Protracted course and larger lesions
3. Secondary syphilis
   a. Not pruritic
   b. Often a history of prior genital lesions
   c. Positive serology
   d. More common on palms and soles
4. Psoriasis
   a. Found predominantly on the extremities and scalp
   b. Rash has a whitish, thicker scale.
   c. A more chronic course
5. Seborrheic dermatitis
   a. A chronic clinical course
   b. Irregular, greasy scales
   c. On the sternum and other hairy areas
   d. No "herald patch"
6. Lichen planus
   a. More papular and violaceous
   b. Involving mucosa of the mouth and lips
7. Kaposi's sarcoma
   a. Oval, violaceous plaques
   b. May have a "Christmas tree" pattern
   c. No scaling
8. Nummular eczema
   a. Usually not confined to the trunk
   b. Round lesions
   c. More chronic than PR

Treatment

1. Keep as mild as possible to prevent complications. Avoid soap, wool, and sweating; minimize irritation.

2. Sunlight and ultraviolet (UV) therapy modestly helpful

Medications

1. Used mainly to control pruritus
   a. Oatmeal collodial bath, every day or every other day
   b. Calamine lotion
   c. Oral antihistamines
   d. Topical steroids in a hydrophilic cream base
2. Systemic steroids for severe pruritus
   a. Prednisone, 20 to 40 mg daily, taper over 1 to 2 weeks
   b. Triamcinolone acetonide, 40 mg intramuscularly

Patient Education

Very important to reassure patient that
1. PR is essentially noncontagious.
2. No other organs are involved.
3. The rash should resolve completely.
4. Recurrences are rare (3 per cent of cases).

Key Treatment

Primary	Alternative
• Exposure to sunlight	• UV therapy
• Oatmeal collodial baths	• Prednisone, 20 to 40 mg, taper over 1 to 2 weeks
• Calamine lotion	
• Oral antihistamines	• Triamcinolone acetonide, 40 mg intramuscularly
• Topical steroids in hydrophillic base	

Bibliography

Bjornberg A: Pityriasis rosea. *In* Fitzpatrick TB, Eisen AZ, Wolff K, Freeberg IM, Austen KF (eds): Dermatology in General Medicine, 4th ed. New York, McGraw-Hill, 1993, pp 1117–1123.

Fitzpatrick TB, Johnson RA, Polano MK, et al: Pityriasis rosea, in Color Atlas and Synopsis of Clinical Dermatology: Common and Serious Diseases, 2d ed. New York, McGraw-Hill, 1992, pp 58–61.

Gibson LE, Perry HO: Papulosquamous eruptions and exfoliative dermatitis. *In* Moschella SL, Hurley HJ (eds): Dermatology, 3d ed. Philadelphia, WB Saunders, 1992, pp 622–625.

Sauer GC: Manual of Skin Diseases, 6th ed. Philadelphia, JB Lippincott, 1991, pp 139–143.

Vidimos AT, Camisa C: Tongue and cheek: Oral lesions in pityriasis rosea. Cutis 1992;50:276–280.

264 Vitiligo

Marc A. Darr

Etiology and Epidemiology

1. Etiology is uncertain. Vitiligo is thought to be autoimmune in nature, because it is often seen in conjunction with other autoimmune disorders (thyroid disease, diabetes mellitus, Addison's disease, and pernicious anemia).
2. Affects both sexes equally but more noticeable in dark-skinned persons
3. Incidence is approximately 1 per cent.
4. Vitiligo is an acquired condition; congenital cases are extremely rare. Incidence peaks between 10 and 30 years.
5. Approximately 30 per cent of patients have a family member with the disease. Exact inheritance pattern is unclear.

Symptoms

1. White spots on skin
2. Patient may have a history of premature graying of hair.
3. Patient may have a history of alopecia.

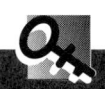

Key Symptom

- White spots on skin

Clinical Findings

1. Hypopigmented macule(s) ranging from 1 mm to several centimeters in diameter
   a. Usually white, but may be off-white or tan in color
   b. Tend to be circular or oval-shaped
   c. Accentuated by viewing with Wood's lamp, especially in light-skinned patients
   d. Often have scalloped edges
   e. May be focal, segmental, or generalized
   f. Generalized vitiligo usually occurs in a very symmetrical pattern.
   g. Common sites include extensor surfaces (knees, elbows, back of hands), body folds (axilla, genitalia), and skin around body orifices (mouth, eyes, nostrils, nipples, umbilicus).
   h. Macules also occur frequently at sites of skin trauma (elbows, collar, waistband) and previously sunburned areas. This is known as the "Koebner phenomenon."
2. Other skin findings may include
   a. Leukotrichia
   b. Halo nevi
   c. Alopecia areata
3. Iritis is seen in 10 per cent of patients with vitiligo.
4. Patients may have associated signs of hyperthyroidism, diabetes, pernicious anemia, or Addison's disease.

Key Signs

- White, oval-shaped macules
- Symmetrical pattern
- Lack of other skin changes
- Lesions accentuated by Wood's lamp
- Koebner phenomenon

Laboratory Tests

1. Diagnosis is usually made by history and physical examination. Laboratory tests are rarely necessary.
2. If performed, skin biopsy reveals normal skin, except for an absence of melanocytes.
3. Once diagnosis of vitiligo is established, the clinician should consider screening for vitiligo-associated conditions:
   a. T_4 and thyroid-stimulating hormone (TSH) for thyroid disease
   b. Complete blood count (CBC) for pernicious anemia
   c. Fasting blood sugar for diabetes
   d. Na^+, K^+, and/or cortisol level for Addison's disease

Differential Diagnosis

1. Tinea versicolor
2. Tuberous sclerosis
3. Pityriasis alba
4. Postinflammatory hypopigmentation
5. Leprosy
6. Lupus erythematosus
7. Chemical leukoderma
8. Nevus anemicus

Treatment

1. The patient's need/desire for treatment must be determined.

952

a. Vitiligo is primarily of cosmetic and social concern. The significance of vitiligo is much greater in darker-skinned individuals. In some cultures, the social stigmata attached to vitiligo can be devastating.

b. Vitiligo tends to be stable initially and then slowly progresses over several years.

c. Untreated vitiligo lesions usually remain for life, but some individuals develop spontaneous repigmentation.

Treatment Options

a. Education and reassurance often are all that is necessary in mild cases.

b. Sunscreens (SPF >30) should be used by all patients with vitiligo. Sunscreen will diminish tanning; tanning makes hypopigmented areas more noticeable. Sunscreen also decreases the risk of koebnerization and actinic damage.

c. Cosmetics: Makeups, skin dyes, and instant-tanning preparations may provide good results.

d. Repigmentation

(1) Topical steroids for isolated lesions

(2) Topical or oral PUVA photochemotherapy for more extensive disease

e. Depigmentation: useful for patients with extensive disease. This procedure involves "bleaching" the remaining normal skin with monobenzylether of hydroquinone (monobenzone [Benoquin]). This provides a permanent, uniform, and usually highly satisfactory result. Patients will, however, be at increased risk of sunburn after this procedure.

Medication

1. Topical steroids as noted above. Use hydrocortisone (1% or 2.5%) on the face and skin folds, more potent steroids elsewhere. Interrupted schedule should be used if steroids are given for more than 6 to 8 weeks. Follow closely for evidence of steroid atrophy.

2. Topical psoralen (methoxsalen [Oxsoralen]) for isolated macules. Topical psoralen is highly phototoxic. Patients must avoid sunlight for 3 days after treatment.

3. Oral psoralen is effective treatment for widespread vitiligo.

WARNING

Oral psoralens should not be used in children under age 12.

---

4. Monobenzone as above for depigmentation.

Diet

No special dietary measures.

Activity

Full

Patient Education

1. Benign nature of disease should be explained.

2. Patient should be instructed to use high-SPF sunscreens.

3. Avoid sun exposure at midday.

4. Risks and benefits of repigmentation and depigmentation should be explained to patients considering these therapies.

Key Treatment

- Drug of choice depends on severity of disease.
- Reassurance
- Sunscreen
- Cosmetics
- Repigmentation with steroids, psoralen plus ultraviolet A radiation (PUVA)
- Depigmentation with monobenzone

Follow-Up

1. Follow-up varies depending on the treatment plan.

2. Most patients with mild disease will require only periodic skin examinations as part of their overall health care maintenance.

3. Patients on repigmentation/depigmentation regimens will require multiple visits over several months to years.

4. All patients should have an eye examination by an ophthalmologist.

 ## Bibliography

Arnold HL, Odom RB, James WD: Andrew's Diseases of the Skin: Clinical Dermatology, 8th ed. Philadelphia, WB Saunders, 1990, pp 1000–1003.

Bernstein JE: Pigmentary disorders of the skin. In Rakel RE (ed): Conn's Current Therapy. Philadelphia, WB Saunders, 1994, pp 821–822.

Fitzpatrick TB, et al: Color Atlas and Synopsis of Clinical Dermatology: Common and Serious Diseases, 2d ed. New York, McGraw-Hill, 1992, pp 630–635.

Habif TP: Clinical Dermatology: A Color Guide to Diagnosis and Therapy. St Louis, CV Mosby, 1985, pp 395–397.

Mosher DB, et al: Disorders of pigmentation. In Fitzpatrick TB et al (eds): Dermatology in General Medicine, 4th ed, vol 1. New York, McGraw-Hill, 1993, pp 923–933.

265 Herpes Simplex Infection

Arthur R. Slaughter

Etiology

1. Herpes simplex virus types 1 and 2 (HSV-1 and HSV-2) are herpes DNA viruses that cause either recognized or unrecognized primary infection most often as herpes labialis or gingivostomatitis (HSV-1) or genital herpes (HSV-2); each type can infect any site; digital and eye herpetic infections usually are caused by HSV-1.

2. Thereafter, either type may reactivate off and on throughout life to cause annoying and infectious skin disease.

3. HSV-1 does confer some partial immunity to HSV-2.

4. Disseminated simplex and simplex encephalitis may occur.

Symptoms

1. Primary infection begins with lesions 2 to 21 days after topical inoculation.

2. In addition to oral area sores and sore throat, herpes labialis often begins with fever, headache, myalgia, and cervical lymphadenopathy.

3. Primary genital herpes may present as painful urination, burning vulvar, scrotal, or penile pain, local swelling, erythema, fatigue, backache, or joint, abdominal, or suprapubic pain.

4. Reactivation of labial lesions may come at times of stress or excess sun exposure as extended painful lips for several days, with single or multiple lesions, often limited to an area involving the mucocutaneous borders of the lips.

5. Reactivation of genital herpes may be preceded by hours or days with genital pain, paresthesia, or numbness; the lesions tend to be unilateral; the degree of discomfort varies but is less than with primary infection.

6. Herpetic whitlow (HSV on finger), herpetic keratoconjunctivitis, and a poxlike eruption in atopic dermatitis (one cause of Kaposi's varicelliform eruption) are other ways primary or reactivated HSV may appear.

Key Symptoms

- Local discomfort
- Grouped lesions

Clinical Findings

1. In HSV-1, clusters of small, clear vesicles on the lips, face, buccal mucosa, soft palate, floor of the mouth,

and throat; within 1 to 3 days the vesicles break and leave painful ulcers that take 4 to 14 days to crust.

2. In HSV-2, typical grouped vesicles, pustules, and painful erosions or ulcers may then appear, sometimes with a vaginal discharge.

Key Signs

- Clustered vesicles
- Painful erosions or ulcers
- Local swelling
- Regional lymphadenopathy

Laboratory Tests

1. Tzanck smear (scrape base of a lesion, smear on a slide, and stain with Wright's or Giemsa's) can be done in the office; shows multinucleated giant cells often with inclusion bodies; does not distinguish between varicella-zoster (VZV) and herpes simplex virus (HSV).

2. Viral culture taken by Dacron swab from scraped base of lesion into special media takes 2 to 14 days for results.

3. Antibody testing of sera is positive if fourfold or greater rise between acute and convalescent (at 2 weeks) samples.

Key Tests

- Tzanck smear
- HSV culture
- Antibody testing

Differential Diagnosis

1. Impetigo
2. Aphthous stomatitis
3. Herpangina
4. Syphilitic chancre
5. Stephens-Johnson syndrome
6. Varicella, coxsackievirus, or HSV may cause Kaposi's varicelliform eruption.

Treatment

1. May use topical Campho-Phenique for recurrent herpes labialis for local relief

2. Occasionally children with severe gingivostomatitis may require intravenous hydration.

954

3. If patient is unable to void because of periurethral involvement, suggest sitting in warm bath or pouring cup of warm water over genitals to urinate.

4. Topical cool compresses with Burow's solution for 15 minutes four to five times daily may be soothing.

5. Women with a history of genital herpes or who have a sex partner with genital herpes should have HSV cultures obtained at delivery to aid in decisions for the newborn. Women with active genital lesions at the time of labor should have cesarean section; the neonate should be cultured and treated with intravenous acyclovir if cultures are positive or clinical disease develops.

Medication

1. Drug of choice: Acyclovir (Zovirax) is indicated orally for primary or recurrent genital herpes and intravenously for severe initial genital herpes, HSV encephalitis, and HSV in immunocompromised patients and neonates.

   a. Acyclovir for initial genital HSV: 200 mg orally every 4 hours five times daily for 5 days

   b. Acyclovir for recurrent genital HSV

      (1) Continuous suppressive: 400 mg orally twice daily (or 200 mg orally three to five times daily) for 1 year and re-evaluate need for continuation

      (2) Episodic: 200 mg orally every 4 hours five times daily for 5 days taken early during recurrences

   c. Acyclovir for severe initial genital HSV in normal host or any HSV in immunocompromised: 5 mg/kg (250 mg/m^2 for age <12 years) intravenously over 1 hour every 8 hours for 5 days.

   d. Acyclovir for HSV encephalitis, neonatal HSV, or disseminated HSV: 10 mg/kg (500 mg/m^2 for age <12 years) intravenously over 1 hour every 8 hours for 10 days.

   e. Patients require adequate hydration during intravenous acyclovir administration and dosage adjustment for renal insufficiency.

   f. Acyclovir is not indicated for primary or recurrent herpes labialis, although its use is reported.

   g. Because of unproven safety, acyclovir's systemic use in pregnancy is reserved for intravenous treatment of severe or complicated HSV; the manufacturer and Centers for Disease Control and Prevention maintain a registry (1-800-722-9292, ext. 58465) that should be notified in these cases.

2. Alternative drugs

   a. Vidarabine (Vira-A) may be used for HSV encephalitis (15 mg/kg/day for 10 days), neonatal infections (30 mg/kg/day for 10 days), and keratitis (3% ointment five times daily for 7 to 21 days), but its greater toxicity and lesser efficacy lend preference to acyclovir except for topical ophthalmic use.

   b. Foscarnet (Foscavir), 40 mg/kg intravenously every 8 hours, has been more helpful and less toxic than vidarabine in immunocompromised patients who develop episodic acyclovir resistance.

Diet

1. Normal diet usually

2. Nonacid solids or liquids for HSV gingivostomatitis

Patient Education

1. Avoid kissing or sexual intercourse until lesions are crusted.

2. Encourage use of condoms for all sexual intercourse that is not mutually monogamous, whether or not lesions are present.

3. Avoid contact with immunocompromised persons or neonates while lesions are active (not crusted).

4. Wash hands often both to prevent spread to others and to prevent autoinoculation of other sites.

5. Inform of widespread prevalence of HSV (>90 per cent of population) to put problem into perspective for the patient.

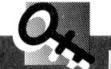

Key Treatment

- Topical compresses

Follow-Up

1. Have patient return if complications are suspected (such as pneumonia) or if disease severity warrants more aggressive intervention.

2. For patients with significant recurrences of genital HSV on chronic acyclovir suppression, monitor at least annually; try drug-free intervals and/or reduce the dose to least that remains effective in reducing recurrences.

Bibliography

Arbesfeld DM, Thomas I: Cutaneous herpes simplex infections. Am Fam Physician 1991;43:1655–1664.

Centers for Disease Control and Prevention: 1993 sexually transmitted diseases treatment guidelines. MMWR 1993;42:1–102.

Dwyer DE, Cunningham AL: Herpes simplex virus infection in pregnancy. Ballieres Clin Obstet Gynecol 1993;7:75–105.

Glickman FS: Herpes simplex virus infection. Fam Pract Recertif 1993;15:21–32.

Vestry JP, Norval M: Mucocutaneous infections with herpes simplex virus and their management. Clin Exp Dermatol 1992;17:221–237.

266 Herpes Zoster Infection

Arthur R. Slaughter

Etiology

Varicella-zoster virus (VZV), a herpes DNA virus, causes a primary infection (*varicella,* or chickenpox), most often during childhood; after dormancy for months to years in the sensory ganglia, VZV then may cause *herpes zoster* (shingles) when reduction in cellular immunity allows the latent virus to spread along a dermatome, usually in adulthood.

Symptoms

1. Herpes zoster often has prodrome of burning, itching sensations in skin or boring or sharp pains lasting hours to days before rash occurs.

2. Lesions appear along a specific dermatome, unilaterally.

3. These begin as red papules that become clustered vesicles, often with malaise, fatigue, or low-grade fever.

4. Vesicles become pustular or hemorrhagic by days 3 to 4.

5. Dry crusting occurs by 7 to 10 days and resolves by days 14 to 21, often leaving scars of varying pigmentation.

6. Pain usually resolves with the rash, but in about 15 per cent an irritating postherpetic neuralgia may persist for over 1 month after the rash, especially in persons over age 40 (in 50 per cent over age 60).

7. Herpetic neuralgia may occur without clinical evidence (zoster sine herpete).

8. Motor neuralgias occasionally occur with paralysis or paresis of the involved areas; these usually resolve within one year with minimal residua.

9. Immunocompromised persons may have lesions more diffusely and more severely.

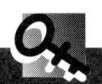

Key Symptoms

- Painful prodrome
- Dermatome, unilateral
- Afebrile or low-grade fever

Clinical Findings

1. Zoster may present initially with no signs, with dysesthesia within a dermatome unilaterally, or with typical lesions.

2. Lesions start as small papules and then become vesicles, often in groups, all within a dermatome on one side.

3. Occasionally, one to three lesions may cross the midline or appear in remote sites.

4. By 3 to 4 days lesions are pustular or hemorrhagic; dry crusts form by 7 to 10 days and resolve by 2 to 3 weeks, often with scars of varying pigmentation.

5. Zoster ophthalmicus, involving the first division of the trigeminal nerve, requires ophthalmologic evaluation and therapy to optimally treat potential ocular involvement (in 50 per cent), especially if the nasociliary branch is involved (in 33 per cent), with lesions visible on the tip of the nose.

Key Signs

- Papules, vesicles, pustules
- Clear or cloudy appearance
- Umbilication, excoriation, crusting
- Dermatome, unilateral
- Afebrile or low-grade fever

Laboratory Tests

1. Tzanck's smear from scraping of base of vesicle takes minutes and is positive in 75 per cent; a positive Tzanck's smear shows multinucleated giant cells but does not differentiate between varicella-zoster (VZV) and herpes simplex virus (HSV).

2. Viral culture from scraped base of lesion may require up to 2 weeks and is positive in 44 per cent.

3. Polymerase chain reaction technique, when clinically available, can be final in 24 hours and positive in 97 per cent; may be done on unstained slide made for Tzanck's smear.

4. Antibody testing, although useful for establishing cause, usually takes too long for clinical impact on contemporaneous diagnosis and treatment.

Key Tests

- Tzanck's smear
- Viral culture
- Antibody testing

Differential Diagnosis

1. Kaposi's varicelliform eruption
2. Dermatitis herpetiformis
3. Herpes gestationis (in pregnant patients)
4. Insect bites

Treatment

1. Soothing baths with baking soda added to water or topical compresses with Burow's solution applied 15 minutes four times daily may give symptomatic relief.

2. Nonnarcotic analgesics such as acetaminophen may reduce pain of zoster.

3. For postzoster neuralgia, capsaicin cream (0.025%) applied three to five times daily may begin to decrease pain after 14 days.

4. Low-dose amitriptyline, begun at 10 to 25 mg daily, may reduce postzoster discomfort.

Medication

1. Drug of choice

   a. *Acyclovir* (Zovirax), given orally within 48 hours of onset of zoster in the usual host (800 mg orally every 4 hours five times daily for 7 to 10 days), may attenuate the duration and severity of zoster and also may decrease the occurrence and duration of postherpetic neuralgia.

   b. *Intravenous acyclovir* is indicated for patients with zoster who are severely immunocompromised. Therapy at doses of 10 mg/kg every 8 hours (500 mg/m² every 8 hours in children) for 7 to 10 days, started within 48 hours of onset; acyclovir can reduce the likelihood of deterioration, time to full healing, and time to end of new lesion formation.

2. Alternative drugs

   a. Famciclovir (Famvir) was recently released for oral treatment of zoster (at 500 mg three times daily for 7 days). Compared with acyclovir, famciclovir has longer duration and stronger concentration of active drug in cells, but these agents were equivalent in accelerating cutaneous healing, loss of acute pain, safety, and efficacy in one study.

   b. Foscarnet (Foscavir) may be considered for immunocompromised persons who do not respond to acyclovir.

   c. Vidarabine (Vira-A) occasionally is used (at 15 mg/kg/day over 12 hours intravenously for 7 days) in immunocompromised patients, but it is less efficacious and more toxic than acyclovir.

   d. Leukocyte interferon may decrease severity and number of days of new lesions but also can decrease granulocyte counts and cause fever and neurasthenia.

   e. Varicella vaccine administration recommendations may be forthcoming. The vaccine does bolster cell-mediated immunity in geriatric populations, but side effects include rash and zoster. Uncertainties are the unknown duration of immunity and booster dose requirements, whether more serious primary varicella may occur as an adult, and whether zoster may be prevented many years later.

Diet

No restrictions

Activity

1. Strict isolation is indicated for cases occurring in a hospital.

2. Health care workers who have no immunity and who have been exposed to an active case of varicella or active herpes-zoster lesions should stay away from immunocompromised patients from days 10 to 21 after exposure (days 10 to 28 if varicella immune globulin is given).

Patient Education

Warn patients to avoid exposure to all immunocompromised individuals and pregnant women who are not immune to varicella-zoster virus.

Key Treatment

- Baths or compresses
- Antipruritics
- Avoid aspirin
- Analgesics: acetaminophen
- Acute medications: acyclovir, famciclovir
- Postzoster neuraliga: capsaicin, amitriptyline

Follow-Up

Follow zoster patients until pain has resolved; on rare occasions of motor impairment, follow until improved significantly (usually by 1 year).

Bibliography

Carmichael JK: Treatment of herpes zoster and postherpetic neuralgia. Am Fam Physician 1991;44:203–210.

Gnann JW: New antivirals with activity against varicella-zoster virus. Ann Neurol 1994;34:S69–S72.

Liesegang TJ: Diagnosis and therapy of herpes zoster ophthalmicus. Ophthalmology 1991;98:1216–1229.

Ljungman P: Herpes virus infections in immunocompromised patients: Problems and therapeutic interventions. Ann Med 1993;25:329–333.

Nahass GT, Goldstein BA, Zhu WY, et al: Comparison of Tzanck smear, viral culture, and DNA diagnostic methods in detection of herpes simplex and varicella-zoster infection. JAMA 1992;268:2541–2544.

267 Warts and Nevi

Virginia E. Robertson

Warts and nevi are generally benign skin lesions; however, certain subclasses of each are associated with premalignant conditions.

Warts

Etiology

1. All *verruca vulgaris* (warts) are caused by human papilloma viruses (HPV).
2. Over 60 different types of HPV are known. Different types will be associated with different clinical manifestations, but there is overlap.
3. Some HPV types are found to have oncogenic potential.
   a. *Cervical intraepithelial neoplasia* (CIN) is associated especially with HPV types 16 and 18, as well as types 31, 33, and 35.
   b. Benign HPV lesions may become associated with neoplasia in immunosuppressed hosts.
4. *Epidermodysplasia verruciformis* is a rare inherited disease that yields numerous HPV papules and macules.
   a. Degeneration into malignant lesions is common.
   b. It is believed to be autosomal recessive.

Symptoms

1. The cosmetic effect may be of most concern to the patient, depending on the size and location of the wart.
2. The patient will note a painless papule or a cluster of papules, generally asymptomatic, that are skin-toned.
3. *Plantar warts* may be painful or present as a foreign-body sensation in ambulatory patients.
4. Hoarseness may be prominent in patients with laryngeal warts.

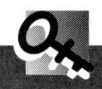

Key Symptom

- Papular skin lesion

Clinical Findings

1. *Common warts* appear most often on the distal extremities and the face.
   a. Variably sized from 1 or 2 mm to 1 cm
   b. Firm, solid, nontender lesion
   c. Dome-shaped, sessile papule or nodule
   d. Hyperkeratotic, corrugated surface
   e. Skin-colored, with black punctae evident on close inspection, representing capillary loops

f. Singular or clustered with satellite lesions from local spread. Clusters may become dense and matted.
2. *Flat warts* or *verruca plana* also may appear on the extremities and face, notably the eyelids but may be less noticeable.
   a. Slightly raised, sessile lesions
   b. Smooth, flat-topped
   c. Skin-colored or slightly darker
3. *Plantar warts* occur on the sole of the foot, most often at high pressure points such as the heel or metatarsal heads.
   a. Endophytic papule, partially or fully inverted (in nonmobile patients, may be more exophytic)
   b. Covered by thick callus
   c. Black punctae evident on close inspection (capillary loops) or after callus removed
   d. Tender with pressure
4. *Anogenital warts* or *condyloma acuminata* appear on the anogenital mucosal surfaces in women and men.
   a. A sexually transmitted disease
   b. Can resemble common warts in appearance or soft, pedunculated, moist lesions
   c. Single or clustered
   d. Skin-colored or hyperkeratotic (leukoplakia)
   e. On cervical epithelium, HPV can induce subclinical changes that may be noted only on Pap smear, colposcopy, or biopsy.
5. *Laryngeal warts* are most often found in infants and children and may cause obstruction, necessitating emergent care.
   a. Hoarseness, stridor, and signs of respiratory distress

Key Signs

- Skin-colored papules
- Hyperkeratosis
- Black punctae

Laboratory Tests

1. Diagnosis can usually be based on clinical findings.
2. Consider biopsy of suspect skin or mucosal lesions, including those resistant to therapy.
3. Pap smears often document HPV-associated histology of the cervix.
4. Colposcopy with biopsy may be indicated when there

are cervical squamous cell changes (atypia, intraepithelial lesions).

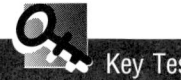

Key Test

- None or skin biopsy

Differential Diagnosis

1. Simple plantar corns may be mistaken for plantar warts. Corns do not have black punctae and have a central translucency when the lesion is pared away.
2. Skin tags or seborrheic keratoses
3. Epidermal nevi and nevus sebaceus
4. Occasionally, premalignant and malignant lesions, including actinic keratoses and squamous cell carcinoma, may be mistaken for warts.

Treatment

A wide range of treatment options exists, all with side effects and none with a guaranteed cure. Treatment choice(s) depend on the type, location, size, responsiveness, cosmetic effect, and premalignant potential of the lesion and the side effects of the treatment.

1. *Watch and wait* may be acceptable for small common or flat warts, as a certain percentage of these will disappear without intervention over time.
2. *Chemical destruction* can be done in home or office:
   a. Pre-soak lesion in warm water for 5 minutes.
   b. Rub away loose wart with an emery board, pumice stone, or scalpel.
   c. Avoiding normal skin, apply agent to wart and cover with plaster or tape to improve penetrance.
   d. Repeat daily or b.i.d. for 2 to 3 months until response is adequate.
   e. Agents and side effects include
      (1) Topical salicyclic acid 15 to 40 per cent; local irritation may be relieved by temporary cessation of therapy.
      (2) Topical formalin, especially for plantar warts; drying and fissuring of skin with occasional allergic reaction
      (3) Weekly office application of caustic agents such as trichloroacetic acid 50 per cent, washed off after 2 hours; occasional scarring of surrounding tissue
3. *Cryotherapy* by the clinician with liquid nitrogen or CO_2 can be used for any type of wart.
   a. Soak the lesion, then scrape excess keratin with scalpel blade.
   b. Using a cotton-tipped swab or spray attachment, apply agent directly and continuously to wart until a whitened halo of 1 to 2 mm appears around the base of the lesion.

c. After the lesion has thawed, reapply a second time.
d. Initially, the lesion will have an erythematous ring, then a blister may form with clear, cloudy, or hemorrhagic fluid. Patient may use a sterile needle to puncture the blister if painful or in an awkward location.
e. The blister or wart will crust and fall off after one week; reapply cryotherapy if needed in 2- to 3-week cycles until adequate effect is achieved.
f. Burning and throbbing, especially during the thaw phase, are uncomfortable but generally well tolerated by most patients.
g. Side effects include occasional scarring, depigmentation or hyperpigmentation, and sensory loss depending on site.

4. *Pharmacologic agents* may be applied topically by clinician or patient or intralesionally by the clinician.
   a. Podophyllin, 25% resin solution, can be applied weekly by the clinician to plantar or anogenital warts. Systemic absorption can yield side effects when large surface areas are covered. Side effects include nausea and vomiting, seizures, peripheral neuropathy, and coma.
   b. Purified podophyllotoxin, 0.5% solution (Condylox), is available for home application by patients for anogenital warts. Side effects are milder, generally only local erythema and irritation.
   c. Cantharidin, 0.7% collodion solution (Cantharone) for common and plantar warts
      (1) Application is followed by occlusion for 24 hours.
      (2) A blister forms, which heals within a week.
      (3) Major side effects are pain from the blister or formation of a ring wart (treatable).
   d. Retinoic acid, 0.05% solution or 0.5% cream for flat warts
      (1) Apply daily until desquamation occurs.
      (2) Local irritation is the major side effect.
   e. 5-fluorouracil 5% for recalcitrant flat warts
   f. Interferon intralesional injections
   g. Bleomycin intralesional injections
5. *Surgery* is reserved for recalcitrant warts.
   a. Electrosurgery
   b. CO_2 laser
6. *Immunotherapy* also would be reserved for recalcitrant warts.
   a. Dinitrochlorobenzene

Patient Education

1. Careful counseling about treatment options, side effects, time course, and expected outcomes should occur before any therapy is begun.
2. For patients with anogenital warts, STD counseling is advisable, including recommendations for condom

use, partner notification, and testing for other STDs as appropriate. Partners should be examined and treated.

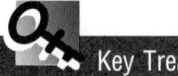

Key Treatment

- Watch and wait
- Topical chemical agents
- Cryotherapy
- Topical podophyllin and other pharmocologic agents

Nevi

Etiology

Clustering of melanocytic nevus cells in the skin causes nevi or *moles.* Sun exposure is a key factor.

Symptoms

1. Generally asymptomatic, with patients noticing the presence or appearance of lesions in various locations. New nevi commonly form through middle age, especially in sun-exposed areas, but tend to regress in later years.
2. If itching or morphologic changes are noted, the clinician needs to consider whether malignant features are present.

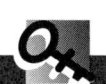

Key Symptom

- Presence of macule/papule

Clinical Findings

1. *Common acquired melanocytic nevi* are benign lesions that are subdivided into three classes, based on the location of the nevus cells in the skin. They have little potential for malignant degeneration.
   a. Junctional nevi
      (1) Pinpoint to few mm macules
      (2) Well-circumscribed
      (3) Uniform in color; typically brown-black
      (4) Widely distributed but especially sun-exposed areas
   b. Compound nevi
      (1) Slightly elevated or dome-shaped
      (2) Uniform in color; may have a hypopigmented "halo"
      (3) Smooth surface but may become rough with age
   c. Dermal nevi
      (1) Dome-shaped, polypoid, pedunculated
      (2) Skin-colored to black
      (3) A variant is called a *blue nevus,* given its characteristic color

2. *Congenital nevi* may be premalignant lesions, especially giant congenital melanocytic nevi.
   a. Present at birth, can be found on any skin surface
   b. Variably sized but may cover entire body parts
   c. Medium-dark brown, variegated color across lesion
   d. Rough or lobulated surface, increasingly so with age
   e. Coarse hair growth
   f. May involve leptomeninges if lesion occurs on head
3. *Dysplastic nevi* can occur sporadically or following a familial, autosomal dominant pattern. These have premalignant potential.
   a. 5 to 10 mm or larger macules or papules
   b. Most often on trunks and limbs
   c. Variegated in color within lesion: pink, tan, brown
   d. Irregular border and surface

Key Signs

- Pigmented macule/papule
- Generally well circumscribed
- Other appearances, depending on type

Laboratory Tests

1. Clinical diagnosis of nevus/nevi is usually adequate.
2. Biopsy may be done for confirmation of initial diagnosis or for lesions with malignant characteristics.

Key Test

- None or skin biopsy

Differential Diagnosis

1. Malignant melanoma
2. Squamous or basal cell carcinomas
   a. Dermal nevi may be indistinguishable from basal cell carcinoma.

Treatment

Many nevi require no treatment. Those with malignant potential require careful monitoring for changes. Excision with adequate margins may be recommended for some nevi with high malignant potential, especially giant congenital melanocytic nevi.

Patient Education

1. Advise patient to look for possible indications of malignant changes.
   a. Change in borders (e.g., less distinct, asymmetric, larger)

b. Change in pigmentation (e.g., more varied or stippled)

c. Crusting or bleeding, erosion

d. Pruritus, pain, tenderness

2. Adequate protection from sun exposure should be encouraged.

Key Treatment

- Monitor for changes

- Excision of some nevi

Follow-Up

Yearly complete skin examinations, more frequently (every six months or more) in patients with dysplastic nevi or other nevus conditions with high malignant potential.

Bibliography

For general text and atlas, see
Fitzpatrick TB, Eisen AZ, et al: Dermatology in General Medicine, 4th Ed. New York, McGraw-Hill, 1993.

For more on cervical HPV and dysplasia, see
Kitchener KC: The role of HPV in the genesis of cervical cancer. Cancer Treat Res 1994;70:29–41.

For a review of melanocytic nevi, see
Marghoob AA, Orlow SJ, Kopf AW: Syndromes associated with melanocytic nevi. J Amer Acad Dermatol 1993;29(3):373–388.

For self-treatment of genital warts, see
Syed TA, Lundin S, Ahmad SA: Topical 0.3% and 0.5% podophyllotoxin cream for self-treatment of condylomata acuminata in women. A placebo-controlled, double-blind study. Dermatology 1994;189(2):142–145.

For a discussion of atypical mole recognition and management, see
Williams ML, Sagebiel RW: Melanoma risk factors and atypical moles. Western J Med 1994;160(4):343–350.

Procedure **Cryosurgery and Electrocautery of Skin Lesions** *Irving D. Wolfe*

Cryosurgery

Indications
1. Treatment of warts and seborrheic and actinic keratoses
2. Treatment of epitheliomas should not be attempted without thermocouple temperature control apparatus and experience in this technique.

Contraindications
1. Melanocytes and neural tissues are more susceptible to cold injury than other anatomic structures.
2. Cryosurgery of skin lesions in African-Americans and other dark-skinned individuals can result in permanent depigmentation of the area.
3. Cryosurgery must be avoided over superficially situated motor nerves including the ulnar nerve at the ulnar groove and the common peroneal nerve at the fibular condyle.
4. Cryosurgery over the digital nerves at the fingerwebs and lateral fingers *usually* results in temporary sensory deficit.

Preparation
1. Informed consent
2. Selection of appropriate lesions
3. Cleansing of the site; not a sterile technique

Equipment
1. Source of liquid nitrogen: Most dermatology offices have a tank of liquid nitrogen that is refilled when necessary by a supplier via tank truck.

2. Application apparatus
   a. Cotton swabs: applicator stick with extra cotton most commonly used with a Styrofoam cup or metal-insulated flask with vented cap. If the metal (i.e., not disposable) flask is used, each swab should be dipped in only once to avoid blood contamination. Glass-lined vacuum flasks should not be used because of danger of explosion.
   b. Spray apparatus (e.g., Cry-Ac) is more efficient and eliminates danger of contamination of nitrogen.
   c. Eye shields

Anesthesia
1. Anesthesia is usually not necessary.
2. Topical anesthesia is not very helpful.
3. Local anesthesia may be administered (e.g., 1% plain lidocaine) to prevent pain.
4. Local anesthesia can be used to elevate a lesion separating it from underlying nerves (e.g., over the lateral fingers).

Precautions
1. See Contraindications.
2. Cryosurgery near the frontal and temporal hairlines can induce headache.
3. Skin on penile shaft should be pouted to avoid freeze of corpora cavernosa, which is very painful.
4. Eyes must be protected, particularly from cryospray injury, with eye shields or with cones to prevent spread of nitrogen. Cones can be purchased from manufacturers of the spray apparatus.

Technique

1. The swab is applied or the spray directed at the center of the lesion and the lesion frozen until a 1-mm halo of hard freeze is achieved.

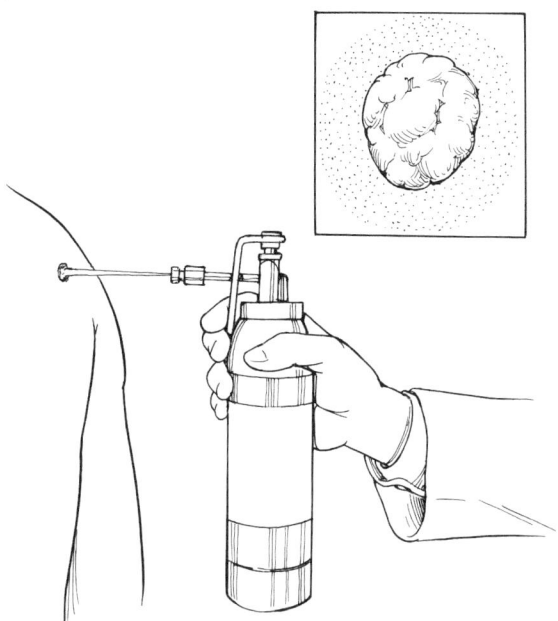

The "C" tip is useful for most applications. Tiny 1- to 2-mm lesions are most accurately treated with a pointed cotton swab. Thicker lesions require longer times to achieve complete freezing. Larger-diameter lesions require that the nitrogen be applied to more than one spot.

2. The lesion is allowed to thaw and the procedure is repeated once.

Follow-Up

1. A blister will ensue, frequently a hemorrhagic one.
2. Blister should be left intact in most instances and allowed to dry and slough in 10 to 14 days.
3. A very tense painful bulla can be punctured in the office or at home with a sterile needle.
4. Progressive spread of blisters, usually on the dorsal hand of elderly patients with atrophic skin, can be handled as described in Item 2.
5. If blister opens or is drained, the lesion must be treated as an open wound with Bacitracin, mupirocin, or povidone-iodine and dressing to prevent infection.
6. Analgesia usually is not necessary, but pain may persist for as long as a day, particularly on digits. Acetaminophen, aspirin, or ibuprofen can be used.

Electrosurgery

Indications

1. Destruction of benign skin lesions including verrucae, benign keratoses, and skin tags
2. With curettage, destruction of appropriately selected small epitheliomas previously subjected to biopsy
3. Adjunctive after shave biopsy or shave excision of *benign* melanocytic nevi for control of bleeding

Contraindications

1. Allergy to local anesthesia
2. Presence of a pacemaker
3. Suspicion of malignant melanoma
4. Large epithelioma
5. Epitheliomas not amenable to eletrosurgical eradication (e.g., morpheaform basal cell carcinomas, many squamous cell carcinomas, tumors near tissue planes)
6. Lesions in areas where depressed scarring is likely (e.g., ala nasae [a relative contraindication])

7. Lesions in areas where hypertrophic scarring is likely (a relative contraindication)
8. Surgery over nail matrix should be done with great caution to avoid injury.
9. Surgery near eyes should be done with caution to avoid ectropion, eye trauma.

Preparation

1. Informed consent
2. Selection of appropriate lesions
3. Cleansing of site, usually done in clean, not sterile, setting

Equipment

1. Gloves: examination gloves adequate
2. Mask with visor for eye protection or additional goggles
3. Waterproof gown
4. Alcohol or povidone-iodine prep pads
5. Anesthesia in disposable syringe with disposable fine 27- to 30-gauge needle
6. No. 15 disposable scalpel blade for biopsy and biopsy container with formalin
7. 3 × 3 gauze pads or applicator sticks
8. Dermal curette, disposable or sterile
9. Appropriate electrosurgical instrument (e.g., Birtcher hyfrecator, Bovie with disposable tip or autoclaved tip and sleeve for working electrode)

Anesthesia

1. 1% or 2% lidocaine plain or with 1:100,000 epinephrine
2. Isotonic saline can be used for brief procedures in the event of history of "caine" allergy.
3. Epinephrine should be avoided in patients with arrhythmia, with significant hypertension, and those taking β-blockers.

Precautions

1. Patient should be in supine position.
2. Patient should not be in contact with ground (i.e., metal table parts).
3. See Contraindications; Anesthesia

Technique

1. Operative area is cleaned, lesion to be removed is anesthetized, and area is draped if appropriate.
2. Eyes and mouth are protected where appropriate.
3. Shave biopsy or excision is performed when indicated (see Indications).
4. Machine is set: a low setting appropriate for small lesions or those in close proximity to eyes; higher setting for larger lesions.
5. Electrode is brought in close proximity (fulguration) or in contact (desiccation) with the lesion or wound.

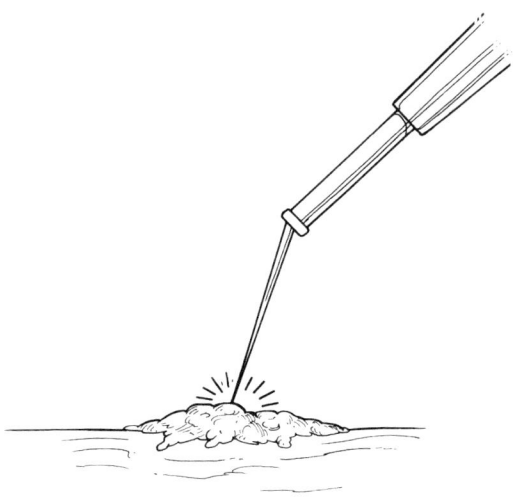

6. Foot or hand switch is depressed and held until lesion has been destroyed and bleeding stopped.
7. Curettage is performed on base of now dry wound until lesion removal is complete.

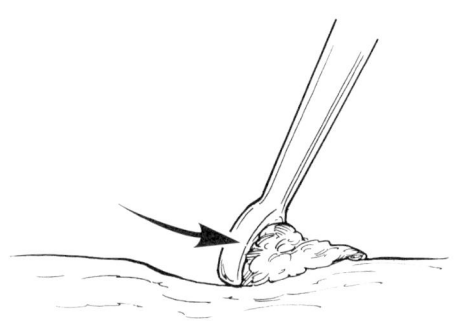

8. Desiccation/fulguration is again performed until hemostasis is complete. Electrosurgery instruments are ineffective in grossly bloody field. Wound can be kept from filling with blood by pressure with gauze pad or applicator stick, which is slowly withdrawn laterally as the wound or lesion is desiccated.

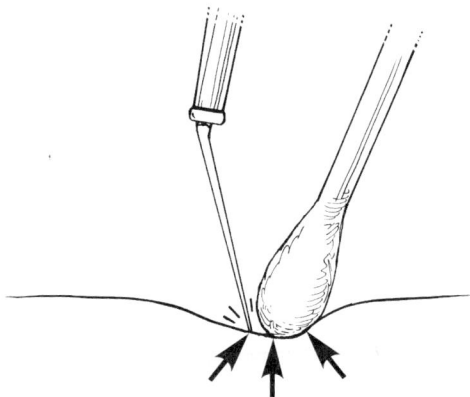

9. Wound is dressed with gauze and Bacitracin ointment or other suitable topical antiseptic or antibiotic.

Follow-Up

1. Wound care instructions: daily dressing change, application of Bacitracin, mupirocin, povidone-iodine, or similar ointment and bandage.
2. Occlusive dressings enhance comfort and speed re-epithelialization in wound healing studies.
3. Most facial wounds re-epithelialize in 10 to 14 days, trunk and extremity lesions in 14 to 21 days.
4. If biopsy is benign, no further follow-up is required.
5. Development of hypertrophic scars is possible in upper trunk electrosurgery, and patient should be so advised. Intralesional steroid injection is sometimes necessary.

Bibliography

Dawler RPR, Walker NPJ: Physical and surgical therapy. *In* Champion RH, Burton JL, Ebeling FJ (eds): Rook's Textbook of Dermatology, 5th ed. Boston, Blackwell, 1992, pp 3113–3114.

Dawler RPR, Walker NPJ: Physical and surgical therapy. *In* Champion RH, Burton JL, Ebeling FJ (eds): Rook's Textbook of Dermatology, 5th ed. Boston, Blackwell, 1992, pp 3109–3111.

Guidelines of American Academy of Dermatology on Cryotherapy. Dermatology World, Supplement, Aug 1993.

Kuflik EG: Cryosurgery updated. J Am Acad Dermatol 1994; 31:925–944.

Rock M: Warts. *In* Provost TT, Farmer ER: Current Therapy in Dermatology-2. Philadelphia, BC Decker, 1988, pp 216–217.

268 Condyloma Acuminata

Anne Cather Cutlip

Etiology

1. Human papillomavirus (HPV) types 6 and 11 usually cause condyloma acuminata or genital warts, a sexually transmitted disease. The natural history of the virus has not been well established. Condyloma may recur or persist after therapy, undergo malignant transformation, or regress spontaneously. There are strong links between certain types of HPV and cancer of the cervix, vagina, vulva, penis, and anus.

2. Children may develop condyloma via
   a. Vertical transmission (born to infected mothers)
      (1) Laryngeal papillomatosis, oral and skin condyloma
      (2) Usually manifested within the first year
   b. Horizontal transmission (raises the question of sexual abuse)
      (1) Typical condyloma in anogenital area
      (2) Usually manifested after the first year

3. Risk factors associated with HPV infection include
   a. Sex with an infected partner
   b. Multiple sexual partners
   c. Previous sexually transmitted diseases
   d. Cigarette smoking
   e. Lack of condom use
   f. Oral contraceptives

4. The majority of persons whose sexual partner has condyloma will themselves develop condyloma within 3 months. An even larger percentage of persons is believed to develop subclinical infection. Autoinoculation is possible.

5. The average incubation period between infection and appearance of condyloma is 3 months but can be as early as 6 weeks.

6. An area of clinically apparent disease may only represent a small amount of the actual infected area. (If condyloma is seen in one part of anogenital tract, probably it is elsewhere.)

Symptoms

1. Condylomata are most often asymptomatic.
2. Patients may feel a "bump" or palpable lesion in the anogenital region, sometimes pruritic.
3. Occasionally a patient complains of urethral obstruction.

Clinical Findings

1. Pink to flesh-colored, papillomatous, pedunculated or sessile mass in the anogenital area or other moist areas. May be pigmented

2. Single or multiple lesions. Initially small but may grow, become confluent, and form a cluster or "cauliflower" mass. Giant condylomata, flesh to brown colored, have uncertain malignant potential.

3. Males commonly develop condyloma on the penile shaft, coronal sulcus, frenulum, prepuce, and glans (less commonly on scrotum, meatus, and anus).

4. Females commonly develop condyloma on the posterior introitus, fourchette, and labia minora. (Can also be found on clitoris, vagina, cervix, urethra, and anus)

Key Signs

- Pedunculated or sessile
- Pink or flesh-colored
- Located in anogenital area
- Single or multiple
- Small to giant size

Laboratory Tests

1. Diagnosis is usually made clinically, based on typical appearance and location.
   a. A magnifying glass helps detect small lesions.
   b. Colposcopy provides better visualization of the genital tract.
   c. Anoscopy also should be available.
   d. Application of 3% to 5% acetic acid typically produces an "acetowhitening" of the condyloma within several minutes. This is not diagnostic but aids identification.

2. There are no current serology tests or culture methods available.

3. Histology and cytology can confirm the diagnosis. Typical histologic features include
   a. Koilocytes: large epithelial cell with small, dense nucleus and clear perinuclear area or "halo"
   b. Hyperkeratosis, dyskeratosis, or acanthosis

4. Other methods available to detect HPV in tissues (often time-consuming and expensive)
   a. DNA hybridization (e.g., dot blot, in situ hybridizations)
   b. Electron microscopy
   c. Immunoperoxidase staining

5. Viral typing may be used to identify which lesions may be at a greater risk for progressing to cancer.

Differential Diagnosis

1. Verruca vulgaris: Occurs anywhere, tends to be thicker, drier, and hyperkeratotic

2. Molluscum contagiosum: Smooth, round papule with central umbilication; occurs anywhere

3. Seborrheic keratoses: multiple, waxy, rough, hyperpigmented papules

4. Condyloma latum: moist, rounded, white papule of syphilis

5. Pearly penile papules: smooth, uniform, small (1 to 2 mm), at the corona

6. Vestibular papillae: female equivalent of pearly penile papules, on both sides of the vulva

7. Bowenoid papulosis: Flat, multicentric, resembles warts; may regress or progress to squamous cell carcinoma; biopsy recommended

8. Bowen's disease: Flat, whitish plaque with well-defined borders; not uncommonly ulcerated

9. Hemorrhoid

10. Nonpigmented nevi

Treatment

1. Before treatment, biopsy is important to rule out malignancy in suspicious lesions.
   a. Giant or rapidly growing condylomata
   b. Pigmented, friable, ulcerated, or confluent hyperkeratotic lesions
   c. Previous treatment failure or recurrent condylomata
   d. Flat, acetowhite lesions

2. Examine entire anogenital tract due to widespread nature of HPV. Consider testing for other sexually transmitted diseases (frequently coexist with human papillomavirus).

3. Treatment modalities vary in the number of office visits, expense, response, and recurrence rates.
   a. Chemical treatments
      (1) Trichloroacetic acid (TCA) or bichloroacetic acid (BCA): 50% to 80% acid in 70% ethyl alcohol applied with cotton applicator (by physician or patient) once or twice a day for 3 days and then none applied for 4 days; repeat until clear. Can be used on the vagina or cervix
      (2) Podophyllin: 20% to 25% topical solution of podophyllotoxin compounded with tincture of benzoin. Applied with cotton swab or applicator stick by physician weekly until clear. Patient must wash off after 3 to 6 hours. Can cause severe skin irritation and be toxic if absorbed systemically. Avoid use on large areas of tissue, in vagina, or in pregnancy.
      (3) Podofilox (Condylox): 0.5% topical solution (purified podophyllotoxin) applied to external warts twice daily for 3 days and then off for 4 days; continue for 6 to 8 weeks. More potent, less irritating, and less toxic than podophyllin. Avoid use in perianal or mucous membrane areas. Patients may apply.
      (4) 5% 5-fluorouracil (5-FU) cream: Most often used for vaginal or periurethral warts or as prophylaxis after ablation. Typically one-third to one-half vaginal applicator once a week for 8 weeks. Recheck every 2 weeks. Can cause extensive erosions and scarring of vaginal and vulvar tissues and urethral strictures. Avoid in pregnancy.
   b. Physical treatments (tend to have lower failure and recurrence rates)
      (1) Cryotherapy: liquid nitrogen or nitrous oxide freezes until iceball extends several millimeters beyond base of lesion. Repeat every 1 to 2 weeks until clear. Few complications. May need local anesthesia. Safe in pregnancy
      (2) Excision: simple or punch biopsy with local anesthesia. Easy and available in most offices.
      (3) Electrosurgery: cautery or desiccation with local anesthesia. Wear mask to avoid viral particles in plume.
      (4) Laser vaporization: requires expert skills, with local or general anesthesia. Not used as an initial treatment. Expensive. Wear mask to avoid viral particles in plume.
   c. Immunoenhancing treatments
      (1) Interferon-α group (alfa-2b [Intron A], alfa-n3 [Alferon N]) multiple intralesional injections several times a week. Use for refractory warts, not first-line therapy. Major side effect is flulike symptoms. Expensive
      (2) Autovaccination and dinitrochlorobenzene injections are not well documented and without controlled studies. Not recommended

Diet

No specific diet has been recognized to prevent or treat condyloma.

Activity

Patients should abstain from sexual activity while being treated; otherwise, activity as tolerated. Advise patients to practice ''safe'' sex (use of a condom is not 100 per cent effective).

Patient Education

The physician should educate patients about the nature of condyloma. Because patients will continue to carry the virus and have a potential for neoplasms, they should be encouraged to have regular examinations and quit smoking. Prevention would be ideal, but once patients have condyloma, they should be encouraged to practice safe sex.

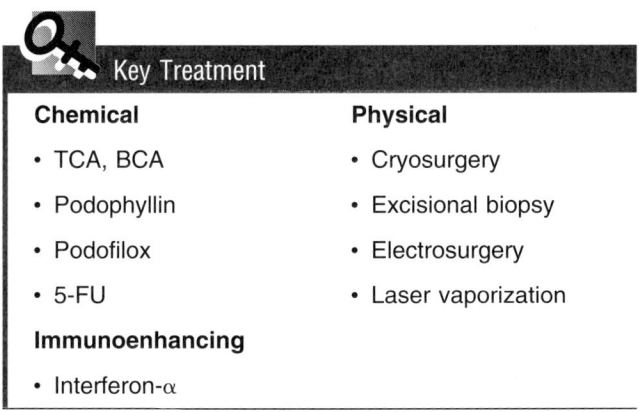

Key Treatment

Chemical	Physical
• TCA, BCA	• Cryosurgery
• Podophyllin	• Excisional biopsy
• Podofilox	• Electrosurgery
• 5-FU	• Laser vaporization
Immunoenhancing	
• Interferon-α	

Follow-Up

1. Treat until all condylomata are gone.
2. Due to the tendency for widespread infection, patients

with condyloma should be thoroughly examined (including Pap smears) every 6 to 12 months initially. Some recommend a screening colposcopy once the diagnosis is made.

Bibliography

Goldfarb MT, Reid R, eds: Dermatologic Clinics: Human Papillomavirus Infection, vol 9, no 2. Philadelphia, WB Saunders, 1991.

Greene I: Therapy for genital warts. *In* Lupton GP, Fitzpatrick JE (eds): Dermatologic Clinics, vol 10, no 1. Philadelphia, WB Saunders, 1992, pp 253–267.

Ling MR: Therapy of genital human papillomavirus infections: II. Methods of treatment. Int J Dermatol 1992;31(11):769–776.

Moscicki AB: Human papillomavirus infections. *In* Barness LA (ed): Advances in Pediatrics, vol 39. Philadelphia, Mosby–Year Book, 1992, pp 257–281.

Steinberg JL, Cibely LJ, Rice PA: Genital warts: Diagnosis, treatment, and counseling for the patient. Curr Clin Top Infect Dis 1993;13:99–122.

269 Leukoplakia and Erythroplasia   *John G. Spangler*

Etiology

1. Cigarette or smokeless tobacco use
2. Repetitive oral trauma (malpositioned teeth, ill-fitting dentures, habitual cheek biting)
3. Long-term, excessive alcohol consumption
4. Oral infections; unproven roles of herpes simplex virus and human papillomavirus
5. Rarely, metabolic disturbances (e.g., avitaminosis A)
6. Betel nut chewing, lime-tobacco mixtures (Southeast Asia)
7. Large percentage of idiopathic cases

Symptoms

1. Usually asymptomatic (over 95 per cent of cases)
2. "Roughness" at site of lesion occasionally noticed
3. Pain or ulceration rare but strongly associated with malignancy

Key Symptoms

- Usually asymptomatic
- Roughness
- Pain (rare)

Clinical Findings

1. Leukoplakia: white surface mucosal lesions that do not wipe off
   a. Clinical appearance varies and may be
      (1) Thin, almost nonpalpable or thick, dense lesions
      (2) Faintly translucent white or speckled red and white or opaque gray colors
      (3) Single lesion (large or small) or scattered lesions with or without adjacent ulcerations
      (4) Associated with candidal superinfection (unfavorable sign but unknown if etiologic agent)
   b. Location
      (1) Fifty per cent of cases occur on tongue, mandibular alveolar ridge, and buccal mucosa; less frequently, palate, maxillary alveolar ridge, floor of mouth, retromolar regions
      (2) In smokeless tobacco or betel nut chewers, lesions usually occur at habitual site of quid placement.
      (3) Tongue and floor of mouth lesions have highest incidence of malignant transformation.
   c. Patient characteristics
      (1) Incidence unknown, but peak onset in fourth decade of life
      (2) May occur in youths who use tobacco heavily (especially smokeless forms)
      (3) Male/female ratio greater than 2:1
      (4) Leukoplakia in nonusers of tobacco has highest rate of malignant transformation (24 per cent).
   d. Histology ranges from hyperkeratosis, to dysplasia, to invasive carcinoma.
   e. Clinical course
      (1) One-third regress with time.
      (2) Between 2 and 15 per cent (average 5 per cent) progress to carcinoma.
      (3) Rest remain essentially unchanged.
   f. Malignant transformation more likely if
      (1) Tongue or floor of mouth location
      (2) Any redness to lesion (see below)
      (3) Papillomatous or verrucous appearance
      (4) Leukoplakia in tobacco nonuser
      (5) Continued exposure to irritants
      (6) Possible increased risk if there is overlying candidal infection
2. Erythroplasia: bright red mucosal plaques or erosions
   a. Often associated with leukoplakia (erythroleukoplakia)
   b. Malignant potential greatly increased with any red component to leukoplakic lesion; 90 per cent of erythroleukoplakia is dysplastic or worse.

Key Signs

White Lesions	Increased Malignant Potential if
- Do not wipe off	- Tongue or floor of mouth location
- Single or multiple lesions	- Any redness
- Nonpalpable or thick	- Papillomatous features
- Red component (erythroplakia)	- Nonuser of tobacco
	- Candidal superinfection

Laboratory Tests

1. Biopsy
   a. Necessary for definitive diagnosis
   b. Biopsy lesions at high risk for malignancy, such as lesions on tongue, lesions with overlying candi-

diasis, and verrucous or papillary lesions, and all red areas.

   c. Toluidine blue (tolonium chloride), a vital stain, helps direct biopsy to areas most likely to contain dysplasia or malignancy.

   d. If biopsy of small lesions suspected to be malignant will distort appearance, or if lesions are in areas difficult to access (e.g., base of tongue, piriform fossa), then physician who will perform definitive treatment should see lesion and preferably perform biopsy.

   e. Both incisional and punch biopsy techniques are acceptable.

   f. Large lesions may require multiple biopsies.

2. Cytologic smears

   a. Not a replacement for biopsy; helps to confirm clinical suspicion only, but cannot treat cancer on basis of cytologic smear alone

   b. Analogous to Papanicolaou smears in collection and staining

Key Tests

- Biopsy for definitive diagnosis
- Toluidine blue to highlight dysplastic areas
- Cytologic smears (not a substitute for biopsy)

Differential Diagnosis

1. Lichen planus: frequently symptomatic, especially if erosive
2. Oral hairy leukoplakia: lingual manifestation of AIDS
3. Systemic lupus erythematosus
4. White sponge nevus
5. Hereditary keratosis

Treatment

1. Remove or correct chronic irritants to allow inflammatory processes to heal; treat *Candida* infection if KOH smear is positive for yeast; follow-up in 2 weeks.
2. Biopsy lesion positive for *Candida* if lesion persists at follow-up
3. All lesions with histopathologic dysplasia must be totally excised.

   a. Carbon dioxide laser (most effective and frequently used)

   b. Electrodesiccation

   c. Cryotherapy

   d. Knife excision

Medication

Vitamin A derivatives show promise but as yet are not routinely recommended; antifungal agents will not remove true leukoplakia.

Patient Education

1. Patients must understand 2 to 15 per cent potential for malignant transformation even of relatively benign-appearing lesions.
2. Importance of cessation of tobacco, alcohol, or other etiologic factors must be stressed, as well as follow-up.

Key Treatment

- Remove irritants
- Treat *Candida* if present
- Excise all dysplastic lesions
  - CO$_2$ laser
  - Electrodesiccation
  - Cryotherapy
  - Knife excision
- Follow-up regularly

Follow-Up

Regular follow-up is mandatory to detect appearance of dysplastic change or new lesions.

Bibliography

Abbey LM: Precancerous lesions of the mouth (review). Curr Opin Dent 1991;1:773–776.

Allen CM, Camisa C: Diseases of the mouth and lips. *In* Sams WM, Lynch PJ (eds): Principles and Practice of Dermatology. New York, Churchill-Livingstone, 1990, pp 932–934.

Holmstrup P, Pindborg JJ: Oral mucosal lesions in smokeless tobacco users. CA 1988;38:230–235.

Kaugars GE, Silverman S Jr, Lovas JG, et al: A review of the use of antioxidant supplements in the treatment of human oral leukoplakia (review). J Cell Biochem Suppl 1993;17F:292–298.

Silverman S Jr, Bhargava K, Mani NJ, et al: Malignant transformation and natural history of oral leukoplakia in 57,518 industrial workers of Gujarat, India. Cancer 1976;38:1790.

Silverman S Jr: Oral Cancer, 3d ed. Atlanta, American Cancer Society, 1990, pp 14–28.

270 Calluses and Corns

Janet L. Purkey

Calluses

Etiology

1. Structural defects
   a. Excessive pronation causing abnormal pressure on the metatarsal heads
   b. Hammer toes, subluxation, and trauma
   c. Change in weight bearing such as associated neuropathy
2. Improperly fitted footwear
   a. High heels, dancers (especially ballet), and athletes who wear poorly fitted shoes
   b. Proper footwear with abnormal weight bearing (see above)

Symptoms

1. Pain on weight bearing
2. Pruritus
3. Burning sensation

Clinical Findings

1. A circumscribed area of hypertrophied and keratinized skin on the plantar surface primarily over the metatarsophalangeal joints
2. Callus may be noted on any area of the forefoot.
3. Soft surfaces are often the sites with structural abnormalities.

WARNING

The diabetic patient needs special attention to the foot examination because ulceration and infection involving callus increase morbidity.

Laboratory Tests

None

Differential Diagnosis

1. Plantar keratosis is usually an inherited condition of hyperkeratosis.
2. Plantar wart is differentiated in that it is not histologically similar and usually does not occur over the metatarsophalangeal joints.

Treatment

1. Educating the patient on home care
   a. Weekly use of a pumice stone
   b. An emery board is also useful
   c. Care must be taken not to disrupt the healthy epithelium

d. Softening the callus in a warm soak may prove helpful.
   e. The diabetic patient must *not* damage healthy skin or cause the callus to bleed.
   f. A small amount of callus must be left to provide protection.
2. Office care for painful callus
   a. Immediate improvement can be obtained by debridement with surgical blades.
   b. Paring the callus with small parallel strokes allows for safe debridement.
   c. May be needed as often as every 2 or 3 months
3. Preventing calluses requires replacement of offending footwear.
   a. The patient should be educated about proper footwear.
   b. An appropriate fit involves not only proper length and width, but the patient also should examine the shoe's "toe box" for depth and placement of the seam.
   c. Low-heeled and soft-soled shoes provide benefit.
   d. Custom footwear is an investment in foot care.
   e. Diabetic patients should wear leather enclosed-toe footwear.
      (1) Maximum foot protection
      (2) Best aeration to prevent maceration
3. Padding around pressure points
   a. A comma-shaped pad or "cookie" will provide support over the metatarsal pad.
   b. Special insoles also can relieve pressure points.
   c. Moleskin is easily shaped for added comfort.
4. Topical keratolytic therapy
   a. May be applied on the recalcitrant callus. (This is more commonly done on plantar warts than on pressure calluses.)
   b. Diabetic patients should not use any keratolytic agent because it may damage adjacent healthy skin.
5. Referral to an orthopedist or podiatrist
   a. Surgical correction of structural defects
      (1) The malaligned metatarsal head can be corrected.
      (2) Other bony prominences may be reduced surgically.
      (3) Procedures that will lessen or eliminate excessive pronation
   b. Referral to a foot specialist may be for nonsurgical treatment as well.

(1) Debridement of patients with diabetes mellitus, peripheral vascular disease, rheumatoid arthritis

(2) These specialists provide many of the special metatarsal pads, insoles, and molds that will enhance nonsurgical therapy.

Follow-Up

1. Patients should be encouraged to use the pumice stone at home on a regular basis and purchase appropriate footwear.

2. If these measures fail to eliminate a painful callus, patients should be followed in the office often for debridement.

3. Referral to an orthopedist or podiatrist should be based on the response to conservative measures.

Corns

Etiology

1. "Corns" or "clavi" refer to callus formation over a bony prominence.

   a. Hard corns are usually seen on the dorsal aspect of the lesser toes and lateral aspect of the fifth toe.

   b. Soft corns are found in the web space between the toes.

      (1) The pressure point lies between two adjacent phalanges.

      (2) The maceration of the corn in a web space makes it "soft."

   c. Seed corns or plantar clavi are found on the plantar surface.

2. Ill-fitting shoes are a primary cause of the epidermal buildup.

3. Structural deformities

   a. Hammer toes with exostosis

   b. Other abnormal bony prominences

Symptoms

1. Corns produce pain when the foot is placed in a tightly fitted shoe.

2. Plantar corns produce pain when weight bearing.

Key Symptoms

Calluses

• Pain on weight bearing

• Pruritus

• Burning sensation

Corns

• Pain when foot is placed in a tightly fitted shoe

• Pain on weight bearing (plantar corns)

Clinical Findings

1. Hard corns are keratotic lesions most commonly observed on the lateral aspect of the fifth toe.

2. Soft corns are most commonly observed in the fourth web space.

3. Plantar corns are conical-shaped hyperkeratotic epidermal lesions with a central portion extending toward sensitive subcutaneous tissue.

Key Signs

Calluses

• Circumscribed area of hypertrophied and keratinized skin on plantar surface primarily over metatarsophalangeal joints

• May be noted on any area of the forefoot

• Soft surfaces are often the sites with structural abnormalities.

Corns

• Hard corns most commonly observed on lateral aspect of fifth toe

• Soft corns most commonly observed in fourth web space

• Plantar corns are conical-shaped and have a central portion extending toward sensitive subcutaneous tissue.

Laboratory Tests

None

Differential Diagnosis

1. Plantar warts look like hyperkeratosis; however, they are quite vascular compared with corns.

2. Foreign bodies with secondary keratosis

3. In diabetics, ulcerations and infection must be ruled out.

Treatment

1. Debriding the excessive buildup of epidermis is crucial to treatment (see Calluses).

2. Enucleation of the apex or central portion of the plantar corn

3. Corn pads reduce pressure over bony prominences.

4. Footwear with adequate length, width, and depth in the "toe box"

5. Liquid nitrogen and salicylic acid can be useful in plantar corns that are recalcitrant to other therapy. (This should be reserved for nonsurgical candidates.)

6. Referral to an orthopedist or podiatrist when above measures fail

Key Treatment

Calluses

- Educating patient concerning home care
  - Weekly use of pumice stone
  - Emery board also useful
  - Soften callus in a warm soak

- Office care for painful callus
  - Debridement with surgical blades

- Topical keratolytic therapy

- Surgical correction of structural defects

Corns

- Debridement of excessive buildup of epidermis

- Enucleation of apex or central portion of plantar corn

- Corn pads reduce pressure over bony prominences.

- Adequate footwear

- Liquid nitrogen and salicylic acid

Follow-Up

Same as under Calluses.

Bibliography

Brahms MA: The small toes. *In* Jahss MH (ed): Disorders of the Foot and Ankle, 2d ed. Philadelphia, WB Saunders, 1991.

George DH: Management of hyperkeratotic lesions in the elderly patient. Clin Podiatr Med Surg 1993;10:69–77.

Gordon GM: Exercise and the aging foot. South Med J 1994;87:36–41.

Richards RN: Calluses, corns, and shoes. Semin Dermatol 1991;10:112–114.

Silfverskiold JP: Common foot problems. Postgrad Med 1991;89:183–187.

271 Lipoma

Lawrence H. Miller

Etiology

1. Definition: a benign neoplasm of fatty origin usually found in the subcutaneous tissue plane. Lipomas tend to be soft, lobulated, and freely movable within surrounding tissues. Although they are benign and may be indistinguishable from surrounding fatty tissue, most lipomas can be tissue-typed into three abnormal cytogenetic subgroups.

2. Epidemiology: Focal, remote trauma is frequently considered an initiating factor, but this is not proven.

Symptoms

1. Typically, lipomas are soft painless masses in the subcutaneous tissue.

2. Pain can be a primary presentation with angiolipoma, a lipoma with an intertwining vascular network.

3. Disfigurement or pressure symptoms may occur with some lipomas that grow to such large size that they interfere with surrounding anatomy or restrict items of apparel (belts, sleeves, collars).

Key Symptoms

- Abnormal skin contour
- Local pressure
- Disfigurement
- Pain

Clinical Findings

1. On physical examination, one might find a soft, well-circumscribed, lobulated, freely movable, nontender subcutaneous mass.

2. Lipomas are most often located on the trunk and upper arms. However, some can be found beneath fascia, which makes them feel firmer, or even subgaleal, in which case they may be confused with bone tumor.

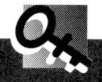

Key Sign

- Soft, lobulated, movable nontender mass

Laboratory Tests

1. The diagnosis can usually be made by careful history and physical examination. There are no specific laboratory tests, although some physicians employ ultrasonography to distinguish lipomas from cysts or abscesses.

2. Postexcision pathologic analysis may be prudent, because some lipomas undergo malignant degeneration.

Key Test

- Ultrasonography

Differential Diagnosis

1. Sebaceous cyst, cysts of fat necrosis, panniculitis, herniation of fat lobules, insulin lipohypertrophy, liposarcoma

2. Careful history, physical findings of firmness and immobility of the mass, local heat, and pain may help to differentiate other conditions from lipoma. Excision and/or tissue pathology may be needed to identify other possibilities.

Treatment

1. Once the diagnosis is made, treatment of lipomas may be no more involved than reassuring the patient. It is a benign condition, and if the mass is not changing, observation over time may be the most prudent management.

2. Large or multiple lesions can be treated with liposuction.

3. Most lipomas can be approached using simple excision or enucleation. This is done by incising the skin over the mass, after appropriate cleansing and local anesthesia. Then, with either a blunt instrument or the operator's finger, the lipoma is "shelled-out" of the surrounding tissue. The resulting cavity should be closed before approximating skin edges to avoid the development of seroma or hematoma.

4. Caution must be exercised in removal of very superficial lipomas, lest the excision process cause compromise to skin vasculature.

5. Some lipomas are deeper than they appear to be—particularly those of the neck and back. They may originate and/or extend beneath fascia and deep into muscles, making removal more complex.

> **WARNING**
>
> **Subcutaneous lipoma excision is simple, but deeper extension through fascia and muscle calls for more extensive surgical technique and expertise.**

Medication
There is no drug treatment for lipoma.
Diet
No dietary intervention has been shown to affect lipoma, either in growth or in regression.

Activity

Minimizing skin trauma would seem prudent but impractical.

Patient Education

1. Give reassurance as to the benign nature of the disorder.

2. Because most lipomas are multiple, educate the patient to recognize lipomas.

Key Treatment

- Reassurance

- Excision/enucleation

- Liposuction

Follow-Up

1. Once removed, lipomas tend not to recur—unless excision is incomplete.

2. Follow-up is limited to appropriate postoperative local wound care.

3. Complications of lipoma are limited to the mode of removal—wound infection, hematoma, seroma, wound dehiscence.

Bibliography

Digregario F, et al: Pleomorphic lipoma. Case reports and review of the literature. J Dermatol Surg Oncol 1992;18(3):197–202.

Molver W, Price MB: Management of complications associated with an excision of a lipoma from the ankle. J Am Podiatr Med Assoc 1992;82(7):388–391.

Mrozak K, et al: Chromosome breakpoints in lipogenic tumors. Cancer Res 1993;53(7):1670–1675.

Rowley JD: Principles of molecular cell biology of cancer. *In* DeVita VT, et al (eds): Cancer Principles and Practice of Oncology, 4th ed, vol 1. Philadelphia, JB Lippincott, 1993, pp 78–79.

Shelley WB, Shelley ED (eds): Advanced Dermatologic Diagnosis. Philadelphia, WB Saunders, 1992, pp 839–841.

Procedure | **EXCISION OF A SEBACEOUS (EPIDERMAL) CYST** | *John W. Ely*

Indications

1. Unsightly or bothersome
2. Recurrent infections or inflammation
3. Increasing size
4. Foul-smelling discharge
5. Pain or tenderness

Contraindications

1. Acute inflammation (requires incision and drainage, if fluctuant, followed by excision after inflammation has resolved)
2. Bleeding disorder

Preparation

1. Obtain informed consent.
2. Assemble equipment.
3. Prepare container for pathology specimen.

Equipment

1. Small procedure tray
   a. 4 × 4 gauze sponges
   b. Small curved scissors (Metzenbaum or iris scissors)
   c. Scalpel handle and No. 15 blade
   d. Small curved hemostats (2)
   e. Needle holder
   f. Small-toothed (Adson) forceps
   g. Fenestrated sterile drape
2. Povidone-iodine swabs
3. Syringe (6 cc) and needles (20- and 27- or 30-gauge)
4. Sterile gloves
5. Surgical masks
6. Face shield or goggles (universal precautions for HIV)
7. Lidocaine, 1% (with epinephrine unless contraindicated)
8. Suture, 3-0 or 4-0 absorbable (chromic, Dexon), 4-0 or 5-0 nylon
9. Single-tooth skin hooks (2)
10. Specimen bottle with formalin
11. Dressing materials (Telfa, 2 × 2 gauze sponges, tincture of benzoin, 1-inch paper tape)

Anesthesia

1. 1% lidocaine (with epinephrine unless contraindicated)
2. Use lidocaine *without* epinephrine in "end circulation" areas such as fingers, toes, ears, nose, and penis.
3. Do not use more than 20 ml of 1% lidocaine.

Precautions

1. Patients should be asked about allergy to local anesthetics, iodine, and tape.
2. Be certain that adequate resuscitation equipment is available.

WARNING

A common error is to rupture the cyst in the mistaken belief that sebaceous cysts are *subcutaneous* structures. Sebaceous cysts are *intradermal* structures and the incision must be very superficial in the region directly over the cyst.

Technique

1. Prepare the skin with povidone-iodine and apply a sterile fenestrated drape.
2. Inject 1% lidocaine (with epinephrine unless contraindicated) using a 27- or 30-gauge needle. Inject the anesthetic so that it dissects the cyst away from the surrounding tissue.

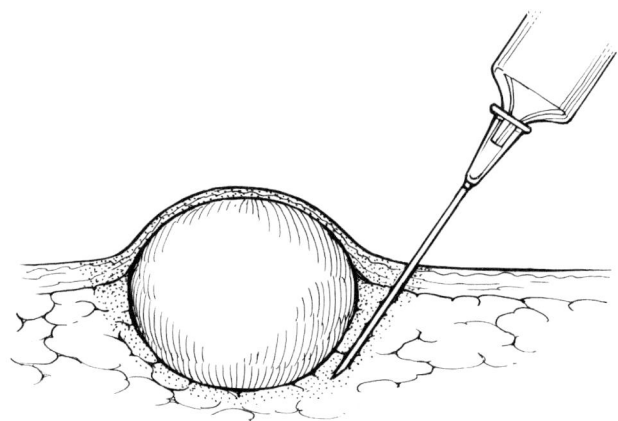

Do not inject into the cyst itself.

3. Make an elliptical incision that surrounds the central opening and is slightly longer than the diameter of the cyst.

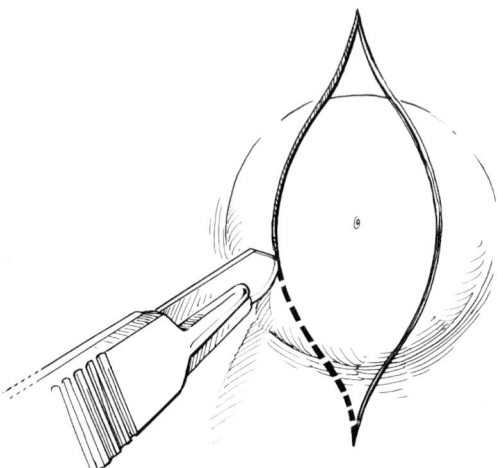

Make the incision parallel to the skin lines.

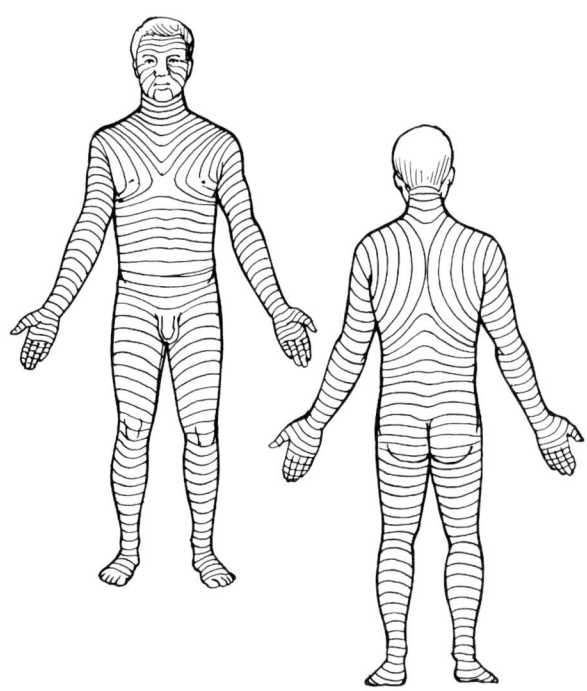

4. Incise the skin very superficially when directly over the cyst. The easiest way to avoid rupturing the cyst is to include, with the cyst, an ellipse of skin around the central opening where the skin is most adherent to the cyst wall.

5. Dissect into the subcutaneous tissue at the ends of the incision where the cyst is not as close to the

surface. Grasp one corner of the skin that is to be removed with the cyst and apply upward traction. Use sharp and blunt dissection to carefully locate the fragile cyst wall.

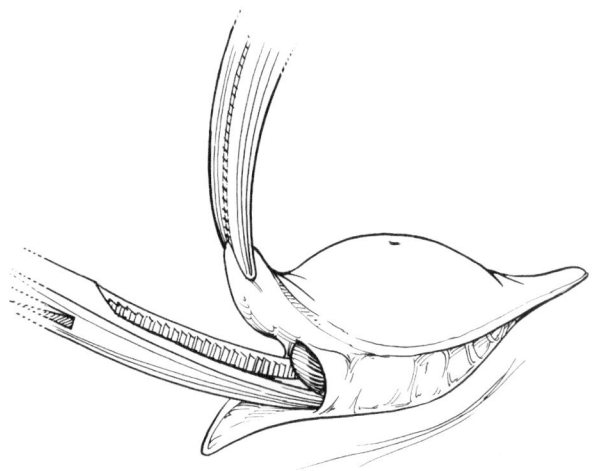

6. Develop a plane between the cyst wall and the surrounding tissue. This dissection is best accomplished by carefully spreading a hemostat or small curved scissors. Use the scissors to cut tissue adherent to the cyst wall.

7. If the cyst ruptures, remove as much keratinous material as possible. Then remove the entire cyst wall using a toothed forceps and scissors. If part of the wall remains, a new cyst may form.

8. Continue the dissection until the cyst is completely free of the underlying tissues, and send it for pathologic examination.

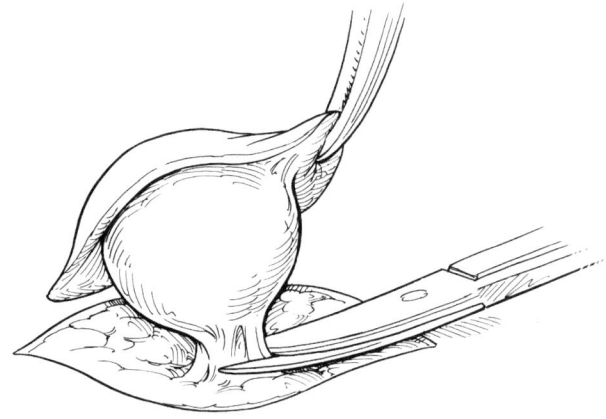

9. Obtain hemostasis with pressure, cautery, or suture ligation if necessary.

10. If the cyst was large, eliminate the dead space by approximating the subcutaneous tissue with absorbable sutures.

11. Close the skin with interrupted nylon sutures.

12. Apply a dressing.

Follow-Up

1. Instruct the patient to keep the wound covered and dry for at least 24 hours.

2. Explain the signs of wound infection to the patient.

3. Remove the sutures after 7 days. Sutures in the back or the extensor surface of joints should remain for 12 to 14 days and sterile adhesive strips applied after removal, because such wounds are prone to dehiscence.

Bibliography

English GM: Ear, nose, throat and sinuses. *In* Hill GJ (ed): Outpatient Surgery, 3rd ed. Philadelphia, WB Saunders, 1988.

Goldstein BG, Goldstein AO: Practical Dermatology. St. Louis, Mosby-Year Book, 1992, pp 34–38.

Goodnight JE: Tumors. *In* Wolcott MW (ed): Ambulatory Surgery and the Basics of Emergency Surgical Care, 2nd ed. Philadelphia, JB Lippincott, 1988.

McGowan GJ: Removing a skin cyst. *In* Driscoll CE, Rakel RE (eds): Procedures for Your Practice, 2nd ed. Los Angeles: Practice Management Information Corporation, 1991.

Schultz B, McKinney, P: Office Practice of Skin Surgery. Philadelphia, WB Saunders, 1985, pp 137–141.

Procedure | PERCUTANEOUS INCISION AND DRAINAGE OF ABSCESS

Charleen Isé

Definition: Abscess: a collection of purulent material in a circumscribed closed cavity. The treatment objective is to create an open wound that will drain infected fluid, devitalized tissue, or foreign body and will heal by secondary intent.

Indications

1. An abscess that is not healing spontaneously or shows clinical worsening (enlargement, cellulitis, lymphangitis, systemic symptoms)
2. The timing is correct: a "ripe" abscess is one that is localized, fluctuant, tender, erythematous; the abscess needs to be ripe for best results
3. The area is reachable percutaneously.
4. There is failure of conservative therapy (heat, antibiotics).

Contraindications

1. Absolute
   a. Location is such that specialist referral is indicated
   b. Lack of patient consent
   c. Incorrect diagnosis (e.g., herpetic whitlow)
2. Relative
   a. Not yet "ripe," not localized
   b. Coagulopathy
   c. Immunosupression
   d. Severe underlying medical problems requiring attention first

Preparation

1. Appropriate history and physical, including allergy
2. Informed consent items to mention should include allergic reaction to local anesthetic leading to death and scarring, bleeding, infection, poor results, no results.

Equipment

1. On a minor surgical tray
   a. Sterile drape
   b. Hemostat, plain forceps, surgical scissors
   c. Culturette aerobic and anaerobic
   d. Iodoform gauze packing 1/4 and 1/2 inch or plain
   e. Local anesthetic
   f. Dressings 4 × 4 inch gauze and adhesive tape
   g. Irrigation solution; saline
   h. Needles: 18 gauge for aspiration and irrigation, 25 to 27 gauge for anesthesia
   i. Syringe 6 cc injection, 25 cc for irrigation
   j. Scalpel blade: No. 11 pointed
   k. Antiseptic cleanser of skin: Povidone-iodine (Betadine) solution, 70% ethyl alcohol, hexachlorophene (pHisoHex)
2. Sterile gloves, protective eye gear and clothing when appropriate

Anesthesia

1. Topical: Ethyl chloride spray: note that it is flammable and not to be used with cautery
2. Local: dosages should not exceed maximal allowable for size of patient
   a. 1% lidocaine with epinephrine
   b. 1% procaine (Novocaine) for amide allergy
   c. 0.25% bupivacaine (Marcaine) for longer duration of analgesia
   d. Add 8.4% sodium bicarbonate into same syringe as anesthetic in a 1:10 dilution to decrease pain of injection by increasing pH of anesthetic.
3. Oral: sodium pentobarbital 100 mg or diazepam 5 to 10 mg or meperidine hydrochloride 100 mg 1 hour before procedure
4. Intravenous and general anesthetic is generally not needed except for very large abscesses (perirectal), or very uncooperative patients (young children). Physicians must follow governmental regulations regarding conscious sedation.

Precautions

1. Use sterile technique to avoid contamination.
2. Avoid squeezing as may rarely lead to bacteremia.
3. Make incision large enough so it will stay open and abscess does not recur.

Technique (Under Local Anesthesia)

1. Place patient in a comfortable position with area well exposed.
2. Clean area with antiseptic agent and allow to dry.
3. Drape as needed.
4. Infiltrate area subcutaneously with local anesthetic where incision is to be made.

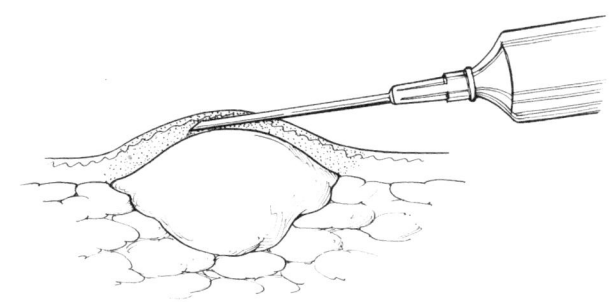

5. Following skin tension lines (see Procedure of Excision of Sebaceous Cyst), make stab incision and extend down to pus cavity.

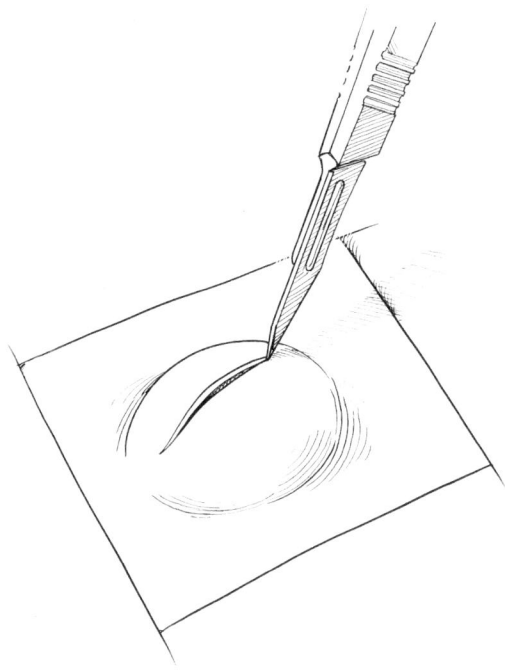

6. Extend incision enough to allow full drainage, widening as necessary.

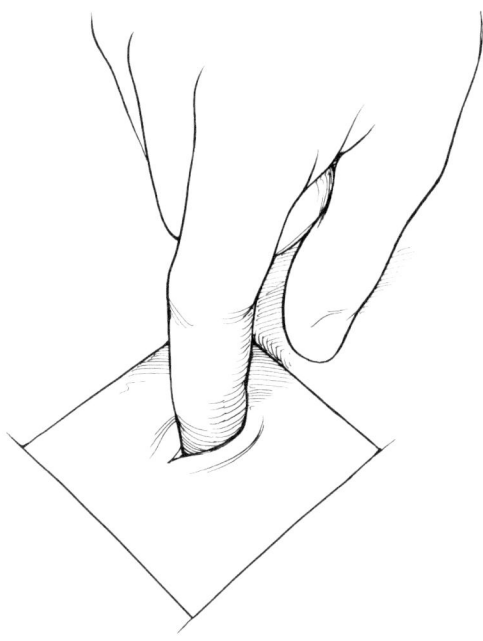

9. Irrigate cavity, especially if foreign material is present.

10. Hemostasis with packing or pressure; cautery is rarely necessary.

11. Insert iodoform gauze if indicated and pack lightly, leaving one end outside of skin acting as a wick.

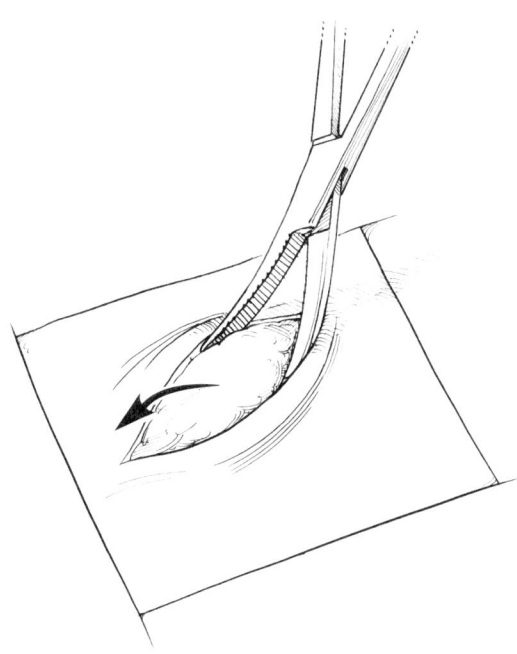

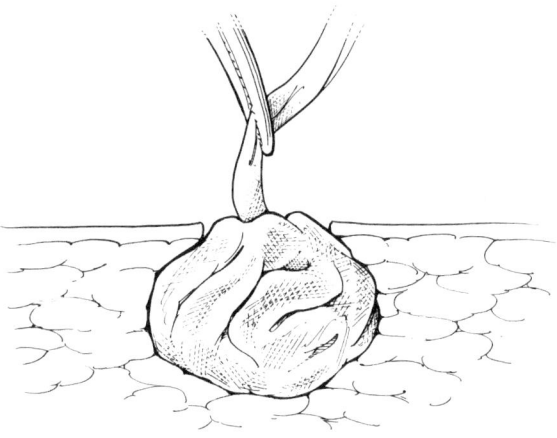

12. Apply sterile dressing.

Follow-Up

1. Elevate area if possible.

2. Apply heat: water soaks for 20 min four times daily for 5 to 7 days

3. Expect area to heal slowly by secondary intent over the next 5 to 7 days.

4. Antibiotics for surrounding cellulitis, lymphangitis, systemic symptoms

7. If desired, take culture (can also irrigate with saline and aspirate for culture).

8. Break adhesions/loculations within abscess cavity with gloved finger or blunt instrument.

5. Follow-up visit can be in 1 to 3 days but sooner for problems.
6. If packing used, expect to change daily.

B Bibliography

Hill, GJ: Outpatient Surgery, 3rd ed. Philadelphia, WB Saunders, 1988, pp 80–82.

Lawrence, CM, Cox, NH: Physical Signs in Dermatology: Color Atlas and Text. London, Mosby-Year Book Europe Limited, 1993; p 221

Mayhew, E, Rodgers, A: Basic Procedures in Family Practice: An Illustrated Manual. Bethany, CT: Fleschner Publishing Co., 1984, pp 1–5.

Micromedex Inc, Local Anesthetic Buffering Efficacy and Stability. Vol 81, 1994.

Pories, WJ, TFT, Office Surgery For Family Physicians. Boston, Butterworth Publishers, 1985, pp 48–49.

272 Hair Disorders

Joan B. Martin

Male Androgenic Baldness

Etiology
1. Inherited condition that is either autosomal dominant or polygenetic
2. Thought to be the result of androgen effects in genetically predetermined individuals.

Symptoms
Hair loss is the only symptom. Loss of hair is premature and accelerated over that of the normal aging process.

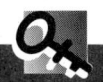
Key Symptom
- Hair loss

Clinical Findings
1. Loss of hair generally occurs first in the temporofrontal region and then the frontal region and vertex. Coarse terminal hairs are replaced with fine vellus hairs.
2. Not associated with any disease, nor does it cause scarring or inflammation

Key Signs
- Pattern of baldness
- Absence of associated disease

Laboratory Tests
If accompanied by signs of virilization, endocrine workup is warranted. In women with accompanying hirsutism, do serum testosterone and dehydroepiandrosterone sulfate levels.

Differential Diagnosis
Can be differentiated from other causes of alopecia by typical pattern and lack of scarring or inflammation; other nonscarring causes of alopecia that may have similarities include
1. Telogen effluvium: Physiologic stress converts hairs to inactive telogen phase, and then they are shed. Diffuse loss can occur rapidly after childbirth, weight loss, illness, drug use, or stress.
2. Drugs: antimitotic agents, heparin, indomethacin, lithium, nitrofurantoin, propranolol, allopurinol
3. Endocrine disorders: Hypothyroidism and hyperthyroidism may cause diffuse thinning of hair.
4. Iron deficiency: diffuse thinning

Treatment
1. Minoxidil
2. Hair transplants
3. Scalp reduction and flaps

Medication
Minoxidil (Rogaine), 2% solution: 1 cc applied to affected areas of dry scalp twice daily. Best for those under age 40 with less than 5 years of hair loss. Requires a minimum of 4 months to show effects, usually 8 to 12 months. Must be used continuously or patient returns to untreated state.

Diet
No effect
Activity
No effect
Patient Education
1. There is no permanent and safe method to stop or reverse male androgenic baldness.
2. Multiple options exist for the patient who chooses to combat this condition. Physician referral to reputable transplantation or graft surgeons is important if requested.

Key Treatment
Drug of Choice
- Minoxidil in selected patients

Follow-Up
Monitor patients on minoxidil for tachycardia, fluid retention, or other systemic effects.

Alopecia Areata

Etiology
1. Uncertain etiology, possibly autoimmune. No proven relationship to stressful events
2. May be associated with atopy, vitiligo, pernicious anemia, thyroiditis, Addison's disease, systemic lupus erythematosus (SLE), ulcerative colitis, and Down syndrome

Symptoms
1. Asymptomatic except for hair loss. Hair loss occurs rapidly.
2. Spontaneous remissions and exacerbations occur.
3. Most commonly occurs under 25 years of age.

981

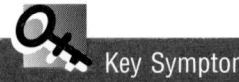

Key Symptom

• Rapid hair loss

Clinical Findings

1. Hair loss initially patchy. Usually occurs in the scalp but may appear in eyebrows, beard, or elsewhere on the body. May progress to include all the scalp (alopecia areata totalis) or entire body (universalis)

2. Hair loss is total within a sharply defined area that is usually round. When the hair loss process is completed, the skin appears smooth, pale, and completely bald. No scarring or inflammation occurs, though early lesions may have mild erythema and tenderness.

3. Nail changes may be present: pitting and longitudinal striations.

4. "Exclamation point" hairs may be found at the margins of early lesions; they have a clubbed bulb, narrow base, and normal upper shaft.

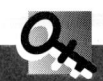

Key Sign

• Rapid hair loss in circumscribed areas

Laboratory Tests

Skin biopsy if any question of diagnosis. Syphilis serology, CBC, thyroid profile

Differential Diagnosis

1. Begins in circumscribed areas and can differentiate from those conditions which cause general thinning.

2. At times difficult to differentiate from cicatricial (scarring) forms of alopecia in their early stages.

   a. Discoid lupus erythematosus usually has scaling and atrophy and occurs in patches.

   b. Scleroderma or morphea produces linear scars.

   c. Lichen planus: Follicular papules occur with inflammation.

   d. Physical/chemical agents: burns, mechanical trauma, radiodermatitis

   e. Neoplasms: metastatic disease or cutaneous neoplasms

   f. Fungus: scaling, advancing border, boggy

   g. Secondary syphilis: "moth-eaten" appearance

   h. Iron deficiency: diffuse thinning

   i. Hypothyroidism: diffuse thinning

   j. Trichotillomania: patchy

Treatment

1. No curative treatment

2. Medications may be of value in limited disease.

3. Psoralen with ultraviolet A light (PUVA) therapy: methoxsalen in combination with long-wave ultraviolet light. Moderately effective, but high relapse rate.

4. Surgical methods not useful.

5. Wigs are an important therapeutic modality; prescribe as "hair prosthesis" for insurance coverage.

Medication

1. Intralesional steroids: local injection of triamcinolone acetonide, 2.5 to 10 mg/ml, may be repeated every 4 weeks but may cause skin atrophy. Does not alter the course of the disease. Use in patients with a few small areas to be treated who request treatment due to anxiety or cosmetic need.

2. Systemic steroids: prednisone, 20 to 40 mg/day. Not recommended due to serious side effects and because disease tends to recur when treatment is stopped.

3. Minoxidil (Rogaine), 2% solution: 1 cc applied to dry scalp twice daily. Cosmetically acceptable results in 10 to 30 per cent. Does not alter the course of the disease.

4. Squaric acid dibutylester or anthralin is used topically to induce contact dermatitis or irritant dermatitis. Patient should be referred to a physician familiar with treatment; moderately effective.

5. Immunomodulators such as inosiplex, topical cyclosporine, and topical nitrogen mustard have been used with some success.

Diet

No recommendations

Activity

No recommendations

Patient Education

1. No universally effective treatment

2. Prognosis is excellent in cases of limited disease. Prognosis is poor in totalis and universalis.

3. New hair may grow back white or of finer texture.

4. Regrowth generally occurs spontaneously within months to 3 years. Recurrences are common.

5. Refer for information and support groups to the National Alopecia Areata Foundation, 714 C Street, Suite 216, San Rafael CA 94901; phone: 415-383-3444.

Key Treatment

Drug of Choice

• Intralesional triamcinolone

Alternative Drug

• Minoxidil

Follow-Up

As required by treatment choice

Bibliography

Burke KE: Hair loss: What causes it and what can be done about it. Postgrad Med 1989;85(6):52–58.

Habif TP: Clinical Dermatology, 2d ed. St Louis, CV Mosby, 1990, pp 598–615.

Nielsen TA, Reichel M: Alopecia: Diagnosis and Management. Am Fam Physician 1995;5(6):1513–1522.

Rosenfield RL, Luck AW: Acne, hirsutism, and alopecia in adolescent girls: Clinical expressions of androgen excess. Endocrinol Metab Clin North Am 1993;22(3):507–532.

Sawaya ME: Biochemical mechanisms regulating human hair growth. Skin Pharmacol 1994;7(1-2):5–7.

Tosi A, Misciali C, Piraccini BM, et al: Drug-induced hair loss and hair growth: Incidence, management and avoidance. Drug Safety 1994;10(40):310–317.

273 Diseases of the Nails

Michael P. Temporal

Onychomycosis

Etiology

This common nail infection, which affects 15 to 25 per cent of the population, is a fungal infection caused by dermatophytes (*Trichophyton, Microsporum* species) or *Candida.*

Symptoms

Usually there are no symptoms, but there may be tenderness and pain from pressure on a thickened nail bed. More commonly it presents as an unsightly nail.

Clinical Findings

The disease may begin anywhere on the nail bed. The initial site of invasion is associated with thickening and discoloration of the nail surface. The nail develops discoloration, erosion, and pitting and has a chalky, dull appearance with yellow-white crumbling debris.

Key Signs

- Thickened nail
- Discolored nail

Laboratory Tests

A 10% KOH preparation confirms hyphae typical of *Trichophyton* infection. Budding or microspores also can be seen. Definitive diagnosis is obtained by culture of nail and debris on Sabouraud's agar.

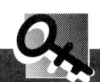

Key Tests

- KOH prep
- Culture

Differential Diagnosis

This nail infection must be distinguished from psoriasis, which has more pitting of nail, periungual inflammation, and typical skin manifestations. Periungual redness and inflammation can be associated with candidal infection, but bacterial infection should be ruled out.

Treatment

Therapy is plagued by a prolonged treatment course and frequent (5 to 20 per cent) recurrence. Treatment of hand onychomycosis is more satisfactory than that of the foot.

1. Topical antifungal agents: These can provide temporary benefit, but their use as sole treatment should be discouraged; usually they are not able to penetrate nail matrix unless the nail is removed.
2. Systemic therapy: mainstay of treatment

   a. Griseofulvin (Grisactin, Gris-PEG, Fulvicin), 750 mg to 1.0 gm microsize (660 to 750 mg ultramicrosize) per day in divided doses: The typical duration of treatment 6 to 12 months for the hand and up to 18 months for the foot. Initial monitoring for neutropenia and alteration of liver function is important.

   b. Ketoconazole (Nizoral): This drug can be used if griseofulvin fails as it has broader antifungal coverage. The dose, 200 mg/day, must be closely supervised as hepatotoxicity has been reported.

   c. Itraconazole (Sporanox): Initial success has been reported at 200 mg/day for 3 to 6 months with fewer side effects than ketoconazole. Pulse therapy of 200 mg b.i.d. for 1 week every month for 3 to 4 months may be tried. Do not give with terfenadine (Seldane).

   d. Terbinafine (Lamisil): This agent will soon be available in the United States as oral preparation. Given at a dose of 250 mg/day for 12 weeks, it has shown a high rate of clinical cure.

3. Nail avulsion: Removal of the nail in severe infection may allow treatment of the nail matrix with a topical agent. This can be accomplished by topical application of 30% salicyclic acid, 40% urea, or 50% potassium iodide applied for 1 week to soften the nail. Alternatively, the nail can be surgically removed.

Patient Education

Tolerating the condition may be preferred to treatment. Good hygiene, comfortable nonbinding shoes, and avoidance of trauma to the nail can aid in prevention. Women may choose to cover nails with enamel rather than treat.

Key Treatment

- Griseofulvin
- Ketoconazole
- Itraconazole

Onychocryptosis (Ingrown Toenail)

Etiology

Most commonly affecting the great toenail, this condition is characterized by a free nail edge penetrating soft tissue of nail fold.

Symptoms

Early presentation is not associated with pain, but as nail penetration progresses it causes a foreign body reaction with swelling and pain. Local skin infection may be noted.

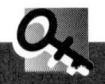

Key Symptoms

- Pain
- Local skin infection

Clinical Findings

The nail edge penetrates the overlying nail skin fold with granulation tissue formation and causes a foreign body reaction—swelling, redness, hyperhidrosis. A progressive case can be exquisitely painful and associated with seropurulent discharge and fetid odor.

Key Signs

- Swelling
- Redness
- Hyperhidrosis

Differential Diagnosis

The ingrown toenail should be differentiated from paronychia (local abscess), trauma (by history and associated subungual hematoma), subungual exostosis (visible on radiograph), and globus tumor of subungual or periungual surface (not associated with nail plate deformity and very tender). Accompanying skin reaction must be differentiated from a squamous cell carcinoma.

Treatment

Removal of offending nail edge is best done with partial onychectomy (see Ingrown Toenail Procedure) and removal of granulation tissue. Early ingrown nails may be treated with local nail edge elevation with cotton and foot soaks for 20 to 30 minutes t.i.d. Oral antibiotics may be indicated for associated cellulitis, such as amoxicillin, 500 mg t.i.d., cephalexin, 500 mg b.i.d., erythromycin, 500 mg q.i.d. for 1 week.

Patient Education

Prevention is key. Proper nail cutting habits should be reviewed, straight across toenail rather than rounded as is done for fingernail. Proper shoes that are nonbinding should be worn, as well as socks and hose that discourage hyperhidrosis.

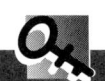

Key Treatment

- Partial onychectomy

Brittle Nails

Etiology

An acquired condition common in the elderly, owing to an alteration in the nail plate or matrix

Symptoms

Dry, irregular nails that feel rough. Unlike onychomycosis, thickening and separation of nail from nail bed usually are not seen.

Clinical Findings

Dehydrated nail with excessive longitudinal ridging and horizontal layering of the distal nail plate and a rough, irregular nail edge

Key Symptoms and Signs

- Dry, irregular nails with rough, irregular nail edge

Differential Diagnosis

This condition should be distinguished from onychomycosis, and may be associated with systemic disease (hyper- and hypothyroidism) and the use of cosmetics (especially frequent application and removal of nail enamels and cuticle removers).

Treatment

Rehydration of the nail can be initiated with foot soaks in lukewarm water at bedtime, followed by application of a moisturizer such as lactic acid lotion, mineral oil, or urea cream. Oral and topical gelatin has been suggested but does not penetrate nail plate. Although the frequent application and removal of nail enamel contributes to this condition, use only once per week can still slow evaporation of water from the nail plate.

Key Treatment

- Rehydration by means of foot soaks
- Application of moisturizer

Bibliography

Bergus CE, Johnson JS: Superficial tinea infections. Am Family Phys 1993;48:259–268.

Cohen PR, Scher RK: Geriatric nail disorders: Diagnosis and treatment. J Am Acad Dermatol 1992;26:521–531.

Lesher J, Levine N, Treadwell P: Fungal skin infections: Common but stubborn. Patient Care 1994;28:16–44.

Midgeley G: Mycology of nail disorders. J Am Derm Assoc 1994;31:568–574.

Pierard GE, et al: Treatment of onychomycosis: Traditional approaches. J Am Acad Dermatol 1993;29:S41–S45.

Procedure INGROWN TOENAIL

Robert L. Bass

Indications
1. Stage I: Erythema and swelling of lateral nail fold
2. Stage II: Infection with edema and drainage
3. Stage III: Formation of granulation tissue with hypertrophy of lateral nail fold

Preparation
Soaks and antibiotics for acute infection

Equipment
1. Straight mosquito hemostat
2. Straight scissors
3. Septal elevator
4. ⅜-inch Penrose drain or sterilized rubberband
5. Dermal curette
6. Needle holder
7. Fresh phenol solution
8. Electrofulgurator unit with insulated probe
9. No. 15 bladed scalpel

Anesthesia
1. 1–2% lidocaine, 2 ml for field block
2. 1% Marcaine, 1–1.5 ml for wing block with or without lidocaine

May be used to prolong postoperative pain relief.

Precautions
1. Rule out osteomyelitis by radiography of infected digits
2. Monitor for circulatory embarrassment and infection in
   a. Diabetes mellitus
   b. Immunocompromised patients
   c. Patients with circulatory disease

Technique

1. Apply field block of toe and wait 10 minutes to ensure anesthesia. Infected ingrown toenails are tender; time may be needed for good anesthesia.

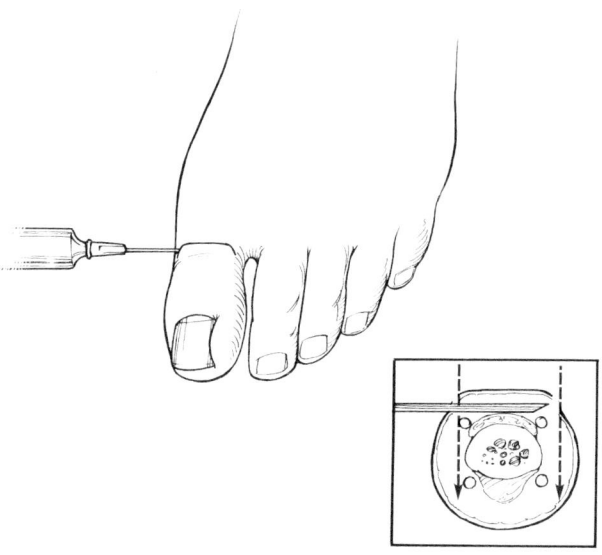

2. Prepare skin with povidone-iodine or Hibiclens.
3. Apply few layers of gauze to base of toe to protect digital neurovascular bundles, followed by Penrose tourniquet, held with hemostat to ensure bloodless field.
4. Free portion of nail plate from nail bed and matrix with septal elevator or straight mosquito hemostat. Plan to remove at least ⅛ to ¼ inch of nail.

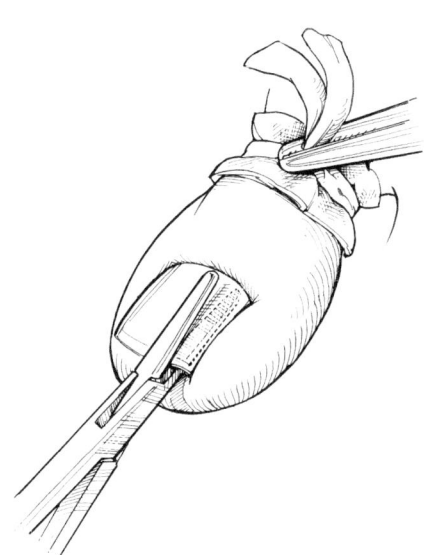

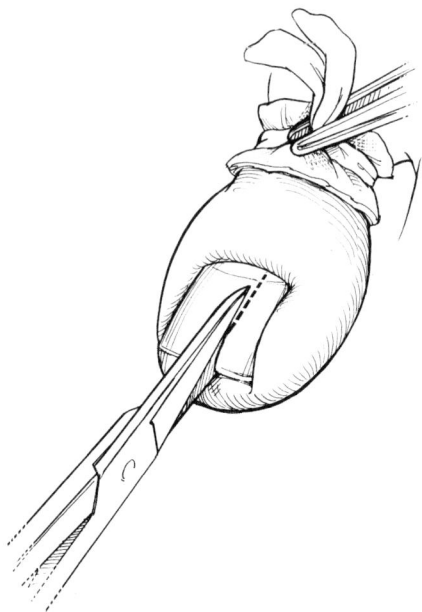

5. Grasp spicule with hemostat and avulse by rotation toward main nail plate.
6. Curette proximal nail matrix and any granulation tissue present.
7. *Phenol method*: Protect surrounding skin with antibiotic ointment. Apply fresh phenol (88% carbolic acid) to base of nail to ablate any remaining matrix and assist in hemostasis. Use three soaked applicator sticks for 1 minute each (with pressure).

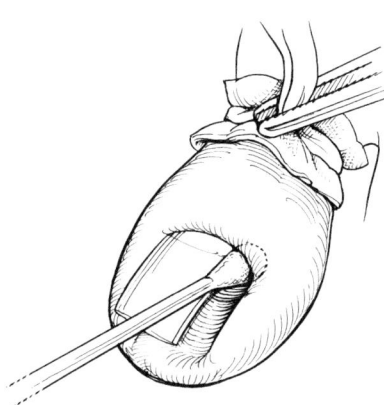

8. Electrocautery of matrix with insulated probe is a good alternative.

9. Remove hypertrophic nail fold by wedge excision if indicated, and suture skin edge to remaining nail plate.

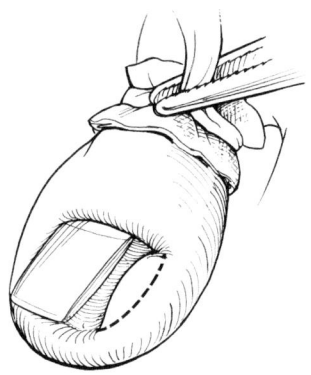

Follow-Up

1. Remove tourniquet, apply antibiotic ointment to wound followed by a nonadherent pressure dressing.
2. Elevate foot and apply ice initially for bleeding and pain.
3. Prescribe acetaminophen with codeine for first 2 to 3 days.
4. First redressing in 4 to 7 days, or as needed for bleeding
5. Serous drainage from phenol treatment is to be expected
6. Healing usually complete in 4 weeks

WARNING

Significant numbers of spicule regrowth have been reported in the literature, regardless of the method of nail removal, often requiring a second lesser procedure.

B **Bibliography**

Daniel CR III: Basic nail plate avulsion. J Dermatol Surg Oncol 1992;18:685–688.

Leahy AL, Timon CI, Craig A, Stephens RB: Ingrowing toenails: improving treatment. Surgery 1990;107:566–567.

Murtagh J: Patient education. Ingrowing toenails. Aust Fam Physician 1993;22(2):206.

Siegle RJ, Stewart R: Recalcitrant ingrowing nails: surgical approaches. J Dermatol Surg Oncol 1992;18:744–752.

VanDerHam AC, Hackeng CAH, Tik Ien Yo: The treatment of ingrowing toenails. J Bone Joint Surg (Br) 1990;72–B:507–509.

274 Stasis Ulcer

David E. Trachtenbarg

Etiology

Underlying causes of stasis ulcers include venous insufficiency, incompetence of the deep vein valves, and deep vein thrombosis.

Symptoms

1. Patients usually present with an ulcer on the lower leg that will not heal in the "gaiter area" between the knee and the foot.
2. The ulcer is usually not painful unless infected.
3. There is often associated aching and swelling of the lower leg aggravated by prolonged standing.
4. There may be a previous history of trauma or vascular surgery or a history of deep vein thrombosis, venous valvular incompetence, or varicosities.

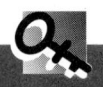

Key Symptom

- Painless ulceration of lower leg

Clinical Findings

1. Stage of ulcer
   a. Stage I: erythema not resolving within 30 minutes of pressure relief with intact epidermis
   b. Stage II: partial-thickness ulcer not extending through the dermis
   c. Stage III: full-thickness ulcer extending through the dermis
   d. Stage IV: ulcer extending through subcutaneous tissue to fascia, muscle, or bone. Staging cannot be confirmed unless the wound base is visible.
2. Untreated ulcers usually have a purulent exudate. There may be pain or tenderness in the wound or surrounding tissue.
3. The exudate is usually serosanguineous or purulent; a fecal odor is a sign of secondary infection.
4. The surrounding skin often has edema, brownish discoloration, or dermatitis. Varicosities are usually present.
5. Watch for signs of significant local or systemic infection, including marked surrounding erythema, copious purulent exudate, and fever.

Key Signs

- An ulcer in the "gaiter area" above the foot and below the knee
- Edema and brownish discoloration of surrounding skin

Laboratory Tests

1. Cultures usually show polymicrobial flora, and bacteria isolated do not correlate with clinical response.
   a. Perform a culture if a systemic infection or significant surrounding cellulitis is suspected.
   b. Cultures should be done following cleansing of the wound base.
2. Consider the possibility of underlying osteomyelitis for stage III and IV ulcers
3. Venous Doppler testing is useful for selected patients, particularly if surgery is contemplated.

Key Tests

- Cultures are generally not helpful.
- Venous Doppler testing in selected patients

Differential Diagnosis

1. The diagnosis is usually straightforward.
2. Consider a mixed ulcer or an arterial ulcer if there is arterial peripheral vascular disease.

> **WARNING**
>
> **Consider biopsy if the ulcer is not healing or there are other signs of disease to rule out carcinoma.**

Treatment

1. Necrotic tissue must be removed to promote healing.
   a. Wet-to-dry dressings are often the most cost-effective way of doing this.
   b. Other options include
      (1) Transparent dressings that enhance leukocyte migration and cause autolysis for shallow wounds (Op-Site, Tegaderm)
      (2) Enzymatic debridement (Travase, Elase, Santyl, Biozyme C)
      (3) Surgical debridement for wounds with a large amount of necrotic tissue
2. Maintain a moist environment. Options include the following:
   a. Saline dressings are the most cost-effective for most patients.
   b. Hydrocolloid dressings (Comfeel, DuoDERM) and transparent dressings (Op-Site, Tegaderm) are useful for selected patients because they may be left in place for several days.

c. Remove excess wound exudate by thorough cleansing at each dressing change.

(1) The solution of choice is normal saline, which does not destroy tissue.

(2) Betadine, hydrogen peroxide, Dakin's solution (potassium hypochlorite), and acetic acid can inhibit wound healing by destroying cells.

d. Hydrocolloid dressings will absorb moderate amounts of exudate (Comfeel, DuoDERM).

3. Eradicate clinical infection.

a. Use systemic antibiotics if cellulitis or systemic infection is present. Common organisms are *Staphylococcus aureus, Streptococcus pyogenes,* and *Pseudomonas aeruginosa.*

b. Topical agents such as silver sulfadiazine (Silvadene) and polymyxin B–bacitracin–neomycin (Neosporin) also may be useful, but topical antibiotics have not consistently been shown to promote wound healing. Watch carefully for signs of sensitization, especially with polymyxin B–bacitracin–neomycin (Neosporin).

4. Eliminate edema (venous compression).

a. Possible choices for venous compression include

(1) Elastic stockings

(2) Zinc oxide bandages (Unna boot); change weekly

(3) Elastic wraps (Ace wrap)

(4) Colloid wrap (DuoDERM); change weekly

b. When using venous compression, monitor patient for circulatory compromise, including swelling, color changes, and temperature changes.

5. Give appropriate nutritional support to provide protein, calories, vitamins, and minerals essential for healing.

6. Maintain adequate circulation and oxygenation to the wound bed. Correct peripheral vascular disease when possible or use an agent such as Trental to improve the circulation if arterial disease is present.

7. Surgery is indicated for selected patients who do not respond to nonsurgical therapy.

Patient Education

1. Keep legs elevated above the heart when lying down.

2. Avoid sitting with the legs crossed.

3. Avoid standing for prolonged periods.

4. Ambulate intermittently throughout the day.

5. Avoid constrictive clothing.

6. Use a moisturizer such as Eucerin or Alpha Keri to keep surrounding skin clean and pliable.

7. Avoid heating pads, hot water bottles, heat lamps, hot solutions, cold solutions, and ice packs to prevent thermal trauma.

8. Reportable symptoms

a. Change in color

b. Change in temperature

c. Pain or other change in sensation

d. Change in drainage or odor

9. Inspect feet and legs daily.

Key Treatment

- Moist wound surface promotes wound healing.

- Venous compression to reduce venous stasis and edema

- Topical treatment of choice for most ulcers is wet-to-dry dressing to remove necrotic tissue followed by moist saline dressings.

Follow-Up

Stasis ulcers heal very slowly. Office visits more often than every 1 to 2 weeks are usually not necessary unless an acute infection is being treated.

Bibliography

Burton CS: Venous ulcers. Am J Surg 1994;167(1A suppl):37S–41S.

Field CK, Kerstein MD: Overview of wound healing in a moist environment. Am J Surg 1994;167(1A suppl):2S–6S.

International Association of Enterostomal Therapy: Standards of care: Dermal wounds: Leg ulcers. J Enterostomal Ther 1988;15(3):102–117.

Leigh IH: Pressure ulcers: Prevalence, etiology, and treatment modalities. Am J Surg 1994;167(1A suppl):25S–30S.

Rowland J: Pressure ulcers: A literature review and a treatment scheme. Aust Fam Physician 1993;22(10):1819–1827.

275 Decubitus Ulcer

David P. Losh

Etiology

1. Pressure over a bony prominence
2. Friction, such as pulling patient across a bed sheet
3. Shear forces, such as partial reclining position
4. Moisture, such as incontinence
5. Contributing factors
   a. Decreased mobility
   b. Decreased sensation
   c. Poor nutrition
   d. Dementia

Symptoms

1. Pain over a bony prominence in stage 1 or 2
2. Relatively pain free in stage 3 or 4

Key Symptom

- Often unnoticed in early stages

Clinical Findings

1. Location: 90 per cent over lower extremities—ischial tuberosities, trochanters, sacrum, heels
2. Clinical staging
   a. Stage 1: Nonblanching erythema lasting over 30 minutes after relief of pressure. Epidermis intact
   b. Stage 2: Partial-thickness skin loss. Extends into but not through the dermis
   c. Stage 3: Full-thickness through the dermis and into subcutaneous tissue. Shallow crater that may include eschar, exudate, infection, necrotic tissue, undermining, or sinus tracts
   d. Stage 4: Deep penetration to fascia or bone

Key Signs

- Erythema
- Exudate
- Ulcer crater
- Necrotic tissue

Laboratory Tests

1. Cultures of ulcer indicated *only* if signs of systemic infection or deep lesions with purulent or foul-smelling drainage
2. Tests for malnutrition
   a. Serum albumin (3.5 gm/dl or lower)
   b. Complete blood count, hemoglobin < 12 gm/dl in men, < 10 gm/dl in women, lymphocytes below 1500/mm^3)
   c. Serum transferrin (< 200 mg/dl)

3. Screening tests for osteomyelitis
   a. White blood cell count ($> 15,000$/mm^3)
   b. Westergren sedimentation rate (> 100 mm/hr)
   c. Plain radiograph (lytic lesions, reactive bone formation, periosteal elevation)

Key Tests

- Serum albumin
- Complete blood count

Differential Diagnosis

1. Venous stasis ulcer—edema, hyperpigmentation, lower extremity
2. Diabetic ulcer—most on forefoot and toes, neurotrophic or ischemic origin
3. Ulceration from arterial insufficiency, resting pain, pale atrophic skin, hair loss, nail dystrophy
4. Ecthyma gangrenosum, *Pseudomonas* infection and neutropenia, gluteal or perineal ulcers
5. Skin cancer—basal cell, squamous cell, other
6. Pyoderma gangrenosum—underlying inflammatory or malignant disease, purple margin
7. Self-induced (factitial) ulcers—underlying psychosocial disorder, geometric, straight margins, only on reachable skin

Treatment

Prevention

1. Identify high-risk patients
   a. Elderly
   b. Recent hospitalization
   c. Immobile
   d. Incontinent
   e. Poor nutrition
   f. Quadriplegia or paraplegia
2. Reduce pressure. Repositioning on side at a 30-degree angle more frequently than every 2 hours. Consider pressure-relief devices.
   a. Special mattresses and overlays
      (1) Static foam mattresses, sheepskin fleeces
      (2) Alternating air pressure pads
   b. Chair cushions, splints, heel protectors, cradle boots
   c. Air-fluidized beds
3. Reduce friction. Use draw sheets for patient transfer.
4. Reduce shearing. Avoid partially reclining bed position.

5. Reduce moisture.

   a. Regular toileting and incontinence treatment

   b. Barrier ointments and absorptive products

Medication and Dressings

1. Debriding methods

   a. Wet-to-damp saline and gauze dressings: used for early debridement, but may cause epithelial damage if allowed to dry.

   b. Enzymatic ointments or creams (Travase, Elase, Santyl, Granulex, Panfil)

   c. Whirlpool soaks

   d. Irrigation, normal saline

   e. Surgical debridement for thick eschars or deep necrotic tissue

2. Lotions, ointments, creams, and topical antibiotics

   a. Emollients aid in good skin care (Eucerine lotion, Keri lotion, others).

   b. Silver sulfadiazine or Neosporin ointment for superficial infections

   c. Avoid antiseptic agents that are toxic to granulation tissue such as chlorhexidine, povidone-iodine, acetic acid, and hydrogen peroxide.

3. Synthetic dressings

   a. Semipermeable transparent film dressings (OpSite, Tegaderm, Bioclusive): best for stage 1 to 3 without heavy exudate.

   b. Hydrocolloid and occlusive dressings (DuoDERM, Restore, Comfeel): best on low- to moderate-exudate wounds. Difficult on areas of irregular contour.

   c. Hydrogels (Vigalon, Geliperm, IntraSite): best on moist, granulating, nonexudative, non–weight-bearing surfaces. Requires daily changes.

   d. Calcium alginate (Kaltostat): for stage 2 to 3 exuding ulcers before re-epithelization. Contraindicated in dry ulcers.

4. Antibiotics: if treating systemic infection or deep purulent lesions, use a broad-spectrum β-lactam antibiotic or combination to cover aerobic and anaerobic organisms. Specific therapy should be guided by culture results from soft-tissue aspirate, blood culture, or bone biopsy.

5. Growth factors: topically applied autologous platelet-derived wound factors. Available in some settings. May increase healing rate in selected chronic ulcers.

Diet

1. Identify signs of malnutrition: nonvolitional weight loss, hypoalbuminemia.

2. Begin nutritional support early. Set realistic treatment goal of at least 35 kcal/kg/day. Use team approach, including nutritionist.

3. Supplement with multivitamin and mineral preparation. Consider vitamin C supplementation, 500 mg twice daily.

Activity

Encourage ambulation, frequent repositioning, and physical therapy if appropriate.

Key Treatment

- Reduce pressure, moisture, shearing, friction
- Use debridement method least damaging to tissue
- Keep well humidified and protected with appropriate dressing

Follow-Up

A preventive regimen and plan of therapeutic interventions should be based on the patient's and family's overall goals and should involve a team including the physician, nurses, nutritionist, and physical and/or occupational therapists.

Bibliography

Bryant RA, Shannon ML, Pieper B, et al: Pressure ulcers. *In* Bryant RA (ed): Acute and Chronic Wounds: Nursing Management. St Louis, Mosby–Year Book, 1992, pp 105–152.

Jeter K, Tintle T: Wound dressings of the nineties: Indications and contraindications. Clin Podiatr Med Surg 1991;8(4):799–816.

Kertesz D, Chow A: Infected pressure and diabetic ulcers. Clin Geriatr Med 1992;8(4):835–852.

Spoelhof GD, Ide K: Pressure ulcers in nursing home patients. Am Fam Physician 1993;47(5):1207–1215.

U.S. Department of Health and Human Services, Public Health Service Agency for Health Care Policy and Research: Pressure Ulcers in Adults: Prediction and Prevention, Clinical Practice Guideline Number 3, May 1992.

276 Scabies

Cynthia M. Pearman

Etiology

1. Scabies is caused by infestation with the mite *Sarcoptes scabiei*. Endemic in many countries, scabies occurs in pandemics in North America in 20- to 30-year cycles. The mite is spread by close contact among family members, sexual contacts, day care centers, and institutional settings. All social levels are affected. Poor hygiene is not a causative factor, although hygiene may affect the extent of the rash. Fomites are unlikely to spread the mite, except in institutional settings (e.g., nursing homes).

2. The adult female mite, barely visible to the naked eye, burrows into the epidermis, where she lives for about 30 days, laying two or three eggs daily. The eggs hatch in 3 to 5 days; the larvae move to the surface, and develop into adults in 10 to 14 days. The new adults breed on the skin surface, and the cycle continues. The incubation period in an affected person is usually 2 to 3 weeks but may be much longer.

3. A hypersensitivity response by the host is probably responsible for much of the clinical findings. Because of prior sensitization, reinfestations will have little or no incubation period; also, symptoms of scabies often persist for weeks after scabecide treatment. Administration of topical or systemic steroids empirically may mask symptoms and confuse the diagnosis (so-called scabies incognito).

Symptoms

1. Extreme pruritus, worse at night
2. Urticaria may occur
3. Scaly skin and crusting in severe cases, especially in those immunocompromised

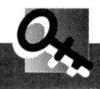

Key Symptom

- Severe pruritus, worse at night

Clinical Findings

1. Typical lesions are inflammatory papules, with raised burrows and tiny vesicles, in a characteristic distribution. The mite may be seen as a tiny dark speck at the end of the burrow.

   a. In normal adults, lesions are usually seen in interdigital spaces, at wrists, elbows, anterior axillary folds, waistline, lower buttocks, the periareolar area in women, and on the genitals in men. The head and face are usually spared in adults but may be involved in tropical climates or in immunocompromised hosts.

   b. In infants, lesions also may be on the scalp, palms, and soles of feet.

2. In the elderly and immunocompromised, a variation called Norwegian (crusted) scabies occurs, with atypical lesions and distribution. In these individuals, the lesions are widespread and crusted, with generalized hyperkeratosis, nail dystrophy, lymphadenopathy, and eosinophilia.

3. A persistent form, nodular scabies, manifests as reddened itchy nodules, often on the male genitalia, waist, and groin. Mites are usually not found in these lesions, which may persist for months.

4. Evidence of secondary bacterial infection may be common, especially in children or in patients with predisposing conditions such as atopic dermatitis.

5. Scabies may be present but overlooked in persons with chronic eczematous dermatoses and should be considered in exacerbations.

6. Scabies is infrequent in African Americans, for uncertain reasons, but when seen will have typical appearance and distribution.

Key Signs

- Inflammatory papules
- Burrows
- Tiny vesicles
- Excoriations
- Typical distribution: interdigital areas, wrists, flexor surfaces, axillae, breasts, penis, skin folds

Laboratory Tests

1. Diagnosis may be made clinically based on a characteristic rash in the appropriate setting, but demonstration of the mite, egg, or mite feces is definitive. The mite or its products can be difficult to find, even with experience.

2. Normal adult hosts may have up to 10 to 20 mites but often less than 10. Best sites for recovery are interdigital areas, hands, wrists, elbows, ankles, feet, and penis.

3. To find a mite, look for a typical burrow. If the mite is visible at the end, it may be lifted out with a sewing needle or injection needle (25 or 26 gauge) that has been moistened with oil (immersion or mineral oil). The mite is placed on a microscope slide, covered with oil, and viewed with scanning (10×) power.

4. Alternatively, the burrow may be scraped vigorously or shaved with a No. 15 scalpel moistened with oil. The material is placed on a slide as outlined above. The mite, egg, or feces (reddish brown) may be visible under 10× magnification.

5. Because the burrows may be few in number and difficult to find, the *burrow ink test* is a useful technique for locating a burrow. To do this, areas of skin likely to have mites, such as finger webs, hands, and wrists, are first painted with blue or black ink (such as fountain pen ink), with attention given to any obvious burrows. The ink is then removed from the surface with alcohol wipes. The ink will seep into burrows and make them readily visible. The burrow can then be scraped or shaved as described above.

6. The diagnosis is sometimes made incidentally on skin biopsy.

Key Tests

- Needle extraction, shaving, or scraping
- Microscopic visualization of mite
- Burrow ink test

Differential Diagnosis

1. Flea bites or other insect infestations
2. Atopic dermatitis
3. Nummular eczema
4. Irritant or contact dermatitis
5. Dermatitis herpetiformis and other autoimmune diseases
6. Lichen planus
7. Folliculitis
8. Syphilis
9. Seborrheic dermatitis
10. Nodular prurigo
11. Pruritic urticarial papules and plaques of pregnancy (PUPPP)
12. Scabies must always be considered as an underlying factor in bacterial skin infections (such as pyoderma or impetigo) or as a complicating factor in eczematous dermatoses (such as atopic dermatitis).

Treatment

1. Scabecides are applied to all areas of skin, traditionally from the neck down. The head and face (sparing eyes, nose, and mouth) should be treated in infants, severe cases, immunocompromised hosts, in warm climates, and in recurrent cases.

   a. Permethrin 5% (Elimite), a synthetic pyrethrin, has become the drug of choice because it is safe and effective even in one treatment. One dose of 30 g or 1 oz of cream will treat one adult. Retreatment is unnecessary unless reinfection occurs, because permethrin kills adults and eggs.

   b. Lindane 1%, or gammabenzene hexachloride (Kwell), was the main treatment before introduction of permethrin. Lindane should not be used in pregnancy or in nursing mothers, infants, or small children, because there have been reports of neurotoxicity, usually from overuse. Recently, concerns have arisen about lindane resistance. Because it is not ovicidal, lindane is usually used as two treatments 1 week apart.

   c. Crotamiton (Eurax) was the preferred treatment for pregnant women and infants before permethrin. It has a higher rate of failure and need for retreatment. It is usually used for two or three successive nights and may be repeated a week later.

   d. Other treatments include sulfur (5% to 15%) in petrolatum and benzyl benzoanate (25%). Both of these, along with lindane, have a significant incidence of irritant or hypersensitivity dermatitis, especially with overuse.

2. Treatment of contacts

   a. All symptomatic family members must be treated concurrently, and most clinicians prefer to treat all household members regardless of symptoms. Extended family and friends should be questioned for symptoms and treated accordingly.

   b. Sexual contacts must be treated, preferably at the same time. Appropriate evaluation for other sexually transmitted diseases (STDs) should be done.

   c. In institutional settings, roommates should be treated, and all caretakers should be treated if symptomatic. Norwegian scabies is a special concern because it is highly contagious owing to large numbers of mites on affected patients.

3. Environmental factors

   a. Underwear, clothing, sheets, and towels used in the 48 hours before treatment must be laundered.

   b. Furniture and other fomites are not a concern because the mite lives up to 48 hours at most away from a human host. Norwegian scabies is the exception, again because of the huge number of mites on the host, which may be transmitted on bed linens and furniture.

4. Symptomatic treatment

   a. Steroids: A midpotency topical steroid, such as triamcinolone 0.1% cream or ointment, is helpful to reduce the symptoms that persist after scabecide treatment. This is usually given in a 2- to 3-week tapered regimen. A lower-potency steroid may be used on the face or in infants. Hydrocortisone 2.5% lotion (Hytone) is useful in widespread rash, since it contains no alcohol. In severe cases or with underlying dermatoses, a tapered course of oral steroids may be needed.

b. Antipruritics: Antihistamines, such as diphenhydramine (Benadryl) or hydroxyzine (Atarax or Vistaril), are helpful, especially at bedtime.

c. Skin moisturizers are useful in winter months or in patients with dry skin or atopic dermatitis. An unscented, alcohol-free type is preferable, such as Eucerin, Moisturel, or Nutraderm.

d. Exfoliatives may be needed in Norwegian scabies because the crust and scale interfere with scabecide effectiveness.

5. Secondary infection

a. Secondary infection with *Staphylococcus* species or *Streptococcus pyogenes* is common in children, in warm climates, in atopic individuals, and in long-standing scabies infestations.

b. Oral antibiotics are indicated unless the secondary infection is minimal and clears with scabecide treatment. Erythromycin, first- or second-generation cephalosporins, or penicillinase-resistant penicillins may be used.

c. The possibility of poststreptococcal glomerulonephritis must be considered in children. In the immunocompromised, secondary infection may lead to septicemia.

Patient Education

1. Persistence of symptoms (bumps and itching) for weeks after treatment must be discussed with instructions for adequate symptomatic treatment. Caution patients not to overuse scabecides: persistent symptoms do not necessarily mean persistent infection.

2. Discuss notification and treatment of all close contacts, including household members, sexual partners, and any symptomatic contacts.

3. Discuss proper use of medications and instructions for linens and clothing.

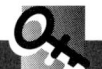

Key Treatment

Drug of Choice	Alternative Drug
• 5% Permethrin (Elimite)	• 1% Lindane (Kwell), crotamiton (Eurax)

Symptomatic

• Topical or systemic steroids

• Antihistamines

• Emollients

Follow-Up

1. It is advisable to see patients again in 2 weeks after treatment. Those with persistent symptoms after 2 weeks should be examined for evidence of persistent infestation (treatment failure) or reinfestation. Many of these will clear with retreatment.

2. If no evidence of persistent infestation (burrows and mites), advise the patient on antipruritics and topical or oral steroids, if not already being used. Review correct use of current medications.

3. Severe or refractory cases or infestations in the immunocompromised or hosts with underlying skin diseases should be followed until clear.

Bibliography

Brodell RT, Helms SE: The scabies preparation. Am Fam Physician 1991;44:505–508.

Burgess I: *Sarcoptes scabiei* and scabies. Adv Parasitol 1994;33:235–292.

Moschella SL, Hurley HJ, eds: Dermatology, 3d ed., vols 1 and 2. Philadelphia, WB Saunders, 1992, pp 200–201, 220, 238, 327, 455, 496, 643, 1002–1003, 1011–1012, 1960–1967, 2199.

Paller AS: Scabies in infants and small children. Semin Dermatol 1993;12(1):3–8.

Sterling GB, Janniger CK, Schwartz RA, et al: Scabies. Am Fam Physician 1992;46:1237–1241.

277 Head, Pubic, and Body Lice

Charles I. Zucker

Etiology

1. Pediculosis, or lice infestation, is caused by two species of Anoplura. Head lice and body lice are subspecies of *Pediculosis humanus. P. humanus capitus* causes head lice, whereas *P. humanus corpora* causes body lice. *Phthirus pubis* is the cause of pubic lice.

2. Nymphs and adult lice feed on human blood. Nits (eggs) are generally found on the hair shafts in the case of head lice and pubic lice. Body lice lay their nits along the seams of clothing.

3. Nymphs and adult lice will die within 48 hours if separated from the host. Nits hatch within 7 to 10 days.

4. Head lice occur most frequently in school-age children or children in day care. Girls are more commonly affected than boys. Crowded conditions with person-to-person contact and sharing of combs, brushes, and hats all contribute to the spread of head lice. Head lice infestation among blacks is rare in the United States. Body lice are prevalent in conditions of poor hygiene such as wartime or homelessness. Pubic lice are spread by sexual contact.

5. There are 6 to 12 million cases of head lice in the United States each year.

6. Body lice have been associated with epidemics of typhus, trench fever, and louse-borne relapsing fever.

Symptoms

1. Intense pruritus is a common symptom in head, body, and pubic lice infestation.

2. Secondary infection from excoriation may occur and cause crusting and scabbing. Secondary infection is particularly common with body lice infestation, which may present with generalized impetigo.

3. Systemic manifestations from secondary infection or immune reaction may include fatigue and low-grade fever.

4. Regional lymphadenopathy can occur from secondary infection or immune reaction.

5. With head lice, the nits are often seen by the patient or family members.

Key Symptoms

- Pruritus
- Excoriation

Clinical Findings

1. Head lice can be diagnosed by the presence of nits along the hair shaft. The nits are cemented to the hair shaft with a chitin bond and therefore cannot be moved. The nit is brown in appearance prior to hatching and white after hatching occurs. Nits and lice tend to be seen predominantly behind the ears and along the back of the neck. The distance the nits are found up the hair shaft is a good measure of how long the infestation has been present. The eggs are laid next to the scalp, and hair grows at about 1 cm per month.

2. Body lice are most readily identified by an examination of the patient's clothing. Nits are usually found hidden in the seams of the clothing.

3. Pubic lice, "crabs," can be identified by nits on the pubic hair. Occasionally, the lice can be seen as yellow-brown or gray specks against the skin. Maculae ceruleae are 1- to 2-cm gray-blue macules that occur with pubic lice and are of uncertain etiology.

Key Signs

Head Lice

- Nits
- Lymphadenopathy

Body Lice

- Nits on clothes
- Lymphadenopathy
- Excoriation

Pubic Lice

- Nits
- Lymphadenopathy
- Maculae ceruleae

Laboratory Tests

1. Nits can be observed with a hand-held magnifying glass or a low-power microscope.

2. Nits fluoresce under Wood's lamp.

3. With pubic lice infestation, strong consideration should be given to testing for other sexually transmitted diseases such as human immunodeficiency virus (HIV), gonorrhea, syphilis, chlamydia, and hepatitis B.

Key Test

- Observation of nits

Differential Diagnosis

1. Diagnosis of head lice and pubic lice is usually clear when nits are observed. The following can be mistaken for nits:

   a. Pilar casts: these can be slid along the hair shaft; nits cannot.

   b. Seborrheic scale: these can be slid along the hair shaft; nits cannot.

   c. Trichomycosis axillaris: an infection of *Corynebacterium tenius* on the axillary hairs. Concretions coat the hairs and are not localized like nits.

   d. Piedra: microscopic examination will show the presence of fungal elements.

   e. Trichonodosis: knotted hair; more common in blacks.

   f. Monilethrix: beads form along hair shaft; no nits present on microscopic examination.

2. Diagnosis of body lice infestation must be made from an examination of the patient's clothes. The rash seen with body lice is nonspecific and caused by the generalized pruritus. This leads to excoriation, often with secondary bacterial infection. The differential would include

   a. Scabies: often present as well; generally involves the hands and feet, areas that are spared by body lice.

   b. Impetigo: examination of clothing would not show nits.

Treatment

1. *Head and pubic lice:* Several options exist for the treatment of head lice and pubic lice. Some are not effective in killing nits and must be repeated in 7 days. The nits of pubic lice are more resistant, and repeat application in 7 days is recommended.

   a. Permethrin (Nix): a synthetic pyrethrin, probably the most effective remedy available. Does not need to be repeated for head lice due to residual killing activity. Permethrin is available without a prescription.

   b. Pyrethrins (Rid, R and C, A-200, Pronto): inexpensive and available without a prescription. These agents must be reapplied in 7 days to kill hatching nits.

   c. Malathion (Ovide): very effective and has residual killing activity. Only one application is necessary, but it must be left on the hair for 8 to 12 hours. Should be repeated in 7 days for pubic lice infestation.

   d. Lindane (Kwell): the standard therapy for many years. It is available by prescription only and requires reapplication in 7 days to kill hatching nits. Probably not as effective as many of the other products available and has the possibility of neurotoxicity when misused, especially in children.

   e. Trimethoprim-sulfamethoxazole (Bactrim, Septra): One tablet twice daily for 3 days will effectively kill head lice. Useful with severe infestations but has no effect on nits and must be repeated in 10 days when the unaffected nits hatch.

2. *Body lice:* Best treated by discarding infested clothes and improving hygiene. The following medications are effective in combination with hygienic measures:

   a. Lindane (Kwell): a single application of the lotion is effective.

   b. Malathion (Ovide): a single application is effective.

   c. Permethrin (Elimite): the 5% strength of permethrin is formulated to treat scabies but should be very effective in a single application.

3. Eyelash infestation can occur in either head lice or pubic lice infestation and can be treated as follows:

   a. Petrolatum jelly can be rubbed into the eyelashes three times a day for 5 days. Baby shampoo can be used similarly.

   b. Fluorescein drops are immediately toxic to lice.

   c. Physostigmine ointment (Eserine) should be applied twice daily for 3 days; can cause pupillary constriction.

4. Other medications, such as oral hydroxyzine or diphenhydramine, can be useful to treat the pruritus that accompanies lice infestation. Topical steroids can be used to reduce inflammation. If there is superimposed bacterial infection in body lice or severe head lice infestation, an antistaphylococcal antibiotic should be administered.

Diet
No special dietary requirements

Activity
Children can return to school after application of a pediculocide. Some schools enforce a "no nit" policy, which does ensure that treatment has been given.

Patient Education

1. Parents should be advised that head lice infestation does not indicate poor hygiene.

   a. Nits can be removed with a fine-tooth comb that is included with many of the pediculocide preparations.

   b. When nits are very extensive, removal can be facilitated by wetting with vinegar or formic acid (step 2) for 10 minutes before removal.

2. Personal items such as combs or brushes should be soaked in hot water with a pediculocide for 15 minutes.

3. Clothes and bedding should be washed with hot water and dried in the dryer or dry-cleaned. Alternatively, the items can be placed in a plastic bag for 10 days, and the lice will die from lack of food.

4. Household members and close contacts of patients with head lice should be examined carefully for head lice and treated if any suspicion of infestation exists.

Persons sharing a bed with the patient should be treated prophylactically.

5. Patients with pubic lice should notify their sexual contacts of the infection and be counseled regarding sexually transmitted disease screening and prevention.

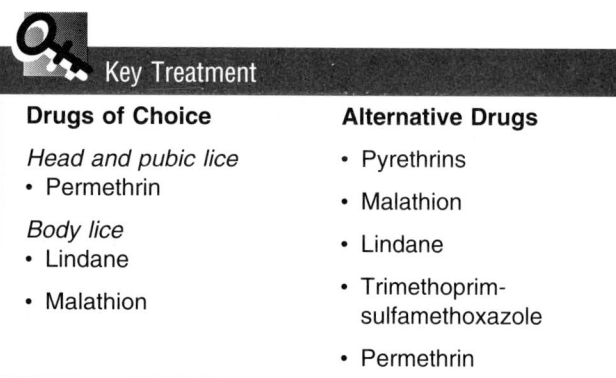

Key Treatment	
Drugs of Choice	**Alternative Drugs**
Head and pubic lice	• Pyrethrins
• Permethrin	
	• Malathion
Body lice	
• Lindane	• Lindane
	• Trimethoprim-sulfamethoxazole
• Malathion	
	• Permethrin

Follow-Up

1. All patients should be carefully re-examined 1 week after the final treatment to make sure no lice remain.

2. In cases of recurrent lice infestation, all household members and close contacts should be treated.

Bibliography

Elgart ML: Pediculosis. Dermatol Clin 1990;8(2):219–228.

Habif TP, Clinical Dermatology: A Color Guide to Diagnosis and Therapy, 2d ed. St Louis, CV Mosby, 1990, pp 378–381.

Hogan DJ, Schachner L, Tanglertsampan C: Diagnosis and treatment of childhood scabies and pediculosis. Pediatr Clin North Am 1991;38(4):941–957.

Peter G, Lepow ML, McCracken GH, Phillips CF, eds: Report of the Committee on Infectious Diseases, 22nd ed. Elk Grove Village, Ill, American Academy of Pediatrics, 1991, pp 352–354.

278 Fungus Infections of the Skin
David M. Adelson

Etiology

1. Fungus infections of the skin are usually caused by dermatophytes or fungi of the genus *Candida* or *Malassezia*.

2. Dermatophytes are of three genera, *Microsporum, Trichophyton,* and *Epidermophyton.* These aerobic organisms parasitize keratin of the skin, hair, and nails. Deeper penetration occurs with local or systemic immunosuppression.

   a. Geophylic dermatophytes normally are found in the soil but can infect humans or animals, zoophilic dermatophytes are found on animals but can infect humans, and anthropophilic dermatophytes have humans as their only host.

   b. Certain species more commonly infect specific areas. *Microsporum* species generally invade the hair and glabrous skin. *Epidermophyton* infection usually involves the groin or feet. *Trichophyton* species infect the hair, skin, and nails.

   c. Transmission is from direct contact with infected persons, animals, or fomites.

3. *Candida albicans* is usually responsible for cutaneous candidiasis but non-*albicans* candidal organisms can cause infection. The mucosal epithelium or stratum corneum is invaded in areas of maceration or in patients with decreased cell-mediated immunity. Antibiotic therapy, diabetes, pregnancy, and the use of oral contraceptives can increase the risk of candidiasis.

4. *Malassezia furfur* causes tinea versicolor, a common superficial fungal infection, and *Malassezia (Pityrosporum)* folliculitis. This organism can exist in two yeast forms called *P. ovale* and *P. orbiculare.*

Symptoms

1. Dermatophyte infections may be pruritic or asymptomatic. Occasionally, there are tenderness and inflammation. Other symptoms depend on location.

   a. Scalp (tinea capitis): alopecia, scaling, occasionally swelling, occasionally purulent discharge

   b. Feet (tinea pedis): scaling, thickened soles, occasionally small blisters

   c. Nails (onychomycosis): thickening, brittleness, and subungual debris

2. Candidiasis: itching and burning. Swelling, redness, scaly, creamy exudate

3. *Malassezia* infections

   a. Tinea versicolor: usually asymptomatic but occasionally pruritic. Often hypopigmented macules, especially in summer. Mild scale with scratching

   b. *Malassezia* folliculitis: asymptomatic or pruritic acne-like rash

Key Symptoms

- Itching
- Inflammation
- Scaling
- Tenderness
- Alopecia
- Blisters (rare)

Clinical Findings

Clinical findings depend on the organism and location of the infection.

1. Dermatophyte infections

   a. Scalp (tinea capitis)

   (1) Noninflammatory form: one or multiple scaly patches or plaques, broken hair and/or stubs (black dots). Alopecia with minimal inflammation

   (2) Inflammatory form: papular or nodular erythematous plaque. Alopecia. Can develop into a boggy purulent nodule often with a surface yellow crust (kerion)

   b. Body (tinea corporis): Erythematous plaque with central clearing and sharp margins. There is an advancing scale and an erythematous papular edge trailing this scaling. Occasionally intense inflammation with or without pustules

   c. Groin (tinea cruris): similar morphology to infections on the body. Papules, vesicles, or pustules may stud the border. The scrotum and penis are usually spared.

   d. Feet (tinea pedis): The most frequent form of cutaneous fungal infection. There are three common forms of presentation.

   (1) Interdigital tinea pedis: macerated, red, and scaly toe web space. Often associated fissuring. The fourth web space is most commonly involved.

   (2) Moccasin type: dry scaly thick skin on soles and sides of feet. Soles are erythematous. May be seen on two feet and one hand or one foot and two hands

   (3) Vesicular type: erythema, vesicles, and scaling, usually of the instep. The vesicles may coalesce into larger bullae.

   e. Hands (tinea manus): scaly palms, occasionally dorsal, often unilateral

   f. Nails (onychomycosis): Three clinical variants of dermatophyte nail infection exist.

(1) Distal subungual onychomycosis: thickening of the nail and collection of debris under the distal edge of the nail. The thickened nail becomes brittle and crumbles. The disease progresses from the distal edge proximally.

(2) Proximal subungual onychomycosis: thickening and crumbling of the nail begins at the proximal nail fold, with disease progressing toward the tip

(3) Superficial white onychomycosis: white chalky adherent plaques on the surface of the nail

2. Candidal infections

a. Intertrigo: Body fold such as the axillae, groin, gluteal folds, inframammary skin, interdigital spaces, corners of mouth, and retroauricular skin are involved. The area is intensely red, moist, and edematous. The edge is sharply marginated, and there are usually surrounding satellite pustules or papules. With severe maceration the pustules are usually absent, and there is a cheesy exudate. In the groin, the scrotum is often involved.

b. Paronychia: erythema and edema around nail fold. The cuticle is lost. Subsequent dystrophic nail transverse ridging occurs, which may progress to a thickened and brittle nail. Purulent exudate is often expressed from the proximal nail fold.

c. Diaper candidiasis: maceration, intense erythema, involving the skin folds, and satellite pustules. Papular and nodular lesions can occur.

d. Oral candidiasis: whitish patches loosely adherent to the mucosa. Red beefy tongue at times. Smooth patch with loss of papillae in central tongue

e. Balanitis: red pinpoint pustules or papules on the glans and foreskin

3. *Malassezia* infections

a. Tinea versicolor: small red, tan brown, or hypopigmented macules with fine scale. Usually seen on the sternal skin, back, lateral chest, and sides of neck. Facial lesions can occur on infants and children.

b. *Malassezia* folliculitis: pruritic acne-like papules and pustules on the chest or back

Key Signs	
• Annular plaque	• Alopecia
• Erythema and scale	• Broken hairs
• Dry, thickened soles	• Thickened nails
• Satellite pustules (*Candida*)	• Cheesy exudate (*Candida*)

Laboratory Tests

1. Potassium hydroxide (KOH) preparation: Skin or nail scrapings or hair plucks from the edge of the involved sites are obtained. KOH 10% to 20% is placed on a glass slide, a cover slip is applied, and it is gently heated. The slide is viewed microscopically for fungus.

a. Chlorozol black E is a stain that combines KOH and a fungal stain and stains fungus a blue-black color. It contains DMSO; therefore, heating is not necessary.

b. Hyphae seen in dermatophyte infections, pseudohyphae in candidal infections, and short fat hyphae and/or yeast in diseases caused by *Malassezia*

2. Wood's light (black light) shone on the affected area in a pitch-black room:

a. Yellow or green-yellow fluorescence of hair shafts suggests fungal infection.

b. Coral-red fluorescence is seen in primary or secondary erythrasma (see Differential Diagnosis).

3. Fungal culture: skin scrapings, nail clippings, or hair plucks from the involved area

a. Sabouraud's dextrose agar: standard in mycology laboratories

b. Dermatophyte test medium (DTM) contains a pH color indicator. Dermatophyte growth raises the pH of the medium, changing the color to red.

4. Skin biopsy: rarely necessary. However, fungal infections can be diagnosed when not expected initially. Histologic fungal stains will show the organism.

Key Tests
• KOH preparation
• Fungal culture

Differential Diagnosis

1. Dermatophyte infection

a. Tinea capitis: psoriasis, seborrheic dermatitis, alopecia areata, trichotillomania

b. Tinea corporis: psoriasis, nummular eczema, pityriasis rosea, secondary syphilis

c. Tinea cruris: psoriasis, seborrheic dermatitis, erythrasma, intertrigo, candidal intertrigo

d. Tinea pedis

(1) Interdigital type: erythrasma and mixed intertriginous infection caused by secondary bacterial infection

(2) Moccasin type: psoriasis, irritant foot dermatitis, keratoderma, secondary syphilis

(3) Vesicular type: dyshidrotic eczema, palmoplantar psoriasis

e. Onychomycosis: nail psoriasis, traumatic nail dystrophy

2. Candidal infection
   a. Intertrigo: same as above (tinea cruris)
   b. Paronychia: bacterial paronychia, usually staphylococcal
   c. Diaper candidiasis: irritant diaper dermatitis, seborrheic dermatitis, psoriasis. Rare: histiocytosis X, congenital syphilis, acrodermatitis enteropathica
   d. Oral candidiasis: lichen planus, leukoplakia, oral hairy leukoplakia
   e. Balanitis: herpes genitalis, lichen planus, psoriasis
3. *Malassezia* infections
   a. Tinea versicolor: pityriasis rosea, seborrheic dermatitis, secondary syphilis, vitiligo
   b. *Malassezia* folliculitis: bacterial folliculitis, acne vulgaris

Treatment

1. Keep infected area clean and dry.
2. When used as a single agent, topical antifungals are ineffective in treating fungal infections of the scalp, beard area, or nails.
3. An oral agent is also preferred if extensive body areas are infected.

Medication

A. By categories
   1. Topical antifungals
      a. Imidazole compounds: effective in treating dermatophyte, *Candida,* and *Malassezia* infections. Low cost and wide spectrum make them the drug of choice for uncomplicated, limited disease. Included in this group are clotrimazole (Lotrimin), miconazole (Monistat), ketoconazole (Nizoral), econazole (Spectazole), sulconazole (Exelderm), oxiconazole (Oxistat), and terconazole (Terazol).
      b. Allylamines include naftifine (Naftin) and terbinafine (Lamisil), which have a wide spectrum and are fungicidal for dermatophytes and fungistatic for *Candida.*
      c. Ciclopirox olamine (Loprox) is an effective broad-spectrum fungicidal agent.
      d. Nystatin is a polyene antibiotic that is only effective in *Candida* infections.
   2. Oral antifungals
      a. Griseofulvin is effective in dermatophyte but ineffective in candidal or *Malassezia* infections. Some reports of resistant dermatophytes
      b. Oral imidazoles have broad spectrum of activity and include ketoconazole, fluconazole, and itraconazole.
B. By infections
   1. Dermatophyte infection
      a. Tinea capitis: adult: griseofulvin (ultramicrosize), 250–375 mg/day. Pediatric: griseoful-

vin (ultramicrosize), 5.5 to 7.3 mg/kg/day. Treat for 6 weeks. Alternative: itraconazole* (Sporanox), 100 mg/day for 6 weeks
   b. Tinea corporis
      (1) Limited: topical imidazole for 2 to 3 weeks. Medication should continue for at least 1 week after clinical cure.
      (2) Extensive or in beard area: griseofulvin (ultramicrosize), 250 to 375 mg/day. Treat for 4 weeks. Alternative: fluconazole* (Diflucan), 150 mg/week for 4 weeks; itraconazole,* 100 mg/day for 15 days
   c. Tinea cruris: topical imidazole for 2 to 3 weeks. Medication should continue for at least 1 week after clinical cure. Alternative: griseofulvin (ultramicrosize), 250 to 375 mg/day for 2 to 4 weeks; fluconazole, 150 mg/week for 4 weeks; itraconazole, 100 mg/day for 15 days
   d. Tinea pedis: topical imidazole for 4 weeks. Alternative: griseofulvin (ultramicrosize), 250 to 375 mg twice daily for 4 to 8 weeks; fluconazole,* 150 mg/week for 4 weeks; itraconazole,* 100 mg/day for 4 weeks
   e. Onychomycosis: griseofulvin (ultramicrosize), 375 to 500 mg twice daily for 9 months (fingernails) or 18 months (toenails). Alternative: itraconazole,* 200 mg twice daily for 7 days; repeat monthly for 3 months (fingernails) or 4 months (toenails). Fluconazole, 150 mg/week for 12 months
2. Candidal infection: topical imidazole, nystatin, ciclopirox, or allylamine. Alternative: if recalcitrant, oral ketoconazole, 200 mg/day, fluconazole, 100 mg/day, or itraconazole, 100 mg/day
3. *Malassezia* infections
   a. Tinea versicolor
      (1) Limited: selenium sulfide 2.5% lathered on for 5 minutes and then rinsed, or topical imidazole. Alternative: 50% propylene glycol twice daily for 2 weeks
      (2) Extensive: ketoconazole, 400 mg in a single dose, repeated in 1 week; fluconazole, 400-mg single dose
   b. *Malassezia* folliculitis: selenium sulfide 2.5% lathered on for 5 minutes and then rinsed

Diet
No restrictions

Activity
No restrictions

Patient Education

1. Reinfection is common, so avoid sharing personal

---

*Fluconazole and itraconazole are not FDA approved for the treatment of dermatophyte infection. Because medication dosages often change, check all dosages before dispensing.

hygienic tools, kitchen utensils, shoes, or clothing with others.

2. With tinea pedis, avoid occlusive footwear; wear shower shoes in shower shared with public, that is, health club or hotel.

3. Others in the family should be evaluated for infection, particularly with tinea capitis.

Key Treatment

Drugs of Choice	Alternative Drugs
• Topical imidazole (body)	• Topical allylamine
• Griseofulvin (scalp, nails)	• Topical ciclopirox
	• Oral itraconazole
	• Oral fluconazole

Follow-Up

1. Persistent or recurrent infections should be re-evaluated.

2. A post-therapy fungal culture should be obtained in patients with tinea capitis.

Bibliography

Degreef HJ, DeDoncker PRG: Current therapy of dermatophytosis. J Am Acad Dermatol 1994;31:S25–S30.

Elgart ML, Warren NG: The superficial and subcutaneous mycoses. *In* Moschella SL, Hurley HJ (eds): Dermatology, 3rd ed, vol 1. Philadelphia, WB Saunders, 1992, pp 869–912.

Faergemann J: *Pityrosporum* infections. J Am Acad Dermatol 1994;31:S18–S20.

Gupta AK, Sauder DN, Shear NH: Antifungal agents: An overview, part I. J Am Acad Dermatol 1994;30:677–698; and Gupta AK, Sauder DN, Shear NH: Antifungal agents: An overview, part II. J Am Acad Dermatol 1994;30:911–933.

Odds FC: Pathogenesis of *Candida* infections. J Am Acad Dermatol 1994;31:S2–S5.

279 Burns

Geoffrey Peter Gustavsen

Etiology

1. Burns are tissue damage caused by agents such as heat, chemicals, mechanical abrasion, sunlight, electricity, or nuclear radiation. Fire, scalding liquids, and steam are the most common causes of severe burns.

2. The skin is the largest organ in the body and has many functions, two of the most important being to keep microorganisms out and moisture and electrolytes in. These functions are lost with significant burns.

3. The skin is composed of two layers, the epidermis and the dermis.
   a. The epidermis is the thin outer layer made up of epithelial cells.
   b. The dermis is a thicker layer that contains nerve endings, blood vessels, collagen, elastin fibers, and the epidermal appendages (hair follicles, sebaceous glands, and sweat glands).
   c. The epidermal appendages are crucial in burn healing because they are lined with epithelial cells. This relatively sheltered lining is the source of re-epithelization for any burned area.

4. Burns are classified by their extent of damage as either first, second, or third degree.
   a. First- and second-degree burns are considered partial-thickness burns.
   b. Third-degree burns are considered full-thickness burns.

Symptoms

First- and second-degree burns are very painful, while the deeper damage of a third-degree burn destroys nerves and makes tissue insensitive to pain.

Key Symptoms

- First- and second-degree burns: hypersensitive and painful
- Third-degree burns: anesthetic

Clinical Findings

1. First-degree burns: erythema, tenderness, often edematous
2. Second-degree burns
   a. Same as first-degree burns with some measure of blistering
   b. The entire epidermis is destroyed, but the dermis is largely intact.

3. Third-degree burns
   a. Total skin necrosis
   b. The skin is charred with a leathery surface that is insensitive to pain or touch. If pressure is applied to the burn, the surface will not blanch or refill because the blood vessels are thrombosed.

Key Signs

- First-degree burns: erythema
- Second-degree burns: blisters, shiny, weeping
- Third-degree burns: nonblanching, hard, leathery

Assessment

1. Determining burn severity is important for triage (inpatient versus outpatient) and initial fluid resuscitation.
2. Estimation of body surface area (BSA) burned
   a. The "rule of nines" divides the surface of the adult body into areas that are a multiple of 9 per cent.
   b. The patient's palm represents about 1 per cent of BSA and gives another rough estimate of burn size.
3. Triage
   a. Minor burn: outpatient treatment
      (1) Second-degree burns < 15 per cent of BSA
      (2) Third-degree burns < 2 per cent of BSA
      (3) Burns that spare face, hands, feet, and perineum
   b. Moderate/major burns: inpatient treatment
      (1) More extensive burns
      (2) Chemical or electrical burns
      (3) Associated inhalation injury or major trauma
      (4) Patients with significant medical problems

Treatment

1. First-degree burns
   a. Cooling
      (1) Immerse in cold water or apply cold wet towels.
      (2) Warm blankets to rest of body as needed to avoid systemic hypothermia
   b. Mild analgesics, a covering, or an emollient eases the pain early on.
   c. Topical anesthetics may decrease pain but can be sensitizing.

d. First-degree burns will heal spontaneously without scarring in 3 to 4 days

2. Second-degree burns

a. Debridement: Intact blisters can be left for 3 to 4 days if no sign of infection. Bulky blisters can be decompressed, and devitalized skin removed.

b. Gentle cleansing with antiseptic or mild soap

c. Topical antibiotics

(1) Bacitracin: Apply to very limited second-degree burns.

(2) Silver sulfadiazine (Silvadene) is preferred for larger or deeper burns.

d. Dressings

(1) Nonadherent gauze next to the skin covered by a bulky dressing

(2) Wounds of face and ears may be easier to treat without bandages.

(3) Daily dressing changes (premedication may be required)

e. Tetanus prophylaxis

(1) Tetanus toxoid, 0.5-cc subcutaneous booster

(2) Tetanus immune globulin (Hyper-Tet), 250 U intramuscularly plus toxoid if never immunized.

f. Second-degree burns heal spontaneously in 2 to 3 weeks without scarring.

3. Third-degree burns

a. Usually require skin grafting

b. Can take months to heal. Scarring occurs.

4. Extensive burns (>15 per cent of BSA) may require fluid resuscitation. A rough guide: 2 to 4 ml × wt (kg) × per cent second-degree and third-degree burns/24 hours. Administer first half over 8 hours and the second half over the next 16 hours.

Diet

Additional vitamins C (500 mg) and A (10,000 U) daily

Activity

1. If burn overlies a joint, attempt full range of motion at least three times daily.

2. Elevation of burned part as often as possible to limit edema

Patient Education

Management of minor burns does not require a lot of expertise, but it is time-consuming for the caregiver and painful for the patient.

Key Treatment

• First-degree burns: cooling and covering

• Second-degree burns: cleansing and debridement; topical antibiotics and dressings; tetanus prophylaxis

• Third-degree burns: same as second-degree burns. Usually require skin grafting.

Bibliography

American Burn Association: Hospital and prehospital resources for optimal care of patients with burn injury: Capital guidelines for development and operation of burn centers. J Burn Care Rehabil 1990;11:98.

Clark WR: Burns. *In* Rakel RE (ed): 1994 Conn's Current Therapy. Philadelphia, WB Saunders, 1994, pp 1133–1138.

Curreri PW, Luterman A: Burns. *In* Schwartz SI (ed): Principles of Surgery, 5th ed. New York, McGraw-Hill, 1989, pp 285–305.

Dimick AR: Burns and electrical injuries. *In* Tintinalli JE (ed): Emergency Medicine: A Comprehensive Study Guide, 3rd ed. New York, McGraw-Hill, 1992, pp 691–694.

280 Rosacea

Elizabeth E. Brownell

Etiology

1. Rosacea is a chronic episodic skin disorder with onset between the ages of 30 and 50 years. It affects women three times more than men.
2. The cause of rosacea is unknown. There are many postulated causes, several of which include
   a. Genetic predisposition
   b. Hypertension
   c. *Demodex folliculorum* mites
   d. Gastrointestinal disease
3. Known contributing factors to rosacea are
   a. Persons predisposed to flushing and blushing
      (1) Dietary and environmental precipitation
      (2) Menopause
      (3) Vasodilator drug therapy
   b. Exposure to sunlight and heat

Symptoms

1. Excessive flushing and blushing with persistence of facial heat and redness
2. Sensitive skin that may sting and burn after use of lotions, cosmetics, or astringents
3. Persistent painful papules and cysts unresponsive to antiacne therapy

Key Symptoms

- Facial heat and redness
- Sensitive skin
- Painful papules and cysts

Clinical Findings

1. Rosacea affects the central face, especially the forehead, cheeks, chin, nose, and glabella. The hallmarks of rosacea, after an episode of flushing, are erythema, telangiectasias, papules, and papulopustules. Comedones are classically *absent*.
2. Rosacea occurs as intermittent but progressively more severe episodes.
   a. Mild erythema lasting for hours to days and a few scattered telangiectasias
   b. Moderate erythema, more telangiectasias, papules, and pustules that may persist for weeks
   c. Bright erythema, networks of telangiectasias, papules, and pustules. Variable patches of edema affect primarily the cheeks and nose.
3. Characteristic of more severe rosacea are chronic inflammation, connective tissue hypertrophy with col-

lagen deposition, and diffuse sebaceous gland hyperplasia. Disfiguring deformities resulting from these tissue changes are the "phymas." The most characteristic is rhinophyma, a gross deformity of the nose primarily affecting men.

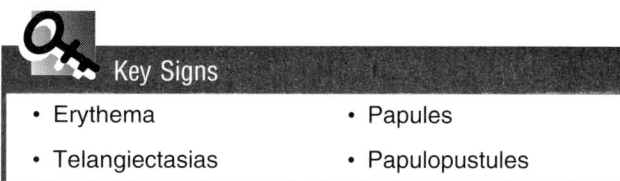

Key Signs

- Erythema
- Telangiectasias
- Papules
- Papulopustules

Laboratory Tests

1. The diagnosis of rosacea is based on clinical findings. There are no definitive laboratory tests.
2. Histopathology is variable, and a combination of findings may support the diagnosis of rosacea, but biopsies are not routinely performed for diagnoses.

Differential Diagnosis

1. Acne vulgaris
2. Perioral dermatitis
3. Seborrheic dermatitis
4. Contact dermatitis
5. Lupus erythematosus
6. Carcinoid flush
7. Cutaneous tuberculosis

Treatment

1. Rosacea can be treated, but complete cure is usually not possible.
2. Treatment is based on the predominant clinical findings and severity of the disease. Options include topical therapy, systemic therapy, and dietary and environmental modifications.

Medication

A. Topical therapy
   1. Topical antibiotics can be effective against papulopustular rosacea: Tetracycline, erythromycin, or clindamycin in a 0.5 to 2.0% concentration applied twice daily.
   2. Metronidazole (0.75% MetroGel) applied twice daily
      a. Greatest effect on papules and pustules
      b. Little effect on erythema and telangiectasias
   3. Drying lotions applied once or twice daily
      a. Benzoyl peroxide
      b. Sulfur-containing lotions
   4. 1% Hydrocortisone cream may be useful in decreasing the erythema and inflammation of rosa-

cea. Fluorinated steroids should *not* be used. Although initially effective, prolonged use causes a rebound worsening of rosacea symptoms.

5. Telangiectatic vessels may be treated by superficial electrodesiccation or laser surgery.

6. Soft tissue hypertrophy in rhinophyma is most effectively treated with CO_2 laser surgery, dermabrasion, or electrosurgery.

B. Systemic therapy

1. Systemic antibiotics are effective in treating the inflammatory lesions (papules and pustules) of rosacea.

   a. Tetracycline, 250 mg orally four times daily, until symptoms diminish and then taper or discontinue the medication.

   b. Erythromycin or minocycline, 50 to 100 mg daily, is an alternative if tetracycline is ineffective.

   c. Metronidazole, 250 mg twice daily, may be as effective as tetracycline in a first-line approach or as an alternative if tetracycline is ineffective.

2. Isotretinoin (13-*cis*–retinoic acid) (Accutane)

   a. Isotretinoin may be effective in severe rosacea or rosacea unresponsive to other forms of therapy.

   b. Standard dose: 0.5 to 1.0 mg/kg/day for 15 to 20 weeks. Used primarily in refractory rosacea. Adverse effects can limit course of treatment. Low dose: 0.1 to 0.2 mg/kg/day. Improvement may take longer than standard dose. Fewer adverse effects
   Minidose: 2.5 to 5 mg daily (*not* adjusted for body weight). Improvement may take up to 6 months. Adverse effects are minimal.

   c. Adverse effects are dose-related.

      (1) Ocular

         (a) Blepharitis

         (b) Dry eyes

      (2) Hepatotoxicity

      (3) Teratogen: contraindicated in pregnant women

Diet
Avoid any foods that might cause vasodilation of blood vessels and therefore facial flushing, including hot liquids, alcohol, tea, spicy foods, coffee, and tobacco.

Activity
Avoid extremes of weather: prolonged sun exposure, heat, wind, and cold.

Patient Education

1. See Diet above.

2. Sunscreens with a sun protection factor (SPF) of 15 or higher

3. Use a mild, nondrying soap.

4. Avoid local skin irritants: alcohol-based facial cleansers, peeling agents, abrasive facial cleansers, topical medications.

5. Stress management may be helpful.

Key Treatment

- Topical therapy
- Systemic therapy

Follow-Up
Determined by individual treatment and severity of disease.

Bibliography

Arndt AA: Rosacea and periorifacial (perioral) dermatitis. *In* Bernhardt MS (ed): Manual of Dermatologic Therapeutics, 5th ed. Boston, Little, Brown, 1995, pp 160–163.

Habif TP: Acne, rosacea and related disorders. *In* Klein EA, Menczer BS (eds): Clinical Dermatology: A Color Guide to Diagnosis and Therapy, 2nd ed. St Louis, CV Mosby, 1990, pp 136–137.

Moschella SL, Hurley HJ: Rosacea. *In* Fletcher J (ed): Dermatology. 3d ed, vol 2. Philadelphia, WB Saunders, 1992, pp 1487–1491.

Plewig G: Rosacea. *In* Fitzpatrick TB, Eisen AZ, Wolff K, et al: (eds): Dermatology in General Medicine, 4th ed, vol 1. New York, McGraw-Hill, 1993; pp 727–735.

Wilken JK: Rosacea: Pathophysiology and treatment. Arch Dermatol 1994;130:359–362.

281 Tattoos

Mark Wells

History

Human flesh has served as a canvas for artistic expression since the dawn of time. Modern puncture tattooing probably dates back to 8000 B.C. and remains common today. Tattoos traditionally have been a male bastion, with approximately 9 per cent of men and 1 per cent of women in the United States bearing such ornamentation. Recent reports suggest that more women may be seeking them, paralleling their emancipation from conventional roles.

Etiology

1. *Amateur tattoos:* Self-inflicted tattooing is easily accomplished by dipping the point of a needle in ink and pricking the skin repeatedly. These tattoos are characterized by irregular pigment depth, making removal much more problematic.

2. *Professional tattoos:* These tattoos are characteristically performed under antiseptic conditions using an electric needle, repetitively puncturing the skin at rates up to 50 times per second. Pigment is deposited at a relatively constant depth within papillary dermis.

3. *Post-traumatic tattoos:* Foreign bodies are embedded within the dermis after an abrasion to the skin. The epithelial elements regenerate, resulting in permanent entrapment of the debris within the dermis.

4. *Medical and cosmetic tattoos:* Historically, tattooing has been used medically to camouflage vascular malformations of the skin. Generally, these efforts have failed. Recently, tattooing has been used successfully to create the areola following mastectomy and breast reconstruction. Additionally, the cosmetic industry has utilized tattooing to apply permanent lip and eye liner as well as brow pigmentation to its customers, often with disastrous consequences.

Histopathology

A. *Initial reaction*
   1. Wheal and flare reaction with edema
   2. Nonspecific inflammation
   3. Superficial crusting and loss of the epidermis
   4. Some loss of pigment as it extrudes through needle punctures

B. *Over months*
   1. Unassimilated granules remain between collagen bundles within the dermis permanently
   2. Some pigments may be transported to adjacent lymph nodes

C. *Over years*
   1. Mild perivascular lymphocytic inflammation causes dermal fibrosis and loss of tattoo definition.
   2. Colors begin to fade.
   3. Process is accelerated by sun exposure.

Complications

A. *Pyogenic infections*
   1. Superficial
      a. Impetigo
      b. Ecthyma
   2. Deep infections
      a. Furunculosis
      b. Erysipelas
      c. Cellulitis

B. *Nonpyogenic infections*
   1. Syphilis
   2. Hepatitis B
   3. Tetanus
   4. ? Human immunodeficiency virus
   5. Molluscum contagiosum
   6. Tuberculosis cutis
   7. Leprosy

C. *Cutaneous disease that localizes in tattoos*
   1. Vaccinia
   2. Verruca vulgaris
   3. Herpes simplex and zoster
   4. Psoriasis
   5. Lichen planus
   6. Darier's disease
   7. Chronic diskoid lupus erythematosus
   8. Keratoacanthoma

D. *Acquired tattoo pigment sensitivity*
   1. Mercury (red)
   2. Chromium (green)
   3. Cadmium (yellow)
   4. Cobalt (blue)

E. *Miscellaneous reactions*
   1. Hypertrophic scarring
   2. Keloids
   3. Sarcoidal granulomas
   4. Lymphadenopathy
   5. Localized scleroderma
   6. Erythema multiforme

Treatment

The skepticism that society at large holds toward people with tattoos parallels the ambivalence of the tattooee toward his or her own dermal ornamentation. Tattoos most commonly subject to removal include names, obscene subjects, or antisocial messages. Additionally, tattoos on the hand and face are more likely to require subsequent removal. Despite many practitioners' claims, there is no technique that can remove a tattoo without the risk of scarring or pigmentary changes.

1. *Overtattooing:* tattoo artists are often requested to modify unacceptable tattoos. Their methods include overtattooing or retattooing with a lighter pigment in an attempt to mask a dark tattoo. Alternatively, older, unacceptable tattoos can be incorporated into new ones, albeit at the cost of a larger tattoo.

2. *Cauterization:* numerous do-it-yourself methods have been recommended, including cauterization with cigarettes or hot coat hangers. The third-degree burns caused by these methods are associated with a major incidence of unacceptable scarring.

3. *Salabrasion:* the technique consists of applying an irritating substance to the tattoo for several days, after which table salt is rubbed into the tattoo site. The result is epidermal abrasion with underlying inflammation. Pigment is leached out during the healing phase. Often the process must be repeated several times to be effective. Scarring, which is sometimes hypertrophic, is not uncommon.

4. *Dermabrasion:* a small area of the tattoo is anesthetized and abraded with a high-speed mechanical wheel. Only the epidermis and part of the papillary dermis are removed. As soon as the tattoo pigment appears in dermis, the process is stopped. The epidermis is allowed to regenerate from the residual adnexal structures dermis. Often a significant scar results. Alternatively, dermabrasion has been combined with the application of caustic chemicals to enhance pigment extrusion. Tannic acid and silver nitrate or trichloroacetic acid are applied following abrasion of the epidermis. The resultant eschar is then allowed to separate, along with a portion of the underlying pigment and dermis.

5. *Cryosurgery:* freon, carbon dioxide, liquid oxygen, and liquid nitrogen have all been used, the result being epidermal and partial dermal necrosis with sloughing of a portion of the pigment. This technique has generally been abandoned because of poor results.

6. *Acids:* caustic substances such as nitric acid have been advised for the removal of tattoos. Some authors have had satisfactory results even though the risk of hypertrophic scarring remains significant.

7. *Surgery:* small tattoos may be amenable to surgical excision and direct closure; larger ones are more difficult. Serial excision of the tattoo in two or three stages allows removal of a larger area than would otherwise be possible in one stage. Another approach is tissue expansion. By progressively stretching the normal skin adjacent to a tattoo over several months with a temporary inflatable prosthesis, it may be possible to excise the tattoo and resurface the region with a local advancement flap. This technique has the advantage of covering the tattooed region with tissue of similar texture and quality. However, a major disadvantage is time required for the expansion and need for multiple stages. Additionally, expander extrusion or infection is not uncommon.

Some professional tattoos may be amenable to tangential excision if the pigment is in a superficial plane within the dermis. The epithelial elements are allowed to regenerate from the remaining dermal structures over a period of a week to 10 days. Alternatively, if the excision extends into the subcutaneous fat, split- or full-thickness skin grafting can be performed to resurface the wound.

8. *Laser:* the newest technique to remove tattoos involves the use of lasers to vaporize the intradermal pigment. Early studies utilized the CO_2 and argon lasers. Both these devices cause disruption of the epidermis with exposure of the pigment-laden dermis. These lasers rely on the tattoo pigment being carried away in the post-treatment exudate as well as dermal sclerosis to obscure residual deeper pigment. Their use has been associated with variable degrees of hypertrophic scarring and hypopigmentation.

More recently, the Q-switched ruby laser has been used with some success. Q-switching is a mechanism used to control the light output by concentrating all the energy into a single, intense pulse of light. In the Q-switched ruby laser, high-intensity flashlamps are used to excite the ruby crystal to produce red photons with nanosecond pulse durations and extremely high peak power at a wavelength of 694 nm. Normally, hemoglobin and melanin of the skin absorb light in the wavelengths from 400 to 600 nm. By using longer wavelengths, it was hoped to specifically target the tattoo pigments while selectively sparing the surrounding dermal structures. Results with this laser have been promising; however, patients often need multiple treatments. The newest laser to be advocated is the Q-switched alexandrite laser. Results have generally been similar to those of the ruby laser.

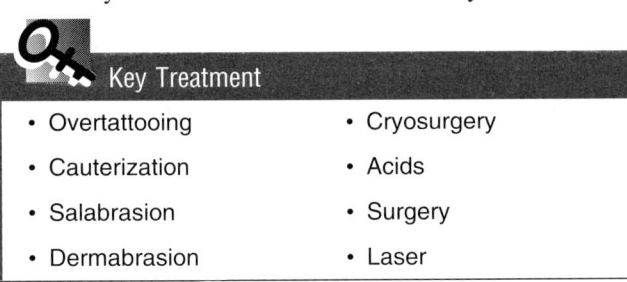

Key Treatment	
• Overtattooing	• Cryosurgery
• Cauterization	• Acids
• Salabrasion	• Surgery
• Dermabrasion	• Laser

B Bibliography

Horowitz J, Nicter LS, Stark D: Dermabrasion of traumatic tattoos: Simple, inexpensive, effective. Ann Plast Surg 1988;21:257.

Lowe NJ, Luftman D, Sawcer D: Q-switched ruby laser: Further observations on treatment of professional tattoos. J Dermatol Surg Oncol 1994;20:307–311.

Milroy BC: Tattoos and their removal. Med J Aust 1993;15:717–719.

Nelson JS: Lasers: State of the art in dermatology. Dermatol Clin 1993;11:15–26.

Sperry K: Tattoos and tattooing: II. Gross pathology, histopathology, medical complications, and applications. Am J Forensic Med Pathol 1992;13:7–17.

Procedure | **WOUND MANAGEMENT** | *Thomas J. Zuber*

Goals

1. Maintain or return tissue to its prior condition and function.
2. Enhance the local wound environment to promote healing.
3. Close the wound primarily without interference to nearby structures or tissues.
4. Approximate straight, sharply incised, vertical wound edges.
5. Undermine skin edges to close the wound under low tension.
6. Spare tissue whenever possible, but excise jagged or devitalized tissue that will interfere with healing.
7. Create the most cosmetically acceptable scar.

Note: See the next procedure, Wound Revision, for preparation and follow-up.

Equipment

1. A minor surgery tray can be used to manage most wounds.
2. Equipment for administering local anesthesia can be included in the minor surgery tray, if desired.
3. Instruments include
   a. Needle holders
   b. Adson forceps with and without teeth
   c. A skin hook
   d. Metzenbaum scissors
   e. Iris scissors
   f. A scalpel blade handle
   g. Two hemostats
4. Materials include
   a. A pack of sterile 4-in by 4-in gauze
   b. Suture materials for subcuticular and skin closure
   c. A No. 15 scalpel blade
   d. Povidone-iodine solution to clean the skin surface
   e. Sterile saline for irrigation
   f. Sterile gloves

Anesthesia

1. Most wounds can be managed with a local or a field block.
2. Administer anesthesia into the subcuticular tissue to lessen the discomfort.
3. Consider nerve block when appropriate (i.e., facial wounds).
4. Materials include
   a. 10-cc syringe
   b. 18-gauge needle to draw up solution from the anesthetic bottle
   c. 27- or 30-gauge needle to administer the anesthetic solution
   d. 1 to 2% lidocaine with or without epinephrine
   e. Nonsterile gloves for anesthetic administration. Change to sterile gloves for wound closure.
   f. Alcohol or povidone-iodine wipes to clean the skin surface

Precautions

1. Never close a wound until the function of the underlying tendons, nerves, and vessels has been ensured.
2. Undermine at a level just below the dermal-fat junction to avoid vessels and nerves that may be in the deep tissue.
3. Do not place povidone-iodine or other toxic solutions into a wound because they interfere with wound healing.
4. Create good hemostasis in all wounds to prevent excess scar formation or scar retraction after the resolution of a hematoma.
5. Do not close tangential wounds without creating vertical wound edges.
6. Do not use skin sutures to pull displaced tissue edges together because excessive stress causes suture marks (railroad tracks).

Technique

1. Thoroughly inspect all wounds.
   a. Ensure proper function of the underlying tendons, nerves, and vessels prior to wound closure.
   b. All foreign bodies or foreign material should be removed from the wound.
   c. Whenever possible, irrigate the wound with copious amounts of sterile saline.
   d. Avoid placing povidone-iodine or other toxic substances directly into the wound.
2. All wounds should have adequate hemostasis.
   a. Applying hemostats to a bleeding vessel for a brief period usually is adequate.
   b. Electrocautery can be used in a wound base for hemostasis.
   c. Deep buried sutures will close dead space below the skin surface and often provide adequate hemostasis.

d. If a vessel continues to bleed, grasp the site with the hemostat tip and place a "figure of 8" absorbable suture into the tissue.

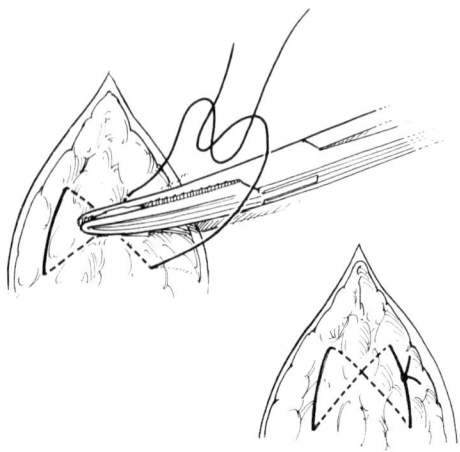

3. Prepare skin edges.
   a. It is advantageous to close sharp, straight, vertical wound edges.
   b. Ragged edges can be trimmed with a No. 15 scalpel or with scissors.

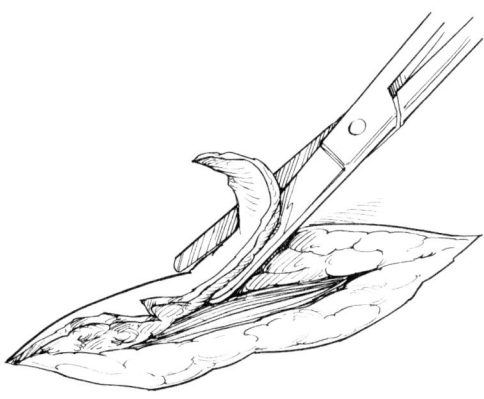

   c. Wound edges should be vertical. Tangential wounds create depressed, noticeable scars when they retract after healing. Tangential wound edges should be transformed into vertical wound edges.

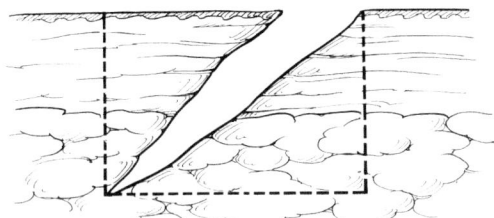

4. Facial wounds are best managed by sparing as much tissue as possible.
   a. Z-shaped or zigzag wounds can be closed by reapproximating angled skin edges.
   b. If the wound edge is too irregular, crushed, or devitalized, consider excising the entire wound and transforming it into a fusiform excision for closure.

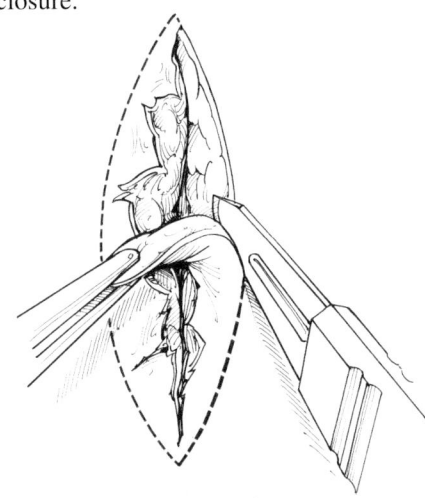

5. Undermining lateral skin edges frees up tissues for closure under reduced tension.
   a. Undermining is useful in areas where natural tension exists in the skin, such as the scalp or lower legs.
   b. The optimal level for undermining generally is just below the dermal-fat junction, since nerves may be found in deeper tissue.
   c. Undermining can be achieved with scissors or a scalpel.

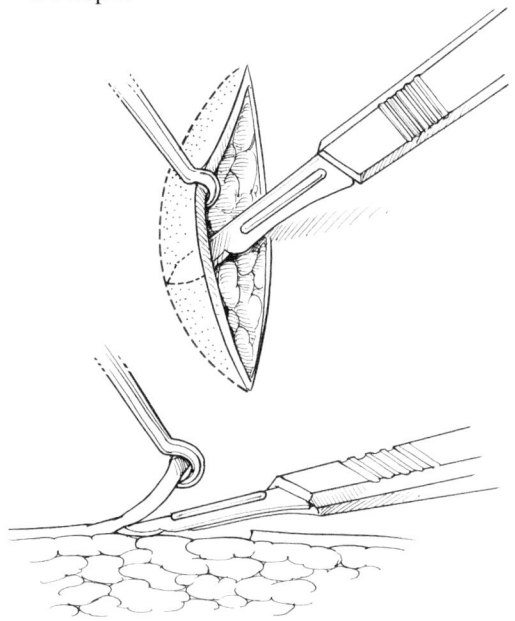

 Bibliography

Pfenninger JL, Fowler G: Procedures for Primary Care Physicians. St Louis, Mosby–Year Book, 1994.

Pories WJ, Thomas FT: Office Surgery for Family Physicians. Boston, Butterworth, 1985.

Swanson NA: Atlas of Cutaneous Surgery. Boston, Little, Brown, 1987.

Trott A: Wounds and Lacerations: Emergency Care and Closure. St Louis, Mosby–Year Book, 1991.

Zuber TJ, DeWitt DE: The fusiform excision. Am Fam Physician 1994;49:371–376.

Goals

1. Whenever possible, orient the wound in the direction of the skin lines (least skin tension).
2. Create wounds that lie flat, and avoid elevated corners that have a boat appearance, known as "dog-ears."
3. Repair dog-ears when they are large or create a cosmetic problem.
4. Redirect wounds that cross flexion creases using Z-plasty technique.
5. Close defects using local tissue or advancement flap technique.

Indications

1. Wounds crossing flexor creases
2. Wounds oriented perpendicular to the lines of least skin tension
3. Wounds with large tissue defects
4. Wounds with cosmetically unacceptable dog-ear defects at the end of the wound

Contraindications

1. Wounds that are more than 12 to 24 hours old (relative contraindication)
2. Wounds that are infected
3. Complicated wounds, with injury to deep structures, or wounds that are beyond the expertise of the treating physician
4. Coagulopathy or bleeding disorder
5. Uncooperative patient or one unable to care for his or her wound

Preparation

1. Cleanse the skin surface with povidone-iodine solution.
2. Keep antibacterial solutions or other toxic solutions out of the wound.
3. Irrigate the wound with copious amounts of sterile saline.
4. Inspect the wound for injury to underlying tendons, nerves, or vessels.
5. Confirm proper function of the injured body part.
6. Anesthetize with local or field block.

Note: See the preceding procedure, Wound Management, for equipment and anesthesia.

Technique

1. The lines of least skin tension often coincide with wrinkles or age lines.
   a. A scar that is parallel to or oriented in the direction of the lines of least skin tension will heal with a thin, more cosmetically acceptable scar.
   b. Whenever possible, orient the wound in the direction of the lines of least skin tension.

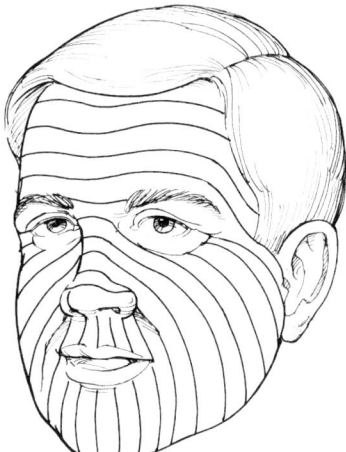

2. Properly repaired wounds lie flat.
   a. When a wound is pulled together centrally, elevated tissue may result at the corners of the wound.
   b. The elevated corners make the wound appear boat-shaped or with dog-ears.
3. Large dog-ear defects can create unacceptable scars.
   a. Many methods of dog-ear repair exist.
   b. A simple repair can be achieved by creating an elliptical excision at the corner of the wound that continues in the same direction as the wound.

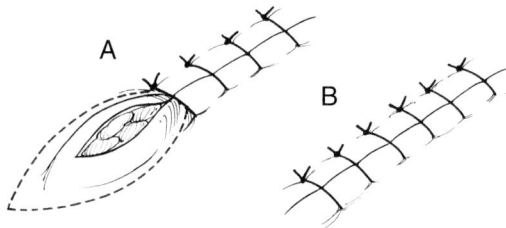

   c. This repair extends the length of the final wound.
4. Wounds that cross a flexion crease can create large scars that contract and interfere with function.
   a. These wounds can be redirected using Z-plasty technique.
   b. Incisions are created at each end of the wound that are directed at an angle of 60 degrees to the wound.

c. Each incision is made on opposite sides of the original wound.

d. The skin is undermined, creating two triangular flaps of tissue.

e. The corners of the triangular flaps are transposed.

f. The wound is repaired with the central axis of the Z-plasty at 90 degrees to the original direction of the wound.

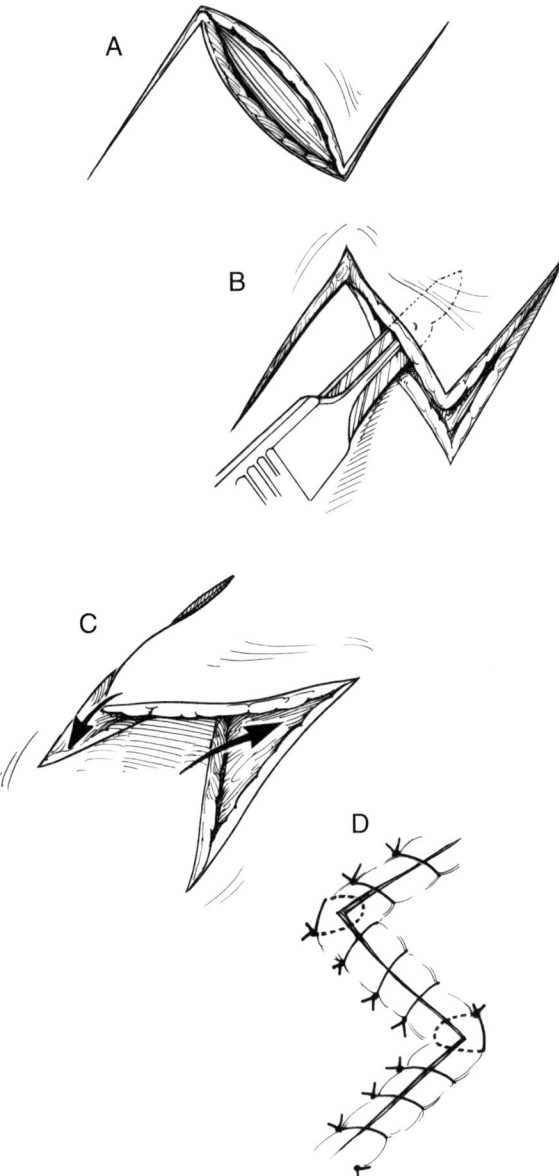

5. Large defects may require extensive tissue undermining to permit proper closure.

a. Local tissue can be rearranged to close a defect.

b. Creating a flap from nearby skin (advancement flap) can facilitate closure of the defect.

c. As the flap of skin is pulled over the defect, dog-ears will develop unless triangles of tissue (Burow's triangles) are excised from the outside skin edges at the far end of the flap.

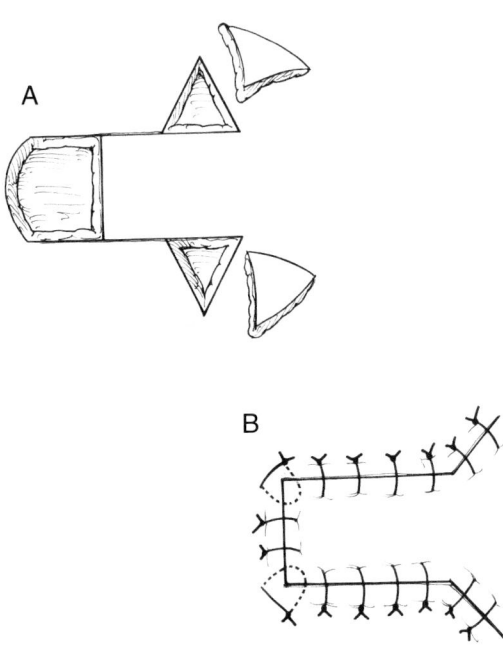

d. The final result should appear as a flat wound.

Follow-Up

1. Apply antibiotic cream to the wound daily until healed.

2. Apply direct pressure to the surgical site for the first 2 hours after the procedure.

3. Examine wounds promptly if there are signs of infection or hematoma.

4. Remove sutures after an interval appropriate for the repair and body site (see Laceration Repair).

Bibliography

Borges AF: Dog-ear repair. Plast Reconstr Surg 1982;69:707–713.

Parish LC, Lask GP: Aesthetic Dermatology. New York, McGraw-Hill, 1991.

Stegman SJ, Tromovitch TA, Glogau RG: Basics of Dermatologic Surgery. Chicago, Year Book Medical Publishers, 1982.

Swanson NA: Atlas of Cutaneous Surgery. Boston, Little, Brown, 1987.

Procedure LACERATION REPAIR

John L. Pfenninger

Indications

1. Laceration
2. Incision/excision repair

Contraindication

1. Contaminated wound
2. Disrupted nerves or tendons (refer?)

Preparation

1. Copious irrigation (laceration) with saline or lactated Ringer's
2. Proper debridement as necessary to remove devitalized tissue
3. Betadine wash
4. Anesthetic
5. Draping
6. Inform patient of procedure, risks of scarring, infection, discomfort

Equipment

1. 27-gauge, 1½-inch needle and syringe
2. Needle holders
3. Fine tissue scissors
4. Suture scissors
5. No. 15 blade and scalpel handle
6. Sterile gloves
7. Two sterile drapes (one fenestrated)
8. 4 × 4 sterile gauzes
9. 5-0 or 6-0 nylon or Prolene suture for face
10. 3-0 or 4-0 nylon or Prolene suture for trunk, extremities
11. 3-0 or 4-0 Vicryl or Dexon for buried suture
12. Possible Steri-Strips

Anesthesia

See Procedures on local and regional anesthesia (Chapters 42 and 196). If repairing a laceration, enter through the laceration.

Precautions

1. Use antistaphylococcal antibiotics for prophylaxis in immune-suppressed, diabetic, and elderly patients, and when there is vascular-compromised tissue.
2. Check tetanus status.
3. Before repairing a laceration, document intact neurovascular and tendon structures.
4. Do not use epinephrine with the lidocaine in "dirty wounds" or in the fingers, nose, penis, toes, or earlobes.
5. Close all dead spaces in wound.
6. Approximate but do not strangulate wound edges.
7. Make deeply buried stitches support any wound tension so that skin margins are slightly tented up but without tension.

Technique

1. Simple interrupted

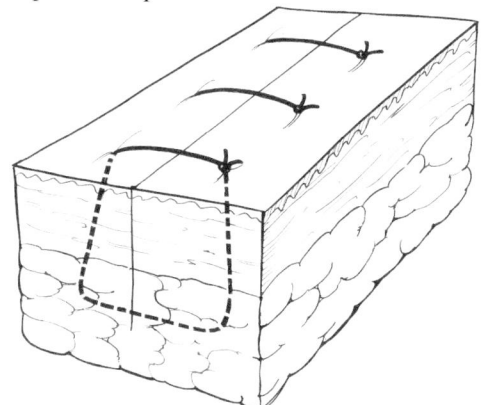

   a. The shape of the path of the suture should look like an Erlenmeyer flask.
   b. The closer the sutures, the less wound tension and thus less scarring. Sutures should be placed as far apart as they traverse across the wound.
   c. The levels of tissue should be approximated to the same levels on the opposite side. This closure can be used for most wounds.

2. Running stitch

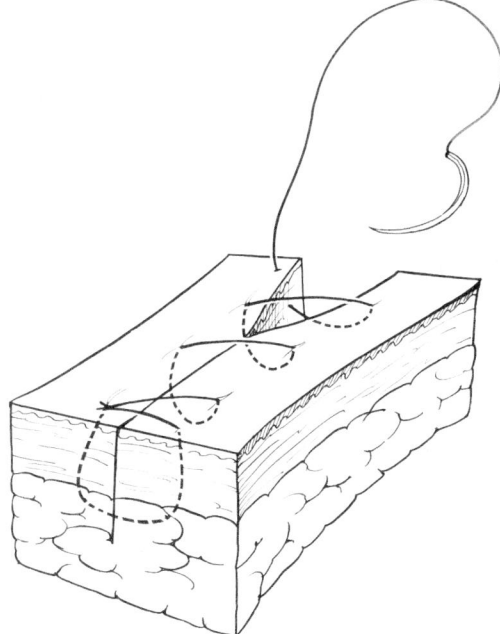

Advantages are that this closure is quick and provides some hemostasis. Use where scarring is not that important (e.g., scalp).

3. Two-layered closure—deep inverted stitch

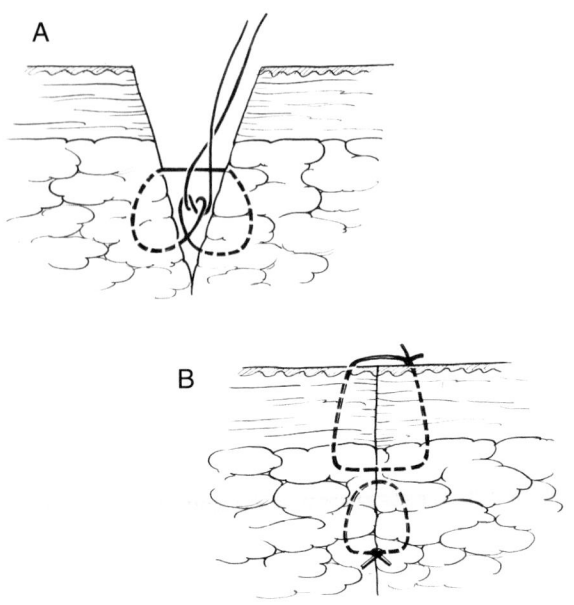

Use with deep wounds, in conjunction with undermining to close wounds under tension or with a significant gap of wound margins. Remember "bottoms up" to obtain an inverted knot—start at the bottom of the wound, go up, across, and then down. The knot ends up at the bottom of the wound, where it will cause less inflammation.

4. Subcuticular closure

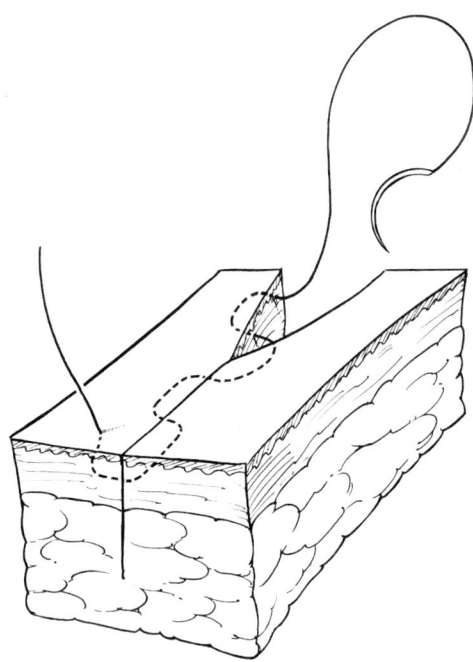

Use only if skin margins lie opposed without tension. Real advantage is minimal scarring. May be left in place 2 weeks or more. Use Prolene—it is more slippery and stronger than nylon.

5. Mattress sutures

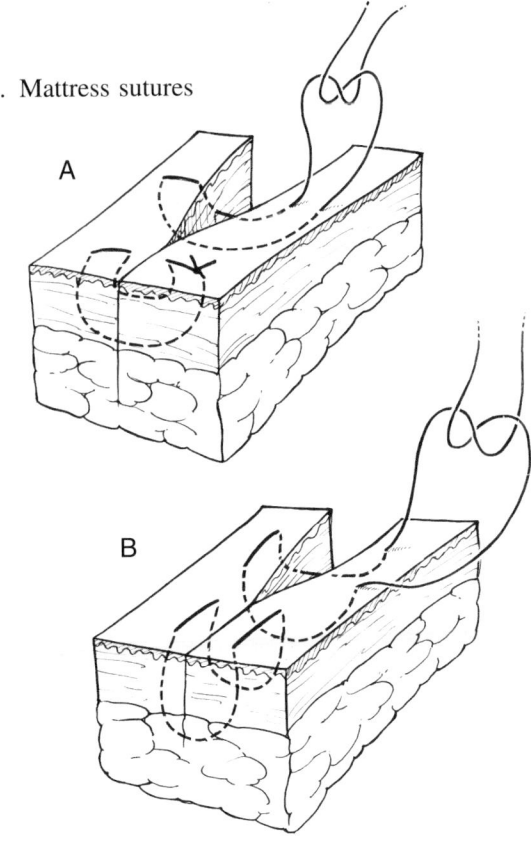

Use where there is significant wound tension or with very thin or very thick skin.

Follow-Up

1. Keep area dry for 24 hours, and then wash gently with mild soap and water three to four times a day. May cover with antibiotic ointment.
2. Report redness, drainage, or persistent pain (indications of infection).
3. Use Tylenol or ibuprofen for pain.
4. Rest as appropriate; possible elevation and/or ice.
5. Antibiotics as indicated
6. Suture removal according to the following:
   a. Face, 4 to 7 days
   b. Trunk, 10 to 12 days
   c. Extremities, 10 to 14 days

Method of Suture Removal

Cut near knot where suture enters skin. Pull suture across wound edge to avoid pulling "dirty" suture through the wound; pressure tends to pull wound edges together.

Bibliography

Leversee J, McCall MW, Salascke SJ: Office excision of facial lesions. Patient Care 1990;Feb:26–41.

Moy RL, Lee A, Zalka A: Commonly used suturing techniques in skin surgery. Am Fam Physician 1991;44(5):1625–1634; and 1991;44(6):2123–2128.

Snell G: Laceration repair. *In* Pfenninger JL, Fowler GC (eds): Procedures for Primary Care Physicians. St Louis, Mosby–Year Book, 1994.

Swanson NA: Atlas of Cutaneous Surgery. Boston, Little, Brown, 1986.

Zuber TJ, DeWitt DE: The fusiform excision. Am Fam Physician 1994;49(2):371–378.

Zuber TJ, Pfenninger JL: The Reimbursement Manual for Office Procedures. Midland, MI, The National Procedures Institute, 1994.

Zuber TJ, Purvis JR: Coding and reimbursement of primary care biopsy and destruction procedures. J Fam Pract 1992;35:433–441.

282 Common Neurologic Symptoms

Dizziness is one of the most elusive and difficult symptoms to evaluate and manage, yet its incidence is second only to that of fatigue among nonpain symptoms reported by outpatient clinics. While generally defined as a disturbed state of spatial awareness, in clinical practice, it is often a vague complaint encompassing many varying disease processes. Despite the vast differential, dizziness is often self-limiting; even chronic dizziness is not associated with an increased incidence of serious disease such as tumor or cerebrovascular accident (CVA).

Differential Diagnosis

Drackman's classic study has led to the classification of four types:

1. Vertigo (about 50 per cent)
2. Presyncope (5 per cent)
3. Disequilibrium (5 per cent)
4. Light-headedness (20 per cent)

Idiopathic causes may constitute 10 to 15 per cent.

Refer to Ch. 283, Stroke; Ch. 288, Migraine Headache; and Ch. 303, Meniere's Disease.

Vertigo

Defined as sensation of abnormal movement, often spinning of the surroundings or of the body. This is the most common cause of dizziness.

1. *Peripheral vertigo*
   a. Benign positional vertigo: the most common cause of peripheral vertigo. Described as brief, episodic vertigo associated with changes of head position, especially while recumbent.
   b. Labyrinthitis: intense constant vertigo for a few days, resolving within 1 to 2 weeks, often accompanied by hearing loss. This is often further subdivided by cause.
      (1) Viral: most common
      (2) Bacterial: severe, seen in the setting of bacterial meningitis
      (3) Serous: associated with otitis media
   c. Vestibular neuronitis: unilateral vestibular dysfunction without hearing loss
   d. Meniere's disease: episodic vertigo with spells occurring for hours, recurring over months to years.

Accompanied by hearing loss, tinnitus, and a feeling of pressure in the affected ear.

2. *Central vertigo:* These disorders are less common than peripheral vertigo and are frequently manifested by other disorders, with dizziness being a secondary complaint. Examples:
   a. Vertebrobasilar insufficiency, often associated with other symptoms such as ataxia, diplopia, or facial weakness
   b. Tumors. Acoustic neuromas are tumors of the eighth cranial nerve associated with asymmetric hearing loss.

Vertigo is usually mild and not the presenting complaint. Other less frequent causes of central vertigo include multiple sclerosis, cerebellar or lateral medullary infarction, and migraine headaches.

History

It is important to focus on the duration, episodic nature, severity, and affective position, along with hearing loss and other associated symptoms such as weakness and ataxia.

1. Physical examination: The ear should be examined to rule out cerumen impaction or otitis media. A gross hearing screen can be helpful. Specific attention should be placed on a thorough neurologic examination. Probably the most useful test is the Hallpike maneuver, in which the patient's head is rotated to one side and then lowered slowly to 30 degrees below the horizontal. The patient is observed for nystagmus (either rotational or vertical) and reproduction of the vertigo symptoms. In benign positional vertigo, the patient experiences rotational nystagmus and often severe vertigo, but usually on only one side. Also, the response resolves quickly and cannot be reproduced after two to three repetitions; this is known as "fatigability." In contrast, central lesions may cause vertical nystagmus, usually of a longer duration and with the absence of fatigability.

2. Further testing: usually only necessary to confirm a suspected diagnosis, as suggested by a thorough history and physical examination.
   a. Audiometry may be particularly useful. If asymptomatic hearing loss is noted, consider brain stem auditory evoked response. If consistent with a unilateral eighth nerve lesion, an imaging study is warranted to rule out a tumor, especially acoustic neuroma. Magnetic resonance imaging is the imaging modality of choice; however, if it is not

available, computed tomography with contrast is adequate.

b. If vertigo persists or there is uncertain diagnosis, further testing, usually in consultation with a neurotologist, may be warranted. These tests may include electronystagmography, rotational chair, dynamic posturagraphy, and a neurotologic examination.

Management

1. *Benign positional vertigo:* Pharmacologic therapy usually is not helpful. Habituation exercises that recreate the symptoms may lessen the severity and frequency of vertigo. However, many patients may not be able to tolerate the intense vertigo associated with this reproduction.

2. *Acute labyrinthitis:* vestibular neuronitis. Treat with

   a. Meclizine, 25 to 50 mg orally q 6 hr

   b. Dimenhydrinate, 50 mg orally q 6 hr

   c. Promethazine, 25 to 50 mg orally q 6 hr

3. *Meniere's disease:* Difficult to treat. Sodium restrictions and diuretics (i.e., HCTZ, 25 mg, triamterene, 50 mg) may decrease the frequency of attacks. For chronic disabling disease, ablative surgery also can be considered.

Presyncope

Usually associated with cardiovascular disease. Described as a feeling of impending faint or loss of consciousness but no true syncope.

1. *Cardiac:* Usually accompanied by other symptoms such as chest pain, shortness of breath, or dyspnea on exertion.

   a. *Mechanical:* Consider valvular disease (aortic stenosis), outflow obstruction (hypertrophic obstructive cardiomyopathy), or poor cardiac output.

   b. *Electrical:* Arrhythmias.

2. *Vascular:* More common than cardiac causes and usually benign. Patients may describe orthostatic symptoms related to position change. There are multiple causes, including vasovagal response, medications, dysautonomia, and decreased baroreceptor sensitivity associated with aging.

History

Focus on the medications (e.g., phenothiazines, nitrates, α_1 blockers), position effect on symptoms, and accompanying symptoms consistent with cardiovascular disease.

1. Physical examination: orthostatic blood pressure and pulse measurements in the lying, sitting, and standing positions may be useful. Careful cardiovascular examination to evaluate for poor cardiac output or valvular disease.

2. Additional testing: May need an electrocardiogram, echocardiogram, or chest radiograph to further evalu-

ate cardiovascular disease. Holter monitoring may be useful if arrhythmia is suspected.

Management

Management depends on the underlying disorder.

Disequilibrium

Usually seen in elderly patients with multiple concomitant illnesses. The hallmark of this disorder is an unsteady gait.

History

Should focus on any illnesses that may be reversible to improve patient function. Direct questioning toward visual acuity (cataracts), neuromuscular (history of CVA with residual deficit or peripheral neuropathy, central nervous system disease such as Parkinson's), or a history of degenerative joint disease.

1. Physical examination should encompass a careful examination of gait and static balance. It is important to evaluate muscle strength, reflexes, proprioception, and coordination. Visual acuity and fields also may be important.

2. Further testing: If peripheral neuropathy is suspected, vitamin B_{12} and folate levels, VDRL, blood glucose, and thyroid function tests may be useful.

Management

This is usually limited, because the disease processes are frequently chronic and irreversible. May consider physical therapy for strength improvement. It is important to increase safety in the home environment (no loose rugs or long staircases). A walker or other supportive device also may be helpful.

Light-headedness

Often very vague and difficult to evaluate. Light-headedness is often associated with underlying psychiatric disorders such as anxiety, depression, stress reactions, and substance abuse. The hyperventilation syndrome also can cause dizziness but is often accompanied by other symptoms, including headache, palpitations, chest pain, and weakness.

History

Should focus on thorough social history, including substance abuse, as well as questions regarding depression and anxiety. Physical examination is often normal. Hyperventilation may reproduce symptoms; however, this is nonspecific, since it also may cause dizziness in patients with a vestibular disorder.

Management

Supportive with reassurance of benign and self-limited

nature of this condition. It is important to address any underlying psychiatric disorder if present.

Bibliography

Drackman DA, Hart CW: An approach to the dizzy patient. Neurology 1972;22:323–334.

Kroenke K: Dizziness: Practical office workup and recommendations. Consultant 1993;1:80–90.

Kroenke K, Lucas CA, Rosenberg ML, et al: Causes of persistent dizziness: A prospective study of 100 patients in ambulatory care. Ann Intern Med 1992;117:898–904.

Stein J, et al: Textbook of Internal Medicine, 3rd ed. Boston, Little, Brown, 1990, pp 928–930.

Warner EA, Wallach PM, Adelman HM, Sahlin-Hughes K: Dizziness in primary care patients. J Gen Intern Med 1992;7:454–463.

Symptom	**Tremor**	*Thomas R. Pellegrino*

1. *Tremor* is defined as a rhythmic, oscillating, involuntary movement that may involve the extremities, the trunk, or the head and neck. Like other involuntary movements, it may be temporarily suppressed by the patient and is absent during sleep. Tremor is frequently worsened by anxiety or fatigue and by a wide variety of medications. Tremor may present as an isolated phenomenon or may be a symptom of some underlying disease.

2. Most individuals have experienced tremor at some time, usually when anxious or fatigued or following excess use of caffeine, alcohol, or over-the-counter medications; such tremors are self-limited and usually cause no impairment of function, so such persons rarely seek medical attention.

3. In some persons, tremor may be virtually constant and may cause significant embarrassment or annoyance; tremor also may cause serious impairment of function. Handwriting and other fine movements are often affected, but some patients may experience difficulty with speech, eating, or working.

Differential Diagnosis

Tremors traditionally are characterized as either resting or action tremors depending on when they are most evident, but this distinction is not absolute. In addition, more than one kind of tremor may be present in a given patient.

1. Action tremors: typically increased with muscle activity and reduced or absent at rest.

   a. Physiologic tremor: most evident in extremities held in fixed position against gravity. Usually of low amplitude, fast (6 to 12 Hz). Most evident in fingers and hands; little functional impairment.

   b. Essential tremor: most evident during active use of affected muscles. Low or moderate amplitude, fast (6 to 12 Hz). May involve extremities or head and neck. May cause significant functional impairment.

   c. Cerebellar tremor: classic "intention" tremor. Moderate or high amplitude, relatively slow (3 to 5 Hz). Often causes severe functional impairment.

2. Resting tremors: typically maximal when the involved extremities are at rest and relieved or absent during voluntary activity. Parkinsonian tremor may be associated with idiopathic Parkinson's disease or with parkinsonism of some other cause.

The most important diagnostic distinction is between parkinsonian tremor and essential tremor; note that *both* may be present in a given patient. Parkinsonian tremors, as noted, are typically most evident at rest; they may be asymmetrical and involve the extremities, sparing the head and neck. The typical movement is alternation of pronation and supination of the forearm or "pill-rolling" movements of the fingers. Essential tremor, on the other hand, is most evident during activity; it is usually symmetrical and may involve the head and neck as well as the extremities. The typical movement is flexion-extension.

> Refer to Ch. 296, Parkinson's Disease.

History: Key Questions to Ask

1. Is the tremor present primarily at rest or with activity?

2. Which parts of the body are affected? Does the tremor affect both sides of the body equally?

3. What makes the tremor better or worse? Ask about the effects of any drugs, caffeine, alcohol.

4. Does the patient use any regular drugs (with or without medical advice)? What about alcohol?

5. How does the tremor affect the patient? Is the effect only cosmetically limiting, or does the tremor impair specific activities?

6. Are there other symptoms of neurologic disease? Ask specifically about weakness, "stiffness" or slowness of movement, impaired gait or balance, slurred speech, and altered handwriting.

7. Is there any family history of tremor?

Clinical Findings

1. Is the tremor present primarily at rest or with activity? What parts of the body are affected?

2. Is the movement flexion-extension or pronation-supination? Is "pill-rolling" present?

3. Is muscle tone normal or increased? Is cogwheel rigidity present?

4. Is there any abnormality of speech, gait, or posture?

The clinical examination is helpful to clarify the details of the history and to look for other signs of neurologic disease that may not have been reported by the patient. In most patients presenting for evaluation of tremor, a fairly comprehensive neurologic examination will be necessary.

Tests

In most cases, the diagnosis of a specific tremor is based entirely on the history and clinical examination. There are no specific laboratory or imaging studies needed unless the clinical evaluation suggests some underlying disease.

Management

1. Physiologic tremor
   a. Reassure patient that no "disease" is present.
   b. Avoid caffeine and other stimulants.
   c. Anxiolytics for *occasional* use in specific stressful situations
   d. *Propranolol* in small doses (10 to 20 mg t.i.d.) is sometimes helpful.
2. Essential tremor
   a. Avoid caffeine and other stimulants.
   b. Alcohol in small amounts frequently is very helpful but should be recommended with *great caution*.
   c. Either *propranolol* or *primidone* may be helpful.

If one drug is ineffective or not tolerated, try the other. Doses:
   (1) Propranolol, 20 mg t.i.d. to start; increase as needed and tolerated.
   (2) Primidone, 50 mg at bedtime to start; gradually increase to 250 to 300 mg/day in divided doses.
3. Cerebellar tremor: usually very difficult to treat unless underlying disease can be treated. In some patients, physical or occupational therapy can be helpful. No specific drug therapy available.
4. Parkinsonian tremor
   a. Stop or reduce any drugs that might exacerbate parkinsonism.
   b. In patients with Parkinson's disease, use standard treatment regimens.

Bibliography

Calne DB: Treatment of Parkinson's disease. N Engl J Med 1993;329:1021–1027.

Friedman JH: Essential tremor. *In* Johnson RT, Griffen JW (eds): Current Therapy in Neurologic Disease, 4th ed. St. Louis, Mosby–Year Book, 1993, pp 273–276.

Koller WC, Busenbark K, Miner K: The relationship of essential tremor to other movement disorders: A report on 678 patients. Ann Neurol 1994;35:717–723.

Stern MB: Parkinson's disease. *In* Johnson RT, Griffen JW (eds): Current Therapy in Neurologic Disease, 4th ed. St. Louis, Mosby–Year Book, 1993, pp. 242–246.

Weiner WJ, Lang AE: Movement Disorders: A Comprehensive Survey. Mt. Kisco, NY, Futura, 1989, pp 221–256.

| Symptom | **Paresthesias** | *James P. McKenna* |

Paresthesias are abnormal sensations arising spontaneously without an apparent stimulus. These sensations have been described variously as tingling, pins and needles, prickling, electric, burning, vibrating, buzzing, or crawling. Paresthesias often arise from compression of peripheral nerves but also may result from ectopic foci in the peripheral or central nervous system. Brief paresthesias occurring from resting on the sciatic, peroneal, or ulnar nerve may be experienced as the limb "falling asleep" and have no significance; however, persistent paresthesias warrant further evaluation.

Differential Diagnosis

A. Most common
   1. Entrapment neuropathies
      a. Carpal tunnel syndrome—median nerve at the wrist
      b. Cubital tunnel syndrome—ulnar nerve at the elbow
      c. Peroneal neuropathy—peroneal nerve lateral at the head of the fibula
      d. Meralgia paresthetica—lateral femoral cutaneous nerve at the inguinal ligament
   2. Radiculopathy
      a. Cervical—C5, C6, or C7
      b. Lumbosacral—L5 or S1
   3. Restless legs syndrome
   4. Diabetic polyneuropathy
   5. Vitamin B_{12} deficiency
B. Less common
   1. Multiple sclerosis
   2. Guillain-Barré syndrome
   3. Medication (isoniazid, vincristine, diuretics, nonsteroidal anti-inflammatory drugs [NSAIDs])
   4. Hypocalcemia
   5. Carcinomatous neuropathy (breasts and lung cancer)

Carpal tunnel syndrome, the most common compression mononeuropathy, is often bilateral, with the dominant hand more severely affected. Median nerve entrapment is usually idiopathic or occupational but may be secondary to pregnancy, hypothyroidism, rheumatoid arthritis, sequelae of injury, and rarely due to amyloidosis, acromegaly, or multiple myeloma. B_{12} deficiency is most often due to pernicious anemia but may be secondary to gastric disease (gastrectomy, tumor) or small intestine malabsorption (Crohn's disease, celiac sprue, blind loop). Rare causes of paresthesias include leprosy, polycythemia vera, tumors of peripheral nerves, rabies, focal sensory seizures, and other causes of neuropathy, including less common entrapment neuropathies.

> Refer to Chs. 159 and 160, Diabetes Mellitus; Ch. 212, Carpal Tunnel and Other Nerve Entrapments; Ch. 299, Multiple Sclerosis; and Ch. 304, Guillain-Barré Syndrome.

History: Key Questions to Ask

1. What is the distribution of the paresthesias?
2. How long have the sensations been present?
3. Does any position or activity alter those sensations?
4. Does pain, numbness, weakness, stiffness, or clumsiness exist?
5. Have there been any recent changes in medication?

Paresthesias that occur only in the distribution of single peripheral nerves are most often secondary to entrapment neuropathies. Pain, numbness, and weakness, if present, are confined to the distribution to the nerve and usually are of gradual onset. Pain from radiculopathy, usually due to degenerative disk disease, is typically abrupt in onset, increased by twisting and bending, and exacerbated by heavy lifting or the Valsalva maneuver. The restless legs syndrome manifests as uncomfortable, crawling, dull, tingling sensations in the lower legs that occur at rest, especially at night, and produce an irresistible urge to move the legs. Distal sensory polyneuropathy is the most common diabetic neuropathy and occurs in about 40 per cent of diabetics whose illness has spanned 25 years. Symptoms may include paresthesias, numbness, and severe aching, deep pain. About 70 per cent of patients with neurologic symptoms from B_{12} deficiency experience paresthesias, typically in a glove and stocking distribution. Twenty per cent of patients with multiple sclerosis present with paresthesias. Paresthesias are the earliest symptom in most cases of Guillain-Barré syndrome, followed by rapidly progressing ascending weakness.

Clinical Findings

1. Tinel's sign (percussing an entrapped nerve heightens distal paresthesias) may be present in carpal tunnel and cubital tunnel syndromes.
2. Phalen's sign (flexion of the wrists enhancing median nerve paresthesias) may be present with carpal tunnel syndrome.
3. Sensory abnormalities in common entrapment syndromes
   a. Carpal tunnel syndrome—palmar surface of radial three and one-half fingers
   b. Cubital tunnel syndrome—ulnar side of the fourth finger and fifth finger
   c. Peroneal nerve—lateral aspect of the leg
   d. Meralgia paresthetica—anterolateral thigh
4. Radiculopathy may cause decreased strength, sensation, and reflexes in the corresponding affected nerve root.
5. Physical findings in restless leg syndrome occur only in cases secondary to iron or folate deficiency or uremia.
6. Diabetic polyneuropathy is predominantly sensory with bilateral loss of sensation for pain, touch, temperature, and proprioception distally with minimal weakness.
7. B_{12} deficiency may cause paresthesias only early in the course of the illness or may occur with anemia, glossitis, abnormal position and vibrations, weakness, spasticity, decreased deep tendon reflexes, and a wide variety of psychiatric features ranging from mood and personality changes to psychosis and delirium.
8. Multiple sclerosis manifestations may be protean and depend on the locations of the plaques (see Ch. 299, Multiple Sclerosis).
9. Guillain-Barré syndrome is characterized by an ascending paralysis and hyporeflexia with much less significant or absent sensory disturbance.
10. Lhermitte's sign (flexion of the neck causing paresthesias radiating from the neck into the limbs) is classically present in cervical cord disease due to multiple sclerosis but may be present with other cervical cord lesions.
11. Paresthesias may occur with no abnormal physical findings early in B_{12} deficiency, multiple sclerosis, Guillain-Barré syndrome, and entrapment neuropathies.

Tests

1. In most cases of paresthesias, a careful history and physical examination will reveal the cause of the paresthesias.
2. Electromyography (EMG) and nerve conduction studies help identify the source of the abnormality.
3. Glucose and glycosylated hemoglobin levels demonstrate the degree of control in diabetes.
4. Vitamin B_{12}. If a deficiency exists, the levels are usually less than 200 pg/ml. Schilling tests locate the malabsorption site.
5. Polysomnography demonstrates periodic movements of sleep in restless legs syndrome but are rarely necessary.
6. Magnetic resonance imaging is the most reliable imaging study in multiple sclerosis.

7. Cerebrospinal fluid demonstrates rising serum protein in Guillain-Barré syndrome and oligocolonal banding in multiple sclerosis.

8. Normal values of ferritin, blood urea nitrogen (BUN), creatinine, bicarbonate, and folate exclude secondary causes of restless legs syndrome.

9. Normal serum calcium levels exclude hypocalcemia.

Management

1. Entrapment neuropathies

   a. Carpal tunnel syndrome—wrist cock-up splint, anti-inflammatory medication, surgical decompression

   b. Cubital tunnel syndrome—elbow splint to prevent elbow flexion, surgical decompression if necessary

   c. Peroneal nerve—Avoid crossing legs.

   d. Meralgia paresthetica—Avoid compression, weight loss, hydrocortisone injections.

2. Radiculopathy—Avoid activities that increase pain, physical therapy, NSAIDs, limited bed rest; surgery if unresponsive.

3. Diabetes—Improve diabetic control; amitriptyline or desipramine from 10 to 25 mg at bedtime up to 125 to 150 mg for painful neuropathy.

4. Vitamin B_{12} deficiency—1000 μg intramuscularly weekly for 1 month and then once a month for life

5. Guillain-Barré syndrome—Initiate plasmapheresis early.

6. Multiple sclerosis—ACTH, methylprednisone, and prednisone have been demonstrated in clinical trials to benefit.

Follow-Up

Follow-up is essential to ensure that the causes of paresthesias have been appropriately evaluated.

PEARLS

- Transient paresthesias do not suggest a neurologic lesion.

- If paresthesias persist and no abnormality is found, re-examine the patient.

- Neurologic abnormalities may precede hematologic abnormalities in vitamin B_{12} deficiency.

 Bibliography

Diseases of the peripheral nerves. *In* Adams RD, Victor N (eds): Principles of Neurology, 5th ed. New York, McGraw-Hill, 1993, pp 1117–1169.

Feasby TE: Inflammatory demyelinating polyneuropathies. Neurol Clin 1992;10:651–670.

Jeddy TA, Berridge DC: Restless legs syndrome. Br J Surg 1994;81:49–50.

Posner JB: Disorders of sensation. *In* Bennett JC, Plum F (eds): Cecil Textbook of Medicine, 20th ed. Philadelphia, WB Saunders, 1996.

Thompson HG, Roland LT: Pain and paresthesias. *In* Roland LT (ed): Merritt's Textbook of Neurology, 8th ed. Philadelphia, Lea & Febiger, 1989, pp 28–30.

283 Stroke

Douglas C. McCrory

Etiology

A. Ischemic (75 per cent of all strokes)
   1. Thrombus related to atherosclerosis of carotid or large intracranial arteries (30 per cent of ischemic strokes)
   2. Embolus from cardiac source (20 per cent of ischemic strokes); secondary hemorrhage may follow embolic stroke.
   3. Lacunar (small vessel) (20 per cent of ischemic strokes)
   4. Unknown, multiple, or uncommon causes (30 per cent of ischemic strokes)

B. Intracerebral hemorrhage (15 per cent of all strokes)—bleeding directly into brain parenchyma
   1. Amyloid angiopathy in the elderly
   2. Hypertensive arterial disease
   3. Arteriovenous malformations (AVMs)
   4. Anticoagulant drugs or bleeding diatheses

C. Subarachnoid hemorrhage (SAH) (10 per cent of all strokes)—bleeding around the brain
   1. Ruptured congenital (''berry'') aneurysm (80 per cent of SAHs)
   2. Amyloid angiopathy in the elderly
   3. Inflammatory or infectious processes or drug abuse

Symptoms

A. Focal symptoms
   1. Focal or multifocal neurologic deficit persisting for more than 24 hours
   2. Carotid (anterior circulation) system symptoms can involve the upper and/or lower extremity and/or face on the opposite side, the opposite visual field, or the eye on the same side.
      a. Motor dysfunction
         (1) Dysarthria
         (2) Weakness
         (3) Clumsiness
      b. Sensory symptoms
         (1) Numbness
         (2) Paresthesia
      c. Loss of vision
         (1) Monocular blindness (same side eye)
         (2) Homonymous hemianopia (opposite visual field)
      d. Aphasia
      e. Hemispatial neglect
   3. Vertebrobasilar (posterior circulation) system symptoms can involve any combination of upper and lower extremities and face, left and/or right sides.
      a. Motor dysfunction
         (1) Dysarthria
         (2) Weakness
         (3) Clumsiness
      b. Sensory symptoms
         (1) Numbness
         (2) Paresthesia
      c. Loss of vision
         (1) Monocular blindness (same side eye)
         (2) Homonymous hemianopia (opposite visual field)
      d. Loss of balance, ataxia, vertigo, diplopia, or dysphagia

B. Nonfocal symptoms suggest increased intracranial pressure (ICP) and are common in subarachnoid hemorrhage, hypertensive cerebral hemorrhage, or major ischemic stroke with cerebral edema.
   1. Headache
   2. Vomiting
   3. Impaired level of consciousness (restlessness, drowsiness, coma)
   4. Cranial nerve palsies

Key Symptoms

Focal	Nonfocal
• Aphasia	• Headache
• Dysarthria	• Coma
• Hemiparesis	
• Monocular blindness	

Clinical Findings

1. Physical examination clues to cause
   a. Carotid bruit—systolic murmur heard over the mid to upper neck
   b. Hollenhorst plaque—atheromatous emboli visible in retinal arterioles on ocular fundus examination
2. Anatomic localization (see Symptoms)
   a. Sidedness of neurologic deficits
   b. Pattern of neurologic deficits

Key Signs

• Carotid bruit

• Hollenhorst plaque

Laboratory Tests

1. Computed cerebral axial tomography (CT scan)
   a. Distinguishes ischemic and hemorrhagic stroke
   b. Should be performed within 24 hours
2. Carotid artery duplex Doppler ultrasonography—in carotid area symptoms to screen for carotid stenosis
3. Echocardiography—identifies intracardiac thrombi (source of embolus)
4. Cerebral angiography
   a. Determines the degree and location of a known carotid stenosis
   b. Necessary prior to carotid endarterectomy
   c. Identifies aneurysm or AVM suspected from CT scan in hemorrhagic stroke

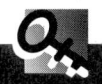

Key Tests

- CT scan
- Carotid artery duplex Doppler ultrasound
- Transthoracic echocardiography

Differential Diagnosis

1. Migraine prodrome
2. Subdural hematoma
3. Brain tumors
4. Seizure disorder
5. Arteritis
6. Multiple sclerosis
7. Central nervous system infection

Treatment

1. Perform serial neurologic examinations to recognize progressing stroke.
2. Control excessively high systemic blood pressure. Aggressive control may be dangerous except in the setting of hypertensive encephalopathy or acute myocardial infarction.
3. Avoid hypotonic fluids (e.g., D_5W), which may exacerbate cerebral edema.
4. Avoid prolonged use of intravenous and indwelling urinary catheters.

Medication

1. Low-dose heparin is used to prevent thrombophlebitis in acute stroke.
2. Aspirin is useful for secondary prevention of ischemic stroke.
3. Ticlopidine (Ticlid) is an alternative to aspirin when it fails or patients are aspirin-intolerant
4. Anticoagulant drugs—high-dose heparin (short term), warfarin (long term)
   a. Should be used only after hemorrhage has been ruled out by CT scan
   b. Acute treatment for progressive ischemic stroke
   c. Secondary prevention of cardiogenic emboli

Surgery

1. Carotid endarterectomy is useful for secondary prevention of ischemia in patients with anterior circulation nondisabling strokes and an ipsilateral carotid stenosis of more than 70 per cent.
2. Craniotomy for intracranial aneurysm or AVM

Diet

1. Nothing by mouth for the first 24 hours
2. Clinically assess swallowing to exclude aspiration before initiating diet.
3. Begin enteral nutrition (e.g., via nasoduodenal tube or gastrostomy tube) within a week if unable to take oral feeding.

Activity

1. Frequent turning and appropriate bedding for immobile patients
2. Range-of-motion exercises to avoid contracture
3. Early physical therapy to improve bed mobility, transfers, ambulation, ability for activities of daily living

Patient Education

1. Discuss expectations for recovery with patient and family.
2. Begin planning for intermediate care in rehabilitation facility, nursing home, or home.

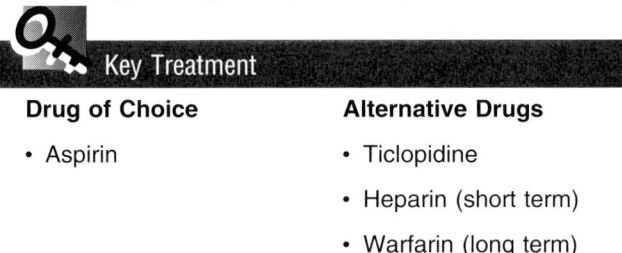

Key Treatment

Drug of Choice	Alternative Drugs
• Aspirin	• Ticlopidine
	• Heparin (short term)
	• Warfarin (long term)

Follow-Up

1. Monitor for depression, common following stroke.
2. Rehabilitation at home or specialized facility
3. Risk factor modification
   a. Hypertension
   b. Smoking
   c. Diabetes mellitus
   d. Heavy alcohol use
   e. Hypercholesterolemia

Bibliography

Adams HP Jr, Love BB: Medical management of aneurysmal subarachnoid hemorrhage. *In* Barnett HJM, Mohr JP, Stein BM, Yatsu FM (eds): Stroke: Pathophysiology, Diagnosis, and Management, 2nd ed. New York, Churchill Livingstone, 1992, pp 1029–1054.

Goldstein LB, Matchar DB: Clinical assessment in the evaluation of stroke. JAMA 1994;271:1114–1120.

Gresham GE: Rehabilitation of the stroke survivor. *In* Barnett HJM, Mohr JP, Stein BM, Yatsu FM (eds): Stroke: Pathophysiology, Diagnosis, and Management, 2nd ed. New York, Churchill Livingstone, 1992, pp 1189–1201.

Marshall RS, Mohr JP: Current management of ischaemic stroke. J Neurol Neurosurg Psychiatry 1993;56:6–16.

Matchar DB, McCrory DC, Barnett HJM, Feussner JR: Medical treatment for stroke prevention. Ann Intern Med 1994; 121(1):41–53.

284 Transient Ischemic Attack

Robert J. Wityk

Etiology

1. A transient ischemic attack (TIA) is defined as a neurologic deficit caused by focal ischemia that resolves completely within 24 hours. The risk of subsequent stroke is 5 to 10 per cent per year and is highest in the first month after TIA. Transient monocular blindness (TMB), also called amaurosis fugax, may represent in some cases a TIA involving the eye.
2. Causes of TIA/TMB include
   a. Large-artery atherosclerosis (e.g., carotid stenosis, intracranial stenosis)
   b. Small-vessel disease (lacunar TIA)
   c. Embolism: cardiac source, aortic arch atheroma, intravenous drug abuse
   d. Hematologic disorders: coagulopathy (e.g., antiphospholipid syndrome), thrombocytosis, leukemia, polycythemia, sickle cell disease
   e. Nonatherosclerotic vasculopathy: arterial dissection, vasculitis (e.g., Takayasu's arteritis), fibromuscular dysplasia, moyamoya

Symptoms

1. Most TIAs last between 10 and 20 minutes, and the majority last less than 1 hour. TIAs due to large-vessel atherosclerosis are often hemodynamic in nature and occur as stereotyped, repetitive spells. Cardioembolic TIAs tend to last longer and may present as a major neurologic deficit that resolves over an hour or two.
2. TMB can occur as a shade obscuring the upper or lower half of vision in one eye. Some patients report complete loss of vision in the eye or a "graying" of vision.
3. A list of carotid-, vertebrobasilar-, and lacunar-related symptoms is shown in Table 284–1.

Key Symptoms

• Hemiparesis	• Dysarthria
• Aphasia	• Visual loss
• Paresthesias	• Diplopia

Clinical Findings

1. Most patients with TIA are neurologically intact. Examination should include auscultation for carotid, supraclavicular, and orbital bruits. Neurologic examination may reveal signs of previous strokes or acute neurologic deficit of which the patient is unaware (e.g., unilateral neglect or visual field loss).
2. Patients with TMB should be examined for temporal artery tenderness, optic nerve lesions, and retinal emboli. Patients should be referred for complete ophthalmologic evaluation, including dilated fundus examination and measurement of intraocular pressure.

Key Signs

- Carotid bruit
- Retinal emboli

Laboratory Tests

1. Routine laboratory tests include
   a. Complete blood count (CBC), platelets, coagulation tests (PT/aPTT)
   b. Electrolytes, glucose, and calcium
   c. Sedimentation rate (particularly for TMB if temporal arteritis is suspected)
   d. In selected patients: antinuclear antibodies (ANA), syphilis serology, toxicology screen
2. Head computed tomographic (CT) scan should be obtained because 10 to 20 per cent of patients with TIA have an infarct in the territory of the brain relevant to their symptoms. Magnetic resonance imaging (MRI) is more sensitive than CT and is preferred for patients with lacunar or vertebrobasilar TIAs or when vascular territory is not well defined.
3. Vascular evaluation includes carotid duplex studies for patients with TMB or carotid territory TIA. Transcranial Doppler studies of the intracranial vertebrobasilar system are useful screening tests for patients with brain stem TIA.
4. Magnetic resonance angiography (MRA) is an alternative to ultrasound studies. MRA is performed without infusion of contrast material and can be obtained concurrent with an MRI. The specificity and sensitivity of MRA appear to be equal to or better than those of ultrasound. Although the role of MRA is evolving, it is a good noninvasive means for assessment of both intra- and extracranial vessels.
5. Echocardiography and Holter monitoring are used to look for cardiac sources of emboli. Transesophageal echocardiography (TEE) with a bubble study (looking

TABLE 284–1.   SYMPTOMS OF TIA

Carotid Territory	Vertebrobasilar
Paresthesia/weakness of hand, arm, and face	Dysarthria
Aphasia (dominant hemisphere)	Vertigo, ataxia
Dysarthria	Diplopia
Unilateral neglect	Visual field loss
	Perioral paresthesias
Lacunar	Acute confusional state
Hemibody sensory loss or paresthesia	Profound general weakness
Pure motor hemiparesis	

for intracardiac shunting) is preferred in young patients. TEE is also useful in older patients with unexplained TIAs to evaluate for aortic arch atheroma.

6. Angiography also should be considered in patients with
   a. Carotid stenosis and TIA who are potential candidates for carotid endarterectomy
   b. Intracranial large-vessel disease suggested by noninvasive tests in whom long-term anticoagulant use is considered
   c. Recurrent TIAs and inconclusive noninvasive evaluation
   d. Suspected carotid or vertebral artery dissection
7. Other tests to be considered, particularly if no clear etiology is found, include
   a. Detailed coagulation studies (e.g., antiphospholipid antibodies, Russell's viper venom time for lupus anticoagulant)
   b. Lumbar puncture for signs of meningeal inflammation

Key Tests

- Sedimentation rate
- Carotid duplex
- Head CT scan

Alternative

- MRI with magnetic resonance angiography

Differential Diagnosis

1. Migraine with aura typically presents with visual scintillations and scotoma and can occur in the absence of headaches and for the first time in later life.
2. Focal seizures may produce focal or migratory sensory symptoms. Postictal weakness (Todd's paralysis) can mimic TIA if the history is unclear.
3. Other considerations in the differential diagnosis include
   a. Brain lesions: tumor, subdural hematoma, arteriovenous malformation
   b. Metabolic: hypoglycemia, hypercalcemia, hyperventilation
   c. Peripheral nerve disorder: carpal tunnel, radiculopathy
   d. Cardiac arrhythmia, cardiac syncope
   e. Vertigo from labyrinthitis or Meniere's disease
4. The differential diagnosis of TMB should specifically include
   a. Temporal arteritis
   b. Optic nerve disorders: optic neuritis, ischemic optic neuropathy, papilledema (including pseudotumor cerebri)
   c. Ocular disorders: glaucoma, branch retinal artery occlusion, central retinal vein occlusion, retinal detachment, retinal artery vasospasm

Treatment

1. Carotid disease: Carotid territory TIA with 70 to 99 per cent carotid stenosis is an indication for carotid endarterectomy in patients who are a good surgical risk. The value of surgery in patients with less than 70 per cent stenosis or an ulcerated plaque is uncertain. Medical treatment is aspirin, 325 mg daily. Patients with acute carotid artery occlusion may benefit from 4 to 6 weeks of anticoagulant therapy followed by aspirin. Patients with chronic carotid occlusion and TIA often respond to improving cerebral perfusion by hydration, prevention of orthostatic hypotension, and reduction of antihypertensive medications.
2. Vertebrobasilar disease: Patients with vertebrobasilar stenosis or occlusion often improve with anticoagulants. The long-term benefit of anticoagulation is uncertain. Patients with less severe disease should be treated with aspirin.
3. Lacunar TIA: Aspirin, 325 mg daily, is the treatment of choice.
4. Cardiac emboli: Heparin followed by warfarin is recommended. Patients with prosthetic valves and TIAs on warfarin may benefit from the addition of dipyridamole or aspirin.
5. Arterial dissection: Anticoagulation with warfarin is used for 3 to 6 months to prevent artery-to-artery embolism. Many patients have spontaneous healing of the dissection and can then be switched to aspirin.
6. Recurrent symptoms on aspirin: Higher doses of aspirin are helpful (325 mg twice or three times daily). Ticlopidine (Ticlid), 250 mg twice daily with meals, is an alternative treatment for patients who are aspirin-intolerant or who have recurrent TIAs on aspirin. Diarrhea is a common side effect, and patients must be monitored with biweekly blood counts for leukopenia (generally reversible on stopping the drug).

Key Treatment

- Treatment depends on the suspected underlying etiology.

Follow-Up

1. Patients with TIA have a high incidence of coronary artery disease (often silent) and may need further cardiac evaluation as well as risk-factor reduction.
2. Young patients with a negative evaluation tend to have a benign prognosis.

 ## Bibliography

Barnett HJ, Eliasziw M, Meldrum HE: Drugs and surgery in the prevention of ischemic stroke. N Engl J Med 1995;332:238–248.

Brass LM, Fayad PB, Levin SR: Transient ischemic attacks in the elderly: Diagnosis and treatment. Geriatrics 1992;47(5): 35–53.

Brown RD, Evans BA, Wiebers DO, et al: Transient ischemic attack and minor ischemic stroke: An algorithm for evaluation and treatment. Mayo Clin Proc 1994;69:1027–1039.

The Amaurosis Fugax Study Group: Current management of amaurosis fugax. Stroke 1990;21:201–208.

van Gijn J: Aspirin: Dose and indications in modern stroke prevention. Neurol Clin 1992;10:193–207.

285 Falls in the Elderly

James T. Pacala

Falls and injurious sequelae of falls are increasingly common with age. About one third of community-dwelling individuals over age 75 fall at least once in a given year; half fall multiple times. Approximately 5 per cent of falls result in a fracture; 1 per cent cause a hip fracture.

Etiology

The cause of most falls is multifactorial. Risk factors for falls can be divided into intrinsic (i.e., characteristics of the faller) and extrinsic (i.e., characteristics of the faller's environment) factors.

A. Intrinsic factors
1. Neurologic disorders arising from a number of conditions (e.g., Alzheimer's, stroke, Parkinson's)
   a. Vestibular dysfunction
   b. Proprioceptive dysfunction
   c. Cognitive impairment
2. Musculoskeletal disorders commonly caused by deconditioning, arthritis, or paralysis
   a. Muscular weakness
   b. Joint pain
   c. Foot problems
3. Sensory impairment
   a. Visual disturbance
   b. Hearing impairment
4. Cardiovascular disorders
   a. Postural hypotension
   b. Cardiac arrhythmia
5. Acute medical illness
6. Medications (can adversely affect all the above)
7. Risky behaviors
   a. Hurrying or running (especially while carrying a heavy object)
   b. High-risk activities (e.g., standing on the back of a chair to reach a high object)
B. Extrinsic factors
1. Environmental obstacles
2. Slippery surfaces
3. Ill-fitting clothes and footwear
4. Poor lighting
5. Inappropriate furniture

Risk Assessment

1. Assess risk for falling by inquiring about conditions listed above as risk factors.
2. In those who have fallen, characterize the fall:
   a. Type: Did the patient fall due to

(1) Stumbling over an object?
(2) Slipping (what type of surface)?
(3) Weakness ("legs gave out")?
(4) Loss of balance?
(5) Loss or near loss of consciousness?

b. Location: room in home, other building, outside
c. Activity just before fall: walking, standing still, arising from bed or chair, climbing stairs, hurrying
d. Level of consciousness: light-headedness, dizziness

Key Symptoms

- Light-headedness
- Loss of equilibrium
- Loss of consciousness (prior to fall)
- Slip
- Stumble or trip
- Weakness, especially in lower extremities

Clinical Findings

1. Abnormal balance
   a. Loses balance after sternal nudge from behind
   b. Unsteady gait on
      (1) Flat surfaces: vestibular dysfunction
      (2) Uneven surfaces: proprioceptive dysfunction
      (3) Turning: proprioceptive, sensory, muscular problems
2. Abnormal gait: decreased step height, festination
3. Cognitive deficit on mental status testing
4. Muscle weakness: difficulty getting up from and sitting down in a chair, paralysis, weakness on examination
5. Foot problems: bunions, calluses
6. Vision problems: cataract, field cut, decreased acuity
7. Hearing problems: cerumen impaction, presbycusis
8. Postural hypotension
9. Contributing medications
   a. Antidepressants
   b. Barbituates
   c. Benzodiazepines
   d. Diuretics
   e. Phenothiazines
10. Extrinsic hazards on home or institutional assessment, including poor lighting, throw rugs, deep-pile carpet, absence of grab bars in shower and toilet, electrical cords and loose items on the floor, poorly fitting shoes

1023

Key Signs

- Abnormal balance
- Abnormal gait
- Muscle weakness
- Risky medical regimen
- Environmental hazards
- Postural hypotension

Laboratory Tests

1. Performance-based balance and gait testing is essential.
   a. The easiest test is to have the patient get up from a chair, walk down a hallway, turn, walk back, and sit down again.
   b. Other, more quantitative tests can be easily accomplished in the office setting, for example, the "get-up and go" test (see Mathias reference).
   c. Formal balance and gait testing can be performed at referral centers.
2. Other tests should be guided by history and physical examination. Examples:
   a. Electrocardiogram and Holter monitoring should be obtained if there was dizziness, light-headedness, or loss of consciousness before the fall.
   b. Vitamin B_{12} and glucose testing is indicated if peripheral neuropathy is present.

Key Test

- Simple balance and gait assessment: Have patient rise from a chair, walk down a hall, turn, walk back, and sit again; evaluate step height, symmetry, path deviation, and balance.

Differential Diagnosis

1. Remember that most falls are caused by several factors.
2. The challenge for clinicians is figuring out which risk factors are implicated.
3. Although rare, it is important to exclude arrhythmia and aortic stenosis if there has been loss or near-loss of consciousness.

Treatment

Medications

1. *Reduction* or *discontinuation* of medicines that can contribute to falls is essential.
2. In cases of postural hypotension, fludrocortisone can be useful as part of the therapeutic regimen.

Diet

1. Adequate caloric intake to help prevent muscular weakness
2. Adequate hydration to minimize postural hypotension

Activity

1. Balance training
2. Gait training
3. Muscle strengthening
4. Correction of vision and hearing problems
5. Correction of foot problems
6. Treatment of acute medical illnesses
7. Elimination of environmental hazards
   a. Remove electrical cords, loose items from floors
   b. Use shallow-pile carpet or nonskid wax on floors
   c. Grab bars in bathroom (toilet and shower)
   d. Properly fitting shoes
   e. Improve lighting, eliminate glare

Patient Education

1. Instruction in risk factors for falls
2. Counsel regarding behavioral risk factors
3. Home safety checklist

Key Treatment

- A multidisciplinary team approach (physician, physical therapist, podiatrist, home assessment nurse) works best to detect and treat all intrinsic and extrinsic risk factors.

Follow-Up

1. After a fall, patients should be seen monthly for 3 months and then quarterly to follow status of risk factors.
2. Many older adults underreport falls. Having them keep a falls diary can be of help.

Bibliography

Malmivaara A, Heliovaara M, Knedt P, et al: Risk factors for injurious falls leading to hospitalization or death in a cohort of 19,500 adults. Am J Epidemiol 1993;138:384–394.

Mathias S, Nayak US, Isaacs B: Balance in elderly patients: The "get-up and go" test. Arch Phys Med Rehabil 1986;67:387–389.

Rubenstein LZ, Robbins AS, Josephson KR, et al: The value of assessing falls in an elderly population: A randomized clinical trial. Ann Intern Med 1990;113:308–316.

Studenski S, Duncan PW, Chandler J, et al: Predicting falls: The role of mobility and nonphysical factors. J Am Geriatr Soc 1994;42:297–302.

Tinetti ME, Speechley M: Prevention of falls among the elderly. N Engl J Med 1989;320:1055–1059.

286 Altered Mental State/Dementia (Delirium)

F. Allan Martin

Etiology

1. Often goes undiagnosed and is associated with a 20 to 30 per cent mortality rate
2. Predisposing factors
   a. Young age but more commonly advanced age
   b. Prior history of dementia or other primary degenerative brain disease
   c. Multiple coexistent medical problems
   d. Presence of polypharmacy, especially psychoactive drugs, but almost any drug or combination can be related to delirium in susceptible persons
   e. Abuse of alcohol or other drugs
3. Frequently the heralding symptoms of underlying major medical or surgical pathology
4. Multiple possible causes exist, and several causes may coexist in any individual patient with delirium (Table 286–1).

Symptoms

1. Multiple areas of possible dysfunction may be variably affected in delirium (Table 286–2).
2. Delirium seems to correlate best with the symptom complex of suddenness of onset and fluctuating course over time with prominent impairment in attention.

Clinical Findings

1. Evaluation of a patient's cognitive status is essential but may be difficult to obtain.

TABLE 286–1. FREQUENT CAUSES OF DELIRIUM

Drugs, dehydration
Electrolyte imbalances, environmental changes (e.g., location, extremes of temperature, etc.)
Liver disease (e.g., encephalopathy), lungs (hypoxia)
Infection (especially urinary tract infection and pneumonia), immune system dysfunction, intracranial lesions
Retention (urinary or fecal)
Ischemia (cerebral or cardiac), intoxication, intestinal obstruction
Uremia
Myocardial disease (e.g., infarction, arrhythmia, congestive heart failure), metabolic abnormalities

2. Key clinical signs usually can be elicited from an interview and thorough physical examination of the patient combined with data from the patient's family and nursing staff. Especially important is the record of all medication use, both prescribed and over-the-counter.
3. No single set of diagnostic criteria exists for all patients.
4. Physical findings usually correlate with the underlying disease processes that caused the delirium.
5. A few nonspecific physical findings may suggest the presence of delirium in an acutely confused patient.
   a. Autonomic dysfunction, such as tachycardia, bradycardia, flushing, pallor, hyper- or hypotension, impairment of pupillary or sweating function
   b. New onset of asterixis, tremor, or seizure

TABLE 286–2. CLINICAL FEATURES OF DELIRIUM, DEMENTIA, AND ACUTE FUNCTIONAL PSYCHOSIS

	DELIRIUM	DEMENTIA	ACUTE FUNCTIONAL PSYCHOSIS
Onset	Sudden	Insidious	Sudden
Course over 24 hours	Fluctuating, with nocturnal exacerbation	Stable	Stable
Consciousness	Reduced	Clear	Clear
Attention	Globally disordered	Normal, except in severe cases	May be disordered
Cognition	Globally disordered	Globally impaired	May be selectively impaired
Hallucinations	Usually visual or visual and auditory	Often absent	Predominantly auditory
Delusions	Fleeting, poorly systematized	Often absent	Sustained, systematized
Orientation	Usually impaired, at least for a time	Often impaired	May be impaired
Psychomotor activity	Increased, reduced, or shifting unpredictably	Often normal	Varies from psychomotor retardation to severe hyperactivity, depending on the type of psychosis
Speech	Often incoherent, slow or rapid	Patient has difficulty finding words, perseveration	Normal, slow, or rapid
Involuntary movements	Often asterixis or coarse tremor	Often absent	Usually absent
Physical illness or drug toxicity	One or both are present	Often absent, especially in Alzheimer's disease	Usually absent

Reprinted with permission from Lipowski ZJ: Delirium in the elderly patient. N Engl J Med 1989;320:580.

Key Signs

Altered mental status with evidence of the following:
- Acute onset and fluctuating course over the day

- Inattention

- Disorganized thinking

- Altered level of consciousness

Presence of the first two plus either the third or the fourth strongly suggests delirium.

From Inouye SK: Clarifying confusion: The confusion assessment method. Ann Intern Med 1990;113:947.

Laboratory Tests

1. Should be directed by history and physical examination
2. Screening laboratory examinations
   a. Chemistry profile to include electrolytes, magnesium, calcium, liver, renal, and thyroid function tests, albumin, glucose, vitamin B_{12}, and folate levels.
   b. Complete blood count and differential, clotting studies, arterial blood gases
   c. Urinalysis with cultures of blood and urine
   d. Serum levels of ingested drugs, though even therapeutic levels may cause delirium
   e. Screen for illicit drugs and alcohol level as indicated.
   f. Chest radiograph and electrocardiogram
3. Tests possibly indicated if preceding not diagnostic
   a. Electroencephalogram looking for a diffuse slow-wave pattern, common in delirium
   b. Computed tomography or magnetic resonance imaging of head may be indicated, especially with history of head trauma or focal/abnormal neurologic examination
   c. Lumbar puncture with cerebrospinal fluid evaluation if meningitis/encephalitis is suspected, especially if patient has potential for immunosuppression

Key Tests

- No pathognomonic laboratory tests available

Differential Diagnosis

1. Must first distinguish delirium from other neuropsychiatric disorders (see Table 286–2)
2. After delirium is recognized, then pursuit of likely medical/surgical cause can proceed.

Treatment

1. Specifically targeted at correction of medical disorder
2. Attempt nonpharmacologic therapy initially, such as well-lighted room, avoidance of over- or understimulating environment, gentle one-on-one interaction, attempt to reorient patient, and close communication with family.
3. Restraints may be used in the short term if patients' behavior compromises medical care or presents a significant threat to themselves or others.
4. Attempt to withdraw, reduce, or stop all nonessential medications.

Medication
1. Benzodiazepines have benefits of rapid onset of action with relatively few side effects during short-term use (Table 286–3).
2. Antipsychotics are particularly effective in patients with hallucinations, delusions, and paranoia (see Table 286–3).

Diet
1. Maintain adequate nutrition, either intravenously or orally.
2. Provide adequate vitamins and minerals as indicated, especially folate, thiamine, magnesium, and multivitamins.

Activity
1. Very close observation until delirium clears
2. Resolution of delirium may take longer than improvement or resolution of precipitating metabolic abnormalities.

Patient Education
1. Avoidance of precipitating factors, such as alcohol and illicit drugs

TABLE 286–3. DRUGS USEFUL IN SYMPTOMATIC TREATMENT OF DELIRIUM

Targeted Symptoms	Drug	Dosing*	Maximum Daily Dose
Acute agitation with or without psychosis	Lorazepam (Ativan)†	0.5–1.0 mg q 1–2 hr IV, IM, PO	10 mg
Acute agitation with prominent psychosis	Haloperidol (Haldol)‡	2–5 mg q 30–60 min IM, PO	100 mg
Alcohol withdrawal	Chlordiazepoxide (Librium)†	50–100 mg q 2–4 hr IV, PO	Titrated to sedation

*Should decrease dose to one-quarter to one-half of these doses in elderly or debilitated patients.
†Benzodiazepines may further impair attention.
‡Close monitoring for onset of extrapyramidal effects is indicated.

2. Disease-specific information for patients and families to maximize self-care and recognition of recurrence

Key Treatment

- Supportive care
- Treat underlying precipitating illnesses
- Drug therapy as indicated

Follow-Up

1. Once delirium clears, follow-up can be tailored to the precipitating medical or surgical causes and the age of the patient.

2. Geriatric patients who survive an episode of delirium have a higher likelihood of institutionalization and mortality. They may therefore need more stringent aftercare.

3. In delirious patients, there probably exists a more fragile metabolic homeostasis and tenuous reserve capacity, with the onset of delirium merely a marker for such.

Bibliography

Alessi CA: Delirium. *In* Reuben DB, Yoshiikawa TT (eds): Geriatrics Review Syllabus Supplement, 1993–94 ed. New York, American Geriatrics Society, 1993, pp 69S–73S.

Brown MM, Hachinski VC: Acute confusional states and delirium. *In* Isselbacher KJ, Braunwald E (eds): Harrison's Principles of Internal Medicine, 13th ed. New York, McGraw-Hill, 1994, pp 139–141.

Diagnostic and Statistical Manual of Mental Disorders, 4th ed. Washington, American Psychiatric Association, 1994.

Inouye SK, van Dyck CH, Alessi CA, et al: Clarifying confusion: The confusion assessment method, a new method for detection of delirium. Ann Intern Med 1990;113:941–948.

Lipowski ZJ: Delirium in the elderly patient. N Engl J Med 1989;320:578–582.

287 Headache

Manthani J. Reddy

Epidemiology and Etiology

1. Headache is an almost universal symptom among human populations. References have been found in Sumerian and Roman texts to headache. Epidemiologic studies across cultures show lifetime rates of up to 93 per cent of the population in the previous 12 months.

2. Studies of health care delivery have found headache to be one of the presenting symptoms for a high percentage of primary-care visits. There are approximately 42 million patient visits to physicians annually for headache.

3. Although the majority of these common headaches are benign, it is crucial to be vigilant for causes of headache that can be life-threatening and require immediate recognition and intervention (Table 287–1).

4. Traditionally, headache has been divided by symptomatology into distinct headache syndromes, such as migraine, cluster, and tension-type. These types were further elaborated by the International Headache Society in 1988 in a hierarchical classification system with operational diagnostic criteria for the distinct types (Table 287–2). More recent research has questioned the physiologic basis for distinguishing vascular from muscle tension causes for headache.

5. In patients referred to a headache clinic, 10 per cent of headaches were found to be secondary to an organic disorder. The remaining 90 per cent were found to be due to vascular, tension, and other causes.

6. A conceptual model distinguishing three categories of headache is proposed: those presenting acutely as new or uniquely severe ("new-onset headache"), headache that occurs as intermittent discrete attacks ("recurrent headache"), and chronic persistent headache that may occur daily ("chronic headache").

History

The importance of a good history cannot be overemphasized; a purely psychogenic cause for headache is rare. Differentiation between headache causes is most often accomplished via empathic listening by the physician.

1. Key information that should be elicited:
   a. Severity (scale from 0 to 10, getting worse?)
   b. Onset (How long have you had it?)
   c. Frequency, duration, intensity
   d. Location, quality (throbbing or constant?)
   e. Precipitators (Does anything make the headache worse or better?)
   f. Associated symptoms, such as neurologic symptoms
   g. Any similar episodes previously?
   h. Worst headache ever?

2. Medical and family history, including history of trauma, recent lumbar puncture

3. Environmental and social history, environmental exposures, stressors

4. Analgesic or other substance use and abuse

5. Age: In elderly patients a new headache presenting with burning pain and tenderness in the temporal area may represent temporal arteritis. Other characteristic manifestations in addition to polymyalgia rheumatica include jaw or tongue claudication, burning or pain in the temporal area, and an elevated sedimentation

TABLE 287–1. CRITICAL CAUSES OF ACUTE HEADACHE

CAUSE	ADVERSE OUTCOMES	SIGNS	DIAGNOSTIC TESTS
Acute angle closure glaucoma	Blindness	Ocular HTN, dilated pupils, eye pain	Ocular HTN, C/D ratio in fundus
Temporal arteritis	Blindness	Tenderness, temporal area, older pt >50, sx of polymyalgia rheumatica	Sed. rate (>50), temporal art. biopsy, at least 5 cm required
Meningitis	Increased morbidity and mortality	Nuchal rigidity, fever, Kernig's, Brudzinsky's	LP, rapid antibiotic therapy
CVA	Mortality, neurologic deficits	Neurologic signs	Clinical or radiologic
CNS mass lesion: tumor, abscess	Mortality, neurologic deficits	Papilledema, mental status change	CT scan/MRI
Subarachnoid hemorrhage	Mortality, neurologic deficits	Worst ever	CT scan/LP
Malignant HTN	End-organ damage	Papilledema, elevated bp systolic >210, diastolic >120	Vital signs, funduscopy, UA micro, ECG, cardiologic examination
Pheochromocytoma	End-organ damage	Classic presentation	CT of adrenals, urinary metanephrines
Toxic exposure	—	Confusion, nausea	See env/occ chart
HIV	Increased morbidity	HIV risks, opportunistic inf: crypto, CMV, toxo	HIV test, LP, CT/MRI
Acute sinusitis	Intracranial extension	Fever, toxic, sinus tenderness	Sinus radiographs, CT

TABLE 287-2. INTERNATIONAL HEADACHE SOCIETY CLASSIFICATION

PRIMARY CODE	HEADACHE TYPE
1	Migraine
2	Tension-type headache
3	Cluster headache and chronic paroxysmal hemicrania
4	Misc. headache unassociated with structural lesion
5	Headache associated with head trauma
6	Headache associated with vascular disorders
7	Headache associated with nonvascular intracranial disorder
8	Headache associated with substances or withdrawal
9	Headache associated with noncephalic infection
10	Headache associated with metabolic disorder
11	Headache or facial pain associated wtih disorder of face/cranium
12	Cranial neuralgias
13	Headache not classifiable

rate. If there is high clinical suspicion, the patient should be started on high-dose corticosteroids while awaiting definitive diagnosis by temporal artery biopsy.

6. HIV status: Patients infected with the HIV virus may have all the common or unusual causes of headache, but specific causes should be considered (see above).

7. Occupation: Eyestrain often associated with video display terminals can cause headache with workplace exposure. Other occupational toxic exposures may first manifest with headache (Table 287–3).

Tests

1. Physical examination
   a. Blood pressure in both arms
   b. Auscultation of the head for bruits
   c. General physical examination
   d. Neurologic examination (to rule out critical causes below)
2. Laboratory tests
   a. Routine laboratory tests, including complete blood count, chemistry panel, urinalysis, and drug screen should be done when indicated.
   b. Lumbar puncture (LP) if infection/meningitis/encephalitis, pseudotumor cerebri, or meningeal cancer is suspected.

c. Radiology—when to order:
   (1) Consider computed tomography (CT) for acute bleed, mass effect, or neurologic deficit. Magnetic resonance imaging is useful for soft tissue and posterior fossa defects.
   (2) Electroencephalogram to rule out epileptic equivalent headache in children and for encephalitis
   (3) Chest radiograph if malignancy is suspected
   (4) Sleep study if sleep apnea is suspected

Differential Diagnosis

1. New-onset headache: Consider specific critical causes when patients present with a new or different headache. Although uncommon, critical causes of headache may lead to significant morbidity and mortality and should be excluded (see Table 287–1).
   a. Ocular disorders: acute angle closure glaucoma usually presents at 25 to 40 years. Commonly patients have prominent eye pain and headache. Examination shows dilated pupils, narrow anterior chamber, ocular hypertension (usually >40 Hg), and increased cup-to-disk ratio (>0.6 in vertical diameter). Treatment should be started while awaiting ophthalmalogic consultation. Treatment choices include osmotic diuretics, acetazolamide, topical β-blockers (e.g., Timoptic), and cycloplegics (pilocarpine ophthalmic).
   b. Infectious causes: Causes of headache include acute sinusitis and meningitis, the latter manifested by nuchal rigidity, fever, and positive Kernig's (with flexion of hip, unable to extend at knee) and Brudzinsky's signs (flexion at neck causes flexion at hip and knees). Lumbar puncture should be performed followed by empirical therapy with broad-spectrum coverage. Delaying the tap and treatment sequence for even 30 minutes may worsen the outcome. Examination of the skin should be done for petechiae in meningococcemia.
   c. Central nervous system mass lesion: patient may present with increased intracranial pressure (ICP) and headache. Papilledema may be present on funduscopy. Other clues are altered mental status and neurologic deficits.

TABLE 287-3. ENVIRONMENTAL/OCCUPATIONAL FACTORS IN HEADACHE

TOXIC AGENT	OTHER SYMPTOMS	DIAGNOSIS/THERAPY
Carbon monoxide (truck, cab driver, firefighter, burn victim)	Confusion, somnolence, cherry-red skin, blebs in dark skin	Carboxyhemoglobin, O_2, hyperbaric chamber
Heavy metal (lead)	Irritability, fatigue, impaired psychomotor function	Lead level
Video display terminal (eyestrain)	Sore eyes, blurring	Vision correction, change display or lighting
Physical agents (cold)	History	Avoidance
Drugs (cimetidine, vasodilators, oral contraceptives, analgesics)	Drug history	Check reference source (e.g., PDR), modify medication
Altitude (acute mountain sickness)	Insomnia, dyspnea, anorexia, fatigue, mental status changes	History, O_2, calcium channel blocker
Other substances: MSG, mushrooms	Nausea, liver toxicity	History

d. Subarachnoid hemorrhage (SAH): Diagnosis may be suggested by a "thunderclap" headache described as the worst headache ever. Other suggestive symptoms are transient loss of consciousness, stiff neck, nausea, vomiting, photophobia, seizures, pupillary dilation, and pain located over the eye. The time from onset to maximum intensity is usually less than 5 minutes. Headache is a prominent symptom in over half the cases. Headache beginning during exertion or straining may be a sign of a leaking berry aneurysm with increased ICP. Most aneurysms bleed after the patient reaches age 35. The initial bleeding (sentinel/warning bleeding) is usually small (<5 ml). Cerebrospinal fluid (CSF) reaction causes increased pressure and stops the bleeding; rebleeding is hazardous. Diagnosis of SAH is by CT and lumbar puncture: xanthochromia (initial tap only), and may have elevated CSF pressure. Photometric studies for hemoglobin and its breakdown products will clinch the diagnosis. The recommended treatment is to start the patient on a calcium channel blocker (nimodipine) to prevent cerebral vasospasm and refer for surgical clipping.

e. HIV: A study of 46 cases of headache among HIV patients at a referral clinic identified cryptococcal meningitis, progressive multifocal leukoencephalopathy, encephalitis, and generalized sepsis as the most common diagnoses. Along with drug reactions, these causes occurred more frequently in this population than migraine or tension headache. This was particularly true when patients presented with nausea or diffuse headache. MRI/CT imaging and LP may be required for diagnosis.

f. Metabolic causes to be considered include hyponatremia (check serum electrolytes), uremia (BUN, Cr), hypoglycemia (glucose), carbon monoxide poisoning (carboxyhemoglobin), and hypercapnia/COPD/sleep apnea (CO_2).

g. When there is a change in established headache pattern, critical causes should be ruled out.

2. Recurrent headache

a. Among the types of headaches occurring intermittently, migraine and cluster-type occur most commonly. Migraine, which occurs in 10 per cent of the population, is often unilateral, lasting hours to days, and is associated with nausea, vomiting, photophobia, or phonophobia. This headache type may evolve years later into daily chronic tension-type headache plus migraine (see Chapter 288).

b. Cluster headaches are also called "suicide headaches" because of the pain intensity. Unlike the migraine sufferer who seeks a quiet, dark place alone to sleep, the cluster patient paces restlessly. More common in middle-aged men, the ocular/periocular pain lasts 20 minutes to 2 hours and

occurs in clusters of days or weeks. Associated symptoms include ipsilateral rhinorrhea, nasal congestion, lacrimation-conjunctival injection, and occasionally, Horner's syndrome. Systemic symptoms of migraine are rare. Alcohol or daytime napping may precipitate an attack. Treatment options include prednisone plus methysergide at start of cluster sequence, oxygen by mask, ergot formulations, lithium, or anesthesia of the sphenopalatine fossa.

c. Facial neuralgias, especially trigeminal neuralgia (tic douloureux), should be considered. Severe pain occurs in the distribution of the affected nerve. Clinically, trigger points can be identified. Some patients may need rhizotomy of the trigeminal ganglion for relief.

d. Headaches that are new-onset or recurrent may be due to environmental exposures at home or in the workplace (see Table 287–3).

e. Although critical causes most commonly present as new-onset acute headaches, they may present as recurrent headache when not immediately diagnosed (subarachnoid hemorrhage, pheochromocytoma).

f. Acute exertional headache occurs suddenly, related to coughing, sneezing, straining, running, or orgasm. It can last for ½ hour and should be distinguished from subarachnoid hemorrhage (consider CT).

3. Chronic headache: Tension-type headaches (also termed "muscle contraction" or "stress headaches") are commonly encountered in general practice. Tension-type headaches are described as bilateral, dull, constant pain in a bandlike distribution. They may be associated with tiredness, anorexia, pericranial muscle tenderness, and fatigue. Chronic headaches may be divided into episodic or chronic daily types. The latter may have characteristics of migraine and thus are called "mixed tension-vascular headaches." Chronic daily headaches paradoxically may be caused by the excessive use of analgesics, which leads to rebound headache.

Treatment

Medication
See Table 287–4.
Diet
Special dietary restrictions are useful only in migraine.
Activity
A relaxing, enjoyable form of exercise can be suggested.
Patient Education
During attacks, a hot compress can be applied to the forehead. Massage of the scalp may be helpful. Avoidance of trigger factors should be discussed.

Follow-Up

1. Reasons for concern (consider immediate neurologic consult):

TABLE 287–4. TREATMENT FOR TENSION-TYPE HEADACHES

CONSERVATIVE MODALITIES	PHARMACOLOGIC THERAPY	DOSAGE
Warm/cold compress	Acetaminophen	Acetaminophen, 325–650 mg q 4–6 hr prn
Stress reduction	Aspirin or NSAID (acute)	ASA, 325–650 mg q 4–6 hr prn
Exercise	Antidepressant (for chronic headache or depression)	Amitriptyline, 25–50 mg q h s initial
Consider drug reduction (postanalgesic headache syndrome)	Consider anxiolytic or muscle relaxant (short course)	Short-acting agent for brief periods
Biofeedback, relaxation therapy		

TABLE 287–5. DANGER SIGNALS IN HEADACHE

DANGER SIGNALS	POSSIBLE CAUSES
Headache during exertion/straining	Leaking berry aneurysm, increased ICP
Headache with fever	Meningitis, encephalitis
Headache when neck is not perfectly supple	Meningitis, encephalitis
Headache in a drowsy, confused patient	Increased ICP (encephalitis, meningitis, metabolic)
Headache with abnormal examination (pupil size, fundus, EOM reactivity, facial asymmetry, reflexes)	Subdural
Headache in a patient who looks ill	Critical causes

a. Headache with transient or lasting focal neurologic signs or symptoms

b. Progressive worsening of headache

c. New-onset headache without obvious cause

d. Orthostatic headache (low CSF pressure)

e. Headache of dramatic onset, suggesting subarachnoid hemorrhage, even if CT and LP negative

f. Headache of any type that fails to respond to treatment

g. Headache presenting with seizures

2. Tension-type headaches may require frequent, brief visits. At each visit, positive progress should be reinforced with teaching emphasized (see Table 287–4).

3. There should be easy access to the physician for acute attacks (Table 287–5).

Bibliography

Brew BJ, Miller J: Human immunodeficiency virus–related headache. Neurology 1993;43(6):1098–1100.

Couch JR: Headache to worry about. Med Clin North Am 1993;77:141–163.

Silberstein SD: Differential diagnosis of headache. Hosp Med 1994;30:49–60.

Solomon GD: Concomitant medical disease and headache. Med Clin North Am 1991;75:631–638.

Stevens MB: Tension-type headaches. Am Fam Physician 1993;47:799–804.

288 Migraine Headache

Michael B. Stevens

Etiology

1. Cerebral blood flow studies suggest a "spreading oligemia" from the occipital to the frontal lobe during migraine headache. Extracranial blood flow increases.

2. Changes in serotonergic neurotransmission and plasma serotonin levels have been implicated in the pathogenesis of migraine headaches.

Symptoms

1. Specific symptoms often vary with the specific type of migraine headache. The "basic types" of migraine headaches as proposed by the Headache Classification Committee of the International Headache Society are in Table 288–1.

2. Before the onset of the actual headache, some patients may experience a prodrome, or "aura," of visual, sensory, motor, or affective manifestations. Visual auras and especially "scintillating scotoma" (shimmering vision or flashing lights) are the most common.

3. Following the aura (if present), the patient develops a deep, throbbing, and often debilitating headache. The pain may be unilateral or bilateral.

4. Associated symptoms may be nausea, photophobia, and phonophobia. Vomiting may occur.

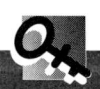
Key Symptoms

- Aura, usually visual (if present)
- Deep, throbbing headache on one or both sides
- Nausea, photophobia

Clinical Findings

1. Patients may have an ill appearance and pallor.
2. Physical examination, including funduscopic and neurologic examination, is unremarkable. Meningismus is absent.

TABLE 288–1. BASIC TYPES OF MIGRAINE HEADACHES

CLASSIFICATION NO.	NAME
1.1	Migraine without aura
1.2	Migraine with aura
1.3	Ophthalmoplegic migraine
1.4	Retinal migraine
1.5	Childhood periodic syndromes
1.6	Complications of migraine
1.7	Other migraine disorders

Headache Classification Committee of the International Headache Society.

1032

Key Signs

- Other than an ill appearance, the physical findings are *normal*.

Laboratory Tests

1. Given a medical history consistent with migraine and a normal physical examination, laboratory testing is not helpful or cost-effective.

2. Laboratory testing, especially brain imaging studies (computed tomography [CT] or magnetic resonance imaging [MRI]), is useful and necessary in patients who have historical details or physical markers (except meningismus) for serious pathology.

3. If meningismus is present, a lumbar puncture is indicated.

Key Tests

- Laboratory and radiographic testing is useless, except for the exclusion of other disease.

Differential Diagnosis

1. Before making the diagnosis of migraine, other serious systemic illnesses must be considered and excluded. These are cerebral hemorrhage, cerebral infarction, encephalitis, intracranial mass, meningitis, and others.

2. During the history and physical examination, the physician should be watchful for any symptoms and signs of possible serious disease (see below [Warning box]). In their absence, the physician may safely make the diagnosis of migraine if supported by the patient's historical and physical findings.

WARNING

Symptoms and Signs of Possible Serious Disease
- **Patients whose frequent headaches begin after age 30**
- **Frequent headaches localizing to one area**
- **Headaches associated with altered mental status, meningismus, neurologic deficits, or seizure**
- **Headaches *caused by* bending over, coughing, or sneezing**
- **Headaches refractory to first-line treatment**

Treatment

Medication

1. The treatment of migraine headache is a three-faceted approach: *abortive* (at the *immediate* onset of the headache), *interval* (during the headache), and *prophylactic* (to prevent the headache).

2. Abortive therapy is *only* useful during the aura (if present) or start of the migraine headache. Abortive medications include the various ergot compounds (e.g., Cafergot) and sumatriptan (Imitrex).

3. Interval therapy is directed at treating the migraine headache. These medications include analgesics and antiemetics to provide relief of symptoms or sumatriptan to resolve the migraine.

4. Prophylactic therapy is used to prevent or reduce the frequency and/or severity of migraines. The commonly used medications are the β-blockers, calcium channel blockers, and antidepressants. The new selective serotonin-reuptake inhibitor (SSRI) antidepressants may have a theoretical yet unproven advantage over other antidepressants.

5. Sumatriptan, if not contraindicated by coronary artery disease or pregnancy, is the drug of choice.

Diet

Numerous foods and food additives (Table 288–2) can precipitate a migraine headache in those susceptible.

Activity

1. Rest is an important mainstay of therapy.

2. The frequency and severity of migraine headaches may be reduced with regular exercise, sexual activity, and proper sleep habits.

3. Heat or cold applications, relaxation therapy, biofeedback, and hypnotherapy may be used as adjunctive therapies.

4. If stress or depression is a major inciter of migraine headache, individual or family counseling may be helpful.

Patient Education

1. The best treatment for migraines is preventive.

2. Patients who are prone to migraine headaches should

TABLE 288–2. FOOD/FOOD ADDITIVE PRECIPITANTS OF MIGRAINE

SUBSTANCE	MAJOR FOOD SOURCE
Nitrates/nitrites	Reddened (colored with additives) meats (e.g., hot dogs)
Phenylethylamines (e.g, tyramine)	Aged cheeses, red and blush wines, champagne, chocolates, certain nuts
Monosodium glutamate (MSG)	Many prepared foods, Oriental foods
Caffeine (by withdrawal)	Coffee, tea, sodas, and cola beverages
Other	Fruits, dairy products, shellfish

be encouraged to adopt a lifestyle that will help to eliminate or reduce migraine headaches by reducing inciting agents or activities. These lifestyle changes include avoiding known precipitants, exercising regularly, and maintaining good sleep habits.

Follow-Up

1. Patients with migraine headaches should be followed up according to their degree of frequency and severity: A more frequent or severe headache demands a more urgent follow-up.

2. Headache journals (records of the date and severity [e.g., 1 to 10 scale] of headaches) are useful to determine a baseline, to determine if therapy is working, and to discover precipitants (e.g., menses in women).

 Bibliography

Headache Classification Committee of the International Headache Society: Classification and diagnostic criteria for headache disorders, cranial neuralgias and facial pain. Cephalalgia 1988; 8(suppl 7):1–96.

Hoffert MJ: Treatment of migraine: A new era. Am Fam Physician 1994;49(3):633–638.

Lance JW: The pathophysiology of migraine. *In* Dalessio DJ, Silberstein SD (eds): Wolff's Headache and Other Head Pain, 6th ed. New York, Oxford University Press, 1993, pp 59–95.

Robbins LD: Management of Headache and Headache Medications. New York, Springer-Verlag, 1994, pp 1–63.

Silberstein SD, Saper JR: Migraine: Diagnosis and treatment. *In* Dalessio DJ, Silberstein SD (eds): Wolff's Headache and Other Head Pain, 6th ed. New York, Oxford University Press, 1993, pp 96–170.

289 Seizure Disorder

Andrew D. Massey

Etiology

1. No cause can be found in 40 to 70 per cent of patients with seizures.
2. Seizures can be caused by a variety of nonspecific acute or chronic central nervous system (CNS) injuries or disorders:
   a. CNS infections
   b. Head trauma
   c. Brain tumor
   d. Stroke
   e. Birth injury
   f. Degenerative diseases of the CNS
   g. Genetic disorders
   h. Cerebral malformations
   i. Metabolic disorders
   j. Drug or alcohol withdrawal
   k. Toxins

Symptoms

1. An epileptic seizure is a sudden objective or subjective temporary change in behavior usually lasting several seconds or minutes and accompanied by various motor, sensory, psychic, or autonomic changes.
2. Consciousness is often affected with amnesia afterward.

Key Symptoms

- Consciousness usually affected
- Motor, sensory, psychic, or autonomic changes
- Amnesia following the seizure

Clinical Findings

1. Seizures are classified according to the behavioral changes of the seizure and electroencephalographic (EEG) findings.
2. Behavioral and EEG changes of primary generalized seizures indicate initial involvement of both cerebral hemispheres, while partial seizures indicate involvement of only one or part of one cerebral hemisphere.
3. Primary generalized tonic-clonic seizure: sudden loss of consciousness, violent generalized tonic muscle contraction giving way to rhythmic clonic jerking movements, sometimes associated with tongue biting and incontinence, followed by period of deep drowsiness. Usually lasts 1 to 2 minutes.
4. Absence seizure: sudden loss of consciousness with motionless stare lasting 5 to 10 seconds, occasionally longer. May exhibit rhythmic eye blinking or automa-

---

The International Classification of Epileptic Seizures

I. Primary generalized seizures
  A. Generalized tonic-clonic
  B. Absence
  C. Myoclonic
  D. Atonic
II. Partial seizures
  A. Simple partial
  B. Complex partial
  C. Partial with 2° generalization
III. Unclassified epileptic seizures

---

tisms such as lip smacking, chewing, swallowing, or fumbling hand movements. Seizure ends suddenly with patient fully alert afterward.

5. Myoclonic seizure: sudden, brief, irregular involuntary contractures of limbs, trunk, or facial muscles usually without loss of consciousness.
6. Atonic seizure: sudden loss of postural tone that may result in a fall, is extremely short in duration, and may or may not occur with loss of consciousness.
7. Partial seizure: sometimes initiated with an aura such as an unpleasant taste or unexplained fear. If patient remains alert, it is termed a "simple partial seizure"; if there is an alteration or complete loss of consciousness, it is termed a "complex partial seizure." Automatisms may occur, and the seizure usually ends with the patient amnestic for the event. Partial seizure may progress to generalized tonic-clonic seizure (i.e., partial seizure with second-degree generalization.

Laboratory Tests

1. Diagnosis is based on a description of the seizure behavior.
2. EEG is the most important test and helps differentiate partial from primary generalized seizures; i.e., focal EEG abnormality indicates a partial seizure disorder, generalized abnormality indicates primary generalized seizure.
3. 24-Hour ambulatory EEG monitoring, or continuous in-hospital monitoring with video recording can distinguish epileptic seizures from nonepileptic events.

WARNING

A normal EEG does not rule out a seizure disorder. An abnormal EEG does not necessarily confirm the diagnosis. Diagnosis is primarily based on a consistent clinical history.

---

4. Other laboratory studies help determine if a cause for the seizure exists and are obtained when clinically indicated.

   a. CT or MRI head scan

   b. Cerebral angiogram

   c. Lumbar puncture

   d. Blood work: complete blood count (CBC), electrolytes, Ca^{2+}, Mg^{2+}, phosphorus, glucose, renal and liver functions, arterial blood gases (ABGs), antinuclear antibody

   e. Other: urinalysis, drug screen

Key Tests

- EEG
- MRI or CT
- Lumbar puncture
- CBC and ABGs
- Chemistry profile
- 24-hour EEG monitoring
- Drug screen
- Blood cultures
- Urinalysis

Differential Diagnosis

1. Cardiac syncope: dysrhythmia, valvular heart disease, vasovagal attack, or orthostatic hypotension

2. Sleep disorders: narcolepsy/cataplexy or night terrors

3. Psychiatric disorders: panic attacks, rage attacks, fugue state, and psychogenic (nonepileptic) seizures

4. Any other condition causing a sudden, temporary behavioral change: transient ischemic attacks, migraine, and childhood breath-holding spells

Treatment

Medication

1. Choice of anticonvulsant depends on the type of seizure and the patient's ability to tolerate the side effects.

2. Start with single drug and slowly increase the dose until seizures are controlled or intolerable side effects occur.

3. If seizures not adequately controlled and other disorders that may mimic epileptic seizures have been eliminated, the patient may be a candidate for seizure surgery.

Patient Education

1. If seizures are uncontrolled, avoid operating heavy equipment, swimming, heights, and driving.

2. Seizure-free period of 6 to 12 months required by most states before a patient with epilepsy can legally drive.

Follow-Up

1. Periodic office visit every 3 to 6 months to evaluate seizure control and side effects to anticonvulsants.

2. Serum anticonvulsant levels help assess patient compliance and guide dosage requirements.

Bibliography

For more information on classification of epileptic seizures, see

Commission on Classification and Terminology of the International League Against Epilepsy: Proposal for revised clinical and electroencephalographic classification of epileptic seizures. Epilepsia 1981; 22:489–501.

For more information on clinical features and management of childhood seizures, see

O'Donohoe NV (ed): Epilepsies of Childhood, 3rd ed. Boston, Butterworth-Heinemann, 1994.

For more information on when to treat first seizures, see

So EL: Update of epilepsy. Med Clin North Am 1993; 77(1):203–214.

For more information on the initial evaluation of seizures, see

Pellegrino TR: An emergency department approach to first-time seizures. Emerg Med Clin North Am 1994; 12(4):925–939.

For more information on long-term management of seizures, see

French J: The long-term therapeutic management of epilepsy. Ann Intern Med 1994; 120(5):411–422.

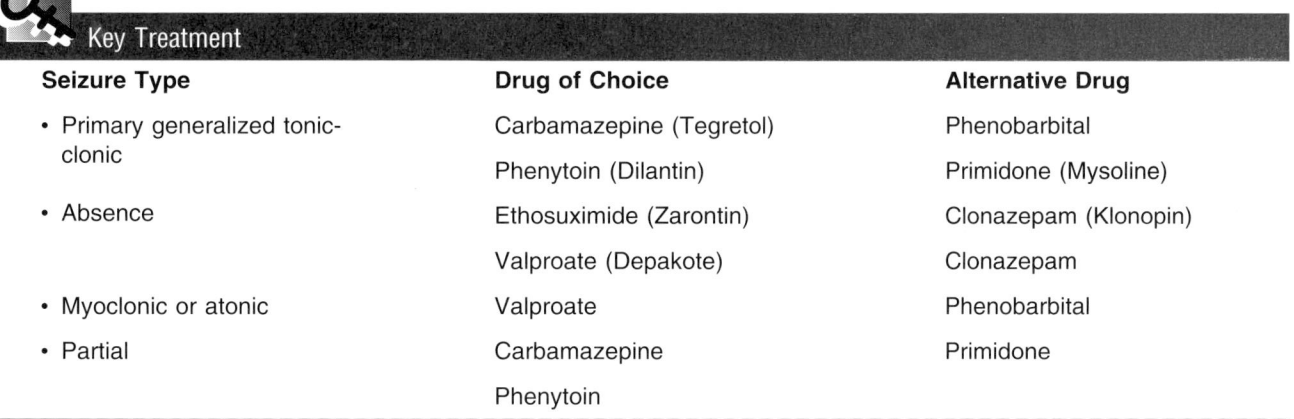

Key Treatment

Seizure Type	Drug of Choice	Alternative Drug
• Primary generalized tonic-clonic	Carbamazepine (Tegretol)	Phenobarbital
	Phenytoin (Dilantin)	Primidone (Mysoline)
• Absence	Ethosuximide (Zarontin)	Clonazepam (Klonopin)
	Valproate (Depakote)	Clonazepam
• Myoclonic or atonic	Valproate	Phenobarbital
• Partial	Carbamazepine	Primidone
	Phenytoin	

Etiology

Dyslexia is a primary reading disorder. Although no cause has been defined, current theories have suggested the following correlations:

1. Genetic: 40 per cent of dyslexic children have an immediate relative with a similar problem.
2. Neuroanatomic: symmetry or reversal of asymmetry of the planum temporale, with the right greater than the left
3. Neurophysiologic: Visual evoked potentials seem to indicate altered rapid visual processing. Another finding, through bielectrical mapping, shows altered left hemisphere function.

Popular Misconceptions

There are several findings that have been linked commonly with dyslexia. Despite the lack of scientific evidence, they have retained popularity and are worth mentioning.

1. Visual-spatial deficits underlie dyslexia.
2. Backward writing and letter reversals are characteristic.
3. Uncertain hand preference is characteristic.

Although these findings may be present in the dyslexic child, they are frequently present in normal children as well.

Symptoms

1. Poor school performance
2. Reading skills below normal or "expected" for age. Because children usually begin reading in first grade, evaluation of the child is more accurate after the third grade.
3. Inability to decipher the phonetics of a word
4. Inability to interpret whole words
5. Frequent spelling errors
6. Reading/writing backward
7. Misinterpreting number sequences
8. Frequent errors with simple mathematical tasks
9. Social problems with school mates
10. Poor school behavior

Key Symptoms

- Poor reading skills
- Repetitive errors in simple mathematical tasks
- Difficulty with the usage and/or interpretation of the written language.
- Antisocial behavior

Clinical Findings

A complete physical examination must be performed. This ought to include a psychosocial assessment to rule out some of the secondary causes of learning disability. The evaluation may be completely normal. However, there may be soft neurologic findings, which are often related to learning disabilities.

1. Motor
   a. Arms extended: may drop or spread
   b. Head rotation: arms drop or spread
   c. Unable to hop, stand on one foot
   d. Finger and foot tapping slow
   e. Presence of choreiform movements
2. Cerebellar
   a. Finger-nose-finger dysmetria
   b. Tandem inadequate
   c. Dysdiadochokinesia (impairment of ability to perform rapid alternating movements in opposite directions, such as the quick pronation and supination of the hand)
3. Sensory
   a. Copy of finger movement inadequate (inability to imitate gestures or signs with the indicated hand; inability to construct figures with fingers such as the bow using the thumbs and index fingers of opposite hands)
   b. Finger agnosia: loss of ability to perceive a stimulus applied to the fingers
4. Cranial nerves
   a. Head moves with extraocular muscles
   b. Strabismus
   c. Inability to hold lateral gaze
   d. Grimace, unable to raise eyebrow
   e. Tongue waggle irregular
   f. Impaired speed or speech repeating (inability to repeat sounds in a sequence with the given speed) Sounds commonly used are *la la, da da, pa ta ka.*

Key Signs

- Normal child: no major neurologic or psychiatric findings

Laboratory Tests

Although there are no biochemical tests, a wide array of neuropsychological tests are available for the assessment of specific impairments that may be present in a dyslexic child. Some of the tests are listed below.

1. Naming tasks: Boston Naming Test, Oldfield Naming Test, Rapid Automatized Naming

2. Language comprehension: Token Test, stories, relational sentences

3. Repetition tasks: words, Spreen Benton sentences

4. Auditory discrimination tasks: Goldman-Fristoe-Woodcock Auditory Skills Test battery

5. Sound-blending tasks, articulation tasks, segmentation tasks

6. Visual-motor tasks: Bender Gestalt test, Rey complex figure, Draw-a-person

7. Sequencing tests: rote series

8. Memory: paired association test, digit span

9. Visual-perceptive tasks: Ravens matrices, Motor Free Test

10. Reading tests: Gray Oral Reading Test, silent/oral with and without comprehension, wide range Achievement Test

11. Spelling tests: Wide Range Achievement Test-revised (WRAT-R)

12. Math tests: WRAT-R, Key Math

13. Intelligence test: Wechsler Intelligence Scale for Children-revised (WISC-R)*

The WISC-R and the WRAT-R tests are used for the initial screening. The other tests are then used for the assessment of specific deficits.

Key Tests

- WISC-R
- WRAT-R

Differential Diagnosis

Causes of secondary reading disorders

1. Mental retardation, cerebral palsy, genetic defects

2. Delayed maturation (late bloomer)

3. Emotional or psychiatric disorders such as depression, family conflicts, child abuse

4. Educational or emotional deprivation

5. Physical disorders such as neurologic deficits (visual, auditory), chronic illnesses, trauma

6. Behavior disorders such as attention-deficit hyperactivity disorder (ADHD), autism

Treatment

1. The family physician may be the first to see a child with a learning disability. Although not qualified to treat, it will be his or her task to perform the initial

*Text material (Nos. 1–13) has been borrowed from Nass R: Rapid assessment of the mental status exam of the child. Emerg Clin North Am 1987; 739–750; and Developmental dyslexia: An update. Pediatr Rev 1992;13:231–235.

evaluation and coordinate needed evaluations by specialists (neurologists, neuropsychiatrists, educators). Educational and tutoring plans and proper school placement will provide the family with invaluable support. This also will facilitate the continuity of care of the child by the family physician.

2. Dyslexia requires a team approach. Physicians will address health issues that may arise. Personal tutoring and individualized educational programs will be necessary to meet the particular needs of the child. A wide range of activities and exercises is available to help a child to either circumvent or correct a deficit.

3. Psychologists may be of assistance in helping with family and personal issues that often appear. These may take the form of altered affect and/or behavior. A support network of parents and counselors is especially important because of the low self-esteem these children are susceptible to, which in turn may further undercut their educational process.

4. Successful remediation may occur, but it requires a long-term commitment from the family, the child, and the professionals involved.

Patient Education

Resources for the patient and family

1. The Orton Dyslexia Society
   Suite 382
   8600 La Salle Road
   Baltimore, MD 21204-6020
   1-800-ABCD-123

2. The National Center for Learning Disabilities
   99 Park Avenue
   New York, NY 10016
   (212) 687-7211

3. Learning Disabilities Association of America, Inc.
   4156 Liberty Rd.
   Pittsburgh, PA 15234
   (412) 341-1515

Key Treatment

- Individualized tutoring
- Exercises to correct the deficit
- Counseling
- Supportive parents

Bibliography

David R (ed): Pediatric Neurology for the Clinician. Princeton, NJ: Appleton & Lange, 1991.

Hume C, Snowling M: The classification of children with reading difficulties. Dev Med Child Neurol 1988;30:398–402.

Keys M: The pediatrician's role in reading disorders. Pediatr Clin North Am 1993;40:869–879.

Nass R: Developmental dyslexia: An update. Pediatr Rev 1992;13:231–235.

Rumsey JM: The biology of developmental dyslexia. JAMA 1992;268:912–915.

Narcolepsy

Etiology

The cause of narcolepsy is unknown. Altered sleep and rapid eye movement (REM) sleep mechanisms underlie the symptoms. For example, cataplexy has the appearance of REM-like atonia of skeletal muscle outside the context of a REM period. Dopaminergic and noradrenergic neural transmission is likely defective. There is a strong linkage with certain HLA subtypes of DR-2 and Dqw1, but not all cases are familial. Onset is usually in adolescence or young adulthood.

Symptoms

1. Sleepiness is the primary symptom, sometimes in the form of sleep attacks. Although sleep and sleepiness occur at times outside the habitual sleep period (night), the total amount of sleep attained by narcoleptics in a 24-hour day is not increased compared with normal individuals. Daytime naps are usually refreshing. "Automatic behavior" refers to waking activity of which the patient may not be aware, such as driving home without memory of such or acting strangely. Presumably, automatic behavior is the result of microsleeps invading waking activities.
2. Cataplexy is pathognomonic for the classic syndrome and consists of partial or total loss of muscle tone without loss of consciousness, usually provoked by anticipatory emotion. Laughter, surprise, and their anticipation are the most common inciting emotions. Injury to the patient can occur, and this symptom can be disabling depending on the patient's occupation and goals.
3. Sleep paralysis is the experience of being awake but unable to move, usually occurring near sleep onset or offset, and usually quite frightening. The attack usually lasts for seconds. Eye movements remain intact, and some patients use them to help abort the spell.
4. Hypnogogic hallucinations are vivid dream-like experiences which the patient cannot distinguish from reality. These may occur during daytime naps.
5. Disturbed nocturnal sleep is common in narcoleptics, especially older narcoleptics. This problem compounds the daytime sleepiness and contributes to disability.

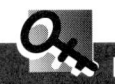

Key Symptoms

- Sleepiness
- Cataplexy
- Sleep paralysis
- Hypnogogic hallucinations
- Disturbed nocturnal sleep

Clinical Findings

1. The examination is normal, by definition, except perhaps for manifest sleepiness.
2. Cataplexy can be diagnosed by observing loss of deep tendon reflexes during an attack and the prompt resumption of reflexes after.

Key Sign

- Cataplexy

Laboratory Tests

1. The diagnosis is confirmed by an overnight sleep study followed by a multiple sleep latency test (MSLT). This test is a series of daytime naps with measurement to EEG-defined sleep and will show a mean sleep latency of under 7 minutes with at least two sleep-onset REM periods.
2. HLA typing is useful only in occasional cases that do not fit a standard pattern. The associated phenotypes are common in the general population, but their absence is evidence against classic narcolepsy with cataplexy.

Key Tests

- Overnight polysomnogram and multiple sleep latency test (MSLT)
- MSLT should show both sleepiness and sleep-onset REM periods.

Differential Diagnosis

1. Sleep apnea, even mild forms in which snoring disturbs sleep without frank apnea, can cause sleepiness. Nocturnal myoclonus also can present as sleepiness. These conditions are ruled out by the overnight polysomnogram. Idiopathic hypersomnolence is a syndrome of sleepiness but without the REM-related symptoms of narcolepsy. Psychiatric conditions may cause complaints of sleepiness, fatigue, and altered sleep and dream content. Antisocial personality disorders might manifest with periods of inactivity or withdrawal that can occasionally be confused with true sleepiness. Medical conditions causing sleepiness, such as hypothyroidism or hydrocephalus, also must be ruled out.

2. Cataplexy must be distinguished from seizures and ischemic vertebrobasilar drop attacks.

Treatment

Treatment of the sleepiness consists primarily of stimulant medication. When cataplexy is mild, the stimulants can sometimes control it effectively. Cataplexy and the other REM-related symptoms are treatable with REM-suppressant agents such as the tricyclic antidepressants.

Medication

1. A variety of stimulant agents can be used successfully, and individuals vary greatly in their responses and needs.
   a. Pemoline (Cylert), 37.5 to 150 mg daily in one or two divided doses
   b. Methylphenidate (Ritalin), 20 to 60 mg daily in two or three divided doses—available in regular and sustained-release forms
   c. Dextroamphetamine or methamphetamine, 20 to 60 mg daily in one or two divided doses—available in regular and sustained-release forms
2. REM-related symptoms such as cataplexy can be controlled with agents that increase central nervous system (CNS) synaptic norepinephrine.
   a. Tricyclic agents, especially clomipramine (Anafranil), 25 to 75 mg daily, and protriptyline (Vivactil), 5 to 20 mg daily, are effective, although their use is sometimes limited by anticholinergic side effects.
   b. Fluoxetine (Prozac), 20 to 80 mg daily, is an alternative.

Patient Education

Planned naps after lunch and after work can be helpful. Often, a brief nap before a drive is as effective as a take-as-needed stimulant. Patients should avoid shifts in their sleep schedule. Patients must be warned to respect the dangers of their sleepiness when involved in activities such as driving.

Key Treatment

- Stimulant agents, such as pemoline, methylphenidate, or dextroamphetamine

Restless Legs Syndrome and Nocturnal Myoclonus

Etiology

1. Restless legs syndrome (RLS) is a condition in which patients experience an unpleasant and hard to describe feeling in the limbs when they are at rest, particularly in the evening. It often interferes with sleep onset. Nocturnal myoclonus, also called periodic limb movement disorder (PLMS), is a related condition of repetitive, periodic, and stereotypical movements of the limbs, usually the legs, during quiet waking or non-REM sleep. About 85 per cent of patients with RLS have PLMS, but many patients with PLMS do not have restless legs and may present instead with insomnia or excessive daytime sleepiness.
2. The cause of both conditions is unknown. Because PLMS is common, often asymptomatic, and its prevalence increases with age, it can be difficult to establish its pathogenic significance. There is speculation that venous or arterial insufficiency contributes to RLS, and there is some evidence that lumbar disk disease predisposes to PLMS. However, neurochemical deficiencies probably underlie RLS—alterations in dopamine or perhaps endogenous opioid systems. It is not known what level of the nervous system is abnormal, although electrophysiologic studies suggest an alteration in mechanisms at the pontine level or higher. RLS is familial in about one half of cases, but no clear-cut genetic pattern or gene defect has been established. Certain medications, such as tricyclic antidepressants or lithium, can precipitate RLS.

Symptoms

1. RLS is diagnosed on the basis of the symptoms and history. The sensation should be bilateral, very disagreeable, but not painful. It is often described as a tingling, prickling, tense, or "creepy-crawly" feeling. As mentioned, it is most notable when the patient is at rest, particularly in the evening. The urge to rub or to move the affected limbs is irresistible. Dyskinesias, myoclonic jerking, and marching in place are not uncommon. Most patients with RLS also have PLMS, which usually emerges during sleep.
2. PLMS is diagnosed on the basis of sleep-related repetitive, periodic, and stereotypical movements of the limbs, usually the legs. These take a form similar to a triple-flexion response with Babinski's sign and have both jerky and sustained components, last 0.5 to 5 seconds, and occur every 20 to 40 seconds. They may be disruptive to sleep or to a bedpartner's sleep. The symptom produced is either insomnia or excessive daytime sleepiness, and this condition should be considered in any patient with these complaints.

Key Symptoms

- Irresistible restless sensation of the limbs, especially the legs
- Repetitive and periodic leg movements during sleep causing insomnia or sleepiness

Clinical Findings

By definition, the examination is normal in idiopathic RLS with PLMS.

Laboratory Tests

Nocturnal polysomnography is capable of demonstrating PLMS. Certain specific variations of these sleep studies can sometimes quantitate RLS as well. Considering that the available treatments have significant potential risks, documentation of the condition is desirable.

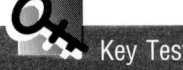
Key Test

- Nocturnal polysomnography

Differential Diagnosis

1. RLS and PLMS have been associated in small series with many medical conditions, including pregnancy, uremia, neuropathy, myelopathy, amyloidosis, and anemias, but no definitive studies show a clear increased prevalence in any medical disease. Chronic obstructive pulmonary disease (COPD), Isaacs syndrome, Huntington's disease, and leukemias also have been reported in patients with RLS or PLMS. These conditions should be considered when evaluating a patient.

2. RLS and PLMS should be distinguished from other sleep-related movements, such as hypnic jerks. Myoclonic epilepsy and partial seizures might be confused with the jerky motions of PLMS. RLS should be distinguished from neuropathic pain and from akithesia. Akithesia produces a similar restless sensation and is often caused by neuroleptic use or by dyskinetic movement disorders. REM behavior disorder and sleep apnea are significant conditions with an increased prevalence of PLMS and should be ruled out prior to treatment. For example, arousals from apneas may appear to be leg-induced arousals to a casual observer.

Treatment

Treatment is aimed at either reducing the dysesthesia of RLS or at improving sleep quality in PLMS to eliminate insomnia or daytime sleepiness.

Medication

1. Dopaminergic agents are effective in up to 70 per cent of patients with RLS, and the benefit can be sustained for several years. L-Dopa with carbidopa is most often used, but direct dopamine agonists also appear to be effective. Both the subjective dysesthesias and the number of leg movements in sleep are reduced. Carbidopa/levodopa (Sinemet) is usually given in doses of 25/100 mg or 50/200 mg at bedtime with a repeat dose in the middle of the night if needed. The continuous-release form is also useful

because of the sustained action. Side effects have been minor, such as nausea or dizziness. Daytime rebound of the sensation occurs in about one third of patients, often leading to daytime use of L-dopa. Since use of these agents is not approved by Food and Drug Administration (FDA) for the indication of RLS, insomnia, or pain, caution is advised. Consideration should be given to reserving this treatment for refractory cases or for elderly patients.

2. Benzodiazepines, particularly temazepam (Restoril) and clonazepam (Klonopin), have been shown to improve sleep quality and to aid sleep onset in patients with RLS and PLMS. Their effect on the number of leg movements is less than that of L-dopa, but the arousals associated with the movements are reduced. Clonazepam is usually used in doses of 0.5 to 2.0 mg at bedtime; temazepam in doses of 15 to 30 mg. Tolerance and escalation of effective doses are sometimes encountered, as well as morning sedation.

3. Opioids, particularly propoxyphene and oxycodone, have been shown to relieve RLS and to decrease the number of leg movements, but the effect is not as robust as with L-dopa. Nonetheless, these agents are useful in many patients, and long-term side effects are better defined. Propoxyphene (Darvon) is used in doses from 65 to 195 mg at bedtime.

Key Treatment

- Dopaminergic agents, such as L-dopa

- Benzodiazepines, such as temazepam and clonazepam

- Opioids, such as propoxyphene and oxycodone

Bibliography

Becker PM, Jamieson AO, and Brown WD: Dopaminergic agents in restless legs syndrome and periodic limb movements of sleep: Response and complications of extended treatment in 49 cases. Sleep 1993;16:713–716.

Culebras A: The neurology of sleep. Neurology 1992;42(suppl 6):1–94.

Kryger MH, Roth T, Dement WC: Principles and Practice of Sleep Medicine, 2nd ed. Philadelphia, WB Saunders, 1994, pp 589–595, 549–561.

Mitler MM, Aldrich MS, Koob GF, Zarconc VP: Narcolepsy and its treatment with stimulants. Sleep 1994;17(4):352–371.

Thorpy MJV (ed): Handbook of Sleep Disorders. New York, Marcel Dekker, 1990, pp 197–216, 457–478.

292 Bell's Palsy

Roger R. Hesselbrock

Etiology

1. Postinfectious: thought to be secondary to nerve compression from edema, classically associated with an upper respiratory infection
2. Viral: as seen with herpes zoster (Ramsay-Hunt syndrome) or HIV infections
3. Bacterial: syphilis, Lyme disease
4. Inflammatory: sarcoidosis
5. Demyelinating diseases such as multiple sclerosis or postinfectious demyelination
6. Diabetes is a predisposing factor; up to fourfold increased incidence compared with nondiabetics.
7. Hypertension is possibly predisposing; recovery rate is lower compared with normotensives.
8. Pregnancy: higher incidence, particularly in the third trimester or if preeclampsia is present
9. Idiopathic: a diagnosis of exclusion

Symptoms

1. Sudden weakness of the lower motor neuron type: involves both the upper and lower face
2. Postauricular pain: often seen in postinfectious cases
3. Ipsilateral lacrimation
4. Hyperacusis: if the stapedial nerve is affected
5. Ipsilateral dysgeusia
6. Subjective facial numbness

Key Symptoms

- Subacute to acute facial weakness of the lower motor neuron type involving the upper and lower facial musculature
- Postauricular pain
- Lacrimation

Clinical Findings

1. Facial weakness, lower motor neuron type, both upper and lower face. This is generally ipsilateral but may involve the contralateral side with Lyme disease or sarcoidosis. Corneal protection should be assessed on examination.
2. Normal facial sensation
3. Normal ocular movements
4. Normal reflexes and coordination
5. Vesicular lesions seen on the tympanic membrane and external auditory canal in zoster-related facial paralysis

Key Sign

- Facial weakness, lower motor neuron type, upper and lower face involved. Corneal protection may be inadequate and should be assessed on examination.
- The remainder of the neurologic examination is normal.

Laboratory Tests

1. Routine blood work, such as complete blood count (CBC) and chemistry studies, is normal.
2. Varicella zoster titer may be increased in zoster-related facial palsy.
3. Lyme titer is increased in Lyme disease–associated facial paresis.
4. Spinal fluid examination may show increased protein and mononuclear pleocytosis in inflammatory or infectious causes.
5. Magnetic resonance imaging (MRI) may show edema or enhancement of the facial nerve in inflammatory or postinfectious cases, will reveal mass lesions in the cerebellopontine angle region, and can show demyelinating lesions of multiple sclerosis.

Key Tests

- Complete blood count and erythrocyte sedimentation rate (ESR)
- Chemistry panel: electrolytes, glucose, blood urea nitrogen (BUN), creatinine, hepatic enzymes
- Syphilis serology: RPR or VDRL *and* FTA-ABS or MHA-TP
- HIV serology if at increased risk by history
- Lyme titer if at risk by history
- Angiotensin-converting enzyme level if sarcoidosis is suspected: may be falsely elevated if the patient is a smoker
- MRI scan with gadolinium contrast, with attention to the facial nerve and posterior fossa
- Spinal fluid examination in inflammatory or nonviral infectious cases: cultures, cell count, protein, glucose, VDRL, IgG index, oligoclonal bands, Lyme or HIV titers if suspected. Exclude mass lesions with MRI before performing lumbar puncture.
- Nerve conduction studies after 5 to 7 days can assess the degree of degeneration; serial studies may predict if surgical correction may be beneficial.

6. Nerve conduction studies show abnormalities of conduction latency and stimulation threshold starting about 5 days after onset of symptoms. Serial studies may be useful to determine the extent of damage and select surgical candidates.

7. Needle electromyographic (EMG) studies do not reveal denervation changes for 14 to 21 days after symptom onset.

Differential Diagnosis

1. Trauma: usually apparent on presentation but may see delayed weakness after injury
2. Herpes zoster infection
3. Neurosyphilis
4. Sarcoidosis
5. Lyme disease
6. HIV infection
7. Neoplasms: usually in the cerebellopontine angle region, primary or metastatic
8. Demyelinating disease
9. Diabetic-related
10. Hypertension-related
11. Pregnancy-related

Treatment

1. Supportive care: Protect the eye with artificial tears during the daytime and ocular lubricant ointments at night, and consider taping lids if poor corneal coverage is noted.
2. Surgical decompression: Consider if nerve conduction response amplitude decreases to 10 per cent or less of the unaffected side on serial testing; if so, recovery with decompression is up to 90 per cent satisfactory compared with about 50 per cent when treated medically.

Medication

1. Corticosteroids: If no contraindications, oral prednisone, 1 mg/kg daily for 3 to 5 days, with rapid taper and total course of about 10 days. Best used when started within 4 days of the onset of symptoms. Monitor for electrolyte disturbances and hyperglycemia.
2. Acyclovir (Zovirax): useful in zoster-associated facial palsy if begun within 72 hours of onset of symptoms; 10 mg/kg intravenously every 8 hours for 7 days is recommended.

Patient Education

1. Attention to eye protection is crucial (see above); patients should report ocular pain, drainage, or discharge.
2. Approximately 70 per cent likelihood of complete recovery, with better recovery if weakness is incomplete and if signs of recovery are seen within 6 weeks after symptom onset.

3. Recurrence rate of about 10 per cent; weakness may recur contralaterally.

Key Treatment

Drug of Choice	Alternative Drugs
• Prednisone, 1mg/kg/d orally for 3 to 5 days, with rapid taper and a total course of about 10 days	• Acyclovir, 10 mg/kg intravenously every 8 hours for 7 days, in herpes zoster–related facial paralysis

Follow-Up

1. Serial examinations are useful to document progress or deterioration.
2. Serial nerve conduction studies are useful if moderate to complete facial weakness is present and may help select those patients who are candidates for surgical decompression.
3. Side effects of any medications used should be monitored.
4. Refer to an ophthalmologist for
   a. Persistent ocular pain
   b. Corneal abrasion or ulceration
5. Refer to a neurologist or otolaryngologist when
   a. Progressive symptoms occur
   b. Hearing loss or other otologic symptoms occur
   c. Abnormalities other than facial weakness are documented on neurologic examination
   d. Weakness is recurrent
   e. Abnormalities are found on MRI scanning or spinal fluid examination

The opinions and assertions contained herein are the private views of the author and are not to be construed as the official policy or position of the U.S. government, the Department of Defense, or the Department of the Air Force.

Bibliography

Hughes GB: Practical management of Bell's palsy. Otolaryngol Head Neck Surg 1990;102:658–663.

Karnes WE: Diseases of the seventh cranial nerve. In Dyck PJ et al (eds): Peripheral Neuropathy, 3rd ed, vol 2. Philadelphia, WB Saunders, 1993, pp 818–836.

Niparko JK, Mattox DE: Bell's palsy and herpes zoster oticus. In Johnson RT, Griffin JW (eds): Current Therapy in Neurologic Disease, 4th ed. St Louis, Mosby–Year Book, 1993, pp 355–361.

Petruzzelli GJ, Hirsch BE: Bell's palsy: A diagnosis of exclusion. Postgrad Med 1991;90:115–127.

293 Trigeminal Neuralgia

Howard Tung

Etiology

1. The etiology of trigeminal neuralgia is thought to be related to compression of the trigeminal nerve at some point between the gasserian ganglion and the pons.
2. Frequently, a vascular loop at the level of the root entry zone where the trigeminal nerve enters the pons (root entry zone) is found to be the etiologic factor for trigeminal neuralgia.
3. Other common causes of trigeminal nerve root compression include benign tumors (meningioma, epidermoid cyst, acoustic neuroma) or plaque formation in multiple sclerosis.

Symptoms

1. Trigeminal neuralgia, or tic douloureux, is a symptom characterized by paroxysms of intense, stabbing pain within the distribution of the trigeminal nerve. The pain is often described as lancinating or shocklike in quality, lasting a few seconds to a minute or two.
2. A patient may suffer from one or two attacks per day to as many as 10 or 20 attacks per hour. The pain is typically more pronounced during the day, with markedly fewer episodes experienced at night. Many times, "trigger points" such as touching of the face, wind blowing across the face, or hot or cold liquids may initiate the pain. The pain also may begin spontaneously or with innocuous facial movements such as speaking, chewing, or swallowing.
3. In general, the pain syndrome is usually unilateral, involving the second or third divisions of the trigeminal nerve and rarely involving the ophthalmic division.
4. The majority of patients are over age 50, with women affected more often than men.

Key Symptoms

- Paroxysms of stabbing pain on one side of the face
- Attacks last only seconds to a minute or two

Clinical Findings

1. Most often, examination of the sensory and motor components of the fifth cranial nerve is normal in idiopathic trigeminal neuralgia.
2. Association of the cranial nerve abnormalities suggests other pathology such as a cerebellopontine angle mass.

Laboratory Tests

Neuroradiologic workup including magnetic resonance imaging (MRI) of the head is usually normal but important in excluding tumors or substantiating other neurologic disease processes (e.g., multiple sclerosis) that may present with trigeminal neuralgia.

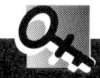

Key Tests

- None (MRI to rule out tumor or diagnose multiple sclerosis)

Differential Diagnosis

The diagnosis of trigeminal neuralgia rests mainly on strict clinical criteria and is usually readily distinguishable from other craniofacial neuralgias or pain arising from the jaw, teeth, or sinuses. The differential diagnosis includes

1. Multiple sclerosis
2. Glossopharyngeal neuralgia
3. Postherpetic neuralgia
4. Raeder's paratrigeminal syndrome
5. Atypical facial neuralgia
6. Chronic cluster syndrome (Horton's cephalgia)
7. Cluster headaches
8. Post-traumatic facial neuralgia
9. Temporomandibular joint pain
10. Pain secondary to disease of dental, sinus, or orbital origin

Treatment

Medical therapy is the treatment of choice for idiopathic trigeminal neuralgia, and a number of medications have proven effective in the relief of pain.

1. Approximately 80 per cent of patients will obtain pain relief with the anticonvulsant carbamazepine (Tegretol), while phenytoin (Dilantin) will improve up to 50 per cent of patients. Begin the Tegretol dose gradually with an initial dose of 200 mg/day. The dose may then be increased slowly (e.g., 100 to 200 mg every 2 or 3 days) until pain relief is achieved or drug toxicity develops. A typical dose may be 600 to 800 mg/day in three divided doses, but doses as high as 1200 to 1800 mg/day may be required to achieve pain relief in some. It is important for patients to have their complete blood count and liver function tests followed periodically because carbamazepine may cause hematosuppression or liver dysfunction.
2. Baclofen (Lioresal) and clonazepam (Klonopin) also have proven useful but overall are less effective than

carbamazepine or phenytoin and are considered secondary forms of medical therapy.

3. Surgical therapy also has proven to be effective in the treatment of trigeminal neuralgia. Surgical treatment is reserved for patients refractory to medical treatment or for those who develop untoward side effects to medical therapy. In general, surgical treatment for trigeminal neuralgia is divided into percutaneous trigeminal neurolysis and microvascular decompression.

   a. Percutaneous trigeminal neurolysis

     (1) Percutaneous approaches to the gasserian ganglion have proven excellent in obtaining relief for the pain of trigeminal neuralgia. These techniques utilize placement of a needle or electrode through the foramen ovale to the trigeminal cistern of Meckel's cave with a subsequent procedure to destroy the gasserian ganglion and retrogasserian rootlets.

     (2) The major advantages of percutaneous procedures include avoidance of general anesthesia as compared with open microvascular decompression, short hospital stays (one day), and the procedure may be repeated easily if necessary.

     (3) In our series of over 500 patients with glycerol injection, initial pain relief has been achieved in over 85 per cent. Reported recurrence rates are variable in the literature, but generally, 20 to 25 per cent may experience recurrence of pain in 2 to 3 years, which is consistent with my experience. Side effects include sensory numbness in many patients, but this is usually well tolerated. Rarely, corneal anesthesia (without keratitis) or hyperesthesia may occur, but I have found this to be transient.

     (4) Radiofrequency thermocoagulation lesions offer similar results to glycerol injections. Instead of chemical destruction of the gasserian ganglion and rootlets with glycerol, thermocoagulation of the ganglion is carried out with a temperature-monitoring electrode. I have found the side effects with radiofrequency lesions similar to those of glycerol injections, except that the sensory disturbances tend to be more severe, with severe dysesthesias and anesthesia dolorosa occurring rarely. When surgical treatment has been successful, patients then are slowly tapered off their medical regimen.

   b. Microvascular decompression

     (1) The frequent finding of vascular compression of the root entry zone of the trigeminal nerve in patients with trigeminal neuralgia was first commented on by Dandy in 1934. Clinical and anatomic studies of patients with trigeminal neuralgia have supported this finding. However, the fact that vascular decompression is not the sole cause of trigeminal neuralgia is attested to by the observation that compression is not found in as many as 10 to 15 per cent of patients at surgery.

     (2) Microvascular decompression is suitable for patients with typical trigeminal neuralgia intractable to medical therapy and who are otherwise healthy and without excessive anesthesia risks. Presently, I perform microvascular decompression through a small retromastoid craniectomy with mobilization of the offending vascular structure (usually the superior cerebellar artery) away from the root entry zone of the trigeminal nerve and subsequent placement of a Teflon pledget between the artery and nerve.

     (3) Advantages of microvascular decompression include treating the apparent cause of pain, which can be curative and usually affords longer pain-free periods compared with percutaneous procedures. The procedure is nondestructive, sparing the nerve, and generally carries fewer of the sensory disturbances noted with other procedures. Risks of microvascular decompression include the need for general anesthesia and retromastoid craniectomy with increased potential for serious complications (e.g., meningitis, hemorrhage, cerebrospinal fluid leak, cranial nerve deficit).

Therapeutic Approach to Patients with Trigeminal Neuralgia

1. When first evaluating a patient with trigeminal neuralgia, there is no substitute for an accurate and careful history and physical examination. If the patient appears to have typical trigeminal neuralgia, diagnostic studies (e.g., MRI with and without contrast) are indicated to rule out the possibility of a posterior fossa tumor or lesion. If these are negative, medical treatment is indicated with Tegretol. Dilantin is later used if maximal doses of Tegretol are unsuccessful. If medical therapy fails or untoward side effects occur, surgical treatment is considered.

2. In elderly, medically infirm patients, we recommend percutaneous trigeminal neurolysis procedures. In my hands, glycerol injections have proven highly effective in relieving trigeminal neuralgia pain with fewer side effects versus trigeminal radiofrequency rhizotomy. This procedure also has been attractive to patients for its short hospital stay, with patients often returning to work the next day with a high rate of success. In addition, I have found this procedure also useful for trigeminal neuralgia related to multiple sclerosis.

3. In younger patients, a careful discussion of microvascular decompression and percutaneous trigeminal

neurolysis, with expected results and possible risks of each procedure, is undertaken and a choice made by the patient. Although curative in a majority of cases, if the condition recurs after microvascular decompression, it can then be treated by percutaneous technique or re-exploration with partial division of the trigeminal sensory root.

 Bibliography

Fujimaki T, Fukushima T, Miyazaki S: Percutaneous retrogasserian glycerol injection in the management of trigeminal neuralgia: Long-term follow-up results. J Neurosurg 1990; 73:212–216.

Hamlyn PJ, King TT: Neurovascular compression in trigeminal neuralgia: A clinical and anatomical study. J Neurosurg 1992;76:948–954.

Jannetta PJ: Observations on the etiology of trigeminal neuralgia, hemifacial spasm, acoustic nerve dysfunction and glossopharyngeal neuralgia: Definitive microsurgical treatment and results in 117 patients. Neurochirurgia 1977;20:145–154.

Lunsford LD, Apfelbaum RI: Choice of surgical therapeutic modalities for treatment of trigeminal neuralgia: Microvascular decompression, percutaneous retrogasserian thermal or glycerol rhizotomy. Clin Neurosurg 1985;32:319.

Waltz TA, Dalessio DJ, Copeland B, Abbott G: Percutaneous injection of glycerol for the treatment of trigeminal neuralgia. Clin J Pain 1989;5:195–198.

294 Peripheral Neuropathy

Jerry M. Earll

Etiology

1. The anatomic diagnosis of peripheral neuropathy usually can be described accurately, while the actual cause is identifiable only 50 to 80 per cent of the time.
2. The etiology is broad, and it is helpful to classify by predominant pathologic features.
   a. Axonal: neuronal neuropathies
   b. Paranodal: segmental demyelination
3. The exact cause of metabolic and toxic neuropathies is not always clear and frequently involves combinations.
4. Diabetes is the leading cause of polyneuropathy and is the most common complication in the more than 5 million diabetics in the United States.
   a. Glucose toxicity role suspected since neuropathy occurs
      (1) In both insulin-dependent (IDDM) and non–insulin-dependent diabetes mellitus (NIDDM)
      (2) In diabetes associated with pancreatitis, pancreatic trauma, and hemochromatosis
      (3) Sixty per cent less often in the tight-control arm of the DCCT (Diabetes Control and Complications) study
   b. Associated metabolic derangements
      (1) Increased glycosylated proteins and advanced glycosylation end products
      (2) Increased sorbitol and decreased myoinositol
   c. Autoimmune and vascular abnormalities contribute.

Symptoms

1. In polyneuropathies, sensation is frequently affected disproportionately more than motor function.
2. Longer nerves are usually affected first so that symptoms begin in the toes and feet. Descriptions such as "feet feel like wood" or "walking on egg shells" are common.
3. Impaired sensation can result in unsteady gait and complaints of falling, especially in the dark.

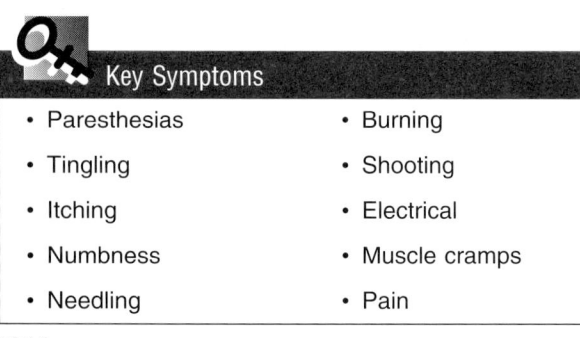

Key Symptoms

• Paresthesias	• Burning
• Tingling	• Shooting
• Itching	• Electrical
• Numbness	• Muscle cramps
• Needling	• Pain

Clinical Findings

Somatic neuropathies can be divided into three major subdivisions, although there are some overlaps.

1. Symmetrical distal polyneuropathy
2. Focal or mononeuropathy
3. Proximal sensorimotor neuropathy

Key Signs

• Skin dryness and hair loss	• Stocking and glove hypalgesia and anesthesia
• Decreased stretch reflexes	• Decreased pain and temperature
• Muscle weakness, foot drop	• Decreased touch and pressure
• Decreased vibration	
• Foot ulcers and deformity	

Laboratory Tests

1. Nerve conduction tests may be indicated for those neuropathies that are not readily explainable.
   a. Axonal neuropathies: Conduction is normal or mildly reduced. Electromyography reveals muscle denervation.
   b. Demyelinating neuropathies: Conduction is slowed without electromyographic denervation.
   c. In many cases there is a combination of demyelination and axonal neuropathy.
2. Semmes-Weinstein monofilament testing can be done easily by primary care providers to assess change and risk of foot injury; failure to detect pressure from 5.07 monofilament is associated with high risk.
3. Nerve biopsy indicated in diagnosing some multiple mononeuropathy syndromes such as vasculitis, sarcoidosis, amyloidosis, and leprosy.

Key Tests

• Complete blood count	• Thyroid function
• Sedimentation rate	• Immunoglobulins and electrophoresis
• Electrolytes	
• Blood sugar	• B_{12} and folate
	• Chest radiograph

Differential Diagnosis

1. Wide spectrum of diseases: toxic, bacterial, viral infections, nutritional, chemical, hereditary, metabolic

2. Common diseases that manifest with neuropathy
   a. Axonal
      (1) Diabetes
      (2) Toxic and alcohol
      (3) B_{12} deficiencies
      (4) Paraneoplastic
      (5) Hereditary, type II
      (6) Dysproteinemias and paraproteinemias
      (7) Drugs: Dilantin, Antabuse, pyridoxine, nitrofurantoin, amiodarone, metronidazole, vincristine, cisplatinum, Taxol, isoniazid
   b. Demyelinating
      (1) Diabetes
      (2) Guillain-Barré syndrome
      (3) Chronic inflammatory neuropathy
      (4) Dysproteinemias and paraproteinemias
      (5) Hereditary, Type I
      (6) Drugs as above
   c. Focal and multifocal
      (1) Diabetes
      (2) Entrapment
      (3) Vasculitis
      (4) Infections: herpes zoster, syphilis, Lyme, AIDS, leprosy

Treatment

1. Specific treatments for documented infections, nutritional deficiencies, hereditary diseases, uremia, and the withdrawal from toxins, drugs, and alcohol are standard.
2. Helpful physical measures include warm baths, high-quality skin care with nondrying lotions to seal in moisture, light body stockings to reduce physical stimulation in hyperesthesia, and transcutaneous nerve stimulation techniques.

Medication

1. Drug treatment is primarily aimed at relief of symptoms.
2. Blocking the sorbitol pathway with aldose reductase inhibitors and blocking the production of advanced glycosylation end products with aminoguanidine look promising.
3. Resist use of benzodiazepines. They lower pain thresholds and are addicting.

Diet

1. Emphasize good nutrition, including the importance of consuming five fruits and vegetables per day.
2. Vitamin and nutritional therapy is not established as beneficial but is safe and is often used as "insurance." This includes folate, 1 mg, a multiple-vitamin tablet daily, plus vitamin B_{12} injections intra-muscularly, 100 μg/week or 1000 μg/month, for at least 3 months. Inositol is available over the counter and is frequently given orally in an effort to restore depleted myoinositol.

Activity

Activity is encouraged with careful observation for pressure points, trauma, infections, ulcers, and arthritic deformities.

Patient Education

1. Instruction in basic care of underlying disease and importance of compliance with programs and vigilance for injury
2. Emphasize alcohol avoidance, glucose control, and prompt care for complications; daily foot inspection.

Key Treatment

- Analgesics: aspirin, acetaminophen, NSAIDs
- Topical: capsaicin for burning and hypersensitivity
- Tricyclic antidepressants: amitriptyline, nortriptyline with fluphenazine (Prolixin)?
- Serotonin reuptake inhibitors: paroxetine (Paxil), fluoxetine (Prozac)
- Anticonvulsants: carbamazepine (Tegretol), valproic acid (Depakene)
- Other: clonidine (Catapres), clonazepam (Klonopin)

Follow-Up

1. Antidepressant medications are often effective analgesics in smaller doses than those required for major depression.
2. Increase each class of medication to maximum tolerated dose before changing medication; combinations are frequently more effective and reduce side effects.
3. Emphasize that neuropathy symptoms usually improve with time. Explain that symptoms sometimes appear to worsen as nerves repair themselves and become more functional.

Bibliography

Adams RD, Victor M (eds): Diseases of the Peripheral Nerves: Principles of Neurology, 5th ed. New York, McGraw-Hill, 1993, pp 1117–1169.

Greene DA, Sima AAF, Stevens MJ, et al: Complications: Neuropathy, pathogenetic considerations. Diabetes Care 1992; 15:1902–1925.

Ross MA: Neuropathies associated with diabetes. Med Clin North Am 1993;77:111–129.

The Diabetes Control and Complications Trial Research Group 1993: The effect of intensive diabetes treatment on the development and progression of long-term complications in insulin-dependent diabetes mellitus. N Engl J Med 1993;329:977–986.

Vinik AI, Holland MT, LeBeau JM, et al: Diabetic neuropathies. Diabetes Care 1992;15:1926–1975.

295 Reflex Sympathetic Dystrophy

Robert Jay Schwartzman

Etiology

1. Definition: Reflex sympathetic dystrophy (RSD) is a syndrome consisting of five major components

   a. Burning pain

   b. Autonomic dysfunction

   c. Edema

   d. Movement disorder

   e. Dystrophy and atrophy

   It is initiated primarily by damage to a major nerve or C-nociceptive and A-delta pain fibers in affected soft tissue.

2. Epidemiology: All age groups are susceptible. Particular injuries that are associated with RSD are

   a. Brachial plexus traction injuries

   b. Carpal tunnel surgery

   c. Arthroscopic knee surgery

   d. Fractures with concomitant nerve injury

   e. Radiculopathy and soft tissue injury

3. Risk factors: A few families have been reported with RSD. There appears to be no genetic predisposition. Fifty per cent of all patients with RSD have been casted. Most of these patients have had sprains, Colles' fracture, or trimalleolar ankle fractures. A completely severed nerve does not cause RSD. Damage to blood vessel walls and nerves from electrical injury, from ergotamine toxicity, or from vein stripping may incite the process.

Symptoms

All features of RSD may be present in the affected extremity while the contralateral extremity demonstrates subtle subclinical signs and symptoms of specific components of the syndrome. The process in its early stages is sympathetically maintained but with time becomes sympathetically independent. It may spread to the entire body surface and can involve the visceral autonomic nervous system and bone.

1. Pain: characterized by *hyperalgesia* (lower pain threshold with enhanced pain perception), mechanical and thermal *allodynia* (pain induced by innocuous mechanical or thermal stimuli) and *hyperpathia* (increased pain threshold that once exceeded induces severe pain that reaches maximum intensity explosively and continues when the stimulus is withdrawn).

2. Hypoesthesia: Some patients with RSD are hypoesthetic in the affected area. The pain spreads both proximally and distally and does not respect a nerve or dermatomal distribution. It frequently is more severe on extensor surfaces.

Key Symptoms

- Pain out of proportion to injury
- Burning pain
- Deep ache
- Allodynia
- Hyperalgesia

Clinical Findings

1. Edema: Edema is seen in both early and late stages of the illness at the site of injury, distal to it and at times over major areas of the body. The edematous skin has a brawny, reddened quality.

2. Autonomic dysfunction: Autonomic dysfunction is present in all stages of RSD. Early in the illness the involved extremity may be warm, suffused, red, and dry but with time becomes pale, cool, hyperhidrotic, and cyanotic. Temperature changes from warm to cool may vary within a short period of time in stage I disease. Generalized capillary circulatory dysfunction occurs in all fingers and toes of the affected extremity rather than in a nerve or dermatomal distribution.

3. Movement disorder: All patients with RSD manifest some aspects of its concomitant movement disorder. These features are

   a. An inability to initiate movement rapidly

   b. Dystonia

   c. Weakness

   d. Spasm

   e. Hyperactive reflexes

   f. Tremor

4. Dystrophy and atrophy: Early in the course of the illness the nails become thickened, ridged, and brittle. Hair becomes darker and grows more rapidly. Edematous areas demonstrate brawny, reddened, thickened skin. In later stages, nails break, hair is lost in the affected area, and the skin becomes shiny and atrophic. There is profound muscle atrophy; bone demonstrates periarticular resorption, and tendon and cartilage degeneration is present.

Key Signs

- Swelling
- Abnormal temperature
- Hyperhidrosis
- Cyanosis
- Livedo reticularis
- Dystonia
- Tremor
- Atrophy of muscle
- Shiny skin
- Dystrophic nails

Laboratory Tests

The underlying cause of the illness must be identified.

1. Thermography identifies small fiber abnormalities (sympathetic and C-fiber in several dermatomes in the affected areas in a characteristic pattern).

2. A triple-phase bone scan may demonstrate abnormal pooling and increased periarticular uptake in 30 per cent of patients.

3. Sympathetic blockade of the affected area will afford dramatic relief of pain if the process is still sympathetically maintained. If the process is sympathetically independent, it will not relieve pain.

4. An intravenous phentolamine test (α_1-adrenergic antagonist) will be positive (pain relief) if the process is still sympathetically maintained.

5. Plain radiographs reveal clear periarticular and cystic bone changes in late-stage disease.

Key Tests

- Thermogram
- Triple-phase bone scan
- Response to sympathetic blockade
- Plain films

Differential Diagnosis

1. Autonomic dysfunction, edema, and pain from underlying soft tissue injury or fracture
2. Thrombophlebitis
3. Ergotism

Treatment

1. Diagnosis and treatment of the underlying injury
2. Sympathetic blockade of the upper extremity
   a. A series of five superior ganglion blocks followed by intensive physical therapy
   b. Sympathetic blockade of the lower extremity: a series of paravertebral sympathetic blocks followed by weight-bearing, stretching, and strengthening exercises
   c. If both lower extremities are involved, a 3- to 5-day epidural 0.25% Marcaine block
3. Elavil for sleep and diflunisal (Dolobid), 250 mg t.i.d., for pain in early stages
4. In sympathetic independent pain, a dorsal column stimulator is placed. In refractory single-extremity problems, a combination of nerve and dorsal column stimulation is utilized.
5. In generalized RSD that is refractory to all other forms of treatment, a morphine intrathecal pump is utilized. Approximately 35 mg/day relieves most patients.

Key Treatment

- Relieve underlying cause
- Sympathetic blockade
- Intense physical therapy
- Dorsal column stimulation
- Morphine pump

Bibliography

Abram SH: Incidence and epidemiology. *In* Stanton-Hicks M, Janig W, Boas RA (eds): Reflex Sympathetic Dystrophy. Boston, Kluwer Academic Publishers, 1990.

Blumberg H, Griesser HJ, Hornyak ME: Mechanisms and role of peripheral blood flow dysregulation in pain sensation and edema in reflex sympathetic dystrophy. *In* Stanton-Hicks M, Janig W, Boas RA (eds): Reflex Sympathetic Dystrophy. Boston, Kluwer Academic Publishers, 1990.

Bonica JJ: Causalgia and other reflex sympathetic dystrophies. *In* Bonica JJ, Liebeskind JC, Albe-Fessard DG (eds): Advances in Pain Research and Therapy. New York, Raven Press, 1979.

Schwartzman RJ: Reflex sympathetic dystrophy. *In* Frank HL (ed): Spinal Cord Trauma. Amsterdam, Elsevier, 1992.

Schwartzman RJ, McLellan TL: Reflex sympathetic dystrophy, a review. Arch Neurol 1987; 44:555–561.

296 Parkinson's Disease

John T. Slevin

Etiology

A. Anatomy, biochemistry, pathology
   1. Parkinson's disease (PD) is an *idiopathic* condition resulting from neuronal degeneration and loss in pigmented brain stem nuclei.
   2. Losses are prevalent in the zona compacta of the substantia nigra, a pigmented nucleus containing dopaminergic neurons projecting (via the *nigrostriatal pathway*) to the putamen and caudate nuclei. Functionally, this loss of inhibitory dopaminergic input is thought to account for much of the hypokinetic motor symptoms of PD.
   3. The Lewy body, an eosinophilic intracytoplasmic neuronal inclusion, is considered the *sine qua non* of idiopathic PD but has been reported in several other neurologic diseases.
   4. Recent evidence lends support to an *oxidant theory*: PD may result from either an extrinsic mechanism (oxidation of a protoxin, e.g., methylphenyltetrahydropyridine [MPTP]) or an intrinsic mechanism whereby free radicals are generated by dopamine metabolism.

B. Biometric data
   1. The most common movement disorder in clinical practice—prevalence: 100 cases per 100,000 population; incidence: 20 cases per 100,000 population per year
   2. Onset between ages 40 and 70 (peak onset in mid-50s)
   3. No definite gender, ethnic, geographic, or socioeconomic predispositions are known.
   4. Rare families may be predisposed to PD with apparent autosomal dominant inheritance.

Symptoms

1. Slowness of movement; leads to difficulties in grooming, dressing, and feeding
2. Stiffness: affects both flexors and extensors of limbs and axial muscles, with patients complaining that they feel "wooden" or are moving against great resistance
3. Tremor: Usually unilateral at onset, it can progress to involve the face and lower extremities; exaggerated by anxiety, absent in sleep.
4. Posture/gait abnormalities: Patients assume a stooped posture and develop a disturbance of equilibrium leading to frequent falls.
5. Other: autonomic disturbances, including orthostatic hypotension, constipation, hyperhydrosis; muscle cramps and aching; micrographia; slurred, hypo-phonic, monotonous speech. Ultimately, dementia is seen in over half of patients.

Clinical Findings

1. Bradykinesia: patient sits immobile on the examining table. Appearance of *masked facies,* or poker face, with decreased eyeblink
2. Rigidity, usually *cogwheel rigidity,* wherein passive movement of a joint causes sequential catches as in turning a ratchet; resistance is uniform throughout range of motion. Rigidity becomes increasingly prominent in later stages of the disease.
3. Gait disturbance: An initial lack of arm swing with walking evolves into a propulsive, or *festinating,* shuffling, small-stepped gait with en bloc, or whole-body, turning.
4. A resting, *pill-rolling* tremor of 3 to 6 Hz that diminishes with movement is an initial symptom in 70 per cent of patients.
5. Exaggerated *glabellar reflex* (Myerson's sign: blinking that does not reduce or stop with repeated tapping on the forehead)
6. Mild orthostatic hypotension; sialorrhea; moist, greasy face with seborrheic dermatitis

Key Symptoms/Signs

Cardinal	Secondary
• Akinesia/bradykinesia	• Dysarthria
• Postural/gait abnormalities	• Micrographia
	• Seborrhea
• Rigidity	• Sialorrhea
• Tremor	

Laboratory Tests

1. PD is a clinical diagnosis with no definitive test(s).
2. Computed tomography and magnetic resonance imaging are either normal or show nonspecific atrophy.
3. Electroencephalogram, blood, and cerebrospinal studies are typically normal.

Differential Diagnosis

1. Isolated depression: manifested mainly as psychomotor retardation, major depression may be confused with PD, with which a reactive depression is not uncommon. Evidence suggests a primary depression in PD due to the diminution of biogenic amines.
2. Essential tremor: characterized by a postural and ki-

netic (not resting) tremor of the hands and head without bradykinesia and rigidity. It frequently decreases temporarily with ingestion of ethanol, and more than 50 per cent of patients respond to propranolol or primidone. Frequently positive family history

3. Parkinson plus syndromes: differentiated from idiopathic PD by the presence of various associated signs and symptoms

a. Parkinsonism + disturbances of ocular motility: Progressive supranuclear palsy

b. Parkinsonism + cerebellar signs and symptoms: Olivopontocerebellar degenerations

c. Parkinsonism + severe autonomic insufficiency: Shy-Drager syndrome

4. Secondary parkinsonism

a. Head trauma (e.g., from professional boxing)

b. Metabolic disorders, especially hypoparathyroidism

c. Postviral encephalitis: rare, sporadic cases

d. Toxins and industrial exposure (especially consider in the younger patient): carbon tetrachloride, carbon monoxide, carbon disulfide, cyanide, manganese, methanol, MPTP (the by-product of a street drug, this agent creates an animal model of idiopathic PD)

e. Drugs (the most common cause of secondary parkinsonism, which itself is the most common drug-induced movement disorder)

(1) Neuroleptics, especially haloperidol, fluphenazine

(2) Antiemetics, especially prochlorperazine, metoclopramide

(3) Reserpine

(4) α-Methyldopa (rarely)

(5) Lithium carbonate (rarely)

Treatment

1. PD is relentlessly progressive; no treatment modalities have been shown to categorically slow disease progression. Treatment is palliative and directed at relieving symptoms.

2. Several surgical procedures are currently under evaluation. Thalamotomy (reduces tremor) and pallidotomy (reduces tremor, rigidity, and bradykinesia) are in revival. Implantation of human fetal nigral cells and installation of trophic factors are under investigation.

3. Choice of medication(s) depends on stage (see below) of illness; all are oral preparations only.

Medication

A. Dopaminergic agents

1. All act by enhancing activity at central dopamine receptors, and all have common side effects, including

a. *Anorexia, vomiting, dizziness*

b. *Dyskinesia:* usually choreiform movements; the effect is dose dependent and usually occurs after prolonged therapy.

c. *Psychotic episodes, dementia, depression:* half of patients on chronic dopamine replacement therapy develop psychiatric side effects. Visual hallucinations and vivid nightmares are frequent early signs. Psychotic episodes usually take the form of paranoid delusions. Symptoms usually improve with reduction of dopaminergic agents.

2. Levodopa and carbidopa (Sinemet, Atamet): *precursor therapy*

a. Levodopa crosses the blood-brain barrier and is then converted to dopamine.

b. Additional side effects

(1) *Cardiac arrhythmia:* rare in preparations including carbidopa, which blocks the peripheral decarboxylation of levodopa to dopamine.

(2) *Orthostatic hypotension:* usually transient; occurs early in treatment and resolves

c. Dosing: carbidopa/levodopa (10 mg/100 mg, 25 mg/100 mg, and 25 mg/250 mg) and carbidopa/levodopa extended-release (50 mg/200 mg and 25 mg/100 mg) tablets. Initial dose 25 mg/100 mg tablet three times daily. Extended-release preparations are helpful in patients who show excessive symptomatic fluctuations.

3. Bromocriptine (Parlodel): *direct receptor agonist* (primarily D_2 dopamine receptors)

a. Permits use of lower dosages of levodopa with improvement in side effect profile (including dyskinesia) and fewer symptomatic fluctuations

b. Additional side effects: exacerbation of peptic ulcer disease and *erythromelalgia*, a painful reddish skin discoloration

c. Dosing: initially, 2.5 mg/day; increase by additional 2.5 mg/week as tolerated. Little improvement beyond 20 mg/day in most patients.

4. Pergolide (Permax): *direct receptor agonist* (D_1 and D_2 dopamine receptors)

a. Benefit and side effect profile similar but not identical to that of bromocriptine

b. Dosing: initially, 0.05 mg/day for 3 days and increase in 0.05-mg increments every 3 days and by 0.125 mg after higher doses reached. Average greatest response 0.75 to 1.5 mg/day.

5. Selegiline (Eldepryl): *MAO-B inhibitor*

a. Increases level of intrinsically/extrinsically derived dopamine by blocking catabolism. It has been suggested that drugs of this class may help slow the progression of PD; to date, studies have shown little significant effect in this regard.

    b. Additional side effects: *insomnia*; will potentiate side effects of levodopa

  6. Amantadine (Symmetrel): *indirect agonist* (and an anti-A₂ viral agent)

    a. Used in early PD; useful in treating tremor; can delay need for levodopa

    b. Additional side effects: congestive heart failure, urinary retention, livedo reticularis

B. Anticholinergic agents

  1. Blocking the cholinergic overactivity provides relief for some patients. First choice in treatment of patients with primarily tremor. Little effect on hypokinesia or rigidity.

  2. Side effects: dry mouth, constipation, and blurred vision common; urinary retention in men; may cause confusion in older patients; be alert to signs of closed-angle glaucoma

  3. Most commonly used: benztropine (Cogentin), trihexiphenidyl (Artane)

Rational Treatment Strategy and Problems

For the treatment of early and midcourse PD, the therapeutic index (efficacy/side effects) may be optimized by the use of multiple medications at lower doses (e.g., levodopa/carbidopa plus direct agonist) rather than high-dose monotherapy.

Treatment problems include

1. Dyskinesias: see side effects of dopaminergic agents above

2. On-off phenomenon: marked, rapid fluctuations between a parkinsonian state and normal or dyskinetic state that do not directly correlate with time of dosing

3. Loss of efficacy: patients lose response to medications as PD progresses, usually not before the fifth year of overt symptoms.

Diet

Some patients exhibit a significant delay or occasionally no response after levodopa dosing. Efficacy may be improved by dosing *before* meals or by reducing dietary protein (especially breakfast and lunch). Patients who have more trouble with the peripheral side effects of levodopa (nausea and vomiting) often improve with dosing *after* meals.

Activity

Patients with PD, like everyone, should participate in a regular exercise program. They should focus on maintaining range of mobility and muscle strength. A physical therapist familiar with PD often can help individualize an exercise program.

Patient Education

1. Encourage participation in local support groups.

2. Encourage membership in a national support group, most of which provide newsletters.

3. Be aware of various publications ("bibliography," for example).

Key Treatment

- No treatment modality has categorically slowed disease. Treatment is palliative and aimed at relieving symptoms.

Follow-Up

1. One must know the interval between levodopa dosing and the clinical examination and whether the patient feels *off* or *on* when examined to determine if a change in therapy is necessary, usually at two to three yearly visits.

2. Of many rating scales used for PD, the Hoehn-Yahr staging scale has been in use for over 25 years:

  a. Stage 0 = no signs of disease

  b. Stage I = unilateral disease

  c. Stage II = bilateral or midline involvement

  d. Stage III = stage II + impaired balance

  e. Stage IV = severe disability, inability to walk

  f. Stage V = wheelchair-bound/bedridden

Bibliography

Hubble JP, Cao T, Hassanein RES, et al: Risk factors for Parkinson's disease. Neurology 1993;43:1693–1697.

Jankovic J, Marsden CD: Therapeutic strategies in Parkinson's disease. *In* Jankovic J, Tolosa E (eds): Parkinson's Disease and Movement Disorders, 2nd ed. Baltimore, Williams & Wilkins, 1993, pp 115–144.

Lieberman AN, Williams FL: Parkinson's Disease: The Complete Guide for Patients and Caregivers. New York, Simon & Schuster, 1993.

Paulson GW: Therapy of patients with Parkinson's disease. Arch Neurol 1994;51:754–756.

Payami H, Larsen K, Bernard S, Nutt J: Increased risk of Parkinson's disease in parents and siblings of patients. Ann Neurol 1994;36:659–661.

297 Alzheimer's Disease

Robert J. Moss

Epidemiology

1. Major public health problem affecting over 4 million persons
2. Fourth leading cause of death, with 46,000 deaths per year
3. Costs may exceed $50 billion per year
4. Major risk factors
   a. Advanced age
   b. Family history of dementia in first-degree relative
   c. Family history of Down syndrome

Etiology

1. Histopathologic changes (frontal, temporal, and parietal lobes)
   a. Intracellular neurofibrillary tangles
      (1) Abnormal filamentous accumulation in cytoplasm of neurons
      (2) Major ultrastructural unit is paired helical filament
   b. Extracellular neuritic plaques: Abnormal nerve processes with central β amyloid protein core. β-Amyloid derived from amyloid precursor protein (APP).
2. Cholinergic hypothesis
   a. Cholinergic neurons are selectively vulnerable to injury with retrograde degeneration of subcortical nuclei.
   b. Choline acetyltransferase and acetylcholine are decreased.
   c. Degree of cognitive impairment directly related to loss of cholinergic neurons and neurotransmitters
3. Genetic hypothesis
   a. Older persons with Down syndrome have high incidence of Alzheimer's disease
   b. Genetic studies have linked familial Alzheimer's disease (FAD) with mutations on chromosomes 21, 14, and 19.
   c. The gene for APP is located on chromosome 21.
   d. Early-onset FAD is associated with chromosome 14.
   e. Late-onset FAD is associated with chromosome 19.
   f. Apolipoprotein E gene is on chromosome 19. Two alleles of APOE-ε4 increase the risk and decrease the age of onset for Alzheimer's disease (AD).
4. Aluminum: Associated with plaques, but relevance unknown
5. Viral: Little evidence for

Symptoms

1. Progressive memory loss (short and long term)
2. Impairment in at least one other area of cognitive function
   a. Abstract thinking
   b. Judgment
   c. Visual-spatial function
   d. Language
   e. Apraxia
   f. Agnosia
   g. Personality change
3. Impairment in social functioning (home, job, activities of daily living)
4. Consciousness not clouded (absence of delirium)

Key Symptoms

- Progressive memory loss
- Impairment in at least one other area of cognitive functioning
- Impaired social functioning
- Clear sensorium

Clinical Findings

1. Abnormal mental status screening examination (such as Folstein Mini-Mental Status Exam)
2. Physical and neurologic examinations fail to identify other causes of dementia.

Key Sign

- Normal physical and neuromuscular examinations support the diagnosis of a dementia of the Alzheimer's type.

Laboratory Tests

1. Thyroid-stimulating hormone (TSH) to exclude hyper- or hypothyroidism
2. Erythrocyte sedimentation rate (ESR) to exclude underlying inflammatory disease
3. Chemistry profile to exclude metabolic, renal, or hepatic disease
4. Urinalysis (UA) to exclude renal disease
5. Complete blood count (CBC) to exclude anemia
6. Folate and vitamin B_{12} to exclude nutritional deficiency

7. Fluorescent treponemal antibody absorption test for syphilis to exclude tertiary syphilis

8. Human immunodeficiency virus (HIV) titer to exclude HIV infection for individuals at risk

9. Lumbar puncture to rule out slow viral or fungal disease if fever or nuchal rigidity present

10. Neurodiagnostic imaging (yield is 3.5 per cent for pathologic abnormalities)

    a. Electroencephalogram to rule out underlying seizure disorder

    b. Computed tomographic (CT) brain scan to exclude tumor, subdural hematoma, stroke, normal-pressure hydrocephalus

    c. Magnetic resonance imaging (MRI) is more sensitive to small-vessel disease.

    d. Positron-emission tomography scan used experimentally to determine functional abnormalities that predict cognitive changes

    e. SPECT scan used for the same with characteristic pattern of decreased uptake in temporoparietal areas seen in AD.

11. Brain biopsy is the only definitive test for diagnosis.

Key Laboratory Tests

• TSH	• Folate
• CBC	• B$_{12}$
• UA	• FTA-ABS
• Chemistry profile	• CT or MRI brain scan

Differential Diagnosis

1. Delirium

    a. Acute onset with fluctuating levels of consciousness

    b. High mortality secondary to underlying cause

2. Depression

    a. Fluctuating cognitive loss with depressed mood

    b. "I don't know" answers

3. Other dementia syndromes

    a. Multiple-infarct dementia

       (1) Stepwise decline with multiple cardiovascular risk factors

       (2) Focal neurologic signs

    b. Medications: sedatives, antihypertensives, antidepressants, neuroleptics

    c. Alcohol

    d. Normal-pressure hydrocephalus: triad of urinary incontinence, dementia, and gait ataxia

    e. Toxic, metabolic, nutritional, infectious, and other neurologic causes

Treatment

Medication

1. Drugs to augment acetylcholine: cholinesterase inhibitors

    a. Tetrahydroaminoacridine (tacrine HCl [Cognex])

       (1) Approved for mild to moderate AD

       (2) A subgroup of AD patients show modest improvement.

       (3) Twenty per cent develop reversible increase in transaminases.

    b. Agonists (bethanechol) not shown to be effective

    c. Precursors (lecithin) not shown to be effective

2. Nootropil or metabolic enhancers (piracetam) not shown to be effective

3. Vasodilators (Hydergine) approved but not shown to improve memory

4. Future medications

    a. Nerve growth factor

    b. Drugs that affect beta-amyloid metabolism and APP

    c. Drugs that affect APOE-ε4

Behavioral Syndromes

1. Depression can occur in 20 per cent of patients with AD. Consider antidepressants with low anticholinergic effect.

2. Anxiety: behavioral program and short-acting anxiolytics

3. Agitation: low anticholinergic neuroleptic medications or short-acting benzodiazepines

Diet

1. Weight loss is seen commonly.

2. Patients need to be reminded to eat.

3. May need home-delivered meals.

4. May need supervised or hand-fed meals.

5. May need soft foods, thick liquids, enteral tube feedings.

Activity

Supervised activity such as walking will help maintain muscle tone and improve sleep.

Patient Education

1. Explain diagnosis

2. Caregiver support

    a. Respite

    b. Support groups, live-in help, day care

3. Financial planning

4. Anticipate home care and placement needs

5. Review behavior syndromes (include falls, incontinence, sleep disturbance, and wandering)

6. Discuss advance directives, guardianship, and other ethical issues

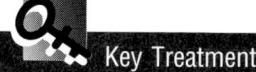

Key Treatment

- Drugs that augment acetylcholine, such as cholinesterase inhibitors

Follow-Up

1. Should be seen every 4 to 6 months
2. Document cognitive decline and behavior.
3. Health maintenance to optimize function
4. Assess caregiver burden

Bibliography

Diagnostic and Statistical Manual of Mental Disorders, 4th ed. Washington, American Psychiatric Association, 1994.

Mullan M, Crawford F, Buchanan J: Technical feasibility of genetic testing for Alzheimer's disease. Alzheimer Dis Assoc Disord 1994;8:102–115.

Winkler MA: Tacrine for Alzheimer's disease: Which patient, what dose? JAMA 1994;271:1023–1024.

Winograd CH, Jarvik LF: Physician management of the demented patient. J Am Geriatr Soc 1986;34:295–308.

Yankner BA, Mesulam MM: β-Amyloid and the pathogenesis of Alzheimer's disease. N Engl J Med 1991;325:1849–1857.

298 Myasthenia Gravis

John J. Hart

Etiology

1. Myasthenia gravis (MG) is an autoimmune disease caused by antibody and T-cell attack on the nicotinic acetylcholine receptors (AChR) of the muscle endplate.

   a. Between 85 and 95 per cent of MG patients have antibodies to their AChRs.

   b. T-cell immunity is theorized to occur after sensitization in the thymus to a protein similar or identical to the embryonic AChR.

2. MG age classification and respective etiologies

   a. Adult MG: autoimmune etiology as described above

   b. Childhood MG

   (1) Transient neonatal MG: MG mothers passively transfer antibodies to 10 to 20 per cent of their children.

   (2) Congenital MG: caused by a variety of neuromuscular junction defects and *is not* autoimmune-mediated

   (3) Juvenile MG: etiology identical to adult MG, earlier onset

Symptoms

1. Voluntary muscle weakness and increased fatigability
2. Diplopia
3. Dysphagia
4. Jaw weakness while chewing
5. Choking
6. Fluid regurgitation through nose when swallowing
7. Difficulty maintaining volume of voice

Key Symptoms

- Easily fatigued, weak muscles
- Diplopia

Clinical Findings

1. Muscle weakness initially is transitory.
2. Weakness is exacerbated with continuous use, warmer surroundings, at the end of the day, and with physiologic and psychosocial stress.
3. Order of muscle group involvement from most to least common: ocular, bulbar, neck, limb girdle, and distal extremity
4. Forty per cent of MG patients eventually develop bulbar muscle problems.
5. Ninety per cent of MG patients develop ocular findings (ptosis, acquired strabismus). Of those whose symptoms stay localized to the eyes for 1 year, 90 per cent will have ocular MG.

6. Clinical classification

   a. Ocular only

   b. Generalized

   (1) Mild: ocular with gradual progression to skeletal and bulbar muscles, no respiratory symptoms

   (2) Moderate: more rapid and involved progression, no respiratory symptoms

   (3) Severe

   (a) Acute fulminating

   (b) Late severe: severe symptoms after approximately 2 years

Key Signs

- Ptosis
- Muscle weakness
- Dysarthria

Laboratory Tests

1. AChR antibody assay: Antibody is elevated up to 95 per cent of the time in generalized MG but less with ocular MG.

2. Edrophonium (Tensilon) test: This anticholinesterase is administered intravenously and the patient is observed for improvement.

   a. Children heavier than 75 pounds and adults: 2 mg edrophonium is given intravenously over 15 to 30 seconds. The test is positive if muscular strength increases. If a positive response does not occur, an additional 8 mg of edrophonium is given and muscular strength is again evaluated. Decreased doses are used for infants and children less than 75 pounds.

   b. False-negative results occur, especially with ocular MG. It is sometimes combined with other ocular tests to better diagnose ocular MG.

   c. False-positive results have been reported.

3. Electromyogram

   a. A decremental response is seen with MG.

   b. Repetitive nerve stimulation tests have been improved to newer, more sensitive, stimulated single-fiber electromyography.

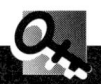

Key Tests

No single test is adequate for diagnosis; all three are used, that is:

- Acetylcholine antibody assay
- Edrophonium test
- Electromyogram

Differential Diagnosis

1. Eaton-Lambert syndrome
2. Muscular dystrophies
3. Brain tumors
4. Endocrine myopathies
5. Amyotrophic lateral sclerosis
6. D-Penicillamine administration (may induce AChR antibodies)

Treatment

1. Thymectomy has become accepted as improving all MG, although less with ocular MG.
2. Plasmapheresis and plasma exchange give short-term improvement and are useful in acute situations.

Medication

1. Acetylcholinesterase inhibitors
   a. Pyridostigmine (Mestinon)
   b. Neostigmine bromide (Prostigmin)
2. Immunosuppressive medicines
   a. Prednisone
   b. Cyclophosphamide (Cytoxan)
   c. Cyclosporine (Sandimmune)
   d. Azathioprine (Imuran)

Diet

Monitor for metabolic abnormalities secondary to prednisone and correct, such as potassium supplementation, caloric restriction.

Activity

Overexertion may exacerbate MG.

Patient Education

1. Physiologic and emotional stress may exacerbate MG.
2. Many common medicines exacerbate MG.
   a. Antibiotics: aminoglycosides, polymyxins, tetracyclines
   b. Cardiac drugs: verapamil, β blockers
   c. Others: phenytoin, chlorpromazine
3. Side effects of key medicines used to treat MG
   a. Pyridostigmine (Mestinon): diarrhea, bradycardia, sweating, salivation
   b. Prednisone: subclinical presentations of infections

Key Treatment

Drugs of Choice

- Pyridostigmine (Mestinon)
- Prednisone

Follow-Up

1. Progression of weakness
2. Thyroid function studies
3. Watch and screen for other autoimmune diseases.

Bibliography

Afiki AK, Bell WE: Tests for juvenile myasthenia gravis: Comparative diagnostic yield and prediction of outcome. Child Neurol 1993;8(4):403–411.

Conti-Tronconi BM, McLane KE, Raftery MA, et al: The nicotine acetylcholine receptor: Structure and autoimmune pathology. Crit Rev Biochem Mol Biol 1994;29(2):69–123.

Drachman DB: Myasthenia gravis. N Engl J Med 1994; 330(25):1797–1810.

Engel AG: Congenital myasthenic syndromes. Neurol Clin 1994;12(2):401–437.

Sommer N, Melms A, Weller M, Dichgans J: Ocular myasthenia gravis: A critical review of clinical and pathological aspects. Doc Ophthalmol 1993;84(4):309–333.

299 Multiple Sclerosis

Michael D. Kaufman

Etiology

1. Theories of pathogenesis
   a. Autoimmune disease directed against myelin proteins, oligodendroglia cells, or other antigens
   b. Chronic infection of the central nervous system (CNS)
2. Increasingly prevalent in the United States and Europe
3. Environmental determinants
   a. More common as distance from the equator increases
   b. Outbreaks suggest transmission of an agent that induces disease
   c. Susceptibility depends on childhood residence
4. Genetic contributions: multiple genes involved
   a. High prevalence in whites (90 to 95% of U.S. patients)
   b. Increased incidence among family members (Table 299–1)
   c. Gender: three females to one male

Symptoms

1. Primarily affects young adults, usually starting unilaterally or focally but eventually becoming bilateral, disseminated, and progressive
2. Common: limb weakness, numbness and paresthesia, chronic aching pain, monocular impairment of vision, double vision, slurred speech, imbalance, vertigo, urgency, constipation, impotence, depression, fatigue, cool extremities, radiating paresthesias associated with neck flexion, heat intolerance
3. Less common: radicular pains, facial weakness, hearing loss, trigeminal neuralgia, euphoria, confusion, oscillating vision, paroxysmal symptoms lasting seconds to minutes
4. Uncommon: severe apraxias or aphasia, extrapyramidal movement disorders, seizures, perineal pains, hypersomnolence, hemianopsia
5. Symptoms may be vague and precede recognizable signs, falsely suggesting somatization or hysteria.
6. Course
   a. Benign: 10 to 30 per cent

TABLE 299–1. MS RISK WHEN FAMILY MEMBER AFFECTED

RELATIONSHIP	LIFETIME MS RISK
General Caucasian population	<0.2%
Sibling or parent with MS	1–3%
Dizygotic twin with MS	2–5%
Monozygotic twin with MS	17–40%

   b. Relapsing-remitting/secondary progressive: more than 50 per cent
   c. Primary progressive: 10 to 20 per cent; often affects spinal cord; no exacerbations
   d. Less common patterns: optic neuritis and myelitis, recurrent optic neuritis, acute MS, associated with diseases of known etiology

> ### WARNING
>
> **Some patients report what appears to be a benign course for years, only then to experience rapid progression. Therefore, prediction of a benign outcome at almost any time is inappropriate.**

Key Symptoms

- Neurologic symptoms lasting days to weeks in a young adult
- Numbness, weakness, and ataxia, often appearing together
- Monocular visual blurring or binocular diplopia
- Worsening symptoms with vigorous activity or heat
- Bowel, bladder, and sexual dysfunction

Clinical Findings

1. Common: asymmetrical weakness most often of the legs, patchy sensory loss, pale optic disks, internuclear ophthalmoplegia, nystagmus, hyperreflexia with Babinski's signs, spastic gait, ataxia, diminished visual acuity
2. Less common: hyporeflexia, well-defined sensory levels, writhing facial muscles, oscillating eye movement, afferent pupillary defect, deafness, atrophy of muscle, significant dementia
3. Uncommon: homonomous hemianopsia, choreoathetosis, aphasia, apraxia

Key Signs

- Signs often bilateral
- Weakness in an upper motor neuron pattern
- Ataxia or abnormal gait
- Internuclear ophthalmoplegia
- Diminished visual acuity

Laboratory Tests

1. No tests are pathognomonic.
2. Magnetic resonance imaging (MRI): relatively specific, but false-positive and false-negative results
   a. Ovoid high-intensity areas on T_2-weighted scan involving white matter of brain and spinal cord. Three characteristic lesions preferred. Enhancement suggests acute inflammation.
   b. Serial MRIs have shown that the majority of high-intensity areas (about 80 per cent) appear without clinical exacerbation.
3. Cerebrospinal fluid (CSF): findings in MS are relatively specific
   a. Cell count: less than 40 white blood cells (WBCs), predominantly lymphocytes
   b. Protein: under 100 mg/dl; usually normal
   c. Oligoclonal immunoglobulin bands, (+) CSF, (−) serum
   d. IgG index: above 0.70
      IgG index = CSF (IgG/albumin)/serum (IgG/albumin)
4. Evoked potentials: relatively nonspecific; includes visual, brain stem, somatosensory, cortical motor evoked potentials and blink reflex
   a. Can find subclinical areas of disease
   b. Visual evoked potentials can be relatively specific and helpful if no history of optic neuritis

Key Tests

- MRI scans
- CSF oligoclonal immunoglobulin bands and IgG index

WARNING

MS is diagnosed only when physiologically consistent symptoms and signs and laboratory tests converge to suggest involvement of white matter projections from multiple areas within the CNS. Signs and symptoms fluctuate with time. No other pathology can exist to explain the complaints and findings. The diagnosis is not secure without appropriate positive laboratory findings.

Differential Diagnosis

1. Differential diagnosis varies with the patient's symptoms and with the duration of disease. Most difficult diagnostic problems arise with initial exacerbations, progressive myelopathies, and uncommon patterns.
2. MS can be mimicked by and can mimic conversion reactions.

Treatment

1. Many disease-specific therapies now investigational
2. Symptomatic therapy often multidisciplinary

Medication

A. Symptomatic treatment (Table 299–2)
B. Disease-specific
   1. Exacerbations: new or reappearance of previous symptom(s) evolving over days or weeks (range minutes to months) not due to a metabolic disturbance and preceded by at least 30 days of stability.
      a. Methylprednisolone, 1 gm intravenously daily for 3 to 5 days; may speed recovery from and possibly delay further exacerbations. Follow with tapering, low dose of steroid.
      b. ACTH, intravenously or intramuscularly
   2. Relapsing-remitting/secondary progressive
      a. Betaseron (interferon-beta$_{1b}$) results in fewer exacerbations and brain MRI lesions. FDA approved for fully ambulatory patients with recent exacerbations
      b. COP-I (Copolymer I) may soon receive FDA approval.
   3. Primary and secondary progressive (treatment not universally accepted)
      a. Cyclophosphamide and methylprednisolone in monthly intravenous boluses appear helpful in patients under age 40.
      b. Low-dose azathioprine and methotrexate show a trend toward stability.
      c. Cladribine is under study.

Diet

No specific diet recommended

Activity

1. Physical therapy: restorative and maintenance
2. Occupational therapy: energy conservation and adaptive devices
3. Aquatic therapy for the more impaired

Patient Education

1. Patients need to understand that treatment is palliative and the course is unpredictable.

TABLE 299–2. SYMPTOMATIC THERAPY

SYMPTOM	TREATMENT
Fatigue	Amantadine and stimulants; look for depression
Depression	Antidepressants and counseling
Spasticity	Baclofen; treat if loss of spasticity does not compromise ability to stand, transfer, etc.
Urgency	Anticholinergics if bladder spastic; intermittent catheterization if bladder will not empty
Constipation	Fiber, softeners, suppositories, enemas, oral lactulose
Neuralgic pain	Carbamazepine and phenothiazines
Chronic aching pains	Antidepressants and phenothiazines
Dysmetria	High-dose isoniazid and clonazepam; hard to treat
Postural tremor	Propranolol

2. Address social, insurance, and employment issues early.

3. Treatments that are expensive and potentially dangerous require extensive informed consent and patient cooperation.

4. National MS Society provides supplementary patient education.

Follow-Up

1. Regular thorough examinations to assess patient's condition

2. Interferon beta-1b may cause a depression of the white blood count and elevation of liver function tests. Follow monthly for 3 months and then every 3 months. Persistent elevations of liver transaminase functions should prompt withdrawing treatment until liver tests are normal; then reinstitution at half the dose. Watch for symptoms of depression; suicides reported.

3. Pseudoexacerbations due to fever and infection should be treated appropriately, not with methylprednisolone or ACTH.

Bibliography

Matthews WB (ed): McAlpine's Multiple Sclerosis, 2nd ed. New York, Churchill Livingstone, 1991.

Offenbacher H, Fazekas F, Schmidt R, et al: Assessment of MRI criteria for a diagnosis of MS. Neurology 1993;43:905–909.

Rudick RA, Goodkin DE: Treatment of Multiple Sclerosis: Trial Design, Results and Future Perspectives. New York, Springer-Verlag, 1992.

Rudick RA, Schiffer RB, Schwetz KM, Herndon RM: Multiple sclerosis: The problem of incorrect diagnosis. Arch Neurol 1986;43:578–583.

300 MRI or CT in CNS Imaging

David E. King

Emergency Imaging

1. In most central nervous system emergencies, including head trauma and suspected subarachnoid hemorrhage, or if the patient is in unstable condition or without a reliable medical history, non–contrast-enhanced computed tomography (CT) is the modality of choice. At present, CT is faster than magnetic resonance imaging (MRI), poses less risk, and interferes less with monitoring of the patient. Patients cannot be placed in an MR scanner if they have intracranial aneurysm clips in place, ferrous intraocular foreign bodies, certain types of prosthetic heart valves, or any type of pacemaker or implanted electromechanical device such as pumps and osteostimulators. MRI is insensitive to subarachnoid hemorrhage and less reliable than CT at detecting intraparenchymal cerebral hemorrhage, two findings that alter the emergency management of the stroke patient. Although subdural and epidural hemorrhages, acute ischemic strokes, and intracranial masses are shown somewhat more vividly with MRI than with CT, the sensitivity of CT is adequate in the emergency situation. The two are equivalent in evaluation of acute hydrocephalus, but MRI underperforms CT at demonstrating foreign bodies and fractures. Neither CT nor MRI consistently detects meningitis.

2. In acute spinal fracture and dislocation, CT should be chosen and directed to the area of interest. MRI is much more sensitive and efficient for surveying the entire spinal canal for intraspinal masses (neoplastic, inflammatory, or traumatic) and intrinsic abnormalities of the spinal cord and nerve roots (demyelination, neoplasm, syrinx, arteriovenous malformation, infarct, metastasis).

Nonemergency Imaging

1. If the patient has no unsafe internal metal, can tolerate being placed in the MR scanner, and can remain motionless for the requisite periods of several minutes at a time to complete the MR examination, the inherently greater tissue contrast in MRI makes it the imaging study of choice for the brain, meninges, pituitary gland, cranial nerves, spinal cord, and nerve roots. However, calcifications in the brain, typical of prenatal infections, are not reliably shown with MRI. Lesions of the face, sinuses, and orbits, of the calvarium, temporal bones, and skull base, and of the spinal column itself are complementarily imaged by MR and CT. High-resolution CT surpasses MRI for bone detail, whereas MRI excels with soft tissue and bone marrow.

2. Advanced MR and CT installations are both capable of producing angiographic images of vascular abnormalities such as aneurysms, arteriovenous malformations, and large-vessel stenoses and occlusions, although CT angiography (CTA) requires infusion of intravenous contrast material, but MR angiography (MRA) does not.

TABLE 300–1. MR vs CT IN CENTRAL NERVOUS SYSTEM IMAGING

BRAIN	MR vs CT
Abscess	MR or CT
Acoustic neuroma	MR
AIDS (infection, tumor)	MR
Alzheimer's disease	CT or MR
Aneurysm (*not clipped*)	MR and MRA
Arteriovenous malformation	MR and MRA
Bell's palsy	MR
Brain tumor	MR
Cavernous sinus lesion	MR
Coma (emergency)	CT
Congenital infection	CT
Congenital malformation	MR
Dementia	CT
Dissection (carotid, vertebral)	MR and MRA
Dizziness	MR
Guillain-Barré syndrome	MR
Headache	MR
Hydrocephalus	CT or MR
Meniere's disease	MR or CT
Meningitis	MR or CT
Multiple sclerosis	MR
Myasthenia gravis	MR
Neurodegenerative disorder	MR
Paresthesia	MR
Parkinson's disease	MR
Pituitary tumor	MR
Radiation necrosis	MR
Seizure disorder	MR
Stroke—rule out hemorrhage	CT
—all other situations	MR or CT
Subarachnoid hemorrhage	CT
Subdural hemorrhage	CT or MR
Transient ischemic attack	MR and MRA
Trauma	CT
Tremor	MR
Trigeminal neuralgia	MR

SPINE	MR vs CT
Arteriovenous malformation	MR
Compression fracture	CT or MR
Disk herniation	MR
Diskitis	MR
Epidural abscess or hematoma	MR
Hemangioma (vertebral)	MR or CT
Hemorrhage into spinal cord	MR
Infarction of spinal cord	MR
Metastasis	MR
Multiple sclerosis	MR
Osteomyelitis	MR
Postoperative scar	MR
Spinal cord tumor	MR
Spondylosis	MR or CT
Syringomyelia	MR
Transverse myelitis	MR
Trauma	CT and MR

Table 300–1 contains a list of common symptoms and diagnoses, with the specific modality most useful for each.

Bibliography

Bazan C: Imaging of lumbosacral spine neoplasms. Neuroimaging Clin North Am 1993; 3(3):591–608.

Cohen WA, Hayman LA: Computed tomography of intracranial hemorrhage. Neuroimaging Clin North Am 1992; 2(1):75–87; and Watanabe AT, Mackey JK, Lufkin RB: Imaging diagnosis and temporal appearance of subarachnoid hemorrhage. Neuroimaging Clin North Am 1992; 2(1):53–59.

Masters LT, Zimmerman RD: Imaging of supratentorial brain tumors in adults. Neuroimaging Clin North Am 1993; 3(4):649–669.

Sklar EM, Post JD, Lebwohl NH: Imaging of infection of the lumbosacral spine. Neuroimaging Clin North Am 1993; 3(3):577–590.

Takahashi M, Shimomura O, Sakae T: Comparison of magnetic resonance imaging with myelography and computed tomography-myelography in the diagnosis of lumbar disc herniation. Neuroimaging Clin North Am 1993; 3(3):487–498.

301 Meningitis

Dawn Schissel

Etiology

A. Aseptic
1. Viral
   a. Enteroviruses—Coxsackievirus, echovirus
   b. Adenoviruses
   c. Mumps virus
   d. Epstein-Barr virus
   e. Herpes-simplex virus
2. Fungal—found most commonly in the immuno-compromised
   a. *Candida albicans*
   b. *Coccidioides immitis*
   c. *Cryptococcus neoformans*
3. Tuberculosis
   a. *Mycobacterium tuberculosis*
4. Syphilis

B. Bacterial (in order of prevalence)
1. Neonates
   a. Group B streptococcus
   b. *Escherichia coli*
   c. *Listeria monocytogenes*
2. Infants and toddlers: Highest incidence of meningitis in this age group (3 months to 2 years)
   a. *Haemophilus influenzae*
   b. *Neisseria meningitidis*
   c. *Streptococcus pneumoniae*
3. Older children and adolescents
   a. *S. pneumoniae*
   b. *N. meningitidis*
   c. *H. influenzae*
4. Adults
   a. *S. pneumoniae*
   b. *Listeria monocytogenes*
   c. *N. meningitidis*
   d. *H. influenzae*

Symptoms

1. Headache: sudden onset, severe, frontal
2. Fever: less than 40° C if aseptic; often greater than 40° C if bacterial
3. Photophobia
4. Stiff neck
5. Nausea and vomiting
6. Viral prodrome common in aseptic meningitis
7. Neonates present with decreased feeding, lethargy, increased irritability, and respiratory distress.

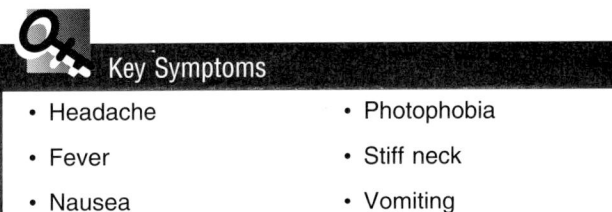

Key Symptoms

- Headache
- Fever
- Nausea
- Photophobia
- Stiff neck
- Vomiting

Clinical Findings

Meningeal signs
1. Nuchal rigidity
2. Kernig's sign: Patient lies supine, flexes knee and hip, and then extends knee. If pain occurs, positive sign.
3. Brudzinski's sign: Patient lies supine, bends neck forward. If knees flex spontaneously, positive sign.
4. Purpura or petechiae
5. Fever, tachycardia
6. Altered sensorium, ranges from confusion to coma
7. Increased white blood cell (WBC) count on complete blood count (CBC) with a predominance of neutrophils and immature cells

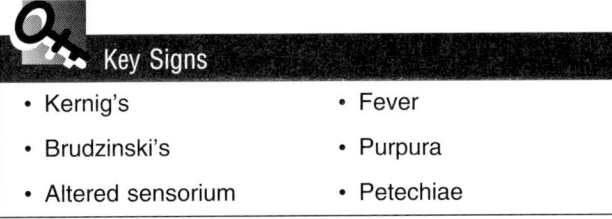

Key Signs

- Kernig's
- Brudzinski's
- Altered sensorium
- Fever
- Purpura
- Petechiae

Laboratory Tests

A. Aseptic
1. Cerebrospinal fluid (CSF) evaluation
   a. No growth on cultures
   b. Negative Gram's stain
   c. Latex agglutinins negative
   d. WBC less than 1000, predominantly mononuclear cells
   e. Protein: normal to slightly elevated
   f. Glucose: normal to slightly decreased
2. Clinical evaluation

B. Bacterial
1. CSF evaluation
   a. Increased opening pressure of more than 180 mm Hg
   b. Decreased glucose: less than 40 mg/dl
   c. Increased protein: greater than 50 mg/dl
   d. WBC count greater than 1000; less than

10,000/mm³, primarily polymorphonuclear cells

e. Gram's stain positive for organisms 70 to 90 per cent of the time.

f. Latex agglutinin studies for *S. pneumoniae, H. influenzae,* and *N. meningitidis* available

2. Blood culture: positive in 50 per cent of cases

3. Clinical evaluation

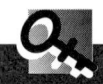

Key Test

• Lumbar puncture for CSF evaluation

Differential Diagnosis

1. Brain abscess: abnormalities seen on CT scan, focal neurologic deficits

2. Subarachnoid hemorrhage: Lumbar puncture is persistently bloody.

3. Epidural abscess: Neurologic deficits are generally focal.

Treatment

A. Aseptic

1. Uncomplicated, mild: Symptomatic treatment with intravenous or oral fluids, pain relief, rest, acetaminophen

2. Severely ill: Treat empirically with intravenous antibiotics.

a. Ceftriaxone (Rocephin) adults, 1 gm every 12 hours; children, 50 mg/kg every 12 hours

b. Cefotaxime (Claforan) adults, 1 gm every 8 hours; children, 50 mg/kg/day in divided doses every 12 hours

c. May add a penicillin, e.g., ampicillin, adults 2 gm every 6 hours; children 100 mg/kg/day in divided doses every 6 hours

3. If unclear, hospitalize and observe for 24 hours. Consider repeat lumbar puncture and watch for WBC shift from polymorphonuclear cells to mononuclear cells.

B. Bacterial

1. Antibiotic treatment (intravenous) must be initiated emergently, and agent must cross the blood-brain barrier. Hospitalize patient.

2. Neonates

a. Ampicillin, 100 to 200 mg/kg/day in divided doses every 6 hours *plus*

b. Gentamicin, 7.5 mg/kg/day every 8 hours, or cefotaxime, 50 to 100 mg/kg/day in divided doses every 12 hours

3. Children and adolescents

a. Ampicillin, 100 to 200 mg/kg/day in divided doses every 6 hours *plus*

b. Third-generation cephalosporin

(1) Cefotaxime, 50 to 100 mg/kg/day in divided doses every 12 hours

(2) Ceftriaxone, 50 mg/kg every 12 hours

4. Adults

a. Ampicillin, 2 gm every 6 hours *plus*

b. Third-generation cephalosporin

(1) Cefotaxime, 1 gm every 8 hours

(2) Ceftriaxone, 1 gm every 12 hours

(3) If *Pseudomonas* is suspected, ceftazidime, 1.5 gram every 8 hours

5. Treatment consists of intravenous antibiotics for 10 to 14 days unless pathogen is a gram-negative bacillus, then intravenous therapy is 21 days in duration.

6. Repeat lumbar puncture is not necessary if patient is responding clinically to therapy.

7. Intravenous fluids should be limited in neonates and children to no more than two-thirds maintenance to decrease risk of cerebral edema.

C. Tuberculosis

1. Isoniazid, 15 to 20 mg/kg/day (maximum 500 mg/day) in children and 8 to 10 mg/kg/day (maximum 300 mg/day) in once- or twice-daily doses

2. Rifampin, 15 to 20 mg/kg/day (maximum 600 mg/day) in adults or children in once- or twice-daily doses

Key Treatment

• Ampicillin

• Third-generation cephalosporin

• Acetaminophen

Follow-Up

1. Adults need no follow-up, because permanent neurologic sequelae are rare when meningitis is treated promptly.

2. Children should have hearing tested when treatment is complete and clinical picture has normalized.

Bibliography

Bradley JS: Meningitis. Hosp Pract 1993;28(suppl 2):15–19.

Choi C: Bacterial meningitis. Clin Geriatr Med 1992;8:889–902.

Feigin R, McCracken G, Klein J: Diagnosis and management of meningitis. Pediatr Infect Dis J 1992;11:785–814.

Lefrock JL, Shapiro ED, Wenger J: Meningitis: Find it early, treat it fast. Patient Care December 15, 1991;25:133–163.

Polito JM, Stollerman GH: Aseptic meningitis: A case for clinical experience. Hosp Pract May 30, 1992;27:27–39.

Indications

1. Central nervous system (CNS) infection
   a. Bacterial meningitis (characterized by fever, headache, and stiff neck): lumbar puncture (LP) is essential to diagnosis.
   b. Consider fungal, syphilitic, tuberculosis, viral, and aseptic meningitis as diagnostic possibilities too.
   c. LP is less sensitive in detecting ventriculoperitoneal shunt infections.
2. Subarachnoid hemorrhage (SAH)
   a. LP is the most sensitive diagnostic tool to diagnose SAH.
   b. If feasible, do computed tomography (CT) first; LP not indicated if SAH is diagnosed on CT.
3. Carcinomatous meningitis: especially with lymphoma, leukemia, melanoma, and breast and lung cancer
4. Various inflammatory conditions: multiple sclerosis, Guillain-Barré syndrome
5. Miscellaneous conditions (the LP may be therapeutic as well as diagnostic): pseudo-tumor cerebri, normal-pressure hydrocephalus
6. Introduction of diagnostic and therapeutic substances: contrast media, antibiotics, anesthetics, chemotherapy, radionuclides.

Contraindications

1. Evidence of increased intracranial pressure (ICP) from mass lesions such as neoplasm, abscess, or parenchymal hemorrhage. Consider raised ICP if
   a. Papilledema is present.
   b. Focal neurologic signs are detected.
   c. Computed tomography or magnetic resonance imaging (MRI) findings suggest raised ICP.

2. Infection in skin or other tissue overlying the anticipated lumbar puncture site
3. Anticoagulated state
   a. Bleeding diathesis (e.g., prolonged prothrombin time)
   b. Thrombocytopenia (e.g., platelets less than 50,000)

Preparation

1. Explain procedure fully to patient and/or family.
2. Obtain signed informed consent.
3. A full-length examination table (preferred), firm flat bed or stretcher, well-lighted room

Equipment

1. Antiseptic solutions, such as povidone-iodine, alcohol
2. Sterile drapes, gloves, gauze, Band-Aid.
3. 20- to 22-gauge spinal needle with stylet
4. Manometer, three-way stopcock, four labeled collection tubes

Anesthesia

1. 3- to 5-cc syringe with 22- to 25-gauge long needle
2. 1 to 3 cc plain lidocaine, 1% to 2%

Precautions

1. Computed tomography or magnetic resonance imaging before LP unless bacterial meningitis is strongly suspected, because delay in this diagnosis substantially increases morbidity and mortality
2. Reverse anticoagulation at least 1 hour before LP

Technique

1. Patient position
   a. Lateral recumbent position on a firm mattress or examination table is preferred.
      (1) Neck, trunk, hips, and knees are flexed, but avoid respiratory embarrassment.
      (2) Axis of spine is parallel to the floor, but hips and shoulders are perpendicular to the bed or table.
   b. Patient sitting curled forward initially may help locate landmarks in an obese patient or infant.
2. Select puncture site low enough to avoid puncturing spinal cord (cord ends at L1–L2).
   a. Palpate superior aspects of iliac crests; an imaginary line between these two points selects the appropriate lumbar interspace in adults (L3–L4, L4–L5).

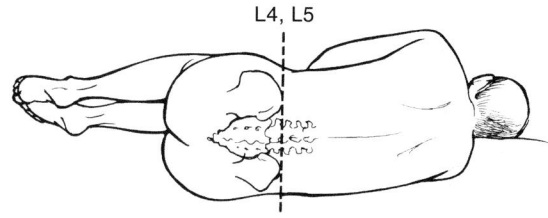

   b. Use lower interspaces in infants, since their spinal cord ends at L3.

3. Prepare puncture site.

   a. Glove, cleanse area with povidone-iodine, wipe with alcohol, and then place sterile drapes.

   b. Reglove to avoid iodine contamination of LP needle.

4. Anesthetize interspace subcutaneously and into deeper tissues with lidocaine.

5. Needle insertion

   a. Insert the needle with stylet in place in midpoint of selected interspace.

   b. Direct needle 10 to 20 degrees cephalad, that is, toward umbilicus; bevel parallel to the long axis of the spine to separate, not transect, dural fibers and nerve roots.

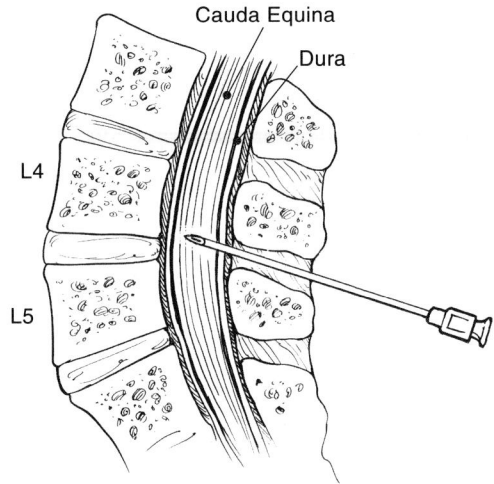

Cauda Equina

Dura

L4

L5

   c. Withdraw stylet after penetrating the dura, characterized by a pop. Check for spinal fluid.

     (1) If no pop is felt or needle has been advanced 3 to 6 cm without fluid, the stylet should be removed and replaced every 2 to 3 mm as the needle continues to slowly advance.

     (2) If the tap is dry, rotate needle 90 to 180 degrees.

     (3) If hard resistance is met, check to ensure midline interspace position. Withdraw needle with stylet and either redirect needle angle or restart procedure.

     (4) Very obese or spondylotic patients may be done under fluoroscopy via paramedian approach by experienced clinicians only.

     (5) Lateral C1 to C2 or cisterna magna puncture may be required if the LP is unsuccessful or the lumbar area is infected.

6. Cerebrospinal fluid (CSF) pressure measurement and sample collection

   a. Replace the stylet until the manometer or three-way stopcock is attached.

   b. Extend neck and legs, thereby preventing an artificially raised opening pressure.

   c. Open the stopcock to the manometer, and record the opening pressure (normal <200 mm H₂O).

   d. Close the stopcock to the manometer, and collect 1 to 2 cc of CSF in each of four labeled tubes.

7. Withdrawing LP needle

   a. Replace the stylet, and withdraw slowly to avoid aspiration of nerve roots.

   b. Apply a Band-Aid to the puncture site.

Follow-Up

1. Have the patient lie supine for 2 to 3 hours after procedure to avert a spinal headache.

2. Order CSF studies

   a. Obtain a cell count (see Table 301–1) and differential (perform on first and fourth collection tubes if a traumatic tap is suspected), Gram's stain, bacterial cultures, and CSF and serum glucose.

TABLE 301–1. TYPICAL CEREBRAL SPINAL FLUID (CSF) CHARACTERISTICS IN VARIOUS DIAGNOSES*

Condition	Appearance	Pressure	Glucose (mg/dl)	Protein (mg/dl)	Cell Count (per mm³)
Normal	Clear Colorless	Normal <200 mm H₂O	60–70% of peripheral glucose	15–45 mg/dl	≤5 leukocytes/mm³ (mononuclear)
Meningitis					
Bacterial	Cloudy	↑	↓	↑	↑ 500–10,000, neutrophils predominate
Tuberculosis, fungal	Clear, maybe cloudy	↑	N or ↓	↑	predominate
Viral/asceptic	Clear	N or ↑	N	Slightly ↑ N or ↑	↑ 10–500, lymphocytes predominate >6, lymphocytes predominate
Other Conditions					
Meningeal carcinomatosis	Clear	↑	N or ↓	N or ↑	10–500, lymphocytes predominate
Subarachnoid hemorrhage (SAH)	Bloody, does not clot, xanthochromic supernatant	↑	N	↑	1000–3.5 × 10⁶ RBCs, RBC:WBC ratio higher than ratio in peripheral blood
Traumatic tap	Blood clots, supernatant is not xanthochromic	N	N	↑	No. of RBC in CSF = no. of RBCs in peripheral blood; fewer RBCs in collection tube 4 than in tube 1
Multiple sclerosis	Clear	N	N	N or ↑	0–20 lymph
Guillain-Barré syndrome	Clear or xanthochromic	N or ↑	N	↑↑	N
Pseudotumor cerebri	Clear	↑	N	N	N

*↑ = increase; ↓ = decrease; N = normal.

303 Meniere's Disease

Stephen L. Nelson

Etiology

Pathophysiologically, patients demonstrate hydrops of the membranous labyrinth of the inner ear, which damages the delicate vestibular and cochlear hair cells. The cause of this excess fluid and pressure, however, is unknown. Approximately one third of cases have an allergic factor that responds to treatment. Other postulated causes include metabolic disorders, vascular anomalies, viral and syphilitic infections, and trauma.

Symptoms

1. Spontaneous, intermittent attacks of vertigo, tinnitus, low-frequency hearing loss, and ear fullness
2. Severe whirling vertigo with associated nausea and vomiting lasting 15 minutes to several hours (up to 24 hours) with long periods of remission (weeks to months or years)
3. Tinnitus is low pitched, and although continuous, it fluctuates in intensity (often worsens preceding an attack).
4. Hearing loss often persists during remission, although auditory symptoms fluctuate (worsens preceding an attack).
5. Recruitment of loudness (an abnormally rapid increase in loudness in the affected ear causing sudden loud noises to be painful)
6. Other vagal symptoms may appear (abdominal pain, bradycardia, pallor, sweating).
7. Usually unilateral (~70 per cent): Bilateral involvement often indicates allergic or metabolic cause.
8. Onset usually occurs at age 20 to 50+ (especially in fifth decade), but it can happen at any age.

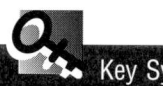
Key Symptom

- Intermittent attacks of severe vertigo, tinnitus, low-frequency hearing loss, and ear fullness

Clinical Findings

1. Nystagmus during "attacks"
2. Diplacusis (perception of a single auditory stimulus as two separate sounds, resulting in poor speech discrimination)
3. Weber test: lateralizes to unaffected ear
4. Rinne test: air conduction >bone conduction (normal pattern prevails)

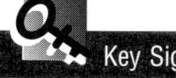
Key Sign

- Nystagmus (horizontal) and diplacusis

Laboratory Tests

1. Thyroid studies, syphilis serology, and lipid studies to rule out thyroid disease, syphilis, and hyperlipidemia, respectively
2. Impedance audiometry demonstrates recruitment of loudness (i.e., an abnormally rapid increase in loudness in the affected ear indicating end organ or cochlear pathology).
3. Audiogram shows low-frequency sensorineural hearing loss (may progress to include all tones and may become total).
4. Electronystagmography (ENG): caloric testing hypoactive
5. Auditory brain stem response (ABR): separates cochlear from retrocochlear (as in acoustic neuroma)
6. Magnetic resonance imaging (MRI) if ABR does not rule out acoustic neuroma

Key Tests

- Impedance audiometry
- Audiogram
- ABR
- MRI (if necessary)

Differential Diagnosis

1. Allergic cause is treatable in one third of cases, especially if bilateral
2. Hypo/hyperthyroidism
3. Hyperlipidemia
4. Viral labyrinthitis
5. Benign positional vertigo
6. Acoustic neuroma
7. Syphylitic vertigo
8. Labyrinthine fistula
9. Vestibular granuloma
10. Temporal bone fracture
11. Multiple sclerosis

Treatment

Medical except in about 10 per cent who have severe refractory vertigo and require surgery

Medication

Divided into acute and maintenance therapy

1. Drugs of choice
   a. *Acute*
      (1) Atropine, 0.2 to 0.4 mg intravenously
      (2) Diazepam (Valium) 5 mg intravenous (slow push); may repeat as needed

(3) Meclizine (Antivert), 25 to 100 mg daily or in divided doses

(4) Scopolamine patch (Transderm-Scōp)

  b. *Maintenance*

(1) Meclizine, 12.5 to 25 mg t.i.d. or q.i.d.

(2) Diazepam, 1 to 2 mg b.i.d. or q.i.d.

(3) Thiazide diuretics (25 to 50 mg hydrochlorothiazide per day) in conjunction with low-salt diet (70 per cent effective according to some sources)

2. Alternative drugs

  a. *Acute*

(1) Dimenhydrinate (Dramamine), 50 mg intramuscularly or slow intravenous q 4–6 hr

(2) Promethazine (Phenergan), 25 to 50 mg intramuscularly or intravenously q 4–6 hr

(3) Cyclizine (Marezine), 50 mg orally q 4–6 hr

(4) Diphenhydramine (Benadryl), 25 to 50 mg intravenously

  b. *Maintenance*

(1) Promethazine, 25 mg orally q 4–6 hr

(2) Diphenhydramine, 25 mg orally q 4–6 hr

Surgical

The surgical procedure may be endolymphatic sac shunt (60 per cent cure) or vestibular nerve section (99 per cent cure: used especially in cases of total hearing loss) if medical treatment fails.

Diet

Low-salt diet is recommended but has been of unproven value.

Activity

Strict bed rest is advised during attacks; otherwise there are no restrictions.

Patient Education

1. Avoid ototoxic drugs.
2. Avoid significant noise exposure.
3. Over time the vertigo improves, but the hearing loss worsens.

Follow-Up

Initially follow-up is frequent for patient education; then it is carried out as needed to monitor the course of the disease and to evaluate for progressive hearing loss.

 Bibliography

Baloh RW: Approach to the dizzy patient. Baillieres' Clinical Neurology 1994;3:453–465.

DeWeese DD, Saunders WH: Textbook of Otolaryngology, 6th ed. St. Louis, CV Mosby, 1982, pp 401–405.

Gantz, Bruce J. and Moore, Dennis M.: Differential Diagnosis and Management of the Dizzy Patient. *In* American Academy of Otolaryngology - Head and Neck Surgery Foundation: Common Problems of the Head and Neck, 1993. Philadelphia, WB Saunders, 1993, pp 204–205.

Paparella MM: Pathogenesis and pathophysiology of Meniere's disease. Acta Otolaryngol (Supplement) 1991;485:26–35.

Ruckenstein MJ, Rutka JA, Hawke M: The treatment of Meniere's disease: Torok revisited. Laryngoscope 1991; 101:211–218.

304 Guillain-Barré Syndrome

Kishore J. Harjai

Etiology

1. Guillain-Barré syndrome (GBS) is an acute, inflammatory polyradiculoneuropathy, characterized primarily by symmetrically progressive muscle weakness and areflexia. The first clear description was offered in 1916 by Guillain, Barré, and Strohl.

2. Epidemiology

   a. With the virtual elimination of poliomyelitis, GBS has become the most common cause of acute generalized paralysis in developed countries, with average annual incidence rates varying from 0.4 to 1.7 per 100,000 population.

   b. While estimates vary, it is thought to be more common in women than in men.

   c. It occurs at all ages, with a minor peak frequency in young adults and a second, larger one in the fifth through eighth decades of life. Overall, it is more common in older than in younger people.

   d. Seasonal difference in incidence has been reported, but is not universally accepted.

3. Causes

   a. The exact cause of GBS is unknown, but it is thought to be due to a cell-mediated immunologic reaction directed at peripheral nerve.

   b. Precipitating factors include

      (1) Infection: Antecedent respiratory or gastrointestinal (GI) infection is reported to occur in 60 per cent of patients in the four weeks preceding the onset of symptoms of GBS; viral (*Cytomegalovirus,* Epstein-Barr, herpesviruses simplex and zoster, influenza A, measles, mumps, rubella, adenovirus, ECHO, Coxsackie, hepatitis B, HIV) and bacterial (*Mycoplasma, H. pylori, B. burgdorferi*) infections have been associated with the onset of GBS.

      (2) Surgery (in 5 to 10 per cent of patients with GBS) and use of spinal or epidural anesthesia

      (3) Vaccines (antirabies vaccines containing central nervous system tissue, and possibly, swine influenza and oral polio vaccines)

   c. Incidence is increased in lymphoma (Hodgkin and non-Hodgkin), pregnancy, postpartum period, and systemic lupus erythematosus.

Symptoms

1. Paresthesias and weakness: onset is usually acute, with paresthesias in the fingertips and toes. Weakness typically starts in the legs, and progresses to the arms, face, and oropharynx in a few days. Symptoms plateau in 2 to 3 weeks, and then improve in a few weeks.

2. Pain in the lower extremities, flank, or back.

3. Onset may be subacute, simulating chronic inflammatory demyelinating polyneuropathy (CIDP). Some patients may have a "stuttering" course with a series of stages of progression and plateau.

Key Symptoms

- Ascending weakness
- Pain
- Distal paresthesias
- Antecedent infection/ illnesses

Clinical Findings

1. Symmetric weakness, initially in the legs, progressing to involve the upper extremities

2. Areflexia or hyporeflexia

3. Minimal objective sensory loss

4. Respiratory failure occurs in 30 per cent

5. Autonomic dysfunction (disturbances of heart rate, blood pressure, or sweating; cardiac arrhythmias, abnormal hemodynamic responses to drugs, pupillary dysfunction, gastrointestinal dysfunction, urinary retention, flushing) is seen in 65 per cent of all patients with GBS.

6. Variant presentations (in up to 15 per cent of cases)

   a. Fisher's syndrome: ophthalmoplegia, ataxia, and areflexia, with little weakness; most common variant; accounts for about 5 per cent of all cases

   b. Pure motor weakness without any sensory disturbances

   c. Isolated weakness of the arm and oropharynx, or of the leg

   d. Bilateral facial weakness with distal paresthesias

   e. Severe ataxia and sensory loss

   f. Acute pandysautonomia: an autonomic neuropathy often combined with sensory features

   g. "Axonal" GBS: rapid, almost complete paralysis, with electrically inexcitable motor nerves

Key Signs

- Progressive symmetric weakness in both arms and both legs
- Minimal sensory signs
- Autonomic dysfunction
- Decreased/absent reflexes
- Cranial nerve involvement, especially bilateral facial weakness
- Respiratory failure

Laboratory Tests

1. Nerve conduction studies: Evidence of demyelination is the most sensitive and specific laboratory finding in GBS, and occurs earlier and more frequently than elevation of cerebrospinal fluid (CSF) protein. Early demyelination is seen as a reduction in the amplitude of the muscle action potential after stimulation of the distal as compared with the proximal nerve. Abnormal late responses that indicate abnormalities in proximal nerves or roots may be seen.

2. CSF analysis

   a. Increase in protein concentration >0.55 gm per liter occurs after the first week, peaking at 4 to 6 weeks; a protein concentration above 2.5 gm per liter should make one suspect spinal cord compression.

   b. Few or no cells in CSF (<10 cells per cubic millimeter)

   c. Normal opening pressure

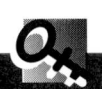

Key Tests

- Nerve conduction studies
- CSF analysis

Differential Diagnosis

1. Poliomyelitis: purely motor, asymmetric, areflexic paralysis; epidemic occurrence

2. Acute myelopathy: sensorimotor paralysis below affected level; sphincter paralysis

3. "Locked-in" syndrome: secondary to basilar artery thrombosis or embolism; preserved tendon reflexes; Babinski sign; abnormal pupillary reflexes

4. Acute myasthenia gravis: no sensory symptoms; tendon reflexes preserved

5. Botulism: consistent bradycardia; early loss of pupillary reflexes

6. Tick paralysis: no sensory loss; normal CSF protein

Treatment

1. Early hospitalization and good ancillary care

2. Respiratory care

   a. Ventilatory muscle weakness is suggested by increased respiratory rate, decreased tidal volume, and paradoxic inward movement of the abdomen during inspiration. Abnormalities of arterial blood gases (i.e., hypoxia, hypercarbia, and acidosis) occur late. Risk for ventilatory insufficiency is high in patients with an inspiratory force <20 cm H_2O and vital capacity <15 ml/kg.

   b. Assess strength of cough and ability to maintain airway patency.

   c. Endotracheal intubation and mechanical ventilation: Perform early in patients with deteriorating respiratory function to minimize pulmonary complications. Synchronized intermittent mandatory ventilation or pressure support ventilation may be used. Endotracheal intubation alone may be necessary to protect the airways, clear them, or institute continuous positive airway pressure.

   d. Early tracheostomy: generally desirable, especially in patients who have severe GBS with evidence of axonal involvement together with ventilatory failure and dysautonomia.

3. Cardiovascular care

   a. Continuous electrocardiographic and blood pressure monitoring: for all patients admitted to the ICU

   b. Temporary pacing: for patients with complete heart block or symptomatic bradycardias

   c. Pulmonary artery catheterization: for hemodynamic monitoring and to guide fluid therapy

4. General measures

   a. Maintain joint mobility: physiotherapy, occupational therapy

   b. Prophylaxis against deep venous thrombosis

   c. Chest physiotherapy for bedridden patients

   d. Routine cultures of urine and tracheal secretions in ICU patients

   e. Skin care to prevent decubitus ulcer and eye care in patients with facial weakness to prevent corneal ulceration

   f. Maintenance of adequate nutrition: Enteral feeding is preferred but may be precluded by delayed gastric emptying, ileus, or diarrhea. Institute parenteral nutrition, if indicated.

   g. Care of tracheostomy, if present

   h. Psychosocial support

   i. Pain management: using nonsteroidal anti-inflammatory agents, antidepressants (for paresthetic pain), or narcotic analgesics

5. Medical management

   a. Early plasmapheresis (250 ml/kg of plasma removed in four to six sessions), used in patients with severe GBS, shortens hospital stay, duration of assisted ventilation, and time to achieve independent walking. As replacement fluid, albumin is as effective as fresh frozen plasma. Due to high cost and incidence of adverse effects, and lack of data in mild cases, this modality should be reserved for patients who are unable to walk or who are rapidly worsening.

   b. Intravenous immune globulin (400 mg/kg/day for 5 consecutive days) given in the first 2 weeks of the disease was found to be as effective as plasmapheresis in a large multicenter trial. If these results are duplicated in other trials, intravenous immune globulin may be preferred over plasmapheresis, because it is easy to administer, easily available, and without the risks of extracorporeal circulation.

   c. The use of steroids is not beneficial and currently lacks justification.

6. Management of complications: nosocomial infections, hypotension, cardiac arrhythmias

Key Treatment

- Plasmapheresis or intravenous immune globulin
- Respiratory care
- Good nursing and ancillary care
- Maintain hemodynamic stability
- Psychologic support

Prognosis

1. Mortality: 3 per cent; due to cardiac arrest, adult respiratory distress syndrome, pulmonary embolism and infections
2. Residual disability: severe in 10 per cent; mild or none in the rest
3. Recurrences of acute neuropathy or development of chronic neuropathy in 3 per cent
4. Poor prognosis indicated by old age, need for assisted ventilation, and electromyogram findings of severely reduced amplitudes of muscle action potential and widespread denervation. Early plasmapheresis shortens the time to achieve independent walking and the time a patient stays on a ventilator.

Follow-Up

1. Continued psychosocial support and patient education: The Guillain-Barré Syndrome Foundation International is an excellent source.
2. Continued physiotherapy and occupational therapy, if indicated

 Bibliography

Alter M: The epidemiology of Guillain-Barré syndrome. Ann Neurol 1990;27(suppl):S7–S12.

Guillain-Barré Syndrome. *In* Adams RD, Victor M (eds): Principles of Neurology, 5th ed. New York, McGraw-Hill, 1993, pp 1126–1130.

Hund EF, Borel CO, Cornblath DR, Haley DF, et al: Intensive management and treatment of severe Guillain-Barré syndrome. Crit Care Med 1993;21:433–446.

Ropper AH: The Guillain-Barré syndrome. N Engl J Med 1992; 326:1130–1136.

Tenorio G, Ashkenasi A, Benton JW: Guillain-Barré syndrome. *In* Scheld WM, Whitley RJ, Durack DT (eds): Infections of the Central Nervous System. New York, Raven Press, 1991, pp 259–282.

305 Head Injuries in Sports

Aaron Rubin

Etiology

Most commonly caused by a forceful blow to the head.

1. Head injuries are common injuries in contact sports such as football, hockey, rugby, soccer, boxing, and wrestling, as well as "noncontact" sports such as basketball, baseball, cycling, auto racing, motocross, and gymnastics. Head injuries include minor head injuries (concussions), severe head injuries, and second-impact syndrome (SIS).

   a. It has been estimated that up to 20 per cent of high school football players (over 250,000) suffer a concussion in a given year.

   b. Severe head injuries include cerebral contusion, intracranial hemorrhage, epidural hematoma, and subdural hematoma. These are fortunately rare in sports. Most severe head injuries are readily recognizable by immediate and prolonged (greater than 5 minutes) loss of consciousness (LOC).

   c. Second-impact syndrome (SIS) is rapid development of diffuse brain swelling and herniation following a second head injury. These may be seemingly minor injuries but with devastating consequences. The National Center for Catastrophic Sports Injury Research in Chapel Hill, North Carolina, identified 51 cases of head injury death between 1980 and 1991. Of these, 29 appear to be due to SIS.

2. Biomechanical forces and mechanism of head injury

   a. Blow to resting movable head usually produces maximal injury beneath the point of impact (coup injury).

   b. Moving head contacting a nonmobile object results in maximal injury to opposite side of brain injury (contrecoup injury).

   c. Epidural hematoma commonly occurs with a temporal skull fracture tearing the middle meningeal artery. The patient may have a lucid interval after the injury until the hematoma expands, leading to mass effect and eventual brain herniation. The underlying brain is generally not significantly injured, and rapid evaluation and treatment have good results.

   d. Acute subdural hematoma is often associated with a higher degree of brain damage and swelling and a poor prognosis even with rapid evaluation and treatment.

   e. Intracerebral hematoma is associated with severe acceleration injury with prolonged LOC. Mortality varies depending on the location of the lesion and level of consciousness at the time of presentation.

   f. Subarachnoid hemorrhage results from rupture of a congenital vascular lesion like an aneurysm or arteriovenous malformation that may occur in conjunction with trauma.

   g. SIS is probably due to lack of autoregulation of the brain leading to vascular engorgement and edema of the brain with herniation and coma. *This is a major reason for careful evaluation of the head-injured athlete and caution with return to play.*

   h. Minor head injuries (concussions) are by far the most common of head injuries. There are various grading systems for concussions (Table 305–1). Concussion has been defined by the Congress of Neurological Surgeons as "an immediate and transient impairment of neural function such as alteration of consciousness, disturbance of vision, equilibrium, and other similar symptoms."

Symptoms

1. Loss of consciousness (LOC) and headache are the primary signs of head injury. Serious head injury is usually associated with LOC.

2. Symptoms include headache, dizziness, difficulty concentrating, amnesia (posttraumatic as well as retrograde), irritability, confusion, hyperexcitability, and LOC.

3. Concussion may have mild symptoms and at times may only be noted with careful neuropsychiatric testing. Even mild concussion may impair attention and information processing.

4. Postconcussion syndrome may follow mild head injury.

   a. Common symptoms (reported in greater than 20 per cent): headache (muscle contraction, migraine, cluster), dizziness, fatigue, nonspecific psychological symptoms (irritability, anxiety, depression), mild memory loss, difficulty concentrating

   b. Less common (1 to 20 per cent): benign, positional vertigo, hearing loss, anosmia, photophobia, sleep disturbance, hyperacusis

TABLE 305–1. GRADING SYSTEMS FOR CONCUSSION

GRADE	CANTU (1986)	COLORADO (1991)
1	No LOC, dazed, HA, post-traumatic amnesia <30 min	No LOC, confusion without amnesia
2	LOC <5 min or post-traumatic amnesia >30 min	No LOC, dazed, confusion with amnesia
3	LOC > 5 min or post-traumatic amnesia >24 hours	LOC (any period of time)

LOC, loss of consciousness; HA, headache.

c. Rare problems (less than 1 per cent): delayed subdural and epidural hematoma, seizure disorder, transient global amnesia, movement disorder, Parkinson's disease, torticollis.

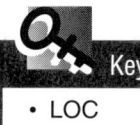

Key Symptoms

- LOC
- Headache
- Amnesia
- Difficulty concentrating
- Dizziness
- Irritability
- Confusion

Clinical Findings

1. Evaluation of airway, breathing, and circulation (ABCs) and the cervical spine is performed initially.
2. Initial evaluation should include an estimate of the Glasgow coma scale (Table 305–2) or the AVPU system (alert, responds to verbal, responds to pain, unresponsive)
3. History of mechanism of injury, complaints of headache, tinnitus, blurred vision, nausea, unsteadiness, problems concentrating, or emotional lability should be obtained as well as history of previous head injury.
4. Neurologic examination should be performed, including pupillary response, Romberg's test, heel-to-toe gait, finger to nose, extraocular motion, concentration (digits repeated backward, months in reverse order), memory (details of injury, previous games, president, governor).
5. History and examination should be repeated 5, 10, and 20 minutes after injury. Before return to play, examination should be repeated with provocative maneuvers such as a short sprint, push-ups, and sit-ups. Symptoms or neurologic findings should prevent return to play.

Key Signs

- Memory loss
- Inability to concentrate
- Gait disturbance
- Abnormal Glasgow score
- Abnormal pupillary response

Laboratory Tests

1. Radiographs are generally not considered helpful in mild head injuries. They do not predict intracranial trauma. They should be used in suspected cases of skull fracture.
2. Computed tomography (CT) is helpful in diagnosing intracranial pathology. This should generally be reserved for patients with Glasgow coma scale less than 15, abnormal mental status, or focal neurologic deficits.
3. Magnetic resonance imaging (MRI) is more sensitive than CT but is more expensive, less available, and not been found to affect clinical outcome. MRI is better at finding contusions, providing some information on diffuse axonal injury, and possibly predicting delayed traumatic intracerebral hematoma, but not in influencing surgical intervention over CT.
4. Electroencephalography (EEG) has limited sensitivity and specificity in minor head injuries but may be helpful when a post-traumatic seizure disorder is suspected.
5. Auditory brain stem response (ABR) may be abnormal after mild head injury. Again, the clinical usefulness is uncertain.
6. Neuropsychiatric testing is helpful in evaluating and following individuals with head injury.

Key Tests

- CT scan
- MRI

Differential Diagnosis

1. In the comatose individual: subdural hematoma, epidural hematoma, subarachnoid bleed, intracerebral hematoma, drug or alcohol overdose, and metabolic disease
2. Minor head injuries and postconcussion syndrome: migraines, psychiatric disorder, drug and alcohol abuse, and underlying learning disorders

Treatment

1. Planning for the evaluation and care of the seriously head-injured athlete should occur prior to the event. An emergency plan should be in place for all athletic practices and games.

TABLE 305–2. GLASGOW COMA SCALE*

I. Best Motor Response		II. Verbal Response		III. Eye Opening	
Obeys	6	Oriented	5	Spontaneous	4
Localizes	5	Confused conversation	4	To speech	3
Withdraws from pain (flexion)	4	Inappropriate words	3	To pain	2
Abnormal flexion	3	Incomprehensible sounds	2	None	1
Abnormal extension (decerebrate posturing)	2	None	1		
None	1				

*I + II + III = coma score: 13–15 (minor), 9–13 (moderate), less than 8 (coma), 5–8 (severe).

a. Initial assessment of the head-injured athlete should be performed by a certified athletic trainer or the team physician. All coaches and other supervisors should be made aware of the seriousness of head injury for events when the athletic trainer or physician is not available.

b. Cervical spine injury should be assumed in any unconscious athlete. Initial assessment should be performed without moving the athlete. As always, *airway, breathing, and circulation* (ABCs) should be addressed. The athlete should be carefully moved to his or her back with control of the cervical spine only by appropriately trained persons. Removing a football helmet is not recommended due to unnecessary movement of the C-spine and problems managing the C-spine in a player with shoulder pads. Face mask should be removed by cutting the attachments with an instrument designed to do such. This should be practiced by all appropriate personnel. Airway should be maintained by jaw thrust and oxygen given to all comatose individuals. The athlete should be placed on a spine board and the C-spine stabilized for transport to the nearest neurosurgical emergency facility.

c. Intubation should be considered in the comatose athlete with hyperventilation to decrease the P_{CO_2}. Blood pressure should be maintained near normal. Hypotonic intravenous fluids should be avoided. There have not been satisfactory studies to support the routine use of corticosteroids in management of closed head injury.

d. Evaluation of the C-spine and further evaluation of coma should be carried out at the neurosurgical facility.

2. Sideline management of minor head injury also should be planned.

a. The athlete who is conscious and without neck pain or tenderness may be removed from the playing field for evaluation on the sidelines or in the locker room. Worsening symptoms or examination may require initiation of the emergency action plan.

b. The athlete should remain under observation with repeat examinations at regular intervals every 5 to 10 minutes.

c. If the athlete is agitated, he or she should be moved to a quiet place with rapid access to the medical team. If any concern about the degree of injury is present, the athlete should be transported to the emergency room for further observation.

d. If the player does remain on the sideline, care should be taken to prevent his or her premature return to the contest. This may occur as a result of the athlete's denial about the potential seriousness of the injury, confusion due to the injury, or in the "heat of the battle."

e. If the athlete is allowed to return home, a responsible adult should be instructed in the care of the athlete with written instructions.

3. Treatment of postconcussion syndrome is often in the realm of family physicians.

a. Recognition of the preceding symptoms is the first step. Patients with symptoms of fatigue, headache, tinnitus, problems concentrating, and the like should be questioned about previous head injuries.

b. Postconcussion headaches have been treated with amitriptyline, nonsteroidal anti-inflammatory drugs, muscle relaxants, propranolol, calcium channel blockers, as well as transcutaneous electrical nerve stimulation (TENS) and biofeedback.

c. Teachers should be made aware of possible learning difficulties, problems with concentration and focus, and emotional lability that may occur after a minor head injury.

d. Family should be counseled about the problem and its treatment and prognosis.

Key Treatment

- Basic life support with cervical spine caution
- Oxygen
- Intubation with hyperventilation
- Transport to neurosurgical emergency hospital

TABLE 305-3. RETURN TO PLAY BASED ON COMMON GRADING SYSTEMS

GRADE	CANTU (1986)	COLORADO (1991)
1	Asymptomatic for 1 week 2nd—may return in 2 weeks if asymptomatic for 1 week 3rd—terminate season	May return after 20 minutes if asymptomatic, CT/MRI* 2nd in same contest—remove 3rd—terminate season (at least 3 months off)
2	Asymptomatic for 1 week 2nd—minimum of 1 month; may return if asymptomatic for 1 week, consider terminating season 3rd—terminate season	Asymptomatic for 1 week, CT/MRI* 2nd—1 month off 3rd—terminate season
3	Minimum of 1 month; may return then if asymptomatic for 1 week 2nd—terminate season	Minimum of 1 month if asymptomatic for at least 2 weeks; conditioning drills may resume if asymptomatic after 2 weeks, CT/MRI

*Consider CT or MRI if symptoms persist longer than 1 week.

Follow-Up

1. Follow-up should continue until symptoms have resolved. Do not forget about postconcussion syndrome and the potentially long course it may take.
2. Return-to-play issues are difficult. Two guidelines are provided (Table 305–3). These are only guidelines, and all have limitations. Many athletes with mild head injury have limited or no symptoms. The goal of limiting return to play is to avoid the disaster of the second-impact syndrome and morbidity due to repeated head injury.

Bibliography

Cantu RC: Cerebral concussion in sport. Sports Med 1992; 14(11):64–74.

Colorado Medical Society: Guidelines for the Management of Concussion in Sports. 1990 (revised 1991). P.O. Box 17550, Denver, CO 80217-0550; phone: (303) 779-5455.

Evans RW: The postconcussion syndrome and the sequelae of mild head injury. Neurol Clin 1992;10(4):815–845.

Henderson JM, Browning DG: Head trauma in young athletes. Med Clin North Am 1994;78(2):289–303.

Lehman LB, Ravich SJ: Closed head injuries in athletes. Clin Sports Med 1990;9(2):247–261.

306 Postconcussion Syndrome

Randolph W. Evans

Etiology

1. Definition: a constellation of symptoms and signs that may occur alone or in combination following usually mild head injury. Loss of consciousness does not have to occur for the postconcussion syndrome to develop. Mild head injury is defined as an injury resulting in an initial Glasgow coma scale score of 13 to 15.

2. Epidemiology
   a. The annual incidence of mild head injury per 100,000 population is about 150.
   b. Mild head injury accounts for about 75 per cent of all head trauma.
   c. Estimates of the relative causes of head trauma in the United States are as follows: motor vehicle accidents, 45 per cent; falls, 30 per cent; occupational accidents, 10 per cent; recreational accidents, 10 per cent; and assaults, 5 per cent.
   d. Perhaps 50 per cent of patients with mild head injury will develop the postconcussion syndrome.

3. Neuropathology
   a. Damage to the scalp, skull, and meninges can lead to scalp lacerations, skull fractures, and subdural and epidural hematomas.
   b. Damage to brain parenchyma by coup and contrecoup injuries can lead to brain contusions, lacerations, and hemorrhages.
   c. Diffuse axonal injury may account for many aspects of the postconcussion syndrome.
   d. A neurochemical substrate of mild head injury may consist of release of excitatory neurotransmitters such as acetylcholine and glutamate.

Symptoms

1. A multitude of symptoms and signs can follow mild head injury (Table 306–1).

2. Headaches have been variably reported as occurring in 30 to 90 per cent of patients who are symptomatic. The most common type is muscle-contraction headaches often associated with greater occipital neuralgia. This headache type also can be due to neck and temporomandibular joint injuries. Much less often, migraine and, rarely, cluster-type headaches may develop after mild head injury.

3. Dizziness is reported by 53 per cent of patients within 1 week of the injury. The different causes include labyrinthine concussion, benign positional vertigo, and rarely a perilymph fistula. Occasionally, sensorineural hearing loss and tinnitus can result.

4. Fourteen per cent of patients report blurred vision

most often due to convergence insufficiency. Occasionally, third, fourth, and sixth cranial nerve palsies occur, resulting in diplopia.

5. About 5 per cent of patients report decreased smell and taste. The olfactory filaments can be damaged by mild head injury. About 10 per cent report light and noise sensitivity.

6. Over 50 per cent report nonspecific psychological symptoms including irritability, personality change, anxiety, and depression. Fatigue and sleep disturbance are less commonly reported. A post-traumatic stress disorder also can develop following mild head injury.

7. Four weeks after the injury, about 20 per cent of patients complain of memory problems and difficulty

TABLE 306–1. KEY SYMPTOMS: SEQUELAE OF MILD HEAD INJURY

Headaches
  Muscle contraction type
  Migraine
  Cluster
  Greater occipital neuralgia
  Supraorbital and infraorbital neuralgia
  Secondary to neck injury
  Secondary to temporomandibular joint syndrome
  Owing to scalp laceration or local trauma
  Mixed
Cranial nerve symptoms and signs
  Dizziness
  Vertigo
  Tinnitus
  Hearing loss
  Blurred vision
  Diplopia
  Convergence insufficiency
  Light and noise sensitivity
  Diminished smell and taste
Psychologic and somatic complaints
  Irritability
  Anxiety
  Depression
  Personality change
  Fatigue
  Sleep disturbance
  Decreased libido
  Decreased appetite
Cognitive impairment
  Memory impairment
  Impaired concentration and attention
  Slowing of reaction time
  Slowing of information processing speed
Rare sequelae
  Subdural and epidural hematomas
  Seizures
  Transient global amnesia
  Tremor
  Dystonia

From Evans RW: Postconcussion syndrome. *In* Evans RW, Baskin DS, Yatsu FM (eds): Prognosis of Neurological Disorders. New York, Oxford University Press, 1992, with permission.

with concentration. Deficits in cognitive functioning that may occur include a reduction in speed of information processing and attention, prolonged reaction time, and decreased memory for new information.

Clinical Findings

1. There may be no physical findings on examination.

2. In cases of greater occipital neuralgia, the symptoms are reproduced with palpation over the greater occipital nerve, which is located approximately midway between the inion and posterior mastoid just below the occipital crest.

3. Rotatory nystagmus may be present in patients with vertigo due to peripheral vestibular dysfunction.

Laboratory Tests

1. Skull radiographs are usually not necessary to evaluate patients with mild closed head injury.

2. A computed tomographic (CT) scan, when indicated, is the preferred imaging modality for evaluation of acute head trauma. In patients who have had a mild head injury and have a normal neurologic examination, the yield of CT scans is quite small. After mild head injury, the incidence of neurosurgical complications is between 1 and 3 per cent. A subdural hematoma occurs in less than 1 in 5000 patients who are seen in the hospital after mild head injury.

3. MRI is more sensitive than CT scan in evaluating extra-axial and intra-axial lesions in the acute and chronic stages following head injury but rarely affects outcome.

4. EEG studies are usually not indicated for evaluating mild head injury because of limited sensitivity and specificity. However, an elctroencephalogram (EEG) is helpful when a post-traumatic seizure disorder is suspected. Brain mapping and auditory brain stem response studies are not indicated for the evaluation of mild head injury.

5. Electronystagmography (ENG) studies may be helpful in evaluating dizziness. Audiograms are indicated in patients with hearing complaints.

6. In patients with prominent visual complaints, formal visual field testing is part of the evaluation.

7. In patients with significant cognitive complaints, neuropsychological testing is often worthwhile

Key Tests

When indicated:

- CT scan or MRI of the head
- EEG
- ENG
- Audiogram
- Visual fields
- Neuropsychological testing

Differential Diagnosis

1. In patients with progressive clinical symptoms or an abnormal neurologic examination, consider a delayed or chronic subdural or epidural hematoma.

2. With time, postconcussion syndrome will generally not worsen. In cases where structural pathology has been excluded, consider possibilities such as depression, anxiety, hysteria, somatiform disorder, compensation neurosis, and malingering.

Treatment

1. Treatment is individualized after each of the problems is properly diagnosed.

2. Muscle-contraction-type headaches may respond to simple analgesics, barbiturates-narcotics (with caution), nonsteroidal anti-inflammatory drugs, antidepressants (particularly tricyclics), and muscle relaxants. For greater occipital neuralgia, a nerve block may be helpful. Biofeedback, physical therapy, and TENS units may help intractable headaches.

3. Migraines may respond to the usual prophylactic and symptomatic medications.

4. The treating physician or, if indicated, a psychologist or psychiatrist should provide the patient with psychological support. When psychological symptoms are prominent, psychotropic medications may be used.

Activity

1. Patients usually can return to normal activities within a few weeks. Some patients have prolonged disability.

2. Return to contact sports is discussed in Ch. 305.

Patient Education

1. Education of the patient and family members is essential and in many cases is the most important part of treatment.

2. The general public may be misled by the "Hollywood head injury myth" into believing that mild head injuries should not cause persistent symptoms. Head injuries are presented in two contexts in the movies or on television. In the first, in action, detective, martial arts, western, and boxing films, the injuries may appear serious but do not result in significant sequelae. The public is led to overestimate how much head injury a person can withstand. In the second context, in slapstick and cartoons, head trauma not only is not serious but can be very funny. Counterexamples such as knockouts and the "punch drunk" state in boxers may be helpful in patient education.

Key Treatment

- Individualize for each symptom
- A number of treatments are available for each headache type.
- Psychological support and education of the patient are crucial.

Follow-Up

1. Prevention: Encourage your patients to use helmets for activities such as bike or motorcycle riding.

2. Monitoring: periodic follow-up visits for patients with persistent symptoms even if only for psychological support

3. Prognosis

    a. Symptoms persist more often in patients who are women, over age 40, or with a prior history of head injury.

    b. Although headaches resolve in about 50 per cent of patients by 3 months, some 20 per cent may still complain of headaches 3 years after the injury.

    c. Cognitive impairment usually resolves within 3 to 6 months after the injury. A small percentage of patients have deficits that may persist indefinitely.

    d. Some physicians believe that patients who sustain injuries resulting in litigation have persistent symptoms due to compensation neurosis or malingering. Although this is true for a small number, most plaintiffs still symptomatic at the time of litigation are not cured by a verdict. Litigants have similar symptoms, improving with time, and similar cognitive test results as nonlitigants.

Bibliography

Alves W, Macciocchi SN, Barth JT: Postconcussive symptoms after uncomplicated mild head injury. J Head Trauma Rehabil 1993;8:48–59.

Duus BR, Lind B, Christensen H, Nielsen OA: The role of neuroimaging in the initial management of patients with minor head injury. Ann Emerg Med 1994;23:1279–1283.

Evans RW: The postconcussion syndrome and the sequelae of mild head injury. Neurol Clin 1992;10(4):815–847.

Fisher JM, Williams AD: Neuropsychologic investigation of mild head injury: Ensuring diagnostic accuracy in the assessment process. Semin Neurol 1994;14(1):53–59.

McAllister TW: Neuropsychiatric sequelae of head injuries. Psychiatr Clin 1992;15(2):395–413.

307 Subdural Hematoma

Erol Taşdemiroğlu

Subdural hematoma or hemorrhage is characterized by a collection of blood between the dura mater and the arachnoid membranes of the central nervous system. Depending on the rapidity of bleeding and the size of the blood vessel that is torn, subdural hematomas are classified as acute, subacute, or chronic. Acute and subacute hematomas are associated with contusion and laceration of the cerebral parenchyma and are sometimes called "complicated subdural hematomas." Infantile subdural effusions are considered a separate entity. The source of bleeding may be arterial or venous. If a rupture of the arachnoid membrane accompanies the formation of a hematoma, the condition is called a "complex subdural hygroma." Subdural hematomas can be located in the supratentorial region (convexity, interhemispheric, subtemporal, or suboccipital hematomas), the infratentorial region (posterior fossa subdural hematomas), or the spine.

Etiology

1. Trauma (birth trauma, physical child abuse)
2. Coagulopathy (secondary to cancer chemotherapy, hepatic and hematologic diseases, hemophilia, anticoagulant therapy, vitamins C or K, hypovitaminosis)
3. Arteriovenous malformation or rupture of an aneurysm into the subdural space
4. Ventricular shunting procedures or lumbar puncture
5. Neoplasms (primary neoplasms or metastases to the subdural space)
6. Other (alcoholism, hypertension, hemodialysis, infusion of osmotic diuretics, intracranial operations, infections)

Symptoms

A. Acute subdural hematomas: Symptoms occur within the first 24 hours of injury. Acute subdural hematomas generally extend over large portions of the brain. Two types of traumatic acute subdural hematomas have been described:

 1. Bleeding is associated with cortical and parenchymal lacerations. Usually the underlying primary brain injury is severe. The size of the hematoma is insignificant. Often there is no lucid interval.
 2. This type of hematoma is characterized by massive hemorrhage caused by a tear in large bridging veins or the dural sinuses. Primary brain damage is less severe, and a lucid interval may occur. Acute subdural hematomas are occasionally caused by birth trauma.

B. Subacute subdural hematomas: Clinical symptoms occur within an interval of 3 to 21 days after injury. Signs and symptoms are usually similar to those of chronic subdural hematomas.

C. Chronic subdural hematomas: Symptoms start at least 3 weeks after head injury. Symptoms can mimic transient ischemic attacks (TIAs) and may show fluctuations.

Bilateral chronic subdural hematomas are seen in 15 to 20 per cent of patients.

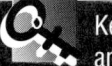

Key Signs and Symptoms: Subacute and Chronic Subdural Hematomas

- Dull headaches, seizures
- Changes in personality and mental status
- Hemiparesis, dysphasia, hemisensory changes
- Papilledema, retinal hemorrhage, photophobia

D. Subdural hematoma in infants and children: Chronic subdural hematomas or subdural effusions are seldom seen in patients more than 2 years of age unless a shunt procedure was carried out; they rarely occur in adolescents less than age 20. Chronic infantile subdural collections are usually bilateral and frequently communicate under the falx.

Calcified chronic subdural hematomas are usually bilateral and may remain asymptomatic for years. They only manifest themselves when seizure activity or mental retardation becomes apparent.

Key Signs and Symptoms: Subdural Hematomas in Infants and Children

- Increased intracranial pressure (abnormal width and tension of the fontanelle, palpable separation of the cranial sutures, "cracked-pot" percussion sound of the skull, irritability and vomiting)—in 60 per cent
- Seizures (local or generalized)—in 40 per cent
- Macrocrania (characterized by biparietal enlargement and distention of superficial scalp veins)
- Retinal or subhyaloid hemorrhage
- Anemia
- Generalized hypertonicity of the extremities
- Lateralizing or focal motor deficits

E. Spinal subdural hematomas: Spinal subdural hematomas can complicate lumbar puncture (therapeutic or diagnostic) or may occur spontaneously. This type of hematoma is most commonly located in the lower thoracic or thoracolumbar regions. Clinical symptoms often include sphincter dysfunction, paralysis of the lower extremities, and back pain.

F. Posterior fossa subdural hematomas: Posterior fossa subdural hematomas constitute fewer than 1 per cent of all subdural hematomas. These hematomas are usually acute in nature and characterized by bleeding from torn bridging veins or posterior fossa dural sinuses.

G. Subdural hygroma: Subdural hygromas appearing during the post-traumatic period are characteristically subdural fluid collections that are crystal clear or mildly xanthochromic. Subdural hygromas are called "simple" if they occur alone or "complex" when they are associated with parenchymal injuries. These hygromas are also seen after monitoring and vigorous treatment of increased intracranial pressure in patients with Reye's syndrome. The clinical manifestations are similar to those of subdural hematomas.

Diagnosis

1. Skull radiographs may reveal skull fracture line, shift of physiologic midline calcifications (falx cerebri and pineal gland), and calcified subdural hematoma membrane.

2. Subdural tap is another procedure used to diagnose infantile chronic subdural effusions. In newborns, the results of taps of the subdural space through the fontanelle or the coronal suture may be misleading, because the hematoma is usually coagulated and solid.

3. Cerebral angiography is characterized by biconvex avascular extracerebral mass.

4. Electroencephalogram (EEG): may be abnormal; diffuse reduction of voltage and/or unilateral suppression of alpha rhythm on the side where the hematoma is located.

5. Radioisotope brain scan shows increased activity over the cortex on the side where the hematoma is located.

6. B-mode ultrasonography is a relatively easy, harmless, noninvasive, and economic way to diagnose and follow chronic infantile subdural hematomas.

7. Computed tomographic (CT) scan (Table 307–1): Cerebral edema is frequently seen. Acute subdural hematomas are hyperintense on CT scans (Fig. 307–1) and are usually localized over the convexity. Whereas subacute subdural hematomas are 70 per cent isointense on axial CT scan, chronic subdural hematomas are 76 per cent hypointense (Fig. 307–2) and 16 per cent isointense on axial CT scans. However, layering phenomena and repeated episodes of hemorrhage may produce hematomas of variable attenuation and size (Fig. 307–3).

8. Magnetic resonance imaging (MRI) (Table 307–1): The MRI appearance of subdural hematoma shows an evolving pattern of variable signal intensity. When recurrent bleeding occurs in a subdural hematoma, the different events may be distinguishable by the variable signal intensities on MRI (Fig. 307–4)

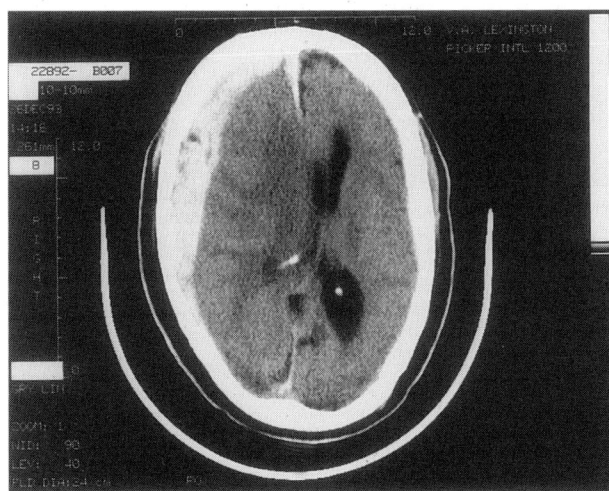

Figure 307–1 Axial CT scan of the head without contrast enhancement shows supratentorial large hyperdense acute subdural hematoma and cerebral edema with mass effect resulting in midline shift.

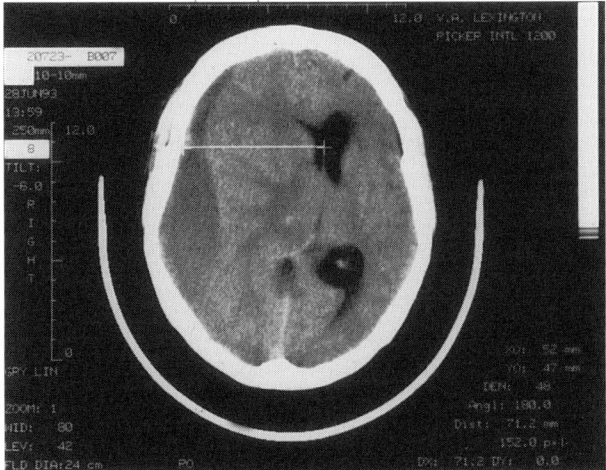

Figure 307–2 Axial CT scan of the head without contrast enhancement shows large hypodense fluid collection over the right hemisphere with significant midline shift.

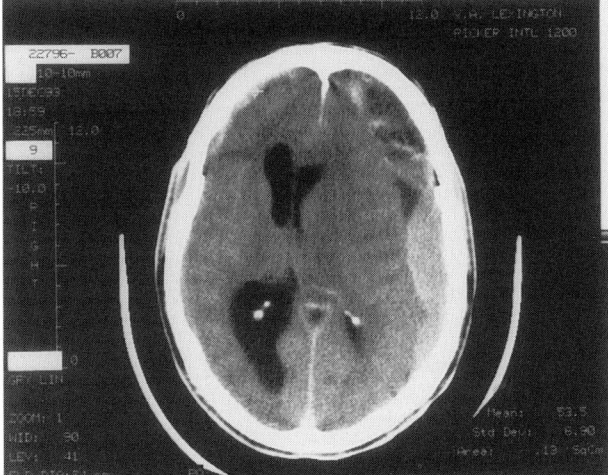

Figure 307–3 Axial CT scan of the head shows large subdural hypo- and hyperdense fluid accumulation characterized by rehemorrhage into the subdural space.

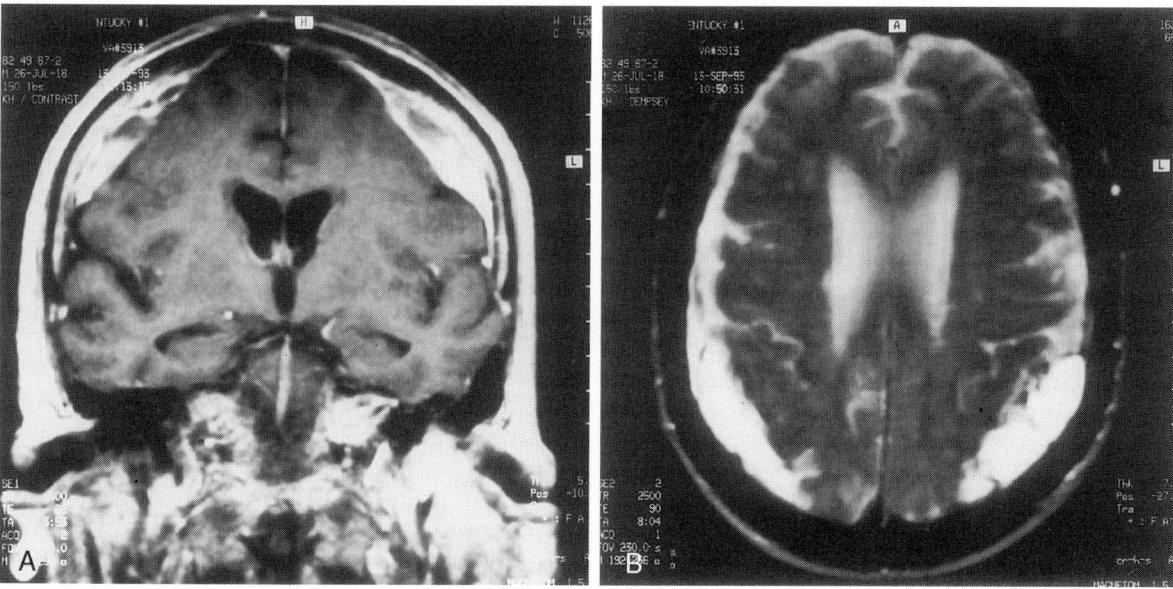

Figure 307–4 Gadolinium enhanced coronal T_1-weighted *(A)* and axial T_2-weighted *(B)* MRI images show inhomogeneous subdural fluid collection that represents different ages of the blood products within.

TABLE 307–1. SUBDURAL HEMATOMA DENSITY CHANGES ON CT AND MRI WITH TIME

STAGE	CT SCAN	MRI		
		Hemoglobin	T_1-Weighted	T_2-Weighted
Hyperacute (<24 hr)	Hyperdense Intracellular iron	Oxyhemoglobin	Hypointense to brain parenchyma	Hyperintense (CSF density) to brain parenchyma
Acute (1–3 d)	Hyperdense Intracellular iron	Deoxyhemoglobin	Isointense to brain parenchyma	Hypointense to brain
Early subacute (3–7 d)	Isodense Intracellular iron	Methemoglobin	Hyperintense to brain (+)	Hypointense to brain
Late subacute (>7 d)	Isodense Extracellular iron	Methemoglobin	Hyperintense to brain (+ +)	Hyperintense to brain
Chronic (>3 wk)	Hypodense Extracellular iron	Methemoglobin	Hyperintense to brain (+)	

Treatment

Surgery

1. Acute and subacute subdural hematomas: If the collection of blood in a symptomatic hematoma is thicker than 1 cm at its thickest point, rapid surgical evacuation should be considered. Hematomas characterized by massive hemorrhage should be evacuated rapidly. The primary treatment of subacute subdural hematomas is also surgical drainage.

2. Chronic subdural hematoma: Surgical evacuation of the hematoma is indicated for symptomatic lesions with maximum thickness greater than about 1 cm. If a significant recollection is demonstrated, a short course of dexamethasone, 2 to 4 mg four times daily for a period of ranging from 7 to 14 days, is instituted. Only when this regimen fails to improve the situation is reoperation considered. Residual subdural collections after treatment are common and may require up to 6 months for complete resolution. Persistent fluid collections, especially those evident on CT scan dur-

ing the first 20 postoperative days, should not be re-evacuated unless they increase in size, as demonstrated by CT scan, or the patient shows no signs of recovery or deteriorates neurologically.

3. Calcified subdural hematoma: Calcified subdural hematoma is not responsible for seizures or mental retardation. The surgical indications for treating such a lesion are progressive mental retardation, an increase in the number of seizures, or other progressive neurologic deficit.

4. Spinal subdural hematoma: A laminectomy should be performed as soon as possible after the diagnosis is made so that the amount of neurologic damage can be held to a minimum.

5. Subdural hygroma: Surgical evacuation is unnecessary for the patients who are clinically improving or stable.

Medication

Because the development of chronic subdural hematoma is an inflammatory process, inhibition of inflammatory re-

TABLE 307–2. GRADING OF CHRONIC SUBDURAL HEMATOMA

GROUP	DESCRIPTION
0	Neurologically normal
1	Alert and oriented; mild symptoms, including headache, reflex asymmetry, seizure
2	Lethargic or disoriented with variable neurologic deficits such as hemiparesis
3	Stuporous but responds appropriately to noxious stimuli; severe focal signs such as hemiplegia
4	Comatose; decerebrate or decorticate posturing

Reprinted with permission from Markwalder TM, Steinsiepe KF, Rohner M, et al: The course of chronic subdural hematomas after burr-hole craniostomy and closed-system drainage. J Neurosurg 1981;55:390–396.

action would be beneficial. Glucocorticoids have been shown to inhibit neomembrane formation and neovascularization in experimental subdural hematomas. Intravenous hyperosmolar agents such as mannitol with or without steroids are the cornerstone of medical treatment. Small and mildly symptomatic chronic subdural hematomas could be treated with steroids. Seizure prophylaxis is considered.

Prognosis and Outcome

1. The mortality rate associated with acute subdural hematomas is 50 to 90 per cent, but these rates are higher for aged patients (60 per cent) and for patients who use anticoagulants (90 per cent). The mortality rate drops to 30 per cent if surgery is performed within 4 hours of the injury. Subacute subdural hematomas carry a much better prognosis than acute subdural hematomas. However, in posterior fossa, subdural hematoma prognosis is related to the patient's neurologic condition and the severity of the head injury.

2. The mortality rates after treatment of a chronic subdural hematoma are reported at less than 10 per cent in large series, and approximately 75 per cent of patients are able to resume normal functioning. The mortality rate drops to 5 per cent in patients who are alert or drowsy (grades 0 to 2; see Table 307–2).

3. After treatment of chronic subdural effusions, although approximately 75 per cent of infants show normal development, 5 per cent show some degree of psychomotor retardation.

Bibliography

Becker DP, Gade GF, Young HF, Feuerman TF: Diagnosis and treatment of head injury in adults. *In* Youmans JR (ed): Neurological Surgery: A Comprehensive Guide to the Diagnosis and Management of Neurosurgical Problems, 3d ed, vol 3. Philadelphia, WB Saunders, 1990, pp 2017–2148.

Bradley WG Jr: Hemorrhage and brain iron. *In* Stark DD, Bradley WG Jr (eds): Magnetic Resonance Imaging, 2d ed, vol 1. St. Louis, Mosby–Year Book, 1992, pp 721–69.

Drapkin AJ: Chronic subdural hematoma: Pathophysiological basis for treatment. Br J Neurosurg 1991;5:467–473.

Hamilton MG, Frizzell JB, Tranmer BI: Chronic subdural hematoma: The role of craniotomy re-evaluated. Neurosurgery 1993;33:67–72.

Keller TS, Schneider RC: Craniocerebral trauma. *In* Schneider RC, Kahn EA, Crosby EC, Taren JA (eds): Correlative Neurosurgery, 3d ed, vol 2. Springfield, Ill, Charles C Thomas, 1982, pp 1301–1414.

308 Common Behavioral Symptoms

Insomnia is the most common sleep complaint. It is a symptom of patients experiencing a variety of diseases, and it must be investigated with a careful history and usually a brief examination to arrive at a diagnosis and appropriate therapy. Insomnia is the perception by patients that their sleep is inadequate or abnormal; however, patients may use the term insomnia to indicate problems of fatigue, night awakenings not resulting in daytime dysfunction, daytime sleepiness, or mood disturbances.

Differential Diagnosis

1. Psychophysiologic insomnia
   a. *Transient psychophysiologic insomnia* is of less than 3 weeks' duration and is usually the result of some identifiable environmental event such as a change in life circumstance, grief, altered schedule, or withdrawal from a drug or medication. It responds to maintenance of sleep hygiene, avoidance of stimulants, and a brief supervised use of benzodiazepines.
   b. *Chronic psychophysiologic insomnia* lasts more than 3 weeks and commonly more than 3 months. Some physicians believe that inadequate management of transient insomnia leads to the chronic state via a sleeplessness phobia and sleep performance anxiety.
2. *Secondary insomnias* are caused by medical, psycho-

logical, or painful conditions or misuse of substances (Table 308–1).
3. *Primary insomnias* are much less common and include those disorders which can be identified by polysomnography.
   a. *Sleep apneas,* both the common obstructive type and the rare central type, are characterized by periods of apnea often associated with desaturation, dysrhythmia, and partial arousal from sleep. Sedatives make this problem worse.
   b. *Periodic limb movement* causes stereotyped repetitive movements of legs and occasionally arms.
   c. *Rapid eye movement (REM) sleep disorder,* though actually a parasomnia, can present with active, sometimes violent movements which interestingly are more disturbing to the partner than the patient. It is more common in men in their fifties and older.
   d. *Sleep phase asynchronies* cause mismatching of the biologic sleep clock and the environment. It can result from time zone shifts or varied sleep schedules or be idiopathic. Adolescents tend to have delayed sleep phase, with sleepiness occurring after midnight, while elders tend to have the opposite problem, falling asleep and arousing too early.
   e. *Childhood-onset insomnia* is a rare insomnia probably related to a developmental defect in the sleep-wake circuitry. History usually suggests this problem since birth, but most children who sleep poorly suffer from environmental stress or dysfunctional parenting.

Refer to Ch. 51, Sleep Apnea; Ch. 60, Chronic Heart Failure; Ch. 313, Depression; Ch. 316, Generalized Anxiety Disorder; Ch. 319, Alcoholism; and Ch. 321, Substance Abuse.

TABLE 308–1. COMMON MEDICAL AND PSYCHIATRIC CAUSES OF INSOMNIA

Nocturnal Dyspnea	**Affective Disorders**
Asthma/COPD	Depression
Congestive heart failure	Mania
Gastrointestinal reflux	
Obstructive sleep apnea	**Anxiety Disorders**
	Generalized anxiety disorder
Nocturia	Pain disorder
Urinary tract infection	Obsessive-compulsive disorder
Benign prostatic hypertrophy	Post-traumatic stress disorder
Hyperglycemia	
Diuretic therapy	**Cognitive disorders**
	Psychosis
Trunkal Discomfort	Dementias
Acid peptic disease	
Gallbladder disease	**Somatization Disorders**
Angina	Somatoform pain disorders
Intestinal ischemia	Subjective insomnia*
Limb Discomfort	**Organic Causes of Anxiety**
Nocturnal leg cramps	Hyperthyroidism
Degenerative arthritis	Alcohol abuse
Peripheral vascular disease	Stimulant abuse
Neuropathic pain	Drug abstinence

*DSM-IV does not categorize this as a somatization disorder but it has features of a distorted perception of sleep without any objective findings.

History

1. Onset of problem, frequency of occurrences, course or change over time
2. Time to bed, time to sleep, time awakened
3. Nocturnal awakening for what cause: dyspnea, nocturia, discomfort, disturbing thoughts/dreams
4. Total hours in bed, total hours asleep

5. Daytime naps, daytime sleepiness
6. Partner notes: restless movements, loud snoring, periods of apneas, change in mood, change in consumption of alcohol, caffeine, drugs
7. Medications, drugs, alcohol, nicotine, caffeine
8. Background psychiatric and situational history
9. Review of systems referable to medical and psychiatric causes (see Table 308–1)

Clinical Findings

A few physical findings are important to search for in the evaluation of insomnia.

A. *Obstructive sleep apnea*
1. Obesity usual, sometimes morbid, but not an absolute feature
2. Small oropharyngeal space with difficulty visualizing the retropharynx
3. In extreme cases, somnolence, pulmonary hypertension, cor pulmonale (pickwickian syndrome)
4. Sedatives *accentuate* this problem.

B. *Pulmonary disease* or *congestive heart failure*
1. Rales, wheezes, decreased expiratory force evident on pulmonary examination
2. Cardiomegaly, extrasystolic gallop, jugular venous distention, dependent edema
3. Polycythemia, hypercarbia, hypoxemia, hyperbicarbinatemia, right-sided heart strain or hypertrophy by electrocardiogram (ECG) (may also indicate advanced obstructive sleep apnea).

C. *Affective or anxiety disorders*
1. Depression is associated with early morning awakening; anxiety with difficulty falling asleep.
2. Somatic hyperawareness or preoccupation
3. Sympathetic arousal with tachycardia, midriasis, fine tremor, palmar sudation (exclude thyroid disease and stimulant use)

D. *Substance abuse/abstinence*
1. Hypertension, tachycardia, fine tremor
2. Elevated liver function tests, uric acid, or mean corpuscular volume suggest occult heavy alcohol use.
3. Urine toxicology screen for amphetamines, cocaine, opiates

Tests

1. *Sleep diary,* an inexpensive, simple technique for quantifying insomnia complaints, records bedtime, time until sleep, arising time, awakenings, daytime naps, and qualitative assessment of sleep and daytime alertness. It has the drawback of potential subjective distortion.
2. *Polysomnography* is the primary means of evaluating complicated or recalcitrant chronic insomnias. It is not indicated in the evaluation of all insomnias. Usually it is carried out in a sleep laboratory, which requires overnight evaluation on one or several occasions. Simultaneous recordings of ECG, electroencephalography, respiratory muscle activity, pulse oximetry, nasal airflow, general muscle tone, and visual observation provide information to classify the insomnia.
3. *Continuous overnight pulse oximetry* has been found useful as a screening tool for obstructive sleep apnea. Brief desaturations below the baseline suggest apnea spells; this is particularly true if saturations drop below 90 per cent, but positive studies should be confirmed with a formal sleep study. Normal nocturnal oximetry without periodic desaturations decreases the likelihood of obstructive sleep apnea.
4. *Therapeutic trial of oxygen or Continuous Positive Airway Pressure (CPAP)* may improve quality of sleep for patients with respiratory diseases. Third-party payors may require some demonstration of need (arterial blood gas or polysomnography) before approving this, but some will allow a trial therapy.

Management

Therapy should be directed at the underlying cause of insomnia, if one can be found. This is particularly important if a medical or psychiatric cause is suspected. Indiscriminate use of sedatives at the least may mask a symptom of a potentially treatable illness and at worst may cause the patient to deteriorate.

A. *General measures*
1. *Sleep hygiene* should be taught to all insomniacs (Table 308–2).
2. *Stimulus-control instructions* are used for chronic insomniacs because many have developed behavioral responses to sleeping or their sleeping environment which preclude sleep and perpetuate the insomnia (Table 308–3).

TABLE 308–2.   SLEEP HYGIENE

Do's	Don'ts
Consistent awakening time	Nap during the day
Achieve aerobic fitness	Take caffeine, alcohol, CNS-acting drugs before bedtime
Regular dietary habits and mealtime	Eat large meals before bedtime
Comfortable sleeping place	Engage in difficult emotional or physical activity immediately before bedtime
Develop a sleep ritual	

Data from Regestein QR: Sleep Disorders. *In* Stoudemire A (ed): Clinical Psychiatry for Medical Students. Philadelphia, JB Lippincott, 1990, p 578.

TABLE 308–3.   STIMULUS CONTROL INSTRUCTIONS

1. Lie down to sleep only when you are sleepy.
2. Use your bed only for sleep or sexual activity.
3. If you are unable to fall asleep after 10 minutes, get up and leave the bedroom.
4. Repeat Step 3 as often as necessary.
5. Get up at the same time each morning.
6. Do not nap during the day.

From Bootzin RR, Perlis ML: Nonpharmacologic treatments of insomnia. Clin Psychiatry 1992; 53(suppl): 37–45; permission granted. Copyright 1992, Physicians Postgraduate Press.

3. *Relaxation* is a commonly recommended therapy for insomnia. It can take the form of progressive muscle relaxation, self-hypnosis, yoga, or biofeedback response.

4. *Cognitive therapy* is occasionally useful for insomnia. This is particularly true if insomnia is associated with affective or anxiety disorder. Brief therapy by the clinician on time management, appropriate self-expectation, and problem-solving skills can go a long way to help the overly busy achiever adjust lifestyle.

B. *Specific management*

1. *Obstructive sleep apnea*

a. *Sleeping position* may affect the apnea frequency, and if patients can sleep on their side or stomach, ventilation may improve. Some clinicians have suggested sewing tennis or Ping-Pong balls to pajama backs to discourage supine sleeping.

b. *Nasal CPAP* or the modified *biphasic positive airway pressure (BiPAP)* greatly improves ventilation in selected patients. Drawbacks including discomfort of face mask, headache, dry nasal passages, and noise decrease compliance to this therapy.

c. *Nasal oxygen* correcting nocturnal hypoxemia often gives patients with cardiopulmonary disease an improved sense of sleep satisfaction and daytime energy.

d. *Protriptyline,* an alerting tricyclic antidepressant, in a dose of 5 to 10 mg at bedtime, has been found useful in some patients by decreasing the depth of non-REM sleep where apneas more commonly occur.

e. *Oral orthoses* can maintain an open airway by advancing the mandible and increasing the posterior airway space during sleep. Dental referral is required.

f. *Uvulopalatopharyngoplasty (UPPP) or tracheostomy* is rarely needed in patients with severe obstructive sleep apnea unresponsive to usual therapy. The pharyngeal airway is enlarged by resection of soft tissue (UPPP).

2. *Sleep phase asynchronies*

a. *Chronotherapy* or delaying bedtime is a technique used primarily for delayed sleep phase insomnia. It consists of successively delaying sleep by 3 hours each night until bedtime occurs at the desired time.

b. *Phototherapy* uses bright light (7000 to 12,000 lux) in the spectral range of sunlight for 30 to 60 minutes to treat circadian rhythm disturbances. The timing of the light will shift the sleep phase, with early morning exposure causing a phase advance and early evening exposure a phase delay.

C. *Pharmacologic:* If treatment with a sedative-hypnotic drug is chosen, one should observe some general principles. The lowest effective dose should be tried. Doses should be reduced in the elderly or renal or hepatic disease patients and used with great caution in respiratory disease patients. All sedative-hypnotics are indicated only for short-term use in the treatment of insomnia, most induce habituation and withdrawal, and all can cause rebound insomnia upon abrupt cessation.

1. *Benzodiazepines* are the most widely used in the treatment of insomnia (Table 308–4). All are DEA schedule intravenous drugs with potential for dependence and abuse. All are nonselective agonists of GABA neuroreceptors, and all suppress the deeper stages of sleep. Selection of agents may be influenced by duration of effect. Longer-acting agents have less rebound insomnia in the early morning but cause more next-day sedation. Patients with difficulty initiating sleep may benefit from a shorter-acting agent. Patients with difficulty sleeping after midsleep arousal are better suited for a longer-acting agent. Profound antegrade amnesia has occurred with triazolam, but any of the benzodiazepines may cause this. Short-

TABLE 308–4. COMPARISON OF BENZODIAZEPINES APPROVED FOR INSOMNIA THERAPY

Drug Name	Trade Name	Onset	Duration	Available Strengths	Usual Daily Dosage	Cost*
Flurazepam	*Generic*	Rapid to intermediate	Long	15 mg, 30 mg	30 mg	$1.42
	Dalmane (Roche)			15 mg, 30 mg		$3.76
Temazepam	*Generic*	Intermediate to slow	Intermediate	15 mg, 30 mg	30 mg	$1.59
	Restoril (Sandoz)			7.5 mg, 15 mg, 30 mg		$4.19
Triazolam	*Generic*	Intermediate	Short	0.125 mg, 0.25 mg	0.25–0.5 mg	$4.26
	Halcion (Upjohn)			0.125 mg, 0.25 mg		$4.52
Quazepam	*Doral* (Wallace)	Rapid	Long	7.5 mg, 15 mg	15 mg	$6.09
Estazolam	*ProSom* (Abbott)	Rapid to intermediate	Intermediate	1 mg, 2 mg	2 mg	$5.96
Zolpidem†	*Ambien* (Searle)	Rapid	Short	5 mg, 10 mg	10 mg	$8.72

*Average Wholesale Price for one week's treatment with the lowest starting dosage recommended by the manufacturer according to manufacturer's listing in Drug Topics Red Book 1995.
†Chemically unrelated to benzodiazepines, but binds the same receptors.
Data from The Medical Letter.

and intermediate-acting agents may cause withdrawal more than longer-acting agents. It is best to taper doses when discontinuing. Table 308–4 lists those approved for use in insomnia, although any benzodiazepine will have sedative effects.

2. *Nonbenzodiazepine GABA-receptor agonist* recently became commercially available. Zolpidem (Searle), 10 mg, is the first, but others may soon be available. Advances in GABA neuropharmacology have identified subclasses of receptors to which this agent may have some selective affinity. It appears to have little effect on sleep stages, but the sleep EEG with treatment is similar to that for benzodiazepines.

3. *Tricyclic antidepressants* in low dose are used by some clinicians. They appear to decrease the incidence of α-wave intrusion into non-REM sleep, a phenomenon that decreases the restorative quality of sleep. They, too, are limited in use by side effects, primarily anticholinergic and daytime sedation. Amitriptyline, 10 to 25 mg, and nortriptyline, 25 to 50 mg, are commonly used agents. If insomnia is secondary to depression, full doses of antidepressants are indicated. One may choose an agent with a sedating side effect such as amitriptyline, nortriptyline, imipramine, doxepin, or trazadone. Among the newer class of *selective serotonergic reuptake inhibitors (SSRIs),* sertraline appears to be the most sedating.

4. *Antihistamines* are commonly used in over-the-counter sedative medications. Diphenhydramine, 25 to 50 mg, is the most commonly prescribed. Anticholinergic side effects are marked, and caution should be used in elderly patients or those with obstructive uropathy.

D. *Other sedatives*

1. *Choral hydrate* is an effective hypnotic in short-term use, but its effectiveness disappears within 2 weeks despite maintaining physical dependence.

2. *L-Tryptophan* was used with some success for insomnia, but the appearance of eosinophilic-myalgia syndrome associated with a particular pharmaceutical lot caused this drug to be pulled from the market. It is believed this disease was caused by a contaminant formed in the chemical process. Possibly L-tryptophan will again be available when contamination can be eliminated.

3. *Barbiturates* are rarely used now because of the induction of hepatic enzymes, the risk of abuse, and their narrow therapeutic-toxic dose range.

4. *Alcohol* is used by many individuals for treatment of insomnia. This action should be discouraged because it can suppress REM sleep temporarily with rebound REM-disrupting sleep.

PEARLS

- Insomnia is a symptom with many causes.

- Most insomnia is due to an affective disorder.

- All insomniacs should be instructed on sleep hygiene techniques regardless of etiology.

- Pharmacotherapy is indicated for brief periods of psychophysiologic insomnia.

B **Bibliography**

American Academy of Family Physicians: Patient Information: Insomnia and What You Can Do To Sleep Better. Am Fam Physician 1994;49:1423–1424.

Kryger MH, Roth T, Dement WC (eds): Principles and Practice of Sleep Medicine. Philadelphia, WB Saunders, 1989.

Mendelson WB: Human Sleep: Research and Clinical Care. New York, Plenum, 1987.

Mendelson WB: Insomnia and Related Sleep Disorders. Psychiatr Clin North Am 1993;16:841–851.

Thawley SE (ed): Sleep Apnea Disorders. Med Clin North Am 60/6, 1985.

Symptom	**Fatigue**	*Anthony L.-T. Chen*

Fatigue, also called "lassitude" or "tiredness," may be offered as a primary complaint or as a feature accompanying other symptoms. It is not a diagnosis but a symptom, a nonspecific, subjective sensation of ill-being that reflects emotional, social, or physical dysfunction.

For the patient, fatigue creates significant morbidity by degrading quality of life and productivity. For the primary-care physician, fatigue is a challenge to use a broad approach that incorporates clinical reasoning, negotiation, and interpersonal skills.

Differential Diagnosis

1. Mood disorder, especially depression

2. Stress, whether social or physical

3. Infection, especially viral

4. Endocrine disorder, especially thyroid disease and diabetes

5. Medication side effect

6. Cardiovascular disease

7. Lifestyle, including sleep, diet, exercise, work, and substance use habits

---

Refer to Ch. 60, Chronic Heart Failure; Ch. 61, Cardio-myopathy; Chs. 141–145, The Anemias; Chs. 225–243, Infectious Diseases; Ch. 313, Depression; Ch. 316, Generalized Anxiety Disorder; and see Ch. 312, procedure on BATHE Technique.

Etiology

Most complaints of fatigue will have a nonorganic cause. Fifty to sixty per cent will be functional or psychological in origin, and 40 to 50 per cent will be physical; depression is the most common diagnosis and occurs in 20 to 30 per cent of cases. The role of stress and lifestyle factors is unknown but can be expected to be large. More exhaustive lists of physical diagnoses can be found in the Bibliography.

History

1. Patient concerns and expectations
2. Duration of symptoms: less than 4 weeks more likely to be physical, while more than 4 months more likely to be psychosocial
3. Character of symptoms
   a. Progressive instead of fluctuating suggests physical.
   b. Worse in morning suggests psychosocial.
   c. Nonspecific and multiple symptoms suggest psychosocial.
4. Symptoms that suggest alternate diagnostic algorithms
   a. Fever
   b. Organ- or system-specific symptoms (e.g., dyspnea on exertion)
   c. Menstrual abnormality (i.e., pregnancy or menopause)
5. Symptoms of depression (mood, sleep, appetite, social activity)
6. Symptoms of anxiety and other psychiatric disorders
7. Social context
   a. Stressors and supports (family, economic/financial, school/work)
   b. Family transitions (birth, marriage, divorce, death, illness)
   c. BATHE questions (see Ch. 312, procedure on the BATHE technique)
8. Medications
9. Lifestyle
   a. Sleep, diet, activity, and work habits
   b. Substance use and habits; consider CAGE questions (see Table 319–3)
10. Patient's theory of disease (illness explanatory model)

Duration and character of symptoms may help differentiate physical from psychosocial causes. Because of their high incidence, depression and psychosocial causes must be screened for. Using a problem-solving approach, the presence of certain symptoms, such as fever or weakness, would suggest alternate diagnostic algorithms; a history of risk factors would prompt additional evaluation. Establishing patient concerns, expectations, and illness explanatory model allows the physician and patient to negotiate the extent and pace of evaluation and treatment.

Clinical Findings

1. General appearance: ill suggests physical, while anxious or depressed suggests psychosocial.
2. Weakness suggests physical.
3. Mental status examination may be abnormal.

There are no specific signs for fatigue, but the preceding may suggest the cause. A complete physical examination may reveal clues to a physical diagnosis.

Tests

1. Complete blood count
2. Glucose
3. Thyroxine (T_4) and thyroid-stimulating hormone (TSH)
4. Urinalysis
5. Sedimentation rate (ESR)
6. Appropriate routine cancer screening (e.g., Pap smear, fecal occult blood)
7. Consider psychological screening tests (e.g., Beck, Zung, Center for Epidemiologic Studies Depression Scale [CES-D], Minnesota Multiphasic Personality Inventory [MMPI]).
8. Consider screening tests for support and stress (e.g., Duke Social Support and Stress Scale [DUSOCS], family APGAR, family circle, genogram).

Cost-effectiveness evaluations of laboratory testing have markedly reduced the number of tests now recommended in the absence of an obvious physical diagnosis. Abnormal tests occur no more than 25 per cent (and often less than 10 per cent) of the time and frequently do not influence the diagnosis. The high frequency of psychosocial causes of fatigue suggests that psychological and social screening tests may be useful.

Management

1. Treat underlying medical illness, if present.
2. Initiate brief counseling or make referral for psychotherapy, if indicated.
3. Establish therapeutic relationship: listen, reassure, and provide empathy.
4. Formulate plan to reduce or manage stressors.

Medication

1. Withdraw any suspected medications.

2. Consider an empirical trial of antidepressants.

Diet

1. Encourage a balanced, low-fat, high-fiber diet and regular meals.

Activity

1. Prescribe moderate exercise.

2. Consider recommending a diary of symptoms.

Patient Education

1. Explain the interaction of psychosocial and somatic functioning (mind-body connection).

2. Provide guidance and support appropriate for life stage.

3. Teach or recommend resources for stress and personal management skills.

Follow-Up

1. Schedule a complete physical examination in follow-up of brief initial examination.

2. Review interval history for evolution of symptoms that may make the cause more apparent ("test of time").

3. Review compliance with exercise, diet, stress reduction, and other interventions.

4. If a physical problem was present, monitor appropriate parameters.

5. At each visit, negotiate the extent and pace of evaluation and treatment based on patient concerns and expectations.

6. Continue to build on therapeutic relationship.

7. Schedule frequent, regular visits for those with multiple somatic complaints or many concerns.

8. Avoid excessive tests or procedures.

PEARLS

- Fatigue is a nonspecific symptom, not a diagnosis.

- The majority will have a nonorganic cause; depression is the most common diagnosis.

- Diagnosis is mostly based on history and an understanding of the epidemiology; routine laboratory testing should be minimized.

- Duration of symptoms less than 4 weeks and a progressive deterioration suggest a physical cause.

- Duration of symptoms more than 4 months, peak symptomatology in the morning, and nonspecific and multiple symptoms suggest a psychosocial cause.

- Physician-patient negotiation, a therapeutic relationship, and a broad approach are cornerstones of successful management.

Bibliography

Elnicki DM, Shockcor WT, Brick JE, Beynon D: Evaluating the complaint of fatigue in primary care: Diagnoses and outcomes. Am J Med 1992;93:303–306.

McGee SR: Fatigue. *In* Fihn SD, McGee SR (eds): Outpatient Medicine. Philadelphia, WB Saunders, 1992, Ch 21, pp 72–74.

Ridsdale L, Evans A, Jerrett W, et al: Patients with fatigue in general practice: A prospective study. Br Med J 1993; 307:103–106.

Solberg LI: Lassitude: A primary care evaluation. JAMA 1984;251:3272–3276.

Valdini AF: Fatigue of unknown aetiology—a review. Fam Pract 1985;2(1):48–53.

| Symptom | **Irritability** | *Debra Feldman* |

Irritability is defined as both hyperexcitability to a stimulus and impatience. The symptom of irritability may be present in a wide range of medical illnesses, neurologic conditions, and psychiatric disorders. Irritability also may be an appropriate reaction to a stressful situation, such as psychological stress or pain and discomfort. As such, this symptom may require no specific assessment or treatment other than measures to alleviate the underlying stressors. If no such stressor can be identified, or if the degree of irritability appears excessive, an evaluation should be undertaken. Because of the nonspecific nature of irritability, a patient who presents with this symptom must be evaluated extensively to uncover other more specific symptoms and signs.

Differential Diagnosis

1. Mood disorders, especially those with manic features, such as bipolar disorder (also seasonal affective disorder)

2. Personality disorder, such as antisocial personality, borderline personality, and passive aggressive personality

3. Anxiety disorder

4. Hyperactive attention disorder

5. Menopause

6. Premenstrual syndrome

7. Hyperthyroidism

8. Vitamin deficiency, such as vitamin B_{12}, niacin, riboflavin

9. Substance abuse and substance abuse withdrawal syndromes (includes withdrawal from alcohol, nicotine, and controlled substances)

10. Dementia
11. Frontal lobe syndrome
12. Postconcussion syndrome
13. Medications, such as glucocorticoids, androgens, theophylline
14. Sleep disorders and sleep deprivation
15. Electrolyte abnormalities, such as hypercalcemia, acidemia, hypoglycemia

> Refer to Ch. 108, Menopause; Ch. 171, Hypercalcemia; Ch. 172, Hypoglycemia; Ch. 291, Sleep Disorders; Ch. 311, Personality Disorders; Ch. 313, Depression; Ch. 315, Panic Disorder; Ch. 316, Generalized Anxiety Disorders; and Ch. 321, Substance Abuse.

History: Key Questions to Ask

1. What is the age of the patient?
2. What is the pattern of onset of the irritability? Was it sudden or gradual? Is there a temporal pattern? Are there specific stimuli that induce the irritability?
3. What relieves or diminishes the symptoms?
4. Are there any associated neurologic symptoms?
5. What has been the impact of the symptoms on the patient's daily activities?
6. What is the patient's ability to function in daily activities like?
7. Is there any use of prescription medications?
8. Is there any alcohol or other type of substance abuse?
9. Is there any history of head trauma?
10. Are there any stressors in the patient's life prior to and during the onset of the symptom of irritability?
11. Are there any concurrent medical conditions?

The history taken from the patient should be complete but should include the specific questions listed above to help narrow down the differential diagnosis.

Clinical Findings

1. Vital signs may show tachycardia, tachypnea, and mild hypertension consistent with adrenergic stimulation, especially when the irritability is due to hyperthyroidism, substance abuse, or withdrawal syndromes.
2. Oral findings of chelosis and glossitis may be present with vitamin-deficiency states.
3. Evidence of head trauma may be present in postconcussive disorder.
4. Abnormalities of the neurologic examination may be present, as in vitamin B_{12} deficiency; loss of vibratory sense, proprioception, and touch sensation are early findings. In dementia, altered mental status will be present, as well as other abnormalities associated with

frontal lobe deterioration and Parkinson's and Huntington's diseases.

Many of the conditions associated with the symptom of irritability will show no findings on physical examination, especially the psychiatric syndromes, premenstrual syndrome, menopause, and sleep deprivation. Other conditions will show nonspecific physical examination findings, such as signs of adrenergic stimulation.

Tests

1. Electrolytes and glucose, calcium, magnesium
2. Blood count with indices
3. Mini-Mental Status Exam
4. Vitamin B_{12} level
5. Thyroid function tests
6. Toxicology screen

The clinical tests performed will depend on the likelihood of uncovering the cause of irritability by performing the test. All patients with irritability that cannot be easily explained on the basis of the history and physical examination should probably get electrolytes, blood count, and mental status examination. The other tests on the list would only be appropriate if indicated by the history and physical examination. Under specific circumstances more testing may be appropriate; for example, if dementia is uncovered, the physician should search for reversible causes. If a sleep disorder is suspected, a sleep study should be considered.

Management

There is no single treatment for irritability because of the many possible causes of the symptom. Management should be directed at treating the underlying condition. Physicians may be tempted to treat irritability with sedative or anxiolytic medications, but this treatment should be avoided unless it is aimed at treating a specific condition. Referral to a psychiatrist may be indicated if no underlying medical condition is uncovered.

> ### PEARLS
>
> - Irritability is a nonspecific symptom of many varied causes that result in impatience or hyperexcitability to stimuli.
>
> - Irritability may occur as an appropriate reaction to psychological stress, pain, or discomfort. In that setting, no extensive evaluation is required, and treatment should be aimed at relieving the stressors.
>
> - Excessive irritability should be evaluated by taking a complete history and performing a complete physical examination.
>
> - Treatment of irritability should be aimed at the causative condition.

Bibliography

American Psychiatric Association: Diagnostic and Statistical Manual of Mental Disorders, 3rd ed. revised. Washington, American Psychiatric Association, 1987, pp 97–254.

Maly RC: Early recognition of chemical dependence [published erratum appears in Prim Care 1993; 20(2):x]. Primary Care 1993;20(1):33–50.

Pariser SF: Women and mood disorders: Menarche to menopause. Ann Clin Psychiatry 1993;5(4):249–254.

Shattil S, Cooper R: Anemia, weakness and pallor, and Vitter R: Sore tongue and sore mouth. *In* Blacklow RS (ed): MacBryde's Signs and Symptoms. Philadelphia, JB Lippincott, 1983, pp 569–570, 123–124.

Wartofsky L: Diseases of the thyroid. *In* Isselbacher ED, et al (eds): Harrison's Principles of Internal Medicine, 13th ed, vol 2. New York, McGraw-Hill, 1994, pp 1941–1943.

309 Marital Discord

Ray Pastorino

The issues underlying marital discord are as diverse and multifaceted as the people involved in those conflicts. Each marriage is psychologically unique, as is each conflict. The content or subject matter of the discord is not as important as the following constants: how well and clearly the parties and/or family system communicates or goes about attempting to resolve conflict, the stress level and pain existing within the marriage, attitudes toward the resolution of conflict, and the options and resources available to couples for resolving discord.

Etiology

1. The most common features underlying marital discord are conflict and distress. Conflict may be engaged or stress generated through factors either internal or external to the marriage. The *DSM-IV,* code 61.1 (1994), defines partner relational problems as a category that should be used "when the focus of clinical attention is a pattern of interaction between spouses or partners characterized by negative communication (e.g., criticisms), distorted communication (e.g., unrealistic expectations), or noncommunication (e.g., withdrawal) that is associated with clinically significant impairment in individual or family functioning or the development of symptoms in one or both partners." Other factors that may be seen as contributing to the discord schema include the following:

   a. Transiting developmental stages of life (e.g., the newly married couple, the advent of children, children going to school, adolescence, children leaving home, the empty nest, retirement). Such developmental stages of life and the stress experienced transiting them may be further amplified by divorce, single parenting, death of a family member or partner, remarriage (blended family configurations), history of childhood abuse, and the use of dominant paradigm win-lose problem-solving and communication styles.

   b. Symptom-, illness-, or disability-focused families may include the child-centered family, families configured around an alcohol/drug-dependent, asthmatic, or disabled or mentally ill member, sexual dysfunction or abuse. Where sexual abuse is reported and founded, the child victim will commonly be removed from the home, frequently leading to divorce. Illness or the death of a child may well create the greatest strain on a marriage. Where a child has died of illness or accident, more than 50 per cent end in divorce.

   c. The couple's ability or inability to negotiate and resolve universal issues such as time spent together or apart, housekeeping chores and upkeep, fiscal management of the new family, and both interactions and limit setting with extended families. The marital relationship alters the individual's sense of control, however well or poorly realized, that existed prior to marriage. As a result, the marriage becomes the crucible within which conflicts over power and control arise. All marriages, particularly those which produce children, will have to address these issues. Absent specific parent effectiveness training, the effect of normal problems will be escalated.

   d. Marital discord also will be found more prevalent in couples whose own parents were divorced and in couples who were married as teenagers. Differences in socioeconomic background also may lead to discord, as will issues emanating from the family of origin (e.g., unrealistic expectations by one spouse for the partner to be either an all-giving mother or all-protective father figure may lead to disappointment when expectations are not met).

   e. Choice of conflict-resolution modalities may serve to amplify both conflict and distress. Adults have not typically been taught cooperative/collaborative problem-solving skills. As children, significant difference and conflict among peers is first encountered during the latency stage, specifically third grade, when simultaneous efforts to master social skills occur. This becomes a crucial time for children to learn nonadversarial communication skills. Typically this does not happen, and children learn the options that are available to them: adversarial (legal) and authoritarian-based processes (dependent on third-party decision makers), aggression, avoidance, and triangulation. These options commonly lead to further escalation of conflict and separation of the parties rather than resolution and reconciliation. These options also prestructure attitudes regarding conflict resolution, thus establishing lifelong patterns of problem solving grounded in authority and competition versus cooperation and collaboration.

2. Attitudes toward conflict in the United States tend to prefigure the manner in which conflict is experienced. Conflict is typically eschewed by most and certainly not normatively seen as an opportunity for positive change and growth. The language and semantic structuring of conflict is that of "war," witnessed by the attitudes and strategies felt toward and used against one's "adversary."

Symptoms

1. Symptoms of marital discord will be found either overtly or covertly. Overt symptoms may include direct verbal reference to intermarital conflict and dissatisfaction as well as direct displays of anger, anxiety, and depression. Covert symptoms may appear through substance abuse or dependence, infidelities, reduction in the patient's normal performance at work, increased withdrawal from normal activities, sexual dysfunction, eating disorders, and acting-out behavior on the part of one or more children. Children's behavior that may actually signal marital problems may include siblings fighting among themselves or with others at school, diminished school performance, truancy, and suspensions from school.

2. Evidence of domestic violence highlights both individual pathology and marital discord. Marital discord, if left unaddressed, may trigger escalating levels of domestic violence. Indicators of abuse include the following:

   a. Repeated injuries difficult to account for as accidental

   b. Vague complaints or acute anxiety with no reported injuries

   c. Strokes in young women: Consider blows to head or strangulation.

   d. Isolation of the women with concomitant fear of partner's anger or of harm

   e. Reluctance to speak or disagree in presence of abuser

Key Symptoms

- Direct reference to discord
- Marital focused depression/anxiety
- Decrease in work performance
- Withdrawal from normal activity
- History of domestic violence
- Substance abuse/ dependence
- Parent-child problems
- Infidelities

Differential Diagnosis

1. Diagnosis of marital problems may be uncomplicated when overt symptoms are demonstrated. However, when exploring covert symptomatology (e.g., passive and bruised patient, acting-out children) or in choosing a treatment modality, a thorough history and construction of an extended family genogram will be useful. Couples unwilling or unable to approach resolving discord through cooperative procedures or those also experiencing substance abuse, chronic depression, or domestic violence will require specific interventions/referrals prior to marital counseling or mediation.

2. Healthy marriages that continue to grow evidence equality and shared power, with open and honest communication between spouses. Individuals in these marriages seek to resolve conflicts (versus winning and being right), and both realize and accept that the marriage will require commitment and hard work. These couples will be open to collaborative, win-win approaches to problem solving.

Treatment

1. Preventive education and counseling: Preventive education in the form of premarital counseling and guidance, parenting classes, and the development of conflict-resolution skills is always useful for individuals and couples contemplating marriage, as are prenuptial agreements. Working with a trained professional, therapist, or communication specialist early in life and at least before or early in a marriage allows a couple to safely explore their compatibility and learn basic and effective communication skills. Frequently, marital discord presents when already beyond the point of no return. Therefore, it becomes helpful, instructive, and therapeutic to encourage couples to seek the help of a therapist or mediator when interpersonal conflicts first appear in order to constructively manage what are frequently very normal differences and learn new skills to address these problems.

2. Mediation and conflict management: Referring couples to mediation and conflict-resolution specialists has become popular and promising. Mediative approaches carry neither the stigmas of the courtroom, disease, or the psychotherapist. These approaches offer a safe context within which both collaborative problem solving and authentic encounter of human likeness and difference may be creatively met, experienced, and resolved. Perhaps more effective long-range prevention may be initiated by physicians through their encouragement of peer-conflict management programs in local schools (grades 3 through 12). Children begin to encounter difference and engage in conflict in the second to third grade. Providing win-win conflict-resolution skills at this critical juncture potentiates better communication and problem-solving life skills. With systemic change at this level, family and cultural systems are unable to remain static.

3. Primary-care couples/family counseling or referral: The physician who is interested may elect to counsel or mediate for couples and/or families directly. If so, the physician will want to obtain additional information and training in the area of conflict resolution or systemic couples or family therapy (see Note, next page). The latter may be conducted either in brief or multiple-couples forms. In the alternative, referral to qualified mental health professionals and conflict managers is recommended.

Key Treatment

Treatment of Choice	Alternative Treatment
• Preventive education/ counseling	• Primary-care counseling
• Mediation/conflict resolution	• Referral to professional

Bibliography

American Psychiatric Association: Diagnostic Criteria from Diagnostic and Statistical Manual, 4th ed. Washington, American Psychiatric Association, 1994

Fisher R, Ury W: Getting to Yes: Negotiating Agreement Without Giving In. New York, Penguin Books, 1991.

Pastorino R: A ''user''-designed mediation approach: Fostering evolutionary consciousness and competence. World Futures 1993;36:155–164.

Ury W: Getting Past No: Negotiating With Difficult People. New York, Bantam Books, 1991.

Note: For more detailed information and networking concerning conflict resolution, you may contact the Institute for Conflict Analysis and Resolution at George Mason University, Fairfax, Virginia, or the Institute for Multi-Track Diplomacy, 1133 20th Street, NW, Suite 321, Washington DC 20036.

310 Domestic Violence

Howard A. Holtz

Etiology

1. Power imbalance in intimate adult relationships often reflects historical and present-day gender bias. Subjugation of women or misogyny in society can be reflected in interpersonal relationships; that is, the private may mirror the public.

2. Male moral development and socialization are marked by absolute principles (right and wrong), taking control, and action, while women typically develop more contextual ethics and collaborative and emotional processing skills. These differences may help explain why women are so often the recipients and men the perpetrators of domestic violence.

3. Despite these important sex differences, female-to-male and homosexual domestic violence does occur. However, male-to-female domestic violence is the major public health problem.

4. Observing violence in one's family or community or in repeated cultural exposures may model behavior or even teach that violence often works to achieve one's goals.

5. Alcohol and other drugs may be a permissive factor and are commonly associated with episodes of domestic violence but are not thought to be causal.

Symptoms

1. The main risk factor is being a woman; females most frequently experience the effects of domestic violence perpetrated by men. Because domestic violence is so common (3 to 4 million adult women battered every year in the United States) and the symptoms so varied, all women should be asked about physical, emotional, and sexual abuse in the social history.

2. The response to domestic violence may manifest as chronic pain, headaches, functional gastrointestinal (GI) or gynecologic symptoms (irritable bowel, pelvic pain), or musculoskeletal complaints. These somatic presentations are thought to occur more commonly in battered women because of the stress of living in violent relationships. Sensorineural hearing loss, bruises, soft-tissue swelling, fractures, and "spontaneous" abortions may result directly from physical abuse. Before *any* psychiatric diagnosis is given to a woman, especially panic disorder, post-traumatic stress disorder, depression, personality disorder, dysthymia, generalized anxiety disorder, or somatization disorder, one must ask about a history of domestic violence. The diagnosis often changes from "major depression" to "major depression secondary to domestic violence."

Key Symptoms

- Chronic pain
- Headache
- Functional GI, gynecologic, musculoskeletal complaints

Clinical Findings

There are no pathognomonic physical signs. Most injuries are non-life-threatening soft-tissue injuries. The lack of findings to support an organic disease process should prompt the physician to ask about domestic violence as an underlying social cause of the patient's complaints.

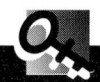

Key Sign

- None or repeated soft-tissue injuries

Laboratory Tests

1. Occasionally, occult trauma can be detected radiographically (i.e. healed fractures, bony fragments, or calcification from previous internal bleeding); however, the most useful diagnostic tests are questions in the history.

2. Screening questions: Does your partner ever lose his temper? What happens when he does? Have you ever been slapped, hit, or kicked by your partner? Are you ever afraid to speak your mind with your partner? Have you ever been forced to engage in sexual activity? Have you ever had to call the police or obtain a restraining order against your partner?

3. Case-finding questions: I see many women who have problems similar to yours who have been humiliated or beaten at home; has this ever happened to you? Did someone do this to you?

Key Test

- Radiograph (or none)

Differential Diagnosis

1. Accidental trauma
2. Migraine or tension headache
3. Fibromyalgia
4. Irritable bowel syndrome, functional dyspepsia
5. Affective and anxiety disorders
6. Somatoform disorders, personality disorders

7. Dyspareunia, pelvic pain, endometriosis
8. Disorders associated with recurrent "spontaneous" abortion
9. Substance abuse (may be associated problem in abuser or victim)

Treatment

Medication

Do not overprescribe psychotropic drugs if domestic violence is the primary problem; occasionally, temporary symptom control with anxiety-reducing drugs or antidepressants is required. Make it clear in the medical record that the *primary* problem is domestic violence and not psychiatric.

Patient Education

ABCDES

1. *A* stands for *alone.* Acknowledge the loneliness and isolation your patient has most likely experienced. Tell her how common a problem violence against women is and how commonly you identify it in your practice. Validate the anguish that she and other women in abusive relationships endure in facing the problem alone.

2. *B* stands for *belief.* This is your belief that the violence is wrong, that it is a crime inside as well as outside the home. Articulate your conviction that violence is the responsibility of the batterer. Regardless of specific problems in a relationship, violence is not an acceptable solution. If her self-esteem has been seriously eroded by the abuser, this statement of belief correctly defines the problem. It categorizes the violence as a problem of the abuser and begins the process of empowering the woman.

3. *C* stands for *confidentiality.* Adult domestic violence is not child abuse, where the legal and developmental incompetence of the victim requires providers to report to public protective agencies. Let the patient know that it is important to document the findings regarding domestic violence in the chart but that the information will not be released or disclosed without her permission. Explain that as a "medicolegal" document, her medical record can be very helpful in child custody and divorce proceedings, in obtaining restraining orders, or in criminal prosecutions, if pursued in the future.

4. *D* stands for *documentation.* As noted above, the medical record can be pivotal in future court decisions. Even when women are unable to admit that they have been battered, it is appropriate to make an assessment of battering if this is the most likely diagnosis:

   "The pattern and frequency of injuries, as well as the anxiety demonstrated by the patient when discussing her husband, are characteristic of battered women syndrome."

   Avoid pejorative negative descriptors and psychiatric labels, such as "hysterical" or "borderline." The emotional reaction of being out of control is a logical reflection of what the woman experienced. Women may more accurately be described as frightened, trembling, angry, anxious, crying, or re-experiencing a traumatic event, but most important, it must be described as secondary to the domestic violence.

5. *E* stands for *education.*
   a. It is imperative that women be given referrals to community resources. Battered women's shelters often provide much more than emergency shelter. They often provide 24-hour hotline numbers, nonresident counseling and support groups, programs for children who have witnessed their mother's abuse, and programs for batterers. Some provide legal advocacy for victims and community education for professionals and their staffs. Women's organizations, coalitions for battered women, hospital-based programs, and government-sponsored victim's assistance programs also may provide these and other services.
   b. Referrals to private mental health providers must be based on their expertise and appreciation of the dynamics of domestic violence. The consultants' professional group (social worker, counselor, psychologist, psychiatrist) is less important than their knowledge of domestic violence. Couples counseling is generally inappropriate and a potentially dangerous therapy in relationships characterized by power imbalance. If a shelter or coalition cannot recommend a counselor/therapist, it is important to question potential consultants about their approach to domestic violence victims. Do they express a strong *belief,* as noted above, or do they tend to practice a form of victim blaming by exploring the victim's personality to look for provocative or facilitating traits?
   c. Legal options, such as the availability of temporary restraining orders, also can be discussed. Excellent patient education pamphlets are available and can be displayed in waiting rooms, bathrooms, and examining areas.

6. *S* stands for *safety.*
   a. A safety plan is an essential aspect of the patient encounter. A quick escape plan should be rehearsed, similar to a fire drill. If it is feasible, advise the woman to hide important documents, money, an extra set of car keys, clothes, and meaningful items for the children for quick getaways. Risk increases when there is concomitant sexual abuse, threats of death, a pattern of escalating violence, or when weapons are available. However, it is the woman who can best assess the potential for serious injury or death. If she tells you her husband will not respect a temporary restraining order and will attack her on the courthouse steps, believe her. Too many women have

died because professionals have underestimated how an abuser will react to a changing domestic situation or legal restraints.

b. If emergency shelter is not available, you can admit a patient to the hospital. The ICD diagnosis and code are Battered Adult Syndrome: 995.81. The following safeguards should be in place to protect a victim admitted to the hospital: visitor restriction, patient information blackout, notification of hospital security, and contacting local police.

Follow-Up

Women often cannot extricate themselves from violent relationships because abusers continue to stalk them or threaten worse abuse if they leave; other reasons include financial or emotional barriers. Do not become angry and judgmental if a woman does not leave a violent relationship on your time schedule. Include domestic violence as a chronic problem and ask about it on follow-up visits; leave your door open as an informed advocate who can help her when she is ready to make changes.

 Bibliography

Flitcraft AH, Hadley SM, Hendriks-Matthews MK, et al: Diagnostic and Treatment Guidelines on Domestic Violence. Chicago, American Medical Association, 1992.

Holtz HA, Esposito CN, Podhorin R: A domestic violence primer for clinicians. NJ Med 1994;91(12):848–850 (part 1), 853–854, (part 2).

Parker B, McFarlane J, Soeken K: Abuse during pregnancy: Effect on maternal complications and birth weight in adult and teenage women. Obstet Gynecol, 1994;84(3):323–328.

Scarinci IC, McDonald-Haile J, Bradley LA, et al: Altered pain perception and psychosocial features among women with gastrointestinal disorders and a history of abuse: A preliminary model. Am J Med 1994;47:108–118.

Sugg NK, Invi T: Primary care physicians' response to domestic violence: Opening Pandora's box. JAMA 1992;267(23):3157–3160.

311 Personality Disorders (Borderline, Dependent)
Robert M.A. Hirschfeld

Borderline Personality Disorder

Etiology

A. Psychodynamic theories
   1. Excessive aggression
      a. Unstable identity development
      b. Unstable development of affective tolerance
   2. Maternal withdrawal
      a. Incomplete differentiation of child from mother
      b. Dual and inconsistent image of mother
         (1) Rewarding and gratifying in response to dependency
         (2) Punitive and withdrawing in response to autonomy
      c. Child rejects attention to reality in order to maintain relationship with the mother.
   3. Introjective failure: child's failure to internalize sense of self
B. Biogenetic theories
   1. Affective dysregulation
      a. Inability to modulate emotional responses to environmental events (e.g., easy to rage, quickly to sadness)
      b. Secondary to defect in brain catecholamine metabolism
   2. Neurologic dysfunction
      a. Due to genetic predisposition or "early organic insult"
      b. Low threshold for activation of the limbic structures

Symptoms

A. Frantic efforts to avoid real or imagined abandonment
B. A pattern of unstable and intense interpersonal relationships characterized by alternating between extremes of idealization and devaluation
C. Identity disturbance: persistent and markedly disturbed, distorted, or unstable self-image or sense of self
D. Impulsivity in at least two areas that are potentially self-damaging (e.g., spending, sex, substance abuse, reckless driving, binge eating)
E. Recurrent suicidal behaviors, gestures, or threats, or self-mutilating behavior
F. Affective instability due to a marked reactivity of mood (e.g., intense episodic dysphoria, irritability, or anxiety usually lasting a few hours and only rarely more than a few days)
G. Chronic feelings of emptiness
H. Inappropriate, intense anger or lack of control of anger (e.g., frequent displays of temper, constant anger, recurrent physical fights)
I. Transient, stress-related paranoid ideation or severe dissociative symptoms

Differential Diagnosis

A. Often co-occurs with other disorders, such as mood disorders
   1. Symptoms must occur in absence of mood symptoms
   2. Personality pattern must be early onset and long-standing
B. Differential diagnosis of other personality disorders
   1. Histrionic personality disorder
      a. Histrionic patients
         (1) Exhibit more pure attention seeking from everyone
         (2) Exhibit more superficial behavior
      b. Borderline personality disorder patients
         (1) Exhibit self-destructiveness
         (2) Exhibit angry disruptions in close relationships
         (3) Exhibit chronic feelings of deep emptiness and loneliness
   2. Schizotypal personality disorder
      a. Common symptoms: paranoid ideas and illusions
      b. Differences: Common symptoms are much more transient, interpersonally reactive, and responsive to external structuring in borderline personality disorder.
   3. Paranoid personality disorder: Characteristics of paranoid personality disorder distinguishable from borderline personality disorder
      a. Relative stability of self-image
      b. Lack of self-destructiveness
      c. Lack of impulsivity
      d. Lack of abandonment concerns
   4. Narcissistic personality disorder: Characteristics of narcissistic personality disorder distinguishable from borderline personality disorder
      a. Relative stability of self-image
      b. Lack of self-destructiveness
      c. Lack of impulsivity

d. Lack of abandonment concerns

5. Antisocial personality disorder

a. Common symptoms: manipulative behavior

b. Differences

(1) Borderline personality disorder patients are manipulative to gain nurturance.

(2) Antisocial personality disorder patients are manipulative for material gratification, power, or profit.

Treatment

A. Psychodynamic psychotherapy

1. Establish secure attachment and trusting alliance with patient to establish sense of safety.

2. Provide stable treatment framework with clear patient-physician boundaries, schedules, and rules and fairness.

3. Therapist must actively identify, confront, and direct the patient's behaviors; establish connection between actions and feelings.

4. Set limits on behaviors that threaten safety of the patient or therapist or the continuation of therapy.

5. Make self-destructive behaviors ungratifying.

B. Supportive psychotherapy: Aim to improve patient's adaptation to life circumstances and diminish self-destructive responses to interpersonal conflicts.

C. Cognitive therapy

1. Develop a collaborative relationship with specific goals.

2. Select initial goals or target areas.

3. Minimize noncompliance through adhering to treatment framework.

4. Make the patient aware of dichotomous thinking (review experience along continuum rather than absolute right or wrong behavior) and work to identify and decrease it.

5. Increase control over emotions.

6. Improve impulse control.

7. Strengthen sense of identity.

8. Develop alternative nondestructive strategies to combat sense of emptiness and threat of abandonment.

D. Dialectical behavior therapy: combination of individual and group therapy

1. Group focuses on behavioral coping skills.

2. Individual focuses on six hierarchically set goals

a. Suicidal behaviors

b. Therapy-interfering behaviors

c. Behaviors that interfere with quality of life

d. Behavioral skill acquisition

e. Post-traumatic stress behavior

f. Self-respect behavior

E. Group therapy

1. Peers confront maladaptive and impulsive patterns without being perceived as controlling to the patient.

2. Dependent or maladaptive gratifications are more easily made undesirable.

3. Group demonstrates a number of different coping methods.

4. Network of support

F. Pharmacotherapy

1. Tricyclic antidepressants and selective serotonin reuptake inhibitors

2. Monoamine oxidase inhibitors

3. Lithium carbonate and anticonvulsants: control angry impulses.

4. Neuroleptics: low-dose effects in reducing depression, anxiety, hostility, and psychotic-like symptoms (depersonalization, derealization, illusions, and ideas of reference)

5. Anxiolytics: Use cautiously.

Follow-Up

A. Sustained long-term psychotherapy for 3 to 5 years

B. Compliance

C. Monitor effectiveness and judge side effects of pharmacotherapy.

Bibliography

American Psychiatric Association: Diagnostic and Statistical Manual of Mental Disorders, 4th ed. Washington, DC, American Psychiatric Association, 1994.

Gunderson JG: Borderline Personality Disorder. Washington, DC, American Psychiatric Press, 1989.

Gunderson J, Links P: Treatment of borderline personality disorders. *In* Gabbard GO (ed): Treatment of Psychiatric Disorders: The DSM-IV Edition. Washington, DC, American Psychiatric Association, 1995.

Tasman A, Hales RE, Frances AJ: Review of Psychiatry, vol 8, sec I. Eds: Washington, DC, American Psychiatric Press, 1989.

Treatments of Psychiatric Disorders, vol 3, sec 26. Washington, DC, American Psychiatric Association, 1989.

Dependent Personality Disorder

Etiology

A. Primary symptoms are predominantly submissive, reactive, and clinging behavior.

B. Psychoanalytic theory: drawn to others to satisfy instinctual drive of dependency

C. Social psychological theory

1. Dependency is a learned behavior, a drive secondary to primary drives such as hunger or thirst, acquired with experience.

2. Dependency displayed in the mother-child relationship is generalized to other interpersonal relationships.

D. Ethologic theory

1. Dependency is a form of attachment (i.e., emotional bonds between people).

2. Wish to be close to and in contact with the dependent object; upset if separation occurs

Symptoms

A. Is unable to make everyday decisions without an excessive amount of advice and reassurance from others

B. Needs others to assume responsibility for most major areas of his or her life

C. Has difficulty expressing disagreement with others because of fear of loss of support or approval

D. Has difficulty initiating projects or doing things on his or her own because of a lack of self-confidence in judgment or abilities rather than because of a lack of motivation or energy

E. Goes to excessive lengths to obtain nurturance and support from others, to the point of volunteering to do things that are unpleasant

F. Feels uncomfortable or helpless when alone, because of exaggerated fears of being unable to care for himself or herself

G. Urgently seeks another relationship as a source of care and support when a close relationship ends

H. Unrealistic preoccupation with fears of being left to take care of himself or herself

Differential Diagnosis

A. Borderline personality disorder

1. Common symptoms of fear of abandonment

2. Differences

a. Characteristic of borderline personality disorder

(1) Reacts to abandonment with feelings of emotional emptiness, rage, and demands

(2) Unstable and intense relationships

b. Characteristic of dependent personality disorder

(1) Reacts to abandonment with increasing appeasement and submissiveness

(2) Urgently seeks a replacement relationship to provide caregiving and support

B. Histrionic personality disorder

1. Common symptoms

a. Appears childlike and clinging

b. Has a strong need for reassurance and approval

2. Differences

a. Characteristic of histrionic personality disorder

(1) Flamboyant

(2) Actively demands attention

(3) Gregarious and charming behavior

b. Characteristic of dependent personality disorder

(1) Self-effacing

(2) Docile

C. Avoidant personality disorder

1. Common symptoms

a. Feelings of inadequacy

b. Hypersensitivity to criticism

c. Need for reassurance

2. Differences

a. Characteristic of avoidant personality disorder: such a strong fear of humiliation and rejection that these patients withdraw unless they are certain that they will be accepted

b. Characteristic of dependent personality disorder: pattern of seeking and maintaining connections to important others rather than avoiding and withdrawing from relationships

D. Dependency as a consequence of Axis I disorders

1. Present in other disorders

a. Mood disorders

b. Panic disorders

c. Agoraphobia

2. Characteristic of dependent personality disorder

a. Early onset, chronic course, and symptoms that do not occur in Axis I patients

b. Traits that are inflexible, maladaptive, and cause significant functional impairment or subjective distress

Treatment

A. Individual psychodynamic psychotherapy

1. Develop trusting relationship with the patient and allow the patient to transfer dependent wishes onto the therapist

2. Encourage expression of real feelings and wishes, endurance of the anxiety of making decisions, acceptance of pleasurable experiences

3. Allow the patient to make own decisions

4. Conceptualize goals and encourage commitment to attaining these goals

5. Limit sessions and self-empower the patient

B. Cognitive behavior therapy

1. Form techniques to foster accurate self-appraisal and independent decision-making behavior.

2. Define goals and set agendas for sessions.

3. Challenge dichotomous thinking of the patient.

4. Encourage in vivo exposure to anxiety-provoking situations.

5. Develop positive behavior schemas and constructive substitute behaviors to replace old dependency habits.

6. Encourage use of relaxation, assertiveness training, role playing as adjunctive treatment.

C. Pharmacotherapy
Some improvement in symptoms of concurrent Axis I disorders but overall full recovery is unlikely.

Follow-up

A. Long-term treatment of 3 to 5 years

B. Tapering number of sessions but still making them available

Bibliography

American Psychiatric Association: Diagnostic and Statistical Manual of Mental Disorders, 4th ed. Washington, DC, American Psychiatric Association, 1994.

Frances AJ, Hales RE (eds): Psychiatric Update: American Psychiatric Association Annual Review, Vol 5. Washington, DC, American Psychiatric Press, 1986.

Perry C: Treatment of dependent personality disorder. *In* Treatment of Psychiatric Disorders: DSM-IV Edition. in press.

Treatments of Psychiatric Disorders, Vol 3, Section 26. Washington, DC, American Psychiatric Association, 1989.

312 Somatoform Disorders

Dale A. Matthews

Etiology

1. Predisposing factors
   a. Frequent or severe illness during childhood
   b. Overprotective parents
   c. Personal or family histories of psychiatric illness, alcoholism and drug addiction, physical and sexual abuse, divorce, and antisocial behavior
   d. Lower educational attainment and socioeconomic class
2. Precipitating factors
   a. Stressful life events (e.g., bereavement, acute physical illness or injury)
   b. Overwork or strenuous activity prior to the illness (i.e., "burnout")
3. Perpetuating factors
   a. Development and maintenance of the "sick role"
   b. Poor self-esteem, impaired social and occupational skills, ongoing disability claims (and other forms of "secondary gain")
   c. Physicians' somatization through excessive diagnostic testing or an unwillingness to explore psychosocial concerns

Symptoms

Recurrent somatic symptoms in multiple organ systems unexplained by medical illness or known pathophysiologic mechanisms, or if disease is present, the symptoms are in excess of what would be expected.

Key Symptoms

• Chest pain	• Dizziness
• Abdominal pain	• Palpitations
• Back pain	• Nausea
• Headaches	• Vomiting
• Dysmenorrhea	• Anorexia
• Fatigue	• Food intolerance
• Weakness	• Sexual indifference
• Paralysis	

Clinical Findings

1. Multiple, diffuse or vague complaints, fear and conviction of serious illness, and preoccupation with or exaggeration of bodily symptoms.
2. Usually seen in general medical or surgical settings: Patients generally eschew psychiatrists. Extensive use of medical care system. Many doctors are consulted (often concurrently), and patients undergo many types of diagnostic tests and treatments (including multiple medications and surgeries) to little avail. Iatrogenic illness (e.g., increased side effects from medications) is common.
3. Often, a histrionic personality style is found with dramatic, emotional, seductive, and/or shallow affect and vague inconsistent and/or contradictory histories.
4. A low pain threshold, heightened sensitivity to stimuli, an excessive fear of illness, aging, and death, and overconcern about appearance may be found. Self-esteem is low. Many are overly self-conscious, vulnerable to stress, prone to excessive self-criticism and feelings of shame and guilt, and believe they deserve punishment. They tend to be anxious, depressed, hostile, and dependent.
5. The illness or symptom may have a symbolic meaning (e.g., deafness after "hearing bad news"), thereby serving as a means of communicating distress. Alexithymia (inability to express emotion in verbal terms) may be present. Patients may vigorously deny the role of psychological factors in the development of symptoms.

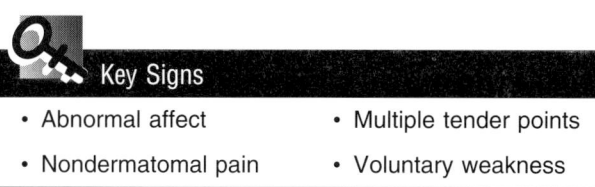

Key Signs

• Abnormal affect	• Multiple tender points
• Nondermatomal pain	• Voluntary weakness

Laboratory Tests

1. No laboratory findings are pathognomonic, although extensive testing is common. If minor abnormalities are found, symptoms may be in excess of the usual clinical findings for that laboratory test. If significant abnormalities are found, organic illness must be considered.
2. Diagnostic restraint is advisable: Tests should be done only when classic presentations of illness or objective signs of disease are found.

Differential Diagnosis

1. The somatoform disorders include
   a. Body dysmorphic disorder (preoccupation with some imagined defect in appearance)
   b. Conversion disorder (loss or impairment of functioning suggestive of a physical disorder that is instead an expression of a psychological conflict or need)

1105

c. Hypochondriasis (preoccupation with fear of having a serious disease)

d. Somatization disorder (a long-standing history of recurrent and multiple somatic complaints or belief that one is sickly)

e. Pain disorder (preoccupation with pain in the absence of adequate physical findings to account for the pain or its intensity)

2. Other psychiatric illnesses to consider

a. Mood and anxiety disorders (particularly major depression and panic disorder)

b. Substance abuse

c. Personality disorders (e.g., histrionic, borderline, passive-dependent, narcissistic)

d. Schizophrenia

3. Medical illnesses to consider

a. Myasthenia gravis

b. Multiple sclerosis

c. Systemic lupus erythematosus

d. Acute intermittent porphyria

e. Endocrine disorders (hypothyroidism/hyperthyroidism, hypocortisolism/hypercortisolism, and hyperparathyroidism)

Treatment

1. Listen patiently to the "organ recital" of complaints, taking each symptom seriously, negotiating which symptoms to evaluate during the visit, and performing a brief, focused physical examination at each visit.

2. Accept and acknowledge the symptoms as genuine expressions of suffering, thereby giving "permission" to the patient to receive the care he or she desperately needs. Do not dispute the reality of the complaint, but do not promise quick relief or cure. The goal is to minimize disability and maximize functional capacity and the patient's sense of control over the symptom.

3. Gently and gradually begin to encourage (by selective attention and reinforcement) verbal expression of problems and feelings in lieu of new somatic symptoms. Recognize and reward any incipient personal insights and growth and healthy behaviors and coping mechanisms.

4. Do not just "rule out" organic illness, but "rule in" treatable psychiatric illness using standard psychiatric criteria. However, do not prematurely assume that the complaint reflects psychologic stress and not treatable organic illness.

5. Use a multimodal approach, incorporating fitness training, relaxation, and other stress-management approaches.

6. Find something to admire and respect in the patient (e.g., ability to endure despite prolonged and severe discomfort). Empathize and try to understand his/her

point of view. Discover the patient's model of illness and expectations regarding care, and negotiate together an acceptable explanation of the illness and treatment plan. Address conflicts explicitly.

7. Validate and legitimize the need for continued medical attention and ensure long-term continuity and availability. Focus on establishing a long-term, trusting relationship. Use referral sparingly. Find a psychiatrist adept in the medicine-psychiatry interface to use as needed. Encourage group therapy.

8. Be realistic about the goals of treatment. Set appropriate personal and professional limits. Obtain support from colleagues to avoid building frustration and resentment.

Medication
Treat depression, anxiety, or other concomitant psychiatric disorders as needed; otherwise try to avoid drugs.

Diet
1. No specific diet is necessary, but a healthy, well-balanced diet tailored to individual needs is a useful adjunct.

2. In a desperate search to get well, some try a great variety of dietary regimens or other self-help methods with little success. Unusual "fad" diets with extravagant claims (and price tags) should be discouraged.

Activity
General conditioning and aerobic exercise are a useful general aid to health by building self-esteem and confidence.

Patient Education
Patients should be notified whenever tests and examinations do not reveal evidence of significant medical illness. They should always be told that their symptoms and their suffering are real (i.e., not "all in their head") and that they have increased sensitivity to painful stimuli, but that no serious or life-threatening illness is present. They also should be informed that continued careful observation is advisable.

 Key Treatment

- Establish long-term relationship of trust and mutual respect.
- Validate symptoms and need for ongoing treatment
- Use psychotropic medicine for symptoms of depression and anxiety.

Follow-Up

1. To ensure careful follow-up and to prevent the patient from feeling rejected or abandoned, follow-up appointments should always be scheduled on a regular basis (e.g., every 1 to 4 weeks at the beginning) and not made contingent on the development of new symptoms.

2. The appointments can be brief (15 to 20 minutes) and

should always include a brief physical examination tailored to the patient's presenting complaints.

 Bibliography

For details of classification of somatoform disorders, see
American Psychiatric Association (Committee on Nomenclature and Statistics): Diagnostic and Statistical Manual of Mental Disorders, 4th ed. Washington, DC, American Psychiatric Association, 1994.

For comprehensive reviews of the subject from a psychiatric perspective, see
Kellner R: Somatization: Theories and research. J Nerv Ment Dis 1990;178:(3):150–160; and Kellner R: Diagnosis and treatments of hypochondriacal syndromes. Psychosomatics 1992; 33(3):278–289.

For comprehensive reviews of the subject from a primary-care perspective, see
Kaplan C, Lipkin M, Gordon G: Somatization in primary care: Patients with unexplained and vexing medical complaints. J Gen Intern Med 1988;13:177–190; and Smith RC: Somatization disorder: defining its role in clinical medicine. J Gen Intern Med 1991;6(2):168–175.

For an important trial demonstrating the cost-effectiveness of training physicians in diagnosing and treating somatoform disorders, see
Smith GR, Monson RA, Ray DC: Psychiatric consultation in somatization disorder. N Engl J Med 1986;314:1487–1493.

For techniques on how to care for patients with somatization, see
Morrison J: Managing somatization disorder. Dis Mon 1990;36(10):537–591; Bass C, Benjamin S: The management of chronic somatization. Br J Psychiatry 1993;162:472–480; and Creed F, Guthrie E: Techniques for interviewing the somatising patient. Br J Psychiatry 1993;162:467–471.

Procedure THE BATHE TECHNIQUE

Marian R. Stuart

The BATHE technique is a verbal procedure consisting of a series of four questions followed by an empathic response.

B: Background: What is going on in your life?
A: Affect: How do you feel about that?
T: Trouble: What troubles you about that?
H: Handling: How are you handling that?
E: Empathy: That must be very difficult.

Indications

1. To answer the question "Why is the patient here now?" as part of constructing a medical history
2. To establish personal rapport with patients
3. To serve as a rough screening test for anxiety or depression
4. To probe for possible psychosocial precipitants related to somatic complaints
5. To operationalize the biopsychosocial model by establishing the context of the patient's illness
6. To help patients connect their physical symptoms with their emotional responses and the circumstances of their lives
7. To explore a patient's reaction to a diagnosis
8. To handle an unexpected psychosocial revelation at the end of an interview
9. To explore lack of compliance, requests for inappropriate referrals, or other difficult situations in the doctor-patient relationship
10. As a structure for a brief counseling session or a family interview

Contraindications

1. Patients in severe pain or life-threatening circumstances
2. Resistance on the part of the patient, expressed as suspiciousness or hostility

3. Not sufficient in itself for suicidal patients, battered spouses, sexual abuse victims, or substance abusers
4. Psychosis. Also, may be ineffective with personality-disorder patients, especially borderline patients.
5. Modifications may need to be made for patients with developmental disorders, physical handicaps, of different cultural backgrounds, or when language is a barrier.

Preparation

The BATHE technique needs little preparation. In the routine patient interview, it follows the exploration of the reason for the visit. Patients can be BATHEd repeatedly during a visit as relevant history emerges.

Equipment

None required. The physician should sit, make eye contact, listen attentively, and refrain from taking notes or otherwise distracting the patient.

Precautions

1. Try to say nothing except the BATHE questions.
2. Do not allow patients to elaborate at length on the circumstances or details of their situations. Do summarize briefly, and ask the next question.
3. Do not analyze or interpret patients' responses.
4. Avoid giving advice.
5. When patients fail to answer the "affect" question and provide more background information, intervene quickly by repeating, "Yes, but how do you *feel* about that?" until you get a response.
6. When patients express positive feelings, do not assume that there is nothing "troubling" them. Modify the T question accordingly.
7. Recognize that it is not your job to fix the patient's problems, only to provide support and clarification.

Technique

1. *B* = background. "What is going on in your life?" ascertains the context of the visit. If the patient has already discussed this, go directly to affect.
2. *A* = affect. "How do you feel about that?" elicits the patient's emotional response. It is therapeutic for the patient to label the feeling(s).
3. *T* = trouble. "What troubles you the most about that?" gets at the symbolic meaning for the patient.
4. *H* = handling. "How are you handling that?" helps to assess his or her resources and response to the situation.

5. *E* = empathy. "That must be very difficult for you" acknowledges reasonable coping responses. Ideally you would
   a. State the feeling of the patient, that is, "You are really angry. . . ."
   b. Paraphrase your understanding of the circumstances, that is, "Your wife decided. . . ."
   c. Then state that you *can* understand that this must be difficult. Anyone would be upset by that situation. This normalizes the patient's reaction.
6. In a family conference, each member in turn is

BATHEd. This provides information and opens communications.

Follow-Up

1. When a psychosocial problem is uncovered, the patient is asked to return to discuss the situation further.
2. At the return visit, the opening BATHE question becomes, "Tell me what's been happening since I saw you."
3. For further information and additional techniques, see *The Fifteen-Minute Hour.*

Bibliography

Bloom BL: Stuart and Lieberman's fifteen minute hour. *In* Planned Short-Term Psychotherapy: A Clinical Handbook. Boston, Allyn & Bacon, 1992, pp 273–277.

Lieberman JA III, Stuart MR: Practicing biopsychosocial medicine. *In* RE Rakel (ed.): Textbook of Family Practice, 5th ed. Philadelphia, WB Saunders, 1995.

Stuart M, Lieberman JA III: Finding time for counseling in primary care. Patient Care, November 15, 1994;118–127.

Stuart MR, Lieberman JA III: The Fifteen-Minute Hour: Applied Psychotherapy for the Primary Care Physician, 2d ed. Westport, CT, Praeger, 1993.

Stuart MR, Simko MD: A technique for incorporating psychological principles into the nutrition counseling of clients. Top Clin Nutr 1991;6(4):32–39.

313 Depression

Denis F. Darko

Etiology

1. Organic: Depression can be a part of, even a presenting symptom of, medical illness, such as stroke or cancer. Common medical causes of depression are listed below.

2. Psychosocial: Troublesome social circumstances or emotional losses, or childhood emotional loss or trauma, conspire to facilitate depression. It is often an emotional response to loss (death, divorce, job loss), perceived loss (fear of disability or death with the onset of a major medical illness), or a history of a major loss (loss of a parent in childhood) combined with current stressful life circumstances (stressful job, difficult marriage). Depression can develop in response to chronic pain or disability. Medical illness is one of the most severe forms of stress.

3. Heredity: Depression with or without psychosocial precipitants often occurs in individuals with a family history of depression or related illnesses, such as anxiety disorders, bipolar disorder (manic depressive disorder), panic attacks, agoraphobia (fear of being in open spaces), alcoholism or other substance abuse, obsessive compulsive disorder, or anorexia nervosa. This familial association is less relevant in depression caused by medical illness or medication.

4. A brain-based illness: In depression, changes in brain neurochemistry and function can be demonstrated by research methods, including sleep electroencephalographic studies, positron-emission tomography, single-photon-emission computed tomography, or cerebrospinal fluid (CSF) catecholamine metabolite levels.

Symptoms

1. Patients feel sad, down, or depressed most of the day, nearly every day, and lose interest or pleasure in previously enjoyed activities (anhedonia).

2. Decrease or increase in appetite, weight loss or gain, insomnia or hypersomnia, anxiety, daily fatigue, loss of energy, and mental or motor agitation or slowing are other common symptoms.

3. Further possible symptoms are feelings of worthlessness, excessive guilt, diminished ability to think or concentrate, and indecisiveness. Thoughts of death and recurrent suicidal ideation, with or without a plan, may be present. A suicide plan may progress to an actual suicide attempt.

4. Depression in childhood and adolescence can look much different from that in the adult, with onset of behavioral problems, anger, rebelliousness, falling school grades, deterioration of friendships, and emotional distance from parents.

Key Symptoms

- Sadness
- Appetite changes
- Sleep changes/fatigue
- Feels worthless
- Thoughts of death
- Anhedonia
- Anxiety/nervousness
- Difficulty thinking/ concentrating
- Inappropriate guilt
- Suicidal ideation

Clinical Findings

1. The patient presents as discouraged, tired, slowed down, irritable, or angry. Some patients deny that much is wrong and focus solely on physical illness, such as headaches, backache, upset stomach, constipation, or other aches, pains, discomforts, or disability.

2. An alternate clinical presentation is worry, nervousness, perhaps even agitation and pacing in the office. Some patients are demanding, impulsive, or self-dramatizing when depressed.

3. Medical evaluation may find little or no physical pathology.

4. If medical pathology is present (arthritis, low back pain, cardiac arrhythmia), the depressed patient's preoccupation with the illness may be out of proportion to its severity.

Key Signs

- Discouraged, sad
- Nervous/anxious
- Agitated or slowed
- Self-effacing or demanding
- Grumpy/complaining
- Irritable/angry
- Gives a vague history
- Comments about death

Laboratory Tests

1. While laboratory tests confirming depression are not yet available, laboratory tests to rule out other diseases that may present as depression are necessary.

2. Thyroid function studies, complete blood count (CBC) with differential cell count, sedimentation rate, a blood chemistry panel, and urinalysis are needed to support the diagnostic impression by ruling out occult medical illness.

3. Above age 45, an electrocardiogram (ECG) is helpful to rule out arrhythmias or cardiac ischemia as cause

attempt when depressed or a psychotic decompensation with depression that rendered them unable to pursue personal hygiene, good health practices, and activities of daily living.

Bibliography

For more information on mood disorders, see

Kaplan HI, Sadock, BJ: Synopsis of Psychiatry, 6th ed. Baltimore, Williams & Wilkins, 1991, pp 363–388.

For more information on depression in childhood and adolescence, see

Shafii M, Shafii SL (eds): Clinical Guide to Depression in Children and Adolescents, Washington, DC, American Psychiatric Press, 1992.

For more information on diagnostic criteria, see

The Diagnostic and Statistical Manual of Mental Disorders, 4th ed. Washington, DC, American Psychiatric Association, 1994.

For information on the American Psychiatric Association's ''Let's Talk Facts About . . .'' series of pamphlets for patient education, contact

American Psychiatric Press, Inc., 1400 K Street, N.W., Suite 1101, Washington DC 20005; telephone: 1-800-368-5777.

For more information on both the psychopharmacology and psychotherapy of mood disorders, see

Dunner DL (ed): Current Psychiatric Therapy. Philadelphia, WB Saunders, 1993.

for anergy, fatigue, and functional cardiac disability with resultant irritability or discouragement.

4. Test for HIV seropositivity if risk factors, signs, or symptoms indicate.

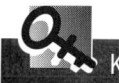

Key Tests

- Thyroid function
- Electrolytes
- Blood urea nitrogen (BUN), creatinine
- ECG
- Complete blood count with differential
- SGOT, LDH, gamma GT
- Sedimentation rate
- HIV

Differential Diagnosis

1. Bipolar mood disorder is probable if the patient has ever had a manic episode (elation or irritability, rapid speech, high energy, racing thoughts, decreased need for sleep, social intrusiveness, poor judgment).

2. Neurologic disorders that may present as depression include dementia (Alzheimer's or multi-infarct), stroke, Parkinson's disease, multiple sclerosis, or temporal lobe epilepsy.

3. Endocrine illnesses that may present as depression include menses-related mood changes, hypothyroidism, apathetic hyperthyroidism, diabetes mellitus, parathyroid disorders, Cushing's disease, Addison's disease, and postpartum endocrine changes.

4. Infectious or inflammatory illnesses may present as or be accompanied by depression, including pneumonia, arthritis, arteritis, lupus, mononucleosis, hepatitis, tuberculosis, HIV, and other viral infections.

5. Other causes of depression include many antihypertensive (e.g., angiotensin-converting enzyme inhibitors, β blockers) and other cardiac medications (e.g., calcium channel blockers, digoxin), alcoholism or other drug abuse, steroid or opiate use, or medications used to treat Parkinson's disease.

6. Further medical illnesses that may present as depression are cardiopulmonary disease, especially that associated with hypoxia, anergy, or anemia (e.g., congestive heart failure, myocardial infarction), cancer, uremia, sleep apnea, a history of severe head injury, and vitamin deficiencies, including folate, B_{12}, and thiamine deficiency. Depression can be associated with any severe medical illness.

> **WARNING**
>
> **Suicidal plan or intent demands immediate intervention to prevent the patient from completing a suicide.**

Treatment

1. Severe depression can be a rapidly fatal illness. Half of all suicides in the United States follow the onset

of a major depression. The most important principle in treatment of depression is to ensure the safety of a suicidal patient, usually with hospitalization.

2. The second important principle in treatment is to discover all contributing or etiologic medical illnesses and pursue vigorous treatment of each.

3. Depression with or without a known organic component is treated most successfully with a combination of an antidepressant (perhaps with an anxiolytic) medication and psychotherapy. Many organic depressions (e.g., depression from prednisone use) can improve when treated with antidepressant medications, despite continuance of the medical cause.

4. Psychotherapy helps the patient cope with the illness and with the need to take medications and tolerate the side effects and to repair disrupted family ties, careers, and friendships. The psychotherapy should at first be supportive in nature (active, encouraging). Several approaches, including psychodynamic, interpersonal, cognitive, and behavioral, have been successful. Success with previous depressed patients, experience, and training of the therapist are important.

5. Psychotherapy may be done by an internist, family physician, pediatrician, or gynecologist, if trained and experienced in psychotherapy, although the time necessary for extended office visits may make this impractical. For some patients, couples therapy, group psychotherapy, or family therapy may be helpful.

Medication

1. The selective serotonin reuptake inhibitors (SSRIs) are the medications of first choice, balancing effectiveness with side effects and patient acceptance. They are not superior to tricyclics in efficacy or onset of action. It is prudent to begin with a low dose for a few days to judge a patient's sensitivity to side effects (headache, dizziness, nausea, nervousness, insomnia, sedation, diarrhea). A typical starting dose may be sertraline, 50-mg tablet, ½ tablet daily. Dose may be increased ½ or 1 tablet each morning after 4 to 7 days if side effects are not uncomfortable for the patient. A typical final effective dose is 50 to 200 mg daily. The available SSRIs are:

   a. Sertraline (Zoloft), 50- and 100-mg scored tablets; paroxetine (Paxil), 20-mg scored and 30-mg tablets; fluoxetine (Prozac), 10- and 20-mg capsules, and 20 mg per 5 ml liquid.

   b. Liquid Prozac may be helpful in the elderly, who respond to and have side effects with small dosages and who may have difficulty splitting tablets. One-eighth teaspoon, containing 2.5 mg, is a good starting dose.

2. If side effects are problematic or the SSRI chosen is not effective at high dose, the medication should be stopped. When stopping any psychotropic medication that has been taken for more than a few weeks, it is safer and more comfortable to the patient to taper the medication slowly. A trial of bupropion (Wellbutrin),

trazodone (Desyrel), nefazodone (Serzone), or one of the tricyclics (desipramine, imipramine) is a reasonable next step. A typical starting dose is bupropion, 75-mg tablet, ½ tablet each morning. Dose may be increased to 1 tablet each morning after 4 to 7 days if side effects (same as with the SSRIs) are not uncomfortable for the patient. The maximum dose is 150 mg three times daily.

3. The usual procedure is to slowly increase the dose of a selected antidepressant (an increment every week) until a good antidepressant response is attained (usually 3 to 6 weeks after the appropriate dose is reached) or problematic side effects develop, preventing further dosage increases.

4. If the patient has bipolar disorder (a history of both manic and depressive episodes), lithium carbonate, carbamazepine, and valproic acid are necessary medications in the treatment regimen to prevent a manic episode. A typical starting dose of lithium is 300 mg daily or twice daily, with dosage adjustments over time based on blood levels (therapeutic range is 0.5 to 1.0 mEq/L) and side effects (tremor, nausea, diarrhea, malaise).

5. While the monoamine oxidase inhibitors (MAOIs) are safe and effective when used properly, the dietary and medication restrictions add complexity to their use. They are best used by physicians who have time for and interest in this further effort and when depression has been refractory to other medications combined with psychotherapy.

Diet

1. While specific diets have not been found helpful in the treatment of depression, healthy diet is a component of treatment. The anorexia of depression can cause weight loss and poor nutrition, while the hyperphagia of depression can cause weight gain and unhealthy diet (high fat, high sodium, low fiber). Poor diet may augment the anergy and malaise of depression.

2. Healthy and appropriate diet to maintain a medically appropriate weight should be strongly encouraged. As with any therapeutic intervention with depressed patients, the physician may need to present the recommendation with enthusiasm and clarity to aid compliance.

Activity

1. Exercise, like diet, is not independently efficacious in the treatment of depression. Many depressed patients with anergy, malaise, apathy, and daytime fatigue find that they are incapable of pursuit of even an easy exercise regimen.

2. To the extent that the patient can comply, exercise can help promote recovery from depression. The physician should recommend that the patient adopt an exercise regimen, even if as minimal as a 15-minute walk on 3 alternate days each week. Encouragement

from the personal physician may help with m tion.

Patient Education

1. Many people do not understand major depr as a medical, brain-based illness, as opposed occasional mood of depression (feeling down) t experience at times. Many attach a stigma to r illness, including depression, and some even b that major depression is a moral weakness or c ter flaw. Patient and family education are the most important.

2. Physician education time can be made effici patient education brochures. The American Psy ric Association publishes the "Let's Talk Facts . . ." series of pamphlets on many topics, inc depression, mental health in the elderly, and hood disorders.

3. Education on medication use is often nec Many patients view medication use with the ": for a headache" approach and are unfamiliar w use and efficacy pattern of antidepressants. Th to take medication daily for weeks and tolera effects while awaiting benefit needs both edt and supportive encouragement.

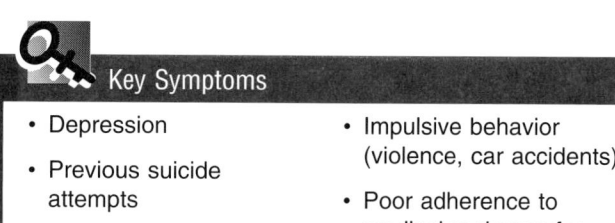

Key Treatment

Drugs of Choice	Alternative Drugs
• Sertraline	• Bupropion
• Paroxetine	• Desipramine
• Fluoxetine	• Nortriptyline
• Trazodone	• Imipramine

Follow-Up

1. It is best to have the initial follow-up visit w week to evaluate medication side effects an encouragement. Weekly or biweekly visits w often suffice for 6 weeks while medications ar adjusted and evaluated. Monthly or bimonthl can be scheduled once the patient has becon depressed, is familiar with the medication, gaining emotional support from family, frie support groups. Patients should be seen by th sicians at least quarterly as long as they are o cation.

2. Since the natural course of a depressive ill typically 6 months to 2 years, the patient sho on medication for at least 6 months after the sion is fully treated before a slow taper fr medication is attempted.

3. For patients with a history of several severe e of major depression, it may be advisable to o medication a lifetime necessity, like insuli diabetic. Examples are a history of serious

---

314 Suicide Assessment

Robert Maurer

Extent of the Problem

1. Over 30,000 Americans complete suicides annually.
2. Eighth leading cause of death among all ages
3. Second leading cause among youth; between 1960 and 1993 there has been a 200 per cent increase in teenage suicide.

Etiology

1. Experience of loss
2. Depression
3. Experience of severe rejection in childhood

Symptoms

1. Depression
2. Grief
3. Nonadherence with regimens for life-threatening disease. Examples: diabetics who overeat or drink, cardiac patients who smoke
4. Excessively giving and preoccupied with pleasing others. Patients who experience childhood rejection may spend their lives making it up to their parents and then their friends, boss, doctor, by always being kind, giving, and generous without ever accepting help or favors themselves. The more extreme the giving, the greater is the risk of suicide.
5. Extreme need to excel (perfectionism)
    a. Patients at any age who are outstanding in everything they do may be compensating for an overwhelming feeling of being unworthy.
    b. Often compulsively competitive in work and sport
    c. May be accompanied by excessive giving; may appear as a model in the community
6. History of multiple childhood accidents

Key Symptoms

• Depression	• Impulsive behavior (violence, car accidents)
• Previous suicide attempts	
• Alcoholism/drug abuse	• Poor adherence to medical regimens for life-threatening diseases

Clinical Findings

1. Suicide may be a childhood-onset disorder.
    a. It may be primarily due to early childhood experiences of rejection or neglect.
        (1) Suicidal adults recount stories told them by their parents, such as

• "Your mother or father had a nervous breakdown when you were born."
• "Your father or mother left when you were born."
• "If it weren't for you, I'd have left your mother/father years ago."
• Repeated stories of the pain of childbirth
• Parents abandoning the child to surrogates

    (2) Children "build in" a voice of rejection and guilt over being born.
    b. There are three common strategies that children develop to deal with the feeling that they are not wanted, are a burden, or are an imposition on their parents, and it is these strategies rather than the suicidal behavior that is likely to be present in the physician's office.
        (1) *Giving* is used by children who discover that when they are helpful and attentive to a parent's needs, they are rewarded. Thus, by cleaning the house, cooking, becoming a parent's confidant, the child feels valuable and is acting more or less like a thoughtful house guest, not wanting to impose or be a bother. As adults, when the giving is thwarted, such as when a mate leaves, they may then become suicidal.
        (2) *Perfectionism* is related to giving, in that children perceive that if they do everything right at home and in the world, they can justify their existence. They become model children, excellent students, and successful at everything. The strategy can be interrupted by any significant failure in academic, athletic, work, or romantic endeavor.
        (3) *Aggression.* If children perceive they are not wanted, and particularly if a parent is physically abusive, children may decide to hate the messenger. These angry children frequently get into fights, are highly disruptive, perform illegal acts, or are absent from school. As they begin to improve their behavior, they may become more suicidal.
2. Overwhelming loss
3. Major depression
4. Alcoholism or drug abuse

Treatment

1. Identify patients at risk and ask them about suicidality even if no symptoms are present. Use any pretext the patient offers, such as stress or relationship difficulties.

2. When a patient is in crisis, rule out suicide as soon as possible in the interview.

a. As early as possible in the interview say, "I'm glad that you are telling me what happened. I need to know more, but before you do, can I ask a question? What is the pain like at its worst? How bad does it get?"

b. The answer will usually be nondescript. Follow with, "Does the pain ever get so bad that you wish you didn't wake up the next morning?" This will elicit many "false positives." Suicidal ideation does not always mean the patient is actually a suicide risk.

c. You have now switched the focus of the interview from the details of the precipitating event to the crucial agenda of whether the patient will stay alive long enough to get help.

d. If the patient answers yes, ask, "Do you feel you could actually act out the wish to hurt or kill yourself?"

e. Any answer other than "No, absolutely not" should be considered a yes. An answer of "I don't think so" or "I'm too much of a coward to do it" or "I guess not" requires that you pursue the doubts.

3. If the patient indicates that suicide is an option, thank him or her for confiding in you. Proceed to determine intensity of the suicidality by asking

a. "How often do you think about it? How recent?"

b. "Do you have a plan?"

c. "Do you have the means to carry out the plan?"

4. Begin the "suicide contracting" process or hospitalize.

5. Offer immediate counseling assistance. One way of doing so is to say, "I am glad you are being honest with me. I know that is not easy. Would you like some help with the pain? Would you be willing to see a doctor who specializes in this kind of pain, who can help you so you won't have to feel this bad? Would you go see that counselor once, then come back (or call me) and tell me if you think it can help? I can get you an appointment today or tomorrow."

6. If the patient agrees to go, ask if he or she will "contract" to stay alive until the appointment with the mental health professional. A request such as this is suggested: "Here is the name and phone number of the counselor I think can help you. I'd like to ask one more important question, since I know you are hurting: will you guarantee that you will not hurt yourself, not kill yourself until you have seen the counselor, no matter how much it hurts? You'll call me if you need help, but you'll stay alive and free of accidents until you've seen the doctor."

7. If the patient is hesitant, add, "I understand your doubts that anyone can help. Would you go just once? What do you have to lose? If you are right, that the counseling cannot help, you have only postponed your decision. If you are wrong and you do find help and comfort there, you'll have the peace and happiness you deserve."

8. If the patient agrees, ask him or her to sign an agreement just to reinforce the power of the decision. The nonsuicide contract is written as follows: "Under no conditions will I accidentally or purposefully take my life for [fill in a time period long enough to allow the patient time to get to the psychotherapist, usually 24 to 48 hours]."

9. Have the patient sign the contract, and place a copy in the medical chart.

10. If the patient has a specific plan and the means to carry it out, negotiate about giving up the means. One way of explaining this is: "By giving up your pills, it makes it easier to live up to the contract . . . just as it is easier to diet if you don't have your favorite food in the house."

a. If the preferred method is pills, have the patient surrender the lethal dose, and prescribe small amounts.

b. If the preferred method is a firearm, have the patient give it to a friend who will not return it.

11. Encourage the patient to stay with a friend for a few days or nights. Suicidal people often have good friends but are reluctant to "bother" them.

12. If the patient will not agree to the contract, he or she should be considered acutely suicidal and hospitalized.

Follow-Up

1. Have the patient call you, preferably see you, after the first visit. While this is not clinically necessary, it is a strong message to the patient that you are not abandoning him or her.

2. If the patient is not seeing the counselor until the following day, have the patient call you during the evening to provide additional support.

B Bibliography

Drye R, Goulding R, Goulding M: No-suicide decision: patient monitoring of suicidal risk. Am J Psychiatry 1973;130:171–174.

Isometsa MD, Henriksson MM, Aro HM, et al: Suicide in major depression. Am J Psychiatry 1994;151:530–536.

Lepine JP: Suicide attempts in patients with panic disorders. Arch Gen Psychiatry 1993;50:144–149.

Patterson WM, Dohn H, Bird J, Patterson G: Evaluation of suicidal patients: The sad person scale. Psychosomatics 1983;24:343–352.

Pfeffer CR: The Suicidal Child. New York, Guilford Press, 1986.

315 Panic Disorder

Joseph B. Selby

Etiology

1. The cause of panic disorder has been postulated to be neurophysiologic, with a pathologic low threshold response to the "fight or flight mechanism."
2. Some investigators suggest that early life experiences may predispose one to personality factors that lead to the development of panic disorder.
3. Panic disorder is more common among first-degree biological relatives with panic disorder. The concordance rate for monozygotic twins in one 1983 study using *DSM-III* criteria was 31 per cent as compared with no concordance for dizygotic twins.

Epidemiology

1. The lifetime prevalence of panic disorder is 1.5 to 2.0 per cent of the population.
2. Panic disorder without agoraphobia is equally common in males and females.
3. Panic disorder with agoraphobia has a female-to-male ratio of 2:1.
4. Two thirds of agoraphobic patients have panic disorder as well.
5. Panic disorder most commonly presents in young adulthood, the mean age at presentation being 24 to 26 years of age.
6. There is an increase in the onset of panic attacks observed at ages 15 to 19. The onset of panic disorder after the age of 40 is rare.
7. In clinical settings, panic disorder with agoraphobia is much more common than panic disorder without agoraphobia.

Symptoms

1. The symptoms experienced during a panic attack include dyspnea, choking sensation, syncope, palpitations, tachycardia, chest pain, diaphoresis, nausea, trembling, paresthesias, hot flashes, and chills.
2. In addition to the physical symptoms, patients often experience depersonalization, fear of dying, fear of going crazy, or fear of doing something uncontrolled or uncharacteristic during the attack.

Key Symptoms

- Dyspnea
- Dizziness
- Chest pain
- Depersonalization
- Abdominal distress
- Palpitations
- Fear of going crazy

Clinical Findings

1. The initial panic attack is hallmarked by its spontaneous presentation. The unexpected nature of the panic attack is an essential feature of the disorder.
2. Panic attacks occasionally follow excitement, emotional trauma, or exertion and do not necessarily represent panic disorder.
3. Ingestion of caffeine, alcohol, or nicotine may precede a panic attack. Other drugs likely to induce panic attacks are amphetamines, cocaine, anticholinergics, amyl nitrate, theophylline, and hallucinogens.
4. The typical panic attack begins with a 10- to 15-minute period of accelerating symptoms. The entire attack lasts for about 30 minutes.
5. It is not unusual for a patient to develop a phobic avoidance of certain situations coincidental with the panic attack. The environmental cues may then become associated with and a stimulus for panic attacks.
6. A common associated feature in panic disorder is anticipatory anxiety.
7. Because of the somatic features of panic disorder, otherwise young, physically healthy adults frequently present to emergency rooms with cardiac and respiratory complaints.
8. *DSM-IV* diagnostic criteria for panic disorder with or without agoraphobia
   a. Both (1) and (2)
      (1) Recurrent unexpected panic attacks
      (2) At least one of the attacks has been followed by at least 1 month of one or more of the following:
         (a) Concern about additional attacks
         (b) Worry about the implications or consequences of an attack
         (c) A significant change in behavior related to the attacks
   b. Absence or presence of agoraphobia
   c. The panic attacks are not due to direct physiologic effects of a substance.
   d. The panic attacks are not better accounted for by another mental disorder.

Key Signs

- Spontaneous presentation
- Duration of attack 30 minutes or less
- Phobic avoidance
- Anticipatory anxiety

Laboratory Tests

1. The symptoms of anxiety and panic are nonspecific and can occur in many disease states. Some basic laboratory tests and studies are needed to rule out associated disease: thyroid studies, serum electrolytes (sodium, potassium, calcium), blood glucose, 12-lead ECG, chest radiograph.
2. Other tests may be needed based on clinical judgment. They are usually not done as screening tests and are obtained when clinically indicated: Urine studies for vanillylmandelic acid (VMA), meta-nephrines, 5-hydroxyindoleacetic acid (5HIAA), B_{12}, heavy metal screen, CT or MRI of the brain, cortisol levels.

Differential Diagnosis

1. Endocrine disorders must be considered.
   a. Hyperthyroidism
   b. Hypercortisolism
   c. Hypoglycemia
   d. Carcinoid
   e. Premenstrual syndrome
   f. Hypothyroidism
   g. Pheochromocytoma
   h. Addison's disease
   i. Hypoparathyroidism
2. Other medical conditions can give symptoms that mimic panic attacks and thus panic disorder.
   a. Chronic obstructive pulmonary disease (COPD)
   b. Myocardial infarction
   c. Collagen-vascular diseases
   d. Brain tumor
   e. Demyelinating disease
   f. Pulmonary embolism
   g. Brucellosis
   h. B_{12} deficiency
   i. Heavy metal intoxication
   j. Aspirin intolerance
3. Substance-induced anxiety disorders must be ruled out.
   a. Intoxication from caffeine, cocaine, and amphetamine
   b. Alcohol, sedative, opiate, and antihypertensive withdrawal
4. Anxiety and fear are associated with other psychiatric illnesses, and they, too, should be ruled in or ruled out.
   a. Major depression
   b. Other anxiety disorders
   c. Mood disorder due to a general medical condition
   d. Anxiety disorder due to a general medical condition
   e. Somatization disorder
   f. Simple phobia

Treatment

1. Psychological treatment for panic disorder
   a. Relaxation training is used to reduce arousal and to control anxiety before it escalates to panic.
   b. Exposure therapy is used in panic disorder with agoraphobia as a tool for desensitization to phobic situations.
   c. Cognitive therapy appears to be the single most effective psychological treatment.
2. Pharmacological treatment for panic disorder
   a. Antidepressants are effective in treating panic disorder and are the agents of choice. Monoamine oxidase inhibitors seem to have antiphobic activity. Imipramine has been shown to give improvement in symptoms in 70 to 90 per cent of patients *after 6 weeks of therapy.* Desipramine, nortriptyline, doxepin, amitriptyline, fluoxetine, sertraline, and paroxetine have all been reported to be clinically effective. Maprotiline, trazodone, and amoxapine are less effective. While some patients may respond to small doses of antidepressants, full therapeutic antidepressant doses are most often required.
   b. Benzodiazepines are effective at reducing anticipatory anxiety. Alprazolam (Xanax) results in marked improvement in 50 per cent of patients, with an additional 40 per cent showing moderate improvement. Studies have shown that efficacy in treatment of anxiety with benzodiazepines does not diminish, and the drug remains effective without escalation of dose. Recent studies on dose indicate that 6 mg/day of alprazolam is more effective than 2 mg/day, but drug dependence is a significant risk.
   c. The usefulness of β-adrenergic blockers in treatment of panic disorder is questionable. They are effective in treatment of autonomic symptoms associated with panic attacks but are generally less effective in treating the disorder than other agents.
   d. The most effective form of treatment for panic disorder is likely a combination of a pharmacologic agent and cognitive behavioral therapy.

Diet

Patients should avoid caffeine, nicotine, and alcohol. Care should be exercised in the use of medications that contain anticholinergics.

Activity

1. Specific activities related to exposure therapy and desensitization should be conducted at the discretion of the patient and therapist.
2. Care may need to be used when driving or operating equipment if drowsiness occurs with benzodiazepine therapy or with antidepressant use.

Patient Education

There are excellent workbooks available for patient education, e.g., Barlow reference below.

Key Treatment

- An antidepressant with or without a benzodiazepine

- Provide or arrange for cognitive behavioral therapy in conjunction with medical treatment.

- Continue antidepressant treatment for at least 6 months.

- As an antidepressant is titrated, short-term use of benzodiazepines (4 to 6 weeks) to control acute panic attacks is often very effective.

- Relapse in the first 2 years can be 30 to 80 per cent.

- Most patients respond to reinstitution of treatment.

- Patients with a history of drug abuse/dependence or antisocial personality disorder should probably not receive benzodiazepines.

Follow-Up

1. Close weekly follow-up during initiation of drug therapy is warranted.

2. Monthly follow-up once therapeutic doses are reached is practical.

3. Weekly follow-up may again be needed when titration off medication occurs.

4. Arrangement for follow-up and emergency calls on an as-needed basis is necessary.

 Bibliography

Barlow DH, Graske MG: Mastery of Your Anxiety and Panic. Albany, NY, Graywind Publications, 1989.

First MB (ed): Text and Criteria: Diagnostic and Statistical Manual of Mental Disorders, 4th ed. Washington, DC, American Psychiatric Association, 1994, pp 393–444.

Kaplan H, Sadock B: Synopsis of Psychiatry, Behavioral Sciences Clinical Psychiatry, 7th ed. Baltimore, Williams & Wilkins, 1994, pp 573–616.

Papp L, Klein D, Gorman J: Carbon dioxide hypersensitivity, hyperventilation, and panic disorder. Am J Psychiatry 1993;150(8):1149–1157.

Sandler M, Schildkraut J: Abstracts from Panic and Anxiety: A Decade of Progress. An International Conference June 19–22, 1990, Geneva, Switzerland. J Psychiatr Res 1990;24(Suppl 1)–103.

316 Generalized Anxiety Disorder   *Thomas L. Leaman*

Etiology

1. May result from unresolved adjustment disorder with anxious mood
2. In 50 per cent of cases a precipitating emotional stressor can be identified.
3. In the other 50 per cent no stressor can be identified; a disturbance of the neurotransmitters is presumed to be the cause.

Symptoms

1. Worry and anxiousness over multiple real or projected problems. The worry is out of proportion to the situation and out of control.
2. At least three of the following symptoms
   a. Restlessness
   b. Fatigue
   c. Trouble concentrating
   d. Irritability
   e. Sleep disturbance
   f. Muscle tension
3. Frequently characterized by episodes of severe autonomic symptoms
   a. Cardiac: chest pain, palpitations, tachycardia, tachypnea
   b. Pulmonary: hyperventilation, smothering sensations, dyspnea
   c. Gastrointestinal: globus hystericus, indigestion, abdominal pains, flatulence, diarrhea, constipation
   d. Genitourinary: frequency, menstrual irregularities, sexual dysfunction
   e. Dermatologic: paresthesias, sweating, hot flushes, chills, pruritus

Key Symptoms

- Worry
- Fatigue
- Chest pain, palpitations
- Smothering sensation
- Indigestion

Clinical Findings

Consider in any patient with the underlying symptoms described above, especially if accompanied by episodes of autonomic symptom clusters.

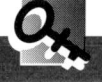

Key Signs

- Agitation
- Sweating, tremor
- Scattered mentation
- Hyperventilation

Tests

Instruments useful in helping to confirm or refute the diagnosis:

1. Sheehan Patient Rated Anxiety Scale: Self-administered, 35 questions. Useful both for diagnosis and monitoring response to treatment. Scores may be tabulated directly by patient.
2. Hopkins Symptom Checklist (SCL90): Lengthy questionnaire, requires training in interpretation.
3. Hamilton Anxiety and Depression Scales: Both are physician administered but require some training.
   a. HAM-A (anxiety) consists of 14-item checklist of anxiety symptoms.
   b. HAM-D (depression) is a 17-item, interview-based scale.
4. Zung Anxiety Self-Assessment Scale: Self-administered scale; interpretation requires physician analysis.
5. Covi Anxiety and Raskin Depression Scales: Three items on each scale; interpreted by physician; useful in differentiating between anxiety and depression.

Key Tests

- Hamilton Anxiety and Depression Scales
- Covi Anxiety and Raskin Depression Scales

Differential Diagnosis

1. Somatic diseases. None of the symptoms of generalized anxiety disorder is pathognomonic, and all may be caused by a wide variety of other diseases. Among the most prominent are endocrine disorders (especially hyperthyroidism), cardiac diseases (especially coronary artery disease), and pulmonary disorders (especially chronic obstructive pulmonary disease). It is not necessary, or even possible, to rule out every conceivable disease that could be responsible for the symptoms exhibited. Rather, it is important to rule out those that are most dangerous or most likely. The diagnosis should be suspected on the basis of the pattern of symptoms over time. The somatic symptoms tend to occur in clusters, usually subsiding

within a few weeks. They tend to recur in a variable period of time, involving the same organ system again or an entirely different system or even multiple systems.

2. Mental diseases. The diagnosis is not made if the patient has a psychosis or bipolar disease or is under the effects of drugs (abuse or medication).

3. Other anxiety disease. The diagnosis is not made if the patient has another anxiety disease.

4. Depression. Most people with generalized anxiety disorder (GAD) have symptoms of depression at some stage in their disease. It is usually possible to determine which is the primary disease on the basis of a careful history.

    a. Symptoms common to both anxiety and depression
      (1) Fatigue
      (2) Tearfulness
      (3) Eating disturbances
      (4) Irritability
      (5) Excessive worry
      (6) Difficulty concentrating

    b. Symptoms especially characteristic of anxiety
      (1) Difficulty falling asleep or staying asleep
      (2) Pain syndromes: tends to be acute, sharp
      (3) Patients often complain of nervousness, want help.
      (4) Mood may be elevated.
      (5) Autonomic symptoms prominent

    c. Symptoms especially characteristic of depression
      (1) Early morning awakening
      (2) Pain syndromes: tends to be chronic, dull
      (3) Patients often unaware of their illness, want to be left alone
      (4) Mood may be depressed.
      (5) Anhedonia
      (6) Suicidal thoughts

Treatment

There are three treatment modalities: psychotherapy, pharmacotherapy, and patient education. Most people with GAD require both of the first two; all need the last.

1. Psychotherapy
    a. In many patients with GAD there is an identifiable stress factor in the cause of the disease. Any such stressors should be sought and the patient's coping mechanisms explored. In anyone who has GAD, particularly if it has gone undiagnosed or misdiagnosed for a prolonged period of time, the disease itself may serve as a perpetuating stressor.

    b. Supportive counseling, cognitive therapy, psychodynamic psychotherapy, family therapy, or various behavior therapies are most frequently used in GAD.

    c. Other techniques that may be helpful adjuncts, but not necessarily of proven value, include exercise, meditation, progressive relaxation, biofeedback, yoga, and t'ai chi.

2. Pharmacotherapy. Three groups of drugs have proven useful in the management of GAD: azipirones, benzodiazepines, and tricyclic antidepressants.

    a. Azipirones. Currently, there is only one approved drug in this group, buspirone (BuSpar). This is generally considered to be the drug of choice in the initial treatment.
      (1) Advantages: well tolerated, does not interact with alcohol or benzodiazepines, and does not cause drug dependency
      (2) Disadvantages: very slow to work (2 to 4 weeks), not always effective, and in some people can cause the side effects of dizziness, drowsiness, nausea, and headache

    b. Benzodiazepines. Benzodiazepines are usually grouped according to their duration of action; the long-acting (up to 100 hours), the intermediate, and the short-lasting (5 to 15 hours).
      (1) Advantages: effectiveness, prompt action, side effects tend to diminish with time, rarely addictive
      (2) Disadvantages: may cause drug dependency; symptoms of withdrawal may mimic anxiety symptoms; abrupt withdrawal of the short-acting benzodiazepines after prolonged high dosage may cause convulsions; slow, tapered withdrawal essential
      (3) Possible side effects: sedation, dizziness, and ataxia

    c. Tricyclic antidepressants
      (1) Often used with antianxiety agents
      (2) Occasionally effective alone for GAD

Patient Education

Crucial in the management of anxiety diseases

1. Anxiety disorders are "closet" diseases, often not openly discussed.

2. Patients tend to blame themselves.

3. Anxiety patients have trouble concentrating, remembering.

Key Treatment

- Counseling
- BuSpar, benzodiazepines, tricyclic antidepressants
- Patient education

Follow-Up

GAD is a chronic disease with many somatic manifestations. Patients should be encouraged to remain under continuous monitoring.

Bibliography

Leaman TL: Healing the Anxiety Diseases. New York, Plenum Press, 1992.

McGlynn TJ, Metcalf HL: Diagnosis and Treatment of Anxiety Disorders: A Physician's Handbook. 2nd ed. Washington, DC, American Psychiatric Press, 1992.

Walley EJ, Beebe DK, Clark JL: Management of common anxiety disorders. Am Fam Physician 1994;50:1745–1752.

Weekes C: Hope and Help for Your Nerves. New York, Hawthorne Books, 1969.

Wyshak G, Barsky AJ: Relationship between patient self-ratings and physician ratings of general health, depression, and anxiety. Arch Fam Med 1994;3:419–424.

Procedure | **DEEP MUSCLE RELAXATION EXERCISES** | *Robert A. DiTomasso*

Indications

1. Maladaptive levels of stress, anxiety, anger, and hostility
2. Important component in treatment of generalized anxiety disorder, panic disorder, simple phobia, speech anxiety, and test anxiety
3. Anxiety and maladaptive arousal as causative factors in onset or exacerbation of stress-related physical disorders: essential hypertension, migraine headache, tension headache, low back pain, bruxism, temporomandibular joint syndrome, Raynaud's disease
4. Component in preparation of patients for stressful medical procedures and distress following surgery
5. For prevention and treatment of anticipatory nausea and vomiting as side effects of cancer chemotherapy
6. Component in treatment of acute pain and chronic pain syndromes
7. Primary insomnia

Contraindications

1. Intervention is generally very safe with rare side effects; when they occur, side effects tend to be mild and generally present early in the process.
2. Avoid use with psychotic patients, since may precipitate psychotic episode.
3. Beware of underlying organic problems that may mimic anxiety (such as hyperthyroidism, pheochromocytoma, withdrawal reactions) or cause physical symptoms (such as headache caused by brain tumor), which if left medically untreated could endanger health of patient.
4. Avoid applying to problems for which no efficacy has been demonstrated.

Preparation

1. Rule out organic causes for patient's symptoms.
2. Conduct biopsychosocial formulation of presenting problem based on interview, observation, past history, self-report measures, and physiologic measures; pinpoint how maladaptive arousal or anxiety is implicated in problem manifested.
3. Determine need for alternative pharmacologic and/or psychosocial intervention instead of, or in conjunction with, deep muscle relaxation.
4. Present problem formulation to patient, and educate patient about causative role of stress, anxiety, or arousal in problem.
5. Provide treatment rationale for deep muscle relaxation; why it would be expected to help without overstating case.

6. Foster positive expectation for change, and nurture and bolster motivation.
7. Explore and address fears, concerns, myths, and anticipations about relaxation therapy.
8. Identify prior experiences, if any, with relaxation-based techniques: type, duration, and outcome.
9. Present relaxation as skill to be acquired through practice.
10. Present it as an active coping strategy for patient to use in the future.
11. Outline the specific muscle groups, and explain concept of tension-relaxation cycle.
12. Demonstrate a tension-relaxation cycle for each muscle group, and emphasize need to relax only one group at a time.
13. Screen for present or past injuries to muscle groups that may interfere with tension-relaxation cycles.
14. Teach patient use of self-monitoring chart to track symptoms during baseline, treatment, and follow-up as a measure of efficacy.
15. Provide patient with relaxation chart to facilitate reminder for practice and promote adherence.

Equipment

1. Physical environment free of distractions and interruptions and conducive to relaxation
2. A comfortable chair able to provide full support of body (e.g., recliner)
3. Dimmed lighting to create relaxing atmosphere

Precautions

1. Although rare, watch for precipitation of "relaxation-induced anxiety" in patients who fear the following: loss of control, the physical feelings accompanying the relaxed state, feelings possibly associated with prior traumas, feelings of floating, and the letting go experience.
2. With patients prone to excessive cognitive worriment, consider use of relaxing imagery.
3. Overcontrolled perfectionistic patients with obsessive-compulsive tendencies who "try hard" to relax
4. Hypervigilant patients excessively focused on physical sensations
5. Patients with unrealistic expectations about relaxation
6. Patients with past or present physical injuries where tensing muscles may cause discomfort

Technique

1. Instruct patient to settle back into the recliner and close eyes.
2. Follow outline provided in Table 316-1 and conduct two tension-relaxation cycles for each muscle group.
3. Repeatedly focus the patient's attention to slowing breathing rate during the exercise.
4. Provide explicit instruction and suggestions to enhance the relaxation and active "letting go" of tension by patient.

TABLE 316–1. OUTLINE FOR ADMINISTERING DEEP MUSCLE RELAXATION

MUSCLE	INSTRUCTIONS FOR TENSING	INSTRUCTIONS FOR FOCUSING ON SENSATIONS (8–10 s)	INSTRUCTIONS FOR RELAXING (RELEASING TENSION)	INSTRUCTIONS FOR FOCUSING ON RELAXATION AND THE CONTRAST
Right hand	Make a fist as tightly as you can . . . tighter and tighter	Hold the tension and concentrate on tension in your fist	Let go of the tension. Allow your hand to relax letting your fingers go loose. Actively relax the tension away	Focus on relaxing sensations in your hand and examine the contrast between tension and relaxation
Left hand	Make a fist as tightly as you can . . . tighter and tighter	Hold the tension and concentrate on tension in your fist	Let go of the tension. Allow your hand to relax letting your fingers go loose. Actively relax the tension away	Focus on relaxing sensations in your hand and examine the contrast between tension and relaxation
Right/left forearms	Press arms downward on the arm of the recliner (Alternative: Lift arms and place them straight out in front of you away from your body, making them straighter and straighter, as straight as possible)	Hold the tension and concentrate on the tension in your forearms	Let your arms relax and rest comfortably on your lap	Focus on the relaxing sensations in your forearms noticing the difference between tension and relaxation
Right/left arms	Bring your arms toward your shoulders bending at the elbow	Hold the tension and focus on the tension in your arms	Allow your arms to relax and rest comfortably	Focus on the relaxing feelings in your arms once again noticing the difference
Toes	Curl your toes as tightly as you can	Hold the tension in your toes and examine it	Let go of the tension in your toes and let your toes rest comfortably	Concentrate on the relaxing sensations and examine the difference
Calves	Lift both feet slightly off the ground and point your toes away from you	Hold the tension there and examine the feelings of tension in your calves	Let your legs rest comfortably now and feel the relaxing sensations	Focus on the relaxing sensations in your calves and take notice of the difference between tension and relaxation
Thighs	Tighten your thigh muscles by pressing the heels of your feet into the floor as hard as you can	Hold the tension there and pay attention to the sensations of tension in your thighs	Now, just let the tension go	Focus on those relaxed feelings and focus on the difference
Abdomen	Tighten your abdominal muscles tighter and tighter	Hold the tension there	Gradually release the tension in your abdomen by letting go	Concentrate on the relaxing sensations and the difference
Chest	Take a deep breath and fill up your lungs as much as you can	Hold your breath and concentrate on the sensations of tension in your chest	Gradually exhale while saying the word "relax" to yourself	As you are exhaling focus on the relaxing sensations that accompany letting go. Now, focus on the difference between tension and relaxation
Neck	Bend your head forward and let your chin touch your chest	Keep your head forward and hold the tension in your neck	Bring your neck back to its normal position	Just focus on the relaxed feelings in your neck and note the difference
Jaw	Clench your jaw as tightly as you can . . . tighter and tighter	Hold the tension there and concentrate on the tension there	Now, just let your jaw relax comfortably	Focus on the relaxing feelings in your jaw and focus on the difference
Lips	Press your lips together as tightly as possible, tighter	Hold your lips pressed together	Let your lips relax	Concentrate on the relaxing sensations in your lips and notice the difference
Eyes	With eyes closed, close your eyes tighter and tighter	Hold the tension around your eyes and focus on the tension	Now, just let your eyes relax	Concentrate on the relaxation and study the difference
Forehead	Wrinkle your forehead by raising your eyebrows as high as you can	Keep your forehead wrinkled and concentrate on the tension there	Now, relax your forehead by smoothing it out as much as you can . . . smoother and smoother	Notice the difference between tension and relaxation

Adapted from Barlow and Cerney, 1988; Clum, 1990; Masters et al., 1987; Poppen, 1988.

5. Teach patient to associate the relaxed state with the cue word "relax" by repeatedly pairing the word "relax" with exhalation and relaxed sensations throughout.

6. At conclusion of the total tension-relaxation exercise, instruct patient to follow path of relaxation through each muscle group from toes to forehead as in the accompanying table with added suggestions of sensations of relaxation, warmth, and heaviness.

7. Finally, at end of entire exercise, instruct patient, when ready, to count backward from 5 to 1; open eyes at count of 1 with suggestion to feel relaxed, alert, and refreshed.

8. The entire exercise is administered by physician, who observes patient for signs of increased relaxation.

9. Formal sessions are conducted once a week until patient is proficient at inducing relaxed state on own.

10. Clinician may audiotape a relaxation session for home use by patient.

11. Patient is encouraged to practice technique once or twice daily.

Follow-Up

1. Track improvements in patient's symptoms through patient and physician monitoring.

2. Provide continued reinforcement for practice of relaxation.

3. Incorporate and plan relapse-prevention strategies designed to prevent tension from reaching maladaptive levels.

4. Gradually increase intervals between sessions to foster practice and generalization.

5. Remind patient to use tension as a cue to relax.

6. Plan periodic booster sessions to foster maintenance of gains.

 Bibliography

Barlow DH, Cerney JA: Psychological Treatment of Panic. New York, Guilford Press, 1988, pp 96–119.

DiTomasso RA, Mills O: The behavioral treatment of essential hypertension: Implications for medical psychotherapy. Med Psychother 1990;3:125–134.

Clum GA: Coping with Panic: A Drug-Free Approach to Dealing with Anxiety Attacks. Pacific Grove, CA, Brooks/Cole Publishing, 1990, pp 69–91.

Masters JC, Burish TG, Hollon SD, Rimm DC: Behavior Therapy Techniques and Empirical Findings, 3d ed. Fort Worth, Harcourt Brace Jovanovich, 1987, pp 36–77.

Poppen R: Behavioral Relaxation Training and Assessment. New York, Pergamon Press, 1988.

317 Hyperventilation Syndrome

Randolph W. Evans

Etiology

1. Definition: A syndrome characterized by a variety of somatic symptoms induced by physiologically inappropriate hyperventilation and usually reproduced in whole or in part by voluntary hyperventilation.

   a. Acute hyperventilation with obvious rapid breathing accounts for only 1 per cent of all cases.

   b. Chronic hyperventilation without obvious rapid breathing is responsible for 99 per cent of cases. May occur with a small imperceptible increase in tidal volume or a mild increase in resting respiratory rate or both. Once established, an occasional deep breath will keep the P_{CO_2} low.

2. Epidemiology

   a. Occurs in about 6 to 11 per cent of the general patient population

   b. Occurs two to seven times more frequently in females

   c. Most patients range in age between 15 and 55 years, but can occur in childhood and in the elderly.

3. Pathophysiology

   a. Hyperventilation produces a reduction in arterial P_{CO_2} resulting in alkalosis.

   b. Respiratory alkalosis produces the Bohr effect, a left shift of the oxygen dissociation curve with increased binding of oxygen to hemoglobin and reduced oxygen delivery to tissues.

   c. Alkalosis also causes a reduction in plasma Ca^{2+} concentration. Hypophosphatemia may occur due to intracellular shifts of phosphorus caused by altered glucose metabolism. In chronic hyperventilation, bicarbonate and potassium levels may be decreased due to increased renal excretion.

   d. Stress can trigger a hyperadrenergic state that may trigger hyperventilation due to β-adrenergic stimulation.

   e. Cerebral blood flow can be reduced by 30 to 40 per cent by low P_{CO_2}-induced cerebral vasoconstriction. Coronary vasoconstriction can occur in patients with occlusive disease or Prinzmetal's angina.

4. Mechanisms of symptom production

   a. Chest pain may arise from the intercostal or anterior chest muscles, occasionally from angina.

   b. Shortness of breath or difficulty getting a good breath may be due to overinflation of the chest.

   c. Dry mouth, bloating, belching, flatulence, and epigastric fullness may be due to aerophagia.

   d. Dizziness, headache, visual disturbance, tinnitus, ataxia, syncope, and various psychological symptoms may be produced by diminished cerebral blood flow.

   e. The cause of paresthesias is not certain. Possibilities include decreased cerebral perfusion and increased peripheral nerve axonal excitability.

   f. Muscle spasms and tetany may be due to respiratory alkalosis and hypocalcemia.

   g. In chronic hyperventilation, hypophosphatemia may result in tiredness, dizziness, poor concentration, disorientation, and paresthesias. Hypokalemia can cause muscle weakness and lethargy.

   i. A hyperadrenergic state with anxiety may result in tremor, tachycardia, anxiety, and sweating.

5. Pathogenesis

   a. Acute hyperventilation may be triggered by acute stress, anxiety, or emotional upset.

   b. Chronic hyperventilation may be a bad habit of exaggerated thoracic breathing with episodes triggered by any physical or emotional disturbance that produces increased ventilation.

Symptoms

1. The symptoms and signs are protean and can occur alone or in various combinations. Dizziness, dyspnea, chest pain, and paresthesias are the most frequent.

2. Include general, cardiovascular, gastrointestinal, neurologic, psychological, and respiratory manifestations

3. Paresthesias may be symmetrical, involving one or various combinations of sites, including the face, especially periorally, and the extremities, especially the hands and feet. Unilateral paresthesias also can occur affecting the left side of the face and body more often than the right.

4. Unusual psychological complaints may be reported such as feelings of unreality and hallucinations.

1125

Key Symptoms

- General:
    Fatigability, exhaustion, weakness, sleep
    disturbance, nausea, sweating

- Cardiovascular:
    Chest pain, palpitations, tachycardia, Raynaud's
    phenomenon

- Gastrointestinal:
    Aerophagia, dry mouth, pressure in throat,
    dysphagia, globus hystericus, epigastric fullness
    or pain, belching, flatulence

- Neurologic:
    Headache, pressure in the head, fullness in the
    head, head warmth
    Blurred vision, tunnel vision, momentary flashing
    lights, diplopia
    Dizziness, faintness, vertigo, giddiness,
    unsteadiness
    Tinnitus
    Numbness, tingling, coldness of face, extremities,
    trunk
    Muscle spasms, muscle stiffness, carpopedal
    spasm, generalized tetany, tremor
    Ataxia, weakness
    Syncope and seizures

- Psychologic:
    Impairment of concentration and memory
    Feelings of unreality, disorientation, confused or
    dream-like feeling, déjà vu
    Hallucinations
    Anxiety, apprehension, nervousness, tension, fits of
    crying, agoraphobia, neuroses, phobic, panic

- Respiratory:
    Shortness of breath, suffocating feeling, smothering
    spell, unable to get a good breath or breathe
    deeply enough, frequent sighing, yawning

Reprinted with permission from Evans RW: Neurologic aspects of hyperventilation syndrome. Semin Neurol 1995;15(2). Copyright Thieme Medical Publishers, Inc.

Clinical Findings

1. With acute hyperventilation, tachypnea is present; with chronic, there may be no obvious signs.
2. Tetany and carpopedal spasm occur rarely.

Key Signs

- Tachypnea in acute hyperventilation

- Rarely tetany or carpopedal spasm

Laboratory Tests

1. The diagnosis depends on reproducing some or all of the symptoms with the hyperventilation test and excluding other possible causes by either clinical reasoning or laboratory testing when indicated.

2. The hyperventilation test can be performed with either an increased ventilation rate of up to 60 breaths per minute or simply deep breathing for 3 minutes.

   a. The hyperventilation test should not be performed in patients with ischemic heart disease, cerebrovascular disease, pulmonary insufficiency, hyperviscosity states, significant anemia, sickle cell disease, and uncontrolled hypertension.

   b. Dizziness, unsteadiness, and blurred vision commonly develop within 20 to 30 seconds, especially with the patient in the standing position; paresthesias usually start later. Chest pain is reported by 50 per cent of patients after 3 minutes of hyperventilation and by all by 20 minutes.

   c. For clinical purposes, measurement of arterial or end-tidal volume P_{CO_2} is not necessary. There is no clear correlation between arterial P_{CO_2} and neurologic manifestations.

   d. For some patients with hyperventilation syndrome, symptoms cannot be reliably reproduced during the hyperventilation test. The provocation test lacks test-retest reliability. Antecedent anxiety and stress may need to be present to reproduce symptoms.

3. Hyperventilation can produce electrocardiogram changes including T-wave inversion, ST-segment depression, and ST-segment elevation in patients without coronary artery disease.

Key Test

- Hyperventilation provocation test

Differential Diagnosis

1. Salicylism, caffeinism, and other drug effects
2. Cirrhosis and hepatic coma; acute pain such as with a myocardial infarction, splenic flexure syndrome, cholecystitis, fever and sepsis, dissecting aortic aneurysm, respiratory dyskinesia, pulmonary embolism, pneumothorax, interstitial lung disease, asthma, heat and altitude acclimatization, and a variety of neurologic conditions including brain stem strokes and intracranial hypertension.
3. Similar transient neurologic and psychological symptoms may occur in migraine aura, partial and partial complex seizures, multiple sclerosis, transient ischemic attacks, and panic attacks.

Treatment

1. There is a lack of well-controlled treatment trials for the various approaches available.
2. Patient education and breathing instructions for attacks are the most important and often only treatment necessary.
3. Medications may be helpful in selected cases.

4. Breathing exercises and diaphragmatic retraining may be helpful for some patients.

5. Biofeedback and hypnosis may help patients who do not respond to usual treatments.

6. Psychological and psychiatric referral may be necessary in patients with significant anxiety, depression, or panic disorder.

Medication

1. β-blockers may reduce palpitations, tremor, and anxiety.

2. Benzodiazepines may be helpful for anxious patients when prescribed for a short period of time.

3. Antidepressant medications may be helpful in patients with underlying depression or panic disorder.

Patient Education

1. An explanation of the difference between acute and chronic hyperventilation should be provided. Many patients with the chronic form will protest that they do not breathe rapidly as in the hyperventilation test. Explain how breathing a little too fast or too deep can cause a drop in P_{CO_2}. Then explain briefly how the symptoms may be produced by physiologic changes.

2. Reassuring patients that they do not have a serious condition is crucial. If the diagnosis is clear-cut, avoid laboratory testing.

3. Explain how anxiety and various emotional states might trigger symptoms. Alternatively, if a patient chronically hyperventilates because of stress or out of habit, explain this connection.

4. Once the patient understands the pathophysiology, then treatment of an acute episode by elevating the P_{CO_2} makes sense. Suggest that if the patient has additional episodes, he or she should try a breathing treatment. Options include holding the breath and counting to 10, followed by breathing every 6 seconds for a minute or so or breathing into a lunch bag placed over the nose and mouth for up to several minutes.

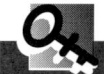

Key Treatment

Treatment of Choice	Alternative Treatment
• Patient education	• Medications
• Instruction in "breathing treatment"	

Follow-Up

1. Monitoring

   a. Have the patient check with you by telephone a week or so after the initial visit.

   b. If the symptoms persist, a follow-up visit and discussion of additional treatment may be necessary.

2. Prognosis: For most patients, education, reassurance, and instruction in "breathing treatment" will lead to resolution of episodes.

Bibliography

Evans RW: Neurologic aspects of hyperventilation syndrome. Semin Neurol 1995;15(2):115–125.

Gardner WN: Hyperventilation syndromes. Respir Med 1992;86:273–275.

Lum LC: Hyperventilation syndromes in medicine and psychiatry: A review. J R Soc Med 1987;80:229–231.

Magarian GJ: Hyperventilation syndromes: Infrequently recognized common expressions of anxiety and stress. Medicine 1982;61:219–236.

Smith CW: Hyperventilation syndrome: Bridging the behavioral-organic gap. Postgrad Med 1985;78:73–84.

318 Phobia

Robila Ashfaq

1. *Definition:* an irrational fear resulting in a conscious avoidance of the specific feared object, activity, or situation. It can be divided into three major categories
   a. Social phobia is the fear of humiliation or embarrassment in public places. Social phobia includes phobias about eating in restaurants, public speaking, and public musical performances.
   b. Agoraphobia is the fear of being alone in public places, especially in situations in which a rapid exit would be difficult.
   c. Specific phobia is a residual category that includes specific phobias not covered under social phobias or agoraphobia. The feared objects in simple phobias are animals, storms, heights, illness, injury, and death.

Epidemiology
1. Social phobia: affects 3 to 5 per cent of the population. Males and females are equally represented. Social phobias usually occur in the early to late teens, although they can begin at any age.
2. Simple phobias: are more common among women than men. The six-month prevalence varies from 5 to 12 per cent.
3. Agoraphobia: occurs in the middle to late twenties. Agoraphobia is more common in women. The onset is usually reported after a traumatic event. The lifetime prevalence is 0.6 per cent; at least two thirds of agoraphobic patients actually have concomitant panic disorder.

Etiology
1. Psychoanalytic factors: Classically, Freud viewed the phobic disorder as a result of conflicts centered on an unresolved childhood oedipal situation. The primary ego defense mechanism being involved is displacement, which arouses affects such as signal anxiety, thus avoiding the oedipal genital drives and castration anxiety. More recent psychodynamic issues are related to shame, aggression, trauma, and unresolved grief in the origin of social phobia, with shame being considered the most important dynamic. Fear of public humiliation derives from an inner conviction of one's basic defenses, incompetence, and deficiency and may mask reaction formation, sexual anxieties, conflicts over pride, competition, dependency, narcissism, and struggles with aggression.
2. Family studies: A study of a sample of female twins found that concordance for social phobia was greater for monozygotic (24 per cent) than for dizygotic twins (15 per cent), suggesting a genetic contribution, although specific phobic attitudes and behaviors may be transferred.
3. Biological factors: Biological challenge studies, such as those with sodium lactate, have demonstrated specificity in promoting panic attacks only in patients in panic disorders, thereby showing a greater behavioral sensitivity to a wide variety of precipitating factors. In contrast, social phobia patients have a normal sensitivity to lactate, and react less severely to the factors.
4. Behavioral factors: Behavioral factors have shifted from the traditional pavlovian stimulus-response model of the conditioned reflex to the more recent operant conditioned theory, whereby anxiety is viewed as a drive that motivates to abort painful affect. When applied to the phobias, such avoidance behavior becomes fixed as a stable symptom because of its effectiveness in protecting the patient from phobic anxiety.
5. Sleep studies: The subjective and EEG patterns of patients with social phobias are normal, whereas panic disorder patients report a lifetime rate of insomnia and sleep panic attacks.

Symptoms/Clinical Findings
1. Social phobia: In social phobias, exposure to specific phobic stimulus (or stimuli) almost invariably provokes an immediate anxiety response. Nonetheless, this anxiety reaction may be experienced as subjective (e.g., distress, apprehensiveness, or discomfort) or somatic (e.g., trembling, sweating, palpitations, or blushing), a combination of these responses, or a full-blown panic attack. The anxiety response of social phobia seems to be gradual rather than immediate. When panic attacks occur in social phobia, they are generally associated with a phobic situation (i.e., stimulus bound), but when phobias are comorbid with panic disorder, "spontaneous" panic attacks occur.
2. Agoraphobia: Patients experience symptoms of dizziness, difficulty breathing, weakness in limbs, fainting episodes, and buzzing or ringing in the ears. Specific autonomic symptoms such as palpitations, trembling, sweating, and blushing are particularly characteristic of social phobia patients. Significantly more patients with panic disorder than those with social phobia report palpitations, chest pains, tinnitus, blurred vision, headaches, and fear of dying. Help-seeking behavior also clearly distinguishes social phobia patients. Patients with social phobias feel more comfortable when alone, whereas agoraphobic patients feel less anxiety when accompanied by familiar figures. Only 5.4 per cent of social phobia patients

seek services from mental health practitioners, in contrast to the 72 per cent of the panic disorder patients.

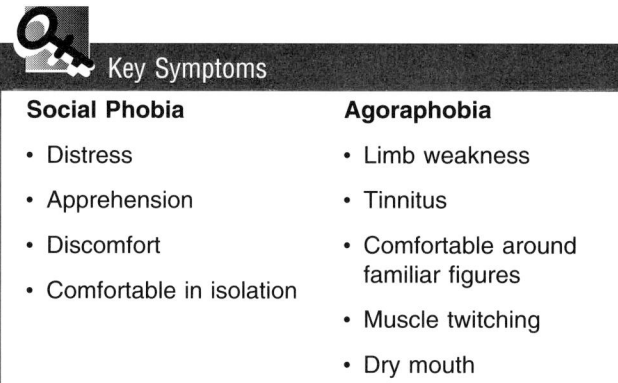

Key Symptoms

Social Phobia	Agoraphobia
• Distress	• Limb weakness
• Apprehension	• Tinnitus
• Discomfort	• Comfortable around familiar figures
• Comfortable in isolation	• Muscle twitching
	• Dry mouth

Key Signs

Social Phobia	Agoraphobia
• Blushing	• Dizziness
• Sweating	• Difficulty breathing
• Trembling	• Fainting
• Palpitations	

Differential Diagnosis

1. Organic disorders: Isolated symptoms of phobia are rare in concurrence with organic disorders, although possible with certain tumors or cerebrovascular accidents, substance abuse, especially alcohol dependence, hallucinogens, and sympathomimetic drugs. Evidence suggests that patients with social phobias are more than twice as likely to have alcohol problems as are nonpatients. Social phobia is nine times more likely to be present in persons with alcohol dependence.

2. Psychiatric Disorders

   a. Anxiety disorders are present in 47 per cent of cases of social phobia.

   b. Obsessive compulsive disorder is present in 10 per cent of cases of social phobia.

   c. Simple phobia is present in 25 per cent of cases and panic disorder with agoraphobia in 17 per cent of cases.

   d. Patients with phobia have a high rate of major depression and suicidal ideation. These individuals often come to family physicians with psychosomatic symptoms, depression, or phobias.

   e. Avoidant personality disorder is commonly seen in phobias.

   f. Schizoid personality disorder is seen in social phobics.

   g. Paranoid personality disorder is seen in simple phobias.

Differential Diagnosis

Psychiatric D/D	Organic D/D
Anxiety disorder	Substance abuse
• Panic disorders	• Alcohol dependency
• Agoraphobia	• Hallucinogens
• Generalized anxiety	• Sympathomimetics
• Obsessive compulsive	Tumors (rare)
• Social/simple phobia	Cerebrovascular accident
Mood disorders	
• Major depressive episode	
• Dysthymia	
Schizophrenia	
Personality disorders	
• Schizoid	
• Avoidant	
• Paranoid	

Treatment

Treatment interactions include psychopharmacologic, psychodynamic, and cognitive behavioral approaches. The course of illness becomes chronic and pervasive when other comorbid conditions exist. Severity also increases in comorbid situations because of association itself, the decreased responses to treatment, decreased help-seeking behavior, and frequent association with self-medication. This difficulty in recognizing phobias poses particular treatment challenges.

1. Pharmacologic

Pharmacotherapy includes agents from different classes with different mechanisms of action, including

   a. Antidepressants: monoamine oxidase inhibitors (MAOIs), selective serotonin reuptake inhibitors, and reversible inhibitors of MAO-A. MAOIs (e.g., phenelzine [Nardil]) in particular are used to prevent anticipatory anxiety in social phobias and panic attacks. Tricyclic antidepressants are also used. Treatment might need to be continued for 6 to 12 months since symptoms reappear after discontinuation.

   b. High-potency benzodiazepines: alprazolam (Xanax) might show improvement in avoidant personality traits. Clonazepam (Klonopin) is also being used. β-adrenergic blocking drugs, such as propranolol, are used for performance anxiety (e.g., in public speakers and musicians) to block the physiological signs of anxiety, such as tachycardia and tremors.

2. Behavioral Techniques

a. Systematic desensitization is a technique in which the patient is exposed serially to graded anxiety-provoking stimuli, from the least to most frightening, and is used in phobia treatment. Patients are taught to self-induce a state of relaxation in the face of each anxiety-provoking stimulus.

b. Flooding: Patients are exposed to the phobic stimuli, actual or through imagery, for as long as they can tolerate until they can no longer feel it.

c. Insight-oriented psychotherapy: This focuses on

helping patients to understand their unconscious meaning of anxiety and to seek alternative ways to deal with the phobic stimulus.

Other Therapy

Hypnosis and family therapy are also used as adjunctives to the more traditional treatments.

Course and Prognosis

Most patients are able to live relatively normal lives in spite of phobic disorders because phobic objects or situations are easily avoidable. Social phobias may have a chronic course, although some evidence indicates that they decrease after middle age. Simple phobias that begin in childhood regress spontaneously.

Key Treatment

Pharmacologic

• Antidepressants

• High-potency benzodiazepines

Behavioral Therapy

• Systematic desensitization

• Flooding

• Insight-oriented psychotherapy

• Hypnosis

Bibliography

American Psychiatric Association: Diagnostic and Statistical Manual of Mental Disorders, 4th ed. Washington, DC, American Psychiatric Association, 1994.

Gabbard GO: (1992) Psychodynamics of panic disorders and social phobia. Bull Menninger Clinic 1992;56:A3–A13.

Kaplan HI, Sadock BJ: Anxiety disorders. *In* Social and Simple Phobias Etiology. Baltimore, Williams & Wilkins, 1993, pp 400–401.

Liebowitz MR: Pharmocotherapy of social phobia. J Clin Psychiat 1993;25:31–35.

Marshall JR: The psychopharmacology of social phobia. Bull Menninger Clinic 1994;56:A43–A49.

319 Alcoholism

Warren G. Thompson

Etiology

1. Genetic: Sons of alcoholics are four times as likely to be alcoholic as sons of nonalcoholics, whether they are raised by biological or adoptive parents. The data from adoption studies on daughters of alcoholics are less clear, but a recent twin study in women found higher concordance in monozygotic twins, suggesting that heredity is also important in women. Studies of genetic markers and of a specific gene for alcoholism are inconclusive.

2. Ethnicity and culture: Rates among American Indians are very high, while rates among Asian-Americans appear to be lower than the general population. France has a much higher prevalence of alcoholism than Italy, even though the per capita alcohol consumption in Italy is slightly higher.

3. Occupations: bartenders, painters, and physicians

4. Social influences: Rates of alcoholism decline when the price of alcohol is increased substantially. Legal restrictions on alcohol also decrease the rates of alcoholism.

5. Sex: Rates are much higher in men than in women. Women living with a substance-abusing male are at high risk.

Natural History

1. The majority of young male heavy drinkers reduce drinking to nonproblem drinking as they get older without intervention.

2. The typical onset of problem drinking in females occurs later than in males (after age 25). However, progression is more rapid, and females usually enter treatment earlier. Women are more likely to abuse prescription drugs with alcohol.

3. The spontaneous remission rate of alcoholism is 10 to 30 per cent.

4. In a study (J Stud Alcohol 1982;43:273–288) of the natural history of seeking help, only 31 per cent of men with a self-defined drinking problem sought help from a physician. These men often did not reveal they had a problem with drinking, and only 50 per cent were asked about their alcohol intake. Only 25 per cent of the problem drinkers were either encouraged to reduce their intake or warned about the health hazards of drinking, and only 3 per cent of these heavy drinkers were referred to a treatment program by their physician. Physicians need to learn to screen effectively for alcoholism (Table 319–1).

Diagnosis

Medical symptoms, clinical findings, and laboratory tests are neither sufficiently sensitive nor sufficiently specific to

TABLE 319–1. WHY SCREEN FOR ALCOHOLISM

The problem is common (between 10 and 20 per cent in general medical outpatient populations).
Effective screening tests are available.
If one does not screen, the diagnosis is likely to be missed (50 to 90 per cent of alcohol problems are missed in the office).
Effective treatments are available (especially if diagnosis is early).
Early identification can prevent physical and psychosocial problems from developing in the patient, family, and society.

Adapted with permission from Bigby JA (ed): Substance Abuse Education in General Internal Medicine: A Manual for Faculty. Washington, DC, Society of General Internal Medicine, 1993.

be useful in the diagnosis of alcoholism. Screening and diagnosis require an assessment of the consequences of alcoholism in several domains (see below).

Symptoms

1. Patients with alcoholism may complain of abdominal pain, diarrhea, weight loss, palpitations, sexual dysfunction, memory loss, depression, blackouts, and seizure or give a history of gastrointestinal (GI) bleeding.

2. The patient may present with symptoms of the consequences of alcoholism (holiday heart syndrome, cirrhosis, alcoholic hepatitis, Wernicke's encephalopathy).

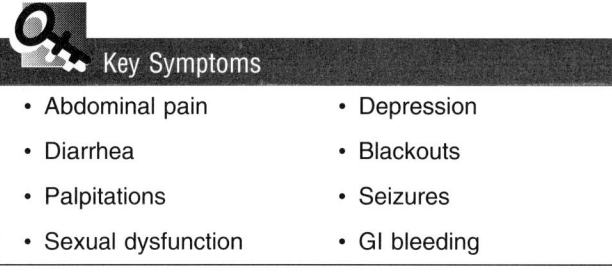

Key Symptoms	
• Abdominal pain	• Depression
• Diarrhea	• Blackouts
• Palpitations	• Seizures
• Sexual dysfunction	• GI bleeding

Clinical Findings

Patients with alcoholism may present with gynecomastia, testicular atrophy, spider angiomas, hepatomegaly, abdominal tenderness, and evidence of cerebellar dysfunction or hypertension.

Key Signs
• Alcohol odor on breath
• Bilateral parotid gland enlargement
• Unexplained tremulousness

Laboratory Tests

1. No laboratory test is sufficiently sensitive to be relied on as a screening test for alcoholism.

2. Gamma-glutamyltransferase (GGT) and mean corpuscular volume (MCV) are the most sensitive laboratory tests.

3. Aspartate aminotransferase, other liver function tests, the complete blood count, creatinine kinase, amylase and lipase, magnesium, phosphorus, uric acid, and triglycerides also may provide clues to the diagnosis.

Key Test

- The blood alcohol level (Table 319–2) is the most specific and most underutilized test for the diagnosis of alcoholism.

Screening

The most practical, sensitive, and specific screening tool is the CAGE questionnaire (Am J Psychiatry 1974; 131:1121–1123). The CAGE has been validated in several general medical populations, including the elderly. The literature suggests that patients who respond to all four questions positively are more than 100 times as likely to have alcoholism as the general population. Those who respond with 3, 2, 1, and 0 positive responses are 20 times, 6 times, 1½ times, and ⅟₇ as likely, respectively. Table 319–3 contains a set of questions that are practical for office use and which will pick up most patients presenting with alcoholism. In addition, these questions provide the main tools needed to make the diagnosis of alcoholism.

Formal Diagnosis

1. *The Diagnostic and Statistical Manual of Mental Disorders (DSM-IV)* defines alcohol abuse as continued use despite familial or occupational consequences or recurrent use in hazardous situations (driving while intoxicated) over a 12-month period; the patient does not meet the criteria for physical dependence.

2. The diagnosis of alcohol dependence requires three or more of the following seven symptoms:
   a. Continued drinking despite physical or psychological consequences caused or exacerbated by alcohol
   b. Neglect of other activities
   c. Inordinate time spent drinking and recovering
   d. Drinking more or over a longer period than intended
   e. Inability to control drinking

TABLE 319–2. BLOOD ALCOHOL LEVELS DIAGNOSTIC OF ALCOHOLISM

Blood alcohol level > 300 mg/dl at any time
Blood alcohol level > 150 mg/dl if not obviously intoxicated
Blood alcohol level > 100 mg/dl on a routine office visit

TABLE 319–3. SCREENING FOR ALCOHOLISM

1. Do you drink alcohol at all? (If yes, go to questions 2 to 5.)
   If no: Have you ever had a drinking problem?
       Has anyone in your family had a drinking problem?
2. Have you ever been concerned about your drinking?
3. CAGE questionnaire: Follow-up on positive questions with questions about the circumstances and the reasons:
   Have you ever felt the need to *C*ut down on your drinking?
   Have people *A*nnoyed you by criticizing your drinking?
   Have you ever felt bad or *G*uilty about your drinking?
   Have you ever had a drink first thing in the morning to steady your nerves or get rid of a hangover? (*E*ye-opener)
4. Has anyone in your family ever had problems with alcohol?
5. Other questions that are often useful:
   When was your last drink? (Less than 24 hours is a red flag.)
   Do you ever get preoccupied with drinking or have an irresistible craving for alcohol?
   Have you had blackouts or memory loss after drinking?
   Is your drinking different now than 5 years ago?
   Have you ever been arrested for drinking, such as for driving under the influence?
   Have you ever gotten in trouble at work because of drinking?
   Have you neglected your family, work, or obligations for 2 or more days in a row because you were drinking?
   Have you ever been to an AA meeting?

Adapted with permission from Bigby JA (ed): Substance Abuse Education in General Internal Medicine: A Manual for Faculty. Washington, DC, Society of General Internal Medicine, 1993.

   f. Tolerance (increased amounts needed for effect)
   g. Withdrawal symptoms on cessation or drinking to relieve or avoid withdrawal symptoms

Treatment

Medication

No drugs have been shown to improve the outcome of alcoholic patients in large, controlled trials. The largest trial of disulfiram (Antabuse) showed very little benefit.

Patient Education

1. It is easy for the physician to get discouraged, but even brief physician advice makes a difference.

2. A trial period of controlled drinking with careful follow-up may be appropriate for a diagnosis of alcohol abuse. Complete abstinence is the only treatment for alcohol dependence.

3. The physician should present the diagnosis in a nonjudgmental fashion that emphasizes the consequences of alcohol on that patient's life and the need for complete abstinence. The word "alcoholic" should be avoided.

4. The value of inpatient versus outpatient rehabilitation continues to be debated. Patients should be hospitalized if there is a history of delirium tremens or if the patient has ongoing serious medical problems. Consideration of inpatient treatment should be given when there is poor social support or the patient has significant psychiatric problems or a history of relapse after treatment.

5. Alcoholics Anonymous (AA) should be strongly recommended. Physicians should have literature about AA available to patients. The address is AA General Service, P.O. Box 459, Grand Central Station, New York, NY 10163. One does not have to be religious

to go to AA. Patients should attend at least five different meetings in order to find the meeting most compatible with them (an inner-city resident may be uncomfortable at a suburban meeting, and vice versa). Women may do better at meetings open only to women. Hospitalized patients should be encouraged to call from the hospital (AA will send someone to talk to him/her if the patient makes the contact). Patients need to attend meetings regularly (daily at first) and for a sufficient length of time (usually 2 years or more) because recovery is a difficult and lengthy process.

6. In the beginning, patients should remove alcohol from their home and avoid bars and other establishments where there is strong pressure to drink.

7. If the patient has an antisocial personality (severe problems with family, peers, school, and police before age 15 and before the onset of alcohol problems), recovery is unlikely, and the doctor should not spend a great deal of time with these patients (until an effective treatment for antisocial personality is devised). If the patient has a primary depression (the depression must antedate the problems with alcohol, or it must be a significant problem during long periods of sobriety), this problem should be addressed.

8. Family members of alcoholics should be strongly encouraged to contact Alanon and Alateen. The address is Alanon Family Group Headquarters, P.O. Box 182, Madison Square Garden Station, New York, NY 10159-0182.

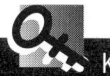

Key Treatment

- Patient education

Follow-Up

1. Frequent follow-up is essential to support the patient in recovery. The patient should be asked about attendance at AA meetings and about his or her relationship with his or her sponsor.

2. The key step for the patient is to realize that treatment does not end with sobriety. Recovery means that

TABLE 319-4. RELAPSE PREVENTION

1. Learning to say no to drinking in social situations
2. Handling heavy-drinking friends who will try to undermine the patient's sobriety
3. Handling stress (do not ignore symptoms of anxiety)
4. Avoid boredom (patients have previously been spending a great deal of time drinking and recovering, and now they have time on their hands)
5. Learning to get along again with family and close friends (family problems often increase when drinking stops)
6. Identify other situations that can lead to drinking again and develop ways to cope with these situations

Adapted from Schuckit MA: Treatment of alcoholism in office and outpatient settings. *In* JH Mendelson, NK Mello (eds): Medical Diagnosis and Treatment of Alcoholism. New York, McGraw-Hill, 1992, p 381.

patients can handle the stresses of everyday life without alcohol. Therefore, the patient must develop and *rehearse* strategies to cope with high-risk situations (Table 319–4). Attending to these situations is essential for both treatment and follow-up.

 Bibliography

For more information on diagnosis, see
American Psychiatric Association: Diagnostic and Statistical Manual of Mental Disorders, 4th ed. Washington, DC, American Psychiatric Association, 1994.

For more information on improving skills in diagnosis and treatment and on teaching about alcoholism, see
Bigby JA (ed): Substance Abuse Education in General Internal Medicine: A Manual for Faculty. Washington, DC, Society of General Internal Medicine, 1993.

For more information on diagnosis and treatment of alcoholism, see
Mendelson JH, Mello NK (eds): Medical Diagnosis and Treatment of Alcoholism. New York, McGraw-Hill, 1992.

For documentation of the utility of the CAGE questionnaire, see
Buchsbaum DG, Buchanan RG, Centor RM, et al: Screening for alcohol abuse using CAGE scores and likelihood ratios. Ann Intern Med 1991;115:774–777.

For documentation of the importance of early recognition and physician advice to stop drinking, see
Walsh DC, Hingson RW, Merrigan DM, et al: The impact of a physician's warning on recovery after alcoholism treatment. JAMA 1992;267:663–667.

320 Fetal Alcohol Syndrome

Margo K. Anderson

Etiology

1. A diagnosis of fetal alcohol syndrome (FAS) or fetal alcohol effects (FAE) requires a history of maternal drinking.
2. A medical diagnosis of FAS is characterized by
   a. Growth deficiency
   b. A pattern of specific physical anomalies, including characteristic facial features
   c. Central nervous system (CNS) dysfunction
3. Fetal alcohol effects (FAE) are characterized by "... children whose mothers drank alcohol and who have two of the three characteristics of FAS."

Incidence

1. FAS is the leading known cause of mental retardation in the Western world and has a worldwide incidence of 1.9 in 1000 live births. FAS afflicts 1 in 700 to 750 live births in the United States.
2. Fetal alcohol syndrome occurs in all racial groups according to the proportion of alcohol-abusing mothers.
3. Approximately one third to one half of alcoholic mothers who drink during pregnancy have babies with FAS.

Symptoms

1. Growth deficiency
2. Physical anomalies
3. Behavioral and learning problems owing to CNS dysfunction

Key Symptoms

- Growth deficiency
- Physical anomalies
- Behavioral and learning problems owing to CNS dysfunction

Clinical Findings

1. FAS/FAE exhibits a specific pattern of malformation seen only in babies of women who consume alcohol during their pregnancy.
2. Alcohol produces a spectrum of defects, the severity of which is proportional to the amount of maternal drinking.
3. Growth deficiency
   a. Intrauterine growth retardation (IUGR)
   b. Infancy and childhood: fifth to tenth percentile weight for height
   c. Adolescence

(1) Females—normal weight for height
(2) Males—underweight for height; height most severely affected

4. Specific physical anomalies
   a. Craniofacial characteristics (Fig. 320–1)
      (1) Short palpebral fissure
      (2) Smooth philtrum (diminished to absent)
      (3) Flat/elongated midface (midface and mandibular growth deficiencies)
      (4) Increased inner-canthal distance
      (5) Thin vermilion of upper lip
      (6) Associated visual malformations include ptosis, strabismus, optic nerve hypoplasia, myopia, and increased tortuosity of retinal vessels.
      (7) Tooth malformation secondary to malocclusion due to jaw malformation
   b. Skeletal characteristics
      (1) Scoliosis
      (2) Pectus excavatum
      (3) Joint alterations: congenital hip dislocation, limited movement of fingers, elbows, and/or wrists
      (4) Altered palmar crease
      (5) Short fifth finger
   c. Heart anomalies (30 to 40 per cent affected)
      (1) Atrial septal defect
      (2) Ventricular septal defect
   d. Other
      (1) Conductive hearing loss
      (2) Immunologic deficiency
      (3) Cleft lip and/or cleft palate
      (4) Protuberant ears
      (5) Strawberry hemangioma
      (6) Hypoplastic labia majora

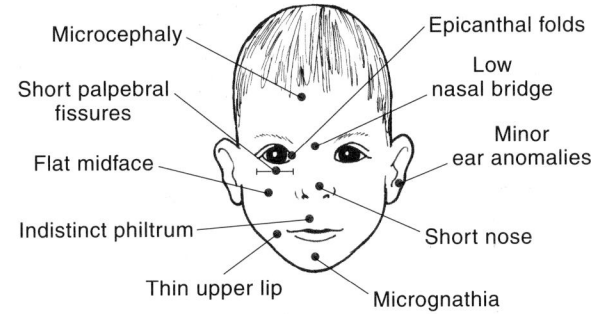

Figure 320–1. Facies in fetal alcohol syndrome. Modified from Streissguth AP, LaDue RA, Randels SP: A manual on adolescents and adults with fetal alcohol syndrome with special reference to American Indians. Indian Health Service, Public Health Service, U.S. Dept. of Health and Human Services, 1988, p 7.

5. CNS dysfunction
  a. Intellectual/academic
    (1) Average IQ is 65 (wide range of IQ scores from low-average to mild and moderate retardation).
    (2) Average reading level is fourth grade.
    (3) Average spelling level is third grade.
    (4) Average math level is second grade.
  b. Behavior/CNS dysfunction
    (1) Infancy: tremulousness, irritability, feeding difficulties (weak suck), failure to thrive, hypotonia, and developmental delays
    (2) Preschool: hyperactive, alert, outgoing, excessively friendly, increased need for bodily contact, lacks richness of speech, thought, and grammatical complexity, problems with coordination
    (3) Early school age: increasing difficulty with math (reading and writing may be equal to other children), attention deficit disorder (ADD), emotional lability, memory deficits, social intrusiveness, sexual exploration, and hostility and destructiveness
    (4) Middle school age and adolescence: school achievement at a maximum, poor attention, good verbal skills (often masks seriousness of situation), decreased motivation and attendance, problems with abstract learning, memory difficulties, lack of social inhibition, increased risk of sexual abuse and pregnancy

Laboratory Tests

1. None specific for FAS/FAE. Usual workup for failure to thrive and maternal alcoholic screening tests (Michigan Alcohol Screening Test/MAST, CAGE, TACE) may be useful.
2. Psychological and/or neurologic tests may be helpful to determine extent of CNS dysfunction.

Differential Diagnosis

1. Rule out other causes for growth deficiencies.
2. Rule out failure to thrive.
3. Possible referral to dysmorphologist about deformities

WARNING

There is no known safe amount of alcohol that can be consumed by expectant mothers. Therefore, only total abstinence can prevent FAS/FAE.

Treatment

1. Accurate and early diagnosis of FAS/FAE is essential for optimal treatment.
  a. Identifying at-risk patients in the community through community health nurses, school teachers, social workers, and other health care professionals as well as an examination by dysmorphologist or medical geneticist
  b. Family physicians are in a unique position to identify those at risk, knowing the family's history of alcoholism, maternal history, and newborn status.
2. Case management: Must be individualized due to the wide spectrum of affected patients.
  a. Complete periodic physical examinations for follow-up of associated birth defects
  b. Complete psychological testing including professional intervention for depression, drug abuse, and behavior management
  c. Early intervention for special educational needs, including infant stimulation programs, preschool language programs, individualized education planning emphasizing adaptive functioning instead of IQ (i.e., vocational training)
  d. Medical: proper workup and follow-up of failure to thrive and ADD. Necessity for effective birth control because they are easily victimized
  e. Counseling: individual, family, and group
  f. Increased adolescent services due to difficulties with onset of puberty
3. Caregiver considerations
  a. Adequate education concerning FAS/FAE
  b. Arrangements for respite care
  c. Access to local support groups and agencies (caseworkers, state developmental disability funds, Supplemental Social Security income)
  d. Parental/family counseling with support groups
  e. Appropriate alcohol-abuse treatment if the caregiver is the birth mother, including counseling to reduce maternal guilt

 Key Treatment

- Identify at-risk patients through family history, maternal history, and newborn status
- Complete periodic physical examinations
- Complete psychological testing

Follow-Up

1. Prevention
  a. Counseling patients regarding the danger of alcohol intake during pregnancy, including identifying at-risk patients

b. Educating the community and other health care professionals about FAS/FAE

2. Continuity of medical care through infancy, childhood, adolescence, and adulthood

3. Assistance with school and community resources

 Bibliography

Jones KL: Diagnosis and management of fetal alcohol syndrome. Pediatr Rounds 1993;2(3):5–8.

Kleinfeld J, Wescott S: Fantastic Antone Succeeds (FAS)! Anchorage, University of Alaska Press, 1993.

Lewis DD, SE Woods: Fetal alcohol syndrome. Am Fam Physician 1994;50(5):1025–1032.

Olson HC, Burgess DM, Streissguth AP: Fetal alcohol syndrome (FAS) and fetal alcohol effects (FAE): A lifespan view, with implications for early intervention. *In* Zero to Three: National Center for Clinical Infant Programs, vol 13, no. 1, 1992, pp 24–29.

Streissguth AP, Aase JM, Clarren SK, et al: Fetal Alcohol Syndrome in adolescents and adults, JAMA 1991;265(15): 1961–1967.

321 Substance Abuse

Ernest Frugé

Etiology

1. There are a number of competing theories of etiology (e.g., biological, psychodynamic, sociopolitical).
2. Substance abuse is best conceptualized as a biopsychosocial disease resulting from an interplay of physical, psychological, and social factors unique to each patient.
3. It is most important to determine for each patient what factors may maintain drug use, motivate quitting, and precipitate relapse following treatment.

Definition of Key Terms

1. Substance abuse: The use of a substance in a way that is not medically or socially (e.g., legally) sanctioned and/or causes harm to self or others
2. Addiction: Repeated use despite negative physical, psychological, or social consequences
3. Tolerance: Diminishing effect of a drug with regular use. Significant increase over time in amount of drugs needed to produce the desired results
4. Dependence: Physical adaptation so that rapid removal of the drug causes a withdrawal syndrome
5. Withdrawal: Reduction in amount of substance taken in. Depending on the rate of reduction and class of drug, a drug-specific withdrawal syndrome can occur, ranging from mild flulike symptoms to severe reactions (e.g., seizures, cardiovascular collapse).
6. Overdose: Toxic or lethal amount of substance
7. Detoxification: Management of withdrawal symptoms by administering declining doses of the substances or of a cross-tolerant drug
8. Relapse: Return to substance abuse after a period of abstinence

Epidemiology

1. About 35 to 40 per cent of the U.S. population will use illicit drugs at some time in their lives, and 6 to 8 per cent will meet the formal criteria for dependence. These percentages do not include the abuse of alcohol or prescription drugs.
2. It is likely that an individual will abuse more than one substance simultaneously.
3. Particular populations present greater risks for substance abuse. Keeping substance abuse in mind when dealing with these populations is important.
   a. Adolescents and young adults. Children are experimenting with drugs at earlier ages. Between 40 and 50 per cent of high school seniors admit some use of illicit drugs. Use of alcohol and smoking cigarettes are correlated with the use of illicit drugs. It is likely that drugs often play a role in accidents and injuries (including homicide and suicide), the leading causes of death in this age range.
   b. Neonates. Drug use during pregnancy is correlated with birth complications and defects. Exposure can be particularly damaging if it occurs within the first trimester. Infants born to addicted mothers also may be addicted.
   c. Elderly. At risk for self-overmedication or polypharmacy due to lack of coordination between multiple physicians involved in their care. Symptoms of substance abuse may be hidden by family members, misdiagnosed as other medical conditions, or mistakenly viewed as simply a by-product of "aging" (e.g., problems in attention).
   d. Disadvantaged populations. This includes ethnic and racial minorities, homeless individuals, and the disabled.

Symptoms and Clinical Findings

1. Arylcyclohexylamines
   a. Examples: phencyclidine (PCP), ketamine
   b. Effects
      (1) Desired effects include altered sensory perceptions and reduced inhibition.
      (2) Tolerance develops in high-dose users.
      (3) Dependence and withdrawal have not been conclusively documented.
   c. Signs of overdose: disorientation, coma, catatonia, nystagmus, hypertension, and seizures
2. Hallucinogens
   a. Examples: lysergic acid diethylamide (LSD), mescaline, methylene dioxyamphetamine (MDA), methylene dioxymethamphetamine (MDMA), 1-(2,5-dimethoxy-4-methylphenyl)-2-aminopropane (DOM/STP), trimethoxyamphetamine (TMA), N,N-dimethyltryptamine (DMT), N,N-diethyltryptamine (DET), psilocybin.
   b. Effects
      (1) Desired effects include altered sensory perception and stimulation.
      (2) Tolerance develops rapidly.
      (3) Dependence and withdrawal do not occur.
   c. Signs of overdose: disorientation, dilated pupils, nausea, rambling speech, perceptual distortions, seizures (severe cases)
3. Cannabis (marijuana)
   a. Examples: hashish, tetrahydrocannabinol (THC)
   b. Effects

(1) Desired effects include euphoria, central nervous system (CNS) depression.

(2) Tolerance and dependence develop with high-dose use.

(3) Withdrawal is mild and does not appear for 8 to 10 days due to long half-life. Symptoms may include anxiety, insomnia, and nausea.

4. Opiates

   a. Examples: heroin, morphine, methadone, codeine, pentazocine, butrophanol, meperidine, buprenorphine, hydromorphone, propoxyphene

   b. Effects

      (1) Desired effects include euphoria, CNS depression, analgesia.

      (2) Tolerance develops rapidly to euphoria and CNS depression, less rapidly to analgesia.

      (3) Dependence develops rapidly to short-acting drugs (morphine, heroin, and methadone) and less rapidly to long-acting drugs (codeine and partial agonist drugs).

   c. Signs of overdose: decreased respiration, miotic pupils, bradycardia, hypotension, pulmonary edema, coma

5. Sedative-hypnotics

   a. Examples: barbiturates, benzodiazepines, sleeping pills, muscle relaxants, "minor tranquilizers"

   b. Effects

      (1) Desired effects include euphoria and CNS depression.

      (2) Tolerance develops more rapidly to desired effects than to therapeutic effects and more rapidly to therapeutic effects than to lethality, except for benzodiazepines, where lethal doses are rare. Cross-tolerance exists for all sedative-hypnotics.

      (3) Dependency develops more rapidly to short-latency, short-acting drugs and less rapidly to the long-acting drugs.

      (4) Withdrawal may be life-threatening.

   c. Signs of overdose: respiratory depression, nystagmus, depressed deep tendon reflexes, hypotension, dysarthria, coma

6. Solvents (inhalants)

   a. Examples: gasoline, halogenated hydrocarbons (Freon), nitrous oxide, toluene, carbon tetrachloride, airplane glue, amyl nitrite, butyl nitrite

   b. Effects

      (1) Desired effects include euphoria, CNS depression, "rush" of blood pressure, and respiration changes.

      (2) Tolerance may develop with prolonged use.

      (3) Dependence and withdrawal not well-documented

   c. Signs of overdose: disorientation, odor of solvent, arrhythmia, hypoxia

7. Stimulants

   a. Examples: amphetamines, prescription diet pills, methylphenidate, cocaine, caffeine

   b. Effects

      (1) Desired effects include stimulation of the CNS, euphoria, and appetite control.

      (2) Tolerance develops rapidly, particularly the anorexiant effect.

      (3) Dependence is now thought to develop; however, withdrawal symptoms are relatively mild.

   c. Signs of overdose

      (1) Acute signs include hyperactivity, diaphoresis, dilated pupils, tremor, tachycardia, hypertension, hyperpyrexia, stereotypical behavior, seizures, and paranoia.

      (2) Within 24 to 36 hours, patient may experience hypersomnolence, hyperphagia, and EEG changes. After several weeks, insomnia and depression

8. Anabolic steroids

   a. Examples

      (1) Oral: ethylestrenol (Maxibolin), fluoxymesterone (Halotestin), methyltestosterone (Android-5, Virilon)

      (2) Injectable: nandrolone deconoate (Deca-Durabolin), testosterone cypionate (Depo-Testosterone), testosterone enanthate (Testaval 90/4)

   b. Effects

      (1) Desired effects include increased muscle mass, strength, and fighting ability. Desired effects also include decreased healing time following injury and decreased recovery time following weight training.

      (2) Adverse effects include psychiatric disorders such as depression, mania, psychosis, and marked aggressiveness.

      (3) Unclear evidence for physical dependence and withdrawal, but psychological dependence develops, compounded by the social reinforcement linked with enhanced appearance and performance.

   c. Signs of overuse

      (1) Short-term signs include rapid increase in size, behavioral and mood alterations (particularly increased aggressiveness), and excessive acne.

      (2) Chronic signs of overuse include hypercalcemia, diabetes, testicular atrophy, impotence, virilization and voice changes in females, arthritis, hyperlipidemia, liver tumors, hepatic cholestasis, jaundice, and hepatocellular carcinoma.

Diagnosis

1. General considerations in diagnosis

a. Early detection and intervention are associated with better treatment outcomes.

b. Scanning for drug use should be incorporated into routine history taking and should focus on problems that are often associated with substance abuse.

c. Early indicators are typically behavioral, psychological, and social.

d. Medical complications are usually associated with chronic abuse and overdose.

e. Other psychiatric disorders (e.g., anxiety, depression, personality disorders) often coincide with substance abuse.

2. Leading psychosocial indicators

a. Psychological/behavioral: anxiety, depression, distractibility, mood swings, irritability, violence, poor judgment, memory loss, psychosis (e.g., hallucinations, delusions)

b. Work/school: declining and/or disrupted performance, frequent absences or tardiness, frequent job changes

c. Family and social relations: spouse or child abuse, emotional and behavioral disorders in patient's children, loss of friends (or development of antisocial friends in children and adolescents), neglect of children's welfare

d. Legal and financial: crime (including delinquency), arrests for DUI, theft, public intoxication or disturbing the peace, financial mismanagement (e.g., defaulted loans), selling possessions

3. Medical complications potentially associated with substance abuse

a. Cardiovascular: arrhythmias, arteritis, cardiomyopathy, cor pulmonale, endocarditis, hypertension, myocardial infarction, myocarditis, thrombophlebitis, vasculitis

b. Pulmonary: abscess, cellulitis, hemorrhage, edema, pneumothorax, reduced pulmonary function, respiratory depression, foreign-body reactions

c. Gastrointestinal: abdominal cramping and diarrhea, anorexia, cirrhosis, chronic constipation

d. Neurologic: ataxia, delirium, ischemia, peripheral nerve lesions, seizures, stroke, coma

e. Reproductive: impaired sperm production, complications in pregnancy (intrauterine growth retardation), congenital abnormalities, infertility, irregular menses, neonatal distress, sexually transmitted disease, testicular enlargement or atrophy

f. Septicemia and infections: fungal ophthalmitis, hepatitis, renal disease, HIV infection, tetanus

g. Other physical examination findings: conjunctivitis, hepatomegaly, increased sweating, jaundice, malnutrition, miosis, muscle weakness or wasting, mydriasis, nystagmus, poor hygiene, repeated injuries, rhinorrhea, scleral icterus

h. Seeking to obtain psychoactive drugs from the physician without clear medical indications

Laboratory Tests and Detection

1. Toxicology screens with combining procedures such as immunoassays and chromatographic assays are useful in determining which drugs are involved in emergency situations.

2. Drug testing is of limited use in general practice due to the limited amount of time reflected in the tests.

Differential Diagnosis

1. Primary mental disorder (e.g., mental disorders due to a general medical condition, dementia, psychosis, mood disorders, anxiety disorders)

2. Nonpathologic substance use (e.g., medical or recreational purposes)

3. Dual psychiatric diagnosis (e.g., anxiety, depression)

Treatment

1. General considerations

a. Selection of treatment strategies is determined by the severity of the problem and cooperation of the patient.

b. It is crucial that the physician maintain confidentiality and a supportive, nonjudgmental stance, focusing on the physical health and well-being of the patient.

c. Patients often deny or distort their drug-use pattern.

(1) If substance abuse is suspected, generally assume that patients are underestimating or denying substance use unless proved otherwise.

(2) Use collateral sources of information (e.g., spouses, parents) whenever possible and appropriate.

(3) Some patients, however, may exaggerate use (e.g., adolescents attempting to shock their parents).

d. Moving from physical findings and implications for health and competence (e.g., sexual difficulties) may be a doorway to increase motivation.

e. Early identification, education, and brief interventions can have very positive effects. Once substance abuse is discovered, it is important to determine the following:

(1) Range and patterns of substances used over time and currently (e.g., types, duration, frequency, routes of administration)

(2) Current (and predicted future) negative consequences of continued use/abuse

(3) Incentives for continued use/abuse and incentives for quitting

(4) Personal vulnerabilities, sources of support, resources and strengths

f. A frank discussion of use patterns and the short- and long-term negative consequences along with suggestions on how to modify habits may promote change or set the stage for future treatment efforts.

g. In severe cases the physician may be asked to coordinate or participate in a meeting of significant others in the patient's social network (e.g., spouse, children, employer, friends).

   (1) The aim of this type of meeting (termed an "intervention") is to overcome a patient's denial of substance abuse or dependency and secure an agreement by the patient to pursue treatment.

   (2) The participants rehearse and then present specific evidence of the negative consequences of the problem both present and future (e.g., a spouse may announce the intention to divorce). Such presentations should be done in a compassionate, matter-of-fact manner, not judgmental, guilt-inducing, or threatening.

2. General rules for treatment of withdrawal and overdose

a. Withdrawal

   (1) Withdrawal (detoxification) often can be managed on an outpatient basis but requires clear commitment to abstinence by the patient, a reliable caregiver, and daily monitoring by the physician.

   (2) Inpatient detoxification is indicated for sedatives (and alcohol), when there are serious medical complications (e.g., sepsis, history of seizures), or when the conditions for patient compliance and daily physician monitoring are not present.

   (3) Use long-acting drugs showing cross-dependence with the drug of abuse.

   (4) Withdraw drugs in blind fashion using fixed-volume dosages.

   (5) All drugs that produce dependence lead to a protracted abstinence syndrome that lasts for months.

b. Overdose

   (1) Ensure adequate airway and respiration.

   (2) Maintain the cardiovascular system.

   (3) Assess the patient's level of consciousness.

   (4) Draw appropriate blood studies before starting an intravenous line.

   (5) Administer a 50% glucose solution and naloxone, 2 mg.

c. Drugs taken orally

   (1) Determine the amount of time since the drug was taken.

   (2) If the patient is fully conscious, administer an emetic and activated charcoal.

   (3) In comatose patients, perform a gastric lavage with an endotracheal tube in place to prevent aspiration. Then administer activated charcoal through a nasogastric tube.

3. Treatment programs

a. Formats for treatment can range from outpatient programs, partial hospitalization (day or evening), inpatient programs, and residential programs (e.g., "therapeutic communities").

b. At this time, there is no evidence that one format of treatment for substance abuse (e.g., inpatient versus outpatient) is generally better than any other.

c. Referral to more expensive, restrictive inpatient programs should be determined by factors such as the following:

   (1) Repeated failure of prior outpatient or partial hospital treatment efforts

   (2) Serious medical or psychiatric concurrent conditions (e.g., high suicidal risk)

   (3) Lack of (or seriously disturbed) social support system

d. Choice of treatment modalities is often limited by the patient's ability to pay.

e. Physicians should become familiar with the local range of programs available in both the public and private sectors, refer based on the best estimate of fit with patient characteristics, and evaluate program effectiveness over time.

f. Physicians can begin to evaluate programs by asking program representatives the following questions:

   (1) What is the program's theoretical model, basic structure, and staffing?

   (2) How does the program evaluate outcome?

   (3) What is the cost of treatment?

   (4) What is the scope and content of the assessment and treatment plan?

   (5) Does the program include detoxification?

   (6) What is the nature and cost of the relapse-prevention strategies and aftercare programs (postdischarge components)?

   (7) What is the relationship between the program and referring physician?

4. Self-help groups

a. Twelve-step programs:

   (1) There are a number of nonprofit programs derived from the fundamental model of Alcoholics Anonymous which focus on other substances of abuse (e.g., Narcotics Anonymous, Cocaine Anonymous).

   (2) These programs offer the addicted patient an opportunity to overcome the denial and develop new principles for life without drugs in

an atmosphere of mutual support and anonymity.

(3) The groups emphasize the spiritual aspects of recovery yet are not religious organizations.

(4) The twelve-step programs designed to help the families of addicted patients (e.g., Al-Anon) can be of substantial help to both loved ones and the patient.

b. Other resources

(1) Additional self-help programs may be available in your area.

(2) Most local and state governments have offices dealing with drug abuse and can provide additional information.

Follow-Up

1. General

a. Recovery is a long-term process requiring extensive personal changes and often involving several relapses.

b. Continuity of compassionate care by the primary care physician for both the identified patient and his or her family can be a crucial element in maintaining the process of recovery.

2. Primary prevention

a. Physicians can have positive effects through education of their child and adolescent patients and involvement in the community as well (e.g., school-based programs on the health risks of drugs and alcohol).

b. Substance abuse cuts across all socioeconomic, racial, and ethnic groups. There are additional factors that can create vulnerability to substance abuse, including poverty, family disruption, negative peer influence, and parents with a history of substance abuse.

c. The National Clearinghouse for Alcohol and Drug Abuse Information has validated the Problem Oriented Screening Instrument for Teenagers (POSIT) as a method for screening for substance abuse and developmental risk factors.

Bibliography

American Academy of Family Physicians: Diagnosis and Treatment of Drug Abuse in Family Practice. American Family Physician Monograph, Summer, 1994.

Augenstein WL (ed): Emergency aspects of drug abuse. Emerg Med Clin North Am 1990;8(3):467–730.

Blondell RD (ed): Clinics in office practice: Substance abuse. Primary Care 1993;20(1):1–276.

Diagnostic and Statistical Manual of Mental Disorders, 4th ed. Washington, DC, American Psychiatric Association, 1994.

Lange WR, White N, Robinson N: Medical complications of substance abuse. Postgrad Med 1992;92(3):205–214.

322 Nicotine Dependence

Jack L. Cox

Epidemiology

1. More than 50 million United States adults were tobacco users in 1991, including 46 million cigarette smokers and 5.3 million smokeless tobacco users (Table 322–1).

2. Adult cigarette use

   a. A total of 25.7 per cent of U.S. adults were current smokers in 1991; 43.5 million adults were former smokers.

   b. By the year 2000, an estimated 21.7 per cent (43 million) of U.S. adults will be smokers, including 22.7 per cent of women and 19.9 per cent of men.

3. Adult smokeless tobacco use

   a. In 1991, 2.9 per cent of U.S. adults were current smokeless tobacco users; 7.9 million adults were former smokeless tobacco users.

   b. The rate of smokeless tobacco use has tripled from 1972 to 1991.

4. Adolescent tobacco use

   a. Around 89 per cent of adult smokers started smoking before age 18 years and 60 per cent before age 14.

   b. Approximately 3000 adolescents begin smoking each day; 750 of these will die from tobacco-related diseases.

   c. A total of 75 per cent of smoking adolescents have at least one parent who smokes; 70 per cent of high school dropouts smoke.

   d. In 1991, 17.7 per cent of high school seniors were frequent smokers, and 11.9 per cent were frequent smokeless tobacco users.

Morbidity and Mortality

1. In 1990, 419,000 deaths were directly attributable to smoking. One out of every 5 deaths in the United States is directly related to smoking.

   a. Smoking kills more U.S. adults each year than all

TABLE 322–1. ADULT TOBACCO USE PREVALENCE (1991)

	CIGARETTES, PER CENT OF POPULATION	SMOKELESS TOBACCO, PER CENT OF POPULATION
Men	28.1 (24.0 million)	5.6 (4.8 million)
Women	23.5 (22.2 million)	0.6 (533,000)
White	25.5	3.1
Black	29.2	2.3
<12 years education	32	4.6
≥15 years education	13.6	1.4

TABLE 322–2. SMOKING-RELATED DEATHS

Cardiovascular 　Ischemic heart disease (myocardial infarct) 　Cerebrovascular disease (stroke) 　Hypertension 　Atherosclerosis	180,000 deaths
Neoplasms (cancer) 　Cervix uteri 　Esophagus 　Kidney 　Larynx 　Lip, oral cavity, pharynx 　Lung 　Pancreas 　Urinary bladder	150,000 deaths
Respiratory disease 　Pneumonia/influenza 　Emphysema/chronic bronchitis	84,000 deaths

deaths caused by alcohol, illicit drugs, homicide, suicide, car accidents, fires, and AIDS combined. Most deaths from smoking are cardiovascular-related, neoplasm-related, or respiratory-related (Table 322–2).

   b. Average life expectancy for a 30-year-old man who smokes 1 pack per day is 64.8 years; for a 30-year-old man who never smoked it is 82.7 years.

   c. An individual who quits smoking at any time in his or her life increases the quality and quantity of life. For example, an individual who quits smoking before 50 years of age decreases overall mortality by 50 per cent over the next 15 years.

   d. Cigarette smoking is related to increased risk for complications in pregnancy (low birth weight, ectopic pregnancy frequency, spontaneous abortion, premature birth, placenta abruption), osteoporosis in women, cataract formation, and respiratory infections.

2. Environmental tobacco smoke (ETS) accounts for approximately 53,000 deaths annually: 37,000 from cardiovascular disease, 3700 from lung cancer, and 12,000 from other neoplasms.

   a. ETS has been labeled a class A carcinogen by the Environmental Protection Agency (EPA).

   b. ETS has been associated with an increased frequency of sudden infant death syndrome (SIDS), an increased incidence of pneumonia, asthma, upper respiratory symptoms in childhood, and increased respiratory symptoms in adults.

3. Smokeless tobacco users are at an increased risk of oropharyngeal cancer, teeth/gum disease, coronary artery disease, and peptic ulcers.

TABLE 322–3. WITHDRAWAL SYMPTOMS

Anxiety/irritability	Nicotine craving
Headaches	Restlessness
Impaired concentrating	Sleep disturbance
Increased hunger	Somnolence

Why People Use Tobacco

Addiction

1. Nicotine in tobacco products is at least as addictive as cocaine or heroin and is the reason most people use tobacco.
   a. Eighty per cent of smokers attempting to quit "cold turkey" undergo physiologic withdrawal symptoms. These symptoms usually peak in 48 to 72 hours and last for up to 4 to 6 weeks (Table 322–3).
   b. Nicotine withdrawal is the primary reason for relapse for smoking early on in attempted cessation.
2. Nicotine dependence is high if a smoker smokes within 30 minutes of awakening, smokes more than 20 cigarettes per day, or has had significant withdrawal symptoms with a previous quit attempt.

Psychosocial

1. Most smokers start smoking in response to peer, sibling, or parental smoking.
2. Smokers use tobacco for stress reduction, relaxation, and/or reward. Stress is the most common reason for late relapse in quit attempts. Coping mechanisms must be addressed for the quitting smoker in order to prevent relapse.
3. There is a higher incidence of underlying depression in smokers versus nonsmokers.

Habit

1. There are many cues that may precipitate craving for tobacco. These include the smell of coffee or cigarette smoke, seeing someone smoke, and after meals and with alcohol use.
2. These cues can be used to help a smoker quit by recognizing which cues are important and formulating plans for avoiding or handling them.

Treatment

Pharmacologic

1. Nicotine polacrilex and nicotine transdermal patches (nicotine withdrawal therapy, NWT) are the only pharmacologic therapies that have been shown to be consistently helpful in smoking cessation. There are not enough studies as of now on NWT in smokeless tobacco cessation (Table 322–4).
2. Clonidine, inderal, benzodiazepines, silver acetate, and lobeline have not been shown to consistently improve 1-year smoking cessation rates versus placebo.
3. The more intensive the behavioral intervention, the more successful abstinence; NWT doubles 1-year success rates of any behavioral intervention.

4. Other NWTs that are currently investigational include nicotine nasal spray, nicotine oral inhaler, and the nicotine oral lozenge.

Behavioral Approaches

(Adapted from the National Cancer Institute's manual "How to Help Your Patients Stop Smoking.")

1. Ask about each patient's smoking status at every opportunity: former, current, never, or passive smoke exposure.
   a. About 70 per cent of smokers visit a physician's office at least once per year, yet 54 per cent of smokers in one study reported not being asked if they smoked nor told to quit.
   b. Simply asking a patient if he or she smokes and telling him or her to quit increases chances for abstinence.
2. Advise all smokers to quit in a supportive, caring, nonjudgmental way, and let them know that if they have problems quitting, you will help them. Cutting down is a step in the right direction, but complete abstinence should be the goal.
3. Assess motivation to quit (J. O. Prochaska's model for behavioral change).
   a. Precontemplators are individuals not currently interested in quitting.
   b. Contemplators are thinking of quitting within the next 6 months.
   c. Smokers in preparation are considering quitting within the next month and actively looking at strategies to quit.
   d. Smokers in the action phase are involved in changing their behavior and environment to quit.
   e. Patients in the maintenance phase have quit for over 6 months and are addressing ways to prevent relapse.
4. Assist smokers in quitting.
   a. Precontemplators may need clear information on the hazards of smoking and the benefits of quitting to move them into the contemplation phase.
   b. Contemplators need advice on strategies to help them quit: group programs versus self-help programs and the benefits of NWT.
   c. Individuals in the preparation and action phases

TABLE 322–4. AVAILABLE NICOTINE WITHDRAWAL THERAPIES

Nicotine polacrilex
  Nicorette (2 mg gum), Marion Merrell Dow, Inc.
  Nicorette DS (4 mg gum), Marion Merrell Dow, Inc.
Nicotine transdermal patches
  Nicoderm (21 mg, 14 mg, 7 mg; 24-hour patch), Marion Merrell Dow, Inc.
  Habitrol (21 mg, 14 mg, 7 mg; 24-hour patch), Basel-Ciba-Geigy Corporation
  ProStep (22 mg, 11 mg; 24-hour patch), Elan/Lederle Laboratories
  Nicotrol (15 mg, 10 mg, 5 mg; 16-hour patch), McNeil Consumer Products

need reassurance in their ability to quit and stay quit. Most smokers have made three to seven attempts at quitting before being successful. Setting a quit date greatly increases long-term success.

d. Individuals in the maintenance phase benefit from positive feedback and advice on relapse prevention.

e. Most smokers who are highly nicotine dependent (see above) will benefit from concurrent NWT.

5. Arrange follow-up for all smokers attempting to quit, preferably at 1 week, 1 month, and 3 months after the quit date, or individualize. If a smoker relapses, identify the reason, and encourage another attempt to quit or continue abstinence.

Bibliography

For a more in-depth discussion on smoking and smoking cessation, including the risk and benefits, see
Fiore M (ed): Cigarette smoking. Med Clin North Am 1992;76:289–539. Cigarette smoking among adults: United States, 1992, and changes in definition of smoking. MMWR 1994;43:342–346.

For more information on NWT, see
Glover ED (ed): Special issue: Nicotine withdrawal therapy. Health Values 1993;17:4–79; or Benowitz NL: Nicotine replacement therapy: What has been accomplished—Can we do better? Drugs 1993;45:157–170.

For more information on stages of quitting, see
Prochaska JO, DiClemente CL, Norcross JC: In search of how people change: Applications to addictive behaviors. Am Psychol 1992;47:1102–1114.

323 Schizophrenia

Linda B. Andrews

Etiology

1. One per cent lifetime prevalence; men and women equally affected; average age of onset, late teens to early adulthood; similar prevalence worldwide

2. Specific etiology not known

3. Stress-diathesis model: Both neurophysiologic and psychosocial factors appear to be important. An individual has specific vulnerability or genetic predisposition, which, when acted on by stressors, allows the development of symptoms of schizophrenia.

4. Dopamine hypothesis: Hypoactive dorsolateral prefrontal cortex (DLPFC) dopamine neurons (secondary to problems in migration of neural tissue in early development) cause hyperactive limbic system dopamine neurons. Adolescence triggers the need to use one's DLPFC as higher cognitive functions develop.

5. Genetics: The closer the genetic relationship to the proband, the higher the risk of developing schizophrenia (i.e., monozygotic twins, 47 per cent; dizygotic twins, 12 per cent; general population, 1 per cent). Similar incidence in twins separated at birth and reared in different environments

Symptoms

1. Psychotic symptoms (active phase) for at least *1 month* (a, b, or c)

    a. Prominent hallucinations (hallucination is a perception of an external stimulus when no external stimulus is present)

    b. Bizarre delusions (delusion is a false belief not shared by others who have the same knowledge, experience, or cultural background that is firmly maintained even though it is contraindicated by social reality)

    c. Two of the following: delusions, hallucinations, disorganized speech (frequent loosening of associations [LOA] or incoherence), grossly disorganized or catatonic behavior, or negative symptoms (flat affect, poverty of speech, lack of initiative)

These are sometimes called the "positive symptoms of schizophrenia" and may be related to the hyperactive limbic system dopamine neurons.

2. Some symptoms (chronic phase) for at least *6 months* (i.e., isolation, withdrawal, decreased work performance, peculiar behavior, poor hygiene, flat affect, speech changes, odd beliefs, unusual perceptions, lack of initiative, interest or energy)

These are sometimes called the "negative symptoms of schizophrenia" and may be related to the hypoactive DLPFC dopamine neurons.

3. Decreased level of functioning (work, social, self-care)

4. No prominent mood symptoms (i.e., no prominent symptoms of depression or mania)

5. No "organic" cause for symptoms

6. Subtypes of schizophrenia

    a. Paranoid: prominent paranoid ideations, best prognosis and generally later onset

    b. Catatonic: significant psychomotor changes, including stupor, negativism, rigidity, excitement, or posturing

    c. Disorganized: loosening of associations, disinhibition, and grossly disorganized behavior

    d. Undifferentiated: not clearly one of the preceding three subtypes

    e. Residual: no active phase symptoms but has two or more of the chronic-phase symptoms

Key Symptoms

- Hallucinations

- Delusions

- Decreased level of functioning

- Not attributable to another medical or psychiatric condition

Clinical Findings

1. Premorbid history: often a history of being a quiet, passive, withdrawn child, few friends, introverted, loner, daydreamer

2. Often positive family history of schizophrenia

3. Chronic deteriorating course of exacerbations and remissions

4. Positive symptoms: hallucinations, delusions, LOA. Negative symptoms: isolation, withdrawal, poor hygiene, flat affect, lack of initiative, interest, or energy

5. Fifty per cent attempt suicide; 10 per cent succeed.

6. Mental status examination

    a. Orientation: usually alert and oriented with clear sensorium and no fluctuation in level of consciousness

    b. Motor activity: may fluctuate between agitation and psychomotor retardation

    c. Affect and mood: The most common affective presentations are either blunted emotional re-

1145

sponsiveness or overly labile/inappropriate emotions. The blunted affect can represent symptoms of the illness or parkinsonian side effects of medications used to treat the illness.

d. Thought process/content: when psychotic, often illogical, not goal-directed, may include loosening of associations, flight of ideas, thought blocking, or delusions (persecutory, grandiose, religious, somatic or thought-control, thought-broadcasting, thought-withdrawal)

e. Perception: when psychotic, often prominent hallucinations (usually auditory)

f. Insight: often poor

g. Judgment: when psychotic, poor; when not psychotic, adequate

h. Memory and abstraction: often impaired

7. Physical examination findings: Frequently soft neurologic symptoms, abnormal eye movements (increased rate of blinking, abnormal rapid eye movements, and decreased ability to follow an object through space with smooth eye pursuit), tics, stereotypes, grimacing, impaired fine motor skills, abnormal motor tone, but no physical findings are diagnostic or pathognomonic.

8. CT scan: Static ventricular enlargement, indicative of decreased cortical mass, is present at onset of illness in 10 to 50 per cent of patients (not diagnostic). PET scan: decreased frontal lobe metabolism, especially during psychological tests that stress this area of the brain

9. EEG findings: Significant number of patients have abnormal records with some tendency toward left-sided abnormalities (not diagnostic).

10. Psychological testing: when psychotic, projective tests (Rorschach) abnormal

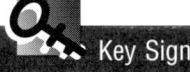

Key Signs

- Hallucinations
- Delusions
- Positive family history of schizophrenia
- Chronic deteriorating course

Laboratory Tests

1. There are no laboratory tests that definitively diagnose schizophrenia.

2. The workup to evaluate schizophrenia should include tests necessary to exclude other medical conditions that can present with psychotic symptoms (toxicology screens, CBC, RPR, CHEM-20, thyroid function tests, CT scan, EEG).

3. Mental status examination

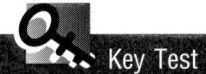

Key Test

- Mental status examination

Differential Diagnosis

1. Medical disorders or substance abuse (intoxication or withdrawal) that present with psychotic symptoms

2. Schizophreniform disorder: diagnosed if the patient has had symptoms for less than 6 months

3. Brief psychotic disorder: diagnosed if the symptoms have been present at least 1 day but less than 1 month

4. Schizoaffective disorder: diagnosed if depressive or manic symptoms are at least as prominent as the psychotic symptoms

5. Mood disorders with psychotic symptoms: diagnosed if the psychotic symptoms are brief relative to the mood symptoms. Cross-sectionally, mania can mimic schizophrenia.

6. Delusional disorder: diagnosed if the patient has non-bizarre delusions for at least 6 months and does not have any of the other symptoms of schizophrenia

7. Personality disorders: Patients with borderline, paranoid, schizoid, and schizotypal personality disorders all may have brief periods of psychotic symptoms.

Treatment

First assess whether or not the patient needs to be hospitalized for diagnostic purposes, stabilization on medications, patient's safety (i.e. suicidal ideations), or patient's lack of ability for self-care.

Medication

1. Guidelines

a. Define target symptoms to be treated.

b. Choose an antipsychotic medication that has worked for the patient or family member in the past, if one exists.

c. Make choices based on side-effect profile.

d. Give patient an adequate trial (4 to 6 weeks on medication) at adequate doses.

e. If patient does not respond, try medications from different chemical classes.

f. Maintenance doses may be lower than those required to treat acute episodes.

g. Monitor for compliance.

2. Antipsychotic medications (previously called "neuroleptics" or "major tranquilizers") are the medications of choice for schizophrenia.

a. Newer atypical antipsychotics such as clozapine (Clozaril) or risperidone (Risperdal) may be more effective. Clozapine does have a serious potential side effect of agranulocytosis.

b. All traditional antipsychotics are equally efficacious. Traditional antipsychotics can generally be grouped based on high or low affinity for blocking D_2 (dopamine) receptors.

    (1) High-potency

        (a) Haloperidol (Haldol)

        (b) Fluphenazine (Prolixin)

        (c) Trifluoperazine (Stelazine)

    (2) Low-potency

        (a) Chlorpromazine (Thorazine)

        (b) Thioridazine (Mellaril)

c. Acute episodes of psychotic symptoms generally respond to 5 to 30 mg of high-potency antipsychotics or 300 to1000 mg of low-potency antipsychotics.

d. Side effects for high-potency antipsychotics include extrapyramidal symptoms (acute dystonic reactions, akathisia-restlessness, induced parkinsonism) and neuroleptic malignant syndrome (fever, rigidity, autonomic instability, altered mental status), a life-threatening side effect that occurs in 0.5 to 1 per cent of patients treated with these medications. Anticholinergic medications (diphenhydramine [Benadryl], benztropine [Cogentin]) can be used to treat acute dystonic reactions.

e. Side effects for low-potency antipsychotics include anticholinergic side effects (dry mouth, blurred vision, urinary retention, constipation), postural hypotension, and sedation.

f. Most antipsychotics also can cause weight gain and impotence. A long-term and usually irreversible side effect of all antipsychotics is tardive dyskinesia. Tardive dyskinesia occurs in 15 to 20 per cent of patients treated with antipsychotics.

g. Atypical antipsychotics combine dopamine and serotonin blockade and may cause less extrapyramidal symptoms.

Patient Education

1. Patient and family education about schizophrenia is crucial for compliance (Alliance for the Mentally Ill is a national referral resource: 1-800-950-NAMI).

2. Supportive group therapy also may be useful to reduce social isolation and improve reality testing.

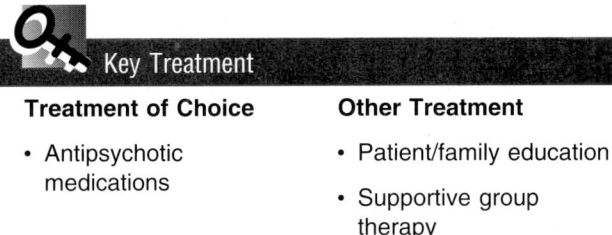

Key Treatment	
Treatment of Choice	**Other Treatment**
• Antipsychotic medications	• Patient/family education
	• Supportive group therapy

Follow-Up

1. Decisions to maintain patients on antipsychotics are based on the severity of the illness as well as the availability of family and community support.

2. Greater than two thirds of patients relapse within the first 6 months following the discontinuation of antipsychotic medication. Therefore, the patient can be instructed that he or she may need this medication indefinitely. Once stabilized, the patient can be followed as an outpatient as frequently as weekly or as infrequently as every 3 to 6 months depending on symptom stability.

Bibliography

Andreasen NC: Schizophrenia: From Mind to Molecule, 1st ed. Washington, DC, American Psychiatric Press, 1994.

Davis KL, Kahn RS, Ko G, Davidson M: Dopamine and schizophrenia: A review and reconceptualization. Am J Psychiatry 1991;148:1474–1486.

Diagnostic and Statistical Manual of Mental Disorders (DSM-IV). Washington, DC, American Psychiatric Association, 1994, pp 273–304.

Hyman SE, Nestler EJ: The Molecular Foundations of Psychiatry, 1st ed. Washington, DC, American Psychiatric Press, 1993, pp 141–150.

Kaplan H, Saddock B: Synopsis of Psychiatry, 7th ed. Baltimore, Williams & Wilkins, 1994, Ch 13, pp 457–486.

324 Obsessive Compulsive Disorder

Norman H. Rasmussen

Obsessive compulsive disorder (OCD) is characterized by recurrent and intrusive thoughts, ideas, impulses, or images (*obsessions*) and/or by the presence of stereotyped repetitive behaviors (*compulsions*). Obsessive compulsive disorder is a generally chronic and often disabling condition with a lifetime prevalence of 2 to 3 per cent based on recent epidemiologic studies. The disorder affects males and females equally. Approximately one third of adult cases are of childhood onset.

Etiology

1. The specific cause of OCD is unknown.
2. Genetic evidence
   a. Recent twin studies indicate a concordance rate in the 50 to 90 per cent range for monozygotic (MZ) twins as compared with the 40 per cent range for dizygotic (DZ) twin pairs.
   b. In family studies of OCD probands, up to 25 per cent of the fathers and 9 per cent of the mothers have OCD. When subclinical OCD is included, approximately 35 per cent of all first-degree relatives are affected.
3. Neurobiologic basis for OCD
   a. Neuroimaging studies (positron emission tomography, single positron emission computed tomography, magnetic resonance imaging) of nontreated and treated OCD patients have revealed neurophysiologic abnormalities in primarily three brain areas: orbital frontal cortex, cingulate cortex, and head of the caudate.
   b. Although there are no published postmortem studies in OCD, the morphology of the brain in living patients, as evidenced primarily on computed tomography (CT) findings, reveals no consistent evidence of structural pathology.
   c. Neurotransmitter dysfunction or specifically a serotonergic mechanism (i.e., serotonin uptake blockade) is implicated.
4. Psychosocial causes
   a. Freudian psychodynamic factors based primarily on the ego-defense mechanisms of reaction formation, isolation, and undoing
   b. Learning theory views obsessions as a conditioned stimulus to anxiety and compulsions as an anxiety-reduction response.
5. To summarize, the cause of OCD is poorly understood, but the extant research suggests multiple determinants, including neurophysiologic abnormalities, heredity, and learning history. Overall, it appears that genetic and neurobiologic factors constitute the primary etiologic roles with psychosocial determinants exacerbating the OCD disorder.

Symptoms

1. The essential sign is either recurrent obsessions or compulsions.
   a. Obsessions
      (1) Recurrent and persistent thoughts, ideas, images, or impulses viewed as intrusive and senseless
      (2) Attempts are made to suppress, ignore, or neutralize the obsession with some other thought or an action.
   b. Compulsions
      (1) Intentional and repetitive behavior performed in response to an obsession or in a stereotyped ritualistic manner according to certain rules
      (2) The purpose is to neutralize or prevent anticipated distress or a dreaded event, but the compulsive act is not connected in a realistic way to what it is designed to prevent or neutralize.
   c. There are patients who are purely obsessional or purely ritualizers, but the most common pattern (approximately 75 per cent) is a combination of the two essential features.
2. Obsessions and compulsions share several common features
   a. The thought or impulse to act persistently invades the person's conscious awareness.
   b. The thought or impulse to act is ego-dystonic or ego-alien.
   c. The thought or impulse to act is recognized as irrational, but the person is unable to prevent it.
   d. There is a strong desire to resist the idea or impulse.
   e. The obsessions and compulsions are time-consuming and lead to fatigue.
3. The obsessions and compulsions significantly interfere with the patient's normal routine, work performance, or social functioning due to the marked distress and/or excessive time (i.e., take more than 1 hour per day) involved.
4. Onset of symptoms
   a. Mean age of onset is 20 years of age.
   b. Over 50 per cent experience the onset of symptoms before age 24 and 80 per cent by age 35.
   c. Approximately one third of cases in adults have their onset in childhood.

5. Associated features frequently include depression, anxiety, and personality disorders.

Key Symptoms

- Obsession of contamination followed by washing compulsion

- Obsession of doubt followed by a compulsion of checking

- Obsessional slowness or taking excessive time to carry out activities of daily living

Clinical Findings

1. The OCD patient is frequently embarrassed or ashamed of his or her symptoms and therefore will not confide in the physician during a regular office visit. Thus the physician must be alert to recognize associated physical and/or psychological signs.
   a. Possible physical indicators
      (1) Chapped or eczematoid-appearing hands from frequent washings.
      (2) Gum lesions from excessive teeth brushing
   b. Possible psychological indicators
      (1) Depressed mood
      (2) Insistent concerns or firm belief that she or he has an infectious disease, e.g., acquired immune deficiency syndrome (AIDS)
2. Brief office-based screening index
   a. If the physician is suspicious of possible OCD based on physical and/or psychological indicators, ask the following brief questions:
      (1) Do you overly worry about contamination from dirt or other environmental substances?
      (2) Do you have to wash your hands repeatedly?
      (3) Do you have the need to repeatedly check locks or switches?
   b. If the patient answers yes to any of the screening questions, there is a strong possibility of OCD.

Key Signs

- Acknowledgment or observation of excessive handwashing or other cleaning rituals

- Acknowledgment or observation of repeating rituals, such as going in and out of a door

- Acknowledgment or observation of checking rituals, such as locked doors, appliances, or car brakes

Laboratory Tests

1. Neuroimaging studies such as CT are not yet routinely indicated because the findings do not clearly lead to a differential treatment plan.
2. Formal personality testing on instruments such as the Minnesota Multiphasic Personality Inventory (MMPI) and the Millon Clinical Multiaxial Inventory (MCMI-II) is indicated for several reasons.
   a. The high prevalence (i.e., 60 to 70 per cent) of concomitant personality disorders in OCD patients
   b. There are relationships between the personality subtype and treatment participation, compliance, and outcome; for example, patients with no evident personality pathology and those with dependent qualities demonstrate the best outcome, whereas schizotypal personality disorder consistently predicts a poorer outcome.
3. Formal clinician-rated testing on the Yale-Brown Obsessive Compulsive Scale (Y-BOCS) is important for making treatment decisions and assessing treatment progress related to
   a. Content and severity of specific OCD symptoms
   b. Degree of self-control over specific OCD symptoms

Key Tests

- Minnesota Multiphasic Personality Inventory (MMPI)

- Millon Clinical Multiaxial Inventory (MCMI-II)

- Yale-Brown Obsessive Compulsive Scale (Y-BOCS)

Differential Diagnosis

1. Major neurologic disorders to consider in the differential diagnosis
   a. Tourette's syndrome
   b. Chronic motor or vocal tic disorder
   c. Transient tic disorder
   d. Temporal lobe epilepsy
2. Primary psychiatric disorders that need to be differentiated from OCD
   a. Schizophrenia
      (1) In schizophrenia, the symptoms are generally more bizarre.
      (2) The OCD patient has more insight into his or her disorder as compared with the schizophrenic.
   b. Depression
      (1) The obsessing in depression is milder and of the brooding and ruminative type as compared with the severe, persistent, and intrusive egodystonic obsessional thinking in OCD.
      (2) The presence or absence of other symptoms (e.g., recurrent thoughts of death) indicative of major depression can help to make this differentiation.
   c. Phobias
      (1) In the phobias, the avoidance behavior is generally of a more circumscribed nature.

(2) OCD patients tend to be less successful in avoiding the feared object than are phobic patients.

d. Obsessive compulsive personality disorder

(1) There are no true obsessions or compulsions in obsessive compulsive personality disorder.

(2) The degree of social and occupational impairment is significantly greater in OCD.

3. Other medical conditions

a. Postpartum onset

b. Sydenham's chorea

Treatment

1. Interdisciplinary treatment including both behavioral therapy and psychopharmacology is indispensable for several reasons.

a. Each treatment has differential therapeutic effects on symptoms and types of patients.

b. Some patients who obtain no therapeutic benefit with behavior therapy improve on medication, and vice versa.

c. Patients who refuse one of the treatments may use the other as an alternative.

d. Patients who are noncompliant with one may adhere to the other.

2. Behavior therapy

a. Between 65 and 75 per cent of OCD patients improve on behavioral therapy.

b. Appears to be the most beneficial on the compulsive rituals with a secondary effect on the associated obsessions

c. There are neurophysiologic changes (e.g., decreased cerebral glucose metabolism in the right caudate region) on PET similar to that produced by fluoxetine (Prozac) treatment.

d. The behavioral treatment of choice is exposure and response prevention (ERP).

(1) Exposure: deliberately facing the feared and avoided thought, situation, place, or object

(2) Response prevention: delaying, diminishing, or preventing the anxiety-reducing compulsive rituals

(3) The rationale for ERP: The obsession creates a high level of discomfort and a parallel urge to engage in a compulsive ritual or to avoid the feared stimulus; avoidance and/or compulsive rituals are self-reinforcing because they produce a partial anxiety reduction; exposure and response prevention break this self-reinforcing chain and chronic pattern because the anxiety is gradually diminished (habituation) when the patient refrains from performing the compulsive ritual in response to the anxiety-evoking stimulus; the urge to perform the

compulsive ritual or avoidance behavior is progressively decreased.

e. Behavioral group therapy and individual behavioral therapy are equally effective, although individually based treatment usually results in more rapid reductions in OCD symptom severity.

3. Pharmacotherapy

a. Medications generally produce a 30 to 90 per cent reduction in OCD symptoms.

b. The drugs of choice are the antidepressants, particularly those with prominent serotonergic reuptake blocking properties.

(1) Clomipramine (Anafranil)

(2) Fluoxetine (Prozac)

(3) Sertraline (Zoloft)

(4) Fluvoxamine (Luvox)

(5) Paroxetine (Paxil)

c. Augmenting agents for treatment-resistant OCD patients

(1) Buspirone (BuSpar)

(2) Clonazepam (Klonopin)

(3) Trazodone (Desyrel)

(4) Alprazolam (Xanax)

(5) Lithium carbonate (Lithane)

(6) Clonidine (Catapres)

(7) Fenfluramine (Pondimin)

(8) Methylphenidate (Ritalin)

(9) Tryptophan (L-tryptophan)

WARNING

L-Tryptophan has been implicated in an increased incidence of eosinophilia-myalgia syndrome.

---

4. Psychodynamic psychotherapy has not been demonstrated to be an effective first-line treatment.

5. Psychosurgery (e.g., bimedial lukotomy that produces lesions in the thalamofrontal connections) should be considered only if the patient, despite adequate treatment trials, remains severely disabled.

6. Most effective treatment: exposure and response prevention (ERP) behavior therapy combined with serotonergic reuptake inhibitors (SRIs).

Key Treatment

- Exposure and response prevention (ERP) behavior therapy

- Serotonergic reuptake inhibitors (SRIs)

Follow-Up

1. Most patients treated with a combination of behavioral therapy and medication can expect significant long-term symptom improvement but not complete remission.

2. Common reasons for treatment failure

   a. Misdiagnosis, such as schizophrenia

   b. Inadequate treatment, such as medication trial too short or medication dosage too low

   c. Treatment noncompliance, such as patient refuses medication due to a fear of long-term effects or inability to tolerate the initial increased anxiety associated with behavioral therapy

3. Preliminary evidence indicates a relapse rate of over 90 per cent soon after medication-only treatment.

4. Family counseling is useful in preventing the avoidant behavior that is a serious complication of OCD.

Bibliography

For a comprehensive and detailed treatise on the diagnosis and treatment of OCD, see
Jenike MA, Baer L, Minichiello WE (eds): Obsessive-Compulsive Disorders: Theory and Management, 2nd ed. Chicago, Year Book Medical Publishers, 1990.

For patient education, see
Foa E, Wilson R: Stop Obsessing! How to Overcome Your Obsessions and Compulsions. New York, Bantam, 1991.

For more information on treatment-resistant patients, see
Goodman WK, McDougle CJ, Barr LC, et al: Biological approaches to treatment-resistant obsessive compulsive disorder. J Clin Psychiatry 1993; 54(suppl)6:16–26.

For an overview of OCD, see
Hales RE, Yudofsky SC, Talbott JA (eds): Textbook of Psychiatry, 2nd ed. Washington, DC, American Psychiatric Press, 1994, pp 532–544.

For more information on the pharmacologic treatment of OCD, see
Lydiard RB: Obsessive-compulsive disorder: A new perspective in diagnosis and treatment. Int Clin Psychopharmacol 1994; 9(suppl 3):33–37.

325 Common Poisoning Symptoms

Symptom	Abdominal Pain	*Jonathan L. Temte*

Abdominal pain can result from a vast array of underlying medical and psychological problems. In the context of poisoning and environmental problems, however, one must consider the wide range of possible ingestions and exposures and then narrow the field using the more probable ingestions or exposures.

Differential Diagnosis

1. Food poisoning
   a. Bacterial toxins: Cases of food poisoning present with abdominal pain, nausea, vomiting, and diarrhea and are often associated with outbreaks. Patients are usually afebrile.
      (1) Staphylococcal poisoning results from improperly prepared and stored protein-containing foods.
      (2) *Clostridium* toxin can be found in cooked meats.
      (3) *Bacillus cereus* toxin is often associated with fried rice.
      (4) Scombroid fish poisoning occurs with ingestion of tuna or mackerel.
      (5) Paralysis may occur in neurotoxic seafood poisoning (NSP) and botulism.
   b. Mushrooms and plants
      (1) Poisonous mushrooms, especially those of the genus *Amanita*
      (2) Toxalbumin-producing plants, such as jequirty bean and rosary bean
2. Drug and household chemical ingestion: A great number of pharmaceutical products can cause symptoms of abdominal pain when excessive dosages are ingested.
   a. Common drugs
      (1) Digoxin
      (2) Theophylline
      (3) Iron (Fe) supplements
      (4) Erythromycin can cause abdominal pain in therapeutic doses.
   b. Other medications. Abdominal pain often occurs in eosinophilia-myalgia syndrome (EMS) caused by contaminated L-tryptophan supplements. Intake of iodine-containing topical solutions also may cause abdominal pain.
   c. Household chemicals. The ingestion of household chemicals and cleaning products can be a common problem, especially with young children.
      (1) Caustics (e.g., acids, alkalis, bleach) cause abdominal pain through direct irritant effect.
      (2) Halogenated hydrocarbons found in solvents, floor waxes, and adhesive cements
      (3) Pesticides
      (4) Arsenic (As) containing products, such as insecticides, rodenticides, and wood preservatives
3. Occupational and environmental exposures
   a. Occupational exposures. Exposures to hazardous materials from manufacturing and industry can cause abdominal pain in employees working directly in these settings and in people living and working nearby. Agricultural chemicals can affect farm laborers and may contaminate groundwater supplies.
      (1) Heavy metals such as lead (Pb), arsenic (As), mercury (Hg), and thallium (Tl)
      (2) Other exposures include benzene, formaldehyde, pesticides (e.g., flouride salts, organophosphates [OP], pentachlorophenol [PCP], phosphorus), and polychlorinated biphenyls (PCBs).
   b. Environmental exposures. Other environmental exposures resulting in abdominal pain include
      (1) Carbon monoxide.
      (2) Agent orange (AO) and phenoxy herbicides.
      (3) Lead (Pb).
      (4) Chemical warfare agents (similar in action to organophosphate pesticides).
4. Effects of the physical environment. Decreased partial pressures of oxygen and increased 2,3-DPG at high altitudes can promote sickling of erythrocytes in people with sickle cell anemia, resulting in abdominal pain. In rare cases, abdominal angina can occur at high elevations due to lowered oxygen tensions, especially in the postprandial setting. These patients usually have underlying atherosclerosis or vasculitis.

Refer to Ch. 77, Appendicitis; and Ch. 326, Poisoning, Acute and Chronic

History

1. Possible exposures
   a. Foods. Ask about recent picnics, dining out, recent seafood consumption, and home canning.

TABLE 325–1. SYMPTOMS COMMONLY ASSOCIATED WITH POISONINGS THAT CAUSE ABDOMINAL PAIN

SYMPTOM	FOOD POISONING	MEDICATIONS	CAUSTICS AND HYDROCARBONS	PESTICIDES	HEAVY METALS	PCBS AND AGENT ORANGE
Nausea and vomiting	+	+		+	Fe, As, Hg	AO
Diarrhea	+	+		+	Tl, Fe, As, Hg	AO
Constipation					Pb	
Anorexia		Digoxin			As	AO
Oral irritation	Plants		+			
Stomatitis					As	
Metallic taste					Hg	
Salivation				OP	Hg	
Breath odor				Phosphorus	As	
Skin rash	Scombroid				As	+
Hair loss					As, Tl	
Sweating				OP		
Wheezing				OP		
Visual changes		Digoxin				
Peripheral neuropathy					Pb, As	
Incontinence				OP		
Tremors/fasciculations		Theophylline		Fluorides, OP		
Paralysis	Bot., NSP				Tl	AO
Cognitive changes			Hydrocarbons		Pb	AO, PCB
Headache					Pb	AO, PCB
Anxiety		Theophylline				

Symptoms related to a general category are indicated by "+." Specific agents are identified by name or symbol.
See text for explanation of abbreviations.

b. Medications: What medications are available to the patient in his or her household?

c. Occupational exposures: Ask about exposure to heavy metals, pesticide production, agricultural practices, and ventilation.

d. Travel: Ask about recent travel to areas where water may be contaminated, pesticides used, or exotic plants available.

e. Household exposures: What cleaning products and insecticides are used? Where are they kept? Is there pealing or cracking paint on the walls? What is the age of the dwelling?

2. Duration of abdominal pain

a. Acute pain: Effects are seen almost immediately with caustics and usually occur within 1 to 24 hours after ingestions of contaminated foods, poisonous plants, and mushrooms.

b. Chronic pain: Chronic pain is more common with medical therapy (e.g., digoxin or theophylline toxicity) and household or occupational exposures to heavy metals, PCBs, and carbon monoxide.

3. Associated symptoms: Symptoms (Table 325–1) can help narrow the field of possible exposures.

4. Concomitant medical problems: Include in the past medical history information on atherosclerosis, hepatic and renal dysfunction, pulmonary disease, sickle cell disease, and multiple transfusions.

Clinical Findings

1. General (Table 325–2)

a. Hyperpyrexia with possible pesticide exposure suggests pentachlorophenol poisoning.

b. Dehydration is commonly found in food poisoning and also with arsenic toxicity.

c. Hypotension can result from dehydration or bradycardia or effects of iron, thallium, and arsenic.

d. Mental status changes are associated with hydrocarbon, carbon monoxide, and lead toxicity.

2. Cardiovascular

a. Bradycardia may be found in digitalis toxicity and organophosphate poisoning.

b. Tachycardia is associated with theophylline toxicity and mushroom poisoning.

3. Respiratory

a. Bronchorrhea and wheezing are commonly found in organophosphate poisoning.

b. Pulmonary edema can be found in organophosphate or pentachlorophenol poisoning.

4. Skin

a. A rash associated with recent seafood ingestion may indicate scombroid.

b. Follicular or eczematous dermatitis can be found in chronic arsenic poisoning.

c. Chloracne, characterized by cysts filled with straw-colored liquid, is highly suggestive of PCBs.

5. Neurologic signs

a. Miosis occurs with organophosphate poisoning due to cholinergic stimulation.

b. Extensor muscle weakness may occur with lead toxicity.

c. Fasciculations suggest theophylline toxicity or poisoning with organophosphates or fluoride salts.

TABLE 325–2. CLINICAL PRESENTATIONS AND SIGNS COMMONLY FOUND IN POISONINGS THAT CAUSE ABDOMINAL PAIN

CLINICAL SIGNS	FOOD POISONING	MEDICATIONS	CAUSTICS AND HYDROCARBONS	PESTICIDES	HEAVY METALS	PCBs AND AGENT ORANGE
General						
Dehydration	+				As	
Hypotension	+	+			Fe, As, Tl	
Hyperpyrexia				PCP		
Mental status changes			Hydrocarbons		Pb	+
Cardiovascular						
Tachycardia	Mushrooms	Theophylline				
Bradycardia		Digoxin		OP		
Respiratory						
Wheezing				OP		
Pulmonary edema				PCP, OP		
Skin						
Rash	Scombroid					
Follicular dermatitis					As	
Chloracne						+
Neurologic						
Miosis				OP		
Extensor weakness					Pb	
Fasciculations		Theophylline		OP, Fluorides		
Paralysis	Bot., NSP			Fluorides		
Musculoskeletal						
Myalgias		EMS				
Renal						
Acute tubular necrosis					Hg	

Signs occurring in general categories are indicated by ''+.'' Specific agents are identified by name or symbol.
See text for explanation of abbreviations

d. Paralysis occurs in botulism, neurotoxic seafood poisoning (NSP), and poisoning from fluoride salts and thalium.

6. Musculoskeletal: Incapacitating myalgias are the hallmark of esosinophilia-myalgia syndrome.

7. Renal: Acute tubular necrosis may occur in mercury poisoning.

Tests

1. Food poisoning
   a. Food contamination: Culture food, vomitus, or stool. Bioassay of food and serum for toxin if botulism or NSP is suspected.
   b. Mushroom poisoning: Follow renal and hepatic function tests and prothrombin times.

2. Medications
   a. Digitalis toxicity: Electrocardiogram (ECG), electrolytes (especially potassium), and serum digoxin level
   b. Theophylline: ECG, serum theophylline level, serum glucose, and consider serum pH
   c. EMS: Obtain complete blood count (CBC) with differential if eosinophilia-myalgia syndrome is suspected.

3. Caustics and hydrocarbons
   a. Caustics. Consider upper gastrointestinal (GI) endoscopy to define extent of tissue damage for all ingestions of caustic material, including acids, alkalis, and formalin. Obtain chemistry survey and blood gases to assess possible hypocalcemia, hyperkalemia, and metabolic acidosis.
   b. Hydrocarbons. Follow liver function tests.

4. Pesticides. Assess plasma and erythrocyte cholinesterase activity levels. These will be lowered to less than 50 per cent of normal levels in organophosphate poisoning. Follow calcium levels if fluoride salt poisoning.

5. Heavy metals. Consider abdominal radiographs if ingestion of iron tablets or elemental lead is suspected.
   a. Iron: Obtain serum iron, total iron-binding capacity, and ferritin levels. Also, consider serum glucose and pH.
   b. Lead: Obtain levels of serum lead, blood urea nitrogen (BUN), creatinine, and free erythrocyte protoporphyrin. Also obtain CBC with differential (microcytic anemia with basophilic stippling).
   c. Arsenic: 24-hour urine for arsenic. Check CBC for signs of anemia.
   d. Mercury: Serum and urine Hg level. Look for active urine sediment.

6. Carbon monoxide: Obtain carboxyhemoglobin level. Consider ECG.

Management

1. Basic life support
2. Discontinuation or limitation of exposure
   a. Ingestions

(1) Dilute caustics and carefully lavage (consider early endoscopy before lavage).

(2) Eliminate others using *emesis, lavage, activated charcoal,* and *cathartics* (ELACC).

b. Topical absorption of organophosphate pesticides: Health care providers should be gowned and gloved. Remove patient's clothing, shampoo hair, and clean all skin surfaces.

WARNING

High risk for secondary contamination of health care workers by organophosphate pesticides

---

c. Inhalations: Remove from place of exposure. Displace carbon monoxide using 100 per cent oxygen. Assisted ventilation may be necessary. Also consider use of hyperbaric chamber.

3. Specific interventions

WARNING

Call the nearest poison control center for current recommendations on treatment.

---

a. Food poisoning

(1) Food poisoning is usually self-limited. Public health department should be notified of outbreak.

(2) Paralysis (e.g., botulism, NSP) may require hospitalization and mechanical ventilation.

(3) Treat mushroom poisoning as above (ELACC). Institute vigorous intravenous fluid rehydration with forced diuresis (>300 cc/hr of urine output). Penicillin, silymarin, and cimetidine may be useful. With severe hepatic toxicity, liver transplantation is a final option.

b. Medications: Decrease absorption as above.

(1) Digoxin: Symptomatic bradycardia may be treated with atropine (0.5 to 2.0 mg intravenously). Lidocaine may be used for other dysrhythmias. Digoxin antibody may be given in extreme cases.

(2) Theophylline: Intravenous esmolol (25 to 50 μg/kg/min) or propranolol (0.5 to 1.0 mg) may be given for symptomatic tachycardia.

(3) EMS: Glucocorticoids may be of some benefit.

c. Caustics

(1) Acids and formalin: Dilute with water or milk. *Do not induce emesis.* Consider early upper GI endoscopy. Provide supportive care with correction of metabolic acidosis.

(2) Halogenated hydrocarbons: Emesis and lavage are controversial because of risk of aspiration pneumonitis. Consider possible hemodialysis.

(3) Others: Follow management for ingestions above.

d. Pesticides

(1) Organophosphates: Support respiration and follow management above. Use atropine (0.02 to 0.05 mg/kg intravenously every 15 minutes) until some effects are manifested. Administer pralidoxime (20 to 50 mg/kg intravenously every 2 to 12 hours).

(2) Fluoride salts and phosphorus: Dilute with milk or calcium gluconate. Follow management for ingestions above. Then administer intravenous solution of 10% calcium gluconate to maintain serum calcium. Supportive care.

(3) Pentachlorophenol: Avoid atropine. *Lower body temperature.* Supportive care.

e. Heavy metals: If acute ingestion, follow management for ingestions above.

(1) Iron: Administer deferoxamine (10 to 15 mg/kg/hr intramuscularly or intravenously) until serum iron less than 250 μ/dl.

(2) Lead: Chelation with CaEDTA (50 mg/kg/day intravenous infusion for 5 days)

(3) Arsenic: Administer dimercaprol (BAL) (2.5 to 3.0 mg/kg intramuscularly as 10% solution in oil, then 2 to 3 mg/kg intramuscularly every 4 hours for 2 days). Then administer oral penicillamine (25 mg/kg/day every 6 hours for 7 days, max. 2 gm/day).

(4) Mercury: Dimercaprol as above. Maintain appropriate urine output.

(5) Thalium: Administer potassium chloride and Prussian blue (potassium ferrichexacyanoferrate). Consider hemodialysis.

PEARLS

• The telephone numbers of the 42 regional poison control centers certified by the American Association of Poison Control Centers are listed in the back of the *Physicians' Desk Reference.* The trained personnel at these centers are available 24 hours per day and are invaluable sources of information in the management of poisoning and overdose.

• The federal Hazardous Substances Act requires content labeling of hazardous household products.

Bibliography

For more information on treatment of drug overdose, see
Haddad LM, Winchester JF (eds): Clinical Management of Poisoning and Drug Overdose, 2d ed. Philadelphia, WB Saunders, 1990.

For overview of poisoning and drug overdose, see
Lovejoy FH, Kayser DL: Acute poison and drug overdose. *In* Isselbacher KJ, Braunwald E, Wilson JD, et al (eds): Harrison's Principles of Internal Medicine, 13th ed, vol 2. New York, McGraw-Hill, 1994, pp 2441–2461.

For more information on occupational chemical exposures, see
National Institute for Occupational Safety and Health: Pocket Guide to Chemical Hazards. DHSS (NIOSH) publ no. 85-114, 1987.

For more information on wide spectrum of poisoning, see
Olson KR, Becker CE: Poisoning. *In* Saunders CE, Ho MT (eds): Current Emergency Diagnosis and Treatment, 4th ed. Norwalk, CT, Appleton & Lange, 1992, pp 730–768.

For more information on occupational and environmental exposures, including heavy metals, see
Rom WN (ed): Environmental and Occupational Medicine, 2d ed. Boston, Little, Brown, 1992.

Many forms of poisoning and environmental exposures present with vomiting and/or diarrhea. A wide variety of overdoses, toxic chemicals, metals, plants, and infections cause gastrointestinal (GI) symptoms. Most poisonings in children are accidental ingestions, whereas most adult poisonings occur as intentional drug abuse or suicide attempts, accidental industrial exposures, or accidental overdose of prescription drugs. The history of the present illness is often the key in determining the cause. Clinical evaluation of the patient, combined with consultation with a local poison control center, when appropriate, will determine the best treatment options.

Differential Diagnosis

1. Medications that commonly involve vomiting at toxic levels include theophylline (>20 μg/ml), lithium, digoxin, quinine, quinidine, colchicine, fluoride, phenytoin, acetaminophen, and salicylates. Laxative abuse, quinidine, and digoxin are common sources of chronic diarrhea.

2. Heavy metals ingestions of iron, lead, arsenic, cadmium, mercury, tin, zinc, and nickel may cause vomiting and diarrhea. Vomiting in iron overdose is predictive of severe toxicity. Arsenic poisoning also may present with massive diarrhea. Mercury poisoning is often accompanied by mucus-like diarrhea and hemorrhagic colitis.

3. Alcohol intoxication often presents with vomiting. Cocaine abuse may cause vomiting and diarrhea. Significant opiate or benzodiazepine withdrawal presents with these symptoms, accompanied by hyperactive bowel sounds.

4. Organophosphate poisoning, petroleum ingestion, and ingestion of household cleaners and soaps, as well as a number of other chemical exposures, can present with GI disturbance.

5. Carbon monoxide inhalation causes nausea and vomiting at levels of 30 to 40 per cent carboxyhemoglobin saturation.

6. Ingestion of many types of mushrooms, plants, shellfish, and deep sea fish often causes vomiting.

7. Causes of infectious diarrhea, which often afflicts travelers, include enterotoxigenic *Escherichia coli* (most common cause), *Salmonella, Campylobacter, Shigella, Yersinia, Staphylococcus aureus, Clostridium difficile, Vibrio parahaemolyticus,* and less commonly *Entaemoeba histolytica* and *Plesiomonas shigellosis.* Noninflammatory agents causing infectious diarrhea include rotavirus, Norwalk virus, adenovirus, *Giardia, Cryptosporidium, Vibrio cholerae,* toxigenic *E. coli, Clostridium,* and *Acromonas.* These agents are ingested in contaminated food and water.

8. Other infections which may present with vomiting and/or diarrhea include HIV, malaria, hepatitis A, hepatitis C, strongyloidiasis, fish tapeworm, botulism, schistosomiasis, Lyme disease, Rocky Mountain spotted fever, and snake envenomations.

9. Contamination of water can occur in natural disasters such as floods or earthquakes, subjecting a population to exposures similar to those which occur with traveler's diarrhea.

Refer to Ch. 326, Poisoning, Acute and Chronic, and Part V, Gastrointestinal Disease (Chs. 72 to 86).

History: Key Questions to Ask

1. How long ago was the ingestion? Was it accidental or intentional? When did the symptoms begin?

2. Can you identify what substance caused these symptoms?

3. How many episodes of vomiting and/or diarrhea have occurred?

4. What is the consistency and color of vomitus? See Table 325–3 for a list of drug ingestions that discolor vomit in characteristic ways.

5. What makes the symptoms increase or decrease?

6. What is the color and consistency of the diarrhea? Is there any blood in it?

7. Are there any associated symptoms, including fever, sweats, nausea, abdominal pain, or cramping?

8. Identify which medications the patient has been taking, all known allergies, the patient's age and weight, and all other medical problems.

Clues to diagnosis also may come from a diet, work, or travel history. It will be useful to know whether other household members or coworkers have similar symptoms

TABLE 325–3. DISCOLORATION OF VOMITUS BY DRUGS

SIGN OR SYMPTOM	POISON
Colored material in gastric lavage or vomitus	
Pink or purple	Potassium permanganate
Blue, green	Copper salts, chemical dyes added to fluorides or mercury bichloride
Green	Nickel salts
Pink	Cobalt salts
Yellow	Picric acid, nitric acid
Bright red	Mercurochrome, nitric acid
Black, coffee-like grounds	Sulfuric acid, oxalic acid, nitric acid
Brown	Hydrochloric acid
Luminescent in dark	Yellow phosphorus
Discolored, bloody (hematemesis)	Alkalis, acids, fluoride, phosphorus, salicylates, iron

From Arena JM, Drew RH: Poisoning: Toxicology, Symptoms, Treatment, 5th ed. Springfield, Ill, Charles C Thomas, 1986. Courtesy of Charles C Thomas Publishers, Springfield, Illinois.

and any medications they take. If routine history is unhelpful, have the patient describe all activities over the past few days, since this may reveal a forgotten exposure.

Clinical Evaluation

1. Assess level of consciousness and ABCs—airway, breathing, and circulation.
2. Vital signs, including orthostatic blood pressure and pulse measurements
3. Examine oral mucosa and skin turgor for hydration.
4. Perform a thorough abdominal examination, with special attention to bowel sounds, tenderness over the liver, and liver size.
5. A rectal examination also should be done, especially to check for the quality of any stool and the presence of blood.

Tests

1. On all patients obtain
   a. STAT serum glucose in suspected poisoning cases
   b. Complete blood count (CBC) to screen for infection or anemia
   c. Electrolytes and anion gap
   d. Urinalysis
2. Consider also ordering
   a. Urine toxicologic screen to look for drug ingestions
   b. Liver function tests to rule out hepatic/biliary dysfunction
   c. Abdominal radiographs to screen for agents that are radiopaque (arsenic, chloral hydrate, lead, iron, tricyclic antidepressants, phenothiazines, and enteric and slow-release capsules) and to aid in clinical evaluation
   d. Electrocardiogram if cardiotoxicity is suspected
   e. Chest radiograph and pulmonary function tests if pulmonary involvement is suspected
   f. Examination of stool for leukocytes, ova, parasites, and culture if infectious causes are suspected

Management

1. Vomiting and diarrhea due to poisoning
   a. Do not give agents to suppress these symptoms. Treat the patient supportively and make efforts to decrease further absorption of the ingested agent. Resuscitation should be provided as necessary with intravenous fluids, oxygen, thiamine, glucose, and Narcan in patients with decreased mental status. Treatment of hypovolemia may be the main therapy needed by an alert patient.
   b. For the home management of poisoning in a conscious patient, the administration of syrup of ipecac may be appropriate; however, a physician, pharmacist, or poison center should be consulted first by phone. The recommended doses are 10 cc in infants 9 to 12 months of age, 15 cc in children, and 30 cc in adults. This should be followed by 8 to 12 oz of clear liquid for adults and proportionately less for children. Do not administer ipecac to infants less than 9 months of age, and use with great caution in those younger than 1 year. These doses may be repeated once within 30 minutes if emesis has not yet occurred. Ipecac is generally not used in the hospital setting because activated charcoal is now believed to be more effective.
   c. The use of emetics is contraindicated in patients with decreased mental status, impaired gag reflex, those who are seizing, and when ingestion of caustic agents or petroleum agents is suspected.
   d. Gastric lavage should be performed for ingestion of toxins known to be of serious toxicity (e.g., tricyclic antidepressants) or when emesis is contraindicated.
   e. Activated charcoal (AC) should be administered after lavage or instead of lavage (in cases of less severe toxic potential) in order to adsorb toxins. AC adsorbs ipecac and therefore should be given after vomiting from ipecac has occurred, if it has been used. Ideally, a dose 10 times the mass of the ingested poison is given. General doses recommended are 50 to 100 gm for adults, 25 to 50 gm for children, and 1 gm/kg for infants. One level tablespoon of AC contains 5 to 6 grams. Mix the charcoal for 30 seconds before administration. The aqueous slurry form of activated charcoal is safer to use than sorbitol-containing forms because it causes less fluid and electrolyte loss. Agents that are poorly adsorbed by AC include methanol, iron, lithium, and strong acids and bases.
   f. Administer cathartics after giving activated charcoal. Recommended doses are 1 to 1.5 gm/kg of sorbitol or 3 to 4 ml/kg of magnesium citrate (which works more slowly). Use cautiously or in limited quantity if multiple doses of activated charcoal are used. Irritant cathartics such as aloes, cascara, or oil-based cathartics (e.g., castor oil) are generally not recommended.
   g. Administer specific antidotes for specific ingestions, as directed by a poison control center.
   h. Ingestion of petroleum agents must be managed cautiously. Emesis should not be induced routinely, because aspiration of volatile hydrocarbons can cause severe pulmonary damage. Removal of these substances by lavage with protection of the airway by endotracheal intubation may be necessary.
   i. Stable patients who may have ingested poisons that have delayed toxicity (e.g., mushrooms, methanol, acetaminophen) or which are enter-

ically recycled (e.g., tricyclic antidepressants) must be followed for hours to days after the initial evaluation.

j. All patients who attempted suicide should be evaluated for future suicide risk prior to release from the emergency department.

2. Traveler's vomiting and diarrhea or food poisoning

a. Fluid and electrolyte replacement with nonalcoholic, noncaffeinated beverages is the treatment of choice for all cases. Most cases are self-limited to 1 to 5 days' duration.

b. Individuals afflicted with mild cases of nonbloody diarrhea (without fever or dysentery) can use bismuth subsalicylate—2 tablets every 4 to 6 hours p.r.n. or 30 cc every 30 minutes for up to eight doses. Alternatively, loperamide (Imodium) can be used in the following doses: 4 mg initially, followed by 2 mg after each stool, up to 16 mg/day. Do not use loperamide in moderate to severe cases or when antibiotics are being given.

c. Empirical use of antibiotics may be appropriate. Please refer to the Bibliography for detailed recommendations.

Prevention

1. The routine prescription of medications in child-resistant containers reduces pediatric overdoses. All medications and toxic chemicals should be kept out of the reach of children and within locked cabinets. Medicines and chemicals should be stored in their original containers so that their contents can be readily identified in the event of an ingestion.

2. Prevention of travel-related exposures must focus on avoidance of potentially contaminated food and beverages. Safe foods are generally those served after being cooked and still hot or fruits or vegetables that are peeled by the traveler. Safe beverages are those served in a sealed container, purified by the traveler, boiled or pasteurized milk products, or alcoholic beverages in an intact container. Chemoprophylaxis is generally not recommended but is discussed in the pertinent Bibliography articles.

PEARLS

- Initial efforts should focus on resuscitation and stabilization of the patient and management of hypovolemia.

- Rapidly collect serum and urine specimens prior to the initiation of therapy.

- Once you have a suspected agent in any case of poisoning, call the nearest poison control center for the most current information on treatment.

- Remember to consider the usual differential diagnosis of vomiting and diarrhea in your initial evaluation.

Bibliography

For more information on toxic plants, see

Lamp KF: AMA Handbook of Poisonous and Injurious Plants. Chicago, Review Press, 1985.

For more information on traveler's diarrhea, see

DuPont HL, Ericsson CD: Prevention and treatment of traveler's diarrhea. N Engl J Med 1993; 328(25):1821–1827.

For more information on poisoning, refer to the following references:

Eilers MA, Garrison TE: General management principles. *In* Rosen P, Barkin RM (eds): Emergency Medicine—Concepts and Clinical Practice, 3d ed, vol 3. St Louis, Mosby–Year Book, 1992, pp 2470–2503.

Goldfrank LR, Flomenbaum NE, Lewin NA, et al: Goldfrank's Toxicologic Emergencies. E Norwalk, CT, Appleton & Lange, 1990.

Haddad LM, Winchester JF: Clinical Management of Poisoning and Drug Overdose. Philadelphia, WB Saunders, 1994.

Krenzelok EP, Dunmire SM: Acute poisoning emergencies— Resolving the gastric decontamination controversy. Postgrad Med 1992;91(2):179–186.

326 Poisoning, Acute and Chronic

J. Gregory Rosencrance

Etiology

1. In 1992, 1,864,188 poisonings were reported to poison centers in the United States.

2. Over 90 per cent of all poisonings occur in the home. Over 85 per cent of poisonings reported to poison centers are accidental. Children <6 years of age account for approximately 60 per cent of reported poisonings.

3. Drugs most frequently involved in suicide attempts are the tricyclic antidepressants and acetaminophen.

4. Chronic overdoses most frequently involve digoxin, theophylline, and salicylates.

Symptoms

1. In children, physical evidence such as tablet or plant fragments, smell of cleaning products or chemicals, non-food stains, and opened bottles or containers may be more suggestive than symptoms.

2. Interviews of family, friends, or medical personnel transporting the patient may reveal information to suggest that an overdose has occurred.

3. Lack of immediate symptoms does not rule out a significant ingestion with acetaminophen, iron, tricyclic antidepressants, and calcium channel blockers. Following some poisonings, symptoms may be delayed for up to 8 hours—longer if sustained-release preparations have been ingested.

4. Some common toxic syndromes, or "toxidromes," include

    a. Anticholinergic agent ingestions: dry mucous membranes, flushed skin, dilated pupils, hyperthermia, urinary retention, decreased bowel sounds, tachycardia, and lethargy. Seizures and hallucinations may occur in severe cases.

    b. Opiate (narcotic) ingestions: miosis, respiratory depression, coma

    c. Cholinergic agent ingestions: salivation, lacrimation, urinary and fecal incontinence, vomiting, diaphoresis. In severe cases, CNS depression, pulmonary edema, weakness, brachycardia or tachycardia, muscle fasciculations, and seizures may occur.

    d. Sympathomimetic agents/drugs of abuse: tachycardia (reflex bradycardia), hypertension (may precede hypotension), hyperpyrexia, hyperreflexia, delusions, paranoia. Seizures and profound hyperpyrexia may follow larger overdoses.

Clinical Findings

1. The physical examination should include an evaluation for evidence of trauma and a thorough neurologic examination.

2. The skin should be evaluated for needle marks. Lesions or rashes may indicate dermal contact with a toxin.

3. The presence of certain odors may aid in making the diagnosis; however, the absence of an odor is not reliable in excluding any intoxications.

4. Important components of the neurologic examination include

    a. Mental status

    b. Observation for evidence of seizure activity

    c. Pupillary size

        (1) Common causes of *mydriasis* include anticholinergics, meperidine, mushrooms, sympathomimetics, and glutethimide.

        (2) Common causes of *miosis* include cholinergics, clonidine, mushrooms, insecticides, nicotine, narcotics, phenothiazines, and phencyclidine.

    d. Gag reflex

    e. Focal neurologic signs should prompt consideration of nontoxicologic medical conditions.

    f. Drugs are occasionally transported in the rectum, vagina, or gastrointestinal tract. An unexpected cardiac or respiratory arrest in a patient suspected of transporting drugs should prompt an examination of these areas along with abdominal radiography.

    g. The combination of history and physical examination is usually all that is needed (and available) to guide the initial management of the patient.

Key Symptoms

• Arrhythmias	• Respiratory depression
• CNS depression	• Seizures
• Confusion	• Nausea/vomiting/ diarrhea

Key Signs

- Needle marks
- Trauma
- Focal neurologic signs

Laboratory Tests

1. Electrocardiography can provide evidence of arrhythmias or conduction delays. This is especially important in the case of tricyclic antidepressants.

2. Electrolytes are helpful in evaluating metabolic abnormalities, especially metabolic acidosis.

   a. The anion gap $[Na^+ - (HCO_3^- + Cl^-)]$ normal (8 to 12 mEq), if elevated in the presence of a metabolic acidosis, is associated with *A*lcohol, *M*ethanol, *U*remia, *D*iabetic Acidosis, *P*araldehyde, *I*ron, *I*soniazid, *L*actic Acidosis, *E*thylene Glycol, *S*alicylates, carbon monoxide, cyanide, and toluene.

   b. A small anion gap (<6 mEq) may indicate bromism or lithium toxicity.

   c. The osmolar gap is helpful in making the diagnosis of exogenous toxins.

      (1) Osmolar gap = measured osmolarity minus the calculated osmolarity

      (2) Calculated osmolarity = $2Na^+ + GLUCOSE/18 + BUN/2.8$

      (3) If the osmolar gap is greater than 10 mosm/L, consider ethanol, ethylene glycol, isopropanol, methanol, propylene glycol, glycerol, mannitol, sorbitol, acetone, and diatrizoate.

      (4) An osmolar gap that is <10 mosm/L does not exclude these toxins reliably.

3. Toxicologic laboratory screening

   a. Random comprehensive urine drug screens are seldom helpful in the emergency setting.

   b. The history and physical examination should guide the ordering of drug screens.

   c. Quantitative rather than qualitative drug levels are crucial when dealing with acetaminophen, salicylates, methanol, ethylene glycol, isopropyl alcohol, anticonvulsants, digoxin, theophylline, iron, and lithium.

   d. Limitations of toxicology screening include

      (1) Time delay in obtaining the results

      (2) Is there correlation between the drug identified and the effects observed?

      (3) Has the patient taken the agent over the long term?

   e. Comprehensive drug screens should be ordered only when the results will change the treatment that the patient is already receiving.

Key Tests

- Electrolytes
- Anion gap
- Electrocardiogram

Treatment

Gastric Decontamination

1. Syrup of ipecac: most efficacious if given within 30 to 45 minutes following the ingestion.

   a. Syrup of ipecac (SI) is contraindicated following ingestions of caustics, hydrocarbons, drugs known to cause abrupt loss of consciousness or seizures, foreign bodies, and nontoxic ingestions.

   b. Ipecac is contraindicated in unconscious patients, patients in seizure, or those with increased potential for decreased levels of unconsciousness. It should not be used after intentional ingestions because the substances ingested, the amount ingested, and the time of ingestion cannot be ascertained.

   c. Dose

      (1) Infants (6 to 12 months): 10 ml

      (2) Children (1 to 12 years): 15 ml

      (3) Adults: 30 ml

      These doses are repeated in 20 to 30 minutes if emesis has not occurred. Dose may be given with any liquid. Milk and carbonated beverages do not interfere with the effectiveness of ipecac.

2. Gastric lavage

   Gastric lavage is performed before administration of activated charcoal.

   a. Tube diameter

      (1) Adults: 34 to 40 French orogastric tube

      (2) Children: 24 to 28 French orogastric tube

   b. Fluid volume

      (1) Adults: 150 ml to 200 ml aliquots (5 to 10 L total) of warm water or normal saline

      (2) Children: 50 ml to 100 ml aliquots of normal saline

3. Activated charcoal (AC)

   a. AC adsorbs a wide variety of toxins preventing their absorption from the gastrointestinal tract but does not absorb heavy metals (iron, lithium), alcohols, highly ionized compounds, caustics, and cyanide.

   b. Dose

      (1) Children: 1 to 2 gm/kg

      (2) Adults: 50 to 100 gm

   c. May be given with a cathartic, either sorbitol or magnesium citrate. Other cathartics interfere with the adsorptive capacity of AC and should not be used.

4. Multiple-dose activated charcoal (MDAC)

   a. MDAC regimens may enhance the excretion of theophylline, phenobarbital, phenytoin, and carbamazepine.

   b. The clinical efficacy of MDAC following ingestions of tricyclic antidepressants, salicylates, and digoxin is questionable.

c. Dose: 50 gm every 4 hours (adults). A cathartic should be given no more frequently than every third dose. 10 gm every hour may be given if the larger doses are not tolerated.

5. Whole bowel irrigation (WBI)

   a. WBI utilizes a polyethylene glycol electrolyte lavage solution (PEG-ELS) to hasten removal of ingested substances.

   b. Possible indications are patients who present late following an ingestion, ingestion of sustained-release pharmaceuticals, toxins not adsorbed by AC, and foreign bodies.

   c. WBI is most commonly utilized for iron, lithium, cocaine packets, and sustained-release calcium channel blockers.

   d. Dose

   (1) Adults: 2 L/hr for 5 hours

   (2) Children: 500 ml/hr

   e. End point of therapy: This includes documentation of passage by radiographs (in the case of iron tablets or cocaine packets), decreasing drug levels, clear rectal effluent if patient has clinically improved and drug levels are falling. *Note:* Clear rectal effluent is not an end point for removal of foreign bodies or cocaine packets.

Antidotes

1. Specific antidotal therapy is available for very few toxins and is not always needed.

2. The duration of the antidote may be shorter than the duration of action of the toxin.

3. Antidotal therapy does not replace gastric decontamination.

TABLE 326–1. ANTIDOTES COMMONLY USED WITHIN THE FIRST HOUR OF TREATMENT

TOXIN	ANTIDOTE	DOSE AND COMMENTS*
Opiates	Naloxone	Starting dose 2 mg. More may be needed for overdoses of some synthetic narcotics; less may be used in addicts to avoid precipitating withdrawal.
Methanol, ethylene glycol	Ethanol	Loading dose 10 ml I.V. of 10% solution per kilogram of body weight, maintenance dose 1.5 ml per kilogram per hour. Increase the maintenance dose during dialysis. Titrate to a blood ethanol level of 22 mmol per liter (100 mg per deciliter).
Anticholinergic	Physostigmine	1 to 2 mg intravenously over 5 minutes. Use only for severe delirium. May be useful to treat seizures or tachydysrhythmias, but strong clinical evidence is lacking.
Organophosphate or carbamate insecticides	Atropine	Test dose 2 mg intravenously. Repeat in larger increments until drying of pulmonary secretions occurs.
Isoniazid	Pyridoxine	Give in gram-per-gram equivalent doses to what was ingested. If amount ingested is unknown, start with 5 gm intravenously.
β-blockers	Glucagon	Starting dose 5 to 10 mg intravenously. Titrate to response (normalization of vital signs). Maintenance dose of 2 to 10 mg per hour may be used.
Tricyclic antidepressant	Bicarbonate	1 to 2 mmol per kilogram intravenously for substantial cardiac conduction delay or ventricular dysrhythmias. Titrate to response and arterial pH of 7.45–7.50.
Digitalis glycosides	Digoxin-specific antibodies	Equimolar to ingestion: the number of milligrams of digoxin ingested divided by 0.6 is the number of vials required. If amount of digoxin ingested is unknown and the patient has life-threatening dysrhythmias, give 10 to 20 vials intravenously. If steady state serum digoxin concentration is known, the number of vials to administer equals: $$\frac{\text{concentration (in ng/ml)} \times 5.6 \times \text{weight in kg}}{600}$$
Benzodiazepines	Flumazenil	0.2 mg over 30 seconds. If there is no response after 30 seconds, give 0.3 mg over 30 seconds. If there is no response after 30 seconds, give 0.5 mg over 30 seconds at 1-minute intervals up to a total dose of 3 mg. *Contraindicated* in serious overdose from coingestion of tricyclic antidepressants or if taking benzodiazepines for the control of seizures.
Calcium channel blockers	Calcium	1 gm calcium chloride given over 5 minutes by intravenous infusion with continuous cardiac monitoring. May be repeated often in life-threatening situations, but the serum calcium level should be monitored after the third dose. Currently there are no data to support this form of treatment.
Acetaminophen	*N*-Acetyleysteine	140 mg/kg loading dose orally, then 70 mg/kg every 4 hours for a total of 17 doses. If the 4-hour acetaminophen level is toxic, all 17 doses must be given.

*Doses given are for adults.
Adapted by permission from Kulig K: Initial management of ingestion of toxic substances. N Engl J Med 1992;326:1679.

4. The primary means of treating toxic exposures remains stabilization of the cardiopulmonary status along with supportive care.

5. Suggested empiric therapy for patients with altered mental status includes

   a. Dextrose

   b. Oxygen as necessary

   c. Naloxone

   d. Thiamine

6. Antidotes should not be administered indiscriminately since they may be harmful if used inappropriately. Consultation with a regional poison center is extremely helpful in guiding antidotal therapy (Table 326–1).

Key Treatment

- Gastric decontamination
- Specific antidotal therapy
- Supportive care

Follow-Up

1. Response to initial treatment and antidotes should not create a false sense of security; ingestions are often multiple, and toxicity from unsuspected compounds may be delayed.

2. Suicide attempts and gestures are often multiple; proper care to prevent repetitions is paramount.

3. Poisoning in children should prompt a dedicated educational effort in the home and perhaps a home assessment.

Bibliography

Ellenhorn MJ, Barceloux DG: Medical Toxicology Diagnosis and Treatment of Human Poisoning. New York, Elsevier, 1988, pp 42–51.

Goldfrank LR, Flomenbaum NE, et al: General management of the poisoned or overdosed patient, In Goldfrank's Toxicologic Emergencies, 4th ed. E Norwalk, CT, Appleton & Lange, 1990, pp 5–20.

Gossell TA, Bricker JD: Principles of Clinical Toxicology, 3rd ed. New York, Raven Press, 1994.

Kulig K: Initial management of ingestions of toxic substances, N Engl J Med 1992; 326:1677–1681.

327 Food Poisoning

John N. Aucott

Foodborne disease results from ingestion of either food or water contaminated with pathogenic microorganisms, microbial toxins, or chemicals or from consumption of naturally occurring plant and animal toxins. The diagnosis of foodborne disease should be considered when an acute illness with gastrointestinal and/or neurologic manifestations affects two or more persons who have previously shared a meal. Outbreaks are divided by the Centers for Disease Control and Prevention (CDC) into four subgroups according to the incubation period: 1 hour, probable chemical poisoning; 1 to 7 hours, probable *Staphylococcus* food poisoning; 8 to 14 hours, probable *Clostridium perfringens* food poisoning; and more than 14 hours, probable other infectious or toxic agents. In addition to the incubation period, the differential diagnosis is based on the following clinical syndromes.

History

1. *Food ingestion*
   a. Fish and shellfish: scombroid, ciguatera, anisakiasis, neurotoxic shellfish poisoning, *Vibrio* spp., hepatitis A, Norwalk virus
   b. Chinese food: MSG, fried rice (*Bacillus cereus* emetic syndrome)
   c. Meats: *C. perfringens,* eggs/chicken (*Salmonella*), beef (toxoplasmosis, *Escherichia coli*), pork/bear (trichinosis), ham (*S. aureus*)
   d. Water: *Giardia, Cryptosporidium,* Norwalk virus, hepatitis A, chemicals/metals
   e. Beverages: heavy metals
   f. Fruits/vegetables: insecticides, potato toxins, wild/ornamental plant toxins
2. *Host factors*
   a. Immunosuppressive disorders: HIV, cirrhosis, immunosuppressive medications
   b. History: sexual exposure, travel history, recent antibiotic use

Symptoms

1. *Gastrointestinal symptoms*
   a. Nausea
   b. Vomiting
   c. Diarrhea
   d. Abdominal cramping
   e. Weight loss
2. *Neuromuscular and systemic symptoms*
   a. Botulism: dysphagia, diplopia, dysarthria, weakness, blurred vision, dyspnea
   b. Mushrooms: (depending on species) hepatic and renal failure, seizures, coma, disulfiram-like symp-

toms, cholinergic effects, anticholinergic effects, hallucinations
   c. Fish/shellfish: paresthesias, cutaneous flushing/burning, headache, dizziness/ataxia
   d. Chemicals: cholinergic symptoms (cholinesterase inhibitors)
   e. Trichinosis: muscle pain, eosinophilia

The history should identify high-risk patients based on food consumption, underlying illnesses, and behaviors. Important symptoms include the presence or absence of vomiting and the differentiation of inflammatory from noninflammatory diarrhea. Recognizing neurologic and systemic symptoms is critical to diagnosing the rare life-threatening case of botulism, fish toxin, cholinesterase inhibitor insecticides, or mushroom ingestion.

Key Symptoms

- Nausea, vomiting
- Abdominal pain, diarrhea
- Neurologic symptoms

Clinical Findings

1. Nausea, vomiting, and watery diarrhea with dehydration
2. Inflammatory diarrhea with tenesmus, fever, abdominal pain, blood or leukocytes in stool
3. Neuromuscular or systemic symptoms

Preformed heat-stable toxins (*S. aureus* and *B. cereus*) result in a short-incubation illness with vomiting. Heat-labile toxins produced in vivo (*C. perfringens* and long-incubation *B. cereus*) result in a longer incubation period and noninflammatory, watery diarrhea. Organisms capable of tissue invasion and causing inflammatory diarrhea have a longer incubation period and include *Salmonella, Shigella* spp., invasive *E. coli,* and *Campylobacter.* Neurotoxins associated with botulism and fish poisoning result in motor or sensory symptoms.

Key Signs

- Absence of peritoneal signs
- Fever unusual (except in inflammatory diarrhea)
- Neurologic signs

Laboratory Tests

1. Stool examination for blood, fecal leukocytes, and parasites

2. Bacterial culture of stool, emesis, and food

3. Viral identification by PCR or electron microscopy

4. Toxin testing for botulism, fish toxins, chemicals, and some bacterial toxins

A presumptive diagnosis usually can be made based on the incubation period, predominant symptoms, and epidemiology of outbreak. Specific diagnostic evaluation is indicated in high-risk patients with neurologic or systemic symptoms or those with symptoms for more than 1 to 2 days' duration, severe dehydration, fever, bloody diarrhea, unexplained abdominal pain, or weight loss. In these patients, further evaluation may identify an agent requiring specific therapy. Tests that must be specifically requested include identification of pathogenic *E. coli*, Norwalk virus identification, acid-fast staining for *Cryptosporidium*, and most assays for bacterial, plant, or animal toxins.

Key Tests

- Stool examination for blood
- Fecal leukocytes

Differential Diagnosis

1. *Upper gastrointestinal symptoms of nausea and vomiting:* staphylococcal food poisoning, heavy metals, Norwalk virus, *B. cereus* emetic syndrome, mushrooms, anisakis and other fish tapeworms

2. *Upper small bowel symptoms with noninflammatory watery diarrhea: C. perfringens,* Norwalk virus, enterotoxigenic *E. coli, B. cereus* diarrheal syndrome, *Giardia, Cryptosporidium*

3. *Inflammatory diarrhea: Salmonella, Shigella, Campylobacter,* enteroinvasive *E. coli, Vibrio parahaemolyticus, Yersinia, E. histolytica, V. vulnificus*

4. *Neuromuscular or systemic symptoms with/without gastrointestinal symptoms:* botulism, trichinosis, hemolytic uremic syndrome due to *E. coli* 0157:H7, fish/shellfish toxins (histamine-like scombrotoxin, ci-

guatera, neurotoxic shellfish poisoning), chemicals (cholinesterase inhibitor pesticides, monosodium glutamate [MSG], toxic oils), plants (mushrooms, fava beans, water hemlock, herbal remedies)

The differential diagnosis of food poisoning should consider a combination of the specific symptoms including the presence of neurologic or systemic symptoms and the incubation period (Table 327–1).

Treatment

1. Replace gastrointestinal fluid losses with oral or parenteral electrolyte solutions; supportive therapy for neurologic manifestations.

2. Antiemetics are contraindicated. Emesis may be induced if it has not occurred spontaneously.

3. Antiperistaltic agents should be avoided in cases of inflammatory diarrhea.

4. Specific therapy for botulism, inflammatory bacterial infections, and parasitic infections is warranted.

Management of foodborne disease is based on recognizing that the majority of illness is self-limited and therapy nonspecific and supportive. The clinical course of *S. aureus, B. cereus, C. perfringens,* viral gastroenteritis, and most other bacterial gastroenteritis is not shortened by antibiotic therapy, and rarely do these illnesses result in significant morbidity or mortality. Specific treatment is only indicated for high-risk patients or for serious disease due to botulism, parasitic infections, and invasive bacterial disease. Empirical therapy for patients with febrile dysenteric illness also may be indicated.

Patient Education and Prevention

1. Proper food storage or holding temperature, personal hygiene of the food handler, adequate cooking, and use of uncontaminated equipment

2. Identification of safe food sources is necessary to prevent outbreaks of fish/shellfish, mushroom, and chemical poisoning.

3. Avoidance of raw fish, shellfish, meats, and eggs, especially in patients with cirrhosis or immunosuppression

TABLE 327–1.   CLINICAL DIAGNOSIS OF FOODBORNE ILLNESS BY INCUBATION PERIOD AND SYMPTOMS

PREDOMINANT SYMPTOMATOLOGY	INCUBATION PERIOD			
	<2 hours	1–7 hours	8–14 hours	>14 hours
Upper intestinal, nausea/vomiting	Heavy metals Chemicals Mushrooms	*S. aureus B. cereus Anisakis*	*Anisakis*	Norwalk agent
Noninflammatory diarrhea, no fecal leukocytes			*C. perfringens B. cereus*	Enterotoxigenic *E. coli V. cholerae Giardia lamblia* Norwalk agent
Inflammatory ileocolitis				*Salmonella, Shigella, Campylobacter,* invasive *E. coli, V. parahaemolyticus, E. histolytica*
Extragastrointestinal, neurologic	Insecticides, mushroom, and plant toxins, MSG, shellfish scombroid	Ciguatera, shellfish		Botulism *E. coli* 0157:H7 Associated hemolytic-uremic syndrome

4. Use of proper storage containers to prevent heavy metal contamination

5. Use of properly filtered and treated water supplies

Key Treatment

• Oral or parenteral electrolyte solutions for fluid losses

• Supportive therapy for neurologic manifestations

• Emesis may be induced if it has not occurred spontaneously.

Bibliography

Bean NH, Griffin PM: Foodborne disease outbreaks in the United States, 1973–1987: Pathogens, vehicles, and trends. J Food Prot 1990;53:804–817.

Eastaugh J, Shepherd S: Infectious and toxic syndromes from fish and shellfish consumption. Arch Intern Med 1989;149:1735–1740.

Guerrant RL, Bobak DA: Bacterial and protozoal gastroenteritis. N Engl J Med 1991;325:327–340.

Hedberg CW, MacDonald KL, Osterholm MT: Changing epidemiology of food-borne disease: A Minnesota perspective. Clin Infect Dis 1994;18:671–682.

Herwaldt BL, Craun GF, Stokes SL, Juranek DD: Waterborne-disease outbreaks, 1989–1990, CDC: Surveillance summaries, December 1991. MMWR 1991:40(no. SS3):1–22.

328 Lead Poisoning

George E. Kikano

Etiology

1. Lead poisoning (plumbism) is a major public health problem in the United States and is preventable. All U.S. children are considered at risk for lead poisoning. In 1991, the Centers for Disease Control and Prevention lowered the definition of safe blood lead level (BLL) to less than 10 μg/dl of whole blood. Previously, a BLL of 25 μg/dl was considered acceptable, but growing evidence has linked lower levels to significant adverse effects.

2. Most cases of lead poisoning occur either through ingestion or inhalation. Sources of lead exposure are

   a. Paint (major source): interior and exterior

   b. Drinking water

   c. Contaminated soil

   d. Airborne and dust

   e. Industrial and hobbies (ceramics, stained glass)

   f. Other: folk remedies, cosmetics, food, retained bullets

3. Children are at increased risk for lead poisoning because of

   a. Repeated hand-to-mouth activity

   b. Higher gastrointestinal absorption of lead

   c. Pica (ingestion of nonfood products)

Symptoms

1. Most people with lead poisoning are asymptomatic. With mild to moderate exposure, nonspecific symptoms can occur: abdominal discomfort, fatigue, myalgias, anorexia, headache, paresthesias, irritability. Symptomatic lead poisoning is considered a medical emergency.

2. With continuous exposure or high levels, affected individuals can have symptoms related to many organ systems:

   a. Gastrointestinal (GI): abdominal pain, vomiting, constipation

   b. Central nervous system (CNS): lethargy, irritability, decreased hearing, seizures, acute encephalopathy and coma (with levels >100 μg/dl)

   c. Renal: hypertension and renal failure in affected adults

3. Neurodevelopmental deficits in children: change in behavior, decreased intelligence, reduced attention span, poor school performance. Children with either prenatal or postnatal exposure to lead scored lower on mental developmental scales and had lower IQ scores.

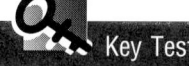

Key Symptoms

- Mostly asymptomatic
- Abdominal pain
- Myalgias
- Cognitive deficits
- Lethargy
- Irritability
- Seizures
- Encephalopathy

Clinical Findings

1. Physical examination is generally not helpful in diagnosing lead poisoning.

2. Affected children may exhibit the following:

   a. Be pale secondary to anemia

   b. Be irritable

   c. Show cognitive deficit

   d. Have congenital abnormalities with severe prenatal exposure.

3. Since all U.S. children are considered to be at risk, physicians should routinely screen for lead poisoning.

   a. Questions at each well child visit to assess child's risk

   b. Blood lead levels starting at 1 year of age for low-risk children and at 6 months of age for high-risk ones.

Laboratory Tests

1. Measurement of venous blood lead level (BLL) is the most accurate test for diagnosing lead poisoning. Capillary lead level, when available, is an alternative test if done properly. Erythrocyte protoporphyrin (EP) used to be the test of choice for lead screening. However, with lowered acceptable BLL, EP has poor sensitivity.

2. Other tests that should be either obtained or considered for children with lead poisoning.

   a. Iron studies: Fe, total iron-binding capacity, ferritin

   b. CaEDTA provocative chelation test

   c. Plain films of the abdomen may show recently ingested lead chips.

   d. "Lead lines" may be seen on radiographs of long bones in some cases.

Key Test

- Venous blood lead level (BLL) is the preferred test.

Differential Diagnosis

Depending on the presenting symptoms, if any, lead poisoning may be confused with other causes of

1. Neurologic diseases and seizures
2. Developmental delay and behavioral problems
3. Anemia
4. GI disorders

WARNING

- **All U.S. children are considered to be at risk for lead poisoning and should be screened routinely.**
- **Public health efforts are targeted to primary prevention of lead poisoning.**

Treatment

1. The source of lead exposure should be identified and affected individuals removed from that source to prevent further exposure. Local public health authorities should be notified.
2. All symptomatic cases should receive immediate chelation therapy. Management of asymptomatic children depends on their BLL:
   a. <10 μg/dl: routine screening
   b. 10–19 μg/dl: Recheck in 3 to 4 months. Environmental investigation.
   c. >19 μg/dl: complete medical and environmental evaluation. The effectiveness of chelation for BLL of 25 to 44 μg/dl has not been established.
   d. >45 μg/dl: chelation therapy and environmental evaluation
   e. >70 μg/dl: Hospitalize for chelation therapy.

Medication

Chelating agents are used to reduce the body burden of lead. They can be used singly or in combination depending on the BLL. Chelating agents include

1. Edetate calcium disodium (Calcium EDTA)(Calcium Disodium Versenate), intravenous. Renal and hepatic function should be monitored during treatment. Dosage is 35 to 75 mg/kg/day in divided doses every 8 to 12 hours for 3 to 5 days.
2. Dimercaprol (BAL in oil), intramuscular. It should not be used in children allergic to peanuts or those who have G6PD deficiency. Dosage is 3 to 4 mg/kg every 4 hours for 5 to 7 days.
3. D-Penicillamine (Cuprimine), oral. It is contraindicated in children allergic to penicillin. Commonly used for treatment of lead poisoning but not FDA approved for this condition. The usual dose is 25 to 35 g/kg/day.

4. Succimer (DMSA) (Chemet), oral. Used for outpatient chelation

Diet

The diet of children with lead poisoning should have adequate amounts of iron, calcium, zinc, and proteins.

Activity

Parents should try to minimize pica activity of children at high risk.

Patient Education

1. All parents should be educated about potential sources of lead poisoning.
2. Providers also should review with parents probable symptoms of lead poisoning and potential complications.
3. Parents should be aware of ways to prevent or decrease the risk of exposure, e.g., renovation and remodeling techniques, wet mopping, food storage.
4. Household members of affected individuals should be screened.

 Key Treatment

- In children, the course of treatment with succimer is usually for 3 weeks. The initial dose is 10 μg/kg every 8 hours for the first 5 days, then 10 μg/kg every 12 hours for 14 days.
- Remove lead sources
- Reduce exposure
- Chelating agents

Follow-Up

1. Providers should make sure that the sources of lead exposure have been identified and abated. This can be done in collaboration with public health agencies. Abatement should be completed before children are allowed to return to their environment.
2. BLL of children treated with chelating agents should be rechecked 7 to 21 days after therapy. This will help evaluate for rebound increases in levels and guide further treatment.

 Bibliography

Agency for Toxic Substances and Disease Registry: Special Issue on Lead Toxicity, vol 2, no 1. January-February 1992.

American Academy of Pediatrics: Lead Poisoning: From Screening to Primary Prevention. Committee on Environmental Health, The American Academy of Pediatrics, 1993 (RE 9307).

Centers for Disease Control and Prevention: Preventing Lead Poisoning in Young Children. Statement, Centers for Disease Control, Atlanta, GA, 1991.

National Lead Information Center, 1019 19th Street, NW, Suite 401, Washington, DC 20036-5105.

Needleman HL, Schell A, Bellinger D, et al: The long-term effects of exposure to low doses of lead in childhood: An 11-year follow-up report. N Engl J Med 1990;3222:83–88.

329 Animal Bites

James R. Blackman

Etiology

1. Between 1 and 3 million mammalian bites to humans occur annually in the United States; 1 million seek medical attention (1 to 2 per cent of emergency department visits). Most occur indoors.

2. Dog bites represent 70 to 90 per cent of all bites. The dog frequently belongs to family or a close neighbor. More than half of victims are children, a result of poorly supervised animal-child interaction.

3. Cat bites represent 5 to 20 per cent of mammalian bites, have a higher incidence of infection (deep puncture wounds), and are more common in women.

4. Human and rodent bites make up most of the remainder of mammalian bites.

5. Predisposing factors include
   a. Youth
   b. Disturbing a sleeping, feeding, injured, or unfamiliar animal
   c. Teasing, kissing, or playing recklessly with an animal
   d. Separating fighting animals
   e. Chasing wild animals
   f. Fist-fighting (human)
   g. Occupations such as animal control, police work, postal work, veterinary medicine, farming, and hunting
   h. Unprovoked attacks from feral (wild) dogs and cats, and sick or injured wild animals such as skunks, squirrels, or bats; some may have rabies

Symptoms

The following information should be recorded in any animal bite history

1. Concerning the animal
   a. Type of animal (including breed if known)
   b. Relationship of the animal to the victim
   c. Circumstances of the bite (provoked or unprovoked)
   d. Time and location of the incident
   e. Vaccination and health status of the animal (if known)
   f. Current location of animal (if known)

2. Concerning the victim
   a. First aid measures given
   b. Tetanus immunization status
   c. Past history of diseases of immunologic compromise
   d. Symptoms of musculoskeletal, neurologic, or vascular compromise

Clinical Findings

1. The extremities are involved in 75 per cent of cases when victims handle or attempt to avoid the animal. Head and neck injuries are the next most common.

2. Serious problems may result from
   a. Skull penetration following a bite to the cranium in a small child
   b. Bites over a joint
   c. Puncture wounds
   d. Lip and face bites in children

3. Wounds (abrasions, crush injuries, lacerations, and punctures) should be described as to size, location, and type. Include diagrams. If infected, describe adenopathy and diagram extent of cellulitis.

4. Wounds should be classified as high risk or low risk, facilitating management as regards suturing and empiric antibiotic therapy.
   a. High-risk wounds include all human and cat bites, hand and foot wounds (including closed fist injuries), wounds surgically debrided, puncture wounds, wounds involving joints, ligaments, tendons, and bones, bites with treatment delay exceeding 12 hours, and bites in immunocompromised individuals (primary immunologic disorder, HIV, chronic alcoholism, asplenium, diabetes mellitus, presence of prosthetic valves or joints, immunosuppressive therapy).
   b. Low-risk wounds include lacerations involving the extremities, face, and body.

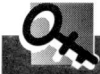

Key Signs

- Large hematoma
- Motor weakness
- Decreased capillary refill
- Decreased sensation
- Loss of function

Laboratory Tests

For most mammalian bites, laboratory tests and radiographs are unnecessary.

1. If significant blood loss is expected, hematocrit may be indicated, followed by type and crossmatch.

2. Cultures of wounds are necessary only in those cases in which an immunocompromised patient is infected, when there is evidence of sepsis, or when empiric antibiotic therapy fails. Organisms come from animal oral flora and human skin and include aerobes and anaerobes.

Key Organisms

Human Bites	Animal Bites
• Staphylococcal species	• Staphylococcal species
• Streptococcal species	• Streptococcal species
• *Eikenella*	• *Pasteurella multocida*
	• Variety of aerobic and anaerobic bacteria

3. Gram's stains and cultures on fresh, uninfected wounds correlate poorly with subsequent infections and waste financial resources.

4. Radiographs are indicated when bony penetration is suspected: hands, wrists, feet, head (skull films or cranial computed tomography).

Key Complications

• Neurovascular damage	• Musculotendinous injury
• Bony or joint penetration with infection	• Severe crush injury
• Compartment syndrome	• Meningitis and cerebral abscess
• Cellulitis	• Prosthetic valve and joint infection
• Septic shock	• Scarring and disfiguration

Treatment

1. Control airway, breathing, and circulation, and inspect for major crush injury or penetrating trauma.

2. Provide meticulous wound care.

   a. Inspect carefully for depth and extent of injury and neurovascular and musculoskeletal integrity. Bite wounds may be more severe than they appear.

   b. Debride and irrigate wound.

   (1) Provide mechanical cleansing and careful excision of devitalized tissues; crushed, devitalized tissue is particularly common with dog bites (do not soak).

   (2) Keep debridement to a minimum for facial lacerations.

   (3) Leave enough tissue to close the wound and preserve function.

   (4) Irrigate with 18- or 19-gauge needle on a 15- or 20-cc syringe using normal saline or, preferably, 1% povidone-iodine solution. If high risk of rabies transmission, use 20% soap and water or ethyl alcohol for at least 10 minutes followed by 1% benzalkonium chloride. More potent antiseptics devitalize tissue. Finish irrigation with normal saline to remove antiseptic.

   c. Repair.

   (1) Meticulous irrigation and debridement may allow wound closure.

   (2) Low-risk wounds may be sutured primarily.

   (3) High-risk wounds should be closed secondarily.

   (4) Wounds of questionable risk may be managed with delayed primary closure (some hand wounds).

3. Empiric antibiotic therapy is indicated for all high-risk wounds. Regimens are based on the most likely offending organisms. Give one parenteral dose prior to ER care.

4. Treat established wound infections aggressively.

   a. Provide adequate surgical debridement and drainage.

   b. Perform Gram's stain and culture.

   c. Hospitalize those with severe blood loss, sepsis, open fracture, osteomyelitis, severe hand injury, and deep tissue injury; provide parenteral antibiotics covering gram-positive and gram-negative aerobes and anaerobes.

   d. Follow-up bite wounds frequently in office to evaluate for infection and wound healing (24 and 48 hours).

5. Provide tetanus prophylaxis in standard manner (Table 329–1).

6. Review rabies postexposure prophylaxis guidelines. Exposure is defined as an open bite or wound in contact with body fluids.

   a. Wild animals

   (1) Provide prophylaxis for bites from rabies-endemic species (bats anywhere in the United States; raccoons, skunks, foxes, based on local public health recommendations).

   (2) Provide prophylaxis for bites from wild carnivores (e.g., coyotes, bobcats) and groundhogs living in a rabies-endemic area.

   (3) No treatment is necessary for provoked exposure from animals where rabies is not endemic in the species involved or in other animals in the area (e.g., rodents, rabbits, and many wild animals).

   b. Domestic animals

   (1) No treatment is indicated if animal is immunized or healthy and available for 10 days of observation.

   (2) Treatment indicated

   (a) Dogs in most developing countries and in the United States along Mexican border

   (b) Animal rabid or suspected rabid

   c. If health or immunization status is unknown at time of exposure, consult public health officials for current recommendations.

TABLE 329–1. TETANUS PROPHYLAXIS

NEED FOR TETANUS TOXOID AND TETANUS IMMUNE GLOBULIN BASED ON HISTORY OF IMMUNIZATIONS	LOW RISK*		HIGH RISK†	
	Toxoid‡	TIG§	Toxoid	TIG
Not known	Yes	No	Yes	Yes
Zero	Yes	No	Yes	Yes**
One	Yes	No	Yes	Yes**
Two	Yes	No	Yes	Yes
Three or more				
Last booster <5 year	No	No	No	No
Last booster <10 year	No	No	Yes	Yes
Last booster >10 year	Yes	No	Yes	Yes

*Low risk: Clean, little devitalized tissue, easily debrided (and irrigate).
†High risk: Dirty, deep, much devitalized tissue, difficult to debride (and irrigate).
‡Toxoid: Adult, 0.5 ml dT I.M.
      Child <5, 0.5 ml DPT I.M.
      Child >5, 0.5 ml DT I.M.
§TIG (tetanus immune globulin): 250–500 U IM in limb opposite of toxoid.
**Plus completion of immunization (three injections) with booster doses, at 30 and 60 days after initial injection.

d. Consult state or local health departments for any questions.

7. Specific treatment recommendations

   a. In previously vaccinated individuals with documented antibody response give two doses of human diploid cell vaccine (HDCV) or rabies vaccine adsorbed (RVA), 1.0 ml intramuscularly (deltoid), one each on days 1 and 3. Rabies immune globulin (RIG) should not be given.

   b. In unvaccinated individuals give RIG, 20 IU/kg, one half infiltrated into wound and remainder intramuscularly (gluteal); then five doses of HDCV or RVA, 1.0 ml intramuscularly (deltoid), one each on days 1, 3, 7, 14, and 28.

8. Review for possibility of hepatitis B or C transmission in human bites and provide immunoprophylaxis for hepatitis B if indicated (administer hepatitis B immune globulin, 0.06 ml/kg intramuscularly, immediately and repeat in 30 days).

9. Precautions should be taken if human bite is by a known HIV carrier.

Patient Education

1. Animals are territorial and will not attack unless territory is entered.

2. Virtually all animals give some kind of warning sign.

3. Children should never be left alone with an animal.

4. Wild animals are never safe, and pet ferrets are particularly dangerous.

5. Foster attitudes of animal love and respect.

6. Provide obedience training in companion animals.

7. Keep animals under control.

8. Do not run if confronted by a threatening dog.

Key Treatment

Human Bites

• Nafcillin followed by dicloxacillin plus penicillin

• If penicillin-allergic, tetracycline (but not in children and during pregnancy)

Cat Bites

• Nafcillin followed by dicloxacillin or penicillin G followed by penicillin V

• If penicillin-allergic, erythromycin

Dog Bites

• Nafcillin followed by dicloxacillin or cefazolin followed by cephalexin

• If penicillin-allergic, erythromycin

Bibliography

Anderson CR: Animal bites. Guidelines to current management. Postgrad Med 1992;92:134–136.

Callanan ML, French SP: Bites and injuries inflicted by mammals. In Auerbach PS: Management of Wilderness and Environmental Emergencies. 3rd ed. St. Louis, Mosby–Year Book, 1995, pp 927–993.

Groleau G: Rabies. Emerg Med Clin North Am 1992;361–368.

Ruskin JD, et al: Treatment of mammalian bite wounds of the maxillofacial region. J Oral Maxillofac Surg 1993;51:174–176.

Stewart CE: Bites and stings. Part 2 of Mammalian Bites. In Stewart CE: Environmental Emergencies. Baltimore, Williams & Wilkins, 1990, pp 194–206.

330 Insects and Spiders

Thomas C. Michels

Etiology

1. Bites: insects (fleas, bed bugs, flies, mosquitoes) and others (spiders, ticks, chiggers)
2. Stings: hymenoptera (honeybee, wasp, yellow jacket, hornet, fire ant) and scorpions

Symptoms

1. Local minor reactions
   a. Normal reaction following any sting or bite
      (1) Immediate local pain with swelling; subsides in 1 to 2 hours
      (2) Early pruritus that may persist for several days
      (3) Ticks cause itching and local wheal, can transmit tick bite fever, tick paralysis, Rocky Mountain spotted fever, and Lyme disease.
   b. Large local reaction
      (1) Swelling extending from sting site over large area, such as entire extremity
      (2) Peaks at 48 hours, may last up to a week
2. Local major (dermonecrotic) reactions
   a. Prototype is bite of brown recluse spider (*Loxosceles reclusa*): cutaneous loxoscelism.
   b. Bite may go unnoticed, or victim may feel mild stinging or burning.
   c. May note a papule at the site with pain and tenderness 24 to 72 hours later
   d. Necrotic ulcer later develops and may take weeks to heal.
3. Anaphylaxis
   a. Most commonly with hymenoptera envenomation; can occur with other bites or stings
   b. Same symptoms as with anaphylaxis from any cause
4. Systemic toxic reactions: most commonly due to neurotoxins in arthropod venom
   a. Systemic loxoscelism
      (1) Symptoms start 24 to 72 hours after bite of brown recluse spider.
      (2) Fever, malaise, rash, arthralgias, nausea, and vomiting; may progress to collapse
   b. Latrodectism: bite of the black widow spider (*Latrodectus mactans*) or its relatives
      (1) Bite often unnoticed, but victim may feel a pinprick sensation.
      (2) In 20 to 30 minutes, limb and lymph node pain, local swelling, itching, or hives develop.
      (3) May progress to crampy pain in thighs, abdomen, and chest, with sialorrhea, nausea, and vomiting.
   c. Scorpion stings
      (1) Most bites in United States are due to bark scorpion (*Centuroides sculpturatus*), endemic to Southwest but can be transported anywhere
      (2) Shortly after bite victim may note local itching, regional paresthesias, then diaphoresis, dyspnea, sialorrhea, lacrimation, muscle pain, nausea, vomiting.

Key Symptoms

- Stinging, burning
- Extremity pain or paresthesias

If severe:
- Abdominal pain
- Sialorrhea
- Nausea and vomiting

Clinical Findings

1. Local minor reactions
   a. Normal reaction has small papule or wheal, with or without evidence of excoriation.
   b. Papular urticaria described after fleas bites and others
   c. Painful wheals followed by vesicles and pustules typical for fire ant bite in southeastern United States
   d. Large local reaction has wheal at bite site; may have regional edema and erythema.
2. Local major (dermonecrotic) reactions
   a. Early: red, edematous, or blanched area surrounding bite
   b. Later: hemorrhagic blister surrounded by irregular purpura
   c. Eschar forms days later; necrotic ulcer that may take months to heal; more extensive in areas with subcutaneous fat (thighs, abdomen, buttocks)
3. Anaphylaxis
4. Systemic toxic reactions
   a. Systemic loxoscelism: fever, hypotension, shock, scarlatiniform rash, splenomegaly
   b. Latrodectism
      (1) Hypertensive, restless patient; flushed, sweating face, contorted with spasm or pain

(2) Prominent muscle rigidity, including abdominal muscles

c. Scorpion stings

(1) Initially tachycardia, hypertension; can progress to hypotension with shock

(2) Involuntary motor activity; can progress to seizures, cranial nerve dysfunction

Key Signs

- Erythematous papules
- Central punctum
- Hemorrhagic blister

If severe:
- Hypertension or hypotension
- Muscle rigidity
- Involuntary movement

Laboratory Tests

1. Few specific diagnostic tests: venom-specific IgE in serum of patient with anaphylaxis indicates specific allergy
2. Tests search for complications or monitor supportive care
3. Leukocytosis and hyperglycemia usual in stress reactions
4. Severe reactions: elevated creatine phosphokinase (CPK) or renal failure; loxoscelism may show hemoglobinuria or disseminated intravascular coagulation (DIC).

Key Tests

- None (glucose, white blood cell count, blood urea nitrogen, creatinine, coagulation studies useful in severe cases)

Differential Diagnosis

1. History of exposure and bite; have patient bring the offending organism in for identification.
2. Local minor reactions: Many ''bug bites'' have similar presentation.
   a. Ask for history of travel, exposure to outdoor or unhygienic environments, pets, or others with same condition.
   b. Papules grouped on exposed surfaces or snug spots in clothing suggest infestation or flea bites.
   c. Examination should look for urticarial papules with a central punctum.
   d. Chigger (harvest mite) bites (southern United States): discrete, bright-red papules of legs and waist with hemorrhagic puncta and intense pruritus

e. Differential diagnosis includes atopic dermatitis, allergic or irritant contact dermatitis, and viral or drug eruption.
3. Dermonecrotic reactions: Early differential includes vasculitis, purpura, or Lyme disease; later, pyoderma.
4. Anaphylaxis
5. Systemic toxic reactions
   a. Systemic loxoscelism: Severe reactions can present as acute renal failure or disseminated intravascular coagulation (DIC) from any cause.
   b. Latrodectism
      (1) Severe reactions can present as acute abdomen; history of bite, abrupt onset, and patient writhing in pain help distinguish.
      (2) Differential includes tabic crisis, acute psychosis, meningitis, or acute renal failure.
   c. Scorpion stings: Severe reactions may present as insecticide poisoning.

Treatment

A. Minor local reactions: cool compresses, topical lotions such as calamine, camphor-menthol
   1. Secondary infection requires antibiotic treatment as with cellulitis.
   2. Large local reactions: antihistamines (e.g., chlorpheniramine 4 to 8 mg or diphenhydramine 50 mg every 6 hours) or steroids (e.g., prednisone, 40 mg once daily for 2 to 3 days)
B. Dermonecrotic reactions
   1. Initial management: Immobilize limb, apply cold compresses.
   2. Consider Sawyer extractor: extracts venom with negative pressure.
   3. Hospital care: Carefully cleanse wound; tetanus prophylaxis; avoid local injections into wound and steroids; antibiotics only for secondary infection.
   4. Dapsone for adults with rapidly progressive, severe bite; 50 to 500 mg/day, divided twice daily for 2 weeks.
   5. Colchicine advocated by some: 1.2 mg initially, then 0.6 mg every 2 hours for 2 days, then 0.6 mg every 4 hours for 2 days.
   6. Corrective surgery delayed 8 weeks for adequate tissue demarcation of necrosis.
C. Anaphylaxis: Refer for allergy testing and desensitization therapy.
D. Systemic toxic reactions
   1. Identification of biting or stinging arthropod crucial if specific antivenom considered.
   2. General supportive measures important: ABCs of resuscitation; intravenous volume expansion; monitoring; oxygen.

3. Systemic loxoscelism: general supportive measures; treat acute renal failure or DIC if present.

4. Latrodectism

  a. Cool compresses to bite site; consider Sawyer extractor.

  b. General supportive measures.

  c. Muscle relaxants provide symptomatic relief.

    (1) Diazepam: 5 to 10 mg intramuscularly or intravenously, may repeat in 3 to 4 hours; children 1 month to 5 years: 1 to 2 mg per dose; larger doses for severe spasm

    (2) Methocarbamol: 15 mg/kg slowly intravenously, followed by oral therapy

    (3) Calcium gluconate 10% solution, 1 to 2 ml/kg up to 10 ml per dose; often affords more striking relief, although transient

  d. Tetanus prophylaxis

  e. Antivenin available from Merck & Co. (West Point, PA) in severely affected patients.

5. Scorpion stings

  a. General supportive measures

  b. Local compresses, analgesics; consider Sawyer extractor.

  c. Tetanus prophylaxis

  d. Treat hypertension, tachycardia with β blockers.

  e. Specific antivenin available for severe cases from Arizona State University, Tempe, AZ.

Patient Education

1. Patients with hymenoptera sensitivity

  a. Minimize exposure: no bare feet outdoors, wear long pants, gloves when gardening; avoid perfumes, hair sprays, and bright, pastel, or white clothing.

  b. Self-administration of epinephrine; commercially available kits (ANA-Kit, EpiPen)

2. Avoidance measures for patients with outdoor exposure

  a. Wear work gloves when cleaning up debris.

  b. Consider use of pesticides in heavily infested areas.

  c. Brush off, do not swat, something crawling on body.

  d. Check outdoor clothing, shoes before putting them on.

  e. Insect repellents useful against many insects and ticks.

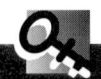

Key Treatment

- Cool compresses
- Antihistamines
- Tetanus prophylaxis
- Muscle relaxants
- Specific antivenin in severe cases

Follow-Up

1. Most patients with sting or bite reactions have self-limited course.

2. Ongoing desensitization therapy for hymenoptera sensitivity.

3. Follow-up to determine if debridement or excision is necessary in dermonecrotic reaction.

4. Follow-up for those with systemic toxic reactions determined by specific clinical syndrome.

Bibliography

For an overview of common bites and stings with differential features, see

Dershewitz RA (ed): Ambulatory Pediatric Care, 2nd ed. Philadelphia, JB Lippincott, 1993, pp 275–278.

For details on hymenoptera sensitivity and other reactions, see

Reisman RE: Stinging insect allergy. Med Clin North Am 1992; 76:883–894.

For a detailed review of spider and scorpion envenomation, including photographs, see

Allen C: Arachnid envenomations. Emerg Med Clin North Am 1992;10:269–288.

For a broad overview briefly covering many insects and arachnids, see

Stawiski MA: Insect bites and stings. Emerg Med Clin North Am 1985;3:785–808.

331 Snakebite

Peter DeMartino

Etiology

1. Poisonous snakes are responsible for approximately 8000 to 10,000 snakebites annually, resulting in 10 to 15 deaths. United States southeastern and gulf states have the highest bite rate per 100,000 population. Most bites occur between April and October, with peak months being July and August.

2. There are two families of poisonous snakes in the United States, coral snakes (Elapidae) and pit vipers (Crotalidae).

   a. Coral snakes are found in southern states, eastern coral snakes in southeastern and gulf states, and Arizona coral snakes in Arizona and New Mexico. They are small, shy, nocturnal snakes with brightly colored red, yellow, and black rings. They rarely bite humans; however, when startled or threatened, they can strike using short fixed fangs; they inject a potent neurotoxin using successive chewing movements.

   b. Pit vipers account for 99 per cent of all snakebite poisonings in the United States. They are named for heat-sensitive pits between their nostrils and eyes. The family of Crotalidae is made up of rattlesnakes, copperheads, cottonmouths, and massasaugas.

      (1) There are 16 species of rattlesnakes. They are found in almost every state, accounting for the majority of venomous snakebites, as well as most fatalities. The eastern and western diamondbacks are the largest and most dangerous.

      (2) Cottonmouths, or water moccasins, are small aquatic snakes found in southeastern and southwestern states. They are aggressive, with moderately toxic venom.

      (3) Copperheads are widely distributed throughout the lower 48 states, occurring most commonly on mountains and wooded hillsides. Their venom is less toxic and rarely fatal but can cause significant injury.

3. Snake venom is a highly complex mixture of enzymes and toxic proteins.

   a. Pit viper venom contains numerous proteolytic enzymes that cause significant local soft tissue necrosis, as well as hemolysis and hemorrhage.

   b. Coral snake venom is predominantly neurotoxic, causing neuromuscular blockade with respiratory and bulbar paralysis.

Symptoms

1. Clinical presentation is important in determining the severity of envenomation and planning a treatment strategy.

2. Pit viper envenomation results in the rapid development of severe burning pain locally, followed by swelling, erythema, and ecchymoses. Systemic symptoms include fever, nausea, vomiting, disorientation, delirium, convulsions, muscle cramps, perioral paresthesias, and bleeding. Severe envenomation may result in shock and circulatory collapse 30 minutes or more after the bite.

3. Coral snake envenomations typically have little or no local symptoms. Systemic symptoms will usually develop within 5 hours of the bite and reflect the potent neurotoxic nature of the venom. Typical manifestations include numbness and weakness in the region of the bite, followed by salivation, ataxia, dysphagia, and dysarthria secondary to palatal and pharyngeal paralysis. Respiratory paralysis, seizures, coma, and death may follow within 8 to 72 hours of a severe envenomation.

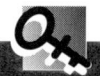

Key Symptoms

- Local burning pain (numbness if coral snake)
- Fever, nausea, vomiting, disorientation

Clinical Findings

1. Important clinical manifestations suggestive of a pit viper bite include fang puncture marks with local tissue destruction, swelling, ecchymoses, and hemorrhagic bullae. Destruction may be extensive with local necrosis, gangrene, secondary infection, and/or development of a compartment syndrome. Severe envenomation with ensuing hypotension and circulatory collapse may be accompanied by disseminated intravascular coagulation (DIC) with hematemesis, hematuria, and hemorrhage. Acute renal failure may develop as a result, with acute tubular necrosis or cortical necrosis.

2. Coral snake bites usually appear as multiple shallow fang punctures. Other signs include ptosis, mydriasis, loss of deep tendon reflexes, and respiratory depression.

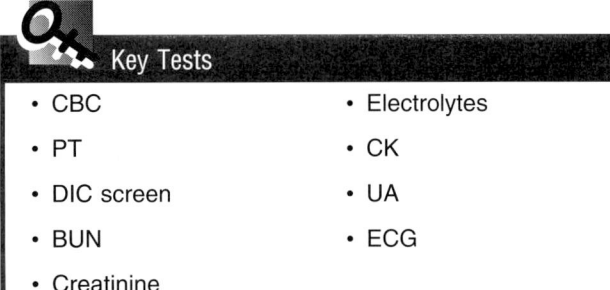

Key Signs

- Local tissue destruction, edema, ecchymoses, bullae
- Hemorrhage, hematuria, hematemesis
- Acute renal failure
- Ptosis, mydriasis, loss of deep tendon reflexes

Laboratory Tests

1. The following laboratory tests should be performed on all patients suspected of venomous snakebite:
   a. Complete blood count (CBC) with platelets and differential
   b. Prothrombin time (PT), partial thromboplastin time (PTT), and DIC panel
   c. Type and cross
   d. Blood chemistries, including blood urea nitrogen (BUN), creatinine, electrolytes, transaminases, bilirubin, and creatine kinase (CK)
   e. Urinalysis (UA)
   f. 12-lead electrocardiogram

2. In cases of severe envenomation, common laboratory abnormalities include progressive hemolytic anemia, leukocytosis (20,000 to 30,000/mm^3), thrombocytopenia, DIC with prolonged PT, PTT, and hypofibrinogenemia. Proteinuria, hematuria, and acute renal failure with azotemia also may occur.

Key Tests

• CBC	• Electrolytes
• PT	• CK
• DIC screen	• UA
• BUN	• ECG
• Creatinine	

Treatment

1. First aid in the field should consist of calming and reassuring the patient as well as immobilization of the affected extremity. Exertion will only increase systemic absorption of venom. The victim should be transported to the nearest hospital promptly. ICU admission, close monitoring, and supportive care are mandatory in all suspected envenomations.

2. Use of tourniquets and incision and suction is controversial; however, most authors strongly discourage this practice. Wide constriction bands can be used if anatomically possible; however, they should not be tighter than to allow one finger beneath without difficulty. This will impede lymphatic drainage and systemic absorption of venom without further compromising blood flow to damaged tissues.

3. Antivenin is the only specific therapy for snake bites. The patient should have two large-bore peripheral intravenous lines started, the first for administration of antivenin and the second for fluid, blood products, and other medications as necessary.

4. Antivenin should be administered intravenously. Local injection of antivenin at the bite site is not recommended.

5. Skin testing is necessary prior to intravenous administration; however, this does not rule out the possibility of anaphylaxis.

6. Dosage of antivenin can be estimated based on the clinical grading of envenomation. It should be diluted in 500 ml of saline or dextrose and given over 1 to 2 hours. For pit viper bites:
   a. Grade 0: no envenomation, no local or systemic findings, no antivenin necessary
   b. Grade 1: minimal envenomation, local pain, and edema, no systemic symptoms, 1 to 5 vials of antivenin
   c. Grade 2: moderate envenomation, local as well as mild systemic and/or laboratory findings, 5 to 15 vials of antivenin
   d. Grade 3: severe envenomation, severe local, systemic, and laboratory abnormalities, 20+ vials of antivenin

7. Additional infusions should be repeated every 2 hours until progressive signs and symptoms and laboratory abnormalities have resolved.

8. Eastern coral snake or Arizona coral snake antivenin should be administered to anyone suspected of envenomation from these particular snakes regardless of absence of signs or symptoms, since symptoms may progress rapidly once they appear.
   a. 3 to 5 vials of antivenin, if suspect envenomation and no signs or symptoms present
   b. 6 to 10+ vials if systemic symptoms exist

9. Tetanus toxoid and/or tetanus immune globulin should be given if not immunized.

10. Broad-spectrum antibiotics should be given if a wound infection is suspected. Snake oral flora contain gram-negative and gram-positive rods.

11. Fasciotomy and surgical debridement should be reserved for massive necrosis, gangrene, or decompression of a compartment syndrome.

12. Cryotherapy, ice packs, or ice water has no place in the treatment of snakebites. Evidence suggests that this treatment may increase damage to already ischemic tissue. In addition, vasoconstriction prevents antivenin from penetrating bite region.

13. Complications of treatment are generally related to reactions to antivenin.
    a. Hypersensitivity reactions with anaphylaxis may occur in as many as 25 per cent of patients receiving antivenin.

b. Serum sickness develops in 50 to 75 per cent of patients receiving antivenin. Symptoms of fever, malaise, arthralgias, lymphadenopathy, and morbilliform rash usually develop within 7 to 14 days.

WARNING

- **Cryotherapy is not indicated.**
- **Incision and suction have no benefit; may cause more damage.**

Patient Eduction

1. Prevention is the most important aspect of patient education.
2. Avoid snake-infested areas.
3. Wear protective clothing, such as boots, heavy trousers, and gloves, when walking in snake-inhabited regions.

Key Treatment

- Antivenin is the only specific treatment.
- Immobilization and rapid transport to local hospital
- Supportive care
- Surgical debridement/fasciotomy when indicated

Bibliography

Davidson TM, Schafer SF: Rattlesnake bites: Guidelines for aggressive treatment. Postgrad Med 1994;96:107–114.

Forks TP: Evaluation and treatment of poisonous snakebites. Am Fam Physician 1994;50:123–130.

Gold BS, Barish, RA: Venomous snakebites. Emerg Med Clin North Am 1992;10:249–267.

Gold BS, Wingert WA: Snake venom poisoning in the United States: A review of therapeutic practices. South Med J 1994; 87:579–589.

Russell F: When a snake strikes. Emerg Med 1990;22:21–43.

332 Heat Exhaustion and Stroke

Laramie C. Triplett

Etiology

1. Heat exhaustion (HE): Heat illnesses occur when the body is unable to maintain cooling in the face of increased environmental temperatures and humidity. The cardiovascular system figures prominently in the regulation of body temperature: When body temperature becomes elevated, cardiac output increases markedly, the skin's blood vessels dilate, and blood is shunted to the periphery of the body. Most commonly, heat illness occurs in individuals who are poorly acclimatized to a hot environment and/or who are in poor physical condition. The elderly, especially those taking diuretics, are more prone to develop heat illness.

2. Exertional heat injury (EHI): A relatively milder form of heat stroke may occur in athletes and other individuals who routinely engage in exertional activities out-of-doors. The classic example often cited is the runner. Predisposing factors for the development of exertional heat injury include
   a. Environmental temperature greater than 80° F
   b. Relatively high humidity
   c. Insufficient acclimatization
   d. Poor conditioning
   e. Obesity
   f. Improper hydration
   g. Age
   h. Previous heatstroke

3. Classic heatstroke (CHS): Heat stroke is a life-threatening illness and must be treated as a true medical emergency. Classic heatstroke is most common in elderly persons with pre-existing chronic medical illness.
   a. Predisposing factors
      (1) Ambient temperature greater than 90° F
      (2) Poorly ventilated dwelling
      (3) Lack of air conditioning
      (4) High humidity
      (5) Age (infants, children, elderly)
   b. Predisposing illnesses
      (1) Arteriosclerosis, myocardial dysfunction, valvular heart disease, peripheral vascular disease
      (2) Diabetes mellitus
      (3) Alcoholism
      (4) Dementia
      (5) Ectodermal dysplasia
      (6) Absence of sweat glands
      (7) Severe scleroderma

   c. Predisposing medications and drugs
      (1) Diuretics
      (2) Anticholinergics
      (3) Phenothiazines
      (4) Antihistamines
      (5) Antiparkinsonians
      (6) Antidepressants (primarily tricyclic)
      (7) Laxatives (abuse)
      (8) Amphetamines
      (9) Cocaine
      (10) Barbiturates
      (11) Hallucinogens

Symptoms

Symptoms common to HE, EHI, and CHS include headache, extreme weakness, nausea and vomiting, vertigo, and faintness.

1. Heat exhaustion: The picture may resemble that of a flu-like illness. Symptoms include the above; anorexia and the urge to defecate are common.

2. Exertional heat injury: Symptoms overlap those of heat exhaustion and heatstroke.

3. Classic heatstroke: In addition to the above, one may see tremor, dyspnea, paresthesias, and confusion or irrational behavior.

 Key Symptoms

Heat Exhaustion
- Copious sweating
- Headache

Exertional Heat Injury
- Headache
- Muscle cramps
- Chills

Clinical Findings

Findings common to HE, EHI, and CHS include tachycardia, hypotension, and pallor.

1. Heat exhaustion
   a. Normal or subnormal temperature
   b. Skin pallor
   c. Cold, clammy skin
   d. Dilated pupils

2. Exertional heat injury
   a. Piloerection on trunk and upper extremities
   b. Tachypnea
   c. Ataxia
   d. Incoherent speech
   e. Loss of consciousness
3. Classic heatstroke
   a. Core temperature greater than 106° F
   b. Hot, dry skin
   c. Lethargy, stupor, or coma
   d. Flaccid muscles
   e. Decreased deep tendon reflexes

Key Signs

Heat Exhaustion

- Normal or subnormal temperature
- Skin pallor
- Cold, clammy skin
- Dilated pupils

Exertional Heat Injury

- Freely sweating
- Temperature of 102° to 104° F

Classic Heatstroke

- High temperature (>106° F)
- Altered mental status
- Anhidrosis

Laboratory Tests

1. Heat exhaustion: In most cases, no laboratory tests are required for diagnosis, provided that an appropriate history is obtainable. If this is not the case, it may be helpful to obtain some basic laboratory studies when any of the three illnesses being discussed are suspected.
   a. Complete blood count (CBC), electrolytes, urinalysis
   b. Electrocardiogram
2. Exertional heat injury: Data usually show hemoconcentration, hypernatremia, elevated liver function tests and muscle enzymes, hypocalcemia, hypophosphatemia, and occasionally hypoglycemia. Less often there are additional abnormalities such as thrombocytopenia, disseminated intravascular coagulation (DIC), hemolysis, rhabdomyolysis, and myoglobinuria; acute tubular necrosis (ATN) is a potential complication. Obtain the laboratory tests noted above plus

   a. Prothrombin time
   b. Blood urea nitrogen (BUN), creatinine, liver and muscle enzymes, calcium, phosphorus, and glucose
   c. Urine osmolality and urine sodium concentration. Osmolality will be less than 350 mOsm/kg, and sodium concentration will be greater than 40 mEq/L in ATN.
3. Classic heatstroke: While urine and blood studies and other investigations may be essentially unremarkable, several abnormalities are common. In addition to previously mentioned laboratory tests, obtain
   a. Clotting time, bleeding time, fibrinogen, fibrin split products, serum lactic acid
   b. Arterial blood gases—respiratory alkalosis (CHS) or metabolic acidosis (EHI)
   c. ECG—tachycardia, sinus arrythmia, ST-segment depression, flattened or inverted T waves, acute myocardial infarction

Differential Diagnosis

1. Heat exhaustion
   a. Heatstroke—Only core body temperature can differentiate heat exhaustion from heatstroke.
   b. Sepsis or other severe infection
   c. Myocardial infarction
2. Exertional heat injury: Above, plus
   a. Heatstroke
   b. Neuroleptic malignant syndrome (NMS)
3. Classic heatstroke: All of the above.

Treatment

Initial treatment consists of moving the patient to a cool environment for rest and hypotonic fluid replacement.
1. Heat exhaustion
   a. Rest should be in a recumbent position to allow spontaneous recovery.
   b. Fluid replacement can be accomplished with oral fluids; rarely are intravenous fluids necessary.
2. Exertional heat injury
   a. Cool the patient promptly and replace lost body fluids. Placing the patient on wet sheets (on a slotted gurney, if possible) and massaging with ice packs may be sufficient for cooling.
   b. The patient should be hospitalized for 24 to 48 hours for observation.
3. Classic heatstroke: Treatment must be prompt and aggressive to prevent serious complications and death.

Medication

1. If oliguria and ATN are present, a single dose of mannitol, 12.5 gm intravenously, may be given.

2. If adequate intravenous fluids have been given, a single dose of furosemide, 200 mg intravenously, may be given in an effort to promote renal blood flow and urine output.

3. Persistent oliguria may necessitate early dialysis.

4. Dantrolene sodium, which may be beneficial in the treatment of neuroleptic malignant syndrome, is of no benefit in the treatment of heat exhaustion or heatstroke.

Diet

There are no specific dietary interventions or changes.

Activity

1. Heat exhaustion and exertional heat injury

   a. The patient should initially be put at rest as described above.

   b. The precipitating activity and other strenuous activities should be avoided for several days until complete recovery occurs.

2. Classic heatstroke

   a. Limit activity to necessary activities of daily living after the patient recovers and is able to leave the hospital.

   b. Some elderly patients may require home health services or (temporary) nursing home placement.

   c. Other limitations and postdischarge activities and instructions will depend on pre-existing illnesses or complications of heatstroke.

Patient Education

1. Heat exhaustion

   a. Patients should be instructed to acclimatize slowly to hotter environments, particularly if relative humidity is high.

   b. Patients also should be instructed to drink adequate amounts of fluids during times of increased heat and humidity.

2. Exertional heat injury can be avoided by

   a. Performing strenuous activities early in the morning when temperature and relative humidity are likely to be lower.

   b. Maintaining hydration by drinking adequate amounts of water (250 to 300 ml) before and during activity.

   c. Avoiding alcohol before and during activity.

3. Classic heatstroke: Patients must be educated as to the precipitating factors leading to their heatstroke and should be made aware of shelters and other living arrangements that may be available to them during heat waves.

Key Treatment

Heat Exhaustion

- Recumbent positioning

- Rest in cool environment

- Hypotonic fluid replacement

Exertional Heat Injury

- Apply cold packs or fluids to lower core body temperature to 100° F

- Massage extremities

- Infuse hypotonic fluids with glucose

Classic Heatstroke

- Place patient in cool environment and provide adequate ventilation.

- Immerse patient in ice water under supervision of nurse or physician.

- Monitor core temperature and discontinue active cooling efforts when core temperature reaches 101° to 102° F.

- Massage skin to stimulate return of cooled blood to central organs and brain.

- Hydrate with hypotonic crystalloids.

- Watch closely for signs of congestive heart failure and pulmonary edema.

Follow-Up

1. All patients should be seen again within 1 week to ensure that complete recovery has taken place and that the patient understands appropriate preventive measures.

2. For victims of classic heatstroke, follow-up also will depend on pre-existing illnesses and any sequelae of the heatstroke.

Bibliography

Bross MH, Nash BT, Carlton FB: Heat emergencies. Am Fam Physician 1994;50:389–396.

Petersdorf RG: Hypothermia and hyperthermia. *In* Harrison's Principles of Internal Medicine, 13th ed. New York, McGraw-Hill, 1994, pp 2473–2477.

Simon HB: Hyperthermia and heatstroke. Hosp Pract 1994; 29:65–80.

Tek D, Olshaker JS: Heat illness. Emerg Med Clin North Am 1992;10:299–311.

Tom PA, Garmel GM, Auerbach PS: Environment-dependent sports emergencies. Med Clin North Am 1994;78:311–315.

333 Frostbite

Frank S. Celestino

Etiology

1. Tissue injury and destruction are due to freezing. Extracellular ice crystals increase the extracellular osmotic gradient leading to cell death. Progressive vascular ischemic thrombosis and occlusion occur via red cell sludging, platelet aggregation, endothelial injury, and the local generation of prostaglandins and thromboxanes causing vasoconstriction.

2. Risk factors
   a. Prolonged exposure to cold climate
   b. Previous frostbite injury
   c. Inappropriate or wet clothing
   d. Immobility
   e. Impaired cognition
   f. Extremes of age
   g. Malnutrition
   h. Smoking
   i. Psychiatric illness
   j. Sedative and alcohol use
   k. Hypothyroidism
   l. Pre-existing cardiac or vascular disease
   m. Lack of acclimatization
   n. Skin damage
   o. Extremes of temperature and wind chill factor
   p. Cold exposure at high altitude

Symptoms

1. Superficial injury (partial to complete skin involvement only)
   a. Paresthesias, tingling, and moderate numbness
   b. Burning, throbbing, or aching discomfort
   c. Prickly or itchy sensations
   d. Painful dysesthesias and burning on rewarming
2. Deep injury (skin plus varying involvement of subcutaneous tissue, muscle, bone)
   a. Profound numbness/anesthesia
   b. Stiffness and immobility
   c. Heaviness and "block of wood" feeling
   d. Joint pains/arthralgias

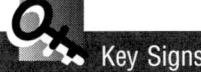

Key Symptoms

Superficial	Deep
• Paresthesias, tingling	• Numbness
• Burning or aching	• Stiffness

e. Burning, throbbing, tingling, aching, or shooting pains on rewarming

Clinical Findings

1. Most often involves fingers, toes, nose, and ears.
2. Superficial injury
   a. Cold, frozen, white, nonblanchable, and waxy-appearing skin
   b. Soft, pliable, and resilient subcutaneous tissue before thawing
   c. Erythema, mild to moderate edema, bleb formation, and occasional desquamation on thawing
   d. No permanent tissue loss occurs
3. Deep injury
   a. Icy, hard, and wooden skin
   b. Nonresilient and hard subcutaneous tissue
   c. Intense hyperemia, marked edema, cyanosis, hemorrhagic blisters, skin necrosis, gangrene, and even mummification after thawing
   d. Permanent tissue loss occurs

Key Signs

Superficial Injury
- Nonblanchable, waxy-appearing skin
- Soft, resilient subcutaneous tissue before thawing

Deep Injury
- Icy, hard, and wooden skin/limb
- Hard, nonresilient subcutaneous tissue before thawing

Laboratory Tests

1. Complete blood count (CBC)
2. Serial radionuclide angiography and/or triple-phase bone scans are useful in deep frostbite injuries to help with the identification and debridement of nonviable tissue
3. Wound and blood cultures if superimposed infection is suspected
4. Other laboratory tests and radiographs are needed only to detect and manage multisystem complications of any concomitant systemic hypothermia

Key Tests

- Serial radionuclide angiography and/or bone scanning for deep injuries

Differential Diagnosis

1. Frostnip: transient, localized, very superficial skin cooling without sequelae
2. Chilblain (pernio): nondestructive, cold-induced, chronic hypersensitivity (vasculitic) skin reaction causing itching, burning, violaceous discoloration, mild edema
3. Immersion foot (trench foot): nonfreezing pedal tissue injury due to prolonged exposure to wet and cold conditions
4. Systemic hypothermia: cold-induced decrease from average homeothermic core body temperature (37° C) to less than 35° C because of environmental exposure or immersion

Treatment

1. Protect involved part from mechanical trauma; no rubbing or massaging.
2. Avoid rewarming if there is *any* risk of refreezing, even if this means walking on frozen feet.
3. Admit to the hospital all patients except those with the most superficial and localized injuries.
4. Initiate treatment for any associated systemic hypothermia.
5. Begin rapid but controlled rewarming by immersing the frozen body part in circulating warm water bath heated to 40° to 42° C (*not any warmer*). A flushed appearance of the involved part, usually occurring after 20 to 30 minutes, signals reperfusion and the need to cease rewarming.
6. Early (within 36 to 72 hours) regional sympathectomy is controversial.
7. Subsequent supportive measures include protection of the limb from infection and trauma, twice daily hydrotherapy in a warm (33° to 37° C) water/disinfectant bath, nicotine avoidance, limb elevation, and use of sterile dressings.

Medication

1. Narcotics are given as needed for pain, especially during rewarming.
2. Unless contraindicated, give ibuprofen (minimum of 12 mg/kg orally per day) for 1 week to combat prostaglandin-mediated ischemia and inflammation.
3. Tetanus prophylaxis as indicated
4. Prophylactic antibiotics are controversial. In one non-randomized trial using 500,000 units of penicillin every 6 hours intramuscularly, treated patients had less tissue loss and a lower amputation rate. Subsequent antibiotics are based on culture results.
5. Debride blisters and cover with aloe vera gel every 6 hours.
6. Thrombolytic therapy is experimental. A very small recent trial using recombinant tissue plasminogen activator infused directly into the involved limb showed promising results.

Diet

As tolerated.

Activity

1. Protect injured body part.
2. Initiate physical therapy once edema significantly lessens.

Patient Education

1. Regarding risk factors for frostbite and early signs and symptoms
2. Establishment of buddy system during wilderness exploration
3. Concerning possible sequelae
   a. Hypersensitivity with painful dysesthesias, especially on re-exposure to cold
   b. Hyperhydrosis
   c. Skin discoloration
   d. Joint pain
   e. Growth plate abnormalities in children
   f. Vasomotor instability
   g. Muscle atrophy
   h. Gangrene and tissue loss

Key Treatment

- Do not rewarm if there is *any* risk of refreezing.
- Admit almost all patients to the hospital.
- Rapid controlled rewarming in warm water bath (40° to 42° C) for 20 minutes.
- Subsequent elevation, protection, daily hydrotherapy, surveillance for infection.

Follow-Up

1. Escharotomy may be necessary if impaired circulation or movement. Fasciotomy occasionally needed to alleviate a compartment syndrome due to extensive tissue edema.
2. Because early prediction of the extent of nonviable tissue is difficult in frostbite, amputation should not be considered until it is definitively established that tissues are dead. Aphorisms such as "frostbite in January, amputate in July" illustrate this principle. Autoamputation of digits involved in deep frostbite may avoid surgical intervention and help limit the amount of tissue that would have been removed.
3. Only indication for early debridement is uncontrolled infection. Otherwise, delay debridement for 1 to 3 months until the level of gangrene is demarcated.
4. Researchers are exploring the use of serial radionuclide scintigraphy to allow earlier assessment of ulti-

mate tissue viability and the need for debridement/amputation.

 Bibliography

Britt DL, Dascombe WH, Radriguez A: New horizons in the management of hypothermia and frostbite injury. Surg Clin North Am 1991;71:345–370.

Foray J: Mountain frostbite: Current trends in prognosis and treatment. Inter J Sports Med 1992;13(suppl 1):S193–196.

Harvey CK: An overview of cold injuries. J Am Podiat Med Assoc 1992;82:436–438.

Mills WJ Jr, O'Malley J, Kappes B: Cold and freezing: A historical chronology of laboratory investigation and clinical experience. Alaska Med 1993;35:89–116.

Pulla RJ, Pickard LJ, Carnett TS: Frostbite: An overview with case presentations. J Foot Ankle Surg 1994;33:53–63.

334 Altitude Sickness

Paul J. Hughes

Etiology

1. Acute exposure to altitudes above 8000 feet (2438 m) can result in a constellation of symptoms referred to as "altitude sickness" (AS). Although these symptoms may be similar to many other illnesses, the history of high-altitude exposure separates this entity from the other items in the differential diagnosis. Entities included in AS include acute mountain sickness (AMS), high-altitude cerebral edema (HACE), and high-altitude pulmonary edema (HAPE).

2. The principal physiologic insult from high-altitude exposure is hypoxia. The partial pressure of oxygen decreases with increasing altitude, and primary response to this hypoxia is an increase in minute ventilation. This increase in ventilatory rate causes a drop in the partial pressure of carbon dioxide in the alveoli, resulting in a respiratory alkalosis.

3. There are other physiologic responses to high-altitude exposure. There is a decrease in plasma volume, an increase in erythropoietin, and a bicarbonate diuresis. There is also an increase in sympathetic activity, causing an increased heart rate, pulmonary vasoconstriction, and increased cerebral blood flow.

4. Physical conditioning does not appear to affect the occurrence of AMS. The limiting factor with exercise at altitude is lung function.

Signs and Symptoms

A. Acute mountain sickness
1. History of rapid ascent to altitude higher than 8000 feet
2. Shortness of breath
3. Headache
4. Anorexia
5. Dizziness
6. Nausea
7. Insomnia
8. Lassitude, difficulty concentrating

B. High-altitude pulmonary edema
1. Most often occurs on the second night at altitude
2. Early signs and symptoms
   a. Dyspnea
   b. Dry cough
   c. Decreased exercise tolerance
   d. Confusion
3. Late signs and symptoms
   a. Dyspnea at rest
   b. Cyanosis
   c. Crackles
   d. Pink frothy sputum
   e. Tachycardia
   f. Tachypnea

C. High-altitude cerebral edema
1. Uncommon below 12,000 feet
2. Early signs and symptoms essentially the same as AMS
3. Late signs and symptoms
   a. Increasing confusion
   b. Ataxia
   c. Seizures

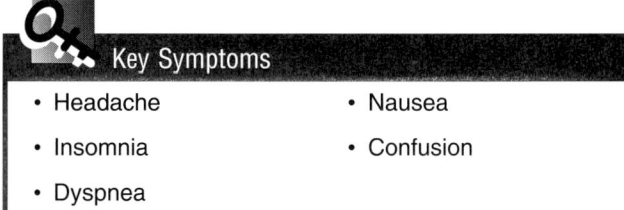

Key Symptoms

- Headache
- Insomnia
- Dyspnea
- Nausea
- Confusion

Clinical Findings

1. There are no specific clinical findings.

2. In advanced HACE and HAPE, the development of central nervous system (CNS) signs and signs of pulmonary congestion become manifest. However, early in the development of AMS, HAPE, and HACE, the findings are nonspecific and therefore not particularly useful. The emergence of symptoms in the proper setting and a high index of suspicion are the most important diagnostic factors.

Laboratory Tests

1. There are no particularly useful laboratory studies for the evaluation of AMS, HAPE, or HACE.

2. The chest radiograph may show pulmonary congestion and/or some patchy, fluffy infiltrates. However, patients with no symptoms may have a similar radiographic picture. Therefore, most diagnostic information comes from the history and physical examination in the proper clinical setting.

Treatment

A. At altitude
1. Early recognition is paramount.
2. The primary therapy for all forms of altitude sickness is to "go down."

3. A descent of at least 2000 feet, preferably to an altitude of less than 10,000 feet, is imperative if symptoms are severe. Descend early while the patient is able to assist in the descent.

4. Supplemental oxygen is useful in relieving hypoxia-related symptoms. This is especially helpful with sleep-aggravated hypoxia. Oxygen bottles are cumbersome, however, and therefore are not usually carried on many treks.

5. A Gamow bag can be used to temporarily increase the ambient pressure. This portable hyperbaric chamber can simulate descent and together with supplemental oxygen is useful in buying time until a descent is possible.

6. Nifedipine (Procardia, Adalat) may be effective in HAPE. It reduces pulmonary artery pressure and improves oxygenation. It is dosed 10 mg sublingually (open or pierce the capsule) and 20 mg orally every 6 to 8 hours until descent is possible.

B. In hospital
1. Primary hospital care consists of high-flow, continuous oxygen and bed rest.

2. Diuretics are not indicated.

3. Assisted-ventilation methods are not indicated and in some cases may slow improvement.

4. A decrease in tachycardia, tachypnea, and dyspnea and an improvement in mental status are indications of resolution.

Key Treatment

- Descent is the definitive treatment.
- Supplemental oxygen

Prevention

1. Fitness. Good physical conditioning improves exercise tolerance, although this may not prevent altitude-related illness. An improved hemodynamic response to exercise may be of some benefit in preventing HAPE and HACE.

2. Good health. Poorly controlled hypertension, diabetes, or other chronic diseases will have an effect.

3. Control of the rate of ascent.
   a. Begin below 8000 feet. Travel by automobile rather than air, if possible. This provides time to acclimate.
   b. Rest the first day.
   c. Ascend about 1000 feet per day. If symptoms start, descend.

4. Climb high, sleep low.

5. Avoid alcohol.

6. Keep well hydrated.

7. Acetazolamide (Diamox), 250 to 1000 mg/day, starting 12 to 24 hours before arrival and continuing for 3 to 4 days can significantly reduce the severity of AMS symptoms.

Bibliography

Bracker MD: Acute Mountain Sickness, Surviving Conference at 9,000 Feet. Ninth Annual Wilderness Medicine Conference Syllabus, University of California, San Diego School of Medicine, Snowmass, Colorado, August 1993.

McMurray SJ: High altitude medicine for family physicians. Can Fam Physician 1994;40:711–718.

Sutton JR: Mountain sickness. Neurol Clin 1992;10(4):1015–1030.

Tom PA, Garmel GM, Auerbach PS: Environment-dependent sports emergencies. Med Clin North Am 1994;78(2):305–325.

Tso E: High-altitude illness. Emerg Med Clin North Am 1992;10(2):231–247.

335 Aquatic Injuries

Bruce Flareau

Jellyfish Stings

Etiology

The tentacles of the jellyfish contain thousands of venom-containing stinging cells known as nematocysts. These remain active for several days after the creature's death such that injuries may result from brushing against live or dead tentacle fragments.

Symptoms

Abrupt development of painful erythematous eruptions in linear welts or patches.

Differential Diagnosis

1. Cousins of the jellyfish, the Portuguese man-of-war and the blue bottle, are found off the coasts of Florida and Hawaii, respectively. Symptoms are similar to those produced by jellyfish, but more severe, with fever, wheezing, vomiting, or even paralysis. These lesions may require steroids and supportive care.

2. Sea anemones also possess nematocysts that may cause mild stings if brushed against.

Treatment

1. Immediate application of vinegar to deactivate any remaining undischarged nematocysts.

2. After 3 to 5 minutes, the tentacles may be scraped off.

3. Jellyfish stings should not be rinsed in fresh water because this may cause the nematocyst to discharge.

4. In the Chesapeake Bay area, the most common jellyfish is the sea nettle, which has unique vinegar-resistant nematocysts. In these waters, a saltwater paste of baking soda should be applied.

Stingray Lacerations

Etiology

Stingrays are usually found burrowed in the sand in shallow water and will hurl their barbed "tail" upward in a defensive response to being stepped on or disturbed. The resulting wound may be both a laceration and a venomous puncture.

Symptoms

1. The victim usually presents with disproportionally painful lesions.

2. The sharp, shooting pain of a stingray laceration usually peaks in a few hours and, if untreated, resolves within a few days.

3. These lesions may cause nausea, weakness, and even respiratory distress.

Tests

Marine puncture wounds should be routinely radiographed for retained fragments.

Differential Diagnosis

Like the stingray, bony fish (i.e., lion, weaver, scorpion, cat, and stone fish) can inject venom using their spines. The toxin remains potent for 24 to 48 hours such that one can sustain injuries after the death of the animal, even with refrigeration.

Treatment

1. Stingray and bony fish lesions should be soaked in water as hot as can be tolerated (115 to 120° F) for 60 to 90 minutes in order to inactivate the heat-labile toxins. The wound should be thoroughly cleansed and debrided. Retained fragments should be removed when possible, and surgical removal may be necessary.

2. As with any puncture wound, tetanus prophylaxis is recommended. Antibiotics are optional depending on the physician's level of suspicion for infection (see "Marine Infections" below)

Marine Infections (Cutaneous)

Etiology

1. Streptococci and staphylococci are the common infecting organisms.

2. Of concern, however, are the marine-specific bacteria such as *Erysipelothrix, Mycobacterium marinum, Pseudomonas* species, and the halophilic (salt-loving) *Vibrio* species. Of these, *Vibrio* appears to be the most prevalent.

Symptoms

Patients typically complain of pain, swelling, tenderness, or loss of function.

Clinical Findings

Patients may present with nonhealing abrasions, granulomas, painful red swollen lesions of acute cellulitis, or a more maculopapular, nonvesiculating infection of the hands.

Laboratory Tests

Wound cultures may be performed with attention to halophilic bacteria and atypical *Mycobacterium* culture media.

Differential Diagnosis

1. Fish handlers' disease is caused by infection with *Erysipelothrix* bacteria. It is a rash-like infection of the palmar surfaces of the hands most commonly seen in those who handle or prepare fish.

2. Wound granulomas may be caused by infection with *M. marinum*; however, coral cuts or other retained foreign matter such as sea urchin spines or sponge spicules may present as granulomas. Empiric antibiotic therapy, cultures, and occasionally wound biopsies may be necessary to arrive at a diagnosis.

Treatment

1. Cleanse the wound to remove foreign debris and reduce the possibility of granuloma formation.

2. Tetanus prophylaxis should be administered as with any tetanus-prone wound.

3. Antibiotic selection

    a. Resistant to penicillins and cephalosporins, the *Vibrio* species require quinolones, sulfa agents, or tetracycline for adequate treatment. Due to photosensitivity, the tetracyclines are poorly tolerated in the Sunbelt, and for this reason, the quinolones (Cipro or Floxin) or trimethoprim-sulfamethoxazole (Bactrim or Septra) are often the selected agents. Any marine infection not responding to a penicillin derivative should be given a trial with one of these agents. Remember that quinolone antibiotics are poor coverage for streptococcal infections and thus may not be the best first-line treatment.

    b. Fish handlers' disease should be treated with penicillin, erythromycin, or a cephalosporin, or based on culture sensitivity results.

    c. *M. marinum* infection is a difficult infection to eradicate and may require surgical excision for definitive therapy. Antibiotic selection may include minocycline, trimethoprim-sulfamethoxazole, or rifampin plus ethambutol.

Marine Ingestions

Etiology

Ingestion of marine life may result in a variety of food poisonings. Causes range from endogenous poisons within the fish itself, to animal ingested toxins, and to bacterial decomposition. Focus is on the latter two in this discussion of scombroid and ciguatera poisoning.

Scombroid

Scombroid poisoning is the result of decaying fish being ingested. The amino acid histadine is converted to histamine by bacteria, and the individual has a massive histamine exposure that presents much like anaphylaxis.

Symptoms

Flushing, headaches, dizziness, nausea, diarrhea, and vomiting may begin within minutes to hours of the ingestion.

Clinical Findings

May include bronchospasm, respiratory distress, palpitations, supraventricular tachycardia, and mild hypotension.

Laboratory Tests

None commercially available

Differential Diagnosis

Any disorder presenting with gastrointestinal symptoms, including gastroenteritis, hepatitis

Treatment

Cardiovascular support and antihistamine (H_1 and H_2) therapy. Symptoms usually resolve within 12 to 24 hours.

Ciguatera

Ciguatera is acquired by ingesting fish which themselves have ingested the offending dinoflagellate. Thought to be a type of reef flora, it concentrates up the food chain until a critical mass is ingested by the patient. The majority of implicated fish are grouper, snapper, jack, and barracuda, although almost any fish can be involved. The offending agent, known as ciguatoxin, is tasteless and unaffected by refrigeration or cooking.

Symptoms

1. Within 6 hours of ingestion the victim may experience gastrointestinal and neurologic symptoms.

2. Initially, gastrointestinal symptoms predominate with abdominal cramps, nausea, vomiting, and diarrhea. These usually resolve within 24 to 48 hours and may be followed by neurologic symptoms on the third to fifth day.

3. The hallmark of this illness is the reversal of hot-cold sensation, which may last for months.

4. Severe cases may be complicated by bradycardia, shock, respiratory failure, and rarely death.

Treatment

Treatment is supportive but may involve diphenhydramine for concomitant pruritus and mannitol for neurologic symptoms. Mannitol doses of up to 1 gm/kg at a rate of 500 ml/hr have been used with success in small studies. Fortunately, the disease is usually self-limited and treatment other than prevention unnecessary.

Prevention

Recurrent episodes tend to have increased severity, and thus victims should eliminate fish and fish derivatives from their diet. Other foods such as nuts and alcohol may precipitate recurrence and should be avoided for at least 6 months.

Bibliography

For more information on scombroid poisoning, see
Lange WR: Scombroid poisoning. AFP, April 1988;163–168.

For more information on ciguatera poisoning treatment with mannitol, see

Palafox NA, Jain LG, Pingo AZ, et al: Successful treatment of ciguatera fish poisoning with intravenous mannitol. JAMA 1988;259:2740–2742.

For more information on ciguatera poisoning, see
Lange WR: Ciguatera toxicity. AFP, April 1987;177–182.

For more information on marine injuries, see
Auerbach PS: Marine envenomations: Review article. N Engl J Med 1991;325:486–493; and Flareau B: Hazardous marine animals. *In* Rakel RE (ed): Conn's Current Therapy. Philadelphia, WB Saunders, 1994.

Reference Intervals* for the Interpretation of Laboratory Tests

William Z. Borer

Introduction

Most of the tests performed in a clinical laboratory are quantitative in nature. That is, the amount of a substance present in blood or serum is measured and reported in terms of concentration, activity (e.g., enzyme activity), or counts (e.g., blood cell counts). The laboratory must provide reference values to assist the clinician in the interpretation of laboratory results. These reference ranges comprise the physiologic quantities of substance (concentrations, activities, or counts) to be expected in healthy individuals. Deviation above or below the reference range may be associated with a disease process, and the severity of the disease process may be associated with the magnitude of the deviation. Unfortunately there is rarely a sharp demarcation between physiologic and pathologic values, and the transition between these two is often gradual as the disease process progresses.

The terms "normal" and "abnormal" have been used to describe the laboratory values that fall inside or outside of the reference range respectively. Use of these terms is now discouraged because it is virtually impossible to define normality and because "normal" may be confused with the statistical term "Gaussian." Reference ranges are established from statistical studies in groups of healthy volunteers. While these study subjects must be free of disease, they may have lifestyles or habits that result in subtle variations in their laboratory values. Examples of these variables include diet, body mass, exercise, and geographic location. Age and gender may also affect reference values. When the data from a large cohort of healthy subjects fit a Gaussian distribution, the usual statistical approach is to define the reference limits as two standard deviations above and below the mean. By definition, the reference range excludes the highest and the lowest 2.5 per cent of the population. Although non-Gaussian distributions are handled by different statistical methods, the result is similar in that the reference range is defined by the central 95 per cent of the population. In other words, the odds are 1 in 20 that a healthy individual will have a laboratory result that falls outside the reference range. If 12 laboratory tests are performed, the odds increase to about 1 in 2 that at least one of the results will be outside the reference range. This means that all healthy individuals are likely to have a few laboratory results that are unexpected. The physician must then integrate those data with other clinical information such as the history and physical examination to arrive at the appropriate clinical decision. The reference range for many tests (especially enzyme and immunochemical measurements) varies with the method used. It is important that each laboratory establish reference ranges appropriate for the methods that it employs.

SI Units

During the past decade a concerted effort has been made to introduce SI units (le Système International d'Unités). The rationale for conversion to SI units is sound. Laboratory data are scientifically more informative when the units are based on molar concentration rather than on mass concentration. For example, the conversion of glucose to lactate and pyruvate or the binding of a drug to albumin is more easily understood in units of molar concentration. Another example is illustrated as follows:

Conventional Units

1.0 gram of hemoglobin
    combines with 1.37 ml of oxygen
    contains 3.4 mg of iron
    forms 34.9 mg of bilirubin

SI Units

4.0 mmol of hemoglobin
    combines with 4.0 mmol of oxygen
    contains 4.0 mmol of iron
    forms 4.0 mmol of bilirubin

Another advantage of SI units involves the standardization of nomenclature to facilitate global communication of medical and scientific information. The units, symbols, and prefixes in the International System are shown in Tables 1, 2, and 3.

Unfortunately, problems have arisen with the implementation of SI units in the United States. Their introduction in 1987 prompted many medical journals to report laboratory values in both SI and conventional units in anticipation of complete conversion to SI units in the early 1990s. The lack of a coordinated effort toward this goal has forced a retrenchment on the issue. Physicians continue to think and

---

*Some of the values included in the tables have been established by the Clinical Laboratories at Thomas Jefferson University Hospital, Philadelphia, PA and have not been published elsewhere. Other values have been compiled from the sources cited above. These tables are provided for information and educational purposes only. They are intended to complement data derived from other sources, including the medical history and physical examination. Users must exercise individual judgment in using the information provided in this appendix.

practice using laboratory results expressed in conventional units, and few if any United States hospitals or clinical laboratories exclusively use SI units. It is not likely that complete conversion to SI units will occur in the foreseeable future, yet most medical journals will probably continue to publish both sets of units. For this reason the tables of reference ranges in this appendix are given in both conventional units and SI units.

B Bibliography

AMA Drug Evaluations, 6th ed. Chicago, American Medical Association, 1992.

Bick RL (ed): Hematology: Clinical and Laboratory Practice. St. Louis, Mosby-Yearbook, 1993.

Borer WZ: Selection and Use of Laboratory Tests. *In* Tietz NW, Conn RB, Pruden EL (eds): Applied Laboratory Medicine. Philadelphia, WB Saunders, 1992, pp 1–5.

Campion EW: A retreat from SI units. N Engl J Med 1992; 327:49.

Friedman RB, Young DS: Effects of Disease on Clinical Laboratory Tests. 2nd ed. Washington, AACC Press, 1989.

Henry JB: Clinical Diagnosis and Management by Laboratory Methods, 18th ed. Philadelphia, WB Saunders, 1991.

Hicks JM, Young DS: DORA '92–93: Directory of Rare Analyses. Washington, AACC Press, 1992.

Jacobs DS, Kasten BL, Demott WR, Wolfson WL: Laboratory Test Handbook, 2nd ed. Baltimore, Williams & Wilkins, 1990.

Kaplan LA, Pesce AJ: Clinical Chemistry: Theory, Analysis, and Correlation, 2nd ed. St. Louis, CV Mosby, 1989.

Kjeldsberg CR, Knight JA: Body Fluids: Laboratory Examination of Amniotic, Cerebrospinal, Seminal, Serous and Synovial Fluids. 3rd ed. Chicago, ASCP Press, 1993.

Laposata M: SI Unit Conversion Guide. Boston, NEJM Books, 1992.

Scully RE, McNeely WF, Mark EJ, McNeely BU: Normal Reference Laboratory Values. N Engl J Med 1992;327:718–724.

Speicher CE: The Right Test: A Physician's Guide to Laboratory Medicine, 2nd ed. Philadelphia, WB Saunders, 1993.

Tietz NW (ed): Clinical Guide to Laboratory Tests, 2nd ed. Philadelphia, WB Saunders, 1990.

Wallach J: Interpretation of Diagnostic Tests: A Synopsis of Laboratory Medicine, 5th ed. Boston, Little, Brown, 1992.

Young DS: Implementation of SI units for clinical laboratory data. Ann Intern Med 1987;106:114–129.

Young DS: Determination and validation of reference intervals. Arch Pathol Lab Med 1992;116:704–709.

Young DS: Effects of Drugs on Clinical Laboratory Tests, 3rd ed. Washington, AACC Press, 1990.

TABLE 1. BASE SI UNITS

Property	Base Unit	Symbol
Length	meter	m
Mass	kilogram	kg
Amount of substance	mole	mol
Time	second	s
Thermodynamic temperature	kelvin	K
Electric current	ampere	A
Luminous intensity	candela	cd
Catalytic amount	katal	kat

TABLE 2. DERIVED SI UNITS AND NON-SI UNITS RETAINED FOR USE WITH THE SI

Property	Unit	Symbol
Area	square meter	m^2
Volume	cubic meter	m^3
	liter	L
Mass concentration	kilogram/cubic meter	kg/m^3
	gram/liter	g/L
Substance concentration	mole/cubic meter	mol/m^3
	mole/liter	mol/L
Temperature	degree Celsius	$C = K - 273.15$

TABLE 3. STANDARD PREFIXES

Prefix	Multiplication Factor	Symbol
yocto	10^{-24}	y
zepto	10^{-21}	z
atto	10^{-18}	a
femto	10^{-15}	f
pico	10^{-12}	p
nano	10^{-9}	n
micro	10^{-6}	μ
milli	10^{-3}	m
centi	10^{-2}	c
deci	10^{-1}	d
deca	10^{1}	da
hecto	10^{2}	h
kilo	10^{3}	k
mega	10^{6}	M
giga	10^{9}	G
tera	10^{12}	T

REFERENCE VALUES FOR HEMATOLOGY

	CONVENTIONAL UNITS	SI UNITS
Acid hemolysis (Ham test)	No hemolysis	No hemolysis
Alkaline phosphatase, leukocyte	Total score 14–100	Total score 14–100
Cell counts		
Erythrocytes		
Males	4.6–6.2 million/mm^3	4.6–6.2 $\times$ 10^{12}/L
Females	4.2–5.4 million/mm^3	4.2–5.4 $\times$ 10^{12}/L
Children (varies with age)	4.5–5.1 million/mm^3	4.5–5.1 $\times$ 10^{12}/L
Leukocytes, total	4500–11,000/mm^3	4.5–11.0 $\times$ 10^9/L
Leukocytes, differential*		
Myelocytes	0%	0/L
Band neutrophils	3–5%	150–400 $\times$ 10^6/L
Segmented neutrophils	54–62%	3000–5800 $\times$ 10^6/L
Lymphocytes	25–33%	1500–3000 $\times$ 10^6/L
Monocytes	3–7%	300–500 $\times$ 10^6/L
Eosinophils	1–3%	50–250 $\times$ 10^6/L
Basophils	0–1%	15–50 $\times$ 10^6/L
Platelets	150,000–350,000/mm^3	150–350 $\times$ 10^9/L
Reticulocytes	25,000–75,000/mm^3 (0.5–1.5% of erythrocytes)	25–75 $\times$ 10^9/L
Coagulation tests		
Bleeding time (template)	2.75–8.0 min	2.75–8.0 min
Coagulation time (glass tube)	5–15 min	5–15 min
D-dimer	<0.5 μg/ml	<0.5 mg/L
Factor VIII and other coagulation factors	50–150% of normal	0.5–1.5 of normal
Fibrin split products (Thrombo-Welco test)	<10 μg/ml	<10 mg/L
Fibrinogen	200–400 mg/dl	2.0–4.0 g/L
Partial thromboplastin time (PTT)	20–35 s	20–35 s
Prothrombin time (PT)	12.0–14.0 s	12.0–14.0 s

*Conventional units are percentages; SI units are absolute counts.

Table continues on the opposite page

REFERENCE VALUES FOR HEMATOLOGY *Continued*

	CONVENTIONAL UNITS	SI UNITS
Coombs' test		
Direct	Negative	Negative
Indirect	Negative	Negative
Corpuscular values of erythrocytes		
Mean corpuscular hemoglobin (MCH)	26–34 pg/cell	26–34 pg/cell
Mean corpuscular volume (MCV)	80–96 μm^3	80–96 fL
Mean corpuscular hemoglobin concentration (MCHC)	32–36 g/dl	320–360 g/L
Haptoglobin	20–165 mg/dl	0.20–1.65 g/L
Hematocrit		
Males	40–54 ml/dl	0.40–0.54
Females	37–47 ml/dl	0.37–0.47
Newborns	49–54 ml/dl	0.49–0.54
Children (varies with age)	35–49 ml/dl	0.35–0.49
Hemoglobin		
Males	13.0–18.0 g/dl	8.1–11.2 mmol/L
Females	12.0–16.0 g/dl	7.4–9.9 mmol/L
Newborn	16.5–19.5 g/dl	10.2–12.1 mmol/L
Children (varies with age)	11.2–16.5 g/dl	7.0–10.2 mmol/L
Hemoglobin, fetal	<1.0% of total	<0.01 of total
Hemoglobin A_{1C}	3–5% of total	0.03–0.05 of total
Hemoglobin A_2	1.5–3.0% of total	0.015–0.03 of total
Hemoglobin, plasma	0–5.0 mg/dl	0.0–3.2 μmol/L
Methemoglobin	30–130 mg/dl	19–80 μmol/L
Sedimentation rate (ESR)		
Wintrobe, Males	0–5 mm/hr	0–5 mm/hr
Females	0–15 mm/hr	0–15 mm/hr
Westergren, Males	0–15 mm/hr	0–15 mm/hr
Females	0–20 mm/hr	0–20 mm/hr

REFERENCE VALUES* FOR CLINICAL CHEMISTRY (BLOOD, SERUM, AND PLASMA)

	CONVENTIONAL UNITS	SI UNITS
Acetoacetate plus acetone		
Qualitative	Negative	Negative
Quantitative	0.3–2.0 mg/dl	30–200 μmol/L
Acid phosphatase, serum (Thymolphthalein monophosphate substrate)	0.1–0.6 U/L	0.1–0.6 U/L
ACTH (see Corticotropin)		
Alanine aminotransferase (ALT, SGPT), serum	1–45 U/L	1–45 U/L
Albumin, serum	3.3–5.2 g/dl	33–52 g/L
Aldolase, serum	0.0–7.0 U/L	0.0–7.0 U/L
Aldosterone, plasma		
Standing	5–30 ng/dl	140–830 pmol/L
Recumbent	3–10 ng/dl	80–275 pmol/L
Alkaline phosphatase (ALP), serum		
Adult	35–150 U/L	35–150 U/L
Adolescent	100–500 U/L	100–500 U/L
Child	100–350 U/L	100–350 U/L
Ammonia nitrogen, plasma	10–50 μmol/L	10–50 μmol/L
Amylase, serum	25–125 U/L	25–125 U/L
Anion gap, serum, calculated	8–16 mEq/L	8–16 mmol/L
Ascorbic acid, blood	0.4–1.5 mg/dl	23–85 μmol/L
Aspartate aminotransferase (AST, SGOT), serum	1–36 U/L	1–36 U/L
Base excess, arterial blood, calculated	0 ± 2 mEq/L	0 ± 2 mmol/L
Bicarbonate		
Venous plasma	23–29 mEq/L	23–29 mmol/L
Arterial blood	21–27 mEq/L	21–27 mmol/L
Bile acids, serum	0.3–3.0 mg/dl	0.8–7.6 μmol/L
Bilirubin, serum		
Conjugated	0.1–0.4 mg/dl	1.7–6.8 μmol/L
Total	0.3–1.1 mg/dl	5.1–19.0 μmol/L
Calcium, serum	8.4–10.6 mg/dl	2.10–2.65 mmol/L
Calcium, ionized, serum	4.25–5.25 mg/dl	1.05–1.30 mmol/L
Carbon dioxide, total, serum or plasma	24–31 mEq/L	24–31 mmol/L
Carbon dioxide tension (P_{CO_2}), blood	35–45 mm Hg	35–45 mm Hg
β-Carotene, serum	60–260 μg/dl	1.1–8.6 μmol/L
Ceruloplasmin, serum	23–44 mg/dl	230–440 mg/L
Chloride, serum or plasma	96–106 mEq/l	96–106 mmol/L
Cholesterol, serum or EDTA plasma		
Desirable range	<200 mg/dl	<5.20 mmol/L
LDL cholesterol	60–180 mg/dl	1.55–4.65 mmol/L
HDL cholesterol	30–80 mg/dl	0.80–2.05 mmol/L
Copper	70–140 μg/dl	11–22 μmol/L
Corticotropin (ACTH), plasma, 8 A.M.	10–80 pg/ml	2–18 pmol/L
Cortisol, plasma		
8 A.M.	6–23 μg/dl	170–630 nmol/L
4 P.M.	3–15 μg/dl	80–410 nmol/L
10 P.M.	<50% of A.M. value	<50% of A.M. value
Creatine, serum		
Males	0.2–0.5 mg/dl	15–40 μmol/L
Females	0.3–0.9 mg/dl	25–70 μmol/L
Creatine kinase (CK, CPK), serum		
Males	55–170 U/L	55–170 U/L
Females	30–135 U/L	30–135 U/L
Creatine kinase MB isoenzyme, serum	<5% of total CK activity	
	<5% ng/ml by immunoassay	
Creatinine, serum	0.6–1.2 mg/dl	50–110 μmol/L
Ferritin, serum	20–200 μg/ml	20–200 μg/L
Fibrinogen, plasma	200–400 mg/dl	2.0–4.0 g/L
Folate, serum erythrocytes	2.0–9.0 ng/ml	4.5–20.4 nmol/L
	170–700 ng/ml	385–1590 nmol/L
Follicle-stimulating hormone (FSH), plasma		
Males	4–25 mU/ml	4–25 U/l
Females, premenopausal	4–30 mU/ml	4–30 U/L
Females, postmenopausal	40–250 mU/ml	40–250 U/L
γ-glutamyltransferase (GGT), serum	5–40 U/L	5–40 U/L
Gastrin, fasting, serum	0–110 pg/ml	0–110 mg/L
Glucose, fasting, plasma or serum	70–115 mg/dl	3.9–6.4 nmol/L
Growth hormone (hGH), plasma, adult, fasting	0–6 ng/ml	0–6 μg/L
Haptoglobin, serum	20–165 mg/dl	0.20–1.65 g/L
Immunoglobulins, serum (see Immunologic Procedures)		

*Reference values may vary, depending on the method and sample source used.

Table continues on the opposite page

REFERENCE VALUES* FOR CLINICAL CHEMISTRY (BLOOD, SERUM, AND PLASMA) *Continued*

	CONVENTIONAL UNITS	SI UNITS
Insulin, fasting, plasma	5–25 μU/ml	36–179 pmol/L
Iron, serum	75–175 μg/dl	13–31 μmol/L
Iron binding capacity, serum		
Total	250–410 μg/dl	45–73 μmol/L
Saturation	20–55%	0.20–0.55
Lactate, venous blood	5.0–20.0 mg/dl	0.6–2.2 mmol/L
arterial blood	5.0–15.0 mg/dl	0.6–1.7 mmol/L
Lactate dehydrogenase (LD, LDH), serum	110–220 U/L	110–220 U/L
Lipase, serum	10–140 U/L	10–140 U/L
Lutropin (LH), serum		
Males	1–9 IU/L	1–9 U/L
Females		
Follicular phase	2–10 IU/L	2–10 U/L
Midcycle peak	15–65 U/L	15–65 U/L
Luteal phase	1–12 U/L	1–12 U/L
Postmenopausal	12–65 U/L	12–65 U/L
Magnesium, serum	1.3–2.1 mg/dl	0.65–1.05 mmol/L
Osmolality	275–295 mOsm/kg water	275–295 mOsm/kg water
Oxygen, blood, arterial, room air		
Partial pressure (PaO$_2$)	80–100 mm Hg	80–100 mm Hg
Saturation (SaO$_2$)	95–98%	95–98%
pH, arterial blood	7.35–7.45	7.35–7.45
Phosphate, inorganic, serum		
Adult	3.0–4.5 mg/dl	1.0–1.5 mmol/L
Child	4.0–7.0 mg/dl	1.3–2.3 mmol/L
Potassium		
Serum	3.5–5.0 mEq/L	3.5–5.0 mmol/L
Plasma	3.5–4.5 mEq/L	3.5–4.5 mmol/L
Progesterone, serum, adult		
Males	0.0–0.4 ng/ml	0.0–1.3 mmol/L
Females		
Follicular phase	0.1–1.5 ng/ml	0.3–4.8 mmol/L
Luteal phase	2.5–28.0 ng/ml	8.0–89.0 mmol/L
Prolactin, serum		
Males	1.0–15.0 ng/ml	1.0–15.0 μg/L
Females	1.0–20.0 ng/ml	1.0–20.0 μg/L
Protein, serum, electrophoresis		
Total	6.0–8.0 g/dl	60–80 g/L
Albumin	3.5–5.5 g/dl	35–55 g/L
Globulins		
α_1	0.2–0.4 g/dl	2–4 g/L
α_2	0.5–0.9 g/dl	5–9 g/L
β	0.6–1.1 g/dl	6–11 g/L
γ	0.7–1.7 g/dl	7–17 g/L
Pyruvate, blood	0.3–0.9 mg/dl	0.03–0.10 mmol/L
Rheumatoid factor	0.0–30.0 IU/ml	0.0–30.0 kIU/L
Sodium, serum or plasma	135–145 mEq/L	135–145 mmol/L
Testosterone, plasma		
Males, adult	300–1200 ng/dl	10.4–41.6 nmol/L
Females, adult	20–75 ng/dl	0.7–2.6 nmol/L
Pregnant females	40–200 ng/dl	1.4–6.9 nmol/L
Thyroglobulin	3–42 μ/ml	3–42 μg/L
Thyrotropin (hTSH), serum	0.4–4.8 μIU/ml	0.4–4.8 mIU/L
Thyrotropin-releasing hormone (TRH)	5–60 pg/ml	5–60 ng/l
Thyroxine (FT$_4$), free, serum	0.9–2.1 ng/dl	12–27 pmol/L
Thyroxine (T$_4$), serum	4.5–12.0 μg/dl	58–154 nmol/L
Thyroxine-binding globulin (TBG)	15.0–34.0 μg/ml	15.0–34.0 mg/L
Transferrin	250–430 mg/dl	250–430 g/L
Triglycerides, serum, after 12-hr fast	40–150 mg/dl	0.4–15.0 g/L
Triiodothyronine (T$_3$), serum	70–190 ng/dl	1.1–2.9 nmol/L
Triiodothyronine uptake, resin (T$_3$RU)	25–38%	0.25–0.38
Urate		
Males	2.5–8.0 mg/dl	150–480 μmol/L
Females	2.2–7.0 mg/dl	130–420 μmol/L
Urea, serum or plasma	24–49 mg/dl	4.0–8.2 nmol/L
Urea nitrogen, serum or plasma	11–23 mg/dl	8.0–16.4 nmol/L
Viscosity, serum	1.4–1.8 × water	1.4–1.8 × water
Vitamin A, serum	20–80 μg/dl	0.70–2.80 μmol/L
Vitamin B$_{12}$, serum	180–900 pg/ml	133–664 pmol/L

REFERENCE VALUES FOR THERAPEUTIC DRUG MONITORING (SERUM)

	THERAPEUTIC RANGE	TOXIC CONCENTRATIONS	PROPRIETARY NAMES
Analgesics			
Acetaminophen	10–20 µg/ml	>250 µg/ml	Tylenol
			Datril
Salicylate	100–250 µg/ml	>300 µg/ml	Aspirin
			Ascriptin
			Bufferin
Antibiotics			
Amikacin	25–30 µg/ml	Peak >35 µg/ml	Amikin
		Trough >10 µg/ml	
Chloramphenicol	10–20 µg/ml	>25 µg/ml	Chloromycetin
Gentamicin	5–10 µg/ml	Peak >10 µg/ml	Garamycin
		Trough >2 µg/ml	
Tobramycin	5–10 µg/ml	Peak >10 µg/ml	Nebcin
		Trough >2 µg/ml	
Vancomycin	5–10 µg/ml	Peak >40 µg/ml	Vancocin
		Trough >10 µg/ml	
Anticonvulsants			
Carbamazepine	5–12 µg/ml	>15 µg/ml	Tegretol
Ethosuximide	40–100 µg/ml	>150 µg/ml	Zarontin
Phenobarbital	15–40 µg/ml	40–100 ng/ml (varies widely)	
Phenytoin	10–20 µg/ml	>20 µg/ml	Dilantin
Primidone	5–12 µg/ml	>15 µg/ml	Mysoline
Valproic acid	50–100 µg/ml	>100 µg/ml	Depakene
Antineoplastics and Immunosuppressives			
Cyclosporine-A	50–400 ng/ml	>400 ng/ml	Sandimmune
Methotrexate, high dose, 48 hr	Variable	>1 µmol/L 48 hr after dose	Mexate
			Folex
Bronchodilators and Respiratory Stimulants			
Caffeine	3–15 ng/ml	>30 ng/ml	
Theophylline (Aminophylline)	10–20 µg/ml	>20 µg/ml	Accurbron
			Elixophyllin
			Quibron
			Theobid

Table continues on the opposite page

REFERENCE VALUES FOR THERAPEUTIC DRUG MONITORING (SERUM) *Continued*

	THERAPEUTIC RANGE	TOXIC CONCENTRATIONS	PROPRIETARY NAMES
Cardiovascular Drugs			
Amiodarone	1.0–2.0 μg/ml	>2.0 μg/ml	Cordarone
(Specimen must be obtained more than 8 hr after last dose)			
Digitoxin	15–25 ng/ml	>35 ng/ml	Crystodigin
(Specimen must be obtained 12–24 hr after last dose)			
Digoxin	0.8–2.0 ng/ml	>2.4 ng/ml	Lanoxin
(Specimen must be obtained more than 6 hr after last dose)			
Disopyramide	2–5 μg/ml	>7 μg/ml	Norpace
Flecainide	0.2–1.0 ng/ml	>1 ng/ml	Tambocor
Lidocaine	1.5–5.0 μg/ml	>6 μg/ml	Xylocaine
Mexiletine	0.7–2.0 ng/ml	>2 ng/ml	Mexitil
Procainamide	4–10 μg/ml	>12 μg/ml	Pronestyl
Procainamide + NAPA	8–30 μg/ml	>30 μg/ml	
Propranolol	50–100 ng/ml	Variable	Inderal
Quinidine	2–5 μg/ml	>6 μg/ml	Cardioquin
			Quinaglute
Tocainide	4–10 ng/ml	>10 ng/ml	Tonocard
Psychopharmacologic Drugs			
Amitriptyline	120–150 ng/ml	>500 ng/ml	Amitril
			Elavil
			Triavil
Bupropion	25–100 ng/ml	Not applicable	Wellbutrin
Desipramine	150–300 ng/ml	>500 ng/ml	Norpramin
			Pertofrane
Imipramine	125–250 ng/ml	>400 ng/ml	Tofranil
Lithium	0.6–1.5 mEq/L	>1.5 mEq/L	Lithobid
(Obtain specimen 12 hr after last dose)			
Nortriptyline	50–150 ng/ml	>500 ng/ml	Aventyl
			Pamelor

REFERENCE VALUES FOR CLINICAL CHEMISTRY (URINE)*

	CONVENTIONAL UNITS	SI UNITS
Acetone and acetoacetate, qualitative	Negative	Negative
Albumin		
Qualitative	Negative	Negative
Quantitative	10–100 mg/24 hr	0.15–1.5 μmol/d
Aldosterone	3–20 μg/24 hr	8.3–55 nmol/d
δ-aminolevulinic acid (δ-ALA)	1.3–7.0 mg/24 hr	10–53 μmol/d
Amylase	<17 U/hr	<17 U/hr
Amylase/creatinine clearance ratio	0.01–0.04	0.01–0.04
Bilirubin, qualitative	Negative	Negative
Calcium (regular diet)	<250 mg/24 hr	<6.3 nmol/d
Catecholamines		
Epinephrine	<10 μg/24 hr	<55 nmol/d
Norepinephrine	<100 μg/24 hr	<590 nmol/d
Total free catecholamines	4–126 μg/24 hr	24–745 nmol/d
Total metanephrines	0.1–1.6 mg/24 hr	0.5–8.1 μmol/d
Chloride (varies with intake)	110–250 mEq/24 hr	110–250 mmol/d
Copper	0–50 μg/24 hr	0–0.80 μmol/d
Cortisol, free	10–100 μg/24 hr	27.6–276 nmol/d
Creatine		
Males	0–40 mg/24 hr	0–0.30 mmol/d
Females	0–80 mg/24 hr	0–0.60 mmol/d
Creatinine	15–25 mg/kg/24 hr	0.13–0.22 mmol/kg/d
Creatinine clearance (endogenous)		
Males	110–150 ml/min/1.73 m²	110–150 ml/min/1.73 m²
Females	105–132 ml/min/1.73 m²	105–132 ml/min/1.73 m²
Cystine or Cysteine	Negative	Negative
Dehydroepiandrosterone		
Males	0.2–2.0 mg/24 hr	0.7–6.9 μmol/d
Females	0.2–1.8 mg/24 hr	0.7–6.2 μmol/d
Estrogens, total		
Males	4–25 μg/24 hr	14–90 nmol/d
Females	5–100 μg/24 hr	18–360 nmol/d
Glucose (as reducing substance)	<250 mg/24 hr	<250 mg/d
Hemoglobin and myoglobin, qualitative	Negative	Negative
Homogentisic acid, qualitative	Negative	Negative
17-Ketogenic steroids		
Males	5–23 mg/24 hr	17–80 μmol/d
Females	3–15 mg/24 hr	10–52 μmol/d

Table continues on the opposite page

REFERENCE VALUES FOR CLINICAL CHEMISTRY (URINE)* *Continued*

	CONVENTIONAL UNITS	SI UNITS
17-Hydroxycorticosteroids		
Males	3–9 mg/24 hr	8.3–25 μmol/d
Females	2–8 mg/24 hr	5.5–22 μmol/d
5-Hydroxyindole acetic acid		
Qualitative	Negative	Negative
Quantitative	2–6 mg/24 hr	10–31 μmol/d
17-Ketosteroids		
Males	8–22 mg/24 hr	28–76 μmol/d
Females	6–15 mg/24 hr	21–52 μmol/d
Magnesium	6–10 mEq/24 hr	3–5 mmol/d
Metanephrines	0.05–1.2 ng/mg creatinine	0.03–0.70 mmol/mmol creatinine
Osmolality	38–1400 mOsm/kg water	38–1400 mOsm/kg water
pH	4.6–8.0	4.6–8.0
Phenylpyruvic acid, qualitative	Negative	Negative
Phosphate	0.4–1.3 g/24 hr	13–42 mmol/d
Porphobilinogen		
Qualitative	Negative	Negative
Quantitative	<2 mg/24 hr	<9 μmol/d
Porphyrins		
Coproporphyrin	50–250 μg/24 hr	77–380 nmol/d
Uroporphyrin	10–30 μg/24 hr	12–36 nmol/d
Potassium	25–125 mEq/24 hr	25–125 mmol/d
Pregnanediol		
Males	0–1.9 mg/24 hr	0–6.0 μmol/d
Females, proliferative phase	0–2.6 mg/24 hr	0–8.0 μmol/d
luteal phase	2.6–10.6 mg/24 hr	8–33 μmol/d
postmenopausal	0.2–1.0 mg/24 hr	0.6–3.1 μmol/d
Pregnanetriol	0–2.5 mg/24 hr	0–7.4 μmol/d
Protein, total		
Qualitative	Negative	Negative
Quantitative	10–150 mg/24 hr	10–150 mg/d
Protein/creatinine ratio	<0.2	<0.2
Sodium (regular diet)	60–260 mEq/24 hr	60–260 mmol/d
Specific gravity		
Random specimen	1.003–1.030	1.003–1.030
24-hour collection	1.015–1.025	1.015–1.025
Urate (regular diet)	250–750 mg/24 hr	1.5–4.4 mmol/d
Urobilinogen	0.5–4.0 mg/24 hr	0.6–6.8 μmol/d
Vanillylmandelic acid (VMA)	1–8 mg/24 hr	5–40 μmol/d

*Reference values may vary, depending upon the method used.

REFERENCE VALUES FOR TOXIC SUBSTANCES

	CONVENTIONAL UNITS	SI UNITS
Arsenic, urine	<130 μg/24 hr	<1.7 μmol/d
Bromides, serum, inorganic	<100 mg/dl	<10 mmol/L
Toxic symptoms	140–1000 mg/dl	14–100 mmol/L
Carboxyhemoglobin, blood		
Urban environment	<5% (% saturation)	<0.05 (saturation)
Smokers	<12% (% saturation)	<0.12 (saturation)
Symptoms		
Headache	>15% (% saturation)	>0.15 (saturation)
Nausea and vomiting	>25% (% saturation)	>0.25 (saturation)
Potentially lethal	>50% (% saturation)	>0.50 (saturation)
Ethanol, blood	<0.05 mg/dl	
	<0.005%	<1.0 mmol/L
Intoxication	>100 mg/dl	
	>0.1%	>22 mmol/L
Marked intoxication	300–400 mg/dl	
	0.3–0.4%	65–87 mmol/L
Alcoholic stupor	400–500 mg/dl	
	0.4–0.5%	87–109 mmol/L
Coma	>500 mg/dl	>109 mmol/L
	>0.5%	
Lead, blood		
Adults	<25 μg/dl	<1.2 μmol/L
Children	<15 μg/dl	<0.7 μmol/L
Lead, urine	<80 μg/24 hr	<0.4 μmol/d
Mercury, urine	<30 μg/24 hr	<150 nmol/d

REFERENCE VALUES FOR CEREBROSPINAL FLUID

	CONVENTIONAL UNITS	SI UNITS
Cells	<5/mm³; all mononuclear	<5 × 10⁶/L, all mononuclear
Electrophoresis	Albumin predominant	Albumin predominant
Glucose	50–75 mg/dl (20 mg/dl less than in serum)	2.8–4.2 mmol/L (1.1 mmol less than in serum)
IgG		
Children under 14	<8% of total protein	<0.08% of total protein
Adults	<14% of total protein	<0.14% of total protein
IgG index $\left(\dfrac{\text{CSF/serum IgG ratio}}{\text{CSF/serum albumin ratio}}\right)$	0.3–0.6	0.3–0.6
Oligoclonal banding on electrophoresis	Absent	Absent
Pressure, opening	70–180 mmH₂O	70–180 mmH₂O
Protein, total	15–45 mg/dl	150–450 mg/L

REFERENCE VALUES FOR TESTS OF GASTROINTESTINAL FUNCTION

	CONVENTIONAL UNITS
Bentiromide test	6-hr urinary arylamine excretion greater than 57% excludes pancreatic insufficiency
Carotene, serum	60–250 ng/dl
D-Xylose absorption test	5-hr urinary excretion >20% of ingested dose
Fecal fat estimation	
Qualitative	No fat globules seen by high power microscope
Quantitative	<6 g/24hr (>95% coefficient of fat absorption)
Gastric acid output	
Basal	
Males	0–10.5 mmol/hr
Females	0–5.6 mmol/hr
Maximum (after histamine or pentagastrin)	
Males	9.0–48.0 mmol/hr
Females	6.0–31.0 mmol/hr
Ratio: basal/maximum	
Males	0–0.31
Females	0–0.29
Secretin test, pancreatic fluid	
Volume	>1.8 ml/kg/hr
Bicarbonate	>80 mEq/L

REFERENCE VALUES FOR IMMUNOLOGIC PROCEDURES

	CONVENTIONAL UNITS	SI UNITS
Complement, serum		
C3	85–175 mg/dl	0.85–1.75 g/L
C4	15–45 mg/dl	150–450 mg/L
Total hemolytic (CH_{50})	150–250 U/ml	150–250 U/ml
Immunoglobulins, serum, adult		
IgG	640–1350 mg/dl	6.4–13.5 g/L
IgA	70–310 mg/dl	0.70–3.1 g/L
IgM	90–350 mg/dl	0.90–3.5 g/L
IgD	0–6.0 mg/dl	0–60 mg/L
IgE	0–430 ng/dl	0–430 μg/L

Lymphocyte subsets, whole blood, heparinized

Antigen	Cell Type	Percentage	Absolute
CD3	Total T cells	56–77%	860–1880
CD19	Total B cells	7–17%	140–370
CD3 and CD4	Helper-inducer cells	32–54%	550–1190
CD3 and CD8	Suppressor-cytotoxic cells	24–37%	430–1060
CD3 and DR	Activated T cells	5–14%	70–310
CD2	E rosette T cells	73–87%	1040–2160
CD16 and CD56	Natural killer (NK) cells	8–22%	130–500

Helper/Suppressor ratio: 0.8:1.8

REFERENCE VALUES FOR SEMEN ANALYSIS

	CONVENTIONAL UNITS	SI UNITS
Volume	2–5 ml	2–5 ml
Liquefaction	Complete in 15 min	Complete in 15 min
pH	7.2–8.0	7.2–8.0
Leukocytes	Occasional or absent	Occasional or absent
Spermatozoa		
Count	60–150 × 10^6/ml	60–150 × 10^6/ml
Motility	>80% motile	>0.80 motile
Morphology	80–90% normal forms	0.80–0.90 normal forms
Fructose	>150 mg/dl	>8.33 mmol/L

Index

Note: Page numbers in *italics* indicate illustrations; those followed by t indicate tables.

1203

DISEASES AND ICD-9CM CODES *(Continued)*

Finger Dislocations   834.00
Finger Fractures   816.00
First Trimester Bleeding   640.93
Fluid Balance   276.5 and 276.6
Food Allergy   693.1
Food Poisoning   005.9
Foot Fractures   825.20
Frostbite   991.3
Fungus Infections   117.9
Gallstones   574.2
Gastritis   535.5
Gastroesophageal Reflux   530.81
Generalized Anxiety Disorder   300.00
Gestational Hyperglycemia/Diabetes   648.8
Giardiasis   007.1
Glaucoma   365.9
Glomerulonephritis   583.9
Goiter   240.9
Gout   274.9
Guillain-Barré Syndrome   357.0
Gynecomastia   611.1
Hair Disorders   704
Head Injury in Sports   854.0
Head, Pubic and Body Lice   132.3
Headache   784.0
Hearing, Impaired   389.9
Heartburn   787.1
Heat Exhaustion   992.5
Heat Stroke   992.0
Hematuria   599.7
Hemoglobinopathy   282.7
Hemolytic Anemia   282.9
Hemoptysis   786.3
Hemorrhoids   455.6
Hepatitis   573.3
Herpes Simplex Infection   054.9
Herpes Zoster Infection   053.9
Hirsutism   704.1
Histoplasmosis   115.90
HIV Associated Infections   042.0
HIV Infection, Asymptomatic V08
HIV Infection, Early Symptomatic   042
HIV Infection, Late Symptomatic   042
Hodgkin's Disease   441.9
Hookworm Infection   126.9
Hydrocele   603.9
Hyperbilirubinemia   782.4
Hypercalcemia   275.4
Hypercalciuria   275.4
Hyperhidrosis   780.8
Hyperkalemia   276.7
Hyperlipidemia   272.4
Hypernatremia   276.0
Hyperparathyroidism   252.0
Hyperprolactinemia   253.1
Hypertension   401.9
Hyperventilation Syndrome   306.1
Hypocalcemia   275.4

Hypoglycemia   251.2
Hypokalemia   276.8
Hyponatremia   276.1
Hypothyroidism   244.9
Impetigo   684
Impotence   302.72
Inappropriate Secretion of Antidiuretic Hormone   253.6
Indigestion   536.8
Induction of Labor   659.1
Infertility   Male: 606.9; Female: 628.9
Influenza   487.1
Insect and Spider Bites   989.5
Insomnia   780.52
Interstitial Lung Disease   515
Intussusception   560.0
Iron Deficiency Anemia   280.9
Irritable Bowel Syndrome   564.1
Jaundice   782.4
Kaposi's Sarcoma   176.9
Ketoacidosis   276.2
Kidney Cancer   189.0
Laryngitis   464.0
Larynx Cancer   161.9
Lead Poisoning   984.9
Leprosy   030.9
Leukemia   208.9
Leukoplakia   702.8
Lipoma   214.9
Lung Cancer   162.9
Lupus Erythematosus   695.4
Lyme Disease   088.81
Lymphadenopathy   785.6
Lymphoma   202.8
Malaria   084.6
Malnutrition   263.9
Measles   055.9
Melanoma   172.9
Meniere's Disease   386.00
Meningitis   322.9
Menopause   627.2
Metastatic Cancer of Unknown Origin   199.1
Migraine Headache   346.9
Miliaria   705.1
Mononucleosis, Infectious   075
Multiple Sclerosis   340
Myasthenia Gravis   358.0
Myocardial Infarction, Acute   410.9
Myofascial Syndromes   729.1
Nails   703.9
Nerve Entrapments   355.9
Neutropenia   288.0
Nevi   448.1
Nicotine Dependence   305.1
Nongonococcal Urethritis   099.40
Obesity   278.00
Obsessive Compulsive Disorder   300.3
Oliguria   788.5
Optic Neuritis   377.30